Modern Epidemiology

FOURTH EDITION

Modern Epidemiology

FOURTH EDITION

Timothy L. Lash
O. Wayne Rollins Distinguished Professor of Epidemiology
and Chair
Department of Epidemiology
Rollins School of Public Health, Emory University
Atlanta, Georgia

Tyler J. VanderWeele
John L. Loeb and Frances Lehman Loeb
Professor of Epidemiology
Departments of Epidemiology and Biostatistics
Harvard T.H. Chan School of Public Health
Boston, Massachusetts

Sebastien Haneuse
Professor of Biostatistics
Department of Biostatistics
Harvard T. H. Chan School of Public Health
Boston, Massachusetts

Kenneth J. Rothman
Distinguished Fellow, Research Triangle Institute
Research Triangle Park, North Carolina
and
Professor of Epidemiology
Boston University School
of Public Health
Boston, Massachusetts

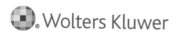 Wolters Kluwer

Philadelphia · Baltimore · New York · London
Buenos Aires · Hong Kong · Sydney · Tokyo

Executive Editor: Sharon Zinner
Development Editor: Sean McGuire
Editorial Coordinator: Cody Adams, Julie Kostelnik
Production Project Manager: Catherine Ott
Design Coordinator: Steve Druding
Manufacturing Coordinator: Beth Welsh
Prepress Vendor: TNQ Technologies

9 8 7 6 5 4 3 2 1

Printed in Mexico

Library of Congress Cataloging-in-Publication Data

ISBN-13: 978-1-4511-9328-2

Cataloging-in-Publication data available on request from the Publisher.

shop.lww.com

QUADM1220

Contents

Preface and Acknowledgments

The fourth edition of *Modern Epidemiology* arrives 35 years after the first edition, which was a much smaller single-authored volume that outlined the concepts and methods of a rapidly growing discipline. The second edition, published 12 years later, was a major transition, as the book grew along with the field. It saw the addition of a second author and an expansion of topics contributed by invited experts in a range of subdisciplines. The third edition, which was published in 2008, saw the addition of a third author and encompassed a comprehensive revision of the content and the introduction of topics that 21st century epidemiologists would find essential.

This fourth edition welcomes insights from two new authors, whose work in the past decade has substantially influenced the design, analysis, and interpretation of epidemiologic research. Like the earlier editions, it encompasses a comprehensive revision of the content, with coverage of methods that have emerged in the interim, such as agent-based modeling, quasi-experimental designs, mediation analysis, and causal modeling. It also updates coverage of methods such as concepts of interaction, bias analysis, and time-varying designs and analysis and continues to cover the full breadth of epidemiologic methods and concepts.

This edition retains the basic organization of the earlier editions, with the book divided into four parts. Part I (Foundations) now comprises six chapters rather than five, with the topic of causation now divided into a conceptual chapter on causal inference and scientific reasoning and a second chapter on formal causal models. We have also moved the introductory chapter on epidemiologic study designs, with validity and efficiency considerations, into the Foundations part of the text. The topic of interaction was Chapter 18 in the second edition, was Chapter 5 in the third edition, and is now Chapter 26 (Part III, Data Analysis) of the fourth edition. We have moved it again to reflect the recent and influential advances in understanding interaction and mediation analyses (now Chapter 27), which require a firm understanding of the fundamentals of epidemiologic research and analysis before they can be fully appreciated. The third edition saw the addition of a new chapter on causal diagrams, which no longer appears as a standalone chapter in the fourth edition. The use of causal graphs to encode assumptions is now so widely incorporated into epidemiologic study design and analysis that the content has been distributed and fully incorporated into the other chapters of the text, including the chapters on causal models. Part II of the text addresses fundamental and advanced aspects of study design and interpretation. In this edition, each of the three major threats to validity—confounding, selection bias and generalizability, and information bias—receives separate treatment in its own chapter. These chapters describe the structures that give rise to the bias, design considerations to reduce the influence of the bias, and simple methods of quantitative bias analysis to estimate the direction, magnitude, and uncertainty attributable to the bias. Also new to this section is a chapter on the use of secondary data, such as registry-based research, which now often serves as the primary source of data, or an ancillary source of data, for many epidemiologic investigations. As in earlier editions, Part II also includes chapters that address cohort designs, case-control designs (including case-crossover and other case-only designs), surveillance, and field methods for data collection. This part concludes with an initial treatment of precision and study size, particularly regarding planning study size.

Part III of this edition addresses data analysis, with updated treatments of conventional approaches to data analysis, such as categorical statistics, stratification, standardization, regression modeling, and dose-response analysis. New content expands on analysis strategies for time-to-event analysis, longitudinal and cluster-correlated analysis, and causal inference with time-varying exposures. As noted above, methods for analyses to address interaction and mediation now appear in Part III. The chapter on bias analysis has been revised, with simple bias analysis methods moved forward to chapters in Part II and with expanded coverage of semi-Bayesian, Bayesian, and empirical bias analysis in its place. The chapter on ecologic analyses has been updated, and we have added a chapter on agent-based modeling and another chapter on instrumental variables and quasi-experimental approaches. The chapter on Bayesian Analysis has been reprinted without revision from the third edition. The chapter's author, Sander Greenland, would have liked to update the chapter, but circumstances did not permit it.

As in the second and third editions, Part IV comprises additional topics that are more specialized than those considered in the first three parts of the book. Prominent authors with substantial experience in each of these topic areas have agreed to write these chapters as an introduction to the topics. Each chapter keeps to a common outline, including (1) a description of the major objectives of the topic area, the history of how it came to be a topic unto itself, and the seminal contributions to public health or medicine; (2) a description of methodologies that are unique to the topic, particularly well suited to the topic, ill advised for the topic area, or otherwise especially relevant to the topic; (3) a description of methodologic challenges that are particularly pertinent to the topic, solutions that have been proposed or implemented, and evaluation of whether these solutions have been adequate; (4) a description of ethical, legal, policy, or social issues that are especially pertinent to the topic; and (5) anticipated directions for the topic, with respect to methodologic developments and content areas for research. For most of the Part IV topics, there are excellent complete textbooks, so our goal with this common outline was to assure that readers would receive an overview of the topic's history, unique challenges, and anticipated directions. Many topics return for the fourth edition, such as social epidemiology, infectious disease epidemiology, genetic and molecular epidemiology, and others, and many new topics have been added, such as psychiatric epidemiology, injury and violence epidemiology, occupational epidemiology, pharmacoepidemiology, and others.

In this text, we hope to acquaint those who wish to understand the concepts and methods of epidemiology with the issues that are central to the discipline and to point the way to key references for further study. The bibliography has been extensively revised and updated, with each chapter now having its own reference list. To make the text easier to read, we now use superscript numerals in text to cite original papers, rather than inserting the paper's authors and publication years as in earlier editions. To facilitate access to all relevant sections of the book that relate to a given topic, we have indexed the text thoroughly. We thus recommend that the index be consulted by those wishing to read our complete discussion of specific topics.

We hope that this new edition provides a resource for teachers, students, and practitioners of epidemiology. We have attempted to be as accurate as possible, but we recognize that any work of this scope will contain mistakes and omissions. We are grateful to readers of earlier editions who have brought such items to our attention. We intend to continue our past practice of posting such corrections on an internet page, as well as incorporating such corrections into subsequent printings. Please consult https://shop.lww.com/Modern-Epidemiology/p/9781451193282 to find the latest information on errata.

We are especially grateful to our colleague Sander Greenland, who was a coauthor of the second and third editions of *Modern Epidemiology*. Although he decided not to join the author group for the fourth edition, much of the text still reflects the ideas and writing that he contributed to the earlier editions. He has not reviewed or approved the text of the fourth edition, but his earlier contributions have been brought forward, revised, and edited by the current authors throughout. As noted above, however, Chapter 23 on Bayesian Analysis appears without revision or updating from the third edition.

We are also grateful to many colleagues who have reviewed sections of the current text and provided useful feedback. Although we cannot mention everyone who helped in that regard, we give special thanks to Catherine Lesko and Penelope Howard for review and comments on Chapter 14 "Selection Bias and Generalizability," to Dana Flanders for review and comments on material in Chapter 6 "Epidemiologic Study Design With Validity and Efficiency Considerations," to James Robins and Miguel Hernán with whom discussions notably influenced the content of Chapter 12 "Confounding and Confounders," to Sara Sauer, Harrison Reeder, and Alexander Levis for review and comments on Chapter 24 "Longitudinal and Cluster-Correlated Data Analysis," and to Rebecca Nash who generated a revised and corrected Figure 29-1 in Chapter 29 "Bias Analysis." Brandon Marshall would like to acknowledge Professors Melissa Tracy and David Savitz for their insightful comments and reviews of Chapter 31 "Agent-Based Modeling." Matthew Fox and Emily Gower would like to acknowledge Dr. Brooke Nichols and Samantha Tulenko for their helpful reviews of Chapter 32 "Infectious Disease Epidemiology." An earlier version of Chapter 23 "Introduction to Bayesian Statistics" appeared in the *International Journal of Epidemiology* (2006;35:765-778), reproduced with permission of Oxford University Press.

Timothy L. Lash
Tyler J. VanderWeele
Sebastien Haneuse
Kenneth J. Rothman

Contributors

James W. Buehler, MD
Clinical Professor & Interim Chair
Department of Health Management & Policy
Dornsife School of Public Health
Drexel University
Philadelphia, Pennsylvania

Stephanie M. Engel, PhD
Professor
Department of Epidemiology
Gillings School of Global Public Health
University of North Carolina at Chapel Hill
Chapel Hill, North Carolina

Matthew P. Fox, DSc, MPH
Professor
Departments of Epidemiology and Global
    Health
Boston University
Boston, Massachusetts

M. Maria Glymour, ScD
Professor
Department of Epidemiology and Biostatistics
University of California, San Francisco
San Francisco, California

Emily W. Gower, PhD
Associate Professor
Department of Epidemiology
University of North Carolina at Chapel Hill
Chapel Hill, North Carolina

Sander Greenland, MA, MS, DrPH, C Stat
Professor Emeritus
Department of Epidemiology and Department
    of Statistics
University of California
Los Angeles, California

Patricia Hartge, MA, ScD
Senior Investigator, Retired
Division of Cancer Epidemiology and Genetics
National Cancer Institute
National Institutes of Health
Bethesda, Maryland

Irva Hertz-Picciotto, MPH, PhD
Professor
Department of Public Health Sciences
University of California, Davis
Davis, California

Richard S. Hopkins, MD, MSPH
Independent Epidemiologist
Middlebury, Vermont

Frank B. Hu, MD, PhD
Professor and Chair
Department of Nutrition
Harvard T.H. Chan School of Public Health
Boston, Massachusetts

Krista F. Huybrechts, MS, PhD
Associate Professor of Medicine and
    Epidemiology
Division of Pharmacoepidemiology,
    Department of Medicine
Brigham and Women's Hospital and Harvard
    Medical School
Boston, Massachusetts

Anne Marie Jukic, PhD
Investigator
Epidemiology Branch
National Institute of Environmental Health
    Sciences
Durham, North Carolina

Jay S. Kaufman, PhD
Professor
Department of Epidemiology, Biostatistics and
    Occupational Health
McGill University
Montreal, Quebec, Canada

Katherine M. Keyes, PhD
Associate Professor
Department of Epidemiology
Columbia University, Mailman School of
    Public Health
New York, New York

Guohua Li, MD, DrPH
Mieczyslaw Finster Professor
Departments of Anesthesiology and
    Epidemiology
Columbia University
New York, New York

Brandon D. L. Marshall, PhD
Associate Professor
Department of Epidemiology
Brown University
Providence, Rhode Island

Stephen W. Marshall, PhD
Professor
Departments of Epidemiology and Exercise
    and Sport Science
University of North Carolina at Chapel Hill
Chapel Hill, North Carolina

Hal Morgenstern, BArch, MRP, PhD
Professor Emeritus
Departments of Epidemiology
Environmental Health Sciences, and Urology
University of Michigan
Ann Arbor, Michigan

Lorelei Mucci, ScD, MPH
Professor
Department of Epidemiology
Harvard T.H. Chan School of Public Health
Boston, Massachusetts

Claire H. Pernar, ScD, MPH
Research Associate
Department of Epidemiology
Harvard T.H. Chan School of Public Health
Boston, Massachusetts

David Richardson, PhD
Professor
Department of Epidemiology
School of Public Health
University of North Carolina at Chapel Hill
Chapel Hill, North Carolina

Sebastian Schneeweiss, MD, ScD
Professor of Medicine and Epidemiology
Division of Pharmacoepidemiology,
    Department of Medicine
Brigham and Women's Hospital and Harvard
    Medical School
Boston, Massachusetts

Sharon B. Schwartz, PhD
Professor of Epidemiology at CUMC
Department of Epidemiology
Columbia University, Mailman School of
    Public Health
New York, New York

Henrik Toft Sørensen, MD, PhD, DMSc
Professor, Chair
Department of Clinical Epidemiology
Aarhus University
Aarhus, Denmark
Adjunct Professor
Department of Epidemiology
Boston University
Boston, Massachusetts

Konrad H. Stopsack, MD MPH
Research Associate
Department of Medicine
Memorial Sloan Kettering Cancer Center
New York, New York

Ezra S. Susser, MD, DrPH
Professor
Departments of Epidemiology and Psychiatry
Columbia University, Mailman School of
    Public Health
New York State Psychiatric Institute
New York, New York

Sonja A. Swanson, ScD
Associate Professor
Department of Epidemiology
Erasmus Medical Center
Rotterdam, Netherlands

Duncan C. Thomas, PhD
Professor and Verna Richter Chair in
    Cancer Research
Department of Preventive Medicine
University of Southern California
Los Angeles, California

**Jan P. Vandenbroucke, MD, PhD, FRCP,
FRCPE**
Emeritus Professor of Clinical Epidemiology
Leiden University Medical Center
Leiden, Netherlands
Professor of Clinical Epidemiology
Aarhus University
Aarhus, Denmark
Honorary Professor
London School of Hygiene and Tropical
    Medicine
London, United Kingdom

Jon Wakefield, PhD
Professor
Departments of Statistics and Biostatistics
University of Washington
Seattle, Washington

Clarice R. Weinberg, PhD
Senior Investigator
Biostatistics and Computational Biology
    Branch
National Institute of Environmental Health
    Sciences
Research Triangle Park, North Carolina

Allen J. Wilcox, MD, PhD
Emeritus Investigator
Epidemiology Branch
National Institute of Environmental Health
    Sciences
Durham, North Carolina

Walter C. Willett, MD, DrPH
Professor
Departments of Nutrition and Epidemiology
Harvard T.H. Chan School of Public Health
Boston, Massachusetts

Lauren A. Wise, ScD
Professor
Department of Epidemiology
Boston University School of Public Health
Boston, Massachusetts

John S. Witte, PhD
Professor
Department of Epidemiology and Biostatistics
University of California San Francisco
San Francisco, California

PART I

Foundations

CHAPTER 1

The Scope of Epidemiology

Kenneth J. Rothman, Timothy L. Lash, Sebastien Haneuse, and Tyler J. VanderWeele

INTRODUCTION

Epidemiology is the science that studies disease occurrence and health states in human populations. Descriptive epidemiology (also known as medical demography) measures how disease frequency and other population health indicators vary with age, gender, geographic location, race/ethnicity, and other characteristics of person, time, and place. Such description can provide critical insights into the potential causes of disease. For example, early in the AIDS epidemic, descriptive epidemiology strongly indicated that AIDS was an infectious disease transmitted through direct contact with body fluids. Descriptive epidemiology also provided early insights into the long latency period of HIV infection, the underlying cause of AIDS.

Etiologic or analytic epidemiology assesses the effect of exposures, which include possible causes, on the occurrence of disease. Exposures can be evaluated on the scale of individual persons, such as behaviors, occupations, environmental hazards, medical history, or personal characteristics such as age. They can also be measured on the microscale, such as a person's genetics, microbiome, or metabolic profile. Finally, exposures can be measured on a macroscale, such as social characteristics like disparities in wealth in one's society or the birth cohort to which one belongs.

Some health and medical events, such as an injury or influenza, may occur within seconds or hours and are said to have rapid or *acute* onset. Others, such as atherosclerosis, neurodegenerative disease, or cancer, may develop gradually over years or decades and are said to have prolonged or *chronic* onset. Categorical distinctions such as macro versus micro level and acute versus chronic onset reflect underlying continuous scales for exposures and outcome events that can be investigated with epidemiologic methods. For example, myocardial infarction is an acute-onset event often arising from the gradual development of atherosclerosis, which has been associated with a person's genetics, lifestyle, social situation, and environmental circumstances. Regular exercise can reduce the risk of this event, but the risk can increase for a short time after an individual episode of vigorous exercise. This example illustrates the complexities of the etiologic relations measured by epidemiologic research and hints at the various methodologic challenges that have been tackled as the science has developed.

The main strength of epidemiology is that it assesses the disease burden, or exposure-disease association, in the human species. The evidence from epidemiologic research is therefore directly relevant to the population of interest. The main limitation is that it is not as easy as it may seem. At its most fundamental level, epidemiology is an exercise in counting within groups. But whom to count, how to count them, when to count them, and how to compare them introduce complexities well beyond what intuition might suggest. Epidemiologic investigations that ignore these complexities can yield misleading measurements, so when would-be epidemiologists use methods that stem from intuition rather than solid training in the principles of epidemiology, important errors are likely to occur. Therefore, until the final part, the focus of this book is on epidemiologic theory and research methods founded on that theory.

ROOTS OF EPIDEMIOLOGY

Epidemiology has its roots in early attempts to understand and improve public health. As agriculture replaced hunting, and small clans began to aggregate into villages and towns, people faced problems such as acquiring a reliable source of freshwater and eliminating human waste from their community. These problems were best dealt with as community projects. Living more densely, they also became more susceptible to epidemic disease, an important threat to any established society. For example, during the middle ages, the growth of cities in Europe was accompanied by epidemics of leprosy, plague, and other scourges. The Black Death was a pandemic of what is believed to be bubonic plague that swept Europe in mid-14th century, killing between one-third and one-half of the population. Travelers from plague-infested areas were often barred entry into communities, and patients were sometimes kept isolated. The term "quarantine" comes from the Italian phrase "quaranta dei," referring to the 40 days during which all goods and travelers were kept in isolation during plague periods in Venice, an important shipping port.

John Snow, an important early figure in the history of epidemiology, conducted research on the communication of cholera, which he believed was spread through exposure to water contaminated with human waste. His "natural experiment" was a study of cholera incidence in relation to the consumption of water from two competing companies, one carrying comparatively clean, Thames water from upstream of London and the other, water that was drawn downstream of London and therefore contaminated with sewage. In some districts of London, the competing water companies piped their water down the same streets, and, on these streets, most residents did not know which company supplied their home. Although Snow's research design was elegant, it failed to sway the medical scientists of the time, most of whom held firmly to the view that cholera was spread through foul air rather than contaminated water.[1]

Snow's work was one of a few examples of excellent epidemiologic investigations that were conducted before the 20th century. These examples are, however, isolated events. A systematized body of principles by which to design and evaluate epidemiology studies began to form only in the second half of the 20th century. These principles evolved in conjunction with an explosion of epidemiologic research, the evolution of which continues today.

Several large-scale epidemiologic studies started in mid-20th century have had far-reaching influences on health. For example, the Framingham Heart Study, initiated in 1948, is notable among several long-term follow-up studies of cardiovascular disease that have contributed importantly to understanding the causes of this public-health problem.[2] By its 70th anniversary, more than 3,700 scientific publications have emerged from this one epidemiologic project. Knowledge from this and similar epidemiologic studies has helped stem the epidemic of cardiovascular disease in the industrialized Western world.[3,4]

Another example of 20th-century epidemiology with far-reaching implications was the Salk vaccine field trial of 1954.[5] With several hundred thousand school children as subjects, this study was for decades the largest formal human experiment ever conducted and provided the first practical basis for the prevention of paralytic poliomyelitis. In the 21st century, the DEVTA trial of vitamin A supplementation and intestinal deworming surpassed the Salk vaccine trial in size by enrolling two million children in India. DEVTA ultimately reported no substantial preventive benefit against childhood mortality associated with either intervention.[6,7]

The 20th century also saw the publication of many epidemiologic studies on the effects of tobacco use. These studies led eventually to the landmark report, Smoking and Health, issued by the US Surgeon General.[8] The report was the first among many on the adverse effects of tobacco use on health issued by the Surgeon General.

Since the time of these important studies, epidemiologic research has steadily attracted greater public attention. Unlike more basic science, epidemiologic research is work with which the public and media can readily connect. Both researchers and news media, boosted by a rising tide of social concern about health and environmental issues, have vaulted many epidemiologic studies to prominence, sometimes well before sufficient evidence had accumulated to merit consideration of policy implications, as in the case of a reported outbreak of Hodgkin disease among high-school students.[9]

Disagreement about basic conceptual and methodologic points led, in some instances, to profound differences in the interpretation of data. An historical example with which students of epidemiology should be familiar involves a controversy that erupted in the mid-1970s about whether exogenous estrogens are carcinogenic to the endometrium. Several case-control studies had reported an extremely strong association, with up to a 15-fold increase in risk.[10-12] One group, Horwitz and Feinstein, argued that a selection bias accounted for most of the observed association,[13] whereas others argued that the alternative design proposed by Horwitz and Feinstein introduced a downward selection bias far stronger than any upward bias it removed.[14-16] Ultimately, the former view lost out to proponents of the latter view. Modern students of epidemiologic methods may be surprised to learn that only 50 years ago such different views were held by prominent and credible epidemiologists on a methodologic topic that they would now so readily understand. Such disagreements about fundamental concepts in the relatively recent past, at least on the time scale of scientific inquiry, suggest that the methodologic foundations of the science had not yet been established and that epidemiology remained young in conceptual terms.

The last third of the 20th century and the beginning of the 21st century have seen rapid growth in the understanding and synthesis of epidemiologic concepts. The main stimulus for this conceptual growth seems to have been accelerated the growth of epidemiologic research, coupled with controversy. The explosion of epidemiologic activity accentuated the need to improve understanding of the theoretical underpinnings. For example, early studies on smoking and lung cancer[17,18] were scientifically noteworthy not only for their substantive findings but also because they demonstrated the efficacy and great efficiency of the case-control study. Controversies about proper case-control design led to recognition of the importance of relating such studies to an underlying source population[19-22] (see Chapter 8). Likewise, analysis of data from the Framingham Heart Study stimulated the development of multiple logistic regression,[23,24] one of the most popular and enduring modeling methods in epidemiology (see Chapters 21 and 22).

In the 21st century, epidemiologic concepts have continued to evolve rapidly, perhaps because the scope, activity, and influence of epidemiology continue to increase. This rise in epidemiologic activity and influence has been accompanied by growing pains, largely reflecting concern about the validity of the methods used in epidemiologic research and the reliability of inferences drawn from the results. The disparity between the results of randomized[25] and nonrandomized[26] studies of the association between hormone replacement therapy and cardiovascular disease provided a high-profile example of hypotheses supposedly established by observational epidemiology and subsequently contradicted.[27,28] The conflicting results, however, may have been reconciled by Hernán et al.,[29] who provided evidence that the discrepancies between the randomized and nonrandomized studies were due to differences in the populations studied and the length of follow-up. Methodologic approaches continue to evolve and to be subject to critical debate. In addition, epidemiologists debate priority areas for their research endeavors. For example, tensions remain between those who advocate for molecularly focused epidemiologic research,[30] behaviorally focused research,[31,32] and socially focused research.[33]

It may be discouraging to practice in a field in which basic concepts are still maturing and in which even prominent practitioners often disagree on conceptual issues. Furthermore, as epidemiology is so often in the public eye, it can be a magnet for criticism. The criticism has occasionally broadened to a distrust of the methods of epidemiology itself, going beyond skepticism of specific findings to general criticism of epidemiologic investigation.[34,35] These criticisms and anxieties, though hard to accept, should nevertheless be welcomed by scientists. We should strive to learn from our mistakes and embrace the challenge of working in so dynamic and prominent a field. There is much that epidemiologists can do to increase the reliability and utility of their findings; providing readers the basis for achieving that goal is an aim of this textbook.

As we prepare to deliver this book to the publisher in mid-2020, we are in the grip of the COVID-19 pandemic. Epidemiology is suddenly a field of broad interest. Week after week there are questions directed at epidemiologists about the Sars-Cov-2 virus, how to control it, and how to treat the disease that it causes. Who is most susceptible and why? Should we wear masks? Should our children attend school? Is it safe to press the elevator button in our building? Should I stop my antihypertensive medication? Will antimalaria drugs prevent infection? Is it safe to see the doctor or go to the hospital? If I recover, can I get reinfected? All of these are questions that epidemiologists can answer, with time, material support, and patience. Unfortunately, decisions have had to be made rapidly, often with uncertain evidence, and with the pervasive influence of politics often weighing as heavily as the science.

In the midst of the pandemic, there has been a flurry of research, some good, some less than adequate, but all done under the pressure of attempting to answer vital questions while a deadly pandemic rages through a susceptible population. Suddenly, the need to understand the principles of epidemiology has become a priority. In the years to come, there will be a lot to learn from the actions taken during the pandemic. The different courses of the pandemic in countries with strict lockdowns—such as Iceland, South Korea, Cuba, and Japan—compared with more lax restrictions— such as Sweden, the US, and Brazil—will provide important lessons. It is already clear that, as has too often been witnessed, individuals and nations with the least resources bear an outsized burden. At the outset of the pandemic, there was little relevant knowledge to guide us. Much will be learned by studying the effectiveness of the widely variant public health and medical responses. Fortunately, for most diseases that we face, we do not have the time urgency of a deadly pandemic that raises fresh questions demanding immediate answers. But whether the questions raised involve treating old scourges such as atherosclerosis or new threats such as COVID-19, the underlying principles that we need to apply to find the answers will be the same. It is those principles that we address in this book.

DESCRIPTIVE VERSUS ANALYTIC EPIDEMIOLOGY

The first steps in constructing a compendium of epidemiologic information in a specific disease area constitute descriptions of the disease epidemiology. This descriptive epidemiology involves assembling measures of disease occurrence for demographic and geographic subpopulations. Contrasts of disease incidence for natalmales and females, by age, by gender identity, by race/ethnicity, by urban or rural residence, and by time period, are examples of descriptive epidemiology. Demographic and geographic patterns in disease occurrence provide information that is useful both for public-health programming and for etiologic understanding. Thus, sex-specific differences in sexually transmitted infections may suggest differences in behaviors or differences in socially patterned use of condoms, age patterns may suggest prenatal or postnatal causes, and geographic patterns may reflect differences in sun exposure and concomitant vitamin D sufficiency. In MacMahon and Pugh's influential textbook of epidemiology,[36] there were separate chapters for "Person," "Place," and "Time," indicating the importance of describing the epidemiology of any disease with regard to these fundamental characteristics.

Some epidemiologists divide epidemiology into "descriptive epidemiology" and "analytic epidemiology." This division is based on the notion that descriptive epidemiology serves to generate hypotheses about the causes of a disease, whereas analytic epidemiology subjects those hypotheses to more focused and rigorous tests to weed out the tenable from the untenable hypotheses. In this book, we do not maintain this division into descriptive and analytic epidemiology because this mindset diminishes the importance of descriptive epidemiology and disease surveillance and because the division is never that clear. The interplay between generating new hypotheses and subjecting those hypotheses to rigorous tests exists, or should exist, at all levels of information, including what is commonly considered descriptive epidemiology. This division, however, raises a more fundamental question: what is the logical process by which we can draw conclusions about the causes of a disease? Below we consider the question of scientific reasoning in science generally and in epidemiology in particular.

SCIENTIFIC REASONING AND THE PHILOSOPHY OF SCIENCE

Because much epidemiologic research is aimed at uncovering the causes of disease, it is useful for epidemiologists to be familiar with the basic issues that underlie scientific reasoning. The most fundamental methodologic questions about interpreting data hinge on long-standing, well-debated principles that have their roots in the philosophy of science. Causal inference, which we address in considerable depth in subsequent chapters, may be viewed as a special case of the more general process of scientific reasoning. The literature on this topic is too broad for us to review thoroughly here, but we will provide a brief overview of certain points relevant to epidemiology, at the risk of some oversimplification.

Inductivism

Modern science began to emerge around the 16th and 17th centuries, when the knowledge demands of emerging technologies stimulated inquiry into the origins of knowledge. An early codification of the scientific method was Francis Bacon's *Novum Organum*, which, in 1620, presented an inductivist view of science. In this philosophy, scientific reasoning is said to depend on making generalizations, or inductions, starting from observed patterns and progressing to general laws of nature; the observations are said to induce the formulation of a natural law in the mind of the scientist. Thus, an inductivist would have said that Jenner's observation of lack of smallpox among milkmaids induced in Jenner's mind the theory that cowpox (common among milkmaids) conferred immunity to smallpox.

Inductivist philosophy was systematized in the canons of John Stuart Mill,[37] which evolved into inferential guidelines that are still in use today, such as those of Bradford Hill.[38] These guidelines are discussed in detail in Chapter 2.

Refutationism

Inductivist philosophy provided numerous important insights. Nonetheless, in the 18th century, the Scottish philosopher David Hume described a disturbing deficiency in inductivism. Hume showed that an inductive argument carried no logical force in the deductive sense familiar in mathematics; instead, such an argument represented an assumption that certain events would in the future follow the same pattern as they had in the past. Thus, to argue that if one threw a ball in the air, it would eventually slow down and reverse course to fall to earth because that had always been observed in the past corresponded to an assumption that the pattern observed to date (objects thrown upward slow down, reverse course, and return to earth) would continue into the future. In the same way, to argue that cowpox caused immunity to smallpox because no one got smallpox after having cowpox corresponded to an assumption that the pattern observed to date (no smallpox after cowpox) would continue into the future.

Hume pointed out that, even for the most reasonable sounding of such assumptions, there was no logical necessity behind the inductive argument. Of central concern to Hume was the issue of causal inference and failure of induction to provide a foundation for it[39]:

> "Thus not only our reason fails us in the discovery of the ultimate connexion of causes and effects, but even after experience has inform'd us of their constant conjunction, 'tis impossible for us to satisfy ourselves by our reason, why we shou'd extend that experience beyond those particular instances, which have fallen under our observation. We suppose, but are never able to prove, that there must be a resemblance betwixt those objects, of which we have had experience, and those which lie beyond the reach of our discovery."

In other words, no number of repetitions of a particular sequence of events, such as the appearance of a light after flipping a switch, can prove a causal connection between the action of the switch and the turning on of the light. No matter how many times the light comes on after the switch has been pressed, the possibility of coincidental occurrence cannot be ruled out. Causal inference based on mere association of events additionally constitutes a logical fallacy known as *post hoc ergo propter hoc* (Latin for "after this therefore on account of this"). This fallacy is exemplified by the inference that the crowing of a rooster is necessary for the sun to rise because sunrise is always preceded by the crowing.

The *post hoc* fallacy is a special case of a general logical fallacy known as the fallacy of affirming the consequent. This fallacy of confirmation takes the following general form: "We know that if H is true, B must be true; and we know that B is true; therefore H must be true." Though a fallacy, this reasoning is often used by scientists in interpreting data. For example, when one argues as follows: "If sewer service causes heart disease, then heart disease rates should be highest where sewer service is available; heart disease rates are indeed highest where sewer service is available; therefore, sewer service causes heart disease." Here, H is the hypothesis "sewer service causes heart disease" and B is the observation "heart disease rates are highest where sewer service is available." The argument is logically unsound, as demonstrated by the fact that we can imagine many ways in which the premises could be true but the conclusion false. For example, economic development could lead to both sewer service and elevated heart disease rates, without any effect of sewer service on heart disease. In this case, however, we also know that one of the premises is not true—specifically, the premise, "If H is true, B must be true." This particular form of the fallacy exemplifies the problem of confounding, which we will discuss in detail in later chapters.

Since the skeptical writings of Hume, philosophers of science have tried either to refute the skepticism or to weave it into their thinking. In the early 20th century, Hume's thesis began to become accepted. Available observations, however, are always consistent with several hypotheses that themselves are mutually inconsistent, which explains why, as Hume noted, scientific theories cannot be deductively proven to be empirical facts. In particular, consistency between a hypothesis and observations is no proof of the hypothesis because we can always invent alternative hypotheses that are also consistent with the observations.

In contrast to the futility of attempting to prove a hypothesis, one school of thought, championed by Popper,[40] noted that a valid observation that is inconsistent with a hypothesis implies that the hypothesis as stated is false. In other words, though proving a scientific hypothesis deductively is impossible, it is claimed that refuting one is not. This refutationist viewpoint was illustrated by Magee,[41] who described a hypothetical research program to learn the boiling point of water. A scientist who boils water in an open flask and repeatedly measures the boiling point at 100°C will never, no matter how many confirmatory repetitions are involved, prove that 100°C is always the boiling point. On the other hand, merely one attempt to boil the water in a closed flask or at high altitude will refute the proposition that water always boils at 100°C.

According to refutationist philosophy, science advances by a process of "conjecture and refutation." Scientists form hypotheses based on intuition, conjecture, and previous experience. Good scientists use deductive logic to infer predictions from the hypothesis and then compare observations with the predictions. Hypotheses whose predictions agree with observations are confirmed only in the sense that they can continue to be used as explanations of natural phenomena. At any time, however, they may be refuted by further observations and might be replaced by other hypotheses that are more consistent with the observations.

One way to rescue the concept of induction is to resurrect it as a psychological phenomenon, as Hume and Popper claimed it was, but one that plays a legitimate role in hypothesis formation. The philosophy of conjecture and refutation places no constraints on the origin of conjectures. Even delusions are permitted as hypotheses and therefore inductively inspired hypotheses are valid starting points for scientific evaluation. This concession does not admit a logical role for induction in definitively establishing scientific hypotheses, but it allows the process of induction to play a part, along with imagination, in the scientific cycle of conjecture and refutation.

The philosophy of conjecture and refutation has profound implications for the methodology of science. The popular concept of a scientist doggedly assembling evidence to support a favorite thesis is objectionable because it encourages scientists to consider their own pet theories as their intellectual property, to be confirmed, proven, and, when all the evidence is in, cast in stone and defended as natural law. Such attitudes hinder critical evaluation, interchange, and progress. The approach of conjecture and refutation, in contrast, encourages scientists to be skeptical, to consider multiple hypotheses, and to seek crucial tests that narrow the pool of competing hypotheses by falsifying one of them.

Ideally, falsification is not personal. Criticism leveled at a theory need not be seen as criticism of the person who proposed it. When used constructively, the refutationist approach can be highly productive. It has been suggested that the reason why certain fields of science have advanced rapidly during certain periods while others languished is that the rapidly advancing fields were propelled by scientists who were busy constructing and testing competing hypotheses; the other fields, in contrast, were described as "sick by comparison because they have forgotten the necessity for alternative hypotheses and disproof."[42]

The refutationist model of science has a number of valuable lessons for research conduct, especially of the need to seek alternative explanations for observations, rather than focus on the chimera of seeking scientific "proof" for some favored theory. Nonetheless, it is vulnerable to criticisms that observations (or their interpretations) are themselves laden with theory (sometimes called the Duhem-Quine thesis).[43] Thus, observations can never provide the sort of definitive refutations that are the hallmark of popular accounts of refutationism. For example, there may be uncontrolled and even unimagined biases that have made our refutational observations invalid; to claim refutation is to assume as true the unprovable theory that no such bias exists. Refutations depend on theories, and therefore their foundation is not completely secure. The net result is that logical certainty about either the truth or falsity of a scientific theory is impossible.[44]

Consensus and Naturalism

Some 20th-century philosophers of science, most notably Kuhn,[45] emphasized the role of the scientific community in judging the validity of scientific theories. These critics of the conjecture and refutation model suggested that the refutation of a theory involves making a choice. Every observation is itself dependent on theories. For example, observing the moons of Jupiter through a telescope seems to us like a direct observation but only because the theory of optics on which the telescope is based is so well accepted. When confronted with a refuting observation, a scientist faces the choice of rejecting either the validity of the theory being tested or the validity of the refuting observation, which itself must be premised on scientific theories that are not certain.[46] Observations that are falsifying instances of theories may at times be treated as "anomalies," with the theory retained in the hope that the anomalies may eventually be explained. Of course, anomalies may lead eventually to the overthrow of current scientific doctrine, just as Newtonian mechanics was displaced (remaining as a useful approximation) by relativity theory.

Kuhn asserted that in every branch of science the prevailing scientific viewpoint, which he termed "normal science," occasionally undergoes major shifts that amount to scientific revolutions. These revolutions signal a decision of the scientific community to discard the scientific infrastructure rather than to falsify a new hypothesis that cannot be easily grafted onto it. Kuhn and others have argued that the consensus of the scientific community determines what is considered accepted and what is considered refuted, and that acceptance and refutation are only meaningful in relation to what is accepted by that community as established knowledge.

A classical view that the ultimate goal of scientific inference is to capture some objective truths about the material world in which we live. This view leads to the notion that any theory of inference should ideally be evaluated by how well it leads us to these truths. Measurement of how well this ideal has been achieved are extremely difficult to validate, however, for we have no way of knowing with certainty that we have found an absolute truth about the world. Thus, knowledge about the world will always be tentative to a greater or lesser degree. This uncertainty may be negligible in some branches of physical science but is so large as to be the motivation for research in health and medical sciences. Truth arguably still remains the goal, but our capacity to arrive at it is limited, regardless of whether consensus beliefs about the truth evolve.

Frequentism

In light of the limits of investigative methods, our inferences and our store of accepted facts will inevitably contain errors to some unknown degree. This conclusion, labeled *fallibilism*, was reached by the American pragmatic philosopher Charles Sanders Peirce in the late 19th century.[47] To address these limitations, the geneticist and statistician R. A. Fisher developed a theory and methodology of inference based on experiments designed to provide known frequencies of results under explicit, ideal conditions.[48,49]

A pivotal requirement of Fisher's *frequentist* methodology was that the experiment incorporate a device or instrument that generated treatment assignments (allocations) in a random fashion, with known frequencies for all possible assignment patterns. This known behavior of the assignment instrument (also known as the allocation mechanism) could then be used to compute the probabilities of subsequent observations under a specific hypothesis about the effect of treatment, which formed the basis of Fisher's statistical tests. Typically, the hypothesis chosen for the computation—the test hypothesis—was that the treatment had no effect, which today is called the causal null hypothesis. Other hypotheses could be used instead, but experimental design and subsequent computations are simplest for this null hypothesis. In Fisher's time, before the advent of electronic computers, this simplicity encouraged a focus on the null hypothesis—a focus that remains, inappropriately, to the present day in most statistics texts and analyses.[50]

Borrowing the terms "statistical significance" and "significance test" from earlier statistical writers—but *not* their meaning of the term—Fisher computed what he called a "level of significance" for the experimental outcome in relation to the hypothesis tested, which in more neutral terms is known as a *P-value*. For simple experiments designed to "test" the null, this *P*-value was the frequency (expressed as a probability) with which one should expect the experimental design to produce an effect estimate as large as observed or larger if in fact there was no effect of the treatment. There are many subtleties and qualifications that should be attached to the *P*-value and this description, which we will review at length in Chapter 15. For now, the most important one, which Fisher also emphasized, is that the *P*-value as Fisher defined it is *not* the probability of the tested hypothesis. Unfortunately, it is often misinterpreted as if it were that probability.

A *P*-value may, however, be viewed as measuring, under ideal conditions, the compatibility or consistency between the experimental outcome and the tested hypothesis, with $P = 1$ indicating that the outcome is exactly what the hypothesis predicted, and $P = 0$ indicating that the outcome is impossible under the hypothesis. In this usage, it is crucial to note that $P = 1$ does *not* mean the hypothesis is correct, for there may be many other hypotheses that are also highly compatible with the outcome. In addition, the results may only reflect departures from the ideal setting assumed by the computation of the *P*-value; the result may have arisen from invalid assumptions, from computing errors, and in the extreme, a clever analyst can manipulate the data or methods to produce a large or small *P*-value.

There were several logical gaps in Fisher's paradigm, especially in regard to how to use the *P*-value to make decisions. These gaps were addressed by the theory of hypothesis testing and confidence intervals developed by the statisticians Jerzy Neyman and Egon Pearson in the 1920s and 1930s. This theory focused on providing explicit error rates for testing and estimation methods under ideal design settings for experiments and surveys and by the 1950s had become the standard approach in much of statistical teaching and analysis. As with Fisher's significance testing theory, the Neyman-Pearson theory does *not* provide probabilities of hypotheses; instead, it seeks decision rules with known acceptable error rates under an assumed allocation or selection mechanism.

Although frequentist statistical methods have become the convention for most analyses, they suffer severe limitations in general and for epidemiology in particular. They seem extraordinarily difficult even for trained statisticians to interpret correctly: The human mind seems wired to seek results phrased as hypothesis probabilities, which frequentist methods simply do not supply, and as a consequence, frequentist results get misinterpreted as such probabilities; see Greenland et al. for a bibliography of references documenting this problem and 25 examples of misinterpretations found in the scientific literature.[51] Another severe problem is that conventional methods assume that the study data were generated under ideal conditions, involving known random assignment and selection mechanisms. Unfortunately, few observational studies come close to satisfying these conditions. Much of this book will be concerned with identifying how these conditions are violated and what can be done to prevent or account for these violations.

Bayesianism

As with frequentism, Bayesian philosophies of inference may hold an objective view of scientific truth and a view of knowledge as tentative or uncertain but focus on measurement of knowledge or information rather than truth.[52] Specifically, and in contrast to frequentist methodologies, Bayesian methods seek to provide hypothesis probabilities. Like refutationism, modern versions of Bayesian philosophy evolved from the writings of 18th-century thinkers: The focal arguments first appeared in an essay by the Reverend Thomas Bayes, for whom the approach was eventually named.[53] Although the renowned French mathematician and scientist Pierre Simon de Laplace first gave it an applied statistical format, modern Bayesian philosophy did not emerge until after World War I.

The central problem addressed by Bayesian philosophies is the following: In classical logic, a deductive argument can provide no information about the truth or falsity of a scientific hypothesis unless you can be 100% certain about the truth of the premises of the argument. Consider the logical argument called *modus tollens*: "If H implies B, and B is false, then H must be false." This argument is deductively valid, but the conclusion follows only on the assumptions that the premises "H implies B" and "B is false" are true statements. If these premises are statements about the physical world, we cannot possibly know them to be correct with 100% certainty because all observations are subject to error. Furthermore, the claim that "H implies B" will often depend on its own chain of deductions, each with its own premises of which we cannot be certain.

For example, if H is "Television viewing causes homicides" and B is "Homicide rates are highest where televisions are most common," the first premise in *modus tollens* regarding the proposition that television viewing causes homicides will be: "If television viewing causes homicides, homicide rates will be highest where televisions are most common." The validity of this premise is doubtful—after all, even if television does cause homicides, homicide rates may be low where televisions are common and leisure time is ample because of socioeconomic advantages in those areas.

Continuing to reason in this fashion, we could arrive at a more pessimistic state than even Hume imagined. Not only is induction without logical foundation, but deduction has limited scientific utility because we cannot ensure the truth of all the premises, even if a logical argument is valid. The personalistic ("subjective") Bayesian answer to this problem is partial in that it makes a severe demand on the scientist and puts a severe limitation on the results. It says roughly this: If you can assign degrees of certainty, or personal probabilities, to the premises of your valid argument, you may use any and all the rules of probability theory to derive a degree of certainty for the conclusion, and this certainty will be a deductively valid consequence of your original certainties. An inescapable fact is that your concluding certainty, or posterior probability, may depend heavily on what you used as your set of initial certainties or prior probabilities. If this set of initial certainties is not the same as that of a colleague, that colleague may very well assign a certainty to the conclusion different from the one you derived. With the accumulation of consistent evidence, however, along with mutual trust among the colleagues, the data can usually force even opinions starting as extremely disparate sets of prior probabilities to converge toward similar posterior probabilities.

Because the posterior probability emanating from a Bayesian inference depends on the person supplying the set of initial certainties and so may vary across individuals, the inferences are subjective. This subjectivity of Bayesian inference is often mistaken for a subjective treatment of truth. Not only is such a view of Bayesianism incorrect, some might view it as diametrically opposed to Bayesian philosophy. The Bayesian approach represents a constructive attempt to deal with the dilemma that scientific laws and facts should not be treated as known with certainty, whereas classic deductive logic yields conclusions only when some law, fact, or connection is asserted with 100% certainty.

A common criticism of Bayesianism is that it diverts attention away from the classic goals of science, such as the discovery of how the world works, toward psychological states of mind called "certainties," "subjective probabilities," or "degrees of belief."[54] This criticism, however, fails to recognize the importance of a scientist's state of mind in determining what theories to test and what tests to apply, the consequent influence of those states on the store of data available for inference, and the influence of the data on the states of mind.

Another reply to this criticism is that scientists already use data to influence their degrees of belief, and they are not shy about expressing those degrees of certainty. The problem is that the conventional process is informal and intuitive and therefore not subject to critical scrutiny. At its worst, it often amounts to nothing more than the experts announcing that they have seen the evidence and here is how certain they are. How they reached this certainty is left unclear or, put another way, is not "transparent." The problem is that no one, even an expert, is very good at informally and intuitively formulating certainties that accurately predict facts and future events.[55-57] Psychologic investigations have found that most people, including scientists, reason poorly in general and especially poorly in the face of uncertainty.[55-57] One reason for this problem is that biases and prior prejudices can easily creep into expert judgments. Bayesian methods force experts to specify explicitly the strength of their prior beliefs, why they have such beliefs, defend those specifications against arguments and evidence and update their degrees of certainty with new evidence in ways that do not violate probability logic.[58]

In any research context, there will be an unlimited number of hypotheses that could explain an observed phenomenon. Some argue that progress is best aided by severely testing (empirically challenging) those explanations that seem most probable considering past research, so that shortcomings of currently "received" theories can be most rapidly discovered. Indeed, much research in certain fields takes this form, as when theoretical predictions of particle mass are put to ever more precise tests in physics experiments. This process does not involve mere improved repetition of past studies; it involves tests of previously unexamined but important predictions of the theory.[59] Moreover, there is an imperative to make the basis for prior beliefs open to criticism and defensible. That prior probabilities can differ among persons does not mean that all such beliefs are based on the same information, nor that all are equally tenable. An important use for subjective Bayesian methods is for reasoning under less than ideal conditions, where the methods can provide many warnings against being overly certain about one's conclusions.[58,60,61] For example, as we shall discuss at greater length in Chapter 30, conventional confidence intervals quantify only random error under often questionable assumptions and so should not be interpreted as measures of total uncertainty, particularly for nonexperimental studies.[62]

Scientific Reasoning for Causal Inference in Epidemiology

Epidemiologic hypotheses may invoke little or nothing in the way of mechanistic concepts, making the hypotheses themselves only qualitative statements about the effect of an exposure on an outcome, such as "poor diet causes cardiovascular disease." These vague hypotheses have only vague consequences, making them difficult to test. To cope with this vagueness, epidemiologists often focus on testing the negation of the causal hypothesis, that is, the null hypothesis that the exposure does not have a causal relation to disease. Then, any observed association can potentially refute the hypothesis, subject to the substantial assumption (auxiliary hypothesis) that biases and chance fluctuations are not solely responsible for the association.

Nonetheless, if the causal mechanism is stated specifically enough, epidemiologic observations can provide crucial tests of competing, nonnull causal hypotheses. For example, when toxic shock syndrome was first studied, there were two competing hypotheses about the causal agent. Under one hypothesis, the cause was a chemical in the tampon, so that women using tampons were exposed to the agent directly from the tampon. Under the other hypothesis, the tampon acted as a culture medium for staphylococci that produced a toxin. Both hypotheses explained the relation of toxic shock occurrence to tampon use. The two hypotheses, however, led to opposite predictions about the relation between the frequency of changing tampons and the rate of toxic shock. Under the hypothesis of a chemical agent, more frequent changing of the tampon would lead to more exposure to the agent and possible absorption of a greater overall dose. This hypothesis predicted that women who changed tampons more frequently would have a higher rate than women who changed tampons infrequently. The culture-medium hypothesis predicts that women who change tampons frequently would have a lower rate than those who change tampons less frequently because a short duration of use for each tampon would prevent the staphylococci from multiplying enough to produce a damaging dose of toxin. Thus, epidemiologic research, by showing that infrequent changing of tampons was associated with an increased rate of toxic shock, refuted the chemical theory in the form presented. There was, however, a third hypothesis that a chemical in some tampons (*e.g.*, oxygen content) improved their performance as culture media. This chemical-promotor hypothesis made the same prediction about the association with frequency of changing tampons as the microbial toxin culture-medium hypothesis.[63]

The toxic shock example illustrates a critical point in understanding the process of causal inference in epidemiologic studies: Many of the hypotheses being evaluated in the interpretation of epidemiologic studies are auxiliary hypotheses in that they are independent of the presence, absence, or direction of any causal connection between the study exposure and the disease. For example, explanations of how specific types of bias could have distorted an association between exposure and disease are the usual alternatives to the primary study hypothesis. Much of the interpretation of epidemiologic studies amounts to the testing of such auxiliary explanations for observed associations.

Causal Criteria Versus Causal Considerations

In practice, how do epidemiologists separate causal from noncausal explanations? Despite philosophic criticisms of inductive inference, inductively oriented considerations are often used as criteria for making such inferences.[64] If a set of necessary and sufficient causal criteria could be used to distinguish causal from noncausal relations in epidemiologic studies, the job of the scientist would be eased considerably. With such criteria, all the concerns about the logic or lack thereof in causal inference could be subsumed: It would only be necessary to consult the checklist of criteria to see if a relation were causal. As indicated from the philosophy reviewed earlier, such a set of sufficient criteria does not exist. Nevertheless, lists of causal criteria have become popular, possibly because they seem to provide a road map through complicated territory and perhaps because they suggest hypotheses to be evaluated in a given problem. A commonly used set of criteria was based on a list of considerations or "viewpoints" proposed by Sir Austin Bradford Hill,[38] which will be discussed in detail in Chapter 2.

Whereas the observations from earlier in this chapter imply that it is detrimental to codify the inferential process based solely on checklist criteria,[65] scientists have continued to refine causal considerations as aids to inference.[66-68] Although it can be argued that causality assessments are better guided by formal modeling frameworks, causal considerations may remain useful as heuristic aids.[69-72] An intermediate, refutationist approach seeks to transform proposed criteria into deductive tests of causal hypotheses.[73-75] Such an approach helps avoid the temptation to use causal criteria simply to buttress preferred theories and instead allows epidemiologists to focus on evaluating competing causal theories using crucial observations.

Regardless of the future of causal considerations, considerable progress has been made since Hill's time in precisely defining and modeling causal effects, leading to more complete understanding of when and how such effects can and cannot be estimated from data sources. These developments have become central to modern epidemiologic methodology and will be the focus of Chapters 2 and 3.

References

1. Vinten-Johansen P. *Cholera, Chloroform, and the Science of Medicine: A Life of John Snow*. Oxford, NY: Oxford University Press; 2003.
2. Tsao CW, Vasan RS. The Framingham Heart Study: past, present and future. *Int J Epidemiol*. 2015;44(6):1763-1766.
3. Stallones RA. The rise and fall of ischemic heart disease. *Sci Am*. 1980;243(5):53-59.
4. Schmidt M, Jacobsen JB, Lash TL, Botker HE, Sorensen HT. 25 year trends in first time hospitalisation for acute myocardial infarction, subsequent short and long term mortality, and the prognostic impact of sex and comorbidity: a Danish nationwide cohort study. *BMJ*. 2012;344:e356.
5. Francis T Jr, Korns RF, Voight RB, et al. An evaluation of the 1954 poliomyelitis vaccine trials. *Am J Public Health Nations Health*. 1955;45(5 pt 2):1-63.
6. Awasthi S, Peto R, Read S, et al. Vitamin A supplementation every 6 months with retinol in 1 million preschool children in north India: DEVTA, a cluster-randomised trial. *Lancet*. 2013;381(9876):1469-1477.
7. Awasthi S, Peto R, Read S, et al. Population deworming every 6 months with albendazole in 1 million pre-school children in North India: DEVTA, a cluster-randomised trial. *Lancet*. 2013;381(9876):1478-1486.
8. United States Department of Health EaW. *Smoking and Health: Report of the Advisory Committee to the Surgeon General of the Public Health Service*. PHS Publ No 1103. Washington, DC: Government Printing Office; 1964.
9. Vianna NJ, Greenwald P, Brady J, et al. Hodgkin's disease: cases with features of a community outbreak. *Ann Intern Med*. 1972;77(2):169-180.
10. Smith DC, Prentice R, Thompson DJ, Herrmann WL. Association of exogenous estrogen and endometrial carcinoma. *N Engl J Med*. 1975;293(23):1164-1167.
11. Ziel HK, Finkle WD. Increased risk of endometrial carcinoma among users of conjugated estrogens. *N Engl J Med*. 1975;293(23):1167-1170.
12. Mack TM, Pike MC, Henderson BE, et al. Estrogens and endometrial cancer in a retirement community. *N Engl J Med*. 1976;294(23):1262-1267.
13. Horwitz RI, Feinstein AR. Alternative analytic methods for case-control studies of estrogens and endometrial cancer. *N Engl J Med*. 1978;299(20):1089-1094.
14. Hutchison GB, Rothman KJ. Correcting a bias? *N Engl J Med*. 1978;299(20):1129-1130.
15. Jick H, Watkins RN, Hunter JR, et al. Replacement estrogens and endometrial cancer. *N Engl J Med*. 1979;300(5):218-222.
16. Greenland S, Neutra R. An analysis of detection bias and proposed corrections in the study of estrogens and endometrial cancer. *J Chronic Dis*. 1981;34(9-10):433-438.

17. Wynder EL, Graham EA. Tobacco smoking as a possible etiologic factor in bronchiogenic carcinoma; a study of 684 proved cases. *J Am Med Assoc*. 1950;143(4):329-336.

18. Doll R, Hill AB. A study of the aetiology of carcinoma of the lung. *Br Med J*. 1952;2(4797):1271-1286.

19. Dorn HF. Tobacco consumption and mortality from cancer and other diseases. *Public Health Rep*. 1959;74(7):581-593.

20. Sheehe PR. Dynamic risk analysis in retrospective matched-pair studies of disease. *Biometrics*. 1962;18:323-341.

21. Miettinen OS. Estimability and estimation in case-referent studies. *Am J Epidemiol*. 1976;103:226-235.

22. Cole P. The evolving case-control study. *J Chronic Dis*. 1979;32(1-2):15-27.

23. Cornfield J. Joint dependence of risk of coronary heart disease on serum cholesterol and systolic blood pressure: a discriminant function analysis. *Fed Proc* 1962;21(4 pt 2):58-61.

24. Truett J, Cornfield J, Kannel W. A multivariate analysis of the risk of coronary heart disease in Framingham. *J Chronic Dis*. 1967;20(7):511-524.

25. Rossouw JE, Anderson GL, Prentice RL, et al. Risks and benefits of estrogen plus progestin in healthy postmenopausal women: principal results from the Women's Health Initiative randomized controlled trial. *J Am Med Am*. 2002;288(3):321-333.

26. Stampfer MJ, Colditz GA. Estrogen replacement therapy and coronary heart disease: a quantitative assessment of the epidemiologic evidence. *Prev Med*. 1991;20(1):47-63.

27. Davey Smith G. Classics in epidemiology: should they get it right? *Int J Epidemiol*. 2004;33:441-442.

28. Prentice RL, Langer R, Stefanick ML, et al. Combined postmenopausal hormone therapy and cardiovascular disease: toward resolving the discrepancy between observational studies and the Women's Health Initiative clinical trial. *Am J Epidemiol*. 2005;162(5):404-414.

29. Hernan MA, Alonso A, Logan R, et al. Observational studies analyzed like randomized experiments: an application to postmenopausal hormone therapy and coronary heart disease. *Epidemiology*. 2008;19(6):766-779.

30. Collins FS, Varmus H. A new initiative on precision medicine. *N Engl J Med*. 2015;372(9):793-795.

31. Willett WC, Stampfer MJ. Current evidence on healthy eating. *Annu Rev Public Health*. 2013;34:77-95.

32. Ford ES, Caspersen CJ. Sedentary behaviour and cardiovascular disease: a review of prospective studies. *Int J Epidemiol*. 2012;41(5):1338-1353.

33. Bayer R, Galea S. Public health in the precision-medicine era. *N Engl J Med*. 2015;373(6):499-501.

34. Taubes G. Epidemiology faces its limits. *Science*. 1995;269(5221):164-169.

35. Maziak W. Is uncertainty in complex disease epidemiology resolvable?. *Emerg Themes Epidemiol*. 2015;12:7.

36. MacMahon B, Pugh TF. *Epidemiology: Principles and Methods*. Boston, MA: Little, Brown; 1970.

37. Mill JSA. *System of Logic, Ratiocinative and Inductive*. 5th ed. London: Parker, Son and Bowin; 1862.

38. Hill AB. The environment and disease: association or causation? *Proc R Soc Med*. 1965;58:295-300.

39. Hume D. *A Treatise of Human Nature*. 2nd ed. Oxford, NY: Oxford Press; 1888.

40. Popper KR. *Logik Der Forschung*. Vienna: Julius Springer; 1934.

41. Magee B. *Philosophy and the Real World: An Introduction to Karl Popper*. La Salle, IL: Open Court; 1985.

42. Platt JR. Strong Inference: certain systematic methods of scientific thinking may produce much more rapid progress than others. *Science*. 1964;146(3642):347-353.

43. Curd M, Cover JA, eds. Section 3: the Duhem-Quine thesis and underdetermination. *Philosophy of Science*. W.W. Norton & Company; 1998.

44. Quine WVO. Two dogmas of empiricism. *The Philosophical Review*. 1951;60:20-43.

45. Kuhn TS. *The Structure of Scientific Revolutions*. 2nd ed. Chicago, IL: University of Chicago Press; 1970.

46. Haack S. *Defending Science – Within Reason. Between Scientism and Cynicism*. Amherst, NY: Prometheus Books; 2003.

47. Peirce CS. *The Philosphical Writings of Peirce*. Mineola, NY: Dover Publications, Inc.; 1955.

48. Fisher RA. *Statistical Methods for Research Workers*. 4th ed. London; 1932.

49. Fisher RA. The logic of inductive inference. *J R Stat Soc Ser A*. 1935;98:39-54.

50. Greenland S. Invited commentary: the need for cognitive science in methodology. *Am J Epidemiol*. 2017;186(6):639-645.

51. Greenland S, Senn SJ, Rothman KJ, et al. Statistical tests, P values, confidence intervals, and power: a guide to misinterpretations. *Eur J Epidemiol*. 2016;31(4):337-350.

52. Howson C. Bayes or bust – a critical-examination of bayesian confirmation theory – earman. *J Nat*. 1992;358(6387):552.

53. McGrayne SB. *The Theory That Would Not Die: How Bayes' Rule Cracked the Enigma Code, Hunted Down Russian Submarines, & Emerged Triumphant From Two Centuries of Controversy*. New Haven, CT: Yale University Press; 2011.

54. Popper KR. *The Logic of Scientific Discovery (In German)*. New York, NY: Basic Books; 1959.

55. Kahneman D, Slovic P, Tversky A. *Judgment under Uncertainty: Heuristics and Biases*. New York, NY: Cambridge University Press; 1982.
56. Gilovich T. *How We Know What Isn't So*. New York, NY: Free Press; 1993.
57. Gilovich T, Griffin D, Kahneman D. *Heuristics and Biases: The Psychology of Intuitive Judgment*. New York, NY: Cambridge University Press; 2002.
58. Greenland S. Probability logic and probabilistic induction. *Epidemiology*. 1998;9(3):322-332.
59. Lash TL. Advancing research through replication. *Paediatr Perinat Epidemiol*. 2015;29(1):82-83.
60. Greenland S. Induction versus Popper: substance versus semantics. *Int J Epidemiol*. 1998;27(4):543-548.
61. Greenland S. Bayesian perspectives for epidemiological research: I. Foundations and basic methods. *Int J Epidemiol*. 2006;35(3):765-775.
62. Morey RD, Hoekstra R, Rouder JN, Lee MD, Wagenmakers EJ. The fallacy of placing confidence in confidence intervals. *Psychon Bull Rev*. 2016;23(1):103-123.
63. Lanes SF, Rothman KJ. Tampon absorbency, composition and oxygen content and risk of toxic shock syndrome. *J Clin Epidemiol*. 1990;43(12):1379-1385.
64. Weed DL, Gorelic LS. The practice of causal inference in cancer epidemiology. *Cancer Epidemiol Biomarkers Prev*. 1996;5(4):303-311.
65. Lanes SF, Poole C. 'Truth in packaging?' The unwrapping of epidemiologic research. *J Occup Med*. 1984;26(8):571-574.
66. Weiss NS. Can the "specificity" of an association be rehabilitated as a basis for supporting a causal hypothesis? *Epidemiology*. 2002;13(1):6-8.
67. Susser M. What is a cause and how do we know one? A grammar for pragmatic epidemiology. *Am J Epidemiol*. 1991;133(7):635-648.
68. Weiss NS. Inferring causal relationships: elaboration of the criterion of "dose-response". *Am J Epidemiol*. 1981;113(5):487-490.
69. Hofler M. Causal inference based on counterfactuals. *BMC Med Res Methodol*. 2005;5:28.
70. Hofler M. Getting causal considerations back on the right track. *Emerg Themes Epidemiol*. 2006;3:8.
71. Phillips CV, Goodman KJ. Causal criteria and counterfactuals; nothing more (or less) than scientific common sense. *Emerg Themes Epidemiol*. 2006;3:5.
72. Glass TA, Goodman SN, Hernan MA, Samet JM. Causal inference in public health. *Annu Rev Public Health*. 2013;34:61-75.
73. Maclure M. Popperian refutation in epidemiology. *Am J Epidemiol*. 1985;121(3):343-350.
74. Weed DL. On the logic of causal inference. *Am J Epidemiol*. 1986;123(6):965-979.
75. Kaufman JS, Poole C. Looking back on "causal thinking in the health sciences". *Annu Rev Public Health*. 2000;21:101-119.

CHAPTER 2

Causal Inference and Scientific Reasoning

Tyler J. VanderWeele, Timothy L. Lash, and Kenneth J. Rothman

INTRODUCTION

This chapter and the next provide an overview of useful concepts and problems in reasoning about and constructing methods for causal inference. It is convenient to divide inferential concepts into two broad classes: those embodied in canonical frameworks, in which causality is a property of an association to be characterized and diagnosed by symptoms and signs (as in classic medical investigations); and those embodied in mathematical models of causation, which form the basis for modern causal-inference methodologies. These are not mutually exclusive approaches, nor do they exhaust all possibilities; rather, they reflect historical traditions that until recently had only limited intersection. This chapter will focus on canonical frameworks and the problems of common intuitive modes of reasoning, while the next chapter will focus on causal models as an approach to addressing these problems.

CANONICAL FRAMEWORKS

Perhaps the oldest of the canonical approaches is traceable to John Stuart Mill in his attempt to lay out a system of inductive logic based on canons or rules that causal associations were presumed to obey.[1] Rather than deal with precise details and debates about how to define core terms like "cause" and "effect," the canonical approach starts with ordinary language use and focuses instead on listing key considerations that arise in evaluating evidence when attempting to draw a causal inference.

Perhaps the most widely cited of such lists are the Austin Bradford Hill considerations[2] (sometimes mischaracterized as "criteria" by later writers), which are discussed critically in numerous sources[3-6] and which will be the focus here. In Hill's own words, these considerations were not meant to be a checklist or set of criteria to be met, but rather "points to consider" when evaluating whether a precisely measured association arose from a causal effect. The considerations listed by Hill refer to various qualities of the association, as follows: (1) strength, (2) consistency, (3) specificity, (4) temporality, (5) biologic gradient, (6) plausibility, (7) coherence, (8) experimental evidence, and (9) analogy. Only consideration (4), proper temporal sequence (cause must precede effect), is a necessary condition for causation. The remaining considerations are not necessary conditions; instead, they are like diagnostic symptoms or signs of causation—that is, properties that an association is assumed more likely to exhibit if it is causal than if it is not.[2,7,8] Thus, the canonical approach makes causal inference more akin to clinical judgment than experimental science, although experimental evidence is among the considerations.[2,5,8] Some of the considerations (such as temporal sequence, strength of association, dose-response or predicted gradient, and specificity) are empirical signs and thus subject to conventional statistical analysis; others (such as plausibility) refer to prior belief and thus (as with disease symptoms) require more extensive familiarity with scientific literature on the topic to evaluate properly.

Hill's list was an expansion of an earlier list published in the landmark US Surgeon General's report Smoking and Health,[9] which in turn relied on the inductive canons of John Stuart Mill[10] and the discussion given by Hume.[11] Subsequently, others, especially Susser, further developed causal considerations.[12] Hill's canonical approach remains widely cited in the health sciences, subject to many variations in detail. Nonetheless, it has been criticized for its incompleteness and informality, and the consequent poor fit it affords to the deductive or mathematical approaches familiar to classic science and statistics.[5]

Although there have been some interesting attempts to reinforce or reinterpret certain canons as empirical predictions of causal hypotheses,[7,13-16] there is no formal or generally accepted mapping of the entire approach to a coherent statistical or inferential methodology; one simply uses standard statistical or logical techniques to test whether empirical considerations are violated. For example, if the causal hypothesis linking X to Y predicts a strictly increasing trend in Y with X, a test of this statistical prediction by a test of trend may serve as a statistical criterion for determining whether the hypothesis meets or fails the dose-response canon. Similarly, if the causal hypothesis linking X to Y predicts that X should be analogously linked to Z, but X and Z are not associated, then the hypothesis fails the analogy canon. Such usage falls squarely in the falsificationist tradition of 20th-century statistics, but leaves unanswered most of the policy questions that drive causal research.[4]

A CRITICAL ANALYSIS OF HILL'S CAUSAL CONSIDERATIONS

Hill suggested using his considerations to distinguish causal from noncausal associations that were such that the associations themselves were already "perfectly clear-cut and beyond what we would care to attribute to the play of chance", which was interpreted by some to mean that a statistical criterion beyond temporality was necessary for causal inference. This implication is highly controversial and we shall return to it in Chapter 15. Notably, Hill also emphasized that causal inferences cannot be based on a set of rules, condemned emphasis on statistical significance testing, and recognized the importance of many other factors in decision making.[4] The view that Hill's considerations should be used as necessary criteria for causal inference remains popular, but misguided. We thus examine the inferential value of each of them in detail, along the lines suggested by Hoggatt et al.,[17] and with allusions to the historical use of the Hill considerations in the evaluation of the evidence for a causal association between cigarette smoking and lung cancer.

Strength

The strength of an association is important because the stronger an association, the harder it is to explain away as artifacts of biases. There is, however, no general rule for how large an association needs to be to meet this consideration or whether it ought to be measured on the difference or ratio scale (see Chapter 5). The apparent preference for evaluating strength of association on the ratio scale may have derived from the very strong risk ratios, but more modest risk differences, associating cigarette smoking with lung cancer.[18] There have been some attempts to set sharp boundaries to identify causal associations, such as at a doubling of risk, but these attempts have been based on legal interpretations, and they invoked fallacious arguments connecting relative risks to causation probabilities (see also Chapter 5).[19,20] Furthermore, there are many weaker associations that are generally agreed to reflect causal effects. These weak associations are considered causal in part because they have been replicated in a variety of populations using different designs and in part because of considerations other than strength. Examples include the associations between air pollution and mortality, between smoking and heart disease, and between environmental tobacco smoke and lung cancer.

Similarly, there are several well-known examples of relatively strong noncausal associations. One example is the association between birth rank and Down syndrome: Maternal aging, which is strongly associated with an infant's birth rank, has since been accepted as explaining the association between birth rank and Down syndrome. Such examples remind us that a strong association is neither necessary nor sufficient for causality and that weakness of an association is neither necessary nor sufficient for absence of causality. A strong association can help to rule out hypotheses that the association is entirely due to confounding or other bias. Bias analysis can be used along with external information to estimate or speculate quantitatively on the extent to which possible bias sources have affected the strength of an observed association (see Chapters 12, 13, and 30).

Consistency

A consistent finding is an association reported across multiple populations, over time, and using different study designs. Although the presence of a consistent result is often taken as a compelling argument for causality, it is not definitive. For example, an inverse association of β-carotene with cancer was seen across epidemiologic studies but was not seen in subsequent randomized trials. Conversely, the absence of consistency does not imply the absence of a causal effect. Acute effects may be submerged in studies that examine only chronic exposure, and some agents may operate only in a small but highly susceptible subpopulation, so their association in the whole population is diluted by the lack of association in the vast majority. Nonetheless, consistency across studies of a similar design helps rule out chance as an explanation for an observed association. Consistency across studies of different designs can provide evidence against specific biases but cannot rule out bias entirely unless all reasonably possible biases have been addressed.

One mistake in evaluating consistency is so common, and yet wrong, that it deserves special mention. It is sometimes claimed that a literature or set of results is inconsistent simply because some results are "statistically significant" and some are not. This sort of evaluation is completely fallacious even if one accepts the use of frequentist significance testing methods. The effect estimates from a set of studies could all be identical even if many were significant and many were not, the difference in statistical significance arising solely because of differences in the standard errors of the estimates of association. Conversely, the estimates of association could be considerably divergent even if all were statistically nonsignificant.

Even without invoking statistical significance, the consistency consideration brings the potential for inferential errors by overreliance on it or misinterpretation of what is consistent evidence. In this regard, it has natural connections to the role of reproducibility in scientific inference, as discussed below.

Specificity

In Hill's formulation, specificity of an association can refer either to a cause having a single effect or an effect having a single cause. The limitations of this form of specificity are apparent even in the case of smoking and lung cancer. Although the smoking and lung cancer association is stronger (on the ratio scale) than the association between smoking and, say, heart disease, there is general agreement today that smoking can increase the risk of many diseases, including heart disease and other cancers. Indeed, many behavioral, environmental, social, and genetic risk factors have been causally linked to more than one health outcome.

Specificity can strengthen a causal inference if a competing noncausal hypothesis would predict a nonspecific association. For example, the strong association reported during the 1980s between estrogen hormone replacement therapy and cardiovascular endpoints was considered important evidence that the connection was causal, but Petitti et al. reported that the association was equally strong for accidents, homicides, and suicides.[21] This lack of specificity shed doubt on the causal interpretation. In a later publication, she suggested that a possible explanation for the nonspecific findings might be compliance with therapy, pointing out that compliance with taking a placebo in randomized trials was strongly related to lower risk of cardiovascular death.[22] The approach of examining associations with other outcomes (or other exposures) that should have no causal effects is sometimes referred to as one of using "negative controls".[23,24] Although such issues can be addressed via randomized trials, the controversy surrounding trials of mammography[25-27] shows that in practice even evidence from randomized trials can be interpreted differently by different stakeholders.

Temporality

Temporality means that a cause must precede its effects, and this is a necessary condition for valid causal inference. Although this positive assertion strikes many as inarguable, an observation that Y preceded possible cause X in a specific study is not an argument against causality in studies where Y followed X. Temporality rules out causality only if we know that X never occurred before Y in studies showing an association between X and Y. Much of Hill's discussion on temporality concerned these questions of potential reverse causation. If X and Y vary over time, it is also possible that there is feedback between them such that both affect each other. If we have measurements of these variables over time, longitudinal causal models can help evaluate such feedback,[28] an issue we return to below and in Chapter 26.

Biologic Gradient

Biologic gradient refers to the presence of a dose-response or exposure-response curve with an expected shape. Although Hill referred to a "linear" gradient, without specifying the scale, the more usual expectation for causal analyses is that the trend will be strictly monotonic (steadily increasing or decreasing). For example, more smoking means more carcinogen exposure and more tissue damage, hence more opportunity for carcinogenesis.

Some causal associations, however, show an approximate threshold effect rather than a strictly monotonic trend. For example, there may be a sharp increase in risk for specific outcomes at low to moderate doses of a given exposure that tapers off at higher doses, or there may be no adverse effect until saturation of detoxification mechanisms is reached, resulting in increased risk only at higher doses. Although some mistakenly treat any nonmonotonic dose-response association as refuting causation, many substances display U-shaped or J-shaped dose-response effects, often in a manner consistent with their hypothesized biologic effects. For example, very low and very high doses of certain vitamins may decrease life expectancies, a fact consistent with the known biologic properties of vitamins that are essential at moderate doses but toxic at high doses.

Conversely, an apparent monotonic dose-response relation may be an artifact of a bias that correlates with dose. For example, if an uncontrolled confounder is monotonically associated with the exposure and monotonically associated with the disease, an apparent dose-response relation between exposure and outcome could simply reflect the dose-response relation between the confounder and outcome.[14] The noncausal relation between birth rank and Down syndrome mentioned earlier shows a strong "biologic gradient" that merely reflects the monotonic relations between maternal age and birth rank and between maternal age and occurrence of Down syndrome. These issues imply that the existence of a monotonic association is neither necessary nor sufficient for a causal relation. A nonmonotonic relation only provides evidence against those causal hypotheses specific enough to predict a monotonic dose-response curve.

Plausibility

A causal explanation is *plausible* if it appears reasonable or realistic within the context in which the hypothesized cause and its effect occur. This context includes not only epidemiologic but also other human studies, animal and tissue studies, and current understanding of the biology, pathology, toxicology, and other mechanisms related to the effect. Plausibility can change as the context evolves and will be misleading when current understanding is misleading or wrong.

For example, in the early 19th century, miasma theory was the leading explanation of disease clusters and outbreaks. The theory that miasmas caused cholera was thus highly plausible at the time, because it was compatible with the observation that cholera occurs in outbreaks. But this high plausibility did not demonstrate that cholera is caused by miasmas, and waterborne transmission, which seemed less plausible before Snow's studies,[29] turned out to be the correct theory.

One Bayesian approach attempts to measure plausibility on a probability scale (0-1), thus equating plausibility with certainty, credibility, or prior belief. This quantification displays the dogmatism or open-mindedness of the analyst in a public fashion, with certainty values near 1 or 0 betraying a strong commitment of the analyst for or against a hypothesis (see Chapter 24). It can also provide a means of testing those quantified beliefs against new evidence.[30-32] Nonetheless, no proposed approach can transform plausibility into an objective condition.

Coherence

Hill used the term "coherence" to mean that the hypothesized causal relation of exposure to disease does not conflict with current understanding of the disease process. Hill emphasized that absence of such coherence was not a strong argument against causality. If an observed association apparently conflicts with current scientific understanding of a disease process, it may be that the understanding is mistaken rather than that the association is noncausal. For example, at the time it was made, the observation that shallow inhalers of cigarette smoke had increased rates of lung cancer relative to deep inhalers seemed to contradict simple mechanically based expectations. Subsequent research on lung cancer, however, found that the cells most affected by cigarette smoke tended to be in the upper respiratory tract, which was in fact consistent with the observed association for shallow inhalers.[33]

Conversely, coherence provides at best only weak support for causality, because many different theories will exhibit such coherence, including most theories that are proposed and eventually refuted. For example, the theory that the inverse association of β-carotene with cancers observed in epidemiologic studies represented a preventive effect was quite coherent with contemporary theories of antioxidants and cancer, but this theory was nonetheless refuted by subsequent randomized trials. The idea that a causal association should be supported by a coherent evidence base has innate appeal. When subjected to critical inspection, however, and consideration of the lack of an objective procedure by which the coherence of an evidence base might be evaluated, it becomes apparent that the consideration of coherence needs to be handled carefully and is potentially subject to abuse.

Experimental Evidence

Experimental evidence may refer to clinical trials, to animal experiments, or to experiments on tissues. These are, however, very different types of evidence, each with different strengths and weaknesses. Evidence from human experiments, when it exists at all, may apply only to volunteer populations with artificial exposure patterns (see Chapter 14). Animal experiments usually involve rodents or other species with susceptibilities potentially different from humans, and typically involve exposure levels different from those that humans experience. Consequently, uncertainty in extrapolations from animals to humans can be a major source of the overall uncertainty in quantitative risk assessments.[34,35]

To Hill, however, experimental evidence meant something else: the "experimental or semiexperimental evidence" obtained from reducing or eliminating a supposedly harmful exposure and seeing if the frequency of disease subsequently declines. Although he called this the strongest possible evidence of causality that can be obtained, such a "before-and-after" time trend analysis can be biased by concomitant secular changes. Such designs are discussed further in Chapter 29.

Analogy

Analogy refers to drawing inferences about the association between a given exposure and disease based on what is known about other exposure-disease relations. For example, based on what is known about the health effects of cigarette smoking, we might expect that inhalation of other combustibles (*e.g.*, marijuana) would have similar effects, even in the absence of studies on the subject. Analogy can be a useful scientific tool for generating new hypotheses about disease processes. Its utility, however, is limited by the breadth of knowledge and imagination of the scientist. Absence of such analogies may reflect only lack of imagination or experience, not falsity of the hypothesis.

Reasoning by analogy is common and often used to argue for the plausibility of a theory. For example, the theory that the association of smoking with cervical cancer was at least partially causal became more plausible once it was accepted that smoking could cause cancer of the bladder, pancreas, and other organs not directly exposed to smoke. Here, however, we see how analogy can be at odds with specificity: The more apt the analogy, the less specific the effects of a cause or the less specific the causes of an effect.

Summary

As is evident, the standards offered by Hill for judging whether epidemiologic evidence reflects a causal association are saddled with reservations and exceptions. Hill himself did not use the word "criteria" in the paper. He called them "viewpoints" or "perspectives." On the one hand, he asked, "In what circumstances can we pass from this observed *association* to a verdict of *causation*?" (emphasis in original). Yet, despite speaking of verdicts on causation, he disagreed that any "hard-and-fast rules of evidence" existed by which to judge causation: "None of my nine viewpoints can bring indisputable evidence for or against the cause-and-effect hypothesis and none can be required as a *sine qua non*."[2]

Actually, as noted above, the fourth viewpoint, temporality, is indeed necessary (a *sine qua non*) for causal explanations of observed associations. But, aside from temporality, interpreted as cause precedes effect, there is no necessary and sufficient criterion for determining whether an observed association is causal. This conclusion accords with the views of Hume and many others that causal inferences cannot attain the certainty of logical deductions. Although some have argued that it is detrimental to cloud the inferential process by considering checklist criteria,[36] there has been continuing refinement of causal considerations as aids to inference.[8] For example, refutationist approaches seek to transform considerations into deductive tests of causal hypotheses.[13,16,37] These approaches avoid the temptation to use causal considerations simply to buttress pet theories at hand and instead allow epidemiologists to focus on evaluating competing causal theories using crucial observations. Although this refutationist approach to causal inference may seem at odds with the common implementation of Hill's viewpoints, it actually seeks to answer the fundamental question posed by Hill, and the ultimate purpose of the viewpoints he promulgated:

> What [the nine viewpoints] can do, with greater or less strength, is to help us to make up our minds on the fundamental question—is there any other way of explaining the set of facts before us, is there any other answer equally, or more, likely than cause and effect?

> **(Hill, 1965,[2] p. 11)**

The crucial phrase "equally or more likely than cause and effect" suggests to us a subjective assessment of the certainty or probability of the causal hypothesis at issue relative to another hypothesis. Although Hill wrote at a time when expressing uncertainty as a probability was unpopular in statistics, it appears from his statement that, for him, causal inference is at least partially a subjective matter of degree of personal belief, certainty, or conviction. In any event, this view is precisely that of subjective Bayesian statistics (Chapter 24).

It is unsurprising that case studies[38] and surveys of epidemiologists[39] show that epidemiologists have not agreed on a set of causal considerations or on how to apply them. In one study in which epidemiologists were asked to employ causal "criteria" to fictional summaries of epidemiologic literatures, the agreement was only slightly greater than would have been expected by chance.[39]

More disturbingly, causal considerations as well as statistical methods are often used to make a case for a position for or against causality that has been arrived at by other, unstated means. Authors sometimes pick and choose among the considerations and definitions they deploy and then weigh them in *ad hoc* ways that depend only on the exigencies of the discussion at hand. In this sense, causal considerations can appear to function less like standards or principles and more like values,[40] which vary across individual scientists and even vary within the work of a single scientist, depending on the context and time. Once again, apart from temporality, universal and objective causal criteria, if they exist, have yet to be identified.

GENERAL PROBLEMS IN SCIENTIFIC INFERENCE AND REPORTING

Although Hill's viewpoints are often discussed in assessing evidence for causality, they are by no means the only considerations that influence causal inferences. In this section, we will discuss some additional considerations used for evaluating scientific evidence. They apply not only to causal inference, but also to prediction, and to descriptive assessments of prevalence, incidence, and distribution of disease and health.

The Problem of "Statistical Significance" and Dichotomized P-Values

We will address the precision of estimates of effect in detail in several later chapters. As alluded to above, however, the role of statistical significance testing in the evaluation of evidence is so widespread, and so frequently erroneously implemented, that it merits preliminary discussion here. Briefly, a statistically significant result is typically defined as one for which the accompanying P-value is less than or equal to a prespecified cutoff value, which is usually denoted by the Greek letter α (alpha) and hence called the *alpha level* of the statistical test. As a source of much confusion, both the P-value and the α-level have at times also been called the "significance level" of the test, even though they are two different concepts. A P-value is the probability that a test statistic computed from the data would be more extreme than or as extreme as its observed value assuming that the test hypothesis is true, the statistical model is correct, and that there is no source of bias in the data collection or analytic processes. In contrast, the α-level is the maximum tolerable type I error rate, where the latter is the probability of rejecting the test hypothesis when it is in fact true.

The common convention is to take the null hypothesis (of no association, or of no effect, depending on the context) as the sole test hypothesis, and to take 0.05 as the α-level, so that $P \le 0.05$ is taken as grounds for claiming the results refute the null hypothesis and $P > 0.05$ is taken as grounds for claiming the results support the null hypothesis. As has been noted for many decades and we will explain at length in Chapter 15, both of these interpretations are erroneous. Despite decades of published objections to these misinterpretations, use of 0.05-level null hypothesis significance testing (NHST)[41,42] continues to unduly influence research practice and interpretations.[39,43,44] Simply put, studies in which there are true causal effects may yield results that are not statistically significant and statistically significant results do not distinguish causal from noncausal effects.

The practice of using $P \le 0.05$ as a criterion to determine "whether or not there is an effect" is particularly problematic and can lead to absurdities. It suggests that $P = 0.04$ implies there is an effect, whereas $P = 0.06$ implies there is no effect. But the P-value is in fact a continuous measure of evidence, and there is no appreciable difference between $P = 0.04$ and $P = 0.06$. Moreover, with a very large study almost every effect, regardless of how small or inconsequential, is likely to have a low P-value. Furthermore, in small studies, even substantial effects might have relatively high P-values simply because the study lacks sufficient precision to discriminate between large associations and small or absent associations. Statistical precision is an essential consideration when interpreting evidence and cannot be gauged from a single P-value. The conclusion that "there is no effect" as a conclusion drawn solely from a P-value above 0.05 is never justified. A P-value is only a measure of the consistency or compatibility of the tested hypothesis with the observations, and even then is a valid measure only under ideal conditions involving (among other things) no unaccounted-for bias in the results.[42-44]

There are several ways to address these shortcomings of hypothesis testing. One approach is to present P-values not only for the null hypothesis, but also for other hypotheses of concern, for example, a test of the doubling of risk. Another approach that generalizes this idea is to present a *confidence interval*, which displays the entire range of associations or effect sizes that would have a P-value greater than the alpha level.[45] Confidence intervals help investigators and readers understand the imprecision (random error) in estimates. For example, before interpreting a $P = 0.80$ as support for no effect, one should examine the accompanying confidence interval to see what other effect sizes would also have large P-values and thus are relatively consistent with the study results. Imprecision will be reflected by a wide confidence interval, which may contain large and important effect sizes even though the interval also contains the null effect.

A deeper problem is that outputs of conventional statistical computations, whether P-values, confidence intervals, or the like, refer only to uncertainty left by random errors after making adjustments for known and measured bias sources. Considerations for drawing inference about causal effects are, however, far more numerous, and include issues of uncontrolled confounding, measurement error and selection bias.[46-48] Neither a P-value nor a confidence interval reflect the uncertainty that should remain from such uncontrolled bias sources. A very low P-value derived from all available studies, along with bias analyses (see Chapter 30), may provide a convincing argument that an observed association is not due entirely to uncontrolled confounding, measurement error, or selection bias and thus provide a basis for inferring with higher certainty that an effect is present. Similarly, a very narrow confidence interval around the null, derived from all available studies, along with a bias analysis, may provide a convincing argument that any effect present is negligible or at least below any reasonable detection threshold. Nonetheless, as we describe in the following section, other issues must also be considered before reaching such conclusions.

Replicability

For Bradford Hill, a consistent finding is one reported across multiple populations, over time, and using different study designs. More recent discussions have pointed out the importance of the narrower concept of *replicability* or *repeatability*, in which one attempts to repeat a study by applying the same design to the same type of subjects but conducted by a different set of investigators. The original study is then said to have been replicated if similar results are obtained in the repeated study. (The same concept is also sometimes called reproducibility, although we will reserve that term for a more specialized concept discussed below.)

There have been few incentives to replicate studies. Public research funding, and therefore publicly funded researchers, has emphasized innovation, which incentivizes studies with new research hypotheses over replication of studies with previously studied hypotheses. But with increasing recognition of the potential importance of replication, this paradoxical incentivization is beginning to change, and some journals now require replication of certain research results before publication. Attempts at replicating results in psychology[49] and in the biological sciences[50] have claimed that results in these fields show low replication rates,[49-51] although these conclusions have been challenged as being based on faulty statistical analyses and for failing to replicate precisely the original study designs.[52] One problem is that replication has sometimes been based on a criterion of statistical significance, which is an inappropriate way to judge whether a result has been replicated.[44,53] Beyond that, differences that explain failure to replicate may arise from following a design different from the original study or from failing to draw subjects from the same underlying population.[52] Such instances seem better described as lack of consistency across designs or populations rather than as failure to replicate results, given that important study features were not in fact replicated. Furthermore, such inconsistency may provide valuable information: Results from different designs may provide important evidence about study biases, while different results from different populations may provide evidence on how exposure effects vary across populations. One could reasonably argue that perfect replication is at best a theoretical construct, because even simple experiments always occur in different places and at different times. One must always ultimately assume that unaccounted-for differences in conditions in the replication study are ignorable.

That said, there are many possible avenues to explain genuine replication failures in addition to different designs and different populations. Discrepancies in the results of an original study and a replication study can arise due to chance variation, so it is important that differences in the original and replication studies are reported with such variation considered. Among less easily handled reasons for discrepancies, it is possible that either in the original study or the replication study, errors were made in the recording or analysis of the data. If the error occurred in the original study, then the replication study can help note and correct such errors. It is even possible that data were manipulated (or even fabricated), although reproducibility studies (discussed below) are more efficient for identifying these explanations. Another possibility is that the researchers selected from among several models or statistical results those that support their prior conception of what the results should look like.[54,55] In this case, the replication study would be less likely to return consistent results.

We wish to emphasize several limitations of study replications:

1. If results differ between the original study and a replication study, it is not necessarily the case that the original study is wrong. It may be that the replication study was incorrectly carried out, or that analytical errors were made, or that it in fact used a different study population. Failure to replicate may indicate the need for further research rather than a definitive judgment on the original study's results.

2. While a replication study with results that closely match the original study may provide further evidence for the original study's conclusions, it certainly does not guarantee the conclusions are correct. It is possible both studies are flawed in the same ways, so that the same set of biases affect them both. This latter point is especially relevant if the replication study does indeed match as closely as possible the design, methods, and population of the original.

3. The resources required to carry out an original study and then replicate it can be considerably greater than those required for carrying out a single study. Replication is desirable in strengthening the evidence for a study's conclusion, but in light of the increased cost, detailed consideration needs to be given as to whether the research question merits the resources required to address replicability.

4. Replication should not be based on statistical significance. Measures of effect may be identical in two studies but statistically significant in one and not the other, and widely different effect estimates from two studies may both be either statistically significant or not.

Reproducibility

A further narrowing of focus, usually requiring far less expenditure than replication, arises in concerns about *reproducibility* of study results, by which we mean the extent to which other investigators can obtain the same results using the data and analysis methods or software used in the original studies (again, some authors use "reproducibility" to refer to what we have termed replicability). Attempts to reproduce results may detect errors or biases in the original data, its management, or analysis and may reveal sensitivity of results to seemingly minor analysis choices.

To address reproducibility, some journals now request or even require that authors submit both data and software analysis code to be stored on journal repositories and to be made publicly accessible so that the results of an analysis can be verified. The provision of such data and code more easily allow for identifying instances in which unintentional coding or analysis mistakes have been made, or when data manipulation or analysis choices might be responsible for what was reported originally. However, weighing against the expectation that authors should provide data and computing code to accompany their studies submitted for publication are data privacy concerns, as well as intellectual property concerns pertaining to statistical computing code.

Selective Reporting

Beyond errors, there is the problem that analyses of all but the simplest data sets require many choices about how to code and analyze the data. Even when these choices are made in an unbiased and transparent manner, they may seriously affect the reported results. Potential sensitivity of results to seemingly innocuous and routine analysis choices is now recognized as a serious problem, especially since such sensitivity provides an avenue for selective reporting of analyses based on results.[56,57] Selective reporting is one of the chief concerns behind calls for reproducibility studies; one proposal for addressing the problem is to have teams of rivals with different views and competing theories analyze the data independently, so as to be able to spot each other's potential errors and biases.[54]

Another level of selection based on results arises when reviewers and editors allow recommendations or decisions for publication to depend on the study results rather than on the soundness of the data collection and analysis methods that produced those results. Preceding these decisions is the authors' decision of whether or not to submit a paper for publication, based on its results, especially if those results are null. This problem of publication bias can distort entire literatures. Proposals to prevent this problem include having studies submitted, reviewed, and accepted for publication based on their methods alone, with reviewers blinded to the results and thus presumably forced to make recommendations without regard to those results[58]—although reviewer blinding may be compromised by preliminary abstracts or presentations of the study. A simpler alternative would be to address the mistaken belief that publication is merited only for results meeting certain criteria, such as statistical significance. Without such beliefs, analysts would be more apt to conduct analyses in accordance with principles that yield the most robust, and hence replicable, result.[44] For this change in beliefs to occur, there would have to be a groundswell change in scientific culture, which seems unlikely to happen soon, but nonetheless there is reason for hope that this might be attained eventually.[59,60]

Preregistration of Research Protocols, Data Availability, and Shared Computing Code

Another measure to limit publication bias is preregistration of studies. In 2004, the International Committee of Medical Journal Editors announced a policy requiring the preregistration of clinical trial protocols in a publicly available repository as a mandatory prerequisite for publication of the trial's results in their journals. The motivation for this announcement focused on the importance of reporting all trial results pertaining to the initial aims of the trial, as an obligation to both participants and to society. The main objective was to counter the suppression of results, primarily to avoid the potential for a new trial to randomize participants to treatments that an earlier study had found to be ineffective, but for which results had not been published.[61,62] Potential new trialists would be able to learn of the earlier trial, and presumably its results, before initiating another study, even if the results of the earlier study had never been published.

Following this model, a working group sponsored by the European Center for Ecotoxicology and Toxicology of Chemicals—an "industry-funded expert not-for-profit think tank whose sole purpose is to enhance the quality of chemicals risk assessment so that chemicals management decisions are informed, reliable and safe"—proposed in 2009 that the same preregistration requirement ought to be implemented for nonrandomized studies. The topic was widely debated in the epidemiologic literature, including different views on the philosophic, theoretical, and practical considerations.[63-66]

The working group and authors of commentaries that supported preregistration of protocols of nonrandomized studies focused mainly on its purported utility in identifying false-positive associations that may arise because of deviations from a priori hypotheses and methods. That is, commentators saw suppression or downweighing of results that were not preregistered as a public good—exactly the opposite of the primary motivation for the trialists' registries. They have focused especially on the notion that preregistered protocols containing preregistered hypotheses provide a safeguard against selective reporting of some results (*e.g.*, statistically significant results) from among many generated results and therefore reduce type I errors. These commentators and others regarded it as self-evident that inferences based on results about prespecified hypotheses are more reliable. However, some literature on the philosophy of science suggests that there is no basis for a large difference in strength of posterior belief when evidence pertains to a prespecified hypothesis versus when it pertains to an equivalent hypothesis specified after viewing the data.[66-69] The reliability of an inference regarding a particular hypothesis is a function of the quality of the designs and analyses of the studies included in the evidence base, in conjunction with the credibility of the associated hypothesis. These have nothing to do with prespecification of the hypothesis, preregistration of the protocol, or how many other hypotheses were simultaneously evaluated.[70]

In 2014, a self-appointed committee promulgated new guidelines called the "Transparency and Openness Promotion Guidelines," which proposed eight standards that could be implemented in whole or part by journals.[71] Journals that adopted the guidelines would choose the level of their implementation for each standard, ranging from level 0, connoting no implementation of the standard, to level 3, connoting full implementation and active policing of the standard by the journal editors. Standards included preregistration of the protocol, as well as public availability of the data and computing code. The stated motivation was to improve the reproducibility of research results by increasing the transparency of the research process and products. This perspective treats each research paper as if its results were right or wrong, as eventually determined by whether its results are reproduced or not. A more thoughtful perspective views each research result as an imperfect measurement of an underlying parameter and allows time for the accumulation of evidence, potentially from many studies, to ultimately yield knowledge that can guide policy.[72]

Research is ultimately a creative process; its regimentation can lead to serious error when (as may be inevitable) the researcher faces a problem which the imposed protocols did not anticipate and were not designed to address.[72] Some regimentation is inevitable, especially to ensure that research is conducted ethically and to enable efficient allocation of scarce resources to support it. Efforts to insist on regimentation to improve the yield, while they may be superficially appealing, may not only diminish creativity, but may also intentionally or unintentionally downweight credible research results viewed as out of compliance with the regulations. Incorporating compliance with needless regimentation into evaluations of research results, and whether the results support a causal inference, thus risks slowing scientific progress by inhibiting creative approaches to research progress. Investigators should pursue a variety of strategies to make clear in advance their analysis plan, but imposing requirements with observational studies has the potential to do more harm than good.

The Human Element

Generating and interpreting epidemiologic evidence is a human endeavor, subject to all of the vagaries of the human condition. Among these are temptations to achieve apparent success through fraud and to manipulate, highlight, or interpret evidence in a fashion more consistent with competing interests or wishful thinking than with classic scientific ideals of pursuit of truth. Examples of such investigator bias are common, and some have harmed public health and welfare. Some manipulations and fraud may come to light by altruistic reporting from a colleague, critical appraisal of results that are too good to be true, and failure of the research result to replicate in studies of sufficiently similar design. Cases of data manipulation and biased evidence interpretation, however, can be more difficult to detect, since the consequences may produce unremarkable results. Such manipulations may be subtle enough to escape detection by reviewers and editors of leading journals, and because there is rarely systematic monitoring of data management and analysis, there is rarely any idea of how many reported results are in fact the product of such manipulation or fraud.

Management of competing interests through required disclosures and institutional management of these disclosures have become widely accepted, although enforcement is weak and the effectiveness of this disclosure and management strategy has been difficult to demonstrate. One strategy to address concerns about evidence affected by competing interest is to stratify studies based on what is known about such interests; this strategy has in fact been applied and has displayed that such interests do predict reported results, although the causal explanation for such findings can be controversial. Stratification allows one to downweight or even discard studies in which clear conflicts of interest exist. Nonetheless, there is no evidence that this downweighting can be done consistently enough or accurately enough to ensure that a weighted evidence summary would be more reliable than comparable summaries that simply stratified on competing interests or ignored the issue altogether.

A second, less often appreciated, influence of investigator biases on the interpretation of evidence is our poor ability to reason in the face of uncertainty, as well documented in cognitive psychology and behavioral economics.[73-75] Economic models once assumed that humans participated in the economy as rational actors. That view was gradually abandoned or curtailed as it emerged that individual economic decision-making does not correspond to the choices predicted by mathematic models of how a rational actor would behave. Humans will, for example, on average behave differently to avoid a possible loss than to achieve a possible gain, even when the financial considerations are mathematically equivalent. While behavioral models have developed to accommodate these predictable and subjective irrationalities, many scientists, journals, and agencies continue to operate under the illusion that there is a single rational scientific method followed by all ethical researchers. Most of the present book is devoted to methods to aid researchers in approaching this ideal, but it should be recognized that even the most sophisticated investigators may fall short of rational evaluation of their own results and the relevant literature, adding yet another dimension of complexity for those interested in obtaining an accurate evaluation of existing evidence.

As we will describe in detail in later chapters, scientific evidence is always subject to unknown degrees of error. Were there no such errors in epidemiologic evidence, there would be no need for the methods covered in this book. These errors are conventionally divided into two components: random errors ("chance variation"), which are assumed to display no consistent direction or structure beyond that described by probability distributions; and systematic errors ("biases"), which do have a consistent direction and structure. Because in a given application both these errors are of uncertain size, interpreting evidence is an exercise in reasoning under uncertainty. All humans, including scientists, make predictable mistakes in such reasoning. Among the most pernicious of these biases are failure to account for baseline information (the "base-rate fallacy") and overconfidence.[55]

The *base-rate fallacy* refers to the observation that, when respondents are asked to estimate the probability of an event on the basis of the background or usual frequency of the event (such as a disease) and specific evidence about whether the event actually occurred in a specific case or patient, respondents systematically focus on the specific evidence and largely ignore the background frequency. One psychological explanation for this observation is that specific evidence is concrete and emotionally interesting, thereby more readily inspiring a mental script to explain its relevance; in contrast, the background frequency is abstract and emotionally uninteresting, so less likely to inspire an explanatory script that contradicts the specific evidence. Regardless, failure to account for the background frequency (risk) of an event may affect inference from epidemiologic results. Consider a conventional point estimate and confidence interval for the association of an exposure with a disease as the specific evidence about whether exposure causes the disease, and the baseline information to be information from other epidemiologic studies. The base-rate fallacy is then manifested when the investigators draw causal conclusions that clearly assign excessive weight to their own results and ignore what others have reported. Bayesian methods, which we discuss in later chapters, provide one quantitative method for addressing this human tendency to favor one's own results over what others have reported.

Overconfidence bias refers to the tendency to set too narrow an uncertainty range around a guess or educated estimate of an unknown quantity and is relevant to most inference and decision-making. An example arises when the conventional frequentist confidence interval for the association of an exposure with a disease is treated as if it captures all the uncertainty about the actual effect of the exposure on the disease frequency. Doing so results in overconfidence because a frequentist confidence interval does not incorporate the uncertainty one should have about uncontrolled bias sources, nor does it necessarily account for all uncertainties one should have about the distribution of random errors. It also does not incorporate prior information. Furthermore, studies of overconfidence indicate that an intuitive inflation of the confidence interval to account for these sources of uncertainty aside from random error will typically be insufficient. This insufficiency further contributes to the human tendency to overinterpret the specific evidence at hand.

Because a confidence interval fails to account for uncertainty beyond random error, it should be considered a minimum description of the true uncertainty, in that it would be sufficient only if the study and analysis were perfect, free of all bias beyond those that were successfully controlled via design and adjustment methods, and with no credible prior information. Explicitly listing sources of uncertainty not accounted for by the interval is one effective strategy to reduce overconfidence. Simply weighing whether the causal hypothesis is true—without specifying alternative explanations—actually increases overconfidence, because we tend to focus more on explanations for why it could be true than for why it could be false. To overcome this tendency, one must actively imagine alternative explanations, which illuminates the causal hypothesis as only one in a set of competing explanations for the observed association.

Problems of Evidence Cumulation and Synthesis

As noted above, a single study is rarely sufficient to reliably draw conclusions about effects of an exposure or intervention. Although exceptions exist (such as the first study linking diethylstilbestrol to female genital tract cancer[76] or when many patients suffer obvious adverse reactions to new drugs), most often multiple studies from independent research groups as well as interlocking lines of evidence are needed to support firm conclusions.[77,78] All of this information takes time to accumulate. While replication can strengthen evidence, a single replication study does not definitively establish a conclusion either. However, as numerous studies with different investigators and potentially different designs are undertaken, the evidence can eventually become more compelling.

Further complications arise in determining at what point, if any, policy action should be taken based on the accumulating evidence. It may be that delaying action until a high degree of certainty is attained will result in costs unacceptable to at least some of the concerned parties, even when acting sooner increases the risk of error. Although there is an extensive literature on risk assessment and decision analysis, there is no generally accepted methodology for making such determinations, especially when multiple lines of evidence (*e.g.*, human, animal, and tissue studies) must be synthesized. Because the issues involved in policy recommendations and action decisions extend well beyond epidemiology and its methods,[79] we will not discuss them in detail. However, the importance of synthesizing evidence from different sources, and different designs (sometimes now referred to as "triangulation"), will remain within epidemiology, and may be the topic of yet further new methodological development concerning causal inference and scientific reasoning.

References

1. Mill JSA. *A System of Logic, Ratiocinative and Inductive*. London: John W. Parker, West Strand; 1843.
2. Hill AB. The environment and disease: association or causation? *Proc R Soc Med*. 1965;58:295-300.
3. Koepsell TD, Weiss NS. *Epidemiologic Methods: Studying the Occurrence of Illness*. New York, NY: Oxford University Press; 2003.
4. Phillips CV, Goodman KJ. The missed lessons of Sir Austin Bradford Hill. *Epidemiol Perspect Innov*. 2004;1(1):3.
5. Rothman KJ, Greenland S. Causation and causal inference in epidemiology. *Am J Public Health*. 2005;95:S144-S150.
6. VanderWeele TJ. Hill's causal considerations and the potential outcomes framework. *Observ Stud*. 2020;6:47-54.
7. Susser M. Falsification, verification and causal inference in epidemiology: reconsideration in the light of Sir Karl Popper's philosophy. In: Rothman KJ, ed. *Causal Inference*. Chestnut Hill, MA: Epidemiology Resources Inc; 1988;33-58.
8. Susser M. What is a cause and how do we know one? A grammar for pragmatic epidemiology. *Am J Epidemiol*. 1991;133(7):635-648.
9. United States Department of Health EaW. *Smoking and Health: Report of the Advisory Committee to the Surgeon General of the Public Health Service*. PHS Publ No 1103. Washington, DC: Government Printing Office; 1964.
10. Mill JSA. *System of Logic, Ratiocinative and Inductive*. 5th ed. London: Parker, Son and Bowin; 1862.
11. Hume D. *A Treatise of Human Nature*. 2nd ed. Oxford, NY: Oxford Press; 1888.
12. Kaufman JS, Poole C. Looking back on "causal thinking in the health sciences". *Annu Rev Public Health*. 2000;21:101-119.
13. Weed DL. On the logic of causal inference. *Am J Epidemiol*. 1986;123(6):965-979.
14. Weiss NS. Inferring causal relationships: elaboration of the criterion of "dose-response". *Am J Epidemiol*. 1981;113(5):487-490.
15. Weiss NS. Can the "specificity" of an association be rehabilitated as a basis for supporting a causal hypothesis? *Epidemiology*. 2002;13(1):6-8.
16. Rosenbaum PR. *Observational Studies*. 2nd ed. New York, NY: Springer; 2002.
17. Hoggatt KJ. Greenland S, VanderWeele TJ. *Causation and causal inference. Oxford Textbook of Global Public Health*. Vol 3. 6th ed. Oxford, United Kingdom: Oxford University Press; 2015;44:591-598.
18. Poole C. On the origin of risk relativism. *Epidemiology*. 2010;21(1):3-9.
19. Greenland S. The relation of the probability of causation to the relative risk and the doubling dose: a methodologic error that has become a social problem. *Am J Public Health*. 1999;89:1166-1169.
20. Greenland S, Robins JM. Epidemiology, justice, and the probability of causation. *Jurimetrics*. 2000;40:321-340.
21. Petitti DB, Perlman JA, Sidney S. Postmenopausal estrogen use and heart disease. *New Engl J Med*. 1986;315(2):131-136.
22. Petitti DB. Coronary heart disease and estrogen replacement therapy. Can compliance bias explain the results of observational studies? *Ann Epidemiol*. 1994;4(2):115-118.
23. Lipsitch M, Tchetgen Tchetgen E, Cohen T. Negative controls: a tool for detecting confounding and bias in observational studies. *Epidemiology*. 2010;21(3):383-388.
24. Weisskopf MG, Tchetgen Tchetgen EJ, Raz R. Commentary: on the use of imperfect negative control exposures in epidemiologic studies. *Epidemiology*. 2016;27(3):365-367.
25. Freedman DA, Petitti DB, Robins JM. On the efficacy of screening for breast cancer. *Int J Epidemiol*. 2004;33(1):43-55.
26. Gotzsche PC. Mammography screening: truth, lies, and controversy. *Lancet*. 2012;380(9838):218.
27. Oeffinger KC, Fontham ET, Etzioni R, et al. Breast cancer screening for women at average risk: 2015 guideline update from the American Cancer Society. *J Am Med Assoc*. 2015;314(15):1599-1614.
28. Robins JM, Greenland S, Hu F. Estimation of the causal effect of a time-varying exposure on the marginal mean of a repeated binary outcome (with discussion). *J Am Stat Assoc*. 1999;94:687-712.
29. Paneth N. Assessing the contributions of John Snow to epidemiology: 150 years after removal of the broad street pump handle. *Epidemiology*. 2004;15(5):514-516.

30. Box GEP. Sampling and Bayes inference in scientific modeling and robustness. *J R Stat Soc Ser A.* 1980;143:383-430.

31. Greenland S. On sample-size and power calculations for studies using confidence intervals. *Am J Epidemiol.* 1988;128(1):231-237.

32. Gelman A, Shalizi CR. Philosophy and the practice of Bayesian statistics. *Br J Math Stat Psychol.* 2013;66(1):8-38.

33. Wald NA. Smoking. In: Vessey MP, Gray M, eds. *Cancer Risks and Prevention.* New York, NY: Oxford University Press; 1985.

34. Freedman DA, Navidi W, Peters SC. On model uncertainty and its statistical implications. In: Dijlestra TK, ed. *On the Impact of Variable Selection in Fitting Regression Equations.* Berlin: Springer-Verlag; 1988;1-16.

35. Crouch EAC, Lester RL, Lash TL, Armstrong SA, Green LC. Health risk assessments prepared per the risk assessment reforms under consideration in the U.S. Congress. *Hum Ecol Risk Assess.* 1997;3:713-785.

36. Lanes SF, Poole C. 'Truth in packaging?' the unwrapping of epidemiologic research. *J Occup Med.* 1984;26(8):571-574.

37. Maclure M. Popperian refutation in epidemiology. *Am J Epidemiol.* 1985;121(3):343-350.

38. Weed DL, Gorelic LS. The practice of causal inference in cancer epidemiology. *Cancer Epidemiol Biomarkers Prev.* 1996;5(4):303-311.

39. Holman CD, Arnold-Reed DE, de Klerk N, McComb C, English DR. A psychometric experiment in causal inference to estimate evidential weights used by epidemiologists. *Epidemiology.* 2001;12(2):246-255.

40. Poole C. Causal values. *Epidemiology.* 2001;12(2):139-141.

41. Stang A, Poole C, Kuss O. The ongoing tyranny of statistical significance testing in biomedical research. *Eur J Epidemiol.* 2010;25(4):225-230.

42. Greenland S. Randomization, statistics, and causal inference. *Epidemiology.* 1990;1(6):421-429.

43. Greenland S, Senn SJ, Rothman KJ, et al. Statistical tests, P values, confidence intervals, and power: a guide to misinterpretations. *Eur J Epidemiol.* 2016;31(4):337-350.

44. Lash TL. The harm done to reproducibility by the culture of null hypothesis significance testing. *Am J Epidemiol.* 2017;186(6):627-635.

45. Rothman KJ. A show of confidence. *N Engl J Med.* 1978;299(24):1362-1363.

46. Lash TL, Fink AK. Semi-automated sensitivity analysis to assess systematic errors in observational data. *Epidemiology.* 2003;14(4):451-458.

47. Greenland S. Multiple-bias modeling for analysis of observational data (with discussion). *J R Stat Soc Ser A.* 2005;168:267-308.

48. Lash TL, Fox MP, MacLehose RF, Maldonado G, McCandless LC, Greenland S. Good practices for quantitative bias analysis. *Int J Epidemiol.* 2014;43(6):1969-1985.

49. Open Science Collaboration. PSYCHOLOGY. Estimating the reproducibility of psychological science. *Science.* 2015;349(6251):aac4716.

50. Begley CG, Ellis LM. Drug development: raise standards for preclinical cancer research. *Nature.* 2012;483(7391):531-533.

51. Ioannidis JP, Allison DB, Ball CA, et al. Repeatability of published microarray gene expression analyses. *Nat Genet.* 2009;41(2):149-155.

52. Gilbert DT, King G, Pettigrew S, Wilson TD. Comment on "Estimating the reproducibility of psychological science". *Science.* 2016;351(6277):1037.

53. Gelman A, Stern H. The difference between "significant" and "not significant" is not itself statistically significant. *Am Statistician.* 2006;60(4):328-331.

54. Nuzzo R. How scientists fool themselves - and how they can stop. *Nature.* 2015;526(7572):182-185.

55. Lash TL. Heuristic thinking and inference from observational epidemiology. *Epidemiology.* 2007;18(1):67-72.

56. Phillips CV. Publication bias in situ. *BMC Med Res Methodol.* 2004;4:20.

57. Gelman A, Loken E. The statistical crisis in science. *Am Scientist.* 2014;102(6):460-465.

58. Chambers CD, Feredoes E, Muthukumaraswamy SD, Etchells PJ. Instead of "playing the game" it is time to change the rules: registered reports at AIMS Neuroscience and beyond. *AIMS Neuroscience.* 2014;1(1):4-17.

59. Wasserstein RL, Assoc AS. ASA statement on statistical significance and P-values. *Am Statistician.* 2016;70(2):131-133.

60. Wasserstein RL, Schirm AL, Lazar NA. Moving to a world beyond "p<0.05". *Am Statistician* 2019;73(sup1):1-19.

61. De Angelis C, Drazen JM, Frizelle FA, et al. Clinical trial registration: a statement from the international committee of medical journal editors. *Croat Med J.* 2004;45(5):531-532.

62. Krleza-Jeric K, Chan AW, Dickersin K, Sim I, Grimshaw J, Gluud C. Principles for international registration of protocol information and results from human trials of health related interventions: Ottawa statement (part 1). *BMJ.* 2005;330(7497):956-958.

63. Editors T. The registration of observational studies – when metaphors go bad. *Epidemiology*. 2010;21(5):607-609.

64. Samet JM. To register or not to register. *Epidemiology*. 2010;21(5):610-611.

65. Lash TL. Preregistration of study protocols is unlikely to improve the yield from our science, but other strategies might. *Epidemiology*. 2010;21(5):612-613.

66. Lash TL, Vandenbroucke JP. Commentary: should preregistration of epidemiologic study protocols become compulsory? Reflections and a counterproposal. *Epidemiology*. 2012;23(2):184-188.

67. Savitz DA. Commentary: prior specification of hypotheses cause or just a correlate of informative studies? *Int J Epidemiol*. 2001;30(5):957-958.

68. Swaen GG, Teggeler O, van Amelsvoort LG. False positive outcomes and design characteristics in occupational cancer epidemiology studies. *Int J Epidemiol*. 2001;30(5):948-954.

69. Lipton P. Testing hypotheses: prediction and prejudice. *Science*. 2005;307(5707):219-221.

70. Cole P. The hypothesis generating machine. *Epidemiology*. 1993;4(3):271-273.

71. Nosek BA, Alter G, Banks GC, et al. SCIENTIFIC STANDARDS. Promoting an open research culture. *Science*. 2015;348(6242):1422-1425.

72. Lash TL. Declining the transparency and openness promotion guidelines. *Epidemiology*. 2015;26(6):779-780.

73. Kahneman D, Slovic P, Tversky A. *Judgment under Uncertainty: Heuristics and Biases*. New York, NY: Cambridge University Press; 1982.

74. Gilovich T, Griffin D, Kahneman D. *Heuristics and Biases: The Psychology of Intuitive Judgment*. New York, NY: Cambridge University Press; 2002.

75. Ariely D. *Predictably Irrational: The Hidden Forces That Shape Our Decisions*. 1st ed. New York, NY: Harper; 2008.

76. Herbst AL, Ulfelder H, Poskanzer DC. Adenocarcinoma of the vagina. Association of maternal stilbestrol therapy with tumor appearance in young women. *N Engl J Med*. 1971;284(15):878-881.

77. Haack S. *Defending Science – Within Reason. Between Scientism and Cynicism*. Amherst, NY: Prometheus Books; 2003.

78. Lawlor DA, Tilling K, Davey Smith G. Triangulation in aetiological epidemiology. *Int J Epidemiol*. 2016;45(6):1866-1886.

79. Lash TL. Truth and consequences. *Epidemiology*. 2015;26(2):141-142.

CHAPTER 3

Formal Causal Models

Tyler J. VanderWeele and Kenneth J. Rothman

To say two variables X and Y are *associated* is to say that information about one variable conveys information about (and thus allows one to partially predict) the other variable. In statistics, the same concept is often described by saying X and Y covary, or are statistically dependent. However, in ordinary language, the term "dependent" suggests one variable affects the other in some causal sense, and yet it is well known that "association is not causation."

If X precedes Y, what distinguishes causation from mere association or predictable covariation of X and Y? Intuitively, we might say that knowing the association of X with Y allows us to predict Y when we see X; thus, association is a relation we can see directly by passive observation of X and Y. In contrast, we may say that knowing the association is causal means that we can further predict what will happen to Y if X were forcibly changed.

This intuitive distinction has ambiguities and shortcomings. Over the past century, several formal models of causation were developed to address some of these problems. In this chapter, we provide a brief overview of four models that have seen use in health applications: potential-outcome (counterfactual) models,[1-7] graphical causal models,[8-13] sufficient-component cause (SCC) models,[14,15] and structural-equations models.[3-6] We focus on special insights facilitated by each approach, translations among the approaches, and the level of detail specified by each approach. Further details of the potential-outcome models are also given in Chapter 5 in discussion of effect measures, further discussion of the sufficient cause framework in Chapter 26 on interaction, and other results on graphical models in Chapter 12 on confounding.

Confounding itself is a central problem of causal inference, and some understanding of the concept is necessary to appreciate the importance of causal modeling. Roughly, confounding refers to mixing up effects of other factors with the effects we wish to study. Thus we say the association of a treatment or exposure with an outcome is *confounded*, or that confounding is present, if the size of the association reflects (at least in part) the effects of other factors on the outcome, rather than the actual effects of the treatment or exposure. The distortion produced by this confounding may be upward or downward and thus may lead to overestimation or underestimation of the effect under study. For example, it may be observed that wearing of dresses instead of pants is associated with breast cancer, but this association does not correctly reflect an effect of wearing dresses; instead, the association is confounded by the effects of sex. More precise characterizations of confounding, along with understanding and extensions of methods to deal with the problem, require the more precise definitions of causation and effects afforded by the causal models described below.

POTENTIAL-OUTCOME (COUNTERFACTUAL) MODELS

Precise deductions about effects typically require a quantitative model that specifies in detail what would happen under alternative possible patterns of interventions or exposures. An important class of quantitative models originating with Neyman and Fisher in the early 20th century[1] are the *potential-outcome* or *counterfactual* models, which form the foundation of most statistical methods for causal inference.[1-4,7] These models formalize notions of cause and effect found in much of philosophy and epidemiology,[7,16,17] such as this passage from MacMahon and Pugh: "… an association may be classed presumptively as causal when it is believed that, had the cause [exposure] been altered, the effect [outcome] would have changed."[17] A key feature of this description is its *counterfactual* element: It refers to what would have happened if, contrary to fact, the exposure had been something other than what it actually was.

Consider the setting in which we are interested in assessing the effect of some exposure X on an outcome Y. Within the "counterfactual" or "potential outcomes" framework,[9,18-23] we let Y_x denote the outcome that would have occurred had X been set to x. If the exposure is binary, then there are two such potential outcomes, Y_0 and Y_1. For each individual, we only get to observe the outcome corresponding to the exposure level that actually occurred for that individual. If the individual actually had exposure level $X = 0$, then we observe Y_0 and we will not in general know the value of Y_1 for that individual. If the individual actually had exposure level $X = 1$, then we observe Y_1 and we will not in general know the value of Y_0 for that individual. That we do in fact observe one of potential outcomes for each individual is sometimes referred to as the "consistency assumption"; stated formally, it is that for an individual who has actual exposure $X = x$, the actual outcome Y is equal to Y_x.

Although we only get to observe one of the potential outcomes for each individual, at least hypothetically we could conceive of both potential outcomes. We could then define the causal effect for an individual as the difference between the two potential outcomes: $Y_1 - Y_0$. We would say that the exposure had an effect on the outcome for that individual if the difference, $Y_1 - Y_0$, were nonzero. Because we generally know only one of the two potential outcomes for each individual, we cannot in general calculate the individual level causal effect. We might hope nonetheless to be able to estimate the average (mean) of the individual effects $Y_1 - Y_0$ in a population, denoted by $E(Y_1 - Y_0)$ ("E" stands for "expectation," a synonym for the population mean of the quantity in the brackets). Even to be able to do this, we need further assumptions; the simplest is to assume that the potential outcomes have the same distribution in each exposure group (*i.e.*, are comparable across the exposure groups). This would be the case on average if the exposure were randomized, but with observational data and nonrandomized exposures, this will usually be an implausible assumption. In such cases, instead we might assume that at least within strata of some set of measured covariates C, the different exposure groups are comparable in their potential outcomes. This assumption is sometimes referred to as an "unconfoundedness" or "no-unmeasured-confounding" assumption or an "exchangeability" assumption (in epidemiology), an "ignorable treatment assignment" assumption (in statistics), or an "exogeneity" assumption (in economics).

More formally, we will say A is independent of B given C (or conditional on C) if within levels of C there is no association of A and B. The no-unmeasured-confounding assumption (again also called "ignorability," "exchangeability," or "exogeneity") can then be stated as: the potential outcomes Y_x are each independent of the exposure or treatment X given the covariates Z—that is, that within strata of the covariates Z the potential outcomes Y_x are not associated with the exposure level actually received. If this were the case, the groups that actually had exposure level $X = 1$ and $X = 0$ would be comparable in their potential outcomes Y_0—that is, in terms of what would have occurred had exposure been set to level 0. Similarly, we would have that the groups that actually had exposure level $X = 1$ and $X = 0$ would be comparable in their potential outcomes Y_1—that is, in terms of what would have occurred had exposure been level 1. Denote the conditional expectation of Y given $Z = z$ by $E(Y|z)$, which is the mean of Y in the subpopulation with $Z = z$. If there is no unmeasured confounding, we can obtain average causal effects from the observed data within strata of covariates as follows:

$$E(Y_1 - Y_0|z) = E(Y_1|z) - E(Y_0|z)$$
$$= E(Y_1|X = 1, z) - E(Y_0|X = 0, z)$$
$$= E(Y|X = 1, z) - E(Y|X = 0, z)$$

where the second equality follows by the no-unmeasured-confounding assumption that Y_x is independent of X given Z and the third equality follows from the consistency assumption that Y_x is the actual outcome when the actual treatment is x. Whereas the quantity $E(Y_1 - Y_0|z)$ is a contrast of potential outcomes, the final expression in the display equation above, $E(Y|X = 1, z) - E(Y|X = 0, z)$, is an empirical quantity we can estimate from the observed data. Under the no-unmeasured-confounding assumption, these two quantities are equal; we can estimate the average causal effect within strata of covariates using just the observed data: $E(Y_1 - Y_0|z) = E(Y|X = 1, z) - E(Y|X = 0, z)$. This is the causal effect within stratum of covariates $Z = z$. If we wanted to estimate the average causal effect for the population, $E(Y_1 - Y_0)$, we could again do this under the no-unmeasured-confounding assumption by standardizing over the covariate distribution in the population (see Chapter 5): $E(Y_1 - Y_0) = \sum_z[E(Y_1 - Y_0|z)P(z)] = \sum_z[E(Y|X = 1, z) - E(Y|X = 0, z)]P(z)$, where $\sum_z$ denotes the sum over the covariates z. Once again this final expression is one that we can empirically estimate from the observed data. This is the effect of the exposure for the population under study; one can also estimate the effect of the exposure for just the exposed, or just the unexposed by appropriate standardization as will be discussed further in Chapter 5.

As noted above, randomization of exposure forces the potential outcomes Y_x to be independent of X, so that the no-unmeasured-confounding assumption holds without conditioning on any covariates at all. In this case, we can estimate the average causal effect just by comparing observed outcomes across the exposure groups: $E(Y_1 - Y_0) = E(Y|X = 1) - E(Y|X = 0)$. With observational data for which the exposure is not randomized, we typically try to collect data on and stratify by, or otherwise control for, a sufficiently rich set of covariates Z so that the no-unmeasured-confounding assumption is plausible (see Chapter 12 on confounding). However, with observational data, we never know whether the assumption is in fact satisfied or how severely it might be violated. Bias analysis or sensitivity analysis techniques, the topic of Chapter 29, can be useful in assessing how strong an unmeasured confounder would have to affect both the exposure and the outcome in order to alter conclusions.

We can also use the potential outcomes framework to provide a causal interpretation of regression coefficients (see Chapters 20 and 21 on regression) under unconfoundedness assumptions. Suppose that the effect of X on Y is unconfounded conditional on covariates Z. Suppose in a linear regression model of a continuous outcome Y on a dichotomous exposure X, we also controlled for covariates Z so that the regression model was:

$$E(Y|X = x, Z = z) = \alpha_0 + \alpha_1 x + \alpha_2' z,$$

To accommodate multiple covariates, z might denote a vector (ordered list) of covariates and α_2 a vector of coefficients, so that $\alpha_2' z$ becomes a sum of coefficients times covariates, for example, with $z = (z_1, z_2)'$ so that $\alpha_2' z = \alpha_{21} z_1 + \alpha_{22} z_2$. Then under the assumption of unconfoundedness conditional on Z, the average causal effect of the exposure X on outcome Y is just given by α_1 since $E(Y_1 - Y_0|z) = E(Y|X = 1, z) - E(Y|X = 0, z) = (\alpha_0 + \alpha_1 1 + \alpha_2' z) - (\alpha_0 + \alpha_1 0 + \alpha_2' z) = \alpha_1$. Thus if the regression model is correctly specified, the regression coefficient for the exposure can be interpreted as the average causal effect if there is no unmeasured confounding conditional on covariates Z. We will return to questions of measures of effect and methods to estimate them in Chapter 12 and to regression models in Chapters 20 and 21.

While the potential outcomes framework is often articulated with a dichotomous exposure X taking values 1 and 0, it is equally applicable to categorical or continuous exposures. In this case, the potential outcome Y_x is simply again the outcome that would have occurred had X been set to level x, but now there are many, not just two, such levels that could be compared. A causal effect is a comparison of two such levels. We could, for example, compare two levels of the exposure, x_1 and x_0, in their effects on an outcome, and the causal effect for this comparison is then $Y_{x_1} - Y_{x_0}$. For example, if the exposure X were cigarettes smoked per day and the outcome Y were some measure of lung function, then we could compare smoking one pack (20 cigarettes) per day to not smoking at all, $Y_{20} - Y_0$; or we could consider smoking two packs per day to not smoking at all, $Y_{40} - Y_0$; or two packs per day to one pack per day, $Y_{40} - Y_{20}$. The framework applies in the same manner with simply replacing 1 with some level x_1 and 0 with some other level x_0.

Several technical and linguistic points are worth noting. Sometimes the terms "potential outcome" and "counterfactual outcome" are used interchangeably, but some authors (*e.g.*, Rubin, 2005[24]) contrast the use of the terms "potential outcome" and "counterfactual outcome" and prefer to use the term "potential outcome" within the context of the outcomes under each of two potential exposures, states, or interventions. If there are two potential exposure states, 0 and 1, then Y_0 would be used to denote the outcome under exposure 0 and Y_1 would be used to denote the outcome under exposure 1. If, in fact, exposure 0 takes place, then the outcome Y_0 occurs; it is what actually occurred; it is not counterfactual or contrary to fact. If the actual exposure was 0, then the outcome that would have taken place under exposure 1, Y_1, is counterfactual; that is, it is the outcome that would have occurred if, contrary to fact, something had taken place, namely the exposure being 1, other than what actually did. If exposure 1 takes place, then the outcome Y_1 occurs; and the outcome that would have taken place under exposure 0, Y_0, is counterfactual. Thus, under Rubin's terminology, only one of the two outcomes is "counterfactual" or contrary to fact. Rubin prefers using the terminology "potential outcomes" because, before any exposure takes place, neither of the outcomes is contrary to fact, and after the exposure takes place, only one outcome is.

Other authors use "counterfactual outcomes" for both Y_0 and Y_1. In this use of terminology, the view is that some exposure, either 0 or 1, will naturally occur and this will lead to the actual outcome Y. The variables Y_0 and Y_1 are viewed as those that would have taken place had there been an *intervention* to set the exposure to 0 or to 1, respectively. Thus, with respect to the outcome that would have naturally occurred, Y, both Y_0 and Y_1, outcomes that would have occurred under some *intervention,* are viewed as "counterfactual." This is because Y_0 and Y_1 are the outcomes that would have taken place if, contrary to fact, there had been an intervention to set the exposure to 0 or 1, respectively. Under this perspective, it is also assumed that if the exposure that naturally occurs is 0, then $Y = Y_0$; and if the exposure that naturally occurs is 1, then $Y = Y_1$—that is, if the exposure naturally takes a particular value, then the actual outcome is equal to the outcome that would have occurred under an intervention to set the exposure for that individual to that value. But it is this "consistency" assumption that ties the counterfactual outcomes to the observed outcomes.

This brings us also to some other subtleties in the notation being employed. The very notation Y_0 and Y_1 effectively presuppose that these potential outcomes are well defined. For these potential outcomes to be well defined an individual's potential outcome must depend only on the treatment or exposure that was received, not on the treatment or exposure status of other individuals. This is sometimes referred to as a "no interference" assumption. It would generally not hold, for example, in an infectious disease setting in which the treatments were someone's vaccination status. It is possible to accommodate violations of this assumption and to allow for interference but the framework then becomes considerably more complex.[25-32] For the potential outcomes Y_0 and Y_1 to be well defined, it is also important that there are not different versions of the exposure that may lead to different outcomes. This would be the case if there were no ambiguity about how to apply any treatment to any individual in the study, or at least that any such ambiguity does not give rise to different outcomes, *i.e.*, that the variation in giving the treatment, for example, is irrelevant for the outcome. This is sometimes referred to as an assumption of "No Multiple Versions of Treatment" or as "Treatment Variation Irrelevance." Further discussion of the assumption and how to handle possible violations is given elsewhere.[25,33-35] The two assumptions required for the potential outcomes to be well defined—the no-inference assumption and the no-multiple-versions-of-treatment assumption—are sometimes together referred to as the Stable Unit Treatment Value Assumption or SUTVA.[25,26] What this ultimately amounts to, however, is that the potential outcomes are well defined.

The strength of the above assumptions has been taken as a weakness of the potential-outcome model.[36] It has been argued, however, that such strong assumptions are inescapable if one wishes to quantify causal effects and are merely hidden by traditional methods that fail to make them explicit.[10,37-45] Adopting the model in fact leads us to recognize central obstacles to causal inference, stemming from the fact that the only potential outcome Y_x that can be observed for an individual is the one corresponding to the treatment actually received by that individual, Y; the remaining Y_x can only be imputed or estimated, not observed. Yet people routinely speculate about such quantities in day-to-day life (*e.g.*, "if I had only bought Microsoft stock when it was first issued, my net worth would be millions of dollars"). Such everyday examples show that the problems attributed to modeling potential outcomes are intrinsic problems of causal inference that are obscured by other approaches. We consider it an advantage of potential-outcome models that they aid inference by making such problems explicit.[7,46]

Certain other criticisms of potential-outcome models can also be addressed by extensions of the framework. For example, potential outcomes are not inherently deterministic, because the Y_x may be values of parameters of probability distributions (*e.g.*, expected age at death) rather than directly observable events (*e.g.*, actual age at death).[46] As another example, potential-outcome models are not limited to person-level analyses; for example, the "individuals" in the model may be social units or aggregates (although the associations observed among these aggregates may be confounded by person-level effects).[47]

One way to summarize the scope of potential-outcome models is that they represent the limit of what one could learn about individual causes and effects from doing only perfect crossover trials, with no knowledge of mechanisms of action. For example, suppose X and Y represent completely reversible exposure and outcome variables, with X indicating a nasal irritant and Y a sneezing probability. We could then estimate an individual's sneezing probabilities when irritant present and absent, Y_1 and Y_0, through a series of trials on the individual that alternated $X = 1$ with $X = 0$, provided there were no carryover effects or temporal variations in the sneezing responses represented by the potential outcomes Y_1 and Y_0. When such trials cannot be performed, as is usual in human health studies, we could still estimate the population distribution of Y_x by applying treatment x to a random sample from that population. By repeating such experiments for various treatment levels (or by randomizing a random sample to different treatment levels) we can estimate how the population outcome distribution would vary with treatment distribution.[1,3,7,46]

Potential-outcome models may encompass purely hypothetical effects as well as actual effects. Consider a trial of the effects of a medication dose x measured in mg/d on an outcome Y which could be diastolic blood pressure in mm Hg after 30 days. A causal model may define values of Y_x for all doses of x, even if the only doses actually given are 0 and 20 mg/d and so the only effects observed involve those doses. We could, however, fit a line through the average outcomes at the two observed doses, and thus extrapolate to the average potential outcome at 30 mg/d and interpolate to the average potential outcome at 10 mg/d. The fitted model may thus provide values for the outcomes for treatment at 30 and 10 mg/d. Nonetheless, because no 30 or 10 mg/d dosing is actually observed, the corresponding potential outcomes are never observed either, and the difference $Y_{30} - Y_{10}$ becomes a purely hypothetical effect, estimated by modeling, of 30 vs. 10 mg/d.

The hypothetical nature of these projections is another source of uncertainty in effect estimates beyond that addressed by conventional statistical methods. In particular, we might obtain a notably different estimate if instead we fit a line through the logarithms of the average outcomes, which raises the problem of model uncertainty (see Chapter 21). Some causal modeling methods attempt to avoid dealing with purely hypothetical potential outcomes by imposing a *treatment positivity* requirement, sometimes expressed by saying there is a positive probability (nonzero chance) of receiving any treatment for which an effect will be estimated. This condition is much stronger than the treatment possibility (*e.g.*, in the above example, it was physically possible to administer 30 mg/d, but was simply not allowed in the study). While positivity is assumed by several important causal modeling techniques, it is insufficient to avoid all problems of hypothetical treatments and outcomes (especially when exposure has many more possible levels than can be observed) and, at the same time, is too restrictive for many purposes.

GRAPHICAL MODELS

Following a long history of informal use in path analysis, causal diagrams (graphical causal models) saw an explosion of theoretical development during the 1990s,[8-10] including elaboration of connections to other methods for causal modeling. The latter connections are especially valuable for those familiar with some but not all methods, as some background assumptions and sources of bias are more easily seen with certain models, whereas practical statistical procedures may be more easily derived under other models.

We begin with a brief summary of terms and concepts of directed-graph theory. After describing concepts for graphs, we will relate these concepts to associations among variables on a graph. We will then further relate associations among variables on a graph to causal relations on a graph. See Spirtes et al. (2001)[8] and Pearl (2009)[10] for more detailed explanations and formal graphical causal models. See Dechter et al. (2010),[48] Richardson and Robins (2013),[49] and Berzuini et al. (2012)[50] for alternative interpretations of such models, including developments such as single world intervention graphs or SWIGs, which constitute an alternative interpretation of causal diagrams.

Figure 3-1 provides the graphs used for illustration below. An *arc* or *edge* is any line segment (with or without arrowheads) connecting two variables; a graph is *directed* if all the arcs in it are arrows pointing in one direction. If there is an arrow from a variable X to another variable Y in a graph, X is called a *parent* of Y and Y is called a *child* of X.

A *path* between two variables X and Y in a directed graph is a sequence of distinct arrows connecting X and Y. A *directed path* is a sequence of edges that follows the direction of the arrows, *i.e.*, such that the child in the sequence is the parent in the next step. If there is a directed path from X to Y, X is called an *ancestor* of Y and Y is called a *descendant* of X. A graph is *acyclic* if no directed

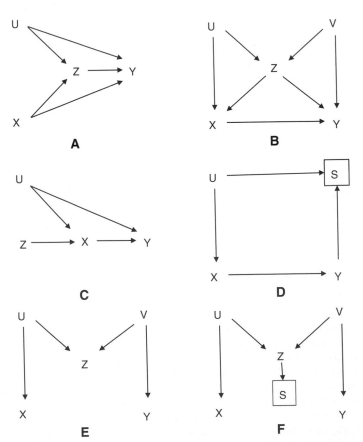

FIGURE 3-1 Four casual diagrams. X and Y are the exposure and outcome variables under study. Different potential confounding structures for the effect of exposure X on outcome Y.

path forms a closed loop, so that no variable is both an ancestor and descendant of another. A graph that is both directed and acyclic is called a *directed acyclic graph* or DAG; each graph in Figure 3-1 is a DAG. Throughout this book, we will use only DAGs for causal graphs, unless stated otherwise.

Association and Graphical Connection

Graphs allow one to reason visually about associations between variables in the graph by examining the paths connecting them. To exploit this feature, we will need some additional terminology. A variable is a *collider* on a particular path if the variables before and after it on the path have arrows going into that variable (*i.e.*, it is the child in a parent-child-parent sequence of variables on the path). Note that a collider is specific to a path. Thus, in Figure 3-1B, the variable Z is a collider on the path U-Z-V, but it is not a collider on the path U-Z-Y.

A noncollider (*i.e.*, a variable that is not a collider on a path) can be one of two types. A *fork* on the path has arrows pointing out to the variables before and after it on the path (*i.e.*, is the parent in a child-parent-child sequence on the path); in Figure 3-1B, Z is a fork on the path X-Z-Y. A *mediator* or intermediate on the path instead has arrows pointing to it and from it along the path (*i.e.*, has a parent before it and a child after it on the path); in Figure 3-1B, Z is a mediator on the path U-Z-Y. Thus, being a collider, fork, or mediator is specific to a path; in Figure 3-1B, Z can be any of those depending on the path under discussion.

A path between two nodes, A and B, is said to be *blocked* or *closed* conditional on a set of variables Z if either (1) no collider on the path is in Z or has a descendant in Z, or (2) at least one noncollider on the path is in Z. Otherwise, the path is said to be *unblocked* or *open* given Z; in other words, the path is unblocked or open given Z if (1) every collider on the path is in Z or has a descendant in Z, and (2) no noncollider on the path is in Z. Two variables in a DAG with no open path between them are said to be *d-separated* (directionally separated); otherwise they are *d-connected*.

DAG models for association assume that, for each graphed variable, conditioning on its parents (and nothing else) will render it independent of any variable that is not a descendant; this requirement is sometimes called the graphical *Markov condition*. It is equivalent to the *connectivity condition*, which is the assumption that d-connection is necessary for association; this can be restated as the assumption that all d-separated variables are unassociated (independent) of one another. This relation between graphical paths and associations is analogous to the relation between electrical wiring and conduction in circuits. Associations between two variables are transmitted through the open paths between them, just as electricity (and hence information) is transmitted between circuit parts via conductive wires. And, just as there is no electrical transmission between two parts if the circuit between them is broken (so no conductor connects them), so two d-separated variables have no open path between them and so must be unassociated; that is, two variables will be independent if every path connecting them is blocked, for then no information can be transmitted between them.

On the other hand, just as presence of a wire does not mean electricity is flowing, the presence of open paths (d-connection) does not automatically lead to an association. For example, the associations transmitted along different pathways may be in opposite directions and thus may balance each other out—although such perfect cancelations would ordinarily not be expected unless created intentionally. The assumption that such graphically invisible independencies are absent (*i.e.*, that d-connection implies association) is the converse of the connectivity condition, and is called the *faithfulness* assumption; because intentional violations are often used in observational study designs, chiefly in the form of cohort matching,[51] we will not use this assumption even though some authors adopt faithfulness as a core assumption.[8]

As noted above, conditioning (stratifying or "controlling") on a collider Z with independent parents U and V can induce an association between the two parents; we can describe this phenomenon by saying that conditioning on Z unblocks or opens the path U-Z-V between its parents, providing an avenue for an association between U and V. An important result is that if one stratifies (conditions) on a descendant Z of two variables U and X, and U and X are independent in the total population, then we should expect U and X to be associated within at least one stratum of Z (exceptions to this rule involve somewhat contrived cancelations of effects).[2,3] Thus in Figure 3-1A even if U and X are unassociated with each other unconditionally, they will (apart from perfect cancelations) be associated within some strata of Z.

Conversely, if Z is a noncollider (whether fork or mediator) on a path between two variables, conditioning on Z blocks or closes that path and thus removes one avenue for an association between the variables. Note that conditioning on a variable or set of variables may open some paths between two variables and close others; thus in Figure 3-1B, conditioning on Z and nothing else closes the path X-Z-Y from X to Y, but opens the path X-U-Z-V-Y.

An easily overlooked feature of statistical DAGs is the presence of implicit "pure noise" variables, also known as "independent random disturbances" or "random effects," one for each graphed variable, with each disturbance connected to other variables only through the variable they perturb. A complete graphical depiction would then show a disturbance ε_x with an arrow to X and no other direct connections; a disturbance ε_y with an arrow to Y and no other direct connections; and so on for every graphed variable. Note that even though ε_y is completely random, it can become associated with ancestors of Y (including other random disturbances) if one conditions on Y (since Y is a collider on every path from ε_x to Y ancestors, including confounders). This conditioning can be a source of bias when Y is the outcome variable and affects selection, as in case-control studies.

The above concepts generalize to analyses of relations among entire sets or groups of variables. Suppose we have three disjoint (nonoverlapping) sets of variables A, B, and C. A path from A to B is one that starts at a variable in A and ends in a variable in B. If all these paths are closed, then A and B are d-separated and A and B are independent (unassociated); otherwise if any of these paths are open, A and B are d-connected. If all paths between A and B are blocked by conditioning on C, then A and B are said to be d-separated by C and will be unassociated conditional on C. As will be described below, this concept of separation by a set C is central to graphical identification of bias sources and sets sufficient for control of bias.

Causal Graphs

DAG models can succinctly encode our information about associations and independencies among variables. They become models that *explain* those associations and independencies when the presence of an arrow is taken to imply the presence of a causal mechanism leading from the parent variable to the child variable. Specifically, a graph is *causal* if every arrow represents the presence of an effect of the parent (causal) variable on the child (affected) variable. All arrows are thus in the temporal direction: A parent variable always occurs before a child variable. To use graphs to reason about confounding control and other forms of bias requires that the representation on the graph be such that there is:

1. No ungraphed confounding: Any variable that affects two or more variables in the graph via distinct direct effects must be shown on the graph as an ancestor of the affected variables, even if it is unmeasured.
2. No ungraphed collider stratification: Any variable that affects selection or is used for stratification and is affected by two or more variables in the graph (including its random disturbance) must be shown on the graph as a descendant of the variables affecting it, even if it is unmeasured.

As may become clear from the descriptions below, these requirements are needed to ensure that any association between two variables in the graph can be attributed solely to open paths between the variables within the graph, and thus can be traced to either variation in graphed causal variables, or conditioning on effects of such variables, or both. Conditions 1 and 2 enforce the connectivity requirement of DAGs by demanding the graph we draw show all variables which can causally explain associations (either as uncontrolled confounders or as controlled colliders), even if those variables are unmeasured or hypothetical.

In a causal graph, a directed path represents a causal pathway, and an X-to-Y arrow represents a direct effect of X on Y within the graph—which is to say, the arrow represents an effect that is not transmitted (mediated) through any other variable in the graph. Each graph in Figure 3-1 summarizes causal relations within a population of individuals, and each variable represents the states or events among individuals in that population. For example, if X is a treatment variable, then the value of X for an individual is the level of treatment received by the individual. Absence of an arrow from X to Y in the graph corresponds to the causal null hypothesis that no alteration of the distribution of X could change the distribution of Y, when all other variables on the graph are fixed.

Confounding in Causal Graphs

Causal graphs are useful for visualizing and reasoning about confounding and selection bias, as both problems can be represented as associations between two variables X and Y arising from open non-directed paths, as opposed to directed paths (causal pathways) from X to Y. In studies of the effects of X on Y, such open nondirected paths are called *biasing paths*, because the associations they transmit can create a discrepancy (bias) between the observed association of X and Y and the association due to the effect of X on Y (which is transmitted only through the directed paths from X to Y).

Confounding may be defined as an association of X and Y that arises from a biasing path from X to Y that begins with an arrow into X and ends with an arrow into Y. In Figure 3-1C, the path from X to U to Y would be a biasing path that constitutes confounding. If there is no confounding path from X to Y, we say their association is *unconfounded* (although as described below it may still be biased by other open nondirected paths). As an illustration, suppose in Figure 3-1A X represents a 6-month weight loss regimen that is randomly assigned within a cohort of cardiovascular patients, with $X = 1$ for regimen assigned and $X = 0$ for not assigned; Z represents a set of clinical coronary heart disease risk factors (serum lipids, blood pressure) measured at regimen completion; Y represents death within the year following completion; and U represents a set of unmeasured genes that affect death risk both directly and through the clinical factors Z. Although U affects Y, there is no open path from X to Y through U, because there is no open path from X to U. This means that U is independent of X and that whatever association we see between X and Y cannot be attributed to effects of U on X and Y; that is, it cannot be attributed to confounding of the X-Y association by U.

As another example, a common approach to analyzing effects of weight on health is to adjust for serum lipids and blood pressure. If weight affects serum lipids and blood pressure, such adjustment cannot be justified as confounding control because it removes that part of the weight effect mediated through serum lipids and blood pressure. It is often thought that such an analysis estimates the direct effect of weight or of a weight-loss regimen. Nonetheless, this rationale fails if the intermediates were also affected by uncontrolled risk factors; it fails even if the treatment X is independent of the uncontrolled factors, so that there is no confounding of the unconditional X-Y association,[52] as in Figure 3-1A. Graph theory shows this fact visually. Because Z is a child of both U and X, one should expect U and X to be associated within at least one stratum of Z; consequently, within strata of Z, U becomes a confounder, even though it was not one to begin with.[13] In general, one should expect control of an intermediate Z to generate bias when Z and Y share causes other than X, as in Figure 3-1A; in such cases, the association of Z with Y is confounded, and so the estimated indirect effect of X on Y being "removed" by Z-adjustment is confounded.[53] Further discussion of assessing direct effects is given in Chapter 27.

Figure 3-1B gives yet another example, which has a counterintuitive quality and had to wait for graph theory for explanation. In this graph we ask, "is it sufficient to stratify only on Z in order to unbiasedly estimate the effect of X on Y?" A common intuitive answer is "Yes," because physically preventing individual variation in Z would block the effects of U on Y and V on X and thus eliminate confounding by U and V (as well as confounding by Z). But in an observational study U and V would ordinarily be associated within some strata of Z, because they both affect Z. Within those strata, U would be associated with Y (through V) as well as with X, and V would be associated with X (through U) as well as with Y; consequently, both U and V would be confounders and one or the other would have to be controlled to remove the confounding.[9,11]

One can recognize the insufficiency of controlling Z alone given Figure 3-1B in more traditional ways: The association of Z with Y given X is confounded by V; because adjustment for Z alone depends on this confounded association, one might conclude correctly that such adjustment could mislead and that adjustment for V as well as Z would remedy the problem. But graphical theory also shows that adjustment for U rather than V would also suffice: because the V-X association produced by Z-adjustment is mediated entirely through U, U-adjustment eliminates confounding by V within Z strata.

Backdoor Paths

A concept useful for identification and control of confounding is that of a *backdoor path*: A path from X to Y is backdoor if its first step is an arrow pointing to X. There is no backdoor path from X to Y in Figure 3-1A, whereas in Figure 3-1C the path X-U-Y is a backdoor path from X to Y. The concept of backdoor path is useful because, if we do not condition on any variable in the graph, the only source of bias of the X-Y association under the null (setting aside differential measurement error) will be via open backdoor paths.[10] In fact, Pearl (1995)[9] showed that if a set of variables Z in a causal DAG blocks all backdoor paths from X to Y, and no variable in Z is a descendant of X (so that there is no selection or conditioning associated with variables in the graph); then controlling for Z suffices to control for confounding for the effect of X on Y. This is sometimes referred to as the backdoor path adjustment criterion. It is an important approach to think about confounding bias on graphs. Nonetheless, as seen in Figure 3-1A and D, selection or conditioning requires we also consider biasing paths that are not backdoor paths.

To illustrate, consider Figure 3-1E. There is no arrow from Z to X or to Y, and so we do not have to adjust for any of U, Z, or V to control for confounding: The only backdoor path from X to Y is X-U-Z-V-Y, which is blocked because Z is a collider on the path. Suppose, however, we condition on Z. This conditioning would open the backdoor path X-U-Z-V-Y and introduce confounding. Thus, it is possible to produce confounding by adjusting for a variable that occurs before the exposure. Bias of this form is sometimes called "M-bias" and is an example of a more general form of bias called *collider stratification bias*, or simply "collider bias"; in Figure 3-1E, the backdoor path can be blocked by further conditioning on either U or V, or both, thus removing the confounding produced by conditioning on Z.

The preceding examples illustrate how causal graphs supply simple visual methods to check for confounding and for sufficiency of confounder adjustment. Some basic results are as follows: (1) an open backdoor path from X to Y can produce an association between X and Y, even if X has no effect on Y, and so can produce confounding; (2) adjustment for certain variables, even those that occur before the exposure, can open backdoor paths, and so produce confounding.[9,10] These results lead to the general criteria for identifying sets of variables sufficient for control of confounding given a graph.[9,10]

Selection Bias

We warn readers that terminology is highly inconsistent, and one especially needs to pay attention to precisely what is meant when reference is made to "confounding" and "selection bias." In particular, the term "selection bias" has been defined in many ways, some so general that they include all of confounding as described above. For example, some econometric literature uses "selection bias" to denote selective treatment assignment, and such nonrandom assignment is a source of confounding. Other definitions are synonyms for collider bias (associations transmitted through colliders that have been conditioned on) and thus include confounding transmitted through colliders, as seen when conditioning on Z in Figure 3-1A and B.

More traditional usage in epidemiology has limited "selection bias" to associations transmitted via the selection indicator S, as in Figure 3-1D. In this usage, selection bias is a special case of collider bias,[54,55] but is of the broadest practical importance because all real analyses are conditional on the individuals and data selected for analysis. This means that selection bias is almost inevitable whenever S is connected to both the exposure and outcome under study. In this book, we will follow traditional usage in which "selection bias" is collider bias arising from the inevitable conditioning on selection. This means that some examples of bias are both confounding and selection bias at once. To illustrate, consider Figure 3-1F, which is the same as Figure 3-1E except with the selection indicator S added and affected by Z. Under this graph, any estimate of the effect will be biased by the association transmitted via X-U-Z-V-Y. In traditional usage, this bias is both confounding, because the association of X with Y can be attributed to an open backdoor path from X to Y; but it is also selection bias, because it arises from a noncausal association of X and Y induced by conditioning on selection S. Furthermore, it is a type of collider bias, specifically M-bias. As in Figure 3-1E, it can be removed by further conditioning on either U or V, or both.

We will revisit these foundational issues in Chapter 12, and much of the design and analysis chapters will be concerned with methods to prevent or reduce confounding and selection bias.

MULTIFACTORIAL CAUSATION AND THE SUFFICIENT-COMPONENT CAUSE MODEL

The sufficient cause framework[14,56,57] conceptualizes causation as a collection of different sufficient conditions or causes for the occurrence of an outcome (effect). Each sufficient condition or cause is usually conceived of as consisting of various (necessary) component causes, with the property that if all components are present the sufficient cause is complete and the outcome occurs. Best known among epidemiologists is Rothman's sufficient-component cause (SCC) model.[14] Rothman conceived of each sufficient cause as representing a mechanism that produces the outcome, such that if all components were present then a mechanistic sequence would be set in motion that would inevitably produce the outcome.

Rothman referred to each component of a sufficient cause as a "component cause" or simply as a "cause." Whereas the principal focus of potential-outcome models is the cause or intervention itself, a sufficient-cause model focuses on the effect. To illustrate the conceptual differences across models, consider the concept of interaction. The graphical and potential-outcome models can be used to portray the presence, though not the mechanics, of causal interactions. Consider, for example, two exposures: phenylketonuria (PKU), which we indicate with X ($X = 1$ if PKU present), and significant phenylalanine consumption (SPC), which we indicate with G ($G = 1$ if SPC present). In some people, these two factors together are both necessary and sufficient to produce brain damage, which we indicate with Y ($Y = 1$ for damage).[17]

In a basic potential-outcome model for this example, there are four potential outcome variables $Y(x,g)$ for every individual, one for every combination of X and G: $Y(1,1)$, $Y(1,0)$, $Y(0,1)$, and $Y(0,0)$. It is sometimes said that synergism is present if $Y(1,1) = 1$ and $Y(1,0) = Y(0,1) = Y(0,0) = 0$, so that actual damage occurs ($Y = 1$) only when both exposures are present ($X = G = 1$). This synergism can be represented in a causal diagram by including the product variable XG, which indicates the presence of both exposures (because $XG = 1$ if and only if $X = G = 1$; otherwise $XG = 0$), then drawing an arrow from XG to Y.[58] We will discuss the topic of causal interaction further in Chapter 26.

Because potential outcomes are quantities specific to individuals in the modeled population, they provide more detail than arrows in graphs. For example, the individuals affected by X and those affected by G may be one and the same, or may not overlap at all. The graph $X \rightarrow Y \leftarrow G$ would hold if the population were composed entirely of individuals with $Y(1,1) = Y(1,0) = Y(0,1) = 1$ and $Y(0,0) = 0$; in this case, if everyone had their actual X and G equal to 0, everyone would be affected by changes in X or changes in G. But the same graph would hold if the population was half individuals with $Y(1,1) = Y(1,0) = 1$ and $Y(0,1) = Y(0,0) = 0$ (individuals affected only by changes in X) and half individuals with $Y(1,1) = Y(0,1) = 1$ and $Y(1,0) = Y(0,0) = 0$ (individuals affected only by changes in G). Like the graph, the potential-outcome model can be extended to include effects of G on X as well as the effects on Y; doing so reveals many distinctions not captured by simply adding an arrow from G to X in the graph.[52] Such examples show that potential-outcome models are logically finer (distinguish more situations) than graphical models of the same variables; this fineness leads to greater notational complexity.

Consideration of causal mechanisms leads to models that are logically finer than either potential-outcome models or graphs. In the sufficient-component cause model,[14] two factors are said to be causal *cofactors* if they are components of the same causal mechanism; the presence of both cofactors is necessary for the mechanism to operate and so produce the outcome under study. This definition refers to mechanisms; thus, the basic units of analysis are the mechanisms that determine the potential outcomes of individuals, rather than the individuals themselves. Many different sets of mechanisms will lead to the same pattern of potential outcomes for an individual; hence, many different SCC models will lead to the same potential-outcome model. As with potential-outcome models, however, SCC models are not inherently deterministic, because the component causes may be random events[59] and because the outcome affected by the completion of a sufficient cause may be a probability distribution rather than an observable event.[60] Further discussion of the formalization and technical details of the SCC model are given elsewhere.[61,62]

The SCC model sometimes employs a pie chart representation of causal mechanisms introduced by Rothman, in which each slice represents a necessary component of the mechanism.[14] To illustrate,

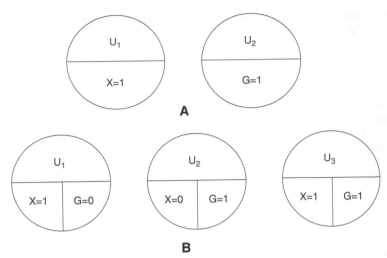

FIGURE 3-2 Two distinct sufficient-component cause (SCC) models for the set of mechanisms within an individual; each leads to the same set of potential outcomes when U_1, U_2, and U_3 are all present. Primary exposures are X and G and additional unknown factors to complete the sufficient causes are U_1, U_2, and U_3.

suppose we are considering mechanisms for angiosarcoma induction in an individual. Figure 3-2 gives an illustration of two distinct SCC models for the disease-causing mechanisms within this individual. The U in the figure represents sets of unmeasured cofactors that would be present regardless of this individual's X or G status. Model (a) posits that there are two mechanisms that can lead to disease in this individual, neither of which involve synergism of X levels and G levels, while model (b) posits three such mechanisms, which show synergism of X levels and G levels. Nonetheless, for individuals for whom U_1, U_2, and U_3 were all present under both models this individual will get the disease unless $X = 0$ and $G = 0$; in other words, under either SCC model the individual's potential outcomes would be $Y(1,1) = Y(1,0) = Y(0,1) = 1$ and $Y(0,0) = 0$. Thus, even if we could conduct a perfect crossover trial on the individual and so observe the individual's outcome under all four combinations of X and G, we would still be unable to determine which SCC model was correct.

As this example and more realistic ones[63-65] show, there are severe limits to the detail about causal mechanisms that can be distinguished using only ordinary ("black-box") randomized trials and epidemiological studies of exposure-disease relations.[63-66] Although discrimination among mechanisms can be important,[65,66] it will usually require direct observations of intermediate steps or of biomarkers for hypothesized mechanisms. We will consider other topics concerning mechanisms in Chapters 26 and 27. For example, we will show that it is sometimes possible to detect the presence of mechanisms that require both of two causes to operate.

The sufficient cause framework has been extended in various ways in the past decade. The theory for empirically testing for sufficient cause interactions has been extended to n-way interactions[62] and to ordinal and continuous exposures.[67,68] The model has been extended to, and used to shed light upon, the phenomena of mediation,[69-71] and attempts have been made to better incorporate time within the sufficient cause framework.[72,73] All of these have been important and valuable advances. Nevertheless, in spite of these advances and the insights that follow from the conceptualization, the model itself continues to be used today principally for teaching and illustrative purposes, rather than in design or analysis.[74]

STRUCTURAL-EQUATION MODELS

Informal use of graphs initially developed as an intuitive aid for structural equations modeling (SEM), in which a web or network of causation is modeled by a system of equations and independence assumptions.[10] Each equation shows how an individual response (outcome, affected, dependent) variable changes as its direct (parent) causal variables change and can thus be viewed as a potential-outcome model for that response.[10] Again, the "individual" may be any unit of interest, such as a person or aggregate. In the system, a variable may appear in no more than one equation as a response variable, but may appear in any other equation as a causal variable. A variable appearing as a response in the system is said to be endogenous (within the system); otherwise it is exogenous.

A causal graph can be viewed as a qualitative schematic for a class of structural-equation models,[10] although, in most interpretations, the equations impose much stronger assumptions than the graph.[45] *Linear* structural-equation models have been very popular in the social sciences and have received some use within epidemiology. These linear system models are often paired with graphical representation of the system of equations as a *path diagram*, which can be viewed as a causal graph specialized to take advantage of the assumed linear relations.[10] In addition to assuming essentially every relationship is linear, many applications of these models further assume that every variable is normally distributed. These are extremely strong assumptions beyond the graphical condition that all sources of confounding and selection bias are visible as biasing paths in the graph (which is usually expressed as an assumption of independent or at least uncorrelated residual variation among the variables in the system).

In parallel with graphs, structural equations models, when interpreted causally, assume that all confounding and collider stratification is correctly represented in the system of equations. This is a stronger requirement than the graphical one, however, for it assumes not only that the necessary confounders and colliders are in the model, but also that the functional forms chosen for the confounder effects and collider causes are correct. Furthermore, a single omitted confounder can bias not just the estimates for the effects it confounds, but also can also bias other effect estimates.

Structural equation models themselves, in their most general context, can be viewed just as an algebraic system for causal graphical models. However, the analytic tools that accompany them, often assuming linearity, normality, and confounding control everywhere, make assumptions that are so strong that they are perhaps best viewed as exploratory tools for hypothesis generation. Interesting hypotheses that emerge from such tools can then be subsequently more rigorously evaluated. Because of their strong assumptions and the extensive technical machinery required for their proper use, we will not cover structural-equation models in greater depth in this book; for further discussion of the interpretative challenges see VanderWeele (2012).[75]

GRAPHICAL VERSUS ALGEBRAIC REPRESENTATIONS

A theme throughout explanation and inference is that different frameworks can provide different insights about the phenomena under study as well as the methods being used to study them. As an illustration that contrasts graphical and algebraic representations of causation, Figure 3-1C diagrams a situation in which Z is an *instrumental variable* or *instrument* for estimating X effects: Z affects X, but is unassociated with the confounder U and is unassociated with Y except through X.[10] We will discuss instrumental variables at greater length in Chapter 28. Such variables are central to randomized trials, in which the instrument Z is the assigned (intended) treatment. Many patients do not fully adhere to their assigned treatment and instead take (or receive) a different level of treatment, X. This nonadherence (noncompliance) with assigned treatment is not random, being susceptible to influence by side effects of treatment and symptoms that may predict the outcome. The concern is then that the received-treatment variable is affected by such unmeasured factors U, which if also risk factors (or close correlates of risk factors) for the outcome under study will confound the relation of actual treatment to the outcome, despite the randomization of treatment assignment.

Standard intent-to-treat analyses examine only the Z association with Y and so are estimating the effect of treatment assignment Z, rather than a physiologic effect of received treatment X. Can we also estimate the latter effect? The answer is yes, provided we can make further (not necessarily unique) quantitative assumptions. The graph makes clear that we should not expect the unconditional X-Y association to equal the X-Y effect, because of confounding by U. The graph also shows, however, that there is no confounding of the Z effects on X or Y (as would be expected if Z was randomized); hence, the unconditional Z-X and Z-Y associations will equal the Z-X and Z-Y effects. We can also see that we might use the Z-Y association to test whether there is an X-Y effect. This is the basic intuition behind an instrumental variable approach. And this is relatively clear from the graph, but if we want to quantify the magnitude of effects, we must turn to other, more algebraic models.

By modeling these effects as potential outcomes, one can put bounds on the X-Y effect.[10] Although one or both bounds may be beyond any plausible range for the X-Y effect,[76] further algebraic modeling assumptions can narrow these bounds sometimes even down to a point that can be estimated from the data.[10] For example, from a linear structural equation modeling perspective, one could obtain the magnitude of the X-Y effect by simply dividing the magnitude of the Z-Y effect by the magnitude of the Z-X effect. Other insights only emerge when we explicitly employ a potential outcomes framework. For example, with binary Z and X, if there is no individual who would take treatment if unassigned, but not take treatment if assigned (an assumption sometimes referred to as "no defiers"), then the ratio of the Z-Y effect to the Z-X effect will in fact give the X-Y effect,[77] but only for the subpopulation of those who comply with their treatment assignment.[76] Different models at different levels of granularity provide different insights.

WHAT IS A CAUSAL VARIABLE?

A controversial issue in all theories of causation is whether a variable must be manipulable to be considered potentially causal. For modeling purposes, some authors would restrict the label "causal" to variables that represent interventions or actions,[78] or at most allow only mutable variables (those susceptible to intervention) as potentially causal.[10] Such restrictions exclude as causal those variables regarded as immutable or defining characteristics of individuals, such as the birth date and genetic sex of persons, but allow as causal such variables as *perceived* age and sex. Even when technology advances enough to allow alteration of a previously immutable characteristic (*e.g.*, through genetic engineering), some authors would only label as "causal" the intervention that alters the characteristic, not the characteristic itself.[78]

In potential-outcome models, the levels of an immutable variable may be represented by strata (*i.e.*, subpopulations) but not by interventions, leaving the potential outcomes and thus effects of the variable undefined. In graphical and structural models, immutable variables may appear as exogenous variables, and so in many formalizations, are not distinguished from manipulable exogenous variables. This practice is arguably more in accord with ordinary usage of "causal"; it is useful because all the graphical rules for assessing bias sources and covariate control continue to apply when including immutable variables.[10] The distinction between mutable and immutable variables remains important, however, as it leads to refinement of vague concepts like "race" into multiple variables that may have very different implications for health outcomes (*e.g.*, mutable variables such as ethnic identification, and immutable variables such as ancestry).[79] Further discussion of these issues is given elsewhere.[80-83] The question of what constitutes a cause or a causal variable and how the potential outcomes framework can be extended remains a matter of debate and discussion within epidemiology.[35,84-90] A more severe problem arises when variables that are not interventions are treated as interventions for planning purposes.[79] A common example is estimation of "the effect" of eliminating a disease (*e.g.*, lung cancer) on life expectancy. This effect is dependent on how the disease is eliminated; for example, if it is eliminated by chemoprevention or vaccination, there may be occasional fatal side effects, or there may be causal or preventive effects on other potentially fatal diseases. Careful consideration of the ambiguities inherent in "disease elimination" should lead instead to estimation of the effect of specific interventions designed to reduce or eliminate the disease burden.

CONCLUSIONS

Each of the four frameworks discussed in this chapter have their strengths and weaknesses. Each is also related to the others, and the principal differences concern the level of granularity at which causation is analyzed. As noted above, graphical models themselves can be interpreted as diagrammatic shorthand for structural equations. Structural equations can be interpreted as sets of counterfactual relations. Sufficient component cause models themselves give rise to potential outcomes and can be graphically represented[91,92] or as a structural equation with the structural equation for a node being the disjunction of its sufficient causes. Again, each of these formal causal models represent various causal relations, but in different ways, and at different level of granularity. See VanderWeele and Robins (2007, 2009)[91,92] for further discussion of relations among these formal frameworks.

Of the four causal modeling methods reviewed here, SCC models stand apart in requiring specification of mechanisms within the individual units under study. There are rarely data to support such detailed specification. In contrast, structural equations have seen extensive analytic application (especially in the social sciences[2,4,5,93]) since the 1920s, as have potential-outcome models.[1] Due to their qualitative form, graphical models can be easily applied in any study to display assumptions of causal analyses and to check whether covariates or sets of covariates are insufficient, excessive, or inappropriate to control given those assumptions.[6,8-13,53] When those assumptions are in doubt, one can still formulate a series of plausible graphs and conduct a corresponding series of analyses.[94] Constructing graphs to accompany conventional statistical analyses of effects can help avoid or spot common mistakes, such as control of intermediates as if they were confounders.[6,13,53]

The frameworks described above help clarify the assumptions needed to move from inferences about associations to inferences about causation. Nonetheless, rarely are all the assumptions known to hold with enough certainty to warrant certainty about deductions based on the models. Much of Part II of this book is devoted to design of studies in ways that will force certain assumptions to hold, or at least make those assumptions more likely to hold to a good approximation. An example is treatment randomization, which if executed correctly ensures that there is no open backdoor path from treatment to any outcome, and thus allows confounding to be treated as a random error. Randomization leaves unaddressed, however, potential problems, such as nonrandom loss to follow-up, treatment crossover, and nonadherence, and does not prevent other biases such as those that arise from conditioning on a variable affected by the treatment. Further details and subtleties about causal inference and formal causal models will be addressed throughout the remainder of the book.

HISTORICAL NOTES

The idea of conceptualizing causation in terms of counterfactuals can be traced at least as far back as Hume (1748)[95] and can be found in subsequent literature on science, philosophy, and law, appearing in epidemiology in MacMahon and Pugh (1967).[17] Mid-20th century developments in modal logic led to full counterfactual theories of causality, as found, for example, in Simon and Rescher (1966)[96] and Lewis (1973)[97]; see also the anthology by Harper et al. (1981).[98] Meanwhile, the basic potential-outcome model was introduced into statistics by Neyman (1923)[18] and Fisher (1935),[99] who applied the model to the analysis of randomized experiments. Over the ensuing decades the framework was used to develop models for such experiments and was sometimes referred to as the "randomization model" (e.g., Welch 1937,[19] Wilk 1955,[20] Cox 1958,[100] and Copas 1973[21]). Rubin popularized the model by coining the term "potential outcome" and by extending the model to include observational (nonexperimental) studies, thus bringing to the fore the problems of unconfoundedness or ignorability and also of no relevant treatment versions and no interference; he also recognized the model's connection to missing-data models (Rubin, 1978).[101] Applications of the model to observational epidemiology emerged soon after, e.g., see Hamilton (1979)[102] and Greenland and Robins (1986).[103] Robins (1986, 1987)[23,104] further extended the basic model to time-varying exposures and covariates. Potential-outcome models have since become the dominant framework for statistical methods in causal inference, especially for observational studies in the health and social sciences.

Graphical models for associations also have a long history and have been applied as part of causal analysis via structural-equation modeling since the pioneering work of Sewall Wright under the heading of path analysis (Wright 1921).[105] The modern form of causal DAG theory, however, began appearing in the 1980s (e.g., Kiiveri et al., 1984[106]); its core foundation in the concepts of d-separation and d-connection was completed by its merging with the theory of Bayesian information networks (Bayes nets) (Pearl, 1988[107]; Verma and Pearl, 1991[108]).

An early simple example of the sufficient cause model can be found in Cayley (1853).[56] Elements of the sufficient cause framework in epidemiology appears in MacMahon and Pugh (1967)[17] and in philosophy in the work of Mackie (1965).[57] Mackie proposed that when we refer to something as a "cause" it is then generally considered to be an "*insufficient* but *necessary* part of a condition which is itself *unnecessary* but *sufficient* for the result." He used the term "INUS condition" as a shorthand for the expression in quotations in the previous sentence, the term "INUS" being derived from the first letter of each of the italicized words. The sufficient cause framework came to popularity in epidemiology principally through the writing of Rothman (1976).[14] Rothman discussed the implications of the framework for epidemiologic research and provided a graphical schematic for the sufficient causes that have informally come to be known as "causal pies."

The sufficient-cause framework has also received attention in the legal literature: Wright (1988)[109] proposed that the equivalent of a component cause or INUS condition be used as a standard for causation in legal reasoning and referred to such a condition as a "NESS factor" where the term "NESS" is derived from the first letter of the italicized words in the expression, "*necessary element* for the *sufficiency* of a *sufficient set*." Similar ideas also appear in the psychology literature (Cheng, 1997[110]; Novick and Cheng, 2004[111]). See VanderWeele (2012)[112] for an overview of the sufficient-cause framework as it has emerged in different disciplines.

References

1. Little RJ, Rubin DB. Causal effects in clinical and epidemiological studies via potential outcomes: concepts and analytical approaches. *Annu Rev Public Health*. 2000;21:121-145.
2. Winship C, Morgan SL. The estimation of causal effects from observational data. *Annu Rev Sociol*. 1999;25:659-706.
3. Greenland S. Causal analysis in the health sciences. *J Am Stat Assoc*. 2000;95:286-289.
4. Sobel ME. Causal inference in the social sciences. *J Am Stat Assoc*. 2000;95(450):647-651.
5. Heckman JJ, Vytlacil EJ. Chapter 70 econometric evaluation of social programs, part I: causal models, structural models and econometric policy evaluation. In: Heckman JJ, Leamer EE, eds. *Handbook of Econometrics*. Vol 6. Amsterdam, The Netherlands: Elsevier; 2007:4779-4874.
6. Kaufman JS, Kaufman S. Assessment of structured socioeconomic effects on health. *Epidemiology*. 2001;12(2):157-167.
7. Maldonado G, Greenland S. Estimating causal effects. *Int J Epidemiol*. 2002;31(2):422-429.
8. Spirtes P, Glymour C, Scheines R. *Causation, Prediction, and Search*. Cambridge, MA: MIT Press; 2001.
9. Pearl J. Causal diagrams for empirical research. *Biometrika*. 1995;82:669-710.
10. Pearl J. *Causality*. 2nd ed. New York, NY: Cambridge University Press; 2009.
11. Greenland S, Pearl J, Robins JM. Causal diagrams for epidemiologic research. *Epidemiology*. 1999;10(1):37-48.
12. Robins JM. Data, design, and background knowledge in etiologic inference. *Epidemiology*. 2001;12(3):313-320.
13. Hernan MA, Hernandez-Diaz S, Werler MM, Mitchell AA. Causal knowledge as a prerequisite for confounding evaluation: an application to birth defects epidemiology. *Am J Epidemiol*. 2002;155(2):176-184.
14. Rothman KJ. Causes. *Am J Epidemiol*. 1976;104(6):587-592.
15. Rothman KJ, Greenland S, Lash TL. *Modern Epidemiology*. Philadelphia, PA: Wilkins; 2008.
16. Levin ML. The occurrence of lung cancer in man. *Acta Unio Int Contra Cancrum*. 1953;9(3):531-541.
17. MacMahon B, Pugh TF. Causes and entities of disease. In: Clark DW, MacMahon B, eds. *Preventive Medicine*. Boston, MA: Little, Brown; 1967.
18. Neyman J. On the application of probability theory to agricultural experiments. Essay on principles: section 9. *Statist Sci*. 1923;5(4):465-472.
19. Welch BL. On the z-test in randomized blocks and Latin squares. *Biometrika*. 1937;29:21-52.
20. Wilk MB. The randomization analysis of a generalized randomized block design. *Biometrika*. 1955;42:70-79.
21. Copas JB. Randomization models for matched and unmatched 2×2 tables. *Biometrika*. 1973;60:467-476.
22. Rubin DB. Estimating causal effects of treatments in randomized and nonrandomized studies. *J Educ Psychol*. 1974;66:688-701.
23. Robins JM. A new approach to causal inference in mortality studies with a sustained exposure period-application to control of the healthy worker survivor effect. *Math Model*. 1986;7:1393-1512.
24. Rubin DB. Causal inference using potential outcomes. *J Am Stat Assoc*. 2005;100(469):322-331.
25. Rubin DB. Randomization analysis of experimental-data – the fisher randomization test comment. *J Am Stat Assoc*. 1980;75(371):591-593.
26. Rubin DB. Statistics and causal inference:comment:which ifs have causal answers. *J Am Stat Assoc*. 1986;81(396):961-962.
27. Hong G, Raudenbush SW. Evaluating kindergarten retention policy. *J Am Stat Assoc*. 2006;101(475):901-910.
28. Rosenbaum PR. Interference between units in randomized experiments. *J Am Stat Assoc*. 2007;102(477):191-200.

29. Hudgens MG, Halloran ME. Toward causal inference with interference. *J Am Stat Assoc.* 2008;103(482):832-842.

30. Vanderweele TJ, Tchetgen EJ. Effect partitioning under interference in two-stage randomized vaccine trials. *Stat Probab Lett.* 2011;81(7):861-869.

31. Tchetgen EJ, VanderWeele TJ. On causal inference in the presence of interference. *Stat Methods Med Res.* 2012;21(1):55-75.

32. VanderWeele TJ. *Explanation in Causal Inference: Methods for Mediation and Interaction.* New York, NY: Oxford University Press; 2015.

33. Hernan MA, VanderWeele TJ. Compound treatments and transportability of causal inference. *Epidemiology.* 2011;22(3):368-377.

34. VanderWeele TJ, Hernan MA. Causal inference under multiple versions of treatment. *J Causal Inference.* 2013;1(1):1-20.

35. VanderWeele TJ. On well-defined hypothetical interventions in the potential outcomes framework. *Epidemiology.* 2018;29(4):e24-e25.

36. Dawid AP. Causal inference without counterfactuals. *J Am Stat Assoc.* 2000;95(450):407-424.

37. Cox DR. Causal inference without counterfactuals: comment. *J Am Stat Assoc.* 2000;95(450):424-425.

38. Casella G, Schwartz SP. Causal inference without counterfactuals: comment. *J Am Stat Assoc.* 2000;95(450):425-427.

39. Pearl J. Causal inference without counterfactuals: comment. *J Am Stat Assoc.* 2000;95(450):428-431.

40. Robins JM, Greenland S. Causal inference without counterfactuals: comment. *J Am Stat Assoc.* 2000;95(450):431-435.

41. Rubin DB. Causal inference without counterfactuals: comment. *J Am Stat Assoc.* 2000;95(450):435-438.

42. Shafer G. Causal inference without counterfactuals: comment. *J Am Stat Assoc.* 2000;95(450):438-442.

43. Wasserman L. Causal inference without counterfactuals: comment. *J Am Stat Assoc.* 2000;95(450):442-443.

44. Dawid AP. Causal inference without counterfactuals: rejoinder. *J Am Stat Assoc.* 2000;95(450):444-448.

45. Robins JM, Richardson TS. Alternative graphical causal models and the identification of direct effects. In: Shrout PE, Keyes KM, Ornstein K, eds. *Causality and Psychopathology: Finding the Determinants of Disorders and Their Cures.* Oxford, NY: Oxford University Press, 2011.

46. Greenland S, Robins JM, Pearl J. Confounding and collapsibility in causal inference. *Stat Sci.* 1999;14:29-46.

47. Greenland S. Ecologic versus individual-level sources of bias in ecologic estimates of contextual health effects. *Int J Epidemiol.* 2001;30(6):1343-1350.

48. Dechter R, Geffner H, Halpern JY. *Heuristics, Probability and Causality. A Tribute to Judea Pearl.* London: College Publications; 2010.

49. Richardson TS, Robins JM. *Single World Intervention Graphs (SWIGs): A Unification of the Counterfactual and Graphical Approaches to Causality.* Center for the Statistics and the Social Sciences, University of Washington Series. Working Paper. 2013;128(30):2013.

50. Berzuini C, Dawid P, Berardinelli L. *Causal Inference: Statistical Perspectives and Applications.* New York, NY: Wiley; 2012.

51. Greenland S, Mansournia MA. Limitations of individual causal models, causal graphs, and ignorability assumptions, as illustrated by random confounding and design unfaithfulness. *Eur J Epidemiol.* 2015;30(10):1101-1110.

52. Robins JM, Greenland S. Identifiability and exchangeability for direct and indirect effects. *Epidemiology.* 1992;3(2):143-155.

53. Cole SR, Hernan MA. Fallibility in estimating direct effects. *Int J Epidemiol.* 2002;31(1):163-165.

54. Hernan MA, Hernandez-Diaz S, Robins JM. A structural approach to selection bias. *Epidemiology.* 2004;15(5):615-625.

55. Hernan MA. Invited commentary: selection bias without colliders. *Am J Epidemiol.* 2017;185(11):1048-1050.

56. Cayley A. *Note on a Question in the Theory of Probabilities.* Vol 6. London: Edinburgh and Dublin Philosophical Magazine; 1853:259.

57. Mackie JL. Causes and conditions. *Am Philo Q.* 1965;2:245-255.

58. VanderWeele TJ, Robins JM. The identification of synergism in the sufficient-component-cause framework. *Epidemiology.* 2007;18(3):329-339.

59. Poole C. Positivized epidemiology and the model of sufficient and component causes. *Int J Epidemiol.* 2001;30:707-709.

60. Vanderweele TJ, Robins JM. Stochastic counterfactuals and stochastic sufficient causes. *Stat Sin.* 2012;22(1):379-392.

61. VanderWeele TJ, Robins JM. Empirical and counterfactual conditions for sufficient-cause interactions. *Biometrika.* 2008;95:49-61.

62. VanderWeele TJ, Richardson TS. General theory for interactions in sufficient cause models with dichotomous exposures. *Ann Stat.* 2012;40(4):2128-2161.

63. Siemiatycki J, Thomas DC. Biological models and statistical interactions: an example from multistage carcinogenesis. *Int J Epidemiol*. 1981;10(4):383-387.

64. Thompson WD. Effect modification and the limits of biological inference from epidemiologic data. *J Clin Epidemiol*. 1991;44(3):221-232.

65. Beyea J, Greenland S. The importance of specifying the underlying biologic model in estimating the probability of causation. *Health Phys*. 1999;76(3):269-274.

66. Greenland S, Robins JM. Epidemiology, justice, and the probability of causation. *Jurimetrics*. 2000;40:321-340.

67. Vanderweele TJ. Sufficient cause interactions for categorical and ordinal exposures with three levels. *Biometrika*. 2010;97(3):647-659.

68. Berzuini C, Dawid AP. Deep determinism and the assessment of mechanistic interaction. *Biostatistics*. 2013;14(3):502-513.

69. Hafeman DM. A sufficient cause based approach to the assessment of mediation. *Eur J Epidemiol*. 2008;23(11):711-721.

70. VanderWeele TJ. Mediation and mechanism. *Eur J Epidemiol*. 2009;24(5):217-224.

71. Suzuki E, Yamamoto E, Tsuda T. Identification of operating mediation and mechanism in the sufficient-component cause framework. *Eur J Epidemiol*. 2011;26(5):347-357.

72. Lee WC. Assessing causal mechanistic interactions: a peril ratio index of synergy based on multiplicativity. *PLoS One*. 2013;8(6):e67424.

73. VanderWeele TJ. Causal interactions in the proportional hazards model. *Epidemiology*. 2011;22(5):713-717.

74. VanderWeele TJ. Invited commentary: the continuing need for the sufficient cause model today. *Am J Epidemiol*. 2017;185(11):1041-1043.

75. VanderWeele TJ. Invited commentary: structural equation models and epidemiologic analysis. *Am J Epidemiol*. 2012;176(7):608-612.

76. Angrist JD, Imbens GW, Rubin DB. Identification of causal effects using instrumental variables (with comments). *J Am Stat Assoc*. 1996;91:444-472.

77. Sommer AS, Zeger S. On estimating efficacy from clinical trials. *Stat Med*. 1991;10:45-52.

78. Holland PW. Statistics and causal inference (with discussion). *J Am Stat Assoc*. 1986;81:945-970.

79. Greenland S. Causality theory for policy uses of epidemiologic measures. In: Murray CJL, Salomon JA, Mathers CD, Lopez AD, eds. *Summary Measures of Population Health*. Cambridge, MA: Harvard University Press/WHO; 2002:291-302.

80. Greiner DJ, Rubin DB. Causal effects of perceived immutable characteristics. *Rev Economics Stat*. 2011;93(3):775-785.

81. VanderWeele TJ, Hernán MA. Causal effects and natural laws: towards a conceptualization of causal counterfactuals for non-manipulable exposures with application to the effects of race and sex. In: Berzuini C, Dawid P, Berardinelli L, eds. *Causal Inference: Statistical Perspectives and Applications*. West Sussex: Wiley and Sons, 2012.

82. VanderWeele TJ, Robinson WR. On the causal interpretation of race in regressions adjusting for confounding and mediating variables. *Epidemiology*. 2014;25(4):473-484.

83. Sen M, Wasow O. Race as a bundle of sticks: designs that estimate effects of seemingly immutable characteristics. *Annu Rev Polit Sci*. 2016;19(1):499-522.

84. Vandenbroucke JP, Broadbent A, Pearce N. Causality and causal inference in epidemiology: the need for a pluralistic approach. *Int J Epidemiol*. 2016;45(6):1776-1786.

85. Krieger N, Davey Smith G. The tale wagged by the DAG: broadening the scope of causal inference and explanation for epidemiology. *Int J Epidemiol*. 2016;45(6):1787-1808.

86. VanderWeele TJ. Commentary: on causes, causal inference, and potential outcomes. *Int J Epidemiol*. 2016;45(6):1809-1816.

87. Robins JM, Weissman MB. Commentary: counterfactual causation and streetlamps. What is to be done? *Int J Epidemiol*. 2016;45(6):1830-1835.

88. Daniel RM, De Stavola BL, Vansteelandt S. Commentary: the formal approach to quantitative causal inference in epidemiology. Misguided or misrepresented? *Int J Epidemiol*. 2016;45(6):1817-1829.

89. Hernan MA. Does water kill? A call for less casual causal inferences. *Ann Epidemiol*. 2016;26(10):674-680.

90. Schwartz S, Gatto NM, Campbell UB. Causal identification: a charge of epidemiology in danger of marginalization. *Ann Epidemiol*. 2016;26(10):669-673.

91. VanderWeele TJ, Robins JM. Directed acyclic graphs, sufficient causes, and the properties of conditioning on a common effect. *Am J Epidemiol*. 2007;166(9):1096-1104.

92. VanderWeele TJ, Robins JM. Minimal sufficient causation and directed acyclic graphs. *Ann Stat*. 2009;37(3):1437-1465.

93. Bowden RJ, TurkingtonDA. *Instrumental Variables*. Cambridge: Cambridge University Press; 1984.

94. Greenland S, Neutra R. Control of confounding in the assessment of medical technology. *Int J Epidemiol*. 1980;9(4):361-367.

95. Hume D. *A Treatise of Human Nature*. 2nd ed. Oxford, NY: Oxford Press; 1888.
96. Simon HA, Rescher N. Cause and counterfactual. *Philos Sci*. 1966;33(4):323-340.
97. Lewis D. Causation. *J Philos*. 1973;70:556-567.
98. Harper WL, Pearce GA, Stalnaker R. *Ifs: Condiitons, Belief, Decision, Chance and Time*. Vol 15. Holland: D. Reidel Publishing Company; 1981.
99. Fisher RA. The logic of inductive inference. *J R Stat Soc Ser A*. 1935;98:39-54.
100. Cox DR. *The Planning of Experiments*. New York, NY: Wiley; 1958.
101. Rubin DB. Bayesian inference for causal effects: the role of randomization. *Ann Stat*. 1978;6:4-58.
102. Hamilton MA. Choosing the parameter for a 2×2 table or a 2×2×2 table analysis. *Am J Epidemiol*. 1979;109(3):362-375.
103. Greenland S, Robins JM. Identifiability, exchangeability, and epidemiological confounding. *Int J Epidemiol*. 1986;15(3):413-419.
104. Robins JM. A graphical approach to the identification and estimation of causal parameters in mortality studies with sustained exposure periods. *J Chronic Dis*. 1987;40(suppl 2):139S-161S.
105. Wright S. Systems of mating: I. The biometric relations between parent and offspring. *Genetics*. 1921;6(111):111-123.
106. Kiiveri HS T, Carlin J. Recursive causal models. *J Aust Math Soc Ser A.*. 1984;36:30-52.
107. Pearl J. *Probabilistic Reasoning in Intelligent Systems*. San Mateo, CA: Morgan Kaufmann; 1988.
108. Verma TPJ. Equivalence and synthesis of causal models. In: Kanal LN; Lemmer JF, eds. *Uncertainty in Artificial Intelligence*. Vol 6. North Holland: Elsevier Science Publishers B V; 1991.
109. Wright RW. Causation, responsibility, risk, probability, naked statistics, and proof: pruning the bramble bush by clarifying the concepts. *Iowa Law Rev*. 1988;73:1001-1077.
110. Cheng PW. From covariation to causation: a causal power theory. *Psychol Rev*. 1997;104(2):367-405.
111. Novick LR, Cheng PW. Assessing interactive causal influence. *Psychol Rev*. 2004;111(2):455-485.
112. Vander Weele TJ. The sufficient cause framework in statistics, philosophy, and hte biomedical and social sciences. In: Berzuini C, Dawid P, Berardinelli L, eds. *Causal Inference: Statistical Perspectives and Applications*. West Sussex: Wilcy and Sons; 2012.

CHAPTER 4

Measures of Occurrence

Timothy L. Lash and Kenneth J. Rothman

In this chapter, we begin to address the basic elements, concepts, and tools of epidemiology. A good starting point is to define epidemiology. Some epidemiologists define it in terms of its methods. Although the methods of epidemiology may be distinctive, it is more typical to define a branch of science in terms of its subject matter rather than its tools. MacMahon and Pugh[1] gave a widely cited definition, which we update slightly: Epidemiology is the study of the distribution and determinants of disease frequency in human populations. A similar subject-matter definition has been attributed to Gaylord Anderson,[2] who defined epidemiology simply as the study of the *occurrence* of illness. Although reasonable distinctions can be made between the terms *disease* and *illness,* we will treat them as synonyms here.

Recognizing the broad scope of epidemiology today, we may further expand the definition of epidemiology to include the study of the distribution of health-related states and events in populations. With this expanded definition, we intend to capture not only disease and illness but physiologic states such as blood pressure, psychologic measures such as depression score, and positive outcomes such as disease immunity. Other sciences, such as clinical or medical research, are also directed toward the study of health and disease, but in epidemiology, the focus is on population distributions.

The objective of most epidemiologic research is to obtain a valid and precise estimate of the frequency of disease occurrence or of the effect of a potential cause on the occurrence of the disease. The first objective is part of the broad field of descriptive epidemiology, including surveillance for patterns of disease occurrence that vary with time, place, or population subgroups. The second objective is part of the field of etiologic epidemiologic research.

For both objectives, disease occurrence is often a binary (either/or) outcome such as "dead/alive." To achieve these objectives, an epidemiologist must be able to measure the frequency of disease occurrence, either in absolute or in relative terms. All measures of disease occurrence must be measured in a population, which is a group of people observed at or over a specific time. We will therefore begin with definitions and descriptions of populations. We will then focus on four basic measures of disease occurrence or frequency.[3] An *incidence time* is the time at which a new case of disease occurs among population members. An *incidence proportion* is the proportion of the population developing disease during a specified period of time. An *incidence rate* is the number of new cases of disease per unit of person-time. A *prevalence* measures the proportion of people who have a disease at a specific time and thus is a measure of status rather than of the newly occurring disease.

Figure 4-1 illustrates the calculation of these four basic measures of disease frequency using a hypothetical population of 10 people observed for 12 months. We will work out the calculations in each of the respective sections. We will also discuss how these measures generalize to outcomes measured on a more complex scale than a dichotomy, such as lung function, lymphocyte count, or antibody titer. Finally, we will describe how measures can be *standardized* or averaged over population distributions of health-related factors to obtain summary occurrence measures.

TYPES OF POPULATIONS

The simplest definition of a population is a group of people who share characteristics or meet criteria that define membership in the population. These defining characteristics inevitably include restrictions to a particular time and usually involve restrictions on the location of population members. Populations are observed at a single point in time (*i.e.*, cross-sectionally) or over the course of time (*i.e.*, longitudinally), where the time scale is measured starting from some event. Calendar time is measured from a conventional historical reference point, but time may instead be measured from an event whose occurrence in calendar time varies across persons; for example, age (which is usually measured from birth date) or time since first employment in an occupation.

Some locations are explicit and easy to define because they change very little over time, such as an island. Locations defined by political boundaries are more susceptible to change, so populations partly defined by residence or citizenship within a particular political boundary will usually also have to incorporate an element of calendar time. Often, however, restrictions by location are not

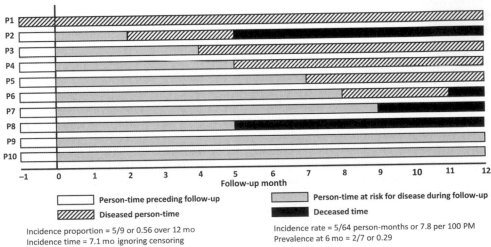

FIGURE 4-1 Illustration of four basic measures of disease frequency using a population of 10 persons (P1-P10) with person-time depicted 1 month before, and 12 months after, the start of follow-up for the occurrence of a disease.

explicit but instead are determined in a nebulous way by the defining characteristics of the population. Consider the geographic boundary of a population that would seek medical care at a particular hospital. This population is no doubt partly determined by geographic proximity of residence but may also be affected by healthcare insurance considerations, familiarity with healthcare providers, and visitors to the area who find themselves in need of medical care.

Membership criteria may change over time. A population limited to tall women likely experiences little emigration out or immigration in over time on the basis of being a tall woman. A population limited to married women is much more likely to experience emigration and immigration over time on the basis of being a married woman. Population definitions can address this migration by defining membership on the basis of satisfying the criterion at a particular point in time (*e.g.*, marital status on January 1, 2015, or on the 30th birthday or at initial entry into the population) or by allowing for changes in membership status in coordination with changes in marital status. All of these considerations are incorporated into the more formal definitions of various types of populations that follow.

Closed Populations

Given a particular timescale, we may distinguish populations according to whether they are *closed* or *open* on that scale. A closed population adds no new members over time and loses members only to death. Some demographers and ecologists use a broader definition of closed population that allows new members to be added but only at birth.

Members of a closed population are those who meet the defining membership criteria, which might include age, sex, geographic locale, calendar time restrictions, exposure circumstances, and consent to participate in a research study. For each person who becomes a member of a closed population, the time when the last entry criterion is met is described as the *index time* or *entry time*. It follows from the definition of a closed population that membership is permanent, except for losses due to death.

A closed population experiencing a constant death rate over time would decline in size exponentially (which is what is meant by the term *exponential decay*). In practice, however, death rates for a closed population change with time because the population is aging as time progresses and the instantaneous rate of death (the hazard, defined below) usually increases with age. Consequently, the decay curve of a closed human population is never exponential. *Life-table methodology*, described below, is a procedure by which the death rate (or disease rate) of a closed population is evaluated within successive small age or time intervals, so that the age or time dependence of mortality can be elucidated. With any method, however, it is important to distinguish age-related effects from those related to other time axes because each person's age increases directly with an increase along any other time axis. For example, a person's age increases with increasing duration of employment, increasing calendar time, and increasing time from the start of follow-up.

Open Populations

In contrast, open populations may gain members over time, through immigration or birth, or lose members over time through emigration or death. Open populations are sometimes called dynamic populations, but "dynamic" means changing over time, and closed populations also change over time. An open population differs from a closed population in that it is open to new members who did not qualify for the population initially. An example is the population of a country. People can enter an open population through various mechanisms. Some may be born into it; others may migrate into it. For an open population of people who must have attained a specific age, persons can become eligible to enter the population by aging into it. Similarly, persons can exit by dying, by aging out of a defined age group, emigrating, or becoming diseased (the latter method of exiting applies only if first occurrences of a disease are being studied). Persons may also exit from an open population and then reenter it, for example, by emigrating from the geographic area in which the population is located and later moving back to that area.

It follows from the definition of an open population that membership is dynamic, which explains why these populations are sometimes called dynamic populations. However long a person satisfies all of the membership criteria for an open population, she is a member of the population. Whenever she fails to satisfy even one of the status criteria, at that point, she is not a member of the population. For large populations, it may become difficult to completely track all potential members with regard to satisfying all status criteria at all times. In this circumstance, sampling may be the most efficient approach, as we will discuss in Chapter 8.

The distinction between closed and open populations depends in part on the time axis used to describe the population, as well as on how membership is defined. All persons who ever used a particular drug would constitute a closed population if time is measured from the start of their use of the drug. These persons would, however, constitute an open population in calendar time because new users might accumulate over a period of time. If, as in this example, membership in the population always starts with an event such as initiation of treatment and never ends thereafter, the population is closed along the time axis that marks this event as the index time for each member because all new members enter only when they experience this event. The same population will, however, be open along most other time axes. If membership can be terminated by later events other than death, the population is open along any time axis.

By the above definitions, any study population with loss to follow-up is open. For example, membership in a study population might be defined in part by being under active surveillance for disease; in that case, members who are lost to follow-up have by definition left the population, even if they are still alive and would otherwise be considered eligible for study. It is common practice to analyze such populations using time from the start of observation, an axis along which no immigration can occur. Such populations may be said to be "closed on the left," and are often called "fixed cohorts," although the term *cohort* is often used to refer to a different concept, which we discuss next.

Populations Versus Cohorts

The term *population* as we use it here has an intrinsically temporal and potentially dynamic element: One can be a member at one time, not a member at a later time, a member again, and so on. This usage is the most common sense of population, as with the population of a town or country. The term *cohort* is sometimes used to describe any study population, but we reserve it for a narrower concept, that of a group of persons for whom membership is defined in a permanent fashion, or a population in which membership is determined by satisfying a set of defining events and so becomes permanent. An example of a cohort would be the members of the graduating class of a school in a given year. The list of cohort members is fixed at the time of graduation and will not increase. Other examples include the cohort of all persons who ever used a drug and the cohort of persons recruited for a follow-up study. In the latter case, the study population may begin with all the cohort members but may gradually dwindle to a small subset of that cohort as those initially recruited die or are loss to follow-up. Those lost to follow-up remain members of the initial-recruitment cohort, even though they are no longer being followed as part of the study population. With this definition, the members of any cohort constitute a closed population along the time axis in which the chronologically last defining event (*e.g.*, birth with Down syndrome or study recruitment) is taken as the index time. A *birth cohort* is the cohort defined in part by being born at a particular time. For example, all persons born in Ethiopia in 1990 constitute the Ethiopian birth cohort for 1990.

Steady State

If the number of people entering a population is balanced by the number exiting the population in any period of time within levels of age, sex, and other determinants of risk, the population is said to be *stationary* or in a *steady state*. Steady state is a property that can occur only in open populations, not closed populations. It is possible, however, to have a population in steady state in which no immigration or emigration is occurring; this situation would require that births perfectly balance deaths in the population. The graph of the size of an open population in steady state, plotted against time on the *x*-axis, is simply a horizontal line.

People are continually entering and leaving a population in steady state in a way that might be diagrammed as shown in Figure 4-2. In the diagram, the symbol > represents a person entering the population, a line segment represents his or her membership time, and the termination of a

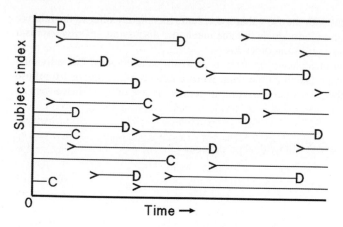

FIGURE 4-2 Composition of an open population in approximate steady state, by time; > indicates entry into the population, D indicates disease onset, and C indicates exit from the population without the disease.

line segment represents the end of his or her membership time. A terminal D indicates that the membership ended because of disease onset, and a terminal C (representing censoring) indicates that the follow-up time (but not the membership time) ended for other reasons leading to loss to follow-up. In theory, any time interval will provide a good measure of disease occurrence in a stationary population.

Additional Terminology

Epidemiologists use many other modifiers to describe populations, and not all of these modifiers are used consistently. Three common terms are *source population, study population,* and *target population.* The *source population* is the population from which persons will be sampled and included in a measurement of disease frequency. For example, the source population of the original Framingham Heart Study included men and women between the ages of 30 and 62 years who were residents of the town of Framingham, Massachusetts, in 1948.[4] The *study population* is the subset, up to a complete census, of the *source population* whose experience is included in a measurement of disease frequency. Not all men and women who were eligible to join the Framingham Heart Study were invited to participate, and not all who were invited to participate agreed to participate. Those who were invited, agreed, and were free of prevalent cardiovascular disease constituted the study population.[4] The *target population* comprises the persons for whom information gleaned by the measurement of disease frequency will be relevant. Information about risk factors for cardiac disease from the Framingham Heart Study has contributed to a nearly 75% decline in mortality related to cardiovascular disease in most industrialized societies.[5]

INCIDENCE PROPORTIONS AND SURVIVAL PROPORTIONS

Given an outcome event or "incident" of interest, within a given interval of time, we can express the incident number of cases in relation to the size of the population at risk. We first measure population size at the start of a time interval, excluding persons who have already had the event of interest. We next count the number of new cases of the outcome event of interest that arise over the given time interval. If no one enters the population (immigrates) or leaves alive (emigrates) after the start of the interval, the proportion of people who become cases among those in the population at the start of the interval is called the *incidence proportion.* The incidence proportion may also be defined as the proportion of a closed population at risk that becomes diseased within a given period of time. The incidence proportion is sometimes called the *cumulative incidence,* but that term is also used for another quantity we will discuss later. A more traditional term for incidence proportion is *attack rate,* but we reserve the term *rate* for person-time incidence rates.

If *risk* is defined as the probability that a disease develops in a person within a specified time interval, then incidence proportion is a measure, or estimate, of the average risk over that time interval for the persons in the closed population. Although this concept of risk applies to individuals, whereas incidence proportion applies to populations, incidence proportion is sometimes called risk. This usage is consistent with the view that individual risks merely refer to the relative frequency of the disease in a group of individuals like the one under discussion. *Average risk* is a more accurate synonym, one that we will sometimes use.

Another way of expressing the incidence proportion is as a simple average of the individual proportions for each person. The latter is either 0 for those who do not have the event or 1 for those who do have the event. The number, A, of people who experience disease onset is then a sum of the individual proportions,

$$A = \sum_{\text{persons}} \text{Individual proportions}$$

and so

$$\text{Incidence proportion} = \frac{\sum_{\text{persons}} \text{Individual proportions}}{\text{Initial size of the population}} = \frac{A}{N}$$

If one calls the individual proportions the "individual risks," this formulation shows another sense in which the incidence proportion is also an "average risk."

Like any proportion, the value of an incidence proportion ranges from 0 to 1 and is dimensionless. It is not interpretable, however, without specification of the time period to which it applies. An incidence proportion of death of 3% means something very different when it refers to a 40-year period than when it refers to a 40-day period.

In Figure 4-1, 10 people are being followed starting at time zero. Of the 10, nine of them, labeled P2-P10, are at risk at the beginning of follow-up. By the end of the 12-month follow-up period, five incident cases of the disease were ascertained. The incidence proportion is therefore 5/9 or 0.56 over the 12 months of follow-up.

A useful measure complementary to the incidence proportion is the *survival proportion,* which may be defined as the proportion of a closed population at risk that does *not* become diseased within a given period of time. If R and S denote the incidence and survival proportions, then $S = 1 - R$. In Figure 4-1, the incidence proportion is 0.56, so its complement equals the survival proportion, $1 - 0.56 = 0.44$. Note that this measure, while called the survival proportion, refers to remaining disease free to the end of the follow-up period and *not* to remaining alive during this interval. Among P2-P10, four persons (P2, P6, P7, and P8) died during the follow-up period, and five survived. With death as the outcome, the incidence proportion would be $4/9 = 0.44$ and the survival proportion would be the complementary, 5/9 or 0.56.

Another measure that is commonly used is the *incidence odds,* defined as $R/S = R/(1 - R)$, the ratio of the proportion getting the disease to the proportion not getting the disease. If R is small, $S \approx 1$ and $R/S \approx R$; that is, the incidence odds will approximate the incidence proportion when both quantities are small. Otherwise, because $S < 1$, the incidence odds will be greater than the incidence proportion and, unlike the latter, it may exceed 1. For example, using the outcome depicted in Figure 4-1, the incidence odds equals $0.56/(1 - 0.56) = 1.27$. Because in this case the incidence proportion is not small, the incidence odds provides a poor approximation to the incidence proportion.

A specific type of incidence proportion is the *case fatality rate,* or *case fatality ratio,* which is the incidence proportion of death among those in whom an illness develops (it is therefore not a rate in our sense, but a proportion). The time period for measuring the case fatality rate is often unstated, but it is always better to specify it.

INCIDENCE TIMES

To measure the frequency of disease occurrence in a population, it is insufficient merely to record the number of people or the proportion of the population that is affected. It is also necessary to take into account the time elapsed before disease occurs, as well as the period of time during which

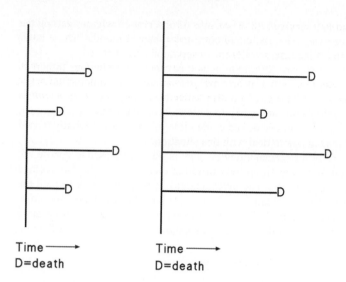

FIGURE 4-3 Two different patterns of mortality.

events were counted. Consider the frequency of death. Because all people are eventually affected, the time from birth to death becomes the determining factor in the rate of occurrence of death. If, on average, death comes earlier to the members of one population than to members of another population, it is natural to say that the first population has a higher death rate than the second. Time is the factor that differentiates between the two situations shown in Figure 4-3. Average incidence time is therefore conceptually the average waiting time for the event to occur. As we will explain below, this conceptualization fits well enough for inevitable events but less well when not everyone in a population develops the outcome for which incidence time is being measured.

In an epidemiologic study, we may measure the time of events in a person's life relative to any index event. When we refer to age, for example, the index event is birth, but we might instead use the start of a treatment or the start of an exposure as the index event. The index event may occur at a time that is unique to each person, as is the case with birth, but it could also be set to a common value, such as a day chosen from the calendar. The time of the index event determines the time origin or *zero time* for measuring the timing of events.

A person's *incidence time* for an outcome is defined as the time span from zero time to the time at which the outcome event occurs, if it occurs. Synonyms for incidence time include *event time, failure time,* and *occurrence time.* A man who experienced his first myocardial infarction in 2015 at age 50 years has an incidence time of 2015 in (Western) calendar time and an incidence time of 50 in age time. A person's incidence time is undefined if that person never experiences the outcome event. There is a convention that classifies such a person as having an incidence time that is not specified exactly but is known to exceed the last time that the person could have experienced the outcome event. Under this convention, a woman who had an appendectomy at age 45 years without ever having had appendiceal cancer is classified as having an incidence time for cancer of the appendix that is unspecified but greater than age 45 years. It is then said that the appendectomy at age 45 years *censored* the woman's appendiceal cancer incidence at age 45 years.

In Figure 4-1, the index event occurs at month 0, which may be synchronized to calendar time if the reference event is a shared exposure, such as inhaling potentially toxic fumes accidentally released from an industrial site. If the index event is the date of a specific surgical procedure, then it is not likely to be synchronized to calendar time. Six of the ten people whose experience is charted in the figure are observed to be diseased before the end of the follow-up, but person 1 (P1) was diseased before the population came under observation. This person's incidence time cannot, therefore, be measured as part of this observation. Incidence times must be measured among those who are disease free at the time of the index event. Five of the nine people who were disease free at time zero became diseased during the 12 months of follow-up (P2 at 2 months, P3 at 4 months, P4 at 5 months, P5 at 7 months, and P6 at 8 months). P7 died at 9 months and P8 died at 5 months, both without ever contracting the disease, so their incidence times are unspecified but greater than

9 or 5 months, respectively. P9 and P10 survived the 12 months of observation without getting the disease or dying, so their incidence times are unspecified but greater than 12 months. These latter two were presumably still at risk to get the disease after the observation period ended.

There are many ways to summarize the distribution of incidence times in populations if there is no censoring. For example, one could look at the mean time, median time, and other summaries. Such approaches are commonly used with time to death, for which the average, or *life expectancy,* is a popular measure for comparing the health status of populations. If there is censoring, however, the summarization task becomes more complicated, and epidemiologists have traditionally turned to the concepts involving *person-time at risk* to deal with this situation.

The term *average age at death* deserves special attention, as it is sometimes used to denote life expectancy but is more often used to denote an entirely different quantity, namely, the average age of those dying at a particular point in time. The latter quantity is more precisely termed the *cross-sectional* average age at death. The two quantities can be very far apart. Comparisons across exposure categories of cross-sectional averages of age at an event (such as death) can be quite misleading when attempting to infer causes of the event.[6] We shall discuss these problems later on in this chapter.

INCIDENCE RATES

Person-Time and Population-Time

Epidemiologists often study outcome events that are not inevitable or that may not occur during the period of observation. In such situations, the set of incidence times for a specific event in a population will not all be precisely defined or observed. One way to deal with this complication is to develop measures that take into account the length of time each individual was in the *population at risk* for the event. This length or span of time is called the *person-time* contribution of the individual.

Suppose we graph the survival experience of a closed population that starts with 1,000 people. Because death eventually claims everyone, after a period of sufficient time, the original 1,000 will have dwindled to zero. A graph of the size of the population with time might approximate that in Figure 4-4. The curve slopes downward because as the 1,000 persons in the population die, the population at risk of death is reduced. The population is closed in the sense that we consider the fate of only the 1,000 persons present at time zero, their entry or index time. The accumulated experience, or person-time, of these 1,000 persons is represented by the area under the curve in the diagram. As each person dies, the curve notches downward; that person no longer

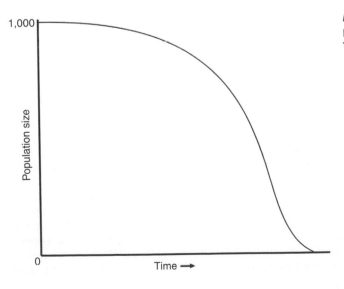

FIGURE 4-4 Size of a closed population of 1,000 people, by time.

contributes to the person-time denominator of the death (mortality) rate. Each person's contribution is exactly equal to the length of time that person is followed from the start to the end of the follow-up. In this example, because the entire population is followed as long as necessary until all have died, the finish for each person is that person's death. In other instances, such as in measuring the incidence rate of a specific disease (see below), the contribution to the person-time experience in the denominator of the rate would continue until either the onset of disease, death from another cause, loss to follow-up, or some arbitrary cutoff time for observation, whichever came soonest. The sum of the person-time over all population members is called the total *person-time at risk* or the *population-time at risk*. This total person-time should be distinguished from clock time in that it is a summation of time that occurs simultaneously for many people, whereas clock time is not. The total person-time at risk merely represents the total of all time during which disease onsets could occur and would be counted as incident events occurring in the population of interest.

Suppose we added up the total person-time experience of this closed population of 1,000 and obtained a total of 75,000 person-years. The death rate would be $(1,000/75,000) \times \text{year}^{-1}$ because the 75,000 person-years represent the experience of all 1,000 people until their deaths. Furthermore, if time is measured from the start of the follow-up, the average death time (incidence time) in this closed population would be the inverse of the death rate, equal to 75,000 person-years/1,000 persons = 75 years.

Population and Individual Rates

We define the *incidence rate* of the population as the number of new cases of disease (incident number) divided by the person-time over the follow-up period,

$$\text{Incidence rate} = \frac{\text{Number of disease onsets}}{\sum_{\text{persons}} \text{Time spent in population}}$$

This rate has also been called the *person-time rate, incidence density, force of morbidity* (or *force of mortality* in reference to deaths), *hazard rate,* and *disease intensity,* although the latter three terms are more commonly used to refer to the theoretical limit approached by an incidence rate as the unit of time measure approaches zero.

When the risk period is of fixed length, Δt, the proportion of the period that a person spends in the population at risk is their amount of person-time during follow-up divided by Δt, which is the maximum follow-up. It follows that the average size of the population over the period is

$$\bar{N} = \sum_{\text{persons}} \frac{\text{Time spent in population}}{\Delta t}$$

Hence, the total person-time at risk over the period is equal to the product of the average size of the population over the period, $\bar{N}$, and the fixed length of the risk period, Δt. If we denote the incident number of disease onsets by A, it follows that the incidence rate equals $A/(\bar{N} \cdot \Delta t)$. This formulation shows that the incidence rate has units of inverse time (per year, per month, per day, etc.). The units attached to an incidence rate can thus be written as year^{-1}, month^{-1}, or day^{-1}.

Outcome events are only eligible to be counted in the numerator of an incidence rate if they occur to persons who are contributing time to the denominator of the incidence rate at the time that the disease onset occurs. Likewise, only time contributed by persons eligible to be counted in the numerator if they suffer such an event should be counted in the denominator. Person-time at risk terminates at the occurrence of the event under study, at death, or at the occurrence of any event that precludes the person from getting the disease. For example, a person is no longer at risk for cancer of the appendix when they have an appendectomy to cure appendicitis. Person-time at risk is censored when a person is lost to follow-up or at the termination of the study's follow-up period. In both cases, the person may still contract the disease, but it will not be eligible to be counted in the numerator of the rate that the study is measuring.

In Figure 4-1, P1 has already had the disease before the study begins so is never at risk during the study's follow-up period. P1 contributes no person-time. P2-P6 get the disease at 2, 4, 7, 8, and 9 months, respectively, after the index event that begins the follow-up period. Person-time terminates for these five persons at the time they get the disease. P7 and P8 contribute person-time until their deaths at 9 and 5 months, at which time their person-time contributions are terminated. P9 and P10 are at risk for the entire 12 months of the study's follow-up period, so contribute this amount of person-time, after which their follow-up is censored by the end of the study's ascertainment protocol. The total person-time at risk is therefore $(2 + 4 + 7 + 8 + 9 + 9 + 5 + 12 + 12) = 64$ months. The incidence rate equals 5/64 months because five incident cases were observed in the 64 months of follow-up, equivalent to a rate of 7.8 cases per 100 person-months.

Another way of expressing a population incidence rate is as a time-weighted average of individual rates. An individual rate is either 0/(time spent in population) = 0, if the individual does not experience the event, or else 1/(time spent in the population) if the individual does experience the event. We then have that the number of disease onsets A is

$$A = \sum_{\text{persons}} \left(\text{Time spent in population}\right)\left(\text{Individual rate}\right)$$

and so

$$\text{Incidence rate} = \frac{\sum_{\text{persons}} \left(\text{Time spent in population}\right)\left(\text{Individual rate}\right)}{\sum_{\text{persons}} \left(\text{Time spent in population}\right)}$$

This formulation shows that the incidence rate ignores the distinction between individuals who do not contribute to the incident number A because they were in the population only briefly, and those who do not contribute because they were in the population a long time but never got the disease (e.g., immune individuals, at least over the follow-up period). In this sense, the incidence rate deals with the censoring problem by ignoring potentially important distinctions among those who do *not* get the disease, such as termination of follow-up by death versus censoring of follow-up by the end of the study's ascertainment protocol.

Although the notion of an incidence rate is a central one in epidemiology, the preceding formulation shows it cannot capture all aspects of disease occurrence. This limitation is also shown by noting that a rate of 1 case/(100 years) = 0.01 year^{-1} could be obtained by following 100 people for an average of 1 year and observing one case, but it could also be obtained by following two people for 50 years and observing one case, a very different scenario. To distinguish these situations, more detailed measures of occurrence are also needed, such as incidence time.

Proper Interpretation of Incidence Rates

Apart from insensitivity to important distinctions, incidence rates have interpretational difficulties insofar as they are often confused with risks (probabilities). This confusion arises when one fails to account for the dependence of the numeric portion of a rate on the units used for its expression.

The numeric portion of an incidence rate has a lower bound of zero and no upper bound, which is the range for the ratio of a nonnegative quantity to a positive quantity. The two quantities are the number of events in the numerator and the person-time in the denominator. It may be surprising that an incidence rate can exceed the value of 1, which might seem to indicate that more than 100% of a population is affected. It is true that at most 100% of persons in a population can get a disease, but the incidence rate does not measure the proportion of a population that gets disease, and in fact it is not a proportion at all. Recall that incidence rate is measured in units of the reciprocal of time. Among 100 people, no more than 100 deaths can occur, but those 100 deaths can occur in 10,000 person-years, in 1,000 person-years, in 100 person-years, or in 1 person-year (if the 100 deaths occur after an average of 3.65 days each, as in a military engagement). An incidence rate of 100 cases (or deaths) per 1 person-year might be expressed as

$$100\frac{\text{Cases}}{\text{Person-year}}$$

It might also be expressed as

$$10,000\frac{\text{Cases}}{\text{Person-century}}$$

$$8.33\frac{\text{Cases}}{\text{Person-month}}$$

$$1.92\frac{\text{Cases}}{\text{Person-week}}$$

$$0.27\frac{\text{Cases}}{\text{Person-day}}$$

The numeric value of an incidence rate in itself has no interpretability because it depends on the selection of the time unit. It is thus essential in presenting incidence rates to give the time unit used to calculate the numeric portion. That unit is usually chosen to ensure that the minimum rate from among a series of rates has at least one digit to the left of the decimal place. For example, a table of incidence rates of 0.15, 0.04, and 0.009 cases per person-year might be multiplied by 1,000 to be displayed as 150, 40, and 9 cases per 1,000 person-years. One can use a unit as large as 1,000 person-years regardless of whether the observations were collected over 1 year of time, over 1 week of time, or over a decade, just as one can measure the speed of a vehicle in terms of kilometers per hour even if the speed is measured for only a few seconds.

Relation of Incidence Rates to Incidence Times in Special Populations

The reciprocal of time is an awkward concept that does not provide an intuitive grasp of an incidence rate. The measure does, however, have a close connection to more interpretable measures of occurrence in closed populations. Referring to Figure 4-4, one can see that the area under the curve is equal to $N \times T$, where N is the number of people starting out in the closed population and T is the average time until death. The time-averaged death rate is then $N/(N \times T) = 1/T$; that is, the death rate equals the reciprocal of the average time until death.

In a stationary population with no migration, the crude incidence rate of an inevitable outcome such as death will equal the reciprocal of the average time spent in the population until the outcome occurs.[7] Thus, in a stationary population with no migration, a death rate of 0.04 year^{-1} would translate to an average time from entry until death of 25 years. Similarly, in a stationary population with no migration, the cross-sectional average age at death will equal the life expectancy. The time spent in the population until the outcome occurs is sometimes referred to as the *waiting time* until the event occurs, and it corresponds to the incidence time when time is measured from entry into the population.

If the outcome of interest is not death but either disease onset or death from a specific cause, the average-time interpretation must be modified to account for *competing risks*, which are events that "compete" with the outcome of interest to remove persons from the population at risk. Even if there is no competing risk, the interpretation of incidence rates as the inverse of the average waiting time will usually not be valid if there is migration (such as loss to follow-up), and average age at death will no longer equal the life expectancy. For example, the death rate for the United States in 1977 was 0.0088 year^{-1}. In a steady state, this rate would correspond to a mean lifespan, or expectation of life, of 114 years. Other analyses, however, indicate that the actual expectation of life in 1977 was 73 years.[8] The discrepancy is a result of immigration and to the lack of a steady state. Note that the no-migration assumption cannot hold within specific age groups, for people are always "migrating" in and out of age groups as they age.

OTHER TYPES OF RATES

In addition to numbers of cases per unit of person-time, it is sometimes useful to examine numbers of events per other unit. In health services and infectious disease epidemiology, epidemic curves are often depicted in terms of the number of cases per unit time, also called the *absolute rate,*

$$\frac{\text{No. of disease onsets}}{\text{Time span of observation}}$$

or $A/\Delta t$. Because the person-time rate is simply this absolute rate divided by the average size of the population over the time span, or $A/\left(\bar{N}\cdot\Delta t\right)$, the person-time rate has been called the *relative rate*[9]; it is the absolute rate relative to or "adjusted for" the average population size.

Sometimes it is useful to express event rates in units that do not involve time directly. A common example is the expression of fatalities by travel modality in terms of passenger-miles, whereby the safety of commercial train and air travel can be compared. Here, person-miles replace person-time in the denominator of the rate. Like rates with time in the denominator, the numerical portion of such rates is completely dependent on the choice of measurement units; a rate of 1.6 deaths per 10^6 passenger-miles equals a rate of 1 death per 10^6 passenger-kilometers.

The concept central to precise usage of the term *incidence rate* is that of expressing the change in incident number relative to the change in another quantity, so that the incidence rate always has a dimension. Thus, a person-time rate expresses the increase in the incident number we expect per unit increase in person-time. An absolute rate expresses the increase in incident number we expect per unit increase in clock time, and a passenger-mile rate expresses the increase in incident number we expect per unit increase in passenger-miles.

Recurrent Events

Incidence proportions and incidence rates often include only the first occurrence of disease onset as an eligible event for the numerator. For the many diseases that are irreversible states, such as multiple sclerosis, cirrhosis, or death, there is at most only one onset that a person can experience. For some diseases that do recur, such as rhinitis, we may simply wish to measure the incidence of "first" occurrence or first occurrence after a prespecified disease-free period, even though the disease can occur repeatedly. For other diseases, such as cancer or heart disease, the first occurrence is often of greater interest for etiologic study than subsequent occurrences in the same person because the first occurrence or its medical therapies affect the rate of subsequent occurrences. For these diseases, research on recurrences and other events that follow the incident diagnosis mostly falls into the realm of clinical epidemiology (see Chapter 35). For these reasons, it is typical that the events in the numerator of an incidence proportion or incidence rate correspond to the first occurrence of a particular disease, even in those instances in which it is possible for a person to have more than one occurrence. In this book, we will assume we are dealing with first occurrences, except when stated otherwise.

As foreshadowed with the explanation of the rate calculation for Figure 4-1, when the events tallied in the numerator of an incidence rate are first occurrences of disease, then the time contributed by each person in whom the disease develops should terminate with the onset of the disease. The reason is that the person is no longer eligible to experience the event (the first occurrence can occur only once per person), so there is no more information about first occurrence to obtain from continued observation of that person. Thus, each person who experiences the outcome event should contribute time to the denominator until the occurrence of the event but not afterward. Furthermore, for the study of first occurrences, the number of disease onsets in the numerator of the incidence rate is also a count of people experiencing the event because only one event can occur per person.

An epidemiologist who wishes to study both first and subsequent occurrences of disease may decide not to distinguish between first and later occurrences and simply count all the events that occur among the population under observation. For example, one might be interested in occurrence of respiratory tract or urinary tract infections, both of which can occur repeatedly in the same person. If so, then the time accumulated in the denominator of the rate would not cease with the occurrence of the outcome event because an additional event might occur in the same person. In this situation, person-time continues to accumulate for each person even after a disease onset occurs, until the end of the study follow-up period. For these outcomes, the rate computed by dividing first and recurrent events by all person-time at risk for first and recurrent events is a more relevant and clinically interpretable measure of disease burden than considering only the first event that occurs.[10] Recurrent events are not, however, independent. One can only have a second event after experiencing the first, and one can only have a third event after the second, and so on. In addition, recurrent events tend to cluster in a subgroup of persons who have many more than the average number of events during a given time period. These and other considerations invalidate standard statistical techniques.[11] Methods are available to account for these concerns in crude and stratified analyses,[10] and regression models for rates of recurrent events are also available.[12,13]

Often, however, there is enough of a biologic distinction between first and subsequent occurrences to warrant measuring them separately. One approach is to define the "population at risk" differently for each occurrence of the event: The population at risk for the first event would consist of persons who have not experienced the disease before (as in the rate calculation for Figure 4-1). The population at risk for the second event (which is the first recurrence) would be limited to those who have experienced the event once and only once, etc. Thus, studies of second cancers are restricted to the population of those who survived their first cancer. A given person should contribute time to the denominator of the incidence rate for first events only until the time that the disease first occurs. At that point, the person should cease contributing time to the denominator of that rate and should now begin to contribute time to the denominator of the rate measuring the second occurrence. If and when there is a second event, the person should stop contributing time to the rate measuring the second occurrence and begin contributing to the denominator of the rate measuring the third occurrence, and so forth.

In Figure 4-1, the first disease onset might provide a new reference event for a study of second occurrence. Assuming no second events occurred, the follow-up time between 2 and 5 months for P2, between 4 and 12 months for P3, between 5 and 12 months for P4, between 7 and 12 months for P5, and between 8 and 11 months for P6 would be person-time at risk for a second occurrence, yielding 30 months total follow-up. Follow-up would terminate for those who died at the time of their death and would be censored at month 12 for those who survived to the end of the ascertainment protocol period. The investigator might choose to include months 0 to 12 as time at risk contributed by P1. However, that person was diagnosed at an unknown date before the study ascertainment protocol began. The person may have had a recurrence between diagnosis and time zero of the ascertainment protocol, meaning that P1 would not be at risk for second occurrence because she has already had a second occurrence, but that event would not have been ascertained. Even if P2 had not had a second occurrence, the instantaneous rate of second occurrence (the hazard, defined below) may depend on time from the first occurrence. Since that time is unknown, it would be unwise to combine months 0 to 12 contributed by P1 with the person-time contributed by the newly diagnosed P2 to P6.

RELATIONS AMONG INCIDENCE MEASURES

For sufficiently short time intervals, there is a very simple relation between the incidence proportion and the incidence rate of a nonrecurring event. Consider a closed population over an interval t_0 to t_1, and let $\Delta t = t_1 - t_0$ be the length of the interval. If N is the size of the population at t_0 and A is the number of disease onsets over the interval, then the incidence and survival proportions over the interval are $R = A/N$ and $S = (N - A)/N$. Now, suppose the time interval is short enough that the size of the population at risk declines only slightly over the interval. Then, $N - A \approx N$, $S \approx 1$, and so $R/S \approx R$. Furthermore, the average size of the population at risk will be approximately N, so the total person-time at risk over the interval will be approximately $N\Delta t$. Thus, the incidence rate (I) over the interval will be approximately $A/N\Delta t$, and we obtain

$$R = A/N = \left(A/N\Delta t \right)\Delta t \approx I\Delta t \text{ and } R \approx R/S$$

In words, the incidence proportion, incidence odds, and the quantity $I\Delta t$ will all approximate one another if the population at risk declines only slightly over the interval. We can make this approximation hold to within an accuracy of $1/N$ by making Δt so short that no more than one person leaves the population at risk over the interval. Thus, given a sufficiently short time interval, one can simply multiply the incidence rate by the time period to approximate the incidence proportion. This approximation offers another interpretation for the incidence rate: It can be viewed as the limiting value of the ratio of the average risk to the duration of time at risk as the latter duration approaches zero. Using the example depicted in Figure 4-1, the incidence proportion $R = 0.56$, the incidence rate $I = 0.078$ per month, and $\Delta t = 12$ months. $I\Delta t$ therefore equals 0.94, which is a poor approximation to R because the incidence proportion is not small (*i.e.*, as noted above, R does not approximately equal R/S).

Disease occurrence in a population reflects two aspects of individual experiences: the amount of time the individual is at risk in the population and whether the individual actually has the focal event (*e.g.*, gets disease) during that time. Different incidence measures summarize different aspects of the distribution of these experiences. Average incidence time is the average time until an event and incidence proportion is the average "risk" of the event (where "risk" is 1 or 0 according to whether or not the event occurred in the risk period). Each is easy to grasp intuitively, but they are often not easy to estimate or even to define. In contrast, the incidence rate can be applied to the common situation in which the time at risk and the occurrence of the event can be unambiguously determined for everyone. Unfortunately, it can be difficult to comprehend correctly what the rate is telling us about the different dimensions of event distributions, and so it is helpful to understand its relation to incidence times and incidence proportions. These relations are a central component of the topics of survival analysis and failure-time analysis in statistics.[14,15]

Product-Limit Formula

There are relatively simple relations between the incidence proportion of an inevitable, nonrecurring event (such as death) and the incidence rate in a closed population. To illustrate them, we will consider the small closed population shown in Figure 4-5. The time at risk (risk history) of each member is graphed in order from the shortest on top to the longest at the bottom. Each history either ends with a D, indicating the occurrence of the event of interest, or ends at the end of the follow-up, at $t_5 = 19$. The starting time is denoted t_0 and is here equal to 0. Each time that one or more events occur is marked by a vertical dashed line, the unique event times are denoted by t_1 (the earliest) to t_4, and the end of follow-up is denoted by t_5. We denote the number of events at time t_k by A_k, the total number of persons at risk at time t_k (including the A_k people who experience the event) by N_k, and the number of people alive at the end of follow-up by N_5.

Table 4-1 shows the history of the population over the 20-year follow-up period in Figure 4-5, in terms of t_k, A_k, and N_k. Note that because the population is closed and the event is inevitable, the

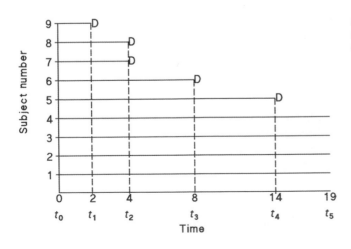

FIGURE 4-5 Example of a small closed population with the end of follow-up at 19 years.

TABLE 4-1

Event Times and Intervals for the Closed Population in Figure 4-5

	Start	Outcome Event Times (t_k)				End
	0	2	4	8	14	19
Index (k)	0	1	2	3	4	5
No. of outcome events series (A_k)	0	1	2	1	1	0
No. at risk series (N_k)	9	9	8	6	5	4
Proportion surviving series (S_k)		8/9	6/8	5/6	4/5	4/4
Length of interval series (Δt_k)		2	2	4	6	5
Person-time ($N_k \Delta t_k$)		18	16	24	30	20
Incidence rate (I_k)		1/18	2/16	1/24	1/30	0/20

number remaining at risk after t_k, N_{k+1}, is equal to $N_k - A_k$, which is the number at risk up to t_k minus the number experiencing the event at t_k. The proportion of the population remaining at risk up to t_k that also remains at risk after t_k is thus

$$S_k = \frac{N_k - A_k}{N_k} = \frac{N_{k+1}}{N_k}$$

We can now see that the proportion of the original population that remains at risk at the end of follow-up is

$$S = \frac{N_5}{N_1} = \frac{N_5}{N_4} \frac{N_4}{N_3} \frac{N_3}{N_2} \frac{N_2}{N_1} = S_4 S_3 S_2 S_1$$

which for Table 4-1 yields

$$S = \frac{4}{5} \frac{5}{6} \frac{6}{8} \frac{8}{9} = \frac{4}{9}$$

This multiplication formula says that the survival proportion over the whole time interval in Figure 4-5 is the product of the survival proportions for every subinterval t_{k-1} to t_k. In its more general form, when there are v subintervals

$$S = \prod_{k=1}^{v} \frac{N_k - A_k}{N_k}$$

[4-1]

This multiplication formula is called the *Kaplan-Meier* or *product-limit* formula.[14,15]

Exponential Formula

Now let t_k be the total person-time at risk in the population over the subinterval from t_{k-1} to t_k, and let $\Delta t_k = t_k - t_{k-1}$ be the length of the subinterval. Because the population is of constant size N_k over this subinterval and everyone still present contributes Δt_k person-time units at risk, the total person-time at risk in the interval is $N_k \Delta t_k$, so that the incidence rate in the time following t_{k-1} up through (but not beyond) t_k is

$$I_k = \frac{A_k}{N_k \Delta t_k}$$

But the incidence proportion over the same subinterval is equal to $I_k\Delta t_k$, so the survival proportion over the subinterval is

$$S_k = 1 - I_k\Delta t_k$$

Thus, we can substitute $1 - I_k\Delta t_k$ for S_k in Equation 4-1

$$S = \left(1 - I_5\Delta t_5\right)\left(1 - I_4\Delta t_4\right)\left(1 - I_3\Delta t_3\right)\left(1 - I_2\Delta t_2\right)\left(1 - I_1\Delta t_1\right)$$

$$= \left[1 - (0)5\right]\left[1 - \left(\frac{1}{30}\right)6\right]\left[1 - \left(\frac{1}{24}\right)4\right]\left[1 - \left(\frac{2}{16}\right)2\right]\left[1 - \left(\frac{1}{18}\right)2\right] = \frac{4}{9}$$

as before.

If each of the subinterval incidence proportions $I_k\Delta t_k$ is small (<0.10 or so), we can simplify the last formula by using the fact that, for small x,

$$1 - x \approx e^{-x}$$

Taking $x = I_k\Delta t_k$ in this approximation formula, we get $1 - I_k t_k \approx \exp(-I_k\Delta t_k)$, so

$$S \approx e^{-I_v\Delta t_v}e^{-I_{v-1}\Delta t_{v-1}}\cdots e^{-I_1\Delta t_1}$$

$$= e^{-I_v\Delta t_v - I_{v-1}\Delta t_{v-1}\cdots - I_1\Delta t_1}$$

$$= e^{-\sum_{k=1}^{v}I_k\Delta t_k}$$

which for Table 4-1 yields

$$e^{-0(5)-\frac{1}{30}(6)-\frac{1}{24}(4)-\frac{2}{16}(2)-\frac{1}{18}(2)} = 0.483$$

not too far from the earlier value of 4/9 = 0.444. Finally, we use the fact that the incidence proportion for the whole period is $1 - S$ to get

$$R = 1 - S \approx 1 - e^{-\sum_{k=1}^{v}I_k\Delta t_k} \qquad \text{[4-2]}$$

Equation 4-2 is cited in many textbooks and is sometimes called the *exponential formula* for relating rates and incidence proportions. The sum in the exponent, $\sum_k I_k\Delta t_k$, is sometimes called the *cumulative incidence*[16] or *cumulative hazard*.[14,15] Confusingly, the term *cumulative incidence* is also often used to denote the incidence proportion. The cumulative hazard, although unitless, is *not* a proportion and will exceed 1.0 when the incidence proportion exceeds $1 - e^{-1} = 0.632$.

We wish to emphasize the assumptions we used to derive the exponential formula in Equation 4-2:

1. The population is closed.
2. The event under study is inevitable (there is no competing risk).
3. The number of events A_k at each event time t_k is a small proportion of the number at risk N_k at that time (*i.e.*, A_k/N_k is always small).

If the population is not very small, we can almost always force assumption 3 to hold by measuring time so finely that every event occurs at its own unique time (so that only one event occurs at each t_k). In Table 4-1, the discrepancy between the true R of 5/9 = 0.556, and the exponential formula value of 1 − 0.483 = 0.517 is rather small considering that A_k/N_k gets as large as 2/8 = 0.25 (at t_2). Dividing the time so finely that every event occurs at its own unique time thus improves the correspondence between R and the exponential value.

We can reduce Δt still further, to as short a time interval as we like, so that the proportion of time intervals that contain outcome or censoring events is negligible compared with the total number of intervals. As the interval Δt shrinks, the fixed number of observed cases A is spread over ever larger number of intervals, until the probability of any one case occurring in an interval becomes proportional to the interval length. Over short enough intervals, that probability for any one person becomes nearly constant from one interval to the next. The ratio of that probability to the interval length is called the *hazard, hazard rate,* or *force of morbidity/mortality* and represents the expected number of events per unit of time for a particular person during a short time interval at a particular time. The *hazard* therefore has units of inverse time. Although they share the same dimensions, the *incidence rate* is a measurable quantity observable in populations, whereas the *hazard rate* is a theoretical quantity pertaining to an individual. The mean *hazard*, averaged over the intervals observed for each person in a population, is expected to equal the population's incidence rate.

Modeling the hazard has advantages, under certain assumptions, and disadvantages,[17] all of which will be discussed in Chapters 20 to 22 and 24 to 25. One important subtlety is the potential for a population's hazard to decline over the course of follow-up when it comprises two or more subpopulations with heterogeneous hazards, neither of which itself declines over the course of follow-up.[18] For example, in a population comprising two subpopulations with constant hazards, the overall hazard will steadily decline over time because of the more rapid depletion of susceptible persons in the subpopulation with the higher hazard. At all times, the hazard is an average of the individual hazards. The size of the subpopulation with a higher hazard diminishes more rapidly than the size of the subpopulation with the lower hazard, so the subpopulation with the lower hazard will receive a growing weight in the overall hazard as time goes by. The overall hazard therefore declines until it reaches the hazard of the subpopulation with the lower hazard, which occurs when all the members of the subpopulation with the higher hazard have had the event. This and other nonintuitive patterns arise from heterogeneous hazards within subpopulations.[17,18]

Assumptions 1 and 2 were also used to derive the product-limit formula in Equation 4-1. These assumptions are rarely satisfied, yet they are often overlooked in presentations and applications of the formulas. Some form of the closed-population assumption (assumption 1) is essential because the incidence proportion is defined only with reference to closed populations. A major use of the product-limit and exponential formulas is, however, in translating incidence-rate estimates from open populations into incidence-proportion estimates for a closed population of interest. By assuming that the incidence rates in the two populations are the same at each time, one can justify substituting the survival proportions $(N_k - A_k)/N_k$ or the incidence rates observed in the open population into the product-limit formula or the exponential formula. This assumption is often plausible when the open population one observes is a subset of the closed population of interest, as in a cohort study with losses to follow-up that are unrelated to risk.

Applications With Competing Risks

When competing risks remove persons from the population at risk, application of the product-limit and exponential formulas requires new concepts and assumptions.[19,20] Consider the subinterval-specific incidence rates for our closed population of interest. When competing risks are present, the product-limit formula in Equation 4-1 for the survival proportion S no longer holds because competing risks may remove additional people between disease-onset times, in which case N_{k+1} will be smaller than $N_k - A_k$. Also, when competing risks occur between t_{k-1} and t_k, the population size will not be constant over the subinterval. Consequently, the person-time in interval k will not equal $N_k \Delta t_k$, and $I_k t_k$ will not equal A_k/N_k. Thus, the exponential formula of Equation 4-2 will not hold if competing risks occur. The amount of error will depend on the frequency of the events that are the competing risks.

We can, however, ask the following question: What would the incidence proportion over the total interval have been if no competing risk had occurred? This quantity is sometimes called the *conditional risk* of the outcome (conditioned on removal of competing risks). One minus the product-limit formula of Equation 4-1 gives an estimate of this quantity under the assumption that the subinterval-specific incidence rates would not change if no competing risk occurred (*independent competing risks*). One minus the exponential formula of Equation 4-2 remains an approximation to the conditional risk if A_k/N_k is always small. The assumption that the rates would not change if competing risks were removed is made by almost all survival-analysis methods for estimating conditional risks, but it requires careful scrutiny. Under conditions that would eliminate competing risks, the incidence rates of the outcome under study may be likely to change. Suppose, for example, that the outcome of interest is colon cancer. Competing risks would include deaths from causes other than colon cancer. Removal of so many risks would be impossible; the concept is useful mainly as a hypothetical. In reality an attempt to reduce the competing risks might involve dietary interventions to prevent deaths from other cancers and from heart disease, but these interventions might also lower colon cancer rates, thus violating the assumption that the specific rates would not change if no competing risk occurred.

Because of the impracticality of reducing competing risks without altering rates of the study disease, many authors caution against interpreting survival estimates based on statistical removal of competing risks as the incidence that would actually occur upon removal of competing risks.[14,15,21-25] An arguably more practical approach is to focus on the risk (probability) of the outcome without removing competing risks, sometimes called the "unconditional risk." This quantity is estimable with no assumption about competing-risk removal.[14,21,26,27]

A more defensible use of the product-limit formula is to estimate survival proportions in the presence of censoring (*e.g.*, loss to follow-up). For this usage, the assumption is made that the censoring is random (*i.e.*, the experience of lost subjects differs only randomly from that of subjects not lost). This assumption is often questionable but is addressable in the design and analysis of a study via measurement and adjustment for factors that affect the censoring and the outcome event.[14]

Relation of Survival Proportion to Average Incidence Time

Returning now to the simpler situation of an inevitable nonrecurring outcome in a closed population, we will derive an equation relating survival proportions to average incidence time. First, we may write the total person-time at risk over the total interval in Figure 4-5 as

$$N_1 \Delta t_1 + \ldots + N_V \Delta t_v = \sum_{K=1}^{v} N_k \Delta t_k = 18 + 16 + 24 + 30 + 20 = 108 \text{ person-years}$$

Thus, the average time at risk contributed by population members over the interval is

$$\frac{1}{N_0} \sum_{K=1}^{v} N_k \Delta t_k = \sum_{k=1}^{v} \left(\frac{N_k}{N_0} \right) \Delta t_k = \frac{1}{9} 108 = 12 \text{ years}$$

Note that N_k/N_0 is the proportion who remain at risk up to t_k, that is, the survival proportion from t_0 to t_k. If we denote this proportion N_k/N_0 by $S_{0,k}$ (to distinguish it from the subinterval-specific proportions S_k), the average time at risk can be written

$$\sum_{l=1}^{v} S_{0,k} \Delta t_k = \left(\frac{9}{9} \right) 2 + \left(\frac{8}{9} \right) 2 + \left(\frac{6}{9} \right) 4 + \left(\frac{5}{9} \right) 6 + \left(\frac{4}{9} \right) 5 = 12 \text{ years}$$

as before. Now suppose that the interval is extended forward in time until the entire population has experienced the outcome of interest, as in Figure 4-4. The average time at risk will then equal the average incidence time, so the average incidence time will be computable from the survival proportions using the last formula. The survival proportions may in turn be computed from the subinterval-specific incidence rates, as described above.

Summary

The three broad types of measures of disease frequency—incidence (and survival) proportion, incidence time, and incidence rate—are all linked by simple mathematical formulas that apply when one considers an inevitable nonrecurring event in a closed population that is followed until everyone has experienced the event. The mathematical relations become more complex when one considers events with competing risks, open populations, or truncated risk periods. Interpretations become particularly problematic when competing risks are present.

LIMITATIONS AND GENERALIZATIONS OF BASIC OCCURRENCE MEASURES

All the above measures can be viewed as types of arithmetic means, with possible weighting. Consequently, it is straightforward to extend these measures to outcomes that are more detailed than all-or-none. Consider, for example, antibody titer following vaccination of persons with no antibody for the target antigen. We might examine the mean number of days until the titer reaches any given level L, or the proportion that reaches L within a given number of days. We might also examine the rate at which persons reach L. To account for the fact that a titer has many possible levels, we could examine these measures for different values of L.

Means cannot capture all relevant aspects of a distribution and can even be misleading, except for some special distributions. For example, we have illustrated how—by itself—an incidence rate fails to distinguish among many people followed over a short period and a few people followed for a long period. Similarly, an incidence proportion of (say) 0.30 over 10 years fails to tell us whether the 30% of persons who had the event all had it within 2 years, or only after 8 years, or had events spread over the whole period. An average incidence time of 2 months among 101 people fails to tell us whether this average was derived from all 101 people having the event at 2 months, or from 100 people having the event at 1 month and 1 person having the event at 102 months, or something between these extremes.

One way to cope with these issues without making assumptions about the population distribution is to focus on how the distribution of the outcome event changes over time. We introduced this idea earlier by constructing survival proportions and incidence rates within time intervals. By using short enough time intervals, we could see clearly how events are spread over time. For example, we could see whether our overall event rate reflects many people having the event early and a few people having it very late, or few having it early and many having it late, or anything between. We can also describe the distribution of event recurrences, such as asthma attacks. Many of these patterns are most easily comprehended by visualizing them using survival or cumulative incidence curves.[17]

We may generalize our notion of event to represent any transition from one state to another—not just from "no disease" to "diseased" but from (say) a diastolic blood pressure of 90 mm Hg in one time interval to 100 mm Hg in the next. We can examine these transitions on a scale as fine as our measurements allow, *e.g.*, in studying the evolution of CD4 lymphocyte counts over time, we can imagine the rate of transitions from count x to count y per unit time for every sensible combination of x and y. Of course, this generalized viewpoint entails a much more complex picture of the population. Studying this complexity is the topic of *longitudinal data analysis* (see Chapters 24 and 25). There are many textbooks devoted to different aspects of the topic; for example, Manton and Stallard[28] provide a population-dynamics (demographic) approach, whereas Diggle et al.[29] cover approaches based on statistical analysis of study cohorts and van der Laan and Robins[30] focus on longitudinal causal modeling.

PREVALENCE

Unlike incidence measures, which focus on new events or *changes* in health states, *prevalence* focuses on existing states. Prevalence of a state at a point in time may be defined as the proportion of a population in that state at that time; thus prevalence of a disease is the proportion of the population with the disease at the specified time. The terms *point prevalence, prevalence proportion,* and *prevalence rate* are sometimes used as synonyms. Prevalence generalizes to health states with multiple levels. For example, in considering cardiovascular health, we could examine the prevalence of different levels of diastolic and systolic resting blood pressure; that is, we could examine the entire blood-pressure distribution, not just prevalence of being above certain clinical cutpoints.

The *prevalence pool* is the subset of the population in the given state. A person who dies with or from the state (*e.g.*, from the disease under consideration) is removed from the prevalence pool; consequently, death decreases prevalence. People may also exit the prevalence pool by recovering from the state or emigrating from the population. Diseases with high incidence rates may have low prevalence if they are rapidly fatal or quickly cured. Conversely, diseases with low incidence rates may have substantial prevalence if they are nonfatal but incurable.

In Figure 4-1, the prevalence of disease at 6 months equals the number of persons alive and diseased at 6 months (P1, P3, and P4) divided by all persons alive at 6 months (all 10 persons except P2 and P8, both of whom died before month 6). In the total population, the prevalence therefore equals 3/8 or 0.38. In the cohort of persons at risk for disease at the index event (time zero), the prevalence at 6 months equals 2/7 or 0.29. P1 is excluded from both the numerator and denominator by the fact that she already had disease at the index event.

Use of Prevalence in Etiologic Research

Prevalence is seldom of direct interest in etiologic applications of epidemiologic research. Because prevalence reflects both the incidence rate and the duration of disease, studies of prevalence or studies based on prevalent cases yield associations that reflect both the causes of disease and the determinants of survival with disease. The study of prevalence can be misleading in the paradoxical situation in which better survival from a disease, and therefore a higher prevalence, follows from the action of a preventive agent that mitigates the disease once it occurs. In such a situation, the preventive agent may be positively associated with the prevalence of disease and so be misconstrued as a causative agent.

Nevertheless, for at least one class of diseases, namely, congenital malformations, prevalence is the measure usually employed. The proportion of babies born with some malformation is a prevalence proportion, not an incidence rate. The incidence of malformations refers to the occurrence of the malformations among the susceptible populations of embryos. Many malformations lead to early embryonic or fetal death that is classified, if recognized, as a miscarriage and not as a birth, whether malformed or not. Thus, malformed babies at birth represent only those fetuses who survived long enough with their malformations to be recorded as births. The frequency of such infants among all births is indeed a prevalence measure, the index event in time being the moment of birth. The measure classifies the population of newborns as to their disease status, malformed or not, at the time of birth. This example illustrates that the index event for prevalence need not be a point in calendar time; it can be a point on another time scale, such as age or time since treatment.

To study causes, it would be more useful and direct to measure the incidence than the prevalence of congenital malformations. Unfortunately, it is seldom possible to measure the incidence rate of malformations because the population at risk—young embryos—is difficult to ascertain, and learning of the occurrence and timing of the malformations among the embryos is equally problematic. Consequently, in this area of research, incident cases are not usually studied, and most investigators settle for the theoretically less desirable but much more practical study of prevalence at birth.

Prevalence is sometimes used to measure the occurrence of degenerative diseases with no clear moment of onset, such as multiple sclerosis, amyotrophic lateral sclerosis, Parkinson disease, and Alzheimer disease. It is also used in seroprevalence studies of infection, especially when the infection has a long asymptomatic (silent) phase that can only be detected by serum testing. Human immunodeficiency virus (HIV) infection is a prime example.[31] Early in the epidemic, incidence of infection was back-calculated from incidence of symptom onset (acquired immune deficiency syndrome or AIDS) and prevalence of infection using assumptions and data about the duration of the asymptomatic phase. In epidemiologic applications outside of etiologic research, such as planning for health resources and facilities and public-health interventions, prevalence may be a more relevant measure than incidence.[32] Prevalence is a measure that may be of interest in animal vectors as well as in humans. Mosquito control measures, for example, are undertaken when the prevalence of mosquitos carrying equine encephalitis virus or West Nile virus exceeds a critical threshold at a particular place and time.

Prevalence, Incidence, and Mean Duration

Often, the study of prevalence in place of incidence is rationalized on the basis of the simple relation between the two measures that hold under certain conditions. We will examine these conditions carefully, with the objective of explaining why they rarely, if ever, provide a secure basis for studying prevalence as a proxy for incidence.

Recall that a stationary population has an equal number of people entering and exiting during any unit of time. Suppose that both the population at risk and the prevalence pool are stationary and that everyone is either at risk or has the disease. Then the number of people entering the prevalence pool in any time period will be balanced by the number exiting from it,

$$\text{Inflow (to prevalence pool)} = \text{Outflow (from prevalence pool)}$$

People can enter the prevalence pool from the nondiseased population and by immigration from another population while diseased. Suppose there is no immigration into or emigration from the prevalence pool, so that no one enters or leaves the pool except by disease onset, death, or recovery. If the size of the population is N and the size of the prevalence pool is P, then the size of the population at risk that feeds the prevalence pool will be $N - P$. Also, during any time interval of length Δt, the number of people who enter the prevalence pool will be

$$I(N-P)\Delta t$$

where I is the incidence rate, and the outflow from the prevalence pool will be

$$I'P\Delta t$$

where I' represents the incidence rate of exiting from the prevalence pool, that is, the number who exit divided by the person-time experience of those in the prevalence pool. Therefore, in the absence of migration, the reciprocal of I' will equal the mean duration of the disease, $\bar{D}$, which is the mean time until death or recovery. It follows that

$$\text{Inflow} = I(N-P)\Delta t = \text{Outflow} = \frac{P\Delta t}{\bar{D}}$$

which yields

$$\frac{P}{N-P} = I\bar{D}$$

$P/(N - P)$ is the ratio of diseased to nondiseased people in the population or, equivalently, the ratio of the prevalence proportion to the nondiseased proportion. (We could call those who are nondiseased healthy except that we mean they do not have a specific illness, which does not imply an absence of all illness.)

The ratio $P/(N - P)$ is called the *prevalence odds*;[32] it is the ratio of the proportion of a population that has a disease to the proportion that does not have the disease. As shown above, the prevalence odds equals the incidence rate times the mean duration of illness. If the prevalence is small, say <0.1, then

$$\text{Prevalence proportion} \approx I\bar{D}$$

because the prevalence proportion will approximate the prevalence odds for small values of prevalence.[32] Under the assumption of stationarity and no migration in or out of the prevalence pool,[33]

$$\text{Prevalence proportion} = \frac{I\bar{D}}{1 + I\bar{D}}$$

which can be obtained from the above expression for the prevalence odds, $P/(N - P)$.

Like the incidence proportion, the prevalence proportion is dimensionless, with a range of 0 to 1. The above equations are in accord with these requirements because, in each of them, the incidence rate, with a dimensionality of the reciprocal of time, is multiplied by the mean duration of illness, which has the dimensionality of time, giving a dimensionless product. Furthermore, the product $I \cdot \overline{D}$ has the range of 0 to infinity, which corresponds to the range of prevalence odds, whereas the expression

$$\frac{I\overline{D}}{1 + I\overline{D}}$$

is always in the range 0 to 1, corresponding to the range of a proportion.

Unfortunately, the above formulas have limited practical utility because of the no-migration assumption and because they do not apply to age-specific prevalence. If we consider the prevalence pool of, say, diabetics who are 60 to 64 years of age, we can see that this pool experiences considerable immigration from younger diabetics aging into the pool and considerable emigration from members aging out of the pool. More generally, because of the very strong relation of age to most diseases, we almost always need to consider age-specific subpopulations when studying patterns of occurrence. Under such conditions, proper analysis requires more elaborate formulas that give prevalence as a function of age-specific incidence, duration, and other population parameters.[8,28,34,35]

Although the relation between incidence and prevalence expressed in the above equation seldom holds exactly, prevalence is clearly a function of incidence. The incidence or occurrence of new diseases feeds the inflow to the prevalence pool and is countered by the outflow due to cure, death, or emigration. Measures of disease incidence and measures of disease prevalence therefore measure related, but very different, concepts, so should not be compared directly with one another.[36]

AVERAGE AGE AT EVENT

Life expectancy is usually taken to refer to the mean age at death of a cohort or a closed population defined by a cohort, such as all persons born in a particular year. As such, life expectancy can only unfold over a time interval from cohort inception until the death of the final surviving cohort member (which may be more than a century). In contrast, average age at death usually refers to the average age of persons dying in a narrow time interval. For example, average age at death among people living in Vietnam as of 2020 represents experiences of persons born from roughly 1910 all the way up to 2020. It is heavily influenced by the size of the population in years that contribute to the calculation and by changes in life expectancy across the birth cohorts contributing to it. Thus, like prevalence, it is a cross-sectional (single-time point) attribute of a population, and the population may be open.

Had the population been in steady state for over a century and continued that way for another century or more, the life expectancy of those born today might resemble the average age at death today. The reality in many locales, however, is that the *number* of births per year increased dramatically over the 20th century, and thus the proportion in younger age groups increased. More recently, many Westernized societies have had birth rates below the replacement rate. The first change pulled the average ages at death downward as they became more weighted by the increased number of deaths from younger age groups. As societies are now aging, their average ages at death are again increasing. Changes in actual life expectancy would exert other effects, in most recent societies also increasing the average age at death. The net consequence is that the average age at death can differ considerably from life expectancy in any year.

These same forces and other similar forces also affect the average age of occurrence of other events, such as the occurrence of a particular disease. Comparisons among such cross-sectional averages mix the forces that affect the rate of disease occurrence with demographic changes that affect the age structure of the population.[6] Such comparisons are therefore inherently biased as estimates of causal associations. The use of average age of occurrence of a health event should therefore be avoided in favor of examining age-specific rates.[37,38]

STANDARDIZATION

The notion of standardization is central to many analytic techniques in epidemiology, including techniques for control of confounding (Chapters 12 and 18) and for summarization of occurrence and effects (Chapters 5 and 18). Thus, standardized rates and proportions will arise at several points in this book, where they will be described in more detail. Standardization of occurrence measures is nothing more than weighted averaging of those measures. Proper use of the idea nonetheless requires careful attention to issues of causal ordering, which we will return to in later discussions. We also note that the term *standardization* has an entirely different definition in some branches of statistics, where it means reexpressing quantities in standard deviation units, a practice that can lead to severe distortions of effect estimates.[39,40]

To illustrate the basic idea of standardization, suppose we are given a distribution of person-time specific to a series of variables, for example, the person-years at risk experienced within age categories 50 to 59 years, 60 to 69 years, and 70 to 74 years, for men and women in Quebec in 2000. Let T_1, T_2, ..., T_6 be the distribution of person-years in the six age-sex categories in this example. Suppose also that we are given the six age-sex-specific incidence rates I_1, I_2, ..., I_6 corresponding to the $v = 6$ age-sex-specific strata. From this distribution and set of rates, we can compute a weighted average of the rates with weights from the distribution,

$$I_s = \frac{I_1 T_1 + \cdots + I_6 T_6}{T_1 + \cdots + T_6} = \frac{\sum_{k=1}^{v} I_k T_k}{\sum_{k=1}^{v} T_k}$$

The numerator of I_s may be recognized as the number of cases one would see in a population that had the person-time distribution T_1, T_2, ..., T_6 and these stratum-specific rates. The denominator of I_s is the total person-time in such a population. Therefore, I_s is the rate one would see in a population with distribution T_1, T_2, ..., T_v and specific rates I_1, I_2, ..., I_v. I_s is traditionally called a *standardized rate*, and T_1, T_2, ..., T_v is called the *standard distribution* on which I_s is based. I_s represents the overall rate that would be observed in a population whose person-time follows the standard distribution and whose specific rates are I_1, I_2, ..., I_v.

The standardization process can also be conducted with incidence or prevalence proportions. Suppose, for example, we have a distribution N_1, N_2, ..., N_6 of persons rather than person-time at risk and a corresponding set of stratum-specific incidence proportions R_1, R_2, ..., R_6. From this distribution and set of proportions with $v = 6$ categories, we can compute the weighted average risk

$$R_s = \frac{R_1 N_1 + \cdots + R_6 N_6}{N_1 + \cdots + N_6} = \frac{\sum_{k=1}^{v} R_k N_k}{\sum_{k=1}^{v} N_k}$$

which is a *standardized risk* based on the standard distribution N_1, N_2, ..., N_6. Standardization can also be applied using other measures (such as mean incidence times or mean blood pressures) in place of the rates or proportions.

By convention, a person at risk for the outcome under observation stops contributing person-time when he or she develops the disease. A group with a higher hazard therefore accumulates less person-time than an otherwise identical group with a lower hazard. The higher hazard generates both more cases of the outcome than the lower hazard and less person-time. Thus, both the numerator of the rate (number of new cases) and the denominator of the rate (total person-time) are affected by changes in the hazard. Because the rates that apply to a population can affect the person-time distribution, the standardized rate is not necessarily the rate that would describe what would happen to a population with the standard distribution T_1, ..., T_v if the specific rates I_1, I_2, ..., I_v were applied to it. An analogous discrepancy can arise for standardized odds. This problem can distort inferences based on comparing standardized rates and odds and will be discussed further in Chapter 5. The problem does not arise when considering standardized risks because the initial distribution $N_1, ..., N_y$, representing the number of people at risk at the beginning of follow-up, cannot be affected by the subsequent risks $R_1, ..., R_y$. A higher risk can only generate more cases of the outcome; it does not affect the number of people at risk at the outset.

References

1. MacMahon B, Pugh TF. *Epidemiology: Principles and Methods*. Boston, MA: Little, Brown; 1970.
2. Cole P. The evolving case-control study. *J Chronic Dis*. 1979;32(1-2):15-27.
3. Greenland S. Interpretation and choice of effect measures in epidemiologic analyses. *Am J Epidemiol*. 1987;125(5):761-768.
4. Dawber TR, Meadors GF, Moore FE Jr. Epidemiological approaches to heart disease: the Framingham study. *Am J Public Health Nations Health*. 1951;41(3):279-281.
5. Schmidt M, Jacobsen JB, Lash TL, Botker HE, Sorensen HT. 25 year trends in first time hospitalisation for acute myocardial infarction, subsequent short and long term mortality, and the prognostic impact of sex and comorbidity: a Danish nationwide cohort study. *Br Med J*. 2012;344:e356.
6. Wilk JB, Lash TL. Risk factor studies of age-at-onset in a sample ascertained for Parkinson disease affected sibling pairs: a cautionary tale. *Emerg Themes Epidemiol*. 2007;4:1.
7. Morrison AS. Sequential pathogenic components of rates. *Am J Epidemiol*. 1979;109(6):709-718.
8. Alho JM. On prevalence, incidence, and duration in general stable populations. *Biometrics*. 1992;48(2):587-592.
9. Elandt-Johnson RC. Definition of rates: some remarks on their use and misuse. *Am J Epidemiol*. 1975;102(4):267-271.
10. Glynn RJ, Buring JE. Ways of measuring rates of recurrent events. *Br Med J*. 1996;312(7027):364-367.
11. Anker SD, McMurray JJ. Time to move on from "time-to-first": should all events be included in the analysis of clinical trials? *Eur Heart J*. 2012;33(22):2764-2675.
12. Rogers JK, Yaroshinsky A, Pocock SJ, Stokar D, Pogoda J. Analysis of recurrent events with an associated informative dropout time: application of the joint frailty model. *Stat Med*. 2016;35(13):2195-2205.
13. Ozga AK, Kieser M, Rauch G. A systematic comparison of recurrent event models for application to composite endpoints. *BMC Med Res Methodol*. 2018;18(1):2.
14. Kalbfleisch JD, Prentice RL. *The Statistical Analysis of Failure-Time Data*. 2nd ed. New York, NY: Wiley; 2002.
15. Cox DR, Oakes D. *Analysis of Survival Data*. New York, NY: Chapman and Hall; 1984.
16. Breslow NE, Day NE. *Statistical Methods in Cancer Research. Vol I: The Analysis of Case-Control Data*. Lyon, France: IARC; 1980.
17. Hernan MA. The hazards of hazard ratios. *Epidemiology*. 2010;21(1):13-15.
18. Vaupel JW, Yashin AI. Heterogeneity's ruses: some surprising effects of selection on population dynamics. *Am Stat*. 1985;39(3):176-185.
19. Andersen PK, Geskus RB, de Witte T, Putter H. Competing risks in epidemiology: possibilities and pitfalls. *Int J Epidemiol*. 2012;41(3):861-870.
20. Varadhan R, Weiss CO, Segal JB, Wu AW, Scharfstein D, Boyd C. Evaluating health outcomes in the presence of competing risks: a review of statistical methods and clinical applications. *Med Care*. 2010;48(6 suppl):S96-S105.
21. Pepe MS, Mori M. Kaplan-Meier, marginal or conditional probability curves in summarizing competing risks failure time data? *Stat Med*. 1993;12(8):737-751.
22. Alberti C, Metivier F, Landais P, Thervet E, Legendre C, Chevret S. Improving estimates of event incidence over time in populations exposed to other events: application to three large databases. *J Clin Epidemiol*. 2003;56(6):536-545.
23. Prentice RL, Kalbfleisch JD. Author's reply. *Biometrics*. 1988;44:1205.
24. Greenland S. Causality theory for policy uses of epidemiologic measures. In: Murray CJL, Salomon JA, Mathers CD, Lopez AD, eds. *Summary Measures of Population Health*. Cambridge, MA: Harvard University Press/WHO; 2002:291-302.
25. Greenland S. Epidemiologic measures and policy formulation: lessons from potential outcomes. *Emerg Themes Epidemiol*. 2005;2:5.
26. Benichou J, Gail MH. Estimates of absolute cause-specific risk in cohort studies. *Biometrics*. 1990;46(3):813-826.
27. Gooley TA, Leisenring W, Crowley J, Storer BE. Estimation of failure probabilities in the presence of competing risks: new representations of old estimators. *Stat Med*. 1999;18(6):695-706.
28. Manton KG, Stallard E. *Chronic Disease Modelling*. London, England: Griffin; 1988.

29. Diggle PJ, Heagerty P, Liang K-Y, Zeger SL. *Analysis of Longitudinal Data.* 2nd ed. New York, NY: Oxford; 2002.

30. Van der Laan M, Robins JM. *Unified Methods for Censored Longitudinal Data and Causality.* New York, NY: Springer; 2003.

31. Brookmeyer R, Gail MH. *AIDS Epidemiology: A Quantitative Approach.* New York, NY: Oxford University Press; 1994.

32. Pearce N. Effect measures in prevalence studies. *Environ Health Perspect.* 2004;112(10):1047-1050.

33. Freeman J, Hutchison GB. Prevalence, incidence and duration. *Am J Epidemiol.* 1980;112(5):707-723.

34. Preston SH. Relations among standard epidemiologic measures in a population. *Am J Epidemiol.* 1987;126(2):336-345.

35. Keiding N. Age-specific incidence and prevalence: a statistical perspective. *J R Stat Soc A.* 1991;154:371-412.

36. Flanders WD, O'Brien TR. Inappropriate comparisons of incidence and prevalence in epidemiologic research. *Am J Public Health.* 1989;79(9):1301-1303.

37. Rothman KJ. Longevity of jazz musicians: flawed analysis. *Am J Public Health.* 1992;82(5):761.

38. Sylvestre MP, Huszti E, Hanley JA. Do OSCAR winners live longer than less successful peers? A reanalysis of the evidence. *Ann Intern Med.* 2006;145(5):361-363; discussion 392.

39. Greenland S, Schlesselman JJ, Criqui MH. The fallacy of employing standardized regression coefficients and correlations as measures of effect. *Am J Epidemiol.* 1986;123(2):203-208.

40. Greenland S, Maclure M, Schlesselman JJ, Poole C, Morgenstern H. Standardized regression coefficients: a further critique and review of some alternatives. *Epidemiology.* 1991;2(5):387-392.

CHAPTER 5

Measures of Effect and Measures of Association

Kenneth J. Rothman, Tyler J. VanderWeele, and Timothy L. Lash

 One common objective of epidemiologic research is to estimate the effect of an exposure on the occurrence of a disease or health condition. For reasons explained below, we can seldom observe or even estimate this effect directly. Most often, we observe an association between the exposure and disease among study subjects, which estimates a population association. The observed association will be a poor substitute for the desired effect if it is a poor estimate of the population association or if the population association is not itself close to the effect of interest. Chapters 12 through 15 address specific problems that arise in connecting observed associations to effects. The present chapter defines effects and associations in populations and the basic concepts needed to connect them.

MEASURES OF EFFECT

Epidemiologists use the term *effect* in two senses. In one sense, any case of a given disease or health condition may be the effect of a given cause. *Effect* is used in this way to mean the end point of a causal mechanism, identifying the type of outcome that a cause produces. For example, we may say that liver cirrhosis is an effect of chronic excessive alcohol consumption. This use of the term *effect* merely identifies liver cirrhosis as one consequence of chronic excessive alcohol consumption. Other effects of the exposure, such as accidental injuries, are also possible.

In a more epidemiologic sense, an *effect* of a factor is a change in a population characteristic that is caused by the factor being at one level versus another. The population characteristics of traditional focus in epidemiology are disease-occurrence measures, as described in Chapter 4. If disease occurrence is measured in terms of incidence rate or proportion, then the effect is the change in incidence rate or proportion brought about by a particular factor. We might say that the effect of chronic excessive alcohol consumption, compared with abstinence from alcohol consumption, is to increase the average risk of liver cirrhosis from 1 in 10,000 in 1 year to 1 in 1,000 in 1 year. Although it is customary to use the definite article in referring to this second type of effect (*the* effect of chronic excessive alcohol consumption), this custom does not imply that this is the only effect of chronic excessive alcohol consumption compared with abstinence. An increase in risk for accidental injury and some types of cancer remains possible, and the increase in risk of liver cirrhosis may differ across populations and time. An effect of some factor is thus relative to the outcomes, to the population, and to the time frame.

In epidemiology, it is customary to refer to potential causal characteristics as *exposures*. Thus, *exposure* can refer to a behavior (*e.g.*, chronic excessive alcohol consumption), a treatment or other intervention (*e.g.*, participation in an Alcoholics Anonymous program), a trait (*e.g.*, a genotype that affects the metabolism of alcohol), a social condition (*e.g.*, neighborhood prevalence of alcohol retail outlets), or even a comorbid disease or health condition (*e.g.*, infection with hepatitis C virus).

Population effects are most commonly expressed as effects on incidence rates or incidence proportions, but other measures based on incidence times or prevalences may also be used. Epidemiologic analyses that focus on survival time until death or recurrence of disease are examples of analyses that measure effects on incidence times. *Absolute effect measures* are differences in occurrence measures, and *relative effect measures* are ratios of occurrence measures.[1] Other measures divide absolute effects by an occurrence measure.

For simplicity, our basic descriptions will be of effects in cohorts, which are groups of individuals. As mentioned in Chapter 4, each cohort defines a closed population starting at the time the group is defined. Among the measures we will consider, only those involving incidence rates generalize straightforwardly to open populations.

Difference Measures

Consider a cohort followed over a specific time or age interval—say, from 2015 to 2020 or from ages 50 to 69 years. If we can imagine the experience of this cohort over the same interval under two different conditions—say, exposed and unexposed—then we can ask what the incidence rate of any outcome would be under the two conditions. Thus, we might consider a cohort of adults with a body mass index (BMI) over 30 kg/m^2 and free of prevalent diabetes and an exposure that consisted of mailing to each cohort member a brochure describing a diet and exercise plan designed to help adults reduce their BMI. We could then ask what the diabetes incidence rate would be in this cohort if we carry out this intervention and what it would be if we do not carry out this intervention. These intervention histories represent mutually exclusive alternative histories for the cohort. The two incidence rates thus represent alternative *potential outcomes* for the cohort.

The difference between the two rates we call the absolute effect of our mailing program on the incidence rate or the *causal rate difference*. To be brief, we might refer to the causal rate difference as the excess rate due to the program (which would be negative if the program prevented some cases of incident diabetes).

In a parallel manner, we might ask what the incidence proportion would be if we carry out this intervention and what it would be if we do not carry out this intervention. The difference between the two proportions we call the *absolute effect* of our treatment on the incidence proportion, or *causal risk difference,* or *excess risk* for short. Also in a parallel fashion, the difference in the average diabetes-free years of life lived over the interval under the treated and untreated conditions is another absolute effect of treatment.

To illustrate the above measures in symbolic form, suppose we have a cohort of size N defined at the start of a fixed time interval and that anyone alive without the disease is at risk of the disease. In our example, these would be N persons with BMI greater than 30 kg/m^2 and free of diabetes. Further, suppose that if every member of the cohort is exposed throughout the interval (receives a diet and exercise brochure), A_1 cases will occur and the total time at risk will be T_1. If no member of the same cohort is exposed during the interval (no one receives the diet and exercise brochure), A_0 cases will occur and the total time at risk will be T_0. Then the causal rate difference will be

$$\frac{A_1}{T_1} - \frac{A_0}{T_0} = I_1 - I_0$$

where $I_j = A/T_j$ is the incidence rate under condition j ($j = 1$ is the exposed condition, so the cohort members received the brochure, and $j = 0$ is the unexposed condition, so the cohort members did not receive the brochure). Comparison of measures of disease occurrence under these two exposure conditions is called a *causal contrast*. The causal risk difference will be

$$\frac{A_1}{N} - \frac{A_0}{N}$$

and the causal difference in average disease-free time will be

$$\frac{T_1}{N} - \frac{T_0}{N} = \frac{T_1 - T_0}{N}$$

When the outcome is death, the negative of the average time difference, $T_0/N - T_1/N$, is called the *years of life lost* as a result of exposure. Each of these measures compares disease occurrence by taking differences, so they are called *difference* measures or absolute measures. They are expressed in units of their component measures: cases per unit person-time for the rate difference, cases per person starting follow-up for the risk difference, and time units for the average-time difference.

Ratio Measures

Effect measures may also be calculated by taking ratios. Examples of such ratio (or relative) measures are the *causal rate ratio*

$$\frac{A_1/T_1}{A_0/T_0} = \frac{I_1}{I_0}$$

the *causal risk ratio*

$$\frac{A_1/N}{A_0/N} = \frac{A_1}{A_0} = \frac{R_1}{R_0}$$

where $R_j = A/N$ is the incidence proportion (average risk) under condition j, and the *causal ratio of disease-free time*

$$\frac{T_1/N}{T_0/N} = \frac{T_1}{T_0}$$

In contrast to difference measures, ratio measures are dimensionless because the units cancel upon division. Estimates of the rate ratio and risk ratio are often called *relative risks*. Sometimes, this term is applied to disease or exposure odds ratios as well, although we would discourage such usage. "Relative risk" may be the most common term in epidemiology. Its usage is so broad that one must often look closely at the details of study design and analysis to discern which ratio measure is being estimated or discussed.

The three causal ratio measures are related by the formula

$$\frac{R_1}{R_0} = \frac{R_1 N}{R_0 N} = \frac{A_1}{A_0} = \frac{I_1 T_1}{I_0 T_0}$$

which follows from the fact that the number of cases equals the disease rate times the time at risk. A fourth relative measure can be constructed from the incidence odds. If we write $S_1 = 1 - R_1$ and $S_0 = 1 - R_0$, the *causal odds ratio* is then

$$\frac{R_1/S_1}{R_0/S_0} = \frac{A_1/(N - A_1)}{A_0/(N - A_0)}$$

Relative Excess Measures

When a causal ratio measure is greater than 1, reflecting an average effect that is causal, it is sometimes expressed as an *excess relative risk*

$$IR - 1 = \frac{I_1}{I_0} - 1 = \frac{I_1 - I_0}{I_0}$$

where $IR = I_1/I_0$ is the causal rate ratio. Similarly, the excess causal risk ratio is

$$RR - 1 = \frac{R_1}{R_0} - 1 = \frac{R_1 - R_0}{R_0}$$

where $RR = R_1/R_0$ is the causal risk ratio. These formulas show how excess relative risks equal the rate difference or risk difference divided by (relative to) the unexposed rate or risk (I_0 or R_0), and so are sometimes called relative difference or relative excess measures.

More often, the excess rate is expressed relative to I_1, as

$$\frac{I_1 - I_0}{I_1} = \frac{I_1/I_0 - 1}{I_1/I_0} = \frac{IR - 1}{IR} = 1 - \frac{1}{IR}$$

where $IR = I_1/I_0$ is the causal rate ratio. Similarly, the excess risk is often expressed relative to R_1, as

$$\frac{R_1 - R_0}{R_1} = \frac{R_1/R_0 - 1}{R_1/R_0} = \frac{RR - 1}{RR} = 1 - \frac{1}{RR}$$

where $RR = R_1/R_0$ is the causal risk ratio. In both these measures, the excess rate or risk attributable to exposure is expressed as a fraction of the total rate or risk under exposure; hence, $(IR - 1)/IR$ may be called the *rate fraction* and $(RR - 1)/RR$, the *risk fraction*. Both these measures are often called *attributable fractions*.

A number of other measures are also referred to as attributable fractions. Especially, the rate and risk fractions just defined are often confused with a distinct quantity called the *etiologic fraction*, which cannot be expressed as a simple function of the rates or risks. We will discuss these problems in detail later, where yet another relative excess measure will arise.

Relative excess measures were intended for use with exposures that have a net causal effect. They become negative and hence difficult to interpret with a net preventive effect. One expedient modification for dealing with preventive exposures is to interchange the exposed and unexposed quantities in the measures. The measures that arise from interchanging I_1 with I_0 and R_1 with R_0 in attributable fractions have been called *preventable fractions* and are easily interpreted. For example, $(R_0 - R_1)/R_0 = 1 - R_1/R_0 = 1 - RR$ is the fraction of the risk under the unexposed condition that could be prevented by exposure. In vaccine studies, this measure is also known as the *vaccine efficacy*.

Dependence of the Null State on the Effect Measure

If the occurrence measures being compared do not vary with exposure condition, the measure of effect will equal 0 if it is a difference or relative difference measure and will equal 1 if it is a ratio measure. In this case, we say that the effect is *null* and that the exposed condition, compared with the unexposed condition, has no effect on the occurrence measure. This null state does not depend on the way in which the occurrence measure is compared (difference, ratio, etc.), but it may depend on the occurrence measure. For example, the 150-year average risk of death is always 100%, and so the 150-year causal risk difference is always 0 for any known exposure; nothing has been discovered that prevents death by age 150 years. Nonetheless, many causal contrasts will change the risk of death by age 60 years, so will have a nonzero 60-year causal risk difference. These exposure conditions will also change the death rate and the average death time, compared with their unexposed conditions. Because they affect the death rate and the average death time by age 60 years, the death rate and average death time will also likely be nonnull if measured to age 150 years.

The Theoretical Nature of Effect Measures

The definitions of effect measures given above are sometimes called *counterfactual* or *potential-outcome* definitions. Such definitions may be traced back to the writings of Hume in the 18th century. Although they received little explication until the latter third of the 20th century, they were being used by scientists (including epidemiologists and statisticians) long before.[2-6]

They are called counterfactual measures because at least one of the two conditions in the definitions of the effect measures must be contrary to fact. The cohort may be exposed or treated (*e.g.*, every member sent a mailing) or unexposed or untreated (no one sent a mailing). If the cohort is treated, then the untreated condition will be counterfactual, and if it is untreated, then the treated condition will be counterfactual. Both conditions may be counterfactual, as would occur if only part of the cohort is sent the mailing. The outcomes of the conditions (*e.g.*, I_1 and I_0, or R_1 and R_0, or T_1/N and T_0/N) remain potentialities until a treatment is applied to the cohort.[3,5-7]

One important feature of counterfactually defined effect measures is that they involve two distinct conditions: an index condition, which usually involves some exposure or treatment, and a reference condition—such as no treatment—against which this exposure or treatment will be evaluated. To ask for *the* effect of exposure is meaningless without reference to some other condition. In the preceding example, the effect of one mailing is defined only in reference to no mailing. We could have asked instead about the effect of one mailing relative to four mailings; this causal contrast is very different from one versus no mailing.

Another important feature of effect measures is that they are never observed separately from some component measure of occurrence. If in the mailing example we send the entire population one mailing, the rate difference comparing the outcome to no mailing, $I_1 - I_0$, is not observed directly; we observe only I_1, which is the sum of that effect measure and the (counterfactual) rate under no mailing, I_0: $I_1 = (I_1 - I_0) + I_0$. Therefore, the researcher faces the problem of separating the effect measure $I_1 - I_0$ from the unexposed rate I_0 upon having observed only their sum, I_1.

Defining Exposure Conditions in Causal Contrasts

Because we have defined effects with reference to a *single* cohort under two distinct conditions, one must be able to describe meaningfully each condition for the one cohort.[5,8-11] Consider, for example, the effect of gender (self-identified men versus self-identified women) on heart disease. For these words to have content, we must be able to imagine a cohort of men, their cardiovascular disease incidence, and what their incidence would have been had the very same men been women instead.

The apparent ludicrousness of this demand reveals the vague meaning of gender effect. To reach a reasonable level of scientific precision, gender effect could be replaced by more precise mechanistic concepts, such as hormonal effects, gender-bias effects, transgender effects, and effects of other gender-associated factors, which explain the association of gender with the incidence of cardiovascular disease. With such concepts, we can imagine what it means for the men to have their exposure changed: hormone treatments, sex-change operations, and so on. That is not to say that the statement "gender has an effect of cardiovascular disease" is meaningless, only that, when we speak of a particular effect measure, we must be more precise as to what the exposure is.

The preceding considerations underscore the need to define the index (exposed) and reference (unexposed) conditions in substantial detail to aid interpretability of results. For example, in a study of the effects of contemporaneous chronic excessive alcohol consumption on the occurrence of liver cirrhosis, a detailed definition of the index condition might account for the amount of alcohol consumed per drinking event (drinks per consumption event), frequency of alcohol consumption (drinking events per week), the duration of excessive consumption (years), and the age at which excessive consumption began. Similarly, definition of the absence of exposure for the reference condition—with regard to dose, duration, and induction period—ought to receive as much attention as the definition of the presence of exposure.[12] While it is tempting to define all persons who fail to satisfy the definition of the exposed condition as unexposed, such a definition might dilute the causal contrast by including former excessive consumers, moderate daily drinkers, occasional drinkers, and lifelong teetotalers in the reference group.

Whether the definitions of the index and reference conditions are sufficiently precise may depend in part on the outcome under study and one's prior understanding of the potential causal mechanisms. For example, a study of the effect of current smoking on lung cancer occurrence would set minimums for the frequency, duration, and induction period of cigarette smoking to define the exposed group and would set maximums (perhaps zero) for these same characteristics to define the unexposed group. Former smokers would not meet either the index or reference conditions. In contrast, a study of the effect of current smoking on the occurrence of injuries in a residential fire might allow any current smoking habit to define the exposed group and any current nonsmoking habit to define the unexposed group, even if the latter group includes former smokers. One might be hesitant to include former smokers in the reference group for a causal contrast with current smoking when the outcome is lung cancer but be willing to include former smokers in the reference group for a causal contrast with current smoking when the outcome is injury in a residential fire. This difference arises from the difference in reasonable prior understanding of the causal mechanisms between cigarette smoking and the risk of lung cancer versus injury in a residential fire.

Effects Mediated by Competing Risks

As discussed in Chapter 4, the presence of competing risks leads to complications when interpreting incidence measures. The complexities carry over to interpreting effect measures. In particular, the interpretation of simple comparisons of incidence proportions must be tempered by the fact that they reflect exposure effects on competing risks as well as individual occurrences of the study disease. One consequence of these effects on competing risks is that exposure can affect time at risk for the study disease. To take an extreme example, suppose that exposure was an antismoking treatment and the "disease" was being hit by a drunk driver. If the antismoking treatment was even moderately effective in reducing tobacco use, it would likely lead to a reduction in the cohort's mortality rate, thus leading to more time alive, which would increase the opportunity to be struck by a drunk driver. The result would be more hits from drunk drivers for those exposed and hence higher risk under the exposed condition than the unexposed condition.

This elevated risk of getting hit by a drunk driver is a genuine effect of the antismoking treatment, albeit an indirect and unintended one. The same sort of effect arises from any exposure that changes time at risk of other outcomes. Thus, smoking can reduce the average risk of accidental death simply by reducing the time at risk for an accident. Similarly, and quite apart from any direct biologic effect, smoking could reduce the average risk of Alzheimer disease, Parkinson disease, and other diseases of the elderly, simply by reducing the chance of living long enough to get these diseases. This indirect effect occurs even if we look at a narrow time interval, such as 2-year risk rather than lifetime risk: Even within a 2-year interval, smoking could cause some deaths and thus reduce the population time at risk, leading to fewer cases of these diseases.

Although the effects just described are real exposure effects, investigators typically want to remove or adjust away these effects and focus on more direct effects of exposure on disease. Rate measures account for the changes in time at risk produced by exposure in a simple fashion, by measuring number of disease events relative to time at risk. Indeed, if there is no trend in the disease rate over time and the only effect of the exposure on disease occurrence is to alter time at risk, the rate ratio and difference will be null. If, however, there are time trends in disease, then even rate measures will incorporate some exposure effects on time at risk; when this happens, time-stratified rate comparisons are needed to account for these effects (survival analysis; see Chapter 21).

Typical risk estimates attempt to "adjust" for competing risks, using methods that estimate the counterfactual risk of the study disease if the competing risks were removed. One objection to these methods is that the counterfactual condition is not clear: How are the competing risks to be removed? The incidence of the study disease would depend heavily on the answer. The problems here parallel problems of defining exposure in effect measures: How is the exposed condition to be changed to the unexposed condition or vice versa? Most methods make the implausible assumptions that the exposure could be completely removed without affecting the rate of competing risks, and that competing risks could be removed without affecting the rate of the study disease. These assumptions are rarely, if ever, justified. A more general approach treats the study disease and the competing risks as parts of a *multivariate* or *multidimensional* outcome. This approach can reduce the dependence on implausible assumptions; it also responds to the argument that an exposure should not be considered in isolation, especially when effects of exposure and competing risks entail very different costs and benefits.[8,9] Finally, some methods attempt to assess disease occurrence effect measures among the latent subpopulation who would have survived throughout follow-up irrespective of the exposure condition they were in,[13-17] but these approaches face numerous methodological challenges.

Owing to the complexities that ensue from taking a more general approach, we will not delve further into issues of competing risks. Nonetheless, readers should be alert to the problems that can arise when the exposure may have strong effects on diseases other than the one under study.

ASSOCIATION AND CONFOUNDING

Because the single population in a causal contrast can only be observed under one of the two conditions in the contrast (and sometimes neither), we face a special problem in effect estimation: We must predict accurately the magnitude of disease occurrence under conditions that did not or will not in fact occur. In other words, we must predict certain outcomes under what are or will become counterfactual conditions. For example, we may observe $I_1 = 50$ cases of diabetes per 10,000 person-years in a target cohort of persons with BMI more than 30 kg/m^2 over a 10-year follow-up and ask what rate reduction would have been achieved had these same persons undertaken the brochures diet and exercise plan at the start of follow-up. Here, we observe I_1 and need I_0 (the rate that would have occurred under complete adoption of the diet and exercise plan) to complete $I_1 - I_0$.

Because I_0 is not observed, we must estimate what it would have been. To do so, we would need to refer to data on the outcomes of unexposed persons, such as data from a cohort that did not receive the brochure. From these data, we would construct an estimate of I_0. Neither these data nor the estimate derived from them are part of the effect measure; they are only components of the estimation process. We use them to construct a measure of *association* that we intend to equal the effect measure of interest.

Measures of Association

Consider a situation in which we contrast a measure of occurrence in *two different* populations. For example, we could take the ratio of thyroid cancer incidence rates among males and females in Canada. This thyroid cancer rate ratio comparing the male and female subpopulations is *not* an effect measure because its two component rates refer to different groups of people. In this situation, we say that the rate ratio is a *measure of association;* in this example, it is a measure of the association of sex with thyroid cancer incidence in Canada.

As another example, we could contrast the incidence rate of thyroid cancer in adolescents within a community in the year before and in the third year after release of radioactive waste following an accident at a nuclear power plant. If we take the difference of the rates in these before and after periods, this difference is *not* an effect measure because its two component rates refer to two different subpopulations, one before the accidental release and one after. There may be considerable overlap among the adolescents present in the before and after periods. Nonetheless, the experiences compared refer to different time periods, so we say that the rate difference is a measure of association. In this example, it is a measure of the association between release of radioactive waste and thyroid cancer incidence in the community.

We can summarize the distinction between measures of effect and measures of association as follows: A measure of effect compares what would happen to *one* population under two possible but distinct life courses or conditions, of which at most only one can occur. It is a theoretical or metaphysical concept insofar as it is logically impossible to observe the population under both conditions at the same time, and, hence, it is logically impossible to see directly the size of the effect.[11] In contrast, a measure of association compares what happens in two distinct populations, although the two distinct populations may correspond to one population in different time periods. Subject to physical and social limitations, we can observe both populations and so can directly observe an association.

Confounding

Given the observable nature of measures of association, it is tempting to substitute them for measures of effect (perhaps after making some adjustments). It is even more natural to give causal explanations for observed associations in terms of obvious differences between the populations being compared. In the preceding example of thyroid cancer, it is tempting to ascribe an increase in incidence following the accidental release of radioactivity to the accident itself. Let us analyze in detail how such an inference translates into measures of effect and association.

The effect we wish to measure is that which the accidental release of radioactivity had on the rate. To measure this effect, we must contrast the actual rate of thyroid cancer that occurred after the accidental release with the rate that would have occurred *in the same time period* had the accidental release of radioactivity *not* occurred. We cannot observe the latter rate, for radioactivity was accidentally released, and so the rate of thyroid cancer in the absence of the accidental release in that time period is counterfactual. Thus, we substitute in its place, or exchange, the rate in the time period before the accidental release of radioactivity. In doing so, we substitute a measure of association (the rate difference before and after the accidental release of radioactivity) for what we are really interested in: the difference between the rate of thyroid cancer after the accidental release of radioactivity and what that rate would have been had there been no accidental release of radioactivity in the same time period.

This substitution will be misleading to the extent that the rate before the accident does not equal—so should not be exchanged with—the counterfactual rate (*i.e.*, the rate that would have occurred in the postaccident period if the accident had not occurred). If the two are not equal, then the measure of association will not equal the measure of effect for which it is substituted. In such a circumstance, we say that the measure of association is *confounded* (for our desired measure of effect). Other ways of expressing the same idea is that the before-after rate difference is confounded for the causal rate difference or that *confounding* is present in the before-after difference.[2,18,19] On the other hand, if the rate before the accident does equal the postaccident counterfactual rate, then the measure of association equals our desired measure of effect, and we say that the before-after difference is *unconfounded* or that no confounding is present in this difference.

The preceding definitions apply to ratios as well as differences. Because ratios and differences contrast the same underlying quantities, confounding of a ratio measure will in general imply confounding of the corresponding difference measure and vice versa. However, there can be cases in which, due to exact cancelations in biases, the contrast on one scale might be confounded, while another might not be, but these are unusual occurrences.[20]

The above definitions also extend immediately to situations in which the contrasted quantities are average risks, incidence times, odds, or prevalences. For example, one might wish to estimate the effect of the accidental release of radioactivity on the prevalence of adolescent survivors of thyroid cancer 3 years after the accident. Here, the needed but unobserved counterfactual is what the prevalence of thyroid cancer survivors would have been 3 years after the accident began, had the accident never occurred. We might substitute for that counterfactual the prevalence of adolescent thyroid cancer survivors at the time of the accident. It is possible (though perhaps rare in practice) for one measure of association to be confounded but not another, if the two associations derive from different underlying measures of disease occurrence.[19] For example, there could, in theory, be confounding of the rate ratio but not the risk ratio or of the 5-year risk ratio but not the 10-year risk ratio. Incidence odds are risk-based measures, and, hence, incidence odds ratios will be confounded under exactly the same circumstances as risk ratios.[18,19,21,22] The causal odds ratio for a whole cohort can, however, be closer to the null than any stratum-specific causal odds ratio. Such *noncollapsibility* of the causal odds ratio is sometimes confused with confounding, even though it has nothing to do with the latter phenomenon;[19] it will be discussed further in a later section.

Confounders

Consider again the example of adolescent thyroid cancer associated with the accidental release of radioactivity. Suppose that in the year before the accident, all adolescents in the community had been screened for prevalent thyroid cancer. If this screening program were effective, then the rate of thyroid cancer in the period before the accident would have been elevated by the screen-detected incidence of thyroid cancer cases that had not yet presented symptomatically, and the postaccident rate would have been diminished by advancing the diagnosis date of these cancers to the period before the accident. Thus, if the accident had not occurred, the thyroid cancer incidence would have been higher in the preaccident period than in the postaccident period. In other words, the screening program alone would have caused the observed preaccident rate to be higher than the counterfactual rate (the rate that adolescents would have had after the date of the accident, had there been no accident) for which it is intended to substitute. As a result, the measure of association (which is the before-after rate difference) must be smaller than the desired measure of effect (the causal rate difference). In this situation, we say the screening program *confounded* the measure of association or that the effects of the accidental release of radiation are confounded with the effect of the screening program in the measure of association. We also say that the screening program is a *confounder* of the association and that the association is confounded by the screening program.

Confounders are factors (exposures, interventions, treatments, etc.) that explain or produce all or part of the difference between the measure of association and the measure of effect that would be obtained with a counterfactual ideal. We provide a more formal definition of confounders below and in Chapter 12. In the present example, the screening program explains why the before-after association understates the accident's effect: The before-after difference or ratio includes the effects of the screening program as well as the effect of the accidental release of radioactivity. For a factor to explain this discrepancy and thus confound, the factor must affect or at least predict the risk or rate in at least one exposure group and not be affected by the exposure or the disease.

A large portion of epidemiologic methods are concerned with avoiding confounding or adjusting (controlling) for confounders. Such methods inevitably rely on the gathering and proper use of confounder measurements. We will return repeatedly to this topic. For now, we note that the most fundamental adjustment methods rely on the notion of *stratification* on confounders. If we make our comparisons within appropriate levels of a confounder, that confounder cannot confound the comparisons. For example, if we could limit our before-after comparison to adolescents who were never offered the thyroid cancer screening, then the screening program could not have had an effect (because no program was present), so could not confound the comparison of thyroid cancer rates in these adolescents before and after the program.

A Simple Model That Distinguishes Causation From Association

We can clarify the difference between measures of effect and measures of association, as well as the role of confounding and confounders, by examining risk measures under a simple potential-outcome model for a cohort of individuals.[12,18,23]

TABLE 5-1

An Elementary Model of Causal Types and Their Distribution in Two Distinct Cohorts Over Fixed Duration of Follow-Up

Type	Response[a] Under Exposed Condition	Response[a] Under Unexposed Condition	Description	Proportion of Types in Cohort 1 (Exposed)	Proportion of Types in Cohort 0 (Unexposed)
1	1	1	Doomed	p_1	q_1
2	1	0	Exposure is causal	p_2	q_2
3	0	1	Exposure is preventive	p_3	q_3
4	0	0	Immune	p_4	q_4

[a]1, gets disease over the course of follow-up; 0, does not get disease over the course of follow-up.
Reprinted from Greenland S, Robins JM. Identifiability, exchangeability and epidemiological confounding. *Int J Epidemiol.* 1986; 15:413-419.

Table 5-1 presents the composition of two cohorts, cohort 1 and cohort 0. Suppose that cohort 1 is uniformly exposed to some agent of interest, such as one mailing of a diet and exercise program, and that cohort 0 is not exposed, that is, receives no such mailing. Individuals in the cohorts are classified by their outcomes (incident diabetes, in this example) when exposed and when unexposed:

1. Type 1 or "doomed" persons, for whom exposure is irrelevant over the course of follow-up because disease occurs by the end of follow-up with or without exposure.
2. Type 2 or "causal" persons, for whom exposure is relevant because disease occurs over the course of follow-up if and only if they are exposed.
3. Type 3 or "preventive" persons, for whom exposure is relevant because disease occurs over the course of follow-up if and only if they are unexposed.
4. Type 4 or "immune" persons, for whom exposure is again irrelevant because disease does *not* occur over the course of follow-up, with or without exposure. Note that type 4 persons are not immune from the outcome in general; epidemiologic studies ordinarily exclude persons for whom it is known in advance of follow-up they are not at risk for the outcome.

Type 1 persons may include some whose disease was caused by the exposed condition.[24] Potential outcomes for a type 1 person might be to complete a sufficient cause (see Chapter 3) containing the exposed condition as a component cause before they would complete a sufficient cause that does not contain the exposed condition as a component cause, and both sufficient causes would be completed during the study's follow-up period. This type 1 person will be diseased by the end of follow-up whether she receives the exposed or unexposed condition. However, receiving the exposed condition will cause the disease to occur earlier than it would have occurred under the unexposed condition. The potential-outcome model described here is relative to a specific time of follow-up in its assignment of causation or prevention to only types 2 and 3. Other work has considered potential-outcome models and sufficient cause models involving time to an event.[25-27]

Among the exposed, only type 1 and type 2 persons get the disease, so the incidence proportion in cohort 1 is $p_1 + p_2$. If, however, exposure had been absent from this cohort, only type 1 and type 3 persons would have gotten the disease, so the incidence proportion would have been $p_1 + p_3$. Therefore, the absolute change in the incidence proportion in cohort 1 caused by exposure, or the causal risk difference, is $(p_1 + p_2) - (p_1 + p_3) = p_2 - p_3$, while the relative change, or causal risk ratio, is $(p_1 + p_2)/(p_1 + p_3)$. Similarly, the incidence odds is $(p_1 + p_2)/[1 - (p_1 + p_2)] = (p_1 + p_2)/(p_3 + p_4)$ but would have been $(p_1 + p_3)/[1 - (p_1 + p_3)] = (p_1 + p_3)/(p_2 + p_4)$ if exposure had been absent; hence the relative change in the incidence odds (the causal odds ratio) is

$$\frac{(p_1 + p_2)/(p_3 + p_4)}{(p_1 + p_3)/(p_2 + p_4)}$$

Equal numbers of causal types (type 2) and preventive types (type 3) in cohort 1 correspond to $p_2 = p_3$. Equality of p_2 and p_3 implies that the causal risk difference $p_2 - p_3$ equals 0, and the causal risk and odds ratios equal 1. These values of the causal effect measures are null but do *not* correspond to no effect. They correspond to a balance between causal and preventive effects. The hypothesis of no effect at all is sometimes called the sharp null hypothesis and here corresponds to $p_2 = p_3 = 0$. The sharp null is a special case of the usual null hypothesis that the risk difference is zero or the risk ratio is 1, which corresponds to causal and preventive effects balancing one another to produce $p_2 = p_3$. Only if we can be sure that one direction of effect does not happen (either $p_2 = 0$ or $p_3 = 0$) can we say that a risk difference of 0 or a risk ratio of 1 corresponds to no effect for any individual; otherwise we can only say that those values correspond to no *net* effect or no average treatment effect. More generally, population effect measures correspond only to net effects: A risk difference represents only the net change in the average risk produced by the exposure.

Among the unexposed, only type 1 and type 3 persons get the disease, so the incidence proportion in cohort 0 is $q_1 + q_3$ and the incidence odds is $(q_1 + q_3)/(q_2 + q_4)$. Therefore, the difference and ratio of the incidence proportions in the cohorts are $(p_1 + p_2) - (q_1 + q_3)$ and $(p_1 + p_2)/(q_1 + q_3)$, respectively, while the ratio of incidence odds is

$$\frac{(p_1 + p_2)/(p_3 + p_4)}{(q_1 + q_3)/(q_2 + qp_4)}$$

These measures compare two different cohorts, the exposed and the unexposed, and so are associational rather than causal measures. They equal their causal counterparts only if $q_1 + q_3 = p_1 + p_3$, that is, only if the incidence proportion for cohort 0 equals the incidence proportion that cohort 1 would have experienced if it had been unexposed. If $q_1 + q_3 \neq p_1 + p_3$, then the quantity $q_1 + q_3$ is not a valid substitute for $p_1 + p_3$ for the purpose of estimating a measure of effect. We say that the quantity $q_1 + q_3$ is not *exchangeable* with $p_1 + p_3$. In that case, the associational risk difference, risk ratio, and odds ratio are confounded by the discrepancy between $q_1 + q_3$ and $p_1 + p_3$, so we say that confounding is present in the risk comparisons. Confounding corresponds to a lack of exchangeability arising from a difference between the desired counterfactual quantity $p_1 + p_3$ and the observed substitute $q_1 + q_3$. This difference in turn arises from differences between the exposed and unexposed cohorts with respect to other factors that affect disease risk, the confounders. Informal definitions of the term "confounder" focus on required associations with the exposure and the outcome or on whether control for the confounder reduces the amount of confounding.[28] More formally, for an exposure at a single point in time, a "confounder" is a preexposure covariate C for which there exists a set of other covariates X such that the effect of the exposure on the outcome is unconfounded conditional on X and C, but such that for no proper subset of X and C is the effect of the exposure on the outcome unconfounded conditional on the subset.[28]

Control of confounding would be achieved if we could stratify the cohorts on a sufficient set of these confounders (as defined in Chapter 12) to produce strata within which the counterfactual incidence proportion $(p_1 + p_3)$ and its substitute incidence proportion $(q_1 + q_3)$ were equal, and therefore exchangeable. Within these strata, no confounding would be present.

The degree of confounding may depend on the cohort for which we are estimating effects. Suppose we are interested in the relative effect that exposure would have on risk in cohort 0. This effect would be measured by the causal ratio for cohort 0: $(q_1 + q_2)/(q_1 + q_3)$. Because cohort 0 is unexposed, we do not observe $q_1 + q_2$, the average risk it would have if exposed; that is, $q_1 + q_2$ is counterfactual. If we substitute the actual average risk from cohort 1, $p_1 + p_2$, for this counterfactual average risk in cohort 0, we obtain the same associational risk ratio used before: $(p_1 + p_2)/(q_1 + q_3)$. Even if this associational ratio equals the causal risk ratio for cohort 1 (which occurs only if $p_1 + p_3 = q_1 + q_3$), it will not equal the causal risk ratio for cohort 0 unless $p_1 + p_2 = q_1 + q_2$. To see this, suppose $p_1 = p_2 = p_3 = q_1 = q_3 = 0.1$ and $q_2 = 0.3$. In cohort 1, there is no net effect ($p_2 - p_3 = 0$), whereas in cohort 0, the net causal effect is causal ($q_2 - q_3 = 0.2$). Then $p_1 + p_3 = q_1 + q_3 = 0.2$, but $p_1 + p_2 = 0.2 \neq q_1 + q_2 = 0.4$. Thus, there is no confounding in using the associational ratio $(p_1 + p_2)/(q_1 + q_3) = 0.2/0.2 = 1$ for the causal ratio in cohort 1, $(p_1 + p_2)/(p_1 + p_3) = 0.2/0.2 = 1$ (no net causal effect), yet there is confounding in using this null associational ratio for the causal ratio in cohort 0, for the latter is $(q_1 + q_2)/(q_1 + q_3) = 0.4/0.2 = 2$. This example shows that the presence of confounding can depend on the population chosen as the target of inference (the target population), as well as on the population chosen to provide a substitute for a counterfactual quantity in the target (the reference population). It may also depend on the time period of follow-up, which might affect whether a person who completes a sufficient cause containing the exposed condition as a component cause may later in the follow-up complete a sufficient cause that does not contain the exposed condition as a component cause.[24] If the follow-up period includes the time at which only the first sufficient cause would be completed, then this person would be type 2. If the follow-up period includes the time at which both sufficient causes would be completed, then this person would be type 1. The difference in apparent type might affect whether the exchangeability condition is satisfied.

In addition to satisfying the exchangeability condition, several other assumptions must be met for a measure of association to equal the targeted measure of effect. First, the exposure has to have the same effect on an individual regardless of how the person came to be exposed,[29] an assumption sometimes referred to as "no multiple versions of treatment."[30,31] Second, the effect of the exposure on the individual must not depend on the exposure status of other individuals,[32] an assumption sometimes referred to as "no interference."[30,32-34] These two assumptions—no multiple versions of treatment and no interference are together sometimes called the "Stable Unite Treatment Value Assumption."[30,35] It is these assumptions that are necessary for ordinary individual-level potential-outcomes notation to be well defined. The assumptions can also be explained using the sufficient component cause model introduced in Chapter 3.[36] The no multiple versions of treatment assumption also entail that individual's potential outcome under an exposure condition must be the observed outcome, sometimes referred to in the literature as the "consistency" assumption.[37] The consistency assumption requires that for each exposure condition, the potential outcomes for an individual take the same value regardless of how the exposure status is set or that there are ways to set the exposure status for which the potential outcomes for an individual equal the observed outcome.[38] While the consistency assumption may seem self-evident, it is this assumption that allows conversion of expressions involving probabilities of counterfactuals to expressions involving conditional probabilities of measured variables.[39] Third, the exposed and unexposed conditions must both be observed within strata of all confounders.[40] This assumption, called the positivity assumption, may be violated when it is impossible for persons with a certain set of confounder characteristics to receive the exposed or unexposed condition. For example, certain patient characteristics may strongly contraindicate receipt of a particular treatment. In addition, the positivity assumption may be violated by chance, possibly because of sparse data, but also possibly because confounders are finely divided.

Finally, any causal inference must rest on the combination of data and external information about the data generating mechanism.[41] Causal diagrams (graphical models) provide visual models for distinguishing causation from association and thus for defining and detecting confounding[42-44] (see also Chapter 3). Potential-outcome models and graphical models can be linked via a third class of causal models, called *structural equations*, and lead to the same operational criteria for detection and control of confounding.[44,45]

RELATIONS AMONG MEASURES OF EFFECT

Relations Among Relative Risks

Recall from Chapter 4 that in a closed population over an interval of length Δt, the incidence proportion R, the rate I, and the odds R/S (where $S = 1 - R$) will be related by $R \approx I\Delta t \approx R/S$ if the size of the population at risk declines only slightly over the interval (which implies that R must be small and $S = 1 - R \approx 1$). Suppose now we contrast the experience of the population over the interval under two conditions, exposed and unexposed, and that the size of the population at risk would decline only slightly under either condition. Then, the preceding approximation implies that

$$\frac{R_1}{R_0} \approx \frac{I_1\Delta t}{I_0\Delta t} \approx \frac{R_1/S_1}{R_0/S_0}$$

where $S_1 = 1 - R_1$ and $S_0 = 1 - R_0$. In other words, the ratios of the risks, rates, and odds will be approximately equal if the size of the population at risk declines only slightly over the interval, implying that R_1 and R_0 are both small, although not necessarily equal. The condition that both R_1 and R_0 are small is sufficient to ensure that both S_1 and S_0 are close to 1, in which case, the odds ratio will approximate the risk ratio.[46] For the rate ratio to approximate the risk ratio, we must have $R_1/R_0 \approx I_1T_1/I_0T_0 \approx I_1/I_0$, which requires that exposure only negligibly affects the person-time at risk (*i.e.*, that $T_1 \approx T_0$). Both conditions are satisfied if the size of the population at risk would decline by no more than a few percent over the interval, regardless of exposure status.

The order of the three ratios (risk, rate, and odds) in relation to the null is predictable. When $R_1 > R_0$, we have $S_1 = 1 - R_1 < 1 - R_0 = S_0$, so that $S_0/S_1 > 1$ and

$$1 < \frac{R_1}{R_0} < \frac{R_1}{R_0}\frac{S_0}{S_1} = \frac{R_1/S_1}{R_0/S_0}$$

On the other hand, when $R_1 < R_0$, we have $S_1 > S_0$, so that $S_0/S_1 < 1$ and

$$1 > \frac{R_1}{R_0} > \frac{R_1}{R_0}\frac{S_0}{S_1} = \frac{R_1/S_1}{R_0/S_0}$$

Thus, when exposure affects average risk, the risk ratio will be closer to the null (1) than the odds ratio.

Now suppose that, as we would ordinarily expect, the effect of exposure on the person-time at risk is in the opposite direction of its effect on risk, so that $T_1 < T_0$ if $R_1 > R_0$ and $T_1 > T_0$ if $R_1 < R_0$. Then, if $R_1 > R_0$, we have $T_1/T_0 < 1$ and so

$$1 < \frac{R_1}{R_0} = \frac{I_1T_1}{I_0T_0} < \frac{I_1}{I_0}$$

and if $R_1 < R_0$, we have $T_1/T_0 > 1$ and so

$$1 > \frac{R_1}{R_0} = \frac{I_1T_1}{I_0T_0} > \frac{I_1}{I_0}$$

Thus, when exposure affects average risk, we would ordinarily expect the risk ratio to be closer to the null than the rate ratio. Under further conditions, the rate ratio will be closer to the null than the odds ratio.[47] Thus, we would usually expect the risk ratio to be nearest to the null, the odds ratio to be furthest from the null, and the rate ratio to fall between the risk ratio and the odds ratio.

Effect-Measure Modification (Heterogeneity)

Suppose we divide our population into two or more categories or strata, defined by categories of a covariate that is a potential modifier. In each stratum, we can compare the exposed with the unexposed by calculating an effect measure of our choosing.[20,48] Often we would have no reason to suppose that these stratum-specific effect measures would equal one another. If they are not equal, we say that the effect measure is *heterogeneous* or *modified* or *varies* across strata of the modifier. If they are equal, we say that the measure is *homogeneous, constant,* or *uniform* across strata of the modifier. Note that what is in view here is how the effect of the exposure varies across strata of the modifier; these variations in the exposure effect may not reflect the effect of the modifier itself but possibly only that of some other variables related to the modifier.[49,50] See Chapter 26 for more complete descriptions of effect modification and effect-measure modification.

A major point about effect-measure modification is that, if effects are present, it will usually be the case that no more than one of the effect measures discussed above will be uniform across strata of the modifier.[20] In fact, if both the exposure and the modifier have an effect on the outcome, then at most one of the risk ratio or risk difference measures of the effect of the exposure can be uniform across strata of the modifier; in such cases, there will thus always be effect-measure modification for either the difference or the ratio scale. As an example, suppose that, among men, the average risk would be 0.50 if exposed but 0.20 if unexposed, whereas among women the average risk would be 0.10 if exposed but 0.04 if unexposed. Then the causal risk difference for men is 0.50 − 0.20 = 0.30, five times the difference for women of 0.10 − 0.04 = 0.06. In contrast, for both men and women, the causal risk ratio is 0.50/0.20 = 0.10/0.04 = 2.5. Now suppose we change this example to make the risk differences uniform, say, by making the exposed male risk 0.26 instead of 0.50. Then, both risk differences would be 0.06, but the male risk ratio would be 0.26/0.20 = 1.3, much less than the female risk ratio of 2.5. Finally, if we change the example by making the exposed male risk 0.32 instead of 0.50, the male risk difference would be 0.12, double the female risk difference of 0.06, but the male ratio would be 1.6 with relative excess ratio of 0.6, which is less than half the relative excess ratio of 1.5 computed from the female ratio of 2.5. Thus, the presence, direction, and size of effect-measure modification can be dependent on the choice of measure.[51,52]

Relation of Stratum-Specific Measures to Overall Measures

The relation of stratum-specific effect measures to the effect measure for an entire cohort can be subtle. For causal risk differences and ratios, the measure for the entire cohort must fall within the bounds of the stratum-specific measures. For the odds ratio, however, the causal odds ratio for the entire cohort can be closer to the null than any of the causal odds ratios for the strata.[19,21,22] This phenomenon is sometimes referred to as *noncollapsibility* of the causal odds ratio and has led some authors to criticize the odds ratio as a measure of effect, except as an approximation to risk and rate ratios.[2,19,21,22]

As an example, suppose we have a cohort that is 50% men, and, among men, the average risk would be 0.50 if exposed but 0.20 if unexposed, whereas, among women, the average risk would be 0.08 if exposed but 0.02 if unexposed. Then the causal odds ratios are

$$\frac{0.50/(1-0.50)}{0.20/(1-0.20)} = 4.0 \text{ for men, and } \frac{0.08/(1-0.08)}{0.02/(1-0.02)} = 4.3 \text{ for women}$$

For the total cohort, the average risk if exposed would be just the average of the male and female average risks, 0.5(0.50) + 0.5(0.08) = 0.29; similarly, the average risk if unexposed would be 0.5(0.20) + 0.5(0.02) = 0.11. Thus, the causal odds ratio for the total cohort is

$$\frac{0.29/(1-0.29)}{0.11/(1-0.11)} = 3.3$$

which is less than both the male and female odds ratios. This noncollapsibility can occur because, unlike the risk difference and ratio, the causal odds ratio for the total cohort is not a weighted average of the stratum-specific causal odds ratios.[22] It should not be confused with the phenomenon of confounding,[19] which was discussed earlier. Causal rate ratios and rate differences can also display noncollapsibility without confounding.[53] In particular, the causal rate ratio for a total cohort can be closer to the null than all of the stratum-specific causal rate ratios. To show this, we extend the preceding example as follows. Suppose that the risk period in the example was the year from January 1, 2015, to December 31, 2015, that all persons falling ill would do so on January 1, and that no one else was removed from risk during the year. Then, the rates would be proportional to the odds because none of the cases would contribute a meaningful amount of person-time. As a result, the causal rate ratios for men and women would be 4.0 and 4.3, whereas the causal rate ratio for the total cohort would be only 3.3.

As discussed earlier, risk, rate, and odds ratios will approximate one another if the population at risk would decline only slightly in size over the risk period, regardless of exposure. If this condition holds in all strata, the rate ratios and odds ratios will approximate the respective risk ratios in the strata, and hence, both measures will be approximately collapsible when the risk ratio is collapsible.

ATTRIBUTABLE FRACTIONS

One often sees measures that attempt to assess the public health impact of an exposure by measuring its contribution to the total incidence under the exposed condition. For convenience, we will refer to the entire family of such fractional measures as *attributable fractions*.[54] The terms *attributable risk percent* or just *attributable risk* are often used as synonyms, although "attributable risk" is also used to denote the risk difference.[55-57] Such fractions may be divided into two broad classes, which we shall term *excess fractions* and *etiologic fractions*, the former being the proportion of disease that could be eliminated by eliminating the exposure and the latter being the proportion actually caused by the exposure.

A fundamental difficulty is that the two classes are usually confused, yet excess fractions can be much smaller than etiologic fractions, even if the disease is rare. Another difficulty is that etiologic fractions are not estimable from epidemiologic studies alone, even if those studies are perfectly valid: Assumptions about the underlying biologic mechanism must be introduced to estimate etiologic fractions, and the estimates will be very sensitive to those assumptions.

Excess Fractions

One family of attributable fractions is based on recalculating an incidence difference as a proportion or fraction of the total incidence under exposure. One such measure is $(A_1 - A_0)/A_1$, the excess caseload due to exposure, which has been called the *excess fraction*,[58] where, as earlier in the chapter, A_1 and A_0 are the number of cases that would have occurred in follow-up had the entire population been exposed or unexposed, respectively. In a cohort, the fraction of the exposed incidence proportion $R_1 = A_1/N$ that is attributable to exposure is exactly equal to the excess fraction:

$$\frac{R_1 - R_0}{R_1} = \frac{A_1/N - A_0/N}{A_1/N} = \frac{A_1 - A_0}{A_1}$$

where $R_0 = A_0/N$ is what the incidence proportion would be under the unexposed condition. Comparing this formula to the earlier formula for the risk fraction $(R_1 - R_0)/R_1 = (RR - 1)/RR$, we see that in a cohort, the excess caseload and the risk fraction are equal.

The rate fraction $(I_1 - I_0)/I_1 = (IR - 1)/IR$ is often mistakenly equated with the excess fraction $(A_1 - A_0)/A_1$. To see that the two are not equal, let T_1 and T_0 represent the total time at risk that would be experienced by the cohort under the exposed and unexposed conditions, respectively, during the interval of interest. The rate fraction then equals

$$\frac{A_1/T_1 - A_0/T_0}{A_1/T_1}$$

If exposure has any effect and the disease removes people from further risk (as when the disease is irreversible), then T_1 will be less than T_0. Thus, the last expression cannot equal the excess fraction $(A_1 - A_0)/A_1$ because $T_1 \neq T_0$, although if the exposure effect on total time at risk is small, T_1 will be close to T_0, and so the rate fraction will approximate the excess fraction.

Etiologic Fractions

Suppose that all sufficient causes of a particular disease were divided into two sets, those that contain the exposed condition as a component cause and those that do not, and that the exposure is never preventive. This situation is summarized in Figure 5-1. C and C' may represent many different combinations of causal components. Each of the two sets of sufficient causes represents

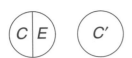

FIGURE 5-1 Two types of sufficient causes of a disease.

a theoretically large variety of causal mechanisms for disease, perhaps as many as one distinct mechanism for every case that occurs. Disease can occur either with or without E, the exposure of interest. The causal mechanisms are grouped in the diagram according to whether or not they contain the exposed condition. We say that exposure can cause disease if exposure will cause disease under at least some set of conditions C. We say that the exposure E caused disease if a sufficient cause that contains E is the sufficient cause that actually brought about the disease.

At first, it seems a simple matter to ask what fraction of cases was actually caused by exposure. We will call this fraction the *etiologic fraction*. Because we can estimate the total number of cases, we could estimate the etiologic fraction if we could estimate the number of cases that were actually caused by E. Unfortunately, this number is not estimable from ordinary incidence data because the observation of an exposed case does not reveal the mechanism that caused the case. Using the potential-outcomes language introduced above, one cannot identify whether a particular exposed case was type 1 or type 2. Type 1 people who have the exposure can develop the disease from a mechanism that does not include the exposure. For example, a smoker may develop lung cancer through some mechanism that does not involve smoking (*e.g.*, one involving asbestos or radiation exposure, with no contribution from smoking). For such lung cancer cases, smoking was incidental; it did not contribute to the cancer causation. There is no general way to tell which factors are responsible for a given case. Therefore, exposed cases include some cases of disease caused by the exposure, if the exposure is indeed a cause (type 2), and some cases of disease that occur through mechanisms that do not involve the exposure (type 1).

The observed incidence rate or proportion among the exposed reflects the incidence of cases in both sets of sufficient causes represented in Figure 5-1. The incidence of sufficient causes containing E could be found by subtracting the incidence of the sufficient causes that lack E. The latter incidence cannot be estimated if we cannot distinguish cases for which exposure played an etiologic role from cases for which exposure was irrelevant.[58,59] Thus, if I_1 is the incidence rate of disease in a population under the exposed condition and I_0 is the rate in that population under the unexposed condition, the rate difference $I_1 - I_0$ does not necessarily equal the rate of disease arising from sufficient causes with the exposure as a component cause and need not even be close to that rate.

To see the source of this difficulty, imagine a cohort in which, for every member, the causal complement of exposure, C, will be completed before the sufficient cause C' is completed. If the cohort is unexposed, every case of disease must be attributable to the cause C'. But if the cohort is exposed from start of the follow-up, every case of disease occurs when C is completed (E being already present), so every case of disease must be attributable to the sufficient cause containing C and E. Thus, the incidence rate of cases caused by exposure is I_1 when under the exposed condition, not $I_1 - I_0$, and thus the fraction of cases caused by exposure is 1, or 100%, even though the rate fraction $(I_1 - I_0)/I_1$ may be very small.

Excess fractions and rate fractions are often incorrectly interpreted as etiologic fractions. The preceding example shows that these fractions can be far less than the etiologic fraction: In the example, the rate fraction will be close to 0 if the rate difference is small relative to I_1, but the etiologic fraction will remain 1, regardless of A_0 or I_0. There are conditions under which the rate fraction and etiologic fraction are equal,[60-62] but these conditions are not testable with epidemiologic data and rarely have any supporting evidence or genuine plausibility.[60,61] One condition sometimes cited is that exposure acts independently of background causes, which will be examined further in a later section. Without such assumptions, however, the most we can say is that the excess fraction provides a lower bound on the etiologic fraction.

One condition that is irrelevant yet is sometimes given is that the disease is rare. To see that this condition is irrelevant, note that the above example made no use of the absolute frequency of the disease; the excess and rate fractions could still be near 0 even if the etiologic fraction was near 1. Disease rarity only brings the case and rate fractions closer to one another, in the same way as it brings the risk and rate ratios close together (assuming exposure does not have a large effect on the person-time); it does not bring the rate fraction close to the etiologic fraction.

Probability of Causation and Susceptibility to Exposure

To further illustrate the difference between excess and etiologic fractions, suppose that at a given time in a cohort, a fraction F of completions of C' was preceded by completions of C. Again, no case can be attributable to exposure if the cohort is unexposed. But if the cohort is exposed, a fraction F of the A_0 cases that would have occurred under the unexposed condition will now be caused by the exposed condition. In addition, there may be cases caused by exposure for whom disease would never have occurred. Let A_0 and A_1 be the numbers of cases that would occur over a given interval under the unexposed and exposed conditions, respectively. A fraction $1 - F$ of A_0 cases would be unaffected by exposure; for these cases, completions of C' precede completions of C. The product $A_0(1 - F)$ is the number of cases unaffected by exposure. Subtracting this product from A_1 gives $A_1 - A_0(1 - F)$ for the number of cases in which exposure played an etiologic role. The fraction of A_1 cases attributable to C (a sufficient cause that requires the exposed condition as a component cause) is thus

$$\frac{A_1 - A_0(1 - F)}{A_1} = 1 - (1 - F)/RR$$

If we randomly sample one case, this etiologic fraction formula equals the probability that exposure caused that case or the *probability of causation* for the case. Although it is of great biologic and legal interest, this probability cannot be epidemiologically estimated if nothing is known about the fraction F.[58,60-63]

For preventive exposures, let F now be the fraction of exposed cases A_1 for whom disease would have been caused by a mechanism requiring the unexposed condition. Then, the product $A_1(1 - F)$ is the number of cases unaffected by exposure; subtracting this product from A_0 gives $A_0 - A_1(1 - F)$ for the number of cases in which exposure would play a preventive role. The fraction of the A_0 unexposed cases that were caused by the unexposed condition (*i.e.*, attributable to a sufficient cause with the unexposed condition as a component cause) is thus

$$[A_0 - A_1(1 - F)]/A_0 = 1 - RR(1 - F) \tag{5-1}$$

As with the etiologic fraction, this fraction cannot be estimated if nothing is known about F.

Returning to a causal exposure, it is commonly assumed, often without statement or supporting evidence, that completion of C and C' occurs independently in the cohort, so that the probability of "susceptibility" to exposure, $\Pr(C)$, can be derived by the ordinary laws of probability for independent events. Now $\Pr(C') = A_0/N = R_0$; thus, under independence

$$\Pr(C \text{ or } C') = A_1/N = R_1$$
$$= \Pr(C) + \Pr(C') - \Pr(C)\Pr(C')$$
$$= \Pr(C) + R_0 - \Pr(C)R_0 \tag{5-2}$$

Rearrangement yields

$$\Pr(C) = \frac{A_1/N - A_0/N}{1 - A_0/N} = \frac{R_1 - R_0}{1 - R_0} \tag{5-3}$$

The right-hand expression is the causal risk difference divided by the proportion surviving under the unexposed condition. Hence, the equation can be rewritten

$$\Pr(C) = (R_1 - R_0)/S_0 = (S_0 - S_1)/S_0 = 1 - S_1/S_0$$

This measure was first derived by Sheps,[64] who referred to it as the *relative difference*. It was later proposed as an index of susceptibility to exposure effects based on the independence assumption.[65] But as with the independence condition, one cannot verify Equation 5-3 from epidemiologic data alone, and it is rarely if ever plausible on biologic grounds.

A Note on Terminology

More than with other concepts, there is profoundly inconsistent and confusing terminology across the literature on attributable fractions. Levin (1953) used the term *attributable proportion* for his original measure of population disease impact,[66] which, in our terms, is an excess fraction or risk fraction. Many epidemiologic texts thereafter used the term *attributable risk* to refer to the risk difference $R_1 - R_0$ and called Levin's measure, an *attributable risk percent*.[55,57] By the 1970s, however, portions of the biostatistics literature began calling Levin's measure an *attributable risk*,[67,68] and unfortunately, part of the epidemiologic literature followed suit. Some epidemiologists struggled to keep the distinction by introducing the term *attributable fraction* for Levin's concept[69,70]; others adopted the term *etiologic fraction* for the same concept and thus confused it with the fraction of cases caused by exposure. Complicating matters further, the fractions we have considered concerned excess and etiologic fractions for the entire population, but one can also consider, as we did with the probability of causation, what proportion of *diseased cases* could be eliminated or are caused by an exposure, and such measures are sometimes also referred to as "attributable fractions." In any case, the term *attributable risk* continues to be used for completely different concepts, such as the risk difference, the risk fraction, the rate fraction, and the etiologic fraction. Because of this confusion, we recommend that the term *attributable risk* be avoided entirely, and that the term *etiologic fraction* not be used for relative excess measures.

GENERALIZING DEFINITIONS OF EFFECT

For convenience, we have given the above definitions for the situation in which we can imagine the cohort of the interest subject to either of two distinct conditions, treatments, interventions, or exposure levels over (or at the start of) the time interval of interest. We ordinarily think of these exposed and unexposed conditions as applying separately to each cohort member. But to study public health interventions, we must generalize our concept of exposure conditions to populations and allow variation in exposure effects across individuals and subgroups. We can therefore also consider the exposure condition of a population as referring to the *pattern* of exposure (or treatment) among the individuals in the population. That is, we can consider the subscripts 1 and 0 to denote different *distributions* of exposure across the population. With this view, effect measures refer to comparisons of outcome distributions under contrasting pairs of exposure patterns across the population of interest.[8,11]

To illustrate this general epidemiologic concept of effect, suppose our population comprises just three members with BMI greater than 30 kg/m^2 at the start of a 5-year interval. Let us give these people identifying numbers, 1, 2, and 3, respectively. Suppose we are concerned with the effect of different distributions (patterns) of mailed diet and exercise programs on the occurrence of diabetes in this population during the interval. One possible exposure pattern is
    Person 1: Mailing at the start of interval and quarterly thereafter.
    Person 2: Mailing at the start of interval and yearly thereafter.
    Person 3: No mailing.
    Call this pattern 0 or the reference pattern. Another possible exposure pattern is
    Person 1: No mailing.
    Person 2: Mailing at the start of interval and yearly thereafter.
    Person 3: Mailing at the start of interval and quarterly thereafter.
    Call this exposure pattern 1 or the index pattern; it differs from pattern 0 only in that the treatment of persons 1 and 3 are interchanged.
    Under both patterns, one-third of the population receives yearly mailings, one-third receives quarterly mailings, and one-third receives no mailing. Yet, it is perfectly reasonable that pattern

0 may produce a different outcome from pattern 1. For example, suppose person 1 would simply discard the mailings unopened, and so under either pattern would retain the same BMI and develop diabetes at year 4. Person 2 receives the same treatment under either pattern; suppose that under either pattern person 2 dies at year 1 of a myocardial infarction. But suppose person 3 would retain the same BMI under pattern 0, until at year 3, she develops diabetes, whereas, under pattern 1, she would read the mailings, successfully improve her diet and exercise habits, and as a consequence never develop diabetes before the end of follow-up.

The total cases of diabetes and accumulated person-time under exposure pattern 0 would be $A_0 = 2$ and $T_0 = 4 + 1 + 3 = 8$ years, whereas the total cases of diabetes and accumulated person-time under exposure pattern 1 would be $A_1 = 1$ and $T_1 = 4 + 1 + 5 = 10$ years. The effects of pattern 1 versus pattern 0 on this population would thus be to decrease the incidence rate from $2/8 = 0.25$ per year to $1/10 = 0.10$ per year, a causal rate difference of $0.10 - 0.25 = 0.15$ per year and a causal rate ratio of $0.10/0.25 = 0.4$; to decrease the incidence proportion from $2/3 = 0.667$ to $1/3 = 0.333$, a causal risk difference of $0.333 - 0.667 = -0.334$ and a causal risk ratio of $0.333/0.667 = 0.5$; and to increase the total years of life lived free of diabetes from 8 to 10. The fraction of diabetes under pattern 0 that is preventable by pattern 1 is $(2-1)/2 = 0.5$, which equals the fraction of diabetes under pattern 0 for whom change to pattern 1 would have etiologic relevance. In contrast, the fraction of the rate "prevented" (removed) by pattern 1 relative to pattern 0 is $(0.25 - 0.10)/0.25 = 1 - 0.4 = 0.6$ and represents only the rate reduction under pattern 1; it does not equal an etiologic fraction.

This example illustrates two key points that epidemiologists should bear in mind when interpreting effect measures and associations meant to estimate them:

1. Effects on incidence rates are not the same as effects on incidence proportions (average risks). Common terminology, such as "relative risk," invites confusion among effect measures. Unless the outcome is uncommon for all exposure patterns under study during the interval of interest, the type of relative risk must be kept distinct. In the preceding example, the rate ratio was 0.4, whereas the risk ratio was 0.5. Likewise, the type of attributable fraction must be kept distinct. In the preceding example, the preventable fraction of diabetes was 0.5, whereas the preventable fraction of the rate was 0.6.
2. Not all individuals respond alike to exposures or treatments. Therefore, it is not always sufficient to distinguish exposure patterns by simple summaries, such as "80% exposed" versus "20% exposed." In the preceding example, both exposure patterns had one-third of the population given quarterly mailings and one-third given yearly mailings, so the patterns were indistinguishable based on exposure prevalence. The effects were produced entirely by the differences in responsiveness of the persons treated.

POPULATION-ATTRIBUTABLE FRACTIONS AND IMPACT FRACTIONS

One often sees *population-attributable risk percent* or *population-attributable fraction* defined as the reduction in incidence that would be achieved if the population had been entirely unexposed, compared with its current (actual) exposure pattern. This concept, due to Levin,[66] who called it an *attributable proportion*, is a special case of the definition of attributable fraction based on the exposure pattern. In particular, it is a comparison of the incidence (either rate or number of cases, which must be kept distinct) under the observed pattern of exposure with the incidence under a counterfactual pattern in which exposure or treatment is entirely absent from the population.

Complete removal of an exposure is often very unrealistic, as with smoking, poor diet, lack of exercise, poverty, and air pollution. Even with legal restrictions, government programs, fitness incentives, and cessation or cleanup programs, many people will continue to expose themselves or to be exposed. A measure that allows for these realities is the *impact fraction*,[71] which is a comparison of incidence under the observed exposure pattern with incidence under a counterfactual pattern in which exposure is only partially removed from the population. Again, this is a special case of our definition of attributable fraction based on the exposure pattern.

STANDARDIZED MEASURES OF ASSOCIATION AND EFFECT

Consider again the concept of standardization as introduced at the end of Chapter 4. Given a standard distribution $T_1, \ldots, T_K$ of person-times across K categories or strata defined by one or more variables and a schedule $I_1, \ldots, I_K$ of incidence rates in those categories, we have the standardized rate

$$I_s = \frac{\sum_{k=1}^{K} T_k I_k}{\sum_{k=1}^{K} T_k}$$

which is the average of the I_k weighted by the T_k. If $I_1{}^*, \ldots, I_K{}^*$ represents another schedule of rates for the same categories, and

$$I_s^* = \frac{\sum_{k=1}^{K} T_k I_k^*}{\sum_{k=1}^{K} T_k}$$

$$IR_s = \frac{I_s}{I_s^*} = \sum T_k I_k \Big/ \sum T_k I_k^*$$

is called a *standardized rate ratio*. The defining feature of this ratio is that the same standard distribution is used to weight the numerator and denominator rate. Similarly,

$$ID_s = \frac{\sum T_k I_k}{\sum T_k} - \frac{\sum T_k I_k^*}{\sum T_k} = \frac{\sum T_k \left(I_k - I_k^* \right)}{\sum T_k}$$

is called the *standardized rate difference*; note that it is not only a difference of standardized rates but is also a weighted average of the stratum-specific rate differences $I_k - I_k^*$ using the same weights as were used for the standardization (the T_k).

Suppose that $I_1, \ldots, I_k$ represent the rates observed or predicted for strata of a given target population if it is exposed to some cause, $T_1, \ldots, T_k$ are the observed person-time in strata of that population, and $I_1{}^*, \ldots, I_k{}^*$ represent the rates predicted or observed for strata of the population under the unexposed condition. The presumption is then that $IR_s = I_s/I_s^*$ and ID_s are the effects of exposure on this population, comparing the overall (crude) rates that would occur under distinct exposure conditions. This interpretation assumes, however, that the relative distribution of person-times would be unaffected by exposure.

If $I_1{}^*, \ldots, I_k{}^*$ represent counterfactual rather than actual rates, say, because the population was actually exposed, then I_s^* need not represent the overall rate that would occur in the population under the unexposed condition. For instance, the change in rates from the I_k to the I_k^* could shift the person-time distribution $T_1, \ldots, T_k$ to $T_1{}^*, \ldots, T_k{}^*$. In addition, as discussed earlier, the exposure could affect competing risks, and this effect could also shift the person-time distribution. If this shift is large, the standardized rate ratio and difference will not properly reflect the actual effect of exposure on the rate of disease.[53]

There are a few special conditions under which the effect of exposure on person-time will not affect the standardized rate ratio. If the stratum-specific ratios I_k/I_k^* are constant across categories, the standardized rate ratio will equal this constant stratum-specific ratio. If the exposure has only a small effect on person-time, then, regardless of the person-time distribution used as the standard, the difference between a standardized ratio and the actual effect will also be small. In general, however, one should be alert to the fact that a special assumption is needed to allow one to interpret a standardized rate ratio as an effect measure, even if there is no methodologic problem with the observations. Analogously, the standardized rate difference will not be an effect measure except when exposure does not affect the person-time distribution or when other special conditions exist, such as constant rate differences $I_k - I_k^*$ across categories.

Incidence proportions have denominators $N_1, \ldots, N_k$ that are not affected by changing rates or competing risks. Thus, if these denominators are used to create standardized risk ratios and differences, the resulting measures may be interpreted as effect measures without the need for the special assumptions required to interpret standardized rate ratios and differences.

Standardized Morbidity Ratios

When the distribution of exposed person-time provides the standard, the standardized rate ratio takes on a simplified form. Suppose $T_1, \ldots, T_k$ are the exposed person time, $A_1, \ldots, A_k$ are the number of cases in the exposed, $I_1, \ldots, I_k$ are the rates in the exposed, and $I_1^*, \ldots, I_k^*$ are the rates that would have occurred in the exposed under the unexposed condition. Then, in each stratum, we have $T_k I_k = A_k$, so the standardized rate ratio becomes

$$\sum T_k I_k \Big/ \sum T_k I_k^* = A_k \Big/ \sum T_k I_k^*$$

The numerator of this ratio is just the total number of exposed cases occurring in the population. The denominator is the number of cases that would be expected to occur under the unexposed condition if the exposure did not affect the distribution of person-time. This ratio of observed to expected cases is called the *standardized morbidity ratio* (SMR), *standardized incidence ratio* (SIR), or, when death is the outcome, the *standardized mortality ratio*. When incidence proportions are used in place of incidence rates, the same sort of simplification occurs upon taking the exposed distribution of persons as the standard: The standardized risk ratio reduces to a ratio of observed to expected cases.

Many occupational and environmental studies that examine populations of exposed workers attempt to estimate SMRs by using age-sex-race categories as strata, and then use age-sex-race specific rates from the general population in place of the desired counterfactual rates $I_1^*, \ldots, I_k^*$. A problem with this practice is that of *residual confounding*. There may be many other differences between the exposed population and the general population besides their age, sex, and race distributions (differences in the prevalence and history of tobacco use, quality of health care, etc.), and some of these differences may confound the resulting standardized ratio. This problem is an example of the more common problem of residual confounding in nonrandomized epidemiology, to which we will return in later chapters.

SMRs estimated across exposure categories or different populations are sometimes compared directly with one another to assess a dose-response trend, for example. Such comparisons are potentially misleading because each exposure category's SMR is weighted by the distribution of that category's person-time or persons, and these weights are not necessarily comparable across the exposure categories. The result is different amounts of residual confounding by the variables used to create the strata within which weights were computed, as well as by unmeasured variables.[72-74] There are, however, several circumstances under which this difference in weights will not lead to important confounding beyond the residual confounding problem discussed earlier.

One circumstance is when the compared populations differ little in their distribution of person-time across the strata within which weights were computed (*e.g.*, when they have similar age-sex-race distributions). Another circumstance is when the stratification factors have little effect on the outcome under study, which is unusual because age and sex are usually among the stratification factors and strongly related to most outcomes. Yet another circumstance is when the stratum-specific ratios are nearly constant across strata within which weights were computed, which corresponds to negligible modification of the ratio by the standardization variables.[73] Although none of these circumstances may hold exactly, the first and last are often together roughly approximated; when this is so, the lack of common standardization weights among compared SMRs will lead to little distortion. Attention can then turn to the many other validity problems that plague SMR studies, such as residual confounding, missing data, and measurement error (see Chapters 12, 13, and 16). If, however, one cannot be confident that the distortion due to comparing SMRs directly is small, estimates should be based on a single common standard applied to the risks in all groups or on a regression model that accounts for the differences among the compared populations and the effects of exposure on person-time.

PREVALENCE RATIOS

In Chapter 4, we showed that the crude prevalence odds, PO, equals the crude incidence rate, I, times the average disease duration, $\bar{D}$, when both the population at risk and the prevalence pool are stationary and there is no migration in or out of the prevalence pool. Restating this relation separately for a single population under exposed and unexposed conditions, or one exposed and one unexposed population, we have

$$PO_1 = I_1 \overline{D_1} \text{ and } PO_0 = I_0 \overline{D_0} \qquad\qquad [5\text{-}4]$$

where the subscripts 1 and 0 refer to exposed and unexposed, respectively. If the average disease duration is the same regardless of exposure, *i.e.*, if $\overline{D_1} = \overline{D_0}$, the crude prevalence odds ratio, POR, will equal the crude incidence rate ratio IR:

$$POR = \frac{PO_1}{PO_0} = \frac{I_1}{I_0} = IR \qquad\qquad [5\text{-}5]$$

Unfortunately, if exposure affects mortality, it will also alter the age distribution of the population. Thus, because older people tend to die sooner, exposure will indirectly affect average duration, so that $\overline{D_1}$ will not equal $\overline{D_0}$. In that case, Equation 5-5 will not hold exactly, although it may still hold approximately.[75]

OTHER MEASURES

The measures that we have discussed are by no means exhaustive of all those that have been proposed. Not all proposed measures of effect meet our definition of effect measure—that is, not all are a contrast of the outcome of a *single* population under two *different* conditions. Examples of measures that are *not* effect measures by our definition include correlation coefficients and related variance-reduction measures.[76,77] Examples of measures that are effect measures by our definition, but not discussed in detail here, include expected years of life lost,[78] as well as risk and rate advancement periods.[79]

Years of life lost, $T_0/N - T_1/N$, and the corresponding ratio measure, T_0/T_1, have some noteworthy advantages over conventional rate and risk-based effect measures. They are not subject to the problems of inestimability that arise for etiologic fractions,[80] nor are they subject to concerns about exposure effects on time at risk. In fact, they represent the exposure effect on time at risk. They are, however, more difficult to estimate statistically from typical epidemiologic data, especially when only case-control data (see Chapter 8) are available, which may in part explain their limited popularity thus far.[81]

References

1. Poole C. On the origin of risk relativism. *Epidemiology*. 2010;21(1):3-9.
2. Greenland S, Morgenstern H. Confounding in health research. *Annu Rev Public Health*. 2001;22:189-212.
3. Greenland S. An overview of methods for causal inference from observational studies. In: Gelman A, Meng XL, eds. *Applied Bayesian Modeling and Causal Inference from an Incomplete-Data Perspective*. New York, NY: Wiley; 2004.
4. Lewis D. Causation. *J Philos*. 1973;70:556-567.
5. Rubin DB. Comment: Neyman (1923) and causal inference in experiments and observational studies. *Stat Sci*. 1990;5:472-480.
6. Greenland S. Causal analysis in the health sciences. *J Am Stat Assoc*. 2000;95:286-289.
7. Rubin DB. Estimating causal effects of treatments in randomized and nonrandomized studies. *J Educ Psychol*. 1974;66:688-701.
8. Greenland S. Causality theory for policy uses of epidemiologic measures. In: Murray CJL, Salomon JA, Mathers CD, Lopez AD, eds. *Summary Measures of Population Health*. Cambridge, MA: Harvard University Press/WHO; 2002:291-302.
9. Greenland S. Epidemiologic measures and policy formulation: lessons from potential outcomes. *Emerg Themes Epidemiol*. 2005;2:5.

10. Hernán MA. Hypothetical interventions to define causal effects—afterthought or prerequisite? *Am J Epidemiol*. 2005;162:618-620.
11. Maldonado G, Greenland S. Estimating causal effects. *Int J Epidemiol*. 2002;31(2):422-429.
12. Hofler M. Causal inference based on counterfactuals. *BMC Med Res Methodol*. 2005;5:28.
13. Frangakis CE, Rubin DB, An MW, MacKenzie E. Principal stratification designs to estimate input data missing due to death. *Biometrics*. 2007;63(3):641-649; discussion 650-62.
14. Hayden D, Pauler DK, Schoenfeld D. An estimator for treatment comparisons among survivors in randomized trials. *Biometrics*. 2005;61(1):305-310.
15. Egleston BL, Scharfstein DO, Freeman EE, West SK. Causal inference for non-mortality outcomes in the presence of death. *Biostatistics*. 2007;8(3):526-545.
16. Rubin DB. Causal inference through potential outcomes and principal stratification: application to studies with "Censoring" due to death. *Statist Sci*. 2006;21(3):299-309.
17. Chiba Y, VanderWeele TJ. A simple method for principal strata effects when the outcome has been truncated due to death. *Am J Epidemiol*. 2011;173(7):745-751.
18. Greenland S, Robins JM. Identifiability, exchangeability, and epidemiological confounding. *Int J Epidemiol*. 1986;15(3):413-419.
19. Greenland S, Robins JM, Pearl J. Confounding and collapsibility in causal inference. *Stat Sci*. 1999;14:29-46.
20. Vander Weele TJ. Confounding and effect modification: distribution and measure. *Epidemiol Method*. 2012;1(1):55-82.
21. Miettinen OS, Cook EF. Confounding: essence and detection. *Am J Epidemiol*. 1981;114(4):593-603.
22. Greenland S. Interpretation and choice of effect measures in epidemiologic analyses. *Am J Epidemiol*. 1987;125(5):761-768.
23. Greenland S, Robins JM. Identifiability, exchangeability and confounding revisited. *Epidemiol Perspect Innov*. 2009;6:4.
24. Gatto NM, Campbell UB. Redundant causation from a sufficient cause perspective. *Epidemiol Perspect Innov*. 2010;7:5.
25. VanderWeele TJ. Causal interactions in the proportional hazards model. *Epidemiology*. 2011;22(5):713-717.
26. Suzuki E, Yamamoto E, Tsuda T. On the relations between excess fraction, attributable fraction, and etiologic fraction. *Am J Epidemiol*. 2012;175(6):567-575.
27. Lee WC. Assessing causal mechanistic interactions: a peril ratio index of synergy based on multiplicativity. *PLoS One*. 2013;8(6):e67424.
28. VanderWeele TJ, Shpitser I. On the definition of a confounder. *Ann Stat*. 2013;41(1):196-220.
29. Hernan MA, VanderWeele TJ. Compound treatments and transportability of causal inference. *Epidemiology*. 2011;22(3):368-377.
30. Rubin DB. Randomization analysis of experimental data: the Fisher randomization test comment. *J Am Stat Assoc*. 1980;75(371):591-593.
31. VanderWeele TJ, Hernan MA. Causal inference under multiple versions of treatment. *J Causal Inference*. 2013;1(1):1-20.
32. Tchetgen EJ, VanderWeele TJ. On causal inference in the presence of interference. *Stat Methods Med Res*. 2012;21(1):55-75.
33. Cox DR. *The Planning of Experiments*. New York, NY: Wiley; 1958.
34. Hudgens MG, Halloran ME. Toward causal inference with interference. *J Am Stat Assoc*. 2008;103(482):832-842.
35. Rubin DB. Statistics and causal inference—which ifs have causal answers. *J Am Stat Assoc*. 1986;81(396):961-962.
36. Schwartz S, Gatto NM, Campbell UB. Extending the sufficient component cause model to describe the stable unit treatment value assumption (SUTVA). *Epidemiol Perspect Innov*. 2012;9:3.
37. Cole SR, Frangakis CE. The consistency statement in causal inference: a definition or an assumption? *Epidemiology*. 2009;20(1):3-5.
38. VanderWeele TJ. Concerning the consistency assumption in causal inference. *Epidemiology*. 2009;20(6):880-883.
39. Pearl J. On the consistency rule in causal inference: axiom, definition, assumption, or theorem? *Epidemiology*. 2010;21(6):872-875.
40. Petersen ML, Porter KE, Gruber S, Wang Y, van der Laan MJ. Diagnosing and responding to violations in the positivity assumption. *Stat Methods Med Res*. 2012;21(1):31-54.
41. Pearl J. An introduction to causal inference. *Int J Biostat* 2010;6(2):Article 7.
42. Pearl J. Causal diagrams for empirical research. *Biometrika*. 1995;82:669-710.
43. Pearl J. *Causality: Models, Reasoning and Inference*. Cambridge, UK: Cambridge University Press; 2000.
44. Greenland S, Pearl J, Robins JM. Causal diagrams for epidemiologic research. *Epidemiology*. 1999;10(1):37-48.

45. Greenland S, Brumback B. An overview of relations among causal modelling methods. *Int J Epidemiol.* 2002;31(5):1030-1037.

46. Cornfield J. A method of estimating comparative rates from clinical data; applications to cancer of the lung, breast, and cervix. *J Natl Cancer Inst.* 1951;11(6):1269-1275.

47. Greenland S, Thomas DC. On the need for the rare disease assumption in case-control studies. *Am J Epidemiol.* 1982;116(3):547-553.

48. Kaufman JS, MacLehose RF. Which of these things is not like the others?. *Cancer.* 2013;119(24):4216-4222.

49. VanderWeele TJ. On the distinction between interaction and effect modification. *Epidemiology.* 2009;20(6):863-871.

50. VanderWeele TJ, Knol MJ. Interpretation of subgroup analyses in randomized trials: heterogeneity versus secondary interventions. *Ann Intern Med.* 2011;154(10):680-683.

51. Berkson J. Smoking and lung cancer: some observations on two recent reports. *J Am Stat Assoc.* 1958;53:28-38.

52. Brumback BA, Berg A. On effect-measure modification: relations among changes in the relative risk, odds ratio, and risk difference. *Stat Med.* 2008;27:3453-3465.

53. Greenland S. Absence of confounding does not correspond to collapsibility of the rate ratio or rate difference. *Epidemiology.* 1996;7(5):498-501.

54. Poole C. A history of the population attributable fraction and related measures. *Ann Epidemiol.* 2015;25(3):147-154.

55. MacMahon B, Pugh TF. *Epidemiology: Principles and Methods.* Boston: Little, Brown; 1970.

56. Szklo M, Nieto FJ. *Epidemiology: Beyond the Basics.* Gaithersburg, MD: Aspen Publishers; 2000.

57. Koepsell TD, Weiss NS. *Epidemiologic Methods: Studying the Occurrence of Illness.* New York, NY: Oxford University Press; 2003.

58. Greenland S, Robins JM. Conceptual problems in the definition and interpretation of attributable fractions. *Am J Epidemiol.* 1988;128(6):1185-1197.

59. Greenland S. The relation of the probability of causation to the relative risk and the doubling dose: a methodologic error that has become a social problem. *Am J Public Health.* 1999;89:1166-1169.

60. Robins JM, Greenland S. Estimability and estimation of excess and etiologic fractions. *Stat Med.* 1989;8(7):845-859.

61. Robins J, Greenland S. The probability of causation under a stochastic model for individual risk. *Biometrics.* 1989;45(4):1125-1138.

62. Beyea J, Greenland S. The importance of specifying the underlying biologic model in estimating the probability of causation. *Health Phys.* 1999;76(3):269-274.

63. Greenland S, Robins JM. Epidemiology, justice, and the probability of causation. *Jurimetrics.* 2000;40:321-340.

64. Sheps MC. Shall we count the living of the dead. *N Engl J Med.* 1958;259(25):1210-1214.

65. Khoury MJ, Flanders WD, Greenland S, Adams MJ. On the measurement of susceptibility in epidemiologic studies. *Am J Epidemiol.* 1989;129(1):183-190.

66. Levin ML. The occurrence of lung cancer in man. *Acta Unio Int Contra Cancrum.* 1953;9(3):531-541.

67. Walter SD. The estimation and interpretation of attributable risk in health research. *Biometrics.* 1976;32(4):829-849.

68. Breslow NE, Day NE. *Statistical Methods in Cancer Research. Vol I: The Analysis of Case-Control Data.* Lyon: IARC; 1980.

69. Ouellet BL, Romeder JM, Lance JM. Premature mortality attributable to smoking and hazardous drinking in Canada. *Am J Epidemiol.* 1979;109(4):451-463.

70. Deubner DC, Wilkinson WE, Helms MJ, Tyroler HA, Hames CG. Logistic model estimation of death attributable to risk factors for cardiovascular disease in Evans County, Georgia. *Am J Epidemiol.* 1980;112(1):135-143.

71. Morgenstern H, Bursic ES. A method for using epidemiologic data to estimate the potential impact of an intervention on the health status of a target population. *J Community Health.* 1982;7(4):292-309.

72. Yule GU. On some points related to vital statistics, more especially statistics of occupational mortality. *J R Stat Soc.* 1934;97:1-84.

73. Breslow NE, Day NE. *Statistical Methods in Cancer Research. Vol II: The Design and Analysis of Cohort Studies.* Lyon: IARC; 1987.

74. Greenland S. Bias in indirectly adjusted comparisons due to taking the total study population as the reference group. *Stat Med.* 1987;6(2):193-195.

75. Newman SC. Odds ratio estimation in a steady-state population. *J Clin Epidemiol.* 1988;41(1):59-65.

76. Greenland S, Schlesselman JJ, Criqui MH. The fallacy of employing standardized regression coefficients and correlations as measures of effect. *Am J Epidemiol.* 1986;123(2):203-208.

77. Greenland S, Maclure M, Schlesselman JJ, Poole C, Morgenstern H. Standardized regression coefficients: a further critique and review of some alternatives. *Epidemiology.* 1991;2(5):387-392.

78. Murray CJL, Salomon JA, Mathers CD, Lopez AD. *Summary Measures of Population Health*. Cambridge, MA: Harvard University Press/WHO; 2002.
79. Brenner H, Gefeller O, Greenland S. Risk and rate advancement periods as measures of exposure impact on the occurrence of chronic diseases. *Epidemiology*. 1993;4(3):229-236.
80. Robins J, Greenland S. Estimability and estimation of expected years of life lost due to a hazardous exposure. *Stat Med*. 1991;10(1):79-93.
81. Boshuizen HC, Greenland S. Average age at first occurrence as an alternative occurrence parameter in epidemiology. *Int J Epidemiol*. 1997;26(4):867-872.

Epidemiologic Study Design With Validity and Efficiency Considerations

Kenneth J. Rothman and Timothy L. Lash

INTRODUCTION

The aim of epidemiologic research is to understand the distribution of disease as well as the causes and noncausal predictors of diseases and disease outcomes in a population. The type of study designs appropriate to a given research problem will depend on the study aims, strengths and limitations of earlier studies of the problem, available resources, and other circumstances.

Epidemiologic study designs comprise both experimental and nonexperimental studies. The scientific experiment is iconic, but what constitutes an experiment? In common parlance, an experiment refers to any trial or test. For example, a professor might introduce new teaching methods as an experiment to see whether students better understand the course materials. For scientists, however, the term has a more specific meaning: An experiment is a set of observations, conducted under controlled circumstances, in which the scientist manipulates the conditions to ascertain what effect, if any, such manipulation has on the observations. Ideally, the experiment will shed light on the underlying principles that govern the events studied. For epidemiologists, the experimenter hopes to gain insight into the effects of an intervention.

This definition of an experiment can be enlarged to include controlled observations without manipulation of the conditions. Thus, the astronomical observations during the solar eclipse of 1919 that corroborated Einstein's general theory of relativity have often been referred to as an experiment. For epidemiologists, however, the word *experiment* usually implies that the investigator implements one or more specific interventions to two or more subsets of participants in the study. The intervention offered to one group may be to carry on their lives without any changes, or something otherwise innocuous, such as to take a placebo medication. Experimental epidemiology is therefore limited to topics for which the exposure condition can be manipulated. Because the subjects who receive these manipulations are human, experimental epidemiology is further limited ethically to studies in which all exposure assignments are expected to cause no harm.

When epidemiologic experiments meet minimal standards of feasibility and ethics, their design is guided by the objectives of reducing variation in the outcome attributable to extraneous factors and accounting accurately for the remaining extraneous variation. Intervention assignments to the two or more intervention subgroups ordinarily come from applying a randomized allocation scheme. The purpose of random allocation is to create groups that differ only randomly at the time of allocation with regard to subsequent occurrence of the study outcome. This random allocation lends meaning to the inferential statistics—such as confidence limits—that often accompany estimates of effect, such as comparisons of risks in the groups, obtained from the study.[1]

Epidemiologic experiments are usually cohort studies (discussed in more general terms later in this chapter) and can be classified into three major types: clinical trials (with patients as subjects), field trials or pragmatic trials (with interventions assigned to individual community members), and community intervention trials (with interventions assigned to whole communities). When experiments are infeasible or unethical, epidemiologists design nonexperimental (also known as observational) studies to emulate what might have been learned had an experiment been conducted.[2,3] In nonexperimental studies, the researcher is an observer rather than an agent who assigns interventions. In addition to the lack of random assignment of the exposure and consequent risk of unbalanced extraneous characteristics between exposed and unexposed individuals, another common challenge of nonexperimental designs is the exposure definition itself. For example, while the meaning of a bariatric surgery intervention in an experimental study is well defined, nonexperimental studies often try to evaluate the effects of poorly defined interventions such as "obesity," for which the corresponding experiment cannot be conducted.[4]

The four main types of nonexperimental epidemiologic studies are cohort studies in which all subjects in a source population are classified according to their exposure status and followed over time to ascertain disease incidence; case-control studies in which cases arising from a source population and a sample of the source population are classified according to their exposure history; cross-sectional studies, including prevalence studies in which one ascertains exposure and disease status as of a particular time; and ecologic studies in which the units of observation are groups of people.

EXPERIMENTAL STUDIES

In a typical experimental study, two or more experimental groups are exposed to different treatments or agents. In a simple two-group experiment, ideally the experimental groups would be identical with respect to extraneous factors that affect the outcome of interest, so that if the treatment had no effect, identical outcomes would be observed for each of the groups. This theoretical objective could only be achieved if one could control all the relevant conditions that might affect the outcome under study. In the biologic sciences, however, this goal is impossible to achieve. The conditions affecting most outcomes are so complex and extensive that they are mostly unknown, and thus cannot be made uniform in the two groups. Hence, there will be variation in the outcome, even in the absence of a treatment effect, and this variation (noise) will make it difficult to observe a treatment effect (signal) when comparing the two groups. For example, even under the most stringent of conditions, the distribution of blood pressure in humans will vary from person to person and within a person from moment to moment. This "biologic variation" reflects variation in the causes that determine the effect and generates the noise that masks the treatment effect's signal. We can think of this as a random error. Of greater concern, if the factors that affect the outcome also affect or are associated with the treatment assignment, then any observed signal from the comparison of the groups is a mixture of the treatment effect, which is the signal of interest, and the effect of the factors that predict both treatment assignment and outcome. These are confounding factors (see Chapter 12), a type of systematic error.

Thus, in biologic experimentation, one rarely, if ever, can create groups across which only the study treatment varies. Instead, the investigator may settle for creating groups in which the net effect of extraneous factors is expected to be small by limiting variability of these factors. For example, it may be impossible to make all animals in an experiment eat the same amount of food. Variation in food consumption could pose a problem if it affected the outcome under study. If this variation could be kept small, however, it might contribute little to variation in the outcome across the groups. The investigator would usually be satisfied if the net effect of extraneous random and systematic factors across the groups were small, relative to the expected effect of the study treatment. Often not even that can be achieved, however. In that case, the experiment must be designed so that the variation in outcome due to extraneous factors can be measured accurately and thus accounted for in comparisons across the treatment groups.

Randomization

One way to reduce the expected variation in the net effect of extraneous factors on the estimate of treatment effects is to achieve balance in those factors across the intervention groups. Thus, food consumption might vary within groups of animals, but if the overall distribution of food consumption was the same across groups, the net effect from food consumption on the comparison of treatment effects should be close to zero. In the early 20th century, R. A. Fisher and others developed a practical basis for experimental designs that accounts accurately for extraneous variability across experimental units (whether the units are objects, animals, people, or communities). This basis is called *randomization* (random allocation) of treatments or exposures among the units. Each unit is assigned treatment by a random assignment mechanism. Such a mechanism is unrelated to the extraneous factors that affect the outcome, so any association between the treatment allocation it produces and those extraneous factors will be random. The variation in the outcome across treatment groups that is not due to treatment effects can thus be ascribed to these random associations and hence can be justifiably called chance variation. Randomization thus has two benefits. First, it breaks the link between extraneous factors and treatment assignment, creating a baseline expectation of no confounding, which addresses the potential for this type of systematic error. Second, because any imbalance of extraneous factors at baseline must therefore arise by chance, it provides a sound rationale for the assignment of a probability distribution to potential data arrangements, which addresses the potential for random error by lending credibility to inferential statistics.[1]

More formally, a hypothesis about the size of the treatment effect, such as the null hypothesis, corresponds to a specific probability distribution for the potential outcomes (see Chapters 3 and 5) under that hypothesis. This probability distribution can be compared with the observed association between treatment and outcomes. The comparison links statistics and inference, which explains why many statistical methods, such as analysis of variance, estimate random outcome variation within and across treatment groups. A study with random assignment of the treatment allows one to compute the probability of the observed association under various hypotheses about how treatment assignment affects outcome. If assignment is random and has no effect on the outcome except through treatment, any systematic (nonrandom) variation in outcome with assignment must be attributable to a treatment effect.

Scientists conducted experiments for centuries before the idea of random allocation crystallized. Experiments that have little extraneous outcome variation, such as those that often occur in physical sciences, have no need of the method. Nonetheless, some social scientists and epidemiologists identify the term *experiment* with a randomized experiment only. Sometimes, the term *quasi-experiment* is used to refer to controlled studies in which exposure was assigned by the investigator without using randomization (see Chapter 28).[5]

Ethical Considerations in Experiments on Human Subjects

In an experiment, those who are exposed to an experimental treatment are exposed because they consented to participate and the investigator assigned the exposure to them. In a purely scientific experiment, the reason for assigning the specific exposure to the particular subject is only to enhance the validity of the study. The steps necessary to reach this goal are operationalized in a study protocol. The primary reason for the assignment is to conform to the protocol, not to meet the needs of the subject.

For example, suppose that a physician treating headache had prescribed a patented drug to her wealthy patients and a generic counterpart to her indigent patients, because the presumed greater reliability of the patented version was in her judgment not worth the greater out-of-pocket cost for those of modest means. Should the physician want to compare the effects of the two medications among her patients, she could not consider herself to be conducting a valid experiment, even though the investigator herself had assigned the exposures. As introduced above, assignment was based in part on extraneous factors that could affect the outcome, such as wealth, so one would expect there to be differences among the treatment groups even if the medications had the same effect on the outcome, that is, one would expect there to be confounding (see Chapters 5 and 12). To conduct a valid experiment, she would have to assign the drugs according to a protocol that would not lead to systematic imbalance of extraneous causes of headache across the treatment groups. The assignment of exposure in experiments is designed to help the study rather than the individual subject. If it is done to help the subject, then a nonexperimental study is still possible, but it would not be considered an experiment because of the confounding that the treatment-assignment criterion might induce.

Because the goals of the study, rather than the subject's needs, determine the exposure assignment, ethical constraints limit severely the circumstances in which valid experiments on humans are feasible. Experiments on human subjects are ethically permissible only when adherence to the scientific protocol does not conflict with the subject's best interests. Specifically, there should be reasonable assurance that there is no known and feasible way a participating subject could be treated better than with the treatment possibilities that the protocol provides. From this requirement comes the constraint that any exposures or treatments given to subjects should be limited to potential preventives of disease or of adverse outcomes from a disease. This limitation alone confines most etiologic research to the nonexperimental variety.

Among the more specific ethical implications is that subjects admitted to the study should not thereby be deprived of some preferable form of treatment or preventive that is not included in the study. This requirement implies that the best available therapy should be included to provide a reference (comparison) for any new treatment. Another ethical requirement, known as *equipoise,* states that the treatment possibilities included in the trial must be equally acceptable, given current knowledge. Equipoise severely restricts the use of placebos. The Declaration of Helsinki states that it is generally unethical to include a placebo therapy as one of the arms of a clinical trial if an accepted remedy or preventive of the outcome already exists, apart from unusual circumstances.[6,7]

Even with these limitations, many epidemiologic experiments are conducted (some of which unfortunately ignore ethical principles such as equipoise). Most are clinical or pragmatic trials, which are epidemiologic studies evaluating treatments for patients who already have acquired disease (*trial* is used as a synonym for *experiment*). Epidemiologic experiments that aim to evaluate primary preventives (agents intended to prevent disease onset in the first place) are less common than clinical trials; these studies are either field trials or community intervention trials.

Clinical Trials

A clinical trial is an experiment with patients as subjects. The goal of most clinical trials is either to evaluate a potential cure for a disease or to find a preventive of disease sequelae such as death, disability, or a decline in the quality of life. The exposures in such trials are not primary preventives, because they do not prevent occurrence of the initial disease or condition, but they are preventives of the sequelae of the initial disease or condition. For example, a modified diet after an individual suffers a myocardial infarction may prevent a second infarction and subsequent death, chemotherapeutic agents given to cancer patients may prevent recurrence of cancer, and immunosuppressive drugs given to transplant patients may prevent transplant rejection.

Subjects in clinical trials of sequelae prevention must be diagnosed as having the disease in question and should be admitted to the study soon enough following diagnosis to permit the treatment assignment to occur in a timely fashion. Subjects whose illness is too mild or too severe to permit the form of treatment or alternative treatment being studied should be excluded. As noted above, treatment assignment should be designed to reduce differences between treatment groups with respect to extraneous factors that might affect the comparison. For example, if some physicians participating in the study favored the new therapy, they could conceivably influence the assignment of, say, their own patients or perhaps the more seriously afflicted patients to the new treatment. If the more seriously afflicted patients tended to get the new treatment, a type of confounding by indication, then valid evaluation of the new treatment would be compromised.[8]

To avoid this and related problems, it is desirable to assign treatments in clinical trials in a way that allows one to account for possible differences among treatment groups with respect to baseline characteristics. As part of this goal, the assignment mechanism should deter manipulation of assignments that are not part of the protocol. Randomization is the best way to deal with concerns about confounding by baseline characteristics and to avoid confounding that arises from treatment assignments based on baseline indications.[1,9–11] The validity of inferences drawn from the trial results depends strongly on having a random assignment protocol as the sole determinant of the treatments received. When this condition is satisfied, confounding due to unmeasured factors can be regarded as random, is accounted for by standard statistical procedures, and diminishes in likely magnitude as the number of subjects randomized increases.[1,12] When the condition is not satisfied, however, unmeasured confounders may bias the statistics, just as in observational studies. Unfortunately, it is difficult to identify a sufficient set of confounders to control adequately for confounding by indication.[8,13]

Given that treatment depends on random allocation, rather than patient and physician treatment decision-making, patients' enrollment into a trial requires their *informed consent*. At a minimum, informed consent requires that participants understand (a) that they are participating in a research study of a stated duration, (b) the purpose of the research, the procedures that will be followed, and which procedures are experimental, (c) that their participation is voluntary and that they can withdraw at any time, and (d) the potential risks and benefits associated with their participation.

Although randomization methods often assign subjects to treatments in approximately equal proportions, this equality is not always optimal. True equipoise provides a rationale for equal assignment proportions, but often one treatment is hypothesized to be more effective based on a biologic rationale, earlier studies, or even preliminary data from the same study. In these circumstances, equal assignment probabilities may be a barrier to enrollment. Adaptive randomization[14] or imbalanced assignment[15] allows more subjects in the trial to receive the treatment expected to be more effective with little reduction in power.

Whenever feasible, clinical trials should attempt to employ *blinding* with respect to the treatment assignment.[16] Ideally, the individual who makes the assignment, the patient, and the assessor of the outcome should all be ignorant of the treatment assignment. Blinding prevents biases that could affect assignment, assessment, or compliance. Most important is to keep the assessor blind, especially if the outcome assessment is subjective, as with a clinical diagnosis. (Some outcomes, such as death, will be relatively insusceptible to bias in assessment.) Patient knowledge of treatment assignment can affect adherence to the treatment regime and can bias perceptions of symptoms that might affect the outcome assessment. Studies in which both the assessor and the patient are blinded as to the treatment assignment are known as *double-blind studies*. A study in which the individual who makes the assignment is unaware which treatment is which (such as might occur if the treatments are coded pills and the assigner does not know the code) may be described as *triple-blind*, though this term is used more often to imply that the data analyst (in addition to the patient and the assessor) does not know which group of patients in the analysis received which treatment.

Depending on the nature of the intervention, it may not be possible or practical to keep knowledge of the assignment from all these parties. For example, a treatment may have well-known side effects that allow the patients to identify the treatment. The investigator needs to be aware of and to report these possibilities, so that readers can assess whether all or part of any reported association might be attributable to the lack of blinding.

If there is no accepted treatment for the condition being studied, it may be useful to employ a placebo as the comparison treatment, when ethical constraints allow it. *Placebos* are inert treatments intended to have no effect other than the psychologic benefit of receiving a treatment, which itself can have a powerful effect. This psychologic benefit is called a *placebo response*, even if it occurs among patients receiving active treatment. By employing a placebo, an investigator may be able to control for the psychologic component of receiving treatment and study the nonpsychologic benefits of a new intervention. In addition, employing a placebo facilitates blinding if there would otherwise be no comparison treatment. These benefits may be incomplete, however, if noticeable side effects of the active treatment enhance the placebo response (the psychologic component of treatment) among those receiving the active treatment.

Placebos are not necessary when the objective of the trial is to compare different treatments with one another. Nevertheless, even without placebos, one should be alert to the possibility of a placebo effect, or of adherence differences, due to differences in formulation or noticeable side effects among the active treatments that are assigned.

Nonadherence to or noncompliance with assigned treatment results in a discrepancy between treatment assigned and actual treatment received by trial participants. Standard practice bases all comparisons on treatment assignment rather than on treatment received. This practice is called the *intent-to-treat* principle, because the analysis is based on the intended treatment, not the received treatment. Although this principle helps preserve the validity of tests for treatment effects, it only estimates the effect of treatment assignment and tends to produce biased estimates of received treatment effects; hence, alternatives have been developed.[17] Nevertheless, alternatives such as the "as treated" or the "per protocol" approaches used in the presence of incomplete adherence and losses of follow-up break the randomization and consequently can also produce biased results.[18] Furthermore, subjects that continue with a treatment years after initiation may be a small subgroup of those initially assigned to the treatment, and may no longer be comparable with the other treatment groups with regard to extraneous factors and risk for the study outcome, even if the randomization produced a balance at the start of follow-up. Adherence may sometimes be measured by querying subjects directly about their compliance, by obtaining relevant data (*e.g.*, by asking that unused pills be returned), or by biochemical measurements. These adherence measures can then be used to adjust estimates of treatment effects using methods in which randomization plays the role of an *instrumental variable* (see Chapter 28).[19–21] Adherence-adjusted treatment effects can also be estimated with inverse probability weighting or G-estimation, which can reduce the bias introduced by nonadherence and loss to follow-up. These methods, however, require time-varying data on confounders and adherence.[22–24]

Most trials are monitored while they are being conducted by a *Data and Safety Monitoring Committee or Board* (DSMB). The primary objective of these committees is to ensure the safety of the trial participants.[25] The committee reviews study results, including estimates of the main treatment effects and the occurrence of adverse events, to determine whether the trial ought to be stopped before its scheduled completion. The rationale for early stopping might be (a) the appearance of an effect favoring one treatment that is so strong that it would no longer be ethical to randomize new patients to the alternative treatment or to deny enrolled patients access to the favored treatment, (b) the occurrence of adverse events at rates considered to be unacceptable, given the expected benefit of the treatment or trial results, or (c) the determination that the reasonably expected results are no longer of sufficient value to continue the trial. The deliberations of the DSMB involve weighing issues of medicine, ethics, law, statistics, and costs to arrive at a decision about whether to continue a trial. Given the complexity of the issues, the membership of the DSMB must comprise a diverse range of training and experiences, and thus often includes clinicians, statisticians, and ethicists, none of whom have a material interest in the trial's result.

The frequentist statistical rules commonly used by DSMB to determine whether to stop a trial were developed to ensure that the chance of Type I error (incorrect rejection of the main null hypothesis of no treatment effect; see Chapter 15) would not exceed a prespecified level (the alpha level) during the planned interim analyses.[26] Despite these goals, DSMB members may misinterpret interim results,[27] and strict adherence to these stopping rules may yield spurious results.[28] Stopping a trial early because of the appearance of an effect favoring one treatment will often result in an overestimate of the true benefit of the treatment.[29] Furthermore, trials that are stopped early may not allow sufficient follow-up to observe adverse events associated with the favored treatment,[30] particularly if those events are chronic sequelae. Bayesian alternatives have been suggested to ameliorate many of these shortcomings.[31–33]

Even when all of the conditions for optimal conduct of a clinical trial are satisfied, the *generalizability* or *transportability* (see Chapter 14) of trial results from the study population to a target population may be affected by selective enrollment. Trial participants (the study population; see Chapter 4) often do not reflect the distribution of sex, age, race, and ethnicity of the target patient population.[34–37] For reasons explained in Chapter 14, representative study populations are not always necessarily or even usually scientifically ideal. However, when treatment efficacy is modified by sex, age, race, ethnicity, or other factors and the study population differs from the target population that would be receiving the treatment with respect to these variables, then the average study effect will differ from the average effect among those who would receive treatment in the target population. In these circumstances, extrapolation of the estimates from the study population to the target population is tenuous or unwarranted, and one may have to restrict the inferences to specific subgroups or, alternatively, standardize the trial results to the target population. In the clinical trial literature, the term "efficacy" is often applied to the estimate of the treatment benefit in the study population, and the term "effectiveness" is often applied to the treatment benefit in the target population.

Practical or pragmatic clinical trials partly address concerns about the generalizability or transportability of clinical trial results by focusing on whether interventions are effective under "real-world" conditions rather than under the controlled "ideal" circumstances of many clinical trials.[38,39] In contrast to more conventional clinical trials, sometimes called "explanatory trials" in this context, pragmatic trials have wide inclusion criteria and few exclusion criteria so as to enroll a diverse population of study participants from a range of clinical practice settings.[40] The goal is to enroll a study population that reflects the range and distribution of patients observed in clinical practice for the particular medical problem, *that is,* a study population that is reasonably representative of the target population. Pragmatic trials are often large and expensive; nesting these trials in existing clinical registries[41] and cluster-randomization (see below) of participating clinical practices are two strategies to improve efficiency.[38] In addition to population-based sampling, registry-based pragmatic trials ordinarily allow rapid consecutive enrollment of patients with the trial indication and sometimes include follow-up for the outcome of interest as part of the registry activities.[42] Although explanatory and pragmatic trials are often compared dichotomously, their characteristics are not so easily binned. Explanatory trials emphasize internal validity by enrolling a restricted patient population in standardized clinical settings and with follow-up for outcomes under direct control of the trial protocol. Pragmatic trials emphasize external validity by enrolling a less-restricted patient population in a range of clinical settings and with follow-up for outcomes that sometimes rely on routine medical records, electronic health records, or registry-based protocols. Although there are these differences in emphasis, both trial designs aim to inform optimal medical care; their design differences might best be evaluated on a continuous rather than a categorical scale.[43–45]

Field Trials

Field trials differ from clinical trials in that their subjects are not defined by the presence of disease or by presentation for clinical care; instead, the focus is on the initial occurrence of disease. Patients in a clinical trial may encounter the outcomes of their disease with high probability during a relatively short time. In contrast, the risk of incident disease among persons free of the disease at the study outset is typically much lower. Consequently, field trials usually require a much larger number of subjects than clinical trials and are usually more expensive. Furthermore, because the subjects are not under active health care and thus do not come to a central location for treatment, a field trial often requires visiting subjects at work, home, or school, or establishing centers from which the study can be conducted and to which subjects are urged to report. These design features add to the cost.

The expense of field trials limits their use to the study of preventives of either extremely common or extremely serious diseases. Several field trials were conducted to determine the efficacy of large doses of vitamin C in preventing the common cold.[46,47] Paralytic poliomyelitis, a rare but serious illness, was a sufficient public health concern to warrant what may have been the largest formal human experiment ever attempted, the Salk vaccine trial, in which the vaccine or a placebo was administered to hundreds of thousands of school children.[48] When the disease outcome occurs rarely, it is more efficient to study subjects thought to be at higher risk. Thus, the trial of hepatitis B vaccine was carried out in a population of New York City male homosexuals, among whom hepatitis B infection occurred with much greater frequency than among all residents of New York.[49] Similarly, the effect of cessation of vaginal douching on the risk of pelvic inflammatory disease was studied in women with a history of recent sexually transmitted disease, a strong risk factor for pelvic inflammatory disease,[50] and the effect of finasteride on the risk of prostate cancer was studied in men at least 55 years old because age is a strong risk factor for prostate cancer.[51]

Analogous reasoning is often applied to the design of clinical trials, which may concentrate on patients at high risk of adverse outcomes. Because patients who had already experienced a myocardial infarction are at high risk for a second infarction, several clinical trials of the effect of lowering serum cholesterol levels on the risk of myocardial infarction were undertaken on such patients.[52,53] It would have been more costly to conduct a trial designed to study the effect of lowering serum cholesterol on the first occurrence of a myocardial infarction, because many more subjects would have to have been included to provide a reasonable number of outcome events to study. The Multiple Risk Factor Intervention Trial (MRFIT) was a field trial of several primary preventives of myocardial infarction, including diet. Although it admitted only high-risk individuals and endeavored to reduce risk through several simultaneous interventions, the study involved 12,866 subjects and cost the equivalent of $700 million 2015 dollars.[54]

As in clinical trials, exposures in field trials should be assigned according to a protocol that limits extraneous variation across the groups, for example, by removing any discretion in assignment from the study's staff. A random assignment scheme is again an ideal choice, but the difficulties of implementing such a scheme in a large-scale field trial can outweigh the advantages. For example, it may be convenient to distribute vaccinations to groups in batches that are handled identically, especially if storage and transport of the vaccine is difficult. Such practicalities may dictate the use of modified randomization protocols such as cluster randomization (explained later). Because such modifications can seriously affect the informativeness and interpretation of experimental findings, the advantages and disadvantages need to be weighed carefully.

Community Intervention and Cluster-Randomized Trials

The community intervention trial is an extension of the field trial that involves intervention on a community-wide basis. Conceptually, the distinction hinges on whether the intervention is implemented separately for each individual. Whereas a vaccine is ordinarily administered singly to individual people, an intervention such as water fluoridation to prevent dental caries is ordinarily administered to individual water supplies. Consequently, when water fluoridation was studied, it was evaluated by community intervention trials in which entire communities were selected and exposure (water treatment) was assigned on a community basis. Other examples of preventives that might be implemented on a community-wide basis include fast-response emergency resuscitation programs, educational programs conducted using mass media, such as Project Burn Prevention in Massachusetts,[55] and school-level interventions to improve access to water, sanitation, and hygiene.[56–58]

Some interventions are implemented most conveniently with groups of subjects that are smaller than entire communities. Dietary intervention may be made most conveniently by family or household. Environmental interventions may affect an entire office, factory, or residential building. Protective sports equipment may have to be assigned to an entire team or league. Intervention groups may be army units, schools, classrooms, vehicle occupants, or any other group whose members are exposed to the intervention simultaneously. The scientific foundation of experiments using such interventions is identical to that of community intervention trials. What sets all these studies apart from field trials is that the interventions are assigned to groups rather than to individuals.

Field trials in which the treatment is assigned randomly to groups of participants are said to be cluster randomized. The smaller the number of groups to be randomized, the less the accomplishment by random assignment. This limitation arises because, although the expectation of no bias is retained by the randomization, the potential for large deviations from the expectation is greater when the number of randomized units is small.[1] If only two communities are involved in a study, one of which will receive the intervention and the other of which will not, such as in the Newburgh-Kingston water fluoridation trial,[59] it cannot matter whether the community that receives the fluoride is assigned randomly or not. Differences in baseline (extraneous) characteristics will have the same magnitude and the same effect whatever the method of assignment is—only the direction of the differences will be affected. It is only when the numbers of groups randomized to each intervention are large that randomization is likely to produce similar distributions of baseline characteristics among the intervention groups. Design and analysis of cluster-randomized trials should thus involve methods that take account of the clustering.[60-65] These methods are essential to estimate properly the amount of variability introduced by the randomization, given a hypothesis about the size of the treatment effects.

NONEXPERIMENTAL STUDIES

The limitations imposed by ethics and costs restrict most epidemiologic research to nonexperimental studies. Although it is unethical for an investigator to expose a person to a potential cause of disease simply to learn about etiology, people often willingly or unwillingly expose themselves to many potentially harmful factors, such as cigarettes:[66]

> [People] choose a broad range of dosages of a variety of potentially toxic substances. Consider the cigarette habit to which hundreds of millions of persons have exposed themselves at levels ranging from almost zero (for those exposed only through smoking by others) to the addict's three or four cigarettes per waking hour...

Beyond tobacco, people in industrialized nations expose themselves, among other things, to a range of exercise regimens from sedentary to grueling, to diets ranging from vegan to those derived almost entirely from animal sources, and to medical interventions for diverse conditions. Each of these exposures may have intended and unintended consequences that can be investigated by observational epidemiology.

Ideally, we would want the strength of evidence from nonexperimental research to be as high as that obtainable from a well-designed experiment, had one been possible. In an experiment, however, the investigator has the power to assign exposures in a way that enhances the validity of the study, whereas in nonexperimental research, the investigator cannot assign the circumstances of exposure. If those who happen to be exposed have a greater or lesser risk for the disease than those who are not exposed, a simple comparison between exposed and unexposed will be confounded by this difference and thus not reflect validly the sole effect of the exposure.

Lack of randomization calls into question the standard practice of analyzing nonexperimental data with statistical methods developed for randomized studies. Without randomization, systematic variation is a composite of all uncontrolled sources of variation—including any treatment effect—but also including confounding factors and other sources of systematic error. As a result, in studies without randomization, the systematic variation estimated by standard statistical methods is not readily attributable to treatment effects, nor can it be reliably compared with the variation expected to occur by chance.[1] Separation of treatment effects from the mixture of uncontrolled systematic variation in nonrandomized studies (or in randomized studies with noncompliance) requires additional hypotheses about the sources of systematic error. In nonexperimental studies, these hypotheses are usually no more than speculations, although they can be incorporated into the analysis as prior distributions in Bayesian analysis or as parameter settings in a bias analysis (see Chapters 23 and 29). In this sense, causal inference in the absence of randomization depends on some speculative elements. The validity of such inference depends on how well the speculations about the effect of systematic errors correspond with their true effect.

Because the investigator cannot assign exposure in nonexperimental studies, he or she must rely heavily on the primary source of discretion that remains: the selection of subjects and the definitions of the conditions defined as "exposed" and "unexposed." If the paradigm of scientific observation is the experiment, then the paradigm of nonexperimental epidemiologic research is the "natural experiment," in which nature emulates the sort of experiment the investigator might have conducted, but for ethical and cost constraints. A renowned example is the elegant study of cholera in London conducted by John Snow. In London during the mid-19th century, there were several water companies that piped drinking water to residents, and these companies often competed side by side, serving similar clientele within city districts. Snow took advantage of this natural experiment by comparing the cholera mortality rates for residents subscribing to two of the major water companies: the Southwark and Vauxhall Company, which piped impure Thames River water contaminated with sewage, and the Lambeth Company, which in 1852 changed its collection point from opposite Hungerford Market to Thames Ditton, thus obtaining a supply of water that was upstream of the sewage of London. As Snow (1855) described it,

> ...The intermixing of the water supply of the Southwark and Vauxhall Company with that of the Lambeth Company, over an extensive part of London, admitted of the subject being sifted in such a way as to yield the most incontrovertible proof on one side or the other. In the subdistricts... supplied by both companies, the mixing of the supply is of the most intimate kind. The pipes of each company go down all the streets, and into nearly all the courts and alleys. A few houses are supplied by one company and a few by the other, according to the decision of the owner or occupier at the time when the Water Companies were in active competition. In many cases a single house has a supply different from that on either side. Each company supplies both rich and poor, both large houses and small; there is no difference in either the condition or occupation of the persons receiving the water of the different companies... it is obvious that no experiment could have been devised which would more thoroughly test the effect of water supply on the progress of cholera than this.

> The experiment, too, was on the grandest scale. No fewer than three hundred thousand people of both sexes, of every age and occupation, and of every rank and station, from gentle folks down to the very poor, were divided into two groups without their choice, and, in most cases, without their knowledge; one group being supplied with water containing the sewage of London, and amongst it, whatever might have come from the cholera patients, the other group having water quite free from impurity.

> To turn this experiment to account, all that was required was to learn the supply of water to each individual house where a fatal attack of cholera might occur...

There are two primary types of nonexperimental studies in epidemiology. The first, the *cohort study* (also called the follow-up study or incidence study), is a direct analog of the experiment. Different exposure groups are compared, but (as in Snow's study) the investigator, rather than assigning subjects to exposure groups, only selects them to observe and classifies them by exposure status. The second, the *case-control study*, employs an extra step of sampling from the source population for cases. Whereas a cohort study would include all persons in the population giving rise to the study cases, a case-control study selects only a sample of those persons and chooses whom to include in part based on their disease status. This extra sampling step can make a case-control study much more efficient than a cohort study of the same population, but it introduces a few subtleties and avenues for bias that are absent in typical cohort studies.

More detailed discussions of both cohort and case-control studies and their variants, with specific examples, are presented in Chapters 7 and 8. We provide here brief overviews of the designs.

Cohort Studies

In the paradigmatic cohort study, the investigator defines two or more groups of people who are free of disease and differ according to the extent of their exposure to a potential cause of disease. These groups are referred to as the study cohorts. When two groups are studied, one is usually thought of as the exposed or index cohort—those individuals who have experienced the putative causal event or condition—and the other is then thought of as the unexposed or reference cohort. There may be more than just two cohorts, but each cohort would represent a group with a different level or type of exposure. For example, an occupational cohort study of chemical workers might comprise cohorts of workers in a plant who work in different departments of the plant, with each cohort being exposed to a different set of chemicals. The investigator measures the incidence times and rates of disease in each of the study cohorts and compares these occurrence measures.

In Snow's natural experiment, the study cohorts were residents of London who consumed water from either the Lambeth Company or the Southwark and Vauxhall Company and who lived in districts where the pipes of the two water companies were intermixed. Snow estimated the frequency of cholera deaths, using households as the denominator, separately for people in each of the two cohorts:[67]

> According to a return which was made to Parliament, the Southwark and Vauxhall Company supplied 40,046 houses from January 1 to December 31, 1853, and the Lambeth Company supplied 26,107 houses during the same period; consequently, as 286 fatal attacks of cholera took place, in the first four weeks of the epidemic, in houses supplied by the former company, and only 14 in houses supplied by the latter, the proportion of fatal attacks to each 10,000 houses was as follows: Southwark and Vauxhall 71, Lambeth 5. The cholera was therefore fourteen times as fatal at this period, amongst persons having the impure water of the Southwark and Vauxhall Company, as amongst those having the purer water from Thames Ditton.

The design of Snow's natural experiment has been long-heralded, but it failed to persuade critics at the time, in part because Snow's data on the number of households supplied by each water company were for all districts of both companies and not restricted to the districts in which the supply of water was intermingled.[68] Nonetheless, despite this imperfection, Snow's concept was elegant and inspirational.

Many cohort studies begin with but a single cohort that is heterogeneous with respect to exposure history. Comparisons of disease experience are made within the cohort across subgroups defined by one or more exposures. Examples include studies of cohorts defined from membership lists of administrative or social units, such as cohorts of doctors or nurses, or cohorts defined from employment records, such as cohorts of factory workers.

Case-Control Studies

Case-control studies are best understood and conducted by defining a source population at the outset, which represents a hypothetical study population in which a cohort study might have been conducted, and by identifying a single disease of interest. If a cohort study were undertaken, the primary tasks would be to identify the exposed and unexposed denominator experience, measured in person-time units of experience or as the number of people in each study cohort, and then to identify the number of cases occurring in each person-time category or study cohort. In a case-control study, these same cases are identified and their exposure status is determined just as in a cohort study, but denominators from which rates could be calculated are not measured. Instead, a control group of study subjects is sampled from the entire source population that gave rise to the cases.

For example, Snow could have identified the 300 fatal attacks of cholera in London and randomly selected 300 controls from among all households served by the two water companies. Among cases, 286 (95%) would have lived in households with water supplied by the Southwark and Vauxhall Company. Suppose that, in the control series, the prevalence of households served by the two companies corresponded to the overall prevalence. For the Southwark and Vauxhall company, one would expect $300 \times 40,046/(40,046 + 26,107) = 300 \times 61\% = \sim182$ controls. For the Lambeth company, one would expect $300 \times 26,107/(40,046 + 26,107) = 300 \times 39\% = \sim118$ controls. From that, one can use the odds ratio (OR) to estimate the relative number of households receiving water from the two companies and calculate the cholera mortality ratio of $(286/182)/(14/118) = \sim13$, a fair approximation to the mortality ratio of 14 (71 per 10,000/5 per 10,000) reported by Snow. The validity of this estimate depends on the assumption that the sample of controls gives a valid estimate of the proportion of households receiving water from the Southwark and Vauxhall company, which in turn would depend on how the sample was identified.

The primary purpose of the control group is to estimate the relative size of the exposed and unexposed denominators within the source population (in the example, this corresponds to 182/118 controls $\sim$ 40,046/26,107 households). Just as we can attempt to measure either risks or rates in a cohort, the denominators that the control series represents in a case-control study may reflect either the number of people in the exposed and unexposed subsets of the source population or the amount of person-time in the exposed and unexposed subsets of the source population (see Chapter 8). From the relative size of these denominators, the relative size of the incidence rates or incidence proportions can then be estimated. Thus, case-control studies yield direct estimates of relative effect measures. Because the control group is used to estimate the distribution of exposure in the source population, the cardinal requirement of control selection is that the controls must be sampled independently of their exposure status.

Prospective Versus Retrospective Studies

Studies are often labeled as either *prospective* or *retrospective*, and these labels strongly connote the study quality.[69] Studies labeled "prospective" are almost uniformly viewed as having a higher quality design than studies labeled "retrospective." Unfortunately, several definitions have been used for these terms, and only one of these definitions merits the strong connotation about design quality.

The first of these definitions corresponds directly to the study design, with *prospective* used to denote cohort studies and *retrospective* used to denote case-control studies.[70,71] Using the terms prospective and retrospective in this way conveys no information beyond the design label and fails to highlight other important aspects of a study design for which the description prospective or retrospective might be illuminating. More importantly, cohort studies are not inherently more valid than case-control studies. Labeling the former as *prospective* and the latter as *retrospective*, when these labels so strongly connote quality, unfairly promotes the inherent quality of cohort studies and unfairly diminishes the quality of case-control studies.

Under the second definition, the terms *prospective* and *retrospective* refer to the timing of the accumulated person-time with respect to the study's conduct.[72] Under this usage, when the person-time accumulates before the study is conducted, it is said to be a *retrospective* study, even if the exposure status was recorded before the disease occurred. When the person-time accumulates after the study begins, it is said to be a *prospective* study. In this situation, the exposure status is ordinarily recorded before disease occurrence, although there are exceptions. For example, job status might be recorded for an occupational cohort at the study's inception and as workers enter the cohort, but an industrial hygienist might assign exposure levels to the job categories only after the study is completed and therefore after all cases of disease have occurred. The potential then exists for disease to influence the industrial hygienist's assignment, unless the industrial hygienist has been effectively blinded to study outcomes. Additional nuances can similarly complicate the classification of studies as retrospective or prospective with respect to the timing of study conduct. For example, cohort studies can be conducted by measuring disease events after the study begins, by defining cohorts as of some time in the past and measuring the occurrence of disease in the time before the study begins, or a combination of the two. Similarly, case-control studies can be based on disease events that occur after the study begins, or events that have occurred before the study begins, or a combination. Thus, both cohort and case-control studies can ascertain events prospectively, retrospectively, or both from the point of view of the time that the study begins.

This second definition breaks the one-to-one link between the labels and the study design. Studies that take advantage of person-time that has already accumulated are not, however, inherently less valid than studies that begin to accumulate person-time only after the project is initiated. Once again, labeling the former as retrospective and the latter as prospective, when these labels so strongly connote quality, unfairly promotes the inherent quality of studies that use future person-time and diminishes the quality of studies that use past person-time.

That said, it is worth noting that access to historical data may affect study validity. Historical ascertainment has implications for selection bias and missing-data bias insofar as records or data may be missing in a systematic fashion. For example, preserving exposure information that has been recorded in the past may depend on disease occurrence, as might be the case if occupational records were destroyed except for workers who have submitted disability claims. In determining whether the information in a study is valid, the possibility that disease could influence either the recording of the data or its entry path into the study should therefore be considered. These concerns more often arise in studies for which the person-time has already occurred, so recording of the data and its entry path into the study is out of the investigator's control. In studies for which the person-time has yet to occur, recording of the data and its entry path into the study is under the investigator's control, so good practices for data collection should prevent selection and missing-data bias.

The third definition of retrospective and prospective highlights a central feature of study design that does correspond to study quality, which is the order in time of the recording of exposure information and the occurrence of disease.[72] In studies where the exposure is measured by asking people about their history of exposure, it is possible that the occurrence of disease could influence the accuracy of recording of exposure and bias the study results, for example, by influencing recall. This concern for differential misclassification does correspond to a threat to validity, so a study based on such recall is one that merits the label retrospective, at least with respect to the recording of exposure information, and perhaps for the study as a whole. Assessing exposure by recall after disease has occurred is a feature of many case-control studies, which may explain why case-control studies are often labeled retrospective. A study with retrospective measurement in this sense is subject to the concern that disease occurrence or diagnosis has affected exposure evaluation. A similar concern would apply to the use of information recorded after disease occurrence, if that information could have been influenced by the diagnosis. For example, the mention of a history of diabetes in a medical record could be influenced by a current diagnosis of myocardial infarction. Not all case-control studies involve recall or recording of information after a case has been diagnosed. For example, case-control studies that evaluate drug exposures have prospective measurement if the information on the exposures and other risk factors was recorded before disease development, even if the record of prescription was not in the hands of the investigator until much later. These case-control studies are more appropriately described as prospective, at least with respect to exposure measurement, provided that the prescription data were not manipulated in reaction to subsequent disease status.

Furthermore, not all study variables need to be measured simultaneously. Some studies may combine prospective measurement of some variables with retrospective measurement of other variables. Such studies might be viewed as being a mixture of prospective and retrospective measurements. A reasonable rule might be to describe a study as prospective if the exposure measurement could not be influenced by the disease and retrospective otherwise. This rule could lead to a study with a mixture of prospectively and retrospectively measured variables being described differently for different analyses, and appropriately so. For each analysis, the labels would accurately correlate to the design quality. Those with exposure information recorded before disease outcome would be labeled prospective, and their validity would not be threatened by the potential for disease status to have affected the accuracy of the exposure information. Those with exposure information recorded after disease outcome would be labeled *retrospective*, and their validity would be threatened by the potential for disease status to have affected the accuracy of the exposure information. Only this definition of the terms corresponds to the strong connotation pertaining to design quality.

These considerations demonstrate that the classification of studies as prospective or retrospective is not straightforward and that these terms do not readily convey a clear message about the study's quality.[69] The most important study feature that these terms might illuminate would be whether the disease could influence the exposure information in the study, and this is the usage that we recommend. Prospective and retrospective will then be terms that could each describe some cohort studies and some case-control studies. Under the alternative definitions, studies labeled as "retrospective" might actually use methods that preclude the possibility that exposure information could have been influenced by disease, and studies labeled as "prospective" might actually use methods that do not exclude that possibility. Because the term *retrospective* often connotes an inherently less reliable design and the term *prospective* often connotes an inherently more reliable design, assignment of the classification under the alternative definitions does not always convey accurately the strengths or weaknesses of the design. Because the terms are used inconsistently, yet so strongly correlate to perceived quality, it might be best to avoid using them at all. Whether or not they are used, it is always good practice to clearly state how, when, and in what order data were collected.[73]

Cross-Sectional Studies

A study that includes as subjects all persons in the population at the time of ascertainment or a representative sample of all such persons, selected without regard to exposure or disease status, is referred to as a *cross-sectional study*. A cross-sectional study conducted to estimate prevalence is called a *prevalence study*. Usually, exposure is ascertained simultaneously with the disease, and different exposure subpopulations are compared with respect to their disease prevalence. Such studies need not have etiologic objectives. For example, delivery of health services often requires knowledge of how many items will be needed (such as number of hospital beds), without reference to the causes of the disease. Cross-sectional studies may sometimes involve sampling subjects differentially with respect to disease status to increase the number of cases in the sample, especially when the disease is rare, with insidious onset, and of long duration. Such studies are sometimes called *prevalent case-control studies,* because their design is much like that of incident case-control studies, except that the case series comprises prevalent rather than incident cases.[74] In addition, periodic cross-sectional studies are sometimes conducted, often using sampling strategies that will allow reweighting of the study population to the target population, to understand trends in measures of population health. Examples include the National Health Nutrition Examination Survey, which is fielded every second year with the primary goal of assessing the health and nutritional status of adults and children in the United States by both interviews and physical examinations. Many other nations and regions field similar periodic health studies. Cross-sectional associations between variables measured by these studies are sometimes reported as estimates of etiologic association. Given that cross-sectional data are so often used for etiologic inferences, a thorough understanding of their potential limitations is essential.

One problem is that such studies often have difficulty in determining the time order of events.[75] Another problem, often called length-biased sampling,[76] is that the cases identified in a cross-sectional study will overrepresent cases with long duration of illness and underrepresent those with short duration of illness. To see this, consider two extreme situations involving a disease with a highly variable duration. A person contracting this disease at age 20 and living until age 70 can be included in any cross-sectional study during the person's 50 years of disease. A person contracting the disease at age 40 and dying within a day has almost no chance of inclusion. Thus, if an exposure does not alter disease risk but causes the disease to be mild and prolonged when contracted (so that exposure is positively associated with duration), the prevalence of exposure will be elevated among cases. As a result, a positive exposure-disease association is expected in a cross-sectional study, even though exposure has no effect on disease risk and would be beneficial if disease occurs. If exposure does not alter disease risk but causes the disease to be rapidly fatal if it is contracted (so that exposure is negatively associated with duration), then prevalence of exposure will be relatively low among cases. As a result, the exposure-disease association observed in the cross-sectional study is expected to be negative, even though exposure has no effect on disease risk and would be detrimental if disease occurs. There are analytic methods for dealing with the potential relation of exposure to duration.[76] These methods require either the diagnosis dates of the study cases or information on the distribution of durations for the study disease at different exposure levels; such information may be available from medical databases.

Despite these limitations, there are circumstances when associations from cross-sectional study designs reliably estimate causal effects. First, the difference in prevalence between two exposure groups can be viewed as a causal effect itself.[77] Prevalence is a widely reported epidemiologic measure, and a cross-sectional study is a natural design to estimate and compare prevalences at a specified point in time. To estimate a causal effect on prevalence, one can conceptualize a follow-up study in which a target population is randomized to an exposure at the start of follow-up. In contrast to a cohort study of disease incidence, the individuals in this target population need not be disease free at baseline. The causal effect of the exposure on prevalence at the cross-sectional study's time point could then be estimated by a prevalence difference or ratio. Flanders et al. described the conditions and assumptions necessary to validly estimate a causal effect on prevalence from such a cross-sectional study,[77] which include the general considerations discussed in Chapter 5. The key additional condition for estimating causal effects on prevalence differences in a cross-sectional study is that subjects are selected from a population that is representative of all survivors from the underlying baseline cohort.

Second, when exposure contrasts from studies of cross-sectional design meet the general criteria discussed in Chapter 5, and additional criteria,[78] the prevalence OR provides a valid estimate of the incidence rate ratio.[78,79] When the criteria are met, these studies estimate the combined effect of the exposure contrast on the incidence of the disease and survival with the disease in the target population at the start of follow-up.[77] This combined effect may be of particular relevance for disabilities and for chronic, incurable diseases of long duration and insidious onset, such as diabetes, chronic obstructive pulmonary disease, and many neurodegenerative diseases. For conditions and diseases of these types, properly interpreted estimates of prevalence differences or ratios could help to elucidate the apparently paradoxical associations described as examples above.

Proportional Mortality Studies

A proportional mortality study includes only dead subjects. The proportions of dead exposed subjects assigned to index causes of death are compared with the proportions of dead unexposed subjects assigned to the index causes. The resulting *proportional mortality ratio* (PMR) is the traditional measure of the effect of the exposure on the index causes of death. Superficially, the comparison of proportions of subjects dying from a specific cause for an exposed and an unexposed group resembles a cohort study measuring incidence. The resemblance is deceiving, however, because a proportional mortality study does not involve the identification and follow-up of cohorts. All subjects are dead at the time of entry into the study.

The premise of a proportional mortality study is that if the exposure causes (or prevents) a specific fatal illness, there should be proportionately more (or fewer) deaths from that illness among dead people who had been exposed than among dead people who had not been exposed. This reasoning suffers two important flaws. First, a PMR comparison cannot distinguish whether exposure increases the occurrence of the index causes of death, prevents the occurrence of other causes of death, or some mixture of these effects.[80] For example, a proportional mortality study could find a proportional excess of cancer deaths among daily aspirin users compared with nonusers of aspirin, but this finding might be attributable to a preventive effect of aspirin on cardiovascular deaths, which compose the plurality of noncancer deaths. Thus, an implicit assumption of a proportional mortality study of etiology is that the overall death rate for categories other than the index is not related to the exposure.

The second major problem in mortality comparisons is that they cannot determine the extent to which exposure causes (or prevents) the index causes of death or worsens (or improves) the prognosis of the illnesses corresponding to the index causes. For example, an association of aspirin use with stroke deaths among all deaths could be due to an aspirin effect on the incidence of stroke, an aspirin effect on the severity of stroke, an aspirin effect on survival duration after a stroke, or some combination of these effects.

The ambiguities in interpreting a PMR are not necessarily a fatal flaw, because the measure will often provide insights worth pursuing about causal relations. In many situations, there may be only one or a few narrow causes of death that are of interest, and it may be judged implausible that an exposure would substantially affect either the occurrence or prognosis of any nonindex deaths. Nonetheless, many of the difficulties in interpreting proportional mortality studies can be mitigated by considering a proportional mortality study as a variant of the case-control study. To do so requires conceptualizing a combined population of exposed and unexposed individuals in which the cases occurred. The cases are those deaths, both exposed and unexposed, in the index category or categories; the controls are other deaths.[81]

The guiding principle of control selection is to choose individuals who represent the source population from which the cases arose, so as to measure the distribution of exposure within that population. Instead of sampling controls directly from the source population, we can sample deaths occurring in the source population, provided that the exposure distribution among the deaths sampled is the same as the distribution in the source population; that is, the exposure should not be related to the causes of death among controls (see Chapter 8).[82] If we keep the objectives of control selection in mind, it becomes clear that we are not bound to select as controls all deaths other than index cases. We can instead select as controls a limited set of reference causes of death, selected on the basis of a presumed lack of association with the exposure. In this way, other causes of death for which a relation with exposure is known, suspected, or highly plausible can be excluded.

Treating a proportional mortality study as a case-control study can thus enhance study validity. It also provides a basis for estimating the usual epidemiologic measures of effect that can be derived from such studies.[83] The same type of design and analysis reappeared in the context of analyzing spontaneously reported adverse events in connection with pharmaceutical use. The US

Food and Drug Administration maintains a database of spontaneous reports, the Adverse Event Reporting System (AERS),[84] which has been a data source for studies designed to screen for associations between drugs and previously unidentified adverse effects using empirical Bayes techniques.[85] Similar databases of adverse event reports are collected elsewhere.[86] It has been proposed that these data should be analyzed in the same way that mortality data had been analyzed in proportional mortality studies,[87] using a measure called the proportional reporting ratio, or PRR, which is analogous to the PMR in proportional mortality studies. This approach, however, is subject to the same problems that accompanied the PMR. As with the PMR, these problems can be mitigated by applying the principles of case-control studies to the task of surveillance of spontaneous report data.[88] More recently, the safety of approved medical products has been monitored by access to distributed databases of millions of health records, enabling rapid design and analysis of prospective cohort studies of potential medical hazards.[89,90]

Ecologic Studies

The study types described thus far share the characteristic that the observations made pertain to individuals. It is possible to conduct research in which the unit of observation is a group of people rather than an individual. Such studies are called *ecologic* or *aggregate studies* (see Chapter 30). The groups may be classes in a school, factories, cities, counties, or nations, or a population observed at two different points in time. The only requirement is that only information on the populations studied is available to measure the exposure and disease distributions in each group; no individual level data are available. For example, incidence or mortality rates are commonly used to quantify disease occurrence in the groups. Exposure may also be measured by an overall index; for example, county alcohol consumption may be estimated from alcohol tax data, information on socioeconomic status is available for census tracts from the US decennial census, and environmental data (temperature, air quality, etc.) may be available locally or regionally. These environmental data are examples of exposures that are measured by necessity at the level of a group, because individual-level data are usually unavailable or impractical to gather.

When exposure varies across individuals within the ecologic groups, the degree of association between exposure and disease need not reflect individual-level associations.[91–97] In addition, use of proxy measures for exposure (*e.g.*, alcohol tax data rather than consumption data) and disease (mortality rather than incidence) further distort the associations.[98] Finally, ecologic studies often suffer from unavailability of data necessary for adequate control of confounding in the analysis when the goal is to estimate the effect of the exposure at the individual level.[95] Even if the research goal is to estimate effects of group-level exposures on group-level outcomes, problems of data inadequacy as well as of inappropriate grouping can severely bias estimates from ecologic studies.[96,97,99] All of these problems can combine to produce results of questionable validity on any level.

Despite these limitations, ecologic studies can be useful for assessing associations of exposure distributions with disease occurrence, because such associations may signal the presence of effects that are worthy of further investigation.[100] Two-stage or hybrid designs that supplement ecologic data with efficiently sampled individual-level data provide protections against the ecologic biases and fallacy.[101,102] There are also other design and analysis strategies that enhance the potential for causal interpretations from ecologic or hybrid study designs. For example, difference-in-difference estimators compare changes in an outcome's risk or rate over time in a population exposed to some intervention with changes in the outcome over time in a comparable but unexposed population (see Chapter 28).[103] Conventional ecologic studies might compare only the postintervention outcome risk with the preintervention outcome risk, but this would ignore changes in outcome risk that might have occurred even without the intervention. Subtracting the postintervention and preintervention difference in outcome risk observed in a comparable population that did not receive the intervention is meant to account for any change in outcome risk that did not arise from the intervention. Causal interpretation of the difference-in-difference estimator requires the strong assumption that the populations exposed and unexposed to the intervention would have had the same changes in outcome risks or rates were it not for the intervention. This assumption might be untenable if factors associated with changes in the outcome risk or rate are unbalanced in the populations exposed and unexposed to the intervention, although analytic strategies may be used to adjust for these imbalances.[103] The conceptual underpinnings of the difference-in-difference design have been extended to related designs—such as the trend-in-trend design[104]—which uses multiple exposure categories, instead of only two, and multiple measurements of the outcome, instead of only two. Thus, ecologic data should often be viewed warily when reaching causal interpretations, but there are design and analysis strategies that reliably overcome what might appear to be inherent limitations of ecologic study designs.

Hypothesis Generation Versus Hypothesis Screening

Studies in which validity to assess causality is less secure have sometimes been referred to as "hypothesis-generating" studies to distinguish them from "analytic studies," in which validity may be better. Ecologic and cross-sectional studies have often been considered as hypothesis-generating studies because of concern about various biases, but as noted above, both study designs can, in some circumstances, yield valid results for the purpose of causal inference. Thus, the distinction between hypothesis-generating and analytic studies is not conceptually accurate. It is the investigator, not the study, that generates hypotheses,[105] and any type of data may be used to test hypotheses.

For example, international comparisons indicate that Japanese women have a much lower age-standardized breast cancer rate than women in the United States.[106] These data are ecologic and subject to the usual concerns about the many differences that exist between cultures. Nevertheless, the finding corroborates a number of hypotheses, including the theories that alcohol consumption, obesity, high-risk physical features of the breast, and high risk reproductive histories (all more prevalent among US women than Japanese women) may be important determinants of breast cancer risk.[106,107] The international difference in breast cancer rates is neither hypothesis generating nor analytic, because the hypotheses arose independently of this finding. Thus, the distinction between hypothesis-generating and analytic studies is one that is best replaced by a more accurate distinction.

A proposal that we view favorably is to refer to preliminary studies of limited validity or precision as *hypothesis-screening studies*. In analogy with screening of individuals for disease, such studies represent a relatively easy and inexpensive test for the presence of an association between exposure and disease. To the extent such an association exists and has potentially important implications for health, it should be subject to more rigorous and costly assessment using a more valid study design, which may be called a confirmatory study. Although the screening analogy should not be taken to an extreme, it does better describe the progression of studies than the hypothesis-generating/analytic study distinction.

DESIGN STRATEGIES TO IMPROVE STUDY ACCURACY

There are a number of design strategies aimed at the overlapping goals of efficient control of confounding and efficient subject selection. We use *efficiency* to refer to both the statistical precision and the cost-effectiveness of the study design.

Design Options to Control Confounding

Various methods are used to help control confounding in the design of epidemiologic studies. One, randomization, is applicable only in experiments. In contrast, restriction is applicable to all study designs. Matching is often treated as another option for control of confounding, but this view is not accurate. The primary benefits of matching (when they arise) are more in the realm of improved *efficiency* in confounder control—that is, an increase in the precision of the confounder-adjusted estimate, for a given study size. Matching is therefore covered in its own section.

Randomization

When it is practical and ethical to assign exposure to subjects, one can in theory create study cohorts that would have an expectation of exchangeable incidences of disease in the absence of the assigned exposure and so eliminate the expectation of confounding. If only a few factors determine incidence and if the investigator knows of these factors, an ideal plan might call for exposure assignment that would lead to identical, balanced distributions of these causes of disease in each group. In studies of human disease, however, there are always unmeasured (and unknown) causes of disease that cannot be forced into balance among treatment groups. Randomization is a method that allows one to limit confounding by unmeasured factors probabilistically and to account quantitatively for the potential residual confounding produced by these unmeasured factors.

As described above, randomization does not lead to identical distributions of all factors, but only to distributions that tend, on repeated trials, to be similar for factors that are not affected by treatment. The tendency increases as the sizes of the study groups increase. Thus, randomization works well to prevent substantial confounding in large studies but is less effective for smaller studies.[108] In the extreme case in which only one randomization unit is included in each group (as in the community fluoridation trial described above, in which there was only one community in each group), randomization is completely ineffective in preventing confounding. As compensation for its unreliability in small studies, randomization has the advantage of providing a firm basis for calculating confidence limits that allow for confounding by unmeasured, and hence uncontrollable, factors. Because successful randomization allows one to account quantitatively for uncontrollable confounding, randomization is a powerful technique to help ensure valid causal inferences from studies, large or small.[1] Its drawback of being unreliable in small studies can be mitigated by measuring known risk factors before random assignment and then making the random assignments within levels of these factors. Such a process is known as *matched randomization* or *stratified* randomization and will be discussed further below.

Restriction

A variable cannot produce confounding if it is prohibited from varying. Restricting the admissibility criteria for subjects to be included in a study is therefore an extremely effective method of preventing confounding. If the potentially confounding variable is measured on a nominal scale, such as race or sex, restriction is accomplished by admitting into the study as subjects only those who fall into specified categories (usually just a single category) of each variable of interest. If the potentially confounding variable is measured on a continuous scale such as age, restriction is achieved by defining a range of the variable that is narrow enough to limit confounding by the variable. Only individuals within the range are admitted into the study as subjects. If the variable has little effect within the admissible range, then the variable cannot be an important confounder in the study. Even if the variable has a nonnegligible effect in the range, the degree of confounding it produces will be reduced by the restriction, and this remaining confounding can be controlled analytically.

Restriction is an excellent technique for preventing or at least reducing confounding by known factors, because it is not only extremely effective but also inexpensive, and therefore it is very efficient if it does not hamper subject recruitment. The decision about whether to admit a given individual to the study can be made quickly and without reference to other study subjects (as is required for matching). The main disadvantage is that restriction of admissibility criteria can shrink the pool of available subjects below the desired level. When potential subjects are plentiful, restriction can be employed extensively, because it improves validity at low cost. When potential subjects are less plentiful, the advantages of restriction must be weighed against the disadvantages of a diminished study group.

As is the case with restriction based on risk or exposure, one may be concerned that restriction to a homogeneous category of a potential confounder will provide a poor basis for generalization of study results. This concern is valid if one suspects that the effect under study will vary in an important fashion across the categories of the variables used for restriction (see Chapter 14). Nonetheless, studies that try to encompass a "representative" and thus heterogeneous sample of a general population are often unable to address this concern in an adequate fashion, because in studies based on a "representative" sample, the number of subjects within each subgroup may be too small to allow estimation of the effect within these categories. Depending on the size of the subgroups, a representative sample often yields unstable and hence ambiguous or even conflicting estimates across categories and hence provides unambiguous information only about the average effect across all subgroups. If important variation (modification) of the effect exists, one or more studies that focus on different subgroups may be more effective in describing it than studies based on representative samples.

Apportionment Ratios to Improve the Study Efficiency

As described in Chapter 15, one can often apportion subjects into study groups by design to enhance study efficiency. Consider, for example, a cohort study of 100,000 men to determine the magnitude of the reduction in cardiovascular mortality resulting from daily aspirin consumption. A study this large might be thought to have good precision. The frequency of exposure, however, plays a crucial role in precision. If only 100 of the men take aspirin daily, the estimates of effect from the study will be imprecise because few cases will likely occur in the mere 100 exposed subjects. A much more precise estimate could be obtained if, instead of 100 exposed and 99,900 unexposed subjects, 50,000 exposed and 50,000 unexposed subjects could be recruited instead.

The frequency of the outcome is equally crucial. Suppose the study had 50,000 aspirin users and 50,000 nonusers, but all the men in the study were between the ages of 30 and 39 years. Whereas the balanced exposure allocation enhances precision, men of this age seldom die of cardiovascular disease. Thus, few events would occur in either of the exposure groups, and as a result, effect estimates would be imprecise. A much more precise study would use a cohort at much higher risk, such as one comprising older men. The resulting study would not have the same implications unless it was accepted that the effect measure of interest changed little with age. This concern relates not to precision, but to generalizability (see Chapter 14).

Consideration of exposure and outcome frequency must also take account of other factors in the analysis. If aspirin users were all 40 to 49 years old but nonusers were all over age 50, the age discrepancy might severely handicap the study, depending on how these nonoverlapping age distributions were handled in the analysis. For example, if one attempted to stratify by decade of age to control for possible age confounding, there would be no information at all about the effect of aspirin in the data, because no age stratum would have information on both users and nonusers.

Thus, we can see that a variety of design aspects affect study efficiency and in turn affect the precision of study results. These factors include the proportion of subjects exposed, the disease risk of these subjects, and the relation of these study variables to other analysis variables, such as confounders or effect modifiers.

Study efficiency can be judged on various scales. One scale relates the total information content of the data to the total number of subjects (or amount of person-time experience) in the study. One valid design is said to be more statistically efficient than another if the design yields more precise estimates than the other when both are performed with the same number of subjects or person-time (assuming proper study conduct).

Another scale relates the total information content to the costs of acquiring that information. Some options in study design, such as individual matching, may increase the information content per subject studied, but only at an increased cost. Cost efficiency relates the precision of a study to the cost of the study, regardless of the number of subjects in the study. Often the cost of acquiring subjects and obtaining data differs across study groups. For example, retrospective cohort studies often use a reference series from population data because such data can be acquired for a price that is orders of magnitude less than the information on the exposed cohort. Similarly, in case-control studies, eligible cases may be scarce in the source population, whereas those eligible to be controls may be plentiful. In such situations, more precision might be obtained per unit cost by including all eligible cases and then expanding the size of the reference series rather than by expanding the source population to obtain more cases. The success of this strategy depends on the relative costs of acquiring information on cases versus controls and the cost of expanding the source population to obtain more cases—the latter strategy may be very expensive if the study cannot draw on an existing case-ascertainment system (such as a registry).

In the absence of an effect and if no adjustment is needed, the most cost-efficient apportionment ratio is approximately equal to the reciprocal of the square root of the cost ratio.[109] Thus, if C_1 is the cost of each case and C_0 is the cost of each control, the most cost-efficient apportionment ratio of controls to cases is $\sqrt{C_1/C_0}$. For example, if cases cost four times as much as controls and there is no effect and no need for adjustments, the most cost-efficient design would include two times as many controls as cases. The square-root rule is applicable only for small or null effects. A more general approach to improving cost efficiency considers the conjectured magnitude of the effect and the type of data.[110] These formulas enable the investigator to improve the precision of the estimator of effect in a study for a fixed amount of resources.

Occasionally, one of the comparison groups cannot be expanded, usually because practical constraints limit the feasibility of extending the study period or area. For such a group, the cost of acquiring additional subjects is essentially infinite, and the only available strategy for acquiring more information is to expand the other group. As the size of one group increases relative to the other group, statistical efficiency does not increase proportionally. For example, if there are m cases, no effect, and no need to stratify on any factor, the proportion of the maximum achievable precision that can be obtained by using a control group of size n is $n/(m + n)$, often given as $r/(r + 1)$, where $r = n/m$. This relation implies that, if only 100 cases were available in a case-control study and no stratification was needed, a design with 400 controls could achieve $400/(100 + 400) = 80\%$ of the maximum possible efficiency.

Unfortunately, the formulas we have just described are misleading when comparisons across strata of other factors are needed or when there is an effect. In either case, expansion of just one group may greatly improve efficiency.[111] Furthermore, study design formulas that incorporate cost constraints usually treat the costs per subject as fixed within study groups.[112,113] Nonetheless, the cost per subject may change as the number increases; for example, there may be a reduction in cost if the collection time can be expanded and there is no need to train additional interviewers, or there may be an increase in cost if more interviewers need to be trained.

MATCHING

Matching refers to the selection of a reference series—unexposed subjects in a cohort study or controls in a case-control study—that is identical, or nearly so, to the index series with respect to the distribution of one or more potentially confounding factors. Early intuitions about matching were derived from thinking about experiments (in which exposure is assigned by the investigator). In epidemiology, however, matching is applied chiefly in case-control studies, where it represents a very different process from matching in experiments. There are also important differences between matching in experiments and matching in nonexperimental cohort studies.

Matching may be performed subject by subject, which is known as *individual matching,* or for groups of subjects, which is known as *frequency matching*. Individual matching involves selection of one or more reference subjects with matching-factor values equal to those of the index subject. In a cohort study, the index subject is exposed, and one or more unexposed subjects are matched to each exposed subject. In a case-control study, the index subject is a case, and one or more controls are matched to each case. Frequency matching involves selection of an entire stratum of reference subjects with matching-factor values equal to that of a stratum of index subjects. For example, in a case-control study matched on sex, a stratum of male controls would be selected for the male cases, and, separately, a stratum of female controls would be selected for the female cases.

One general observation applies to all matched studies: matching on a factor may necessitate its control in the analysis. This observation is especially important for case-control studies, in which failure to control a matching factor can lead to biased effect estimates. With individual matching, often each matched set is treated as a distinct stratum if a stratified analysis is conducted. When two or more matched sets have identical values for all matching factors, however, the sets can and for efficiency should be coalesced into a single stratum in the analysis.[114] That is, the analysis of matched data does not have to follow the design of the matching procedure.[115] For examples, controls may be individually matched by design to cases on three categories of educational attainment. In the analysis, the pair-matched data do not have to be retained, and it would often be statistically inefficient to retain the pair-matched data structure. Instead, educational attainment could be controlled by stratification of the data into the categories of educational attainment (or by the equivalent regression model). Given that strata corresponding to individually matched sets can be coalesced in the analysis, there is no important difference in the proper analysis of individually matched and frequency-matched data.

Purpose and Effect of Matching

To appreciate the different implications of matching for cohort and case-control studies, consider the hypothetical target population of 2 million individuals given in Table 6-1. Both the exposure and natal male sex are risk factors for the disease. Within sex, exposed have 10 times the outcome

TABLE 6-1

Hypothetical Target Population of 2 Million People, in Which Exposure Increases the Risk 10-Fold, Men Have Five Times the Risk of Women, and Exposure is Much More Prevalent Among Men

	Men		Women	
	Exposed	Unexposed	Exposed	Unexposed
No. of cases in 1 y	4,500	50	100	90
Total	900,000	100,000	100,000	900,000
1-y risk	0.005	0.0005	0.0001	0.0001

$$\text{Crude risk ratio} = \frac{(4,500+100)/1,000,000}{(50+90)/1,000,000} = 33$$

risk of the unexposed, and within exposure levels, men have five times the outcome risk of women. There is also substantial confounding, because 90% of the exposed individuals are male and only 10% of the unexposed are male. The crude risk ratio (RR) in the target population comparing exposed with unexposed is 33, considerably different from the sex-specific values of 10.

Suppose that a cohort study draws an exposed cohort from the exposed target population and matches the unexposed cohort to the exposed cohort on sex. If 10% of the exposed target population is included in the cohort study and these subjects are selected independently of sex, we expect approximately 90,000 men and 10,000 women in the exposed cohort. If a comparison group of unexposed subjects is drawn from the 1 million unexposed individuals in the target population independently of sex, the cohort study will have the same confounding as exists in the target population (apart from sampling variability), because the cohort study is then a simple 10% sample of the target population. It is possible, however, to assemble the unexposed cohort so that its proportion of men matches that in the exposed cohort. This matching of the unexposed to the exposed by sex will prevent an association of sex and exposure in the study cohort. Of the 100,000 unexposed men in the target population, suppose that 90,000 (90%) are selected to form a matched comparison group for the 90,000 exposed men in the study, and of the 900,000 unexposed women, suppose that 10,000 (1.1%) are selected to match the 10,000 exposed women.

Table 6-2 presents the expected results (if there is no sampling error) from the matched cohort study we have described. The expected RR in the study population is 10 for men and 10 for women and is also 10 in the crude data for the study. The matching has apparently accomplished its purpose: The point estimate is not confounded by sex because matching has prevented an association between sex and exposure in the study cohort.

TABLE 6-2

Expected Results of a Matched One-Year Cohort Study of 100,000 Exposed and 100,000 Unexposed Subjects Drawn from the Target Population Described in Table 6-1

	Men		Women	
	Exposed	Unexposed	Exposed	Unexposed
Cases	450	45	10	1
Total	90,000	90,000	10,000	10,000
Approximate expected	RR = 10		RR = 10	

$$\text{Crude risk ratio} = \frac{(450+10)/100,000}{(45+1)/100,000} = 10$$

RR, risk ratio.

TABLE 6-3

Expected Results of a Case-Control Study With 4,740 Controls Matched on Sex When the Source Population is Distributed as in Table 6-1

	Exposed	Unexposed
Cases	4,600	140
Controls	4,114	626

Approximate expected crude OR $= \dfrac{4,600(626)}{4,114(140)} = 5.0$

OR, odds ratio.

The situation differs considerably, however, if a case-control study is conducted instead. Consider a case-control study of all 4,740 cases that occur in the source population in Table 6-1 during 1 year. Of these cases, 4,550 are men. Suppose that 4,740 controls are sampled from the source population (case-cohort design, see Chapter 8), matched to the cases by sex, so that 4,550 of the controls are men. Of the 4,740 cases, we expect 4,500 + 100 = 4,600 to be exposed and 4,740 − 4,600 = 140 to be unexposed. Of the 4,550 male controls, we expect about 90%, or 4,095, to be exposed, because 90% of the men in the target population are exposed. Of the 4,740 − 4,550 = 190 female controls, we expect about 10%, or 19, to be exposed, because 10% of the women in the target population are exposed. Hence, we expect 4,095 + 19 = 4,114 controls to be exposed and 4,740 − 4,114 = 626 to be unexposed. The expected distribution of cases and controls is shown in Table 6-3. The crude OR estimate of the RR is much less than the true RR for exposure effect. Table 6-4 shows, however, that the case-control data give the correct result, RR = 10, when stratified by sex. Thus, unlike the cohort matching, the case-control matching has not eliminated confounding by sex in the crude point estimate of the RR.

The discrepancy between the crude results in Table 6-3 and the stratum-specific results in Table 6-4 results from a bias that is introduced by selecting controls according to a factor that is related to exposure, namely, the matching factor. The bias behaves like confounding, in that the crude estimate of effect is biased but stratification removes the bias. This bias, however, is not a reflection of the original confounding by sex in the source population; indeed, it differs in direction from that bias.

The examples in Tables 6-1 to 6-4 illustrate the following principles: in a cohort study without competing risks or losses to follow-up, no additional action is required in the analysis to control for confounding of the point estimate by the matching factors, because matching unexposed to exposed prevents an association between exposure and the matching factors. (As we will discuss later, however, competing risks or losses to follow-up may necessitate analytic control of the matching factors.) In contrast, if the matching factors are associated with the exposure in the source population, matching in a case-control study requires control of the matching factors in the analysis, even if the matching factors are not risk factors for the disease.

TABLE 6-4

Expected Results of a Case-Control Study of 4,740 Cases and 4,740 Matched Controls When the Source of Subjects is the Target Population Described in Table 6-1 and Sampling Is Random Within Sex

	Men		Women	
	Exposed	Unexposed	Exposed	Unexposed
Cases	4,500	50	100	90
Controls	4,095	455	19	171
Approximate expected	OR = 10		OR = 10	

OR, odds ratio.

What accounts for this discrepancy? In a cohort study, matching is of *unexposed* to *exposed* on characteristics ascertained at the start of follow-up, so is undertaken without regard to events that occur during follow-up, including disease occurrence. By changing the distribution of the matching variables in the unexposed population, the matching shifts the risk in this group toward what would have occurred among the actual exposed population if they had been unexposed. In contrast, matching in a case-control study involves matching *nondiseased* to *diseased,* an entirely different process from matching unexposed to exposed. By selecting controls according to matching factors that are associated with exposure, the selection process will be differential with respect to both exposure and disease, thereby resulting in a selection bias[114,116] that has no counterpart in matched cohort studies. The next sections, on matching in cohort and case-control designs, explore these phenomena in more detail.

Matching in Cohort Studies

In cohort studies, matching unexposed to exposed subjects in a constant ratio can prevent confounding of the crude risk difference and ratio by the matched factors because such matching prevents an association between exposure and the matching factors among the study subjects at the start of follow-up. Despite this benefit—outside of registry-based studies (see Chapter 11)—matched cohort studies are uncommon. Perhaps the main reason is the great expense of matching large cohorts without having measurements of the candidate-matched factors on all members of the source population. Cohort studies ordinarily require many more subjects than case-control studies, and matching is usually a time-consuming process. One exception is when registry data or other secondary data are used as a data source. In secondary data studies, an unexposed cohort may be matched to an exposed cohort within the data source relatively easily and inexpensively because the secondary data source has already collected information on the candidate-matched factors, and it is readily accessible in digitized form. This information can be used to match unexposed to exposed with little added expense or effort. When this information must be collected de novo, it is seldom efficient to collect the information needed to accomplish the matching and then to discard members of the source population from the study population simply because they failed to meet matching criteria. It is possible to improve the poor cost efficiency in matched cohort studies by limiting collection of data on unmatched confounders to those matched sets in which an event occurs,[117] but this approach is rare in practice.

Another reason that matched cohort studies are rare may be that cohort matching does not necessarily eliminate the need to control the matching factors in the analysis. If the exposure and the matching factors affect disease risk or censoring (competing risks and loss to follow-up, the original balance produced by the matching will not extend to the persons and person-time available for the analysis. That is, matching prevents an exposure-matching-factor association only among the original counts of persons at the start of follow-up; the effects of exposure and matching factors may produce an association of exposure and matching factors among the remaining persons and the observed person-time as the cohort is followed over time. Even if only pure-count data and risks are to be examined and no censoring occurs, control of any risk factors used for matching will be necessary to obtain valid standard-deviation estimates for the risk-difference and risk-ratio estimates.[118,119]

Matching and Efficiency in Cohort Studies

Although matching can often improve statistical efficiency in cohort studies by reducing the standard deviation of effect estimates, such a benefit is not assured if exposure is not randomized.[120] To understand this difference between nonexperimental and randomized cohort studies, let us contrast the matching protocols in each design. In randomized studies, matching is a type of *blocking*, which is a protocol for randomizing treatment assignment within groups (blocks). In *pairwise blocking,* a pair of subjects with the same values on the matching (blocking) factors is randomized, one to the study treatment and the other to the control treatment. Such a protocol almost invariably produces a statistically more precise (efficient) effect estimate than the corresponding unblocked design, although exceptions can occur.[121]

In nonexperimental cohort studies, matching refers to a family of protocols for subject selection rather than for treatment assignment. In perhaps the most common cohort-matching protocol, unexposed subjects are selected so that their distribution of matching factors is identical to the distribution in the exposed cohort. This protocol may be carried out by individual or frequency matching. For example, suppose that the investigators have identified an exposed cohort for follow-up, and they tally the age and sex distribution of this cohort. Then, within each age-sex stratum, they may select for follow-up an equal number of unexposed subjects.

In summary, although matching of nonexperimental cohorts may be straightforward, its implications for efficiency are not. Classical arguments from the theory of randomized experiments suggest that matched randomization (blocking) on a risk factor will improve the precision of effect estimation when the outcome under study is continuous; effects are measured as differences of means, and random variation in the outcome can be represented by addition of an independent error term to the outcome. These arguments do not carry over to epidemiologic cohort studies, however, primarily because matched selection alters the covariate distribution of the entire study cohort, whereas matched randomization does not.[120] Classical arguments also break down when the outcome is discrete, because in that case the variance of the outcome depends on the mean (expected) value of the outcome within each exposure level. Thus, in nonexperimental cohort studies, matching can sometimes harm efficiency, even though it introduces no bias.

Matching in Case-Control Studies

In case-control studies, the selection bias introduced by the matching process can occur whether or not there is confounding by the matched factors in the source population (the population from which the cases arose). If there is confounding in the source population, as there was in the earlier example, the process of matching will superimpose a selection bias over the initial confounding.[114,116] This bias is generally in the direction of the null value of effect, whatever the nature of the confounding in the source population, because matching selects controls who are more like cases with respect to exposure than would be controls selected at random from the source population. In the earlier example, the strong confounding away from the null in the source population was overwhelmed by stronger bias toward the null in the matched case-control data.

Let us consider more closely why matching in a case-control study introduces bias. The purpose of the control series in a case-control study is to provide an estimate of the distribution of exposure in the source population. If controls are selected to match the cases on a factor that is correlated with the exposure, then the crude exposure frequency in controls will be distorted in the direction of similarity to that of the cases. Matched controls are identical to cases with respect to the matching factor. Thus, if the matching factor were perfectly correlated with the exposure, the exposure distribution of controls would be identical to that of cases, and hence the crude OR would be 1.0. The bias of the effect estimate toward the null value does not depend on the direction of the association between the exposure and the matching factor; as long as there is an association, positive or negative, the crude exposure distribution among controls will be biased in the direction of similarity to that of cases. A perfect negative correlation between the matching factor and the exposure will still lead to identical exposure distributions for cases and controls and a crude OR of 1.0, because each control is matched to the identical value of the matching factor of the case, guaranteeing identity for the exposure variable as well.

If the matching factor is not associated with the exposure, then matching will not influence the exposure distribution of the controls, and therefore no bias is introduced by matching. If the matching factor is indeed a confounder, however, the matching factor and the exposure will be associated. (If there were no association, the matching factor could not be a confounder, because a confounding factor must be associated with both the exposure and the disease in the source population.)

Thus, although matching is usually intended to control confounding, it does not attain that objective in case-control studies. Instead, it superimposes over the confounding a selection bias.[114] This selection bias behaves like confounding, because it can be controlled in the analysis by the methods used to control for confounding. In fact, matching can introduce bias when none previously existed: If the matching factor is unrelated to disease in the source population, it would not be a confounder; if it is associated with the exposure, however, matching for it in a case-control study will introduce a controllable selection bias.

TABLE 6-5

Source Population With No Confounding by Sex and a Case-Control Study Drawn From the Source Population, Illustrating the Bias Introduced by Matching on Sex

	Men		Women	
	Exposed	**Unexposed**	**Exposed**	**Unexposed**
A. Source Population				
Disease	450	10	50	90
Total	90,000	10,000	10,000	90,000
	RR = 5		RR = 5	

$$\text{Crude risk ratio} = \frac{(450 + 50)/100,000}{(10 + 1)90/100,000} = 5$$

B. Case-Control Study Drawn From Source Population and Matched on Sex

Cases	450	10	50	90
Controls	414	46	14	126
	OR = 5		OR = 5	

$$\text{Approximate expected crude OR} = \frac{(450 + 50)/(46 + 126)}{(10 + 90)/(414 + 14)} = 2.0$$

OR, odds ratio; RR, risk ratio.

This situation is illustrated in Table 6-5, in which the exposure effect corresponds to an RR of 5 and there is no confounding in the source population. Nonetheless, if the cases are selected for a case-control study, and a control series is matched to the cases by sex, the expected value for the crude estimate of effect from the case-control study is 2 rather than the correct value of 5. In the source population, sex is not a risk factor because the incidence proportion is 0.001 in both unexposed men and unexposed women. Nevertheless, despite the absence of association between sex and disease within exposure levels in the source population, an association between sex and disease within exposure levels is introduced into the case-control data by matching. The result is that the crude estimate of effect seriously underestimates the correct value.

The bias introduced by matching in a case-control study is by no means irremediable. In Tables 6-4 and 6-5, the stratum-specific estimates of effect are valid; thus, both the selection bias introduced by matching and the original confounding can be dealt with by treating the matching variable as a confounder in the data analysis. Table 6-5 illustrates that, once case-control matching is undertaken, it may prove necessary to stratify on the matching factors, or otherwise control them in the analysis, even if the matching factors were not confounders in the source population.

Matching and Efficiency in Case-Control Studies

It is reasonable to ask why one might consider matching at all in case-control studies. After all, it does not prevent confounding and often introduces a bias. The utility of matching derives not from an ability to prevent confounding, but from the enhanced statistical efficiency that it sometimes affords for the control of confounding (see Rose and van der Laan for a review[122]). Suppose that one anticipates that age will confound the exposure-disease relation in a case-control study and that stratification in the analysis will be needed. Suppose further that the age distribution for cases is shifted strongly toward older ages, compared with the age distribution of the entire source population. As a result, without matching, there may be some age strata with many cases and few controls, and others with few cases and many controls. If controls are matched to cases by age, the ratio of controls to cases will instead be constant over age strata.

Suppose now that a certain fixed case series has been or can be obtained for the study and that the remaining resources permit selection of a certain fixed number of controls. There is a most efficient ("optimal") distribution for the controls across the strata, in that selecting controls according to this distribution will maximize statistical efficiency, in the sense of minimizing the variance of a common OR estimator (such as those discussed in Chapter 8). This "optimal" control distribution depends on the case distribution across strata. Unfortunately, it also depends on the unknown stratum-specific exposure prevalences among cases and noncases in the source population. Thus, this "optimal" distribution cannot be known in advance and used for control selection. Also, it may not be the scientifically most relevant choice; for example, this distribution assumes that the ratio measure is constant across strata, which is never known to be true and may often be false (in which case a focus on estimating a common ratio measure is questionable). Furthermore, if the ratio measure varies across strata, the most efficient distribution for estimating that variation in the effect measure may be far from the most efficient distribution for estimating a uniform (homogeneous) ratio measure.

Regardless of the estimation goal, however, extreme inefficiency occurs when controls are selected that are in strata that have no case (infinite control/case ratio) or when no control is selected in strata with one or more cases (zero control/case ratio). Strata without cases or controls are essentially discarded by stratified analysis methods. Even in a study in which all strata have both cases and controls, efficiency can be considerably harmed if the subject-selection strategy leads to a case-control distribution across strata that is far from the one that is most efficient for the estimation goal.

Matching forces the controls to have the same distribution of matching factors across strata as the cases and hence prevents extreme departures from what would be the optimal control distribution for estimating a uniform ratio measure. Thus, given a fixed case series and a fixed number of controls, matching often improves the efficiency of a stratified analysis. There are exceptions, however. For example, the study in Table 6-4 yields a less efficient analysis for estimating a uniform ratio than an unmatched study with the same number of controls, because the matched study leads to an expected cell count in the table for women of only 19 exposed controls, whereas in an unmatched study no expected cell count is smaller than 50. This example is atypical because it involves only two strata and large numbers within the cells. In studies that require fine stratification whether matched or not, and so yield sparse data (expected cell sizes that are small, so that zero cells are common within strata), matching will usually result in higher efficiency than what can be achieved without matching.

In summary, matching in case-control studies can be considered a means of providing a more efficient stratified analysis, rather than a direct means of preventing confounding. Stratification (or an equivalent regression approach) will still be necessary to control the selection bias and any confounding left after matching, but matching will often make the stratification more efficient. One should always bear in mind, however, that case-control matching on a nonconfounder will usually harm efficiency, for then the more efficient strategy will usually be neither to match nor to stratify on the factor.

If there is some flexibility in selecting cases as well as controls, efficiency can be improved by altering the case distribution, as well as the control distribution, to approach a more efficient case-control distribution across strata. Sometimes, when no effect measure modification of the OR is assumed, it may turn out that the most efficient approach is restriction of all subjects to one stratum (rather than matching across multiple strata). Nonetheless, in these and similar situations, certain study objectives may weigh against use of the most efficient design for estimating a uniform effect. For example, in a study of the effect of occupational exposures on lung cancer risk, the investigators may wish to ensure that there are enough men and women to provide reasonably precise sex-specific estimates of these effects. Because most lung cancer cases in industrialized countries occur in men and most high-risk occupations are held by men, a design with equal numbers of men and women cases would probably be less efficient for estimating summary effects than other designs, such as one that matched controls to a nonselective series of cases.

Partial or incomplete matching, in which the distribution of the matching factor or factors is altered from that in the source population part way toward that of the cases, can sometimes improve efficiency over no matching and thus can be worthwhile when complete matching is not possible.[123] In some situations, partial matching can even yield more efficient estimates than complete matching.[124] There are many more complex schemes for control sampling to improve efficiency beyond that achievable by ordinary matching, such as countermatching; see citations at the end of this section.

Costs of Matching in Case-Control Studies

The statistical efficiency that matching provides in the analysis of case-control data often comes at a substantial cost. One part of the cost is a research limitation: If a factor has been matched in a case-control study, it is no longer possible to estimate the effect of that factor from the stratified data alone, because matching distorts the relation of the factor to the disease. It is still possible to study the factor as a modifier of relative risk (by seeing how the OR varies across strata).[114] If certain population data are available, it may also be possible to estimate the effect of the matching factor.[125,126]

A further cost involved with individual matching is the possible expense entailed in the process of choosing control subjects with the same distribution of matching factors found in the case series. If several factors are being matched, it may be necessary to examine data on many potential control subjects to find at least one that has the same characteristics as the case. Whereas this process may lead to a statistically efficient analysis, the statistical gain may not be worth the cost in time and money.

If the efficiency of a study is judged from the point of view of the amount of information per subject studied (statistical efficiency), matching can be viewed as an attempt to improve study efficiency. Alternatively, if efficiency is judged as the amount of information per unit of cost involved in obtaining that information (cost efficiency), matching may paradoxically have the opposite effect of decreasing study efficiency, because the effort expended in finding matched subjects might be spent instead simply in gathering information for a greater number of unmatched subjects.[114] With matching, a stratified analysis would be more size efficient, but without it, the resources for data collection can increase the number of subjects, thereby improving cost efficiency. Because cost efficiency is usually a more fundamental concern to an investigator than size efficiency, the apparent efficiency gains from matching are sometimes illusory.

Matching that results in discarded data usually harms both statistical efficiency and cost efficiency. Imagine, for example, a case-control study that matches controls to cases on natal sex and three categories of year of birth. These variables are usually easily measured and easily controlled in the analysis by stratification or regression. Now imagine that, for some cases, no control can be matched with the same natal sex and category of year of birth, resulting in the exclusion of that case from the analysis. Cases are information dense (see Chapter 8), so discarding them from the analysis harms the study's statistical efficiency. Because they contribute nothing to the study's results, the resources invested in identifying them, enrolling them into the study, and collecting information about them are wasted, harming the study's cost efficiency. Matching that results in discarded information, particularly when the matched factors can easily be controlled by another method, is the most egregious violation of the intended purpose of matching, which is to improve efficiency.

The cost objections to matching apply to cohort study (unexposed matched to exposed) matching as well as to case-control matching (controls matched to cases). In general, then, a beneficial effect of matching on overall study efficiency, which is the primary reason for employing matching, is not guaranteed. Indeed, the decision to match subjects can result in less overall information, as measured by the expected width of the confidence interval for the effect estimate, than could be obtained without matching, especially if the expense of matching reduces the total number of study subjects. A wider appreciation for the costs that matching imposes and the often meager advantages it offers would presumably reduce the use of matching and the number of variables on which matching is performed.

Another underappreciated drawback of case-control matching is its potential to increase bias due to misclassification. This problem can be especially severe if one forms unique pair matches on a variable associated only with exposure and the exposure is misclassified.[127]

Benefits of Matching in Case-Control Studies

There are some situations in which matching is desirable or even necessary. If the process of obtaining exposure and confounder information from the study subjects is expensive, it may be more efficient to maximize the amount of information obtained per subject than to increase the number of subjects. For example, if exposure information in a case-control study involves an expensive laboratory test run on blood samples, the money spent on individual matching of subjects may provide more information overall than could be obtained by spending the same money on finding more subjects. If no confounding is anticipated, of course, there is no need to match; for example, restriction of both series might prevent confounding without the need for stratification or matching. If confounding is likely, however, matching will ensure that control of confounding in the analysis will not lose information that has been expensive to obtain.

Sometimes one cannot control confounding efficiently unless matching has prepared the way to do so. Imagine a potential confounding factor that is measured on a nominal scale with many categories; examples are variables such as neighborhood, sibship, referring physician, and occupation. Efficient control of sibship is impossible unless sibling controls have been selected for the cases; that is, matching on sibship is a prerequisite to obtain an estimate that is both unconfounded and reasonably precise. These variables are distinguished from other nominal-scale variables such as ethnicity by the inherently small number of potential subjects available for each category. This situation is called a *sparse-data* problem. Although many subjects may be available, any given category has little chance of showing up in an unmatched sample. Without matching, most strata in a stratified analysis will have only one subject, either a case or a control, and thus will supply no information about the effect when using elementary stratification methods. Matching does not prevent the data from being sparse, but it does ensure that, after stratification by the matched factor, each stratum will have both cases and controls.

Although continuous variables such as age have many values, their values are either easily combined by grouping or they may be controlled directly as continuous variables, avoiding the sparse-data problem. Grouping may leave residual confounding, however, whereas direct control requires the use of explicit modeling methods. Thus, although matching is not essential for control of such variables, it does facilitate their control by more elementary stratification methods.

A fundamental problem with stratified analysis is the difficulty of controlling confounding by several factors simultaneously. Control of each additional factor involves spreading the existing data over a new dimension; the total number of strata required becomes exponentially large as the number of stratification variables increases. For studies with many confounding factors, the number of strata in a stratified analysis that controls all factors simultaneously may be so large that the situation mimics one in which there is a nominal-scale confounder with a multitude of categories. There may be no case or no control in many strata and hardly any comparative information about the effect in any stratum. Consequently, if many confounding factors are anticipated, matching may be desirable to ensure that an elementary stratified analysis is informative. But, as pointed out earlier, attempting to match on many variables may render the study very expensive or make it impossible to find matched subjects. Thus, the most practical option is often to match only on age, sex, and perhaps one or a few nominal-scale confounders, especially those with many possible values. Any remaining confounders can be controlled along with the matching factors by stratification or regression methods.

We can summarize the utility of matching as follows: matching is a useful means for improving study efficiency in terms of the amount of information per subject studied, in some but not all situations. Case-control matching is helpful for known confounders that are measured on a nominal scale, especially those with many categories. The ensuing analysis is best carried out in a manner that controls for both the matching variables and unmatched confounders.

Overmatching

A term that is often used with reference to matched studies is *overmatching*. There are at least three forms of overmatching. The first refers to matching that harms statistical efficiency, such as case-control matching on a variable associated with exposure but not disease. The second refers to matching that harms validity, such as matching on an intermediate between exposure and disease. The third refers to matching that harms cost efficiency.

Overmatching and Statistical Efficiency

As illustrated in Table 6-5, case-control matching on a nonconfounder associated with exposure but not disease can cause the factor to behave like a confounder: control of the factor will be necessary if matching is performed, whereas no control would have been needed if it had not been matched. The introduction of such a variable into the stratification ordinarily reduces the efficiency relative to an unmatched design in which no control of the factor would be needed.[128–130] To explore this type of overmatching further, consider a matched case-control study of a binary exposure, with one control matched to each case on one or more nonconfounders. Each stratum in the analysis will consist of one case and one control unless some strata can be combined. If the case and its matched control are either both exposed or both unexposed, one margin of the 2 × 2 table will be 0. As one may verify from the Mantel-Haenszel OR formula (see Chapter 18), such a pair of subjects will not contribute any information to the analysis. If one stratifies on correlates of exposure, one will increase the chance that such tables will occur and thus tend to increase the information lost in a stratified analysis. This information loss detracts from study efficiency, reducing both information per subject studied and information per dollar spent. Thus, by forcing one to stratify on a nonconfounder, matching can detract from study efficiency. Because the matching was not necessary in the first place and has the effect of impairing study efficiency, matching in this situation can properly be described as overmatching.

This first type of overmatching can thus be understood to be matching that causes a loss of information in the analysis because the resulting stratified analysis would have been unnecessary without matching. The extent to which information is lost by matching depends on the degree of correlation between the matching factor and the exposure. A strong correlate of exposure that has no relation to disease is the worst candidate for matching because it will lead to relatively few informative strata in the analysis with no offsetting gain. Consider, for example, a study of the relation between coffee drinking and bladder cancer. Suppose that matching for consumption of cream substitutes is considered along with matching for a set of other factors. Because this factor is strongly associated with coffee consumption, many of the individual strata in the matched analysis will be completely concordant for coffee drinking and will not contribute to the analysis; that is, for many of the cases, controls matched to that case will be classified identically to the case with regard to coffee drinking simply because of matching for consumption of cream substitutes. If cream substitutes have no relation to bladder cancer, nothing is accomplished by the matching except to burden the analysis with the need to control for use of cream substitutes. This problem corresponds to the unnecessary analysis burden that can be produced by attempting to control for factors that are related only to exposure or exposure opportunity,[131] which is a form of *overadjustment.*

These considerations suggest a practical rule for matching: do not match on a factor that is associated only with exposure. It should be noted, however, that unusual examples can be constructed in which case-control matching on a factor that is associated only with exposure improves efficiency.[132] More important, in many situations the potential matching factor will have at least a weak relation to the disease, and so it will be unclear whether the factor needs to be controlled as a confounder and whether matching on the factor will benefit statistical efficiency. In such situations, considerations of cost efficiency and misclassification may predominate.

When matched and unmatched controls have equal cost and the potential matching factor is to be treated purely as a confounder, with only summarization (pooling) across the matching strata desired, we recommend that one avoid matching on the factor unless the factor is expected to be a strong disease risk factor with at least some association with exposure.[129,130,133] When costs of matched and unmatched controls differ, efficiency calculations that take account of the cost differences can be performed and used to choose a design strategy.[134] When the primary interest in the factor is as an effect modifier rather than confounder, the aforementioned guidelines are not directly relevant. Nonetheless, certain studies have indicated that matching can have a greater effect on efficiency (both positive and negative) when the matching factors are to be studied as effect modifiers, rather than treated as pure confounders.[135,136]

Overmatching and Bias

Matching on factors that are affected by the study exposure or disease is almost never warranted and is potentially capable of biasing study results beyond any hope of repair. It is therefore crucial to understand the nature of such overmatching and why it needs to be avoided.

Case-control matching on a factor that is affected by exposure but is unrelated to disease in any way (except possibly through its association with exposure) will typically reduce statistical efficiency. It corresponds to matching on a factor that is associated only with exposure, which was discussed at length earlier, and is the most benign possibility of those that involve matching for a factor that is affected by exposure. If, however, the potential matching factor is affected by exposure and the factor in turn affects disease (*i.e.*, is an intermediate variable), or is affected by both exposure and disease, then matching on the factor will bias both the crude and the adjusted effect estimates.[137] In these situations, case-control matching is nothing more than an irreparable form of selection bias (see Chapter 14).

To see how this bias arises, consider a situation in which the crude estimate from an unmatched study is unbiased. If exposure affects the potential matching factor and this factor affects or is affected by disease, the factor will be associated with both exposure and disease in the source population. As a result, in all but some exceptional situations, the associations of exposure with disease within the strata of the factor will differ from the crude association. Because the crude association is unbiased, it follows that the stratum-specific associations must be biased for the true exposure effect.

The latter bias will pose no problem if the study subjects are not matched on the factor, because then the factor can be ignored in favor of the crude estimate of effect (which is unbiased in this example). If there is inappropriate adjustment for the factor, the estimate will be biased (sometimes called *overadjustment bias*), but this bias can be avoided simply by not adjusting for the factor. If, however, there is matching on the factor, the exposure prevalence among noncases will be shifted toward that of the cases, thereby driving the crude effect estimate toward the null. The stratified estimates will remain biased. With matching, then, both the crude and stratum-specific estimates will be biased, and it will not be possible to obtain an unbiased effect estimate from the study data alone.

It follows that, if (as usual) interest is in estimating the net effect of exposure on disease, one should never match on factors that are affected by exposure or disease, such as symptoms or signs of the exposure or the disease, because such matching can irreparably bias the study data. The only exceptions are when the relative selection probabilities for the subjects under the matched design are known and can be used to adjust the estimates back to their expected unmatched form.

Overmatching and Cost Efficiency

Some methods for obtaining controls automatically entail matching. As noted above, examples include neighborhood controls, sibling controls, and friend controls (see Chapter 8). One should consider the potential consequences of the matching that results from the use of such controls. As an example, in a case-control study it is sometimes very economical to recruit controls by asking each case to provide the names of several friends who might serve as controls and to recruit one or more of these friends to serve as controls. As discussed in Chapter 8, use of friend controls may induce bias under ordinary circumstances. Even when this bias is negligible, however, friendship may be related to exposure (*e.g.*, through lifestyle factors), but not to disease. As a result, use of such friend controls could entail a statistical efficiency loss because such use corresponds to matching on a factor that is related only to exposure. More generally, the decision to use convenient controls should weigh any cost savings against any efficiency loss and bias relative to the viable alternatives (*e.g.*, general population controls). Ordinarily, one would prefer the strategy that has the lowest total cost among strategies that are expected to have the least bias.

The problem of choice of strategy can be reformulated for situations in which the number of cases can be varied and situations in which the numbers of cases and controls are both fixed.[134] Unfortunately, one rarely knows in advance the key quantities needed to make the best choice with certainty, such as cost per control with each strategy, the number of subjects that will be needed with each strategy, and the biases that might ensue with each strategy. The choice will be easy when the same bias is expected regardless of strategy, and the statistically most efficient strategy is also the cheapest per subject. One should simply use that strategy. But in other settings, one may be able to do no better than conduct a few rough, speculative calculations to guide the choice of strategy.

Matching on Indicators of Information Accuracy

Matching is sometimes employed to achieve comparability in the accuracy of information collected. A typical situation in which such matching might be undertaken is a case-control study in which some or all of the cases have already died and surrogates must be interviewed for exposure and confounder information. Theoretically, controls for dead cases should be living, because the source population that gave rise to the cases contains only living persons. In practice, because surrogate interview data may differ in accuracy from interview data obtained directly from the subject, some investigators prefer to match dead controls to dead cases.

Matching on information accuracy is not necessarily beneficial, however. Whereas using dead controls can be justified in proportional mortality studies, essentially as a convenience, matching on information accuracy does not always reduce the overall bias. Some of the assumptions about the accuracy of surrogate data, for example, are unproved.[138] Furthermore, comparability of information accuracy still allows bias from nondifferential misclassification, which can be more severe in matched than in unmatched studies,[127] and more severe than the bias resulting from differential misclassification arising from noncomparability.[139,140]

Alternatives to Traditional Matched Designs

Conventional matched and unmatched designs represent only two points on a broad spectrum of matching strategies. Among potentially advantageous alternatives are partial and marginal matching,[123] countermatching,[141,142] and other matching strategies for improving efficiency.[143] Some of these approaches can be more convenient, as well as more efficient, than conventional matched or unmatched designs. For example, partial matching allows selection of matched controls for some subjects, unmatched controls for others, and the use of different matching factors for different subjects, where the "controls" may be either the unexposed in a cohort study or the noncases in a case-control study. Marginal matching is a form of frequency matching in which only the marginal (separate) distributions of the matching factors are forced to be alike, rather than the joint distribution. For example, one may select controls so that they have the same age and sex distributions as cases, without forcing them to have the same age-sex distribution (*e.g.*, the proportion of men could be the same in cases and controls, even though the proportion of 60-year-old to 64-year-old men might be different).

For both partial and marginal matching, the resulting data can be analyzed by treating all matching factors as stratification variables and following guidelines for matched-data analysis. An advantage of partial and marginal matching is that one need not struggle to find a perfect matched control for each case (in a case-control study) or for each exposed subject (in a cohort study). Thus, partial matching may save considerable effort in searching for suitable controls.

References

1. Greenland S. Randomization, statistics, and causal inference. *Epidemiology*. 1990;1(6):421-429.
2. Hernán MA, Robins JM. Authors' response, Part I. Observational studies analyzed like randomized experiments: best of both worlds. *Epidemiology*. 2008;19(6):789-792.
3. Hernán MA, Robins JM. Using big data to emulate a target trial when a randomized trial is not available. *Am J Epidemiol*. 2016;183(8):758-764.
4. Hernan MA, Taubman SL. Does obesity shorten life? The importance of well-defined interventions to answer causal questions. *Int J Obes (Lond)*. 2008;32(suppl 3):S8-S14.
5. Cook TD, Campbell OT. *Quasi-experimentation*. Chicago, IL: Rand McNally; 1979.
6. Rothman KJ, Michels KB. The continuing unethical use of placebo controls. *N Engl J Med*. 1994;331(6):394-398.
7. Rothman KJ, Michels KB. "When is it appropriate to use a placebo arm in a trial?". In: Guess HA, Kleinman A, Kusek JW, Engel LW, eds. *The Science of the Placebo: Toward an Interdisciplinary Research Agenda*. London: BMJ Books; 2002.
8. Bosco JL, Silliman RA, Thwin SS, et al. A most stubborn bias: no adjustment method fully resolves confounding by indication in observational studies. *J Clin Epidemiol*. 2010;63(1):64-74.
9. Byar DP, Simon RM, Friedewald WT, et al. Randomized clinical trials. Perspectives on some recent ideas. *N Engl J Med*. 1976;295(2):74-80.
10. Peto R, Pike MC, Armitage P, et al. Design and analysis of randomized clinical trials requiring prolonged observation of each patient. I. Introduction and design. *Br J Cancer*. 1976;34(6):585-612.
11. Gelman A, Carlin JB, Stern HS, Rubin DB. *Bayesian Data Analysis*. 2nd ed. New York, NY: Chapman and Hall/CRC; 2003.
12. Greenland S, Robins JM. Identifiability, exchangeability, and epidemiological confounding. *Int J Epidemiol*. 1986;15(3):413-419.
13. Brookhart MA, Wang PS, Solomon DH, Schneeweiss S. Evaluating short-term drug effects using a physician-specific prescribing preference as an instrumental variable. *Epidemiology*. 2006;17(3):268-275.
14. Armitage P. The search for optimality in clinical trials. *Int Stat Rev*. 1985;53:1-13.
15. Avins AL. Can unequal be more fair? Ethics, subject allocation, and randomised clinical trials. *J Med Ethics*. 1998;24(6):401-408.

16. Psaty BM, Prentice RL. Minimizing bias in randomized trials: the importance of blinding. *J Am Med Assoc*. 2010;304(7):793-794.

17. Goetghebeur E, van Houwelingen H, eds. Analyzing non-compliance in clinical trials (special issue). *Stat Med*. 1998;17:247-393.

18. Hernan MA, Hernandez-Diaz S. Beyond the intention-to-treat in comparative effectiveness research. *Clin Trials*. 2012;9(1):48-55.

19. Sommer AS, Zeger S. On estimating efficacy from clinical trials. *Stat Med*. 1991;10:45-52.

20. Angrist JD, Imbens GW, Rubin DB. Identification of causal effects using instrumental variables (with comments). *J Am Stat Assoc*. 1996;91:444-472.

21. Greenland S. An introduction to instrumental variables for epidemiologists. *Int J Epidemiol*. 2000;29(4):722-729.

22. Robins JM. Correcting for non-compliance in randomized trials using structural nested mean models. *Commun Stat Theory Methods*. 1994;23(8):2379-2412.

23. Mark SD, Robins JM. A method for the analysis of randomized trials with compliance information: an application to the Multiple Risk Factor Intervention Trial. *Control Clin Trials*. 1993;14(2): 79-97.

24. Toh S, Hernán Miguel A. Causal inference from longitudinal studies with baseline randomization. *Int J Biostat*. 2008;4(1):22.

25. Wilhelmsen L. Role of the data and safety monitoring committee (DSMC). *Stat Med*. 2002;21(19):2823-2829.

26. Armitage P, McPherson CK, Rowe BC. Repeated significance tests on accumulating data. *J R Stat Soc Ser A*. 1969;132:235-244.

27. George SL, Freidlin B, Korn EL. Strength of accumulating evidence and data monitoring committee decision making. *Stat Med*. 2004;23(17):2659-2672.

28. Wheatley K, Clayton D. Be skeptical about unexpected large apparent treatment effects: the case of an MRC AML12 randomization. *Control Clin Trials*. 2003;24(1):66-70.

29. Pocock SJ, Hughes MD. Practical problems in interim analyses, with particular regard to estimation. *Control Clin Trials*. 1989;10(suppl 4):209S-221S.

30. Cannistra SA. The ethics of early stopping rules: who is protecting whom? *J Clin Oncol*. 2004;22(9):1542-1545.

31. Berry DA. A case for Bayesianism in clinical trials. *Stat Med* 1993;12(15-16):1377-1393; discussion 1395-404.

32. Carlin BP, Sargent DJ. Robust Bayesian approaches for clinical trial monitoring. *Stat Med*. 1996;15(11):1093-1106.

33. Pedroza C, Tyson JE, Das A, et al. Advantages of Bayesian monitoring methods in deciding whether and when to stop a clinical trial: an example of a neonatal cooling trial. *Trials*. 2016;17(1):335.

34. Murthy VH, Krumholz HM, Gross CP. Participation in cancer clinical trials: race-, sex-, and age-based disparities. *J Am Med Assoc*. 2004;291(22):2720-2726.

35. Heiat A, Gross CP, Krumholz HM. Representation of the elderly, women, and minorities in heart failure clinical trials. *Arch Intern Med*. 2002;162(15):1682-1688.

36. Franco S, Hoertel N, McMahon K, et al. Generalizability of pharmacologic and psychotherapy clinical trial results for posttraumatic stress disorder to community samples. *J Clin Psychiatry*. 2016;77(8):e97 5-e981.

37. Kennedy-Martin T, Curtis S, Faries D, Robinson S, Johnston J. A literature review on the representativeness of randomized controlled trial samples and implications for the external validity of trial results. *Trials*. 2015;16:495.

38. Mentz RJ, Hernandez AF, Berdan LG, et al. Good clinical practice guidance and pragmatic clinical trials: balancing the best of both worlds. *Circulation*. 2016;133(9):872-880.

39. Schwartz D, Lellouch J. Explanatory and pragmatic attitudes in therapeutical trials. *J Chronic Dis*. 1967;20(8):637-648.

40. Tunis SR, Stryer DB, Clancy CM. Practical clinical trials: increasing the value of clinical research for decision making in clinical and health policy. *J Am Med Assoc*. 2003;290(12):1624-1632.

41. Christiansen P, Ejlertsen B, Jensen MB, Mouridsen H. Danish breast cancer cooperative group. *Clin Epidemiol*. 2016;8:445-449.

42. Li G, Sajobi TT, Menon BK, et al. Registry-based randomized controlled trials- what are the advantages, challenges, and areas for future research? *J Clin Epidemiol*. 2016;80:16-24.

43. Patsopoulos NA. A pragmatic view on pragmatic trials. *Dialogues Clin Neurosci*. 2011;13(2):217-224.

44. Thorpe KE, Zwarenstein M, Oxman AD, et al. A pragmatic-explanatory continuum indicator summary (PRECIS): a tool to help trial designers. *J Clin Epidemiol*. 2009;62(5):464-475.

45. Ford I, Norrie J. Pragmatic trials. *N Engl J Med*. 2016;375(5):454-463.

46. Karlowski TR, Chalmers TC, Frenkel LD, Kapikian AZ, Lewis TL, Lynch JM. Ascorbic acid for the common cold. A prophylactic and therapeutic trial. *J Am Med Assoc.* 1975;231(10):1038-1042.

47. Dykes MHM, Meier P. Ascorbic acid and the common cold: evaluation of its efficacy and toxicity. *J Am Med Assoc.* 1975;231:1073-1079.

48. Francis T Jr, Korns RF, Voight RB, et al. An evaluation of the 1954 poliomyelitis vaccine trials. *Am J Public Health Nations Health.* 1955;45(5 Pt 2):1-63.

49. Szmuness W, Stevens CE, Harley EJ, et al. Hepatitis B vaccine: demonstration of efficacy in a controlled clinical trial in a high-risk population in the United States. *N Engl J Med.* 1980;303(15):833-841.

50. Rothman KJ, Funch DP, Alfredson T, Brady J, Dreyer NA. Randomized field trial of vaginal douching, pelvic inflammatory disease and pregnancy. *Epidemiology.* 2003;14(3):340-348.

51. Thompson IM, Goodman PJ, Tangen CM, et al. The influence of finasteride on the development of prostate cancer. *N Engl J Med.* 2003;349(3):215-224.

52. Leren P. The effect of plasma cholesterol lowering diet in male survivors of myocardial infarction. A controlled clinical trial. *Acta Med Scand Suppl.* 1966;466:1-92.

53. Detre KM, Shaw L. Long-term changes of serum cholesterol with cholesterol-altering drugs in patients with coronary heart disease. Veterans Administration Drug-Lipid Cooperative Study. *Circulation.* 1974;50(5):998-1005.

54. Kolata G. Heart study produces a surprise result. *Science.* 1982;218(4567):31-32.

55. MacKay AM, Rothman KJ. The incidence and severity of burn injuries following Project Burn Prevention. *Am J Public Health.* 1982;72(3):248-252.

56. Garn JV, Brumback BA, Drews-Botsch CD, Lash TL, Kramer MR, Freeman MC. Estimating the effect of school water, sanitation, and hygiene improvements on pupil health outcomes. *Epidemiology.* 2016;27(5):752-760.

57. Freeman MC, Clasen T, Brooker SJ, Akoko DO, Rheingans R. The impact of a school-based hygiene, water quality and sanitation intervention on soil-transmitted helminth reinfection: a cluster-randomized trial. *Am J Trop Med Hyg.* 2013;89(5):875-883.

58. Freeman MC, Clasen T, Dreibelbis R, et al. The impact of a school-based water supply and treatment, hygiene, and sanitation programme on pupil diarrhoea: a cluster-randomized trial. *Epidemiol Infect.* 2014;142(2):340-351.

59. Ast DB, Smith DJ, Wachs B, Cantwell KT. Newburgh-Kingston caries-fluorine study. XIV. Combined clinical and roentgenographic dental findings after ten years of fluoride experience. *J Am Dent Assoc.* 1956;52(3):314-325.

60. Omar RZ, Thompson SG. Analysis of a cluster randomized trial with binary outcome data using a multilevel model. *Stat Med.* 2000;19(19):2675-2688.

61. Turner RM, Omar RZ, Thompson SG. Bayesian methods of analysis for cluster randomized trials with binary outcome data. *Stat Med.* 2001;20(3):453-472.

62. Spiegelhalter DJ. Bayesian methods for cluster randomized trials with continuous responses. *Stat Med.* 2001;20(3):435-452.

63. Brumback BA, He Z, Prasad M, Freeman MC, Rheingans R. Using structural-nested models to estimate the effect of cluster-level adherence on individual-level outcomes with a three-armed cluster-randomized trial. *Stat Med.* 2014;33(9):1490-1502.

64. Turner EL, Li F, Gallis JA, Prague M, Murray DM. Review of recent methodological developments in group-randomized trials: Part 1-design. *Am J Public Health.* 2017;107(6):907-915.

65. Turner EL, Prague M, Gallis JA, Li F, Murray DM. Review of recent methodological developments in group-randomized trials: Part 2-analysis. *Am J Public Health.* 2017;107(7):1078-1086.

66. MacMahon B. *Strengths and Limitations of Epidemiology. National Academy of Sciences, the National Research Council.* Washington, DC: National Academy of Sciences; 1979.

67. Snow J. *On the Mode of Communication of Cholera.* New Burlington Street, London: John Churchill; 1855.

68. Koch T. Commentary: nobody loves a critic. Edmund A Parkes and John Snow's cholera. *Int J Epidemiol.* 2013;42(6):1553-1559.

69. Vandenbroucke JP. Prospective or retrospective: what's in a name? *Br Med J.* 1991;302(6771):249-250.

70. Doll R. Prospective or retrospective: what's in a name? *Br Med J.* 1991;302(6775):528-529.

71. Last JM. Prospective or retrospective: what's in a name? *Br Med J.* 1991;302(6775):528-529.

72. Morabia A. Prospective or retrospective: what's in a name? *Br Med J.* 1991;302(6775):528-529.

73. Vandenbroucke JP, von Elm E, Altman DG, et al. Strengthening the reporting of observational studies in epidemiology (STROBE): explanation and elaboration. *Epidemiology.* 2007;18(6):805-835.

74. Morgenstern H, Thomas D. Principles of study design in environmental epidemiology. *Environ Health Perspect.* 1993;101(suppl 4):23-38.

75. Flanders WD, Lin L, Pirkle JL, Caudill SP. Assessing the direction of causality in cross-sectional studies. *Am J Epidemiol.* 1992;135(8):926-935.

76. Simon R. Length biased sampling in etiologic studies. *Am J Epidemiol.* 1980;111(4):444-452.

77. Flanders WD, Klein M, Mirabelli MC. Conditions for valid estimation of causal effects on prevalence in cross-sectional and other studies. *Ann Epidemiol.* 2016;26(6):389-394.e2.

78. Reichenheim ME, Coutinho ES. Measures and models for causal inference in cross-sectional studies: arguments for the appropriateness of the prevalence odds ratio and related logistic regression. *BMC Med Res Methodol.* 2010;10(1):66.

79. Pearce N. Effect measures in prevalence studies. *Environ Health Perspect.* 2004;112(10):1047-1050.

80. McDowall M. Adjusting proportional mortality ratios for the influence of extraneous causes of death. *Stat Med.* 1983;2(4):467-475.

81. Miettinen OS, Wang JD. An alternative to the proportionate mortality ratio. *Am J Epidemiol.* 1981;114(1):144-148.

82. McLaughlin JK, Blot WJ, Mehl ES, Mandel JS. Problems in the use of dead controls in case-control studies. I. General results. *Am J Epidemiol.* 1985;121(1):131-139.

83. Wang JD, Miettinen OS. Occupational mortality studies. Principles of validity. *Scand J Work Environ Health.* 1982;8(3):153-158.

84. Rodriguez EM, Staffa JA, Graham DJ. The role of databases in drug postmarketing surveillance. *Pharmacoepidemiol Drug Saf.* 2001;10(5):407-410.

85. DuMouchel W. Bayesian data mining in large frequency tables, with an application to the FDA spontaneous Reporting System (with discussion). *Am Stat.* 1999;53:177-190.

86. Borg JJ, Aislaitner G, Pirozynski M, Mifsud S. Strengthening and rationalizing pharmacovigilance in the EU: where is Europe heading to? A review of the new EU legislation on pharmacovigilance. *Drug Saf.* 2011;34(3):187-197.

87. Evans SJ, Waller PC, Davis S. Use of proportional reporting ratios (PRRs) for signal generation from spontaneous adverse drug reaction reports. *Pharmacoepidemiol Drug Saf.* 2001;10(6):483-486.

88. Rothman KJ, Lanes S, Sacks ST. The reporting odds ratio and its advantages over the proportional reporting ratio. *Pharmacoepidemiol Drug Saf.* 2004;13(8):519-523.

89. Behrman RE, Benner JS, Brown JS, McClellan M, Woodcock J, Platt R. Developing the sentinel system – a national resource for evidence development. *New Engl J Med.* 2011;364(6):498-499.

90. Blake KV, Devries CS, Arlett P, Kurz X, Fitt H; for the European Network of Centres for Pharmacoepidemiology Pharmacovigilance. Increasing scientific standards, independence and transparency in post-authorisation studies: the role of the European Network of Centres for Pharmacoepidemiology and Pharmacovigilance. *Pharmacoepidemiol Drug Saf.* 2012;21(7):690-696.

91. Firebaugh G. A rule for inferring individual-level relationships from aggregate data. *Am Sociol Rev.* 1978;43:557-572.

92. Morgenstern H. Uses of ecologic analysis in epidemiologic research. *Am J Public Health.* 1982;72(12):1336-1344.

93. Richardson S, Stucker I, Hemon D. Comparison of relative risks obtained in ecological and individual studies: some methodological considerations. *Int J Epidemiol.* 1987;16(1):111-120.

94. Piantadosi S, Byar DP, Green SB. The ecological fallacy. *Am J Epidemiol.* 1988;127(5):893-904.

95. Greenland S, Robins J. Invited commentary: ecologic studies – biases, misconceptions, and counterexamples. *Am J Epidemiol.* 1994;139(8):747-760.

96. Greenland S. Ecologic versus individual-level sources of bias in ecologic estimates of contextual health effects. *Int J Epidemiol.* 2001;30(6):1343-1350.

97. Greenland S. A review of multilevel theory for ecologic analyses. *Stat Med.* 2002;21(3):389-395.

98. Brenner H, Savitz DA, Jockel KH, Greenland S. Effects of nondifferential exposure misclassification in ecologic studies. *Am J Epidemiol.* 1992;135(1):85-95.

99. Greenland S. An overview of methods for causal inference from observational studies. In: Gelman A, Meng XL, eds. *Applied Bayesian Modeling and Causal Inference from an Incomplete-Data Perspective.* New York, NY: Wiley; 2004.

100. Savitz DA. Commentary: a niche for ecologic studies in environmental epidemiology. *Epidemiology.* 2012;23(1):53-54.

101. Wakefield J. Ecologic studies revisited. *Annu Rev Public Health.* 2008;29(1):75-90.

102. Wakefield J, Haneuse SJPA. Overcoming ecologic bias using the two-phase study design. *Am J Epidemiol.* 2008;167(8):908-916.

103. Abadie A. Semiparametric difference-in-differences estimators. *Rev Econ Stud.* 2005;72(1):1-19.

104. Ji X, Small DS, Leonard CE, Hennessy S. The trend-in-trend research design for causal inference. *Epidemiology.* 2017;28(4):529-536.

105. Cole P. The hypothesis generating machine. *Epidemiology.* 1993;4(3):271-273.

106. Saika K, Sobue T. Epidemiology of Breast Cancer in Japan and the US. *JMAJ.* 2009;52(1):39-44.

107. Trichopoulos D, Lipman RD. Mammary gland mass and breast cancer risk. *Epidemiology.* 1992;3(6):523-526.

108. Rothman KJ. Epidemiologic methods in clinical trials. *Cancer*. 1977;39(suppl 4):1771-1775.
109. Miettinen OS. Individual matching with multiple controls in the case of all-or-none responses. *Biometrics*. 1969;25(2):339-355.
110. Morgenstern H, Winn DM. A method for determining the sampling ratio in epidemiologic studies. *Stat Med*. 1983;2(3):387-396.
111. Breslow NE, Lubin JH, Marek P, Langholz B. Multiplicative models and cohort analysis. *J Am Stat Assoc*. 1983;78:1-12.
112. Meydrech EF, Kupper LL. Cost considerations and sample size requirements in cohort and case-control studies. *Am J Epidemiol*. 1978;107(3):201-205.
113. Thompson WD, Kelsey JL, Walter SD. Cost and efficiency in the choice of matched and unmatched case-control study designs. *Am J Epidemiol*. 1982;116(5):840-851.
114. Mansournia MA, Jewell NP, Greenland S. Case-control matching: effects, misconceptions, and recommendations. *Eur J Epidemiol*. 2018;33(1):5-14.
115. Pearce N. Analysis of matched case-control studies. *Br Med J*. 2016;352:i969.
116. Pearce N. Bias in matched case-control studies: DAGs are not enough. *Eur J Epidemiol*. 2018;33(1):1-4.
117. Walker AM. Efficient assessment of confounder effects in matched cohort studies. *Appl Stat*. 1982;31:293-297.
118. Weinberg CR. On pooling across strata when frequency matching has been followed in a cohort study. *Biometrics*. 1985;41(1):117-127.
119. Greenland S, Robins JM. Estimation of a common effect parameter from sparse follow-up data. *Biometrics*. 1985;41(1):55-68.
120. Greenland S, Morgenstern H. Matching and efficiency in cohort studies. *Am J Epidemiol*. 1990;131(1):151-159.
121. Youkeles LH. Loss of power through ineffective pairing of observations in small two-treatment all-or-none experiments. *Biometrics*. 1963;19:175-180.
122. Rose S, Laan MJ. Why match? Investigating matched case-control study designs with causal effect estimation. *Int J Biostat*. 2009;5(1):1.
123. Greenland S. Partial and marginal matching in case-control studies. In: Moolgavkar SH, Prentice RL, eds. *Modern Statistical Methods in Chronic Disease Epidemiology*. New York, NY: Wiley; 1986:35-49.
124. Sturmer T, Brenner H. Degree of matching and gain in power and efficiency in case-control studies. *Epidemiology*. 2001;12(1):101-108.
125. Greenland S. Multivariate estimation of exposure-specific incidence from case-control studies. *J Chronic Dis*. 1981;34(9-10):445-453.
126. Benichou J, Wacholder S. A comparison of three approaches to estimate exposure-specific incidence rates from population-based case-control data. *Stat Med*. 1994;13(5-7):651-661.
127. Greenland S. The effect of misclassification in matched-pair case-control studies. *Am J Epidemiol*. 1982;116(2):402-406.
128. Kupper LL, Karon JM, Kleinbaum DG, Morgenstern H, Lewis DK. Matching in epidemiologic studies: validity and efficiency considerations. *Biometrics*. 1981;37(2):271-291.
129. Smith PG, Day NE. Matching and confounding in the design and analysis of epidemiological case-control studies. In: Blithell JF, Coppi R, eds. *Perspectives in Medical Statistics*. New York, NY: Academic Press; 1981.
130. Thomas DC, Greenland S. The relative efficiencies of matched and independent sample designs for case-control studies. *J Chronic Dis*. 1983;36(10):685-697.
131. Poole C. Exposure opportunity in case-control studies. *Am J Epidemiol*. 1986;123(2):352-358.
132. Kalish LA. Matching on a non-risk factor in the design of case-control studies does not always result in an efficiency loss. *Am J Epidemiol*. 1986;123(3):551-554.
133. Howe GR, Choi BC. Methodological issues in case-control studies: validity and power of various design/analysis strategies. *Int J Epidemiol*. 1983;12(2):238-245.
134. Thompson WD, Kelsey JL, Walter SD. Cost and efficiency in the choice of matched and unmatched case-control study designs. *Am J Epidemiol*. 1982;116(5):840-851.
135. Smith PG, Day NE. The design of case-control studies: the influence of confounding and interaction effects. *Int J Epidemiol*. 1984;13(3):356-365.
136. Thomas DC, Greenland S. The efficiency of matching in case-control studies of risk-factor interactions. *J Chronic Dis*. 1985;38(7):569-574.
137. Greenland S, Neutra R. An analysis of detection bias and proposed corrections in the study of estrogens and endometrial cancer. *J Chronic Dis*. 1981;34(9-10):433-438.
138. Gordis L. Should dead cases be matched to dead controls? *Am J Epidemiol*. 1982;115(1):1-5.
139. Greenland S, Robins JM. Confounding and misclassification. *Am J Epidemiol*. 1985;122(3):495-506.
140. Drews CD, Greeland S. The impact of differential recall on the results of case-control studies. *Int J Epidemiol*. 1990;19(4):1107-1112.

141. Langholz B, Clayton D. Sampling strategies in nested case-control studies. *Environ Health Perspect.* 1994;102(suppl 8):47-51.
142. Cologne JB, Sharp GB, Neriishi K, Verkasalo PK, Land CE, Nakachi K. Improving the efficiency of nested case-control studies of interaction by selecting controls using counter matching on exposure. *Int J Epidemiol.* 2004;33(3):485-492.
143. Sturmer T, Brenner H. Flexible matching strategies to increase power and efficiency to detect and estimate gene-environment interactions in case-control studies. *Am J Epidemiol.* 2002;155(7):593-602.

PART II

Study Design and Interpretation

CHAPTER 7

Cohort Studies

Kenneth J. Rothman, Tyler J. VanderWeele, and Timothy L. Lash

This chapter focuses on basic elements for the design and conduct of cohort studies. Further considerations for cohort study design are given in Chapters 12 through 15, and analytic methods applicable to cohort studies are presented in Chapters 17 through 28. Many special aspects of exposure assessment that are not covered here can be found in Armstrong et al.[1]

DEFINITION OF COHORTS AND EXPOSURE GROUPS

The goal of a cohort study is to measure and often to compare the incidence of disease in one or more study cohorts. The word *cohort* designates a group of people who share a common experience or condition. For example, a birth cohort shares the same year or period of birth, a cohort of miners has the experience of their occupational history in common, and a cohort of vegetarians share their dietary habit. Often, if there are two cohorts in a study, one of them is described as the exposed cohort—those individuals who have experienced an event or condition that may affect their risk of one or more health outcomes—and the other is thought of as the unexposed, or reference, cohort. The reference cohort provides the standard against which the change in risk of the exposed cohort is measured. The reference cohort may be defined by the lack of exposure to the index condition, or they may be defined by exposure to a second reference condition. For example, in pharmacoepidemiology, the index condition may be use of a particular pharmaceutical. The reference condition may be lack of use of the particular pharmaceutical, or better yet, use of a second pharmaceutical called the active comparator (see Chapter 43). Analogous index and reference conditions exist for health behaviors, occupations, and other topics of epidemiologic research. If there are more than two cohorts, each may be characterized by a different level or type of exposure. Exposed cohorts and a reference cohort, all defined within a larger cohort, are also sometimes called *subcohorts*. For example, in the Framingham Heart Study,[2] described in detail later in this chapter, the population of the city of Framingham, Massachusetts, is the study cohort, but it comprises many subcohorts whose disease experience has been compared with one another.

Cohorts are established because of some attribute that its members share. Sometimes this common attribute is a shared exposure. It may, however, be only a similar propensity to participate in research and provide accurate information. It might be a shared demographic characteristic, for example, one that is underrepresented in the majority population. In these settings, the cohort is assembled to learn about the prevalence of exposures, the incidence of diseases, or the strength of associations between exposures and diseases in people like those in the cohort. Alternatively, the common attribute may be having experienced a particular health event, such as a stroke or a type of cancer, and the research interest is learning about health outcomes following that event. In all cases, membership in the cohort begins with an investigator's desire to gather information from people who share the common attribute that characterizes the cohort. By assembling cohorts that are defined based on shared exposure or selected demographic characteristics, the investigator can form a study population that is better suited to study exposures, diseases, and their associations than would be possible with a simple random sample of the whole population. The paragraphs below illustrate examples of cohorts established with these various goals in mind.

Exposure-Defined and General-Population Cohorts

An attractive feature of cohort studies is the capability they provide to study a range of possible health outcomes. A mortality follow-up can be accomplished just as easily for all causes of death as for any specific cause. Health surveillance for one disease end point can sometimes be expanded to include many or all end points without much additional work. A cohort study can thus provide a comprehensive picture of the health effects stemming from a given exposure contrast or related to a specific characteristic. Attempts to derive such comprehensive information related to a specific exposure or characteristic motivate the identification of exposure-defined cohorts.

Cohorts Defined by Common Occupation

Occupational cohort studies provide a paradigm for exposure-defined cohorts (see Chapter 41). Rosters of employees or union members are obtained from personnel records and then linked with health records, oftentimes mortality records, to identify the health outcomes. When the outcome is mortality, the cause-of-death information, taken from the death certificate, is often used to provide surrogate information for disease incidence. The reference cohort of unexposed persons may be the geographically overlapping population, restricted to the same age, sex, and calendar period and further standardized to the distribution of these characteristics in the occupational cohort. Although members of the occupational cohort contribute to the general population, and hence appear in both the exposed and unexposed cohorts, the proportion of the general population made up of members of the occupational cohort is usually so small that their influence on the disease or mortality rates of the general population is negligible. Subcohorts may also be created within the occupational cohort, with categorizations based on duration of employment, intensity of exposure to a potentially harmful workplace agent, or an index combining both.

Examples of occupational cohorts that yielded critical public-health information about occupational and environmental hazards include cohorts defined by occupation in asbestos mining and milling,[3] asbestos textile manufacturing,[4] beryllium processing,[5] X-ray imaging,[6] and many others. The occupation of people in these cohorts brought workers in direct contact with a potentially hazardous agent as an inherent part of their work duties. Some occupations bring workers into contact with a hazardous agent as a secondary aspect of their work duties. For example, cohorts of railroad workers[7] and miners[8] working in enclosed spaces with heavy equipment have provided valuable information about the hazards of exposure to diesel exhaust. Finally, some occupational cohorts have been established not so much to study workplace hazards but because the cohort members are expected to have special commitment to research on health and special ability to report health-related information. Examples include the British Doctors Study,[9] which was one of the first cohort studies to report an association between tobacco smoking and lung cancer risk, the Nurses' Health Study,[10] and the Health Professionals Follow-up Study.[11] These latter studies have collected self-reported information about many health behaviors and many health outcomes, relying in part on the participants' commitment to health research and accurate comprehension of the health-related interview questions.

Cohorts Defined by Common Place

Cohorts may also be defined because of shared geographical locale at a particular calendar time. The Framingham Heart Study was initiated in 1948 to study risk factors for heart disease in an adult population.[2] Residents of Framingham, Massachusetts, were invited to join the cohort in part because of the town's proximity to the investigators, who wished to conduct regular physical examinations. Thus, like the healthcare provider cohorts described above, this cohort was created in part to enhance the quality and cost-effectiveness of the data collection efforts. Geographically defined cohorts may also be established to investigate the effects of a known, localized environmental hazard, such as the cohort of residents near Seveso at the time a factory explosion released dibenzodioxins,[12] the cohort of residents exposed to rice oil contaminated with polychlorinated biphenyls and dibenzofurans in Japan[13] and Taiwan,[14] and the cohorts of persons exposed to radiation following the Chernobyl[15] or Fukushima[16] nuclear reactors at the time of their accidental releases of radiation. In these examples, the expected health effects were fairly well understood. Cohorts of residents exposed to natural and man-made catastrophes have also been established to investigate a wide range of health effects, partly because the expected effects are less well understood. Examples include cohorts of residents near Hiroshima and Nagasaki after the atomic bomb attack,[17] residents in Manhattan after the September 11, 2001, terror attack,[18] and of residents affected by flood, isolation, and dislocation after Hurricane Katrina[19] or the major earthquake in Haiti.[20] Finally, some cohorts have been selected to overrepresent geographic regions with high rates of particular diseases or a high prevalence of particular risk factor profiles, in the hopes that oversampling populations in these regions will help to identify public-health interventions to diminish these differences. Examples include the "Reasons for Geographic and Racial Differences in Stroke,"[21] which oversampled residents in the southern stroke belt of the United States, and the "Southern Community Cohort Study,"[22] which oversampled rural residents in the southeastern United States to investigate social and demographic disparities in risk factors for cancer.

Cohorts Defined by Demographic Characteristics

Many cohorts have been enrolled with the goal of studying persons with particular demographic characteristics. The Normative Aging Study has the aim of investigating healthy aging;[23] the Black Women's Health Study was initiated to evaluate the incidence and risk factors for common diseases among a population that had been underrepresented in existing cohorts,[24] and the Singapore Chinese Health study has focused on dietary causes of cancer in an Asian population.[25] There are also cohorts that have oversampled demographic subgroups to ensure adequate representation of various race/ethnicity groups either in the cohort or in the research topic area. Examples include the Jackson Heart Study[26] and the Multi-Ethnic Study of Atherosclerosis.[27]

Cohorts Defined by Health Conditions or Events

In the realm of clinical epidemiology, cohorts are often established by enrolling patients who have had a common health condition or event, with the aim of studying quality of care for the index event or condition, incidence of subsequent events or other health outcomes, and survival. Examples include cohorts of survivors of myocardial infarction,[28] breast cancer,[29] or cirrhosis.[30] More nuanced examples of cohorts established by an index health event are studies of the risk of breast cancer among women who have had an elective abortion,[31] which was the index event, and studies of conception among couples planning a pregnancy,[32,33] in which planning to conceive was the index event. As in earlier illustrations, a health event can also provide an opportunity to enroll people efficiently into a cohort. For example, the KARMA study in Sweden invites women to enroll into the cohort when they attend the age-restricted population-wide mammography screening program.[34] Finally, in the realm of pharmacoepidemiology (see Chapter 43), studies of side effects, rare adverse effects, and late events related to use of prescription medication are often conducted in cohorts established on the basis of having received a prescription for the drug of interest. In these cohorts, the prescription is the index health event, not the health indication for which the medicine was prescribed.

Cohorts Comprising a Sample or a Census of the General Population

Common exposures are sometimes studied through cohort studies that survey a segment of the population that is identified without regard to exposure status. Such "general-population" cohorts have been used to study the effects of smoking, oral contraceptives, diet, and exercise. In nations or political units with centralized registration systems, the dynamic population of residents may be treated as a complete cohort.[35] Given the size of these populations, studies must ordinarily be limited to evaluation of associations between routinely registered exposure information and outcomes, such as routinely recorded employment, socioeconomic status, attained education, and prescription drug information to define the exposure groups, and hospitalized health events as the outcomes. It would be difficult to collect exposure and outcome information from populations of these size by self-report or analysis of biospecimens, for example. Lack of information on health behaviors, bioanalytes, and subclinical health events that are not usually routinely registered is a limitation in cohort studies based on registries[36] (see also Chapter 11).

Cohort Consortiums

Cohorts with sufficient information to evaluate an association sometimes pool data to provide a more precise estimate of the association and to allow dose-response analyses. Such consortiums also allow harmonization of the definitions of exposure, outcome, and covariates.[37] This harmonization provides one advantage over meta-analyses that summarize the estimates of association from the individual cohorts. Data protection guarantees can sometimes present a barrier to pooling, in which case, deidentification or anonymization algorithms[38] and distributed computing solutions have been implemented.[39]

MECHANISMS OF DATA COLLECTION

As described in detail in Chapter 10, data can be collected from cohort members by a wide variety of methods. Cost-efficient methods usually implement linkage with existing registries, such as administrative health records and mortality registries to ascertain outcome information, and personnel records, tax records, census data, and other routinely registered information to ascertain exposure and covariate information. Information on health behaviors, subclinical health outcomes, and more detailed data on routinely registered information must usually be collected directly from individual cohort members. Methods for this collection have evolved with changes to available technology and social norms for interpersonal communication. Many early cohorts collected information by sending paper questionnaires to participants with return postage. Information on returned questionnaires was coded and keyed into databases. These evolved into scannable forms for which most responses could be machine-read, thus eliminating the need for coding or data entry. Cohorts also collected information by telephone interview, in-person interviews, or clinical examinations. The latter two approaches limited cohort enrollment to geographically convenient participants. Interview forms evolved from text to scannable forms in the same fashion as paper questionnaires. Most recently, cohort participants have been able to answer questionnaires via Internet-enabled surveys,[40] which have the advantages of requiring no postage, no interview personnel, and convenience of scheduling.[41]

Collection of data on health outcomes has also evolved over time. Medical record reviews, which are labor intensive and require geographical proximity to the abstractors, provided rich detailed clinical information at a relatively high price. Administrative health records developed to facilitate invoicing for health services allowed identification of some health outcomes, particularly hospitalized events with little ambiguity of diagnosis, such as a cancer surgery. With the advent of electronic medical records, free text searches have been developed to augment or replace use of administrative health records and to collect the same kind of rich health data as previously available only by medical record review. The most labor-intensive and gold-standard method, for collecting data on health is a periodic medical examination. Many cohort studies have regularly invited participants to medical examinations, including even sophisticated and expensive imaging and clinical laboratory testing.

Collection, storage, and analysis of biospecimens have been an important aspect of cohort studies since their inception. Early examples of cohort studies that contributed important public-health information by using biospecimens include the Framingham Heart Study's 1961 report of an association between elevated cholesterol levels and the incidence of myocardial infarction[42] and the studies of the association between blood and dentin lead concentrations and delayed neurodevelopment.[43] Biospecimen collection, storage, and analysis is usually an expensive undertaking, with special protocols required for all aspects of collection, chain-of-custody, preservation, and analysis (see Chapter 36).

Cohort studies that span many years present logistic problems that can adversely affect validity. Whether the study is retrospective or prospective, it is often difficult to locate people or their records many years after they have been enrolled into study cohorts. In prospective studies, it may be possible to maintain periodic contact with study subjects and thereby keep current information on their location. Such tracking adds to the costs of prospective cohort studies, yet the increasing mobility of society warrants stronger efforts to trace subjects. A substantial proportion of subjects lost to follow-up can raise serious doubts about the validity of the study (see Chapter 14). Follow-ups that trace less than about 60% of subjects are generally regarded with skepticism, but even follow-up of 70% or 80% or more can be too low to provide sufficient assurance against bias if there is reason to believe that loss to follow-up may be associated with both exposure and disease.[44] Loss to follow-up is sometimes also called censoring, or more precisely, right-censoring. The complete term "right-censoring" refers to the lack of information about exposure, covariates, and outcomes along a time line with earlier times to the left on a graphical depiction and later times to the right. When follow-up ends, information on the right (later) side of the time line is incomplete and hence censored.

Information preceding the start of follow-up can also affect estimates of disease occurrence and associations of exposure contrasts with disease occurrence within the follow-up period. For example, users of drugs during a time period preceding the start of follow-up may be categorized as "never users" when, in fact, they had been exposed to the drug before information about drug exposures became available.[45] Similarly, adjustment for prevalent comorbid diseases may require a lifetime medical history,[46] which is often unavailable. Persons with a history of myocardial infarction preceding the availability of registry information in a particular cohort might be categorized as having no history of this event. When information is unavailable preceding the start of follow-up or some other date relevant to the collected data, it is called left-censored, again in reference to the usual graphical depiction of timelines with earlier times to the left. The usual solution to left-censoring problems is to require a minimal time period of available information before a person can enter the cohort for follow-up. This minimal time period, sometimes referred to as a "look-back" period, is meant to ensure that accurate information will be available about relevant exposures and events preceding the start of follow-up. Some studies require a minimum look-back period, for example, 1 year, but then use information only from this minimum period for all subjects. Recent work indicates that it may be preferable to use all available information, despite the length of the look-back period varying for different subjects.[47] In cohorts with newly available data sources, such as a new prescription drug registry, left-censoring can be an important threat to validity because there will be incomplete information about prescriptions, exposures, or other disease events preceding the start of follow-up. In addition to incomplete prescription history, left-censoring can be introduced when a cohort has incomplete history of its members' employment before joining an occupational cohort or medical history before joining a clinical cohort, for examples.

CATEGORIZING CASES, PERSONS, AND PERSON-TIME

In principle, a cohort study could be used to estimate average risks, rates, or occurrence times. Except in certain situations, however, average risks and occurrence times cannot be measured directly from the experience of a cohort. Observation of average risks or times of specific events requires that the whole cohort remain at risk and under observation for the entire follow-up period.

Loss of subjects during the study period prevents direct measurements of these averages because the outcome of lost subjects is unknown. Subjects who die from competing risks (outcomes other than the one of interest, see Chapters 4 and 21) likewise prevent the investigator from estimating conditional risks directly (risk of a specific outcome conditional on not getting other outcomes). Thus, average risks and occurrence times can only be accurately measured in a cohort study when there is little or no loss to follow-up and little competing risk. Although some clinical trials provide these conditions, many epidemiologic studies do not. When losses and competing risks do occur, one may still estimate the incidence rate directly, whereas average risk and occurrence time must be estimated using survival (life-table) methods (see Chapter 4).

Average risks are measured with the number of individuals at risk for the outcome at the beginning of follow-up as the denominator, whereas incidence rates have the amount of person-time contributed by these individuals as the denominator. The use of accumulated person-time rather than individuals in the denominator of rates allows flexibility in the analysis of cohort studies. Studies that estimate risk directly are tied conceptually to the identification of specific fixed cohorts of individuals. Studies that measure incidence rates can, with certain assumptions, define the comparison groups in terms of person-time units that do not correspond to specific cohorts of individuals. In these studies, a given individual can contribute person-time to one, two, or more exposure groups in a given study because each unit of person-time contributed to follow-up by a given individual possesses its own classification with respect to exposure status. An individual whose exposure experience changes with time can, depending on details of the study hypothesis, contribute follow-up time to several different exposure-specific rates. In such a study, the definition of each exposure group corresponds to the definition of person-time eligibility for each exposure status.

As a result of this focus on person-time, it does not always make sense to refer to the members of an exposure group within a cohort study as if the same set of individuals were exposed at all points in time. The terms *open population* or *dynamic population* describe a population in which the person-time experience can accrue from a changing roster of individuals (see Chapter 4). Sometimes the term *open cohort* or *dynamic cohort* is used, but this usage conflicts with other usage in which a cohort is a fixed roster of individuals. For example, the incidence rates of cancer reported by a cancer registry come from the experience of an open population. Because the population of residents who would be reported to the registry upon diagnosis of a cancer is always changing, the individuals who contribute to these rates are not a specific set of people who are followed through time.

When the exposure groups in a cohort study are defined at the start of the follow-up, with no movement of individuals between exposure groups during the follow-up, the groups are *fixed cohorts.* The groups defined by treatment allocation in most clinical trials are examples of fixed cohorts. If the follow-up of fixed cohorts suffers from losses to follow-up or competing risks, incidence rates can still be measured directly and used to estimate average risks and incidence times. If no losses occur from a fixed cohort, the cohort satisfies the definition of a *closed population* (see Chapter 4) and is called a *closed cohort*. The term *closed cohort* is also sometimes used to describe what we call a *fixed cohort*; we prefer to keep the terms distinct to make clear the difference. In closed cohorts, unconditional risks (which include the effect of competing risks) and average survival times can be estimated directly.

In the simplest cohort study, the exposure and reference conditions would be permanent and easily identifiable conditions, making the job of assigning subjects to exposed and unexposed cohorts a simple task. Unfortunately, exposures of interest to epidemiologists are seldom constant and are often difficult to measure. Consider the problems of identifying for study a cohort of users of a specific prescription drug. To identify the users requires a method for locating those who receive or who fill prescriptions for the drug. Without a record-keeping system of prescriptions, it becomes a daunting task. Even with a record system, the identification of those who receive or even those who fill a prescription is not equivalent to the identification of those who actually use the drug. Furthermore, those who are users of this drug today may not be users tomorrow and vice versa. Although fixed cohorts of ever and never users of the drug could be identified, a more accurate characterization of exposure status would tie the definition of drug use to time because exposure can change with time. Finally, the effect of the drug that is being studied may be the one that involves a considerable induction period. In that case, the exposure status at a given time will relate to a possible increase or decrease in disease risk only at some later time. Exposure status is then best *lagged* by the length of estimated or assumed induction period. Someone who began to take the drug today might experience a drug-related effect in 10 years, but there might be no possibility of any drug-related effect for the first 5 years after exposure. In that case, the exposure status assigned to person-time lags 5 years behind the follow-up time.

It is tempting to think of the identification of study cohorts as simply a process of identifying and classifying individuals as to their exposure status. The process can be complicated, however, by the need to classify the experience of a single individual in different exposure categories at different times. If the exposure can vary over time, at a minimum, the investigator needs to allow for the time experienced by each study subject in each category of exposure in the definition of the study cohorts. The sequence or timing of exposure could also be important. If there can be many possible exposure sequences, each individual could have a unique sequence of exposure levels and so define a unique exposure cohort containing only that individual.

A simplifying assumption that is common in epidemiologic analysis is that the only aspect of exposure that determines current risk is some simple numeric summary of exposure history. Typical summaries include current level of exposure, average exposure, and cumulative exposure, that is, the sum of each exposure level multiplied by the time spent at that level. Often, exposure is lagged in the summary, which means that only exposure at or up to some specified time before the current time is counted. Although one has enormous flexibility in defining exposure summaries, methods based on assuming that only a single summary is relevant can be severely biased under certain conditions.[48] Specifically, if the exposure is time-varying and a confounder is both affected by prior exposure and also by subsequent exposure and the outcome, then methods described in what follows can be severely biased. We consider appropriate methods for this setting in Chapters 24 and 25. For now, we will assume that a single summary is an adequate measure of exposure (*e.g.*, acute exposure with immediate effects and no carry over). With this assumption, cohort studies may be analyzed by defining the cohorts based on person-time rather than on persons, so that a person may be a member of different exposure cohorts at different times. We nevertheless caution the reader to bear in mind the single-summary assumption when interpreting such analyses.

The time that an individual contributes to the denominator of one or more of the incidence rates in a cohort study is sometimes called the *time at risk,* in the sense of being at risk for development of the disease. Some people and, consequently, all their person-time are not at risk for a given disease because they are immune or they lack the target organ for the study disease. For example, women who have had a hysterectomy and all men are by definition not at risk for uterine cancer because they have no uterus.

Classifying Person-Time

The main guide to the classification of persons or person-time is the study hypothesis, which should be defined in as much detail as possible. If the study addresses the question of the extent to which eating carrots will reduce the subsequent risk of lung cancer, the study hypothesis is best stated in terms of what quantity of carrots consumed over what period of time will prevent lung cancer and in comparison to some equally well-defined reference condition. Furthermore, the study hypothesis should specify an induction time between the consumption of a given amount of carrots and the subsequent effect: The effect of the carrot consumption could take place immediately, begin gradually, or begin only after a delay, and it could extend beyond the time that an individual might cease eating carrots.[49]

In studies with chronic exposures (*i.e.*, exposures that persist over an extended period of time), it is easy to confuse the time during which exposure occurs with the time at risk of exposure effects. For example, in occupational studies, time of employment is sometimes confused with time at risk for exposure effects. The time of employment is a time during which exposure accumulates. In contrast, the time at risk for exposure effects must logically come after the accumulation of a specific amount of exposure because only after that time can disease be caused or prevented by that amount of exposure. The lengths of these two time periods have no constant relation to one another. The time at risk of effects might well extend beyond the end of employment. It is only the time at risk of effects that should be tallied in the denominator of incidence rates for that amount of exposure.

The distinction between time of exposure accrual and the time at risk of exposure effects is easier to see by considering an example in which exposure is very brief. In studies of the delayed effects of exposure to radiation emitted from the atomic bomb,[17] the exposure was nearly instantaneous, but the risk period during which the exposure has had an effect has been very long, perhaps lifelong, although the risk for certain diseases did not increase immediately after exposure. Cancer risk after the radiation exposure increased only after a minimum induction period of several years, depending on the cancer. The incidence rates of cancer among those exposed to high doses of radiation from the bomb, compared with those exposed to nearly no radiation from the bomb, can be calculated separately for different times following exposure, so that one may detect elevations specific to the induction period addressed by the study hypothesis. Without stratification by time since exposure, the incidence rate measured among those exposed to the bomb would be an average rate reflecting periods of exposure effect and periods with no effect because they would include in the denominator some experience of the exposed cohort that corresponds to time in which there was no increased risk from the radiation. Most of this time reflecting little or no increase in risk would have been immediately after the bomb, before radiation-induced cancers began to appear.

How should the investigator study hypotheses that do not specify induction times? For these, the appropriate time periods on which to stratify the incidence rates are unclear. There is no way to estimate exposure effects, however, without making some assumption, implicitly or explicitly, about the induction time. The decision about what time to include for a given individual in the denominator of the rate corresponds to the assumption about induction time. If in a study of delayed effects in survivors of the atomic bombs in Japan, the denominator of the rate included time experienced by study subjects beginning on the day after the exposure, the rate would provide a diluted effect estimate unless the induction period (including the "latent" period) had a minimum of only 1 day. It might be more appropriate to allow for a minimum induction time of some months or years after the bomb explosion.

What if the investigator does not have any basis for hypothesizing a specific induction period? It is possible to learn about the period by estimating effects according to categories of time since exposure. For example, the incidence rate of leukemia among atomic bomb survivors relative to that among those who were distant from the bomb at the time of the explosion can be examined according to years since the explosion. In an unbiased study, we would expect the effect estimates to rise above the null value when the minimum induction period has passed. This procedure works best when the exposure itself occurs at a point or narrow interval of time, but it can be used even if the exposure is chronic, as long as there is a model to describe the amount of time that must pass before a given accumulation of exposure would begin to have an effect.

Chronic Exposures

The definition of chronic exposure based on anticipated effects is more complicated than when exposure occurs only at a point in time. We may conceptualize a period during which the exposure accumulates to a sufficient extent to trigger a step in the causal process. This accumulation of exposure experience may be a complex function of the intensity of the exposure and time. The induction period begins only after the exposure has reached this hypothetical triggering point, and that point will likely vary across individuals. One can measure the induction time for exposure from the time of first exposure, but this procedure involves the often extreme assumption that the first contact with the exposure can be sufficient to produce disease. While this assumption may be reasonable for studies of acute effects of toxic exposures, such as inebriation after consuming substantial alcohol, it would be unreasonable for studies of chronic effects, such as liver cirrhosis associated with chronic alcohol consumption. Whatever assumption is adopted, it should be made an explicit part of the definition of the cohort and the period of follow-up.

Let us consider the steps to take to identify study cohorts when exposure is chronic. First, the investigator must determine how many exposure groups will be studied and determine the definitions for each of the exposure categories. The definition of exposure level could be based on the maximum intensity of exposure experienced, the average intensity over a period of time, or some cumulative amount of exposure. A familiar measure of cigarette smoking is the measure "pack-years," which is the product of the number of packs smoked per day and the number of years smoked. This measure indexes the cumulative number of cigarettes smoked, with one pack-year equal to the product of 20 cigarettes per pack and 365 days, or 7,300 cigarettes. Cumulative indices of exposure and time-weighted measures of average intensity of exposure are both popular methods for measuring exposure in environmental, nutritional, and occupational studies. These exposure definitions should be linked to the time period of an exposure effect, according to the study hypothesis, by explicitly taking into account the induction period.

In employing cumulative or average exposure measures, one should recognize the composite nature of the measures and, if possible, separately analyze the components. For example, pack-years is a composite of duration and intensity of smoking: 20 pack-years might represent half a pack a day for 40 years, one pack a day for 20 years, or two packs a day for 10 years, as well as many other combinations. If the biologic effects of these combinations differ to an important degree, use of pack-years would conceal these differences and perhaps even present a misleading impression of dose-response patterns.[50] Supplemental analyses of smoking as two exposure variables, duration (years smoked) and intensity (packs smoked per day), would provide a safeguard against inadequacies of the pack-years analysis. Other exposure variables that are not accounted for by duration and intensity, such as age at start of exposure, age at cessation of exposure, and timing of exposure relative to disease (induction or lag period), may also warrant separation in the analyses.

Let us look at a simplified example. Suppose the study hypothesis is that smoking increases the risk for lung cancer with a minimum induction time of 5 years. For a given smoking level, the follow-up time experienced by a subject is not "exposed" person-time until the individual has reached that level and then an additional 5 years have passed. Only then is the lung cancer experience of that individual related to smoking according to the study hypothesis. The definition of the study cohort with 20 pack-years of smoking will be the person-time experience of exposed individuals beginning 5 years after they have smoked 20 pack-years. Note that if the cohort study measures incidence rates, which means that it allocates the person-time of the individual study subjects, exposure groups are defined by person-time allocation rather than by rosters of individual subjects.

Note also that all of this depends on the assumption that the effect of smoking on cancer rates is chronic, cumulative, and lagged. A study of the effect of smoking on rate of injury in a house fire would more properly be acute, noncumulative, and instantaneous. It would be a mistake to adopt exposure definitions developed to study the effect of smoking on cancer rates for the study of the effect of smoking on injuries in a house fire. This comparison illustrates the importance of the hypothesis in determining how to categorize person-time as exposed or unexposed, even for fundamentally the same exposure.

Unexposed Time in Exposed Subjects

What happens to the time experienced by exposed subjects that does not meet the definition of time at risk of exposure effects according to the study hypothesis? Specifically, what happens to the time after the exposed subjects become exposed and before the minimum induction has elapsed or after a maximum induction time has passed? Two choices are reasonable for handling this experience. One possibility is to consider any time that is not classified as exposed as unexposed time and to apportion that time to the study cohort that represents the reference, or unexposed, condition. Possible objections to this approach would be that the study hypothesis may be based on guesses about the threshold for exposure effects and the induction period and that time during the exposure accumulation or induction periods may in fact be at risk of exposure effects. To classify the latter experience as person-time in the reference condition may then lead to an underestimate of the effect of exposure (see Chapter 13 for a discussion of misclassification of exposure, in this case resulting from poor construct validity). Alternatively, one may simply omit from the study the experience of exposed subjects that is not at risk of exposure effects according to the study hypothesis. For this alternative to be practical, there must be a reasonably large number of cases observed among subjects with the reference, or unexposed, condition.

For example, suppose a 10-year minimum induction time is hypothesized. For individuals followed from start of exposure, this hypothesis implies that no exposure effect can occur within the first 10 years of follow-up. Only after the first 10 years of follow-up can an individual experience disease due to exposure. Therefore, under the hypothesis, only person-time occurring after 10 years of exposure should contribute to the denominator of the rate among exposed. If the hypothesis were correct, we should assign the first 10 years of follow-up to the denominator of the unexposed rate, presuming that the absence of exposure defines the reference condition. Suppose, however, that the hypothesis were wrong and exposure could produce cases in less than 10 years. Then, if the cases and person-time from the first 10 years of follow-up were added to the unexposed cases and person-time, the resulting rate would be biased toward the rate in the exposed, thus reducing the apparent differences between the exposed and unexposed rates. If computation of the unexposed rate were limited to truly unexposed cases and person-time, this problem would be avoided.

The price of avoidance, however, would be reduced precision in estimating the rate among the unexposed. In some studies, the number of truly unexposed cases is too small to produce a stable comparison, and thus the early experience of exposed persons is too valuable to discard. In general, the best procedure in a given situation would depend on the decrease in precision produced by excluding the early experience of exposed persons and the amount of bias that is introduced by treating the early experience of exposed persons as if it were equivalent to that of people who were never exposed. An alternative that attempts to address both problems is to treat the induction time as a continuous variable rather than a fixed time and model exposure effects as depending on the times of exposure.[51,52] This approach is arguably more realistic insofar as the induction time is allowed to vary across individuals.

Similar issues arise if the exposure status can change from exposed to unexposed. If the exposure ceases but the effects of exposure are thought to continue, it would not make sense to put the experience of a formerly exposed individual in the unexposed category. On the other hand, if exposure effects are thought to be approximately contemporaneous with the exposure, which is to say that the induction period is near zero, then changes in exposure status should lead to corresponding changes in how the accumulating experience is classified with respect to exposure. For example, if individuals taking a nonsteroidal antiinflammatory drug are at an increased risk for gastrointestinal bleeding only during the period that they take the drug, then only the time during exposure is equivalent to the time at risk for gastrointestinal bleeding as a result of the drug. When an individual stops using the drug, the bleeding events and person-time experienced by that individual should be reclassified from exposed to unexposed. Here, the induction time is zero and the definition of exposure does not involve exposure history.

Categorizing Exposure

Another problem to consider is that the study hypothesis may not provide reasonable guidance on where to draw the boundary between exposed and unexposed. If the exposure is continuous, it is not necessary to draw boundaries at all. Instead one may fully use the quantitative information from each individual either by using some type of smoothing method, such as moving averages (see Chapter 19), or by putting the exposure variable into a regression model as a continuous term (see Chapters 20 and 21). Of course, the latter approach depends on the validity of the model used for estimation. Special care must be taken with models of repeatedly measured exposures and confounders, which are sometimes called longitudinal data models (see Chapters 24 and 25).

The simpler approach of calculating rates directly will require a reasonably sized population within categories of exposure if it is to provide a statistically stable result. To get incidence rates, then, we need to group the experience of individuals into relatively large categories for which we can calculate the incidence rates. In principle, it should be possible to form several cohorts that correspond to various levels of exposure. For a cumulative measure of exposure, however, categorization may introduce additional difficulties for the cohort definition. An individual who passes through one level of exposure along the way to a higher level would later have time at risk for disease that theoretically might meet the definition for more than one category of exposure.

For example, suppose we define moderate smoking as having smoked 50,000 cigarettes (equivalent to about 7 pack-years), and we define heavy smoking as having smoked 150,000 cigarettes (about 21 pack-years). Suppose a man smoked his 50,000th cigarette in 2000 and his 150,000th in 2010. After allowing for a 5-year minimum induction period, we would classify his time as moderate smoking beginning in 2005. By 2010, he has become a heavy smoker, but the 5-year induction period for heavy smoking has not elapsed. Thus, from 2010 to 2015, his experience is still classified as moderate smoking, but, from 2015 onward, his experience is classified as heavy smoking. Usually, the time is allocated only to the highest category of exposure that applies. This example illustrates the complexity of the cohort definition with a hypothesis that takes into account both the cumulative amount of exposure and a minimum induction time. Other apportionment schemes could be devised based on other hypotheses about exposure action, including hypotheses that allowed induction time to vary with exposure history.

One invalid allocation scheme would apportion to the denominator of the exposed incidence rate the unexposed experience of an individual who eventually became exposed. For example, suppose that, in an environmental study, exposure is categorized according to duration of exposure to a drinking water contaminant, with the highest exposure category being at least 20 years of exposure. Suppose a resident is exposed to the water for 30 years. It is a mistake to assign the 30 years of experience for that resident to the exposure category of 20 or more years of exposure. The resident only reached that category of exposure after 20 years of living where she was exposed to the water, and only the last 10 years of his or her experience is relevant to the highest category of exposure. Note that if the resident had died after 10 years of exposure, the death could not have been assigned to the 20-years-of-exposure category because the resident would have only had 10 years of exposure.

A useful rule to remember is that the event and the person-time that is being accumulated at the moment of the event should both be assigned to the same category of exposure. Thus, once the person-time spent at each category of exposure has been determined for each study subject, the classification of the disease events (cases) follows the same rules. The exposure category to which an event is assigned is the same exposure category in which the person-time for that individual was accruing at the instant in which the event occurred. The same rule—that the classification of the event follows the classification of the person-time—also applies with respect to other study variables that may be used to stratify the data (see Chapter 18). For example, person-time will be allocated into different age categories as an individual ages. The age category to which an event is assigned should be the same age category in which the individual's person-time was accumulating at the time of the event.

Average Intensity and Alternatives

One can also define current exposure according to the average (arithmetic or geometric mean) intensity or level of exposure up to the current time, rather than by a cumulative measure. In the environmental and occupational settings, the average concentration of an agent in the ambient air would be an example of exposure intensity, although in the occupational setting, one might also have to take into account any protective gear that affects the individual's exposure to the agent. Intensity of exposure is a concept that applies to a point in time, and intensity typically will vary over time. Studies that measure exposure intensity might use a time-weighted average of intensity, which would require multiple measurements of exposure over time. The amount of time that an individual is exposed to each intensity would provide its weight in the computation of the average.

An alternative to the average intensity is to classify exposure according to the maximum intensity, median intensity, minimum intensity, or some other function of the exposure history. The follow-up time that an individual spends at a given exposure intensity could begin to accumulate as soon as that level of intensity is reached. Induction time must also be taken into account. Ideally, the study hypothesis will specify a minimum induction time for exposure effects, which in turn will imply an appropriate lag period to be used in classifying individual experience.

Cumulative and average exposure-assignment schema suffer a potential problem in that they may make it impossible to disentangle exposure effects from the effects of time-varying confounders.[48,53] Methods that treat exposures and confounders in one period as distinct from exposure and confounders in other periods are necessary to avoid this problem[54] (see Chapters 24 and 25).

Immortal Person-Time

Occasionally, a cohort's definition will require that everyone meeting the definition must have survived for a specified period. Typically, this period of immortality comes about because one of the entry criteria into the cohort is dependent on survival. For example, an occupational cohort might be defined as all workers who have been employed at a specific factory for at least 5 years.

There are certain problems with such an entry criterion, among them, that it will guarantee that the study will miss effects among short-term workers who may be assigned more highly exposed jobs than regular long-term employees, may include persons more susceptible to exposure effects, and may quit early because of those effects. Let us assume, however, that only long-term workers are of interest for the study and that all relevant exposures (including those during the initial 5 years of employment) are taken into account in the analysis.

The 5-year entry criterion will guarantee that all of the workers in the study cohort survived their first 5 years of employment because those who died would never meet the entry criterion and so would be excluded. It follows that mortality analysis of such workers should exclude the first 5 years of employment for each worker. This period of time is referred to as *immortal person-time*. The workers at the factory were not immortal during this time, of course, because they could have died. The subset of workers that satisfy the cohort definition, however, is identified after the fact as those who have survived this period.

The correct approach to handling immortal person-time in a study is to exclude it from any denominator, even if the analysis does not focus on mortality. This approach is correct because including immortal person-time will downwardly bias estimated disease rates and, consequently, bias effect estimates obtained from internal comparisons. As an example, suppose that an occupational mortality study includes only workers who worked for 5 years at a factory that 1,000 exposed and 1,000 unexposed workers meet this entry criterion, and that after the criterion is met, we observe 200 deaths among 5,000 exposed person-years and 90 deaths among 6,000 unexposed person-years. The correct rate ratio and difference comparing the exposed and unexposed are then $(200/5,000)/(90/6,000) = 2.7$ and $200/5,000 - 90/6,000 = 25/1,000$ year^{-1}. If, however, we incorrectly include the 5,000 exposed and 5,000 unexposed immortal person-years in the denominators, we get a biased ratio of $(200/10,000)/(90/11,000) = 2.4$ and a biased difference of $200/10,000 - 90/11,000 = 12/1,000$ year^{-1}. To avoid this bias, if a study has a criterion for a minimum amount of time before a subject is eligible to be in a study, the time during which the eligibility criterion is in the process of being met should be excluded from the calculation of incidence rates. More generally, the follow-up time allocated to a specific exposure category should exclude time during which the exposure-category definition is being met.

Immortal person-time bias has arisen in pharmacoepidemiology studies in which prescription drug users must fill one or more prescriptions over some time period.[55] If the outcome is a fatal event, the eligibility periods must be excluded from rate denominators to avoid bias. In cancer survivor studies, immortal person-time bias has sometimes also been called guarantee-time bias,[56] and landmark analysis[57] has been used to denote designs that avoid immortal person-time bias by beginning follow-up at a common time point for all participants and after all enrollment events have been completed. In some pharmacogenetic studies, patients who contribute a biospecimen for genetic analysis after the landmark event, such as a cancer diagnosis, must survive to the time of biospecimen collection.[58] The time between the landmark event and the biospecimen collection is also immortal person-time. In short, any person-time before completion of the chronologically last event for admission into a cohort or subcohort is likely to be immortal person-time, so that person-time and outcome events observed during that person-time should be excluded from the study or otherwise properly treated in the analysis.[56,59]

INDEX EVENT BIAS AND NEW USER DESIGNS

When membership in a cohort is defined by the occurrence of an index health event, such as clinical epidemiology studies of survivors of first myocardial infarction, it has often been observed that risk factors for the index event have little association, or even a protective association, with a recurrent event, such as second myocardial infarction.[60] This pattern of associations may arise from index event bias, a type of collider bias (see Chapters 3 and 14). Studies of survivors are limited to persons who have had the index event, so risk factors for the index event become associated with one another in the survivor population, even if independent of one another in the population giving rise to the population with the index event. This association diminishes the associations between the risk factors and the recurrent event unless a sufficient set of variables are controlled in the analysis (see Chapter 3). Furthermore, if the risk factors also increase the risk of death preceding the index event, then the index event bias can be further amplified.[61]

As an example,[61] obesity is consistently observed to increase the risk of end-stage renal disease and the overall mortality rate, compared with being of normal body mass index. Among persons with end-stage renal disease, obesity is associated with a lower mortality hazard, compared with being of normal body mass index. Studies of the association between obesity and mortality among end-stage renal disease patients must be limited to persons who survived to their diagnosis of end-stage renal disease. Thus, factors that increase the risk of end-stage renal disease or the mortality hazard are associated within one another in cohorts of end-stage renal disease patients, even if independent of one another in the population of persons at risk for end-stage renal disease. The associations between these risk factors and death in the cohort of end-stage renal disease patients may be biased unless all risk factors for end-stage renal disease and death are controlled by design or analysis.[61] This control requires identification of a sufficient set of variables for control (see Chapter 3), and information about these variables before enrollment into the clinical cohort, which can be hampered by left-censoring. When unresolved, this bias is called index event bias because it is induced by restricting (conditioning) the estimate of association on the occurrence of the index event. Alternatively, these biases can be circumvented by studying the effect of current obesity and controlling for obesity prior to end-stage renal disease diagnosis.

A similar consideration applies to studies that can include both prevalent and incident exposed persons. For example, in studies defined by a common occupation, members of the cohort might include those who have worked in the occupation for some time before the study follow-up begins, as well as persons hired only after the study follow-up begins.[62,63] Prevalent employees have been hired and have retained their employment, which requires that they both survive to the start of follow-up and that they and their employers agree to retain their employment. Employees who react poorly to occupational hazards may decide to leave employment, enriching the pool of prevalent employees to those who decide to stay. These employees may react differently physiologically, or may take precautionary measures to avoid occupational hazards more diligently, than those who leave employment. They may, therefore, be selected to have less reaction to occupational hazards than newly employed persons.

In studies of the effect of prescription medications, the same type of consideration applies. At the start of follow-up, prevalent users of the medication might be identified, and over the course of follow-up, new users of the medication might be identified.[64] Prevalent users of the medication have had an indication for the medication and have retained the prescription until the start of follow-up. New users of the medication have only had the indication for the medication. Prevalent users of drugs may be more adherent to prescription medications, more likely to be among those who have the medication's intended benefit, and less likely to be among those who have adverse reactions than new users of the drug, who have not yet experienced any of these selection forces. Prevalent users will also exclude persons who may have died shortly after initiating the drug due to any immediate adverse effects the drug may have upon initiation. It is tempting to increase the size of the exposed group by including both prevalent and incident exposed persons, but prevalent exposed persons are likely to be different than newly exposed persons, and these differences can bias estimates of association. As an example of the differences that can arise from including prevalent users, Danaei et al. (2012) conducted meta-analyses of studies examining the effect of statins on mortality for persons with cardiovascular disease and found that the pooled hazard ratio estimate for prevalent user designs, HR = 0.54 (95% CI: 0.45, 0.66), suggested a considerably larger protective effect than that for incident user designs, HR = 0.77 (95% CI: 0.65, 0.91).[65]

POSTEXPOSURE EVENTS

Allocation of follow-up time to specific categories should not depend on events that occur after the follow-up time in question has accrued. For example, consider a study in which a group of smokers is advised to quit smoking, with the objective of estimating the effect on mortality rates of quitting versus continuing to smoke. For a subject who smokes for a while after the advice is given and then quits later, the follow-up time as a quitter should only begin at the time of quitting, not at the time of giving the advice, because it is the effect of quitting that is being studied, not the effect of advice (were the effect of advice under study, follow-up time would begin with the advice). But how should a subject be treated who quits for a while and then later takes up smoking again?

When this question arose in an actual study of this problem, the investigators excluded anyone from the study who switched back to smoking. Their decision was wrong because, if the subject had died before switching back to smoking, the death would have counted in the study and the subject would not have been excluded. A subject's follow-up time was excluded if the subject switched back to smoking, something that occurred only *after* the subject had accrued time in the quit-smoking cohort. A proper analysis should include the experience of those who switched back to smoking up until the time that they switched back. If the propensity to switch back was unassociated with risk, their experience subsequent to switching back could be excluded without introducing bias. The incidence rate among the person-years while having quit could then be compared with the rate among those who continued to smoke over the same period.

As another example, suppose that the investigators wanted to examine the effect of being an ex-smoker for at least 5 years, relative to being an ongoing smoker. Then, anyone who returned to smoking within 5 years of quitting would be excluded. The person-time experience for each subject during the first 5 years after quitting should also be excluded because it would be immortal person-time.

TIMING OF OUTCOME EVENTS

As may be apparent from earlier discussion, the time at which an outcome event occurs can be a major determinant of the amount of person-time contributed by a subject to each exposure category. It is therefore important to define and determine the time of the event as unambiguously and precisely as possible. For some events, such as death, neither task presents any difficulty. For other outcomes, such as human immunodeficiency virus (HIV) seroconversion, the time of the event can be defined in a reasonably precise manner (the appearance of HIV antibodies in the bloodstream), but measurement of the time is difficult. For others, such as multiple sclerosis and atherosclerosis, the very definition of the onset time can be ambiguous, even when the presence of the disease can be determined unambiguously. Likewise, time of loss to follow-up and other censoring events can be difficult to define and determine. Determining whether an event occurred by a given time is a special case of determining when an event occurred, because knowing that the event occurred by the given time requires knowing that the time it occurred was before the given time.

Addressing the aforementioned problems depends heavily on the details of available data and the current state of knowledge about the study outcome. We therefore will offer only a few general remarks on issues of outcome timing. In all situations, we recommend that one start with at least one written protocol to classify subjects based on available information. For example, seroconversion time may be measured as the midpoint between time of last negative and first positive test. For unambiguously defined events, any deviation of actual times from the protocol determination can be viewed as measurement error (which is discussed further in Chapter 13). Ambiguously timed diseases, such as cancers or vascular conditions, are often taken as occurring at diagnosis time, but the use of a minimum lag period is advisable whenever a long latent (undiagnosed or prodromal) period is inevitable. It may sometimes be possible to interview cases about the earliest onset of symptoms, but such recollections and symptoms can be subject to considerable error and between-person variability.

Some ambiguously timed events are dealt with by standard, if somewhat arbitrary, definitions. For example, in 1993, acquired immunodeficiency syndrome (AIDS) onset was redefined as occurrence of any AIDS-defining illnesses or clinical event (*e.g.*, CD4 count <200/μL). As a second example, time of loss to follow-up is conventionally taken as midway between the last successful attempt to contact and the first unsuccessful attempt to contact. Any difficulty in determining an arbitrarily defined time of an event is then treated as a measurement problem, which can be addressed by the methods described in Chapters 13 and 29. One should recognize, however, that the arbitrariness of the definition for the time of an event represents another source of measurement error, with potential bias consequences that will be discussed in Chapter 13.

EXPENSE

Cohort studies are usually large enterprises. Most diseases affect only a small proportion of a population, even if the population is followed for many years. To obtain stable estimates of incidence requires a substantial number of cases of disease, and therefore the person-time giving rise to the cases must also be substantial. Sufficient person-time can be accumulated by following cohorts for a long span of time. Some cohorts with special exposures (*e.g.*, Japanese victims of atomic bombs)[66] or with detailed medical and personal histories (*e.g.*, the Framingham, Massachusetts, study cohort[67]) have indeed been followed for decades. If a study is intended to provide more timely results, however, the requisite person-time can be attained by increasing the size of the cohorts. Of course, lengthy studies of large populations are expensive. It is not uncommon for cohort studies to cost millions of dollars, and expenses in excess of $100 million have occurred. Most of the expense derives from the need to establish a continuing system for monitoring disease occurrence in a large population. Linking to health registries has provided a cost-efficient method for identifying health outcomes in some population settings.[35,68,69]

The expense of cohort studies often limits feasibility. The lower the disease incidence, the poorer the feasibility of a cohort study, unless public resources devoted to health registries can be productively employed (see Chapter 11). Feasibility is further handicapped by a long induction period between the hypothesized cause and its effect. A long induction time contributes to a low overall incidence because the rate denominators must include the additional follow-up time required to obtain exposure-related cases. To measure any effect, the study must span an interval at least as long as, and in practice considerably longer than, the minimum induction period. Cohort studies are poorly suited to study the effect of exposures that are hypothesized to cause rare diseases with long induction periods. Such cohort studies are expensive in relation to the amount of information returned, which is to say that they are not efficient.

The expense of cohort studies can be reduced in a variety of ways. As mentioned above, one way is to use an existing system for monitoring disease occurrence (see Chapter 11). For example, a regional cancer registry may be used to ascertain cancer occurrence among cohort members. If the expense of case ascertainment is already being borne by the registry, the study will be considerably cheaper.

Another way to reduce cost is to rely on historical cohorts. Rather than identifying cohort members concurrently with the initiation of the study and planning to have the follow-up period occur during the study, the investigator may choose to identify cohort members based on records of previous exposure. The follow-up period until the occurrence of disease may be wholly or partially in the past. To ascertain cases occurring in the past, the investigators must rely on records to ascertain disease in cohort members. If the follow-up period begins before the period during which the study is conducted but extends into the study period, then active surveillance or a new monitoring system to ascertain new cases of disease can be devised.

To the extent that subject selection occurs after the follow-up period under observation (sometimes called retrospective cohort selection; see Chapter 6), the study will generally cost less than an equivalent study in which subject selection occurs before the follow-up period (sometimes called prospective). A drawback of retrospective cohort studies is their dependence on records, which may suffer from missing or poorly recorded information. Another drawback is that entire subject records may be missing. When such "missingness" is related to the variables under study, the study may suffer from selection biases similar to those that can occur in case-control studies (see Chapter 14). For example, if records are systematically deleted upon the death of a cohort member, then all of the retrospective person-time will be immortal and should therefore be excluded.

A third way to reduce cost is to replace one of the cohorts, specifically the unexposed or reference cohort, with general-population information. Rather than collecting new information on a large unexposed population, existing data on a general population are used for comparison. This procedure has several drawbacks. For one, it is reasonable only if there is some assurance that only a small proportion of the general population is exposed to the agent under study. That condition is often met with occupational exposures but may not be met with more prevalent exposures. To the extent that part of the general population is exposed, there is misclassification error that will introduce a bias into the comparison, which is ordinarily in the direction of underestimating the effect (see Chapter 13). Another problem is that information obtained for the exposed cohort may differ in quality from the existing data for the general population. If mortality data are used, the death certificate is often the only source of information for the general population. If additional medical information were used to classify deaths in an exposed cohort, the data thus obtained would not be comparable with the general-population data. This noncomparability may reduce or increase bias in the resulting comparisons.[70] Finally, the exposed cohort is likely to differ from the general population in many ways that are not measured, thus leading to uncontrollable confounding in the comparison. The classical "healthy worker effect" is one example of this problem, in which confounding arises because workers must meet a minimal criterion of health—they must be able to work—that the general population does not.

A fourth way to reduce the cost of a cohort study is to conduct a case-control study within the cohort, rather than including the entire cohort population in the study (Chapter 8). Such "nested" case-control studies can often be conducted at a fraction of the cost of a cohort study and yet produce the same findings with nearly the same precision.

References

1. Armstrong BK, White E, Saracci R. *Principles of exposure measurement in epidemiology.* In: *Principles of Exposure Measurement in Epidemiology. Monographs in Epidemiology and Biostatistics.* Vol 21. New York, NY: Oxford Unviersity Press; 1992.
2. Dawber TR, Meadors GF, Moore FE Jr. Epidemiological approaches to heart disease: the Framingham Study. *Am J Public Health Nations Health.* 1951;41(3):279-281.
3. McDonald JC, Liddell FD, Gibbs GW, Eyssen GE, McDonald AD. Dust exposure and mortality in chrysotile mining, 1910-75. *Br J Ind Med.* 1980;37(1):11-24.
4. Dement JM, Harris RL Jr, Symons MJ, Shy C. Estimates of dose-response for respiratory cancer among chrysotile asbestos textile workers. *Ann Occup Hyg.* 1982;26(1-4):869-887.
5. Mancuso TF, el-Attar AA. Epidemiological study of the beryllium industry. Cohort methodology and mortality studies. *J Occup Med.* 1969;11(8):422-434.
6. Boice JD Jr, Mandel JS, Doody MM, Yoder RC, McGowan R. A health survey of radiologic technologists. *Cancer.* 1992;69(2):586-598.
7. Garshick E, Schenker MB, Munoz A, et al. A retrospective cohort study of lung cancer and diesel exhaust exposure in railroad workers. *Am Rev Respir Dis.* 1988;137(4):820-825.
8. Attfield MD, Schleiff PL, Lubin JH, et al. The Diesel exhaust in miners study: a cohort mortality study with emphasis on lung cancer. *J Natl Cancer Inst.* 2012;104(11):869-883.
9. Doll R, Hill AB. The mortality of doctors in relation to their smoking habits; a preliminary report. *Br Med J.* 1954;1(4877):1451-1455.
10. Belanger CF, Hennekens CH, Rosner B, Speizer FE. The nurses' health study. *Am J Nurs.* 1978;78(6):1039-1040.
11. Rimm EB, Giovannucci EL, Willett WC, et al. Prospective study of alcohol consumption and risk of coronary disease in men. *Lancet.* 1991;338(8765):464-468.
12. Boeri R, Bordo B, Crenna P, Filippini G, Massetto M, Zecchini A. Preliminary results of a neurological investigation of the population exposed to TCDD in the Seveso region. *Riv Patol Nerv Ment.* 1978;99(2):111-128.
13. Onozuka D, Yoshimura T, Kaneko S, Furue M. Mortality after exposure to polychlorinated biphenyls and polychlorinated dibenzofurans: a 40-year follow-up study of Yusho patients. *Am J Epidemiol.* 2009;169(1):86-95.
14. Yu ML, Guo YL, Hsu CC, Rogan WJ. Increased mortality from chronic liver disease and cirrhosis 13 years after the Taiwan "yucheng" ("oil disease") incident. *Am J Ind Med.* 1997;31(2):172-175.
15. Harjulehto T, Aro T, Rita H, Rytomaa T, Saxen L. The accident at Chernobyl and outcome of pregnancy in Finland. *BMJ.* 1989;298(6679):995-997.
16. Yasumura S, Hosoya M, Yamashita S, et al. Study protocol for the Fukushima health management survey. *J Epidemiol.* 2012;22(5):375-383.
17. Kato H. Cancer study on a cohort of atomic bomb survivors. *Natl Cancer Inst Monogr.* 1977;47:31-32.
18. Reibman J, Lin S, Hwang SA, et al. The World Trade Center residents' respiratory health study: new-onset respiratory symptoms and pulmonary function. *Environ Health Perspect.* 2005;113(4):406-411.
19. Uscher-Pines L, Vernick JS, Curriero F, Lieberman R, Burke TA. Disaster-related injuries in the period of recovery: the effect of prolonged displacement on risk of injury in older adults. *J Trauma.* 2009;67(4):834-840.
20. Neuberger A, Tenenboim S, Golos M, et al. Infectious diseases seen in a primary care clinic in Leogane, Haiti. *Am J Trop Med Hyg.* 2012;86(1):11-15.
21. Howard VJ, Cushman M, Pulley L, et al. The reasons for geographic and racial differences in stroke study: objectives and design. *Neuroepidemiology.* 2005;25(3):135-143.
22. Signorello LB, Hargreaves MK, Steinwandel MD, et al. Southern community cohort study: establishing a cohort to investigate health disparities. *J Natl Med Assoc.* 2005;97(7):972-979.
23. Rose CL, Bosse R, Szretter WT. The relationship of scientific objectives to population selection and attrition in longitudinal studies. The case of the normative aging study. *Gerontologist.* 1976;16(6):508-516.

24. Rosenberg L, Adams-Campbell L, Palmer JR. The Black Women's Health Study: a follow-up study for causes and preventions of illness. *J Am Med Womens Assoc*. 1995;50(2):56-58.

25. Hankin JH, Stram DO, Arakawa K, et al. Singapore Chinese Health Study: development, validation, and calibration of the quantitative food frequency questionnaire. *Nutr Cancer*. 2001;39(2):187-195.

26. Sempos CT, Bild DE, Manolio TA. Overview of the Jackson Heart Study: a study of cardiovascular diseases in African American men and women. *Am J Med Sci*. 1999;317(3):142-146.

27. Bild DE, Bluemke DA, Burke GL, et al. Multi-ethnic study of atherosclerosis: objectives and design. *Am J Epidemiol*. 2002;156(9):871-881.

28. Gerber Y, Myers V, Broday DM, Koton S, Steinberg DM, Drory Y. Cumulative exposure to air pollution and long term outcomes after first acute myocardial infarction: a population-based cohort study. Objectives and methodology. *BMC Public Health*. 2010;10:369.

29. Geiger AM, Thwin SS, Lash TL, et al. Recurrences and second primary breast cancers in older women with initial early-stage disease. *Cancer*. 2007;109(5):966-974.

30. Jepsen P, Vilstrup H, Andersen PK, Lash TL, Sorensen HT. Comorbidity and survival of Danish cirrhosis patients: a nationwide population-based cohort study. *Hepatology*. 2008;48(1):214-220.

31. Melbye M, Wohlfahrt J, Olsen JH, et al. Induced abortion and the risk of breast cancer. *N Engl J Med*. 1997;336(2):81-85.

32. Mikkelsen EM, Hatch EE, Wise LA, Rothman KJ, Riis A, Sorensen HT. Cohort profile: the Danish web-based pregnancy planning study – 'Snart-Gravid'. *Int J Epidemiol*. 2009;38(4):938-943.

33. Wise LA, Rothman KJ, Mikkelsen EM, et al. Design and conduct of an internet-based preconception cohort study in north America: pregnancy study online. *Paediatr Perinat Epidemiol*. 2015;29(4):360-371.

34. Skarping I, Brand JS, Hall P, Borgquist S. Effects of statin use on volumetric mammographic density: results from the KARMA study. *BMC Cancer*. 2015;15:435.

35. Frank L. Epidemiology. When an entire country is a cohort. *Science*. 2000;287(5462):2398-2399.

36. Schmidt M, Schmidt SAJ, Adelborg K, et al. The Danish health care system and epidemiological research: from health care contacts to database records. *Clin Epidemiol*. 2019;11:563-591.

37. Psaty BM, Sitlani C. The cohorts for heart and aging research in genomic epidemiology (CHARGE) consortium as a model of collaborative science. *Epidemiology*. 2013;24(3):346-348.

38. El Emam K, Rodgers S, Malin B. Anonymising and sharing individual patient data. *BMJ*. 2015;350:h1139.

39. Toh S, Platt R. Is size the next big thing in epidemiology? *Epidemiology*. 2013;24(3):349-351.

40. Huybrechts KF, Mikkelsen EM, Christensen T, et al. A successful implementation of e-epidemiology: the Danish pregnancy planning study 'Snart-Gravid'. *Eur J Epidemiol*. 2010;25(5):297-304.

41. Ekman A, Litton JE. New times, new needs; e-epidemiology. *Eur J Epidemiol*. 2007;22(5):285-292.

42. Kannel WB, Dawber TR, Kagan A, Revotskie N, Stokes J III. Factors of risk in the development of coronary heart disease – six year follow-up experience. The Framingham Study. *Ann Intern Med*. 1961;55:33-50.

43. Needleman HL, Tuncay OC, Shapiro IM. Lead levels in deciduous teeth of urban and suburban American children. *Nature*. 1972;235(5333):111-112.

44. Greenland S. Response and follow-up bias in cohort studies. *Am J Epidemiol*. 1977;106(3):184-187.

45. Riis AH, Johansen MB, Jacobsen JB, Brookhart MA, Sturmer T, Stovring H. Short look-back periods in pharmacoepidemiologic studies of new users of antibiotics and asthma medications introduce severe misclassification. *Pharmacoepidemiol Drug Saf*. 2015;24(5):478-485.

46. Gilbertson DT, Bradbury BD, Wetmore JB, et al. Controlling confounding of treatment effects in administrative data in the presence of time-varying baseline confounders. *Pharmacoepidemiol Drug Saf*. 2016;25(3):269-277.

47. Brunelli SM, Gagne JJ, Huybrechts KF, et al. Estimation using all available covariate information versus a fixed look-back window for dichotomous covariates. *Pharmacoepidemiol Drug Saf*. 2013;22(5):542-550.

48. Robins JM. A graphical approach to the identification and estimation of causal parameters in mortality studies with sustained exposure periods. *J Chronic Dis*. 1987;40(suppl 2):139S-161S.

49. Rothman KJ. Induction and latent periods. *Am J Epidemiol*. 1981;114(2):253-259.

50. Lubin JH, Caporaso NE. Cigarette smoking and lung cancer: modeling total exposure and intensity. *Cancer Epidemiol Biomarkers Prev*. 2006;15(3):517-523.

51. Thomas DC. Statistical methods for analyzing effects of temporal patterns of exposure on cancer risks. *Scand J Work Environ Health*. 1983;9(4):353-366.

52. Thomas DC. Models for exposure-time-response relationships with applications to cancer epidemiology. *Annu Rev Public Health*. 1988;9:451-482.

53. Robins JM. A new approach to causal inference in mortality studies with a sustained exposure period-application to control of the healthy worker survivor effect. *Math Model*. 1986;7:1393-1512.

54. Robins JM, Mark SD, Newey WK. Estimating exposure effects by modelling the expectation of exposure conditional on confounders. *Biometrics*. 1992;48(2):479-495.

55. Suissa S. Immortal time bias in pharmaco-epidemiology. *Am J Epidemiol*. 2008;167(4):492-499.

56. Giobbie-Hurder A, Gelber RD, Regan MM. Challenges of guarantee-time bias. *J Clin Oncol*. 2013;31(23):2963-2969.

57. Dafni U. Landmark analysis at the 25-year landmark point. *Circ Cardiovasc Qual Outcomes.* 2011;4(3):363-371.
58. Lash TL, Cole SR. Immortal person-time in studies of cancer outcomes. *J Clin Oncol.* 2009;27(23):e55-e56.
59. Rothman KJ, Suissa S. Exclusion of immortal person-time. *Pharmacoepidemiol Drug Saf.* 2008;17(10):1036.
60. Dahabreh IJ, Kent DM. Index event bias as an explanation for the paradoxes of recurrence risk research. *J Am Med Assoc.* 2011;305(8):822-823.
61. Flanders WD, Eldridge RC, McClellan W. A nearly unavoidable mechanism for collider bias with index-event studies. *Epidemiology.* 2014;25(5):762-764.
62. Applebaum KM, Malloy EJ, Eisen EA. Reducing healthy worker survivor bias by restricting date of hire in a cohort study of Vermont granite workers. *Occup Environ Med.* 2007;64(10):681-687.
63. Applebaum KM, Malloy EJ, Eisen EA. Left truncation, susceptibility, and bias in occupational cohort studies. *Epidemiology.* 2011;22(4):599-606.
64. Ray WA. Evaluating medication effects outside of clinical trials: new-user designs. *Am J Epidemiol.* 2003;158(9):915-920.
65. Danaei G, Tavakkoli M, Hernan MA. Bias in observational studies of prevalent users: lessons for comparative effectiveness research from a meta-analysis of statins. *Am J Epidemiol.* 2012;175(4):250-262.
66. Beebe GW. Reflections on the work of the atomic bomb casualty commission in Japan. *Epidemiol Rev.* 1979;1:184-210.
67. Kannel WB, Abbott RD. Incidence and prognosis of unrecognized myocardial infarction. An update on the Framingham study. *N Engl J Med.* 1984;311(18):1144-1147.
68. Steiner JF, Paolino AR, Thompson EE, Larson EB. Sustaining research networks: the twenty-year experience of the HMO research network. *EGEMS (Wash DC).* 2014;2(2):1067.
69. Williams T, van Staa T, Puri S, Eaton S. Recent advances in the utility and use of the general practice research database as an example of a UK primary care data resource. *Ther Adv Drug Saf.* 2012;3(2):89-99.
70. Greenland S, Robins JM. Confounding and misclassification. *Am J Epidemiol.* 1985;122(3):495-506.

CHAPTER 8

Case-Control Studies

Timothy L. Lash and Kenneth J. Rothman

COMMON ELEMENTS OF CASE-CONTROL STUDIES

The use and understanding of case-control studies is one of the most important methodologic developments of modern epidemiology. Conceptually, there are clear links from randomized experiments to nonrandomized cohort studies and from nonrandomized cohort studies to case-control studies. In this chapter, we review case-control study designs and contrast their advantages and disadvantages with cohort designs. We also consider variants of the basic case-control study design.

Conventional wisdom about case-control studies, which antedates the era of modern epidemiology, is that they do not yield estimates of effect that are as valid as measures obtained from cohort studies. According to this conventional wisdom, there is a hierarchy of study designs, with randomized trials considered the most valid, cohort studies less so, and case-control studies even less. Despite the premise that there is a hierarchy of validity inherent to study design, any study of whatever design can have problems with validity; it is only by examining the particulars of a study that an epidemiologist can judge its validity.[1] The idea that case-control studies have inherent validity problems may reflect common misunderstandings in conceptualizing case-control studies, which will be clarified later. One example is that case-control studies are often thought to suffer from recall bias. Recall bias arises when the information on exposure is obtained from interviews after the outcome has occurred, so cases will have reported the exposure information after learning of their diagnosis. Controls would not have had the case-defining diagnosis. The difference in diagnosis status may influence cases to recall or report their exposure history differently than controls. But this possibility is limited to retrospective interview-based case-control studies. If exposure information comes from information recorded before the diagnosis, there will be no recall bias, and even in interview studies, there are methods that can limit recall bias, as explained later.

When designing a nonexperimental cohort study to assess causality, it is often helpful to imagine how we would conduct a hypothetical randomized study of the same exposure contrast.[2-4] Similarly, to design a valid case-control study, it is helpful to imagine what the corresponding cohort study would look like and use it to guide the design. In fact, the best way to conceptualize case-control studies is to consider them as cohort studies with sampling of the denominators to improve study efficiency. Under this conceptualization, for any case-control study, we can envision a corresponding cohort study. In both study designs, the cases would be the same. The source population for the cases in the case-control study, also known as the "study base,"[5] would be the cohort experience (either people or their cumulated person-time) in the corresponding cohort study. However, rather than including all the study base in the case-control study, we sample from it. The sample is the control group. Wacholder described this paradigm of the case-control study as a cohort study with some denominator data missing at random and by design.[6]

As understanding of the principles of case-control studies has progressed, the reputation of case-control studies has also improved. The bad reputation once suffered by case-control studies stems more from instances of poor conduct and overinterpretation of results than from any inherent weakness in the approach. Nonetheless, misperceptions about the inherent validity of the case-control design persist and are even disseminated by prominent clinical journals.[7,8]

Although case-control studies do present more opportunities for bias and concomitant mistaken inference than cohort studies, these opportunities often reflect the relative ease with which a case-control study can be mounted, even by naïve investigators. Properly designed and conducted, case-control studies will yield estimates of effect that are as valid as measures obtained from cohort studies, if the investigators implement certain basic principles. In this chapter, we present these principles and consider common practical elements of designing and conducting case-control studies. We then review the most common variants of case-control study designs and contrast them with cohort designs. We end with a discussion of some common fallacies relating to this design.

PSEUDOFREQUENCIES AND THE ODDS RATIO

If we conceptualize case-control studies to be cohort studies with sampling from the denominators of the cohort study rates or risks, or what we have called the study base, then the primary goal for control selection is that the expectation of the exposure distribution among controls be the same as it is in the source population of cases. If this condition is achieved, then we can use the control series in place of the denominator information in measures of disease frequency to determine the ratio of the disease frequency in exposed people relative to that among unexposed people. This goal will be met if we can sample controls from the source population such that the ratio of the number of exposed controls (B_1) to the total exposed experience of the source population is the same as the ratio of the number of unexposed controls (B_0) to the unexposed experience of the source population, apart from sampling error. For most purposes, this goal needs only to be followed within strata of factors that will be used for stratification in the analysis, such as factors used for restriction or matching (see Chapters 6 and 18). Using person-time to illustrate, the goal requires that B_1 has the same ratio to the amount of exposed person-time (T_1) as B_0 has to the amount of unexposed person-time (T_0), apart from sampling error:

$$\frac{B_1}{T_1} = \frac{B_0}{T_0}$$

Here B_1/T_1 and B_0/T_0 are the control sampling rates—that is, the number of controls selected per unit of person-time. Suppose that A_1 exposed cases and A_0 unexposed cases occur over the study period. The exposed and unexposed rates are then

$$I_1 = \frac{A_1}{T_1} \quad \text{and} \quad I_0 = \frac{A_0}{T_0}$$

We can use the frequencies of exposed and unexposed controls as substitutes for the actual denominators of the rates to obtain exposure-specific case-control ratios or *pseudorates:*

$$\text{Pseudo-rate}_1 = \frac{A_1}{B_1} \quad \text{and Pseudo-rate}_0 = \frac{A_0}{B_0}$$

One can also describe these pseudorates as case-control odds, which is the odds of being a case rather than a control if exposed or if not exposed. The pseudorates have no epidemiologic interpretation by themselves. Suppose, however, that the two control sampling rates, B_1/T_1 and B_0/T_0, are equal to the same value f, as would be expected if controls are selected independently of exposure. If this common sampling fraction f is known, the actual incidence rates can be calculated by simple algebra because, apart from sampling error, B_1/f should equal the amount of exposed person-time in the source population and B_0/f should equal the amount of unexposed person-time in the source population:

$$\frac{B_1}{f} = \frac{B_1}{B_1/T_1} = T_1 \quad \text{and} \quad \frac{B_0}{f} = \frac{B_0}{B_0/T_0} = T_0$$

Therefore, to obtain the incidence rates, we need only to multiply each pseudorate by the common sampling fraction, f.

If the common sampling fraction is not known, which is often the case, we can still compare the sizes of the pseudorates by division. Specifically, if we divide the pseudorate for exposed by the pseudorate for unexposed, we obtain,

$$\frac{\text{Pseudo-rate}_1}{\text{Pseudo-rate}_0} = \frac{A_1/B_1}{A_0/B_0} = \frac{A_1/\left[(B_1/T_1)T_1\right]}{A_0/\left[(B_0/T_0)T_0\right]} = \frac{A_1/(rT_1)}{A_0/(rT_0)} = \frac{A_1/T_1}{A_0/T_0}$$

In other words, the ratio of the pseudorates for the exposed and unexposed is an estimate of the ratio of the incidence rates in the source population, provided that the control sampling fraction is independent of exposure. Because each pseudorate is the case/control odds, we can also say that the ratio of case/control odds, or the odds ratio, is an estimate of the incidence rate ratio. One must therefore keep separate conceptually the computational form of the estimate, called the estimator, and the target quantity it is meant to provide, which is the estimand. In this example, the estimator is the odds ratio and the estimand is the incidence rate ratio. We compute the odds ratio estimator to provide an estimate of the incidence rate ratio estimand.

Thus, using the case-control study design, one can estimate the incidence rate ratio in a population without obtaining information about every subject in the population. Similar derivations given later show that one can estimate the risk ratio by sampling controls from those at risk for disease at the beginning of the follow-up period (case-cohort design) and that one can estimate the risk odds ratio by sampling controls from the noncases at the end of the follow-up period (cumulative case-control design). With these designs, the pseudofrequencies (cases divided by controls) correspond to the risks and risk odds, respectively, multiplied by the sampling rates. For all designs, the estimator is the odds ratio. For case-cohort design, the estimand is the risk ratio and for cumulative case-control design, the estimand is the risk odds ratio.

Sampling the denominators with a control group rather than measuring the person-time experience for the entire source population, as in a cohort study, is intended to enhance study efficiency. There is, however, a statistical penalty for using only a sample of the denominators: The precision of the estimates of the incidence rate ratio from a case-control study will be less than the precision from a cohort study of the entire population that gave rise to the cases (the study base). Nevertheless, the loss of precision that stems from sampling controls will be small if the number of controls selected per case is large (usually four or more). Furthermore, the loss is offset by the cost savings of not having to obtain information on everyone in the source population. The cost savings might allow the epidemiologist to enlarge the study base and so obtain more cases, resulting in a better overall estimate of the incidence rate ratio, statistically and otherwise, than would be possible using the same expenditures to conduct a cohort study. For diseases that are sufficiently rare, cohort studies that require primary data collection become impractical, and case-control studies may be the only practical alternative.

The ratio of the two pseudorates in a case-control study is often written as A_1B_0/A_0B_1 and, in addition to being called the odds ratio, is sometimes called the *cross-product ratio*. It can be viewed as the ratio of cases to controls among the exposed subjects (A_1/B_1), divided by the ratio of cases to controls among the unexposed subjects (A_0/B_0). It can also be viewed as the odds of being exposed among cases (A_1/A_0) divided by the odds of being exposed among controls (B_1/B_0), in which case, it is termed the *exposure odds ratio*. While either interpretation will give the same estimate, viewing this odds ratio estimator as the ratio of case-control ratios shows more directly how the control group substitutes for the denominator information in a cohort study and therefore how the ratio of pseudofrequencies gives the same result as the ratio of the incidence rates, incidence proportion, or incidence odds in the source population (the design-specific estimands), if sampling is independent of exposure.

Defining the Source Population

If the study base is precisely defined before any cases and controls are identified, the case-control study is said to be *population-based* or to have a *primary* base. In a population-based case-control study, the cases are a complete census or a representative sample of all cases and the controls are a random sample from the source population of cases. Random sampling of controls from a well-defined population is usually the most desirable option and may be feasible if a population registry exists or can be compiled. For example, when there is a population-based disease registry and a census enumeration of the population served by the registry, it may be possible to use the census data to sample controls randomly.

If the population within which the case-control study is conducted is a fully enumerated cohort, which allows formal random sampling of cases and controls to be carried out, epidemiologists refer to it as a *nested* case-control study. The term is usually used in reference to a case-control study conducted within an ongoing cohort study, in which further information is obtained on either all or some cases, but for economy is obtained from only a fraction of the remaining cohort members (the controls). For example, when there is an established cohort and exposure ascertainment requires additional data abstraction (*e.g.*, medical record review, genetic test), these data can be collected for cases and for a sample of controls rather than for the full cohort. Cases and controls can be selected from a fixed cohort (*e.g.*, persons born in Sweden in 1970) or from an open (dynamic) population (*e.g.*, persons 18-65 years old alive residing in Sweden between 2010 and 2020).[9]

When it is not possible to identify the source population explicitly, simple random sampling from the source population is not feasible and other methods of control selection must be used. Such studies are sometimes called studies of *secondary* bases because the source population is identified secondarily to the definition of a case-finding mechanism. A secondary source population or "secondary base" is therefore a source population that is defined to correspond to the identification of cases in a given case series. Eligible controls are those persons who would have become cases in the study had they developed the disease.

As an example, consider a case-control study in which the cases are patients treated for severe psoriasis at the Mayo Clinic. These patients come to the Mayo Clinic from all corners of the world. Can we identify the specific source population that gives rise to these cases? To do so, we would have to know exactly who would go to the Mayo Clinic if he or she had severe psoriasis. We cannot enumerate this source population because many people in it do not know themselves that they would go to the Mayo Clinic for severe psoriasis, unless they actually developed severe psoriasis. This secondary study base is a dynamic population, scattered around the world, that comprises those people who would go to the Mayo Clinic if they developed severe psoriasis. The challenge to the investigator is to apply eligibility criteria to the cases and controls so that there is good correspondence between the controls and this source population. For example, cases of severe psoriasis and controls could be restricted to those living within a certain distance of the Mayo Clinic, so that at least a geographic correspondence between the controls and the secondary source population could be assured. The drawback of such a restriction is that it might leave few cases for study.

Unfortunately, the concept of a secondary base is often tenuously connected to underlying realities, and it can be highly ambiguous. For the psoriasis example, whether a person would go to the Mayo Clinic depends on many factors that vary over time, such as whether the person is encouraged to go by his regular physician and whether the person can afford to go. It is not clear, then, how or even whether one could precisely define, let alone sample from, the secondary base. Consequently, it is not clear that one could ensure that controls were members of the base at the time of sampling. For this reason, it is preferable to conceptualize and conduct case-control studies starting with a well-defined source population and then to identify and recruit cases and controls to represent the disease and exposure experience of that population. When one instead takes an arbitrary case series as a starting point, it is incumbent upon the investigator to demonstrate that a source population for those cases can be operationally defined and sampled. Similar considerations apply when one takes a control series as a starting point, as is occasionally done.[10]

Regardless of being primary or secondary, the study base is equivalent to the people who constitute it and the time period through which their experience is assessed (*i.e.*, the study period).[9] In the theoretical cohort or dynamic population that corresponds to the study base, persons with certain inclusion criteria who are at risk for the event would be followed from start date until either the end of the study, a censoring event, or the occurrence of the disease under study. For cases, the period in which the event occurred or disease started is called index time. For controls, the selection of an index time within that person's experience will be discussed later.

Case Selection

In most case-control studies, the design will include all cases within a source population. Recall that case-control studies can be conceptualized as cost-efficient cohort studies. To optimize efficiency, one could imagine assigning some quantity to all potential cases and controls that would measure their information density. This measure would correspond to how much information they contribute to the study's estimate. In general, cases would always have high information density. Therefore, all people in the source population who develop the disease of interest within the study period are ordinarily included as cases in a case-control study. In some designs, cases may not all be information dense. Cases may occur in abundance, for example. It is therefore also permissible to instead examine a subset of the cases in the source population. For example, in a case-control study of the association between a genetic marker and breast cancer recurrence, the source population was stratified into tamoxifen-treated patients with estrogen receptor–positive disease and tamoxifen-untreated patients with estrogen receptor–negative disease.[11] The study hypothesis was that the genetic marker reduced the effectiveness of tamoxifen treatment, so all cases in the tamoxifen-treated estrogen receptor–positive stratum were included. The tamoxifen-untreated estrogen receptor–negative stratum provided a negative control to assure that the genetic marker had no direct effect on recurrence. Cases in that stratum were in abundance and not as information dense as cases in the tamoxifen-treated estrogen receptor–positive stratum, so only a sample of cases in the tamoxifen-untreated estrogen receptor–negative stratum was included.

When sampling cases, the key case-selection requirement is that sampling is independent of the exposure under study, either overall or within strata of factors that will be used for stratification in the analysis. To see this, suppose we take only a fraction, f, of all cases that occurred during the exposed person-time T_1 and unexposed person-time T_0. If this fraction is constant across exposure, and A_1 exposed cases and A_0 unexposed cases occur in the source population, then, apart from sampling error, the rates observed in the study will be fA_1/T_1 and fA_0/T_0, each underestimated by the fraction f. Their ratio will thus be,

$$\frac{fA_1/T_1}{fA_0/T_0} = \frac{A_1/T_1}{A_0/T_0}$$

as in the full cohort. If we wish to estimate the absolute rates and their differences, we would need to divide their study estimates by the case-sampling fraction f. Of course, if fewer than all cases are included, the study precision will be lower. In the example above, cases were sampled at random in the tamoxifen-untreated estrogen receptor–negative stratum within strata of stage and calendar period of diagnosis. Sampling within strata of stage and calendar period of diagnosis allowed frequency matching of cases in the tamoxifen-untreated estrogen receptor–negative stratum to the distribution of these variables among cases in the tamoxifen-treated estrogen receptor–positive stratum. The genetic marker was assayed on biospecimens collected only for selected cases and controls, so the expectation is that it could not have affected the sampling fraction f for either control selection or case selection in the tamoxifen-untreated estrogen receptor–negative stratum. Collecting and assaying the biospecimens were the main study expense; sampling in relation to expected information density introduced substantial cost-efficiency compared with including all patients in the study base.

As in the example, cases can be identified within an established cohort study, yielding a nested case-control study, or from groups that have a common experience or trait (*e.g.*, factory workers), as well as from vital records (*e.g.*, birth certificates), disease registries (*e.g.*, a cancer registry), healthcare databases (*e.g.*, claims files), networks (*e.g.*, patients or medical associations), or from medical records at a clinic or hospital (*e.g.*, discharge diagnoses). Even cases identified in a single clinic or treated by a single medical practitioner are possible case series for case-control studies. The corresponding source population for the cases treated in a clinic is all people who would attend that clinic and be recorded with the diagnosis of interest if they had the disease in question. It is important to specify "if they had the disease in question" because clinics often serve different populations for different diseases, depending on referral patterns and the reputation of the clinic in specific specialty areas. As noted above, without a precisely identified source population, it may be difficult or impossible to select controls in an unbiased fashion.

Control Selection

As a sample of the study base, the control series provides an estimate of the distribution of the exposure and covariates in the source population. There are three primary sampling strategies that can be used to select controls.[12] The first sampling strategy corresponds to a cohort study that calculates incidence rates, using person-time denominators. Because the control series in a case-control study is intended to represent the denominators of the frequency measures in a cohort study, the corresponding case-control strategy involves selecting controls that each represents some number of units of person-time at risk for the study outcome. This approach is called *density-based sampling*. The estimator is the exposure odds ratio, and the estimand is the incidence rate ratio. Some cohort studies measure incidence proportion rather than rates, using person denominators rather than person-time. The second sampling strategy corresponds to these studies; a case-control study that samples controls so that each represents some number of persons at risk for the study outcome. This approach is called *case-cohort sampling*. The estimator is the exposure odds ratio, and the estimand is the risk ratio. The third sampling strategy is similar to a case-cohort design, but it is conducted after the period of risk for the outcome has ended, as might happen after an epidemic. This design is called *cumulative sampling* and involves selecting controls to represent some number of people, but sampling them from among those who did not develop the study outcome during the risk period. The estimator is the exposure odds ratio, and the estimand is the risk odds ratio. These three case-control designs are discussed in greater detail below.

With each control selection strategy, the odds ratio calculation is the same: the estimator is always the odds ratio. But the measure of effect estimated by the odds ratio differs: the estimand depends on the control sampling strategy (Table 8-1). Study designs that implement each of these control selection paradigms will be discussed later, after covering issues that are common to all designs.[13]

Basic Principles for Control Selection

Regardless of the control sampling strategy, there are two basic rules for control selection:

1. Controls should be selected from the same population—the source population—that gives rise to the study cases. If this rule cannot be followed, there needs to be solid evidence that the population supplying controls has an exposure distribution identical to that of the population that is the source of cases, a stringent demand that is rarely demonstrable.

TABLE 8-1

Types of Case-Control Study and the Corresponding Sampling Scheme

		Sampling of Controls, Different Design Names, and Different Estimates			
				Control Selection	
		Case	Density	Case-Cohort	Cumulative
Exposure	Yes	A_1	$B_1 = f(T_1)$	$B_1 = f(N_1)$	$B_1 = f(N_1 - A_1)$
	No	A_0	$B_0 = f(T_0)$	$B_0 = f(N_0)$	$B_0 = f(N_0 - A_0)$

Density sampling: Odds ratio = $(A_1/f\,T_1)/(A_0/f\,T_0) = (A_1/T_1)/(A_0/T_0)$ = Rate ratio.
Case-cohort: Odds ratio = $[A_1/f(N_1)]/[A_0/f(N_0)] = (A_1/N_1)/(A_0/N_0)$ = Risk ratio.
Cumulative: Odds ratio = $[A_1/f(N_1 - A_1)]/[A_0/f(N_0 - A_0)] = [A_1/(N_1 - A_1)]/[A_0/(N_0 - A_0)]$ = Risk odds ratio.

2. Controls should be selected independently of their exposure status, that is, the sampling rate for controls should not vary with exposure (in the complete source population for unmatched studies or within strata of the matched factors for matched studies).

If these two basic rules and the corresponding case rules are met, then the ratio of pseudofrequencies will, apart from sampling error, equal the ratio of the corresponding measure of disease frequency in the source population. If the sampling rate is known, then the actual measures of disease frequency can also be calculated. (If the sampling rates differ for exposed and unexposed cases or controls, but are known, the measures of disease frequency and their ratios can still be estimated using special adjustment formulas.) For a more detailed discussion of the principles of control selection in case-control studies, see Wacholder et al.[14-16]

The second basic rule recognizes that controls are frequently matched to cases on variables expected to be important confounders. Matching was discussed in more detail in Chapter 6. Matching in a case-control study introduces a selection bias meant to improve the statistical efficiency of control for a confounder.[17,18] Fortunately, this selection bias can be removed in the analysis, but its removal may require a different level of precision than required to resolve the confounding. For example, when there is strong confounding by age, 5-year age-groups may be required to adjust for it adequately, even if the matching and resulting selection bias derived from matching used 10-year age groups.[17,18] Analytic control for the selection bias should involve at least as much precision as was involved in the original matching. Removing the selection bias often involves keeping the matched sets together in the analysis (a "matched" or "conditional" analysis) but that is not required.[19] It is also possible to control for the selection bias from matching, and the confounding from the matching factors, with no loss of validity and sometimes with an increase in precision, using an unmatched or unconditional analysis.[17,20]

Can a Person Be Selected Both as a Case and as a Control?

Just as every person contributing to the denominator of a rate or risk measured in a cohort study should be eligible to become a case, every control in a case-control study should also be eligible to become a case (we say that such a person is "at risk"). If such a person, already selected as a control, does become a case, then that person should be included as a case, and therefore would be included as both a control and a case. Note that every case in a cohort study has contributed to the denominator of the rate or risk and that the controls in a case-control study are a sample of those denominators. There is therefore no problem with a person contributing to a case-control study as both a control and a case. One exception to this principle is in a cumulative case-control study, for which controls are sampled only from noncases after the risk period ends. By design, those controls cannot appear as cases. Cumulative case-control studies, however, are inferior to case-cohort studies that sample controls from all who are at risk for disease, as is explained later.

Suppose that in a cohort with a follow-up period that spans 3 years, an at-risk person, free of disease, is selected as a potential control in year 1. Suppose this control develops the disease at year 2 and now becomes a case in the study. How should such a person be treated in the analysis? We want the control group to provide estimates of the relative size of the denominators of the incidence proportions or incidence rates for the compared groups. These denominators include all people who later become cases. Therefore, a person selected as a control who later does develop the disease and is selected as a case should be included in the study both as a control and as a case.[5,21-24] If the controls are intended to represent person-time rather than persons and are selected longitudinally, similar arguments show that a person selected as a control should remain eligible to be selected as a control later and thus might be included in the analysis repeatedly as a control.[23,24] No variance correction is necessary.

SUBTYPES OF THE CASE-CONTROL DESIGN

Sampling From Person-Time (Density Sampling)

The primary type of case-control study, using density sampling,[13] emulates a cohort study that measures rates and therefore uses person-time denominators. In a cohort study using person-time denominators, each person contributes a varying amount of information, as measured by their person-time contribution. Random sampling of controls from that person-time experience does not result in each person having an equal chance of being selected as a control. Rather, the sampling probability of any person as a control should be proportional to the amount of person-time that person spends at risk of disease in the source population. Also, the sampling probability should be independent of exposure. For example, if in the source population, one person contributes twice as much person-time during the study period as another person, the first person would have twice the probability of the second of being selected as a control. This difference in probability of selection is automatically induced by sampling controls at a steady rate per unit time over the period in which cases are sampled (sometimes called *longitudinal sampling*), rather than by sampling all controls at a point in time (such as the start or end of the follow-up period). With longitudinal sampling of controls, a population member contributing person-time for twice as long as another will have twice the chance of being selected. For example, to study the association between use of mobile telephones while driving and risk of car accidents, where only the time driving a car contributes to the person-time at risk, controls would be selected at random driving times and their cell phone use assessed as of those random driving times.

The time during which a subject is eligible to be selected as a control should be the time for which that person is also eligible to become a case, if the disease should occur. Thus, a person in whom the disease has developed or who has died is from that point no longer eligible to be selected as a control. However, that person is eligible to be selected as a control up to that point. This rule corresponds to the contribution of person-time to the denominator of rates in cohort studies (see Chapter 7). Every case that is tallied in the numerator of a cohort study contributes to the denominator of the rate while at risk for disease; the time contribution ends when the person becomes a case (unless repeat occurrences of disease in the same person are allowed) or when the person dies or otherwise drops out of the study base.

One way to sample controls in proportion to their person-time contribution is to use a strategy called *risk-set sampling*.[25,26] Each case that occurs is considered a member of a "risk set," which is the set of study-base members that were at risk for disease at the time that the case occurred. Each case has its own risk set, whose members may overlap those of other risk sets as people enter or leave the study base over time. Risk-set sampling selects controls matched to each case who are in the same risk set as the case, effectively matching on time. The time scale is often calendar time, but it could be time since birth, *i.e.*, age. Because of the matching, if exposure varies over time, the resulting data should be analyzed as matched data.[22] In the mobile telephone example, controls would be selected from among those driving at times of the case accidents and their cell phone use assessed as of those times.

Sampling Persons (Case-Cohort Sampling)

The *case-cohort study* is a case-control study in which the source population is a well-defined cohort, and every person in this cohort has an equal chance of being included in the study as a control, independently of how much time that person has contributed to the person-time experience of the cohort or whether the person developed the study disease. If everyone in the study base has been followed for the same period of time, then the case-cohort study provides an unbiased estimate of the ratio of incidence proportions that would be measured if the entire cohort had been studied.

Case-cohort designs facilitate conduct of a set of case-control studies from a single cohort, all of which use the same control group. A single sample from the cohort at enrollment can be compared with any number of case groups. If matched controls are selected from people at risk at the time a case occurs (as in risk-set sampling), the control series must be tailored to a specific group of cases, and therefore each study outcome would require a different control group. In contrast, the single control group in a case-cohort study, chosen from the list of cohort members at enrollment into the study, can be used to study any outcome, which is one of its key attractions.

One disadvantage is that because of the overlap of membership in the case and control groups (controls who are selected may also develop disease and enter the study as cases), one will need to select more controls in a case-cohort study than in an ordinary case-control study with the same number of cases, if one is to achieve the same amount of statistical precision. Extra controls are needed because the statistical precision of a study is strongly determined by the numbers of distinct cases and noncases. Thus, if 20% of the source cohort members will become cases, and all cases will be included in the study, one will have to select 1.25 times as many controls as cases in a case-cohort study to ensure that there will be as many controls who never become cases in the study. On average, only 80% of the controls in such a situation will remain noncases; the other 20% will become cases. Of course, if the disease is uncommon, the total number of extra controls needed for a case-cohort study will be small.

Cumulative Sampling ("Epidemic" Case-Control Studies)

In some research settings, studies may address a risk that ends before subject selection begins. For example, a case-control study of an epidemic of diarrheal illness after a social gathering may begin after all the potential cases have occurred (because the maximum induction time has elapsed). In such a situation, an investigator might select controls from that portion of the population that remains after eliminating the accumulated cases, that is, one selects controls from among noncases (those who remain noncases at the end of the follow-up) regardless of how much time that person has contributed to the person-time experience of the cohort.

Suppose that the source population is a fixed cohort and that a fraction f of both exposed and unexposed noncases is selected to be controls. Then the ratio of pseudofrequencies will be,

$$\frac{A_1/B_1}{A_0/B_0} = \frac{A_1/f(N_1-A_1)}{A_0/f(N_0-A_0)} = \frac{A_1/(N_1-A_1)}{A_0/(N_0-A_0)}$$

which is the risk odds ratio for the cohort. This ratio will provide a reasonable approximation to the rate ratio, provided that the proportions falling ill in each exposure group during the risk period are low, that is, less than about 10%, and that the prevalence of exposure remains reasonably steady during the study period (see Chapter 4). If the investigator prefers to estimate the risk ratio rather than the incidence rate ratio, the study odds ratio can still be used,[27] but the accuracy of this approximation is only about half as good as that of the odds ratio approximation to the rate ratio.[28] The use of this approximation of the risk ratio by the odds ratio in the cumulative design is the primary basis for the mistaken teaching that a rare-disease assumption is needed to estimate the risk ratio or rate ratio from case-control studies.[12] When the proportion falling in each exposure period is high, 20% or more, the square root of the odds ratio provides a reasonable estimate of the risk ratio.[29] Further transformations of the odds ratio to the risk ratio are available when outcome probabilities are specified to fall in any fixed interval.[30]

Before the 1970s, the standard conceptualization of case-control studies involved the cumulative design, in which controls are selected from noncases at the end of a follow-up period. As discussed by numerous authors,[5,9,21,22] density designs and case-cohort designs have several advantages outside of the acute epidemic setting, including potentially much less sensitivity to bias from exposure-related loss to follow-up.

CASE-ONLY DESIGNS

There are a number of situations in which cases are the only subjects used to estimate or test hypotheses about effects. For example, it may be possible to use theoretical considerations or the past experience of the case herself to construct the expected distribution of exposure in the study base. This expected distribution may be used in place of a separate observed control series. Such situations arise naturally in genetic studies, in which basic laws of inheritance may be combined with certain assumptions to derive a population or parental-specific distribution of genotypes.[31] It is also possible to study certain aspects of joint effects (interactions) of genetic and environmental factors without using control subjects (see more below and in Chapter 37).[32] When the exposure under study is defined by proximity to an environmental source, it may be possible to construct a "specular" (hypothetical) control for each case by conducting a thought experiment. Either the case or the exposure source is imaginarily moved to another location that would be equally likely under the null hypothesis; the case exposure under this hypothetical configuration is then treated as the (matched) "control" exposure for the case.[33] For example, when the exposure under study is defined by proximity to an electric power line, it may be possible to construct a *specular* (hypothetical) control for each case at a symmetrical location.[33] For each case, one considers the mirror image of the residence as if it were across the street. If proximity to electrical wires has no effect on the outcome, then the distribution of distances to the power line would be the same for cases and for imaginary controls living in the hypothetical specular houses. This design would control for general neighborhood environment if residences on the different sides of the street are not systematically different. Similarly, in a study of the relation between farm vehicle crashes and road characteristics, control road segments were matched to cases on postal code, roadway type, and road segment length.[34]

In these examples, the control information comes from examining the exposure experience of the case outside of the *geographic space* in which exposure could be related to the outcome. In other situations, the control information comes from examining the exposure experience of the case outside of the *time* in which exposure could be related to disease occurrence. This type of case-only study is called a case-crossover study.

Case-Crossover

The classic *crossover* randomized trial is a type of experimental cohort study in which two (or more) treatments are compared. In a crossover trial, each subject receives both treatments, with one following the other. Preferably, the order in which the two treatments are applied is randomly assigned for each subject. Enough time should be allocated between the two administrations so that the effect of each treatment can be measured and can subside before the other treatment is given. A persistent effect of the first intervention is called a *carryover effect*. A crossover study is only valid to study treatments for which effects occur within a short induction period and do not persist, *i.e.*, carryover effects must be absent, so that the effect of the second intervention is not intermingled with the effect of the first. The analysis of this crossover study takes into account that the data measured for each of the two exposures are paired within the same person.

The *case-crossover* study is an observational analog of the crossover trial.[35] The method is best suited for studying effects with a sudden onset and exposures that are intermittent and that have short induction periods for the hypothesized effect. For each case, a time window is defined during which the exposure could plausibly have caused the disease onset. The exposure status during this case window is then compared with the exposure status for that same person in one or more control time windows. These control time windows are defined as predisease or postdisease time periods of the same length as the case window and amount to self-matched control periods for each case. If the overall frequency of exposure is known, the expected exposure status during an average control window can be used. For example, Maclure (1991), who introduced the case-crossover design, used it to study the effect of sexual activity on incident myocardial infarction.[35] This topic is well suited to a case-crossover design because the exposure is intermittent and any increase in risk for a myocardial infarction from sexual activity is presumed to be confined to a short time following the activity. In the analysis, Maclure compared the exposure status of cases (*had sex* or *did not have sex* during the 1 hour before the myocardial infarction) with the expected exposure status based on each case's history of sexual activity during the year before the myocardial infarction. If having an event is thought to affect subsequent exposures, the control time windows should all be sampled from before the disease onset. Because a myocardial infarction could affect subsequent sexual activity, the control information in Maclure's study was all taken from before the myocardial infarction.

When the disease of interest cannot affect exposure status, the sampling can be bidirectional with respect to the disease onset. For example, if the study examines the relation between air pollution levels and occurrence of stroke, it would be reasonable to use control information both before and after a case's stroke because having a stroke cannot affect levels of air pollution.

The case-crossover design is a valid and efficient design to study short-term triggering effects. For example, the risk of myocardial infarction may increase during heavy physical exertion,[36] but regular exercise can still reduce the long-term risk of myocardial infarction. Whereas other epidemiologic studies answer the question "why me?," the case-crossover answers the question "why now?"

Because the case window and the control windows necessarily refer to different times, the validity of the case-crossover comparison depends on the assumption that exposure is not changing importantly between these time windows.[37] When only predisease periods are selected as control windows, increasing trends in exposure prevalence between the predisease and the case-exposure periods would result in a larger probability of exposure in the case window from the time trend alone, particularly if there is a long time gap between the windows. When using control windows both before and after the case window (bidirectional sampling), such trends are more like to cancel out if they are monotonic.[38] As noted above, however, postdisease windows should only be used if the outcome cannot affect subsequent exposure. Instead of using discrete time windows, the expected probability of exposure for each case can be estimated from the proportion of time exposed in the last day, week, year, or other relevant period.[39] The analysis of this type of case-crossover study involves using cohort study measures for rate ratios from stratified data, despite the fact that this is not a cohort study.[39] This method is more efficient than categorizing individual time windows as exposed or unexposed, especially if the exposure is rare, although this approach may be more susceptible to time trends in exposure if the exposure data are gathered from a long time interval. It is also possible to adjust case-crossover estimates for bias due to time trends in exposure through use of longitudinal data from a separate nondiseased control group (a case-time-control study).[40] These trend adjustments depend on additional assumptions and may introduce bias if those assumptions are not met.[37,41] This approach assumes controls' exposure trends are a good proxy for the cases' exposure trends, which implies valid selection of control subjects and no recall bias. An alternative strategy to reduce bias from exposure trends over time is to select control windows close in time to the case windows and possibly match them on time of the day or day of the week, or both, to avoid circadian effects or other time patterns.

Although confounding from factors other than time is possible in a case-crossover study, a strength of this design is that each case and its control information is automatically matched on all characteristics, measured or unmeasured, that are stable within individuals (*e.g.*, sex and birth date). Matching coupled with an appropriate analysis of case-crossover data automatically controls for all such fixed confounders, whether or not they are measured. Control for measured time-varying confounders, if necessary, may be possible using modeling methods for matched data.

In addition to controlling for between-person confounding, the case-crossover design avoids the costs and potential biases of selecting and ascertaining a group of control persons. Nonetheless, bias can still be introduced from the selection of cases if exposure around the event affects the selection probability of cases; recall bias can exist if the collection or reporting of information is different for effect and control windows, and within-person confounding can still occur. For example, suppose we are examining whether coffee triggers a myocardial infarction, but smoking is more frequent while drinking coffee; a short-term effect of smoking could confound the coffee effect.[35]

Since its introduction, the case-crossover design has yielded important evidence regarding the triggering relations between air quality and a wide range of causes for hospitalization or mortality,[42] alcohol consumption and injury,[43] pharmaceutical prescriptions and adverse events,[44] vaccination and multiple sclerosis relapse (a null result) and other adverse events,[45,46] and temperature extremes and opioid overdose fatalities,[47] among others. The design has therefore substantially improved the evidence base for understanding triggering conditions of a wide range of exposures and outcomes of public health importance. It is best suited to exposure-outcome hypotheses when the exposure is variable or intermittent over the time periods during which triggering might be relevant, the effect of the triggering exposure on occurrence of the outcome is immediate and then subsides within the time period during which triggering might be relevant, and the outcome occurs abruptly and its occurrence is immediately observable.[48] While the design has been used to study exposure-outcome relations outside these guidelines, there are inevitably concerns about the validity of the case-crossover estimate when departures from this guidance grow large.

Other Case-Only Designs

There are many possible variants of the case-only designs, depending on how control time periods are selected. These variants offer trade-offs among potential for bias, inefficiency, and difficulty of analysis.[49-54] Sometimes, theoretical considerations alone are used to establish the expected distribution of exposure in place of an observed control series. Such situations arise naturally in genetic studies, in which basic laws of inheritance may be combined with certain assumptions to derive a population or parental-specific expected distribution of genotypes.[31] Deviation from the genetic laws would suggest an association with the condition. It is also possible to study certain aspects of joint effects (interactions) of genetic and environmental factors without using control subjects.[32] The goal of this design is not to study effects but to estimate multiplicative interactions between genetic factors and environmental factors, which are assumed to be independent in the study population. Estimates of gene-environment interactions using the case-only design are efficient relative to estimates obtained from an analogous case-control study. In the analogous case-control study, information from the controls would allow analytic control for lack of independence of the genetic factor and environmental factor in the study population. Using the case-only design is therefore cost-efficient because genetic and environmental information is collected only from cases rather than from cases and controls. The case-only design also provides a more statistically efficient estimate of multiplicative interaction than the estimate that would be obtained using the same cases and an equal number of controls. The price for these advantages, however, is the necessity of the strong assumption of independence of the exposure and genetic factor in the study population, which cannot be evaluated using the case-only data and which may be violated more often than realized.[55] The case-only design for studies of genetic interaction will be discussed further in Chapter 37.

A second variant of the case-only design is the *self-controlled case series.*[56] The design was developed for acute adverse events occurring within defined, usually short, time periods after vaccination.[45] Ages at exposure to an acute event are ascertained, and the random variable is the age at event, conditional on its occurrence within a predetermined observation window[45] corresponding to the hypothesized induction period. The requirements for this design are that (1) exposures are transient with short-term effects, (2) outcome events have sudden onset, (3) the outcome does not affect the likelihood of future exposure (*e.g.*, the event is not a contraindication for subsequent exposure), and (4) the outcome does not affect the period of observation (*e.g.*, the outcome event is not death). Unlike the case-crossover design, the self-controlled case series does not require that there be no time trend in the exposure prevalence[45] (although recall that such trends can be taken into account using controls in the case-crossover design). Because the design most often uses electronic health records or administrative claims data (see Chapter 11), it has been used most often to evaluate associations between vaccination[57] or use of pharmaceuticals[58,59] and recurrent or rare adverse events.

Two-Stage Sampling

Another variant of the case-control study uses two-stage or two-phase sampling.[60,61] In this type of study, the control series comprises a relatively large number of people (possibly everyone in the source population), from whom exposure information or perhaps some limited amount of information on other relevant variables is obtained. Then, for a subsample of the controls, more detailed information is obtained on exposure or on other study variables that may need to be controlled in the analysis. More detailed information may also be limited to a subsample of cases. This two-stage approach is useful when it is relatively inexpensive to obtain the exposure information (*e.g.*, from registry or claims data, see Chapter 11), but the covariate information is more expensive to obtain (say, by laboratory analysis). It is also useful when exposure information already has been collected on the entire population (*e.g.*, job histories for an occupational cohort), but covariate information is needed (*e.g.*, genotype). This situation arises in cohort studies when more information is required than was gathered at baseline.

To conduct a "two-stage sampling" design, we first identify the exposure and disease status of all individuals in the study sample and estimate crude exposure effects (stage 1). For the second stage, we select a subset using sampling fractions to improve efficiency or to reduce cost, usually by oversampling exposed cases as this is often the smallest cell in the crude table. After more detailed information is collected from the second-stage sample, the analysis is conducted by taking into account the two-stage sampling. The analysis requires special methods that take into account the second-stage sampling that is not independent of exposure and take full advantage of the information collected at both stages.

SOURCES FOR CONTROL SERIES

The following methods for control sampling apply when the source population is large and dynamic and therefore cannot be explicitly enumerated. Without a roster, one cannot identify all those at risk for disease at the outset of study follow-up, nor those free of disease at the end of study follow-up. Consequently, case-cohort sampling and cumulative sampling of controls are infeasible. Because the population is dynamic, controls should be sampled in proportion to person-time. The case-control odds ratio estimator then provides an estimate of the incidence rate ratio estimand.[9] When the source population is defined secondarily to the case-finding mechanism, the methods below are subject to the reservations about secondary bases described earlier in the chapter.

Neighborhood Controls

If the source population cannot be enumerated, it may be possible to select controls through sampling of residences. This method is not straightforward. Usually, a geographic roster of residences is not available, so a scheme must be devised to sample residences without enumerating them all. For convenience, investigators may sample controls who are individually matched to cases from the same neighborhood. That is, after a case is identified, one or more controls residing in the same neighborhood as that case are identified and recruited into the study. If neighborhood is related to exposure, the matching should be controlled in the analysis.

Neighborhood controls are often used when the cases are recruited from a convenient source, such as a clinic or hospital. Such usage can introduce bias, however, for the neighbors selected as controls may not be in the source population of the cases. For example, if the cases are from a particular hospital, neighborhood controls may include people who would not have been treated at the same hospital had they developed the disease.[15] If being treated at the hospital from which cases are identified is related to the exposure under study, then using neighborhood controls would introduce a bias.

Social Media

Traditional methods of data collection such as paper questionnaires, face-to-face interviews, and phone interviews have been challenged by decreasing participation rates, use of cell phones, privacy, and high cost.[62] With increasing use of internet, the use of web-based self-administered online questionnaires is becoming more common.[63] The penetration of mobile phones in developing countries and the expansion of electronic and mobile health (mHealth) for the practice of medicine allow investigators to consider this methodology to obtain information from populations worldwide (see Chapter 10). These methods are well suited to cohort studies, which often comprise volunteers who once recruited can be followed as effectively or more effectively through the internet as through other means.[64-66] Selective participation concerns may pose a problem for using the internet to sample controls for use in case-controls studies, if self-selection is likely to be related to exposure. This concern is analogous to selective consent to participate among those invited to participate by other methods in secondary base studies.

Hospital- or Clinic-Based Controls

As noted above, the source population for hospital- or clinic-based case-control studies is not often identifiable because it represents a group of people who would be treated in a given clinic or hospital if they developed the disease in question. In such situations, a random sample of the general population will not necessarily correspond to a random sample of the source population. If the hospitals or clinics that provide the cases for the study treat only a small proportion of cases in the geographic area, then referral patterns to the hospital or clinic are important to take into account in the sampling of controls. For these studies, a control series comprising patients from the same hospitals or clinics as the cases may provide a less biased estimate of effect than general-population controls (such as those obtained from case neighborhoods). The source population does not correspond to the population of the geographic area, but only to the people who would seek treatment at the hospital or clinic were they to develop the disease under study. Although the latter population may be difficult or impossible to enumerate or even define very clearly, it seems reasonable to expect that other hospital or clinic patients will represent this source population better than general-population controls. The major problem with any nonrandom sampling of controls is the possibility that they are not selected independently of exposure in the source population. Patients who are hospitalized with other diseases, for example, may be unrepresentative of the exposure distribution in the source population, either because exposure is associated with hospitalization or because the exposure is associated with the other diseases or both. For example, suppose the study aims to evaluate the relation between tobacco smoking and leukemia using hospitalized cases. If controls are people who are hospitalized with other conditions, many of them will have been hospitalized for conditions associated with smoking. A variety of other cancers, as well as cardiovascular diseases and respiratory diseases, are related to smoking. Thus, a control series of people hospitalized for diseases other than leukemia would include a higher proportion of smokers than would the source population of the leukemia cases.

Limiting the diagnoses for controls to conditions for which there is no prior indication of an association with the exposure improves the control series. For example, in a study of smoking and hospitalized leukemia cases, one could exclude from the control series anyone who was hospitalized with a disease known to be related to smoking. Such an exclusion policy may exclude most of the potential controls because cardiovascular disease by itself would represent a large proportion of hospitalized patients. Nevertheless, even a few common diagnostic categories should suffice to find enough control subjects, so that the exclusions will not harm the study by limiting the size of the control series. Indeed, in limiting the scope of eligibility criteria, it is reasonable to exclude categories of potential controls even on the suspicion that a given category might be related to the exposure. If wrong, the cost of the exclusion is that the control series becomes more homogeneous with respect to diagnosis and perhaps a little smaller. But if right, then the exclusion is important to the ultimate validity of the study.

On the other hand, an investigator can rarely be sure that an exposure is not related to a disease or to hospitalization for a specific diagnosis. Consequently, it would be imprudent to use only a single diagnostic category as a source of controls. Using a variety of diagnoses has the advantage of potentially diluting the biasing effects of including a specific diagnostic group that is related to the exposure and allows examination of the effect of excluding certain diagnoses.

Excluding a diagnostic category from the list of eligibility criteria for identifying controls is intended simply to improve the representativeness of the control series with respect to the exposure distribution in the source population. Such an exclusion criterion does not imply that there should be exclusions based on disease history.[23] For example, in a case-control study of smoking and hospitalized leukemia patients, one might use hospitalized controls but exclude any who are hospitalized because of cardiovascular disease. This exclusion criterion for controls does not imply that leukemia cases who have had cardiovascular disease should be excluded; only if the cardiovascular disease was a cause of the hospitalization should the case be excluded. For controls, the exclusion criterion should apply only to the cause of the hospitalization used to identify the study subject. A person who was hospitalized because of a traumatic injury and who is thus eligible to be a control would not be excluded if he or she had previously been hospitalized for cardiovascular disease. The source population includes people who have had cardiovascular disease, and they should be included in the control series. Excluding such people would lead to an underrepresentation of smoking relative to the source population and produce an upward bias in the effect estimates.

If exposure directly affects hospitalization (for example, if the decision to hospitalize is in part based on exposure history), the resulting bias cannot be remedied without knowing the hospitalization rates, even if the exposure is unrelated to the study disease or the control diseases. This problem was in fact one of the first problems of hospital-based studies to receive detailed analysis[67] and is often called Berkson bias; it is discussed further under the topics of selection bias and collider bias (see Chapter 14).

Friend Controls

Choosing friends of cases as controls, like using neighborhood controls, is a design that inherently uses individual matching and needs to be evaluated with regard to the advantages and disadvantages of such matching (see Chapter 6). Aside from the complications of individual matching, there are further concerns stemming from use of friend controls. First, being named as a friend by the case may be related to the exposure status of the potential control.[68] For example, cases might preferentially name as friends their acquaintances with whom they engage in specific activities that might relate to the exposure. Physical activity, alcoholic beverage consumption, and sun exposure are examples of such exposures. People who are more reclusive may be less likely to be named as friends, so their exposure patterns will be underrepresented among a control series of friends. Exposures more common to extroverted people may become overrepresented among friend controls. This type of bias was suspected in a study of insulin-dependent diabetes mellitus in which the parents of cases identified as the controls. The cases had fewer friends than controls, had more learning problems, and were more likely to dislike school. Using friend controls could explain these findings.[69]

A second problem is that, unlike other methods of control selection, choosing friends as controls cedes much of the decision-making about the choice of control subjects to the cases or their proxies (*e.g.*, parents). The investigator who uses friend controls will usually ask for a list of friends and choose randomly from the list, but for the creation of the list, the investigator is completely dependent on the cases or their proxies. This dependence adds a potential source of bias to the use of friend controls that does not exist for other sources of controls.

A third problem is that using friend controls can introduce a bias that stems from the overlapping nature of friendship groups.[70,71] The problem arises because different cases name groups of friends that are not mutually exclusive. As a result, people with many friends become overrepresented in the control series, and any exposures associated with such people become overrepresented as well.

In principle, matching categories should form a mutually exclusive and collectively exhaustive partition with respect to all factors, such as neighborhood and age. For example, if matching on age, bias due to overlapping matching groups can arise from *caliper matching,* a term that refers to choosing controls who have a value for the matching factor within a specified range of the case's value. Thus, if the case is 69 years old, one might choose controls who are within 2 years caliper of age 69 years. Overlap bias can be avoided if one uses nonoverlapping age categories for matching. Thus, if the case is 69 years old, one might choose controls from within the age category 65 to 69 years. In practice, however, bias due to overlapping age and neighborhood categories is probably minor.[71]

Sibling Controls

Matching study subjects with siblings may be used in both cohort and case-control studies to control for shared genetic and environmental factors.[72,73] For example, in a case-control study of breast cancer that included both sister controls and controls sampled from the source population, the two sets of controls differed substantially with regard to many established risk factors for breast cancer, and estimates of associations for established breast cancer risk factors were nearer to expectation using sister controls than population controls.[74] Sibling case-control designs can reduce confounding by shared factors, but they can also increase nondifferential and differential exposure misclassification and potential confounding by nonshared factors.[75,76] For example, imagine a case-control study of oral clefts in which maternal smoking during pregnancy was compared between case infants and their nonmalformed siblings. Within a sibling pair discordant for maternal smoking, the likelihood of the apparently unexposed pregnancy to be actually exposed (*e.g.*, smoking not recorded for one of the pregnancies) would be higher than the overall underrecording probability in the general population of pregnancies because the mother smoked at one point. In addition, the fact that the exposure differs between siblings may be associated with a factor that in turn is associated with the outcome. The discordance for within-sibling confounders would be larger than the discordance when cases are compared with random persons in the population, so the association between the confounder and exposure would be stronger in within-sibling comparisons than in other case-control sampling strategies. If young mothers quit smoking before subsequent pregnancies, smoking would be associated with younger age within-sibling comparisons. If young age were the strongest risk factor for oral clefts, the sibling-matched design could be more biased than a nonsibling approach unless age were controlled in the analysis.

Dead Controls

A dead control cannot be a member of the source population for cases because death precludes the occurrence of any new disease. Suppose, however, that the cases are dead. Does the need for comparability argue in favor of using dead controls? Although certain types of comparability are important, choosing dead controls will misrepresent the exposure distribution in the source population if the exposure causes or prevents death in a substantial proportion of people or if it is associated with an uncontrolled factor that does. If interviews are needed and some cases are dead, it will be necessary to use proxy respondents for the dead cases. To enhance comparability of information while avoiding the problems of using dead controls, proxy respondents can also be used for those live controls matched to dead cases.[15] The advantage of comparable information for cases and controls is often overstated, however, as will be addressed below.

The main justification for using dead controls is convenience, such as in studies based entirely on deaths. Proportional mortality studies were discussed in Chapter 6, where the point was made that the validity of such studies can be improved if they are designed and analyzed as case-control studies. The cases are deaths occurring within the source population. Controls are not selected directly from the source population, which consists of living people, but are taken from other deaths within the source population. This control series is acceptable if the exposure distribution within this group is similar to that of the source population. Consequently, the control series should be restricted to categories of death that are not related to the exposure.

Proxy Controls

It may be impossible to sample controls inside the study base from which case patients arise. In that situation, controls may be sampled from another population that has the same distribution of risk factors as does the study base. This "proxy" source of controls would be valid as long as it has the same exposure distribution as the study base. In the extreme, proxy controls might not be "at risk" of developing the disease. For example, if studying the association between prostate cancer and blood group, one could include females as controls. The blood group distribution of females should be the same as males, but they would be a proxy control group because females are not at risk of developing prostate cancer and are not in the study base.

A good example of an effective proxy control group arose in a study of the causes of an outbreak of electronic-cigarette, or vaping, and product use–associated lung injury (EVALI).[77] In this secondary base case-control study, cases were defined as confirmed or probable cases of EVALI. The case definition required use of e-cigarette or vaping products within 90 days of symptom onset, presence of infiltrates or opacities upon imaging of the lungs, and lack of evidence of other known causes of lung injury or illness. Cases in the study also had to have had a bronchoalveolar lavage biospecimen collected. Bronchoalveolar lavage is an invasive procedure in which a bronchoscope is passed through the mouth or nose into the lungs, fluid is injected into a small part of the lung, and then recovered by vacuum for bioassay. It would be nearly impossible to describe the source population of persons who, were they to develop EVALI, would have appeared as a case in this study. Not only is the source population undefined, but the biospecimen collection adds an additional constraint because there is no representative sample of any source population for which bronchoalveolar lavage specimens are routinely collected. Instead, the study used proxy controls, who were previous participants included in an unrelated research project pertaining to use of tobacco and e-cigarette products.[78] Vitamin E acetate was detected in the bronchoalveolar lavage fluid of 48 of 51 cases and in 0 of 99 controls. No other assay toxicant appeared more than once in any biospecimen of cases or controls. The very strong association between vitamin E acetate and EVALI, and the absence of association with other candidate toxicants, strongly suggested that the presence of vitamin E acetate in vaping products was responsible for the EVALI outbreak. This result, which led to effective interventions, was obtained despite the limitations of the secondary base and proxy control design.

OTHER CONSIDERATIONS FOR SUBJECT SELECTION

Prevalent Cases

The cases in cohort studies are incident cases, and therefore in case-control studies, we aim to include incident cases if possible. When it is impractical to include only incident cases, it may still be possible to enroll prevalent cases of illness. If the prevalence odds ratio in the population is equal to the incidence rate ratio, then the odds ratio from a case-control study based on prevalent cases can estimate the incidence rate ratio without bias. As noted in Chapter 5, however, the conditions required for the prevalence odds ratio to equal the rate ratio are very strong. If exposure is associated with duration of illness (time to death or cure) or migration out of the prevalence pool (loss to follow-up), then a case-control study based on prevalent cases cannot by itself distinguish exposure effects on disease incidence from the exposure association with disease duration or migration, unless the strengths of the latter associations are known. If the size of the exposed or the unexposed population changes with time or there is migration into the prevalence pool, the prevalence odds ratio may be further removed from the incidence rate ratio. Consequently, it is usually preferable to select incident rather than prevalent cases when studying disease etiology. In some instances, one may be interested in the causal effects of an exposure on prevalence.[79]

As discussed in Chapter 4, it is usual to enroll prevalent cases in studies of congenital malformations. In such studies, cases ascertained at birth are prevalent because they have survived with the malformation from the time of its occurrence until birth. For etiological research, it would be preferable to ascertain all incident cases, including affected abortuses that do not survive until birth. Many of these, however, do not survive until ascertainment is feasible, and thus it is virtually inevitable that case-control studies of congenital malformations are based mostly if not entirely on prevalent cases. In this example, the source population comprises all conceptuses, and miscarriage and induced abortion are events that involve the affected individuals exiting the source population before the date when their malformation might be ascertained. Even if an exposure does not affect the duration of survival with a malformation, it may very well affect the risk of miscarriage or abortion.

Other situations in which prevalent cases are commonly used are studies of chronic conditions with ill-defined onset times and limited effects on mortality, such as obesity, Parkinson disease, and multiple sclerosis, and studies of health services utilization.

Representativeness

Some textbooks have stressed the need for representativeness in the selection of cases and controls. The advice has been that cases should be representative of all people with the disease and that controls should be representative of the entire nondiseased population. Such advice can be misleading. A case-control study may be restricted to any type of case that may be of interest: female cases, old cases, severely ill cases, cases that died soon after disease onset, mild cases, cases from Philadelphia, cases among factory workers, and so on. In none of these examples would the cases be representative of all people with the disease, yet perfectly valid case-control studies are possible in each of those situations.[80] The definition of a case can be quite specific as long as it has a sound rationale. Just as cohort studies can be based on special subcohorts rather than on the general population, case-control studies can be based on populations with specific eligibility criteria as well. The main concern is clear delineation of the population that gave rise to the cases.

Ordinarily, controls should represent the source population for cases (within categories of stratification variables), rather than the entire nondiseased population. The latter may differ vastly from the source population for the cases by age, race, sex (e.g., if the cases come from a Veterans Administration hospital), socioeconomic status, occupation, and so on—including the exposure of interest. One of the reasons for emphasizing the similarities rather than the differences between cohort and case-control studies is that numerous principles apply to both types of study but are more evident in the context of cohort studies. In particular, many principles relating to subject selection apply identically to both types of study. For example, it is widely appreciated that cohort studies can be based on special cohorts rather than on the general population. It follows that case-control studies can be conducted by sampling cases and controls from within those special cohorts. The resulting controls should represent the distribution of exposure across those cohorts, rather than the general population, reflecting the principle that controls should represent the source population of the cases in the study, rather than the general population.

Comparability of Information Accuracy

Some authors have recommended that information obtained about cases and controls should be of comparable or equal accuracy, to ensure nondifferentiality (equal distribution) of measurement errors.[14,81,82] The rationale for this principle is the notion that nondifferential measurement error biases the observed association toward the null, and so will not generate a spurious association, and that bias in studies with nondifferential error is more predictable than in studies with differential error.

The comparability-of-information (equal accuracy) principle is often used to guide selection of controls and collection of data. For example, it is the basis for using proxy respondents instead of direct interviews for living controls whenever case information is obtained from proxy respondents. In most settings, however, the arguments for the principle are logically inadequate. One problem, discussed at length in Chapter 13, is that nondifferentiality of exposure measurement error is far from sufficient to guarantee that bias will be toward the null. Such guarantees require that the exposure errors also be *independent* of errors in other variables, including disease and confounders,[83,84] a condition that is not always plausible.[85] For example, it seems likely that people who conceal heavy alcohol use will also tend to understate other socially disapproved behaviors such as heavy smoking, illicit drug use, and so on.

Another problem is that the efforts to ensure equal accuracy of exposure information will also tend to produce equal accuracy of information on other variables. The direction of overall bias produced by the resulting nondifferential errors in confounders and effect modifiers can be larger than the bias produced by differential error from unequal accuracy of exposure information from cases and controls.[86-90] In addition, unless the exposure is binary, even independent nondifferential error in exposure measurement is not guaranteed to produce bias toward the null.[91] Finally, even when the bias produced by forcing equal measurement accuracy is toward the null, there is no guarantee that the bias is less than the bias that would have resulted from using a measurement with differential error.[14,92,93] For example, in a study that used proxy respondents for cases, use of proxy respondents for the controls might lead to greater bias than use of direct interviews with controls, even if the latter results in greater accuracy of control measurements.

The comparability-of-information (equal-accuracy) principle is therefore applicable only under very limited conditions. In particular, it would seem to be useful only when confounders and effect modifiers are measured with negligible error and when measurement error is reduced by using equally accurate sources of information. Otherwise, the bias from forcing cases and controls to have equal measurement accuracy may be as unpredictable as the effect of allowing differential error (unequal accuracy). Quantitative bias analysis (see Chapter 29) allowing for differential misclassification or measurement error will often provide a superior alternative to design strategies aimed at assuring comparability of information accuracy.

Number of Control Groups

Situations arise in which the investigator may face a choice between two or more possible control groups. Usually, there will be advantages for one group that are missing in the other and vice versa. Consider, for example, a case-control study based on a hospitalized series of cases (a secondary base design). Because they are hospitalized, hospital controls would be unrepresentative of the source population to the extent that exposure is related to hospitalization for the control conditions. Neighborhood controls would not suffer this problem but might be unrepresentative of persons who would go to the hospital if they had the study disease. So which control group is better? In such situations, some have argued that more than one control group should be used, in an attempt to address the biases from each group.[94] For example, a matched family control group could reduce confounding by unmeasured genetic characteristics, and a parallel hospital control group could reduce potential differential recall between persons with and without a health event. Gutensohn et al. (1975),[95] in a case-control study of Hodgkin disease, used a control group of spouses as control for environmental influences during adult life but also used a control group of siblings as control for childhood environment and sex. Both control groups are attempting to represent the same source population of cases but have different vulnerabilities to selection biases and match on different potential confounders.

Use of multiple control groups may involve considerable labor and expense so is more the exception than the rule in case-control research. Often, one available control source is superior to all practical alternatives. In such settings, effort should not be wasted on collecting controls from sources likely to be biased. Interpretation of the results will also be more complicated unless the different control groups yield similar results. If the two groups produced different results, one would face the problem of explaining the differences and attempting to infer which estimate was more valid. Logically, then, the value of using more than one control group is limited. If there is more than one control group, the results should be compared, but a lack of difference between the groups shows only that all groups incorporate similar net bias. A difference shows only that at least one is biased but does not indicate which is best or worst.[96] Only external information could help evaluate the likely extent of bias in the estimates from different control groups, and that same external information might have favored selection of only one of the control groups at the design stage of the study.

Timing of Classification and Diagnosis

Chapter 7 discussed at length some basic principles for classifying persons, cases, and person-time units in cohort studies according to exposure status. The same principles apply to cases and controls in case-control studies. If the controls are intended to represent person-time (rather than persons) in the source population, one should apply principles for classifying person-time to the classification of controls. In particular, principles of person-time classification lead to the rule that controls should be classified by their exposure status as of their selection time. Exposures accrued after that time should be ignored. The rule necessitates that information (such as exposure history) be obtained in a manner that allows one to ignore exposures accrued after the selection time. In a similar manner, cases should be classified as of time of diagnosis or disease onset, accounting for any built-in lag periods or induction-period hypotheses. Determining the time of diagnosis or disease onset can involve all the problems and ambiguities discussed in the previous chapter for cohort studies and needs to be resolved by study protocol before classifications can be made.

As an example, consider a case-control study of alcohol use and laryngeal cancer that used neighborhood controls. Suppose that the study examined smoking as a confounder and possible effect modifier and used interviewer-administered questionnaires to collect data. To examine the effect of alcohol and smoking while assuming a 1-year lag period (a 1-year minimum induction time), the questionnaire would have to allow determination of drinking and smoking habits up to 1 year before diagnosis for cases and the date of selection for controls.

Selection time need not refer to the investigator's identification of the control but instead may refer to an event analogous to the occurrence time for the case. For example, the selection time for controls who are selected because they are diagnosed with other diseases can be taken as time of diagnosis for the other disease; the selection time of hospital controls might be taken as time of hospitalization. For other types of controls, there may be no such natural event analogous to the case diagnosis time, and the actual time of selection will have to be used.

In most studies, selection time will precede the time data are gathered. For example, in interview-based studies, controls may be identified and then a delay of weeks or months may occur before the interview is conducted. To avoid complicating the interview questions, this distinction is often ignored and controls are questioned about habits in periods dating back from the interview.

COMMON FALLACIES IN CONTROL SELECTION

A properly designed and executed case-control study is as valid as the corresponding analysis of the full cohort.[97] The essential difference between these two designs is whether they employ 100% samples, as the cohort studies do, or smaller samples of the people or person-time giving rise to the cases, resulting in a case-control study with consequently lower statistical precision than the corresponding cohort study, and requiring a proper sampling of controls. Other than that, the same challenges affect cohort and case-control designs, including defining the etiologically relevant exposure window, dealing with time-dependent variables, obtaining accurate information on exposure and outcome, dealing with confounding, and avoiding a survivor cohort of those with prevalent exposure or other types of selection biases.

Nonetheless, as stated earlier, conventional wisdom about case-control studies is that they do not yield estimates of effect that are as valid as those obtained from cohort studies. This thinking may reflect common misunderstandings in conceptualizing case-control studies, as well as legitimate concern about biased exposure information and subject selection in retrospective case-control studies.

Recall and Record Bias

Concern about recall bias is a common criticism of case-control designs. For example, if exposure information comes from interviews, cases will usually have reported the exposure information after learning of their diagnosis. Diagnosis may affect reporting in a number of ways, for example, by improving memory, thus enhancing sensitivity among cases, or by provoking false memory of exposure, thus reducing specificity among cases. Furthermore, the disease may itself cloud memory and thus reduce sensitivity. These phenomena are examples that lead to *recall bias*. Similarly, the disease can affect the amount and detail of information on past exposures collected in a clinical record. For example, maternal opioid consumption may be more likely to be recorded in neonates that required intensive care unit hospitalization. We could refer to this phenomenon as *recording bias*. The disease cannot affect exposure information collected before the disease occurred, however. Thus exposure information taken from records created before the disease occurs will not be subject to recall bias. Even for case-control studies with self-reported exposure information, recall bias can be limited by using well-designed questionnaires.

Conversely, cohort studies are not immune from problems often thought to be particular to case-control studies. For example, while a cohort study may gather information on exposure for an entire source population at the outset of the study, it still requires tracing of subjects to ascertain exposure variation and outcomes. If the success of this tracing is related to the exposure and the outcome, the resulting selection bias will behave analogously to that often raised as a concern in case-control studies.[98] Similarly, cohort studies sometimes use recall to reconstruct or impute exposure history (retrospective evaluation) and are vulnerable to recall bias if this reconstruction is done after disease occurrence. Thus, although more opportunity for recall and selection bias may arise in retrospective case-control studies than in prospective cohort studies, each study must be considered on its own merits to evaluate its vulnerability to bias, regardless of its design.

Multiple Outcomes

Conventional wisdom also holds that cohort studies are useful for evaluating the range of effects related to a single exposure, whereas case-control studies provide information only about the one disease that afflicts the cases. This thinking conflicts with the idea that case-control studies can be viewed simply as more efficient cohort studies. Just as one can choose to measure more than one disease outcome in a cohort study, it is possible to conduct a set of case-control studies nested within the same population using several disease outcomes as the case series. The case-cohort study (see above) is particularly well suited to this task, allowing one control group to be compared with several series of cases arising in the cohort. Whether or not the case-cohort design is the form of case-control study that is used, case-control studies do not have to be characterized as being limited with respect to the number of disease outcomes that can be studied.

Exposure Opportunity

In cohort studies, the study population is restricted to people at risk for the disease. Some authors have viewed case-control studies as if they were cohort studies done backwards, even going so far as to describe them as "trohoc" studies.[99] Under this view, the argument was advanced that case-control studies ought to be restricted to those at risk for exposure (*i.e.*, those with exposure opportunity). Excluding sterile women from a case-control study of an adverse effect of oral contraceptives and matching for duration of employment in an occupational study are examples of attempts to control for exposure opportunity. If the factor used for restriction (*e.g.*, sterility) is unrelated to the disease, it will not be a confounder, and hence the restriction will yield no benefit to the validity of the estimate of effect. Furthermore, if the restriction reduces the study size, the precision of the estimate of effect will be reduced.[100] There is no need to restrict participants in case-control studies to those who have an opportunity to be exposed.

Inclusion of Healthy Controls

Another principle sometimes used in cohort studies is that the study cohort should be "clean" at start of follow-up, including only people who have never had the disease. Using a false analogy, some have misapplied this principle to case-control design, suggesting that the control group ought to be "clean," and taking that to mean that it should include only people who are healthy. Illness that arises after the start of the follow-up period is not a reason to exclude subjects from a cohort analysis, and such exclusion can lead to bias; similarly controls with illnesses that arose after exposure should not be removed from the control series. Nonetheless, in studies of the relation between cigarette smoking and colorectal cancer, certain authors recommended that the control group should exclude people with colon polyps because colon polyps are associated with smoking and are precursors of colorectal cancer.[101] Such an exclusion actually reduces the prevalence of the exposure in the controls below that in the source population of cases and hence biases the effect estimates upward.[102] Just as in cohort studies, cases with the disease of interest before the start of follow-up should ordinarily be excluded from case-control studies (see the discussion of prevalent cases above). Persons with other health conditions are among those who are at risk for the disease of interest, so they should be eligible to become a case or to be selected as a control. Excluding them from the study introduces a bias. The only exception is when the study excludes some group of people with preexisting conditions for the purpose of addressing its particular hypothesis (*e.g.*, investigators may choose to study tuberculosis using a case-control design and to restrict the study to persons without a history of human immunodeficiency virus [HIV] infection).

References

1. Rothman KJ. Six persistent research misconceptions. *J Gen Intern Med.* 2014;29(7):1060-1064.
2. Hernán MA. Hypothetical interventions to define causal effects—afterthought or prerequisite? *Am J Epidemiol.* 2005;162:618-620.
3. Hernan MA, Taubman SL. Does obesity shorten life? The importance of well-defined interventions to answer causal questions. *Int J Obes (Lond).* 2008;32(suppl 3):S8-S14.
4. Hernan MA. Does water kill? A call for less casual causal inferences. *Ann Epidemiol.* 2016;26(10):674-680.
5. Miettinen OS. Estimability and estimation in case-referent studies. *Am J Epidemiol.* 1976;103:226-235.
6. Wacholder S. The case-control study as data missing by design: estimating risk differences. *Epidemiology.* 1996;7(2):144-150.
7. Irony TZ. Case-control studies: using "real-world" evidence to assess association. *J Am Med Assoc.* 2018;320(10):1027-1028.
8. Blakely T, Pearce N, Lynch J. Case-control studies. *J Am Med Assoc.* 2019;321(8):806-807.
9. Vandenbroucke JP, Pearce N. Case–control studies: basic concepts. *Int J Epidemiol.* 2012;41(5):1480-1489.
10. Greenland S. Control-initiated case-control studies. *Int J Epidemiol.* 1985;14(1):130-134.
11. Lash TL, Cronin-Fenton D, Ahern TP, et al. CYP2D6 inhibition and breast cancer recurrence in a population-based study in Denmark. *J Natl Cancer Inst.* 2011;103(6):489-500.
12. Pearce N. What does the odds ratio estimate in a case-control study? *Int J Epidemiol.* 1993;22(6):1189-1192.
13. Knol MJ, Vandenbroucke JP, Scott P, Egger M. What do case-control studies estimate? Survey of methods and assumptions in published case-control research. *Am J Epidemiol.* 2008;168(9):1073-1081.

14. Wacholder S, McLaughlin JK, Silverman DT, Mandel JS. Selection of controls in case-control studies: I. Principles. *Am J Epidemiol*. 1992;135(9):1019-1028.

15. Wacholder S, Silverman DT, McLaughlin JK, Mandel JS. Selection of controls in case-control studies: II. Types of controls. *Am J Epidemiol*. 1992;135(9):1029-1041.

16. Wacholder S, Silverman DT, McLaughlin JK, Mandel JS. Selection of controls in case-control studies: III. Design options. *Am J Epidemiol*. 1992;135(9):1042-1050.

17. Mansournia MA, Jewell NP, Greenland S. Case-control matching: effects, misconceptions, and recommendations. *Eur J Epidemiol*. 2018;33(1):5-14.

18. Pearce N. Bias in matched case-control studies: DAGs are not enough. *Eur J Epidemiol*. 2018;33(1):1-4.

19. Pearce N. Analysis of matched case-control studies. *Br Med J*. 2016;352:i969.

20. Brookmeyer R, Liang KY, Linet M. Matched case-control designs and overmatched analyses. *Am J Epidemiol*. 1986;124(4):693-701.

21. Sheehe PR. Dynamic risk analysis in retrospective matched-pair studies of disease. *Biometrics*. 1962;18:323-341.

22. Greenland S, Thomas DC. On the need for the rare disease assumption in case-control studies. *Am J Epidemiol*. 1982;116(3):547-553.

23. Lubin JH, Gail MH. Biased selection of controls for case-control analyses of cohort studies. *Biometrics*. 1984;40(1):63-75.

24. Robins JM, Gail MH, Lubin JH. More on "Biased selection of controls for case-control analyses of cohort studies". *Biometrics*. 1986;42(2):293-299.

25. Liddell FDK, McDonald JC, Thomas DC, Cunliffe SV. Methods of cohort analysis: appraisal by application to asbestos mining. *J R Stat Soc Ser A (General)*. 1977;140(4):469-491.

26. Robins JM, Prentice RL, Blevins D. Designs for synthetic case-control studies in open cohorts. *Biometrics*. 1989;45(4):1103-1116.

27. Cornfield J. A method of estimating comparative rates from clinical data; applications to cancer of the lung, breast, and cervix. *J Natl Cancer Inst*. 1951;11(6):1269-1275.

28. Greenland S. Interpretation and choice of effect measures in epidemiologic analyses. *Am J Epidemiol*. 1987;125(5):761-768.

29. VanderWeele TJ. On a square-root transformation of the odds ratio for a common outcome. *Epidemiology*. 2017;28(6):e58-e60.

30. VanderWeele TJ. Optimal approximate conversions of odds ratios and hazard ratios to risk ratios. *Biometrics*. 2019. doi:10.1111/biom.13197.

31. Self SG, Longton G, Kopecky KJ, Liang KY. On estimating HLA/disease association with application to a study of aplastic anemia. *Biometrics*. 1991;47(1):53-61.

32. Khoury MJ, Flanders WD. Nontraditional epidemiologic approaches in the analysis of gene-environment interaction: case-control studies with no controls! *Am J Epidemiol*. 1996;144(3):207-213.

33. Zaffanella LE, Savitz DA, Greenland S, Ebi KL. The residential case-specular method to study wire codes, magnetic fields, and disease. *Epidemiology*. 1998;9(1):16-20.

34. Ranapurwala SI, Mello ER, Ramirez MR. A GIS-based matched case–control study of road characteristics in farm vehicle crashes. *Epidemiology*. 2016;27(6):827-834.

35. Maclure M. The case-crossover design: a method for studying transient effects on the risk of acute events. *Am J Epidemiol*. 1991;133(2):144-153.

36. Mittleman MA, Maclure M, Tofler GH, Sherwood JB, Goldberg RJ, Muller JE. Triggering of acute myocardial infarction by heavy physical exertion. Protection against triggering by regular exertion: Determinants of Myocardial Infarction Onset Study Investigators. *N Engl J Med*. 1993;329(23):1677-1683.

37. Greenland S. Confounding and exposure trends in case-crossover and case-time-control designs. *Epidemiology*. 1996;7(3):231-239.

38. Bateson TF, Schwartz J. Control for seasonal variation and time trend in case-crossover studies of acute effects of environmental exposures. *Epidemiology*. 1999;10(5):539-544.

39. Mittleman MA, Maclure M, Robins JM. Control sampling strategies for case-crossover studies: an assessment of relative efficiency. *Am J Epidemiol*. 1995;142(1):91-98.

40. Suissa S. The case-time-control design. *Epidemiology*. 1995;6(3):248-253.

41. Suissa S. The case-time-control design: further assumptions and conditions. *Epidemiology*. 1998;9:441-445.

42. Carracedo-Martinez E, Taracido M, Tobias A, Saez M, Figueiras A. Case-crossover analysis of air pollution health effects: a systematic review of methodology and application. *Environ Health Perspect*. 2010;118(8):1173-1182.

43. Zeisser C, Stockwell TR, Chikritzhs T, Cherpitel C, Ye Y, Gardner C. A systematic review and meta-analysis of alcohol consumption and injury risk as a function of study design and recall period. *Alcohol Clin Exp Res*. 2013;37(suppl 1):E1-E8.

44. Consiglio GP, Burden AM, Maclure M, McCarthy L, Cadarette SM. Case-crossover study design in pharmacoepidemiology: systematic review and recommendations. *Pharmacoepidemiol Drug Saf.* 2013;22(11):1146-1153.

45. Farrington CP. Control without separate controls: evaluation of vaccine safety using case-only methods. *Vaccine.* 2004;22(15-16):2064-2070.

46. Confavreux C, Suissa S, Saddier P, Bourdes V, Vukusic S; Vaccines in Multiple Sclerosis Study Group. Vaccinations and the risk of relapse in multiple sclerosis. Vaccines in multiple sclerosis study group. *N Engl J Med.* 2001;344(5):319-326.

47. Goedel WC, Marshall BDL, Spangler KR, et al. Increased risk of opioid overdose death following cold weather: a case-crossover study. *Epidemiology.* 2019;30(5):637-641.

48. Maclure M, Mittleman MA. Should we use a case-crossover design? *Annu Rev Public Health.* 2000;21:193-221.

49. Lumley T, Levy D. Bias in the case-crossover design: implications for studies of air pollution. *Environmetrics.* 2000;11:689-704.

50. Vines SK, Farrington CP. Within-subject exposure dependency in case-crossover studies. *Stat Med.* 2001;20(20):3039-3049.

51. Navidi W, Weinhandl E. Risk set sampling for case-crossover designs. *Epidemiology.* 2002;13(1):100-105.

52. Janes H, Sheppard L, Lumley T. Overlap bias in the case-crossover design, with application to air pollution exposures. *Stat Med.* 2004;24:285-300.

53. Janes H, Sheppard L, Lumley T. Case-crossover analyses of air pollution exposure data: referent selection strategies and their implications for bias. *Epidemiology.* 2005;16(6):717-726.

54. Maclure M, Fireman B, Nelson JC, et al. When should case-only designs be used for safety monitoring of medical products? *Pharmacoepidemiol Drug Saf.* 2012;21(suppl 1):50-61.

55. Albert PS, Ratnasinghe D, Tangrea J, Wacholder S. Limitations of the case-only design for identifying gene-environment interactions. *Am J Epidemiol.* 2001;154(8):687-693.

56. Farrington CP. Relative incidence estimation from case series for vaccine safety evaluation. *Biometrics.* 1995;51:228-235.

57. Weldeselassie YG, Whitaker HJ, Farrington CP. Use of the self-controlled case-series method in vaccine safety studies: review and recommendations for best practice. *Epidemiol Infect.* 2011;139(12):1805-1817.

58. Nordmann S, Biard L, Ravaud P, Esposito-Farese M, Tubach F. Case-only designs in pharmacoepidemiology: a systematic review. *PLoS One.* 2012;7(11):e49444.

59. Hallas J, Pottegard A. Use of self-controlled designs in pharmacoepidemiology. *J Intern Med.* 2014;275(6):581-589.

60. Walker AM. Anamorphic analysis: sampling and estimation for covariate effects when both exposure and disease are known. *Biometrics.* 1982;38(4):1025-1032.

61. White JE. A two stage design for the study of the relationship between a rare exposure and a rare disease. *Am J Epidemiol.* 1982;115(1):119-128.

62. Galea S, Tracy M. Participation rates in epidemiologic studies. *Ann Epidemiol.* 2007;17(9):643-653.

63. Ekman A, Litton JE. New times, new needs; e-epidemiology. *Eur J Epidemiol.* 2007;22(5):285-292.

64. Kesse-Guyot E, Assmann K, Andreeva V, et al. Lessons learned from methodological validation research in E-epidemiology. *JMIR Public Health Surveill.* 2016;2(2):e160.

65. Huybrechts KF, Mikkelsen EM, Christensen T, et al. A successful implementation of e-epidemiology: the Danish pregnancy planning study 'Snart-Gravid'. *Eur J Epidemiol.* 2010;25(5):297-304.

66. Topolovec-Vranic J, Natarajan K. The use of social media in recruitment for medical research studies: a scoping review. *J Med Internet Res.* 2016;18(11):e286.

67. Berkson J. Limitations of the application of fourfold table analysis to hospital data. *Biometrics.* 1946;2(3):47-53.

68. Flanders WD, Austin H. Possibility of selection bias in matched case-control studies using friend controls. *Am J Epidemiol.* 1986;124(1):150-153.

69. Siemiatycki J. Friendly control bias. *J Clin Epidemiol.* 1989;42(7):687-688.

70. Austin H, Flanders WD, Rothman KJ. Bias arising in case-control studies from selection of controls from overlapping groups. *Int J Epidemiol.* 1989;18(3):713-716.

71. Robins J, Pike M. The validity of case-control studies with nonrandom selection of controls. *Epidemiology.* 1990;1(4):273-284.

72. Donovan SJ, Susser E. Commentary: advent of sibling designs. *Int J Epidemiol.* 2011;40(2):345-349.

73. Susser E, Eide MG, Begg M. Invited commentary: the use of sibship studies to detect familial confounding. *Am J Epidemiol.* 2010;172(5):537-539.

74. Milne RL, John EM, Knight JA, et al. The potential value of sibling controls compared with population controls for association studies of lifestyle-related risk factors: an example from the Breast Cancer Family Registry. *Int J Epidemiol.* 2011;40(5):1342-1354.

75. Frisell T, Oberg S, Kuja-Halkola R, Sjolander A. Sibling comparison designs: bias from non-shared confounders and measurement error. *Epidemiology*. 2012;23(5):713-720.

76. Keyes KM, Smith GD, Susser E. On sibling designs. *Epidemiology*. 2013;24(3):473-474.

77. Blount BC, Karwowski MP, Shields PG, et al. Lung injury response laboratory working G. Vitamin E acetate in bronchoalveolar-lavage fluid associated with EVALI. *N Engl J Med*. 2020;382(8):697-705.

78. Song MA, Freudenheim JL, Brasky TM, et al. Biomarkers of exposure and effect in the lungs of smokers, nonsmokers, and electronic cigarette users. *Cancer Epidemiol Biomarkers Prev*. 2020;29(2):443-451.

79. Flanders WD, Klein M, Mirabelli MC. Conditions for valid estimation of causal effects on prevalence in cross-sectional and other studies. *Ann Epidemiol*. 2016;26(6):389-394.e2.

80. Cole P. The evolving case-control study. *J Chronic Dis*. 1979;32(1-2):15-27.

81. Miettinen OS. The "case-control" study: valid selection of subjects. *J Chronic Dis*. 1985;38(7):543-548.

82. MacMahon B, Trichopoulos D. *Epidemiology: Principles and Methods*. 2nd ed. Philadelphia, PA: Lippincott Williams & Wilkins; 1996.

83. Chavance M, Dellatolas G, Lellouch J. Correlated nondifferential misclassifications of disease and exposure: application to a cross-sectional study of the relation between handedness and immune disorders. *Int J Epidemiol*. 1992;21(3):537-546.

84. Kristensen P. Bias from nondifferential but dependent misclassification of exposure and outcome. *Epidemiology*. 1992;3(3):210-215.

85. Lash TL, Fink AK. Semi-automated sensitivity analysis to assess systematic errors in observational data. *Epidemiology*. 2003;14(4):451-458.

86. Greenland S. The effect of misclassification in the presence of covariates. *Am J Epidemiol*. 1980;112(4):564-569.

87. Brenner H. Bias due to non-differential misclassification of polytomous confounders. *J Clin Epidemiol*. 1993;46(1):57-63.

88. Marshall JR, Hastrup JL. Mismeasurement and the resonance of strong confounders: uncorrelated errors. *Am J Epidemiol*. 1996;143(10):1069-1078.

89. Marshall JR, Hastrup JL, Ross JS. Mismeasurement and the resonance of strong confounders: correlated errors. *Am J Epidemiol*. 1999;150(1):88-96.

90. Fewell Z, Davey Smith G, Sterne JA. The impact of residual and unmeasured confounding in epidemiologic studies: a simulation study. *Am J Epidemiol*. 2007;166(6):646-655.

91. Dosemeci M, Wacholder S, Lubin JH. Does nondifferential misclassification of exposure always bias a true effect toward the null value? *Am J Epidemiol*. 1990;132(4):746-748.

92. Greenland S, Robins JM. Confounding and misclassification. *Am J Epidemiol*. 1985;122(3):495-506.

93. Drews CD, Greeland S. The impact of differential recall on the results of case-control studies. *Int J Epidemiol*. 1990;19(4):1107-1112.

94. Ibrahim MA, Spitzer WO. The case control study: the problem and the prospect. *J Chronic Dis*. 1979;32(1-2):139-144.

95. Gutensohn N, Li FP, Johnson RE, Cole P. Hodgkin's Disease, tonsillectomy and family size. *N Engl J Med*. 1975;292(1):22-25.

96. le Cessie S, Nagelkerke N, Rosendaal FR, van Stralen KJ, Pomp ER, van Houwelingen HC. Combining matched and unmatched control groups in case-control studies. *Am J Epidemiol*. 2008;168(10):1204-1210.

97. Wacholder S. Bias in full cohort and nested case-control studies? *Epidemiology*. 2009;20(3):339-340.

98. Greenland S. Response and follow-up bias in cohort studies. *Am J Epidemiol*. 1977;106(3):184-187.

99. Feinstein AR. Clinical biostatistics. XX. The epidemiologic trohoc, the ablative risk ratio, and "retrospective" research. *Clin Pharmacol Ther*. 1973;14(2):291-307.

100. Poole C. Exposure opportunity in case-control studies. *Am J Epidemiol*. 1986;123(2):352-358.

101. Terry MB, Neugut AI. Cigarette smoking and the colorectal adenoma-carcinoma sequence: a hypothesis to explain the paradox. *Am J Epidemiol*. 1998;147(10):903-910.

102. Poole C. Controls who experienced hypothetical causal intermediates should not be excluded from case-control studies. *Am J Epidemiol*. 1999;150(6):547-551.

CHAPTER 9

Public Health Surveillance

Richard S. Hopkins and James W. Buehler

BACKGROUND

Public health agencies monitor components of the health of populations over time in support of actions to improve community health. This process is public health surveillance. The World Health Organization's (WHO) definition for surveillance is like those of many other public health organizations: "the ongoing, systematic collection, analysis, and interpretation of outcome-specific data essential to planning, implementing, and evaluating public health practice."[1]

We can carry out surveillance for any of a wide variety of conditions—diseases, injuries, disabilities, or risk characteristics. Sometimes the focus is on monitoring changes in one condition over time and space, or we may want to assess the impact of various conditions over time.[2] We can use surveillance to detect and monitor new conditions (the prime example at the moment being Coronavirus Disease-19, or COVID-19), and also to monitor change in impact of well-known conditions.[3] The surveillance activity might monitor the antecedents or risks of conditions,[4] health events at defined points along the path of their natural history from asymptomatic to end stages,[5–7] or specific manifestations or attributes of conditions (such as clinical severity or responsiveness to treatment). Public health officials might use information from surveillance to identify ill or at-risk individuals or their associates who need interventions or follow-up; identify outbreaks, clusters, or emerging health concerns[8]; illuminate health disparities[9]; identify problems requiring further investigation[10]; or plan or assess public health programs, services, and policies.[11]

Populations under surveillance can be defined narrowly—*e.g.*, people receiving health services at an individual facility—or broadly—*e.g.*, all people within a political jurisdiction or a region or even in the world. Historically, surveillance focused on infectious diseases of public health concern, but surveillance practice now spans the breadth of health problems targeted by public health agencies.

Public health surveillance activities are managed by governmental or international public health agencies with responsibility for protecting and promoting the health of people within geographic boundaries, such as counties, states, nations, or global regions. Such surveillance involves ongoing data collection, management, analysis, interpretation, dissemination, and application. Public health epidemiologists collect data themselves, often from healthcare providers or by carrying out surveys, or they obtain data that were initially collected for other purposes but that can also be used for surveillance. Public health agencies may contract with or delegate to other organizations to complete various surveillance tasks, but they generally cannot delegate the public health responsibility for awareness of their population's health status or for acting on the data generated.[12] The set of functions and networks of people that are needed to monitor a specific condition are referred to as a "surveillance system."

The practice of health-related surveillance is not limited to public health agencies. For example, hospital staff may monitor specific conditions among patients under their care to detect or prevent healthcare-acquired infections or injuries as part of performance management or quality improvement systems.[13] Academic investigators or independent organizations may monitor various conditions among populations of interest to them as part of research activities. Although the same principles that underlie public health surveillance apply to such activities, this chapter will focus on surveillance as conducted by governmental public health agencies.

WHY, WHAT, AND HOW OF PUBLIC HEALTH SURVEILLANCE

We can ask three basic questions about any actual or proposed public health surveillance activity:

Why put a condition under surveillance?
What conditions should be put under surveillance?
How should surveillance be carried out?

The overall shape of any surveillance activity depends on answers to these three questions. The answer to any of these may be influenced by answers to the others. The answers are also subject to resource constraints, as surveillance generally competes for resources with other aspects of disease prevention and control. The incremental cost in staff time, equipment, or goodwill of adding surveillance for one condition to an existing surveillance system, where collection, management, analysis, and/or dissemination costs can be shared, may be small compared with the cost of starting stand-alone surveillance for that condition.

Why Put a Condition Under Public Health Surveillance?

The answer to this question is always the same: to provide timely, appropriate information needed by public health program managers. Information is needed for the operation, planning, or evaluation of any program to prevent disease, injury, disability, or premature death. The shape and scope of the surveillance activity must always have a clear purpose and be driven by programmatic needs. A basic rule of successful surveillance is "Collect only data you are going to use."

Surveillance may be carried out to help make decisions about what conditions should be priorities for disease prevention activities. Many existing health information systems, such as birth and death certificates, hospital discharge records, clinical encounter data, records from hospital emergency department (ED) visits, and general population health surveys, collect information about all diagnoses or multiple health conditions among persons represented within them. They can be used to compare the population impacts of various conditions, or monitor such impacts over time for specific conditions, and to gather information about conditions that do not already have specific surveillance resources dedicated to them.[2]

Surveillance may directly support the operation of a disease control or prevention program. Detection of individual cases of legally reportable diseases (conditions that healthcare providers are required by law, regulation, or administrative policy to report to public health authorities) may prompt immediate public health response (as for tuberculosis, measles, COVID-19 or botulism). Examples of such a response include assuring prompt treatment of people with cases of certain reportable diseases, prophylactic treatment, immunization, assessment, or quarantine of contacts, isolation of cases, separation of people from environmental hazards, or removal of hazards.[14]

Direct support of a disease control or prevention program also includes prompt detection of outbreaks or clusters of disease or changes in patterns of disease that require further investigation or response (as for hepatitis A, salmonellosis, birth defects, injuries, or cancers), through case reporting or other means. Such detection can prompt further investigation to identify the cause or source of an outbreak. Investigation results will inform a community response, such as immunization campaigns, health promotion campaigns, intensified screening or treatment services, or environmental interventions. Response to outbreaks or clusters includes ongoing monitoring of the scope and spread of the event, assessment of the impact of control measures, and documentation of the end of the event, all of which require surveillance data.

Surveillance for newly recognized diseases of unknown etiology can provide insights into possible etiologies and inform initial interventions, and surveillance may be carried out in support of program planning or evaluation even if there is not a public health response to each case or to every outbreak. Thus, surveillance for acquired immunodeficiency syndrome (AIDS) in the early 1980s provided the information about modes of transmission of infection and about at-risk groups that were needed to design and evaluate human immunodeficiency virus (HIV)/AIDS prevention and control programs—even before the HIV was identified as the microbiological cause of AIDS. Surveillance data were later used for HIV/AIDS prevention program evaluation.[15]

Managers of disease control programs need information about the natural history, risk and protective factors, pathophysiology, and effectiveness of prevention and treatment interventions for conditions they are addressing. Such information is usually derived from formal clinical, epidemiologic, and laboratory investigations. They also need information specific to their communities derived from local surveillance: How much disease, exposure, or risk factor is there? Which conditions are causing the most illness, economic impact, and mortality? Is the impact of various health conditions high or low compared with that in other places? Is a condition of interest becoming more common or less? In what population groups and geographic areas are people most at risk? What are the main modes of transmission for infectious agents in this setting? Who is exposed to environmental hazards in this setting, and by what routes? What factors determine behaviors related to disease risk and access to effective care? Are people getting recommended preventive or treatment interventions? What is the impact of the condition on healthcare services and on the workforce, now and in the near future? How much does treatment for this condition cost, and who is bearing the cost?

Surveillance and Research

Surveillance activities can provide important clues for further investigation by researchers. Such research can reinforce, extend, or clarify surveillance findings about high-risk groups, risk factors, and prevention program impacts. Surveillance activities are authorized by law as a core public health function and are constrained by law and by the oversight of public health activities by civil authorities. They are not in themselves considered "research" and do not require review and approval by entities that aim to protect research participants.

Observations about high- and low-incidence subpopulations may prompt further surveillance data collection supplementary to the surveillance system itself and then further analysis to elucidate the reasons for differences. In some surveillance systems, data items collected with each case report, vital record, or survey response allow this kind of analysis internal to the surveillance data themselves. For example, at the individual level, prevalence of tobacco smoking in the Behavioral Risk Factor Surveillance System (BRFSS),[4] a telephone survey conducted by all state health departments in the United States, can be examined in relation to employment status, income, or educational attainment.

At the community level, prevalence of smoking can be examined in relation to community-level interventions taken or not taken, such as tobacco product taxation or comprehensive smoke-free policies, or in relation to differences among communities in the effectiveness of implementation of comparable interventions.[16] When an immunization program is started earlier in one community than another—in the course of ordinary variations in public health practice—rates of vaccination and of the disease intended to be prevented can be monitored and compared over time, to assess the extent to which the actual implementation of the public health program affected disease occurrence. The value and limitations of such time-trend studies have been carefully assessed elsewhere.[17]

Surveillance data can be used to take advantage of "natural experiments" (see also Chapter 28 on quasi-experimental designs). For example, Currie and Walker monitored the rate of adverse pregnancy outcomes in babies born to mothers who lived in neighborhoods near Pennsylvania Turnpike toll plazas,[18] before and after the plazas were switched to electronic toll collection. Each switch eliminated traffic backups and reduced localized air pollution. Rates of preterm delivery and low birth weight, determined from birth certificates, fell near the toll plazas after each switch. This design uses routinely collected surveillance data to address a question never anticipated by those who designed and manage vital statistics systems and helps generate knowledge about the health effects of pollution by vehicle exhaust. In a widely cited article, Case and Deaton also used multiple public health surveillance systems, including mortality and health survey data, to identify and characterize an increase in morbidity and mortality among US middle-aged low-education non-Hispanic Whites after the year 2000.[19]

Surveillance activities can identify and characterize outbreaks and yield information about the cause or source of an outbreak needed to control the outbreak. Analysis of surveillance data often suggests hypotheses about the outbreak that need to be investigated further using cross-sectional, case-control, cohort, or longitudinal studies. Public health officials may carry out a cross-sectional survey of those attending a wedding reception where a foodborne outbreak has occurred, or a case-control study of well and ill participants, to identify a contaminated food item. Laboratory testing of people and food items then follows. If these studies are done in order to solve the immediate outbreak problem, they are part of public health practice, not research, even if they use formal epidemiologic methods and even if observations are made that could be helpful in future outbreak investigations. If investigations are undertaken primarily to advance knowledge more generally, they would generally be considered research and thus subject to regulations that govern research, including human subjects research.

What Conditions Should Be Put Under Surveillance?

Today, surveillance is carried out for almost any condition for which public health disease control or prevention efforts are undertaken. A disease control program may have several or many elements in addition to public health surveillance. They may include:

- specific interventions directed at individual people who have been exposed to infectious agents or other hazards,
- pre- or postexposure immunization of target groups, individuals at risk, or the general population,
- treatment of the sick to improve their outcomes,
- treatment of the sick to render them noninfectious,
- physician education or training,
- laboratory services in support of treatment and disease control interventions,
- isolation of the sick (including use of protective equipment by healthcare workers),
- quarantine of exposed people who remain well,
- screening and follow-up diagnostic testing,
- patient education,
- public education,
- policy changes such as tobacco taxes or bans on smoking in public places,
- safety requirements for seatbelt use in cars or smoke detectors in homes,
- improvements in vehicle and roadway designs,
- elimination or mitigation of environmental hazards,
- environmental or occupational inspection and regulation,

- measures to assure safe water, milk, and food,
- planning, and
- evaluation.

These program elements are combined in ways that reflect our understanding of disease epidemiology, natural history, pathogenesis, preventability, and treatment, exposure to hazards, and, for infectious diseases, modes of transmission. The various elements are combined to achieve reductions in disease risk, morbidity, disability, and/or premature death. Frieden identifies choice of "a technical package of a limited number of high-priority, evidence-based interventions that together will have a major impact" as one of six key elements in a successful public health program.[20] As each element consumes resources, program managers must understand the likely effect of various intervention strategies and their interactions. Some degree of public health surveillance should be an element of every disease control program, but the resources that can be devoted to it must be in proportion to both information needs and resources available for other program elements. Exactly what is put under surveillance, and how, will be shaped by the program elements in place or under consideration.

Thus, the decision to put a condition under surveillance is closely tied to the decision to implement a control program for that condition or to gather the information needed to formulate a disease control strategy and design a program. Such decisions are typically based on factors like[21]:

- the burden of mortality, hospitalization, disability, and acute disease caused by the condition;
- whether it can be prevented or controlled with existing or promising methods;
- the economic impact of the disease and its treatment, absolutely and in relation to the likely cost and effectiveness of a control program; and
- public interest in and concern about the disease.

Given that the decision has been made to put a condition under surveillance, one must still decide on which stage of the natural history of the condition to focus, and how timely, specific or sensitive the surveillance needs to be. For example, if one is interested in understanding a severe infectious disease in a very resource-limited setting, one might focus only on cases that result in hospitalization or death. In a different setting, one might focus on all cases with a laboratory diagnosis, on all cases diagnosed, on all cases suspected by physicians in outpatient or inpatient settings, or even on all persons presenting for medical care with a certain combination of symptoms. For influenza or COVID-19 surveillance, depending on resources available and the types of preventive interventions being implemented, one might focus on deaths or hospitalizations (all or in selected facilities) of persons with suspected or confirmed infection; outpatient visits for influenza-like or COVID-19-like illness in sentinel practices or emergency departments; laboratory detections of influenza or SARS-CoV-2; reports of absenteeism or other disruption in schools, workplaces, prisons, and other settings; whether the circulating virus strains reflect those in the current vaccine; or the antiviral susceptibility of circulating strains. In some instances, information needs for a prevention program might require that several different facets of the condition and its risk factors be put under surveillance, as is done in many countries for influenza.[16]

A well-thought-out public health program should have a clear logic model, which does not have to be complex. Such a model makes explicit the relationships between program activities, one or more levels of intermediate effects of those activities, and the ultimate goals of the public health program. Examining such a logic model can help identify what parameters should be monitored in the population to shed light on the need for, or effectiveness of, the public health program. For example, a program to reduce or eliminate deaths from cervical cancer might, depending on the program model, monitor the percentage of men or women in certain age groups who have received the human papillomavirus (HPV) vaccination or the percentage of women in certain age groups who have received Pap smears at recommended intervals. Additional surveillance outcomes that inform publication health action might include patterns in HPV vaccination uptake or Pap smear findings; trends in the stage at diagnosis of cervical cancer; or trends in cervical cancer hospitalization or mortality. Any of these approaches would fall under the general heading of surveillance directed at cervical cancer, but programs in different jurisdictions with different population age structures or different resources and program elements are likely to make different choices about what aspect(s) of the spectrum of disease to put under surveillance. At a national level, a composite based on insights from multiple different surveillance approaches might be useful.

What is put under surveillance and how surveillance is carried out will often be chosen in tandem. Surveillance does not always require complete ascertainment of the events of interest. For example, it may be cost-effective to carry out surveillance for a disease by counting just people hospitalized with the disease at certain facilities, rather than at all hospitals within a defined area. One may then make inferences about population disease burden based on reasonable assumptions (perhaps based on pilot data collection) about what percentage of the events of interest result in hospitalization at the facilities participating in the surveillance.

If the purpose of surveillance is the prompt detection, characterization, or monitoring of outbreaks, clusters, or important changes in disease patterns then it may make sense for at least one aspect of surveillance to be rapid, as close to instantaneous monitoring of indicator events as possible. Such a strategy would not depend on counting laboratory-confirmed cases of the disease. This is the rationale for putting relatively nonspecific health-related behaviors or events under surveillance—a general strategy often called syndromic surveillance.[22] An increase or change in the occurrence of such events is likely to correlate with increases or changes in the occurrence of specific diseases of interest. The general principle is to monitor relatively nonspecific health-related behaviors or events for which an increase might provide an early and rapid indication of a disease outbreak that will require further investigation and possibly a public health response. Such events might include:

- hospital emergency department (ED) visits or admissions for a syndrome defined by patients' symptoms,
- calls to a nurse hotline for certain combinations of symptoms,
- purchases of antipyretic or antiemetic medications sold in drugstores, or
- trends in Internet searches or mentions for terms suggesting the symptoms or diagnosis of a condition of interest.

Once further investigation has confirmed that an increase in such events corresponds to an actual outbreak or cluster (such as an outbreak of influenza, injuries after an ice storm, drug overdoses due to specific drugs, or asthma), then continued surveillance for the broad, less-specific condition can serve to monitor the spread, magnitude, and eventual end of the outbreak. In a flexible syndromic surveillance system, the search terms used to find health events of interest can also be refined quickly once an outbreak has been documented and applied both retrospectively and prospectively. When an epidemic disease has a very large number of cases, and many or most infected people do not get laboratory diagnoses, then methods like these may be the best solution for monitoring the course and impact of the epidemic, rather than counting cases or laboratory tests.

For some conditions or events for which surveillance is needed, it is essential to monitor the antecedents or early manifestations of diseases because those are the targets of prevention programs. For example, surveillance indicators for tobacco-related disease itself might include mortality, hospitalization, or outpatient medical visits for certain diagnoses, while indicators for the risks of tobacco-related disease might include the prevalence and pattern of tobacco use, aggregate sales of tobacco products (from excise taxes collected), or the presence or absence of policy measures (such as levels of taxation or smoking restrictions). Monitoring current and former tobacco use itself (in total and by subgroup) requires use of a population-based sample survey, since total population counts are impractical. The "what?" of tobacco-use surveillance then consists of answers to questions asked in person, over the telephone, or through Internet-based surveys about self-reported current and former tobacco use, along with demographic and other information. The "what?" of surveillance is influenced by the methods, as questions and answer choices are affected by the mode of administration of a survey.

How Should Surveillance Be Carried Out?

Key topics, including system design, data acquisition, management, analysis, and dissemination, will be addressed in some detail once we have examined some important attributes of a working surveillance system, their relationships to each other, and a brief history of public health surveillance.

Attributes of Surveillance

Working or proposed surveillance systems can be conceptualized as having certain attributes that are functions of the why, what, and how of surveillance. Because improvements in some attributes are often offset by degradations in others, the utility and cost of surveillance depend on how well the mix of attributes is balanced to meet information needs. The attributes defined in the Centers for Disease Control and Prevention (CDC) Updated Guidelines for Surveillance System Evaluation are[23]:

Sensitivity. To what extent does the system identify all targeted events (cases of disease, people with certain behaviors, outbreaks, clusters)? High sensitivity is required if urgent public health action is needed in response to every case to prevent additional cases. For trend monitoring, consistent sensitivity may be more important than high sensitivity. To assess the impact of a health problem, either high sensitivity or enough information to correct for underascertainment is required.

Timeliness. How promptly does information flow through the cycle of surveillance, from health event occurrence to information collection to dissemination to action? The requisite timeliness of data availability depends on the public health urgency of a problem and the types of interventions that are available or planned. Timeliness of surveillance may be important both for a cancer and for an acute infectious disease but may be assessed in months for the former and in days or even hours for the latter. The key issue is whether the information is available *in time* to be useful for disease prevention and control.

Positive predictive value (PPV). To what extent are detected events, either individual cases or suspected outbreaks, really the events that were being sought? Does surveillance measure what it aims to measure? Low positive predictive value leads to noisy data and, when ascertained events prompt further assessments, can lead to wasted effort on follow-up of events that are not of interest. On the other hand, efforts to maximize PPV may jeopardize sensitivity or timeliness. For a given surveillance system, PPV will reflect both the criteria used to define the condition of interest, *i.e.*, the surveillance case definition, and the prevalence of the condition in the targeted population. For a given case definition, the PPV of surveillance will increase as the prevalence of a condition increases. For a given prevalence of the condition, the PPV will increase as the case definition is made more specific.

Representativeness. To what extent do events detected through the surveillance system represent persons with the condition of interest in the target population, with respect to specified characteristics of interest? With respect to any such characteristic, representativeness can be defined as comparable sensitivity for all values of that characteristic (*e.g.*, age group, race, educational level, access to health care). A lack of representativeness may lead to misdirection of health resources toward those who are overrepresented.

Data quality. In a narrow sense, this refers to the accuracy and completeness of record-level data in case reports, surveys, or information systems, including the accuracy and completeness of information entered about various aspects of each event or person for which information is captured and the elimination of duplicate records. In a broad sense, however, data quality is also a function of timeliness, sensitivity, positive predictive value, and representativeness, and of suitability of the data for the purposes for which it is being collected.

Simplicity. Experience has shown that simple systems are more reliable than complex ones, since there are fewer potential points of failure. When assessing an existing or proposed surveillance system, one should ask whether surveillance procedures and processes are as simple as they can be, whether forms are easy to complete and data collection has been kept to a necessary minimum, whether software is user-friendly, systems are easy to maintain, and Internet web pages are easy to navigate, and whether reports are presented in an easily understood manner.

Flexibility. A flexible system can readily adapt to new circumstances, such as changes in the way a disease is diagnosed or treated, changes in the way information is represented electronically, changes in information needs, marked changes in the frequency of a condition, or a need to adjust sensitivity, positive predictive value, or timeliness.

Acceptability. Surveillance systems can only perform optimally when all stakeholders realize their value. When designing, operating, or assessing a surveillance system, one should understand the extent to which participants are enthusiastic about it, whether their effort yields information that is useful to them, whether the systems for assuring privacy and confidentiality are sufficient, and sufficiently transparent and well-explained, and whether the public supports allowing public health agencies access to personal health information for the surveillance purposes. Such support may be encoded in laws or regulations, which ultimately depend upon political support, or in agency procedures.

An additional attribute of importance is *data interoperability*. Can data obtained from various sources, and about various conditions and risk factors, be compared with or combined with each other to detect or characterize cases or events and to support analysis? Formats and standards for vocabulary, data collection, and record transmission in the surveillance information system should be compatible with those of the health information systems from which the information will come. Records should be able to be readily shared with systems in neighboring jurisdictions or at regional or national levels. Krishnamurthy and Conde provide a more complete and technical discussion.[24]

Taken together, these attributes strongly influence the utility of a public health surveillance system: the extent to which it meets the purposes for which it was initiated and can support decision-making in and about a disease prevention or control program. Efforts to optimize these attributes also influence the cost to build and maintain such a system.

Certain attributes are likely to be mutually reinforcing. For example, greater simplicity is likely to enhance acceptability. Others are likely to be competing. Improving timeliness may require compromises in sensitivity, positive predictive value, or data quality, or investments in improving those parameters. Efforts to assure complete ascertainment of events of interest (high sensitivity) may result in inclusion of some events that are not actually due to the disease of interest (false positives), lowering positive predictive value. Efforts to assure that all events entered in the system are actual events of the type sought (high positive predictive value) may result in a loss of sensitivity or timeliness. This balance of attributes is relevant both to detection of individual events and to early detection and characterization of epidemics. For example, statistical thresholds might be lowered to increase sensitivity for timely and complete detection of epidemics and of changes in their characteristics over time. Such a change is likely to result in lower positive predictive value and more frequent "false alarms." Sensitivity, timeliness, and positive predictive value are also in tension with each other as data are being prepared and analyzed for program planning and evaluation purposes. Disease prevention programs often employ a mix of surveillance approaches that have complementary strengths.

Historical Perspective

Surveillance methods used to assess population health and the major causes of death are at the foundation of epidemiology as a discipline. At their origins in the 17th through 19th centuries in Scandinavia[25] and the United Kingdom, and then the United States and elsewhere, antecedents of modern surveillance methods were used for two broad purposes: (1) to monitor changes in cause-specific and total mortality and morbidity over time and by population subgroup (time, place, and person) and (2) to identify people with cases of dangerous infectious diseases so that isolation, quarantine, and other prevention efforts could be initiated.[26,27] Thus, counts of deaths (all-cause, for certain broad categories like stroke, epilepsy, cancer, and injury, and for certain distinctive infectious diseases) were obtained, initially from log books of burial grounds; and physicians and sometimes others were required to report to local authorities cases of a small number of serious infectious diseases with distinct clinical presentations, such as leprosy, smallpox, yellow fever, plague, or cholera. These two separate strands of surveillance are still visible in today's surveillance practice, represented by vital statistics and population-based surveys on the one hand and case reporting on the other. The growing practice of monitoring and comparing the frequency of diseases among different population groups, particularly in burgeoning cities during the industrial revolution, prompted awareness of the strong connection between poverty and disease and helped to fuel the social hygiene movement. Surveillance today continues to illuminate health disparities.

During the 20th century, the body of practice called "surveillance" expanded beyond infectious diseases to address the growing array of health problems targeted by public health agencies. The modern concept of surveillance has been shaped over several hundred years by evolution in how health information has been gathered and how it has been used to guide public health practice.[28] The pace of technological change has increased over time. There have been repeated innovations in what and how population-level health data can be collected and analyzed, reflecting changes in how healthcare professionals think about disease diagnosis, in the information technologies used in clinical practice and public health, in public health interventions available, and in methods of statistical analysis.

In the mid to late 1800s and early 1900s, health authorities in multiple countries began to require that physicians and others report specific communicable diseases to enable local prevention and control activities, such as quarantine of exposed persons or isolation of affected persons. The modern relevance of this approach is emphasized by the response to COVID-19 in 2020, when infected people were isolated, contact tracing and quarantine were scaled up, and in many localities essentially the entire population was put in quarantine. Eventually, local reporting systems coalesced into national systems for tracking certain endemic and epidemic infectious diseases, and the term *surveillance* evolved to describe a population-wide approach to monitoring health and disease.

Important refinements in the methods of notifiable disease reporting occurred in response to specific information needs and evolving information technology. In the late 1940s, concern that cases of malaria were being overreported in the southern United States led to a requirement that case reports be accompanied by documentation of clinical findings and laboratory results. This change in surveillance procedures revealed that malaria was no longer endemic in the southern United States, permitting a shift in public health resources and demonstrating the utility of specific surveillance case definitions.[29]

In the 1950s, the usefulness of outreach to physicians and laboratories by public health officials to identify cases of disease and solicit reports (active surveillance) was demonstrated by poliomyelitis surveillance during the implementation of a national poliomyelitis immunization program in the United States.[30] As a result of these vigorous surveillance efforts, polio surveillance was complete and timely, and cases of vaccine-associated poliomyelitis were reliably shown to be limited to recipients of vaccine from one manufacturer. This finding enabled a targeted vaccine recall, calming of public fears, and continuation of the program.[31] The usefulness of an active approach to surveillance was further demonstrated during the smallpox-eradication campaign, when analysis of surveillance data led to a redirection of vaccination efforts away from mass vaccination to highly targeted vaccination of identified persons who were close contacts of those with detected cases.[32]

During the late 20th century, alternatives to disease reporting were developed to monitor diseases and a growing spectrum of public health problems. These methods now included health surveys, disease registries, networks of "sentinel" physicians, and use of computerized administrative and diagnostic health databases. In 1988, the Institute of Medicine in the United States defined three essential functions of public health: assessment of the health of communities, policy development based on a "community diagnosis," and assurance that necessary services are provided. Fully implementing each of these depends on or can be informed by surveillance.[12]

In the 1980s, the advent of inexpensive microcomputers revolutionized surveillance practice, enabling decentralized data management and analysis, automated data transmission via telephone lines, and electronic linkage of participants in surveillance networks, as pioneered in France.[33] This automation of surveillance was accelerated in the 1990s and early 2000s by advances in the science of informatics and growth in the use of the Internet, wide access to inexpensive computing, and ever-increasing capacity to handle large datasets.

In the United States in the early 1990s, CDC transitioned from collecting weekly telegraphed or faxed tallies from states of reported cases of nationally notifiable diseases to collecting data from states as brief individual nonidentified computer records.[34] This project grew into CDC's National Telecommunications System for Surveillance or NETSS. In a parallel development, state health departments began requiring laboratories to report findings indicative of the presence of a case of a reportable disease, and gradually computerized this process. In the early 2000s, the increasing threat of bioterrorism provided an impetus in several countries for the growth of systems that emphasized the earliest possible detection of epidemics, which is necessary for a timely and effective public health response. This effort included support for web-based state-level systems for acquiring, managing, and transmitting case reports as part of the National Electronic Disease Surveillance System; of electronic laboratory-result surveillance for reportable diseases; and of semiautomated syndromic surveillance. All of these systems continue to undergo improvements to reflect opportunities and challenges presented by new technologies and patterns of clinical care—for example, CDC's NEDSS Modernization Initiative[35] and the National Syndromic Surveillance Program.[36] The systems will likely never be in a fully finished state since their context is so dynamic. While this account emphasizes the US experience, the technology of surveillance is likewise advancing rapidly in many countries.[37]

Similar evolution has occurred in processes for surveillance of noninfectious diseases. Cancer registries, for example, began with requirements for physicians to submit paper case reports. Specially trained registrars used the indexes of hospitals' paper discharge registries to find people with cancer diagnoses and then carefully extracted needed information from their hospital charts. Hospitals began to build their own registries and to computerize them, largely as a result of initiatives of the American College of Surgeons, which required hospitals to use registries to assess cancer treatment outcomes as a condition of accreditation.[38] It then became possible to use records in hospital registries as the basis for records in centralized cancer registries. Most records in central cancer registries are now generated through receipt of digital records from hospital registries, supplemented by identification of likely cases from death certificates and records of radiation therapy centers, pathology laboratories, surgical centers, and hospitals, taking advantage of aggregation of discharge records in state hospital discharge information systems.

The next stage in this process is the automated generation of public health case reports for a wide range of infectious and noninfectious conditions directly from electronic medical records. These systems will result in the progressive automation of nearly the entire process of surveillance, including identifying people with a combination of findings in their electronic health records that define a reportable case, applying jurisdiction-specific case definition criteria to the resulting electronic reports, managing the resulting data, analyzing data statistically to detect aberrant trends, displaying results publicly on the Internet, and returning useful information rapidly to clinicians who are managing the care of people with cases of reportable conditions. Progress has depended critically on development of consensus data vocabulary, messaging standards, and electronic representations of reporting criteria and case classifications. Despite this emphasis on informatics, the interpretation of results and the decision to act on information received through surveillance still requires human judgment.[39]

A parallel process occurred with improvements in vital registration in developed countries. Worldwide, countries are at many stages of development of uniform birth and death registration. Birth and death certificates serve civil purposes as well as public health purposes. For example, birth certificates often serve as proof of age, place of birth, and parentage. Likewise, a death certificate may be necessary for burials and to substantiate claims for life insurance and other death benefits. In some countries, these two uses are implemented with different documents and data systems.

In the United States, the Bureau of the Census took a leadership role in the period 1890 to 1940 in establishing standards across the states for the quality and timeliness of birth and death registration. Achieving compliance with uniform standards was a long process. A uniform Death Registration Area was first established in 1880, which by 1902 included 10 states and the District of Columbia. It gradually expanded its coverage until all states were included by 1933. A similar uniform Birth Registration Area, started in 1915, also had full coverage by 1933.[40] Responsibility was moved into the US Centers for Disease Control and Prevention in 1987.

Vital registration practice in the United States was until quite recently totally dependent on completion of paper forms by various healthcare providers, public health officials, and funeral directors, even though the information on those forms was being key-punched into large data systems starting in the 1960s. Fully computerized real-time state-specific systems for completion of birth and death certificates in hospitals and funeral homes have come into wide use more recently.[41] This improvement has allowed monitoring of deaths from conditions like opioid poisoning or other public health events to be carried out in very close to real time.[42,43]

Advances in biotechnology and informatics, applied in tandem, have allowed the design of systems for detection of outbreaks due to strains of microorganisms, identified through an evolving series of microbiologic techniques. This process started with speciation of microorganisms, dividing one species into several (so that *Shigella sonnei* is distinguished from *Shigella flexneri*, for example), then serogrouping (so that meningococcal infections can be grouped into serogroups such as A, C, and W-135) and serotyping (hundreds of serotypes of *Salmonella enterica*), then pulsed-field gel DNA electrophoresis (many thousands of pulse-field gel electrophoresis [PFGE] patterns for Salmonella isolates), then classification based on nucleic acid sequences (such as extended multilocus sequence typing or MLST).[44] Other advances have allowed immune responses to more and more specific subgroups of infectious agents to be distinguished from each other and detection of nucleic acid specific to particular organisms in the serum and tissues of ill persons. Advances of this type are certain to continue. More fine-grained characterization of infectious agents allows cases that are related to each other (by common exposure or by person-to-person transmission) to be identified, so that investigative effort in a community outbreak is not diverted to background cases that are not part of the outbreak.

Epidemiologists can now monitor a large number of genetically related strains of microorganisms to detect changes in incidence and time-space clustering. Matches between isolates from a hypothesized common source such as a food item and isolates from ill people become more convincing as the strain of the infecting organisms can be defined more and more precisely. As infecting agents get characterized in a more granular way, improved statistical techniques are needed to identify clusters or trends in incidence. Management of very large volumes of data requires advance planning and investments in infrastructure. Improvements in informatics are needed to gain the full value of the improvements in microbiological techniques.[45]

Evolving technologies have also allowed collection of data using hand-held devices, such as mobile telephones, with field editing built-in, and rapid transmission of the data to a central location as attachments to text messages or e-mails, or by direct file transfer. Data transfer can also occur via phone keyboard responses to a standard script implemented centrally. Recording responses to questionnaires and case and contact interviews can be implemented with no need for pencil and paper or for key-punch of data at a central office. During the West African Ebola outbreak of 2014, extensive use of smart devices by well-trained and effectively deployed field teams has been credited as a key element of the successful rapid termination of spread of Ebola infection in Nigeria after only a few cases.[46,47]

Many countries conduct periodic national health surveys. Examples include the surveys conducted by CDC's National Center for Health Statistics[48] in the United States and the Health Survey for England.[49] The United States Agency for International Development and other international aid agencies support demographic and health surveys in multiple countries.[50] Various national surveys are conducted by networks of multinational organizations. National and subnational governments and in-country experts conduct periodic health surveys, as exemplified by surveys conducted in India.[51]

In some countries with incomplete or unreliable registration of vital events, surveys provide the best measures of births and deaths. To the extent that surveys are conducted annually or periodically, they are surveillance systems that provide information that can be used to monitor a wide variety of conditions. National surveys may be complemented by regional- or state-level surveys. For example, in the United States, CDC's Behavioral Risk Factor Surveillance System provides state-level health data and can also be used to make regional and national estimates. It is conducted by states using standard methods with CDC's support and coordination, allows comparison of data between jurisdictions and over time, and supports national aggregation of data.

Automated compilation of text selected from online sources related to possible outbreaks of acute diseases, such as news stories, blog posts, social media posts, online videos, and other online text, has been used for early identification of outbreaks.[52,53] This approach can be used by agencies with a broad geographic focus to identify emergent health threats in advance of local or in-country recognition or confirmation.[54]

SURVEILLANCE BASED ON CASE REPORTING

The core method for infectious disease surveillance has historically been to require physicians, hospitals, and laboratories (and sometimes others) to make case reports to their local public health jurisdiction when a patient with a case of a reportable disease, or a laboratory result indicative of the presence of a reportable disease, comes to their attention. For the past century and more, such requirements have been enshrined in law in most countries, with details of reporting methods, time frames, and criteria specified in law or in public health agency rules or regulations.

A key component of any surveillance system is a "surveillance case definition." Surveillance case definitions establish criteria for what should trigger an initial report, for what will be classified as "a case," and often for classification of cases by level of certainty of diagnosis. For reportable acute diseases, case definitions usually rely on combinations of patient symptoms, clinical observations (such as rash or shortness of breath), clinical signs (such as fever), exposure history (exposure to an infected person, a tick bite with appropriate timing in relation to onset of symptoms, or travel to an epidemic area), and results of diagnostic procedures (microbiology, radiology). Illnesses may be classified as suspected cases based on less stringent criteria than those used for probable or confirmed cases.

For surveillance systems based on case reporting, case definitions might be linked to reporting criteria that include several levels of urgency: some diseases require immediate reporting by telephone even upon preliminary suspicion before diagnostic confirmation, while others require reporting within 24 hours, by the next business day, or within a week. The necessary level of diagnostic certainty before a case report is required should be specified: should a case be reported based on clinical findings or suspicion alone, or should it be reported only when laboratory confirmation is in hand? Levels of urgency in reporting requirements reflect the "windows of opportunity" for public health intervention. Expected rapidity of disease progression, expected timing of infectiousness, time constraints on the effectiveness of prophylaxis for exposed contacts, adverse consequences of missed opportunities for prevention, and possible wasted effort when reported cases turn out not to have the disease of concern can influence the triggers for case reporting.

Surveillance case definitions need to be feasible in the settings where they are used, considering standards of care, access to diagnostic testing, and the capacity of public health staff to implement their use. In resource-poor settings, case definitions may be broad (*e.g.*, fever with headache may be counted as malaria unless another diagnosis is obvious), and usually fewer conditions are made reportable. For example, in places where definitive diagnostic tests are not readily available, WHO has developed guidelines for "syndromic" diagnosis and treatment of sexually transmitted diseases based on observations that can be made in clinics; surveillance criteria follow from such clinical diagnostic classifications.[55]

The content of a case report should also be specified. Initial case reports typically require:

- identification information about the ill person (such as name, age, address, telephone number),
- selected demographic characteristics of importance to the jurisdiction, such as age and gender, as well as other characteristics. For example, in the United States, data on race and ethnicity (Hispanic or not) are usually collected, while, in Australia, Indigenous status is an important variable,
- information about the reporting entity,
- critical dates for the episode of illness (such as dates of exposure, onset of symptoms, clinical contact, diagnosis, laboratory testing, treatment, hospital admission, or death),
- pertinent clinical details and laboratory test results that allow the public agency to assess certainty of diagnosis vis-à-vis the case definition,
- treatment administered so far, and
- outcome (admitted, discharged, died)

The rationale for collecting surveillance data by race—as has been done in the United States for many decades— is often not clearly articulated. Historically, race was apparently conceived as representing biological differences in risks of disease that were not amenable to public health intervention. The best current interpretation is that race is much more a social category than a biological one. Poorer health in persons of minority or marginalized race or ethnicity reflects the direct effects of a lifetime of living with racism day in and day out, the effects of social and economic deprivation driven by institutional racism, and intergenerational effects possibly mediated by epigenetic as well as cultural mechanisms.[56] Collecting and analyzing data by race (as socially defined) allows documentation of health differentials by race, prompts elucidation of the mechanism of those differentials, and allows documentation of progress toward their elimination.

In the United States, there has usually been a two-phase process for infectious disease case reporting to local and state health departments. A brief initial case report can serve as the basis for deciding whether further investigation or other immediate action is needed and can help in outbreak detection. A more complete disease-specific case report form is usually completed days to weeks later for each case of selected diseases, with more detail to assist the health department in documenting risk factors, sources of infection, modes of spread, and/or adequacy of treatment. A case report form for legionellosis, for example, might ask about exposure to sources of hot water or aerosols. If several reported legionellosis cases are found to have such an exposure in common, an epidemiologic and environmental investigation will usually follow, which can lead to control measures to prevent future exposures. That investigation will likely include both microbiologic assessment of the water that is epidemiologically implicated and a search for additional related cases, including people who may not yet have been diagnosed with legionellosis because their disease has been misdiagnosed or its physical manifestation is subclinical.

When several categories of reporters are required to make case reports (for example, physicians and laboratories), reporters are usually asked to assume that no-one else has made or will make the case report and to make all required reports. The combination of reports from clinicians and from laboratories commonly provides more information than either alone. Reports from laboratories provide essential information regarding diagnostic confirmation but often offer little information regarding clinical, demographic, or exposure details because laboratories usually do not collect this information, which is not needed for their testing. The public health agency will then identify duplicate reports so that each person's case is recorded only once and combine information from multiple sources for each case. Methods for automated deduplication of records are widely available.

In the United States, the legal authority to require hospitals, physicians, and laboratories to make case reports to public health authorities lies with the states. The Council of State and Territorial Epidemiologists (CSTE), with the advice of CDC and other federal public health authorities, maintains a list of Nationally Notifiable Diseases (NND). Placement of a condition on this list by a vote of the states through CSTE includes specification of the surveillance case definition (what combinations of findings are necessary for a confirmed, probable or suspected case), criteria for suspecting cases in health records, the needed urgency of case reporting, and recommended standard methods for case detection and reporting. By placing a condition on the NND list, CSTE is recommending to the states that they implement surveillance using the specified methods, and that they share deidentified notifications of cases with CDC. Some states do not make all conditions on the NND list reportable. States' decisions depend on their assessment of their public health needs and resources and on regional variations in the incidence of certain conditions. State health department officials generally want to support national disease prevention and control efforts, resources permitting.

In other countries, similar requirements may be issued by national public health authorities directly. Countries or regions with federal systems have had to develop processes that balance needs and autonomy of the larger entity and of constituent units. In Europe, standardized case definitions for select reportable diseases are maintained by the European Center for Disease Control and Prevention (ECDC), but not all diseases are reportable in all countries.[57] In the Canadian Notifiable Disease Surveillance System, the ten provinces and three territories voluntarily submit notifiable disease data. Since 1987, decisions about placing diseases on the list have been based on federal/provincial/territorial consensus using set criteria. In Australia, the list of nationally notifiable diseases is established by the federal minister of health in consultation with state Ministers of Health after an extensive consensus development process. Reporting practices vary among the six states and two territories and not all states collect data about all the nationally notifiable diseases.[58]

Multiple studies have shown that voluntary reporting of cases by physicians, hospitals, and laboratories is often inconsistent, incomplete, and slow.[59,60] In these passive systems, reporters are informed of their obligations and the methods for reporting, and the public health agency then waits for case reports. Such reporting is reasonably sensitive for diseases that physicians perceive as clearly urgent from a public health perspective, such as botulism, meningococcal meningitis, or tuberculosis, but is very insensitive for many others. Up until the 1980s, such passive reporting was by far the predominant mode of infectious disease surveillance in the United States. Reporters were typically asked to send in postcards with case reports, to make telephone calls for urgent cases, and later to fax one-page case reports to their local health department.

Health departments responded to this incomplete and slow reporting in multiple ways that illustrate a spectrum of more active approaches to surveillance. Some initiated weekly telephone calls from local health departments to offices of all physicians who were likely to treat cases of reportable diseases, like primary care pediatricians, asking for case reports and providing information about disease trends in the community.[61] Similar active measures were undertaken with laboratories in some jurisdictions. US agencies that accredit and license hospitals and laboratories have included compliance with all applicable state laws and regulations as a criterion for approval since the mid-1960s.[62] In many jurisdictions, a small number of laboratories carry out most clinical testing. Focusing surveillance outreach efforts on these laboratories is an efficient means to improve the sensitivity and timeliness of surveillance, even though follow-up with clinicians is often necessary to obtain necessary details about people with reportable conditions.

Health departments identified hospital infection control practitioners (ICPs) as key sources of information about people hospitalized with cases of reportable diseases, as ICPs were consistently involved in decisions about isolation of patients with communicable diseases in their facilities. Health departments reached out to ICPs through their local, state, and national organizations to build partnerships, which were enhanced by ICPs' roles in helping their facilities meet accreditation requirements.

In the context of outbreak or cluster investigations, epidemiology field teams often enhance routine surveillance procedures by contacting physicians, hospitals, and laboratories actively, on a more frequent schedule, to stimulate recognition and reporting of cases of illness that were likely to be part of the outbreak. For example, as part of the epidemiologic response to the first anthrax-by-mail case in Palm Beach County, Florida, in 2001, a team member telephoned every hospital in the county and an adjacent county every morning to identify any people admitted to their intensive care units with respiratory distress and fever in the preceding 24 hours. If there were any such admissions, the team member visited that ICU to perform a record review, looking for possible unrecognized or early-stage pulmonary anthrax.[63]

Starting in the early 1980s, surveillance case definitions for more and more diseases had come to require laboratory confirmation for classification as confirmed cases. As the low and inadequate sensitivity of traditional passive case reporting was becoming more evident, US health departments increasingly implemented requirements for licensed clinical laboratories to report every positive laboratory finding on a list determined by their health department as indicating the presence of a case of a reportable disease. Laboratories were implementing automated laboratory testing equipment and laboratory information management systems (LIMS) and soon started sending printouts of results meeting reporting criteria and in some cases electronic media with the same information.

By the early 1990s, it had become clear that electronic reporting of required positive laboratory results by laboratories to public health agencies was feasible and, in many instances, preferred by laboratories. Over the next 25 years, accelerating since the anthrax-by-mail, World Trade Center, and Pentagon attacks of 2001, standard vocabularies, messaging formats, and messaging systems have been developed and widely implemented by state health departments in collaboration with CDC and the clinical laboratory industry, so that most case reports of reportable diseases are now received at health departments first as an electronic laboratory result. Health departments have modified their reportable disease surveillance information systems to accept these electronic laboratory reports and incorporate them into their case-reporting workflow.

During the 2010s, the success of electronic laboratory reporting has served as a foundation to implement electronic reporting of cases of reportable diseases (ECR) from hospitals' electronic medical records systems, as well as from outpatient electronic medical records. In the United States, federal investments aimed in part at stimulating the national economy following "the Great Recession" that began in 2008 included substantial funding to incentivize doctors and hospitals to adopt electronic health records (EHRs) and to use their EHRs to electronically transmit case data for reportable conditions to health departments. Related investments supported efforts to develop methods that could automate the entire reporting process, starting with automated recognition of reportable diagnoses. The vision for ECR is that reportable cases will be reported more quickly, more completely, and more accurately than by methods requiring a clinician or an infection preventionist to initiate and complete a case report. In turn, at least ideally, this would reduce time needed for public health staff to solicit reports and manage surveillance data, increasing time available for data analysis and follow-up. Such systems can also return targeted useful information to clinicians about community patterns and about treatment and follow-up recommendations. This return flow of information is expected to both improve patient care and enhance future collaboration between clinicians and public health authorities.[64]

Case-Based Chronic Disease Surveillance

Meanwhile, registries for cases of cancer and for infants with birth defects have been developed. These also depend on individual case reports from healthcare providers to public health agencies, though the mechanisms have been very different. Cancer surveillance in the United States started in Connecticut in the 1930s, and states and some large cities over the next 50 years implemented cancer registries with gradually increasing coverage and sophistication. The only national picture of cancer incidence, however, came from death certificates.[65] In 1973, the National Cancer Institute started the Surveillance, Epidemiology and End Results (SEER) cancer registries by assembling a diverse group of states and regions of states.[66] Taken together, the data from these states and regions provided a detailed picture of cancer incidence, stage at diagnosis, course of treatment, and outcome that could be cautiously extrapolated to the country as a whole. There were and are noticeable state and regional variations in all these parameters, in the SEER states, and presumably in the remaining states. In 1993, the Centers for Disease Control and Prevention initiated the National Program of Cancer Registries (NPCR), which eventually supported cancer incidence registries in every state, in coordination with SEER.[67] Similar efforts were made by CDC to support an increasingly complete and representative group of state-level birth defects registries.[68]

Both cancer registries and birth defects registries depend largely on data collected for other purposes: registry staff also review and search for probable cases in electronic representations of birth certificates, death certificates, hospital discharges, emergency department visits, and patient visit and billing data maintained by dermatologists, geneticists, specialty pediatricians, outpatient surgical centers, and radiation therapy facilities. Cancer registries have relied on mandatory reporting; some birth defects registries do also, but others are built entirely by assembling data from other data sources such as hospital discharge records, birth and death certificates, and healthcare claims databases, as well as reporting by clinicians likely to treat children with birth defects (such as pediatric cardiologists).

Incidence registries for selected other chronic diseases have been piloted and, in some cases, implemented in selected regions of the United States. Some serve to identify priority populations for interventions, some to monitor intervention effectiveness on a population level, and others to guide follow-up with affected individuals and their families. Pilot amyotrophic lateral sclerosis (ALS) registries were developed by identifying doctors who are likely to treat people with ALS and asking them voluntarily to fill in a case report form for every existing or new patient with an ALS diagnosis meeting case definition criteria. A national approach was later implemented that combines ascertainment of likely cases of ALS from hospital discharge registries with self-reporting by patients.[69] In countries with electronic records systems of national scope, such an approach is more directly feasible for surveillance of various chronic diseases and conditions than in the United States. For example, Public Health England prepares annual chronic disease profile reports for diabetes, heart disease, kidney disease, and stroke resolved to small geographic areas.

Stroke surveillance is difficult because the number of illness events likely to meet the surveillance case definition is large, and each identified candidate case needs to be carefully reviewed to ascertain whether it is an acute stroke (and not, for example, new recognition of an old stroke, a result of trauma, or the result of a malignancy). Stroke registries as part of the US Paul Coverdell National Acute Stroke Registry Program were implemented in several states.[70] These registries' primary purpose is to support improvements in the quality of care for acute stroke. The surveillance model here was reporting of acute strokes meeting a surveillance case definition by a representative sample of hospitals in each state.

Surveillance for incident cases of diabetes using medical records or administrative datasets is difficult for similar reasons.[71] Diabetes is common, but many cases remain unrecognized for long periods of time. Clinical criteria for the diagnosis of diabetes for surveillance purposes can be complex. Persons may be hospitalized or die of complications of diabetes, such as stroke or heart attack, without mention of diabetes in discharge diagnoses. Surveillance for prevalence of diabetes diagnoses is more straightforward, for example, using sample surveys such as the US Behavioral Risk Factor Surveillance System (BRFSS) or National Health Interview Survey (NHIS) and other nations' counterparts.[72,73] Sentinel surveillance (that is, surveillance conducted at a selected number of locations) for incident cases of type 1 diabetes in children and adolescents has been carried out successfully using networks of clinicians to whom children with diabetes are likely to be referred or in the context of an integrated healthcare plan such as Kaiser Permanente.[74] Use of members of such a healthcare plan may often raise concerns about representativeness, as discussed above. Because effective control of diabetes can prevent serious complications and represents a shared clinical and public health concern, surveillance for HbA1c levels—a marker of diabetes control—can be useful in clinical and public health collaborations aimed at reducing diabetes-related morbidity.[75]

Surveillance for Outbreaks or Clusters

Detection of outbreaks is an often-cited purpose of surveillance. In practice, astute clinicians very commonly detect or strongly suspect outbreaks before public health agencies receive and analyze formal information such as case reports and recognize aberrant trends. Reports from other people with knowledge of a possible outbreak are also important—for example, persons responsible for a group meal, school nurses, coworkers, or employers. Regardless of how outbreaks are detected, surveillance systems can be used to confirm that there is an outbreak and then monitor the progression of an outbreak initially brought to public health attention in such ways. Clusters of cases of new diseases and of diseases that are not individually reportable—such as influenza or norovirus infection—are by definition not detectable through reporting of cases of reportable diseases. Many jurisdictions have a provision that clinicians must report cases or clusters of all diseases of public health significance regardless of whether it is listed by name in the state's regulations.[76,77] The first recognized outbreaks of toxic shock syndrome, legionnaires' disease, and AIDS were all detected through this mechanism.

Assessing sensitivity of a system for outbreak detection requires knowing how many outbreaks (meeting the formal definition) really occurred and of those how many were detected. It can be hard to know about events that should have been detected but were not. Assessing positive predictive value of a system for outbreak detection requires knowing how many outbreaks apparently meeting a formal outbreak definition were recognized and investigated, and then how many of those turned out not in fact to be the kind of event being sought. To compare the sensitivity and positive predictive value of systems for outbreak detection in two or more different jurisdictions, great effort would have to be put into making definitive lists of outbreaks that actually occurred, using the same criteria, for comparison with those detected by the system. Alternatively, the sensitivity of statistical algorithms for outbreak detection can be tested using historical or synthetic trend data.

Outbreaks of infectious and toxic diseases are sometimes detected by examination of patterns and trends in reported cases of reportable diseases, but there are important limitations to such an approach. Clusters of cancers and of birth defects and other adverse pregnancy outcomes also can be detected by regular systematic examination of routinely collected case reports and vital statistics data. Limitations of surveillance in detecting outbreaks include:

1. Many outbreaks of public health significance are due to well-known and common diseases of which cases are not individually reportable, such as *Clostridium perfringens* food poisoning, norovirus gastroenteritis, or influenza.
2. Outbreaks of diseases that are new, or previously unrecognized, cannot be recognized through case reports of reportable diseases.
3. Depending on case reports of diagnosed or even suspected cases of disease for outbreak recognition may be too slow to allow effective public health response because of the time needed for diagnostic tests to be completed or for reports to be made.
4. Outbreaks might be geographically dispersed with too few cases in individual jurisdictions to result in a recognizable increase in cases. Such recognition requires collation of data at regional or national levels. This kind of dispersed outbreak might happen if disease is associated with a widely distributed product or if people exposed to a point source of infection disperse after being exposed.

Thus, there is a need for rapid methods to detect and monitor outbreaks or other urgent public health events using information about people who are early in their course of illness, perhaps even before they seek medical attention, and also for systems to encourage recognition and reporting of possible outbreaks by diverse partners in the community. Contacts between health departments and clinicians that occur in the course of routine surveillance activities, including dissemination of surveillance data to clinicians, can increase the likelihood that clinicians will inform health departments when they suspect that outbreaks or clusters are occurring. The initial case of pulmonary anthrax in Palm Beach County, Florida, in the 2001 anthrax-by-mail outbreak, was recognized promptly because the local health officer was well known and trusted by physicians in her community. A concerned clinician had a low threshold for calling her to talk about an unusual case in his practice, which she in turn recognized as a possible public health emergency.[63]

Detection of outbreaks by review of case reports of reportable diseases is carried out in many ways. In a setting where one person reviews all case reports received, a change in the pattern of case reports may be immediately evident based on personal experience. For example, in a community where an average of one case report of salmonellosis is received per month, receipt of four cases in 1 week would prompt further investigation. In a very populous jurisdiction, automated space-time cluster detection algorithms may be applied to case report data[78] to allow detection of patterns in the data that would be very difficult to detect by relying on manual review of reportable disease case reports. Methods that depend largely on human pattern recognition can be aided by regular (daily, weekly, monthly) organization of data into graphic displays of cases by time period, with a baseline of adequate length, with expected values displayed adjacent to actual values. Similarly, spot maps of reported cases by time period by disease can aid in cluster detection. In between methods that depend mostly on human pattern recognition and fully automated detection of space-time clusters are methods that flag unusual occurrences (compared with historical baselines of various lengths) by disease by geographic unit and/or demographic subgroup for human investigation.

Some outbreaks may not be recognized if cases are few or widely spread out geographically. In such instances, surveillance systems that collate information obtained on a broad geographic basis may detect outbreaks. Such detection may be enhanced if isolates of organisms of public health interest are routinely examined in public health laboratories to detect subtypes, whether as serotypes, serogroups, PFGE patterns, or genetic subtypes that depend on DNA sequencing. An early example of such detection occurred in 1983 in Minnesota, where laboratory-based surveillance of salmonella infections detected an increase in isolates of a particular serotype, *Salmonella enterica subsp enterica serovar Newport.* Subsequent investigation of these cases documented a specific pattern of antibiotic resistance in these isolates and a link to meat from cattle that had been fed subtherapeutic doses of antibiotics to promote growth.[79] The results of this investigation, which was triggered by findings from routine surveillance in one state, contributed to a national reassessment of policies in the United States regarding the use of antibiotics in animals raised for human consumption and also stimulated further development of molecular outbreak detection methods.

Syndromic surveillance systems are designed to detect possible epidemics as quickly as possible, to help characterize recognized epidemics, and to monitor the course of epidemics over time and space. They use automated tracking of disease indicators, changes in which may herald the onset of an epidemic. These systems are used to monitor nonspecific syndromes (*e.g.*, respiratory illness, gastrointestinal illness, febrile rash illness) and other measures (*e.g.*, purchase of over-the-counter or prescription medications, school or work absenteeism, ambulance dispatches) that may increase before clinicians recognize an unusual pattern of illness or before illnesses are diagnosed and reported. As these systems have matured, they increasingly are valued for situational awareness during a recognized public health emergency—providing rapid information about any changes in geographic spread or target groups in the population.[80]

Systems for outbreak detection can be evaluated using similar criteria to those used for other surveillance systems.[81] In order to assess important aspects of surveillance for outbreaks (such as sensitivity, positive predictive value, timeliness), a clear definition of what constitutes an event of interest is needed. The decision about whether an event is an outbreak or cluster of the type being sought in the surveillance system, and therefore requires full investigation, usually results from an iterative winnowing process. Epidemiology staff statistically assess large numbers of possible events detected by or in the system, narrow their focus to a few that warrant careful evaluation, and then fully work up those that appear to be real outbreaks.

Across the world, national programs are at various stages of implementation.[37] Having such a national capacity depends critically on investments in standardizing terminology, syndrome definitions, and the structure and content of notification messages across multiple locally managed systems. In the United States, CDC is expanding its capacity to acquire ED-visit-based syndromic surveillance data from many different locally operated systems. These data, accessed with permission from those systems, allow CDC to have a regional and national picture of what syndromes are being seen commonly in EDs across the country.[36]

A local analyst reviewing daily tallies of ED visits by syndrome can interpret the data in the light of local knowledge about events and can promptly initiate further queries of the data or of clinicians at the front lines. For example, such an analyst can interpret ED visits for certain kinds of injuries or intoxications in light of a local street festival well known for its extravagant alcohol consumption. An analyst at a state or regional level might not have access to this information and thus put unnecessary effort into follow-up. On the other hand, a local analyst may not have any way to know that a local spike in visits for respiratory illness is matched by similar spikes in adjacent jurisdictions. Effective operation of a multilevel surveillance system like this requires trust between analysts and program managers at various levels of the system and in various juris-dictions. Such trust can be supported with well-designed protocols for mutual consultation before data are released or acted upon.

Many types of data can be examined in near-real-time using a syndromic surveillance approach to supplement and illuminate observations from ED visits, which remain the mainstay of this approach. Each day's experience is compared with expected values using various statistical approaches, and alerts at various levels of statistical improbability are generated for analysts to prompt further examination of the data. Examples include poison center consultations, calls to nurse hotlines, absenteeism rates in schools and workplaces (especially useful if reason for absence is recorded), emergency medical services run reports, 911 calls for emergency health assistance, sales of selected prescription and over-the-counter drugs, mentions of specific words in social media posts, and searches for selected terms in Internet search engines. A related approach involves automated monitoring and mapping of mentions of diseases or outbreaks of likely public health importance in large numbers of online media: blogs, newspapers, chat rooms, list serves, maga-zines, and social media. This latter approach can enable public health agencies with a national, regional, or global focus to monitor for signs of disease without being wholly dependent on vari-able surveillance capacities in different jurisdictions.[54]

POPULATION-BASED SURVEILLANCE USING SAMPLE SURVEYS OF INDIVIDUALS

For surveillance of many conditions of public health interest—especially risk factors and health-related behaviors—population-based sample surveys are of great value. Many population-based surveys are carried out for research purposes or to provide one-time answers to specific questions. Characteristics of surveys whose purposes include surveillance include:

- Well-defined sampling schemes that allow inference to whole populations and to subpopula-tions defined by important stratification variables such as age, sex, race or ethnicity, income level, education, or geographic area,
- Questionnaire content that provides information needed to plan or evaluate public health interventions,
- Use of standard methods and questionnaires that allow regional-level data to be compared among regions and to be aggregated at a wider (*e.g.*, national) level, and
- Continuous or repeated administration to allow monitoring of any changes in the prevalence of a condition over time.

In countries with less-developed vital registration systems, or in settings where public health and healthcare systems are disrupted by warfare, civil strife, or natural disasters, population-based sample field surveys are often used to estimate mortality, including infant and child mortality,[82] vaccine coverage, birth rates, fertility, and other population parameters.[83] They have their greatest value when surveys with comparable methods are repeated periodically.[84]

Public health officials may cooperate with university or voluntary agency partners to design such surveys to help with targeting and evaluation of emergency or ongoing preventive or health-care services. Random-sample surveys may also be carried out in more circumscribed populations like residents of a camp for displaced persons. Cluster sample methods originally developed for measurement of immunization coverage[85] are now widely used for other purposes when rapid sur-veillance information is needed.[86] They can be used even when reliable population denominators are not available; aerial or satellite photographs or field surveys can be used for sampling frames.

POPULATION-BASED SURVEILLANCE USING SENTINEL SURVEILLANCE SITES

For some conditions, it makes sense to collect data about events of interest from a random, a systematic, or even (for some purposes) a convenience sample of sites where these events are recorded. A well-understood example of the latter has been ILI-Net,[16] in which states recruit a diverse convenience sample of primary care practices from which they obtain weekly counts of total office visits and of visits for a syndrome of influenza-like illness, stratified by age group and gender. When influenza is active in a community, the percentage of office visits that are due to influenza-like illness rises, and thresholds for considering influenza to be epidemic in a community are derived from many years of experience with this type of data collection. As medical offices become computerized, opportunities have arisen to collect the same data from electronic health records in participating practices. While this approach allows gathering data about more patients, from more practices, the data still represent a convenience sample of office visits.

This approach has been extended to monitoring hospital admissions for persons with a laboratory diagnosis of influenza in select hospitals in select states. The Emerging Infections Program at CDC funds a network of states and localities that carry out active surveillance for selected bacterial pathogens using a common protocol. Data from this network have provided key information for setting national disease control policy, for example, for meningococcal disease vaccine.[11] As noted above, the SEER cancer registry program at the National Cancer Institute maintains high-quality, active cancer incidence, treatment, and outcome surveillance in a diverse sample of about a dozen states and localities.[66] Results of SEER surveillance can, with caution, be considered representative enough of the United States to allow results to apply to the whole country. A conceptually similar approach is to carry out more active surveillance for a condition on a periodic basis, not continuously. When one of us worked at the Colorado Department of Health in the early 1980s, we carried out active searches for cases of congenital rubella syndrome and of rheumatic fever in children at 3-year intervals, to confirm (or refute) the observation that these conditions appeared to have become very rare.

SOURCES, QUALITY AND MANAGEMENT OF DATA

Data Sources

A vast array of data sources has been useful for public health surveillance. As technologies and medical practice continue to change, new data sources are likely to be identified. Each data source has its own characteristics that must be thoroughly understood by a surveillance analyst who proposes to work with the data. Examples of data sources available in the US, by no means complete, include:

For case-based surveillance:

1. Spontaneous case reports of reportable diseases by clinicians, received by telephone, fax, e-mail, or through a web portal ("passive" from the point of view of the public health agency).
2. Cases found by manual review of clinical or laboratory records (*e.g.*, for a cancer or birth defects registry, or in an outbreak setting) ("active" surveillance).
3. Cases or candidate cases found through scheduled or ad-hoc queries of electronic medical records in hospitals or physicians' offices (*e.g.*, electronic laboratory reporting or electronic case reporting or as part of an outbreak investigation).
4. Candidate cases ascertained from administrative records, like hospital discharge or billing records, for comparison with existing case reports and to generate queries for information about not-yet-reported cases.
5. Candidate cases ascertained from ancillary electronic health records that contain a diagnosis field, such as those maintained by pharmacies, radiation therapy centers, diagnostic radiology services, or outpatient surgical facilities.
6. Cases ascertained from death or birth certificates.
7. Both deaths and hospitalizations can be reviewed for case detection purposes using any mention of a cause of interest (such as diabetes, asthma, or an opioid drug) or using the assigned underlying cause for each death or first-mentioned reason for hospitalization (such as myocardial infarction, HIV/AIDS, or drug overdose due to a specific drug). The former is likely to be more sensitive, the latter to have a higher positive predictive value.
8. Cases found through targeted community or facility screening.

For syndromic surveillance:

1. Electronic emergency department records—using chief complaints, nurse triage notes, coded diagnoses, and/or the literal text of diagnoses to assign visits to syndromes.
2. Admission records to hospitals, using free-text "reason for admission" fields and/or coded admission diagnoses to assign admissions to syndromes.

3. "Reason for visit" records maintained by physician offices, either on paper or in electronic health records, binned into syndromes.
4. Purchases of key prescription medications that might indicate the presence of a syndrome of interest.
5. Over-the-counter medications sold, where an increase in sales of "cold and flu" medications or thermometers might be an indicator of an influenza outbreak.
6. Calls to nurse hotlines, assigned to syndromes based on patient's complaint or on nurse's clinical impression.
7. Internet queries for certain search terms, where an increase in such searches might be an early indicator of an outbreak of a particular syndrome or disease.
8. Mentions of key terms on social media platforms—whether symptoms, medications, or diagnoses—where an increase in such mentions might be an early indicator of an outbreak of a particular syndrome or disease.

For risk factor surveillance:

1. Recurring or continuous population-based surveys can provide a means to monitor risk or protective factors such as seatbelt use, smoke detector presence in the household, smoking behavior, alcohol consumption, or receipt of a Pap smear.
2. Consumption data, *e.g.*, tobacco sold, estimated from tax collections, or morphine milligram equivalents of opiate prescription drugs sold, collected from wholesalers by the Drug Enforcement Administration.
3. Social media mentions, for example, of binge alcohol drinking.[87]
4. Real-time electronic measures of population mobility during an infectious disease epidemic, for example by monitoring distances traveled by individuals' cell phones.

For chronic disease surveillance:

1. Administrative records, like hospital discharge registries or billing systems, that contain information about diagnoses, dates of care, and demographics for patient visits to emergency departments as well as hospital admissions.
2. Population-based surveys that gather information about diagnoses (Has a healthcare professional ever told you that you have diabetes?) as well as risk and preventive behaviors.
3. Death certificates—either underlying cause or any mention.
4. High-coverage community systems for sharing of electronic health records that support queries (periodic or ad hoc) or periodic reports about outpatient visits for various diagnoses and allow deduplication within and across providers.
5. Pharmacy claims data.[88]

For injury surveillance:

1. Injury crash data assembled from police reports[89]
2. National Institute for Occupational Safety and Health (NIOSH) fatal occupational injury data system
3. Poison center consultations for poisonings, accidental and intentional
4. Death certificates
5. Coroner/medical examiner reports
6. Police reports
7. ED visit data from electronic medical records
8. Administrative claims data for patient visits[90]

For environmental and occupational health surveillance:

1. Air quality monitoring
2. Water quality monitoring, including coliform counts
3. Employee monitoring data, as done for blood lead in workers with known lead exposure risk on the job, or for workers at risk for radiation exposure
4. Results of inspections in abattoirs and in food processing, wholesaling, storage, and sales operations and in food service operations
5. Results of inspections in other settings

Population denominators for most forms of surveillance:

1. Census data, which provide information on the numbers and demographic characteristics of residents within defined geographic areas. In some settings, population estimates may be based on sample surveys
2. Hospital admissions
3. Survey respondents

Content and Quality of Records

In resource-poor environments, surveillance data may remain paper-based as they move up several administrative levels after the original record is recorded on a paper form. Simplicity in the data fields collected is particularly important in such environments. When one of us (RSH) was first starting out in a small US state health department in the late 1970s, all reportable disease surveillance was done manually. Case reports were received as mailed-in cards from doctors and from health departments or laboratory report forms from the state public health laboratory. Duplicates were identified by visual inspection. Missing data in critical fields generated telephone follow-back to the reporting entity. Case reports were entered in log books with a page for each disease, a row for each case, and columns for name, date of onset, county of residence, age, sex, and race. The columnar data were easy to scan by eye to identify missing or anomalous data and to identify patterns that would suggest outbreaks. For example, several reported cases of shigellosis in children and young adults with the same last name from the same county suggested a family outbreak, while an increase in cases in people with different last names suggested a community outbreak.

In general, epidemiologists prefer more data to less. In particular, the ability to estimate disease rates according to numerous demographic and risk factor parameters is useful when planning and targeting public health programs and when searching for plausible prevention interventions. In an era of electronic health records, the marginal cost of extracting more data from a file of patient data is very small. It is thus tempting to collect as many data items about each person with a suspected or reported case as possible. By contrast, when data items on a case report form must be collected by a local investigator, likely from multiple sources (patient interview, patient's family and social associates, electronic and paper medical records, a laboratory, and one or several physicians), the marginal cost of adding data items can be substantial. In population-based surveys, there are also practical limits to how long questionnaires can be, both because interviewers must be paid by the hour and because respondent fatigue sets in with long questionnaires and leads to early termination of the interview and loss of potentially valuable data.

Apart from the expense of gathering case reports or other records for use in surveillance, adding fields requires additional attention to efforts to assure data quality. Some degree of quality assurance is needed for every field in the record layout, and the more fields there are, the more opportunities there are for errors and nonresponse. This is a specific reason for the dictum that you should not collect data you are not going to use. Data quality efforts should be focused on those fields that will in fact be used. Absent evidence that reported data are used and useful, the motivation to report and to report carefully is diminished, reducing overall data quality. If it is known at the time the data collection system is implemented that certain fields will often be left blank, those fields should not be in the data collection instrument, as the data will not be useable.

Many surveillance information systems have implemented automated processes that operate during the collection process to help assure data quality. For example, if a reporting source has not submitted any data in a particular cycle, when at least some reports would have been expected, this may generate an automated alert to the analyst. If this happens several times within a few cycles, it may generate a more urgent alert. The appearance of a novel code in a particular field (*e.g.*, a new diagnostic code never used before) may generate an alert. Investigation might show that the sending entity has changed coding systems, is putting codes in unexpected locations in the record or is making data entry errors. Records can have internal consistency checks, for example, to assure that seniors are not diagnosed with premature birth, that date of diagnosis precedes date of report, or that date of onset is later than date of birth. Automated processes to merge multiple records on the same person, whether from the same or different sources (*e.g.*, case reports from two physicians, or a physician case report, and an electronic laboratory report), are essential to modern high-volume real-time surveillance systems.

Method of Acquisition of Data

Methods of acquisition of surveillance data are undergoing rapid change, and the rate of change is expected only to increase. For this reason, we will focus here on considerations in choice of such methods, rather than on the methods themselves.

- Solicitation of case reports from clinicians and others with knowledge of cases of the condition of interest is a time-tested way to acquire data and has well-known advantages and disadvantages. From the public health agency's point of view, it requires little effort and is inexpensive, but data quality may be poor. For diseases widely understood to be public health threats, it can be very sensitive and timely, with quite adequate positive predictive value. If kept simple, and clearly justified by urgent public health needs, it can have wide acceptability. It may be the method of choice in early stages of a high-profile outbreak investigation. It is also likely to be slow, insensitive, and have a low positive predictive value for most conditions under surveillance that are important but not urgent. Such reporting can be improved through attention to detail by the receiving public health agency: courteously remind clinicians frequently about their obligations; communicate findings regularly to those who are asked to make reports; act promptly, ethically, and effectively on information received; be available and responsive; make the reporting process simple. In the current environment, simplicity may mean allowing clinicians to make reports by encrypted e-mail, through a dedicated secure website, or using newer communication methods.

- Electronic submission of computerized laboratory results by clinical laboratories, for infectious and toxic diseases and for cancer. This fairly mature technology has several key elements: specification of reportable laboratory findings, including specification of LOINC,[91] SnoMED,[92] or other similar codes that correspond to such findings; development of a standardized vocabulary and message structure for transmission of records to public health agencies; development of a secure method for transferring the records from laboratories to public health agencies; at the receiving agency, development of a method for deduplicating the reports and adding the information to a new or existing record. The relative maturity of this technology reflects the fact that it has been under development and gradual implementation for about 20 years. Currently, the majority of case reports of reportable diseases received by public health agencies are first received as laboratory results. Case reports from clinicians may be faster than electronic laboratory reporting when clinicians are making urgent reports of suspected cases of serious diseases like botulism or meningococcal disease. Electronic laboratory reporting is also not useful for diseases of which cases are not usually laboratory confirmed, such as varicella, tetanus, or staphylococcal food poisoning.

- Electronic case reporting, including automated recognition of cases of reportable conditions through "packaging" and transmission of a case report, is being developed partly on the model of electronic laboratory reporting. It also has parallels in the identification of cases for quality improvement review or for clinical trials. At this writing, the technology is being tested on a few diseases in a few locations. The actual performance of this new surveillance technology in operation remains to be determined. Key elements of the technology are similar to those for electronic laboratory reporting: specification of the conditions to be included in the system; specification of findings (physical findings, vital signs, laboratory results, radiology results, diagnoses, etc), or combinations of findings, in clinical records that would prompt generation of a case-report record; specification of the codes used in electronic health records that would correspond to these findings; development of a standard vocabulary and message structure for case report records; development of a secure methodology for transmission of the record to public health agencies; development of a second-level screen, customized by public health agencies, to identify records for inclusion in the agency's surveillance information system, with the desired sensitivity and positive predictive value; development of systems for inclusion of such electronic case reports in agencies' surveillance information systems, accounting for duplicate and updated reports on the same person or the same episode of illness. The sensitivity and positive predictive value of automated detection of probable cases of reportable diseases remain to be measured in diverse public health and clinical settings. Those parameters can be expected to vary by disease; and the desired balance of sensitivity and PPV also will vary by disease. The incremental value of this technology compared with electronic laboratory reporting alone also remains to be determined in production settings.

- Reports by people in the community who are aware of or who suspect outbreaks and clusters are the most common method by which public health officials learn about outbreaks. In 2018, for example, 683 nonfoodborne acute disease outbreaks were identified by Florida local health departments and reported to the state health department, of which 634 had a reporter type listed. Two-thirds of these outbreaks were due to suspected or confirmed influenza, and the vast majority were due to agents of which cases are not individually reportable, including hand-foot-and-mouth disease and norovirus gastroenteritis. Of these 364, 36% were brought to public health attention by nursing homes or long-term care facilities, 24% by child care facilities, 21% by schools, and only 1.9% (12 outbreaks) were detected by review of reportable disease or syndromic surveillance data. Even among 41 nonfoodborne outbreaks caused by diseases of which individual cases were reportable, only 7 (23.3%) were detected by such review. Among 98 food- and waterborne outbreaks, 22 (22.4%) were detected by review of formal surveillance data, while for over half the outbreaks, the public health agency was alerted by a concerned person or medical provider. (Personal communication, Leah Eisenstein, Florida Department of Health.) Considering the importance of this channel of information, it is important for health departments to have systems to track citizen calls and complaints and to link together multiple citizen reports that are related to each other. More than one telephone call or message may be received about the same event, but if they are received by different staff members, there may be delayed recognition of the relationship. One call may be about discolored or bad-tasting water in an area and another about an increase in diarrhea cases in the same neighborhood, but if they are received in different branches of the public health agency, it may be hard to make the connection that there is a possible waterborne diarrhea outbreak in progress. Similarly, multiple independent reports of illness related to the same food service establishment need to be linked, even if received by more than one channel.[93,94]
- Population-based surveys have become essential to public health planning and evaluation and are further discussed below. They permit the comparison of the magnitude and burden of various health conditions and their precursors to each other in ways that disease-specific surveillance cannot. Data collection methods include survey instruments administered to random or purposive samples by telephone, mail, and door-to-door contact.
- Several kinds of panels for surveillance are increasingly being used for sample surveillance, as telephone surveys have become increasingly impractical in the United States and some other countries. These panels may consist of groups of workers in various settings or people enrolled in a system of health care. Panels may also consist of lists of individuals, assembled by research firms, who can be reliably reached through the Internet, in person, by mail, or by telephone, and who have agreed to participate when asked. Respondents can be weighted to be the representative of the general population.
- Sentinel provider-based surveillance. Enrolling a sample of surveillance sites (medical practice sites, laboratories, hospitals) to provide periodic reports of the occurrence of health events of interest can be very cost-effective compared to attempting to ascertain the events from all providers. Staff time can be invested in developing two-way relationships with a limited set of providers, and these relationships can help assure compliance with surveillance protocols and reduce missing data, site drop-out, and other threats to the integrity of surveillance. This is a setting in which active outreach by public health agency staff may be worth the investment. It is important to do the necessary groundwork to gain confidence that patterns of disease in the patients treated at the sentinel sites are sufficiently representative of those in the population, and that the relationship between patients treated at the sentinel sites and those in the total population is stable over time. Examples of such surveillance systems include the venerable US ILI-Net and systems elsewhere with similar designs,[16] surveillance for hospitalizations for influenza and for stroke,[70] and respiratory and enteric virus surveillance.[95]

Data Security, Confidentiality, Privacy

While the proper balance between privacy rights and governments' access to personal information for disease monitoring has been debated for over a century, the increasing automation of health information, both for medical care and public health uses, has led to heightened public concerns about potential misuse.[96,97] Individuals expect that personal health information is not revealed to, or accessible by, others without their assent. In the context of public health surveillance, this means government public health agencies. Privacy is in tension with the authority that governments are granted to access such information for public health purposes. Confidentiality concerns expectations that governmental public health agencies authorized to access and hold private health information use that information only for authorized purposes and do not disclose that information to others. Security is critical to assuring confidentiality of information in public health surveillance systems by protecting against unauthorized access to personal health information.[98]

In the United States, the 2003 Privacy Rule of the Health Insurance Portability and Accountability Act of 1996 aims to protect privacy by strictly regulating the use and disclosure of identifiable personal health data and yet to allow for legitimate access for public health surveillance and other public health uses.[99] In the United Kingdom, Section 251 of the National Health Service Act 2006, as implemented in Health Service Regulations,[100] fills this role, as does the General Data Protection Regulation in the European Union.[101] Many countries have similar provisions in law or policy. Controversies regarding the balance between public health objectives and individual privacy are likely to increase in parallel with the capacity to automate public health surveillance.[102]

Historically, the practice of surveillance has largely been a government function, but the concept is being applied in an expanding array of settings, and innovations in surveillance approaches are arising from entities outside governmental public health agencies. Public health approaches are reflected in the concept of "population health management" in health care, which involves using healthcare and health insurance data to characterize patient populations, track providers' adherence to care standards, and monitor the achievement of healthcare delivery targets. "Crowd sourcing" approaches are used to solicit online reporting of symptoms to track seasonal illness.[103] Social networks organized by patients with various diseases are being used not just for advocacy but also to assess and monitor health outcomes (*e.g.*, Patients Like Me[104]). Data about Internet searches are being explored to assess whether queries related to specific diseases or symptoms might be useful in detecting changes in illness trends. The concept of health policy surveillance has been advanced by academic investigators supported by private foundations.[105] Academic investigators are advancing the development of analytic methods for surveillance.[80]

With the COVID-19 pandemic, university-based teams and major national media outlets have led efforts to aggregate data from national and state governments, WHO, and other sources; describe epidemiologic patterns; make forecasts; and display data in innovative ways. In the US, the result has been that universities and major news organizations have often eclipsed CDC as public sources of information, including about "hot spots" and racial and ethnic disparities.

ANALYSIS, INTERPRETATION, AND PRESENTATION OF SURVEILLANCE DATA

Analysis and Interpretation

The analysis of surveillance data is generally descriptive and straightforward, using standard epidemiologic techniques. Analysis strategies used in other forms of epidemiologic investigation are applicable to surveillance, including standardizing rates for age or other population attributes that may vary over time or among locations, controlling for confounding when making comparisons, taking into account sampling strategies used in surveys, addressing problems related to missing data or unknown values, and assessing changes in temporal or temporal/spatial trends. In addition to these approaches used in many epidemiologic analyses, there are special situations that require approaches specific to the analysis and interpretation of surveillance data.

Attribution of Date

In analyzing trends, a decision must often be made whether to examine trends by the date that events occurred, were diagnosed, or were reported. Using the date of report is easier but subject to irregularities in reporting. Using the date of diagnosis provides a better measure of disease occurrence. Analysis by date of diagnosis, however, will underestimate incidence in the most recent intervals if there is a relatively long delay between diagnosis and report. Thus, it may be necessary to adjust recent counts for reporting delays, based on previous reporting experience.[106,107]

Attribution of Place

It is often necessary to decide whether analyses will be based on where the ill person was when the relevant exposure occurred, where the person lives, or where health care was provided. These may all differ. For vector-borne diseases, the geographic location of exposure to a vector is often more important than where the ill person normally resides. The place where care is provided may be more important in a surveillance system that monitors the quality of health care, whereas the place of residence would be important if surveillance were used to track the need for preventive or curative services in different areas. In the United States, census data, the primary source for denominators in rate calculations, are based on place of residence, and thus place of residence is commonly used in surveillance analyses.[108] For notifiable disease-reporting systems, this requires cross-jurisdiction (*e.g.*, state-to-state) reporting among health departments when an illness in a resident of one area is diagnosed and reported in another.

Use of Geographic Information Systems

Geographic coordinates (latitude and longitude) for the location of health events or place of residence can be calculated automatically from a street address, allowing automated generation of maps using Geographic Information Systems (GIS) computer software. By combining geographic data on health events with data on the location of hazards, environmental exposures, or preventive or therapeutic services, GIS can facilitate the study of spatial associations between exposures or services and health outcomes.[109] Given the importance of maps for presenting surveillance data, it is not surprising that the use of GIS has grown rapidly in surveillance practice.

Detection of a Change in Trends

Surveillance analysts use a wide array of statistical measures to detect increases (or decreases) in the numbers or rates of events beyond expected levels. The selection of a statistical method depends on the underlying nature of disease trends (*e.g.*, presence or absence of seasonal variations, gradual long-term declines or increases), the length of time for which historical reference data are available, the urgency of detecting an aberrant trend (*e.g.*, detecting a 1-day increase vs. assessing weekly, monthly, or yearly variations), and whether the objective is to detect temporal aberrations or both temporal and geographic clustering.[110,111] For example, to identify unusually severe influenza seasons, CDC uses time-series methods to define expected seasonal counts for deaths attributed to "pneumonia and influenza" and to determine when observed numbers of deaths exceed threshold values.[112] Automated systems aimed at detecting the early onset of bioterrorism-related epidemics have drawn on statistical techniques developed for industrial quality control monitoring, building on methods such as the CUSUM method employed in the CDC's Early Aberration Reporting System.[113]

In assessing a change detected by surveillance, the first question to ask is, "Is it real?" There are multiple artifacts that can affect trends, including changes in staffing among those who report cases or manage surveillance systems, changes in the use of healthcare services or reporting because of holidays or other events, changes in clinicians' interest in or awareness of a disease, changes in surveillance procedures, changes in screening or diagnostic criteria, changes in the availability of screening, diagnostic, or care services, and changes in public interest or publicity about the condition. The second question to ask is, "Is it meaningful?" Regardless of whether an increase in disease is recognized informally or because a statistical threshold was surpassed, judgment is required to determine whether the observation reflects a potential public health problem and the extent and aggressiveness of the next-step investigations. These may range from taking a "wait and see" position with close reexamination in subsequent days to launching a full-scale epidemiologic investigation. This judgment is particularly important for systems that monitor nonspecific syndromes that may reflect illness that could be of little public health importance or could be the earliest stage of potentially severe disease. "False alarms" may be common if statistical thresholds are set too low, increasing the likelihood that alarms are triggered by random variations. Such artifacts emphasize the importance of being familiar with how data are collected and analyzed and with the local context of healthcare services.

Assessing Completeness of Surveillance

If two independent surveillance or data systems are available for a particular condition and if records for individuals represented in these systems can be linked to one another, then it is possible to determine the number in both systems and the number included in each but not the other. Using capture-recapture analysis, the number missed by both can be estimated, in turn allowing an estimate of the total number of cases in the population and calculation of the proportion identified by each.[114] The accuracy of this approach depends on the likelihood of detection by one system being independent of detection by the other. Violations of this assumption may lead to an underestimation of the total number of cases in a population and to an overestimation of the completeness of surveillance.[115]

This approach also depends on the accuracy of record linkages, which in turn depends on the accuracy and specificity of the identifying information used to make linkages. If names are not available, proxy markers for identity, such as date of birth combined with sex, may be used. Even if names are available, they can change, be misspelled, or be listed under an alias. Software that converts names to codes or accepts fuzzy matches can aid in avoiding linkage errors from spelling and punctuation. Nonetheless, other errors in recording or coding data can lead to false matches or nonmatches. In addition to matches based on complete alignment of matching criteria, standards should be set and validated for accepting or rejecting near matches. Although computer algorithms can accomplish most matches and can provide measures of the probability that matches are correct, manual validation of at least a sample of matched and nonmatched records is advisable.

Smoothing

Graphic plots of disease numbers or rates by small units of time or small geographic area may yield an erratic or irregular picture owing to statistical variability, obscuring visualization of underlying trends or geographic patterns. To solve this problem, a variety of temporal or geographic "smoothing" techniques may be used to clarify trends or patterns.[116]

Protection of Confidentiality

In addition to suppressing data when reporting a small number of cases or events that could enable recognition of an individual, statistical techniques may be used to introduce perturbations into data in a way that prevents recognition of individuals but retains overall accuracy in aggregate tabulations or maps.[117,118] In using geographic information systems that attach measures of latitude and longitude to individuals' addresses of residence, the presentation of electronically generated maps can inadvertently reveal the identity of people represented within maps, and care must be taken in the use of such electronic files to avoid disclosing addresses.[119]

Presentation

Because surveillance data have multiple uses, it is essential that they be widely and effectively disseminated, not only to those who participate in their collection, but also to everyone who can use them, ranging from public health epidemiologists and program managers to the media, clinicians, the public, and policy-makers. The mode of presentation should be geared to the intended audience. Tabular presentation is suitable for audiences with the time and interest to review the data in detail. In contrast, well-designed graphs or maps can immediately convey key points.

In addition to issuing published surveillance reports, public health agencies use the Internet to post reports, allowing for more frequent updates and widespread access. Interactive Internet-based utilities can allow users to obtain customized surveillance reports, based on their interest in specific tabulations.

Depending on the nature of surveillance findings and the disease or condition in question, the release of surveillance reports may attract media and public interest. This eventuality should be anticipated. In collaboration with a media communications expert, develop a plan for media inquiries, identify and clarify key public health messages that arise from the data (respecting both the strengths and limits of data), and draw attention to related steps that program managers, policy-makers, or members of the public can take to promote health.

EVALUATION

Operation of surveillance systems consumes resources, and like all disease prevention or control program components, surveillance must be evaluated periodically. Investments in surveillance must be evaluated ultimately in terms of their utility for operation, planning, and evaluation of programs to improve health and prevent disease, disability, and premature death. Several public health organizations have published frameworks or guidelines for surveillance system evaluation, and a systematic review of such guidelines was published in 2015.[120] Guidelines or frameworks have been published by the US CDC,[23] Public Health Canada,[121] and the European Centers for Disease Control and Prevention.[122] Related guidelines have been published for outbreak detection.[81] Most of these identify attributes of a surveillance system that can be formally evaluated, derived at least partially from CDC's original 1988 Guidelines for Evaluation of Surveillance Systems.[123]

The details of surveillance evaluations differ depending on the type of data used (*e.g.*, case reporting vs. population-based sample surveys) and the purpose of surveillance. The relative importance of surveillance attributes can differ according to the purposes of surveillance.[124] For example, for case-based surveillance of botulism, sensitivity and timeliness are more important than positive predictive value. The negative consequences of failing to detect a true case in a timely way are more than enough to justify the effort required to investigate reported cases that turn out not to be botulism. Conversely, for surveillance of Lyme disease in the northeastern United States, where it is common, a high positive predictive value is desired for reported cases[125] as the staff time required to identify noncases among numerous reported laboratory results and cases can be substantial, and there is no public health response required in response to most individual cases.

Published guidelines for surveillance system evaluation generally do not contain quantitative standards for the adequacy of various attributes. For example, what level of sensitivity or timeliness is sufficient for case reporting? Each program manager who carries out a surveillance system evaluation is expected to determine whether the measured performance is acceptable or is sufficient to meet information needs, and how to improve performance when it is not acceptable. Quantitative standards may be set by agencies that fund or make decisions about disease control or prevention programs. An agency that funds emergency preparedness, for example, may set standards for the timeliness and sensitivity of detection of key reportable conditions. Standardized methods for calculation of surveillance system attributes such as sensitivity, positive predictive value, or timeliness, which would allow comparison of jurisdictions to each other, are rarely available. Some of the recommended attributes, such as acceptability, require qualitative assessment.

The Florida Department of Health scores its county-level branches annually on key measures of reportable disease record-level completeness and timeliness. For example, fewer than 25% of reported cases of 32 high-priority diseases can be missing data on any of 11 key demographic and case classification fields; and the interval from receipt of initial case report at the county level to report to the state epidemiology office must be 14 days or less for at least 80% of reported cases of 50 medium and high priority diseases (Personal communication, Leah Eisenstein, Florida Department of Health).

CONTRIBUTIONS

Public health interventions rest on a basis of surveillance—either because surveillance data are used to identify the nature and scope of the health problem, because the data are used in the operation of the program, or because they are used to plan and evaluate the program. For example, in CDC's series of articles in the MMWR about 10 Great Public Health Achievements of the 20th century and for the period 2001 to 2010,[126,127] all achievements were documented through use of public health surveillance data.

Improvements over time in surveillance technology and processes, as described above, have resulted in improved ability to understand the health status of populations in a timely way and thus made it possible for public health officials and policy-makers to make more data-based decisions about priorities. Having good population health data in hand is not a goal in itself—the contributions of public health surveillance are seen in effective public health programs. As stated by former CDC director William Foege in a 1976 article, "The reason for collecting, analyzing, and disseminating information on a disease is to control that disease. Collection and analysis should not be allowed to consume resources if action does not follow."[128]

Managers and policy-makers making decisions about how to allocate public health resources (among diseases, among populations, and among intervention strategies) need information that is obtained in several ways. Much information comes from a knowledgebase built on laboratory, clinical, and planned epidemiologic studies. The latter include the types of studies addressed in depth elsewhere in this book: cohort studies, case-control studies, longitudinal cohort studies, population-based surveys, and so on. Public health surveillance addresses questions that cannot be addressed by this type of research. The specific contribution of surveillance to public health decision-making is in providing timely and credible answers to such key questions with a sustained population-wide perspective.

ISSUES

The practice of public health surveillance is constrained in several important ways, some of which have been mentioned above. Public health officials design surveillance systems to optimize the utility of often imperfect options, make the best use of available resources, and assure that surveillance systems meet ongoing information needs.

- Surveillance consumes programmatic resources. It is always in competition with public health intervention activities. Public health program managers must balance other programmatic needs with information needs.
- Many surveillance activities involve access by government employees to identifiable personal health information about individuals, as well as sometimes sensitive information about schools, businesses, or other organizations. Public health staff might make direct contact with individuals for interviews about very personal matters, sometimes to the surprise of those who are contacted. Public health managers must balance programmatic and information needs on one hand with legitimate privacy concerns on the other. The importance of the latter concern is reflected in security policies for data held by public health agencies, in policies about allowable sharing and public release of identifiable and nonidentifiable data, as well as in codified acceptable behavior by public health staff.
- Public health agencies are expected to recognize and respond to health threats—whether due to infectious diseases, toxins, cancers, birth defects, injuries, or other conditions—quickly and effectively. This response requires acquisition and use of timely, detailed, correct information both as part of surveillance and in rapidly implemented epidemiologic studies, and the response often cannot wait for persons to give consent for their information to be obtained or shared. Public health laws typically authorize public health agencies to obtain personal information from healthcare providers without requiring patients' consent, in order to carry out statutory responsibilities. Agencies must be transparent about what they are collecting and why, what authorities they are relying on, and how data will be stored and, if appropriate, eventually destroyed.
- Methods of quantifying the impact of an epidemic often need to change as the scale of the epidemic changes. In the 2020 COVID-19 pandemic, for example, a reportable disease paradigm was initially the only surveillance strategy. As the epidemic grew, and it became clearer that many infected people were not sick or not sick enough to seek medical attention, the proportion of infections captured by case-reporting fell and additional approaches more similar to those used for influenza surveillance became necessary. Such a change can be difficult for media, political actors and a highly engaged public to adapt to.
- During acute public health events, ad hoc surveillance systems are often established that meet the needs of the response team. Transitioning surveillance to sustainable long-term systems when the condition continues to occur after the acute event is over is often a challenge.
- The public and politicians are often surprised by how much or how little information public health agencies have. Members of the public may—depending on the situation—be alternately concerned about intrusive public health access to information about themselves or about how little public agencies actually know.
- The health information landscape is in constant evolution. Public health agencies face a considerable challenge keeping up with changes in how health information is stored and shared in clinical settings. It is increasingly necessary for them to acquire and maintain expertise in health informatics. This expertise is needed not only to take full advantage of the information opportunities available to them but also to avoid investments in technologies that cannot evolve to take advantage of new opportunities.

- Many important health conditions (like cigarette use or receipt of Pap smears) are best monitored through ongoing or periodic population-based surveys. Changes in consumer technologies (*e.g.*, progressive abandonment of home landline telephone service and increasing use of cellular telephones), in public attitudes about participation in government surveys, and in willingness to accept telephone calls from unknown persons have made survey methods that were viable for many years increasingly impractical or statistically unreliable. Replacement survey methodologies are being studied intensively but face the dual challenges of providing current valid estimates of population parameters and of supporting long-term comparability (backward to previous methods and forward as technology continues to change) in the frequency of the parameters being monitored.

- Surveillance surveys cost money that could alternatively be spent on disease prevention programs. More subjects would mean tighter confidence limits around estimates for the whole population and allow reasonably precise estimates for more subpopulations. More data items would mean a richer dataset for analysis. Both of these desirable characteristics increase the expense of the data collection. Program managers have to decide how many subjects and how long a questionnaire they can afford and must be strategic about what kinds of surveillance information are critical to the success of their prevention programs.

- Rapid changes in information technology are providing numerous new opportunities to monitor population health parameters and to detect emerging issues and concerns about health. Public health practitioners tend to be conservative about what data they use as the basis for public health decisions and want to understand fully the characteristics of any data source that they use. In the first part of the 21st century, there was great interest in using Google Flu Trends to detect influenza activity early and to characterize influenza impact, by counting the number of Google Internet searches using certain search terms. Public health epidemiologists were cautious in adopting this methodology partly because the methods were proprietary and not readily accessible. After several years of availability, the usefulness of Google Flu Trends was called into question by careful analysis. It failed to correctly characterize the 2009 H1N1 pandemic,[129] and for that and other reasons, the data were taken off-line. Public health practitioners could be faulted for failing to use new information sources that could improve detection and characterization of public health issues but could also be faulted for basing important decisions in important part on data that are not yet thoroughly vetted.

- When surveillance systems collect and maintain personally identifiable information as part of individual case records, particularly for diseases that might be stigmatizing, public acceptability depends on the ongoing ability of public health agencies to protect the security of surveillance data and to use the data only for intended public health purposes.

- Surveillance systems often collect data on covariates such as sex, race, ethnicity, national origin, religion, immigration status, and sexual orientation. Our social understanding of what these covariates mean may change over time, classification systems may change, and implementation of categories may change. In 2020, high-profile events that seem to be products of systemic racism have prompted closer examination of health data by race and ethnicity and new explanations of observed patterns. Also, introduction of multiracial categories has reduced comparability of data over time. Similarly, some surveillance data systems now collect more categories of gender than male and female.

- Boundaries of political and census units may change over time.

- Classification systems for diseases may change over time.

READING A REPORT BASED ON SURVEILLANCE DATA

Surveillance data are used in a wide variety of reports, documents, and research reports. Most reports are descriptive: regular frequent surveillance summaries about specific diseases in specific locations, or annual summaries of reportable or notifiable diseases at the city, state, regional, national, or even global level. Some marshal surveillance data in support of the planning or evaluation of public health programs. Especially when used for program evaluation, surveillance data may be used in a hypothesis-testing fashion. For example, an analysis may compare rates in different populations, or time trends in different populations, to determine whether public health programs are being effective or where control resources should be focused.

Whenever reading a paper or report based on surveillance data—whether the data are being used descriptively, for evaluation, or for hypothesis testing—there are several questions one should ask:

1. What are the known properties of the surveillance data, as far as timeliness, sensitivity, positive predictive value, representativeness, and data quality?
2. Given these properties, or the absence of information about these properties, are the data suitable to use for the purpose in the report?
3. If case-based surveillance data show a change in incidence over time, or changes in the risk profile by population subgroup, have the authors considered and examined the possibility of artifact as the reason for the change?—for example,
   a. Changes in case definitions

   b. Changes in use of diagnostic techniques (*e.g.*, adoption of nonculture diagnostic methods for infectious diseases)

   c. Changes in data collection methods, including changes in coding of relevant fields in electronic health records at the sending facilities

   d. Changes in staff at some facilities responsible for providing data

   e. Changes in patterns of use of healthcare facilities, as might occur with opening or closing of facilities, or changes in payment systems

   f. Changes in which facilities are participating in the surveillance system

   g. Changes in coding systems (*e.g.*, ICD9 to ICD10 transition) that have not been accounted for or are happening unevenly

4. If syndromic surveillance data show a change in incidence over time, or changes in the risk profile by population subgroup, have the authors considered and examined the possible role of artifact in causing this change?—for example
   a. Changes in which facilities are participating in the data collection

   b. Changes in how facilities record reason for visit—for example, in a chief complaint field, from free text to choosing from a drop-down menu

   c. Changes in facility-specific abbreviations used in free-text fields that are used to assign free-text chief complaints to syndromes

   d. Changes in syndrome classification algorithms

5. Have the authors examined facility-specific data to assure themselves that observed trends are not due to changes at just one or a few facilities?
6. If survey-based data show a change in incidence or prevalence over time, or changes in the risk profile by population subgroup, have the authors considered and examined the possible role of artifact in causing this change?—for example
   a. Changes in the sampling method (*e.g.*, addition of stratified sampling)

   b. Changes in technology available to potential subjects (*e.g.*, cell phones, Internet, landline telephones)

   c. Changes in public acceptance of surveys

   d. Changes in the way questions are worded

   e. Changes in question order

   f. Changes in what languages are used for the survey instrument or interviews or in the translations of items

   g. Changes in availability of bilingual interviewers

7. Does the system have an ongoing process for quality control of the data?
8. Does the analysis use a reasonable population denominator? Are population estimates reliable at the level of analysis being used (*e.g.*, postal code, census tract, block group)? How old are the most recent population estimates, and are they appropriate for use with numerator data that are used?

9. Are various categories—*e.g.*, race or ethnicity—collected the same way for the numerator data (*e.g.*, cancer cases in a registry) as for the denominator (*e.g.*, a national census)?

10. How close to population-based are the counts of cases or health conditions? Is it reasonable to consider them to be close enough to population-based, so that census denominators can be used to calculate incidence rates?

11. Are known external events accounted for in the analysis of the data?

For many of these questions, especially those related to case and death counts and rates, the COVID-19 pandemic, with widespread media and political attention to surveillance data, has brought to public attention questions about the meaning of such data that have long been the province of epidemiologists. While this attention to the strengths and limitations of surveillance data is welcome, the data can also be misunderstood, or even misused for political rather than public health purposes.

CONCLUDING COMMENTS

Public health surveillance is applied epidemiology. Public health officials use epidemiologic methods to generate information necessary to operate, plan, or evaluate public health activities or to direct further investigation. All public health programs require appropriate local data about the condition being addressed in the program; they also require information generated from more formal clinical, epidemiologic, and laboratory research. The practice of surveillance is dynamic, responding to changes in the relative importance of various health conditions, the technology used to document health care provided to members of the community, healthcare-seeking behavior, funding of healthcare and public health services, the technology available to acquire, transfer, manage, and analyze data, the training and capability of public health staff, and the capability to handle very large volumes of data. Beyond being used for day-to-day program operations, surveillance methods can be used to target preventive interventions to appropriate population subgroups and to assess the reach and effectiveness of such interventions in the population. Analysts of surveillance data must be intimately familiar with the processes that have generated the data they use, and consumers of reports and papers based on surveillance data should also be sure they understand the strengths and possible limitations of the data on which they rely.

References

1. World Health Organization. *Communicable Disease Surveillance and Response Systems*. Geneva, Switzerland: Monitoring and Evaluation; 2006.
2. James SL, Abate D, Abate KH, et al. Global, regional, and national incidence, prevalence, and years lived with disability for 354 diseases and injuries for 195 countries and territories, 1990-2017: a systematic analysis for the Global Burden of Disease Study 2017. *Lancet*. 2018;392(10159):1789-1858.
3. Florida Department of Health. *Florida Influenza Surveillance Reports*. 2019.
4. Pickens CM, Pierannunzi C, Garvin W, Town M. Surveillance for certain health behaviors and conditions among states and selected local areas – behavioral risk factor surveillance system, United States, 2015. *MMWR Surveill Summ*. 2018;67(9):1-90.
5. Centers for Disease Control and Prevention. *Pap Tests*. Maryland ,MD: National Center for Health Statistics Fast Stats; 2017.
6. Canadian Cancer Statistics Advisory Committee. *Cervical Cancer. Canadian Cancer Statistics 2018*. Toronto, ON: Canadian Cancer Society; 2018.
7. New Mexico Department of Health. *New Mexico Substance Abuse Epidemiology Profile*. 2016.
8. Buckeridge D. Outbreak detection through automated surveillance: a review of the determinants of detection. *J Biomed Inform*. 2007;40(4):370-379.
9. Frieden TR; Centers for Disease Control and Prevention (CDC). CDC health disparities and inequalities report – United States, 2013. Foreword. *MMWR Suppl*. 2013;62(suppl 3):1-2.
10. Friedman-Kien AE, Laubenstein L, Marmor M, et al. Kaposis sarcoma and Pneumocystis pneumonia among homosexual men–New York City and California. *MMWR Morb Mortal Wkly Rep*. 1981;30(25)305-308.
11. Cohn AC, MacNeil JR, Harrison LH, et al. Changes in Neisseria meningitidis disease epidemiology in the United States, 1998-2007: implications for prevention of meningococcal disease. *Clin Infect Dis*. 2010;50(2):184-191.
12. Institute of Medicine. *The Future of Public Health*. Washington, DC: National Academy Press; 1988.
13. Kimble LE, Massoud MR, Heiby J. Using quality improvement to address hospital-acquired infections and antimicrobial resistance. *AMR Control, 2019 Overcoming Global Antimicrobial Resistance*. 2017.

14. Ontario Ministry of Health and Long-Term Care. *Infectious Diseases Protocol.* 2018.

15. Centers for Disease Control (CDC). A cluster of Kaposi's sarcoma and Pneumocystis carinii pneumonia among homosexual male residents of Los Angeles and Orange Counties, California. *MMWR Morb Mort Wkly Rep.* 1982;31(23):305-307.

16. Centers for Disease Control and Prevention. *FluView: A Weekly Influenza Surveillance Report Prepared by the Influenza Division.* 2019. Available at https://gis.cdc.gov/grasp/fluview/main.html. Accessed March 12, 2019.

17. Lipsitch M, Jha A, Simonsen L. Observational studies and the difficult quest for causality: lessons from vaccine effectiveness and impact studies. *Int J Epidemiol.* 2016;45(6):2060-2074.

18. Currie J, Walker R. Traffic congestion and infant health: evidence from E-ZPass. *Am Econ J Appl Econ.* 2011;3:65-90.

19. Case A, Deaton A. Rising morbidity and mortality in midlife among White non-Hispanic Americans in the 21st century. *Proc Natl Acad Sci USA.* 2015;112(49):15078-15083.

20. Frieden TR. Six components necessary for effective public health program implementation. *Am J Public Health.* 2014;104(1):17-22.

21. Glassman A, Chalkidou K, Giedion U, et al. Priority-setting institutions in health: recommendations from a Center for Global Development Working Group. *Glob Heart.* 2012;7(1):13-34.

22. National Syndromic Surveillance Program Community of Practice. *Syndromic Surveillance 101.* November 29, 2018. Available at https://knowledgerepository.syndromicsurveillance.org/updated-syndromic-surveillance-101-introductory-course-syndromic-surveillance. Accessed June 25, 2020.

23. German RR, Lee LM, Horan JM, et al; Guidelines Working Group Centers for Disease Control and Prevention. Updated guidelines for evaluating public health surveillance systems: recommendations from the Guidelines Working Group. *MMWR Recomm Rep* 2001;50(RR-13):1-35;quiz CE1-7.

24. Krishnamurthy R, Conde JM. Art and science of interoperability to create connections. In: McNabb S, Conde M, Ferland L, eds. *Transforming Public Health Surveillance.* Amman, Jordan: Elsevier Health Sciences; 2016:267-275.

25. Irgens LM. The fight against leprosy in Norway in the 19th century. *Michael.* 2010;7:307-320.

26. Declich S, Carter AO. Public health surveillance: historical origins, methods and evaluation. *Bull World Health Organ.* 1994;72(2):285-304.

27. Langmuir AD. Evolution of the concept of surveillance in the United States. *Proc R Soc Med.* 1971;64:681-684.

28. Thacker SB, Qualters JR, Lee LM; Centers for Disease Control and Prevention. Public health surveillance in the United States: evolution and challenges. *MMWR Suppl.* 2012;61(3):3-9.

29. Andrews JM, Quinby GE, Langmuir AD. Malaria eradication in the United States. *Am J Public Health Nations Health.* 1950;40(11):1405-1411.

30. Langmuir AD. The surveillance of communicable diseases of national importance. *N Engl J Med.* 1963;268:182-192.

31. Offit PA. The Cutter incident, 50 years later. *New Engl J Med.* 2005;352(14):1411-1412.

32. Fenner F, Henderson DA, Arita I. *Smallpox and its Eradication.* Geneva, Switzerland: World Health Organization; 1988.

33. Valleron AJ, Bouvet E, Garnerin P, et al. A computer network for the surveillance of communicable diseases: the French experiment. *Am J Public Health.* 1986;76(11):1289-1292.

34. Graitcer PL, Burton AH. The epidemiologic surveillance project: a computer-based system for disease surveillance. *Am J Prev Med.* 1987;3:123-127.

35. Richards CL, Iademarco MF, Anderson TC. A new strategy for public health surveillance at CDC: improving national surveillance activities and outcomes. *Public Health Rep* 2014;129(6):472-476.

36. Centers for Disease Control and Prevention. National Syndromic Surveillance Program. Available at https://www.cdc.gov/nssp/index.html. Accessed February 26, 2019.

37. Triple S. *Assessment of Syndromic Surveillance in Europe.* London, England: Lancet; 2011.

38. Cancer AC. *Cancer Program Standards: Ensuring Patient-Centered Care.* Chicago, IL: American College of Surgeons; 2016.

39. Buehler JW, Berkelman RL, Hartley DM, Peters CJ. Syndromic surveillance and bioterrorism-related epidemics. *Emerg Infect Dis.* 2003;9(10):1197-1204.

40. Lunde AS. *The Organization of the Civil Registration System of the United States.* Rockville, MD: International Institute for Vital Registration and Statistics; 1980.

41. Centers for Disease Control and Prevention. *National vital statistics system improvements. NCHS Fact Sheet.* 2015.

42. Atkinson D. *Modernizing the Mortality Data System – Capturing Opioid-Related Death Information to Enhance Data Dissemination and Research: National Center for Health Statistics Slide Set Prepared.* 2018.

43. Sandberg J, Santos-Burgoa C, Roess A, et al. All over the place? differences in and consistency of excess mortality estimates in Puerto Rico after Hurricane Maria. *Epidemiology.* 2019;30(4):549-552.

44. Nadon C, Van Walle I, Gerner-Smidt P, et al; FWD-NEXT Expert Panel. PulseNet International: vision for the implementation of whole genome sequencing (WGS) for global food-borne disease surveillance. *Euro Surveill.* 2017;22(23):30544.

45. Aarestrup FM, Brown EW, Detter C, et al. Integrating genome-based informatics to modernize global disease monitoring, information sharing, and response. *Emerg Infect Dis.* 2012;18(11):e1.

46. Bleiber J, West DM. *Three Ways mobile Helped Stop the Spread of Ebola in Nigeria.* Washington, DC: Brookings; 2015.

47. Sacks JA, Zehe E, Redick C, et al. Introduction of mobile health tools to support Ebola surveillance and contact tracing in Guinea. *Glob Health Sci Pract.* 2015;3(4):646-659.

48. National Center for Health Statistics. *Surveys and Data Collection Systems.* 2018.

49. National Health Service. Health Survey for England 2016. Published December 2018;13.

50. Pullum TW. *Strategies to Assess the Quality of DHS Data.* DHS Methodological Reports No. 26. Rockville, MD: ICF, 2019.

51. Dandona R, Pandey A, Dandona L. A review of national health surveys in India. *Bull World Health Organ.* 2016;94:286-296A.

52. Brownstein JS, Freifeld CC, Reis BY, Mandl KD. Surveillance sans frontières: internet-based emerging infectious disease intelligence and the HealthMap project. *PLoS Med.* 2008;5(7):e151.

53. Brownstein JS, Freifeld CC, Madoff LC. Digital disease detection – harnessing the web for public health surveillance. *N Engl J Med.* 2009;360(21):2153-2157.

54. Centers for Disease Control and Prevention. Global Health Protection and Security: Global Disease Detection (GDD) Program. Available at https://www.cdc.gov/globalhealth/healthprotection/gdd/index.html. Accessed March 2, 2019.

55. World Health Organization. *Guidelines for the Management of Sexually Transmitted Infections.* Geneva, Switzerland: World Health Organization; 2003.

56. Williams DR, Lawrence JA, Davis BA. Racism and health: evidence and needed research. *Annu Rev Public Health.* 2019;40:105-125.

57. European Center for Disease Control and Prevention. EU Case Definitions. Last update 2018.

58. NNDSS Annual Report Working Group. Australia's notifiable disease status, 2014: annual report of the national notifiable diseases surveillance system. Part 1. *Commun Dis Intell Q Rep.* 2016;40(1):E48-145.

59. Doyle TJ, Glynn MK, Groseclose SL. Completeness of notifiable infectious disease reporting in the United States. An analytical literature review. *Am J Epidemiol.* 2002;155:866-874.

60. Jajosky RA, Groseclose SL. Evaluation of reporting timeliness of public health surveillance systems for infectious diseases. *BMC Public Health.* 2004;4(29).

61. Rothenberg R, Bross DC, Vernon TM. Reporting of gonorrhea by private physicians: a behavioral study. *Am J Public Health.* 1980;70:983-986.

62. McGeary MGH. *Medicare conditions of participation and accreditation for hospitals.* In: *Institute of Medicine (US) Committee to Design a Strategy for Quality Review and Assurance in Medicare.* Washington, DC: National Academies Press US; 1990. chap 7.

63. Traeger MS, Wiersma ST, Rosenstein NE, et al. First case of bioterrorism-related inhalational anthrax in the United States, Palm Beach county, Florida 2001. *Emerg Infect Dis.* 2002;8(10):1029-1034.

64. Office of National Coordinator for Health Information Technology. Improving Clinical Care and Public Health With Electronic Case Reporting. Presentation made January 17, 2017. Available at https://www.cdc.gov/ehrmeaningfuluse/docs/ehr-vendors-collaboration-initiative/2017-01-17-digitalbridge_cdc_ehr_-vendor_final.pdf. Accessed March 2, 2019.

65. Mason TJ, McKay FW, Hoover R, Blot W. *Atlas of Cancer Mortality for US Counties 1950-1969.* Washington, DC: US Government Printing Office; 1975.

66. Hankey BF, Ries LA, Edwards BK. The surveillance, epidemiology, and end results program: a national resource. *Cancer Epidemiol Biomarkers Prev.* 1999;8(12):1117-1121.

67. Wingo PA, Howe HL, Thun MJ, et al. A National framework for cancer surveillance in the United States. *Cancer Causes & Control.* 2005;16(2):151-170.

68. Kirby RS, Browne ML. Connecting the circle from surveillance to epidemiology to public health practice. *Birth Defects Res.* 2019;111(18):1327-1328. doi:10.1002/bdr2.1602.

69. Mehta P, Kaye W, Raymond J, et al. Prevalence of amyotrophic lateral sclerosis–United States, 2014. *MMWR Morb Mortal Wkly Rep.* 2018;67(7):216-218.

70. Reeves MJ, Broderick JP, Frankel M, et al; Paul Coverdell Prototype Registries Writing Group. The Paul Coverdell national acute stroke registry: initial results from four prototypes. *Am J Prev Med.* 2006;31(6):S202-S209.

71. Wareham NJ, Forouhi NG. Is there really an epidemic of diabetes? *Diabetologia.* 2005;48(8):1454-1455.

72. Mokdad AH, Ford ES, Bowman BA, et al. Diabetes trends in the US: 1990-1998. *Diabetes Care.* 2000;23(9):1278-1283.

73. Beckles GL. Disparities in the prevalence of diagnosed diabetes–United States, 1999-2002 and 2011-2014. *MMWR Morb Mortal Wkly Rep.* 2016;65(45):1265-1269.

74. Liese AD, D'Agostino RB Jr, Hamman RF; Youth Study Group SEARCH. The burden of diabetes mellitus among US youth: prevalence estimates from the SEARCH for Diabetes in Youth Study. *Pediatrics*. 2006;118(4):1510-1518.

75. Chamany S, Silver LD, Bassett MT, et al. Tracking diabetes: New York city's A1C registry. *Milbank Q*. 2009;87(3):547-570.

76. NSW Health. *Disease Notification*. 2018. Available at https://www.health.nsw.gov.au/Infectious/Pages/notification.aspx. Accessed March 8, 2019.

77. Florida Department of Health. *Health Care Practitioner Reporting Guidelines for Reportable Diseases and Conditions in Florida*. 2014.

78. Weiss D, Boyd C, Rakeman JL, et al. A large community outbreak of Legionnaires' disease associated with a cooling tower in New York City; 2015. *Public Health Rep*. 2017;132(2):241-250.

79. Holmberg SD, Osterholm MT, Senger KA, Cohen ML. Drug-resistant Salmonella from animals fed antimicrobials. *N Engl J Med*. 1984;311(10):617-622.

80. Hopkins RS, Tong CC, Burkom HS, et al. A practitioner-driven research agenda for syndromic surveillance. *Public Health Rep*. 2017;132(suppl 1):116S-126S.

81. Buehler JW, Hopkins RS, Overhage JM, Sosin DM, Tong V; CDC Working Group. Framework for evaluating public health surveillance systems for early detection of outbreaks: recommendations from the CDC Working Group. *MMWR Recomm Rep*. 2004;53(RR-5):1-11.

82. Roberts L, Lafta R, Garfield R, Khudhairi J, Burnham G. Mortality before and after the 2003 invasion of Iraq: cluster sample survey. *Lancet*. 2004;364(9448):1857-1864.

83. Alfaro S, Myer K, Ali I, Roberts L. Estimating human rights violations in south kivu province, democratic republic of the Congo: a population-based survey. *Vulnerable Child Youth Stud* 2012;7(3):201-210.

84. Hagopian A, Flaxman AD, Takaro TK, et al. Mortality in Iraq associated with the 2003-2011 war and occupation: findings from a National cluster sample survey by the University Collaborative Iraq Mortality Study. *PLoS Med*. 2013;10(10):e1001533.

85. World Health Organization. *Vaccination Coverage Cluster Surveys: Reference Manual, Version 3*. 2015.

86. Centers for Disease Control and Prevention. *Community Assessment for Public Health Emergency Response. Overview*. 2018.

87. Das M, Kim NJ. Using Twitter to survey alcohol use in the San Francisco Bay area. *Epidemiology*. 2015;26(4):e39-e40.

88. Guy GP Jr, Zhang K, Bohm MK, et al. Vital signs: changes in opioid prescribing in the United States, 2006-2015. *MMWR Morb Mortal Wkly Rep*. 2017;66(26):697-704.

89. National Highway Traffic Safety Administration. Fatality Analysis Reporting System. Available at https://www.nhtsa.gov/research-data/fatality-analysis-reporting-system-fars. Accessed March 9, 2019.

90. Zogg CK, Haring RS, Xu L, et al. The epidemiology of pediatric head injury treated outside of hospital emergency departments. *Epidemiology* 2018;29(2):269-279.

91. LOINC from Regenstrief. Available at loinc.org. Accessed June 27, 2020.

92. SNOMED International: Leading Healthcare Terminology, Worldwide. Available at snomed.org. Accessed June 27, 2020.

93. Krause G, Altmann D, Faensen D, et al. SurvNet electronic surveillance system for infectious disease outbreaks, Germany. *Emerg Infect Dis*. 2007;13(10):1548-1555.

94. World Health Organization. *Foodborne Disease Outbreaks: Guidelines for Investigation and Control*. Geneva, Switzerland: World Health Organization; 2008.

95. Centers for Disease Control and Prevention. The National Respiratory and Enteric Viruses Surveillance System (NREVSS). Available at https://www.cdc.gov/surveillance/nrevss/index.html. Accessed June 27, 2020.

96. Bayer R, Fairchild AL. Public health. Surveillance and privacy. *Science*. 2000;290(5498):1898-1899.

97. Hodges JG, Gostion LO, Jacobson PD. Legal issues concerning electronic health information: privacy, quality, and liability. *J Am Med Assoc*. 1999;282:1466-1471.

98. Prater VS. *Confidentiality, Privacy and Security of Health Information: Balancing Interests*. Chicago, IL: Biomedical and Health Information Sciences; 2014.

99. Centers for Disease Control, Prevention. HIPAA privacy rule and public health. Guidance from CDC and the US Department of Health and Human Services. *MMWR Morb Mortal Wkly Rep*. 2003;52(suppl 1-17):19-20.

100. National Health Service, England and Wales. The Health Service (Control of Patient Information) Regulations, 2002.

101. Donnelly M, McDonagh M. Health research, consent and the GDPR exemption. *Eur J Health Law*. 2019;26(2):97-119.

102. Mariner WK. Mission creep: public health surveillance and medical privacy. *BUL Rev*. 2007;87(347):347-395.

103. Baltrusaitis K, Brownstein JS, Scarpino SV, et al. Comparison of crowd-sourced, electronic health records based, and traditional health-care based influenza-tracking systems at multiple spatial resolutions in the United States of America. *BMC Infectious Diseases*. 2018;18(1):403.

104. Patients Like Me: About Us. Available at https://www.patientslikeme.com/about. Accessed June 27,2020.

105. Lawatlas. The Policy Surveillance Program. Available at http://lawatlas.org/. Accessed June 27, 2020.

106. Karon JM, Devine OJ, Morgan WM. Predicting AIDS incidence by extrapolating from recent trends. In: Castillo-Chavez C, ed. *Mathematical and Statistical Approaches to AIDS Epidemiology*. Berlin: Springer-Verlag, 1989;58-88.

107. Painter I, Eaton J, Lober W. Using change point detection for monitoring the quality of aggregate data. *Online J Public Health Inform*. 2013;5(1):e186.

108. Council of State and Territorial Epidemiologists (CSTE). *Revised Guidelines for Determining Residency for Disease Notification Purposes*. Position statement 11-SI-04 adopted at 2011 CSTE annual meeting, Pittsburgh, PA. Available at https://cdn.ymaws.com/www.cste.org/resource/resmgr/PS/11-SI-04.pdf. Accessed June 27, 2020.

109. Cromley EK. GIS and disease. *Annu Rev Public Health*. 2003;24:7-24.

110. Janes GR, Hutwagner L, Cates W, Stroup DF, Williamson GD. Descriptive epidemiology: analyzing and interpreting surveillance data. In: Teutsch SM, Churchill RE, eds. *Principles and Practice of Public Health Surveillance*. 2nd ed. Oxford, NY: Oxford University Press; 2000:112-167.

111. Waller L. Detecting disease clustering in time or space. In: Brookmeyer R, Stroup DF, eds. *Monitoring the Health of Populations: Statistical Principles and Methods for Public Health Surveillance*. Oxford, NY: Oxford University Press; 2004:167-201.

112. Armstrong GL, Brammer L, Finelli L. Timely assessment of the severity of the 2009 H1N1 influenza pandemic. *Clin Infect Dis*. 2011;52(suppl 1):S83-S89.

113. Hutwagner L, Browne T, Seeman GM, Fleischauer AT. Comparing aberration detection methods with simulated data. *Emerg Infect Dis*. 2005;11(2):314.

114. Sekar CC, Deming WE. On a method of estimating birth and death rates and the extent of registration. *J Am Stat Assoc*. 1949;44(245):101-115.

115. Hook EB, Regal RR. Capture-recapture methods in epidemiology: methods and limitations. *Epidemiol Rev*. 1995;17(2):243-264.

116. Devine O. Exploring temporal and spatial patterns in public health surveillance data. In: Brookmeyer R, Stroup DF, eds. *Monitoring the Health of Populations: Statistical Principles and Methods for Public Health Surveillance*. Oxford, NY: Oxford University Press; 2004:71-98.

117. Civil Rights USO. *Guidance Regarding Methods for De-identification of Protected Health Information in Accordance with the Health Insurance Portability and Accountability Act (HIPAA). Privacy Rule*. 2012.

118. US Office of Management and Budget. Implementation guidance for title V of the E-government act, confidential information protection and statistical efficiency act of 2002 (CIPSEA). *Fed Regist*. 2007;72(115):33362-33367.

119. US Council National Research. *Putting People on the Map: Protecting Confidentiality with Linked Social-Spatial Data*. Washington, DC: National Academies Press; 2007.

120. Calba C, Goutard FL, Hoinville L, et al. Surveillance systems evaluation: a systematic review of the existing approaches. *BMC Public Health*. 2015;15:448.

121. Health Surveillance Coordinating Committee; Health Canada. *Framework and Tools for Evaluating Health Surveillance Systems*. Ottawa, ON: Health Canada; 2004.

122. European Centre for Disease Prevention and Control. *Data Quality Monitoring and Surveillance System Evaluation – A Handbook of Methods and Applications*. Stockholm: ECDC; 2014.

123. Klaucke DN, Buehler JW, Thacker SB, Parrish RG, Trowbridge FL. Guidelines for evaluating surveillance systems. *MMWR Morb Mortal Wkly Rep*. 1988;6(S-5):1-18.

124. Hopkins RS. Design and operation of local and state infectious disease surveillance systems. *J Public Health Management Pract*. 2005;11(3):184-190.

125. Lukacik G, White J, Noonan-Toly C, DiDonato C, Backenson PB. Lyme disease surveillance using sampling estimation: evaluation of an alternative methodology in New York state. *Zoonoses Public Health*. 2018;65(2):260-265.

126. Centers for Disease Control and Prevention (CDC). Ten great public health achievements–United States, 1900-1999. *MMWR Morb Mortal Wkly Rep*. 1999;48(12):241-243.

127. Centers for Disease Control and Prevention. Ten great public health achievements–United States, 2001-2010. *MMWR Morb Mortal Wkly Rep*. 2011;60(24):814-818.

128. Foege WH, Hogan RC, Newton LH. Surveillance projects for selected diseases. *Int J Epidemiol*. 1976;5(1):29-37.

129. Olson DR, Konty KJ, Paladini M, Viboud C, Simonsen L. Reassessing Google Flu Trends data for detection of seasonal and pandemic influenza: a comparative epidemiological study at three geographic scales. *PLoS Comput Biol*. 2013;9(10):e1003256.

CHAPTER 10

Field Methods

Lauren A. Wise and Patricia Hartge

This chapter discusses primary data collection, also known as field methods, which may be defined as the operationalization of study design. Field methods encompass all phases of study implementation, from the recruitment of study participants, through the collection of all data and materials, to the creation and management of databases for analysis. Primary data collection affects a study's validity, precision, cost efficiency, and ultimate value for research. With the use of increasingly large data sets, epidemiologists today tend to have less training in and experience with field methods than their predecessors.[1-3] Whether those who analyze data from a specific study were directly involved in the field methods, appropriate analysis and interpretation of epidemiologic data require a thorough understanding of the field methods employed.

SETTING AND SUPERVISION

Characteristics of the underlying study population inform every feature of the field methods used in an epidemiologic investigation. For example, methods for studies in resource-poor nations often differ markedly from those in wealthy nations. Methods useful in populations that are completely enumerated (*e.g.*, with national registration) differ from those in populations that can be defined but lack accessible rosters. Language, culture, health status, and social class all influence field design choices. Strategies for recruiting participants depend not only on the general study design but also on the specific design elements, including any requirements for future contact, access to family or colleagues, use of invasive procedures, need for corroborating documents or retrospective exposure assessment. In all studies, ethical requirements, privacy protections, and logistical considerations constrain the choices. Incentives or other methods to increase motivation may be needed to achieve adequate response rates.[4]

In many epidemiologic studies, data collection includes questioning the participant in person, via email, on the telephone, in writing, or via the Internet ("questionnaires"). Many studies also include search and extraction of data from external documents, such as certificates or birth or death, medical records, or employment records ("abstracts"). Many epidemiologic studies also include the measurement of biological markers ("biospecimens") or measures from the environment ("environmental samples"). Virtually all studies now employ the Internet in various ways, including for advertising the study, recruitment, data collection, study management, and documentation. Randomized trials and other experimental studies include another major element, the assignment (*e.g.*, to the intervention or to control). Selected examples of epidemiologic trials and large cohort studies are shown in Tables 10-1 and 10-2.

The principal investigators obtain human participants' approval for the study, as well as for any pilot studies that precede it or subsidiary studies conducted later. For large or complex studies, a study coordinator typically directs daily operations; in multicenter studies, each center may have its own study coordinator as well. Powerful, user-friendly Internet-based software and smaller, lighter, varied hardware are widely available, giving multiple users access to updated data. An experienced and capable study coordinator benefits the operation of the study but the principal epidemiologist still bears the primary responsibility for the implementation. Modern study management systems allow the epidemiologist to monitor the implementation closely.

Epidemiologists work to ensure the quality of the field operations in many ways. First, they try to anticipate the potential challenges of the study, based on previous work by other investigators or preliminary work carried out by the research team (*e.g.*, via pilot testing of standard and alternative methods). Many studies now post detailed study protocols, manuals, and procedures on a study website, providing access to methods that have been tested elsewhere. Epidemiology, other biomedical, and survey research journals publish useful reports on field methods, information that helps the investigator to select appropriate methods and anticipate the likely direction and magnitude of potential study biases.

Second, the principal investigators participate actively in testing the study instruments and procedures.[4,26] To assess the utility of a new method, a major adaptation of a standard method, or a standard method used in a challenging setting, investigators often conduct separate preliminary studies ("pilot study") before finalizing the study procedures. Investigators also employ a wide variety of techniques to pretest the data collection in realistic settings. They may conduct a few interviews, abstract records or collect biospecimens and environmental samples. Often, the investigators will observe study staff at work, watching directly or through one-way mirrors, listening to recorded interviews, monitoring online as Internet-based questionnaires are completed, and talking with participants after data collection.

Third, the investigators are responsible for the documentation of study operations and procedures, including all quality-control plans. The study protocols, manuals, and procedures, are critical for all users of the data and helpful to investigators designing other studies. These need to be kept up to date, especially for complex or long-running studies. The quality-control plans, which are key to monitoring the study as it is being conducted, cover all phases of the study (training, data collection, data entry, coding and analysis). Effective quality-control plans assure protocol adherence, support standardization, and aid in staff retention. In part, a study's degree of complexity and its overall goals determine the quality control plan. The primary goal remains collection of reliable and valid data; a secondary goal is to gather additional information on that reliability and validity in order to inform the analysis.

RECRUITMENT AND PARTICIPATION

In studies conducted in industrialized countries, investigators rely on nearly universal telephone service, widespread access to the Internet, and high rates of literacy. Furthermore, some countries (*e.g.*, in Scandinavia) have complete population rosters and registries, which have been used extensively for research purposes.[27-30] Similar types of studies can sometimes be accomplished within closed populations that are completely covered by rosters, for example, within health maintenance organizations.[31-33] Access to such databases is usually restricted to prevent violation of privacy from the linkage of personal information across databases.

In resource-limited settings, study methods are adapted to the technologies that are locally accessible. Other factors to be addressed include cultural differences (language, traditions, beliefs) and global logistics (protocol approval, specimen shipment, specimen storage, training, local laws, communication). For example, in cultures where women typically give birth at home, study staff can measure birth characteristics by keeping close track of due dates and visiting the home on the birth date with a scale and tape measure.[34] A village elder may decide whether the entire community will participate in a study.[35] Mobile phones, laptop computers, and other portable devices that are not common in the community still may be feasible if they are easily maintained, provide an incentive for participation, or offer improvements in data collection. Translating questionnaires into different languages and dialects are options, and cross-cultural adaptation and validation may be necessary to improve scientific vigor and response.[36,37] Back translation of questionnaires can increase validity.[38]

General principles govern the protection of human participants in research. Historical events that prompted concern about freedom of consent, disclosure of risks, and adequacy of treatment have spurred the evolution of principled statements such as the Nuremberg Code (http://way-back.archive-it.org/4657/20150930181802/http://www.hhs.gov/ohrp/archive/nurcode.html), the Declaration of Helsinki (https://www.wma.net/policies-post/wma-declaration-of-helsinki-ethical-principles-for-medical-research-involving-human-subjects/), the Belmont Report (https://www.hhs.gov/ohrp/regulations-and-policy/belmont-report/read-the-belmont-report/index.html), and the Common Rule (https://www.hhs.gov/ohrp/regulations-and-policy/regulations/finalized-revisions-common-rule/index.html), which then yielded special regulations and guidelines for researchers to follow in the protection of human participants. Although the adaptation of these principles and customs vary among study populations, it is important that researchers be aware of them when designing and conducting studies that involve human participants.

Experimental Studies

For experimental studies (including randomized clinical trials), investigators select from existing lists of potential participants, with current contact information, and approach them individually. For example, in a trial to investigate the role of diet in the recurrence of colorectal adenomas, the investigators identified potential participants by obtaining referrals from participating gastroenterologists and by reviewing medical records of participating endoscopy services.[39] A trial examining the effects of α-tocopherol and β-carotene intake on lung cancer targeted male smokers because of their high risk of disease.[40] Physicians were targeted for a trial of the effect of low-dose aspirin and β-carotene on multiple health outcomes, not because of their risk of disease but because of their interest and likely compliance with the experimental regimen.[41] In a trial of postmenopausal hormone use and diet in relation to breast cancer and other outcomes, investigators targeted women at elevated risk of developing breast cancer.[42,43]

When there is no list from which to recruit participants for intervention studies, investigators often use public notices or advertisements in a variety of settings, including television, radio, newspapers, magazines, and traditional settings (*e.g.*, doctors' offices, university postings, local shops, and restaurants), or the Internet (*e.g.*, social media and health-related websites). Epidemiologists often solicit sponsorship or endorsement by prominent people and community members or medical organizations to increase interest. Many trials and clinic-based studies offer reimbursement for parking or other minor costs of participation. If the time commitment or physical demands of the study are large (*e.g.*, if the study involves biospecimen collection over time points), financial compensation may be necessary. Ultimately, recruitment succeeds by persuading the participants of the value of the intervention study to themselves (*e.g.*, they may receive a free medical examination) and to society.

Typically, randomization follows recruitment. After satisfying all of the eligibility criteria and consenting to participate, participants are randomly assigned to one of the trial arms. Because randomization cannot guarantee a balance of risk factors across the intervention arms, particularly if the study size is small, the investigator should measure a wide range of potential confounders on a baseline questionnaire. The investigator should also collect contact information on the participants until the end of the follow-up period (*e.g.*, names, home address, work address, email address, and

TABLE 10-1

Selected Trials

Name of Study	Years of Study	Characteristics of Study Population	Study Intervention	Key Methods Paper	Link to Study Website (if Available)
Effects of Aspirin in Gestation and Reproduction (EAGeR)	2007-2011	• 1,228 females with one or two previous pregnancy losses • Aged 18-40 y • Trying to get pregnant • Four US medical centers	Daily aspirin (81 mg/d) plus folic acid versus placebo plus folic acid	5	https://www.nichd.nih.gov/about/org/diphr/officebranch/eb/effects-aspirin
Effect of Vitamin D and Calcium Supplementation on Cancer Incidence in Older Women	2009-2015	• 2,303 healthy females • Postmenopausal • Aged ≥55 y • Nebraska	• Vitamin D3 (2000 IU) and calcium (1,500 mg) daily vs. placebo pills	6	
The Learning Early about Peanut Allergy (LEAP) trial	2006-2009	• 640 infants from the United Kingdom with severe eczema, egg allergy, or both. • Aged 4-11 mo at randomization	• Consumption or avoidance of peanuts until 60 mo of age	7	http://www.leapstudy.co.uk/
The Prostate, Lung, Colorectal, and Ovarian Cancer Screening Trial (PLCO)	1993-2011	• 37,000 females and 37,000 males • Aged 55-74 y • No history of cancer or cancer treatments • No colonoscopy, sigmoidoscopy, or barium enema in past 3 y • United States	• Screening with flexible sigmoidoscopy • Screening with chest X-ray • Screening men with digital rectal examination plus serum prostate-specific antigen • Screening women with CA125 and transvaginal ultrasound	8	https://prevention.cancer.gov/major-programs/prostate-lung-colorectal

Study	Years	Population	Intervention(s)	Reference
Promotion of Breastfeeding Intervention Trial (PROBIT)	1996-1998	• 17,046 mother-infant pairs • Singleton full-term infants weighing at least 2,500 g and at least 37 wk gestation • Republic of Belarus (31 maternity hospitals)	• Baby-Friendly Hospital Initiative of WHO/UNICEF, which emphasizes healthcare worker assistance with initiating and maintaining breastfeeding and lactation and postnatal breast-feeding support, vs. usual infant feeding practices and policies [9]	
Women's Health Initiative (WHI)	1993-2005 (extension studies: 2005-2010 and 2010-2020)	• 161,808 females • Aged 50-79 y • Postmenopausal • Intending to reside in the area for at least 3 y • United States	• Hormones (0.625 mg estrogen + 2.5 mg progestin vs. placebo) • Dietary modification (no diet change vs. diet change) • Calcium and vitamin D (1000 mg calcium + 400 IU vitamin D3 daily vs. placebo) [10]	https://www.whi.org/SitePages/WHI%20Home.aspx
Women's Health Study (WHS)	1992-2004	• 39,876 female health professionals • Aged 45 y or older • No history of cancer, cardiovascular disease, or other major chronic illness	• Aspirin (100 mg every other d) versus placebo pill • Vitamin E (600 IU every other d) vs. placebo pill	Aspirin paper[11]: Vitamin E paper[12]: http://whs.bwh.harvard.edu/

TABLE 10-2

Selected Large Cohort Studies

Name of Study	Years of Study	Characteristics of Study Population	Number and Type of Questionnaires	Type of Data Collected	Key Methods Paper	Link
Black Women's Health Study (BWHS)	1995-present	• 59,000 women who self-identify as Black or African American • Aged 21-69 y • United States	• Baseline self-administered postal questionnaires • Biennial follow-up questionnaires (paper or Internet-based)	• Factors that influence health and disease such as contraception use, cigarette smoking, and diet plus any illnesses participants develop	[13]	https://www.bu.edu/bwhs/
California Teachers' Study (CTS)	1995-present	• 133,479 women • Teachers and administrators in California • Aged 22-104 y • 87% White, 3% Black/African American, 4% Hispanic, 6% other or mixed race	• Six self-administered questionnaires	• Health conditions and risk factors for cancer • California cancer registry linkage • Later projects involve biospecimens collection	[14]	https://www.cal-teachersstudy.org/
Coronary Artery Risk Development in Young Adults (CARDIA)	1985-present	• 5,115 Black and White men and women • Aged 18-30 y • United States (Birmingham AL, Chicago IL, Minneapolis MN, Oakland CA)	• Baseline examination • Follow-up in years 2, 5, 7, 10, 15, 20, 25, and 30	• Physical examination, lifestyle factors, substance use, behavioral and psychological variables, medical history • Laboratory tests • Blood samples	[15]	https://www.cardia.dopm.uab.edu/
Danish National Birth Cohort (DNBC)	1996-present	• Over 100,000 females enrolled in early pregnancy • Denmark	• Four computer-assisted interviews (twice during pregnancy, once when child is 6 mo old, once when child is 18 mo old) • One food frequency questionnaire mid-pregnancy • 6 additional follow-ups	• Lifestyle factors, exposures, medical and reproductive history	[16]	https://www.dnbc.dk/

Study	Dates	Population	Data collection	Measurements	Ref	URL
European Prospective Investigation into Cancer and Nutrition (EPIC) study	1990-present	• Over 521,000 females and males • Males aged 40-63 y and females aged 35-69 y • 10 western European countries	• Initial questionnaire • Follow-up questionnaire every 3-5 y (depending on country)	• Diet, lifestyle characteristics, anthropometric measurements, and medical history • Biospecimens collection	17	https://epic.iarc.fr/
Framingham Heart Study	Original = 1948 to present Offspring = 1971-2014 Third generation = 2002-2019 Omni cohort 1 (1994-2014) and 2 (2003-2019)	• Original cohort: • 5,209 males and females • Aged 30-62 y • Framingham, MA • Offspring cohort: • 5,124 males and females • Offspring of the original cohort and their spouses • Third-generation cohort: • 4,095 males and females • At least one parent in the offspring cohort • Omni cohorts: • 507 males and female • 410 males and females • living in or around Framingham, MA • Black/African American, Hispanic, Asian, Pacific Islander, Native American	• Baseline clinic visit • Check up every 2-6 y (in-person examination) • In between examination cycles, interim postal questionnaires • Same study design applies to all cohorts	• Medical history, physical examination, lifestyle interview, laboratory tests	Initial key methods paper[18]. Methods paper involving all cohorts[19].	https://www.framinghamheartstudy.org/

(Continued)

TABLE 10-2 (Continued)

Selected Large Cohort Studies

Name of Study	Years of Study	Characteristics of Study Population	Number and Type of Questionnaires	Type of Data Collected	Key Methods Paper	Link
Multi-Ethnic Cohort Study (MEC)	1993 to present (funding through 2022)	• 215,000 men and women • Hawaii and California • Aged 45-75 y • Five ethnic groups: White, Japanese American, Native Hawaiian, Black/African American, Latino	• Baseline questionnaire • Follow-up questionnaires every 5 y	• Medical history, family cancer history, lifestyle factors • Biospecimens	[20]	https://www.uhcancercenter.org/mec
Multi-Ethnic Study of Atherosclerosis (MESA)	2000-present	• 6,814 males and females • Aged 45-84 y • Asymptomatic • 38% White, 28% African American, 22% Hispanic, 12% Asian • Six clinics in the United States	• Baseline examination • Five additional examinations • Participants contacted every 9-12 mo	• Physical examination, lifestyle factors, blood samples	[21]	https://www.mesa-nhlbi.org/
Nurses' Health Study (1, 2, and 3)	1. 1976-present 2. 1989-present 3. 2010-present	1. 121,700 married registered female nurses aged 30-55 y living in 11 US states 2. 116,430 registered female nurses who started using oral contraceptives during adolescence, aged 25-42 y in US states 3. 45,000 female and male nurses aged 19-46 y, more diverse ethnic backgrounds, United States and Canada	1. Baseline questionnaire, follow-up questionnaires every 2 y, food-frequency questionnaire every 4 y 2. Baseline questionnaire, follow-up questionnaire every 2 y, food-frequency questionnaire every 4 y 3. 30-min online survey every 6 mo	1. Medical history, lifestyle factors, biospecimen collection 2. Diseases, reproductive history, contraception use, biospecimens collection 3. Medical history, lifestyle factors, reproductive history	[22]	https://www.nurseshealthstudy.org

Study	Dates	Population	Methods	Data collected	References
Pregnancy Study Online (PRESTO)/ Snart Foraeldre (SF)/ Snart Gravid (SG) Internet-based time-to-pregnancy studies	SG: 2007-2011 SF: 2011-present PRESTO: 2013-present	• Females aged 21-45 y; males aged ≥21 y • SG: 6,000 females • SF: 8,000 females, 1,500 males • PRESTO: 12,000 females, 3,000 males • Actively planning a pregnancy • Not using contraception or fertility treatments • United States, Canada, Denmark	• Online baseline questionnaire • Online follow-up questionnaires every 2 mo for up to 12 mo • Online food frequency questionnaire	• Socio-demographics, • Anthropometrics • Medical, reproductive, and contraceptive history • Diet • Blood, urine, vaginal swabs • Semen parameters	SG[23]: PRESTO[24]: http://www.snart-foraeldre.dk/ http://presto.bu.edu
Sister Study	2003-present	• 50,884 females • Aged 35-74 y • Sister(s) had breast cancer • No history of breast cancer at baseline • United States	• Baseline questionnaire • Follow-up questionnaire every 2-3 y or annual brief health update	• Residential and occupational history, sister(s) cancer history, lifestyle, socioeconomic status, anthropometric data, medical history • Biospecimens	[25] https://sisterstudy.niehs.nih.gov/ English/index1.htm

contact information for friends or relatives in the event that the participant cannot be located). Such information is critical because many intervention trials require regular follow-up via clinic visits or mailed questionnaires, with telephone calls to nonrespondents. Newer cost-effective options include the use of online questionnaires, apps, or text messaging to collect follow-up data.

Cohort Studies

Many cohorts intended broadly to reflect the general population have become major platforms for epidemiologic study, leading to hundreds of individual analyses and subsidiary investigations. Such cohorts require substantial investment over a sustained period, and they are increasingly seen as national or international resources that the research community shares. Table 10-2 lists selected cohort studies. Field methods employed in these studies often are described on study websites. The design of a general population cohort entails many trade-offs. For example, a cohort with greater variation in exposure might have lower compliance or quality of reporting than a restricted population.[44]

If a cohort study requires collecting the details of an exposure (timing, intensity, other exposures), the data sources used to characterize exposure may be the same as those needed to assemble the cohort. As the value of large overall study sizes has become clearer, consortia that combine cohorts have been formed.[45-47]

Different goals and challenges affect the assembly of cohorts specifically designed to assess the effects of an uncommon medical, occupational, environmental, or other exposure ("specialty cohorts"). For instance, in an occupational cohort study, the investigator assembles the cohort from the records of a company, a union, or a professional or trade association. Many preliminary studies use union or association records alone. In retrospective studies, these records often permit assembly of a complete cohort but lack the detail on tasks and work locations essential to defining each individual's jobs and exposures. When union and company records are available, both sources may be used to increase completeness. For an inception cohort, to be followed prospectively, the study staff might first recruit employers, then recruit workers within defined job categories, interview them to collect baseline information, and conduct follow-up to measure disease incidence.

At the outset, the study team (typically an epidemiologist, an industrial hygienist, a study manager, and one or more abstractors) examines the possible data sources, including occupation records, payroll ledgers, union rolls, medical records, and life and health insurance systems, both computerized and paper. The separate record systems may be incomplete but together enumerate of the cohort. Investigators may interview potential informants at different job levels, from clerical to managerial. Investigators may need access to record systems no longer maintained or stored separately, such as those from pensioners, workers terminated before pension eligibility, workers involved in litigation, or workers under medical care. It is critical to determine whether lists or records were modified once created, for example, to remove decedents, since failure to recognize modifications to records related to the outcome can induce immortal person-time bias. In sum, the assembly of a complete occupational cohort often requires considerable effort.

In medical specialty cohorts, which follow individuals with a particular medical condition or treatment, the investigators select potential participants from surveillance databases, hospital discharge files, pharmacy records, medical insurance data, birth certificates, or routine activity logs kept by medical practices, clinics, and hospital departments such as pathology, surgery, or obstetrics. As in occupational cohorts, investigators must determine whether any of the needed medical records have been moved, destroyed, or lost. Because medical histories and medical records are complex and variable, investigators generally make several preliminary visits to the hospital, clinic, or practice to investigate the sources and quality of data. Any procedures that will be used to confirm conditions or treatments must be specified in advance. Multiple record sources may be needed to determine whether a participant is eligible (e.g., surgical pathology logs to determine the diagnosis and hospital patient files to obtain demographic data).

Case-Control Studies

In a case-control study, the protocol describes the source population from which the cases and controls derive, as explicitly as possible. The choice of source population is constrained by the overall economic and political setting (e.g., whether national population rosters are available), the frequencies of the disease and exposures under study, and the difficulties in diagnosing and confirming disease. For example, the protocol for a case-control study might define the case group as all women in a given age range residing in a defined geographic area, who were newly diagnosed with pathology-confirmed cancer of the ovary during a specified period. The control group then must represent individuals from the same source population, *i.e.*, women in the age range, with one or both ovaries intact, residing in the defined geographic area during the specified time period. For efficiency, sampling may be stratified according to age, ethnicity, or other factors.

Historically, case-control studies were loosely classified as population-based, hospital-based, or clinic-based, but these distinctions ignore common hybrids, nested designs, and evolving Internet-based designs. The ideal setting for a "population-based case-control study" includes accessible rosters of the source population and an accurate registry of all cases occurring in it.[28-30] Often in the United States and elsewhere, the investigator has no access to a complete population roster but does have access to a complete roster of individuals with a particular disease (*e.g.*, cancer). (Such disease registries facilitate case-control studies, but they may be unsuitable if the disease is rapidly fatal and collection of additional data or new biospecimens are necessary.) Often the source population is well defined (*e.g.*, all residents of a geographic area in which cancers are reported to a central registry), but individual members of the population are not readily identifiable by name and address. In most parts of the United States, where no such population rosters exist, population-based sampling has been approximated with sampling from motor vehicle registries,[48,49] telephone directories or random-digit dialing,[50,51] or census tracts.[52] Once-useful approximations fail as patterns of telephone or motor vehicle use have changed markedly. Friends or neighbors once were used as controls, introducing various unmeasured distortions.[53,54]

In case-control studies based in hospitals, clinics, or medical practices, investigators gain access to a convenient list of potential cases (*e.g.*, from hospital records) not linked to an enumerated underlying population. To approximate a sample of the source population, namely, the people that would have gone to that hospital, clinic, or practice had they developed the medical condition, investigators may choose from the neighborhoods of the cases. Another common strategy is to select controls from among patients in other clinics within the same hospital. The protocol typically specifies which diagnoses are to be excluded from the control group because they are related to the exposures of interest. Additional exclusions often include psychiatric diagnoses or other conditions that compromise data collection. In one design variation, a few diagnostic categories are designated for inclusion rather than selecting from an unspecified mixture of diagnoses.

In hospital-based studies especially, it is important that procedures for case and control selection be defined unambiguously and followed consistently, from day to day and from patient to patient. Study staff assigned to select a patient from a clinic on a certain day should follow an algorithm that dictates which particular patient to pick. Such practices not only guard against unconscious enrollment of particular patient types but also allow routine quality checks. Data on patients who are unavailable or unwilling to be studied ought to be recorded so that nonresponse can be characterized.

Occasionally, a convenient population-based control group exists, but there is no disease registry for case ascertainment. In this situation, the investigator needs to locate the cases occurring in the base population using methods tailored to the nature of the medical condition. If the disease requires hospitalization or medical treatment, the study staff creates a disease registry by reviewing the records of hospitals, pathology laboratories, etc., while accounting for emigration, immigration, and medical care across boundaries.

Cross-Sectional Studies and Other Designs

Cross-sectional studies generally use a mixture of the selection and recruitment strategies needed for trials, cohort studies, and case-control studies. The sampling issues typify those of large population-based surveys.[55] Smaller targeted cross-sectional studies of volunteers continue to play a key role in epidemiology. For example, a study of the relation between family cancer history and the presence of founder mutations in the *BRCA1* and *BRCA2* genes among Ashkenazi Jews began with a recruitment campaign typical of any study of volunteers.[56]

Cost-efficient study designs are becoming increasingly popular in a time of limited funding for epidemiologic research. Because laboratory analyses of biologic samples or review of medical records can be expensive, large cohort studies typically employ case-cohort analyses (*i.e.*, selecting a random subset of participants at baseline and all incident cases) or nested case-control analyses (*i.e.*, selecting smaller sets of controls matched to incident cases on time and other factors). Use of these "nested" study designs increases cost efficiency without compromising statistical efficiency (see Chapter 8). Another cost-efficient study design is the case-crossover study, which is useful in settings where a brief exposure causes a transient change in risk of a rare acute-onset outcome.[57] With this method, each case serves as his or her own control. Self-matching of cases eliminates confounding by time-invariant factors, reduces control-selection bias, and increases efficiency.[57] Finally, cohort studies that involve Internet-based recruitment and follow-up represent another example of a cost-efficient study design, with some reports estimating that such studies can reduce costs by more than 50% per participant enrolled.[24,58]

Obtaining High Response

Obtaining high response rates while maintaining high data quality may well be the largest obstacle in epidemiologic research. Response rates are lower than they were decades ago.[59-62] They continue to vary internationally, often reported as higher in China (80%-90%) than in Europe (70%-80%) or the United States (60%-70%). The specific threats to validity depend on study design. In an experimental or cohort study, loss of target population at recruitment does not threaten validity, but loss during follow-up may, so investigators use methods designed to enhance retention. For case-control studies, investigators focus on reducing losses at first contact and on getting some information on all cases and controls.

Investigators need multiple strategies to persuade potential participants to consent to be enrolled, to gain their cooperation for each component, or to maintain an acceptable response rate in studies with repeated contact.[63] Broadly speaking, the strategies aim to increase motivation and attachment to the study, or reduce respondent burden, or incentivize participation. A large literature in epidemiology and in general survey research demonstrates the wide variety of techniques tried and their evolving efficacy in various settings.[60,63] In general, investigators need to persuade respondents that the study has value to them, their families and communities or society at large. Ideally, the investigators use a clear statement of what participation entails, arguments for electing to participate, and information about the source of study funding and the scientific institution at which the investigators work. Many large studies begin with a general public information campaign in advance of contacting individuals. Investigators may also use advance letters, telephone calls, or other endorsements from participants' physicians, community groups, or government agencies. Investigators increasingly post methods and materials on the study website. It is important to have the investigators and other individuals who can speak for the study readily available. Samples of the introductory materials in recent use are widely available from study websites; for older studies, investigators typically share examples. Investigators pretest all contact materials and procedures in the study setting in advance of study initiation or in a setting similar to the one envisioned for the study.

Burden reduction strategies also remain critical for success, and they all present challenging trade-offs in-depth of information collected.[64-68] Although the strategies vary according to the component (questionnaire, consent to abstract, biospecimen, environmental sample), the general approach is similar: compare the marginal perceived burden to the marginal likely gain in information. Pretesting remains essential. Sampling from the total study group for selected substudies offers options for in-depth collection from some but not all respondents. Similarly, abbreviated data collection from individuals who refuse the larger protocol offers options to get something from nearly everyone, and to gain insight into the nonresponders.

Incentives, financial or in-kind, have been extensively used in epidemiology, with considerable variation in impact.[69-72] In some settings, incentives are prohibited on the grounds that they may coerce response.[73] In some settings, the incentive is a valuable object (*e.g.*, a mobile phone) that is used for the data collection. In many settings, modest cash incentives have gained acceptance, coming to be seen as an appropriate expression of gratitude from the investigator to the responder for her time and inconvenience. The timing at which incentives are offered in prospective cohort studies (at baseline vs. over follow-up) can have important implications for bias and cost efficiency.[4,44]

Given a fixed budget for incentives, to enhance internal validity, incentives are best directed at maximizing follow-up (cohort retention) as opposed to initial recruitment. Proposed incentive plans may be pretested, sometimes with a no-incentive arm for comparison.[74]

Finally, participant motivation and attachment are worth acknowledging and renewing during or after the study, even in studies without repeated contact. Follow-ups for initial nonresponders often pay off. Letters and other messages of thanks are appropriate for participants. Newsletters on study progress are valuable to participants and nonparticipants.

DATA COLLECTION AND DATA CAPTURE

Abstracting Records

Abstracts distill information needed for the study from written records kept for other purposes, such as medical charts or employment records. The "abstract" itself may be in any format (paper, voice recording, website entry, etc.). Mobile computing devices or notebook computers simplify record abstraction, increase flexibility, and automate some quality control checks. Regardless of the platform for collection or the format, the abstract must record the participant's identification, the abstractor's identification, and the dates the abstract began and ended.

The larger and more variable the original record, the harder the abstract is to design. The designer tries to make the layout clear, the wording consistent, and the path through the abstract evident. Typically, abstracts use closed-ended questions, which have a prerecorded set of responses from which to select (e.g., participant's sex). Open-ended questions may be used to capture uncommon or more detailed responses (e.g., participant's health insurance provider), although such questions usually require more work in the analytic phase of the study (e.g., for data analyst to code responses). The abstractor often needs to distinguish between negative findings and absent findings for important items. Medical record abstractors should receive training in the medical terminology pertinent to the study and are not expected to glean from the charts what a physician specialist would. Therefore, the abstract reduces the need for interpretation, even at the expense of collecting some redundant data. Similarly, abstractors should be asked to complete items as similar as possible to the nature of the data found in the original record. Even if expert medical personnel are abstracting the records, record-keeping practices vary among hospitals and clinics, so the investigator may need to review charts in the study sites and to interview participating physicians or other health personnel to understand their recording practices. For some studies, the form needs to be designed to capture a relevant period only, or the entire history, with exclusions made in the analysis. Uniformity of the abstraction process is key to minimizing bias.

Devising good abstract forms may be hard, but testing them is usually easy. The investigator abstracts several records, and then one or more of the abstractors independently abstract the same records to measure interabstractor reproducibility.[75] This exercise can reveal gross errors or oversight in form design.

Questionnaire Administration

Questionnaires remain a mainstay of epidemiologic investigations, now administered in a wide variety of ways. A trained interviewer may ask the questions in person, over the telephone, or via Internet videoconferencing. In the self-administered alternative, the respondent reads the questions or hears them read aloud or both. The answers may be captured by audio or video recording, written on paper or entered on an electronic device (laptop, tablet). Interactive voice response and other automated systems offer additional rapidly evolving platforms.

Comparability between study groups is the overarching consideration in deciding on the methods of questionnaire administration. For example, case-control studies comparing hospitalized cases and hospitalized controls lend themselves to in-person interviews in the hospital. On the other hand, if controls are selected from the general population (to approximate the referral network), interviews conducted at home will be more comparable. If biospecimens are collected and an interview conducted, the protocol might specify one home visit to obtain both, home visits by two different field staff (e.g., an interviewer and a phlebotomist), a telephone interview and a home visit, and a home or telephone interview and the provision of respondent instructions and a mailer for collecting and shipping the specimen.

Standardization of questions and questioning both help increase comparability between study groups, but at a cost in information lost. For example, memory loss presents a serious problem, as many exposures under study did not seem interesting or important to the participant at the time they happened, let alone decades later.[76,77] Many cognitive interviewing techniques[78] improve recollection (*e.g.*, context reinstatement, focused retrieval, multiple representation). They work well for qualitative research but are harder to use in epidemiologic studies, surveys, and other quantitative research. Mixed methods investigations include a qualitative component, using structured investigative interviews, along with the quantitative component from which the measures of effect are estimated.

Staff-administered in-person interviews typically cost more than other modes because of the time needed to schedule appointments, travel between interviews (or pay for participant travel), and administer the interviews. Nevertheless, the greater intimacy of in-person interviews may increase the participant's willingness to participate or continue in the study. In-person interviews also tend to increase accuracy and depth of response, because the interviewer is able to clarify questions that are not clear to the respondent. Videoconference interviews by trained staff are available in some settings, reducing costs of travel and offering some of the advantages of direct in-person interviews.

Staff-administered telephone interviews have a few known disadvantages. Like in-person interviews, they require scheduling (after the participant provides initial consent to be approached). When a list of possible answers is read to them aloud, respondents tend to favor the first answer. Supervisors can monitor interviewing more easily in telephone interviews than in-person interviews because they can listen to the conversation. Some sensitive topics can be difficult to query by telephone, because the respondent may become suspicious of the interviewer or the legitimacy of the study. On the other hand, once the respondent trusts the study and develops rapport with the interviewer, questions about socially undesirable behaviors may be answered more readily over the telephone than in person because of the greater social distance in a telephone call.[79]

Self-administered instruments often cost less than interviewer-administered instruments, but they are also the least easily monitored and the most susceptible to misunderstood or skipped questions. Self-administered questionnaires may be mailed to the participant, sent by email, provided at an Internet site, or delivered in person. Internet-based self-administered questionnaires allow for checks that alert the respondent (in real time) to internal data inconsistencies or skipped questions. Self-administered questionnaires may offer advantages when asking sensitive or embarrassing questions because no interviewer is present.

Visual aids to memory can be incorporated into most modes of questionnaire administration, with the exception of voice-only telephone interviews. Photographs of medications help the respondent recognize individual formulations. Food models illustrate portion sizes in dietary interviews. Maps may be used in questions pertaining to residence or travel. Diaries, timelines, or calendar grids can improve accuracy of lifetime residential, occupational, or reproductive histories.

The investigator choosing among the many modes of questionnaire administration considers the length and nature of the questionnaire; the distribution by age, education, health, vision, and hearing of the participants; and the constraints of budget and staff. If several modes of data collection are available, the investigator may devise a pilot study comparing them.[80]

Content and Wording of Questions

Questionnaire designers grapple with the issues of cooperation, fatigue, meaning, memory, and honesty. Errors can be introduced by either the respondent or the interviewer, and the questionnaire should be designed to reduce both types of error. The design of epidemiologic questionnaires benefits from a vast body of survey research experience and literature.[79,81-83] In addition, hundreds of questionnaires are available online or are easily obtained electronically, including sets of questions on basic demographic data, common medical conditions and treatments, tobacco use, dietary patterns, and physical activity. Some of these instruments are copyrighted, requiring a fee for use.

Framing the questions has appropriately received a large amount of attention in survey research literature.[79,84] Wording matters in all surveys because people construe important and simple words such as *anyone, most, average, never,* or *fairly* in varied ways.[85] Medical terms with precise meanings should be explained simply; therefore, "people related to you by blood" may be clearer than "family" and "Has a doctor ever told you that you had...?" might be clearer than "Have you had...?" Lay terminology for illnesses is used when possible (*e.g.*, "heart attack" instead of "myo-cardial infarction"). On the other hand, "medications" may be less likely than "drugs" to be confused with illicit substances.

Question length also affects response. Short questions usually are clearer, but a longer question may improve respondent cognition. For instance, it is hard to absorb all the details of the question, "How many hours per week do you typically use this product in the summertime on weekdays?" The question may be more intelligible if it can be separated into specific questions to reduce the density of concepts[83] or preceded with a description of some of the concepts (*e.g.*, "I'd like you to think about the summertime. I will be asking you about weekdays separately from weekends.").

How many questions does the investigator need to ask on a topic? One or two questions may not gather enough information for a thorough analysis, particularly if an unexpected association emerges. On the other hand, a long series of questions on a single topic may bore the respondent and result in missing or inaccurate answers after the first few questions. Simply reporting a lifetime occupational history, lifetime residential history, or usual diet can easily take 20 minutes.

The order of questions can also affect response. Many questionnaires begin with questions that are not threatening and not taxing to the memory and, if possible, are interesting to the respondent.[79] Questions about sensitive topics usually follow questions about related but less sensitive topics. Some instruments precede such questions with a prologue that acknowledges the personal nature of the question, reiterates the participant's right not to answer, and states the importance of the question to the survey. The format of answers matters, too. For open-ended numerical responses (*e.g.*, how many years), respondents often show digit preference (for 0 and 5). For closed-ended items with an ordered list (*e.g.*, <5, 5-10, 11-19, ≥20), some respondents may favor a part of the range, often the central part. Questions that require the participant to do extra work (*e.g.*, find a measuring tape to measure waist and hip circumference) increase potential for break-off. When higher risks for break-off can be anticipated, it is useful to think of ways to reduce the risk (*e.g.*, enclosing a measuring tape with the questionnaire).

Often the investigators make small compromises in standardization to avoid losing critical data. For instance, a few telephone interviews may be conducted in an in-person interview study for participants who would not participate otherwise. If participants are incapacitated or deceased, proxy information can be useful. It is important to obtain consent from participants to use proxies and often only the most important exposure and outcome information is asked. Spouses tend to provide more complete and accurate data than other family members.[4]

Differences in the quality of data collection may arise from many sources, so the investigator may compare the rates and the reasons for nonresponse, as well as the length of the interview, the quality of understanding and response as assessed by the interviewer (poor, adequate, excellent), and the responses to questions that are expected not to differ between the groups. For example, a substantially longer interview in one group raises the possibility of differential accuracy or completeness of information.

Questionnaires and Respondent Burden

How much information can the questionnaire elicit? Self-administered instruments vary enormously in length. For staff-administered questionnaires, interviews commonly last 50 to 90 minutes in person and 30 to 60 minutes on the telephone. If participants are able to stop and continue the interview at a later time, some participants tolerate longer questionnaires. Usually, once an interview has begun, the participant continues to the end. On the other hand, longer interviews may increase the risk of break-off.[85] Many epidemiologists find it hard to resist including as many questions as possible, even if the quality of the answers decreases as the interview lengthens. Some investigators place the least critical (and/or most sensitive) questions near the end in case of break-off, but the effects of this practice are not known. Investigators of long-term prospective cohort studies may create participant advisory committees, formed of a subset of active participants (*e.g.*, 10-15 participants), to pilot-test the interpretability and acceptability of questions.

A nice feature of Internet-based self-administered questionnaires (relative to paper questionnaires) is that the investigator can glean useful data about the characteristics and determinants of break-off, specifically the proportion of individuals for whom it occurs and on which pages of the questionnaire. In unpublished data from PRESTO, it was found that of the men who started but did not complete their baseline questionnaires, a large proportion discontinued on the page that asked a particularly sensitive question. When the investigators added a new response option of "prefer not to answer," the break-off rates decreased appreciably. Finally, additional ways to decrease participant fatigue are to include a progress bar ("% questionnaire completed") on Internet-based surveys. Finally, the use of apps may enhance the ease with which participants can provide data.[67,86]

Special considerations arise with longitudinal studies that require repeated interviews. Timing questionnaire arrival on a strict annual schedule tied to the participant's birthday or the beginning of each calendar year may improve the likelihood that participants report only events that occurred since the last contact. Otherwise, it is best to avoid questions that refer to "Since we asked you last…" because of the risk of events being forgotten or repeated. Follow-up questionnaires should be shortened by omitting questions that the participants have already answered in previous follow-ups (*e.g.*, menopausal status and age at menopause).

Interviewing Techniques and Training

Interviewers are trained to apply standard interviewing techniques to the particular questionnaire. In studies with biospecimen collection, environmental sampling, and other components in addition to the interview, formal training sessions typically last 4 to 5 days and are followed by several weeks of practice. For a new interviewer, the interview supervisor checks many of the initial interviews, for instance, by attending the interview or reviewing an audio or video recording of it. After interviewers have mastered the techniques, a fraction of their interviews may be audited at random throughout the study.

The interviewer's first job is to persuade the participant to participate. The introduction should convey the scientific importance of the study and of the participant's participation without making participants with particular histories more or less likely to respond. If the participant refuses at first, the interviewer should make another effort to persuade the participant or learn the reason for refusal. The interviewer may ask the participant to talk to the supervisor or someone else before the participant gives a firm refusal. Interviewers document nonresponses with notes that help the supervisor or another interviewer approach the participant. Whenever possible, the interviewer should be blinded as to the participant's exposure or outcome status (depending on the study design).

After obtaining cooperation, the interviewer proceeds with the interview or arranges an appointment. Before an in-person interview, the interviewer arranges any equipment, memory aids, or materials.[87] The interviewer tries to arrange the setting and timing to minimize interruptions and distractions to the respondent. Occasionally, interviews must be stopped and resumed later. The interviewer must note these and other deviations in the administration of the questionnaire, as well as an assessment of the quality of the responses. In Internet-based studies, an editable questionnaire form should be created, not only for editing completed questionnaires, but for interviewing purposes (*e.g.*, if the participant requests a phone interview). If the interview is being conducted online, a hardcopy version of the questionnaire should be available to the interviewer in the event of unanticipated technical glitches (*e.g.*, the server goes down or is slow to respond). If responses are recorded on a paper questionnaire, they can be entered into the online forms by the interviewer after the interview.

Questions that the respondent does not understand are repeated slowly verbatim, not rephrased. If further clarification is needed, the interviewer follows the instructions given during training and in the study manuals. If the participant's answers are not clear or complete, the interviewer uses neutral probes, scripted clarifications, and definitions of medical or technical terms. When respondents require clarifications that are not scripted, interviewers offer to reread the question and ask participants to answer according to their best understanding. To conclude the interview, the interviewer should quickly review the questionnaire for omissions, thank the respondent, and explain that the supervisor may call the respondent to review the interviewer's work. In some studies, the investigator offers the participants the opportunity to be notified of the findings. For instance, report-back methods in environmental epidemiology studies are becoming commonplace.[88]

Physical Examinations

Epidemiologic studies can include physical examinations to measure blood pressure, assess anthropometrics, perform pelvic examinations or ultrasounds, and so on. The order and content of these examinations is much more explicitly prescribed than in a strictly clinical setting. Participants with no abnormal findings whatsoever (including most controls in case-control studies) may be fully examined and described to ensure comparability in the epidemiologic study. If any of the findings is abnormal, the participant should be notified and referred for clinical evaluation, if appropriate.

Examination forms often have complex logical branching, and the examiner has to be able to follow the branching during the examination. Pretesting and quality control are especially important to reduce variation among clinical observers. Studies of interobserver variation may be necessary when the physical examinations are subtle or complex.[75] For example, training in blood pressure measurement often uses a videotape test as an objective standard.

Physical examinations in epidemiologic studies may be conducted by medical or paramedical personnel, with oversight by a physician or other expert reviewer. If the expert reviewer does not see each participant, the examiner should record whether expert review occurred and distinguish the expert's evaluation from the original one.

Biospecimen Collection

Epidemiologic studies increasingly involve laboratory components requiring collection of urine, blood, or tissue from participants. Many of the experimental studies and cohort studies presented in Tables 10-1 and 10-2 include biospecimen collection. One common problem in biospecimen collection is unrecognized laboratory error. Indeed, epidemiologists usually need to investigate the reproducibility of the assay in a pilot study. Field problems may also arise in applying tests or assays to large-scale epidemiologic studies that previously have been conducted only on a small scale. For instance, laboratories that have developed an assay and can achieve high reproducibility with dozens of specimens may be unable to process the thousands of specimens required in a field study. Another typical problem arises when the investigator wishes to collect specimens for storage without a definite assay in mind, so the particular collection and storage requirements are not certain.

The protocol for collecting, processing, labeling, storing, and shipping the specimens is documented in a manual of operations. The biospecimen collection documentation records the participant identifier, the specimen number, whether the specimen was collected at baseline or a subsequent encounter, results of the collection (e.g., number of tubes drawn, medical complications), and processing and storage details (e.g., in which freezer the specimen is stored). Bar-coded labels reduce handwriting or keying errors, and clear, detailed shipping and storage lists minimize losses in transit and aid in tracking those that occur. If the investigator plans to assay a particular chemical in the biospecimen, special collection materials should be used that avoid contamination by that chemical (e.g., use of phthalate-free collection and storage tubes).

Environmental Samples and Global Positioning Systems

Epidemiologic studies sometimes include taking direct measurements of the participant's home or work environment, including chemicals in drinking water, air, soil, or carpet dust and levels of ionizing radiation, sunlight, or electromagnetic fields. These study components may dramatically improve the accuracy of exposure assessment, if the investigator can overcome the typical hurdles. Such issues include identifying a logistically feasible measurement technique, collecting and analyzing samples at an acceptable cost, obtaining the participant's permission and access to the environment for sampling, and (generally) limiting measurement to the current rather than a past environment.

Feasibility and cost are common challenges, even when toxicologists, industrial hygienists, radiation physicists, or other experts in the environmental exposure have developed reliable measurement techniques. Established exposure indicators are not necessarily suited to the size and settings of epidemiologic research. For example, a high-volume surface-sampler vacuum cleaner can extract carpet dust from which pesticide residues can be measured, but at a cost prohibitive to most studies. A convenient sample of the participant's own used vacuum cleaner bag provides an acceptable alternative.[89] Finding feasible and inexpensive methods that produce valid and reliable environmental measures often requires pilot studies before the field protocol can be finalized. Because field conditions cannot always be tightly controlled in population studies, the sampling technician should record the conditions under which the monitoring occurred.

The timing of the relevant exposure often complicates the interpretation of environmental samples in epidemiologic studies, which typically measure current environments. The levels of exposure at a particular place may have changed over time. The participant may have moved or changed jobs. Occasionally, multiple old sites can be monitored. Sometimes, a cumulative environmental measure can be obtained, such as radiation decay products that leave behind traces on glass mirrors or picture frames. More commonly, the investigator has data on longer-term exposure and links those to the current environmental measures to form various measures of exposure status.

As awareness of environmental hazards has increased, investigators have encountered both a greater willingness to permit environmental sampling and heightened interest in the levels found and their meaning. Epidemiologic investigations routinely notify participants with levels above any existing standards.[88] Most also report levels of any compound to a participant who requests the data, accompanied by a clear statement of any known risks and the level of uncertainty.

Increasingly, epidemiologic studies include the use of inexpensive global positioning systems (GPS) devices to record the latitude and longitude of the participant's home or workplace. The position can be linked to geographic information systems (GIS). Using GIS, the investigator can spatially display environmental and epidemiologic data. Applications for GIS in epidemiologic research include locating participants' addresses through geocoding, mapping the source contaminants, and integrating environmental data with disease outcome. Sometimes it is possible to reconstruct historical exposures. With the availability of an increasing number of environmental databases, GIS and GPS technology allow the investigator to link environmental monitoring data with the study population, providing a better understanding of the environmental contaminants and disease outcomes.[90]

Tracing

Some studies do not require contact with the participant but only a determination of vital status or date and cause of death. In the United States, relevant resources include the National Death Index (NDI), NDI Plus, Social Security Administration files, state mortality data tapes, Pension Benefit Information Services, driver's license and car registration records, and Internet mortality tracing. NDI provides the state where the death was recorded, the date of death, and the death certificate number. NDI Plus provides cause of death in addition to the other information. Cost, coverage, and quality vary among these sources.[91]

In some Western countries, complete population, birth, and death registries greatly simplify tracing. In some resource-poor settings (e.g., rural China), local governments have established a vital registration system to track people for births, deaths, marriage, and migration. Specific study follow-up tracking systems have also been established to trace participants in the Nutrition Intervention Trial and the Shandong Intervention Trial. In these instances, the field station staff worked closely with the local governments to ensure that all endpoints were reported and documented in a timely manner.[92]

If participants are to be questioned about outcomes or exposures (active follow-up), they must first be located. With recent, accurate, detailed information on the participant's name, address, telephone number, Social Security or other identification number, parents' names (for a child), and spouse's name and employer, the investigator may begin by mailing information to the last address or by telephoning the participant. Without such detailed information, the investigator should use methods described below to locate the participant. If many participants have died, a vital status search may be the first step.

The more out of date the last known address is, the more difficult the tracing will be. On the other hand, in many countries, tracing is easier if many cohort members have died. The algorithm for tracing depends on the composition of the cohort. In occupational cohort studies, the investigator often knows the participant's Social Security or other national identification number, which helps in matching to mortality registries and other files. With medical cohorts,[93,94] identifying data are often sparser and less accurate, so many sources may be needed to find a large proportion of the cohort. Additional problems arise in following cohorts of women (*e.g.*, because of changes in surname)[95] or cohorts exposed before or at birth.[96] Studies involving women should always elicit data on maiden and married surnames to enhance participant follow-up and optimize ability for data linkage (*e.g.*, vital records).

Follow-Up Techniques

For studies requiring active follow-up, participant tracing and collection of outcome data are usually conducted in tandem. Procedures for mailing the questionnaires or interviewing by telephone or in person are similar to those in case-control studies. One typical procedure is to mail the follow-up questionnaire once, wait a few weeks for its return, mail a second questionnaire to nonrespondents, and then telephone the remaining nonrespondents. The second mailing and the telephone call both increase response markedly in most studies.

Longitudinal studies require repeated follow-ups and present special problems. In some circumstances, nonrespondents in one wave can be approached in subsequent waves. Subsequent waves usually achieve greater response proportions than the initial wave because those not inclined to participate usually refuse the first time. On the other hand, if the cohort has been followed several times, motivation to answer more questions may wane, especially if the questions are repeated on each follow-up. Participants' willingness to participate can be enhanced with periodic study newsletters, describing study findings and progress. Particularly sensitive questions (*e.g.*, abuse victimization) can be added in subsequent waves, after rapport with participants has been established. Increasingly, investigators develop Internet sites to disseminate study findings, in the hope of encouraging participant participation in the next wave of follow-up. In some studies, participants who refuse are not contacted in subsequent waves. Even with excellent response rates in each wave, the multiple opportunities for nonresponse lower the cumulative response rate.

Often, investigators design a study that requires using data from other sources to confirm outcomes reported by participants or their next of kin on follow-up questionnaires. For instance, once the fact of death is known, the cause of death can be collected from the death certificate. Serious illnesses can also be confirmed and detailed by obtaining additional records. For cancers among residents of an area covered by a tumor registry, the registry can often confirm a cancer reported by the participant or next of kin[97] and provide many additional details regarding tumor characteristics. For other conditions requiring hospitalization, records can be requested from the hospital with permission from the patient. Timing is critical because some hospitals do not honor permission forms that were signed beyond a certain period of time.

Updating Exposure Information

The collection of repeated exposure data over time can provide analytical opportunities to reduce random measurement error and evaluate temporal associations between exposure and disease.[44] Measured changes in exposures over time are a mix of true variation and measurement error. Thus, the comparison of participants whose exposures are consistently high with those whose exposures are consistently low can provide an informative assessment of the effects of cumulative exposure, as well as both long and short induction time.[44] An updated cumulative average of individual exposures maximizes use of all data for disease processes like cardiovascular disease or cancer, for which cumulative exposure is likely to have greater etiologic importance. Another benefit of repeated exposure collection is the ability to add items to the follow-up questionnaires to address new and evolving hypotheses (*e.g.*, H1N1, ZIKV viruses).

Data Capture

Data capture means transforming the research data collected in the field into clean files for data analysis. Since the earlier editions of ME, technology has transformed all aspects of data collection, data editing, data cleaning, and data release. Coding, or data reduction by study staff, still occurs in many studies because the questionnaires, abstracts, and other instruments collect narrative responses that require the assignment of codes either during or after data collection. When coding is necessary, often standardized and tested coding schemes are available (*e.g.*, International Classification of Diseases, Standard Industrial Classification codes). Occasionally special schemes must be devised for the study, and long-standing practices for coding data are described in detail in other texts.[81] The coding manual documents the schemes used to encode the data. Nonautomated coding should be performed by a person blinded to the exposure (if coding disease) or disease (if coding exposure) status of participants.

Historically, data from hard copy forms, or from coders' notes, were digitized ("keyed"), typically twice, with the second data entry clerk blinded to the already-keyed data. For identifiers and other critical items, double entry and other extra quality checks remain worthwhile. Computer-assisted and optically scanned forms do not need coding but require care in handling. Captured data are routinely checked to ensure they fall within a range of plausible answers ("range checks") and that they are internally consistent ("logic checks"). Inconsistent answers given by the respondent should be flagged but not changed. Errors in recording, coding, and keying should be corrected and logged.

The numbers of respondents and nonrespondents (overall and within specific groups) tracked by the management system during the field phase are compared and reconciled to the numbers in the data file to be used for analysis. The response counts and rates, manuals used during the field phase, study logs, and data collection instruments serve as essential reference documents throughout analysis and presentation of findings. Finally, the protocol may specify under what conditions collected data will be corrected after the field phase and data cleaning are complete.

EMERGING ISSUES

Epidemiologists are likely to encounter new challenges and opportunities: implementing procedures for the sharing of resources and data; working on interdisciplinary research teams; evaluating new methods to measure exposures, disease susceptibility, and outcomes; identifying new technologies to collect personal and macro-level data (*e.g.*, mobile health or "m-health," involving the use of apps or "wearables"); increasing use of Internet-based methods and mixed methods; and a greater emphasis on "big data" and precision medicine, community-based participatory research, and implementation science.

With the widespread use of health-related and social media websites by the general population, Internet-based recruitment methods are becoming more popular. Platforms like Facebook, Google, and Twitter can be used to place banner advertisements that target individuals who may be suitable for a specific research study, such as by gender, age, and geographic region.[24,98,99] The cost of Internet-based recruitment has been shown to be substantially lower than traditional methods,[24,58] without sacrificing validity.[100-102] Special caution should be taken when interpreting results from cross-sectional studies that recruit participants using the Internet, as such studies might be particularly susceptible to selection bias.

Mixed methods research is defined as the use of quantitative and qualitative methods in a single study.[103-105] Qualitative methods, which are used to understand individual's beliefs, experiences, attitudes, behavior, and interactions, are increasingly used to inform epidemiologic practice. For example, epidemiologists may perform individual or group interviews (*i.e.*, focus groups) about attitudes and barriers toward participation in research to identify strategies to improve recruitment in cohort studies.[106] Likewise, qualitative data from focus groups have been used to improve the interpretability of survey questions[107] and design more effective interventions in clinical trials.[108]

In the 2010s, "big data" and "precision medicine" research projects are being prioritized by some funding bodies such as the National Institutes of Health.[1] For example, the NIH's All of Us Research Program (https://allofus.nih.gov/) is a large-scale effort established in 2018 to collect data from more than one million individuals living in the United States to accelerate research and improve health.[109] Researchers intend to examine individual differences in lifestyle, biology, and the environment with the goal of delivering precision medicine, defined as the tailoring of health-related practices and treatments to the individual. Tools employed in precision medicine can include molecular diagnostics, imaging, and analytics. As of January 2020, the study has enrolled more than 250,000 participants, with more than 50% self-identifying as racial and ethnic minorities. Big data approaches are supported by the lower costs and greater efficiency of powerful technologies (*e.g.*, whole genome sequencing), and the easy integration of such data with other personal data (*e.g.*, electronic health record systems). New apps on smartphones and other digital health technologies (*e.g.*, smart watches) can collect data from participants in a variety of locations. These new developments facilitate the generation and analysis of large data sets for answers to novel research questions. The emphasis on big data and precision medicine has not gone without criticism by some epidemiologists, however, particularly those who worry that these approaches could come "at the expense of engagement with the broader causal architecture that produces population health."[110]

Community-based participatory research is defined as "systematic inquiry with the participation of those affected by the problem, for the purposes of education and action or affecting social change."[111] Community-based participatory research is not a research method but a perspective on research that emphasizes equitable engagement of partners throughout the research process, from identifying the health problems and generating the research questions of interest, through data collection and analysis, to dissemination and use of findings to inform health care and policy.[112,113]

Implementation science leverages interdisciplinary methods to promote the uptake and dissemination of effective interventions in real-world settings.[114] Implementation strategies include approaches that facilitate and sustain the delivery of evidence-based technologies, practices, or services.[115-117] Qualitative and quantitative methods are often used to measure implementation outcomes, including acceptability, cost, feasibility, adherence, and sustainability.[118-120] Theoretical frameworks to support implementation science include those that guide the translation of research into practice, study the determinants of implementation success, and assess the impact of implementation.[117]

Compared with their peers who used the first three editions of this text, epidemiologic investigators are now more likely to work on teams that encompass other disciplines. The team approach often accompanies an expanded study scope or size. In addition, there may be more than one epidemiologist responsible for overall study design, conduct, and analysis. Indeed, many immensely informative epidemiologic studies, especially cohort studies, have passed to their second or third generation of investigators, with key design decisions having been made decades ago. Data pooling, meta-analysis, multicenter studies, and research consortia all require common data elements (see, for example, the PrePARED consortium of preconception cohort studies[121]: https://sph.tulane.edu/prepared-consortium), with some epidemiologists being required to standardize data collection (see, for example, NIH's ECHO initiative[122]: https://www.nih.gov/research-training/environmental-influences-child-health-outcomes-echo-program). It is now standard practice for research institutions to implement data use agreements to protect all parties engaged in research.

If the epidemiologists are pulled in many directions, the field effort may be the phase most likely to be given short shrift. Fortunately, more survey researchers, clinical collaborators, and laboratory scientists have some specialized training and experience in health studies in general and in epidemiology in particular. Researchers in these disciplines typically have a strong interest in some or all of the field methods of a study. Epidemiologists need to work closely with the rest of the team, and they need to maintain responsibility for the conduct of the study. The "field methods"—as outlined in the study protocol, detailed in the manuals of operations and procedures, and bolstered by quality control activities—still form the central bridge between sound design and credible analysis.

ACKNOWLEDGMENTS

We are grateful to the Jessica Levinson for her editorial assistance. We also thank Jack Cahill for his contributions to earlier versions of this chapter.

References

1. Khoury MJ. Planning for the future of epidemiology in the era of big data and precision medicine. *Am J Epidemiol*. 2015;182(12):977-979.
2. Brownson RC, Samet JM, Chavez GF, et al. Charting a future for epidemiologic training. *Ann Epidemiol*. 2015;25(6):458-465.
3. Ehrenstein V, Nielsen H, Pedersen AB, Johnsen SP, Pedersen L. Clinical epidemiology in the era of big data: new opportunities, familiar challenges. *Clin Epidemiol*. 2017;9:245-250.
4. Hunt JR, White E. Retaining and tracking cohort study members. *Epidemiol Rev*. 1998;20(1):57-70.

5. Schisterman EF, Silver RM, Lesher LL, et al. Preconception low-dose aspirin and pregnancy outcomes: results from the EAGeR randomised trial. *Lancet.* 2014;384(9937):29-36.

6. Lappe J, Watson P, Travers-Gustafson D, et al. Effect of vitamin D and calcium supplementation on cancer incidence in older women: a randomized clinical trial. *J Am Med Assoc.* 2017;317(12):1234-1243.

7. Du Toit G, Roberts G, Sayre PH, et al. Randomized trial of peanut consumption in infants at risk for peanut allergy. *N Engl J Med.* 2015;372(9):803-813.

8. Prorok PC, Andriole GL, Bresalier RS, et al. Design of the prostate, lung, colorectal, and ovarian (PLCO) cancer screening trial. *Control Clin Trials.* 2000;21(suppl 6):273S-309S.

9. Kramer MS, Chalmers B, Hodnett ED, et al. Promotion of breastfeeding intervention trial (PROBIT): a randomized trial in the republic of Belarus. *J Am Med Assoc.* 2001;285:413-420.

10. Hays J, Hunt JR, Hubbell FA, et al. The Women's Health Initiative recruitment methods and results. *Ann Epidemiol.* 2003;13(suppl 9):S18-S77.

11. Cook NR, Lee IM, Gaziano JM, et al. Low-dose aspirin in the primary prevention of cancer. The Women's Health Study: a randomized controlled trial. *J Am Med Assoc.* 2005;294(1):47-55.

12. Lee IM, Cook NR, Gaziano JM, et al. Vitamin E in the primary prevention of cardiovascular disease and cancer. The Women's Health Study: a randomized controlled trial. *J Am Med Assoc.* 2005;294(1):56-65.

13. Rosenberg L, Adams-Campbell L, Palmer JR. The Black Women's Health Study: a follow-up study for causes and preventions of illness. *J Am Med Womens Assoc (1972).* 1995;50(2):56-58.

14. Bernstein L, Allen M, Anton-Culver H, et al. High breast cancer incidence rates among California teachers: results from the California Teachers Study (United States). *Cancer Causes Control.* 2002;13(7):625-635.

15. Friedman GD, Cutter GR, Donahue RP, et al. CARDIA: study design, recruitment, and some characteristics of the examined subjects. *J Clin Epidemiol.* 1988;41:1105-1116.

16. Olsen J, Melbye M, Olsen SF, et al. The Danish National Birth Cohort- its background, structure and aim. *Scand J Public Health.* 2001;29(4):300-307.

17. Riboli E, Kaaks R. The EPIC project: rationale and study design. European prospective investigation into cancer and nutrition. *Int J Epidemiol.* 1997;26(suppl 1):S6-S14.

18. Dawber TR, Meadors GF, Moore FE Jr. Epidemiological approaches to heart disease: the Framingham Study. *Am J Public Health Nations Health.* 1951;41(3):279-281.

19. Tsao CW, Vasan RS. Cohort profile: the Framingham Heart Study (FHS). Overview of milestones in cardiovascular epidemiology. *Int J Epidemiol.* 2015;44(6):1800-1813.

20. Kolonel LN, Henderson BE, Hankin JH, et al. A multiethnic cohort in Hawaii and Los Angeles: baseline characteristics. *Am J Epidemiol.* 2002;151(4):346-357.

21. Bild DE, Bluemke DA, Burke GL, et al. Multi-ethnic study of atherosclerosis: objectives and design. *Am J Epidemiol.* 2002;156(9):871-881.

22. Belanger CF, Hennekens CH, Rosner B, Speizer FE. The nurses' health study. *Am J Nurs.* 1978;78(6):1039-1040.

23. Mikkelsen EM, Hatch EE, Wise LA, Rothman KJ, Riis A, Sørensen HT. Cohort profile: the Danish web-based pregnancy planning study – 'Snart-Gravid'. *Int J Epidemiol.* 2009;38(4):938-943. doi:10.1093/ije/dyn191.

24. Wise LA, Rothman KJ, Mikkelsen EM, et al. Design and conduct of an internet-based preconception cohort study in North America: pregnancy study online. *Paediatr Perinat Epidemiol.* 2015;29(4):360-371.

25. Weinberg CR, Shore DL, Umbach DM, Sandler DP. Using risk-based sampling to enrich cohorts for endpoints, genes, and exposures. *Am J Epidemiol.* 2007;166(4):447-455.

26. White E, Hunt JR, Casso D. Exposure measurement in cohort studies: thechallenges of prospective data collection. *Epidemiol Rev.* 1998;20(1):43-56.

27. Melbye M, Wohlfahrt J, Olsen JH, et al. Induced abortion and the risk of breast cancer. *N Engl J Med.* 1997;336:81-85.

28. Laursen M, Bille C, Olesen AW, et al. Genetic influence on prolonged gestation: a population-based Danish twin study. *Am J Obstet Gynecol.* 2004;190:489-494.

29. Hall P, Adami HO, Trichopoulos D, et al. Effect of low doses of ionising radiation in infancy on cognitive function in adulthood: Swedish population based cohort study. *BMJ.* 2004;328(7430):19.

30. Bergfeldt K, Rydh B, Granath F, et al. Risk of ovarian cancer in breast-cancer patients with a family history of breast or ovarian cancer: a population-based cohort study. *Lancet.* 2002;360:891-894.

31. Corley DA, Levin TR, Habel LA, et al. Surveillance and survival in Barrett's adenocarcinomas: a population-based study. *Gastroenterology.* 2002;122:633-640.

32. Izurieta HS, Thompson WW, Kramarz P, et al. Influenza and the rates of hospitalization for respiratory disease among infants and young children. *N Engl J Med.* 2000;342:232-239.

33. Selby JV, Peng T, Karter AJ, et al. High rates of co-occurrence of hypertension, elevated low-density lipoprotein cholesterol, and diabetes mellitus in a large managed care population. *Am J Manag Care.* 2004;10(2 pt 2):163-170.

34. Christian P, Khatry SK, Katz J, et al. Effects of alternative maternal micronutrient supplements on low birth weight in rural Nepal: double blind randomised community trial. *BMJ.* 2003;326:1-6.

35. Macintyre K, Sosler S, Letipila F, et al. A new tool for malaria prevention? Results of a trial of permethrin-impregnated bedsheets (shukas) in an area of unstable transmission. *Int J Epidemiol*. 2003;32:157-160.

36. Lee J, Jung DY. Measurement issues across different cultures. *Taehan Kanho Hakhoe Chi*. 2006;36(8):1295-1300.

37. Epstein J, Santo RM, Guillemin F. A review of guidelines for cross-cultural adaptation of questionnaires could not bring out a consensus. *J Clin Epidemiol*. 2015;68(4):435-441.

38. Maneesriwongul W, Dixon JK. Instrument translation process: a methods review. *J Adv Nurs*. 2004;48(2):175-186.

39. Schatzkin A, Lanza E, Freedman LS, et al. The Polyp Prevention Trial I: rationale, design, recruitment, and baseline participant characteristics. *Cancer Epidemiol Biomarkers Prev*. 1996;5:375-383.

40. Virtamo J, Pietinen P, Huttunen JK, et al. Incidence of cancer and mortality following alpha-tocopherol and beta-carotene supplementation: a postintervention follow-up. *J Am Med Assoc*. 2003;290:476-485.

41. Hennekens CH, Eberlein K. A randomized trial of aspirin and beta-carotene among U.S. physicians. *Prev Med*. 1985;14(2):165-168.

42. Rossouw JE, Anderson GL, Prentice RL, et al; Writing Group for the Women's Health Initiative Investigators. Risks and benefits of estrogen plus progestin in healthy postmenopausal women: principal results from the Women's Health Initiative randomized controlled trial. *J Am Med Assoc*. 2002;288:321-333.

43. Women's Health Initiative. Study findings: Women's Health Initiative Participant Website. Available at https://www.whi.org/about/SitePages/WHI%20Findings.aspx. Accessed July 14, 2004.

44. Willett WC, Colditz GA. Approaches for conducting large cohort studies. *Epidemiol Rev*. 1998;20(1):91-99.

45. National Cancer Institute. *Current Research: Major Areas of Emphasis – Consortia – Cohorts*. http://epi.grants.cancer.gov/consortia/cohort.html. Accessed July 8, 2004.

46. Riboli E, Hunt KJ, Slimani N, et al. European Prospective Investigation into Cancer and Nutrition (EPIC): study populations and data collection. *Public Health Nutr*. 2002;5(6B):1113-1124.

47. Song M, Rolland B, Potter JD, Kang D. Asia Cohort Consortium: challenges for collaborative research. *J Epidemiol*. 2012;22(4):287-290.

48. Titus-Ernstoff L, Egan KM, Newcomb PA, et al. Early life factors in relation to breast cancer risk in postmenopausal women. *Cancer Epidemiol Biomarkers Prev*. 2002;11:207-210.

49. Church TR, Yeazel MW, Jones RM, et al. A randomized trial of direct mailing of fecal occult blood tests to increase colorectal cancer screening. *J Natl Cancer Inst*. 2004;96:770-780.

50. Casady R, Leplowski J. Stratified telephone survey designs. *Surv Methodol*. 1993;19:103-113.

51. Brick JM, Judkins D, Montaquila J, Morganstein D. Two-phase list-assisted RDD sampling. *J Off Stat*. 2002;18:203-216.

52. Montaquila J, Mohadjer L, Khare M. *The enhanced sample design of the future national health and nutrition examination survey (NHANES)*. In: *Proceedings of the Survey Research Methods Section of the American Statistical Association*. 1998:662-667.

53. Flanders WD, Austin H. Possibility of selection bias in matched case-control studies using friend controls. *Am J Epidemiol*. 1986;124:150-153.

54. Ma X, Buffler PA, Layefsky M, et al. Control selection strategies in case-control studies of childhood diseases. *Am J Epidemiol*. 2004;159:915-921.

55. Miller HW. Plan and operation of the health and nutrition examination survey. United States – 1971-1973. *Vital Health Stat 1*. 1973;(10a):1-46.

56. Struewing JP, Hartge P, Wacholder S, et al. The risk of cancer associated with specific mutations of *BRCA1* and *BRCA2* among Ashkenazi Jews. *N Engl J Med*. 1997;336:1401-1408.

57. Maclure M. The case-crossover design: a method for studying transient effects on the risk of acute events. *Am J Epidemiol*. 1991;133(2):144-153.

58. Huybrechts KF, Mikkelsen EM, Christensen T, et al. A successful implementation of e-epidemiology: the Danish pregnancy planning study 'Snart-Gravid'. *Eur J Epidemiol*. 2010;25(5):297-304. doi:10.1007/s10654-010-9431-y.

59. Czajka JL, Beyler A. *Declining Response Rates in Federal Surveys: Trends and Implications (Background Paper)*. Mathematica Policy Research; 2016.

60. Mindell JS, Giampaoli S, Goesswald A, et al. Sample selection, recruitment and participation rates in health examination surveys in Europe – experience from seven national surveys. *BMC Med Res Methodol*. 2015;15:78.

61. Morton SM, Bandara DK, Robinson EM, Carr PE. In the 21st Century, what is an acceptable response rate? *Aust NZ J Public Health*. 2012;36(2):106-108. doi:10.1111/j.1753-6405.2012.00854.x.

62. Galea S, Tracy M. Participation rates in epidemiologic studies. *Ann Epidemiol*. 2007;17(9):643-653.

63. Fox RJ, Crask MR, Kim J. Mail survey response rate: a meta-analysis of selected techniques for inducing response. *Public Opin Q*. 1988;52(4):467-491. Available at http://dx.doi.org/10.1086/269125.

64. Rhemtulla M, Savalei V, Little TD. On the asymptotic relative efficiency of planned missingness designs. *Psychometrika*. 2016;81(1):60-89.

65. Little TD, Jorgensen TD, Lang KM, Moore EW. On the joys of missing data. *J Pediatr Psychol.* 2014;39(2):151-162. doi:10.1093/jpepsy/jst048.

66. Schembre SM, Liao Y, O'Connor SG, et al. Mobile ecological momentary diet assessment methods for behavioral research: systematic review. *JMIR Mhealth Uhealth.* 2018;6(11):e11170. doi:10.2196/11170.

67. Marcano Belisario JS, Jamsek J, Huckvale K, O'Donoghue J, Morrison CP, Car J. Comparison of self-administered survey questionnaire responses collected usingmobile apps versus other methods. *Cochrane Database Syst Rev.* 2015;(7):MR000042.

68. Hirsch JA, James P, Robinson JR, et al. Using MapMyFitness to place physical activity into neighborhood context. *Front Public Health.* 2014;2:19.

69. Singer E, Bossarte R. Incentives for survey participation: when are they coercive? *Am J Prev Med.* 2006;31:411-418.

70. Doody MM, Sigurdson AS, Kampa D, et al. Randomized trial of financial incentives and delivery methods for improving response to a mailed questionnaire. *Am J Epidemiol.* 2003;157:643-651.

71. Edwards P, Cooper R, Roberts I, Frost C. Meta-analysis of randomised trials of monetary incentives and response to mailed questionnaires. *J Epidemiol Community Health.* 2005;59(11):987-999.

72. Singer E, Ye C. The use and effects of incentives in surveys. *Ann Am Acad Polit Soc Sci.* 2013;645(1):112-141.

73. Cavusgil ST, Das A. "Methodological issues in empirical cross-cultural research: a survey of the management literature and a framework." *MIR Manage Int Rev.* 1997;37(1):71-96.

74. Wise LA, Wang TR, Willis SK, et al. Effect of a home pregnancy test intervention on cohort retention and pregnancy detection. *Am J Epidemiol.* 2020:kwaa027.

75. Cook DA, Beckman TJ. Current concepts in validity and reliability for psychometric instruments: theory and application. *Am J Med.* 2006;119(2):166.e7-16.

76. Croyle RT, Loftus EE. Improving episodic memory performance of survey respondents. In: Tanur JM, ed. *Questions about Questions: Inquiries into the Cognitive Bases of Surveys.* New York, NY: Sage Foundation; 1992.

77. Loftus EF, Smith KD, Klinger MR, Fiedler J. Memory and mismemory for health events. In: Tanur JM, ed. *Questions about Questions: Inquiries into the Cognitive Bases of Surveys.* New York, NY: Sage Foundation; 1992.

78. Fisher RP, Quigley KL. Applying cognitive theory in public health investigations: enhancing food recall with the cognitive interview. In: Tanur JM, ed. *Questions about Questions: Inquiries into the Cognitive Bases of Surveys.* New York, NY: Sage Foundation; 1992.

79. Bradburn NM, Sudman S, Wansink B. *Asking Questions: The Definitive Guide to Questionnaire Design – For Market Research, Political Polls, and Social and Health Questionnaires.* rev ed. New York, NY: Jossey-Bass; 2004.

80. Russell CW, Boggs DA, Palmer JR, Rosenberg L. Use of a web-based questionnaire in the black women's health study. *Am J Epidemiol.* 2010;172(11):1286-1291. doi:10.1093/aje/kwq310.

81. Groves RM, Fowler FJ, Couper MP, et al. *Nonresponse in Sample Surveys. Survey Methodology.* New York, NY: John Wiley; 2004.

82. Biemer PP, Groves RM, Lyberg LE, et al., eds. *Measurement Errors in Surveys.* New York, NY: Wiley; 1991.

83. Tanur JM, ed. *Questions about Questions: Inquiries into the Cognitive Bases of Surveys.* New York, NY: Sage Foundation; 1992.

84. Clark HH, Schober MF. Asking questions and influencing answers. In: Tanur JM, ed. *Questions about Questions: Inquiries into the Cognitive Bases of Surveys.* New York, NY: Sage Foundation; 1992.

85. Groves RM, Barnett V, Bradley RA, et al, eds. *Survey Errors and Survey Costs.* New York, NY: Wiley; 1989.

86. Schmitz H, Howe CL, Armstrong DG, Subbian V. Leveraging mobile health applications for biomedical research and citizen science: a scoping review. *J Am Med Inform Assoc.* 2018;25(12):1685-1695. doi:10.1093/jamia/ocy130.

87. Kim H, Nakamura C, Zeng-Treitler Q. Assessment of pictographs developed through a participatory design process using an online survey tool. *J Med Internet Res.* 2009;11(1):e5.

88. Brody JG, Dunagan SC, Morello-Frosch R, Brown P, Patton S, Rudel RA. Reporting individual results for biomonitoring and environmental exposures: lessons learned from environmental communication case studies. *Environ Health.* 2014;13:40. doi:10.1186/1476-069X-13-40.

89. Colt JS, Zahm SH, Camann DE, Hartge P. Comparison of pesticides and other compounds in carpet dust samples collected from used vacuum cleaner bags and from the high-volume surface sampler. *Environ Health Perspect.* 1998;106:721-724.

90. Nuckols JR, Ward MH, Jarup L. Using geographic information systems for exposure assessment in environmental epidemiology studies. *Environ Health Perspect.* 2004;112:1007-1015.

91. Doody MM, Hayes HM, Bilgrad R. Comparability of National Death Index Plus and standard procedures for determining causes of death in epidemiologic studies. *Ann Epidemiol.* 2001;11:46-50.

92. Li JY, Taylor PR, Li GY, et al. Intervention studies in Linxian, China: an update. *J Nutr Growth Cancer.* 1986;3(4):199-206.

93. Griem ML, Kleinerman RA, Boice JD Jr, et al. Cancer following radiotherapy for peptic ulcer. *J Natl Cancer Inst.* 1994;86:842-849.

94. Inskip PD, Monson RR, Wagoner JK, et al. Cancer mortality following radium treatment for uterine bleeding. *Radiat Res.* 1990;123:331-344.

95. Boice JD Jr. Follow-up methods to trace women treated for pulmonary tuberculosis, 1930-1954. *Am J Epidemiol.* 1978;107:127-139.

96. Nash S, Tilley BC, Kurland LT, et al. Identifying and tracing a population at risk: the DESAD Project experience. *Am J Public Health.* 1983;73:253-259.

97. Wasserman SL, Berg JW, Finch JL, Kreiss K. Investigation of an occupational cancer cluster using a population-based tumor registry and the National Death Index. *J Occup Med.* 1992;34:1008-1012.

98. Christensen T, Riis AH, Hatch EE, et al. Costs and efficiency of online and offline recruitment methods: a web-based cohort study. *J Med Internet Res.* 2017;19(3):e58. doi:10.2196/jmir.6716.

99. van Gelder MMHJ, Merkus PJFM, van Drongelen J, Swarts JW, van de Belt TH, Roeleveld N. The PRIDE Study: evaluation of online methods of data collection. *Paediatr Perinat Epidemiol.* 2020;34(5):484-494. doi:10.1111/ppe.12618.

100. Rothman KJ, Cann CI, Walker AM. Epidemiology and the internet. *Epidemiology.* 1997;8(2):123-125.

101. Parks KA, Pardi AM, Bradizza CM. Collecting data on alcohol use and alcohol-related victimization: a comparison of telephone and Web-based survey methods. *J Stud Alcohol.* 2006;67:318-323.

102. Hatch EE, Hahn KA, Wise LA, et al. Evaluation of selection bias in an internet-based study of pregnancy planners. *Epidemiology.* 2016;27(1):98-104.

103. Östlund U, Kidd L, Wengström Y, Rowa-Dewar N. Combining qualitative and quantitative research within mixed method research designs: a methodological review. *Int J Nurs Stud.* 2011;48(3):369-383. doi:10.1016/j.ijnurstu.2010.10.005.

104. Tariq S, Woodman J. Using mixed methods in health research. *JRSM Short Rep.* 2013;4(6):2042533313479197.

105. Zhang W, Watanabe-Galloway S. Using mixed methods effectively in preventionscience: designs, procedures, and examples. *Prev Sci.* 2014;15(5):654-662. doi:10.1007/s11121-013-0415-5.

106. Tavener M, Mooney R, Thomson C, Loxton D. The Australian longitudinal study on women's health: using focus groups to inform recruitment. *JMIR Res Protoc.* 2016;5(1):e31. doi:10.2196/resprot.5020.

107. Khan SM, Bain RES, Lunze K, et al. Optimizing household survey methods to monitor the Sustainable Development Goals targets 6.1 and 6.2 on drinking water, sanitation and hygiene: a mixed-methods field-test in Belize. *PLoS One.* 2017;12(12):e0189089.

108. Minian N, Penner J, Voci S, Selby P. Woman focused smoking cessationprogramming: a qualitative study. *BMC Womens Health.* 2016;16:17.

109. Collins FS, Varmus H. A new initiative on precision medicine. *N Engl J Med.* 2015;372(9):793-795.

110. Keyes K, Galea S. What matters most: quantifying an epidemiology of consequence. *Ann Epidemiol.* 2015;25(5):305-311.

111. Green LW, George MA, Daniel M, et al. *Study of Participatory Research in Health Promotion: Review and Recommendations for the Development of Participatory Research in Health Promotion in Canada.* Vancouver, British Columbia: Royal Society of Canada; 1995.

112. Leung MW, Yen IH, Minkler M. Community based participatory research: apromising approach for increasing epidemiology's relevance in the 21st century. *Int J Epidemiol.* 2004;33(3):499-506.

113. Minkler M. Linking science and policy through community-based participatory research to study and address health disparities. *Am J Public Health.* 2010;100(suppl 1):S81-S87.

114. Eccles MP, Mittman BS. Welcome to implementation science. *Implement Sci.* 2006;1:1.

115. Proctor EK, Powell BJ, McMillen JC. Implementation strategies: recommendations for specifying and reporting. *Implement Sci.* 2013;8:139. doi:10.1186/1748-5908-8-139.

116. Powell BJ, Waltz TJ, Chinman MJ, et al. A refined compilation of implementation strategies: results from the Expert Recommendations for Implementing Change (ERIC) project. *Implement Sci.* 2015;10:21. doi:10.1186/s13012-015-0209-1.

117. Kemp CG, Jarrett BA, Kwon CS, et al. Implementation science and stigma reduction interventions in low- and middle-income countries: a systematic review. *BMC Med.* 2019;17(1):6. doi:10.1186/s12916-018-1237-x.

118. Proctor E, Silmere H, Raghavan R, et al. Outcomes for implementation research: conceptual distinctions, measurement challenges, and research agenda. *Adm Policy Ment Health.* 2011;38(2):65-76.

119. Lewis CC, Fischer S, Weiner BJ, Stanick C, Kim M, Martinez RG. Outcomes for implementation science: an enhanced systematic review of instruments using evidence-based rating criteria. *Implement Sci.* 2015;10:155.

120. Lewis CC, Weiner BJ, Stanick C, Fischer SM. Advancing implementation science through measure development and evaluation: a study protocol. *Implement Sci.* 2015;10:102.

121. Harville EW, Mishra GD, Yeung E, et al. The preconception period analysis of risks and ExposuresInfluencing health and development (PrePARED) consortium. *Paediatr Perinat Epidemiol.* 2019;33(6):490-502. doi:10.1111/ppe.12592.

122. Gillman MW, Blaisdell CJ. Environmental influences on child health outcomes, a research Program of the national Institutes of health. *Curr Opin Pediatr.* 2018;30(2):260-262. doi:10.1097/MOP.0000000000000600.

CHAPTER 11

Studies Relying on Secondary Data

Krista F. Huybrechts and Sebastian Schneeweiss

Epidemiologic studies can be classified in different ways, such as by the design (*e.g.*, cohort, case-control, self-controlled) or by the timing of the ascertainment of exposure relative to the outcome (*i.e.*, prospective versus retrospective). Another meaningful classification depends on the data source used. Some studies rely on primary data collection where the investigator defines what to measure, how to measure, and when to measure data points. Some use preexisting data that were collected for other research and nonresearch purposes and secondarily used for a research study, and others use a combination of both. Primary and secondary data sources have different strengths and weaknesses, offering different opportunities and posing different challenges for study validity. In this chapter, we will describe the use of secondary data in epidemiologic research.

CHARACTERISTICS OF SECONDARY DATA

What are Secondary Data?

In epidemiology, the distinction between primary and secondary data hinges on the relationship between the team that collected the data and the team that is analyzing them. If the data in question were collected by the research team for the purpose of that specific study, they are *primary data*.[1] The investigators largely control the timing of data collection, the level of detail and the investment in obtaining accurate data.[2] If the data were collected by someone else for the purpose of a different

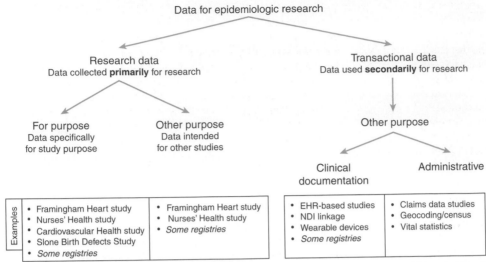

FIGURE 11-1 Data sources for epidemiologic research. EHR, electronic health record; NDI, National Death Index. (Adapted from Franklin JM, Schneeweiss S. When and how can real world data analyses substitute for randomized controlled trials? *Clin Pharmacol Ther*. 2017;102:924-933.)

research study, or if the data are transactional data primarily intended for clinical documentation or administrative purposes but are used secondarily for research, they are considered *secondary data*. The same data can thus be primary data in one study and secondary data in another.[1] The relevance of the data for a specific study may be equally independent of whether they are primary or secondary data, although more often primary data will be more targeted toward a specific study question. Many studies use a combination of both primary and secondary data (Figure 11-1).

Secondary Data for Epidemiologic Research

Below we describe some key secondary data sources that are frequently used in epidemiologic research. While the selected sources are intended to illustrate the spectrum of available data sources, the list is not intended to be exhaustive.

Nationwide Health Registries in the Nordic Countries

The Nordic countries (Denmark, Finland, Iceland, Norway, Sweden) have universal healthcare coverage supported by taxes, with the goal of providing unfettered access to care across all ages and socioeconomic strata. The use of all health services is documented in national health registries; reporting is mandatory and regulated by national laws. Every person is assigned a unique personal identifier at birth or upon immigration. This identifier remains the same until death or emigration and is included in all national registries of a given country allowing linkage among them. These unique characteristics of the national health registries explain the popularity of registry-based epidemiologic studies in the Nordic countries.[4] While we here use the Nordic registries as an example, other nations have similar resources (*e.g.*, provincial administrative health databases in Canada, National Health Insurance Research Database in Taiwan, National Health Information Database in South Korea).

The core Nordic registries are the civil registration systems, medical birth registries, hospital discharge registries, outpatient registries, prescription databases, cancer registries, and cause of death registries. The civil registration systems provide information about the source population, and the medical and other registries document all births and deaths, diagnoses recorded (using the 10th revision of the *International Statistical Classification of Diseases and Related Health Problems*), as well as all diagnostic and therapeutic procedures received. The prescription databases contain information on prescriptions dispensed by pharmacies, along with prescriber and pharmacy data. For each dispensing, the Nordic article number is provided, which is a unique identification code for each drug formulation of a medicinal product with marketing authorization in the Nordic countries. The drugs are classified according to the Anatomical Therapeutic Chemical

(ATC) Classification System and number of defined daily doses (DDD) as defined by the World Health Organization and packages dispensed are recorded in all databases. The databases do not include the indication for the prescription, over-the-counter (OTC) medicines (unless prescribed and dispensed for reimbursement purposes), patient-level data on drug use in inpatient settings, and data on vaccines. Because of the completeness of pharmacy records, the Nordic registries are well suited for postmarketing surveillance of drug use and effects in routine care settings.

The data do have a number of drawbacks, however, owing to the fact that they are transactional data collected for administrative rather than research purposes. For example, filling a prescription does not guarantee that the medication was actually consumed as prescribed, leading to potential misclassification of the exposure. Information about certain lifestyle factors (*e.g.*, smoking, alcohol use) as well as detailed clinical information are not recorded in the registries. From a practical point of view, differences in legal, ethical, technical, and organizational frameworks between countries pose some challenges for trans-Nordic or international collaborative initiatives.[5]

Healthcare Utilization Databases

Healthcare utilization databases (also referred to as "claims databases" or "administrative databases") have much in common with the national health registries in the Nordic countries. They comprise individual-level demographic and insurance enrollment information, as well as data on all physician services, hospitalizations and the accompanying diagnoses and procedures, and all filled outpatient medication prescriptions. They contain the billing codes that healthcare providers submit to payers (*e.g.*, private insurance companies, Medicare, Medicaid).

In contrast to the Nordic registries that include entire country populations, healthcare utilization databases cover specific subsets of the population (*e.g.*, privately insured or publicly insured individuals, geographic region, specific insurance plans). A characteristic that greatly affects the usefulness of a given insurance database is therefore patient turnover rate, known as "churn." Changing life circumstances—such as a drop in income, change in employment status, marriage, or parenthood—can affect health insurance eligibility and contribute to churn. Databases with a high patient turnover rate contain relatively limited information on patient history and longitudinal follow-up, making them less suitable for the study of long-term outcomes or even short-term outcomes if there is concern about substantial confounding by patients' medical history. Healthcare utilization databases throughout the world differ substantially vis-à-vis the representativeness of the general population and patient turnover rates, the scope and depth of the included information, data quality and completeness, and their linkability with data from other sources (*e.g.*, vital statistics, cancer registries, electronic medical records, laboratory results).[2]

Electronic Health Records

Electronic health records (EHRs) have been described as a "repository of patient data in digital form, stored and exchanged securely, and accessible by multiple authorized users."[6] EHRs are transactional data intended for clinical documentation and contain a wide range of patient health-related information, from symptoms, results of physical examinations, laboratory tests and procedures, diagnoses, and treatment to past medical history and social history. Data are obtained from multiple clinicians involved in a patient's care and are composed of both structured and unstructured data. Structured data refer to coded information such as symptom checklists, while unstructured data refer to text in narrative form such as when recording a patient's lifestyle and behaviors or describing the progression of a medical condition.

More than 80% of physicians in the United States use at least a basic electronic medical record system that feeds into the EHR.[7] With the Centers for Medicare and Medicaid Services (CMS) encouraging meaningful use of electronic medical records, the adoption of these systems is on the rise in the United States. EHRs are increasingly used in research as a source for the type of detailed clinical information that tends to be missing from other sources such as healthcare utilization databases. For example, it is relatively quick and easy to extract laboratory values like hemoglobin A1c levels at different time points to study the effect of antidiabetic medications or cholesterol levels when studying the effect of statins.

As for all secondary data, there are limitations of using these data for epidemiologic studies. Only patient health information generated within the network of the providers that maintain the repository will be documented. An incomplete picture will therefore emerge if the patient's care is fragmented and the pertinent information is not transmitted between providers. Second, because the original intention of EHRs is not research but rather support of clinical care, inconsistency in completeness of the record is a common challenge to assuring data quality. In addition, there is no universally adopted standard checklist for the types of data that should constitute EHRs, resulting in heterogeneity between EHR systems. Missing data and between-system heterogeneity in the scope of the records need to be accounted for when designing an epidemiologic study based on EHR data.

The recent emergence of personal health records (PHR) may offer some promise to overcome the EHR limitations in terms of completeness and heterogeneity. The purpose and components of PHRs closely resemble those of EHRs, the key difference being that patients control and manage access to their own health information with PHRs. Patients can choose to share their health data with providers, for example, in cases where patients use home monitoring systems or wearable devices to track the progress of their chronic disease management and activity or document patient-reported outcomes. This flexibility provides physicians with more information to help care for their patients and researchers with more data.[8]

Disease and Exposure Registries

A patient registry uses noninterventional study methods to systematically collect longitudinal information on patients with a particular disease or exposure from multiple data sources such as EHRs, patient self-report, laboratory results, and surveys. However, there is no standard definition for a patient registry, and the term is used interchangeably to refer to disease and exposure registries.

A *disease registry* (or *condition registry*) is "a collection of standardized information about a group of patients who share a condition."[9] It captures, manages, and provides access to condition-specific information for a cohort of patients, including information on diagnostic testing, prognostic testing, therapies offered and received, family history of disease, behavioral and environmental risk factors, symptoms, and disease progression as well as basic demographic information such as age and gender. The specific data collected as well as the length of patient follow-up—which may range from one episode of care to the entirety of the disease progression—are registry-specific, dependent on the main purpose of the registry. Patients may choose to withdraw their participation at any time point.

Disease registries allow medical providers to better manage their patients and address gaps in care, but they are also useful tools for research. A well-known disease registry is the Surveillance, Epidemiology, and End Results (SEER) program[10] that compiles data from multiple cancer registries throughout the United States to assess trends in overall and site-specific cancer incidence, treatment, and survival.

Registries can be sponsored by a government agency (*e.g.*, the national Amyotrophic Lateral Sclerosis [ALS] registry in the United States is congressionally mandated), a nonprofit organization (*e.g.*, Cerebral Palsy registry, managed by the Cerebral Palsy Research Network), a healthcare facility (*e.g.*, Lupus registry at Brigham and Women's Hospital, Boston), or a private company (*e.g.*, National Cooperative Growth Study registry, sponsored by Genentech). Epidemiologic studies using disease registries span a wide range of objectives and methods. The Columbia University Medical Center conducted a prospective cohort study of patients in the ALS registry to examine risk factors for ALS disease progression, in particular oxidative stress.[11] They also conducted a series of case-control studies nested within the registry cohort to evaluate environmental risk factors at different stages of life.[12] The Penn State Medical Center used the registry to study the relationship between psychosocial characteristics and pain from ALS using a cross-sectional approach.[13]

An *exposure registry* is "a collection of standardized information about a group of patients who share an experience."[9] Exposure registries store demographic, employment (in the case of occupational registries), and exposure information and collect health information on exposed individuals. Common types of exposure registries are pregnancy, occupational, environmental, and medical product registries. Pregnancy exposure registries keep records of mothers who take medications or are vaccinated during pregnancy to study the effect on pregnancy outcomes including birth defects.[14] For example, the National Pregnancy Registry for Psychiatric Medications at the Massachusetts General Hospital in Boston enrolls pregnant women between the ages of 18 and 45 years who have taken antipsychotics, antidepressants, or other psychiatric medications during their pregnancy to study the safety of these drugs.[15] Pregnancy registries are a commonly used approach to address the FDA requirements for documenting postmarketing safety of drugs in pregnancy. The Canadian National Dose Registry (NDR) tracks workers with occupational exposure to ionizing radiation and is the largest national registry of its kind in the world.[16] The NDR started collecting data in 1951 and has been used to gain knowledge on health risks from long-term low-level exposure to ionizing radiation through linkage with mortality and morbidity databases. The Veterans Administration (VA) in the United States has established several health registries to monitor the health of veterans who were exposed to specific environmental hazards during military service, including Agent Orange, airborne hazards (*e.g.*, smoke from burn pits, oil-well fires, pollution), and depleted uranium.[17] Registry questionnaire data and deployment information can be linked with VA medical records to study health conditions following these environmental exposures.

Typically, exposure registries lack an internal comparison group free of the exposure, due to the collection of information for only the cohort with a particular exposure. Thus, studies from exposure registries can assess dose-response patterns among the exposure but cannot alone provide a basis for comparative safety or effectiveness of the exposure against its absence.

Well-designed and well-conducted patient registries, especially when linked to other sources to provide a more comprehensive overview of the population's conditions, can be leveraged at different stages in the research process. For example, information from these registries can be useful for developing hypotheses, recruiting patients for clinical trials, monitoring clinical and cost outcomes, and influencing healthcare systems and policy. Because registration is typically voluntary, researchers using these data sources must be mindful of potential self-selection biases and implications for internal validity. Even if the internal validity of the study is sound, because self-selection might not affect compared groups differentially, the self-selection might be important for external validity. For example, patients who are more health conscious might be more likely to volunteer and effects might be weaker or stronger in such patients than in those who are less health conscious.

Vital Records

Vital records refer to records of life events, mainly births, deaths, and marriages or civil unions. This information is collected by the government through civil registration, of which the primary purpose is legal functions in protecting individuals' rights. In the United States, these data are disseminated by the National Center for Health Statistics (NCHS), a division under the Centers for Disease Control and Prevention (CDC), and are widely used as a source of statistical data for public health surveillance.[18] In the Nordic countries, some of these data are integrated in the national health registries.

Researchers are generally interested in the birth and death records. Live birth record data include information on demographics of the parents, the mother's pregnancy history, health status and any medical concerns, and the infant's gestational age, weight, and health status at delivery. Death records primarily collect cause of death information in addition to demographics. Fetal deaths are recorded separately. Data are collected through a multitude of sources such as medical records and questionnaires.

Like all secondary data sources, the information in vital records is not being collected with a specific research question in mind and thus has limitations for use in research. For example, when analyzing vital statistics for perinatal research, investigators may face barriers in accuracy, such as erroneous reporting of medical concerns or omission of medical procedures during delivery.[19] Records may be incomplete, depending on the source. For example, in the United States, death records are available through the Social Security Death Master File (available from the Social Security Administration) and through the National Death Index (available from the CDC). However, since November 2011, the Social Security Administration no longer discloses state death records that it receives through its contracts with the states, as opposed to other sources (*e.g.*, financial institutions, postal authorities, Federal agencies), out of concerns for identity theft. About one-third of all deaths are therefore missing from the Death Master File. The National Death Index continues to be nearly complete, but costs of using this registry may be prohibitive when studying large populations. While vital records are relatively complete in industrialized countries, they tend to be incomplete in countries that do not have well-functioning systems that support the registration of life events, such as some industrializing countries. Finally, there may be practical hurdles accessing the records. Birth records are only available from the state vital statistics offices in the United States, for example, and permission to link these records to other data sources such as claims data needs to be obtained from each individual state.

Integrated Health Systems

The objective of Integrated Delivery Systems (IDSs) is to improve healthcare quality and outcomes and to reduce costs resulting from a fragmented healthcare system with conflicting incentives and lack of coordination. IDSs have been defined as "an organized and collaborative network that links various healthcare providers, via common ownership or contract, to provide a coordinated, vertical continuum of services to a particular patient population or community."[20] They are accountable, both clinically and fiscally, for the health outcomes of the population or community served, and have process improvement systems in place. As such, they differ from insurance systems, which simply pay for the care provided by others. Key to a successful IDS is the availability of comprehensive electronic medical records that are accessible at the point of care and accompany all patient transfers. The electronic medical records are shared by all providers within the system and track the patient's path through the healthcare continuum. They can also be used to enable system-wide evaluation, benchmarking, and improvement.[20]

IDSs are largely an American development. One of the most prominent IDSs is Kaiser Permanente, serving about 10 million enrolled members with about 17,400 physicians in eight states plus the District of Columbia. Kaiser's Division of Research houses multiple data sources, including electronic medical records, disease registries, vital statistics, member health surveys, which collect social and behavioral factors related to health through recurring questionnaires, and records of insurance enrollment. Data can be linked across these sources through a unique member identifier.[21] Given the breadth and depth of information they have available on their members, IDSs are a valuable secondary data source for epidemiologic studies. Other important advantages of these data sources are the ability to interact with providers and members, and to collect biological specimens. Some studies require populations that are larger than a single health plan's and several initiatives have focused on collaborations across IDSs and insurers (e.g., HMO Research Network, Sentinel). An important limitation of using an individual IDS is that the population covered tends to be more homogeneous (i.e., insured employed population), which may limit the possibility to study how effects differ among those of older age or of different insurance or socioeconomic status.[22]

Advantages and Disadvantages of Secondary Data

The use of secondary data in epidemiologic research has important advantages related to study efficiency and feasibility. The most evident advantage is that by using secondary data the research team avoids having to invest time, effort, and money to the collection of new data. As anyone who has been involved in primary data collection can attest, the resources involved in correctly identifying the source population, recruiting participants in an unbiased way, collecting detailed information on exposures, outcomes, potential confounders, and effect modifiers, and creating the dataset can be enormous. Individual researchers seldom have the resources or infrastructure to conduct and regularly repeat large-scale surveys, such as the National Health and Nutrition Examination Survey (NHANES)[23] or the European Health Interview Survey (EHIS).[24] Additionally, secondary data often enable investigators to examine a study question that could not have been addressed were it not for the availability of these data. Drug safety studies are a salient example. As adverse drug outcomes tend to be rare, one typically needs to include thousands of patients exposed to the drug of interest to observe enough outcomes to estimate an effect size with sufficient precision to draw meaningful conclusions. These studies therefore increasingly rely on the use of nationwide health registries, healthcare utilization databases, or integrated health systems that reflect routine care of patients and have the important characteristic that they prospectively record all medication prescriptions or pharmacy dispensings.

Offsetting these advantages are some notable disadvantages of secondary data, which vary according to the data source. These disadvantages stem from the fact that typically the data were collected for a nonresearch purpose or to inform a different research question. The investigator has little or no control over what to measure, how to measure and when to measure the relevant information. The resulting consequences for research applications vary by data source and study question. Not all the variables of interest—e.g., variables that may act as potential confounders or effect measure modifiers—are necessarily included in the source data. Alternatively, the data might be recorded in a suboptimal way for the study at hand. For example, in national health registries or claims data, health outcomes are documented using diagnostic codes, which are attached to the healthcare encounter. Such diagnostic codes might not accurately reflect the disease status (e.g., they might be rule-out diagnoses to justify a certain test procedure), or they might miss some granularity (e.g., severity of the condition). A dataset may include blood pressure as a dichotomous variable (e.g., hypertensive or normotensive), whereas the investigator may be interested in blood pressure measurements as a continuous variable. It may also be the case that the data are available for a somewhat different study population than the investigator would have chosen, with respect to the calendar years covered, the setting (*e.g.*, geographic region, insurance-type), or population characteristics (*e.g.*, patients with atrial fibrillation >65 years versus all patients with atrial fibrillation). The investigator must judge the extent to which such compromises affect the biologic relations studied and limit the generalizability of the results.

The Data Generation Process

To conduct valid research using secondary data, it is crucial to have a deep understanding of how the data were originally collected and for what purpose, as well as potential data quality issues (*e.g.*, response rates, respondent understanding of survey questions, coding errors), and which decisions were made in the creation and cleaning of the dataset. This is true for all secondary data, but in particular for data that were generated for transactional purposes. Such understanding can be attained through collaboration with people that were involved in or are knowledgeable about the different steps in the data generation process.

There are many features of the data generation process that are unique to a given data source and will have repercussions for the study design. For illustrative purposes, we describe a few examples below, mostly drawn from healthcare utilization databases.

Diagnostic and procedure information—documented using coding systems such as the *International Classification of Diseases, Current Procedural Terminology, Read codes, SNOMED Clinical Terms*—is often used to define study outcomes and covariates that may confound or modify an association. Most databases include such information for both outpatient and inpatient encounters, but they differ with respect to the number of diagnoses and procedures attached to each encounter. For instance, a dataset of publicly insured individuals in the United States (*i.e.*, Medicaid Analytic eXtract [MAX]) contains 10 diagnostic fields in the inpatient file and two diagnostic fields in the outpatient file.[25] In a dataset of commercially insured individuals in the United States (*i.e.*, Optum Clinformatics), the inpatient file includes five diagnostic fields, while the number of diagnostic fields in the outpatient file increased from 5 to 25 in 2017. These changes were made to accommodate the specificity of the ICD-10 codes, which were implemented in the United States in October 2015. A similar change was made in British Columbia's hospital discharge database, in which the number of diagnostic fields increased from 16 to 25 in fiscal year 2001/2002, coinciding with changes in their coding systems.[26] However, expanding the number of allocated diagnostic fields does not necessarily improve coding completeness.[27] As only a limited number of diagnostic fields tend to be used, the presence of a chronic comorbid condition among the diagnoses can signify that the patient is relatively healthy since the presence of more serious, acute concerns did not preempt the chronic condition from being listed.[27]

Additionally, in some data sources, the first listed diagnosis is the principal diagnosis, whereas all other diagnoses are considered secondary. Other data sources, however, do not differentiate between principal and secondary diagnoses. Understanding these distinctions is important when developing an algorithm for defining incident outcomes using a particular data source.

Potential challenges in distinguishing between incident and prevalent outcomes are also present when working with inpatient databases. The Premier research database contains the records of about one-sixth of hospitalizations in the United States. Charges for all drugs, procedures, and diagnostic tests during inpatient admissions are date stamped (*i.e.*, charge codes). Patients' discharge diagnoses and discharge status are also recorded.[28] While such an inpatient database is ideal for studying inpatient interventions, it is important to realize that one cannot discriminate between diagnoses that are present on admission and those that emerge at some point during the hospital stay subsequent to the intervention. While typically not a problem for chronic conditions (*e.g.*, dementia), which can reasonably be assumed to be present upon admission, this can be challenging for acute conditions such as delirium, which could be present on admission or could have developed during the hospital stay.

Some data sources may contain an incomplete record of healthcare claims when the beneficiaries have restricted benefits (*e.g.*, pregnancy-related services or prescription drug benefits only) or are enrolled in capitated (risk-based) managed care plans. While encounter records take the place of claims for services provided in capitated managed care plans, these records have been shown to be incomplete in some states (despite Medicaid requiring states to provide this information to the Centers for Medicare and Medicaid Services).[29] It is therefore important to implement strict eligibility criteria based on insurance program provisions and arrangements to increase the completeness of the claim information among individuals included in the study cohort.[30]

In the Nordic national registries, the personal identifier that is assigned at birth or at immigration remains with the individual throughout life. This is not always the case for the member identification number in healthcare utilization databases. Though in some databases, members keep the same identification number when they exit and reenter the insurer's coverage, in others the number will change when they reenter or when they reenter with a different type of coverage. This inconstancy may create challenges when building a longitudinal profile of an individual's medical history.

Apart from these and other features of the data generation process itself, there may also be decisions made by the database holder that change the completeness and interpretation of specific data items over time. Often such changes emanate from concerns over patient confidentiality. The removal of records from the public Death Master File is one such example (see Vital Records). Other examples include the removal of the hospital discharge disposition status for deceased patients in some healthcare utilization databases and omission of codes for external causes of injury (useful when studying intentional self-harm as an outcome) by the billing software used in many hospitals as they have no relevance for hospital payment among most US insurers.

Patient Privacy

Many countries have regulations in place to protect personal health information from inappropriate use or disclosure.[31,32] While the specific options and requirements differ between countries, the general principles are universally applicable. In the United States, the Health Insurance Portability and Accessibility Act (HIPAA) protects so-called protected health information (PHI), individually identifiable health information found in medical records, tests results, and billing information for medical services (among other locations). Under HIPAA regulations, 18 identifiers are generally considered PHI, including names, geographic subdivisions smaller than a state, and dates more specific than a year tied to a particular individual. HIPAA privacy rules permit use or disclosure of PHI by "covered entities" (health plans, clearinghouses, and providers) or their business associates for research under four circumstances.[33]

The first option is for the subject of the PHI to grant written permission, known as informed consent. While feasible for primary data collection, this is usually not viable when using large secondary data sources.

The second option is for an institutional review board (IRB) or privacy board to grant the research team a waiver (or alteration) of consent if it is judged that the PHI use involves no more than a minimal risk to the privacy of individuals, the research could not be conducted without access to the PHI, and the research could not be conducted without the requested waiver or alteration. When submitting the study documentation to the IRB, the team is required to describe in detail the methods that will be used to protect the privacy of subjects and maintain data confidentiality. These typically include substituting codes for names and/or medical record number; removing face sheets or other identifiers from completed questionnaires and surveys; proper disposal of printed computer data; limited access to study data; use of password-protected computer databases; training of research staff in the importance of confidentiality of data; and storing research records in a secure location.

The third option is to use a deidentified dataset. Deidentification can be achieved by removing the 18 identifiers noted above. However, dates are important for ascertaining temporality of events. Time from an index date can be used to substitute for dates, but this option may not be acceptable for epidemiologic studies in which it can be inferred with greater specificity than a year when an event occurred as this would result in violation of patient privacy.[33] Alternatively, an expert can determine that the risk is small that the information to be shared could be used, alone or in combination with other reasonably available information, to identify the subject of the information.

Finally, the information can be released in the form of a limited dataset stripped of certain identifiers. PHI in a limited dataset may include dates (e.g., admission and discharge dates) and more granular elements of addresses than in a deidentified dataset. The covered entity and recipient of a limited dataset must sign a data use agreement specifying the people who have access to the limited dataset and committing the recipient to safeguard the limited dataset and to report unauthorized use or disclosure of it to the covered entity. Most epidemiologic research using secondary data can be conducted using a limited dataset.

Concerns about patient privacy are particularly pertinent for studies that link various data sources. Individual data sources are typically pseudo-deidentified; that is, the data are processed in such a way that they can no longer be attributed to a specific subject without the use of additional information (true deidentification would imply that there is no key that allows reidentification of subjects in a dataset).[5] In order to allow linkage between data sources—such as claims data and EHR, disease registry, or biobank data—that additional information needs to be requested. This request will typically be in the form of a "crosswalk" file that maps the encrypted identifier to the actual personal identifier from the source data (*e.g.*, Social Security Number in the United States, or Personal Identification Number in the Nordic countries). Only the researcher conducting the actual linkage is permitted to have access to the crosswalk key, and as soon as the linkage has been completed, the actual personal identifiers must be stripped from the data, returning the data to pseudo-deidentified form. Methods for conducting studies across multiple data sources that are horizontally or vertically partitioned are available. While they are logistically intricate, they circumvent the need to pool multiple data sources and the resulting privacy concerns.[34,35]

Study Design Considerations

Prospective Versus Retrospective Studies

Studies based on secondary data are often described as retrospective studies by default. This designation is accurate if the prospective/retrospective distinction is used to refer to the timing of the investigator involvement. In studies using secondary data, the subjects are by definition identified after the follow-up period has ended and the study variables have been recorded.

As discussed in Chapter 6, a more useful distinction is when the exposure and covariates were measured relative to the outcome and how this affects the quality and completeness of measurement. By this definition, it becomes evident that studies using secondary data can be either prospective or retrospective. In healthcare utilization databases, for instance, medication use is recorded at the time a prescription is dispensed, which is before disease or adverse events have occurred. Drug safety studies using these data, designed either as a cohort or a nested case-control study, are therefore using prospectively recorded data. In contrast, in the National Birth Defects Prevention Study (NBDPS) conducted by the Centers for Disease Control and Prevention, infants with birth defects and healthy infants without birth defects are identified and mothers are interviewed over the phone about their pregnancy experience and health after they have delivered. Any study based on these data is therefore retrospective, as the exposures are recorded after disease has been diagnosed.

Cohort Study Versus Case-Control Sampling

As described in Chapter 6, cost efficiency is often the main reason for conducting a case-control study as opposed to a cohort study. The efficiency of the case-control design stems from the sampling of controls in place of the complete enumeration of the source population that gave rise to the cases. This begs the question whether a case-control study is ever preferred when working with secondary data, where the source population has already been enumerated and the data have already been collected. The answer is almost never. In nearly all circumstances, a cohort study will be preferred for reasons of statistical efficiency and because this design presents fewer opportunities for bias and mistaken inference due to potential investigator violations against temporality when assessing exposure and confounders (*e.g.*, adjusting for causal intermediates by defining covariates immediately preceding the event).[36] Only when more information is needed than is readily available from the existing records, and it would be expensive to seek this information for everyone in the cohort, will a nested case-control sampling or a case-cohort sampling be preferred. For example, if biospecimens are banked for every member in a registry, then analyzing expression of a biomarker in cases and a sample of the source population will be cost-efficient compared with analyzing expression of the biomarker in every member of the source population, and will also conserve the biospecimens for use in subsequent studies.[37] In this special case, the study will be based on a combination of secondary and primary data.

Matching in Cohort Studies

Matched cohort studies used to be relatively uncommon, the main reason being the great expense of matching large cohorts for primary data collection. This practice has changed in more recent years with the increased availability of large population cohorts from secondary data sources. Matching unexposed to exposed subjects on specific characteristics or on a summary score—such as a propensity score or a disease risk score—is no longer prohibitive given that the entire population is already enumerated and accessible by electronic means. Matching has therefore become a popular option to control confounding in cohort studies based on secondary data. See Chapter 6 for a discussion of matching versus alternatives to control confounding.

RESEARCH APPLICATIONS

Secondary data have been used extensively in epidemiologic research and, in particular, in pharmaco-epidemiologic research. We briefly describe cases of typical use to exemplify the breadth of the research that can be conducted with these data.

Descriptive Epidemiology Studies

Understanding the prevalence and natural history of disease over time and in different populations is important clinical information in itself and can also inform the design of causal inference studies involving a specific exposure (*e.g.*, new intervention or an environmental exposure). Disease registries, such as the SEER cancer registry, are well suited for this purpose.[10] Secondary data sources are also useful to characterize different exposures such as the use of drug therapy, devices, and other medical interventions in routine care. Aspects of particular relevance in such *utilization* studies include the characteristics of new initiators and prevalent users, use for off-label indications, polytherapy, use in vulnerable populations with unknown benefits and risks, and changes in the composition of the patient population over time as guidelines and coverage policies change and experience with a new therapy increases. Secondary data can also be used to assess (1) the level and predictors of primary and secondary *nonadherence* to long-term therapy in routine care, which is an important contributor to increased healthcare spending[38]; as well as (2) physician and institutional *prescribing practices*. By linking the characteristics of providers to data on the prescriptions their patients fill, provider groups that are more likely to prescribe suboptimally can be identified. Information on suboptimal prescribing practices and nonadherence can then be used to target educational and other public health interventions[39] and to inform health systems planning. An in-depth understanding of prescribing practices is also essential in the design of studies using a preference-based instrumental variable to address unmeasured confounding (see Chapter 28).[40]

Comparative Safety and Effectiveness Research

Randomized controlled trials are usually the optimal design for studying efficacy and establish a treatment effect in humans under optimal conditions. They are less well-suited to evaluate rare adverse events, delayed effects, effectiveness (*i.e.*, efficacy in routine care), or effects in vulnerable populations that are typically excluded from clinical trials (*e.g.*, children, pregnant women, frail elderly). Secondary data are therefore commonly used to study the comparative safety and effectiveness of drugs, devices, and procedures.

Hypothesis-Motivated Studies

Because healthcare utilization databases, integrated health systems, and nationwide registries contain virtually complete information on all diagnoses recorded as well as all procedures and prescription medications, they are regularly used to follow-up on a safety signal that may have been detected in a trial setting or through the FDA voluntary Adverse Event Reporting System,[41] EMA's Eudravigilance[42] system, or similar systems in other jurisdictions. For example, following concerns about an increase in the risk of in-hospital death in aprotinin recipients raised in an international study of over 4,000 patients undergoing coronary-artery bypass grafting (CABG), electronic administrative records of an in-hospital claims database in the United States (*i.e.*, Premier Perspective Comparative Database) were used to evaluate the risk of death in hospitalized patients with operating room charges for the use of aprotinin or aminocaproic acid on the day CABG was performed.[43] Patients who received aprotinin were found to have a 1.64-fold higher mortality than patients who received aminocaproic acid, and this finding endured through several approaches to control confounding that were feasible given the large size of the cohort (33,517 patients on aprotinin, and 44,682 patients on aminocaproic acid). This study was one of several that challenged the safety of aprotinin and ultimately resulted in sales being suspended in May 2008. The literature is peppered with examples of similar types of studies, some of which have led to regulatory action (*e.g.*, market withdrawal, labeling changes, restricted use), while others have provided reassurance about the safety of the respective intervention. Comparative effectiveness studies using observational data are much less common than comparative safety studies. This disparity stems largely from confounding by indication that is more likely present in effectiveness studies if a beneficial effect is anticipated based on the findings from randomized controlled trials. Nevertheless, with the appropriate design and analytic approach, secondary data can be used for comparative effectiveness studies as well as comparative safety studies.[41]

Systematic Surveillance Studies

Aprotinin is only one example where a drug remained on the market for many years until epidemiologic studies using secondary data identified safety considerations.[44] In May 2008, the FDA launched the Sentinel Initiative to monitor proactively the safety of FDA-regulated medical products. The Sentinel system draws upon large amounts of electronic administrative and claims data from a diverse group of data partners, and currently includes more than 300 million cumulative patient identifiers. The data from each data partner are converted into a common data structure. Analyses are conducted locally by the data partners using a common analytic program, and the results are submitted to the coordinating center where they are pooled. Such distributed data approach allows for the safeguarding of patient privacy. Efforts are underway to augment the claims data with clinical data, electronic medical records, hospital data, and disease registry data. FDA actively uses the system to monitor the safety of new medications, such as the direct-acting oral anticoagulants[45] and antidiabetic medications (*e.g.*, dipeptidyl-peptidase 4 inhibitors).[46] The evidence generated using this distributed network of secondary data can be used to support a label change, respond to a Citizens Petition, or become part of an Advisory Committee deliberation. It can also provide reassurance to alleviate concern about a particular safety issue and might lead FDA to determine that no regulatory action is necessary based on the available information.[47] While similar initiatives to combine data sources using a distributed network approach have been developed by academic centers in other countries (*e.g.*, Canadian Network for Drug Effect Studies [CNODES], Asian Pharmacoepidemiology Network [AsPEN], European Health Data and Evidence Network [EHDEN]), they are currently not intended for prospective surveillance. Proactive monitoring systems in a single database or across multiple data sources can also be used to monitor the effectiveness of medical products when used in the real-world setting, with the same caveats as described for hypothesis motivated studies.[47]

Studies to Generate Hypotheses

Both hypothesis-motivated and systematic surveillance studies are used to evaluate an exposure-outcome association that is brought into the spotlight by prior evidence. However, large secondary data sources can also be used to screen many exposure-outcome associations to detect previously unknown harmful effects. TreeScan is one example of such an approach. It can be described as "a data mining method that simultaneously looks for excess risk in any of a large number of individual cells [exposure-outcome associations] in a database as well as in groups of closely related cells, taking into account the multiple comparisons inherent in the large number of overlapping groups evaluated."[48] The method is useful for disease surveillance and pharmacovigilance.[48,49] With this approach, the investigator can evaluate whether any of hundreds or thousands of potential adverse events occur with higher probability among exposed versus referent patients. Alternatively, the investigator can evaluate whether a particular disease occurs with higher risk among people exposed to any of hundreds of drugs. In occupational disease surveillance, the approach can be used to evaluate whether certain occupations are at higher risk of dying from a particular disease, such as silicosis.[48,49] Any safety hypothesis generated using this approach will then need to be followed up with a more structured analysis. The subsequent analysis can be done in a separate data source or in the same data source under certain conditions, *i.e.*, quality checks and sensitivity analyses are being conducted to refute the hypothesis, or orthogonal hypotheses are being tested.[50]

Study of Health Policy Changes and Other Events

Health policy changes typically affect subsets of the population (*e.g.*, patients of a given provider, beneficiaries of a given insurer, population of a certain state or province) and constitute a natural experiment anchored in time. Secondary data sources that include detailed longitudinal information on the utilization of healthcare resources in routine care in unselected populations (*e.g.*, claims data, integrated health systems, nationwide health registries) are ideally suited to evaluate the clinical and economic impact of such health policy changes. Birth, death, and chronic disease registries are other routinely collected data that can be used for this purpose.

Longitudinal databases have been widely used to determine the effect of reimbursement policy changes, such as reimbursement caps,[51] curtailment of reimbursement for marginally effective or questionable therapies,[52] prior authorization policies,[53] and reducing medication co-pays.[54] Frequently assessed outcomes are medication use, use of other health services, and clinical measures. Other useful applications include the evaluation of the effect of regulatory warnings on medication use[55] and questions related to equity in access to care.[56] Analyses typically involve segmented regression analyses of interrupted time series data. A control group that is similar to the study group but did not experience the policy intervention can be used to account for secular trends.[10] In addition to health policy changes, the impact of other real-world events (*e.g.*, natural or man-made disasters) can be studied in a similar fashion.

Randomized Trials Embedded in Secondary Data

A novel approach to study beneficial effects or risks of healthcare interventions is to embed randomized controlled trials within national registries or health insurance systems and collect outcome information through claims or other secondary data. This type of pragmatic randomized trial thus combines secondary data with primary data collection. This approach increases the efficiency of trials by leveraging both the infrastructure and the data routinely generated by health insurers. It has been used to address both clinical and policy related questions.[57]

In randomized controlled trials (RCTs), participants are typically identified through the screening of medical records or through active surveillance in inpatient or outpatient care settings. However, beneficiaries of a given health insurer also represent a group of potentially eligible trial participants, and the trial inclusion and exclusion criteria can be implemented in an expedient manner by screening the administrative data. Demographic criteria (*e.g.*, age, gender) can be assessed using the insurance enrollment files, clinical criteria can be assessed based on diagnostic and procedure codes contained in the inpatient and outpatient claims files, and criteria related to earlier medication use can be assessed based on the prescription drug file.[57] For example, the Post-Myocardial Infarction Free Rx Event and Economic Evaluation (MI FREE) trial tested the effect of eliminating copayments for preventive medications (*i.e.*, statins, beta-blockers, angiotensin-converting-enzyme inhibitors, or angiotensin-receptor blockers) after myocardial infarction on medication adherence and cardiovascular outcomes. Among all beneficiaries of Aetna, a large commercial insurer in the United States, the investigators identified patients younger than 65 years who were recently discharged from hospital with a principal or secondary diagnosis code for myocardial infarction and a length of stay between 3 and 180 days.[58] Linking claims data to other types of secondary data, such as laboratory information, can help to further refine the identification of eligible trial participants. The Enhancing Outcomes through Goal Assessment and Generating Engagement in Diabetes Mellitus (ENGAGE-DM) trial, for example, evaluates the effect of a pharmacist intervention on glycemic control for patients with poorly controlled diabetes. The target population consisted of adult patients ($\geq$18 years, according to enrollment file) who filled a prescription for one or more oral hypoglycemic agents in the preceding 12 months (according to outpatient prescription file), and evidence of poor glycemic control within the previous 6 months (HbA1c $\geq$8%, according to linked laboratory test results).[59]

Once the target population has been identified, patients are randomized to the intervention or control arm. Interventions that can be tested in RCTs embedded in claims databases typically involve variations in the design of health insurance, including what services are covered, and the level and method of patient cost sharing (*e.g.*, full coverage versus usual coverage for certain medications[58]). They can also take the form of care management programs targeting patients (*e.g.*, patient engagement strategy using telephone-based pharmacist intervention to improve disease management[60]) or physicians (*e.g.*, providing physicians with educational materials to close the evidence-practice gap[61]).

Routinely collected claims data can also be used to evaluate the study outcomes, rather than relying on information collected from providers during dedicated visits or through telephone outreach as is done in conventional RCTs.[57] The primary outcome in the MI FREE trial, for example, was a composite of the first readmission for a major vascular event or coronary revascularization, and was assessed by applying validated algorithms to healthcare utilization data.[58] The Randomized Evaluation to Measure Improvements in Non-adherence from Low-Cost Devices (REMIND) trial evaluated the impact of three simple reminder devices on medication adherence in patients with common chronic conditions. Administrative pharmacy claims data were used to evaluate adherence based on the medication possession ratio.[62] VALIDATE-SWEDEHEART—a registry-based, multicenter, randomized, controlled, open-label clinical trial to evaluate the use of bivalirudin versus heparin in patients undergoing percutaneous coronary intervention for acute coronary syndromes—used the platform of preexisting healthcare registries for enrollment and randomization, as well as collection of data, and follow-up.[63] The primary endpoint was a composite of death from any cause, myocardial infarction, or major bleeding during 180 days of follow-up.

Claims data may also be used to extend the follow-up in conventional RCTs. The Dialysis Clinical Outcomes Revisited (DCOR) trial compared sevelamer with calcium-based phosphate binders among patients receiving hemodialysis with respect to the risk of mortality and hospitalization.[64] In a companion study, follow-up was extended by linking trial participants to their Medicare claims recorded in the End-Stage Renal Data System from the Centers for Medicare and Medicaid Services.[65] Linkage of claims data to other secondary data, such as the National Death Index, laboratory test result data, and data from electronic health records allows for a broader range of outcomes to be evaluated, including biometric outcomes such as glycated hemoglobin levels.[66]

CONCLUSION

The field of epidemiology has seen rapid growth in the use of secondary data over the last few decades. While secondary data may lack some of the information granularity that can be achieved with primary data collection, they offer many advantages for epidemiologic research. Although the specific scientific value will vary by research context and data source, the range of advantages include large cohort sizes that allow for the evaluation of rare exposures or outcomes, rich and often time-varying information on potential confounding variables and effect modifiers, and longitudinal follow-up. From a practical point of view, their use is cost-efficient. Nevertheless, because the information has not been collected for the purpose of the specific research question at hand, attention needs to be paid to the underlying data generation mechanisms to understand data missingness and misclassification which may lead to residual confounding and misclassification bias. Quantitative bias analysis (see Chapter 29) is advisable if such concerns exist. In addition to enabling the study of important public health questions, the wealth of information available in large secondary data sources has also spurred the advancement of design and analytic approaches to confounding control, including propensity scores and instrumental variables. An in-depth knowledge of the intricacies of the data source used is a fundamental requirement for the validity of studies based upon them.

The integration of horizontally and vertically distributed data offers ever-growing opportunities for epidemiologic research. Integration of horizontally distributed data refers to the pooling of patients from distinct databases (*e.g.*, different registries), which allows for larger and more heterogeneous study populations. Multiple initiatives are already under way in this regard. Integration of vertically distributed data refers to linkage between complementary sources of information on the same patient, including healthcare utilization databases, registries, patient-generated data, and biobanks containing genomic data to enrich the information on each subject. Advancement in technology, such as mobile and wearable devices, offers a promising new source of secondary realworld data. Linkages between multiple sources allow for increased depth of clinical information, and push the boundaries in terms of the range of research questions that can be studied, improvements in confounding control, and opportunities for validation.[34] A linkage of particular relevance in the context of medical interventions is the one between randomized controlled trials and routine healthcare data (*e.g.*, claims data, vital statistics data, disease registry data, census data). Such an approach offers opportunities to enhance both the quality of the randomized controlled trial and of the observational study, at relatively modest investments in time, effort, and money.[67]

References

1. Boslaugh S. *Secondary Data Sources for Public Health: A Practical Guide*. New York, NY: Cambridge University Press; 2007.
2. Schneeweiss S, Avorn J. A review of uses of health care utilization databases for epidemiologic research on therapeutics. *J Clin Epidemiol*. 2005;58:323-337.
3. Franklin JM, Schneeweiss S. When and how can real world data analyses substitute for randomized controlled trials? *Clin Pharmacol Ther*. 2017;102:924-933.
4. Wettermark B, Zoega H, Furu K, et al. The Nordic prescription databases as a resource for pharmacoepidemiological research – a literature review. *Pharmacoepidemiol Drug Safety*. 2013;22:691-699.
5. Ludvigsson JF, Haberg SE, Knudsen GP, et al. Ethical aspects of registry-based research in the Nordic countries. *Clin Epidemiol*. 2015;7:491-508.
6. ISO/TR 20514:2005. Available at https://www.iso.org/standard/39525.html.
7. Office of the National Coordinator for Health Information Technology. Office-based Physician Electronic Health Record Adoption, Health IT Quick-Stat #50. Available at dashboard.healthit.gov/quickstats/pages/physician-ehr-adoption-trends.php. January 2019.
8. Tang PC, Ash JS, Bates DW, Overhage JM, Sands DZ. Personal health records: definitions, benefits, and strategies for overcoming barriers to adoption. *J Am Med Inform Assoc*. 2006;13:121-126.
9. Gliklich RE, Dreyer NA, Leavy MB, eds. *Registries for Evaluating Patient Outcomes: A User's Guide*. Rockville, MD: Agency for Healthcare Research and Quality (US); 2014.
10. Wagner AK, Soumerai SB, Zhang F, Ross-Degnan D. Segmented regression analysis of interrupted time series studies in medication use research. *J Clin Pharm Ther*. 2002;27:299-309.
11. Mitsumoto H, Factor-Litvak P, Andrews H, et al. ALS Multicenter Cohort Study of Oxidative Stress (ALS COSMOS): the study methodology, recruitment, and baseline demographic and disease characteristics. *Amyotroph Lateral Scler Frontotemporal Degener*. 2014;15:192-203.
12. Oskarsson B, Horton DK, Mitsumoto H. Potential environmental factors in amyotrophic lateral sclerosis. *Neurol Clin*. 2015;33:877-888.
13. Centers for Disease Control and Prevention. *ALS Research Notification for Clinical Trials and Studies*. Available at http://www.cdc.gov/als/ALSResearchNotificationClinicalTrialsStudies.html. Accessed July 7, 2020.
14. Food and Drug Administration. *Pregnancy Registries*. Available at http://www.fda.gov/ScienceResearch/SpecialTopics/WomensHealthResearch/ucm251314.htm. Accessed July 7, 2020.
15. Massachusetts General Hospital Center for Women's Mental Health. *National Pregnancy Registry for Psychiatric Medications*. Available at https://womensmentalhealth.org/clinical-and-research-programs/pregnancyregistry/. Accessed July 7, 2020.
16. Government of Canada. *National Dose Registry*. Available at http://www.hc-sc.gc.ca/ewh-semt/occup-travail/radiation/regist/index-eng.php. Accessed July 7, 2020.
17. U.S. Department of Veterans Affairs. *Environmental Health Registry Evaluation for Veterans*. Available at http://www.publichealth.va.gov/exposures/benefits/registry-evaluation.asp. Accessed July 7, 2020.
18. Centers for Disease Control and Prevention National Center for Health Statistics. *National Vital Statistics System*. Available at http://www.cdc.gov/nchs/nvss/about_nvss.htm. Accessed July 7, 2020.
19. Schoendorf KC, Branum AM. The use of United States vital statistics in perinatal and obstetric research. *Am J Obstet Gynecol*. 2006;194:911-915.
20. Enthoven AC. Integrated delivery systems: the cure for fragmentation. *Am J Manag Care*. 2009;15:S284-S290.
21. Enthoven AC. What is an integrated health care financing and delivery system (IDS)? And what must would-be IDS accomplish to become competitive with them? *Health Econ Outcome Res Open Access*. 2016;2:115.
22. Andrade SE, Raebel MA, Boudreau D, et al. Health maintenance organizations/health plans. In: Strom B, Kimmel S, Hennessy S, eds. *Pharmacoepidemiology*. 5th ed. Chichester, West Sussex, United Kingdom: Wiley-Blackwell; 2012:163-188.
23. Centers for Disease Control and Prevention National Center for Health Statistics. *National Health and Nutrition Examination Survey*. Available at http://www.cdc.gov/nchs/nhanes/index.htm. Accessed July 7, 2020.

24. Eurostat. *European Health Interview Survey (EHIS)*. Available at http://ec.europa.eu/eurostat/web/micro-data/european-health-interview-survey. Accessed July 7, 2020.

25. Research Data Assistance Center. Available at http://www.resdac.org/cms-data/files. Accessed July 7, 2020.

26. Population Data BC. Available at http://www.popdata.bc.ca/data/health/dad. Accessed July 7, 2020.

27. Iezzoni LI, Foley SM, Daley J, Hughes J, Fisher ES, Heeren T. Comorbidities, complications, and coding bias. Does the number of diagnosis codes matter in predicting in-hospital mortality? *J Am Med Assoc*. 1992;267:2197-2203.

28. Premier Applied Sciences PI. *Premier Healthcare Database White Paper*. 2018. Available at https://www.premierinc.com/newsroom/education/premier-healthcare-database-whitepaper.

29. Hennessy S, Freeman C, Cunningham F. US government claims databases. In: Strom B, Kimmel S, Hennessy S, eds. *Pharmacoepidemiology*. 5th ed. Chichester, West Sussex, United Kingdom: Wiley-Blackwell; 2012:209-223.

30. Palmsten K, Huybrechts KF, Mogun H, et al. Harnessing the Medicaid Analytic eXtract (MAX) to evaluate medications in pregnancy: design considerations. *PLoS One*. 2013;8:e67405.

31. US Department of Health and Human Services. *HIPAA Privacy Rule*. Available at https://privacyrulean-dresearch.nih.gov/research_repositories.asp. Accessed July 7, 2020.

32. The EU General Data Protection Regulation. Available at https://gdpr.eu/tag/gdpr/. Accessed July 7, 2020.

33. Sarpatwari A, Kesselheim AS, Malin BA, Gagne JJ, Schneeweiss S. Ensuring patient privacy in data sharing for postapproval research. *N Engl J Med*. 2014;371:1644-1649.

34. Bohn J, Eddings W, Schneeweiss S. Conducting privacy-preserving multivariable propensity score analysis when patient covariate information is stored in separate locations. *Am J Epidemiol*. 2017;185:501-510.

35. Toh S, Wellman R, Coley RY, et al. Combining distributed regression and propensity scores: a doubly privacy-protecting analytic method for multicenter research. *Clin Epidemiol*. 2018;10:1773-1786.

36. Schneeweiss S, Suissa S. Discussion of Schuemie et al: "A plea to stop using the case-control design in retrospective database studies". *Stat Med*. 2019;38:4209-4212.

37. Wacholder S. Practical considerations in choosing between the case-cohort and nested case-control designs. *Epidemiology*. 1991;2:155-158.

38. Sokol MC, McGuigan KA, Verbrugge RR, Epstein RS. Impact of medication adherence on hospitalization risk and healthcare cost. *Med Care*. 2005;43:521-530.

39. Avorn J. Academic detailing: "marketing" the best evidence to clinicians. *J Am Med Assoc*. 2017;317:361-362.

40. Brookhart MA, Wang PS, Solomon DH, Schneeweiss S. Instrumental variable analysis of secondary pharmacoepidemiologic data. *Epidemiology*. 2006;17:373-374.

41. Danaei G, Rodriguez LA, Cantero OF, Logan R, Hernan MA. Observational data for comparative effectiveness research: an emulation of randomised trials of statins and primary prevention of coronary heart disease. *Stat Methods Med Res*. 2013;22:70-96.

42. European Medicines Agency. *EudraVigilance*. Available at http://www.ema.europa.eu/ema/index.jsp?curl=pages/regulation/general/general_content_000679.jsp&mid=WC0b01ac05800250b5. Accessed May 4, 2018.

43. Schneeweiss S, Seeger JD, Landon J, Walker AM. Aprotinin during coronary-artery bypass grafting and risk of death. *N Engl J Med*. 2008;358:771-783.

44. Avorn J. *Powerful Medicines: The Benefits, Risks, and Costs of Prescription Drugs*. New York, NY: Penguin Random House; 2005.

45. Toh S, Reichman ME, Graham DJ, et al. Prospective postmarketing surveillance of acute myocardial infarction in new users of saxagliptin: a population-based study. *Diabetes Care*. 2018;41:39-48.

46. Chrischilles EA, Gagne JJ, Fireman B, et al. Prospective surveillance pilot of rivaroxaban safety within the US Food and Drug Administration Sentinel System. *Pharmacoepidemiol Drug Safety*. 2018;27(3):263-271.

47. Schneeweiss S, Eichler HG, Garcia-Altes A, et al. Real world data in adaptive biomedical innovation: a framework for generating evidence fit for decision-making. *Clin Pharmacol Ther*. 2016;100:633-646.

48. Kulldorff M, Dashevsky I, Avery TR, et al. Drug safety data mining with a tree-based scan statistic. *Pharmacoepidemiol Drug Safety*. 2013;22:517-523.

49. Kulldorff M, Fang Z, Walsh SJ. A tree-based scan statistic for database disease surveillance. *Biometrics*. 2003;59:323-331.

50. Wang SV, Kulldorff M, Glynn RJ, et al. Reuse of data sources to evaluate drug safety signals: when is it appropriate? *Pharmacoepidemiol Drug Safety*. 2018;27(6):567-569.

51. Soumerai SB, Ross-Degnan D, Avorn J, McLaughlin T, Choodnovskiy I. Effects of Medicaid drug-payment limits on admission to hospitals and nursing homes. *N Engl J Med*. 1991;325:1072-1077.

52. Soumerai SB, Ross-Degnan D, Gortmaker S, Avorn J. Withdrawing payment for nonscientific drug therapy. Intended and unexpected effects of a large-scale natural experiment. *J Am Med Assoc*. 1990;263:831-839.

53. Fischer MA, Schneeweiss S, Avorn J, Solomon DH. Medicaid prior-authorization programs and the use of cyclooxygenase-2 inhibitors. *N Engl J Med*. 2004;351:2187-2194.
54. Choudhry NK, Fischer MA, Avorn JL, et al. The impact of reducing cardiovascular medication copayments on health spending and resource utilization. *J Am Coll Cardiol*. 2012;60:1817-1824.
55. Block JP, Choudhry NK, Carpenter DP, et al. Time series analyses of the effect of FDA communications on use of prescription weight loss medications. *Obesity*. 2014;22:943-949.
56. Franklin JM, Choudhry NK, Uscher-Pines L, et al. Equity in the receipt of oseltamivir in the United States during the H1N1 pandemic. *Am J Public Health*. 2014;104:1052-1058.
57. Choudhry NK. Randomized, controlled trials in health insurance systems. *N Engl J Med*. 2017;377:957-964.
58. Choudhry NK, Avorn J, Glynn RJ, et al. Full coverage for preventive medications after myocardial infarction. *N Engl J Med*. 2011;365:2088-2097.
59. Lauffenburger JC, Lewey J, Jan S, et al. Rationale and design of the ENhancing outcomes through Goal Assessment and Generating Engagement in Diabetes Mellitus (ENGAGE-DM) pragmatic trial. *Contemp Clin Trials*. 2017;59:57-63.
60. Wennberg DE, Marr A, Lang L, O'Malley S, Bennett G. A randomized trial of a telephone care-management strategy. *N Engl J Med*. 2010;363:1245-1255.
61. Zwarenstein M, Hux JE, Kelsall D, et al. The Ontario printed educational message (OPEM) trial to narrow the evidence-practice gap with respect to prescribing practices of general and family physicians: a cluster randomized controlled trial, targeting the care of individuals with diabetes and hypertension in Ontario, Canada. *Implement Sci*. 2007;2:37.
62. Choudhry NK, Krumme AA, Ercole PM, et al. Effect of reminder devices on medication adherence: the REMIND randomized clinical trial. *JAMA Intern Med*. 2017;177:624-631.
63. Erlinge D, Omerovic E, Frobert O, et al. Bivalirudin versus heparin monotherapy in myocardial infarction. *N Engl J Med*. 2017;377:1132-1142.
64. Suki WN, Zabaneh R, Cangiano JL, et al. Effects of sevelamer and calcium-based phosphate binders on mortality in hemodialysis patients. *Kidney Int*. 2007;72:1130-1137.
65. St Peter WL, Liu J, Weinhandl E, Fan Q. A comparison of sevelamer and calcium-based phosphate binders on mortality, hospitalization, and morbidity in hemodialysis: a secondary analysis of the Dialysis Clinical Outcomes Revisited (DCOR) randomized trial using claims data. *Am J Kidney Dis*. 2008;51:445-454.
66. Choudhry NK, Isaac T, Lauffenburger JC, et al. Rationale and design of the study of a tele-pharmacy intervention for chronic diseases to improve treatment adherence (STIC2IT): a cluster-randomized pragmatic trial. *Am Heart J*. 2016;180:90-97.
67. Najafzadeh M, Gagne JJ, Schneeweiss S. Synergies from integrating randomized controlled trials and real-world data analyses. *Clin Pharmacol Ther*. 2017;102:914-916.

CHAPTER 12

Confounding and Confounders

Tyler J. VanderWeele, Kenneth J. Rothman, and Timothy L. Lash

Confounding is a concern in almost all nonrandomized studies in epidemiology. Epidemiologic analyses are often subject to the criticism that some third factor might be responsible for or negate the relationship between the exposure and the outcome under study. In other words, the concern is that the groups receiving and not receiving the exposure differ from one another with respect to some variable that is also related to the outcome. As a result, considerable effort is often devoted to identifying these confounding variables and to controlling for them in the study design, or to collecting data on them so that they can be controlled in the analysis. The goal is that after such efforts, the groups with and without the exposure will be comparable within strata of controlled covariates.

Formal principles of causal inference and relations to confounding, along with the use of causal diagrams in thinking about confounding control, were described in Chapter 3. Methods for analytic adjustment including stratification, standardization, regression adjustment, and weighting are described in Chapters 18 to 21. In this chapter, we will explore the concepts of confounding and confounders in greater detail. We will review the role of confounding in causal inference, describe distinctions that might be drawn between confounding and selection bias, and consider formal definitions of confounding and confounders as well as principles of confounder selection and issues of confounder timing. We will conclude with a brief description of quantitative bias analysis for unmeasured confounding.

CONFOUNDING AND CAUSAL INFERENCE

In Chapter 3, we said that for an exposure X and outcome Y, the covariates Z suffice to control for confounding for the effect of X on Y if, within strata of the covariates Z, the counterfactual outcomes for Y are independent of the actual exposure received. Said another way, the covariates Z suffice to control for confounding if those with the exposure are comparable in their outcomes to what would have been observed if those without exposure had been exposed, and if those without exposure are comparable in their outcomes to what would have been observed if those with exposure had been unexposed. More formally, as in Chapter 3, if we let Y_x denote the counterfactual outcome or potential outcome that would have been observed for an individual if the exposure X had, possibly contrary to fact, been set to level x, then we can formally define the absence of confounding as follows: We say that the covariates Z suffice to control for confounding if the counterfactuals Y_x are independent of X conditional on Z. We can use the notation $Y_x \perp X \mid Z$ to denote this conditional independence. Again, the definition essentially states that within strata of Z, the group that actually had exposure status $X = x$ is representative of what would have occurred had the entire subpopulation with $Z = z$ been given exposure $X = x$. If this holds, we could use the observed data to reason about the effect of intervening to set $X = x$ for the that subpopulation.

This condition of no confounding for the effect of X on Y conditional on Z is sometimes, in other literatures, described using different terminology. In epidemiology, it is sometimes referred to as "exchangeability"[1] or as "no unmeasured confounding"[2]; in the statistics literature it is sometimes referred to as "weak ignorability" or "ignorable treatment assignment"[3]; in the social sciences it is sometimes referred to as "selection on observables,"[4,5] or as "exogeneity."[5] Whatever the terminology, it is this assumption that justifies the interpretation of associations as causal effects. When the assumption holds and when we also have the technical consistency assumption of Chapter 3, that for those with $X = x$, we have that $Y_x = Y$, then we can estimate causal effects.[6,7] We define causal effects as a contrast of counterfactual outcomes, and under the no unmeasured confounding assumption we can estimate these using the observed data and associations. Specifically we then have that:

$$E\left(Y_1 - Y_0 \mid z\right) = E\left(Y \mid X = 1, z\right) - E\left(Y \mid X = 0, z\right)$$

The left-hand side of the equation is the causal effect of the exposure on the outcome conditional on the covariates $Z = z$. The right-hand side of the equation consists of the observed associations between the exposure and the outcome in the actual observed data. If the effect of X on Y is unconfounded conditional on the measured covariates Z, then these two expressions are equal to each other. We can estimate causal effects from the observed data. Of course this assumption of the absence of confounding is a strong one. With real-world observational data, we can never be certain that it holds. We attempt to control for covariates that are related to both the exposure and the outcome in order to make the assumption as plausible as possible. As described in Chapter 3, causal diagrams can sometimes be helpful in this regard if something is known about the causal structure relating all of the variables. In practice, effort is often made to control for as many covariates as possible that are present before the exposure.[8] We will discuss these and other principles of confounder selection as we proceed through this chapter.

The expression above is for causal effects on a difference scale, but if the effect of the exposure on the outcome is unconfounded conditional on covariates, then one can likewise estimate the causal effect on the ratio scale from the observed data:

$$P\left(Y_1 = 1 \mid z\right) / P\left(Y_0 = 1 \mid z\right) = P\left(Y = 1 \mid X = 1, z\right) / P\left(Y = 1 \mid X = 0, z\right)$$

Again Chapters 18 to 25 consider various statistical approaches for modeling and estimation. Here we will focus on concepts and principles of confounding and confounder selection.

CONFOUNDING VERSUS SELECTION

We have defined the absence of confounding conditional on covariates Z as the condition that $Y_x \perp X|Z$, i.e., that the counterfactual outcomes are independent of actual exposure conditional on the measured covariates. In Chapter 3, we saw that with causal diagrams a sufficient condition for the absence of such confounding was that none of the covariates in Z were themselves affected by the exposure X and that the covariates Z sufficed to block all backdoor paths from the exposure to the outcome.[6] Confounding might then be viewed as a bias that results from any unblocked backdoor path from exposure to the outcome. The classic confounding setting is one in which an unmeasured variable U affects both exposure X and outcome Y and thus will give rise to a nonnull association between X and Y even when there is no effect of X on Y as in Figure 12-1A.

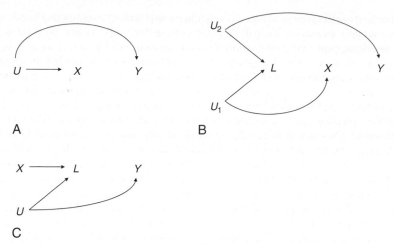

FIGURE 12-1 A, An unmeasured variable *U* that affects both exposure *X* and outcome *Y* creates confounding bias. B, Conditioning on a common effect *L* of two unobserved variables, one of which (*U₁*) is also associated with exposure *X* and the other of which (*U₂*) is associated with outcome *Y* can introduce bias when none was previously present. C, Conditioning on a common effect *L* of exposure *X* and an unmeasured cause *U* of outcome *Y* can introduce selection bias.

A question is sometimes raised as to formal distinctions within epidemiology between "confounding" and "selection bias." Within epidemiology "selection bias" is often used to refer to biases that arise from restricting analysis based on a variable, or stratifying on a variable, related to *selection into the study*. The terminological question regarding distinctions between confounding and selection are difficult because different disciplines often use these terms in different ways. As noted above, many social scientists refer what we have been calling "no confounding" as "selection on observables,"[4,5] and then also refer to the presence of confounding as "selection on unobservables" or as "selection bias." In these social science disciplines, such as economics, the "selection" being referred to is not selection *into the study*, but rather selection into *exposure or treatment groups*. In epidemiology, in contrast, the presence of variables that affect selection in the exposure or treatment groups, that are also related to the outcome, is referred to as "confounding" whereas bias arising from selection *into the study* itself is referred to as "selection bias." But terminology does vary by discipline. Indeed in some fields of study, saying an estimate is "confounded" or that "confounding" is present is synonymous with the presence of bias. That bias would include what epidemiologists would ordinarily call "confounding bias", as well as "selection bias" or bias due to measurement error.

Even within the terminology often used within epidemiology, distinctions between "confounding" and "selection" can be complicated. Consider the causal diagram in Figure 12-1B. Suppose that U_1 affects exposure *X* and variable *L* and U_2 affects outcome *Y* and variable *L*. Here if we do not condition on the variable *L*, there is no confounding for the effect of *X* on *Y* because all backdoor paths from exposure *X* to outcome *Y* are blocked. If we do not condition on any variable, then the backdoor path X-U_1-L-U_2-Y is blocked by *L* because *L* is a collider on the path and we are not conditioning on it. Suppose, however, we want to restrict our estimates of causal effects of *X* on *Y* to the stratum $L = 1$. Hernán et al. give the example of examining the effect of physical activity (*A*) on heart disease (*Y*),[9] with U_1 representing personal attraction to physical activity, U_2 representing parental socioeconomic status, and *L* representing being a firefighter. If we wanted to study the effect of physical activity on heart disease among firefighters, we would condition on $L = 1$. But if we do, we open a backdoor path from *X* to *Y*, namely, X-U_1-L-U_2-Y. The backdoor path becomes open because we are conditioning on a collider on that path, namely *L*. There is sometimes dispute as to whether to call such a phenomenon "confounding" or "selection." On the one hand, the bias results from an unblocked backdoor path from exposure to the outcome, so we might refer to it as "confounding." On the other hand, the bias does result from stratifying on the variable *L* related to selection into the study and so we might refer to it as "selection."

In this book, we will take the perspective that these two terms "confounding" and "selection" need not be mutually exclusive. We will refer to "confounding bias" as any bias that is due to an unblocked backdoor path from exposure to outcome. We will refer to selection bias as any non-causal path from the exposure to the outcome that is unblocked by conditioning on some variable. Said another way, selection bias is an unblocked noncausal path from the exposure to the outcome that is unblocked because of conditioning on a collider or a descendant of a collider. Another way to conceive of this is that selection bias is bias that results from conditioning on a common effect of two variables, one of which is associated with the exposure and the other of which is associated with the outcome.[9] Thus in Figure 12-1B, we would say that the bias introduced by conditioning on L is both "confounding" and "selection." We acknowledge that other authors would refer to this only as "selection" not as "confounding."[10] We here think it is more consistent with ordinary usage to refer to it as both. Otherwise in Figure 12-1B we would have to say that there is bias but that there is no confounding. This terminological approach also has the advantage that "confounding" in the sense defined here comprises all biases that, in expectation, would be eliminated by a randomized trial. The bias that is induced in Figure 12-1B by conditioning on L would not be present in a randomized trial of exposure X because, by randomizing exposure X, U_1 would no longer be related to X, and thus there would no longer be an unblocked backdoor path even when conditioning on L.

The alternative terminological approach, which does not include the bias induced by conditioning on L as confounding, generally defines confounding bias as present only if it is created by a common cause of X and Y.[11] In Figure 12-1B, L is not a common cause of X and Y. The advantage of using such terminology is that there is no overlap between confounding bias and selection bias. The bias in Figure 12-1B could simply be called "selection bias" not "confounding bias." The disadvantage of this approach to terminology, however, is that confounding bias is not as closely related to the concept of randomization. In Figure 12-1B, the bias induced by restricting analysis to a particular stratum of L would be eliminated by randomization of exposure X, but with this alternative terminology, we would still not refer to this as confounding bias. Moreover, the bias induced by conditioning on L can, in some sense, still be thought of as a bias "due to common causes," namely, a common cause U_1 of L and X and a common cause U_2 of L and Y; and it is the conditioning on L that gives rise to bias due to these common causes. Because of these issues we prefer to use the term "confounding bias" here to denote any bias due to an unblocked backdoor path from exposure X to outcome Y, but we emphasize for the reader that these terms may be defined differently by others.

While terminology may be ambiguous in settings such as Figure 12-1B, in other circumstances such terminological complications do not arise. In Figure 12-1A, for example, if data were unavailable on U, the backdoor path X-U-Y is simply an unblocked backdoor path and would be referred to only as confounding. In Figure 12-1C, if we conditioned on the variable L, this would be bias only due to selection. The conditioning on L unblocks the noncausal path X-L-U-Y and thus introduces bias. We will find association between X and Y conditional on L even if there is no causal effect of X on Y. This bias is not due to an unblocked backdoor path from X to Y nor because of a common cause of X and Y, and it would not be eliminated in a randomized trial. It arises simply because conditioning on L unblocks the noncausal path X-L-U-Y.

More important than what we call different types of bias is eliminating them: can we find a set of covariates such that there is no confounding of the effect of the exposure on the outcome conditional on those covariates? The principles of confounding control from Chapter 3, especially if we have knowledge of a causal diagram, can be useful in answering this question. We will also return below to the general principles of confounder selection as we discuss approaches to eliminate confounding bias and avoid selection bias.

OVERADJUSTMENT AND SELECTION

Several papers in the epidemiologic literature on bias have discussed an issue that is sometimes referred to as "overadjustment" bias.[7,12] The classic setting of overadjustment bias concerns settings in which we condition on a variable that is on the pathway from the exposure X to outcome Y, such as the variable L in Figure 12-2A. In this case, our estimates of the causal effect of X on Y will be biased conditional on L because we are blocking some of the effect of X on Y by conditioning on

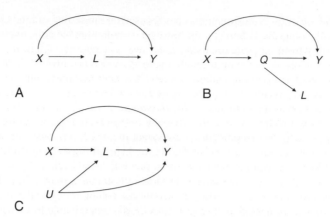

FIGURE 12-2 A, Conditioning on a variable L on the pathway between exposure X and outcome Y is said to be overadjustment bias. B, Conditioning on a variable L that is an effect of a variable Q on the pathway between exposure X and outcome Y gives rise to overadjustment bias. C, Conditioning on a variable L that is both on the pathway between exposure X and outcome Y and also a common effect of exposure X and an unmeasured cause U of outcome Y creates both overadjustment bias and selection bias.

L. Essentially we are adjusting for a variable that should not be controlled. Such "overadjustment" leads to bias. Recall from Chapter 3 that the backdoor path criteria to control for confounding required that the set of variables Z that blocked all backdoor paths from X to Y was not to contain any variable that was a descendant of the exposure X. In Figure 12-2A, the variable L is a descendant of exposure X, and we thus get bias.

However, we had also noted above, in Figure 12-1C, that if we adjusted for the variable L, we would be adjusting for a variable that we should not adjust for and bias would result. We might thus wonder whether there is any distinction between biases due to "overadjustment" versus "selection." Terminology can here again potentially be used in different ways, but there are relevant distinctions that can be drawn. In this book, we will say that overadjustment bias is the bias that results from conditioning on a variable, or a descendant of a variable, that is on a causal pathway from exposure to the outcome.[7,12]

Thus in Figure 12-2A, using the definitions and terminological distinctions above, we would say that by conditioning on L we introduce overadjustment bias because L is on the causal path from X to Y. We would not call this selection bias because there is no noncausal path from X to Y that is unblocked because of conditioning. Likewise in Figure 12-2B, we would say that if we condition on L, we introduce overadjustment bias because L is a variable that is a descendant of a variable Q that is on the causal pathway from X to Y, but again we would not say that this is selection bias. In contrast, in Figure 12-1C, we would say that we introduce selection bias by conditioning on L because, by conditioning on L, we unblock the noncausal path X-L-U-Y. However, we would not say this is overadjustment bias because the variable L is not on a causal path from X to Y nor is it a descendant of such a variable.

In some cases, however, we may have both selection and overadjustment bias. Consider the causal diagram in Figure 12-2C. Here, if we condition on the variable L, we have selection bias because by conditioning on L we have unblocked the noncausal path X-L-U-Y. However, we also have overadjustment bias because L is on the causal pathway from exposure X to outcome Y. Here, then, we have two sources of bias, one from selection and one from overadjustment. We can see that we have two sources of bias because if we had been able to control for U we would eliminate selection bias; there would be no unblocked noncausal path from exposure to outcome as the path X-L-U-Y would be blocked by U even if we conditioned on L. However, we would still have overadjustment bias because the variable L is on the pathway from exposure X to outcome Y. Thus, while there can be settings in which we only have selection bias as in Figure 12-1C and settings in which we have only overadjustment bias as in Figure 12-2A and B, there can also be settings in which conditioning on a variable introduces both selection and overadjustment bias as in Figure 12-2C.

Our discussion here of overadjustment bias has focused on the setting of total causal effects for the exposure X on the outcome Y. Sometimes, however, we might make adjustment for some variable L on the pathway from exposure to outcome, because we are interested in assessing the direct effect of the exposure on the outcome through a path that does not involve L. We will consider this topic in detail in Chapter 27 on mediation analysis. Under certain assumptions, described in Chapter 27, it can be an effective strategy to assess direct effects, and controlling for such a variable may not introduce bias for estimates of *the direct effect*. However, for estimates of the total effect (through all causal pathways from the exposure to the outcome), control for a variable on a pathway from exposure to the outcome, or a descendant of such a variable, will introduce bias in estimates of the total effect, and that bias is what we are here calling overadjustment bias.

While the problem of overadjustment bias may seem clear and relatively straightforward to avoid, in some contexts it can be more subtle. Consider, for example, a study of the effect of physical activity on cardiovascular disease. Suppose detailed measurement of physical activity as the exposure are taken every 4 years, but that body mass index (BMI) is obtainable from medical records on an annual basis. It is not uncommon, when proportional hazards modeling is carried out for the outcome (see Chapter 22), to update the covariate information over time. However, if BMI is updated each year but the prior physical activity measures are used because physical activity is only measured every 4 years, then one will be controlling for covariates that temporally occur after the physical activity exposure and may be affected by it. This too would be an instance of overadjustment bias. Once again, the confounding control principle is not to control for any variable that may be affected by the exposure at the time of its measurement. We will return to these questions further below and also in Chapter 22 in the discussion of the causal effects of time-varying exposures.

In summary, we have the following three types of bias that can result from not adjusting for certain variables that we should adjust for, or that can arise from adjusting for variables that we should not adjust for. These three structural biases concerning variable adjustment can be summarized as:

Confounding bias: The presence of an unblocked backdoor path from exposure to outcome.
Selection bias: A noncausal path from exposure to outcome that is unblocked because of conditioning on some variable.
Overadjustment: The conditioning on a variable that is on, or a descendant of a variable that is on, a causal pathway from exposure to the outcome.

These biases do not exhaust all potential forms of bias. For example, they do not include bias due to measurement error, which is the topic of Chapter 13. Moreover, what precisely we call these biases, and how precisely we distinguish these different biases terminologically, is less important than controlling them. Ultimately, what we want is a set of covariates Z such that the effect of X on Y is unconfounded conditional on Z, *i.e.*, $Y_x \perp X|Z$. We will turn to principles of confounder selection shortly, but first we will consider one more terminological question, the definition of a confounder.

DEFINITION OF A CONFOUNDER

Traditionally, a confounder in epidemiology was understood as a pre-exposure variable that was associated with exposure and was associated also with the outcome conditional on the exposure, possibly conditional also on other covariates.[13] It was also recognized that a confounder should not itself be affected by the exposure,[14] because control for such a variable would most often be an overadjustment. Sometimes the requirement that the covariate was associated with the outcome conditional on the exposure was restricted to an association with the outcome among the unexposed. The developments in causal inference over the past decades, summarized in Chapter 3, have made clear that this definition of a "confounder" is inadequate. It is inadequate because there can be a pre-exposure variable associated with the exposure and the outcome, the control of which introduces, rather than eliminates, bias.[6,15] An example of such a variable is L in Figure 12-1B. Here L is associated with the exposure X; L is also associated with the outcome Y conditional on the exposure X. By the traditional definition, L would be a confounder. However, our estimate of the causal effect of X on Y is unconfounded if we do not condition on L; and if we do condition on L, then we introduce bias in the causal effect of X on Y because of the unblocked backdoor path X-U_1-L-U_2-Y which is unblocked because we are conditioning on the collider L. The traditional definition of a confounder will not suffice.

In this book we will use the term "confounder" in the following way. We will say that a sufficient adjustment set is a set of covariates Z such that the effect of exposure X on outcome Y is unconfounded conditional on Z, *i.e.*, a set of covariates Z such that $Y_x \perp X|Z$. A minimally sufficient adjustment set is a sufficient adjustment set Z such that every member of Z is needed for that set to suffice to control for confounding. In other words, a minimally sufficient adjustment is one such that if we were to remove any covariate or covariates in the set Z, then the reduced set would no longer suffice to control for confounding. We will then, in this book, refer to a confounder as *a member of a minimally sufficient adjustment set.*[16] In other words, if we have a covariate, Z_1, and it is a member of a minimally sufficient adjustment set, so that if Z_1 (or if any other variable) were to be removed from that set then the set would no longer suffice for confounding control, then we will say that Z_1 is a confounder. Said yet another way, we will say that Z_1 is a confounder if there is some other set of variables such that when we include Z_1 among them we can control for confounding, but if we remove Z_1, there is no way to control for confounding with those other remaining variables. There can be causal structures in which there are more than one minimally sufficient adjustment sets. For example, in Figure 12-3A, both (Z_1, Z_3) and (Z_2, Z_3) are minimally sufficient adjustment sets. Either set would suffice to control for confounding. A confounder is just a variable that is a member of at least one minimally sufficient adjustment set. Thus in Figure 12-3A, each of Z_1, Z_2, and Z_3 are confounders; each is a member of a minimally sufficient adjustment set.

Why should we define a confounder in this way? Defining a confounder in this way has two important implications.[16] First, one can show that if we define a confounder in this way, then, on any causal diagram, the set of all confounders will itself suffice to control for confounding.[16] Second, one can show that if a confounder is defined in this way, then for any variable that constitutes a confounder so defined, there will always be some context in which having data on that variable helps to reduce or eliminate bias.

As with other definitional issues, terminology may be used in different ways by different authors, but, surprisingly, other potential definitions that have been put forward in the literature do not in fact have the two properties above! Consider, for example, the traditional definition of a confounder as a variable that is associated with exposure and was associated also with the outcome conditional on the exposure.[13] If we applied this definition to Figure 12-1B then neither U_1 nor U_2 would be considered confounders because U_1 is not associated with Y (the path from U_1 to Y is blocked by L) and U_2 is not associated with X (the path from U_2 to X is blocked by L); however, L would be considered a confounder because L is both associated with X and associated

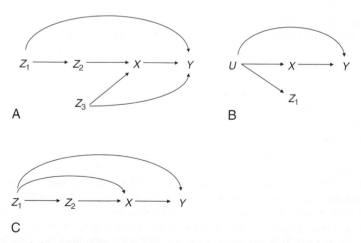

FIGURE 12-3 A, Both (Z_1, Z_3) and (Z_2, Z_3) constitute minimally sufficient adjustment sets to control for confounding of the effect of exposure X on outcome Y. B, A variable Z_1 that can reduce confounding bias due to an unmeasured variable U, but is not itself a member of any minimally sufficient adjustment set may be referred to as a proxy confounder. C, A variable Z_2 may block a backdoor path from exposure X to outcome Y and yet still not help in any context reduce confounding bias regardless of whether adjustment is made for covariate Z_1 or not.

with Y conditional on X. However, if we controlled for L alone we would have bias, whereas if we controlled for no covariates we would not have bias. The traditional definition of a confounder can lead us astray.

Other definitions for a "confounder" that have been put forward also have similar problems. For example, another definition that has been considered for a confounder is a variable for which adjustment is always necessary to avoid confounding bias.[6,11,17] Said another way we might consider defining a confounder as a variable that is a member of every sufficient adjustment set. Although this definition seems appealing upon first glance, it has the awkward implication in Figure 12-3A that neither Z_1 nor Z_2 would be considered confounders. Neither of them is always necessary; we can control for confounding by just controlling for (Z_1, Z_3) so Z_2 is not always necessary; we can also control for confounding by just controlling for (Z_2, Z_3) so Z_1 is not always necessary. Thus according to this alternative definition, neither Z_1 nor Z_2 would be considered confounders; only Z_3 would be considered a confounder because only Z_3 is always necessary. But if we only adjusted for Z_3, we would still have confounding bias because of the unblocked backdoor path X-Z_2-Z_1-Y.

Another potential definition of a confounder that is intuitively appealing is any variable that is useful in reducing the magnitude of the bias.[11,18,19] A downside of this definition is that it is scale-dependent. A variable may be helpful in reducing bias on a risk difference scale but not on the risk ratio scale, or vice versa; a variable under this definition would then be a confounder on the risk difference scale but not a confounder on the risk ratio scale. Another issue with this definition is that it is no longer structural; it cannot be applied simply based on the causal structure relating the variables in a causal diagram, for example; the determination requires instead knowing the numerical values of estimates under different covariate adjustment sets along with the numerical value of the true causal effect. Another consequence of this potential alternative definition is that it may result in a variable being called a confounder even if it is not ever on any backdoor confounding path from exposure to outcome. Consider Figure 12-3B, for example. Here the variable Z_1 may be such that the bias in the causal effect estimate when controlling for Z_1 is less than the bias in the crude completely unadjusted causal effect estimate. However, the variable Z_1 here is not on a backdoor path from exposure to outcome, and is never useful in completely eliminating confounding bias. To eliminate confounding bias we would need to adjust for U, and once we adjust for U, the variable Z_1 is no longer needed. Nevertheless, the property of being useful in reducing the magnitude of bias is an important one. We would thus propose to call a confounder, as above, a member of a minimally sufficient adjustment set; but would propose that we call any variable (such as Z in Figure 12-3B) that is not a member of a minimally sufficient adjustment set but is still helpful in reducing bias (on the effect-measure scale of interest) a "proxy confounder." When we discuss principles of covariate selection we will return again to this notion of a proxy confounder and the consideration of variables that may help reduce, but not completely eliminate, bias.

Another definition of a confounder that might be considered is any variable that blocks a backdoor path from the exposure to the outcome.[11,20] This definition has the advantage of being closely related to the description of confounding bias above as the presence of an unblocked backdoor path. If control is not made for a variable that blocks a backdoor path from exposure to outcome then we might think that confounding bias results. It is possible, however, to construct examples in which a variable blocks a backdoor path from exposure to outcome but in fact is never helpful in either reducing or eliminating bias.[16] Consider the causal diagram in Figure 12-3C. In this diagram, the variable Z_2 blocks a backdoor path from X to Y, namely X-Z_2-Z_1-Y. However, it is possible to construct examples in which controlling for the variable Z_2 in fact increases bias over the crude unadjusted estimate of the association between X and Y.[16] If this is the case, then Z_2 is never helpful in either reducing or eliminating confounding bias. In such an example, if control is not made for Z_1 then controlling for Z_2 only increases the bias; but if control is made for Z_1 then control for Z_2 is not necessary because Z_1 alone suffices to eliminate bias. Thus Z_2 never helps to reduce or eliminate bias; it would thus be odd to call a variable that never helps to reduce or eliminate bias a confounder, but that would be the implication of defining a confounder as a variable that blocks a backdoor path from exposure to outcome. We thus again would maintain that the most conceptually satisfactory definition of a "confounder" is "a member of a minimally sufficient adjustment set." See VanderWeele and Shpitser for further discussion of the properties of this definition,[16] and also of other potential alternative definitions and their potential drawbacks.

An alternative response to the considerations above concerning defining a confounder as a variable that blocks a backdoor path from exposure to outcome is that, in practice, we generally do not know whether a variable such as Z_2 in Figure 12-3C will or will not reduce bias, and that in the absence of such knowledge it may be best to control for any variable that thought to lie on a backdoor path from exposure to outcome. This, however, is more of an argument for a particular principle for covariate selection for confounding control than one concerning concepts and definitions. In the next section, we will consider in some detail practical principles of covariate selection for confounding control. If, however, one were to commit to the principle of controlling for any variable that blocks a backdoor path from exposure to outcome, one might tie the definition of a confounder to this practical principle of covariate selection and thus define a confounder as any variable that blocks a backdoor path from exposure to outcome. For the reasons outlined above, we believe this is, conceptually, a less satisfactory definition than defining a confounder as a member of a minimally sufficient adjustment set. However, as with all of these issues around terminology and definitions, it is difficult to absolutely insist on one definition; the use of the term "confounder" might thus well continue to vary across authors. As we have emphasized throughout, however, the important point is not so much what language is used, but rather whether it is possible to find some set of covariates Z that suffice to control for confounding of the effect of exposure on outcome. This practical task is ultimately of greater importance. Therefore, we now discuss potential principles on which to make decisions about precisely which covariates to adjust for when attempting to control for confounding.

PRINCIPLES OF CONFOUNDER SELECTION

Regardless of how we might formally define a "confounder" we are still left with the practical task of deciding what covariates to adjust for to try to control for confounding. We often must make these decisions without knowing for certain whether adjustment for a particular covariate will reduce bias, and without having much knowledge of the underlying causal structures. We may not know how to represent all covariates on a causal diagram and their relations to each other and to the exposure and outcome. Different principles for deciding which covariates to adjust for to try to control for confounding may require different levels of knowledge regarding the nature of the covariates. If we truly had full knowledge of the structure of a causal diagram that related all of the covariates to each other and to the exposure and outcome then we could make use of the backdoor path criterion in Chapter 3 to determine which covariates would be sufficient to control for confounding bias. However, often such detailed structural information about all of the different possible covariates is not available. Other approaches must then be used.

One principle of covariate selection for confounding control that is sometimes used is what might be referred to as the "pretreatment criterion."[8,21] In this approach one attempts to control for any variable with a value that is set before the treatment or exposure under study begins. Restriction is made to covariates that precede the exposure because otherwise such a covariate might be on the pathway from exposure to outcome and controlling for it might block some of the effect. In principle, one could control for covariates subsequent to the exposure but not affected by the exposure,[6] but as it is difficult to know for sure whether a covariate that is subsequent to the exposure is affected by it, often the restriction is made to covariates temporally prior to the treatment or exposure under study. Any common cause of both the exposure and the outcome must be prior to the exposure and thus such restriction to pre-exposure covariates seems reasonable. Because we often do not know whether a particular covariate in fact affects both the exposure and the outcome, one seemingly reasonable strategy is, whenever possible, to adjust for all available covariates that are temporally prior to the exposure.[8,21]

But is this "pretreatment" approach to confounder selection the best? One problem that arises with the "pretreatment" approach is that in principle one may end up controlling for a pre-exposure covariate that in fact introduces bias.[6,15,22] In the causal diagram in Figure 12-1B, for example, an analysis of the association between X and Y without controlling for any covariate would give valid estimates of causal effects, but in an analysis adjusted for L, there would be bias because of the unblocked backdoor path X-U_1-L-U_2-Y that was unblocked by conditioning on the collider L. Here the "pretreatment" confounder selection approach fails. Its use in fact introduces bias.[6,22]

An alternative approach to confounder selection that requires relatively little knowledge of the underlying causal structure and is used with some frequency in practice is what one might call a "common cause" approach: one adjusts for all pre-exposure covariates that are common causes of exposure and outcome.[23] The application of this criterion requires more knowledge than the application of the "pretreatment" criterion, because for each covariate one must know whether it is a cause of the exposure and of the outcome. Nonetheless, this required knowledge is considerably less than that required to employ the backdoor path criterion, which also requires knowledge of the causal relations between each covariate and every other covariate. The common cause criterion has the advantage that if one is genuinely able to control for all common causes of the exposure and the outcome, then regardless of what the underlying causal diagram might be, control for this set of common causes will suffice to control for confounding for the effect of the exposure on the outcome.[6] A disadvantage of the common cause criterion is that in certain instances, if data on some of the covariates that are common causes of the exposure and the outcome are missing, there might be a different set of covariates that suffices to control for confounding, but that is not captured by the common cause criterion. Consider, for example, the causal diagram in Figure 12-4A and suppose that data on U are not available but that data on Z are available. If the only covariate available were Z, then, as Z is not a common cause of X and Y, the common cause criterion would suggest not to control for it. However, if one did control for Z, even though it is not a common cause of X and Y, this action would suffice to control for confounding. So whereas the "pre-exposure" criterion was too sensitive and could result in control for covariates that create bias, the "common cause" criterion is too specific and may result in not controlling for covariates that in fact would suffice to eliminate bias.

An alternative approach that strikes a balance between these two alternatives is to control for any pre-exposure covariate that is a cause of the exposure, or the outcome, or both. We will refer to this criterion as the "disjunctive cause criterion"[24] because one controls for covariates that are causes of the exposure *or* the outcome (or are causes of both). Like the common cause criterion, this disjunctive cause criterion requires knowledge of whether each covariate is a cause of the exposure and whether it is a cause of the outcome, but it does not require knowledge of the full underlying causal diagram relating each of the covariates to all of the other covariates. The disjunctive cause criterion also has some attractive properties with regard to confounding control. The application of this criterion to Figure 12-1B would result in not controlling for L as L is not a cause of X or Y; the application of the criterion would thus avoid bias generated by controlling for L in Figure 12-1B. Moreover in Figure 12-4A, the disjunctive cause criterion would result in controlling for covariate Z as Z is a cause of X; and the control for covariate Z would then suffice to control for confounding and avoid the bias arising from the common cause criterion that results from not controlling for Z. In fact, it can be shown that, for every causal diagram, if there is any subset of the measured covariates that suffices to control for confounding, then the set selected by the disjunctive cause criterion will suffice as well. This property does not hold for the "pretreatment" as illustrated by Figure 12-1B and does not hold for the "common cause" criterion as illustrated in Figure 12-4A.

A reasoned approach to confounding control, if knowledge is available on whether each covariate is a cause of the exposure and whether each covariate is a cause of the outcome, might then be to apply the disjunctive cause criterion, which selects those covariates that are causes of the exposure, or the outcome, or both. This approach is sensible, but its use in practice would benefit from two further qualifications. First, it has been documented elsewhere that if there is some residual

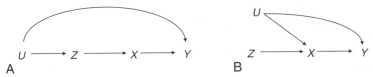

A   B

FIGURE 12-4 A, Controlling for measured covariate Z, even in the presence of unmeasured variable U, eliminates confounding of the relationship between exposure X and outcome Y, even though Z itself is not a common cause of X and Y. B, In the presence of uncontrolled confounding between exposure X and outcome Y induced by unmeasured variable U, controlling for the instrument Z can amplify the bias induced by U.

confounding due to an unmeasured covariate U, then controlling for a variable that is a cause of the exposure, but has no relation to the outcome except through the exposure, can in fact amplify the bias due to U.[25-28] For example, in Figure 12-4B, if U is unmeasured it will generate bias. However, in many cases, the bias will in fact be worse if adjustment is made for Z, than if adjustment is not made for Z.[25-28] Such a variable is a cause of the exposure, but has no relation to the outcome except through the exposure, and is sometimes in other contexts called an "instrument" or an "instrumental variable"[29] and the additional bias that can result from controlling for an instrument in the presence of unmeasured confounding is sometimes called "Z-bias."[26,28] Instrumental variables can sometimes be useful in obtaining estimates of the causal effect through instrumental variable analysis,[29-31] as described in Chapter 28, but controlling for instruments in a regression of the outcome on the exposure has the potential to generate bias. In general, it will often thus be best in practice, if the disjunctive cause criterion is to be used, to omit any variable known to be an instrumental variable from covariate control.[16] In general, the level of knowledge that is required to determine that a variable is an instrumental variable is considerable, as it must be known that it is a cause of the exposure but that it is otherwise unrelated to the outcome. It must be known, then, that the purported instrumental variable is not a cause of the outcome except through the exposure and that it is not related to the outcome through some other covariate. Such substantive knowledge will often not be available, and when instruments are employed in instrumental variable analysis their use is often considered controversial. Thus, while it would be good to discard from covariate selection any covariate known to be an instrument, these settings might, in practice, be quite rare.

A second qualification to the disjunctive cause criterion when used in practice is it might be desirable to adjust for any variable that does not satisfy the disjunctive cause criterion but that may be a proxy for a variable that is a common cause of exposure and outcome.[32] Variable Z_1 in Figure 12-3B is an example. A proxy for a variable that is a common cause of exposure and outcome may be essentially viewed as a confounder that is subject to measurement error, and in most cases, adjustment for such variables will reduce the bias due to confounding.[33-35] However, adjusting for a proxy of a confounder is not always guaranteed to reduce bias as documented also in Chapter 13 on information bias.

PRINCIPLES OF CONFOUNDER SELECTION AND CONFOUNDER TIMING

Another consideration that should be taken into account when making decisions about confounder selection based on substantive knowledge is that of covariate timing. It was noted above that for estimation of total effects (rather than direct effects, see Chapter 27) we do not want to make adjustment for variables that may be on the pathway from the exposure to the outcome. To avoid this, we often refrain from adjusting for covariates that occur subsequent to the exposure. In two-wave longitudinal studies, the exposure and covariates are often all assessed at one time and the outcome is assessed at a subsequent time. However, in many cohort studies, data are collected on all exposures, covariates, and outcomes repeatedly across each wave, perhaps once per year, or once every 2 years. Such designs can allow researchers to examine the effects of time-varying exposures (see Chapter 25), but even when assessing the effects of an exposure at a single point in time, such designs can help make more informed confounder selection decisions based on the temporal ordering of the data. One difficulty with studies in which the exposure and potential confounding covariates are all assessed at the same time is that it can be difficult to determine whether a covariate assessed at the same time as the exposure may in fact be affected by it.

Consider, for example, a study intended to assess the effect of physical activity on cardiovascular disease. BMI might be available as a covariate and it may be thought important to then control for BMI as a confounder. However, it is also conceivable that BMI is on the pathway from physical activity to cardiovascular disease and that control for it may block some of the effect of physical activity. However, it may also be the case that BMI itself affects both subsequent physical activity and subsequent incidence of cardiovascular disease. Someone with a very high BMI may have more difficulty regularly exercising. Thus it is possible that BMI is both a confounder (for the effect of subsequent physical activity) and a mediator on the pathway from prior physical activity to cardiovascular disease. It is thus difficult to know whether or not to adjust for BMI if both BMI and physical activity are measured at the same time. We cannot adequately distinguish in this setting between confounding and mediation. If, however, BMI is available repeatedly over time, then it may be possible to control for BMI in the wave of data prior to the wave that uses exercise as the primary exposure. This approach would better rule out the possibility that the BMI variable used in the analysis is a mediator; if its measurement precedes that of physical activity by a year, then it is more reasonable to interpret it as a confounder. When multiple waves of data are available, it may thus be desirable to control for the covariates in the wave before the primary exposure of interest. As discussed further in Chapter 25, it may also be desirable to control for prior levels of the exposure in the previous wave to rule out additional confounding. This option is not always possible when only two waves of data are available (one for the exposure and covariates and one for the outcome), but when multiple waves of data are available it can be possible to make decisions about covariate timing that allow one to control for confounders while better ruling out the possibility that one might in fact be controlling for a mediator. We will discuss these issues again in Chapter 25 when considering the causal effects of time-varying exposures, but they are relevant even in the context of considering the effects of an exposure at a single point in time. It is also possible to carry out sensitivity analysis of the timing of confounder measurement, and to compare the results when confounders are controlled for contemporaneously with the exposures versus controlled for in the prior wave.[36-39]

STATISTICAL CONFOUNDER SELECTION

The approach described above for covariate selection can be useful when sufficient knowledge is available as to whether each covariate may be a cause of the exposure and/or the outcome. The approach described above essentially involves making decisions about confounder control based on substantive knowledge. Various data-driven statistical approaches to confounder selection have also been proposed. Sometimes, these are motivated by the fact that there is far more covariate data available than is possible to adjust for in a standard regression model, especially when the number of covariates is relatively large and the study size is relatively modest. A statistical covariate selection technique might then be thought to be useful in reducing the number of covariates to achieve a more parsimonious model. Traditionally, this was perhaps the primary motivation for statistical approaches to covariate selection. Even when study sizes are large, however, if the number of covariates is very large, it may be difficult to go through each of the covariates one by one to assess whether they are causes of the exposure and/or outcome. That setting might also motivate a more statistically oriented approach to covariate selection. And, of course, both problems may be present: it may be impractical to substantively go through the covariates one-by-one to assess each, and it may also be the case that the number of covariates may be large relative to the total study size.

Historically, perhaps the most common statistical covariate selection techniques were forward and backward selection. In backward selection, one starts by adjusting for the complete set of covariates and then iteratively discards each covariate unassociated with the outcome conditional on the exposure and the other covariates. Adjustment can be by simultaneous stratification or by regression modeling. If the total set of covariates suffices to control for confounding for the effect of the exposure on the outcome, and if backward selection at each stage does correctly select and discard covariates unassociated with the outcome conditional on exposure and all remaining covariates at that stage, then the final set of covariates selected will also suffice to control for confounding.[24,40] In forward selection, one begins with an empty set of covariates and then examines associations of each covariate with the outcome conditional on the exposure, adding the first covariate that is associated with the outcome, conditional on exposure; then at each stage one examines associations of each covariate with the outcome conditional on the exposure and the covariates already selected, adding the first additional covariate that is thus associated; the process continues until, with the set of covariates selected, all remaining covariates are independent of the outcome, conditional on the exposure and the covariates that have been selected. Again, provided the total set of covariates suffices to control for confounding for the effect of the exposure on the outcome, and that the forward selection at each stage does correctly identify the covariates that are and are not associated with the outcome conditional on exposure and all remaining covariates at that stage, then under some further technical assumptions (that the distribution of the exposure, outcome, and covariates is "faithful" to the underlying causal diagram, see Chapter 3), one can conclude that the final set of covariates selected will also suffice to control for confounding.[24]

While the backward selection and forward selection procedures are intuitively appealing, they do suffer from a number of drawbacks when used in practice. First, when making the determination about whether a covariate is or is not associated with the outcome at each stage, statistical testing using P-values is often used in practice. Such statistical testing in no way ensures that the correct conclusion is reached.[41] The confounding control properties above only hold if, at each stage, the right decision is made. Second, once the final set of covariates is selected using either forward or backward selection, the most common approach is then to fit a final regression model with that set of covariates to obtain estimates and confidence intervals. Unfortunately, if the data have already been used to carry out covariate selection, the estimates and confidence intervals that are obtained following such selection no longer satisfy their strict frequentist definitions.[42] The standard approaches to statistical inference "postselection" break down. Recent work has examined approaches to carry out statistical inference after a data-based covariate selection procedure has been used, but these are no longer as straightforward as simply fitting a final regression model.[43-45]

Alternatively, one might consider doing the covariate selection with half of the data and fitting the final model with the other half of the data. This approach addresses the concerns about valid statistical inference, but results in considerable loss of precision: standard errors are much larger, and confidence intervals much wider, than they would otherwise be. However, a final disadvantage of backward selection when used in practice is that it requires that the study size is sufficiently large to fit the initial model with all covariates included. If one is carrying out covariate selection because the initial set of covariates is very large, then it will not be possible to even begin with such backward selection approaches. Alternatively, if the sample size is sufficiently large that one can fit the initial model with all of the covariates, then it might be sufficient to simply use that model to obtain estimates of the causal effect of the exposure on the outcome. Statistical covariate selection is then not even necessary. For these reasons, these traditional approaches to covariate selection may be of limited use. With many covariates and a smaller dataset, forward selection might be used to try to determine a much smaller set of covariates for which to adjust in the final model, but, because of the postselection statistical inference issues noted above, such analyses are perhaps best viewed as exploratory, rather than as providing a reliable estimate of the causal effect.

A statistical approach to covariate selection closely related to forward and backward selection is what is sometimes called the "change-in-estimate" approach. In this approach, covariate selection decisions are made based upon whether inclusion of a covariate changes the estimate of the causal effect for the exposure by more than some threshold, often 10%.[41] In some ways, this is similar to the forward and backward selection approaches described above in examining empirical associations, but it uses the magnitude of the effect estimates (in particular the magnitude of the change in the exposure effect estimate) rather than the presence or absence of association, or threshold for a P-value, in making covariate selection decisions. Like the forward and backward selection approaches based on associations or P-values, the change in estimate approach still requires that the initial total set of covariates suffice to control for confounding. If used independently one covariate at a time, without consideration of whether the set of covariates suffices to control for confounding, one may be led to control for a covariate that in fact generates bias, such as L in Figure 12-1B. Also, like the forward and backward selection approaches based on associations or P-values, validity of covariate selection with change in estimates requires that the decisions made about these associations are correct, and that sampling variability does not lead to an incorrect decision about association. For example, one may end up with a change in the exposure coefficient with and without a covariate of more than 10%, not because the covariate is a confounder, but simply due to chance variation.

However, the change-in-estimate approach has one further disadvantage that the forward and backward selection procedures do not share: the change in estimate approach is relative to the effect measure and will not work for noncollapsible measures such as the odds ratio or hazard ratio if the outcome is common (see Chapters 4 and 5). For noncollapsible measures such as the odds ratio or hazard ratio with a common outcome, marginal and conditional estimates are not directly comparable. Even in a randomized trial, one can have a true change in an odds ratio after controlling for a covariate, not because of confounding, but because of noncollapsibility.[46] Conversely, an odds ratio estimate may not change even after adjustment for a true confounder because, for example, a downward change in the odds ratio effect measure induced by confounding may be balanced by an upward change in the measure due to noncollapsibility. Thus, even beyond all of the caveats above concerning forward and backward selection, covariate selection based on change-in-estimate approaches is further problematic when noncollapsible effect measures are used. See Chapters 4 and 5 for further discussion.

An alternative approach to covariate selection that has become popular is to use a procedure related to what is now sometimes called a "high-dimensional propensity score."[47,48] In this approach, one covariate at a time, one calculates the risk ratio between that covariate and the outcome, and for a binary covariate, one also examines the prevalence of the covariate comparing the exposed and unexposed. Using these quantities an approximate estimate of the bias that such a covariate might generate is obtained[47,48] and covariates are prioritized in order of this approximate bias. Some portion of the covariates (*e.g.*, 10%) are then chosen based on this ordering of the approximate bias. These might then also be supplemented with certain demographic covariates, or other covariates which, for various reasons, the investigator may want to force into the model. These covariates can then be used in covariate adjustment for the estimation of causal effects either through propensity scores, or through some other modeling approach. Compared with forward and backward selection, this approach has the advantage of making use of information both on the magnitude of association each covariate has with the outcome and with the exposure, and effectively discarding those where one of these two is small. However, compared with the standard forward and backward selection procedures, it has the disadvantage of not sharing the theoretical property that the final resulting set of covariates is guaranteed to suffice to control for confounding if the initial total set suffices (provided the presence of associations is assessed accurately). The "high-dimensional propensity score" (HDPS) does not share this property with the traditional forward and backward selection approaches because with the HDPS, the selection is done one covariate at a time, independent of the others, rather that conditional on the others as with forward and backward selection. Its performance in practice may sometimes be reasonable, but its theoretical properties provide no guarantee. Perhaps most importantly, however, the HDPS approach, like forward and backward selection, makes no adjustment in statistical inference for the fact that the estimate in the final model is obtained "post-selection."

Fortunately, more principled approaches to statistical covariate selection have begun to develop. Some of these involve the use of machine learning algorithms to carry out covariate selection and to carry out flexible modeling between the outcome, exposure, and covariates, and use cross-validation and other approaches to handle inference post-selection. An approach to covariate selection that is flexible and that has been used with some frequency in the biomedical sciences is targeted maximum likelihood estimation.[49-51] This approach uses machine learning algorithms to model both the exposure and the outcome and cross-validation techniques to choose among the best models and covariates. While such approaches may hold promise for statistical covariate selection, more work is needed to understand the study sizes and covariate numbers for which the approach is feasible and has reasonable small-sample properties. While the theoretical properties of these techniques are desirable, they are only applicable asymptotically (requiring large study sizes to be guaranteed to hold), and their performance in smaller studies is sometimes less clear. More practical and simulation-based work is needed to determine in what contexts such approaches to statistical covariate selection work well. Moreover, even with the most sophisticated statistical covariate selection approaches, the initial covariate set itself must include at least one minimally sufficient set, which of course requires some substantive knowledge involving the considerations discussed in the previous sections.[52]

SIMPLE BIAS ANALYSIS FOR UNMEASURED CONFOUNDING

While we may do the best we can at collecting data on, and controlling for, a sufficient set of confounders, the assumption that we have adequately controlled for confounding is always, with observational data, at best approximate. We can never be sure that there is not some other variable that may be related to the exposure and the outcome and confound our estimates. Bias analysis is a type of sensitivity analysis and can be useful in assessing the extent to which an unmeasured variable that affects both the exposure and the outcome would change our effect estimates. Many sensitivity analysis techniques for unmeasured confounding for total effects have been developed.[53-65] Here we will first consider some approaches that have been used with considerable frequency in the literature but impose assumptions to make the sensitivity analysis tractable. We will also discuss some more recent developments that relax these assumptions and can be used more generally. Further discussion of bias analysis, including bias analysis not only for uncontrolled confounding but also for information bias and selection bias, is given in Chapters 13, 14, and 29.

Difference Scale

Suppose we have obtained an estimate of the effect of the exposure X on the outcome Y conditional on measured covariates Z. We can define a bias factor B_{RD} on the additive scale as the difference between (1) the expected differences in outcomes comparing $X = 1$ and $X = 0$ conditional on covariates $Z = z$ and (2) what we would have obtained had we been able to adjust for U as well. The bias factor, B_{RD}, may, under some assumptions, be written as the product of the effect of the unaccounted factor U on the outcome with the degree of association between U and the exposure. If we are willing to assume the effect of U on Y on the difference scale is the same for the exposed and the unexposed (*i.e.*, no interaction between U and X on the additive scale) so that the effect of a one unit increase in U on Y, above and beyond the measured covariates Z, was $\gamma = E(Y|x,z,U = u+1) - E(Y|x,z,U = u)$ then the bias factor is given by[57,66,67]:

$$B_{RD} = \gamma\delta$$

where $\delta = E(U|X = 1,z) - E(U|X = 0,z)$ is simply the average difference in the mean of the unmeasured factor U comparing the exposed and the unexposed with the same value of the covariates Z. If U were binary, then the effect of U on Y is just $\gamma = E(Y|x,z,U = 1) - E(Y|x,z,U = 0)$, and the second term in the expression for the bias factor, δ, is then just $\delta = P(U = 1|X = 1,z) - P(U = 1|X = 0,z)$, the difference in the prevalence of U comparing the exposed and the unexposed. Once we obtain the bias factor B_{RD}, we can obtain a bias-adjusted estimate and confidence interval of what one would have obtained had control been made for U in addition to Z, by simply subtracting the bias factor B_{RD} from the estimate and confidence interval obtained having only adjusted for the measured covariates Z.

This simple result, $B_{RD} = \delta\gamma$, is given in a number of places in the literature[57,66,67] and was shown to hold if the initial estimates were obtained using regression with main effects for X and Z in the regression model. In fact, it can be shown that the result holds more generally and applies irrespective of whether the initial estimate adjusted for Z was obtained by regression, or propensity score analysis, or inverse probability weighting or some other technique, provided the effect of U on Y is the same for both values of the exposure on the additive scale.[65]

We may not believe any particular specification of the parameters, δ and γ, but we could vary these parameters over a range of plausible values to obtain a plausible range of bias-adjusted estimates. This varying of the values assigned to the bias parameters is a sensitivity analysis or a bias analysis; we can carry out an evaluation of the sensitivity of the bias analysis to changes in assumptions. The range of the values over which the bias analysis parameters are varied could be determined by substantive knowledge or other prior studies that may have reported estimates of the associations of the covariates with the outcome. Using this technique, we could also examine how substantial the confounding would have to be to explain away an effect altogether. We could do this for the estimate and confidence interval. We consider such approaches below.

The technique can also be employed for estimates for the effect of the exposure on the exposed (or on the unexposed) with very slight adaptation. For the effect of the exposure on the exposed, the bias analysis parameter is simply specified as the effect of U on Y among the unexposed, *i.e.*, $\gamma = E(Y|X = 0,z,U = 1) - E(Y|X = 0,z,U = 0)$, and then the same approach as described above can be used with the parameter so defined. Likewise, the approach can be used in bias analysis for the effect of the exposure X among those who are actually unexposed, by redefining the bias analysis parameter as the effect of U on Y among the exposed, *i.e.*, $\gamma = E(Y|X = 1,z,U = 1) - E(Y|X = 1,z,U = 0)$. As an example, consider a study by Reinisch et al. that used data from a hospital in Copenhagen to examine the effect of in utero exposure to phenobarbital (X) on intelligence in men as assessed by Danish Military Board Intelligence Test (Y) taken by participants in their early 20s.[68] After adjustment for numerous social, health-related, and demographic covariates, Reinisch et al. obtained an estimate of the effect of the exposure on the exposed of -4.77 test points (95% CI $= -7.96$ to -1.58). However, parental intelligence, which was not measured in the study, may partially confound the analysis. Using the approach above, if we hypothesize an unmeasured confounding variable U of, say, the average of maternal and paternal intelligence measured by the Danish Military Board Intelligence Test, and we assume that if unexposed, a one-point increase in

U would on average result in a 0.5 point increase in Y so that $\gamma = 0.5$, then it follows from the bias factor formula above that $B_{RD} = (0.5)\delta$. It would then require a difference in parental intelligence of $\delta = -4.77/(0.5) = -9.54$ between the parents of the exposed and unexposed on the Danish Military Board Intelligence Test to completely explain away the estimated deficit. Reinisch et al. note that the standard deviation for a national sample of subjects taking the Danish Military Board Intelligence Test was 11.38. Thus nearly a standard deviation difference in parental intelligence between the parents of the exposed and unexposed would be required. This difference is perhaps not entirely implausible, but would constitute fairly substantial unmeasured confounding needed to explain away the estimate of the causal effect.

Ratio Scale

We will now consider the bias factor B_{mult} on the multiplicative scale as the ratio of (1) the risk ratio comparing $X = 1$ and $X = 0$ given only the controlled covariates Z, and (2) what we would have obtained for the risk ratio had we been able to control for both Z and U. We will build on a formula by Schlesselman[54] developed from the work of Bross.[69,70] Related formulas based on different parameterizations can be found in many other sources, including Flanders and Khoury.[56]

To get an easily used formula, we will make the simplifying assumptions that U is binary and that the risk ratios for the effect of U on Y is constant, *i.e.*, no modification of the effects of U on Y on the risk-ratio scale across levels of X. If we let $\gamma_m = P(Y = 1|x,z,U = 1)/P(Y = 1|x,z,U = 0)$ be the effect of U on Y on the risk ratio scale above and beyond the measured covariates Z then

$$B_{mult} = \left[1 + \left(\gamma_m - 1\right)P\left(U = 1 | X = 1, z\right)\right] \Big/ \left[1 + \left(\gamma_m - 1\right)P\left(U = 1 | X = 0, z\right)\right]$$

where $P(U = 1|X = 1,z)$ and $P(U = 1|X = 0,z)$ are simply the prevalence of the unmeasured confounder U among the exposed and unexposed, respectively. We can thus use the bias formula once we specify γ_m, which is the effect of U on Y on the risk ratio scale, and also the prevalence of U among the exposed and exposed. Once we have calculated the bias term B_{mult}, we can obtain a corrected estimate and confidence interval of what would have been obtained had control been made for U in addition to Z, by simply dividing the estimate and confidence interval obtained having only adjusted for the measured covariates Z by the multiplicative bias factor B_{mult}. A similar approach can be used for odds ratios as well if the outcome is rare. Note that to use the multiplicative bias factor, we must now specify the prevalence of the unmeasured confounder in both exposure groups, *i.e.*, $P(U = 1|A = 1,z)$ and $P(U = 1|A = 0,z)$ not just the difference between these two prevalences as with the bias factor for outcomes on the difference scale.

We will illustrate this approach for binary outcomes using analyses presented by Moorman et al. who report on associations between ovarian cancer and breastfeeding.[71] For premenopausal women, with no breastfeeding as a reference group, Moorman et al. report an odds ratio for ovarian cancer of 0.5 (95% CI: 0.3, 0.8) for those women who breast-fed 6 to 12 months versus not at all. Moorman et al. control for a number of covariates but do not control for socioeconomic status (SES), which is often thought to be a confounder in associations between breastfeeding and health outcomes. Let $U = 1$ denote low SES (versus high SES as the reference). Ovarian cancer is a relatively rare outcome, and so the odds ratios approximate risk ratios. Suppose we thought that low SES increased the risk of ovarian cancer by 1.5-fold and that 30% of the 6 to 12 month breastfeeding group was low SES but 70% of the reference group (no breastfeeding) was low SES. From the multiplicative bias factor formula above we would obtain a bias factor of $B_{mult} = [1+(1.5 - 1)(0.3)]/[1+(1.5 - 1)(0.7)] = 0.85$. If we divide the observed estimate and the confidence interval by this bias factor, we obtain a corrected estimate of 0.6 (95% CI: 0.4, 0.9). Suppose instead we thought that low SES increased the risk of ovarian cancer by 2.5 fold and that 30% of the 6 to 12 month breastfeeding group was low SES but 70% of the reference group (no breastfeeding) was low SES. The bias factor would then be $B_{mult} = [1+(2.5 -1)(0.3)]/[1+(2.5 - 1)(0.7)] = 0.71$, and if we divide the observed estimate and confidence interval by this bias factor, we obtain a corrected estimate of 0.7 (95% CI: 0.4, 1.1). The estimate still appears protective but the confidence interval now does contain 1.

One might object to a sensitivity analysis like this because of the assumptions of specifying the strength of the confounding parameters, and furthermore because an investigator could simply choose values parameter values that make the estimate seem robust. A potential remedy would be to provide a large table with different values of the parameters including some which are large, to give readers and researchers a sense as to how sensitive the conclusions are to potential unmeasured confounders. One could also plot all the values of the parameters that suffice to explain away, or reverse, the association. An alternative and arguably simpler approach is to report a metric called the E-value which we describe below.

Bias Analysis and the E-value

The techniques above can be helpful in trying to assess how an uncontrolled confounder of a specified strength might affect estimates of a causal effect. However, sometimes these techniques are criticized as being too subjective, in that whatever estimate is obtained, investigators will choose the sensitivity parameters so that the result looks robust to concerns about uncontrolled confounding. Sometimes these techniques are also criticized on the grounds that they make simplifying assumptions about the unmeasured confounder, such as that the unmeasured confounder is binary, or that there is only one unmeasured confounder, or that there is no interaction between the effects of the unmeasured confounder and the exposure on the outcome. It is possible, however, to address these criticisms of techniques that make assumptions by representing the bias as a function of other parameters (*e.g.*, the confounder associations with exposure and outcome),[72] and to find the values of those other parameters that would be needed to produce the observed association when no effect is present—that is, "explain away" the association, so that it is pure bias.[73] We can also use the techniques to find values of the parameters that would be needed to attenuate the observed effect toward the null from a pre-specified size down to the observed level.

Here and throughout this section, "uncontrolled confounding" refers to the composite confounding attributable to (1) residual confounding, which arises from imperfect measurement of measured and uncontrolled confounders, (2) unmeasured confounding, which arises from variables that would optimally have been measured and controlled, but were not, and (3) unknown confounding, which arises from incomplete specification of the variables that ought to have been included in a minimally sufficient set. This "uncontrolled confounding" is conditional on control for the measured and controlled variables. We begin by describing one such technique and then discuss a metric called the E-value,[73] which is related to this technique.

Suppose after adjustment for a vector of measured covariates Z, we obtain an estimated relative risk of RR, but that we are still concerned about uncontrolled confounding. Suppose that all confounding would be removed if the study could have controlled for one or more unmeasured confounders U, along with Z. Let RR_{UY} denote the maximum risk ratio for the outcome comparing any two categories of the unmeasured confounder, within either exposure group, conditional on Z. Let RR_{XU} denote the maximum risk ratio for any specific level of the unmeasured confounder comparing those with and without exposure, having already adjusted for Z. Both parameters should be specified so that they are greater than 1 (one can take the inverse of those less than 1). Thus RR_{UY} captures how important the unmeasured confounder is for the outcome, and RR_{XU} captures how imbalanced the exposure groups are in the unmeasured confounder U, conditional on control for Z. Once these parameters are specified the maximum relative amount such uncontrolled confounding could reduce an observed risk ratio is given by the following formula[72]:

$$B = RR_{UY} RR_{XU} / (RR_{UY} + RR_{XU} - 1)$$

To obtain the most that this uncontrolled confounding could alter an observed risk ratio and its confidence interval, one simply divides the observed risk ratio and confidence interval by this bias factor B.[72] The formula applies when the observed risk ratio RR is greater than 1. If the observed risk ratio is less than 1, then one multiplies by this bias factor rather than dividing by it.

If we return to the data of Moorman et al. on the relation between maternal breastfeeding and ovarian cancer,[71] in which there was a RR of 0.5 (95% CI: 0.3, 0.8) for those breastfeeding 6 to 12 months compared with no breastfeeding, suppose that the only concern about uncontrolled confounding pertained to the unmeasured confounder of socioeconomic status and that the maximum ratio by which low SES could increase ovarian cancer is $RR_{UY} = 1.5$ and the maximum by which SES differed by breastfeeding status was $RR_{XU} = 2$. The bias factor is then $B = (1.5 \times 2)/(1.5+2-1)$ $= 1.2$. Because the observed risk ratio is less than 1, we multiply the risk ratio by this bias factor to obtain the most that uncontrolled confounding by SES could alter the effect estimate. We thus obtain $RR = 0.5 \times 1.2 = 0.6$. We could also multiply the confidence limits, in which case we obtain (0.36, 0.96). Thus, uncontrolled confounding of this strength would not suffice to explain entirely the effect estimate.

One might object to an analysis like this because of the assumptions of specifying the strength of the confounding parameters, RR_{UY} and RR_{XU}, and, furthermore, because an investigator could simply choose values of RR_{UY} and RR_{XU} that failed to explain away the estimate, or else could choose them to ensure the estimate was explained away. To answer this objection, we can simply report how large these parameters must be to explain away the observed association.

The E-value is the minimum strength of association on the risk ratio scale that an unmeasured confounder, representing a composite of all uncontrolled confounding conditional on control of measured covariates, would need to have with both the exposure and the outcome to explain away an exposure-outcome association. Rather than focusing on whether uncontrolled confounding of a specified strength would suffice to explain away an effect estimate as above, the E-value focuses on the magnitude of the confounder associations that could produce confounding bias equal to the observed exposure-outcome association. The investigator is not choosing the parameters but merely reporting how much the composite bias from uncontrolled confounding, represented by a single unmeasured confounder, would have to be related to the exposure and outcome to explain away an effect estimate. Readers or other researchers can then assess whether confounder associations of that magnitude are plausible. For an observed risk ratio of RR, the E-value can be obtained through a straightforward calculation[72,73]:

$$E\text{-value} = RR + \mathrm{sqrt}\left[RR \times \left(RR - 1 \right) \right]$$

The formula applies to a risk ratio greater than 1; for a risk ratio less than 1, one first takes the inverse of the observed risk ratio and then applies the formula. Thus for the risk ratio above of 0.5, one first takes the inverse $1/0.5 = 2$ and one can obtain the E-value as follows:

$$E\text{-value} = 2 + \mathrm{sqrt}\left[2 \times \left(2 - 1 \right) \right] = 3.41$$

From this E-value we could then conclude that "to explain away the observed risk ratio of $RR = 0.5$, the composite bias from uncontrolled confounding, represented by an unmeasured confounder that was associated with ovarian cancer and with breastfeeding by a risk ratio of 3.4-fold each, above and beyond the measured confounders, could explain it away entirely, but weaker confounding could not fully explain the observed association." The strength of an unmeasured confounder here is understood as the maximum bias that could be generated in the bias formula for B given the confounder associations. Relatively strong uncontrolled confounding associations would be needed to completely explain away this observed exposure-outcome association.

The E-value is a continuous measure of how robust the association is to potential uncontrolled confounding. The lowest possible E-value of 1 (*i.e.*, no unmeasured confounding is needed to explain away the observed association) arises when the observed RR is 1. The higher the RR, the larger the E-value and thus the stronger the confounder associations would have to be to explain away the effect. This inferential approach to evaluation of the potential importance of uncontrolled confounding is in some sense a derivative of the "strength of association" consideration proposed by Bradford Hill.[74] The E-value essentially sets the two parameters, RR_{UY} and RR_{XU}, equal to each other to see the minimum that they would both need to be. If one of the two parameters were smaller than the E-value, then the other would have to be larger. We can also report the

E-value for the limit of the confidence interval closer to the null. One simply calculates, using the formula above, the E-value for the limit of the confidence interval closer to the null.[75] In the case of the ovarian cancer example, the E-value, for the upper limit of the confidence interval (0.8), is obtained by first taking inverses $1/0.8 = 1.25$ and then applying the formula above which produces an E-value for the confidence limit of $1.25 + \text{sqrt}[1.25 \times (1.25 - 1)] = 1.81$. Uncontrolled confounding represented by an unmeasured confounder that was associated with ovarian cancer and with breastfeeding by risk ratios of 1.81-fold each could explain away the upper confidence limit, but weaker confounding could not. The evidence for causality from the E-value thus looks reasonably strong as it would take substantial uncontrolled confounding to reduce the observed association to null.

A similar approach can be used to examine how much confounding would be required to shift an observed risk ratio to any other level by applying the E-value approach and the formula above to the ratio of the specified true risk ratio to the observed risk ratio. For example, if the observed risk ratio were $RR = 3$ and one desired to assess the minimum confounding needed to shift this to a risk ratio of 2, one simply calculates $3/2 = 1.5$ and applies the E-value formula to this quantity to obtain $1.5 + \text{sqrt}[1.5 \times (1.5 - 1)] = 2.36$. If the confounding associations were both $RR_{UY} = RR_{XU} = 2.36$ then this amount of confounding could suffice to shift the risk ratio from 3 to 2 but weaker confounding could not. Likewise if the observed risk ratio were only $RR = 1.03$ and one desired to assess the minimum confounding needed to shift this to a risk ratio of 1.3, one simply calculates $1.03/1.3 = 0.792$ and, taking inverses, one obtains $1/0.792 = 1.26$ and then applying the E-value formula to this quantity gives $1.26 + \text{sqrt}[1.26 \times (1.26 - 1)] = 1.83$. If the confounding associations were both $RR_{UY} = RR_{XU} = 1.83$, then this amount of confounding could suffice to shift the risk ratio from 1.03 to 1.3 but weaker confounding could not.

For risk ratios, E-value calculations are straightforward. For other effect measure scales approximate E-values can be obtained.[73] Software and online E-value calculators are available.[76] The E-value interpretation does, however, depend on context and, in particular, on the measured covariates for which adjustment has been made. The E-value concerns the strength of both of the confounder associations that must be present, *above and beyond the measured covariates*, for an unmeasured confounder representing all uncontrolled confounding to explain away an association. Thus, for example, if two different studies of breastfeeding had the same E-value of 2.5, but one had controlled for multiple indicators of socioeconomic status (educational attainment, income, occupation, home-ownership, wealth), and the other had controlled for only a single binary marker of college education, then the former study would be more robust to uncontrolled confounding, as, in the former study, an unmeasured confounder would have to be associated with both breastfeeding and also the outcome by a risk ratio of 2.5-fold each, through pathways independent of multiple (rather than just one of the) socioeconomic markers.

We emphasize that the E-value results do not guarantee that if there were a confounder with parameters of a particular strength then it necessarily would explain away the effect. They merely indicate that it is possible to construct scenarios in which it could.[72] An unmeasured confounder that has low prevalence in both exposure groups in study population would not bias an estimate as much as a more prevalent confounder.[54,56] If it is known in advance that an unmeasured confounder is rare in both exposure groups, then one may not want to use the E-value approach but rather make use instead of the multiplicative bias factor considered above, which allows one to specify the assumed prevalence of the unmeasured confounder. However, one of the advantages of the E-value approach is that it does not require making assumptions about the prevalence of the unmeasured confounder, or making assumptions about the nature of these unmeasured confounders, such that it is binary.

Routine reporting of E-values for the estimate and confidence interval is straightforward to implement. Reporting of these metrics could strengthen the assessment of evidence for causality in observational studies. The E-value is thus a useful measure of robustness to uncontrolled confounding; however, it needs to be interpreted in context, along with other strengths and weaknesses of a study and design. Principles on reporting E-values are described elsewhere.[77] Reporting more extensive sensitivity analysis for unmeasured confounding beyond the E-value could strengthen the assessment of evidence yet further. Moreover, uncontrolled confounding is not the only source of potential bias in observational studies: measurement error, selection bias, and missing data must also be carefully considered in evaluating evidence. Issues of bias analysis in relation to several sources of bias are discussed further in Chapter 29.

OTHER DISTINCTIONS CONCERNING CONFOUNDING AND CONFOUNDERS

We conclude this chapter with a few further technical points concerning confounding and confounders. Through most of our discussion, we have been considering definitions of confounding related to assessing causal effects of the exposure on the outcome for the entire population, $E(Y_1 - Y_0|Z=z)$, possibly conditional also on covariates, *i.e.*, $E(Y_1 - Y_0|Z=z)$. However, as noted in Chapter 5 and elsewhere, one might also consider estimating causal effects for those actually exposed, $E(Y_1 - Y_0|X=1)$, or alternatively for those actually unexposed, $E(Y_1 - Y_0|X=0)$. These estimates can be obtained by standardizing the outcome difference conditional on measured covariates Z to the distribution of the covariates among either the exposed or the unexposed, respectively, as discussed in Chapter 5. In this case, the counterfactual independence assumptions are somewhat weaker than is required for estimating causal effects for the entire population. In particular, in the discussion at the beginning of the chapter, we said that the covariates Z suffice to control for confounding of the effect of exposure X on outcome Y if the counterfactuals Y_x are independent of X conditional on Z and we used the notation $Y_x \perp X|Z$ to denote this conditional independence. The conditional independence was to apply for all values that we might set the exposure $X = x$ to in the counterfactuals Y_x. For a binary exposure we required that this condition would hold both for Y_1 and for Y_0; that is, we would require both that $Y_1 \perp X|Z$ and that $Y_0 \perp X|Z$. However, if we were only interested in the effect of the exposure among the exposed we would only require $Y_0 \perp X|Z$; we would not need $Y_1 \perp X|Z$. And likewise if we were only interested in the effect of the exposure among the unexposed we would only require $Y_1 \perp X|Z$; we would not need $Y_0 \perp X|Z$. We need both of these conditions if we wanted the effect of the exposure on the entire population $E(Y_1 - Y_0)$.

Also in our discussions above, we stated our assumption for describing confounding as conditional independence of the distribution of counterfactual Y_x and the actual exposure received conditional on covariates Z. This assumption allows for estimation of causal effects on difference scales or ratios scales. For continuous outcomes, it also allows for assessing the distribution of counterfactual outcomes, for example, quantities like, $P(Y_1 > k|Z = z)$ and $P(Y_0 > k|Z = z)$ for each possible k. If, however, all we were interested in were estimating effects on a particular scale, say, the difference scale, then somewhat weaker confounding assumptions would be required. In particular, to estimate average causal effects on the difference scale $E(Y_1 - Y_0|Z=z)$, we do not need independence in the distribution of counterfactual outcomes but only in the mean levels of the counterfactual outcomes. Rather than requiring $Y_x \perp X|Z$, it would be sufficient instead to have $E(Y_x|X=1, Z=z) = E(Y_x|X=0, Z=z)$, which is a somewhat weaker condition. We might refer to conditions like this as absence of confounding for a *particular measure*, rather than *in distribution*.[78] Absence of confounding in distribution implies absence of confounding in any effect measure, but not vice versa. With the presence or absence of confounding in measure, we may have the absence of confounding on one scale (*e.g.*, the risk difference scale) but the presence of confounding on another (*e.g.*, the risk ratio scale). Such instances will in general be unusual but can in principle occur.

In the discussion above, we defined a confounder as a member of a minimally sufficient adjustment set. Robins and Morgenstern put forward a closely related, but not entirely identical definition for a confounder.[79] They were not principally concerned with how the word "confounder" is employed in practice when used in an unqualified sense, but rather with whether a particular variable would still, in some sense, be a confounder if data were also available on other variables. Robins and Morgenstern (Section 2H) say that Z is a confounder conditional on F if causal effects are computable given data on Z and F, but not on F alone.[79] This definition essentially forces the investigator to specify some other set of variables F when stating whether or not the variable is a confounder. It is closely related to the definition of a confounder as a member of a minimally sufficient adjustment set, but the subtle differences between the two point to some important distinctions. The relationship between the two definitions is as follows. In the framework of Robins and Morgenstern,[79] if one were to take as the (unqualified) definition of a confounder that "there exists some set F such that Z is a confounder conditional on F," then this would coincide with the definition of a confounder as a member of a minimally sufficient adjustment set.[16] If their definition of a confounder holds for some context F, then this is the VanderWeele and Shpitser definition[16] as a member of a minimally sufficient adjustment set as well. The VanderWeele and Shpitser definition[16] simply requires that there be some F such that Z is a confounder in the sense of Robins and Morgenstern.[79]

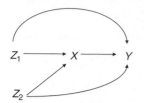

FIGURE 12-5 Neither Z_1 nor Z_2 alone suffice to control for confounding of the effect of exposure X on outcome Y, but it still makes sense to refer to each as a confounder.

The two closely related definitions have different implications, however, with respect to correspondence with ordinary language and epidemiologic practice. Concerning ordinary language, if one were to take the Robins and Morgenstern definition[79] as what epidemiologists mean in ordinary discourse when they use "confounder" in an unqualified sense, it would have some counterintuitive implications. Consider the structure in Figure 12-5. Suppose that an investigator asks, "Is Z_1 a confounder?" Under the definition of Robins and Morgenstern, the answer would either have to be "no" (as the causal effect is not computable with data on Z_1 alone) or, as a perhaps more nuanced response in accordance with the Robins and Morgenstern definition,[79] that "Unless you specify that you are also adjusting for Z_2, then Z_1 is not a confounder." Although this latter response is of course correct, it would be in tension with the way the word "confounder" is ordinarily used in epidemiology. In a context like Figure 12-5, if asked "Is Z_1 a confounder?" we would ordinarily just say "Yes, Z_1 is a confounder." However, Robins and Morgenstern go further than the definition as a member of a minimally sufficient adjustment set in having the investigator explicitly specify the other variables F for which control might be made.[79] Doing so would indeed be useful in practice, though current use of language as to what we refer to as a confounder has not generally adopted this convention.

We might attempt to synthesize these two closely related perspectives, integrating both the insights concerning how epidemiologists ordinarily use language, and that confounding control is always in the context of other variables. We could attempt to do so by drawing the distinction between the ordinary unqualified use of "confounder" and the expression "confounder in the context of control also of some set of variables F." The definition of a confounder as a "member of a minimally sufficient adjustment set"[16] might then be used for "confounder" when used in its unqualified sense as this definition seems to cohere with the ordinary use of the word in epidemiology and with the properties that epidemiologists seem to presuppose a confounder will satisfy. However, the Robins and Morgenstern definition[79] could be used for "confounder" when the context of the other variables is also specified so that a "confounder in the context of F" could be defined as "a variable such that the causal effects are computable given data on Z and F, but not on F alone." Then, in discussions of confounding and confounders, epidemiologists could be encouraged to specify also the context so that more regular reference is made to expressions of the form "confounder in the context of F" as this is generally the more relevant consideration in practice. Proceeding with definitions in this manner using "confounder" in its unqualified sense and "confounder within the context of", then points to important distinctions. The unqualified definition of a confounder as "a member of a minimally sufficient adjustment set"[16] is arguably how the word "confounder" is often used in speech; the contextual definition of Robins and Morgenstern[79] is arguably how discussion about confounding and confounder adjustment ought to proceed in practice. Specifying the context would be useful in making decisions about data collection and confounder control.

However, as noted above, these definitions concerning precisely what is meant by a "confounder" are in some sense secondary, as the goal is ultimately one of confounding control and once we move to confounding control, the principles described above come to the forefront. If one has complete knowledge of a causal diagram, then the backdoor path criterion can be used to identify a set of covariates on backdoor paths from exposure to the outcome that suffices to adjust for confounding.[6] If such knowledge is not available but knowledge is at least available as to which pre-exposure covariates are causes of the exposure or the outcome or both, then the disjunctive cause criterion,[24] or a modification of it, might be used to, as best as possible, select a set of covariates that suffices to control for confounding. The point is not so much whether each covariate is a confounder or not, and in what context, but rather to control for sufficient covariates to eliminate confounding.

References

1. Greenland S, Robins JM. Identifiability, exchangeability, and epidemiological confounding. *Int J Epidemiol*. 1986;15(3):413-419.
2. Robins JM. Estimation of the time-dependent accelerated failure time model in the presence of confounding factors. *Biometrika*. 1992;79:321-334.
3. Rosenbaum PR, Rubin DB. The central role of the propensity score in observational studies for causal effects. *Biometrika*. 1983;70:41-55.
4. Barnow BS, Cain GG, Golberger AS. Issues in the analysis of selectivity bias. In: Stromsdorfer E, Farkas G, eds. *Evaluation Studies*. San Francisco, CA: SAGE; 1980.
5. Imbens GW. Nonparametric estimation of average treatment effects under exogeneity: a review. *Rev Econ Stat*. 2004;86(1):4-29.
6. Pearl J. *Causality*. 2nd ed. New York, NY: Cambridge University Press; 2009.
7. VanderWeele TJ. Concerning the consistency assumption in causal inference. *Epidemiology*. 2009;20(6):880-883.
8. Rubin DB. Should observational studies be designed to allow lack of balance in covariate distributions across treatment groups? *Stat Med*. 2009;28(9):1420-1423.
9. Hernán MA, Hernández-Diaz S, Robins JM. A structural approach to selection bias. *Epidemiology*. 2004;15(5):615-625.
10. Hernán MA, Robins JM. *Causal Inference*. Boca Raton, FL: Chapman & Hall/CRC; 2018.
11. Hernán Miguel A. Confounding. In: Everitt B, Melnick E, eds. *Encyclopedia of Quantitative Risk Assessment and Analysis*. Chichester, West Sussex, United Kingdom: Wiley; 2008.
12. Schisterman EF, Cole SR, Platt RW. Overadjustment bias and unnecessary adjustment in epidemiologic studies. *Epidemiology*. 2009;20(4):488-495.
13. Miettinen O. Confounding and effect-modification. *Am J Epidemiol*. 1974;100(5):350-353.
14. Weinberg CR. Toward a clearer definition of confounding. *Am J Epidemiol*. 1993;137(1):1-8.
15. Greenland S, Pearl J, Robins JM. Causal diagrams for epidemiologic research. *Epidemiology*. 1999;10(1):37-48.
16. VanderWeele TJ, Shpitser I. On the definition of a confounder. *Ann Stat*. 2013;41(1):196-220.
17. Robins JM, Greenland S. The role of model selection in causal inference from nonexperimental data. *Am J Epidemiol*. 1986;123(3):392-402.
18. Miettinen OS, Cook EF. Confounding: essence and detection. *Am J Epidemiol*. 1981;114(4):593-603.
19. Geng Z, Guo J, Fung W-K. Criteria for confounders in epidemiological studies. *J R Stat Soc Ser B Stat Methodol*. 2002;64(1):3-15.
20. Greenland S, Pearl J. Causal diagrams. In: Boslaugh S, ed. *Encyclopedia of Epidemiology*. Thousand Oaks, CA: SAGE Publications; 2007.
21. Rubin DB. For objective causal inference, design trumps analysis. *Ann Appl Stat*. 2008;2(3):808-840.
22. Sjölander A. Propensity scores and M-structures. *Stat Med*. 2009;28(9):1416-1420.
23. Glymour MM, Weuve J, Chen JT. Methodological challenges in causal research on racial and ethnic patterns of cognitive trajectories: measurement, selection, and bias. *Neuropsychol Rev*. 2008;18(3):194-213.
24. VanderWeele TJ, Shpitser I. A new criterion for confounder selection. *Biometrics*. 2011;67(4):1406-1413.
25. Pearl J. On a class of bias-amplifying variables that endanger effect estimates. arXiv preprint arXiv:1203.3503. 2012.
26. Myers JA, Rassen JA, Gagne JJ, et al. Effects of adjusting for instrumental variables on bias and precision of effect estimates. *Am J Epidemiol*. 2011;174(11):1213-1222.
27. Wooldridge JM. Should instrumental variables be used as matching variables? Res Econ. 2016;70(2):232-237.
28. Ding P, VanderWeele TJ, Robins JM. Instrumental variables as bias amplifiers with general outcome and confounding. *Biometrika*. 2017;104(2):291-302.
29. Greenland S. An introduction to instrumental variables for epidemiologists. *Int J Epidemiol*. 2000;29(4):722-729.
30. Hernan MA, Robins JM. Instruments for causal inference: an epidemiologist's dream? *Epidemiology*. 2006;17(4):360-372.
31. Angrist JD, Imbens GW, Rubin DB. Identification of causal effects using instrumental variables (with comments). *J Am Stat Assoc*. 1996;91:444-472.
32. VanderWeele TJ. Principles of confounder selection. *Eur J Epidemiol*. 2019;34(3):211-219.
33. Greenland S. The effect of misclassification in the presence of covariates. *Am J Epidemiol*. 1980;112(4):564-569.
34. Ogburn EL, VanderWeele TJ. On the nondifferential misclassification of a binary confounder. *Epidemiology*. 2012;23(3):433-439.
35. Ogburn EL, Vanderweele TJ. Bias attenuation results for nondifferentially mismeasured ordinal and coarsened confounders. *Biometrika*. 2013;100(1):241-248.

36. Taubman SL, Robins JM, Mittleman MA, Hernan MA. Intervening on risk factors for coronary heart disease: an application of the parametric g-formula. *Int J Epidemiol.* 2009;38(6):1599-1611.
37. Garcia-Aymerich J, Varraso R, Danaei G, Camargo CA Jr, Hernan MA. Incidence of adult-onset asthma after hypothetical interventions on body mass index and physical activity: an application of the parametric g-formula. *Am J Epidemiol.* 2014;179(1):20-26.
38. Danaei G, Pan A, Hu FB, Hernan MA. Hypothetical midlife interventions in women and risk of type 2 diabetes. *Epidemiology.* 2013;24(1):122-128.
39. Lajous M, Willett WC, Robins J, et al. Changes in fish consumption in midlife and the risk of coronary heart disease in men and women. *Am J Epidemiol.* 2013;178(3):382-391.
40. Robins JM. Causal inference from complex longitudinal data. In: Berkane M, ed. *Latent Variable Modeling With Applications to Causality.* New York, NY: Springer-Verlag, 1997;69-117.
41. Maldonado G, Greenland S. Simulation study of confounder-selection strategies. *Am J Epidemiol.* 1993;138(11):923-936.
42. Greenland S Invited commentary: variable selection versus shrinkage in the control of multiple confounders. *Am J Epidemiol.* 2008;167(5):523-529; discussion 530-1.
43. Belloni A, Chernozhukov V, Hansen C. Inference on treatment effects after selection among high-dimensional controls. *Rev Econ Stud.* 2013;81(2):608-650.
44. Chernozhukov V, Hansen C, Spindler M. Valid post-selection and post-regularization inference: an elementary, general approach. *Annu Rev Econ.* 2015;7(1):649-688.
45. Lee JD, Sun DL, Sun Y, Taylor JE. Exact post-selection inference, with application to the lasso. *Ann Statist.* 2016;44(3):907-927.
46. Greenland S, Robins JM, Pearl J. Confounding and collapsibility in causal inference. *Stat Sci.* 1999;14:29-46.
47. Schneeweiss S, Rassen JA, Glynn RJ, Avorn J, Mogun H, Brookhart MA. High-dimensional propensity score adjustment in studies of treatment effects using health care claims data. *Epidemiology.* 2009;20(4):512-522.
48. Rassen JA, Glynn RJ, Brookhart MA, Schneeweiss S. Covariate selection in high-dimensional propensity score analyses of treatment effects in small samples. *Am J Epidemiol.* 2011;173(12):1404-1413.
49. van der Lann MJ, Rose S. *Targeted Learning: Causal Inference for Observational and Experimental Data. Springer Series in Statistics.* New York, NY: Springer-Verlag; 2011.
50. Schuler MS, Rose S. Targeted maximum likelihood estimation for causal inference in observational studies. *Am J Epidemiol.* 2017;185(1):65-73.
51. van der Lann MJ, Rose S. *Targeted Learning in Data Science: Causal Inference for Complex Longitudinal Studies.* New York, NY: Springer Series in Statistics Springer International Publishing; 2018.
52. Hernan MA, Hernandez-Diaz S, Werler MM, Mitchell AA. Causal knowledge as a prerequisite for confounding evaluation: an application to birth defects epidemiology. *Am J Epidemiol.* 2002;155(2):176-184.
53. Cornfield J, Haenszel W, Hammond EC, Lilienfeld AM, Shimkin MB, Wynder EL. Smoking and lung cancer: recent evidence and a discussion of some questions. *J Natl Cancer Inst.* 1959;22(1):173-203.
54. Schlesselman JJ. Assessing effects of confounding variables. *Am J Epidemiol.* 1978;108(1):3-8.
55. Rosenbaum PR, Rubin DB. Assessing sensitivity to an unobserved binary covariate in an observational study with binary outcome. *J R Stat Soc Ser B.* 1983;45(2):212-218.
56. Flanders WD, Khoury MJ. Indirect assessment of confounding: graphic description and limits on effect of adjusting for covariates. *Epidemiology.* 1990;1(3):239-246.
57. Lin DY, Psaty BM, Kronmal RA. Assessing the sensitivity of regression results to unmeasured confounders in observational studies. *Biometrics.* 1998;54(3):948-963.
58. Robins JM, Rotnitzky A, Scharfstein DO. Sensitivity analysis for selection bias and unmeasured confounding in missing data and causal inference models. In: Halloran ME, Berry DA, eds. *Statistical Models in Epidemiology.* New York, NY: Springer-Verlag; 1999:1-92.
59. Rosenbaum PR. *Observational Studies.* 2nd ed. New York, NY: Springer; 2002.
60. Imbens GW. Sensitivity to exogeneity assumptions in program evaluation. *Am Econ Rev.* 2003;93(2):126-132.
61. Greenland S. Basic methods for sensitivity analysis of biases. *Int J Epidemiol.* 1996;25(6):1107-1116.
62. Greenland S. Multiple-bias modeling for analysis of observational data (with discussion). *J R Stat Soc Ser A.* 2005;168:267-308.
63. McCandless LC, Gustafson P, Levy A. Bayesian sensitivity analysis for unmeasured confounding in observational studies. *Stat Med.* 2007;26(11):2331-2347.
64. Lash TL, Fox MP, Fink AK. *Applying Quantitative Bias Analysis to Epidemiologic Data. Statistics for Biology and Health.* New York, NY: Springer; 2009.
65. Vanderweele TJ, Arah OA. Bias formulas for sensitivity analysis of unmeasured confounding for general outcomes, treatments, and confounders. *Epidemiology.* 2011;22(1):42-52.
66. Cochran WG. The omission or addition of an independent variate in multiple linear regression. *Suppl J R Stat Soc.* 1938;5(2):171-176.

67. Marcus SM. Using omitted variable bias to assess uncertainty in the estimation of an AIDS education treatment effect. *J Educ Behav Stat*. 1997;22(2):193-201.

68. Reinisch JM, Sanders SA, Mortensen EL, Rubin DB. In utero exposure to phenobarbital and intelligence deficits in adult men. *J Am Med Assoc*. 1995;274(19):1518-1525.

69. Bross ID. Spurious effects from an extraneous variable. *J Chronic Dis*. 1966;19(6):637-647.

70. Bross ID. Pertinency of an extraneous variable. *J Chronic Dis*. 1967;20(7):487-495.

71. Moorman PG, Calingaert B, Palmieri RT, et al. Hormonal risk factors for ovarian cancer in premenopausal and postmenopausal women. *Am J Epidemiol*. 2008;167(9):1059-1069.

72. Ding P, VanderWeele TJ. Sensitivity analysis without assumptions. *Epidemiology*. 2016;27(3):368-377.

73. VanderWeele TJ, Ding P. Sensitivity analysis in observational research: introducing the E-value. *Ann Intern Med*. 2017;167(4):268-274.

74. Hill AB. The environment and disease: association or causation? *Proc R Soc Med*. 1965;58:295-300.

75. VanderWeele TJ, Ding P, Mathur M. Technical considerations in the use of the E-value. *J Causal Inference*. 2019;7.

76. Mathur MB, Ding P, Riddell CA, VanderWeele TJ. Web site and R package for computing E-values. *Epidemiology*. 2018;29(5):e45-e47.

77. VanderWeele TJ, Mathur MB. Commentary: Developing best-practice guidelines for the reporting of E-values. *Int J Epidemiol*. 2020:dyaa094. doi:10.1093/ije/dyaa094.

78. VanderWeele TJ. Confounding and effect modification: distribution and measure. *Epidemiol Method*. 2012;1(1):55-82.

79. Robins JM, Morgenstern H. The foundations of confounding in epidemiology. *Comp Math Appl*. 1987;14:869-916.

CHAPTER 13

Measurement and Measurement Error

Timothy L. Lash, Tyler J. VanderWeele, and Kenneth J. Rothman

INFORMATION BIAS

As we have emphasized throughout, epidemiologic research is best conceived as an exercise in measurement. The primary objectives of this measurement depend on the nature of the research. For descriptive epidemiology, the objective is usually an estimate of disease occurrence. For analytic epidemiology, the objective is to evaluate the effect of an exposure, compared with an alternative or unexposed condition. At a minimum, both objectives require measurement of the occurrence of the disease. Analytic epidemiology also requires measurement of the exposed and unexposed conditions. Most epidemiologic research studies also require measurement of covariates—potential confounders, modifiers, or mediators—in addition to the outcome and exposure categories. In longitudinal designs, many of these measurements are made more than once. All these measurements are subject to measurement error, and the influence of this error on the primary objective is called *information bias*. In this chapter, we describe the sources of measurement error, their relations to other variables and to one another, the expected direction and magnitude of the resulting information bias, and simple methods to adjust quantitatively for this bias.

Measurement Error, Misclassification, and Bias

Once study subjects have been identified, one must obtain the information about them to use in the analysis. Bias in estimating disease occurrence in descriptive epidemiology or an effect in analytic epidemiology can be caused by measurement errors in the needed information. The direction and magnitude of the resulting information bias depend heavily on whether the distribution of errors for one variable (*e.g.*, exposure or disease) depends on the actual value of the variable, the actual values of other variables, or the errors in measuring other variables.

In this chapter, we reserve the term "measurement error" for application to continuous variables (variables with an infinite number of possible values, at least in theory). For discrete variables (variables with a countable number of possible values, such as indicators for gender), measurement error will be called *classification error* or *misclassification*. Classification error that depends on the actual values of other variables is called *differential misclassification*. Classification error that does not depend on the actual values of other variables is called *nondifferential misclassification*. Classification error that depends on the errors in measuring or classifying other variables is called *dependent error*; otherwise the error is called *independent* or *nondependent error*. *Correlated error* is sometimes used as a synonym for dependent error, but technically it refers to dependent errors that have a nonzero correlation coefficient. More precise definitions of these concepts are given below.

Figure 13-1 uses causal graphs to depict various combinations of differential or nondifferential and dependent or independent misclassification of a dichotomous exposure (X misclassified as X^*) and a dichotomous outcome (A misclassified as A^*).[1] The top left panel of the figure depicts nondifferential and independent misclassification of both the exposure and the outcome. The true value of X influences the measured value X^* and the true value of A influences the measured value A^*. Other factors (U_x) also influence the measured value X^* and a different set of factors

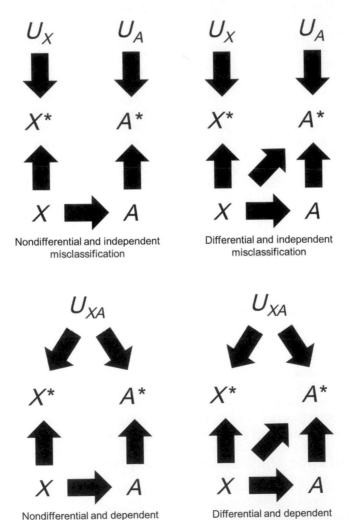

FIGURE 13-1 Graphical depiction of misclassification of a dichotomous exposure (X misclassified as X^*) and a dichotomous outcome (A misclassified as A^*). U represents causes of misclassification.

(U_A) also influence the measured value A^*. There is no open or biasing path between X^* and A^*, indicating that a non-null association between these variables is not expected to arise from this type of misclassification. The top right panel of the figure depicts differential and independent misclassification. The difference between the top right panel and the top left panel is that the true value of the exposure X influences the measured value of the outcome A^*. This situation connotes differential misclassification of the outcome, and now there is an open or biasing path between X^* and A^* ($X^* \Leftarrow X \Rightarrow A^*$), indicating that a non-null association between these variables may arise in whole or in part from this type of misclassification. The bottom left panel of the figure depicts nondifferential and dependent misclassification. The difference between the top left panel and the bottom left panel is that the measured values of X^* and A^* are both influenced by the same set of factors (U_{XA}) that explain their misclassification. This connotes dependent misclassification of the exposure and outcome, and now there is an open or biasing path between X^* and A^* ($X^* \Leftarrow U_{XA} \Rightarrow A^*$). The bottom right panel of the figure depicts differential and dependent misclassification, in which both previously described biasing paths are open.

As with these graphs, much of this chapter will concern misclassification of binary variables, primarily because disease occurrence is usually binary and exposure contrasts often involve comparisons of an exposed condition with an unexposed condition, so are also binary. Data with multiple levels, such as a dose-response analysis, still fit into this structure if each dose is compared with a single unexposed category, although there are important nuances to misclassification of dose categories that are also described below. Outcomes with continuous measures, such as blood pressure, are often categorized into diseased or undiseased states with a threshold to set the boundary, such as the boundary where high blood pressure is said to correspond to the disease "hypertension." Continuously measured exposures or covariates, such as body mass index (BMI), are often also categorized with bounds set based on biologically relevant thresholds or into percentiles. For example, the World Health Organization has set BMI categories that correspond to underweight, normal weight, overweight, obese I, obese II, and obese III. When the outcome, exposure, or a covariate enters the analysis as a continuous variable, measurement error models apply rather than classification error models.

There are many sources from which errors may be introduced into the measurement of a variable. The first level of these sources of error is the conceptual level. Each variable is meant to represent some underlying conceptual construct, and the actual measurement may not correspond well to the conceptual construct (in allied research fields, this incomplete correspondence between the conceptual construct and the actual measurement is called *construct validity*). For example, imagine that a cohort study asked participants how often they consume three or more drinks of alcohol per day. If the association between this measurement of alcohol consumption and the occurrence of liver cirrhosis were to be evaluated in the cohort, the association would probably be non-null. More valid constructs might include more finely divided doses of alcohol and an assessment of the duration in years for different consumption frequencies. This additional information would allow a more accurate estimate of cumulative alcohol consumption, which would likely be more strongly associated with the occurrence of liver cirrhosis. If the association between the original measurement of alcohol consumption and the occurrence of injury in an automobile accident were to be evaluated in the cohort, the association would also probably be non-null. More valid constructs might include the frequency of binge drinking, and even better than that would be to assess the number of alcoholic drinks consumed in the 12 hours preceding the accident. The construct validity of the original measurement may be adequate to study both associations, but the construct validity could be improved in different ways depending on the outcome with which it is to be associated. As another example, consider the measurement of intense physical activity by asking people how many minutes a week are spent in such activity. That measure may have reasonable construct validity when used to assess cardiovascular health, but it may have less construct validity when used to measure overuse injuries that depend on the nature of the activity, such as running versus bicycling. In both examples, the lack of correspondence between measurement and construct arises from incomplete assessment of the exposure information necessary to adequately measure the exposure construct. Poor construct validity can also arise when there is no uniform understanding of what constitutes the exposure itself. For example, there is no consensus understanding of what types of intimate acts constitute "having had sex,"[2] so researchers in this topic area must ask for more complete information to assure adequate construct validity.

The second level of sources of error arises in data collection. Whether data are collected by survey instruments (*e.g.*, mail, telephone, web-based, in-person interview, etc.), by record review (*e.g.*, medical record review or occupational record review), or from registries (*e.g.*, administrative health records, vital statistic registries, or cancer registries), errors in the data are inevitable. Self-reported survey data are subject to errors in recall and reporting. For example, some participants in the cohort example of the previous paragraph may not report accurately the frequency with which they consume three or more alcoholic drinks. Records may contain errors if they are themselves collected by self-report. For example, a medical record annotation of the patient's self-report of the frequency with which they consume three or more alcoholic drinks is subject to the same errors in self-reporting as a survey. Medical records may also contain misdiagnosed conditions or inaccurate information. For example, some patients' blood pressure rises when it is measured at a medical facility. The quality of registry data is only as good as the accuracy of the information supplied to the registry. This information may be inaccurate, for example, if prescriptions for medications were written but not filled, health conditions were not reported in the administrative billing data, or information about behavioral and social confounders were never recorded.[3] Even when all desired variables for an analysis are available, errors may arise by chance in the large datasets analyzed in some registry-based projects. For example, in a study of late effects in natal female long-term survivors of breast cancer, three prostate cancers were recorded.[4]

A third source of error arises in data management and handling. Almost all epidemiologic data are now input to a computer for analysis. The transfer of data from its original source to the analytic dataset is one opportunity for errors of this type, such as keystroke errors. Double data entry, with discrepant values of paired entries flagged by a computing algorithm, is one safeguard against data entry errors. Data transformations are a second opportunity for errors. Many epidemiologic analyses require a measurement of each participant's age. It is much more accurate to ask or extract date of birth and then let the computer calculate age at a particular calendar date, than to ask a person their age or to ask an interviewer to calculate a respondent's age on the date of interview once the respondent has reported their date of birth. In general, it is good practice to collect and enter data at its most fundamental level and then use the computer to make the transformations.

Differential Misclassification

Suppose a cohort study is undertaken to compare incidence rates of emphysema among smokers and nonsmokers. Emphysema is a disease that may go undiagnosed without special medical attention. If smokers, because of concern about health-related effects of smoking or as a consequence of other health effects of smoking (*e.g.*, bronchitis), seek medical attention more often than nonsmokers, then emphysema might be diagnosed more frequently among smokers than among nonsmokers simply as a consequence of the greater medical attention. Smoking does cause emphysema, but unless steps were taken to ensure comparable follow-up, this effect would be overestimated: A portion of the excess of emphysema incidence would not be a biologic effect of smoking, but would instead be an effect of smoking on *detection* of emphysema. This is an example of differential misclassification because underdiagnosis of emphysema (failure to detect true cases), which is a classification error, occurs more frequently for nonsmokers than for smokers.

In the binary classification setting, the *sensitivity* of a disease measurement method is the probability that someone who is truly diseased will be correctly classified as diseased by the method. The *false-negative probability* of the method is the probability that someone who is truly diseased will be incorrectly classified as undiseased; it equals 1 minus the sensitivity. In the example from the preceding paragraph, the sensitivity of disease classification was better for smokers than for nonsmokers. The false-negative probability was therefore higher for nonsmokers than for smokers. The *specificity* of the method is the probability that someone who is truly undiseased will be correctly classified as undiseased. The *false-positive probability* is the probability that someone who is truly undiseased will be incorrectly classified as diseased; it equals 1 minus the specificity. In the example, there was no reason to think that either smokers or nonsmokers without emphysema were incorrectly diagnosed as having the disease. The specificity would therefore be 100% for both and the false-positive probability would be 0% for both. The *predictive value positive* is the probability that someone who is classified as diseased is truly diseased. Finally, the *predictive value negative* is the probability that someone who is classified as undiseased is truly undiseased. All these terms can also be applied to descriptions of the methods for classifying exposure or classifying a potential confounder or modifier. Equations relating these classification parameters to one another will be given below.

In case-control studies of congenital malformations, information is sometimes obtained from interview of mothers after delivery. The case mothers have recently given birth to a malformed baby, whereas most control mothers have recently given birth to an apparently healthy baby. Another variety of differential misclassification, referred to as *recall bias*, can result if the mothers of malformed infants recall or report true exposures differently than mothers of healthy infants (higher sensitivity of exposure recall among cases than controls), or more frequently recall or report exposure that did not actually occur (lower specificity of exposure recall among cases than controls). It is supposed that the birth of a malformed infant serves as a stimulus to a mother to recall and report all events that might have played some role in the outcome. Presumably, such women will remember and report exposures such as infectious disease, trauma, and drugs more frequently than mothers of healthy infants, who have not had a comparable stimulus. An association unrelated to any biologic effect will result from this recall bias.

Recall bias is a possibility in any case-control study that relies on subject memory after the outcome has occurred, because the cases and controls are by definition people who differ with respect to their disease experience at the time of their recall, and this difference may affect recall and reporting. The amount of time elapsed between the exposure and the recall is an important indicator of the accuracy of recall[5]; studies in which the average time since exposure was different for interviewed cases and controls could thus suffer a differential misclassification.

The bias caused by differential misclassification can either exaggerate or underestimate an effect.[6] In each of the examples above, the misclassification ordinarily exaggerates the effects under study, but examples to the contrary can also be found and have been shown to be more common than expected.[7] We include a scenario in which differential misclassification biases toward the null in the worked example later in this chapter.

When the exposure variable enters the analysis as a continuous variable, the equivalent of differential misclassification of a dichotomous exposure variable is differential error in the measurement of the continuous exposure variable. In its simplest form, this error structure assumes that the measured exposure variable is a function of the true exposure and an error term centered on zero and with some variance for controls or undiseased members of a cohort, and a different error term that is not centered on zero and with some variance that is added only to the cases. The fact that the error terms have different means for controls than for cases arises from a differential error generating mechanism, such as recall bias. The expectation of each exposure measurement for controls or undiseased members of a cohort is therefore equal to its true value, but the expectation of each measurement for cases is different than its true value. Depending on the mean of the error term added to the true exposure value for cases, the bias of the estimate of association may be toward or away from the null. In a slightly more complicated form, this differential error structure would have errors centered on different values for controls (or undiseased members of the cohort) and cases, but neither of the means of the error distributions would equal zero.

Nondifferential Misclassification

Nondifferential exposure misclassification occurs when the proportion of subjects misclassified on exposure does not depend on the status of the subject with respect to other variables in the analysis, including disease. Nondifferential disease misclassification occurs when the proportion of subjects misclassified on disease does not depend on the status of the subject with respect to other variables in the analysis, including exposure. We will provide a formal definition below in place of this initial heuristic explanation.

Bias introduced by independent nondifferential misclassification of a binary exposure or disease is predictable in direction, namely, toward or beyond the null value.[8-10] Because of the relatively unpredictable effects of differential misclassification, some investigators endeavor to ensure that the misclassification will be nondifferential, such as blinding of exposure evaluations with respect to outcome status, in the belief that this will guarantee a bias toward the null. Even when blinding is successful, or in cohort studies in which disease outcomes have not yet occurred, collapsing continuous or categorical exposure data into fewer categories can change nondifferential error to differential misclassification.[11,12] And even when nondifferential misclassification is achieved, it may come at the expense of increased total bias.[7,13]

Finally, as will be discussed below, nondifferentiality alone does not guarantee bias toward the null. Contrary to popular misconceptions, nondifferential exposure or disease misclassification can produce bias away from the null if the exposure or disease variable has more than two levels[14,15] or if the classification errors depend on errors made in other variables.[16,17]

Nondifferential Misclassification of Exposure

As an example of nondifferential misclassification, consider a cohort study comparing the incidence of laryngeal cancer among drinkers of alcohol with the incidence among nondrinkers. Assume that drinkers have an incidence rate of 0.00050 per year, whereas nondrinkers have an incidence rate of 0.00010 per year, only one-fifth as great. Assume also that two-thirds of the study population consists of drinkers, but only 50% of them acknowledge it. The result is a population in which one-third of subjects are identified (correctly) as drinkers and have an incidence of disease of 0.00050 per year per, but the remaining two-thirds of the population consists of equal numbers of drinkers and nondrinkers, all of whom are classified as nondrinkers, and among whom the average incidence would be 0.00030 per year rather than the rate of 0.00010 per year among true nondrinkers (Table 13-1). The rate difference has been reduced, by misclassification, from 0.00040 per year to 0.00020 per year, while the rate ratio has been reduced from 5 to 1.7. This bias toward the null value results from nondifferential misclassification of some alcohol drinkers as nondrinkers.

Misclassification can occur simultaneously in both directions; for example, nondrinkers might also be incorrectly classified as drinkers. Suppose that in addition to half of the drinkers being misclassified as nondrinkers, one-third of the true nondrinkers were also misclassified as drinkers. The resulting incidence rates would be 0.00040 per year for those classified as drinkers and 0.00034 per year for those classified as nondrinkers. The additional misclassification thus almost completely obscures the difference between the groups.

This example shows how information bias produced by nondifferential misclassification of a dichotomous exposure will be toward the null value (of no relation) if the misclassification is

TABLE 13-1

Effect of Nondifferential Misclassification of Alcohol Consumption on Estimation of the Incidence Rate Difference and Incidence Rate Ratio for Laryngeal Cancer (Hypothetical Data)

	Incidence Rate ($\times 10^5$ y)	Rate Difference ($\times 10^5$ y)	Rate Ratio
No misclassification			
1,000,000 drinkers	50	40	5.0
500,000 nondrinkers	10		
Half of drinkers classed with nondrinkers			
500,000 drinkers	50	20	1.7
1,000,000 "nondrinkers" (50% are actually drinkers)	30		
Half of drinkers classed with nondrinkers and one-third of nondrinkers classed with drinkers			
666,667 "drinkers" (25% are actually nondrinkers)	40	6	1.2
833,333 "nondrinkers" (60% are actually drinkers)	34		

independent of other errors. If the misclassification is severe enough, the bias can completely obliterate an association and even reverse the direction of association (although reversal will occur only if the classification method is worse than randomly classifying people as "exposed" or "unexposed").

Table 13-2 provides another example. The top panel of the table shows the expected data from a hypothetical case-control study with the exposure measured as a dichotomy. The true odds ratio is 3.0. Now suppose that the exposure is measured by an instrument (*e.g.*, a questionnaire) that results in an exposure measure that has 100% specificity but only 80% sensitivity. In other words, all the truly unexposed subjects are correctly classified as unexposed, but there is only an 80% chance that an exposed subject is correctly classified as exposed, and thus a 20% chance an exposed subject will be incorrectly classified as unexposed. Suppose that the misclassification is nondifferential, which means for this example that the sensitivity and specificity of the exposure measurement method is the same for cases and controls. Let us also assume that there is no error in measuring disease, from which it automatically follows that the exposure errors are independent of disease errors. The resulting data are given in the second panel of the table. With the reduced sensitivity in measuring exposure, the odds ratio is biased in that its approximate expected value decreases from 3.0 to 2.6.

TABLE 13-2

Nondifferential Misclassification With Two Exposure Categories

	Exposed	Unexposed
Correct data		
Cases	240	200
Controls	240	600
	OR = 3.0	
Sensitivity = 0.8		
Specificity = 1.0		
Cases	192	248
Controls	192	648
	OR = 2.6	
Sensitivity = 0.8		
Specificity = 0.8		
Cases	232	208
Controls	312	528
	OR = 1.9	
Sensitivity = 0.4		
Specificity = 0.6		
Cases	176	264
Controls	336	504
	OR = 1.0	
Sensitivity = 0.0		
Specificity = 0.0		
Cases	200	240
Controls	600	240
	OR = 0.33	

OR, odds ratio.

In the third panel, the specificity of the exposure measure is assumed to be 80%, so that there is a 20% chance that someone who is actually unexposed will be incorrectly classified as exposed. The resulting data produce an odds ratio of 1.9 instead of 3.0. In absolute terms, more than half of the effect has been obliterated by the misclassification in the third panel: the excess odds ratio is $3.0 - 1 = 2.0$, whereas it is $1.9 - 1 = 0.9$ based on the data with 80% sensitivity and 80% specificity in the third panel.

The fourth panel of Table 13-2 illustrates that when the sensitivity and specificity sum to 1, the resulting expected estimate will be null, regardless of the magnitude of the effect. If the sum of the sensitivity and specificity is less than 1, then the resulting expected estimate will be in the opposite direction of the actual effect. The last panel of the table shows the result when both sensitivity and specificity are zero. This situation is tantamount to labeling all exposed subjects as unexposed and vice versa. It leads to an expected odds ratio that is the inverse of the correct value. Such drastic misclassification would occur if the coding of exposure categories were reversed during data entry or computer programming.

As seen in these examples, the direction of bias produced by independent nondifferential misclassification of a dichotomous exposure is toward the null value, and if the misclassification is extreme (sum of sensitivity and specificity less than 1.0), the misclassification can go beyond the null value and reverse direction. With an exposure that is measured by dividing it into more than two categories, however, an exaggeration of an association in the middle dose categories can occur as a result of independent nondifferential misclassification.[14,15] This phenomenon is illustrated in Table 13-3.

The correctly classified expected data in Table 13-3 show an odds ratio of 2 for low exposure and 6 for high exposure, both compared with no exposure. Now suppose that there is a 40% chance that a person with high exposure is incorrectly classified into the low exposure category. If this is the only misclassification and it is nondifferential, the expected data would be those seen in the bottom panel of Table 13-3. Note that only the estimate for low exposure changes, it now contains a mixture of people who have low exposure and people who have high exposure but who have incorrectly been assigned to low exposure. Because the people with high exposure carry with them the greater risk of disease that comes with high exposure, the resulting effect estimate for low exposure is biased upward. If some low-exposure individuals had incorrectly been classified as having had high exposure, then the estimate of the effect of exposure for the high-exposure category would be biased downward.

This example illustrates that when the exposure has more than two categories, the bias from nondifferential misclassification of exposure for a given comparison may be away from the null value. When exposure is polytomous (i.e., has more than two categories) and there is nondifferential misclassification between two of the categories and no others, the effect estimates for those two categories will be biased toward one another.[14,18] For example, the bias in the effect estimate for the low-exposure category in Table 13-3 is toward that of the high-exposure category and away

TABLE 13-3

Nondifferential Misclassification With Three Exposure Categories

	Unexposed	Low Exposure	High Exposure
Correct data			
Cases	100	200	600
Controls	100	100	100
		OR = 2	OR = 6
40% of high exposure → 4 low exposure			
Cases	100	440	360
Controls	100	140	60
		OR = 3.1	OR = 6

OR, odds ratio.

from the null value. It is also possible for independent nondifferential misclassification to bias trend estimates away from the null or to reverse a trend.[15] Such examples are unusual, however, because trend reversal cannot occur if the mean exposure measurement increases with true exposure.[19]

It is important to note that the present discussion concerns *expected* results under a particular type of measurement *method*. In a given study, random fluctuations in the errors produced by a method may lead to estimates that are further from the null than what they would be if no error were present, even if the method satisfies all the conditions that guarantee bias toward the null.[20-22] Bias refers only to what is *expected*; if we do not know what the errors were in the study, at best we can say only that the observed odds ratio is probably closer to the null than what it would be if the errors were absent. As study size increases, the probability decreases that a particular result will deviate substantially from its expectation.

A direct consequence is that labeling information biases as "nondifferential" or "differential" reflects an understanding of the mechanisms by which the misclassification errors were introduced and therefore an expectation of how they should act. It does not mean that one can inspect the data themselves and diagnose that the observed data frequencies reflected a nondifferential or differential misclassification of the true data frequencies. For example, if exposure information is collected before an outcome occurs, then one can expect that misclassification of the exposure information would be nondifferential because it is hard to envision how the later occurrence of disease could affect the exposure information before the disease even occurred. The mechanism of exposure misclassification is therefore nondifferential, as in Table 13-1. In this table and other examples, we have shown both the true data frequencies and estimates of association and the expected data frequencies and estimates of association under particular misclassification scenarios. We therefore depict both the true and observed data frequencies, so one can see how a particular misclassification mechanism biased the results. In reality, one would have only the observed data frequencies and an understanding of the mechanisms by which they were obtained, including a hypothesis about whether any misclassification mechanism was likely to have been nondifferential or differential.

When exposure enters the analysis as a continuous variable, the equivalent of nondifferential misclassification of a dichotomous exposure variable is nondifferential error in the measurement of the continuous exposure variable. In its simplest form, this classical error structure assumes that the measured exposure variable is a function of the true exposure and an error term centered on zero and with some variance. The expectation of each measurement is therefore equal to its true value, but the error term introduces noise to the signal and therefore distorts the estimate of association with bias toward the null. BMI, for example, is measured by dividing weight in kilograms by the square of height measured in meters. Errors in BMI can accrue from errors in measuring weight or height. Even for people who maintain a steady weight, it varies throughout the day and is usually measured while wearing some clothes. Height also varies during the day, being greater in the morning. These errors contribute to errors in measuring BMI, which may bias estimates of association between BMI and various health outcomes toward the null. In a somewhat more complicated form of this error structure, the mean of the error distribution does not equal zero, but the error distribution is the same for both controls (or undiseased members of the cohort) and cases.

Nondifferential Misclassification of Disease

The effects of nondifferential misclassification of disease resemble those of nondifferential misclassification of exposure. In most situations, nondifferential misclassification of a binary disease outcome will produce bias toward the null, provided that the misclassification is independent of other errors. There are, however, some special cases, in which such misclassification produces no bias in the risk ratio. In addition, the bias in the risk difference is a simple function of the sensitivity and specificity.

Consider a cohort study in which 40 cases actually occur among 100 exposed subjects and 20 cases actually occur among 200 unexposed subjects. Then, the actual risk ratio is $(40/100)/(20/200) = 4$, and the actual risk difference is $40/100 - 20/200 = 0.30$. Suppose that specificity of disease detection is perfect (there are no false positives), but sensitivity is only 70% in both exposure groups (that is, sensitivity of disease detection is nondifferential and does not depend on errors in classification of exposure). The expected numbers detected will then be $0.70(40) = 28$ exposed cases and $0.70(20) = 14$ unexposed cases, which yield an expected risk-ratio estimate of $(28/100)/$

(14/200) = 4 and an expected risk-difference estimate of 28/100 − 14/200 = 0.21. Thus, the disease misclassification produced no bias in the risk ratio, but the expected risk-difference estimate is only 0.21/0.30 = 70% of the actual risk difference.

What is illustrated above holds more generally: independent nondifferential disease misclassification with perfect specificity will not bias the risk-ratio estimate,[23] but will downwardly bias the absolute magnitude of the risk-difference estimate by a factor equal to the false-negative probability.[24] With this type of misclassification, the odds ratio and the rate ratio will remain biased toward the null, although the bias will be small when the risk of disease is low (<10%) in both exposure groups. This approximation is a consequence of the relation of the odds ratio and the rate ratio to the risk ratio when the disease risk is low in all exposure groups (see Chapter 5).

Consider next the same cohort study, but now with perfect sensitivity of disease detection (no false negatives) and imperfect specificity of 80%. The expected number of apparent cases will then be 40 + (1 − 0.80) (100 − 40) = 52 among the exposed and 20 + (1 − 0.80) (200 − 20) = 56 among the unexposed. Under this formulation, the numerators yield an expected risk-ratio estimate of (52/100)/(56/200) = 1.9 and an expected risk-difference estimate of 52/100 − 56/200 = 0.24. Both measures are biased toward the null, with the expected risk-difference estimate equal to 0.24/0.30 = 80% of the actual value. This example illustrates how independent nondifferential disease misclassification with perfect sensitivity will bias both measures, with the absolute magnitude of the risk-difference estimate downwardly biased by a factor equal to the false-positive probability.[24] If one allows true-positive cases to also be false-positive cases, then the formulation changes. For example, a person might be misdiagnosed initially over the course of follow-up, so a false-positive case, and then correctly diagnosed later in follow-up, so a true case. Under this allowance, the expected number of apparent cases will be 40 + (1 − 0.80) (100) = 60 among the exposed and 20 + (1 − 0.80) (200) = 60 among the unexposed. Under this formulation, the numerators yield an expected risk-ratio estimate of (60/100)/(60/200) = 2.0 and an expected risk-difference estimate of 60/100 − 60/200 = 0.3. The risk ratio is biased toward the null, but the expected risk-difference estimate is unbiased. This example illustrates how independent nondifferential disease misclassification with perfect sensitivity will not bias the risk difference if a false-positive case can subsequently become a true-positive case.

With imperfect sensitivity and specificity, the bias in the absolute magnitude of the risk difference produced by nondifferential disease misclassification that is independent of other errors will be a factor equal to the sum of the false-negative and false-positive probabilities,[24] without allowing for false-positive cases to arise from true-positive cases. The biases in relative effect measures do not have a simple form in this case.

We wish to emphasize that when both exposure and disease are nondifferentially misclassified but the classification errors are dependent, it is possible to obtain substantial bias away from the null,[16,17] and the simple bias relations just given will no longer apply. Dependent errors can arise easily in many situations, such as in studies in which exposure and disease status are both determined from interviews.

When outcome enters the analysis as a continuous variable, the equivalent of nondifferential misclassification of a discrete outcome variable is nondifferential error in the measurement of the continuous outcome variable. The simplest form of the classical error structure again assumes that the measured outcome variable is a function of the true outcome and an error term centered on zero and with some variance. The error term introduces noise to the signal, and while this inflates the variance of the estimate, it does not bias the estimate toward the null. As above, a slightly more complicated form of this error structure allows for the mean of the error distribution to take some value other than zero, but the same distribution applies regardless of exposure status.

Pervasiveness of Misinterpretation of Nondifferential Misclassification Effects

The bias from independent nondifferential misclassification of a dichotomous exposure is always in the direction of the null value, so for a positive effect, one would expect to see a larger estimate if misclassification were absent. As a result, many researchers are satisfied with achieving nondifferential misclassification in lieu of accurate classification. This stance may occur in part because some researchers consider it more acceptable to misreport an association as absent when it in fact exists than to misreport an association as present when it in fact does not exist, and they regard nondifferential misclassification as favoring the first type of misreporting over the latter. Other researchers write as if positive results affected by nondifferential misclassification provide stronger evidence for an association than indicated by uncorrected statistics. There are, however, several flaws in such interpretations.

First, many researchers forget that more than nondifferentiality is required to ensure bias toward the null. One also needs independence of errors in the associated variables and some other constraints, such as the variable being binary. Second, few researchers seem to be aware that categorization of continuous variables (*e.g.*, using quintiles instead of actual quantities of food or nutrients) can change nondifferential to differential error.[11,12]

Even if the misclassification satisfies all the conditions to produce a bias toward the null in the point estimate, it does not necessarily produce a corresponding upward bias in the *P*-value for the null hypothesis.[25,26] As a consequence, establishing that the bias (if any) was toward the null would not increase the evidence that a non-null association was present. Furthermore, bias toward the null (like bias away from the null) is still a distortion and one that will vary across studies. In particular, it can produce serious distortions in literature reviews and meta-analyses, mask true differences among studies, exaggerate differences, or create spurious differences. These consequences can occur because differences in secondary study characteristics such as exposure prevalence will affect the degree to which misclassification produces bias in estimates from different strata or studies, even if the sensitivity and specificity of the classification do not vary across the strata or studies.[27] Typical situations are worsened by the fact that sensitivity and specificity as well as exposure prevalence will vary across studies.[28]

Often, these differences in measurement performance arise from seemingly innocuous differences in the way variables are assessed or categorized, with worse performance arising from oversimplified or crude categorizations of exposure. For example, suppose that taking aspirin transiently reduces risk of myocardial infarction. The word "transiently" implies a brief induction period, with no preventive effect outside that period. For a given point in time or person-time unit in the history of a subject, the ideal classification of that time as exposed or unexposed to aspirin would be based on whether aspirin had been used before that time but within the induction period for its effect. By this standard, a myocardial infarction following aspirin use within the induction period would be properly classified as an aspirin-exposed case. On the other hand, if no aspirin was used within the induction period, the case would be properly classified as unexposed, even if the case had used aspirin at earlier or later times.

These ideal classifications reflect the fact that use outside the induction period is causally irrelevant, and therefore it is not consistent with construct validity. Many studies, however, focus on ever use (use at any time during an individual's life) or on any use over a span of several years. Such cumulative indices over a long time span augment possibly relevant exposure with irrelevant exposure and can thus introduce a bias (usually toward the null) that parallels bias due to nondifferential misclassification arising from lack of construct validity.

Similar bias can arise from an overly broad definition of the outcome. In particular, unwarranted assurances of a null effect can easily emerge from studies in which a wide range of etiologically unrelated outcomes are grouped. In cohort studies in which there are disease categories with few subjects, investigators are occasionally tempted to combine outcome categories to increase the number of subjects in each analysis, thereby gaining precision at the expense of construct validity. This collapsing of categories can obscure effects on more narrowly defined disease categories. For example, in an investigation of the teratogenicity of the drug Bendectin[29]—a drug indicated for nausea of pregnancy—only 35 babies were born with a malformation, so analyses focused on the single outcome, "malformation." But no teratogen causes all malformations; if such an analysis fails to find an effect, the failure may simply be the result of the grouping of many malformations not related to Bendectin with those that are. In fact, despite the authors' claim that "their study provides substantial evidence that Bendectin is not teratogenic in man," their data indicated a strong (though imprecise) relation between Bendectin and cardiac malformations.

Misclassification that has arguably produced bias toward the null is a greater concern in interpreting studies that seem to indicate the absence of an effect. Consequently, in studies that indicate little or no effect, it is crucial for the researchers to attempt to establish the direction of the bias to determine whether a real effect might have been obscured. Occasionally, critics of a study will argue that poor exposure data or poor disease classification invalidates the results. This argument is incorrect, however, if the results indicate a nonzero association and one can be sure that the classification errors biased toward the null, because the bias will be in the direction of underestimating the association. In this situation the major task will instead be in establishing that the classification errors were indeed of the sort that would produce bias toward the null.

Conversely, misclassification that has arguably produced bias away from the null is a greater concern in interpreting studies that seem to indicate an effect. The picture in this direction is clouded by the fact that forces that lead to differential error and bias away from the null (*e.g.*, recall bias) are counterbalanced to an unknown extent (possibly entirely) by forces that lead to bias toward the null (*e.g.*, simple memory deterioration over time). Even with only binary variables, a detailed quantitative analysis of differential recall may be needed to gain any idea of the direction of bias,[7] and even with internal validation data the direction of net bias may rarely be clear.

The importance of appreciating the likely direction of bias was illustrated by the interpretation of a study on spermicides and birth defects.[30,31] This study reported an increased prevalence of several types of congenital disorders among women who were identified as having filled a prescription for spermicides during a specified interval before the birth. The exposure information was only a rough correlate of the actual use of spermicides during a theoretically relevant time period, but the misclassification that resulted was likely to be nondifferential and independent of errors in outcome ascertainment, because prescription information was recorded on a computer log before the outcome was known. One of the criticisms raised about the study was that inaccuracies in the exposure information cast doubt on the validity of the findings.[32,33] These criticisms did not, however, address the direction of the resulting bias, and so are inappropriate if the structure of the misclassification indicates that the bias is downward, for then that bias could not explain the observed association.[31]

As an example, it is incorrect to dismiss a study reporting an association simply because there is independent nondifferential misclassification of a binary exposure, because without the misclassification the observed association would probably be even larger. Thus, the implications of independent nondifferential misclassification depend heavily on whether the study is perceived as "positive" or "negative." Emphasis on quantitative assessment instead of on a qualitative description of study results lessens the likelihood for misinterpretation, and hence we will introduce methods for quantitative assessment below.

Misclassification of Confounders

If a discrete confounding variable is misclassified, or a continuous confounding variable is measured with error, the ability to control confounding in the analysis is hampered.[27,34-38] Independent nondifferential misclassification of a dichotomous confounding variable or independent nondifferential mismeasurement of a continuous confounding variable will ordinarily reduce the degree to which the confounder can be controlled, thus causing a bias in the direction of the confounding by the variable. For a binary confounder, the expected result will lie between the unadjusted association and the correctly adjusted association (*i.e.*, the one that would have obtained if the confounder had not been misclassified), provided that there is no qualitative interaction between the exposure and the confounder.[39] This problem may be viewed as one of residual confounding (*i.e.*, confounding left after control of the available confounder measurements). The degree of residual confounding left within strata of the misclassified confounder will usually differ across those strata, which will distort the apparent degree of heterogeneity (effect modification) across strata.[27] Independent nondifferential misclassification of either the confounder or exposure can therefore give rise to the appearance of effect-measure modification (statistical interaction) when in fact there is none or mask the appearance of such modification when in fact it is present. The misclassification of a confounder that is not binary can result in bias in either direction, even in the absence of qualitative interaction; other sufficient conditions are available[40] for the expected result adjusted for a misclassified categorical confounder to lie between the unadjusted and correctly adjusted associations.

If the misclassification is differential or dependent, the resulting adjusted association may not even fall between the crude and the correct adjusted associations. The problem then becomes not only one of residual confounding but also of additional distortion produced by differential selection of subjects into different analysis strata. Unfortunately, dependent errors among exposure variables are common, especially in questionnaire-based studies. For example, in epidemiologic studies of nutrients and disease, nutrient intakes are calculated from food intakes, and any errors in assessing the food intakes will translate into dependent errors among nutrients found in the same foods. Similarly, in epidemiologic studies of occupations and disease, chemical exposures are usually calculated from job histories, and errors in assessing these histories will translate into dependent errors among exposures found in the same jobs.

If the confounding is strong and the exposure-disease relation is weak or null, misclassification of the confounder can produce extremely misleading results, even if the misclassification is independent and nondifferential. For example, given a causal relation between smoking and bladder cancer, an association between smoking and coffee drinking would make smoking a confounder of the relation between coffee drinking and bladder cancer. Because the control of confounding by smoking depends on accurate smoking information and because some misclassification of the relevant smoking information is inevitable no matter how smoking is measured, some residual confounding by smoking is inevitable.[41] The problem of residual confounding will be even worse if the only available information on smoking is a simple dichotomy such as "ever smoked" versus "never smoked," because the lack of detailed specification of smoking diminishes its construct validity and thereby prohibits adequate control of its confounding. The resulting residual confounding is especially troublesome because it may appear that confounding by smoking has been fully controlled.

The Complexities of Simultaneous Misclassification

Continuing the preceding example, consider misclassification of coffee use as well as smoking. On the one hand, if coffee misclassification were nondifferential with respect to smoking and independent of smoking errors, the likely effect would be to diminish further the observed smoking-coffee association and so further reduce the efficacy of adjustment for smoking. The result would be even more upward residual confounding than when smoking alone were misclassified. On the other hand, if the measurements were from questionnaires, the coffee and smoking errors might be positively associated rather than independent, potentially counteracting the aforementioned phenomenon to an unknown degree. Also, if the coffee errors were nondifferential with respect to bladder cancer and independent of diagnostic errors, they would most likely produce a downward bias in the observed association.

Nonetheless, if the measurements were from a questionnaire administered after diagnosis, the nondifferentiality of both smoking and coffee errors with respect to bladder cancer would become questionable. If controls tended to underreport these habits more than did cases, the resulting differentiality would likely act in an upward direction for both the coffee and the smoking associations with cancer, partially canceling both the downward bias from the coffee misclassification and the upward bias from residual smoking confounding; but if cases tended to underreport these habits more than did controls, the differentiality would likely aggravate the downward bias from coffee misclassification and the upward bias from residual smoking confounding.

The net result of all these effects would be almost impossible to predict given the usual lack of accurate information on the misclassification rates. We emphasize that this unpredictability is over and above that of the random error assumed by conventional statistical methods; it is therefore not reflected in conventional confidence intervals, because the latter addresses only random variation in subject selection and actual exposure and assumes that errors in coffee and smoking measurement are absent (see Chapter 29).

We noted above that independent nondifferential misclassification of the exposure will not bias a trend away from the null if the mean exposure measurement increases with true exposure.[19] Similar conditions pertain also to trends when both the exposure and the disease status are independently nondifferentially misclassified, and even in some cases with dependent and/or differential misclassification.[42] Precise sufficient conditions for the preservation of trends and for the consistency of tests for association under differential and dependent misclassification of the exposure and disease are given elsewhere.[42]

BIAS ANALYSIS OF MISCLASSIFICATION

As noted above, nearly all epidemiologic studies suffer from some degree of measurement error, which is usually referred to as classification error or *misclassification* when the variables are discrete. The effect of even modest amounts of error can be profound, yet rarely is the error quantified.[43] Simple situations can be analyzed, however, using basic algebra,[10,44,45] and more extensive analyses can be done using software that performs matrix algebra (*e.g.*, SAS, GAUSS, MATLAB, R, S-Plus).[46-48] We will focus on basic methods for dichotomous variables; methods pertaining to bias adjustments for misclassification of ordinal or continuous variables are available.[49] Some of this material is repeated in differing detail in Chapter 29, where we then extend the description to methods that allow use of validation study data, in which classification rates are themselves estimated from a sample of study subjects, and to probabilistic and Bayesian bias analysis.

Exposure Misclassification

Consider first the estimation of exposure prevalence from a single observed category of subjects, such as the control group in a case-control study. Define the following quantities in this category:

X	= 1 if exposed, 0 if not
X^*	= 1 if *classified* as exposed, 0 if not
PVP	= probability that someone classified as exposed is truly exposed
	= predictive value of an exposure "positive" = $\Pr(X = 1 \mid X^* = 1)$
PVN	= probability that someone classified as unexposed is truly unexposed
	= predictive value of an exposure "negative" = $\Pr(X = 0 \mid X^* = 0)$
B_1^*	= number classified as exposed (with $X^* = 1$)
B_0^*	= number classified as unexposed (with $X^* = 0$)
B_1	= expected number truly exposed (with $X = 1$)
B_0	= expected number truly unexposed (with $X = 0$)

If they are known, the predictive values can be used directly to estimate the numbers truly exposed (B_1) and truly unexposed (B_0) from the misclassified counts B_1^* and B_0^* via the expected relations.

$$B_1 = PVP \cdot B_1^* + (1 - PVN)B_0^*$$
$$B_0 = PVN \cdot B_0^* + (1 - PVP)B_1^* \qquad\qquad [13\text{-}1]$$

M_0 is not changed by exposure misclassification, so once we have estimated B_1, we can estimate B_0 from $B_0 = M_0 - B_1$. From the preceding equations we can estimate the true exposure prevalence as $P_{e0} = B_1/M_0$. Parallel equations for cases or person-time follow by substituting A_1, A_0, A_1^*, and A_0^* or T_1, T_0, T_1^*, and T_0^* for B_1, B_0, B_1^*, and B_0^* in Equation 13-1. The bias-adjusted counts obtained by applying the equation to actual data are only estimates derived under the assumption that the true predictive values are PVP and PVN and there is no other error in the observed counts (*e.g.*, no random error). To make this clear, one should denote the solutions in Equation 13-1 by $\hat{B}_1$ and $\hat{B}_0$ instead of B_1 and B_0; for notational simplicity, we have not done so.

Equation 13-1 is a bias model that relates the observed data (B_1^* and B_0^*) to the expected true data (B_1 and B_0) through the bias parameters (PVP and PVN). To obtain a solution, one only needs to assign credible values to the two bias parameters. Unfortunately, predictive values are seldom available, and when they are, their applicability is highly suspect, in part because they depend directly on exposure prevalence, which varies across populations and across covariate patterns (see Equations 13-6 and 13-7). Even when available, estimates of PVP and PVN may differ from their true values, which could only be obtained as the proportion of all classified exposed persons who were truly exposed according to the gold standard measurement and the proportion of all classified unexposed persons who were truly unexposed according to the gold standard measurement. But if gold standard were available for all participants, then there would be no misclassification problem to solve. Instead, predictive values are measured in a subset of the study population or a second population, and extrapolation of these measurements to the entire study population may be tenuous. For example, study participants who agree to participate in a much more extensive validation substudy of food intake or medication usage (highly cooperative subjects) may have different patterns of intake and usage than other study participants who were not invited to participate in the validation substudy or who refused the invitation. When one can reliably estimate predictive values in a validation substudy, these estimates must be allowed to vary with disease and confounder levels, because exposure prevalence will vary across these levels. Owing to variations in exposure prevalence across populations and time, predictive values from a second population are even less likely to apply accurately.

These problems in applying predictive values lead to an alternative bias model, which uses bias parameters that do not depend on true exposure prevalence. The following four probabilities, initially defined above, are common examples of such parameters:

Se = probability that someone exposed is classified as exposed
= sensitivity = $\Pr(X^* = 1 | X = 1)$

Fn = probability that someone exposed is classified as unexposed
= false-negative probability = $\Pr(X^* = 0 | X = 1) = 1 - Se$

Sp = probability that someone unexposed is classified as unexposed
= specificity = $\Pr(X^* = 0 | X = 0)$

Fp = probability that someone unexposed is classified as exposed
= false-positive probability = $\Pr(X^* = 1 | X = 0) = 1 - Sp$

The following bias model then relates the expected misclassified counts to the true counts:

$$B_1^* = \text{expected number of subjects classified as exposed}$$
$$= SeB_1 + FpB_0$$

[13-2]

and

$$B_0^* = \text{expected number of subjects classified as unexposed}$$
$$= FnB_1 + SpB_0$$

[13-3]

In most studies, one observes only the misclassified counts B_1^* and B_0^*. If we assume that the sensitivity and specificity are equal to Se and Sp (with $Fn = 1 - Se$ and $Fp = 1 - Sp$), we can estimate B_1 and B_0 by solving Equations 13-2 and 13-3. From Equation 13-3, we get

$$B_0 = \left(B_0^* - Fn\,B_1\right)/Sp$$

We can substitute the right side of this equation for B_0 in Equation 13-2, which yields

$$B_1^* = Se\,B_1 + Fp\left(B_0^* - Fn\,B_1\right)/Sp$$

We then solve for B_1 to get

$$B_1 = \left(Sp\,B_1^* - Fp\,B_0^*\right)/\left(SeSp - FnFp\right)$$
$$= \left(B_1^* - Fp\,M_0\right)/\left(Se + Sp - 1\right)$$
$$B_0 = M_0 - B_1 = \left(B_0^* - Fn\,M_0\right)/\left(Se + Sp - 1\right).$$

[13-4]

From this model, *we* can also estimate the true exposure prevalence as $P_{e0} = B_1/M_0$. Again, the B_1 and B_0 obtained by applying Equation 13-4 to actual data are only estimates derived under the assumption that the true sensitivity and specificity are Se and Sp. These can never be measured with perfect accuracy because they are obtained from a selected subpopulation or a second population.

A sensitivity analysis for the quantitative bias analysis for exposure classification proceeds by applying Equation 13-4 for various pairs of classification probabilities (Se, Sp) to the observed noncase counts $B_1{}^*$ and $B_0{}^*$. This analysis evaluates the sensitivity of the bias analysis results to different assumptions for the values assigned to Se and Sp, the bias parameters of the bias model. To construct a bias-adjusted measure of association, we must also apply an analogous model to estimate A_1 and A_0 from the observed (misclassified) case counts $A_1{}^*$ and $A_0{}^*$:

$$A_1 = \left(A_1^* - \mathrm{Fp}\, M_1\right) \big/ \left(\mathrm{Se} + \mathrm{Sp} - 1\right) \qquad [13\text{-}5]$$

from which we get $A_0 = M_1 - A_1$, where M_1 is the observed case total. These equations may be applied to case-control, closed-cohort, or prevalence survey data. For person-time follow-up data, Equation 13-4 can be modified by substituting T_1, T_0, $T_1{}^*$, and $T_0{}^*$ for B_1, B_0, $B_1{}^*$, and $B_0{}^*$. Mullooly developed a misclassification model specific to person-time data,[50] with extension to simultaneous misclassification of the exposure and outcome variables.

The bias model may be applied within strata of confounders as well. After application of the model, we may compute bias-adjusted stratum-specific and summary effect estimates from the estimated true counts. Finally, we tabulate the bias-adjusted estimates obtained by using different pairs (Se, Sp) and thus obtain a picture of how sensitive the results are to various assumptions about the values assigned to the parameters of the misclassification bias model.

Equations 13-4 and 13-5 can yield negative adjusted counts, which are impossible values for the true counts. One way this can arise is if $Se + Sp < 1$, which implies that the classification is assigning values worse than if they were assigned at random. Imagine that we conduct a coin toss with a probability P of heads to decide whether someone was exposed or not, setting $X^* = 1$ when the coin toss yielded heads (P may be any number between 0 and 1). The sensitivity and specificity of this completely random classification are then P and $1 - P$, respectively, and $Se + Sp = 1$. We will henceforth assume that our actual classification method is better than a coin toss, in the sense that $Se + Sp > 1$.

Even with this assumption, the solution B_1 to Equation 13-4 will be negative if $Fp > B_0{}^*/M_0$, that is, if the assumed false-positive probability exceeds the observed prevalence of exposure in the noncases or, equivalently, if $Sp < B_0{}^*/M_0$. In parallel, B_0 will be negative if $Fn > B_0{}^*/M_1$ (equivalently, $Se < B_1{}^*/M_0$), A_1 will be negative if $Fp > A_1{}^*/M_1$, and A_0 will be negative if $Fn > A_0{}^*/M_1$. A negative result indicates that other errors (e.g., random errors) have distorted the observed counts, the value chosen for Se or for Sp is wrong, or some combination of these problems.

Although sensitivity and specificity do not depend on the true exposure prevalence, they are influenced by other characteristics. Because predictive values are functions of sensitivity and specificity (see Equations 13-6 and 13-7 below), they too will be affected by these characteristics, as well as by any characteristics that affect prevalence. For example, covariates that affect exposure recall (such as age and comorbidities) will alter the classification probabilities for self-reported exposure history and may vary considerably across populations. In such situations, sensitivity and specificity may not generalize well from one population to another.[28] This lack of generalizability is one reason why varying classification probabilities in the equations (sensitivity analysis if the bias analysis) are crucial even when estimates are available from the literature.

Valid variances for adjusted estimates cannot be calculated from the bias-adjusted counts using conventional equations, even if we assume that sensitivity and specificity are known or are unbiased estimates from a validation study. This problem arises because conventional equations do not take account of the data transformations and random errors in the adjustments. Equations that do so are available.[48,51-55] Probabilistic bias analysis (discussed in Chapter 29) can also account for these technical issues and for other sources of bias as well.

If X is a continuous measure of exposure, then regression calibration provides a bias model to adjust for measurement error.[56] Under this bias model,[57] one first models the outcome as a function of the mismeasured continuous variable X^* using, for example, logistic regression

$$\mathrm{logit}\left[\Pr\left(D = 1 \middle| X^*\right)\right] = \beta_0 + \beta X^*$$

where $D = 1$ connotes a case and $D = 0$ connotes a control or undiseased member of the cohort. Next, in a subset of participants for whom both the gold standard (X) and the mismeasured exposure (X^*) have been measured, a linear regression estimates the linear association between X and X^*.

$$\mathrm{E}\left(X\middle|X^*\right) = \alpha + \gamma X^*$$

Finally, one calibrates the first regression coefficient estimate by the second regression coefficient estimate to account for the error introduced by mismeasurement.

$$\hat{\beta}_{RC} = \hat{\beta}\middle/\hat{\gamma}$$

$$\widehat{\mathrm{Var}\left(\hat{\beta}_{RC}\right)} = \frac{\widehat{\mathrm{Var}\left(\hat{\beta}\right)}}{\hat{\gamma}^2} + \frac{\hat{\beta}^2}{\hat{\gamma}^4}\widehat{\mathrm{Var}\left(\hat{\gamma}\right)}$$

The validity of the bias model is conditional on satisfying the usual assumptions of regression models of this form (see Chapters 20 and 21). Because X^* is an imperfect measure of X, the expectation of γ is less than one, so the calibrated estimate of β will be further from the null than the estimate before adjustment for measurement error. If the supposed gold standard (X) is itself subject to measurement error, however, then this regression calibration approach can overcorrect and inflate the estimate too far.[58] Important assumptions of regression calibration include that X and X^* are measured on the same scale, that errors in X (if any) are independent of errors in X^*, that X^* is a linear function of X, and that errors in X^* are nondifferential with respect to D.[59,60] When there is more than one covariate in the logistic regression model, a more general form of the bias model can be applied.[59,61] When the reliability of the mismeasured exposure (X^*) with respect to the true exposure is known (*i.e.*, the proportion of the variance of X^* explained by X, conditional on the measured covariates), then a bias-adjusted estimate can also be obtained directly by division of the estimate by this reliability; alternatively this reliability can be treated as a sensitivity analysis parameter.[62] Regression calibration methods have been extended to outcome models of different forms and to differential measurement error problems.[59,63,64]

Nondifferentiality

In the preceding description, we assumed nondifferential exposure misclassification, that is, the same values of Se and Sp applied to both the cases (Equation 13-5) and the noncases (Equation 13-4). As introduced above, to say that a classification method is nondifferential with respect to disease means that it has identical operating characteristics among cases and noncases, so that sensitivity and specificity do not vary with disease status. We expect this property to hold when the mechanisms that determine the classification are identical among cases and noncases. In particular, we expect nondifferentiality when the disease is unrelated to exposure measurement. This expectation is reasonable when the mechanisms that determine exposure classification precede the disease occurrence and are not affected by uncontrolled risk factors, as occurs in many cohort studies, although even then it is not guaranteed to hold. Thus, to say that there is nondifferential misclassification (such as when exposure data are collected from records that predate the outcome) means that neither disease nor uncontrolled risk factors result in different accuracy of response for cases compared with noncases.

Put more formally, nondifferentiality means that the classification X^* is independent of the outcome D (*i.e.*, the outcome conveys no information about X) conditional on the true exposure X and adjustment variables. This condition may seldom be realized exactly; the expectation of this condition is best examined on the basis of qualitative mechanistic considerations. Intuition and judgment about the role of the outcome in exposure classification errors are the basis for priors about measurement behavior. Such judgments provide another reason to express such priors in terms of sensitivity and specificity, as we will do later, rather than predictive values.

Differentiality should be expected when exposure assessment can be affected by the outcome. For example, in interview-based case-control studies, cases may be more likely to recall exposure (correctly or falsely) than controls, leading to higher sensitivity or lower specificity among cases relative to controls (*recall bias*). When differential misclassification is a reasonable possibility given the mechanisms by which classification errors might arise, we can extend the sensitivity analysis by using different sensitivities and specificities for cases and noncases. Letting Fp_1, Fp_0 be the case and noncase false-positive probabilities and Fn_1, Fn_0 the case and noncase false-negative probabilities, the bias-adjusted odds ratio for a single 2×2 table simplifies to

$$\frac{\left(A_1^* - Fp_1 M_1\right)\left(B_0^* - Fn_0 M_0\right)}{\left(A_0^* - Fp_1 M_1\right)\left(B_1^* - Fn_0 M_0\right)}$$

This equation is sensible, however, only if all four parenthetical terms in the ratio are positive.

Application to an Example

As a numerical example, we shall bias-adjust for misclassification of exposure in a case-control study of use of antidepressants and incident breast cancer among women in western Washington.[65] Women 65 to 79 years old diagnosed with invasive breast cancer during the period 1997 to 1999 while resident in one of three western Washington counties were invited to participate in an interview that collected information on exposure history. Controls were selected from a population-based registry and frequency matched to cases on age, calendar year, and county of residence, and participating controls were similarly interviewed. Among the questions in the interview was participants' self-reported 20-year history of antidepressant use. The crude data are displayed in Table 13-4 and yielded a crude odds ratio of $\dfrac{118/103}{832/884} = 1.21$ (95% CI 0.92, 1.61), which corresponds well to the adjusted odds ratio reported by Chien et al. in the original paper (OR = 1.2, 95% CI 0.9, 1.6). We will therefore bias-adjust the crude results.

The investigators recognized that self-reported history of antidepressant use may be inaccurate and that, given the retrospective design, the accuracy may have differed for cases and controls. They therefore conducted a validation substudy restricted to participants who further consented to access to their pharmacy records and who regularly used one of the pharmacies with available electronic records of filled prescriptions.[66] Twenty years of pharmacy records were not available; we will use validation data comparing the 2-year self-reported history with the same 2-year period of pharmacy records and we will consider the pharmacy records to be a gold standard. Among the 43 cases with a pharmacy record of a filled prescription for antidepressants, 24 self-reported use of an antidepressant, whereas among the 31 controls with a pharmacy record of a filled prescription for antidepressants, 18 self-reported use of an antidepressant. The sensitivity among cases was therefore 24/43 = 56% and among controls was 18/31 = 58%. Among the 146 cases with no pharmacy record of a filled prescription for antidepressants, 144 self-reported no use of an antidepressant,

TABLE 13-4

Crude Data for Case-Control Study of Self-Reported 20-Year History of Antidepressant Use (X^*) and Incidence Breast Cancer (D) Reported by Chien et al.[65]

	$X^* = 1$	$X^* = 0$	Total
Cases ($D = 1$)	$A_1 = 118$	$A_0 = 832$	$M_1 = 950$
Controls ($D = 0$)	$B_1 = 103$	$B_0 = 884$	$M_0 = 987$

Crude odds ratio = (118/103)/(832/884) = 1.21 (95% CI 0.92, 1.61)
From Chien C, Li CI, Heckbert SR, Malone KE, Boudreau DM, Daling JR. Antidepressant use and breast cancer risk. *Breast Cancer Res Treat.* 2006;95(2):131-140.

whereas among the 134 controls with no pharmacy record of a filled prescription for antidepressants, 130 self-reported no use of an antidepressant. The specificity among cases was therefore $144/146 = 99\%$ and among controls was $130/134 = 97\%$.

Table 13-5 displays bias-adjusted data using the validation data exactly as measured. Recall, however, that the validation study was conducted in a select subset of all participants: those who consented to access their pharmacy records and who regularly used one of the pharmacies with available electronic records. We will take account of these sources of uncertainty by conducting a sensitivity analysis of the bias analysis. Chapter 29 describes how to use probabilistic bias analysis or Bayesian methods to further account for these types of uncertainties, as well as others, such as the random error in the measurement of the classification parameters. The first step, though, is to complete the simple bias analysis using the observed crude frequencies from the original study[65] and the 2-year validation data[66] reported for the subset.

From Equations 13-4 and 13-5, we obtain

$$B_1 = \frac{\left[103 - \left(1 - \frac{130}{134}\right)987\right]}{\left[\frac{18}{31} - \left(1 - \frac{130}{134}\right)\right]} = 133.5$$

$$B_0 = 987 - 133.5 = 853.5$$

$$A_1 = \frac{\left[118 - \left(1 - \frac{144}{146}\right)950\right]}{\left[\frac{24}{43} - \left(1 - \frac{144}{146}\right)\right]} = 192.8$$

$$A_0 = 950 - 192.8 = 757.2$$

These yield a bias-adjusted odds ratio of $\dfrac{192.8/133.5}{853.5/757.2} = 1.63$. This value is notably further from the null than the crude odds ratio before bias adjustment of 1.21. Note that we cannot use the bias-adjusted frequencies in conventional equations to compute a variance for this odds ratio because those equations do not take account of the uncertainty in the estimates of the classification parameters. By repeating the preceding calculations with different sets of assumptions about the sensitivities and specificities in cases and controls, we obtain a sensitivity analysis of the bias analysis. Table 13-5 provides a summary of the results of this analysis. Under the nondifferential misclassification scenarios along the descending diagonal, the bias-adjusted odds ratio estimates (1.27, 1.29, 1.32) are always further from the null than the estimate computed directly from the data (1.21, which corresponds to the bias-adjusted estimate one would obtain by assuming $Se = Sp = 1$, so no misclassification). This result reflects the fact that, if the classification mechanism is better than random assignment, exposure is dichotomous, and the misclassification nondifferential and independent of all other errors (whether systematic or random), the bias produced by the exposure misclassification is toward the null. We caution, however, that this rule applies only to the expectation and does not extend automatically to other situations, such as those involving a polytomous exposure, as explained above.

In one form of recall bias, cases recall or report true exposure more completely than do controls, that is, there is higher sensitivity among cases. These combinations of assumed sensitivities are presented despite the fact that the observed sensitivity in cases (56%) was less than the observed sensitivity in controls (58%) for the 2-year history of self-reported antidepressant use validated by comparison with pharmacy records in the validation substudy.[66] The 95% confidence intervals for these proportions overlap substantially (0.41, 0.70 and 0.40, 0.74, respectively), demonstrating that there is a good possibility that the observed rankings are the reverse of the true rankings. Table 13-5 shows that, even if we assume that this form of recall bias is present, bias adjustment may move the estimate away from the null. One example is that when we assume sensitivity of 57% in cases and 55.8% in controls and assume 97.0% specificity in both cases and controls, the bias-adjusted

TABLE 13-5

Bias-Adjusted Antidepressant–Breast Cancer Odds Ratios[a,b] Under Assumptions About the Antidepressant Exposure Sensitivity and Specificity Among Cases and Controls

Case Sensitivity and Specificity		Control Sensitivity and Specificity								
		55.8%	55.8%	55.8%	57.0%	57.0%	57.0%	58.1%	58.1%	58.1%
		97.0%	98.0%	98.6%	97.0%	98.0%	98.6%	97.0%	98.0%	98.6%
55.8%	97.0%	*1.32*	1.17	1.09	1.36	1.20	1.12	1.39	1.14	1.14
55.8%	98.0%	1.46	*1.29*	1.20	1.50	1.33	1.23	1.54	1.26	1.26
55.8%	98.6%	1.55	1.37	*1.27*	1.59	1.41	1.31	**1.63**	1.34	1.34
57.0%	97.0%	1.29	1.14	1.06	*1.32*	1.17	1.09	1.35	1.11	1.11
57.0%	98.0%	1.42	1.26	1.17	1.46	*1.29*	1.20	1.49	1.23	1.23
57.0%	98.6%	1.51	1.33	1.24	1.55	1.37	*1.27*	1.58	1.30	1.30
58.1%	97.0%	1.26	1.11	1.03	1.29	1.14	1.06	*1.32*	1.09	1.09
58.1%	98.0%	1.39	1.23	1.14	1.43	1.26	1.17	1.46	*1.20*	1.20
58.1%	98.6%	1.47	1.30	1.21	1.51	1.34	1.24	1.55	1.27	*1.27*

[a]Bias-adjusted estimates under nondifferential misclassification scenarios, which fall along the descending diagonal, are italicized.
[b]The bias-adjusted estimate corresponding to the sensitivities and specificities for 2-year history of antidepressant use as reported by Boudreau et al[66] and as used in the example computation in the text is bolded.
From Boudreau DM, Daling JR, Malone KE, Gardner JS, Blough DK, Heckbert SR. A validation study of patient interview data and pharmacy records for antihypertensive, statin, and antidepressant medication use among older women. *Am J Epidemiol.* 2004;159(3):308-317.

estimate of the odds ratio is 1.29, which is further from the null than the crude odds ratio of 1.21. This result shows that the association can be diminished by misclassification patterns characteristic of recall bias. To understand this possibly counterintuitive phenomenon, one may think of the classification procedure as having two components: a nondifferential component shared by both cases and controls and a differential component reflecting the recall bias. In many plausible scenarios, the bias toward the null produced by the nondifferential component overwhelms the bias away from the null produced by the differential component.[7]

The example also shows that the uncertainty in results due to the uncertainty about the classification probabilities can be as large as, or in other cases even greater than, the uncertainty conveyed by conventional confidence intervals. The unadjusted 95% confidence interval in the example extends from 0.92 to 1.61, whereas the bias-adjusted odds ratios range from 1.03 to 1.63. Note that this range of uncertainty does not incorporate random error associated with the estimate of the odds ratio, which is the only source of error reflected in the conventional confidence interval, or random error associated with the estimates of the sensitivities and specificities.

Table 13-5 also shows that, in this example, the specificity is a more powerful determinant of the observed odds ratio than is the sensitivity, because the exposure prevalence is low. For example, holding sensitivity constant at 57.0% and allowing specificity to vary yields a bias-adjusted estimate of 1.09 for specificity of 97.0% in cases and of 98.6% in controls and a bias-adjusted estimate of 1.55 for specificity of 98.6% in cases and of 97.0% in controls. Conversely, holding specificity constant at 98.0% and allowing sensitivity to vary yields a bias-adjusted estimate of 1.36 for sensitivity of 55.8% in cases and of 58.1% in controls and a bias-adjusted estimate of 1.23 for sensitivity of 58.1% in cases and 55.8% in controls. The wider range of bias-adjusted estimates yielded when specificity varies, compared with when sensitivity varies, demonstrates that strength of bias is more influenced by specificity than by sensitivity in this example. In general, when exposure prevalence is low, the odds ratio estimate is more sensitive to false-positive error in classifying exposure than to false-negative error, because false positives arise from a larger group and thus can easily overwhelm true positives. Specificity drives the size of the bias adjustment in exposure classification problems when the exposure is rare and drives the size of the bias adjustment in disease classification problems when the disease is rare.[23]

Relation of Predictive Values to Sensitivity and Specificity

Arguments are often made that the sensitivity and specificity of an instrument will be roughly stable across similar populations, at least within levels of disease and covariates such as age, sex, and socioeconomic status. Nonetheless, as mentioned earlier, variations in sensitivity and specificity can occur under many conditions—for example, when the measure is an interview response and responses are interviewer-dependent.[28] These variations in sensitivity and specificity will also produce variations in predictive values, which can be seen from equations that relate the predictive values to sensitivity and specificity. To illustrate the relations, again consider exposure classification among noncases, where $M_0 = B_1 + B_0 = B_1^* + B_0^*$ is the noncase total, and let $P_{e0} = B_1/M_0$ be the true exposure prevalence among noncases. Then, in expectation, the predictive value positive among noncases is

$$
\begin{aligned}
PVP_0 &= \left(\text{number of correctly classified subjects in } B_1^* \right) / B_1^* \\
&= Se\, B_1 / \left(Se\, B_1 + Fp\, B_0 \right) \\
&= Se\left(B_1/M_0 \right) / \left[Se\left(B_1/M_0 \right) + Fp\left(B_0/M_0 \right) \right] \\
&= SeP_{e0} / \left[SeP_{e0} + Fp\left(1 - P_{e0} \right) \right]
\end{aligned}
\tag{13-6}
$$

Similarly, in expectation, the predictive value negative among noncases is

$$
PVN_0 = Sp\left(1 - P_{e0} \right) / \left[FnP_{e0} + Sp\left(1 - P_{e0} \right) \right]
\tag{13-7}
$$

Equations 13-6 and 13-7 show that predictive values are a function of the sensitivity, specificity, *and* the unknown true exposure prevalence in the population to which they apply. When adjustments are based on internal validation data and those data are a random sample of the entire study, there is no issue of generalization across populations. In such situations the predictive value approach is simple and efficient.[67,68] We again emphasize, however, that validation studies may be afflicted by selection bias, or may oversample by design, in both cases violating the randomness assumption needed for this approach and nullifying the expected relations.

Disease Misclassification

Most equations and concerns for exposure misclassification also apply to disease misclassification. For example, Equations 13-1 and 13-4 can be modified to adjust for disease misclassification. For disease misclassification in a closed-cohort study or a prevalence survey, PVP and PVN will refer to the predictive values for disease, and A, B, and N will replace B_1, B_0, and M_0. For the adjustments using sensitivity and specificity, consider first the estimation of the incidence proportion from a closed cohort or of prevalence from a cross-sectional sample. The preceding equations can then be adapted directly by redefining Se, Fn, Sp, and Fp to refer to disease. Let

D $\quad= 1$ if diseased, 0 if not

D^* $\quad= 1$ if classified as diseased, 0 if not

Se $\quad=$ probability someone diseased is classified as diseased

$\quad\quad= $ disease sensitivity $= \Pr(D^* = 1 | D = 1)$

Fn $\quad=$ false-negative probability $= 1{-}Se$

Sp $\quad=$ probability someone nondiseased is classified as nondiseased

$\quad\quad= $ disease specificity $= \Pr(D^* = 0 | D = 0)$

Fp $\quad=$ false-positive probability $= 1{-}Sp$

Suppose that A and B are the true number of diseased and nondiseased subjects, and A^* and B^* are the numbers classified as diseased and nondiseased. Then Equations 13-2 to 13-4 give the expected relations between A, B and A^*, B^*, with A, B replacing B_1, B_0; A^*, B^* replacing B_1^*, B_0^*; and $N = A + B = A^* + B^*$ replacing M_0. With these changes, Equation 13-4 becomes

$$A = \left(A^* - Fp\, N \right) \big/ \left(Se + Sp - 1 \right) \qquad [13\text{-}8]$$

and $B = N - A$. These equations can be applied separately to different exposure groups and within strata, and bias-adjusted summary estimates can then be computed from the bias-adjusted counts. Results of repeated application of this process for different pairs of Se, Sp can be tabulated to provide a sensitivity analysis of the bias analysis. Also, the pair Se, Sp can either be kept the same across exposure groups (nondifferential disease misclassification) or allowed to vary across groups (differential misclassification). As noted earlier, however, special variance equations are required.[48,51-54]

The situation differs slightly for person-time follow-up data. Here, one must replace the specificity Sp and false-positive probability Fp with a different concept, that of the *false-positive rate*, Fr:

$Fr =$ number of false-positive diagnoses (noncases diagnosed as cases) per unit person-time. We then have

$$A^* = Se\, A + Fr\, T \qquad [13\text{-}9]$$

where T is the true person-time at risk. Also, false-negatives (of which there are FnA) will inflate the observed person-time T^*; how much depends on how long the false-negatives are followed. Unless the disease is very common, however, the false negatives will add relatively little person-time and we can take T to be approximately T^*. Upon doing so, we need only solve Equation 13-9 for A:

$$A = \left(A^* - Fr\, T^* \right) \big/ Se \qquad [13\text{-}10]$$

and get an adjusted rate A/T^*. Sensitivity analysis then proceeds (similarly to before) by applying Equation 13-10 to the different exposure groups, computing bias-adjusted summary measures, and repeating this process for various combinations of Se and Fr (which may vary across subcohorts).

The preceding analysis of follow-up data is simplistic, in that it does not account for possible effects if exposure lengthens or shortens the time from incidence to diagnosis. These effects have generally not been correctly analyzed in the medical literature[69,70] (see the discussion of standardization in Chapter 18). In these cases, one should treat time of disease onset as the outcome variable and adjust for errors in measuring this outcome using methods for continuous variables.[62]

Often studies make special efforts to verify case diagnoses, so that the number of false positives within the study will be negligible. If such verification is successful, we can assume that $Fp = 0$, $Sp = 1$, and Equations 13-8 and 13-9 then simplify to $A = A^*/Se$. If we examine a risk ratio RR under these conditions, then, assuming nondifferential misclassification, the observed RR^* will be

$$RR^* = \frac{A_1^*/N_1}{A_0^*/N_0} = \frac{Se\,A_1/N_1}{Se\,A_0/N_0} = \frac{A_1/N_1}{A_0/N_0} = RR$$

In other words, with perfect specificity, nondifferential sensitivity of disease misclassification will not bias the risk ratio, which we noted without proof above. Assuming that the misclassification negligibly alters person-time, the same will be true for the rate ratio[71] and will also be true for the odds ratio when the disease is uncommon. The preceding fact allows extension of the result to case-control studies in which cases are carefully screened to remove false positives.[23]

Suppose now that the cases cannot be screened, so that in a case-control study, there may be many false cases (false positives). It would be a severe mistake to apply the disease misclassification adjustment Equation 13-8 to case-control data if (as is almost always true) Se and Sp are determined from other than the study data themselves,[47] because the use of different sampling probabilities for cases and controls alters the sensitivity and specificity within the study relative to the source population.[72] To see the problem, suppose that all apparent cases A_1^*, A_0^* but only a fraction f of apparent noncases B_1^*, B_0^* are randomly sampled from a closed cohort in which disease has been classified with sensitivity Se and specificity Sp. The expected numbers of apparent cases and controls selected at exposure level j is then

$$A_j^* = Se\,A_j + Fp\,B_j$$

and

$$f \cdot B_j^* = f\left(Fn\,A_j + Sp\,B_j\right)$$

The numbers of true cases and noncases at exposure level j in the case-control study are

$$Se\,A_j + f \cdot Fn\,A_j = \left(Se + f \cdot Fn\right)A_j$$

and

$$Fp\,B_j + f \cdot Sp\,B_j = \left(Fp + f \cdot Sp\right)B_j$$

whereas the numbers of correctly classified cases and noncases in the study are $Se\,A_j$ and $f \cdot Sp\,B_j$. The sensitivity and specificity in the study are thus

$$Se\,A_j/\left(Se + f \cdot Fn\right)A_j = Se/\left(Se + f \cdot Fn\right)$$

and

$$f \cdot Sp\,B_j/\left(Fp + f \cdot Sp\right)B_j = f \cdot Sp/\left(Fp + f \cdot Sp\right)$$

The study specificity can be far from the population specificity. For example, if $Se = Sp = 0.90$, all apparent cases are selected, and controls are 1% of the population at risk, the study specificity will be $0.01(0.90)/[0.1 + 0.01(0.90)] = 0.08$. Use of the population specificity 0.90 instead of the study specificity 0.08 in a bias analysis would produce extremely distorted results. Instead, one can obtain the bias-adjusted estimate of cases as[72]

$$A_j = \frac{A_j^* - (1 - Sp)\left(A_j^* + \dfrac{B_j^*}{f}\right)}{(Se + Sp - 1)}$$

and the bias-adjusted estimate of noncases as

$$B_j = \frac{\dfrac{B_j^*}{f} - (1 - Se)\left(A_j^* + \dfrac{B_j^*}{f}\right)}{(Se + Sp - 1)}$$

The bias-adjusted estimate of controls would be $f \cdot B_j$. In case-control studies with secondary base design (see Chapter 8), f may be unknown, but may be possible to estimate given subject matter knowledge. A sensitivity analysis with a range of values assigned to f would be advisable.

As noted above, when the outcome is a continuous variable, nondifferential measurement error of the outcome inflates the variance of the exposure outcome estimate, but will not introduce bias in the estimate. With differential measurement error of the outcome such that the mean of the error in the outcome measurement depends on the exposure, bias adjustment can be made by subtracting from the observed estimate the direct effect of the exposure on the outcome measurement not through the true outcome.[62,64] Further adjustments may be needed if the differential measurement error in the outcome not only shifts the mean of the outcome measurement but also potentially changes its scale.[62,64]

Confounder Misclassification

The effects of dichotomous confounder misclassification or continuous variable measurement error lead to residual and possibly differential residual confounding.[27] These effects can be evaluated using the methods discussed previously for dichotomous exposure misclassification[36,37,73] or regression calibration.[61] One may apply Equations 13-4 and 13-5 to the confounder within strata of the exposure (rather than to the exposure within strata of the confounder) and then compute a summary exposure-disease association from the adjusted data. The utility of this approach is limited, however, because many confounder adjustments involve more than two strata.

Misclassification of Multiple Variables

So far, our analyses have assumed that only one variable requires adjustment. In many situations, age and sex (which tend to have negligible error) are the only important confounders, the cases are carefully screened, and only exposure remains seriously misclassified. There are, however, many other situations in which not only exposure but also major confounders (such as BMI) are misclassified. Disease misclassification may also coexist with these other problems, especially when studying disease subtypes.

In examining misclassification of multiple variables, it is commonly assumed that the classification errors for each variable are independent of *errors* in other variables. This assumption is different from that of nondifferentiality, which asserts that errors for each variable are independent of the true values of the other variables. Neither, either one, or both assumptions may hold in expectation as a result of design features, and the various combinations have different implications for bias. As mentioned above, the generalization that "nondifferential misclassification of exposure always produces bias toward the null" is false if the errors are dependent or if exposure has multiple levels.

If all the classification errors are independent across variables, we can apply the adjustment equations in sequence for each misclassified variable, one at a time. For example, in a prevalence survey we may first obtain counts bias-adjusted for exposure misclassification from Equations 13-4 and 13-5, then further bias-adjust these counts for disease misclassification using Equation 13-8. If, however, the classification errors are dependent across variables, we must turn to more complex adjustment methods such as those based on matrix adjustment of counts,[47,48,51,52] which we discuss in Chapter 29. Dependent errors most easily arise when the same method, such as an interview or medical record review, is used to ascertain more than one variable involved in the analysis.[74] Matrix methods are also useful for adjustments of polytomous (multilevel) variables. See Chapter 29 for a discussion of the use of validation data for the simple bias adjustment methods described above as well as the matrix methods described in that chapter.

Misclassification and Measurement Error for Other Causal Effects

The focus of this chapter has been on the consequences of misclassification and measurement error on biases of estimates of the causal effect of an exposure on an outcome. Misclassification and measurement error also have consequences for estimates of other causal effects. Nondifferential misclassification of a binary outcome will, for example, bias interaction effect measures on the difference scale toward the null, but classical measurement error of a continuous outcome will not bias interaction measures on the difference scale.[75] Independent nondifferential measurement error of two independent exposures will likewise bias interaction measures on the difference scale toward the null.[76] When two exposures are independent, differential misclassification of a binary exposure that allows misclassification to depend on the outcome will bias measures of multiplicative interaction toward the null.[77] More information on interaction measures and methods is available in Chapter 26.

For direct and indirect effects, nondifferential misclassification of a binary mediator will bias indirect effects toward the null and direct effects away from the null,[78] but this need not hold for a mediator that is not binary.[79] Bias adjustment methods are available for direct and indirect effects when mediators are subject to misclassification or measurement error.[80] Nondifferential misclassification of a binary outcome will bias both direct and indirect effects toward the null, but classical measurement error of a continuous outcome will not bias direct or indirect effects.[81] Misclassification or measurement error of an exposure can bias direct and indirect effects in either direction and must be addressed through bias adjustment techniques.[82] Chapter 27 provides further details about mediation and the estimation of direct and indirect effects.

References

1. Hernan MA, Cole SR. Invited Commentary: causal diagrams and measurement bias. *Am J Epidemiol.* 2009;170(8):959-962; discussion 963-964.
2. Sanders SA, Hill BJ, Yarber WL, Graham CA, Crosby RA, Milhausen RR. Misclassification bias: diversity in conceptualisations about having 'had sex'. *Sex Health.* 2010;7(1):31-34.
3. Funk MJ, Landi SN. Misclassification in administrative claims data: quantifying the impact on treatment effect estimates. *Curr Epidemiol Rep.* 2014;1(4):175-185.
4. Lash TL, Thwin SS, Yood MU, et al. Comprehensive evaluation of the incidence of late effects in 5-year survivors of breast cancer. *Breast Cancer Res Treat.* 2014;144(3):643-663.
5. Klemetti A, Saxen L. Prospective versus retrospective approach in the search for environmental causes of malformations. *Am J Public Health Nations Health.* 1967;57(12):2071-2075.
6. Chen Q, Galfalvy H, Duan N. Effects of disease misclassification on exposure-disease association. *Am J Public Health.* 2013;103(5):e67-73.
7. Drews CD, Greeland S. The impact of differential recall on the results of case-control studies. *Int J Epidemiol.* 1990;19(4):1107-1112.
8. Newell DJ. Errors in the interpretation of errors in epidemiology. *Am J Public Health Nations Health.* 1962;52:1925-1928.
9. Gullen WH, Bearman JE, Johnson EA. Effects of misclassification in epidemiologic studies. *Public Health Rep.* 1968;83(11):914-918.
10. Copeland KT, Checkoway H, McMichael AJ, Holbrook RH. Bias due to misclassification in the estimation of relative risk. *Am J Epidemiol.* 1977;105(5):488-495.
11. Flegal KM, Keyl PM, Nieto FJ. Differential misclassification arising from nondifferential errors in exposure measurement. *Am J Epidemiol.* 1991;134(10):1233-1244.

12. Wacholder S, Dosemeci M, Lubin JH. Blind assignment of exposure does not always prevent differential misclassification. *Am J Epidemiol*. 1991;134(4):433-437.

13. Greenland S, Robins JM. Confounding and misclassification. *Am J Epidemiol*. 1985;122(3):495-506.

14. Walker AM, Blettner M. Comparing imperfect measures of exposure. *Am J Epidemiol*. 1985;121(6):783-790.

15. Dosemeci M, Wacholder S, Lubin JH. Does nondifferential misclassification of exposure always bias a true effect toward the null value? *Am J Epidemiol*. 1990;132(4):746-748.

16. Chavance M, Dellatolas G, Lellouch J. Correlated nondifferential misclassifications of disease and exposure: application to a cross-sectional study of the relation between handedness and immune disorders. *Int J Epidemiol*. 1992;21(3):537-546.

17. Kristensen P. Bias from nondifferential but dependent misclassification of exposure and outcome. *Epidemiology*. 1992;3(3):210-215.

18. Birkett NJ. Effect of nondifferential misclassification on estimates of odds ratios with multiple levels of exposure. *Am J Epidemiol*. 1992;136(3):356-362.

19. Weinberg CR, Umbach DM, Greenland S. When will nondifferential misclassification of an exposure preserve the direction of a trend? *Am J Epidemiol*. 1994;140(6):565-571.

20. Thomas DC. "When will nondifferential misclassification of an exposure preserve the direction of a trend?" *Am J Epidemiol*. 1995;142(7):782-784.

21. Weinberg CR, Umbach D, Greenland S, et al. Weinberg et al. reply. *Am J Epidemiol*. 1995;142:784.

22. Jurek AM, Greenland S, Maldonado G, Church TR. Proper interpretation of non-differential misclassification effects: expectations vs observations. *Int J Epidemiol*. 2005;34(3):680-687.

23. Brenner H, Savitz DA. The effects of sensitivity and specificity of case selection on validity, sample size, precision, and power in hospital-based case-control studies. *Am J Epidemiol*. 1990;132(1):181-192.

24. Rodgers A, MacMahon S. Systematic underestimation of treatment effects as a result of diagnostic test inaccuracy: implications for the interpretation and design of thromboprophylaxis trials. *Thromb Haemost*. 1995;73(2):167-171.

25. Bross I. Misclassification in 2 × 2 tables. *Biometrics*. 1954;10:478-486.

26. Gustafson P, Greenland S. Curious phenomena in Bayesian adjustment for exposure misclassification. *Stat Med*. 2006;25(1):87-103.

27. Greenland S. The effect of misclassification in the presence of covariates. *Am J Epidemiol*. 1980;112(4):564-569.

28. Begg CB. Biases in the assessment of diagnostic tests. *Stat Med*. 1987;6(4):411-423.

29. Smithells RW, Sheppard S. Teratogenicity testing in humans: a method demonstrating safety of bendectin. *Teratology*. 1978;17(1):31-35.

30. Jick H, Walker AM, Rothman KJ, et al. Vaginal spermicides and congenital disorders. *J Am Med Assoc*. 1981;245(13):1329-1332.

31. Jick H, Walker AM, Rothman KJ, et al. "Vaginal spermicides and congenital disorders". *J Am Med Assoc*. 1981;246:2677-2678.

32. Felarca LC, Wardell DM, Rowles B. Vaginal spermicides and congenital disorders. *J Am Med Assoc*. 1981;246:2677-2678.

33. Oakley GP Jr. Spermicides and birth defects. *J Am Med Assoc*. 1982;247(17):2405.

34. Kupper LL. Effects of the use of unreliable surrogate variables on the validity of epidemiologic research studies. *Am J Epidemiol*. 1984;120(4):643-648.

35. Brenner H. Bias due to non-differential misclassification of polytomous confounders. *J Clin Epidemiol*. 1993;46(1):57-63.

36. Marshall JR, Hastrup JL. Mismeasurement and the resonance of strong confounders: uncorrelated errors. *Am J Epidemiol*. 1996;143(10):1069-1078.

37. Marshall JR, Hastrup JL, Ross JS. Mismeasurement and the resonance of strong confounders: correlated errors. *Am J Epidemiol*. 1999;150(1):88-96.

38. Fewell Z, Davey Smith G, Sterne JA. The impact of residual and unmeasured confounding in epidemiologic studies: a simulation study. *Am J Epidemiol*. 2007;166(6):646-655.

39. Ogburn EL, VanderWeele TJ. On the nondifferential misclassification of a binary confounder. *Epidemiology*. 2012;23(3):433-439.

40. Ogburn EL, Vanderweele TJ. Bias attenuation results for nondifferentially mismeasured ordinal and coarsened confounders. *Biometrika*. 2013;100(1):241-248.

41. Morrison AS, Buring JE, Verhoek WG, et al. Coffee drinking and cancer of the lower urinary tract. *J Natl Cancer Inst*. 1982;68(1):91-94.

42. VanderWeele TJ, Hernan MA. Results on differential and dependent measurement error of the exposure and the outcome using signed directed acyclic graphs. *Am J Epidemiol*. 2012;175(12):1303-1310.

43. Jurek AM, Maldonado G, Greenland S, Church TR. Exposure-measurement error is frequently ignored when interpreting epidemiologic study results. *Eur J Epidemiol*. 2006;21(12):871-876.

44. Greenland S. The effect of misclassification in matched-pair case-control studies. *Am J Epidemiol*. 1982;116(2):402-406.

45. Kleinbaum DG, Kupper LL, Morgenstern H. *Epidemiologic Research: Principles and Quantitative Methods*. New York, NY: Van Nostrand Reinhold; 1982.
46. Barron BA. The effects of misclassification on the estimation of relative risk. *Biometrics*. 1977;33(2):414-418.
47. Greenland S, Kleinbaum DG. Correcting for misclassification in two-way tables and matched-pair studies. *Int J Epidemiol*. 1983;12(1):93-97.
48. Greenland S. Statistical uncertainty due to misclassification: implications for validation substudies. *J Clin Epidemiol*. 1988;41(12):1167-1174.
49. Poon WY, Wang HB. Analysis of ordinal categorical data with misclassification. *Br J Math Stat Psychol*. 2010;63(pt 1):17-42.
50. Mullooly JP. Misclassification model for person-time analysis of automated medical care databases. *Am J Epidemiol*. 1996;144(8):782-792.
51. Selén J. Adjusting for errors in classification and measurement in the analysis of partly and purely categorical data. *J Am Stat Assoc*. 1986;81:75-81.
52. Espeland MA, Hui SL. A general approach to analyzing epidemiologic data that contain misclassification errors. *Biometrics*. 1987;43(4):1001-1012.
53. Greenland S. Maximum-likelihood and closed-form estimators of epidemiologic measures under misclassification. *J Stat Plan Inference*. 2007;138:528-538.
54. Gustafson P. *Measurement Error and Misclassification in Statistics and Epidemiology*. Boca Raton, FL: Chapman and Hall; 2003.
55. Greenland S, Gustafson P. Adjustment for independent nondifferential misclassification does not increase certainty that an observed association is in the correct direction. *Am J Epidemiol*. 2006;164:63-68.
56. Rosner B, Willett WC, Spiegelman D. Correction of logistic regression relative risk estimates and confidence intervals for systematic within-person measurement error. *Stat Med*. 1989;8(9):1051-1069; discussion 1071-1073.
57. Spiegelman D, McDermott A, Rosner B. Regression calibration method for correcting measurement-error bias in nutritional epidemiology. *Am J Clin Nutr*. 1997;65(suppl 4):1179S-1186S.
58. Wacholder S, Armstrong B, Hartge P. Validation studies using an alloyed gold standard. *Am J Epidemiol*. 1993;137(11):1251-1258.
59. Fahey MT, Forbes AB, Hodge AM. Correcting for the bias caused by exposure measurement error in epidemiological studies. *Respirology*. 2014;19(7):979-984.
60. Spiegelman D. Approaches to uncertainty in exposure assessment in environmental epidemiology. *Annu Rev Public Health*. 2010;31:149-163.
61. Rosner B, Spiegelman D, Willett WC. Correction of logistic regression relative risk estimates and confidence intervals for measurement error: the case of multiple covariates measured with error. *Am J Epidemiol*. 1990;132(4):734-745.
62. Carroll RJ, Ruppert D, Stefanski LA, Crainiceanu C. *Measurement Error in Nonlinear Models*. Boca Raton, FL: Chapman and Hall; 2006.
63. Thurigen D, Spiegelman D, Blettner M, Heuer C, Brenner H. Measurement error correction using validation data: a review of methods and their applicability in case-control studies. *Stat Methods Med Res*. 2000;9(5):447-474.
64. VanderWeele TJ, Li Y. Simple sensitivity analysis for differential measurement error. *Am J Epidemiol*. 2019;188(10):1823-1829.
65. Chien C, Li CI, Heckbert SR, Malone KE, Boudreau DM, Daling JR. Antidepressant use and breast cancer risk. *Breast Cancer Res Treat*. 2006;95(2):131-140.
66. Boudreau DM, Daling JR, Malone KE, Gardner JS, Blough DK, Heckbert SR. A validation study of patient interview data and pharmacy records for antihypertensive, statin, and antidepressant medication use among older women. *Am J Epidemiol*. 2004;159(3):308-317.
67. Marshall RJ. Validation study methods for estimating exposure proportions and odds ratios with misclassified data. *J Clin Epidemiol*. 1990;43(9):941-947.
68. Brenner H, Gefeller O. Use of the positive predictive value to correct for disease misclassification in epidemiologic studies. *Am J Epidemiol*. 1993;138(11):1007-1015.
69. Greenland S. A mathematic analysis of the "epidemiologic necropsy". *Ann Epidemiol*. 1991;1(6):551-558.
70. Greenland S. The relation of the probability of causation to the relative risk and the doubling dose: a methodologic error that has become a social problem. *Am J Public Health*. 1999;89:1166-1169.
71. Poole C. Exceptions to the rule about nondifferential misclassification (abstract). *Am J Epidemiol*. 1985;122:508.
72. Jurek AM, Maldonado G, Greenland S. Adjusting for outcome misclassification: the importance of accounting for case-control sampling and other forms of outcome-related selection. *Ann Epidemiol*. 2013;23(3):129-135.
73. Savitz DA, Baron AE. Estimating and correcting for confounder misclassification. *Am J Epidemiol*. 1989;129(5):1062-1071.

74. Lash TL, Fink AK. "Neighborhood environment and loss of physical function in older adults: evidence from the Alameda County Study". *Am J Epidemiol.* 2003;157(5):472-473.

75. Jiang Z, VanderWeele TJ. Additive interaction in the presence of a mismeasured outcome. *Am J Epidemiol.* 2015;181(1):81-82.

76. Vanderweele TJ. Inference for additive interaction under exposure misclassification. *Biometrika.* 2012;99(2):502-508.

77. Garcia-Closas M, Thompson WD, Robins JM. Differential misclassification and the assessment of gene-environment interactions in case-control studies. *Am J Epidemiol.* 1998;147(5):426-433.

78. VanderWeele TJ, Valeri L, Ogburn EL. The role of measurement error and misclassification in mediation analysis: mediation and measurement error. *Epidemiology.* 2012;23(4):561-564.

79. Ogburn EL, VanderWeele TJ. Analytic results on the bias due to nondifferential misclassification of a binary mediator. *Am J Epidemiol.* 2012;176(6):555-561.

80. Valeri L, Lin X, VanderWeele TJ. Mediation analysis when a continuous mediator is measured with error and the outcome follows a generalized linear model. *Stat Med.* 2014;33(28):4875-4890.

81. Jiang Z, VanderWeele TJ. Causal mediation analysis in the presence of a mismeasured outcome. *Epidemiology.* 2015;26(1):e8-e9.

82. VanderWeele TJ. *Explanation in Causal Inference: Methods for Mediation and Interaction.* New York, NY: Oxford University Press; 2015.

CHAPTER 14

Selection Bias and Generalizability

Timothy L. Lash and Kenneth J. Rothman

INTRODUCTION

Selection bias arises when the estimate of occurrence or of etiologic effect obtained from a study population differs systematically from the estimate that would have been obtained had information from the source population been available (see Chapter 4 for definitions of source population, study population, and target population). This difference arises from differences between participants at initial study enrollment or from differences between those who continue to participate and those who are lost to follow-up. In studies of disease occurrence, this selection bias arises if the outcome, or ancestors of the outcome, affects participation. In studies of etiologic effects, this selection bias can arise from collider bias,[1] which is a biasing path in a causal graph wherein both the etiologic agent of interest and the outcome of interest are ancestors of initial or continued participation. In studies of etiologic effects, selection bias can also arise if the outcome is associated with the selection and the strength of selection varies in different levels of exposure.[2] Because estimates of occurrence and of etiologic effects are conditioned on participation, the estimates observed in the study population represent a mix of forces that determine participation and forces that determine disease occurrence.

Generalizability and transportability pertain to the question of whether a study's estimate of occurrence or etiologic effect applies to the target population. When a study has poor internal validity, its results will not be generalizable or transportable to the target population. Selection bias is one explanation for why the estimate from a study population may not generalize to the target population, but uncontrolled confounding (see Chapter 12) and information bias (see Chapter 13) are also threats to internal validity and so might also explain lack of generalizability or transportability. It is also possible that different prevalence of effect measure modifiers in the study population and in the target population would cause an estimate (even one with good internal validity) from the study population to be poorly generalizable to the target population. If information on the prevalence of effect measure modifiers in the target population is available, it is possible to standardize the study population to the target population. One strategy to enhance generalizability is to draw a representative sample of the target population to comprise the study population. Although this strategy enhances generalizability, there is often a price to pay with a representative sample in terms of efficiency and validity. For example, studies that oversample persons at high risk for the outcome can enroll fewer participants and achieve the same precision of effect estimates as a representative sample. These efficiencies may then allow a larger share of study resources to be devoted to collecting higher quality information. An investigator will often have to balance generalizability concerns against these efficiency and validity concerns. As noted above, information from study populations that are not representative may still be generalized to the source population and target populations by standardization, for example. Thus, study populations that are not representative may yield more valid results and with greater efficiency, and without any loss of generalizability.

This concept of generalizing to a target population should be distinguished from the concept of generalizability as it is used in many sciences, where generalizability pertains to the extrapolation of information gleaned from a scientific experiment or set of experiments to a broader context. This process is at the heart of scientific inquiry, which involves investigating specific natural phenomena to understand and describe how nature works in a general sense. All these concepts are addressed in greater detail below.

SELECTION BIAS

As noted above, selection biases are distortions in estimates of disease occurrence or of etiologic effect resulting from procedures that influence initial or ongoing study participation. For studies of etiologic effects, it is sometimes possible to disentangle the effects of participation from those of disease determinants analytically using conventional methods for the control of confounding (*e.g.*, standardization or stratification). To employ such analytic control requires, among other things, that the determinants of participation were measured accurately and that participation was not affected by both exposure and disease. When these conditions are not met, analytic control cannot be achieved, but quantitative bias analysis (see Chapter 29) can provide an assessment of the direction, magnitude, and uncertainty about the influence of selection bias, conditional on the accuracy of the bias model.

Some forms of selection bias in case-control studies are described in Chapter 8. Those include use of invalid control groups (*e.g.*, controls composed of patients with diseases that are affected by the study exposure). In Chapter 6, we discussed matching in case-control studies, which intentionally introduces a selection bias to achieve greater statistical efficiency and then controls for that selection bias in the analysis. We consider here some further types of selection bias and then describe quantitative bias analysis methods to address it.

Baseline Participation

Many epidemiologic studies require study subjects to agree to participate. These include most randomized trials, cohort studies, case-control studies, cross-sectional surveys, and studies of other designs. The fundamental reason why study subjects must agree to participate is to provide informed consent, one of the bedrock principles of ethical human subjects research (see Chapter 6). Whenever studies require consent, it is possible that study subjects (those who agree to participate) differ from persons who decline to participate with respect to characteristics related to the study variables. For example, in a retrospective case-control study, eligible persons are usually aware of both their outcome status (case or control) and their exposure history. If both affect the probability of consenting to participate, then selection bias is likely to arise. This type of selection bias can be diagrammed with a simple directed acyclic graph $E \rightarrow P \leftarrow D$, where exposure status is represented by E (exposed or unexposed), disease status (case or control) is represented by D, and participation in the study (yes or no) is represented by P. Estimates of the association between E and D must be obtained by analyzing data provided by the participants (P = yes), so the analyses condition on P, which opens the biasing path $E \rightarrow \boxed{P} \leftarrow D$ that is otherwise blocked by the collider P. The biasing path can be avoided by a design that does not condition on P, such as use of registry or administrative data for which consent to participate is waived and therefore all eligible study subjects are included (see Chapter 11). This solution only applies to the set of hypotheses for which adequate registry data exist. The biasing path can also be avoided by a design for which there is no directed path from D to P, that is, a prospective design. When the disease has not yet occurred at the time when the eligible person is invited to participate, then the disease status cannot affect the decision to participate and the biasing path is avoided. It may be necessary to measure a sufficient set of variables to close other biasing paths, for example, $E \rightarrow P \leftarrow C' \rightarrow D$ and C' has been measured. The sufficient set C' includes risk factors for D that also influence the decision to participate. Finally, the path can also be closed by a design for which it is unlikely that there is a directed path from E to P. For example, in a retrospective case-control study in which E is a genetic factor, E is not likely to be known to participants (except for some hereditary conditions). Consequently, although the case-control design may be susceptible to baseline selection bias, in this case there would be no directed path from E to P and therefore no biasing path.

Loss to Follow-Up

Many epidemiologic studies require study subjects, once enrolled, to agree to continue to participate. These include most randomized trials and cohort studies, as well as case-control studies nested in them. These designs require that participants continue to participate so that they can be regularly followed for information on their outcome status (*e.g.*, diseased or not diseased) and can update their exposures (*e.g.*, potential changes to time-varying exposures such as diet, exercise, comorbid diseases, and use of prescription medications, tobacco, or alcohol). When study subjects who initially agree to participate later end their participation, subsequent information on outcomes and exposures can no longer be collected. The subjects are said to be "lost to follow-up." When the association between an exposure E and an outcome D is estimated in the data, the estimate must be calculated among those who agreed to participate and it must be based upon their experience while they agree to remain participants: $E \rightarrow \boxed{P} \leftarrow D$. This dependence on continued participation opens a biasing path. If both the exposure and factors associated with the risk of the outcome affect participation, then the structure for selection bias due to loss to follow-up would be $E \rightarrow \boxed{P} \leftarrow U \rightarrow D$, in which D does not cause loss to follow-up directly, but some risk factor for D does cause loss to follow-up.

Imagine an observational study of use of statin medications, which are prescribed to prevent hypercholesterolemia and concomitant cardiovascular disease, and the occurrence of dementia. Baseline participants are free of dementia and, under a new user design, also without a history of statin prescription. Over follow-up, some study participants will be prescribed a statin and some will develop dementia. Subjects who are prescribed a statin may elect to continue to participate at greater rates than those who are never prescribed a statin. Also, subjects who develop dementia may be more likely to discontinue participation due to preclinical symptoms than subjects who do not develop dementia. Assuming no association between statin use and the hazard of dementia, the study population will, over time, become more rapidly depleted of nonusers of statins and persons with dementia, and especially depleted of nonusers with dementia. The estimate of association comparing dementia occurrence in statin users with dementia occurrence in nonusers of statins will be greater than the null, but this association will derive from greater losses to follow-up in the nonusers, and especially dementia cases among nonusers. It will not reflect a true effect of statins use on the occurrence of dementia.

Self-Selection Bias

Another source of selection bias is *self-selection*, or *volunteer bias*. This type of bias arises when some or all study subjects initiate the enrollment process to participate in a study (volunteer) rather than study organizers initiating the enrollment process for all participants by inviting them to participate. The concern is that the forces promoting a person to volunteer for a study may include a history of disease occurrence or known factors that place the volunteers at different risks for the disease, and these forces therefore may distort the study estimates. Once again, we have a biasing path $E \leftarrow C' \rightarrow \boxed{P} \leftarrow U' \rightarrow D$ because the exposure E (or more likely predictors of the exposure C') and the disease D (or more likely predictors of the disease U') both affect participation P, and the analysis is conducted only among participants, so we must condition on P. Self-selection bias is therefore a special case of selection bias due to exposure- and outcome-dependent baseline participation, in which the biasing forces affect a subset of the participants (the volunteers). This bias structure can apply more generally to any study for which participants know about the aims of the study at the time they are recruited, and this information affects decisions to participate.

As an example, the Centers for Disease Control investigated leukemia incidence among troops who had been present at the Smoky Atomic Test in Nevada.[3] When the cohort was enrolled, 76% of the troops identified as members of the cohort had known outcomes. Of this 76%, 82% were traced by the investigators, but the other 18% contacted the investigators on their own initiative in response to publicity about the investigation. These volunteers would have known their exposure status (E) and something about the extent of their exposure (C'). They would also have known their disease status (D) at the date of their volunteering to participate and something about their risk of leukemia (U', where the intersection of the set U' and the set C' may not be the empty set). This self-referral of subjects is a threat to validity, because the reasons for self-referral may be associated with both the exposure and the outcome under study among the volunteers.[4] Analysis of the data provided evidence of the volunteer bias. There were four leukemia cases among the $0.18 \times 0.76 = 14\%$ of cohort members who referred themselves and four among the $0.82 \times 0.76 = 62\%$ of cohort members invited by the investigators. These data indicate that volunteer bias was a small but real problem in the Smoky study. If the 24% of the cohort with unknown outcomes had a leukemia incidence like that of the subjects traced by the investigators, we should expect that only $4(24/62) = 1.5$ or about 1 or 2 cases occurred among this 24%, for a total of only 9 or 10 cases in the entire cohort. If instead we assume that the 24% with unknown outcomes had a leukemia incidence like that of subjects with known outcomes, we would calculate that $8(24/76) = 2.5$ or about 2 or 3 cases occurred among this 24%, for a total of 10 or 11 cases in the entire cohort. It might be, however, that all cases among the 38% ($=24\% + 14\%$) of the cohort that was untraced were among the self-reported, leaving no case among those with unknown outcome. The total number of cases in the entire cohort would then be only eight.

Self-selection can also occur before subjects are identified for study. For example, it is routine to find that the mortality of active workers is less than that of the population as a whole.[5,6] This "healthy-worker effect" presumably derives from a screening process, perhaps largely self-selection, that allows relatively healthy people to become or remain workers, whereas those who remain unemployed, retired, disabled, or otherwise out of the active worker population are, as a group, less healthy.[6,7] While the healthy-worker effect had traditionally been classified as a selection bias, one can see that it does not reflect a bias created by conditioning on participation in the study, but rather from the effect of an other factor C' that influences both worker status E and some measure of health D ($E \leftarrow C' \rightarrow D$; see Chapter 12). As such, the healthy-worker effect is an example of confounding rather than selection bias.[1]

Berksonian Bias

Berkson bias, or Berksonian bias, arises in studies of the association between two diseases when the population is limited to a convenience sample, such as hospitalized patients. It was first described by Berkson in 1946.[8] In studies of this type, we have $E \rightarrow \boxed{P} \leftarrow D$, where E is the hypothesized predecessor disease (*e.g.*, diabetes) and D is the hypothesized outcome (*e.g.*, dementia). If both diabetes and dementia increase the risk of hospitalization, and the study population is limited to hospitalized patients as indicated by the box drawn around P, then diabetes and dementia will appear to be associated, even if they are not, because of conditioning on their common consequent of hospitalization. Likewise, causes of diabetes (C') will appear to be associated with dementia ($C' \rightarrow E \rightarrow \boxed{P} \leftarrow D$). Berkson bias is sometimes paradoxical because it can generate a downward bias when both the exposure and the disease increase the chance of selection; this downward bias can induce a negative association in the study population even if the association in the source population is positive but not as large as the bias.

An example of Berksonian bias arose in the early controversy about the role of exogenous estrogens in causing endometrial cancer. Several case-control studies had reported a strong association, with about a 10-fold increase in risk for women taking estrogens regularly for a number of years.[9-12] Most investigators interpreted this increase in risk as a causal relation, but others suggested that estrogens were merely causing the cancers to be diagnosed rather than to occur.[13] Their argument rested on the fact that estrogens induce uterine bleeding. Therefore, the administration of estrogens would presumably lead women to seek medical attention, thus causing a variety of gynecologic conditions to be detected. The resulting bias was referred to as detection bias (a type of information bias, see Chapter 13).

The remedy proposed by Horwitz and Feinstein was to use a control series of women with benign gynecologic diseases.[13] These investigators reasoned that benign conditions would also be subject to detection bias, and therefore using a control series comprising women with benign conditions would be preferable to using a control series of women with other malignant disease, non-gynecologic disease, or no disease, as earlier studies had done. The flaw in this reasoning was the incorrect assumption that estrogens caused a substantial proportion of endometrial cancers to be diagnosed that would otherwise have remained undiagnosed. Even if the administration of estrogens advances the date of diagnosis for endometrial cancer, such an advance in the time of diagnosis need not in itself lead to any substantial bias.[14] Possibly, a small proportion of pre-existing endometrial cancer cases that otherwise would not have been diagnosed did come to attention, but it is reasonable to suppose that endometrial cancer that is not in situ (Horwitz and Feinstein[13] excluded in situ cases) usually progresses to cause symptoms leading to diagnosis.[15] Although a permanent, nonprogressive early stage of endometrial cancer is a possibility, the studies that excluded such in situ cases from the case series still found a strong association between estrogen administration and endometrial cancer risk.[12]

The alternative control group proposed by Horwitz and Feinstein comprised women with benign gynecologic conditions that were presumed not to cause symptoms leading to diagnosis. Such a group would provide an overestimate of the proportion of the source population of cases exposed to estrogens, because administration of estrogens would indeed cause the diagnosis of a substantial proportion of the benign conditions. The use of a control series with benign gynecologic conditions would thus produce a bias that severely underestimated the effect of exogenous estrogens on the risk of endometrial cancer. Another remedy that Horwitz and Feinstein proposed was to examine the association within women who had presented with vaginal bleeding or had undergone treatment for such bleeding.[13] Because both the exposure (exogenous estrogens) and the disease (endometrial cancer) strongly increase bleeding risk, restriction to women with bleeding or treatment for bleeding results in a Berksonian bias so severe that it could easily diminish the observed relative risk by fivefold.[16]

Although the example is now somewhat dated, it provides historical insight into how selection biases came to be understood in the context of an important public health question. Selection biases continue to arise in individual studies, but because of the lessons learned from this example, no more recent example exists in which the selection biases were so thoroughly vetted. A major lesson to be learned from this controversy is the importance of considering selection biases quantitatively rather than qualitatively, using methods described below. Without appreciation for the magnitude of potential selection biases, the choice of a control group can result in a bias so great that a strong association is occluded; alternatively, a null or negligible association could easily be exaggerated. Simple methods for quantitative adjustment for selection biases are discussed below, and more advanced methods are presented in Chapter 29. Another lesson is that one runs the risk of inducing or worsening selection bias whenever one uses selection criteria (e.g., requiring the presence or absence of certain conditions) that are influenced by the exposure under study. If those criteria are also related to the study disease, severe Berksonian bias is likely to ensue.

Distinguishing Selection Bias From Confounding

Selection bias and confounding are two concepts that, depending on terminology, often overlap. For example, in cohort studies, biases resulting from differential selection into exposure groups at the start of follow-up are often called selection bias, but in our terminology, they are examples of confounding, as foreshadowed above in the section on the healthy worker effect. Nonetheless, this terminology is not uniformly applied across scientific disciplines. What epidemiologists call "confounding," economists often refer to as "selection bias." When economists use "selection bias," they understand "selection into treatment groups." When epidemiologists refer to "selection bias," they refer to "selection into study participation."

Consider a cohort study comparing mortality from cardiovascular diseases among longshore-men and office workers. If physically fit individuals (measured by C') self-select or are screened by employment exams into longshoreman work E, we should expect longshoremen to have lower cardiovascular mortality D than that of office workers, even if working as a longshoreman has no effect on cardiovascular mortality ($E \leftarrow C' \rightarrow D$; see Chapter 12). Consequently, the crude esti-mate from such a study could not be considered a valid estimate of the effect of longshoreman work on cardiovascular mortality. Note that this self-selection is not the same as volunteer bias, because self-selection into work as a longshoreman (an exposure group) is not the same as self-selection as a participant in a study.

Suppose, however, that the fitness of an individual who becomes a longshoreman could be measured and compared with the fitness of the office workers. If measurement of fitness factors C' was done accurately on all subjects, the difference in fitness could be controlled in the analysis. Thus, the differences in initial fitness at the time of selection into these two worker exposure groups would be removed by control of the confounders responsible for the bias (assuming positivity). Although the bias results from selection of persons into the worker exposure groups, it is in fact a form of confounding.[1]

Because measurements on fitness at entry into an occupation are generally not available, the investigator's efforts in such a situation could instead focus on the choice of a reference group that would experience the same selection forces as the target occupation. For example, Paffenbarger and Hale conducted a study in which they compared cardiovascular mortality among groups of longshoremen who engaged in different levels of physical activity on the job.[17] They presumed that the selection factors for entering the occupation were similar for the subgroups engaged in tasks demanding high or low activity, because work assignments were made after entering the profession. This design would reduce or eliminate the association between fitness and becoming a longshoreman ($E \quad C' \rightarrow D$). By comparing groups with different intensities of exposure within an occupation (internal comparison), occupational epidemiologists reduce the difference in selec-tion forces that accompanies comparisons across occupational groups, and thus reduce the risk of confounding.

Not all selection forces in cohort studies have the biasing structure of confounding. For example, if exposure affects loss to follow-up and furthermore factors U' related to disease risk also affect loss to follow-up, selection bias occurs because the analysis is conditioned on a common consequence (remaining under follow-up is a descendant of both the exposure and U', which is associated with the outcome). This bias, described in more detail above, could arise in an occupational mortality study if exposure E caused people to leave the occupation early (e.g., move from an active job to a desk job or retirement) and that in turn led to loss to follow-up P. The vector of risk factors U' also predicts loss to follow-up and an increased risk of death D ($E \rightarrow \boxed{P} \leftarrow U' \rightarrow D$). Here, there is no baseline set of covariates (C') creating differences in risk between exposed and unexposed groups; rather, exposure itself is generat-ing the bias. Such a bias would be irremediable without further information on the selection effects, and even with that information, the bias could not be removed by a simple covariate control. Quantitative bias analyses, such as those described below, could be used to estimate the direction and the magnitude of the bias. The possibility of this type of bias, which can arise in randomized studies as well as nonrandomized designs, underscores the need for thorough follow-up in cohort studies, usually requiring a system for outcome surveillance in the cohort (e.g., an insurance claims system). If no such system is in place, the study must implement its own system, which can be expensive.

In case-control studies, the concerns about the choice of a control group focus on factors that might affect selection and recruitment into the study. Although confounding factors also must be considered, they can be controlled in the analysis if they are measured. If selection factors that affect case and control selection are themselves not affected by exposure (e.g., sex), any selection bias they produce can also be controlled by controlling these factors in the analysis. The key, then, to avoiding confounding and selection bias due to pre-exposure covariates is to identify in advance and measure as many confounders and selection factors as is practical. Doing so requires good subject-matter knowledge.

In case-control studies, however, subjects are often selected after exposure and outcome occur (i.e., retrospectively), and hence there is an elevated potential for bias due to combined exposure and disease effects on selection, as occurred in the estrogen and endometrial cancer studies that restricted subjects to patients with bleeding (or to patients receiving specific medical procedures to treat bleeding).

Because many types of selection bias cannot be controlled in the analysis, prevention of selection bias by appropriate control selection can be critical. As described in Chapter 8, selecting all cases and controls from a primary source population is one effective strategy, but may be difficult to achieve if eligible participants must consent to study participation. The alternative design strategy for this prevention then involves selecting a control group that is subject to the same selective forces as the case group, in the hopes that the biases introduced by control selection will cancel the biases introduced by case selection in the final estimates. Meeting this goal even approximately can rarely be assured; nonetheless, it is often the only design strategy available to address concerns about selection bias. This strategy and other aspects of control selection are discussed in Chapter 8. When this design strategy cannot be achieved, quantitative bias analysis can be used to estimate the direction and magnitude of the bias, as described further below.

To summarize, differential selection into exposure groups that occurs before disease leads to confounding and can thus be controlled by adjustments for the factors responsible for the selection differences. In contrast, selection bias as usually described in epidemiology (as well as in the experimental-design literature) arises from selection affected by the exposure under study, is best addressed by study design, is usually irremediable by conventional adjustment methods such as stratification or regression, but may be addressed quantitatively by bias analysis.

QUANTITATIVE BIAS ANALYSIS FOR SELECTION BIAS

Selection bias (including response and follow-up bias) is perhaps the simplest bias to model quantitatively and yet is often the hardest to address convincingly, although attempts have been made.[18-20] The chief obstacle is lack of sufficient information to perform a quantitative analysis. It is thus unsurprising that many subject-matter controversies (such as that described above surrounding exogenous estrogens and endometrial cancer) can be reduced to disputes about selection bias in case-control studies.

An example of controllable selection bias is that induced by matching in case-control studies. As discussed in Chapter 6, one needs to only control the matching factors to remove the bias. Other examples include two-stage studies, which employ biased selection with known selection probabilities and then use those probabilities to adjust for the selection bias.[21-25] Examples of ordinarily uncontrollable bias occur when controls are matched to cases on factors affected by exposure or disease and for which the population distribution is unknown, such as intermediate causal factors or disease symptoms.[16]

Selection bias is controllable when the factors that affect selection are measured on all study subjects, and either (a) these factors are antecedents of both exposure and disease, and so can be controlled like confounders (as described above), or (b) one knows the joint distribution of these factors (including exposure and disease, if they jointly affect selection) in the entire source population, and so can adjust for the bias using methods shown below. A condition equivalent to (b) is that one knows the selection probabilities for each level of the factors affecting selection. Unfortunately, this situation is rare. It usually occurs only when the study incorporates features of a population survey, as in two-stage designs[21,22] and randomized recruitment.[26] In most studies, one can usually only control using estimates of these selection probabilities within collapsed strata and hope that no other factors (such as intermediates or disease symptoms) have influenced selection.

Bias Analysis for Differential Baseline Participation

There is a well-known decomposition for the odds ratio that can be used for quantitative bias analysis of selection bias. Suppose that S_{Aj} and S_{Bj} are the probabilities of case (A) and noncase (B) selection at exposure level j. (For a dichotomous exposure, $j = 1$ for the exposed and $j = 0$ for the unexposed.) Alternatively, in a density-sampled case-control study, let S_{Bj} be the person-time rate of control selection at exposure level j. Then the population case counts can be estimated by A_j/S_{Aj} and the population noncase counts (or person-times) can be estimated by B_j/S_{Bj}. Therefore, the bias-adjusted odds ratio or rate-ratio estimate comparing exposure level j to level 0 is

$$\frac{\left(A_j/S_{Aj}\right)\left(B_0/S_{B0}\right)}{\left(A_0/S_{A0}\right)\left(B_j/S_{Bj}\right)} = \frac{A_j B_0}{A_0 B_j}\left(\frac{S_{Aj} S_{B0}}{S_{A0} S_{Bj}}\right)^{-1} \tag{14-1}$$

For example, see Walker[21] and Kleinbaum et al.[27] In words, a bias-adjusted estimate can be obtained by dividing the sample odds ratio by a selection bias factor $S_{Aj}S_{B0}/S_{A0}S_{Bj}$. Equation 14-1 can be applied within strata of confounders, and the selection bias factor can vary across the strata. Generalizations of this formula to regression settings are also available.[19,28] It can also be applied repeatedly to account for independent sources of selection bias. An alternative conceptualization is to estimate weights within strata of selection factors such that $W_i = 1/S_i$, where S_i is the selection proportion within a stratum. In the above example, there are four strata corresponding to the four combinations of case or noncase (A or B, respectively) with exposure levels j and 0. We can then rewrite Equation 14-1 as.

$$\frac{\left(A_j/S_{Aj}\right)\left(B_0/S_{B0}\right)}{\left(A_0/S_{A0}\right)\left(B_j/S_{Bj}\right)} = \frac{A_j W_{Aj} B_0 W_{B0}}{A_0 W_{A0} B_j W_{Bj}} \tag{14-2}$$

In this conceptualization, the weights inflate the observed frequencies to account for the missing participants. For example, if all eligible cases at exposure level j participate, then $S_{Aj} = 1$ and $W_{Aj} = 1/S_{Aj} = 1/1 = 1$. Each case at exposure level j would count only for itself, because there are no nonparticipants for which to account. If only 50% of eligible cases at exposure level 0 participate, then $S_{A0} = 0.5$ and $W_{A0} = 1/S_{A0} = 1/.5 = 2$. Each case at exposure level 0 would count for itself and for one of the nonparticipant cases at exposure level 0, thus restoring the case count at exposure level 0 to the value it would have had, had all eligible cases at exposure level 0 participated. This reweighting is called "Inverse Probability of Participation Weighting" or "IPPW." The resulting analysis population is called a pseudopopulation, because it is a mixture of the observed population of participants and the nonparticipants obtained by the reweighting. An important and usually unverifiable assumption, discussed in greater detail below, is that the stratification variables used to estimate the weights are sufficient to adjust for the selection bias. It is also important to realize that, although the reweighted frequencies can be used to estimate the bias-adjusted estimate of association, as shown for the odds ratio in Equation 14-2, these reweighted frequencies cannot be used in conventional equations to estimate the variance or other sampling error statistics.

The main obstacle to application of either of these bias models is determining or even getting a vague idea of the selection probabilities S_{Aj} and S_{Bj}. Again, these usually can be estimated only if the study in question incorporates survey elements to determine the true population frequencies. For example, in a retrospective case-control study, one will usually know the overall participation rate of cases and controls (t_A and t_B, respectively). Equations 14-1 and 14-2, however, require the conditional participation rates or selection properties (the S_i). To estimate these, one would need to know the exposure level of both participants and nonparticipants, but as exposure levels are usually obtained from information provided by participants, nonparticipants cannot be assigned to an exposure level, leaving the S_i as nonidentifiable.

One is therefore left to make reasonable guesses, possibly informed by internal or external information and bounding assumptions, to estimate the S_i, as illustrated in the example below. Sensitivity analyses of the quantitative bias models in Equations 14-1 and 14-2 may have to encompass a broad range of possibilities. Equation 14-1 does provide one minor insight: no bias occurs if the selection bias factor is one. One way the latter will occur is if disease and exposure affect selection independently, in the sense that $S_{Aj} = t_A u_j$ and $S_{Bj} = t_B u_j$, where u_j is the marginal selection probability at exposure level j (in density studies, t_B will be the marginal rate of control selection). Occasionally, one may reason that such independence will hold, or independence can be forced to hold through careful sampling. Nonetheless, when refusal is common and subjects know their own exposure and disease status, there may be good reasons to doubt the assumption.[4]

To illustrate these simple methods of bias-adjustment to address selection bias arising from differential baseline participation, we apply them to a case-control study of the relation between mobile phone use and uveal melanoma.[29] Uveal melanoma is a rare cancer of the iris, ciliary body, or choroid, with an age-adjusted incidence of approximately 4.3 cases per million. Given its rarity, it would be difficult to study potential etiologies prospectively in cohort studies; retrospective case-control studies using a secondary study base (see Chapter 8) are far more efficient and feasible, but susceptible to differential participation.

Stang et al. identified 486 incident cases of uveal melanoma between September 2002 and September 2004 at a tertiary care facility. Of these 486 cases, 458 (94%) agreed to participate in the case-control study and completed the interview. One hundred and thirty-six (30%) of the interviewed cases reported regular mobile phone use and 107 (23%) reported no mobile phone use; the remainder used mobile phones irregularly. There were 1,527 eligible population-based controls, of which only 840 (55%) agreed to participate and were interviewed. Two hundred and ninety-seven (35%) of the 840 interviewed controls reported regular mobile phone use and 165 (20%) reported no mobile phone use. The odds ratio associating regular mobile phone use, compared with no mobile phone use, with uveal melanoma incidence equaled 0.71 (95% CI 0.51, 0.97). The difference in participation rates between cases and controls (94% vs. 55%, respectively) raises a concern about the effect of selection bias on this estimate of association.

In anticipation of this concern, Stang et al. asked those who refused to participate whether they would answer a short questionnaire. Their answers would then provide an estimate of the prevalence of mobile phone use among nonparticipants. This type of internal validation project is good practice in the design of epidemiologic research projects. Using study resources (time and money) to gather data to inform quantitative bias analyses is often a better use of these resources than using them to increase the study size, for example.

Of the 27 nonparticipating cases, 10 completed the short questionnaire, and 3 of the 10 (30%) reported regular mobile phone use, which is the same exposure prevalence as measured in the fully participating cases. Of the 663 nonparticipating controls, 284 completed the short questionnaire and 72 (25%) reported regular mobile phone use, which is a lower exposure prevalence than the 35% measured in participating controls. Only two categories were available on the short questionnaire, so those who did not report regular mobile phone use were categorized as nonusers.

Using the data from participants and nonparticipants who completed the short questionnaire, one can see that the odds of participation depend on disease [$OR_{DP} = (243/10)/(462/284) = 14.9$] and on exposure status, which is examined only in the controls [$OR_{EP} = (297/72)/(165/212) = 5.3$]. These associations emphasize the importance of evaluating the influence of selection bias quantitatively.

The crude odds ratio associating regular mobile phone use with uveal melanoma occurrence was $OR_{crude,\ participants} = (136/297)/(107/165) = 0.71$, which also approximately equals the matched odds ratio reported in the study. The matching will therefore be ignored to illustrate the bias-adjustment for selection bias. Among nonparticipants who answered the short questionnaire, the crude odds ratio equaled $OR_{crude,\ short\ q'naire\ participants} = (3/72)/(7/210) = 1.25$, which is in the opposite direction from $OR_{crude,\ participants}$.

To bias-adjust for the selection bias, one could collapse the participant and nonparticipant data, but that would ignore the nonparticipants who did not complete the short questionnaire. Instead, we can assume that this second group of nonparticipants had the same exposure prevalence as those who did agree to participate in the short questionnaire. To apply this assumption, we divide those in the second group of nonparticipants into exposure groups that are in proportion to the exposure prevalence observed among nonparticipating cases and controls who did complete the short questionnaire. For example, multiply the 17 nonparticipant cases by 3/10 to obtain the proportion expected to be regular users. The results are added to the number of observed exposed cases (136) and the number of exposed cases who answered the short questionnaire (3) to obtain an estimate of the number of total exposed cases among those eligible for the study. Similar algebra is applied for the unexposed cases and the exposed and unexposed controls:

$$OR_{bias-adjusted} = \frac{136 + 3 + \dfrac{3}{10}17}{297 + 72 + \dfrac{72}{284}379} \Bigg/ \frac{107 + 7 + \dfrac{7}{10}17}{165 + 212 + \dfrac{212}{284}379} = 1.62$$

[14-3]

As noted above, this solution assumes that the nonparticipants who did not answer the short questionnaire have the same prevalence of mobile phone use, within strata of cases and controls, as the nonparticipants who did answer the short questionnaire. While this assumption cannot be tested empirically with the available data, one could evaluate the effect of violations of the assumption by varying this exposure prevalence assumption (*i.e.*, by conducting a sensitivity analysis of the bias analysis).

This example is unusual in that some data on the exposure prevalence among nonparticipants were available. Ordinarily, only the number of nonparticipating cases and controls would be available, and perhaps the participation rates among eligible cases and controls, but no information about the exposure prevalence among nonparticipants would be known. In this circumstance, one must postulate selection proportions, guided by the participation rates in cases and controls, and bias-adjust the observed odds ratio by multiplying it by the selection bias odds ratio using Equation 14-1 to account for differential initial participation.

Continuing with the example, one can calculate the selection proportions, again assuming that the exposure prevalence among the nonparticipants who answered the short questionnaire equals the exposure prevalence among the nonparticipants who did not answer it. With this assumption, the selection proportions are as follows: $S_{A,j} = 136/(136 + 3 + 3*17/10) = 0.94$, $S_{A,0} = 107/(107 + 7 + 7*17/10) = 0.85$, $S_{B,j} = 297/(297 + 72 + 72*379/284) = 0.64$, and $S_{B,0} = 165/(165 + 210 + 210*379/284) = 0.25$. When these selection proportions are substituted into Equation 14-1, the selection bias odds ratio is 2.28 and the bias-adjusted odds ratio is 1.61.

A second strategy for bias-adjustment would be to use inverse probability of participation weighting. In this example, the weights for exposed cases would be $W_{A,j} = 1/S_{A,j} = 1/0.94 = 1.06$, $W_{A,0} = 1/S_{A,0} = 1/0.85 = 1.18$, $W_{B,j} = 1/S_{B,j} = 1/0.64 = 1.56$, and $W_{B,0} = 1/S_{B,0} = 1/0.25 = 4$. Substituting these weights into Equation 14-2 gives a bias-adjusted odds ratio of 1.63, which, with rounding error, is equivalent to the first bias-adjusted odds ratio.

Bias Analysis for Differential Loss to Follow-Up

When selection bias arises from differential loss to follow-up, quantitative bias analysis requires a bias model to estimate the measure of disease occurrence in the unobserved experience. This unobserved experience is most often person-time, in which case the bias model for a dichotomous exposure can be written:

$$IRD_{bias\text{-}adjusted} = \frac{A_{j,observed} + A_{j,loss\ to\ follow\text{-}up}}{PT_{j,observed} + PT_{j,loss\ to\ follow\text{-}up}} - \frac{A_{0,observed} + A_{0,loss\ to\ follow\text{-}up}}{PT_{0,observed} + PT_{0,loss\ to\ follow\text{-}up}}$$

That is, one must be able to estimate the missing person-time in exposure categories and the number of cases expected to have occurred in that missing person-time.

A worked example derives from a cohort study of the relation between receipt of less than guideline breast cancer therapy and breast cancer mortality over 12 years of follow-up after diagnosis.[30,31] The source population comprised women diagnosed with local or regional breast cancer at eight hospitals between July 1984 and February 1986.[32] Patients' identifying variables were removed from the data set after the enrollment project was completed in accordance with the requirements of the human subjects oversight committee. Patients were reidentified for the follow-up study by matching their characteristics to the cancer registry,[30] which reidentified 390 of the original 449 patients (87%). These 390 patients constitute the study population. The remaining 59 patients (13%) from the source population were lost to follow-up, and it is their person-time that will be modeled for the bias analysis. The probability of reidentification depended strongly on the hospital of diagnosis, because two hospitals participated in the statewide cancer registry for only the latter part of the enrollment period. Patients diagnosed at those hospitals in the first part of the enrollment period were not reported to the cancer registry and so could not be reidentified.

The outcome (breast cancer mortality) was assigned to reidentified patients with a death certificate that listed breast cancer as the underlying cause or a contributing cause of death. Reidentified patients were followed to death or the end of 1996. The crude rate difference associating guideline therapy with breast cancer mortality equaled:

$$IRD_{observed} = \frac{A_{j,observed}}{PT_{1,observed}} - \frac{A_{0,observed}}{PT_{0,observed}} = \frac{40}{687} - \frac{65}{2560} = 3.3/100\,PY$$

The 59 patients lost to follow-up were not reidentified and so could not be matched to the death registry. It was not known, therefore, whether they had died of breast cancer. The hospital where these patients were diagnosed was known, and whether the patients received guideline therapy was known, since this information was ascertained before the identifying variables were deleted from the original data set. To bias-adjust the rate difference for the missing information, one first estimates the amount of missing person-time by multiplying the average follow-up duration among those with ($j = 0$; 2560 PY accrued by 286 patients) and without ($j = j$; 687 PY accrued by 104 patients) guideline therapy by the number of persons missing in each category (46 and 13, respectively).

$$PT_{j,loss\,to\,follow-up} = \frac{687 \cdot 13}{104} = 85.9\ PY \text{ and } PT_{0,loss\,to\,follow-up} = \frac{2560 \cdot 46}{286} = 411.7\,PY$$

This basic model to estimate the missing person-time suffices for illustrative purposes, but could easily be refined. For example, the mechanism by which patients were lost to follow-up was dominated by lack of reporting to the cancer registry early in the enrollment period. Follow-up of all patients was terminated on the same calendar date, so patients enrolled earlier would have had a higher maximum duration of follow-up, and hence a higher average duration of follow-up. The model for missing person-time might, therefore, estimate the amount of missing person-time using the average person-time accrued only by patients diagnosed in the same calendar years as the patients with missing person-time. This average would have been longer than the average calculated above. In addition, the average duration of follow-up is greater for patients with (2560/286 = 9.0 years) than without (687/104 = 6.6 years) guideline therapy, suggesting that patients without guideline therapy may have had different characteristics than those without guideline therapy and that these differences may have affected their time to event. In fact, patients who did not receive guideline therapy more often had advanced stage cancer than patients who received guideline therapy, and advance stage is a risk factor for death from breast cancer, which terminates accrual of person-time. Stage was known for all patients, so implementing the model for missing person-time within stage strata would be feasible. In general, the bias model ought to incorporate this type of prior knowledge about the mechanisms and characteristics of lost person-time.

To estimate the number of missing cases of breast cancer death that occurred in the exposure groups, one multiplies the estimates of missing person-time by educated guesses of the breast cancer mortality rates that would have been observed in them. In this example, a reasonable educated guess would be to use the mortality rates observed among reidentified patients diagnosed at the two hospitals that reported cases to the cancer registry for only part of the study. For reidentified patients without guideline therapy at these two hospitals ($j = j$), there were three breast cancer deaths in 60.8 person-years, giving an incidence rate of 4.9/100 *PY*. For patients with guideline therapy at these two hospitals ($j = 0$), there were five breast cancer deaths in 110.2 person-years, giving an incidence rate of 4.5/100 *PY*. Note that the rate difference at these two hospitals is 0.4/100 *PY*, which is much lower than the estimate of 3.3/100 *PY* computed from all reidentified patients. This observation suggests the possibility of a differential loss to follow-up. The estimates of the number of missing cases of breast cancer death then equal:

$$A_{j,loss\,to\,follow-up} = \frac{85.9\,PY \cdot 4.9}{100\,PY} = 4.2 \text{ and } A_{0,loss\,to\,follow-up} = \frac{411.7\,PY \cdot 4.5}{100\,PY} = 18.7$$

To complete the bias analysis, solve for the bias-adjusted rate difference:

$$IRD_{bias-adjusted} = \frac{40+4.2}{687+85.9} - \frac{65+18.5}{2560+411.7} = 2.9/100\,PY$$

The bias-adjusted incidence rate difference equals 2.9/100 *PY*. This association is nearer the null than the crude incidence rate ratio estimated from the complete data, but not so near the null as the associations observed in just the two hospitals where most women lost to follow-up had been diagnosed. Conditional on the accuracy of the bias model, the bias analysis provides some assurance that the observed association between receipt of guideline therapy and breast cancer mortality was not entirely attributable to differential loss to follow-up.

An alternative analytic bias analysis strategy is to use inverse probability of attrition weighting.[33] In this strategy, the probability of a participant being lost to follow-up is estimated as a function of covariate information. Participants with characteristics like the characteristics of the participants lost to follow-up are then upweighted in the analysis, thereby representing their own contribution to the estimate of association as well as the contribution of the similar participants who were lost to follow-up. Weights can be estimated for individual participants or within strata of participants with similar characteristics. Another alternative is to bound the magnitude of selection bias based on specified associations between factors responsible for selection and the exposure and outcome.[34]

Returning to the earlier example, stratifying by whether patients received guideline care and by whether they were diagnosed at one of the two hospitals where most participants lost to follow-up were diagnosed yields four strata (Table 14-1). Most of the patients diagnosed at the six hospitals that reported to the cancer registry throughout the enrollment period were reidentified and therefore linked to the death registry for follow-up (97% of patients who received guideline therapy and 96% of patients who received less than guideline therapy). The inverse probabilities of attrition weights for these patients are therefore close to one (1.03 and 1.04, respectively). Less than half of the patients diagnosed at the two hospitals that reported to the cancer registry only at the end of the enrollment period were reidentified (45% of patients who received guideline therapy and 27% of patients who received less than guideline therapy). The inverse probabilities of attrition weights for these patients are greater than two (2.25 and 3.69, respectively). The patients diagnosed at these hospitals and followed for breast cancer mortality therefore count more than double the patients diagnosed at the other six hospitals. The IPAW-weighted rates of breast cancer mortality were 5.7/100 person-years for patients who received less than guideline therapy and 2.7/100 person-years for patients who received guideline therapy, yielding an IPAW-weighted rate difference of 3.0/100 person-years.

This IPAW bias-adjusted rate difference is similar to the bias-adjusted rate difference of 2.9/100 person-years computed above. The IPAW method differs slightly in two ways. First, the initial

---

TABLE 14-1

Results of a Study of the Association Between Receipt of Less Than Guideline Breast Cancer Care and Breast Cancer–Specific Mortality, Showing Calculations Used in Inverse Probability of Attrition Weighting (IPAW)[30]

	Received Guideline Therapy		Received Less Than Guideline Therapy	
	Six Hospitals With Complete Registration	Two Hospitals With Incomplete Registration	Six Hospitals With Complete Registration	Two Hospitals With Incomplete Registration
BC deaths/person-years	60/2449.8	5/110.2	37/626.2	3/60.8
Not reidentified/total	11/284	35/48	3/99	10/18
IPAW	1.03	3.69	1.04	2.25
IPAW rate	2.7/100 person-years		5.7/100 person-years	

From Lash TL, Silliman RA, Guadagnoli E, Mor V. The effect of less than definitive care on breast carcinoma recurrence and mortality. *Cancer*. 2000;89(8):1739-1747.

model treated all patients lost to follow-up as if they were diagnosed at the two hospitals with incomplete registration, whereas the IPAW method includes in its bias model an allowance for the few patients who were not reidentified and were diagnosed at one of the other six hospitals. Second, the initial bias-adjusted rate difference applied the observed mortality rate in patients diagnosed and reidentified at the two hospitals to an estimate of the amount of missing person-time based on all reidentified patients. The IPAW model reweights the person-time only from the reidentified patients diagnosed at the two hospitals, with a separate bias-adjustment for the other six hospitals. These slight differences in the bias model account for the small difference in the bias-adjusted estimate. The reweighting assumes that the patients reidentified from among those diagnosed at the two hospitals can stand in for the patients who were not reidentified, even though we know that they were diagnosed earlier in the enrollment period and so had a longer potential follow-up period. This is a shortcoming shared by the first bias model, as noted above. One could more finely divide the strata in which probabilities of attrition were calculated, even to the individual record level, and could then include year of diagnosis as one of the predictors.[35]

GENERALIZABILITY, TRANSPORTABILITY, AND REPRESENTATIVENESS

Generalization in Science

As mentioned earlier, in the wider scientific community, the term "generalization" pertains to the extrapolation of information gleaned from scientific experiments or observation to a broader context. This process broadly speaking involves investigating specific natural phenomena to understand and describe how nature works in a general sense. For example, one can measure the speed of light by many different experimental methods. These experiments, coupled with other earlier results and the theories that grew from them, led to the generalization that the speed of light is constant and to an accepted estimate of this fixed velocity.[36]

This generalization predicts how light will behave in other experiments and thus provides a foundation for further research. Note that the generalization moves from the specific experimental results to an abstract idea about the speed of light. Generalization from specific evidence to foundational laws of nature is the fundamental process of the scientific enterprise. Importantly, the abstract idea that emerges as the scientific generalization is best described as a theory, meaning that it is not a logical deduction but more akin to an informed conjecture. It is therefore subject to further testing, revision, or replacement as new evidence accumulates.

Because generalization does not flow mechanically from scientific observations, it does not follow a prescription or recipe. In epidemiology, there has been some confusion between scientific generalization and the process of extrapolation from a sample to a target population. This type of exercise is often relevant to epidemiology, for the simple reason that sampling reduces the cost that would be incurred by measuring everyone in a population. Inferring a description for a population from a sample of that population is sometimes also described as generalization. Election polling data in advance of Election Day provide a common example. This type of generalization represents a statistical generalization from study population (those who respond to the pollsters) to target population (those who will vote on Election Day), rather than a scientific generalization from the specific evidence provided by a research study to an abstract idea, such as whether an exposure E causes a disease D.

Generalizability and Transportability in Epidemiology

The distinctions between scientific generalization and statistical generalization have not always been kept clear. In more recent literature, largely within the context of population health sciences, the terms generalizability and transportability have been used in relation to the process of applying study results to a larger (target) population than the study population from which the results were obtained. In this context, generalizability pertains to the question of the extent to which a study's estimate of occurrence or association applies to the larger population from which the study population was sampled.[37] This type of generalization, closer to the idea of statistical generalization described above, occurs whenever study results are applied outside the study setting itself.[38] Even if the study population comprises a complete census of the target population, the person-time over which it will be observed for the study is finite and, once analyzed to obtain an estimate of disease occurrence or of an etiologic effect, the resulting estimate must be extrapolated to person-time that had not yet accrued when the result was computed.[39] This extrapolation is one type of generalization, one for which the only assumption is that the person-time that accrues immediately after the observation period is sufficiently like the person-time that had just accrued to apply the result to that subsequent person-time. Barring the population suffering a catastrophic event that widely influences health in the subsequent person-time, this type of generalization is often reasonable. The main point is that there will always be some extrapolation of results from the person-time that was observed to the person-time yet to be observed, even when the study population and the target population comprise exactly the same members.

When the members of the study population are members of the target population, but do not constitute a census of the target population, generalizability in the context of population health sciences is further complicated. The complications include the potential for lack of exchangeability between the study population members and a simple random sample or census of the target population,[40] the potential for the distribution of effect modifiers to be different in the study population and the target population, the potential for different treatment versions in the study population and the target population, and the potential for one person's exposure to affect a second person's outcome (interference) differently in the study population than in the target population.[37] If the prevalence of effect measure modifiers in the study population is different from that in the target population, then even an internally valid estimate of disease occurrence or of an etiologic effect in the study population might be poorly generalizable to the target population from which the sample was drawn, because of the poor representativeness of the sample. This lack of generalizability could be addressed by reweighting, for example, by standardization to the prevalence of effect measure modifiers in the target population, which would require that the effect measure modifiers had been measured in both the study population and the target population or in a sufficient sample of the target population. It is important to note, however, that valid knowledge about disease occurrence or about an etiologic relation may still have public health or medical utility in the target population, even if the estimate from the study population is not readily generalizable to the target population.[41] The defining characteristic of generalizability is that the information obtained from the study sample provides an estimate that can be reliably applied to the whole of the population from which the sample was drawn, either directly or with analytic correction by reweighting or other analytic solutions.[37,42] See Pearl[39] for a more formal treatment.

Transportability is a concept related to generalizability. It pertains to the broader question of the extent to which a study's estimate of occurrence or etiologic effect can be used to derive an estimate for a second population, whose membership was not sampled in the process of enrolling the study population.[37] Lack of internal validity,[38] different prevalence of effect modifiers between the study population and the second population,[43] and the complications described above in the discussion of generalizability can lead to lack of transportability. When the prevalence of effect modifiers has been measured in both the study population and the second population, transportability may be improved by standardization or reweighting. As with generalizability, transportability of study results will depend on the assumption that the person-time of the target population is similar to the person-time in which the effect modifiers have been measured. If the prevalence of effect modifiers changes substantially in the newly accrued person-time, then the standardization to achieve transportability would be imperfect (just as it would be in this instance when generalizing study results). As with generalizability, valid knowledge about disease occurrence or about an etiologic effect may still have public health or medical utility in the target population, even if the estimates from the study population are not readily transportable to the target population.[41] The defining characteristic of transportability is that the information obtained from the study sample provides an estimate that can be reliably used to derive an estimate for a second population that includes no one who was a member of the study population. See Bareinboim and Pearl[44] for a formal treatment.

Although concerns about lack of generalizability and lack of transportability have often been emphasized in the literature, one must not succumb to the idea that as a default, study results are limited to the persons studied and the period over which they were observed.[38] In physics, for example, observations made in one place and time are usually presumed to apply at other places and consistently throughout time, on the assumption that nature exhibits uniformity in its rules. Nonetheless, physicists acknowledge that what we consider to be universal physical laws could vary over time or under boundary conditions and therefore may not be truly universal. The concepts of generalizability and transportability will always involve making assumptions about the domain in which the study results apply. It is good practice to be clear about these assumptions and to avoid becoming paralyzed by them. Public health and medical research are undertaken to improve the human condition, and this goal will always require extrapolation of research results to people and time that have not yet been observed.

Generalizability, Representativeness, and Efficiency

As described above, some epidemiologic studies are designed to enroll a representative sample of subjects from the target population with the goal of enhancing generalizability.[38] This representative sample can be enrolled as a simple random sample or by stratified sampling such that strata with rare combinations of traits are overrepresented. This overrepresentation must be quantifiable, so that it can be corrected by reweighting. Whenever the emphasis of inquiry is on surveillance, representativeness of the study sample, or the ability to reweight, is paramount. Descriptive information on disease occurrence or the prevalence of various exposures is of little utility outside of the study setting when the results cannot be validly extrapolated to another population, and for this reason most surveillance efforts incorporate sampling strategies that allow reweighting of participants to the target population.

Sampling can be effectively incorporated into the design of studies of etiologic effects as well. A straightforward illustration is the nested case-cohort design, in which cases are oversampled in relation to their frequency in the cohort, and controls are undersampled in relation to their frequency in the cohort, perhaps as a simple random sample with known sampling fraction. As noted in Chapter 8, this design is efficient, especially when it is expensive to collect information on the exposure and covariates. Information from all cases is collected, but information from the experience giving rise to the cases—which is abundant in comparison with the information on cases—is only sampled. Because the sampling fraction is known, information on risks in the whole cohort can be recovered by reweighting controls by the inverse of the sampling fraction. More generally, inference to a target population can be obtained by oversampling some subgroups and then standardizing or reweighting the study data to match the target population distribution. Two-stage designs are additional examples of such a strategy.

Sampling to achieve efficiency and representativeness is therefore a critical design element for descriptive research, and sampling to achieve efficiency is also a valuable design element for etiologic research. The importance of sampling to achieve representativeness in etiologic research, however, may depend on the maturity of the research topic.[37] In the earliest research phases, investigators may be willing to trade representative study samples for efficient study samples, such as study samples enhanced in the extremes of the exposure distribution or study samples at particularly high or low risk for the outcome.[38,45] Designs enriched in the exposure, outcome, or both may offer the best opportunity to provide an internally valid and precise estimate of an etiologic effect, even if the design precludes reweighting to a larger population and therefore representativeness. In this setting, selection of participants who are representative of larger populations in the statistical sense will often make it more difficult to make internally valid inferences, for example, by making it more difficult to control for confounding by factors that vary within those populations, more difficult to ensure uniformly high levels of cooperation, and more difficult to ensure uniformly accurate measurements.[38] To reduce these threats to validity, one would select study groups for homogeneity with respect to important confounders, for highly cooperative behavior, and for availability of accurate information, rather than attempt to be representative of the target population. Classic examples include the British Physicians' Study of smoking and health,[46] the Framingham Heart Study,[40,47] and the Nurses' Health Study,[48] none of which were representative of the general population with respect to sociodemographic factors. Their lack of representativeness was presumed to be unrelated to most of the effects studied. If there were doubts about this assumption, they would only become important once it was clear that the associations observed were valid estimates of effect within the studies themselves.

Once the nature and at least the order of magnitude of an effect are established by studies designed to optimize validity, transportability to other unstudied target populations becomes simpler, and ultimately, scientific, rather than statistical, generalization may even be possible.

This process is in large measure a question of whether the factors that distinguish these other target populations from studied populations somehow modify the effect in question. In answering this question, epidemiologic data will be of help and may be essential,[49,50] but other sources of information such as behavioral or other surveillance data and basic pathophysiology may also play a role. For example, although most of the decisive data connecting smoking to lung cancer was derived from observations on men, few doubted that the strong effects observed would carry over at least approximately to women, for the lungs of men and women appear to be similar if not identical in physiologic detail. On the other hand, given the huge sex differences in iron loss, it would seem unwise to generalize freely to natal men about the effects of iron supplementation observed in premenopausal natal women. Such contrasting examples suggest that, perhaps even more than with (internal) inference about restricted populations, statistical generalizability, transportability, and scientific generalizability must bring into play knowledge from diverse branches of science.

References

1. Hernan MA, Hernandez-Diaz S, Robins JM. A structural approach to selection bias. *Epidemiology.* 2004;15(5):615-625.
2. Greenland S. Response and follow-up bias in cohort studies. *Am J Epidemiol.* 1977;106(3):184-187.
3. Caldwell GG, Kelley DB, Heath CW Jr. Leukemia among participants in military maneuvers at a nuclear bomb test. A preliminary report. *J Am Med Assoc.* 1980;244(14):1575-1578.
4. Criqui MH, Austin M, Barrett-Connor E. The effect of non-response on risk ratios in a cardiovascular disease study. *J Chronic Dis.* 1979;32(9-10):633-638.
5. Fox AJ, Collier PF. Low mortality rates in industrial cohort studies due to selection for work and survival in the industry. *Br J Prev Soc Med.* 1976;30(4):225-230.
6. McMichael AJ. Standardized mortality ratios and the "healthy worker effect": scratching beneath the surface. *J Occup Med.* 1976;18(3):165-168.
7. Wang JD, Miettinen OS. Occupational mortality studies. Principles of validity. *Scand J Work Environ Health.* 1982;8(3):153-158.
8. Berkson J. Limitations of the application of fourfold table analysis to hospital data. *Biometrics.* 1946;2(3):47-53.
9. Smith DC, Prentice R, Thompson DJ, Herrmann WL. Association of exogenous estrogen and endometrial carcinoma. *N Engl J Med.* 1975;293(23):1164-1167.
10. Ziel HK, Finkle WD. Increased risk of endometrial carcinoma among users of conjugated estrogens. *N Engl J Med.* 1975;293(23):1167-1170.
11. Mack TM, Pike MC, Henderson BE, et al. Estrogens and endometrial cancer in a retirement community. *N Engl J Med.* 1976;294(23):1262-1267.
12. Antunes CM, Strolley PD, Rosenshein NB, et al. Endometrial cancer and estrogen use. Report of a large case-control study. *N Engl J Med.* 1979;300(1):9-13.
13. Horwitz RI, Feinstein AR. Alternative analytic methods for case-control studies of estrogens and endometrial cancer. *N Engl J Med.* 1978;299(20):1089-1094.
14. Greenland S. A mathematic analysis of the "epidemiologic necropsy". *Ann Epidemiol.* 1991;1(6):551-558.
15. Hutchison GB, Rothman KJ. Correcting a bias? *N Engl J Med.* 1978;299(20):1129-1130.
16. Greenland S, Neutra R. An analysis of detection bias and proposed corrections in the study of estrogens and endometrial cancer. *J Chronic Dis.* 1981;34(9-10):433-438.
17. Paffenbarger RS, Hale WE. Work activity and coronary heart mortality. *N Engl J Med.* 1975; 292(11):545-550.
18. Tang MC, Weiss NS, Malone KE. Induced abortion in relation to breast cancer among parous women: a birth certificate registry study. *Epidemiology.* 2000;11:177-180.
19. Greenland S. The impact of prior distributions for uncontrolled confounding and response bias: a case study of the relation of wire codes and magnetic fields to childhood leukemia. *J Am Stat Assoc.* 2003;98:47-54.
20. Lash TL, Fink AK. Null association between pregnancy termination and breast cancer in a registry-based study of parous women. *Int J Cancer.* 2004;110(3):443-448.
21. Walker AM. Anamorphic analysis: sampling and estimation for covariate effects when both exposure and disease are known. *Biometrics.* 1982;38(4):1025-1032.
22. White JE. A two stage design for the study of the relationship between a rare exposure and a rare disease. *Am J Epidemiol.* 1982;115(1):119-128.
23. Breslow N, Cain K. Logistic regression for two-stage case-control data. *Biometrika.* 1988;75:11-20.
24. Flanders WD, Greenland S. Analytic methods for two-stage case-control studies and other stratified designs. *Stat Med.* 1991;10(5):739-747.

25. Weinberg CR, Wacholder S. The design and analysis of case-control studies with biased sampling. *Biometrics*. 1990;46(4):963-975.
26. Weinberg CR, Sandler DP. Randomized recruitment in case-control studies. *Am J Epidemiol*. 1991;134(4):421-432.
27. Kleinbaum DG, Kupper LL, Morgenstern H. *Epidemiologic Research: Principles and Quantitative Methods*. New York, NY: Van Nostrand Reinhold; 1982.
28. Scharfstein DO, Rotnitsky A, Robins JM. Adjusting for nonignorable drop-out using semiparametric non-response models. *J Am Stat Assoc*. 1999;94:1096-1120.
29. Stang A, Schmidt-Pokrzywniak A, Lash TL, et al. Mobile phone use and risk of uveal melanoma: results of the risk factors for uveal melanoma case-control study. *J Natl Cancer Inst*. 2009;101(2):120-123.
30. Lash TL, Silliman RA, Guadagnoli E, Mor V. The effect of less than definitive care on breast carcinoma recurrence and mortality. *Cancer*. 2000;89(8):1739-1747.
31. Lash TL, Silliman RA. A sensitivity analysis to separate bias due to confounding from bias due to predicting misclassification by a variable that does both. *Epidemiology*. 2000;11(5):544-549.
32. Silliman RA, Guadagnoli E, Weitberg AB, Mor V. Age as a predictor of diagnostic and initial treatment intensity in newly diagnosed breast cancer patients. *J Gerontol*. 1989;44(2):M46-M50.
33. Weuve J, Tchetgen Tchetgen EJ, Glymour MM, et al. Accounting for bias due to selective attrition: the example of smoking and cognitive decline. *Epidemiology*. 2012;23(1):119-128.
34. Smith LH, VanderWeele TJ. Bounding bias due to selection. *Epidemiology*. 2019;30(4):509-516.
35. Greenland S. Quantifying biases in causal models: classical confounding vs collider-stratification bias. *Epidemiology*. 2003;14(3):300-306.
36. Henrion M, Fischhoff B. Assessing uncertainty in physical constants. *Am J Phys*. 1986;54(9):791-798.
37. Lesko CR, Buchanan AL, Westreich D, Edwards JK, Hudgens MG, Cole SR. Generalizing study results: a potential outcomes perspective. *Epidemiology*. 2017;28(4):553-561.
38. Poole C. Commentary: some thoughts on consequential epidemiology and causal architecture. *Epidemiology*. 2017;28(1):6-11.
39. Pearl J. Generalizing experimental findings. *J Causal Inference*. 2015;3(2):259-266.
40. Greenland S. Randomization, statistics, and causal inference. *Epidemiology*. 1990;1(6):421-429.
41. Rothman KJ, Gallacher JEJ, Hatch EE. Why representativeness should be avoided. *Int J Epidemiol*. 2013;42(4):1012-1014.
42. Balzer LB. "All generalizations are dangerous, even this one." - Alexandre Dumas. *Epidemiology*. 2017;28(4):562-566.
43. Keyes KM, Galea S. Commentary. The limits of risk factors revisited: is it time for a causal architecture approach? *Epidemiology*. 2017;28(1):1-5.
44. Pearl J, Bareinboim E. External validity: from do-calculus to transportability across populations. *Stat Sci*. 2014;29(4):579-595.
45. Rothman KJ, Poole C. A strengthening programme for weak associations. *Int J Epidemiol*. 1988;17(4):955-959.
46. Doll R, Hill AB. The mortality of doctors in relation to their smoking habits; a preliminary report. *Br Med J*. 1954;1(4877):1451-1455.
47. Tsao CW, Vasan RS. Cohort profile. The Framingham heart study (FHS): overview of milestones in cardiovascular epidemiology. *Int J Epidemiol*. 2015;44(6):1800-1813.
48. Belanger CF, Hennekens CH, Rosner B, Speizer FE. The nurses' health study. *Am J Nurs*. 1978;78(6):1039-1040.
49. Ebrahim S, Davey Smith G. Commentary: should we always deliberately be non-representative? *Int J Epidemiol*. 2013;42(4):1022-1026.
50. Rothman KJ, Gallacher JEJ, Hatch EE. Rebuttal: when it comes to scientific inference, sometimes a cigar is just a cigar. *Int J Epidemiol*. 2013;42(4):1026-1028.

CHAPTER 15

Precision and Study Size

Kenneth J. Rothman and Timothy L. Lash

We use the term *accuracy* to describe an estimate of an epidemiologic measure that is close to the estimand. Two types of error, systematic and random, detract from accuracy. In earlier chapters, we have considered sources of systematic error, including biases related to selection of study participants, measurement errors of study variables, and confounding. In this chapter, we discuss methods to measure, limit, and account for random error in an epidemiologic study and how to interpret these methods properly.

RANDOM ERROR AND STATISTICAL PRECISION

What is random error? It is often equated with chance or random variation, which itself is rarely well defined. Many people believe that chance plays a fundamental role in all physical and, by implication, biologic phenomena. For some, the belief in chance is so dominant that it vaults random occurrences into an important role as component causes of all we experience. Others believe that causality may be viewed as deterministic, meaning that a full elaboration of the relevant factors in a set of circumstances will lead, on sufficient analysis, to a perfect prediction of effects resulting from these causes. Under the latter view, all experience is predestined to unravel in a theoretically predictable way that follows from the previous pattern of actions. Even with this extreme deterministic view, however, one must face the fact that only rarely could one acquire sufficient knowledge to predict effects perfectly, and then only for trivial cause-effect patterns. The resulting incomplete predictability of determined outcomes makes their residual variability indistinguishable from random occurrences.

A unifying description of incomplete predictability can thus be forged. In this description, random variation equates with a component of ignorance about causes of study outcomes, an ignorance that is inevitable whether the outcome is deterministic or is partly random. For example, predicting the outcome of a tossed coin represents a physical problem, the solution of which is feasible through the application of physical laws. Whether the sources of variation that we cannot explain are actually chance phenomena makes little difference. We treat such variation as being random until we can explain it, and thereby reduce it, by relating it to known factors.

In an epidemiologic study, random variation has many sources, but a major contributor is the process of selecting the specific study participants. This process is usually referred to as *sampling*; the attendant random variation is known as *sampling variation* or *sampling error.* Case-control studies sometimes involve a physical sampling process, whereas cohort studies often do not. Nevertheless, it is a standard practice to treat all epidemiologic studies, including cohort studies, as having sampling error. In this view, the subjects in a study, whether physically sampled or not, constitute a figurative sample of possible people who could have been included in the study or of the different possible experiences the study subjects could have had. Even if all the individuals in a population were included in a study, the study subjects are viewed as a sample of the potential biologic experience of an even broader conceptual population. Under this view, the statistical dictum that there is no sampling error if an entire population (as opposed to a sample of it) is studied does not apply to epidemiologic studies, even if an entire population is included in the study. Conceptually, the actual subjects are always considered a sample of a broader experience of interest—although they seldom actually satisfy the definition of a random sample that underpins the statistical models ordinarily used to measure random variation.[1,2]

Sampling is only one source of random error that contributes to unpredictable inaccuracies in epidemiologic studies. Another source is the unexplained variation in occurrence measures, such as observed incidence rates or prevalence proportions. Sources of systematic errors also abound. For example, when exposure status is not randomly assigned, confounding (see Chapter 12) may lead to deviations of estimated associations from target effects that far exceed what standard statistical models assume probable. Mismeasurement of key study variables also contributes to the overall inaccuracy, in both random and systematic ways. As a result of these extra sources of variation, and because of the weak theoretical underpinnings for conceptualizing study subjects as a sample of a broader experience, the usual statistical tools that we use to measure random variation at best provide minimum estimates of the actual uncertainty we should have about the estimand. One elementary way to improve the quantification of our uncertainty is through *bias analysis,* which we discuss in Chapter 27.

A common measure of random variation in a measurement or estimation process is the *variance* of the process. The *statistical precision of* (or *statistical information in*) a measurement or process is often taken to be the inverse of the variance of the measurements or estimates that the process produces. In this sense, precision is the opposite of random error. Precision of estimation can be improved (which is to say, variance can be reduced) by increasing the size of the study. Precision can also be improved by modifying the design of the study to decrease the variance, given a fixed total number of subjects; this process is called improving the *statistical efficiency* of the study. Perhaps, the most common epidemiologic example of such design improvement is the use of a case-control study rather than a cohort study, because for a fixed study size, the variance of an effect estimate is heavily dependent on the proportion of subjects in the study that are cases, and case-control studies increase this proportion by design.

APPROACHES TO EVALUATING RANDOM ERROR

Statistics and its role in data analysis have undergone a gradual but profound transformation in recent times. There is an essential distinction between a qualitative study objective (to answer a question "yes" or "no") and a quantitative one (to measure something). The recent transformation reflects a growing preference for the latter objective and for statistical methods consistent with it. Until the 1970s, most applications of statistics in epidemiology focused on deciding whether "chance" or "random error" could be solely responsible for an observed association, or equivalently, whether exposure x was related to outcome y. The methods used for this decision were those of classical *significance testing,* predominant in British applications, and those of Neyman-Pearson *hypothesis testing,* predominant in American applications.[3,4] Because of their similarities, the term *significance testing* is often applied to both collections of methods.

These testing applications, which were subject to some early criticism,[5-8] came under growing criticism by epidemiologists and statisticians during the late 20th century, which intensified in the 2010s.[9-12] The critics pointed out that most, if not all, epidemiologic applications need more than a decision as to whether chance alone could have produced an association. More important is the estimation of the magnitude of the association, including an assessment of the precision of the estimation method. The estimation tool used by most authors is the confidence interval, which provides a range of values for the association, under the hypothesis that only random variation has created discrepancies between the true value of the association under study and the value observed in the data.[13] Other authors, while favoring the move toward interval estimation, point out that confidence intervals suffer from some of the flaws associated with significance testing and favor other approaches to interval estimation.[14-17]

Significance Testing and Hypothesis Testing

Nearly 70 years ago, Berkson[6] wrote:

> It is hardly an exaggeration to say that statistics, as it is taught at present in the dominant school, consists almost entirely of tests of significance, though not always presented as such, some comparatively simple and forthright, others elaborate and abstruse.

The ubiquitous use of P-values and references to "statistically significant" findings in the current medical literature demonstrates the dominant role that statistical hypothesis testing still plays in data analysis in some branches of biomedical sciences. Many researchers still believe that it would be fruitless to submit for publication any paper that lacks statistical tests of significance. Until recently, their belief was not entirely ill-founded, because many journal editors and referees relied on tests of significance as indicators of sophisticated and meaningful statistical analysis as well as the primary means of assessing sampling variability in a study.[18] *Statistical significance* is usually based on the P-value (described below): results are considered "significant" or "not significant" according to whether the P-value is less than or greater than an arbitrary cutoff value, usually 0.05, which is called the *alpha level* of the test.

The preoccupation with significance testing derives from the research interests of the statisticians who pioneered the development of statistical theory in the early 20th century. Their research problems were primarily industrial and agricultural, and they typically involved randomized experiments or random-sample surveys that formed the basis for a choice between two or more alternative courses of action. Such studies were designed to produce results that would enable a decision to be made, and the statistical methods employed were intended to facilitate decision-making. The concepts that grew out of this heritage are today applied in clinical and epidemiologic research, and they strongly reflect this background of decision-making.

Statistical significance testing of associations usually focuses on the *null hypothesis,* which is usually formulated as a hypothesis of no association between two variables in a *superpopulation,* the population from which the observed study groups were purportedly sampled in a random fashion. For example, one may test the hypothesis that the risk difference (RD) in the superpopulation is 0 or, equivalently, that the risk ratio (RR) is 1. Note that this hypothesis is about the superpopulation, *not* about the observed study groups. Testing may alternatively focus on any other specific hypothesis, *e.g.,* that the RD is 0.1 or the RR is 2. For non-null hypotheses, tests about one measure (*e.g.,* RD) are not usually equivalent to tests about another measure (*e.g.,* an RR), so one must choose a measure of interest to perform a non-null test.

A common misinterpretation of significance tests[10] is to claim that there is no difference between two observed groups because the null test is not statistically significant, in that P is greater than the cutoff for declaring statistical significance (again, usually .05). This interpretation confuses a descriptive issue (whether the two observed groups differ) with an inference about the superpopulation. The significance test refers only to the superpopulation, not the observed groups. To say that the difference is not statistically significant means only that one cannot reject the null hypothesis that the superpopulation groups are the same; it does *not* imply that the two observed groups are the same.

One needs only to look at the two observed groups to see whether they are different. Significance testing concerns instead whether the observed difference should lead one to infer that there is a difference between the corresponding groups in the superpopulation. Furthermore, even if the observed difference is not statistically significant, the superpopulation groups may be different (*i.e.*, the result does not imply that the null is correct). Rather, the nonsignificant observed difference means only that one should not rule out the null hypothesis if one accepts the statistical model used to construct the test.

Conversely, it is a misinterpretation to claim that an association exists in the superpopulation because the observed difference is statistically significant. First, the test may be significant only because the model used to compute it is wrong (*e.g.*, there may be many sources of uncontrolled bias). Second, the test may be significant because of chance alone; for example, even under perfect conditions, a test using a 0.05 alpha level will yield a statistically significant difference 5% of the time if the null hypothesis is correct.

As we emphasize, the alpha cutoff point is an arbitrary and questionable convention; it can be dispensed simply by reporting the actual *P*-value from the test, which we now discuss in detail. We will then further explore and criticize the theory that led to the widespread use of arbitrary testing cutoffs in research.

P-Values

P-values come in two types: one-tailed and two-tailed. Further, there are two types of one-tailed *P*-values: upper and lower. An *upper* one-tailed *P*-value is the probability that a corresponding quantity computed from the data, known as the *test statistic* (such as a *t*-statistic or a chi-square statistic), will be greater than or equal to its observed value, assuming that (a) the test hypothesis is correct and (b) there is no source of bias in the data collection or analysis processes. Similarly, a *lower* one-tailed *P*-value is the probability that the corresponding test statistic will be less than or equal to its observed value, again assuming that (a) the test hypothesis is correct and (b) there is no source of bias in the data collection or analysis processes (sometimes described by saying that the underlying statistical model is correct). The two-tailed *P*-value is usually defined as twice the smaller of the upper and lower *P*-values, although more complicated definitions have been used. Being a probability, a one-tailed *P*-value must fall between 0 and 1; the two-tailed *P*-value as just defined, however, may exceed 1. The following comments apply to all types of *P*-values. Some authors refer to *P*-values as "levels of significance,"[19] but the latter term is best avoided because it has been used by other authors to refer to alpha levels.

In the classical significance testing paradigm, small *P*-values are supposed to indicate that at least one of the assumptions used to derive it is incorrect, that is, either or both the test hypothesis (assumption a) or the statistical model (assumption b) is incorrect. All too often, the statistical model is taken as given, so that a small *P*-value is taken as indicating a low degree of compatibility between the test hypothesis and the observed data. This incompatibility derives from the fact that a small *P*-value represents a low probability of getting a test statistic as extreme as or more extreme than the observed statistic if the test hypothesis is true and no bias is operative. Small *P*-values, therefore, are supposed to indicate that the test hypothesis is not an acceptable explanation for the association observed in the data. This common interpretation has been extensively criticized because it does not account for alternative explanations and their acceptability (or lack thereof); for example, refer to the study of Berkson[6] and later epidemiologic criticisms by Goodman and Royall,[15] Greenland,[1] Goodman,[4] and Gigerenzer.[3] A less hypothetical and more cautious interpretation is then that a small *P*-value indicates that there is a problem with the test hypothesis or with the study, or with both.[20]

A common but naive misinterpretation of *P*-values is that they represent probabilities of test hypotheses. In many situations, one can compute a Bayesian probability, or credibility for the test hypothesis, but it will almost always be far from the two-tailed *P*-value.[21,22] A one-tailed *P*-value can be used to put a lower bound on the Bayesian probability of certain compound hypotheses,[23] and under certain conditions, it will approximate the Bayesian probability that the true association is the opposite of the direction observed.[24] Nonetheless, a *P*-value for a simple test hypothesis (for example, exposure and disease are unassociated) is not a probability of that hypothesis. That *P*-value is usually much smaller than such a Bayesian probability and so can easily mislead one into inappropriately rejecting the test hypothesis.[15,22]

Another incorrect interpretation is that the *P*-value is the probability of the observed data under the test hypothesis. This probability is known as the likelihood of the test hypothesis, see Goodman and Royall,[15] Royall,[17] Edwards,[25] and the following discussion. The likelihood of a hypothesis is usually much smaller than the *P*-value for the hypothesis, because the *P*-value includes not only the probability of the observed data under the test hypothesis, but also the probabilities for all other possible data configurations in which the test statistic was more extreme than that observed.

A subtle and common misinterpretation of a *P*-value for testing the null hypothesis is that it represents the probability that the data would show as strong an association as observed or stronger if the null hypothesis were correct. This misinterpretation can be found in many methodologic articles and textbooks. The nature of the misinterpretation can be seen in a study of a risk difference (RD). The study might produce an estimate of RD of 0.33 with an estimated standard error (or standard deviation) of 0.20, which would produce a standard normal test statistic of $z = 0.33/0.20 = 1.65$ and a two-tailed $P = 0.10$. The same study, however, might have instead estimated an RD of 0.30 and a standard deviation of 0.15, which would produce a standard normal test statistic of $z = 0.30/0.15 = 2.00$ and $P = 0.05$. The result with the association nearer the null would then produce a smaller *P*-value. The point is that the *P*-value refers to the size of the test statistic (which in this case is the estimate divided by its estimated standard deviation), not to the strength or size of the estimated association.

It is crucial to remember that *P*-values are calculated from statistical models, which are assumptions about the form of study-to-study data variation. Every *P*-value, even "nonparametric" and "exact" *P*-values, depends on a statistical model; it is only the strength of the model assumptions that differs.[26,27] A major problem with the *P*-values and tests in common use (including all commercial software) is that the assumed models make no allowance for sources of bias, apart from confounding by controlled covariates.

Neyman-Pearson Hypothesis Tests

A *P*-value is a continuous measure of the compatibility between a hypothesis and data. Although its utility as such a measure can be disputed,[15,17] a worse problem is that it is often used to force a qualitative decision about rejection of a hypothesis. As introduced earlier, a fixed cutoff point or alpha level, often denoted by the Greek letter α (alpha), is selected as a criterion with which the *P*-value is judged. This point is then used to classify the observation either as "significant at level α" if $P \leq \alpha$, in which case the test hypothesis is rejected, or "not significant at level α" if $P > \alpha$, in which case the test hypothesis is accepted (or, at least, not rejected).

The use of a fixed cutoff α is a hallmark of the Neyman-Pearson form of statistical hypothesis testing. Both the alpha level[28] and the *P*-value[4,29] have been called the "significance level" of the test. This usage has led to misinterpretation of the *P*-value as the alpha level of a statistical hypothesis test. To avoid the error, one should recall that the *P*-value is a quantity computed from the data, whereas the alpha level is a fixed cutoff (usually 0.05) that can be specified without even seeing the data. (As a technical aside, Neyman and Pearson actually avoided use of *P*-values in their formulation of hypothesis tests and instead defined their tests based on whether the value of the test statistic fell within a "rejection region" for the test.)

An incorrect rejection is called a *Type I error*, or alpha error. A hypothesis testing procedure is said to be *valid* if, whenever the test hypothesis is true, the probability of rejection (*i.e.*, the probability that $P \leq \alpha$) does not exceed the alpha level (provided there is no bias and all test assumptions are satisfied). For example, a valid test with $\alpha = 0.01$ (a 1% alpha level) will lead to a Type I error with no more than 1% probability, provided there is no bias or incorrect assumption.

If the test hypothesis is false but is not rejected, the incorrect decision not to reject is called a *Type II,* or beta error. If the test hypothesis is false, so that rejection is the correct decision, the probability (over repetitions of the study) that the test hypothesis is rejected is called the *power* of the test. The probability of a Type II error is related to the power by the equation Pr (Type II error) $= 1 -$ power.

There is a trade-off between the probabilities of a Type I and a Type II error. This trade-off depends on the chosen alpha level. Reducing the Type I error when the test hypothesis is true requires a smaller alpha level, for with a smaller alpha level a smaller *P*-value will be required to reject the test hypothesis. Unfortunately, a lower alpha level increases the probability of a Type II error if the test hypothesis is false. Conversely, increasing the alpha level reduces the probability of Type II error when the test hypothesis is false, but increases the probability of Type I error if it is true.

The concepts of alpha level, Type I error, Type II error, and power stem from a paradigm in which data are used to decide whether to reject the test hypothesis, and therefore follow from a qualitative study objective. The extent to which decision-making dominates research thinking is reflected in the frequency with which the *P*-value, a continuous measure, is reported or interpreted only as an inequality (such as *P* < 0.05 or *P* > 0.05) or else not at all, with the evaluation focusing instead on "statistical significance" or its absence.

When a single study forms the sole basis for a choice between two alternative actions, as in industrial quality-control activities, a decision-making mode of analysis may be justifiable. Even then, however, a rational recommendation about which of two actions is preferable will require consideration of the costs and benefits of each action. These considerations are rarely incorporated into statistical tests. In most scientific and public health settings, it is presumptuous if not absurd for an investigator to act as if the results of his or her study will form the sole basis for a decision. Such decisions are inevitably based on results from a collection of studies, and proper combination of the information from the studies requires more than just a classification of each study into "significant" or "not significant". Thus, degradation of information about an effect into a simple dichotomy is counterproductive, even for decision-making, and can be misleading.

In a classic review of 71 clinical trials that reported no "significant" difference between the compared treatments, Freiman et al.[30] found that in the great majority of such trials, the data either indicated or at least were consistent with a moderate or even reasonably strong effect of the new treatment (Figure 15-1). In all of these trials, the original investigators interpreted their data as indicative of no effect because the *P*-value for the null hypothesis was not "statistically significant." The misinterpretations arose because the investigators relied solely on hypothesis testing for their statistical analysis rather than on estimation. On failing to reject the null hypothesis, the investigators in these 71 trials inappropriately accepted the null hypothesis as correct, which probably resulted in Type II error for many of these so-called negative studies.

Type II errors result when the magnitude of an effect, biases, and random variability combine to give results that are insufficiently inconsistent with the null hypothesis to reject it. This failure to reject the null hypothesis can occur because the effect is small, the observations are too few,

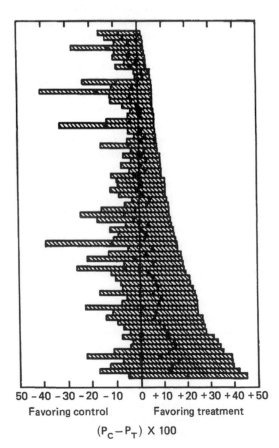

FIGURE 15-1 Ninety percent confidence limits for the true percentage difference for the 71 trials. The vertical bar at the center of each interval indicates the observed difference, P_C-P_π for each trial. (Reproduced with permission from Freiman JA, Chalmers TC, Smith H, et al. The importance of beta, the type II error and sample size in the design and interpretation of the randomized control trial. Survey of 71 "negative" trials. *N Engl J Med.* 1978;299:690-694.)

50 − 40 − 30 − 20 − 10   0   + 10 + 20 + 30 + 40 + 50

Favoring control   Favoring treatment

$(P_C - P_T) \times 100$

or both, as well as from biases. More to the point, however, is that Type I and Type II errors arise because the investigator has attempted to dichotomize the results of a study into the categories "significant" or "not significant." Because this degradation of the study information is unnecessary, an "error" that results from an incorrect classification of the study result is also unnecessary.

Why has such an unsound practice as Neyman-Pearson (dichotomous) hypothesis testing become so ingrained in scientific research? Undoubtedly, much of the popularity of hypothesis testing stems from the apparent objectivity and definitiveness of the pronouncement of significance.[31] Declarations of significance or its absence can supplant the need for more refined interpretations of data; the declarations can serve as a mechanical substitute for thought, promulgated by the inertia of training and common practice. The neatness of an apparent clear-cut result may appear more gratifying to investigators, editors, and readers than a finding that cannot be immediately pigeonholed.

The unbridled authority given to statistical significance in the social sciences has also been attributed to the apparent objectivity that the pronouncement of significance can convey[32]:

> "Let us look and see what is significant" is not too far from the approach of some researchers, and when the data involve perhaps several hundred variables, the practical temptations to use a ready-made decision rule are enormous. . . . [T]he pressure to *decide,* in situations where the very use of probability models admits the uncertainty of the inference, has certain consequences for the presentation of knowledge. The significance test appears to guarantee the objectivity of the researcher's conclusions, and may even be presented as providing crucial support for the whole theory in which the research hypothesis was put forward. As we have seen, tests of significance cannot do either of these things—but it is not in the interests of anyone involved to admit this too openly.

The origin of the nearly universal acceptance of the 5% cutoff point for significant findings is tied to the abridged form in which the chi-square table was originally published.[27] Before computers and calculators could easily give quick approximations to the chi-square distribution, tables were used routinely. Because there is a different chi-square distribution corresponding to every possible value for the degrees of freedom, the tables could not give many points for any one distribution. The tables typically included values at 1%, 5%, and a few other levels, encouraging the practice of checking the chi-square statistic calculated from one's data to see if it exceeded the cutoff levels in the table. In the original formulation of the Neyman and Pearson hypothesis testing, the alpha level was supposed to be determined from contextual considerations, especially the cost of Type I and Type II errors. This more thoughtful aspect of their theory was rapidly lost when the theory entered common scientific use. In fact, the default values assigned to acceptable Type I and Type II errors often run contrary to public health values. Imagine, for example, a study of the effect of a pollution source on the health of a nearby community, designed with acceptable Type I error rate of $\alpha = 0.05$ and with acceptable Type II error rate of $\beta = 0.2$ (80% power). These imply that a Type II error is four times worse than a Type I error. Limiting the Type I error protects the polluter by keeping low the probability of a false-positive result, which would be to declare that it is harmful to the community when it is not. Limiting the Type II error protects the community by keeping low the probability of a false-negative result, declaring no harm when in fact there is harm. Setting a Type II error to be 0.20, four times greater than the Type I error of 0.05, suggests that protecting the pollution source is worth four times as much as protecting the community. It would be a valuable exercise for investigators to write out statements such as these at the design stage to clarify whether they comport with their personal and professional values.

The Alternative Hypothesis

Another hallmark of Neyman-Pearson hypothesis testing, and perhaps one that most distinguishes it from earlier significance-testing paradigms, is that if the test hypothesis is rejected, it is supposed to be rejected in favor of some alternative hypothesis. The alternative hypothesis may be very specific, but more often it is implicit and very broad. For example, if the test hypothesis postulates that there is no association, then the usual (implicit) alternative hypothesis is that there is an association. Such nonspecific alternatives lead to nondirectional tests based on comparing a two-tailed *P*-value from a directional test statistic against the alpha level. Because this *P*-value is sensitive to violations of the test hypothesis in either direction, it is often called a *two-sided P*-value.

Nonetheless, the test and alternative hypotheses can instead be one-sided (directional). For example, the test hypothesis could state that an association is not positive (that is, either null or negative). The alternative is then that the association is positive. Such an alternative leads to use of a *one-sided* test based on comparing an *upper-tailed P*-value from a directional test statistic against alpha. Because this one-tailed *P*-value is sensitive to violations of the test hypothesis in only one direction, it is often called a *one-sided P*-value. An analogous one-sided test that the association was not negative would employ the lower-tailed *P*-value; the alternative for this test is that the association is negative.

Another form of the alternative hypothesis is a finite interval of "equivalence" about the null, for example, that the RD is between −0.1 and +0.1. This alternative is found in comparisons of two treatments (so that the "exposed" are those given one treatment and the "unexposed" are those given another treatment). The bounds of the interval are selected so that any value within the interval is considered close enough to the null for practical purposes. The test hypothesis is then that the two treatments are not equivalent (RD is outside the interval) and is rejected if *P* is less than alpha for all values outside the interval of equivalence. This approach is called *equivalence testing,* and it corresponds to rejecting the test hypothesis when the $1 - \alpha$ confidence interval falls entirely within the equivalence interval.[33]

Note that the alternative hypothesis in all these examples comprises a range of values. For a two-sided test, the alternative comprises every possible value except the one being tested. For epidemiologic effect measures, this two-sided alternative hypothesis will range from absurdly large preventive effects to absurdly large causal effects and include everything in between except the test hypothesis. This hypothesis will be compatible with any observed data. The test hypothesis, on the other hand, corresponds to a single value of effect and therefore is readily consistent with a much narrower range of possible outcomes for the data. Statistical hypothesis testing amounts to an attempt to falsify the test hypothesis. It is natural to focus on a test hypothesis that is as specific as possible because it is easier to marshal evidence against a specific hypothesis than a broad one. The equivalence-testing example shows, however, that in some cases, the alternative may be more specific than the test hypothesis, and the test hypothesis may range from absurdly large preventive effects to absurdly large causal effects.

A major defect in the way all the above alternatives are usually formulated is that they assume the statistical model is correct. Because the model is never exactly correct and is often grossly incorrect, a scientifically more sound formulation of the alternative to the null hypothesis (for example) would be "either the null is false or else the statistical model is wrong."[20] By adding the warning "or else the statistical model is wrong" to the alternative, we allow for the possibility that uncontrolled systematic errors were responsible for the rejection.

Statistical Estimation

If Neyman-Pearson hypothesis testing is misleading, how should results be interpreted and presented? In keeping with the view that science is based on measurement—which leads in turn to quantitative study objectives—the analysis of epidemiologic data can be conceptualized as a measurement problem rather than as a problem in decision-making. Measurement requires more detailed statistics than the simple dichotomy produced by a statistical hypothesis testing. Whatever the parameter that is the target of inference in an epidemiologic study—usually an effect measure, such as a ratio of rates or risks, but it can also be an incidence rate or any other epidemiologic measure—it will be measured on a continuous scale, with a theoretically infinite number of possible values.

The data from a study can be used to generate an estimate of the target parameter. An estimate may be presented as a single value on the measurement scale of the parameter; this value is referred to as a *point estimate.* A point estimate may be viewed as a measure of the extent of the association, or (in causal analyses) the magnitude of effect under study. There will be many forces that will determine the final data values, such as confounding, measurement error, selection biases, and "random" error. It is thus extremely unlikely that the point estimate will equal the true value of the parameter.

It might be tempting to believe that an inferential emphasis on estimation can coexist with an inferential emphasis on testing, but they cannot. Selecting results for attention based on statistical significance distorts the ability to achieve accurate measurement.[11] For example, when power of a study is less than 100%, statistically significant results are more likely to overestimate than to underestimate the true value for the parameter, and results that are not statistically significant are more likely to underestimate than to overestimate the true value for the parameter. This distortion, a mathematical fact, is an inevitable consequence of the selection pressures exerted by the significance testing. Selecting results for attention on the basis of statistical significance also fosters analytic manipulations to achieve statistical significance. "Significance questing" and "P-hacking" describe unplanned changes to study design or analysis implemented to achieve a statistically significant result.[34-36] These changes hinder accurate estimation. In short, selecting results for attention based on statistical significance introduces distortions that preclude the goal of accurate estimation, so the two inferential paradigms cannot coexist.

Confidence Intervals and Confidence Limits

One way to account for random error in the estimation process is to compute P-values for a broad range of possible parameter values (in addition to the null value). If the range is broad enough, we will be able to identify an interval of parameter values for which the test P-value exceeds a specified alpha level (typically 0.05). All parameter values within the range are compatible with the data under the standard interpretation of significance tests. The range of values is called a *confidence interval*, and the endpoints of that interval are called *confidence limits*. The process of calculating the confidence interval is an example of the process of *interval estimation*.

The width of a confidence interval depends on the amount of random variability inherent in the data-collection process (as estimated from the underlying statistical model and the data). It also depends on an arbitrarily selected alpha level that specifies the degree of compatibility between the limits of the interval and the data. One minus this alpha level (0.95 if alpha is 0.05) is called the *confidence level* of the interval and is usually expressed as a percentage.

If the underlying statistical model is correct and there is no bias, a confidence interval derived from a valid test will, over unlimited repetitions of the study, contain the true parameter with a frequency no less than its confidence level. This definition specifies the coverage property of the method used to generate the interval, not the probability that the true parameter value lies within the interval. For example, if the confidence level of a valid confidence interval is 90%, the frequency with which the interval will contain the true parameter will be at least 90%, if there is no bias. Consequently, under the assumed model for random variability (*e.g.*, a binomial model) and with no bias, we should expect the confidence interval to include the true parameter value in at least 90% of replications of the process of obtaining the data. Unfortunately, this interpretation for the confidence interval is based on probability models and sampling properties that are seldom realized in epidemiologic studies; consequently, it is preferable to view the confidence limits as only a rough estimate of the uncertainty in an epidemiologic result due to random error alone. Even with this limited interpretation, the estimate depends on the correctness of the statistical model, which may be incorrect in many epidemiologic settings.[1]

Relation of Confidence Intervals to Significance Tests and Hypothesis Tests

Consider now the relation between the confidence level and the alpha level of hypothesis testing. The confidence level equals 1 minus the alpha level $(1 - \alpha)$ of the test used to construct the interval. To understand this relation, consider the diagram in Figure 15-2. Suppose that we performed a test of the null hypothesis with $\alpha = 0.10$. The fact that the 90% confidence interval does not include the null point indicates that the null hypothesis would be rejected for $\alpha = 0.10$. On the other hand, the fact that the 95% confidence interval includes the null point indicates that the null hypothesis would not be rejected for $\alpha = 0.05$. Because the 95% interval includes the null point and the 90% interval does not, it can be inferred that the two-sided P-value for the null hypothesis is greater than 0.05 and less than 0.10.

The point of the preceding example is not to suggest that confidence limits should be used as surrogate tests of significance. Although they can be and often are used this way, doing so defeats all the advantages that confidence intervals have over hypothesis tests. An interval-estimation procedure does much more than assess the extent to which a hypothesis is compatible with the data. It provides simultaneously an idea of the likely direction and magnitude of the underlying association and the random variability of the point estimate. The two-sided P-value, on the other hand,

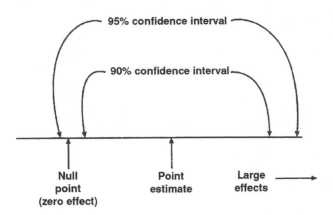

FIGURE 15-2 Two nested confidence intervals, with the wider one including the null hypothesis.

indicates only the degree of consistency between the data and a single hypothesis and thus reveals nothing about the magnitude or even the direction of the association or the random variability of the point estimate.[37]

For example, consider the data in Table 15-1. An exact test of the null hypothesis that the exposure is not associated with the disease gives a two-sided P-value of 0.14. (The methods used to calculate this P-value are described in Chapter 17.) This result might be reported in several ways. The least informative way is to report that the observed association is not significant. Somewhat more information can be given by reporting the actual P-value; to express the P-value as an inequality such as $P > 0.05$ is not much better than reporting the results as not significant, whereas reporting $P = 0.14$ at least gives the P-value explicitly rather than degrading it into a dichotomy. An additional improvement is to report $P_2 = 0.14$, denoting the use of a two-sided rather than a one-sided P-value.

Any one P-value, no matter how explicit, fails to convey the descriptive finding that exposed individuals had about three times the rate of disease as unexposed subjects. Furthermore, exact 95% confidence limits for the true rate ratio are 0.7 and 13. The fact that the null value (which, for the rate ratio, is 1.0) is within the interval tells us the outcome of the significance test: The estimate would not be statistically significant at the $1 - 0.95 = 0.05$ alpha level. The confidence limits, however, indicate that these data, although statistically compatible with no association, are even more compatible with a strong association—assuming that the statistical model used to construct the limits is correct. Stating the latter assumption is important because confidence intervals, like P-values, do nothing to address biases that may be present.

P-Value Functions

Although a confidence interval can be much more informative than a single P-value, it is subject to the misinterpretation that values inside the interval are equally compatible with the data, and all values outside it are equally incompatible. Like the alpha level of a test, however, the specific level of confidence used in constructing a confidence interval is arbitrary; values of 95% or, less often, 99% or 90% are those most frequently used.

A given confidence interval is only one of an infinite number of ranges nested within one another. Points nearer the center of these ranges are more compatible with the data than points farther away

TABLE 15-1

Hypothetical Data From a Cohort Study, Corresponding to the *P*-Value Function in Figure 15-3

	Exposure	
	Yes	No
Cases	9	2
Person-Years	186	128

from the center. To see the entire set of possible confidence intervals, one can construct a *P-value function*.[38-40] This function, also known as a consonance function[41] or confidence-interval function,[42] reflects the connection between the definition of a two-sided *P*-value and the definition of a two-sided confidence interval (*i.e.*, a two-sided confidence interval comprises all points for which the two-sided *P*-value exceeds the alpha level of the interval).

The *P*-value function gives the two-sided *P*-value for the null hypothesis, as well as every alternative to the null hypothesis for the parameter. A *P*-value function from the data in Table 15-1 is shown in Figure 15-3. Figure 15-3 also provides confidence levels on the right and so indicates all possible confidence limits for the estimate. The point at which the curve reaches its peak corresponds to the point estimate for the rate ratio, 3.1. The 95% confidence interval can be read directly from the graph as the function values where the right-hand ordinate is 0.95, and the 90% confidence interval can be read from the graph as the values where the right-hand ordinate is 0.90. The *P*-value for any value of the parameter can be found from the left-hand ordinate corresponding to that value. For example, the null two-sided *P*-value can be found from the left-hand ordinate corresponding to the height where the vertical line drawn at the hypothesized rate ratio = 1 intersects the *P*-value function.

A *P*-value function offers a visual display that neatly summarizes two key components of the estimation process. The peak of the curve indicates the point estimate, and the concentration of the curve around the point estimate indicates the precision of the estimate. A narrow *P*-value function would result from a study with high precision, which derives from a combination of the study size and its efficiency (see Study Efficiency, below). Conversely, a broad *P*-value function corresponds to a study that had low precision.

A confidence interval represents only one possible horizontal slice through the *P*-value function, but the single slice is enough to convey the two essential messages: Confidence limits usually provide enough information to locate the point estimate and to indicate the precision of the estimate. In large-sample epidemiologic statistics, the point estimate will usually be either the arithmetic or the geometric mean of the lower and upper limits. The distance between the lower and upper limits indicates the spread of the full *P*-value function.

The message of Figure 15-3 is that the example data are more compatible with a moderate to strong association than with no association, assuming the statistical model used to construct the function is correct. The confidence limits, when taken as indicative of the *P*-value function, summarize the size and precision of the estimate.[43,44] A single *P*-value, on the other hand, gives no indication of either the size or the precision of the estimate, and, if it is used merely as a hypothesis test, might result in a Type II error if there indeed is an association between exposure and disease.

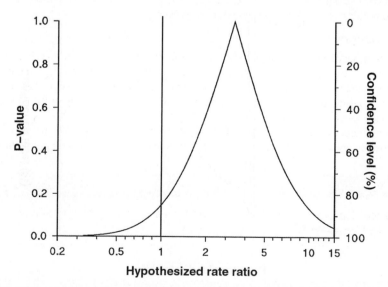

FIGURE 15-3 P-value function, from which one can find all confidence limits, for a hypothetical study with a rate ratio estimate of 3.1 (see Table 15-1).

Evidence of Absence of Effect or Incompatible Results

Confidence limits and *P*-value functions convey information about size and precision of the estimate simultaneously, keeping these two features of measurement in the foreground. The use of a single *P*-value—or (worse) dichotomization of the *P*-value into significant or not significant ones—obscures these features so that the focus on measurement is lost. A study cannot be reassuring about the safety of an exposure or treatment if only a statistical test of the null hypothesis is reported. As we have already seen, results that are not significant may be compatible with substantial effects. Lack of significance alone provides no evidence against such effects.[45]

Standard statistical advice states that when the data indicate a lack of significance, it is important to consider the power of the study to detect as significant a specific alternative hypothesis. The power of a test, however, is only an indirect indicator of precision, and it requires an assumption about the magnitude of the effect. In planning a study, it is reasonable to make conjectures about the magnitude of an effect to compute study-size requirements or power (see below). In analyzing data, however, it is always preferable to use the information in the data about the effect to estimate it directly, rather than to speculate about it with study-size or power calculations.[46-50] Confidence limits and (even more so) *P*-value functions convey much more of the essential information by indicating the range of values that are reasonably compatible with the observations (albeit at a somewhat arbitrary alpha level), assuming the statistical model is correct. They can also show that the data do not contain the information necessary for reassurance about an absence of effect.

Freiman et al.[30] used confidence limits for the RDs to reinterpret the findings from 71 negative clinical trials. These confidence limits indicated that many of the treatments under study were probably beneficial, as seen in Figure 15-1. The inappropriate interpretations of the authors in most of these trials could have been avoided by focusing their attention on the confidence limits rather than on the results of a statistical test.

For a study to provide evidence of lack of an effect, the confidence limits must be near the null value and the statistical model must be correct. In equivalence-testing terms, the entire confidence interval must lie within the zone around the null that would be considered practically equivalent to the null. Consider Figure 15-4, which depicts the *P*-value function from Figure 15-3 on an expanded scale, along with another *P*-value function from a study with a point estimate of 1.05 and 95% confidence limits of 1.01 and 1.10.

The study yielding the narrow *P*-value function must have been large and information dense to generate such precision. The precision enables one to infer that, provided any strong biases or

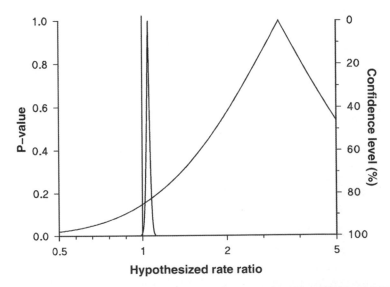

FIGURE 15-4 A *P*-value function from a precise study with a relative risk estimate of 1.05 and the *P*-value function from Figure 15-3.

other serious problems with the statistical model are absent, the study provides evidence against a strong effect. The upper confidence limit (with any reasonable level of confidence) is near the null value, indicating that the data are not readily compatible with large or even moderate effects. Or, as seen from the *P*-value function, the curve is a narrow spike close to the null point. The spike is not centered exactly on the null point, however, but slightly above it. In fact, the data from this large study would be judged as statistically significant by conventional criteria, because the (two-sided) *P*-value testing the null hypothesis is about 0.03. In contrast, the other *P*-value function in Figure 15-4 depicts data that, as we have seen, are readily compatible with large effects but are not statistically significant by conventional criteria.

Figure 15-4 illustrates the dangers of using statistical significance as the primary basis for inference. Even if one assumes no bias is present (*i.e.*, that the studies and analyses are perfectly valid), the two sets of results differ in that one result indicates there may be a large effect, while the other offers evidence against a large effect. The irony is that it is the statistically significant finding that offers evidence *against* a large effect, while it is the finding that is not statistically significant that raises concern about a possibly large effect. In these examples, statistical significance gives a message that is opposite of the appropriate interpretation. Focusing on interval estimation and proper interpretation of the confidence limits avoids this problem.

Numerous real-world examples demonstrate the problem of relying on statistical significance for inference. One such example occurred in the interpretation of a large randomized trial of androgen blockade combined with the drug flutamide in the treatment of advanced prostate cancer.[51] This trial had been preceded by 10 similar trials, which in aggregate had found a small survival advantage for patients given flutamide, with the pooled results for the 10 studies producing a summary odds ratio of 0.88, with a 95% confidence interval of 0.76, 1.02.[52,53] In their study, Eisenberger et al. reported that flutamide was ineffective, thus contradicting the results of the 10 earlier studies, despite their finding an odds ratio of 0.87 (equivalent in their study to a mortality rate ratio of 0.91), a result not very different from that of the earlier 10 studies. The *P*-value for their finding was above their predetermined cutoff for "significance," which is the reason that the authors concluded that flutamide was an ineffective therapy. But the 95% confidence interval of 0.70 to 1.10 for their odds ratio showed that their data were readily compatible with a meaningful benefit for patients receiving flutamide. Furthermore, their results were similar to those from the summary of the 10 earlier studies. The *P*-value functions for the summary of the 10 earlier studies, and the study by Eisenberger et al., are shown in Figure 15-5. The figure shows how the findings of Eisenberger et al. reinforce rather than refute the earlier studies. They misinterpreted their findings because of their focus on statistical significance.

Another example was a headline-generating study reporting that women who consumed moderate amounts of alcohol retained better cognitive function than nondrinkers.[54] For moderate drinkers (up to 15 g of alcohol per day), the authors reported an RR for impaired cognition of 0.81 with 95% confidence limits of 0.70 and 0.93, indicating that moderate drinking was associated with a benefit with respect to cognition. In contrast, the authors reported, "There were no significant associations between higher levels of drinking (15 to 30 g/d) and the risk of cognitive impairment or decline," implying no benefit for heavy drinkers, an interpretation repeated in widespread news reports. Nevertheless, the finding for women who consumed larger amounts of alcohol was essentially identical to the finding for moderate drinkers, with a risk-ratio estimate of 0.82 instead of 0.81. It had a broader confidence interval, however, with limits of 0.59 and 1.13. Figure 15-6 demonstrates how precision, rather than different effect size, accounted for the difference in statistical significance for the two groups. The *P*-value function for moderate drinkers was narrower than the estimate for heavy drinkers. There is more information about moderate drinkers because the prevalence of moderate drinking is higher than the prevalence of heavy drinking. From the data, there is no basis to infer that the effect size differs for moderate and heavy drinkers; in fact, the hypothesis that is most compatible with the data is that the effect is about the same in both groups. Furthermore, the lower 95% confidence limit for the ratio of the RR in the heavy drinkers to the RR in the moderate drinkers is 0.71, implying that the data are also quite compatible with a much lower (more protective) RR in the heavy drinkers than in the moderate drinkers.

These types of inferential errors have contributed to the perceived crisis[55,56] in the reproducibility of scientific research.[11,57] The literature on this perceived crisis has sometimes assessed whether the results of two studies are concordant based on whether their respective results are both statistically

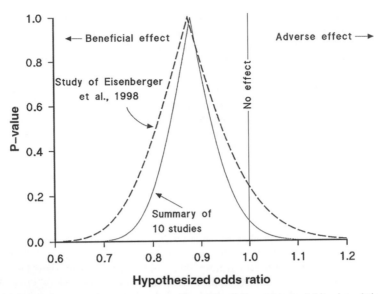

FIGURE 15-5 *P*-value functions based on 10 earlier trials of flutamide (solid line) and the trial by Eisenberger et al. (dashed line), showing the similarity of results and revealing the fallacy of relying on statistical significance to conclude, as did Eisenberger et al., that flutamide has no meaningful effect.

significant or not.[58] This approach has been used to assess reproducibility despite the fact that the idea that two results—one statistically significant and the other not—are necessarily different from one another is a well-known fallacy,[10,59] as described above. Nonetheless, examples of claims of irreproducible results based on *P*-values falling on opposite sides of the commonly accepted Type I error rate are easy to find. In one example, subcutaneous heparin was reported to reduce the risk of deep vein thrombosis compared with intravenous heparin (OR = 0.62, 95% CI 0.39, 0.98);

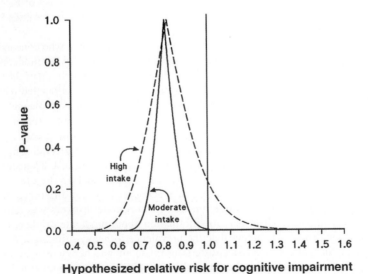

FIGURE 15-6 *P*-value functions for moderate and heavier drinkers of alcohol showing essentially identical negative associations with decline in cognitive function. The authors incorrectly reported that there was an association with moderate drinking, but not with heavier drinking, because only the finding for moderate drinking was statistically significant. (From Stampfer MJ, Kang JH, Chen J, et al. Effects of moderate alcohol consumption on cognitive function in women. *N Engl J Med.* 2005;352:245-253.)

a reanalysis disagreed with the conclusion of a protective effect (OR = 0.61, 95% CI 0.30, 1.25).[60] In a second example, authors concluded that their results (OR = 0.75, 95% CI 0.48, 1.17) did not support previous sparse evidence of a protective effect of statins use against glioma (previous study results were reported to be OR = 0.72; 95% CI 0.52, 1.00 and OR = 0.76; 95% CI 0.59, 0.98).[61] Finally, in a study of the association between antidepressant use during pregnancy and autism spectrum disorder in offspring, the authors reported a meta-analysis of earlier studies (OR = 1.7; 95% CI 1.1, 2.6), a multivariate adjusted hazards ratio in their study (1.59; 95% CI 1.17, 2.17), and an inverse probability of treatment weighted hazards ratio in their study (1.61; 95% CI 0.997, 2.59).[62] They concluded "antidepressant exposure compared with no exposure was not associated with autism spectrum disorder in the child." Examples of this type of misinterpretation abound and likely contribute to the perception that epidemiologic results are poorly reproducible when, at least in these examples, the evidence base is entirely consistent. It is impossible to estimate the degree to which this common misinterpretation has distorted the impression of a reproducibility crisis.[57]

Guidelines for Good Practice

Good data analysis does not demand that P-value functions be plotted routinely. They are especially useful when comparing two or more results. Overlap between the P-value functions will often forewarn against interpreting two results as different when they are not so different at all. For most results, though, it is sufficient to use conventional confidence limits to generate the proper mental visualization for the underlying P-value function. In fact, for large studies, only one pair of limits and their confidence level is needed to sketch the entire function, and one can easily learn to visualize the function that corresponds to any pair of limits. If, however, one uses the limits only to determine whether the null point lies inside or outside the confidence interval, one is only performing a significance test, and all of the biases and inferential errors described above will ensue. It is lamentable to go to the trouble to calculate confidence limits and then use them for nothing more than classifying the study finding as statistically significant or not. One should instead remember that the precise locations of confidence limits are not important for proper interpretation. Rather, the limits should serve to give one a mental picture of the location and spread of the entire P-value function.

The main thrust of the preceding sections has been to argue the inadequacy of statistical significance testing for inference about effects. The view that estimation is preferable to testing has been argued by many scientists in a variety of disciplines, including, for example, economics, social sciences, environmental science, and accident research. There has been a particularly heated and welcome debate in psychology. In the overall scientific literature, hundreds of publications have addressed the concerns about statistical hypothesis testing. Some selected references include Rozeboom,[63] Morrison and Henkel,[64] Wulff,[65] Cox and Hinkley,[19] Rothman,[66] Salsburg,[67] Simon and Wittes,[68] Langman,[69] Gardner and Altman,[70] Walker,[71] Oakes,[72] Ware et al.,[73] Pocock et al.,[74] Poole,[40,43] Thompson,[75] Evans et al.,[76] Anscombe,[77] Cohen,[78] Hauer,[79] Gigerenzer,[3] Ziliak and McCloskey,[80] Batterham and Hopkins,[81] Marshall,[82] the American Statistical Association[9] statement, Lash,[11] and the commentaries in Supplement 1 to Volume 73 (2019) of *The American Statistician*. To quote Atkins and Jarrett[32]:

> Methods of estimation share many of the problems of significance tests—being likewise based on probability model assumptions and requiring "arbitrary" limits of precision. But at least they do not require irrelevant null hypotheses to be set up nor do they force a decision about "significance" to be made—the estimates can be presented and evaluated by statistical *and other* criteria, by the researcher or the reader. In addition, the estimates of one investigation can be compared with others. While it is often the case that different measurements or methods of investigation or theoretical approaches lead to "different" results, this is not a disadvantage; these differences reflect important theoretical differences about the meaning of the research and the conclusions to be drawn from it. And it is precisely those differences which are obscured by simply reporting the significance level of the results.

Indeed, because statistical hypothesis testing promotes so much misinterpretation, we recommend avoiding its use in epidemiologic presentations and research reports. Such avoidance requires that P-values (when used) be presented without reference to alpha levels or "statistical significance" and that careful attention be paid to the confidence interval, especially its width and its endpoints (the confidence limits).[13,44]

Problems With Confidence Intervals

Because they can be derived from P-values, confidence intervals and P-value functions are themselves subject to some of the same criticisms as significance tests.[1,15,16] One problem that confidence intervals and P-value functions share with statistical hypothesis tests is their very indirect interpretations, which depend on the concept of "repetition of the study in a manner identical in all respects except for random error." Interpretations of statistics that appeal to such a concept are called repeated-sampling or *frequentist* interpretations, because they refer to the frequency of certain events (rejection by a test or coverage by a confidence interval) in a series of repeated experiments.

An astute investigator may properly ask what frequency interpretations have to do with the single study under analysis. It is all very well to say that an interval estimation procedure will, in 95% of repetitions, produce limits that contain the true parameter. But in analyzing a given study, the relevant scientific question is this: Does the single pair of limits produced from this one study contain the true parameter? The ordinary (frequentist) theory of confidence intervals does not answer this question. The question is so important that many (perhaps most) users of confidence intervals mistakenly interpret the confidence level of the interval as the probability that the answer to the question is "yes."[83] It is quite tempting to say that the 95% confidence limits computed from a study contain the true parameter with 95% probability. Unfortunately, this interpretation can be correct only for Bayesian interval estimates (discussed later and in Chapter 23), which often diverge from ordinary confidence intervals.

There are several alternative types of interval estimation that attempt to address these problems. We will discuss two of these alternatives in the next two subsections.

Likelihood Intervals

To avoid interpretational problems, a few authors prefer to replace confidence intervals with likelihood intervals, also known as support intervals.[15,17,25] In ordinary English, "likelihood" is just a synonym for "probability." In the likelihood theory, however, a more specialized definition is used: The *likelihood* of a specified parameter value given observed data is defined as the probability of the observed data, given that the true parameter equals the specified parameter value. This concept is covered in depth in many statistics textbooks; for example, see Berger and Wolpert,[84] Clayton and Hills,[85] Edwards,[25] and Royall.[17] Here, we will describe the basic definitions of the likelihood theory.

To illustrate the definition of likelihood, consider again the population in Table 15-1, in which $186/(186 + 128) = 59\%$ of person-years were exposed. Under standard assumptions, it can be shown that, if there is no bias and the true rate ratio is 10, there will be a 0.125 chance of observing nine exposed cases, given 11 total cases and 59% exposed person-years. (The calculation of this probability is beyond the present discussion.) Thus, by definition, 0.125 is the likelihood for a rate ratio of 10, given the data in Table 15-1. Similarly, if there are no biases and the true ratio is 1, there will be a 0.082 chance of observing 9 exposed cases given 11 total and 59% exposed person-years; thus, by definition, 0.082 is the likelihood for a rate ratio of 1, given the data in Table 15-1.

When one parameter value makes the observed data more probable than another value and hence has a higher likelihood, it is sometimes said that this parameter value has higher support from the data than the other value.[17,25] For example, in this special sense, a rate ratio of 10 has higher support from the data in Table 15-1 than a rate ratio of 1, because those data have a greater chance of occurring if the rate ratio is 10 than if it is 1.

For most data, there will be at least one possible parameter value that makes the chance of getting those data highest under the assumed statistical model. In other words, there will be a parameter value whose likelihood is at least as high as that of any other parameter value and so has the maximum possible likelihood (or maximum support) under the assumed model. Such a parameter value is called a *maximum-likelihood estimate* (MLE) under the assumed model. For the data in Table 15-1, there is just one such value, and it is the observed rate ratio $(9/186)/(2/128) = 3.1$. If there are no biases and the true rate ratio is 3.1, there will be a 0.299 chance of observing 9 exposed cases, given 11 total and 59% exposed person-years, so 0.299 is the likelihood for a rate ratio of 3.1, given the data in Table 15-1. No other value for the rate ratio will make the chance of these results higher than 0.299, and so 3.1 is the MLE. Thus, in the special likelihood sense, a rate ratio of 3.1 has the highest possible support from the data.

As has been noted, Table 15-1 yields a likelihood of 0.125 for a rate ratio of 10; this value (0.125) is 42% of the likelihood (of 0.299) for 3.1. Similarly, Table 15-1 yields a likelihood of 0.082 for a rate ratio of 1; this value (0.082) is 27% of the likelihood for 3.1. Overall, a rate ratio of 3.1 maximizes the chance of observing the data in Table 15-1. Although rate ratios of 10 and 1 have less support (lower likelihood) than 3.1, they are still among values that likelihoodists regard as having enough support to warrant further consideration; these values typically include all values with a likelihood above one-seventh of the maximum.[15,17,25] Under a normal model for random errors, such one-seventh likelihood intervals are approximately equal to 95% confidence intervals.[17]

The maximum of the likelihood is the height of the likelihood function at the MLE. A likelihood interval for a parameter (here, the rate ratio) is the collection of all possible values whose likelihood is no less than some specified fraction of this maximum. Thus, for Table 15-1, the collection of all rate ratio values with a likelihood no less than 0.299/7 = 0.043 (one-seventh of the highest likelihood) is a likelihood interval based on those data. Upon computing this interval, we find that all rate ratios between 0.79 and 20 imply a probability for the observed data at least one-seventh of the probability of the data when the rate ratio is 3.1 (the MLE). Because the likelihoods for rate ratios of 1 and 10 exceed 0.299/7 = 0.043, 1 and 10 are within this interval.

Analogous to confidence limits, one can graph the collection of likelihood limits for all fractions of the maximum (1/2, 1/4, 1/7, 1/20, etc.). The resulting graph has the same shape as one would obtain from simply graphing the likelihood for each possible parameter value. The latter graph is called the *likelihood function* for the data. Figure 15-7 gives the likelihood function for the data in Table 15-1, with the ordinate scaled to make the maximum (peak) at 3.1 equal to 1 rather than 0.299 (this is done by dividing all the likelihoods by the maximum, 0.299). Thus, Figure 15-7 provides all possible likelihood limits within the range of the figure.

The function in Figure 15-7 is proportional to

$$\left(\frac{186(\text{IR})}{186(\text{IR}) + 128} \right)^9 \left(\frac{128}{186(\text{IR}) + 128} \right)^2$$

where IR is the hypothesized incidence rate ratio (the abscissa). Note that this function is broader and less sharply peaked than the *P*-value function in Figure 15-3, reflecting the fact that, by likelihood standards, *P*-values and confidence intervals tend to give the impression that the data provide more evidence against the test hypothesis than they actually do.[15]

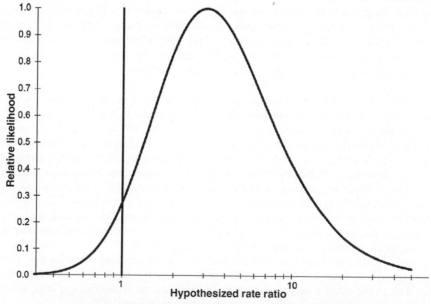

FIGURE 15-7 Relative likelihood function based on Table 15-1.

Some authors prefer to use the natural logarithm of the likelihood function, or *log-likelihood function,* to compare the support given to competing hypotheses by the data.[15,17,25] These authors sometimes refer to the log-likelihood function as the support function generated by the data. Although we find log-likelihoods less easily interpretable than likelihoods, log-likelihoods can be useful in constructing confidence intervals.

Bayesian Intervals

As with confidence limits, the interpretation of likelihood limits is indirect, in that it does not answer the question: "Is the true value between these limits?" Unless the true value is already known (in which case there is no point in gathering data), it can be argued that the only rational answer to the question must be a *subjective* probability statement, such as "I am 95% sure that the true value is between these limits."[86,87] Such subjective probability assessments, or *certainties,* are common in everyday life, as when a weather forecaster predicts 80% chance of rain tomorrow, or when one is delayed while traveling and thinks that there is a 90% chance of arriving between 1 and 2 hours after the scheduled arrival time. If one is *sure* that the true arrival time will be between these limits, this sureness represents a subjective assessment of 100% probability (complete certainty) that arrival will be 1 to 2 hours late. In reality, however, there is always a chance (however small) that one will be delayed longer or may never arrive, so complete certainty is never warranted.

Subjective Bayesian analysis is concerned with producing realistic and rationally coherent probability assessments, and it is especially concerned with updating these assessments as data become available. *Rationally coherent* means only that assessments are free of logical contradictions and do not contradict the axioms of the probability theory (which are also used as axioms for frequentist probability calculations).[86-89]

All statistical methods require a model for data probabilities. The Bayesian analysis additionally requires a *prior probability distribution.* In theory, this means that one must have a probability assessment available for every relevant interval; for example, when trying to study a rate ratio, before seeing the data one must be able to specify one's certainty that the rate ratio is between 1 and 2, and between ½ and 4, and so on. This prior-specification requirement demands that one has a probability distribution for the rate ratio that is similar in shape to Figure 15-3 *before* seeing the data. This is a daunting demand, and it was enough to have impeded the use and acceptance of Bayesian methods for most of the 20th century.

Suppose, however, that one succeeds in specifying in advance a prior probability distribution that gives prespecified certainties for the target parameter. Bayesian analysis then proceeds by combining this prior distribution with the likelihood function (such as in Figure 15-7) to produce a new, updated set of certainties, called the *posterior probability distribution* for the target parameter based on the given prior distribution and likelihood function. This posterior distribution in turn yields posterior probability intervals (posterior certainty intervals). Suppose, for example, one accepts the prior distribution as a good summary of previous information about the parameter and similarly accepts the likelihood function as a good summary of the data probabilities, given various possible values for the parameter. The resulting 95% posterior interval is then a range of numbers that one can be 95% certain contains the true parameter.

The technical details of computing exact posterior distributions can be quite involved and were also an obstacle to the widespread adoption of the Bayesian methods. Modern computing advances have all but eliminated this obstacle as a serious problem; also, the same approximations used to compute conventional frequentist statistics can be used to compute approximate Bayesian statistics.

Another obstacle to Bayesian methods has been that the intervals produced by a Bayesian analysis refer to subjective probabilities rather than objective frequencies. Some argue that, because subjective probabilities are just one person's opinion, they should be of no interest to objective scientists. Unfortunately, in nonexperimental studies, there is (by definition) no identified random mechanism to generate objective frequencies over study repetitions; thus, in such studies, the so-called objective frequentist methods (such as significance tests and confidence intervals) lack the objective repeated-sampling properties usually attributed to them.[1,2,16,26,27,88,90] Furthermore, scientists do routinely offer their opinions and are interested in the opinions of colleagues. Therefore, it can be argued that a rational (if subjective) certainty assessment may be the only reasonable inference we can get out of a statistical analysis of observational epidemiologic data. Some argue that this conclusion applies even to perfect randomized experiments.[14,87,91]

At the least, Bayesian statistics provide a probabilistic answer to questions such as "Does the true rate ratio lie between 1 and 4?" (to which one possible Bayesian answer is "In light of the data and my current prior information, I can be 90% certain that it does"). A more general argument for the use of Bayesian methods is that they can provide point and interval estimates that have better objective frequency (repeated-sampling) properties than ordinary frequentist estimates. These calibrated Bayesian statistics include Bayesian confidence intervals that are narrower (more precise) than ordinary confidence intervals with the same confidence level. Because the advantages of procedures with Bayesian justification can be so dramatic, some authors argue that only methods with a clear Bayesian justification should be used, even though repeated-sampling (objective frequency) properties are also desirable (such as proper coverage frequency for interval estimates).[92-94]

In addition to providing improved analysis methods, the Bayesian theory can be used to evaluate established or newly proposed statistical methods. For example, if a new confidence interval is proposed, we may ask: "What prior distribution do we need to get this new interval as our Bayesian posterior probability interval?" It is often the case that the prior distribution one would need to justify a conventional confidence interval is patently absurd; for example, it would assign equal probabilities to rate ratios of 1 and 1,000,000.[16,88,95] In such cases, it can be argued that one should reject the proposed interval because it will not properly reflect any rational opinion about the parameter after a careful data analysis.[16,93]

Under certain conditions, ordinary (frequentist) confidence intervals and one-sided P-values can be interpreted as approximate posterior (Bayesian) probability intervals.[19,24] These conditions typically arise when little is known about the associations under study. Frequentist intervals cease to have Bayesian utility when much is already known or the data under analysis are too limited to yield even modestly precise estimates. The latter situation arises not only in small studies, but also in large studies that must deal with many variables at once, or that fail to measure key variables with sufficient accuracy.

Summary

Statistics can be viewed as having many roles in epidemiology. Data description is one role, and statistical inference is another. The two are sometimes mixed, to the detriment of both activities, and are best distinguished from the outset of an analysis.

Different schools of statistics view statistical inference as having different roles in data analysis. The hypothesis-testing approach treats statistics as chiefly a collection of methods for making decisions, such as whether an association is present in a source population or "superpopulation" from which the data are randomly drawn. This approach has been declining in the face of criticisms that estimation, not decision-making, is the proper role for statistical inference in science. Within the latter view, frequentist approaches derive estimates by using probabilities of data (either P-values or likelihoods) as measures of compatibility between data and hypotheses, or as measures of the relative support that data provide hypotheses. In contrast, the Bayesian approach uses data to improve existing (prior) estimates in light of new data. Different approaches can be used in the course of an analysis. Nonetheless, proper use of any approach requires more careful interpretation of statistics than has been common.

PRECISION AND STRATIFICATION

In many epidemiologic analyses, the crude data are divided into strata to examine effects in subcategories of another variable or to control confounding. The efficiency of a study can be affected dramatically by stratifying the data. A study that has an overall apportionment ratio that is favorable for precision (which will be a ratio of 1.0 if there is no effect and no confounding) may nevertheless have apportionment ratios within strata that vary severely from low to high values. It is common to see some strata with the extreme apportionment ratios of 0 and infinity (e.g., no cases in some strata and no controls in others). The smaller the numbers within strata, the more extreme the variation in the apportionment ratio across strata is likely to be. The extreme values result from zero subjects or person-time units for one group in a stratum. Small numbers within strata result from having too few subjects relative to the number of strata created. This sparse-data problem can develop even with large studies, because the number of strata required in the analysis increases geometrically with the number of variables used for stratification. Indeed, sparse data are a major limitation of stratified analysis, although the same problem negatively affects regression modeling as well.

When comparisons within strata will be essential and much variation in the apportionment ratio is expected across strata, then matching on the stratification variables (Chapter 6) is one way to improve the efficiency of the apportionment ratio within strata and to reduce sparsity problems without increasing the study size. When matching on all stratification variables is not feasible, increasing the overall number of subjects will at least reduce data sparsity and improve precision, even if only one group (*e.g.*, the controls in a case-control study) can be expanded.

PLANNING STUDY SIZE

Enlarging the size of a study is one of the key ways to reduce random error in an epidemiologic estimate. Practical constraints on resources inevitably limit study size, so one must plan accordingly. One method that is used to plan the size of a study is to calculate the study size based on conventional statistical "sample-size" formulas.[96-100] These formulas relate the size of a study to the study design, study population, and the desired power or precision.

Study-size formulas, being purely mathematical, do not account for anything that is not included as a variable in the formula. At best, they serve only to provide rough guidelines, and in some situations, they may be misleading from a broader perspective. For example, conventional formulas do not weigh the value of the information obtained from a study against its use of resources. Yet a focal problem in planning the study size is determining how to balance the value of greater precision in study results against the greater cost. Solving the problem thus involves a cost-benefit analysis of expending greater effort or funds to gain greater precision. Greater precision has a value to the beneficiaries of the research, but the value is indeterminate because it is always uncertain how many beneficiaries there will be. Furthermore, the potential benefits of the study involve intricacies of many social, political, and biologic factors that are almost never quantified. Consequently, only informal guesses as to a cost-efficient size for an epidemiologic study are feasible. Although study-size determination can be aided by conventional formulas, the final choice must also incorporate unquantified practical constraints and implications of various study sizes.

In this section, we will discuss the considerations that the researcher should weigh in planning the size of a study. The term "sample size" is often used to describe the study size, possibly borrowed from the vocabulary of survey sampling design. We prefer to use "study size" to avoid confusing a study of causal effects with a survey to describe a large population based on a sample from it.

A study size is the primary determinant of the precision of the estimates that come from the study, but better precision—the reduction of random error—is affected not only by the study size but by the study efficiency as well, as described above. Furthermore, the measurement of study efficiency or study informativeness depends on assumptions that are often absent or implicit in statistical discussions, such as what constitutes the most relevant hypotheses and costs.

Study Efficiency

Study efficiency can be thought of as the amount of information that a study produces in relation to its size or cost. Efficiency usually depends on issues such as the ratio of the number of subjects or person-time units across categories of exposure or disease. A study with 1,000,000 people may seem large, but if only 100 of them are exposed and 999,900 are unexposed, it will have considerably less information than a study with an even balance of exposed and unexposed subjects. When the study factor has no effect and no adjustment for confounding is needed, equal apportionment into exposure groups is the most efficient cohort design.[101] In case-control studies, the study efficiency will depend on the balance between case and control groups. As described in Chapter 8, case-control designs are best conceptualized as efficient cohort designs that include all cases and a subset of the cohort giving rise to the cases. This conceptualization rests on the idea of optimizing apportionment of study subjects: cases are usually few in relation to the size of the population giving rise to the cases, so over-representing cases by design is efficient. On the other hand, in cohort studies, it may be costly to engineer a desirable balance of exposure and may lead to inefficiencies in trying to use the data to study a wider range of exposures. In short, if the apportionment of study subjects by categories of exposure or outcome can be manipulated in the study design, it may be advantageous to design the study with a good balance between groups.

The considerations involved in designing an efficient study usually pit the costs of doing so against the benefits, which may be difficult to assess. Nonetheless, it is worth knowing that when the study exposure has no effect and no adjustment is needed, equal apportionment into exposure groups is the most efficient cohort design.[101] For example, when no association is expected for any reason (which is to say, in the absence of any source of association, whether bias or exposure effect), a cohort study of 2,400 persons will be most efficient statistically if it comprises 1,200 exposed and 1,200 unexposed persons for study (a 1:1 exposed-unexposed allocation ratio). Similarly, in a case-control study, when no association is expected, it will be most efficient to have an equal number of cases and controls (a 1:1 case-control allocation ratio). Nonetheless, since we do not know whether an association is present, translating these statistical facts into a directive for study design assumes that the primary goal of the analysis is to evaluate the hypothesis of no association (or, with additional assumptions, no effect).

In the presence of an effect, the statistically most efficient allocation ratio will differ from equal apportionment (1:1) by an amount that depends on the magnitude of the effect.[101] In the cohort example, if priority were instead given to testing the hypothesis that there is a doubling of risk, parallel derivations lead to allocating more of the total to the unexposed, for whom risk is lower than the exposed. For a disease that would occur in no more than a few percent of the cohort, this could lead to a 1:2 allocation ratio (800 exposed and 1,600 unexposed) as more efficient than 1:1 allocation. If equal weight is given to the hypotheses of no association and doubling of risk, the efficient allocation would be nearer 1,000 exposed and 1,400 unexposed than either 1:1 or 1:2 allocation.

Efficiency of a study may be difficult to modify. For example, if exposure is rare, population samples will show a preponderance of unexposed subjects unless special populations are sought. Both cohort studies and case-control studies drawn from a general population tend to be inefficient if exposure has low prevalence. Two-stage (two-phase) sampling designs that account for both exposure and disease frequency are available, although the data they produce requires special analysis methods.

Adjustments for biases such as confounding will also influence study precision, usually diminishing it. In many epidemiologic analyses, the crude data are divided into strata to examine exposure effects within subcategories of another variable, or to control confounding. The efficiency of a study can be affected dramatically by stratifying the data. A study that has an overall apportionment ratio that is favorable for precision, with close to overall balance between the main groups to be compared, may nevertheless have apportionment ratios within strata that vary severely from low to high values. It is not uncommon to see some strata with the extreme apportionment ratios of 0 and infinity (e.g., a case-control study with no cases in some strata and no controls in others). The smaller the numbers within strata, the more extreme the variation in the apportionment ratio across strata is likely to be.

The most extreme values occur when there are zero subjects or person-time units for one group in a stratum. The chance of zero subjects or person-time units for a group in a stratum is increased when there are many strata in relation to the number of study subjects. This sparse-data problem can develop even with studies based on large numbers of subjects. It not only affects study efficiency but can introduce a bias in the estimation of ratio measures. This sparse data bias can be substantial, and is more common than realized, because the number of strata required increases geometrically with the number of variables used for stratification.[102] Indeed, sparse data are a major limitation of stratified analysis, although the problem is not limited to stratified analysis, and can affect regression modeling as well, where it may go unnoticed.[103,104]

When comparisons within strata will be essential and substantial variation in the apportionment ratio is expected across strata, then matching on the stratification variables (see Chapter 6) is one way to improve the efficiency of the apportionment ratio within strata and to reduce sparse-data problems without increasing the overall study size. It is, however, not guaranteed to improve efficiency and may even harm it, especially in case-control studies and especially when matching on variables that are unrelated to the outcome variable. When matching on all stratification variables is not feasible or advisable, increasing the overall number of subjects may mitigate sparse-data problems and improve overall study precision, even if only one group (*e.g.*, the control series) can be expanded.

Study Size

Study size is only adjustable within the constraints of available data and budget. Even when it is not adjustable (*e.g.*, one has only a fixed data base for use), however, study size is usually the largest determinant of study precision. Considerations of study size in the planning stage of a research project are thus essential for investigators and reviewers to assess the potential informativeness of a study.

In planning a study, assessing the informativeness may be addressed in various ways. The typical approaches involve judging the informativeness of a potential study by postulating one or more possible study sizes and calculating a measure of informativeness for each. Often this amounts to calculating the statistical power of the study for a statistical test of a targeted hypothesis (usually but not necessarily a "null" hypothesis) for a range of possible study sizes.

To review briefly these terms and concepts, and their relationships to the study size, we note that conventional statistical hypothesis tests can usually be described as producing a P-value that will be compared to a critical cutoff α. As described above, and subject to all of the limitations already mentioned, the event of $P \leq \alpha$ is usually taken as "rejection" or "statistical significance" at level α, although actual rejection or significance should depend on many other considerations besides the result of a statistical test. The false-positive rate of the test is the probability that $P \leq \alpha$ if the tested hypothesis is correct and is also known as the Type I error rate, alpha error rate, or false-rejection rate. The P-value from the test is said to be valid if the probability that $P \leq \alpha$ equals α (*i.e.*, if the false-positive rate is α). The power of the test for detecting a specific alternative to the tested hypotheses is the probability that $P \leq \alpha$ when the alternative is correct; the value of $1 -$ power is called the false-negative rate, Type II error rate, or beta-error rate, is often denoted by β.

The Imbalance of Power in Traditional Study-Size Computations

There are many formulas that relate study size to power, taking into account design features such as the apportionment ratios of the exposure or outcome groups, whether subjects are clustered by some variable, and what covariates will be controlled analytically. The following problems apply to them all.

The test cutoff α is usually chosen to be 5%, although that choice is rarely explicitly justified. The theory says that α should be chosen to reflect the actual cost of false-positive errors,[105,106] with α being smaller if false positives are costly compared with false negatives and larger in the reverse situation. For a valid test, the chance α of false-positive error and the chance β of false-negative error are inversely related to each other, so in choosing α and β, there is an inevitable trade-off between the risks of the two errors. This alignment of acceptable error rates with values is discussed above but seldom implemented in practice.

Traditional study-size requirements assume that a power of only 80% is acceptable when conducting a test with $\alpha = 5\%$, although (as with $\alpha = 5\%$) that choice is rarely explicitly justified. Although 80% may at first sound high, it means that the false-negative rate β is 20%, which would be wholly unjustified if false negatives were very costly and false positives were not. Adopting such a gross imbalance, allowing the false-negative rate to be four times the false-positive rate, may reflect nothing more than the fact that it results in a much smaller study-size requirement than if both the acceptable false-positive and false-negative rates were set to be 5%.

Complicating matters is that the costs may be radically different for different stakeholders in a problem; for example, in litigation claiming harms from an industrial chemical, false positives are typically very costly for the defendant (*e.g.*, the chemical manufacturer) but beneficial for the plaintiff demanding compensation (*e.g.*, the exposed); conversely false negatives are beneficial for the defendant but costly for the plaintiff. This difference in acceptable error rates means that the tradition of accepting a higher false-negative rate than a false-positive rate when designing studies to test a null hypothesis is a tradition favoring the defendant and more generally favors the null hypothesis over the alternative.

The traditional imbalance in favor of the null in the study design and testing can lead to apparently paradoxical results in which a study with "high power" (*e.g.*, 90%) may fail to reject the null at the 5% level, yet exhibit data that statistically favor the alternative according to other conventional criteria.[107] To avoid such imbalance and its consequences, one may instead seek equal rates of both errors, *e.g.*, by designing a study to have 95% power ($\beta = 5\%$) when using $\alpha = 5\%$. A justification for inequality in terms of error costs may instead be sought, but the justification will not apply to those whose costs differ from the costs assumed by the justification.

Other Drawbacks of Power Calculations

A glaring drawback of power calculations is that they are based on dichotomous statistical testing (technically, Neyman-Pearson hypothesis testing for statistical decisions), and as such they promulgate the "dichotomania" that is characteristic of significance testing, classifying the results of a quantitative exercise into two ultimate categories, significant or not significant. This type of thinking allows divergent conclusions to be drawn from possible study results that might differ little, but with the two results falling on different sides of the demarcation for significance. This critical limitation has been described in detail above.

Relying on power calculations can also lead to overestimation of a study's informativeness. For example, if a study is planned to have 90% power with $\alpha = 5\%$ and the effect is postulated to be a rate ratio of 3.0, the power calculations imply that the study will give statistically significant results with 90% probability, assuming that the statistical model used applies (a tall assumption) and that all other relevant factors, such as control of confounding, are sufficiently taken into account. Imagine that the actual effect is just what was assumed, a rate ratio of 3.0, and the study is conducted at the size that corresponds to 90% power. If the estimated rate ratio had been instead 1.9 or less (which would occur 9% of the time with a true rate ratio of 3), that result would have $P > 0.05$ by the null test and so be easily mistaken for supporting the null (a Type II error). But if the estimate were 1.9, the confidence interval around it would include 3 as well as 1, showing that the result is inconclusive according to the $\alpha = 5\%$ criterion. More generally, a study will be incapable of discriminating between the null and the alternative at a rate equal to the false-negative rate, not the false-positive rate, and thus a study "powerful" by the usual weak standards will often produce results that are ambiguous when interpreted correctly.

Another drawback of power calculations is that they are highly dependent on the alternative chosen for the calculation. Those wanting to claim high power need only use a large value for the alternative, at least up to the point before it becomes obvious they are "gaming" the calculation. Conversely, those wishing to condemn a study as "underpowered" need to only select a small alternative. In reality, the informativeness of a study grows progressively with increasing association or effect size and should be viewed on a continuum. One step toward this goal when planning studies is to plot power against alternatives and do so for different possible study sizes. A power curve graphs study power against effect size and shows the continuous relation between the two.

For all the above reasons and more, power calculations can be misleading when *analyzing study designs and study* data.[47-49,107] These problems lead to considering study precision directly for design as well as for analysis,[100,108] as described next.

Factors Influencing Study Precision

Various factors affect precision of an effect estimate in a study; these are related to study design features and the analytic methods used. For that reason, there are numerous different formulas, mostly based on statistical power, but referred to as "sample size" formulas, that are used to calculate the study size. We do not cover the range of formulas that apply to the entire spectrum of epidemiologic research designs, but below we give a simple general formula to illustrate the inputs needed. Suppose we are planning a cohort study that is intended to measure and compare risk in two groups, so that the denominators are the number of persons in each exposure group. This situation will also include randomized trials that measure outcomes as risks. A simple formula for study size for this type of study was given by Kelsey et al.[109]:

$$N_1 = \frac{\left(Z_{\alpha/2} + Z_\beta\right)^2 p(1-p)(R+1)}{D^2 R}$$

[15-1]

where

N_1 = size of exposed cohort
$R = N_0/N_1$ = ratio of size of unexposed cohort, N_0, to size of exposed cohort, N_1
$Z^{\alpha/2}$ = standard normal deviate corresponding to the alpha level of the hypothesis test
Z^β = standard normal deviate corresponding to the desired study power
p_1 = proportion of exposed cohort hypothesized to develop disease
p_0 = proportion of unexposed cohort expected to develop disease
$p = (p_1 + Rp_0)/(R+1)$
$D = p_1 - p_0$

Notice what must be postulated to compute the study size:

1. the desired power of the study $(1 - \beta)$,
2. an alpha level for a significance test,
3. the relative size of the unexposed and exposed cohorts, R,
4. the risk among unexposed, p_0, and
5. either p_1 or the hypothesized RD, D

If the investigator is interested in estimating an RR from a study instead of an RD, then Equation 15-1 can still be used, by solving $p_1 = RRp_0$. If the cohort study is aiming to measure rates rather than risks, this formula can still be used as a rough approximation by converting the amount of person-time to person denominators N_1 and N_0 by multiplying the person-time by the anticipated average amount of time followed.

Equation 15-1 can also be used to calculate the size of a case-control study. To do so, one would redefine N_1 and N_0 as the size of the case group and control group, respectively, and p_1 and p_0 will be the proportion of cases and controls, respectively, that are exposed. If the study is planned based on an anticipated odds ratio, OR $= p_1(1 - p_0)/[p_0(1 - p_1)]$, then one needs to specify p_0 and the OR and solve for p_1:

$$P_1 = \frac{ORp_0}{1 - p_0 + ORp_0} \qquad [15\text{-}2]$$

When case-control studies involve individual matching retained in the analysis, any matched set that is completely concordant for exposure (that is, if the case and all matched controls have the same exposure value) is effectively lost to the study, as that set contributes no information about the conditional odds ratio. Thus, study size calculations for matched case-control studies are affected by the degree of correlation between the matching factors and the exposure, as well as the ratio of controls to cases. Power and study size formulas for matched case-control data were presented by Miettinen.[110]

Estimating Study Size Based on the Confidence Interval Width

Instead of statistical power, one can plan a study by anticipating the study precision directly.[111] Specifically, one can postulate the desired width of the study confidence interval and examine how that varies with the study size. If we start with the formulas that are used to obtain confidence intervals and set them equal to a desired width, we can solve these equations for the study size. The particular formula to use will depend on which of the three types of data will be involved in the study: (1) risk data with person denominators; (2) rate data with person-time denominators; or (3) case-control data. For each type of data, there will be a formula for a difference measure of effect and another formula for a ratio measure of effect. Case-control studies are an exception, as there is no difference measure.

For difference measures, the asymptotic confidence interval is obtained from

$$\widehat{RD} \pm Z \cdot SD\left(\widehat{RD}\right) \qquad [15\text{-}3]$$

where $\widehat{RD}$ is the point estimate of the risk or rate difference, Z is the value from a standard normal distribution corresponding to the level of confidence (e.g., 1.96 for 95% CI), and $SD\left(\widehat{RD}\right)$ is the standard deviation (also referred to as the standard error) of the estimate.

The corresponding formula for the risk, rate, or odds ratio is

$$e^{\ln(\widehat{RR}) + Z \cdot SD\left[\ln(\widehat{RR})\right]}$$

[15-4]

For a simple approach to estimating study size from these expressions, we can assume that crude data will be the basis for the analysis. This assumption may overstate the precision of the result, as control for confounding often costs some precision. We will also assume that there are no missing data. The effects of these assumptions might need to be considered in the final study planning.

To obtain the study size that corresponds to a given confidence interval width, some design features and other factors must be specified. In a cohort study, these specifications include the following:

1. the risk or rate among unexposed (p_0 for risk, I_0 for rate),
2. the risk or rate among exposed (p_1 or I_1),
3. the relative size of the unexposed and exposed cohorts, R,
4. the desired level of precision, and
5. the confidence level.

For item 2 above, if the rate difference or rate ratio is specified, p_1 or I_1 can be calculated from the difference or ratio and from p_0 or I_0. For item 3, the relative size of the cohorts, R, will be expressed as the ratio of the size of the unexposed cohort to that of the exposed cohort. N_1 will be the size of the exposed cohort and N_0 the size of the unexposed cohort, with $R = N_0/N_1$. For risk data, N_1 will represent people and for rate data, N_1 will represent person-time. The desired level of precision can be expressed in various ways; here we will express precision as the absolute width of the confidence interval for difference measures of effect, and as the ratio of the upper confidence limit to the lower confidence limit for ratio measures of effect. The level of confidence corresponds to Z in the confidence interval formulas above; Z is the value of the standard normal distribution such that the area under the curve from $-Z$ to $+Z$ equals the confidence level. Z is 1.96 for a 95% confidence interval.

For case-control studies, we use a slight variation in the above list. Rather than risk or rates, p_1 and p_0 refer to the respective exposure prevalences among cases and controls. Alternatively, we can specify p_0 and the odds ratio, OR, from which p_1 can be calculated as

$$p_1 = \left. OR p_0 \middle/ \left(1 - p_0 + OR p_0\right)\right.$$

Standard error formulas used for risk and rate differences, risk and rate ratios, and odds ratio are given in Table 15-2. From these, the study size formulas can readily be derived (Table 15-3). As an example, consider a study based on risk data and focused on RD as the measure of interest. Denoting F as the absolute width of the RD that we desire to achieve for a study's confidence interval, we can solve for N_1 as:

$$N_1 = \frac{4Z^2\left[Rp_1\left(1 - p_1\right) + p_0\left(1 - p_0\right)\right]}{RF^2}$$

[15-5]

Suppose that $p_1 = 0.4$ and $p_0 = 0.3$, corresponding to an RD of 0.1. If we plan a study with three times as many unexposed as exposed people ($R = 3$), and we wish the 90% confidence interval to span a distance of 0.08 (so $Z = 1.645$), Equation 15-5 gives a value for N_1 of 524 people and a total for the study size of $524 + 1,573 = 2,097$. With a study of this size, the SD(RD) would be 0.0243, and half of a 90% confidence interval would be equal to $1.645 \times 0.0243 \approx 0.04$, giving a full confidence interval with a width of about 0.08.

Similarly, the same study could be planned with respect to desired precision for the RR. For ratio measures, it is convenient to specify the precision in terms of the magnitude of the ratio of the upper bound to the lower bound, which leads to a constant width on the log scale. For example,

TABLE 15-2

Standard Deviation Formulas for Crude Measures of Epidemiologic Effect

Risk difference
a = exposed cases
b = unexposed cases
N_1 = total exposed people
N_0 = total unexposed people

$$SD\left(\widehat{RD}\right) = \sqrt{\frac{a\left(N_1 - a\right)}{N_1^3} + \frac{b\left(N_0 - b\right)}{N_0^3}}$$

Risk ratio (on log scale)
a = exposed cases
b = unexposed cases
N_1 = total exposed people
N_0 = total unexposed people

$$SD\left[\ln\left(\widehat{RD}\right)\right] = \sqrt{\frac{1}{a} - \frac{1}{N_1} + \frac{1}{b} - \frac{1}{N_0}}$$

Incidence rate difference
a = exposed cases
b = unexposed cases
N_1 = total exposed person-time
N_0 = total unexposed person-time

$$SD\left(\widehat{IRD}\right) = \sqrt{\frac{a}{N_1^2} + \frac{b}{N_0^2}}$$

Incidence rate ratio (log scale)
a = exposed cases
b = unexposed cases
N_1 = total exposed person-time
N_0 = total unexposed person-time

$$SD\left[\ln\left(\widehat{IRR}\right)\right] = \sqrt{\frac{1}{a} + \frac{1}{b}}$$

Odds ratio (case-control study, log scale)
a = exposed cases
b = unexposed cases
c = exposed controls
d = unexposed controls

$$SD\left[\ln\left(\widehat{OR}\right)\right] = \sqrt{\frac{1}{a} + \frac{1}{b} + \frac{1}{c} + \frac{1}{d}}$$

Adapted from Rothman KJ. *Epidemiology, an Introduction.* 2nd ed. New York, NY: Oxford University Press; 2012:chap 9. Formulas 9-2 to 9-6.

the following confidence intervals all have the same precision, with a ratio of upper/lower bound of 2:1.0 to 2.0, 1.5 to 3.0, 0.8 to 1.6, etc. The formula for study size of a cohort study with person denominators giving a fixed value for the ratio of the upper to lower bound for RR confidence interval is

$$N_1 = \frac{4Z^2\left[Rp_0\left(1 - p_1\right) + p_1\left(1 - p_0\right)\right]}{Rp_1p_0\left[\ln\left(F\right)\right]^2} \qquad [15\text{-}6]$$

where F is the desired ratio of upper to lower bound for the confidence interval. If we wish F to be 2, and assuming again that $p_1 = 0.4$ and $p_0 = 0.3$, $R = 3$, and this time using a 95% confidence interval, so that $Z = 1.96$, Equation 15-6 gives a value for N_1 of 73 people and a total study size of 291 people. This size should produce 95% confidence intervals that on the average will have an upper bound that is approximately twice the magnitude of the lower bound. If a study of this size produced results that were equal to the expected risks in the exposed and unexposed groups, we would have 29 exposed cases and 66 unexposed cases, and the 95% confidence interval for the RR would be about 0.93 to 1.86.

Table 15-3 gives all five study size formulas based on the width of the confidence interval, according to the type of data and type of effect measure. Figure 15-8 illustrates the use of the formulas with a graph showing the relation between size of a cohort study measuring risks and the width of a confidence interval for two values of p_0.

Estimating Study Size Based on the Probability That Upper Confidence Bound Stays Below a Level of Concern

Another way to use precision to plan the size of a study arises when the aim is to provide reassurance about the absence of a strong effect. No study can provide evidence for the absence of a small effect, but it is feasible and reasonable to plan a study aimed at indicating the low compatibility between study results and strong effects, when there is a strong prior of little or no effect. In this situation, one can choose an effect level of practical concern and aim to design the study to produce a confidence interval with an upper bound below that demarcation point. Equation 15-7 and equations in Table 15-3, can be used for this calculation, with two small modifications: (1) $4Z^2$ must be replaced with $(Z' + Z)^2$, where Z' is the value of the cumulative normal distribution that corresponds to the desired probability that the upper confidence bound is below the demarcation point chosen and (2) the value of F in the formulas should be the demarcation point, rather than the width of the confidence interval. For example, if one wishes to have 90% probability that the upper

TABLE 15-3

Study Size Formulas Based on the Width of Confidence Interval

Risk data, estimating risk difference

$$N_1 = \frac{4Z^2 \left[Rp_1 (1-p_1) + p_0(1-p_0) \right]}{RF^2}$$

Risk data, estimating risk ratio

$$N_1 = \frac{4Z^2 \left[Rp_0 (1-p_1) + p_1(1-p_0) \right]}{Rp_1 p_0 \left[\ln(F) \right]^2}$$

Rate data, estimating rate difference

$$N_1 = \frac{4Z^2 \left(RI_1 + I_0 \right)}{RF^2}$$

Rate data, estimating rate ratio

$$N_1 = \frac{4Z^2 \left(RI_0 + I_1 \right)}{RI_1 I_0 \left[\ln(F) \right]^2}$$

Case-control data, estimating odds ratio

$$M_1 = \frac{4Z^2 \left[Rp_0(1-p_0) + p_1(1-p_1) \right]}{\left[\ln(F) \right]^2 \left[Rp_1 p_0 (1-p_1)(1-p_0) \right]}$$

N_1 = size of the exposed cohort (persons or person-time).
M_1 = size of case group in the case-control study.
R = size of the unexposed cohort divided by size of the exposed cohort; in the case-control study, size of the control group divided by size of the case group.
p_1 = risk in the exposed cohort; in the case-control study, exposure prevalence in cases.
p_0 = risk in the unexposed cohort; in the case-control study, exposure prevalence in controls.
I_1 = rate in the exposed cohort.
I_0 = rate in the unexposed cohort.
F = width of the desired confidence interval.

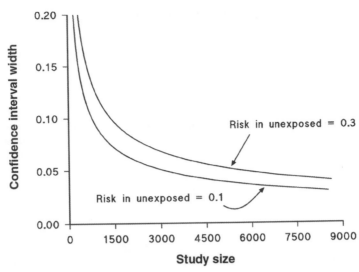

FIGURE 15-8 Study size in relation to 95% confidence interval width for two cohorts of equal size with a risk difference of 0.1.

bound for a rate ratio in a cohort study is below 2.0, assuming that the exposure has no effect, Z' would be 1.282, F would be 2, and the study size for a rate-data study using 95% confidence limits with a rate of 10 cases per 1,000 person-years among unexposed and among exposed, and equal sized exposed and unexposed cohorts, would be 4,374 person-years in each of the two cohorts, for a total of 8,748 person-years. If a study of this size had results equal to the expected value (44 cases in each of the two cohorts), the 95% confidence interval would be about 0.66 to 1.52, with an upper bound well below 2. However, the point estimate will be below 1.3 with 90% probability under the conditions assumed, and the upper bound of the 95% confidence interval would be 2.0 when the point estimate is 1.3.

Summary

Power as a planning tool for study size perpetuates the drawbacks of statistical significance testing. These drawbacks include the temptation to dichotomize study results into qualitative categories that notoriously have led to misinterpreting nonsignificant findings to be support for the null hypothesis and misinterpreting small, precise significant findings to be strong evidence against the null.

The formulas presented here for planning study size are keyed to the anticipated precision of the study and are consistent with the objective of accurate estimation and the inferential goal of interpreting findings as continuous measures that are estimated with varying degrees of precision. Study size is a central determinant of the precision of study results, and it is natural to consider a study's precision in determining or anticipating the size of a study. Given the many unknown elements in implementing an epidemiologic study, the formulas here provide rough approximations, based on a simple crude analysis of data. Consequently, the results are likely to be underestimates of the study size needed for the intended precision in the light of actual data. In particular, control of confounding will usually widen the confidence interval, and missing data will also reduce precision. The degree of loss of precision from these factors will depend on the circumstances of a particular study.

Planning the size of a study requires as input some information that the study itself is intended to elucidate, such as the risk among unexposed and the effect size. This input is needed regardless of whether one is computing study size based on power or on precision. Uncertainty about these values can be addressed by graphing curves for different assumed values of these parameters, as in Figure 15-8. Another possible approach to addressing uncertainty about risks and effects would be to postulate a distribution for these parameters and to use Monte Carlo simulation, drawing repeated samples from the assumed distribution, to estimate study precision. The Monte Carlo method could also be used to extend these formulas, which apply only to dichotomous exposures. Using a Monte Carlo approach, one could assess the precision of more complicated analyses, such as precision in estimating trends in effect over a range of exposure levels, results from stratified analyses, or results affected by systematic errors (see Chapter 29).

References

1. Greenland S. Randomization, statistics, and causal inference. *Epidemiology*. 1990;1:421-429.
2. Greenland S. Multiple-bias modeling for analysis of observational data (with discussion). *J R Stat Soc Ser A*. 2005;168:267-308.
3. Gigerenzer G. Mindless statistics. *J Socioeconomics*. 2004;33:567-606.
4. Goodman SN. P Values, hypothesis tests, and likelihood: implications for epidemiology of a neglected historical debate. *Am J Epidemiol*. 1993;137:485-496.
5. Berkson J. Some difficulties of interpretation encountered in the application of the chi-square test. *J Am Stat Assoc*. 1938;33:526-536.
6. Berkson J. Tests of significance considered as evidence. *J Am Statist Assoc* 1942;37:325-335. Reprinted in *Int J Epidemiol*. 2003;32:687-691.
7. Boring EG. Mathematical versus statistical importance. *Psychol Bull*. 1919;16:335-338.
8. Hogben L. *Statistical Theory*. London: Allen and Unwin; 1957.
9. Wasserstein RL, Lazar NA. The ASA statement on p-values: context, process, and purpose. *Am Stat*. 2016;70(2):129-133. doi:10.1080/00031305.2016.1154108.
10. Greenland S, Senn SJ, Rothman KJ, et al. Statistical tests, P values, confidence intervals, and power: a guide to misinterpretations (2016). *Eur J Epidemiol*. 2016;31:337-350. doi:10.1007/s10654-016-0149-3.
11. Lash TL. The harm done to reproducibility by the culture of null hypothesis significance testing. *Am J Epidemiol*. 2017;186:627-635.
12. McShane BB, Gal D. Statistical significance and the dichotomization of evidence. *JASA*. 2017;112:885-908.
13. Altman DG, Machin D, Bryant TN, Gardner MJ, eds. *Statistics With Confidence*. 2nd ed. London: BMJ Books; 2000.
14. Berger JO, Berry DA. Statistical analysis and the illusion of objectivity. *Am Scientist*. 1988;76:159-165.
15. Goodman SN, Royall R. Evidence and scientific research. *Am J Public Health*. 1988;78:1568-1574.
16. Greenland S. Bayesian perspectives for epidemiologic research. I. Foundations and basic methods (with comment and reply). *Int J Epidemiol*. 2006;35:765-778.
17. Royall R. *Statistical Inference: A Likelihood Paradigm*. New York, NY: Chapman and Hall; 1997.
18. Stang A, Deckert M, Poole C, Rothman KJ. Statistical inference in abstracts of major medical and epidemiology journals 1975-2014: a systematic review. *Eur J Epidemiol*. 2017;32:21-29.
19. Cox DR, Hinkley DV. *Theoretical Statistics*. New York, NY: Chapman and Hall; 1974.
20. Fisher RA. Note on Dr. Berkson's criticism of tests of significance. *J Am Statist Assoc*. 1943;38:103-104. Reprinted in *Int J Epidemiol*. 2003;32:692.
21. Berger JO, Delampady M. Testing precise hypotheses (with discussion). *Stat Sci*. 1987;2:317-352.
22. Berger JO, Sellke T. Testing a point null hypothesis: the irreconcilability of P values and evidence (with discussion). *J Am Stat Assoc*. 1987;82:112-139.
23. Casella G, Berger RL. Reconciling Bayesian and frequentist evidence in the one-sided testing problem. *J Am Stat Assoc*. 1987;82:106-111.
24. Greenland S, Gustafson P. Adjustment for independent nondifferential misclassification does not increase certainty that an observed association is in the correct direction. *Am J Epidemiol*. 2006;164:63-68.
25. Edwards AWF. *Likelihood*. 2nd ed. Baltimore, MD: Johns Hopkins University Press; 1992.
26. Freedman DA. Statistics and the scientific method. In: Mason W, Feinberg SE, eds. *Cohort Analysis and Social Research*. New York, NY: Springer-Verlag; 1985:345-390.
27. Freedman DA, Pisani R, Purves R. *Statistics*. 4th ed. New York, NY: Norton; 2007.
28. Lehmann EL. *Testing Statistical Hypotheses*. 2nd ed. New York, NY: Wiley; 1986.
29. Goodman SN. A comment on replication, p-values and evidence. *Stat Med*. 1992;11:875-879.
30. Freiman JA, Chalmers TC, Smith H, Kuebler RR. The importance of beta, the type II error and sample size in the design and interpretation of the randomized control trial. *N Engl J Med*. 1978;299:690-694.
31. Greenland S. Invited commentary: the need for cognitive science in methodology. *Am J Epidemiol*. 2017;186:639-645.
32. Atkins L, Jarrett D. The significance of "significance tests". In: Irvine J, Miles I, Evans J, eds. *Demystifying Social Statistics*. London: Pluto Press; 1979.
33. Blackwelder WC. Equivalence trials. In: Armitage P, Colton T, eds. *Encyclopedia of Biostatistics*. New York, NY: John Wiley and Sons, Inc; 1998.

34. Motulsky HJ. Common misconceptions about data analysis and statistics. *Br J Pharmacol.* 2015;172:2126-2132.

35. Rothman KJ. Significance questing. *Ann Intern Med.* 1986;105:445-447.

36. Simmons JP, Nelson LD, Simonsohn U. False-positive psychology: undisclosed flexibility in data collection and analysis allows presenting anything as significant. *Psychol Sci.* 2011;22:1359-1366.

37. Bandt CL, Boen JR. A prevalent misconception about sample size, statistical significance, and clinical importance. *J Periodontol.* 1972;43:181-183.

38. Birnbaum A. A unified theory of estimation, I. *Ann Math Stat.* 1961;32:112-135.

39. Miettinen OS. *Theoretical Epidemiology*. New York, NY: Wiley; 1985.

40. Poole C. Beyond the confidence interval. *Am J Public Health.* 1987;77:195-199.

41. Folks JF. *Ideas of Statistics*. New York, NY: Wiley; 1981.

42. Sullivan KM, Foster DA. Use of the confidence interval function. *Epidemiology.* 1990;1:39-42.

43. Poole C. Confidence intervals exclude nothing. *Am J Public Health.* 1987;77:492-493.

44. Poole C. Low P-values or narrow confidence intervals: which are more durable?. *Epidemiology.* 2001;12:291-294.

45. Altman DG, Bland JM. Absence of evidence is not evidence of absence. *Br Med J.* 1995;311:485.

46. Cox DR. *The Planning of Experiments*. New York, NY: Wiley; 1958:161.

47. Goodman SN, Berlin J. The use of predicted confidence intervals when planning experiments and the misuse of power when interpreting results. *Ann Intern Med.* 1994;121:200-206.

48. Hoenig JM, Heisey DM. The abuse of power: the pervasive fallacy of power calculations for data analysis. *Am Stat.* 2001;55:19-24.

49. Senn S. Power is indeed irrelevant in interpreting completed studies. *Br Med J.* 2002;325:1304.

50. Smith AH, Bates MN. Confidence limit analyses should replace power calculations in the interpretation of epidemiologic studies. *Epidemiol.* 1992;3:449-452.

51. Eisenberger MA, Blumenstein BA, Crawford ED, et al. Bilateral orchiectomy with or without flutamide for metastatic prostate cancer. *N Engl J Med.* 1998;339:1036-1042.

52. Prostate Cancer Trialists' Collaborative Group. Maximum androgen blockade in advanced prostate cancer: an overview of 22 randomised trials with 3283 deaths in 5710 patients. *Lancet.* 1995;346:265-269.

53. Rothman KJ, Johnson ES, Sugano DS. Is flutamide effective in patients with bilateral orchiectomy? *Lancet.* 1999;353:1184.

54. Stampfer MJ, Kang JH, Chen J, Cherry R, Grodstein F. Effects of moderate alcohol consumption on cognitive function in women. *N Engl J Med.* 2005;352:245-253.

55. Collins FS, Tabak LA. Policy: NIH plans to enhance reproducibility. *Nature.* 2014;505(7485):612-613.

56. Nosek BA, Alter G, Banks GC, et al. Promoting an open research culture. *Science.* 2015;348(6242):1422-1425.

57. Lash TL, Collin LJ, Van Dyke ME. The replication crisis in epidemiology: snowball, snow job, or winter solstice?. *Curr Epidemiol Rep.* 2018;5:175-183.

58. Open Science Collaboration. Estimating the reproducibility of psychological science. *Science.* 2015;349(6251):aac4716.

59. Gelman A, Stern H. The difference between "significant" and "not significant" is not itself statistically significant. *Am Statistician.* 2006;60:328-331.

60. Rothman KJ, Lanes S, Robins J. Causal inference. *Epidemiology.* 1993;4(6):555-556.

61. Seliger C, Meier CR, Becker C, et al. Statin use and risk of glioma: population-based case–control analysis. *Eur J Epidemiol.* 2016;31(9):947-952.

62. Brown HK, Ray JG, Wilton AS, Lunsky Y, Gomes T, Vigod SN. Association between serotonergic antidepressant use during pregnancy and autism spectrum disorder in children. *J Am Med Assoc.* 2017;317(15):1544-1552.

63. Rozeboom WM. The fallacy of null-hypothesis significance test. *Psych Bull.* 1960;57:416-428.

64. Morrison DE, Henkel RE, eds. *The Significance Test Controversy*. Chicago, IL: Aldine; 1970.

65. Wulff HR. Confidence limits in evaluating controlled therapeutic trials. *Lancet.* 1973;2:969-970.

66. Rothman KJ. A show of confidence. *N Engl J Med.* 1978;299:1362-1363.

67. Salsburg DS. The religion of statistics as practiced in medical journals. *Am Statist.* 1985;39:220-223.

68. Simon R, Wittes RE. Methodologic guidelines for reports of clinical trials. *Cancer Treat Rep.* 1985;69:1-3.

69. Langman MJS. Towards estimation and confidence intervals. *Br Med J.* 1986;292:716.

70. Gardner MA, Altman DG. Confidence intervals rather than P values: estimation rather than hypothesis testing. *Br Med J.* 1986;292:746-750.

71. Walker AM. Reporting the results of epidemiologic studies. *Am J Public Health.* 1986;76:556-558.

72. Oakes M. *Statistical Inference*. Chestnut Hill, MA: ERI; 1990.

73. Ware JH, Mosteller F, Ingelfinger JA. *P values*. In: *Medical Uses of Statistics*. Waltham, MA: NEJM Books; 1986.

74. Pocock SJ, Hughes MD, Lee RJ. Statistical problems in the reporting of clinical trials. *N Eng J Med*. 1987;317:426-432.
75. Thompson WD. Statistical criteria in the interpretation of epidemiologic data. *Am J Public Health*. 1987;77:191-194.
76. Evans SJW, Mills P, Dawson J. The end of the P-value? *Br Heart J*. 1988;60:177-180.
77. Anscombe FJ. The summarizing of clinical experiments by significance levels. *Stat Med*. 1990;9:703-708.
78. Cohen J. The earth is round ($P < 0.05$). *Am Psychol*. 1994;47:997-1003.
79. Hauer E. The harm done by tests of significance. *Accid Anal Prev*. 2003;36:495-500.
80. Ziliak ST, McCloskey DN. Size matters: the standard error of regressions in the American Economic Review. *J Socio-Economics*. 2004;33:527-546.
81. Batterham AM, Hopkins WG. Making meaningful inferences about magnitudes. *Int J Sports Physiol Perform*. 2006;1:50-57.
82. Marshall SW. Commentary on making meaningful inferences about magnitudes. *Sportscience*. 2006;9:43-44.
83. Lash TL, Fox MP, Greenland S, et al. Re: promoting healthy skepticism in the news. Helping journalists get it right. *J Natl Cancer Inst*. 2010;102:829-830.
84. Berger JO, Wolpert RL. *The Likelihood Principle*. 2nd ed. Hayward, CA: Institute of Mathematical Statistics; 1988.
85. Clayton D, Hills M. *Statistical Models in Epidemiology*. New York, NY: Oxford University Press; 1993.
86. DeFinetti B. *The Theory of Probability*. Vol 1. New York, NY: Wiley; 1974.
87. Howson C, Urbach P. *Scientific Reasoning: The Bayesian Approach*. 2nd ed. LaSalle, IL: Open Court; 1993.
88. Greenland S. Probability logic and probabilistic induction. *Epidemiology*. 1998;9:322-332.
89. Savage LJ. *The Foundations of Statistics*. New York, NY: Dover; 1972.
90. Freedman DA. As others see us: a case study in path analysis (with discussion). *J Educ Stat*. 1987;12:101-223.
91. Spiegelhalter DJ, Abrams KR, Myles JP. *Bayesian Approaches to Clinical Trials and Health-Care Evaluation*. New York, NY: Wiley; 2004.
92. Gelman A, Carlin JB, Stern HS, Rubin DB. *Bayesian Data Analysis*. 2nd ed. New York, NY: Chapman and Hall/CRC; 2003.
93. Rubin DB. Bayesianly justifiable and relevant frequency calculations. *Ann Stat*. 1984;12:1151-1172.
94. Rubin DB. Practical implications of modes of statistical inference for causal effects, and the critical role of the assignment mechanism. *Biometrics*. 1991;47:1213-1234.
95. Greenland S. A semi-Bayes approach to the analysis of correlated multiple associations, with an application to an occupational cancer-mortality study. *Stat Med*. 1992;11:219-230.
96. Schlesselman JJ. Sample size requirements in cohort and case-control studies of disease. *Am J Epidemiol*. 1974;99(6):381-384.
97. Rothman KJ, Boice JD. *Epidemiologic Analysis with a Programmable Calculator*. 2nd ed. Newton, MA: Epidemiology Resources; 1982.
98. Greenland S. Power, sample size and smallest detectable effect determination for multivariate studies. *Stat Med*. 1985;4(2):117-127.
99. Greenland S. On sample-size and power calculations for studies using confidence intervals. *Am J Epidemiol*. 1988;128(1):231-237.
100. Greenland S. On sample-size and power calculations for studies using confidence intervals. *Am J Epidemiol*. 1988;128:231-237.
101. Walter SD. Determination of significant relative risks and optimal sampling procedures in prospective and retrospective comparative studies of various sizes. *Am J Epidemiol*. 1977;105:387-397.
102. Rothman KJ, Mosquin PL: Sparse-data bias accompanying overly fine stratification in an analysis of beryllium exposure and lung cancer risk. *Ann Epidemiol*. 2013;23(2):43-48. doi:10.1016/j.annepidem.2012.11.005.
103. Fink AK, Lash TL. A null association between smoking during pregnancy and breast cancer using Massachusetts registry data (United States). *Cancer Causes Control*. 2003;14:497-503.
104. Greenland S, Mansournia MA, Altman DG. Sparse-data bias: a problem hiding in plain sight. *Br Med J*. 2016;353:i1981. doi:10.1136/bmj.i1981.
105. Neyman J. Frequentist probability and frequentist statistics. *Synthese*. 1977;36:97-131.
106. Lakens D, Adolfi FG, Albers CJ, et al. Justify your alpha. *Nat Hum Behav*. 2018;2:168-171.
107. Greenland S. Nonsignificance plus high power does not imply support for the null over the alternative. *Ann Epidemiol*. 2012;22:364-368.
108. Bland JM. The tyranny of power: is there a better way to calculate sample size? *Br Med J*. 2009;339:b3985.

109. Kelsey JL, Thompson WD, Evans AS. *Methods in Observational Epidemiology*. New York, NY: Oxford University Press; 1986:chap 10.
110. Miettinen OS. Individual matching with multiple controls in the case of all or none responses. *Biometrics*. 1969;25:339-355.
111. Rothman KJ, Greenland S. Planning study size based on precision rather than power. *Epidemiology*. 2018;29:599-603.

PART III

Data Analysis

CHAPTER 16

Fundamentals of Epidemiologic Data Analysis

Sebastien Haneuse and Kenneth J. Rothman[*]

ELEMENTS OF DATA ANALYSIS

In Chapter 15, we emphasized that a study may be thought of as a measurement exercise, in which the overall goal is accuracy in estimation. Data analysis is the step in this exercise in which the raw data are initially checked for accuracy and, then, coupled with assumptions about the forces that led to those data, used to compute estimates as well as measures of accuracy (or, equivalently, uncertainty). Toward this, this chapter first describes considerations in data preparation. It then reviews the statistical theory that underpins conventional statistical methods, by which we mean methods that assume all systematic errors are known and accounted for by the adopted statistical model. Such methods focus on accounting for random errors by familiar means such as standard errors, confidence intervals, hypothesis tests, and *P*-values. These methods became the standard of analysis in the early to mid-20th century, in parallel with the ascendance of random sampling and randomization as the "gold standard" of study design.

A good data analysis has several distinct stages. In the first stage, the investigator should review the recorded data for accuracy, consistency, and completeness. This process is often referred to as *data editing* or *data cleaning*. Next, the investigator should summarize the data in a concise form for descriptive analysis, such as contingency tables that classify the observations according to key factors. This stage of the analysis is referred to as data reduction or *data summarization*. Finally, the data are used to estimate measures of epidemiologic interest, typically one or more measures

---

[*]This chapter is based on original material by Sander Greenland and Kenneth J. Rothman.

of occurrence or effect (such as risk or relative-risk estimates), with appropriate confidence intervals. This estimation stage is usually based on smoothing or modeling of the data, which can lead to many philosophical as well as technical issues[1]; see Chapters 19 through 27. Also a part of this stage of analysis is statistical hypothesis testing. As discussed earlier in this book, statistical hypothesis testing is undesirable in most epidemiologic situations. Nevertheless, because the statistical theory and methods of confidence intervals parallel those of statistical hypothesis testing, it is useful to study the theory and methods of statistical hypothesis testing as part of the foundation for understanding the estimation step of data analysis.

The final step of analysis involves properly interpreting the results from the summarization and estimation steps. This step requires consideration of unmeasured factors that may have influenced subject selection, measurement, and risk, as well as issues in statistical inference. These considerations are usually in the form of a description of possible unmeasured factors, along with qualitative judgments about their possible importance and impact. Chapter 29 describes ways in which these considerations can be given a more quantitative form.

DATA EDITING

The first task of data analysis is careful scrutiny of the raw data for errors and correction of such errors whenever possible. Errors find their way into data in a variety of ways; some errors are detectable in editing and some are not. Although often overlooked or minimized, this is an essential step because the quality of the data forms the basis for validity and accuracy of all remaining stages of the analysis.

The data in an epidemiologic study typically come from self-administered or interviewer-administered questionnaires; from existing records that are transcribed for research; or, from electronic databases collected for purposes other than research (such as disease surveillance registries, administrative medical databases, or electronic health records). The data from these sources may be transcribed from this primary form to a code form for machine entry, or they may be electronically loaded directly from one database to a research database.

At the outset coding of responses is often necessary, either preemptively or posthoc. For example, occupational data obtained from interviews need to be classified into a manageable code, as does drug information, medical history, and many other types of data. Data on continuous variables such as age, although often grouped into broad categories for reporting purposes, should be recorded in a precise form rather than grouped because the actual values will allow greater flexibility at later stages in the analysis. For example, different groupings may be necessary for comparisons with other studies. In some settings, the specific choice of coding may be adopted to enhance accuracy. Year of birth, for example, may be preferable to age because it tends to be reported more accurately and does not change with time. Finally, some nominal-scale variables (*i.e.*, those that have only a limited number of possible values) can be precoded on the primary data-collection forms by prespecifying a limited number of response categories. For nominal-scale variables with many possible categories, however, such as country of birth or occupation, precoded questions may not be practical if full detail is desired and respondents may be asked to enter in the specific details.

If all data items can be precoded, it may be feasible to collect the data in a primary form that can be read directly by a machine, for example, by optical scanning. Otherwise, it will be necessary to translate the information on the primary data form before it is stored electronically. Such translation may introduce errors, but it also provides an opportunity to check for errors on the primary form. Alternatively, respondents can be asked to answer questionnaires made available to them on a computer or via the Internet. These data will still need to be edited to code open-response items.

During the coding process, it is desirable to avoid rewriting the data onto a secondary data form since this may generate additional transcription errors. The number of errors may be reduced, however, by coding the data as part of the computer entry process. Moreover, a computer program can be devised to prompt data entry item by item, displaying category codes on a terminal/device screen to assist in coding. If the data are coded and rewritten by hand, they will often require key entry anyway, unless they are coded onto optical-scanning sheets; consequently, direct data entry during coding reduces both costs and errors.

Whenever possible, data entry and data coding should be kept separate. Data entry should follow the original collection form as closely as possible. Computer algorithms should be used to code data from the entries, rather than relying on data entry personnel to perform the coding. For example, if age information is collected as date of birth, it should be entered as date of birth and then age at the study date can be calculated by the computer. Similarly, with fewer rewriting operations between the primary record and the machine-stored version, fewer errors are likely to occur. If rewriting is unavoidable, it is useful to assess the extent of coding errors in the rewritten form by coding a proportion of the data forms twice, specifically by two independent individuals. The information thus obtained can be used to judge the magnitude of any misclassification from coding errors and consequently bias in an analysis.

After entry and coding, basic editing of the data involves checking each variable for impossible or unusual values. For example, gender may be coded 1 for male and 2 for female, in which case, any other recorded value for gender will represent an error or an unknown value. Usually a separate value, such as −1 or 9, is used to designate an unknown value. It is preferable not to use a code of 0 if it can be avoided because nonnumeric codes (such as special missing-value codes) may be interpreted by some programs as a 0. Not assigning 0 as a specific code, not even for unknown information, makes it easier to detect data errors and missing information. Any inadmissible values should be checked against the primary data forms. Unusual values such as unknown gender or unusual age or birth year should also be checked. A good data entry program will provide for detection of such values.

The entire distribution of each variable should also be examined to see if it appears reasonable. In a typical residential population, one expects about half of the subjects to be male; if the subjects have, say, lung cancer, one might expect about 70% to be male; and if the subjects are a typical group of nurses, one might expect relatively few to be male. Deviations from expectations may signal important problems that might not otherwise come to light. For example, a programming error could shift all the data in each electronic record by one or more characters, thereby producing meaningless codes that might not be detected without direct visual inspection of data values. The potential for such errors heightens the need to check carefully the distribution of each variable during the editing of the data.

The editing checks described so far relate to each variable in the data being treated individually. In addition to such basic editing, it is usually desirable to check the consistency of codes for related variables. It is not impossible, but it would be unusual if a person aged 16 years had three children in the data or if an individual 2 m tall weighed less than 50 kg. Furthermore, a man should not have been hospitalized for hysterectomy nor a woman for a vasectomy. Thorough editing will involve many such consistency and logic checks and is best accomplished by computer programs designed to flag such errors,[2] although it can also be done by inspecting cross-tabulations.

It is also important to check the consistency of various distributions, in particular to take advantage of multiple sources of information about related phenomena. If exactly 84 women in a study are coded as "no menopause" for the variable "type of menopause" (coding: no menopause, surgical, drug-induced, natural), then it would be reassuring if exactly 84 are likewise coded as having no menopause for the variable "age at menopause" (for such a variable, the code "no menopause" should take a different code number from that assigned to unknown—e.g., −1 for no menopause and −9 for unknown).

An important advantage of coding and entering data through a computer program is the ability to require all data forms to be entered twice. The data entered in the second pass are compared with the data entered on the first pass, and inconsistencies are flagged and resolved in real time. Double data entry reduces keystroke errors and other data entry errors that affect data quality. A second advantage of entering data through a computer program is the ability to edit the data automatically during the entry process. Inadmissible or unusual values can be screened as they are entered, with the operator alerted accordingly. Related to this is that the data entry program can be written to check for consistency between variables and eliminate some potential inconsistencies by automatically supplying appropriate codes. For example, if a subject is premenopausal, the program can automatically supply the correct code for "age at menopause" and skip the question. On the other hand, it is safer to use the redundancy of the second question to guard against an error in the first. Nonetheless, even with sophisticated editing during data entry, it is still important to check the stored data for completeness and reasonableness of the distribution of each variable.

Even the most meticulous data-collection efforts can suffer from errors that are detectable during careful editing. If editing is planned as a routine part of handling the data, such errors need not cause serious problems. If editing is neglected, however, data errors may undermine subsequent analyses.

DATA DESCRIPTION AND SUMMARIZATION

Data analysis should begin with careful examination of the data distributions of the analysis variables (exposures, diseases, confounders, effect-measure modifiers). This examination can be done with tables, histograms, scatterplots, and/or any other visual aid. We wish to emphasize strongly, however, that these data descriptors should *not* include *P*-values, confidence intervals, or any other statistics designed for making inferences beyond the data. Unfortunately, many statistical packages automatically generate such inferential statistics with all descriptive statistics. This automation is hazardous for a number of reasons, not the least of which is that it invites one to treat inferential statistics as descriptions of the data. With few exceptions, the latter should be avoided because useful and correct interpretations of such statistics require some assumptions or a model about the relation of the data to some population or theoretical structure beyond the data. For example, interpretations of significance tests and confidence intervals refer to the "true value" of the association under study; this value does not exist in the data but in some target population or some theoretical model relating disease to exposure.

If descriptive statistics are not for inference beyond the data, what are they for? First, they can help identify data errors. There may be nothing unusual about having both women younger than 40 years and menopausal women in a dataset. However, if a cross-tabulation of age and menopausal status (premenopausal, natural, surgical) indicates that there are women in the dataset who are younger than 40 years and have had natural menopause, then the correctness of the age and menopausal status data should be (re)checked. Second, descriptive statistics can help anticipate violations of assumptions required by inferential statistics. In epidemiology, most inferential statistics are *large-sample* (asymptotic) statistics, meaning that they require certain numbers of subjects to be "large." For example, a rule of thumb for the validity of the ordinary (Pearson) chi-square (χ^2) test of association for two categorical variables is that expected values for each cell be at least four or five. Suppose, upon examining the observed data, one sees that there are fewer than eight subjects in some categories of an exposure. It is then likely that a cross-tabulation of exposure and disease will result in at least one cell with fewer than four expected subjects, calling into question whether the application of the Pearson χ^2 test will be valid. For such checking purposes, one will often want to return to the descriptive summaries after one has moved on to inferential statistics.

Data Tabulation

In many fields, means, medians, and other continuous measures of centrality are common data summaries. In epidemiology, however, contingency tables, in which the frequency of subjects (or units of observation) with specific combinations of key variable values is tabulated, are often reported. Indeed, such a table may contain essentially all the relevant information in the data, so that it will be all the investigator needs for estimation (see Chapter 17). Even if the table does not contain all relevant information, it can directly display relations among the main study variables. For continuous variables, such as age and diastolic blood pressure, scatterplots and other exploratory visual displays can provide further insights.[3]

Analysis of data in the form of a contingency table essentially assumes that there is at most only a small number of variables that are confounders or effect-measure modifiers. If one must adjust simultaneously for a large number of variables, an analysis based on regression modeling may be necessary. While we defer a broader treatment of regression to Chapters 20, 21, 22 and 24, we note here that examination of contingency tables and scatterplots can reveal whether the number of subjects is adequate for certain types of regression models and can also serve as a check on the validity of the regression analysis. Indeed, proceeding with an abridged analysis based on the contingency table data is essential even if one is certain that the final analysis will be based on a regression model.

Choice of Categories

In order to construct a contingency table, it may be necessary to collapse the edited data into categories. The process can be straightforward for nominal-scale variables, such as religion or ethnicity, which are already categorized. Some categories may be collapsed together when data are sparse, provided these combinations do not merge groups that are very heterogeneous with respect to the phenomena under study. For continuous variables, the investigator must decide how many categories to make and where the category boundaries should be. The number of categories will usually depend on the amount of data available. If the data are abundant, it is nearly always preferable to divide a variable into many categories. On the other hand, the purpose of data summarization is to present the data concisely and conveniently; creating too many categories will defeat this purpose.

For adequate control of confounding, about five categories may often suffice,[4] provided the boundaries are well chosen to reflect the size of the confounder effects expected across and within categories. As discussed later in this chapter and in Chapter 19, use of percentiles to create confounder categories (*e.g.*, using quintiles as boundaries to create five equal-sized categories) may fail to control confounding adequately if the variable is a strong confounder and is unevenly distributed (highly nonuniform) across its range. In that case, one or a few of the resulting confounder-percentile categories are likely to be overly broad, resulting in large confounder effects within those categories (where they will be uncontrolled) and leaving the exposure-effect estimates seriously confounded within those categories.

Similarly, if an exposure variable is categorized to examine effect estimates for various levels of exposure, again about five categories may often suffice, provided the boundaries are well chosen to reflect the size of the effects expected across the range of exposure. As discussed later in this chapter and in Chapter 19, use of percentiles to create the exposure categories may fail to capture exposure effects adequately if the exposure distribution is quite uneven. In that case, one or a few of the resulting exposure-percentile categories are likely to be overly broad, resulting in exposure effects aggregated within those categories (where they may go undetected) and diminished estimates of exposure effects across categories.

In some settings, it may be that the data are so sparse that it is impractical to use as many as five categories for a given variable. When the observations are stretched over too many categories, the numbers within categories become so small that patterns cannot be reliably discerned in the resulting cross-tabulation. Even if the number of categories per variable is only two or three, a large body of data can be spread too thin if the contingency table involves many dimensions, that is, if many variables are used to classify the subjects. As an example, suppose that we create a separate two-way table (or stratum) of a binary exposure and a binary disease for each possible combination of three potential confounders each of which have three. For this setting, this would result in consideration of $3^3 = 27$ confounding strata, for a total of $27 \times 4 = 108$ table cells. With an additional two confounders of three categories each, there will be $3^5 = 243$ strata, for a total of $243 \times 4 = 972$ cells. This will likely be enough to stretch even a considerable body of data quite thinly; a study of 1,000 people will average only about one subject per cell of the multidimensional table! Even more extreme is that if five categories are used for the five confounders, there will be $5^5 = 3,125$ strata, for a total of $3,125 \times 4 = 12,500$ cells.

There is no generally accepted method to decide where to draw the boundary between categories so that decisions must be made on a case-by-case basis. Because of this, a frequently expressed concern is that boundaries might be "gerrymandered," that is modified after a preliminary examination of the effect estimates in such a way that the estimates are altered to provide a desired conclusion. Gerrymandering can occur even when the analyst is attempting to be honest, simply through failure to understand the problems it may engender. For example, conventional statistical methods assume that boundaries were chosen independently of the outcome. Nonetheless, there are legitimate reasons for inspecting the variable distributions when selecting category boundaries. For example, when the cells are large but the data patterns are sensitive to a small shift in the category boundaries, this sensitivity is a finding of potential interest, indicating some special feature of the data distribution. There may be natural categories if the distribution has more than one mode. Nonetheless, it is best to select exposure and outcome categories without regard to the resulting estimates and test statistics; otherwise, the estimates will be biased and *P*-values invalid.

If meaningful category boundaries are inherent in the variable, these should be used whenever possible. For example, in categorizing subjects according to analgesic consumption, relevant categories will contrast the various therapeutic indications for analgesic use, for which the recommended doses can be specified in advance. It is often desirable, especially for an exposure variable, to retain extreme categories in the analysis without merging these with neighboring categories because the extreme categories are often those that permit the most biologically informative contrasts, provided enough subjects fall into these categories.

As mentioned earlier, one common method for creating category boundaries is to set the boundaries at fixed percentiles (quantiles) of the variable. For example, quintile categories have boundaries at the 20th, 40th, 60th, and 80th percentiles of the variable distribution. Although this categorization is sometimes adequate, such an automatic procedure can lead to misleading results in many situations. For example, for many occupational and environmental exposures, such as to electromagnetic fields, most people—over 90%—are exposed in a very narrow range. When this is so, there may be almost no difference in exposure among the first four of the quintile-formed categories, and the fifth high-exposure category may itself contain many persons with exposure little different from the lower categories. As a result, a comparison of risk will reveal no effect across the first four categories, and a diluted effect comparing the fifth to the fourth. The apparent absence of trend produced by such a quintile analysis may be taken as evidence against an effect, when in reality, it is only an artifact of using quintiles rather than biologically or physically meaningful categories.

In a parallel fashion, use of percentiles to create confounder categories can leave serious residual confounding when most of the confounder distribution is concentrated in a very narrow range, but the confounder effect is considerable across its entire range. In that case, there might be almost no difference in the confounder across all but one of the categories, while the remaining category may contain persons with vastly different confounder values. As a consequence, that category may yield a highly confounded estimate of exposure effect and produce bias in any summary estimate of exposure effect.

Another problem in creating categories is how to deal with the ends of the scale. Open-ended categories can provide an opportunity for considerable residual confounding, especially if there are no theoretical bounds for the variable. For example, age categories such as 65+ years, with no upper limit, allow a considerable range of variability within which the desired homogeneity of exposure or risk may not be achieved. Another example is the study of the effects of alcohol consumption on the risk of oral cancer. Control of tobacco use is essential; within the highest category of tobacco use, it is likely that the heaviest alcohol users will also be the heaviest smokers.[5] When residual confounding from open-ended categories is considered likely, we recommend that one place strict boundaries on every category, including those at the extremes of the scale; if sparse categories result, one should use sparse-data analysis methods, such as Mantel-Haenszel methods (see Chapter 17) or modeling (Chapters 20 and 21).

A convenient method of assembling the final categories is to initially categorize the data using a much finer scale than is necessary. A fine categorization will facilitate review of the distribution for each variable; fewer categories for subsequent analyses can then be created by combining adjacent categories. Combining adjacent strata of a confounding variable can be justified if no confounding is introduced by merging the categories. The advantage of starting with more categories than will ultimately be necessary is that the data can be used to help identify which mergings will not introduce confounding. Merging will generally not introduce confounding if the exposure distribution does not vary across strata of the study cohort (in a cohort study) or source population (in a case-control study). It will also not introduce confounding if average risk among the unexposed is constant across strata.

Classification of Subjects and Person-Time

Classification of subjects or person-time into categories of exposure and other covariates is rarely straightforward if the covariate is a time-varying subject characteristic such as an occupational exposure or medication. One specific complication is that the person-time experience classified as "exposed" needs to be defined according to a plausible model for induction time (see Chapters 7 and 16). Before a person becomes exposed, all of that person's time at risk is, naturally, unexposed person-time. If exposure occurs at a point in time and the induction-time model being evaluated calls for a minimum induction time of 5 years, then all the time at risk up to 5 years after the point of exposure for each individual should likewise be treated as unexposed person-time experience rather than exposed. The reason that this time following exposure should be treated as unexposed time is that, according to the induction-time model, any disease that occurs during the period just following exposure relates back to a period of time when exposure was absent.

More generally, tallying persons or person-time units (time at risk) into the appropriate expo-sure categories must be done on subject-by-subject basis, with the assignment into categories pos-sibly involving complicated rules if the exposure itself varies over time. Incident cases are tallied into the same category to which the concurrent person-time units are being added. For example, if the induction-time model specified a minimum induction time of 5 years, an incident case occur-ring 4 years after exposure would not be tallied as an "exposed" case because the person-time for that individual at the time of diagnosis would not be contributing toward "exposed" person-time.

HANDLING OF MISSING VALUES

It will often be the case that some subject records in a data file are incomplete, in that values are missing from that record for some but not all values of study variables. A common way of dealing with such records is simply to delete them from any analyses that involve variables for which the records have missing values. This approach is called *complete-subject analysis*. It has the advan-tage of being easy to implement, and it is easy to understand when it is a valid approach. It will be valid (within the limits of the study) whenever subjects with complete data have been, in effect, randomly sampled from all the subjects in the study; the missing data are then "missing completely at random." It will also be valid if these subjects are randomly sampled within levels of complete variables that are used for stratification.[6]

A major drawback of the complete-subject approach, however, is that it is valid only under lim-ited conditions compared with certain more complex approaches. It can also be inefficient if many subjects have missing values because it discards so much recorded data (it discards all the data in a record, even if only one study variable in the record has a missing value). For these reasons, many alternatives to complete-subject analysis have been developed, as can be found in more advanced statistics books,[6-8] most of which fall into one of two classes. Imputation methods predict and fill in the missing values based on the observed data and the missing-data pattern (the pattern of missing values seen among all records); multiple imputation is a common example.[6,9] Inverse-probability weighted methods only directly analyze those with complete records, as in the complete-subject analysis, but with the contribution of each record weighted on the basis of their estimated proba-bility of completeness (which is obtained from an analysis of the entire dataset).[10,11] All of these methods can be especially valuable when a high proportion of subjects are missing data on a study exposure or a strong confounder. Nonetheless, they assume that the probability that a variable is missing depends only on the observed portion of the data. This "missing at random" condition is weaker than the "missing completely at random" condition but should not be assumed automati-cally, especially when the missing data are responses to sensitive personal questions.

Unfortunately, there are some methods commonly used in epidemiology that can be invalid even if data are missing completely at random. One such technique creates a special missing cate-gory for a variable with missing values and then uses this category in the analysis as if it were just a special level of the variable. In reality, such a category is a mix of actual levels of the variable. As a result, the category can yield completely confounded results if the variable is a confounder[12] and can thus lead to biased estimates of the overall effect of the study exposure. An equivalent method, sometimes recommended for regression analyses, is to create a special "missing-value" indicator variable for each variable, which takes on a value of 1 for subjects whose values are missing and 0 otherwise. This missing-indicator approach is just as biased as the "missing-category" approach.[13] For handling ordinary missing-data problems, both the missing-category and missing-indicator approaches should be avoided in favor of other methods; even the complete-subject method is usually preferable, despite its limitations.

METHODS OF TESTING AND ESTIMATION

As indicated in Chapter 15, there is considerable controversy regarding what are the best or even proper approaches to statistical analysis. Most techniques currently used in epidemiology, how-ever, can be derived from fairly standard methods of significance testing and interval estimation. All such methods require that the analyst (or, by default, the analyst's computer program) make assumptions about the probabilities of observing different data configurations. This is so even if one adopts a "nonparametric" or "distribution-free" approach to data analysis. "Distribution-free" methods involve assumptions (models) about data probabilities just as do other methods; they are distinguished only in that they require weaker assumptions than other methods to be valid. Because these weaker assumptions amount to assuming that sampling was random or exposure was randomized and these assumptions are questionable in observational studies, analysis of epidemiologic data always requires critical examination of the models and assumptions underlying the statistical methods[14]; see also Chapters 20 and 21.

Two broad classes of methods can be distinguished. One comprises *small-sample* (or exact) methods, which are based on direct computation of data probabilities; the other comprises *large-sample* (or asymptotic) methods, which are based on approximations for which the validity and accuracy depends directly on the amount of data available. The latter are often used in settings where exact methods are computationally impractical (*e.g.*, when the analysis involves many subjects or many variables) and because exact methods are not available for all epidemiologic measures. While both sets of approaches will be illustrated later in this chapter, we note that most of this book focuses on large-sample methods.

Test Statistics and P-Values

Recall from Chapter 15 that significance tests begin with a *test statistic*. When choosing a particular test statistic, analysts have many choices including: the Pearson or Mantel-Haenszel χ^2 statistic computed from a contingency table; the Wald statistic, also known as a *Z-ratio* or *Z-value*, which is the estimate of interest (such as an estimated rate difference or estimated log rate ratio) divided by its estimated standard error, and the total number of exposed cases observed in the study, which is used in exact tests.

When considering which statistic to use, it is important to note that they encode different information. A χ^2 statistic, for example, reflects only the absolute distance of the actual observations from what one would expect under the test hypothesis (usually the null) but does not reflect direction of departure. In contrast, both the Z-ratio and the number of exposed cases reflect the direction of departure of the actual observations from what one would expect under the test hypothesis. Wald statistics of -1.92 and 1.92, for example, would represent equal but opposite departures of the actual observations from their expectations under the test hypothesis. Note, in principle, one can compute a nondirectional statistic form a directional statistic, for example, by squaring or taking the absolute value, provided the latter is 0 when the actual observations perfectly conform to what would be expected under the test hypothesis (as with Wald statistics).

To test a hypothesis with a given statistic, one must be able to compute the probability (frequency) distribution, often referred to as the *sampling distribution*, of the statistic over repetitions of the study when the test hypothesis is true. Such computations ordinarily assume the following *validity conditions:* (1) only chance produces differences between repetitions, (2) no biases are operating, and (3) the statistical model used to derive the distribution is correct. The *upper one-tailed P-value* for the observed test statistic is the probability that the statistic would be as high as observed or higher if the test hypothesis and validity conditions were correct; the *lower one-tailed P-value* for the statistic is the probability that the test statistic would be as low as observed or lower if the test hypothesis and validity conditions were correct. In the remainder of this chapter, we will refer to these P-values simply as *upper* and *lower*.

To interpret lower and upper P-values correctly, one must distinguish between *absolute test statistics* and *directional test statistics*. Consider the ordinary χ^2 statistic for a contingency table (Chapter 17). Note the value of this statistic may range from 0 to extreme positive values. Intuitivelty, a very high value of the statistic means that the observations are *far* from what would be expected under the test hypothesis. Thus, a small upper P-value means the observations are unusually *far* from this expectation if the test hypothesis and validity conditions are correct. In contrast, a very low value of the statistic (*i.e.*, close to 0) means that the observations are *close* to this expectation. Thus, a small lower P-value thus means the observations are unusually *close* to this expectation if the test hypothesis and validity conditions are correct. Crucially, for either a small lower P-value or small upper P-value, while we can ascertain that we are either close to or far from the expectation if the test hypothesis and validity conditions are correct, the value of the statistic does not indicate in which direction we are either close to or far from. Thus, the ordinary χ^2 statistic for a contingency table can be considered an absolute test statistic.

Now consider an ordinary Wald statistic, or Z-score, computed from a point estimate and its standard error. This statistic ranges from extreme negative to extreme positive values. A high value of the statistic still means that the observations are far from this expectation, specifically in a positive direction. Now, however, a low value of the statistic (*i.e.*, a large negative number) also means that the observations are far from expected but now in a negative direction. A small lower P-value thus means that the observations are unusually *far* from this expectation if the test hypothesis and validity conditions are correct. In this sense, the Wald statistic is a directional test statistic and we note that the meaning of a lower P-value is different for absolute and directional statistics.

A questionable dual tradition regarding P-values and tests has become firmly established in statistical practice. First, it is traditional to use P-values that refer to absolute departures, regardless of whether the actual scientific, medical, or policy context would dictate concern with only one direction of departure (*e.g.*, a positive direction). This practice is bad enough on contextual grounds. For example, in the legal arena, it has led the use of absolute statistics to determine whether evidence of harm is "significant," even though by the very statement of the problem, the only concern is with a harmful direction of effect. Suppose now, whether from context or tradition, one wishes to use an absolute test. Such a test logically dictates use of an absolute statistic. In a rather strange second tradition, however, it has become common first to compute a directional statistic and from that to compute a nondirectional *two-sided* P-value for the test. This two-sided P-value is usually defined as twice the smaller of the upper and lower P-values. There is, however, a logical problem with two-sided P-values defined in this manner: Unlike one-tailed P-values, they are not necessarily probabilities, as can be seen by noting that they may exceed 1 (as will be shown in a later section). Several different proposals have been made to overcome this problem, one of which (mid-P-values) we discuss later. For now, we use the most common definitions of P-values, in which a one-tailed P-value is always a true probability, but a two-sided P-value is simply twice the smaller of two probabilities and so is not necessarily a probability.

These traditions also have implications for interpreting confidence intervals. Recall that a two-sided 90% confidence interval is the set of all values for the measure of interest that have a two-sided P-value of at least 0.10. It follows that a point is inside the two-sided 90% confidence interval if and only if both its lower and upper P-values are greater than $0.10/2 = 0.05$. Similarly, a point is inside the two-sided 95% confidence interval if and only if both its lower and upper P-values are greater than $0.05/2 = 0.025$. Indeed, these conditions are equivalent to the definitions of 90% and 95% confidence intervals.

Median-Unbiased Estimates

An exact two-sided P-value reaches its maximum at the point where the lower and upper P-values are equal (the peak of the exact P-value function). This point may be taken as a point estimate of the measure of interest and is referred to here as the *median-unbiased estimate*. The name *median unbiased* suggests that the estimate has equal probability of being above the true value as below it. The median-unbiased estimate, as defined here, does not exactly satisfy this condition; rather, it is the point for which the test statistic would have equal probability of being above and below its observed value over repetitions of the study, as well as the peak (maximum) of the exact two-sided P-value function.

Under "large-sample" conditions that will be discussed later, the median-unbiased estimate tends to differ little from the far more common *maximum-likelihood* estimate (MLE), also discussed later. We thus focus on the latter estimate in the ensuing chapters of this book.

Sensitivity and Influence Analysis

Inferential statistics such as P-values and confidence limits must themselves be subjected to scrutiny to complete the statistical portion of the data analysis. Two broad components of this scrutiny are sensitivity and influence analysis.

As mentioned earlier, *all* statistical techniques, even so-called nonparametric or distribution-free methods, are based on assumptions that often cannot be checked with available data.

For example, one may be concerned that the observed association (or lack thereof) was a consequence of an unmeasured confounder, or misclassification, or an undetected violation of the model used for analysis. One way to deal with the issue of possible assumption violations is to conduct a *sensitivity analysis,* in which the statistical analysis is systematically repeated using different assumptions each time to see how sensitive the statistics are to changes in those assumptions. Moreover, one may repeat the analysis with different adjustments for uncontrolled confounding, measurement errors, and selection bias and with different statistical models for computing P-values and confidence limits. Chapter 29 provides an introduction to sensitivity analysis.

It is possible for analysis results to hinge on data from only one or a few key subjects, even when many subjects are observed. *Influence analysis* is a search for such problems. For example, the analysis may be repeated deleting each subject one at a time or deleting each of several special subgroups of subjects, to see if the statistics change to an important extent upon such deletions. Statistical quantities that change little in response to such deletions are sometimes said to be *resistant* to the deletions. When the key estimates of interest are found to be strongly influenced by deletions, it will be necessary to report the influential observations and their degree of influence on the estimates.

Probability Distributions and Exact Statistics

We will illustrate basic concepts of probability distributions and exact statistics in the context of a prevalence survey for human immunodeficiency virus (HIV). Specifically, suppose that we take as our test statistic the number of HIV-positive subjects observed in the sample. It is possible that among 1,000 sampled subjects, 10 would test positive; it is also possible that 4 would test positive; it may also be possible that 100 would test positive. If, however, our sample of 1,000 was drawn randomly from all US Army enlistees, getting 100 positives would be highly improbable (in the sense that we would expect that result to occur rarely), whereas getting 4 positives would not. The reasons are that the US Army will not knowingly enlist high-risk or HIV-positive persons (so such persons tend to avoid enlistment), and HIV prevalence in the general US population is less than a few percent.

Acknowledging that the observed value of the test statistic (*i.e.,* from the data) can potentially take on a range of values, a *probability distribution* is a rule, model, or function that tells us the probability of each possible value. For the present example, suppose that the survey sample consists of 1,000 individuals selected via simple random sampling from the population, and that the true prevalence of HIV in the population is $R = 0.004$. Now let Y be the number of HIV-positive sample subjects. Then the probability of getting $Y = 2$ (*i.e.,* two positives) among the 1,000 surveyed is:

$$\Pr\left(Y = 2 \middle| R = 0.004\right) = 0.146,$$

or about one chance in seven. This probability can be derived as follows. Suppose the subjects are to be selected in sequence, from the first to the 1,000th subject. Assuming that the HIV status of each subject is independent of the status of any other subject, the probability that the first and second subjects are HIV positive and the 998 others are not is:

$$0.004^2\left(1 - 0.004\right)^{998}.$$

Note, the same probability would be obtained if we consider any two distinct subjects (*i.e.,* not just the first and the second but also the first and third or second and fourth) as being positive and the others not. Consequently, to find the total probability that exactly two subjects are positive, we must multiply the above probability by the number of ways, or combinations, in which exactly two of the 1,000 subjects are positive. To find this number of combinations, note that there are 1,000 options for the first of the two subjects and 999 for the second (since whoever is "selected" first is removed from consideration for the second subject). However, viewing the possible combinations through this, we have to note that each unique pair is represented twice: the combination of subject #1 and subject #2 is equivalent, at least in terms of the incidence calculation, to the combination of subject #2 and subject #1. Therefore, the total number of unique combinations of two subjects among the 1,000 is $(1,000 \times 999)/2$. Finally, we can complete the calculation by multiplying this number by the probability above to give:

$$\frac{1,000 \times 999}{2} 0.004^2 (1-0.004)^{998} = 0.146$$

as the probability that exactly two subjects are HIV positive.

The preceding paragraph is an example of a *combinatorial argument.* Such arguments are often used to find sample probabilities when random sampling has been employed in selecting subjects for study. Such arguments also form the foundation of most small-sample statistical methods. In general, the number of unique possible combinations of y subjects taken from N total is given by the expression: $N!/[y! \times (N-y)!]$ In this expression, the exclamation point "!" following a number y is read "factorial" and indicates that one should take the product of all numbers from 1 to y; that is

$$y! = y \times (y-1) \times \cdots 2 \times 1,$$

with 0!, by definition, set equal to 1. Notationally, one often finds that this quantity is expressed in a slightly simplified form, specifically as $\binom{N}{y}$ which can be read as "N choose y." Furthermore, this quantity is referred to as the *combinatorial coefficient* or the *binomial coefficient.* The latter term arises from the fact that $\binom{N}{y}$ appears in the general formula for the binomial distribution (see below). Finally, we illustrate the expression for the combinatorial coefficient by returning to the HIV example to find (again) the number of combinations of $y = 2$ subjects out of $N = 1,000$ is:

$$\binom{1,000}{2} = \frac{1,000!}{2!(1,000-2)!} = \frac{1,000 \times 999 \times 998 \times \cdots \times 2 \times 1}{(2 \times 1)(998 \times 997 \times \cdots \times 2 \times 1)} = \frac{1,000 \times 999}{2}.$$

More generally, we can write down the probability associated with any specific number of positives from the sample. In particular, under the above assumptions, the probability of getting $Y = y$ positives out of $N = 1,000$ subjects, given an HIV prevalence of 0.004, is

$$\Pr(Y = y | R = 0.004) = \binom{N}{y} 0.004^y (1-0.004)^{N-y}. \qquad [16\text{-}1]$$

Equation 16-1 is an example of a probability distribution since it provides a means to calculating the probability for any given number of positives out of the $N = 1,000$ subjects. Formally, it is an example of a *binomial* distribution with a probability *parameter* of 0.004 and a sample size of 1,000.

Now suppose that we carry out the random-sample survey and observe only one positive among 1,000 sampled persons. Using formula 16-1, we can compute the probability of observing $Y \leq 1$ (*i.e.*, one or fewer positives) under the test hypothesis that the HIV prevalence is 0.004 in the sampled population. Because we only need to know the probabilities associated with the events $Y = 0$ and $Y = 1$ to compute the desired quantities, we have:

$$\Pr(Y \leq 1 | R = 0.004) = \Pr(Y = 0 | R = 0.004) + \Pr(Y = 1 | R = 0.004)$$

$$= \binom{1,000}{0} 0.004^0 (1-0.004)^{1,000} + \binom{1,000}{1} 0.004^1 (1-0.004)^{999}$$

$$= (1-0.004)^{1,000} + 1,000 \times 0.004 (1-0.004)^{999}$$

$$= 0.091.$$

Note, this probability is P_{lower}, the traditional (Fisher) lower-tailed exact P-value for the test hypothesis. Here, the number of positives Y serves as the test statistic, and we compute the P-value directly from the exact distribution of Y as given by formula 16-1.

If we repeat our calculation under the test hypothesis that the HIV prevalence is $R = 0.005$, we have to use the following probability distribution to get P-values:

$$\Pr\left(Y = y \mid R = 0.005\right) = \binom{N}{y} 0.005^y \left(1 - 0.005\right)^{N-y}$$

[16-2]

The differences between formulas 16-1 and 16-2 illustrate how the probability distribution for the test statistic changes when the test hypothesis is changed, even though the test statistic Y does not. Formula 16-2 yields a lower P-value of:

$$\Pr\left(Y \leq 1 \mid R = 0.005\right) = \Pr\left(Y = 0 \mid R = 0.005\right) + \Pr\left(Y = 1 \mid R = 0.005\right)$$

$$= \binom{1{,}000}{0} 0.005^0 \left(1 - 0.005\right)^{1{,}000} + \binom{1{,}000}{1} 0.005^1 \left(1 - 0.005\right)^{999}$$

$$= \left(1 - 0.005\right)^{1{,}000} + 1{,}000 \times 0.005 \left(1 - 0.005\right)^{999}$$

$$= 0.040$$

Beyond the lower-tailed exact P-value, by doubling the above quantities, we get two-sided P-values of 0.18 under the hypothesis that the HIV prevalence is 0.004, and 0.08 under the hypothesis that the HIV prevalence is 0.005. To illustrate, recall that a two-sided 90% confidence interval derived from a test comprises all points for which the two-sided P-value from the test is at least 0.10, and the 90% confidence limits are the two points at which the two-sided P-value is 0.10. Because a prevalence of 0.0040 yielded a two-sided P-value greater than 0.10, it must be inside the 90% interval. Because a prevalence of 0.0050 yielded a two-sided P-value less than 0.10, it must be outside the 90% interval. We can interpolate that the upper 90% limit must be roughly (0.10-0.08)/(0.18-0.08) = one-fifth of the way from 0.005 to 0.004, which corresponds to a prevalence of 0.0048. One way to check this interpolation is to compute the lower exact P-value for 0.0048:

$$P_{\text{lower}} = \left(1 - 0.0048\right)^{1{,}000} + 1{,}000 \times 0.0048 \left(1 - 0.0048\right)^{999} = 0.0474.$$

Doubling this lower exact P-value yields a two-sided P-value of 0.095. Because this P-value is just under 0.10, we may conclude that a prevalence of 0.0048 is just outside the 90% interval, and that the upper 90% confidence limit is a little under 0.0048 (the limit is in fact closer to 0.0047).

As indicated earlier, to obtain the median-unbiased point estimate of HIV prevalence, we must find the test hypothesis at which the lower P-value and upper P-value equal one another. We must therefore also calculate the upper exact P-value, P_{upper}, which is the probability that Y is at least as big as the observed value of 1. It is often easier to work with 1 minus this probability, which is the probability that Y is less than its observed value. For example, if we wish to test the hypothesis that the HIV prevalence is 0.001, we use the relation:

$$P_{\text{upper}} = \Pr\left(Y \geq 1 \mid R = 0.001\right) = 1 - \Pr\left(Y < 1 \mid R = 0.001\right).$$

Because 0 is the only possible Y value of less than 1, we have:

$$P_{\text{upper}} = 1 - \Pr\left(Y = 0 \mid R = 0.001\right) = 1 - \left(1 - 0.001\right)^{1{,}000} = 0.63.$$

Using the above calculations, the lower P-value for the same test hypothesis is:

$$P_{\text{lower}} = \left(1 - 0.001\right)^{1{,}000} + 1{,}000 \times 0.001 \left(1 - 0.001\right)^{999} = 0.74.$$

Thus, $P_{upper} < P_{lower}$ for an HIV prevalence of 0.001. If, however, we increase the test hypothesis to 0.0011 and recompute the P-values, we get

$$P_{upper} = 1 - (1 - 0.0011)^{1,000} = 0.67$$

which equals

$$P_{lower} = (1 - 0.0011)^{1,000} + 1,000 \times 0.001(1 - 0.0011)^{999} = 0.67.$$

Thus, 0.0011 is the median-unbiased estimate of the HIV prevalence. Note that this estimate is not quite equal to the sample prevalence of $1/1,000 = 0.0010$. The sample prevalence, however, is not necessarily an ideal estimate in very small samples.[15,16]

A number of comments on this process are worth noting. First, the process of repeated P-value computation typifies many computational approaches for exact analysis, as well as for various approximate methods such as *g-estimation* (Chapter 21). For the preceding simple example, there are formulas that give the exact limits in just one step, but for more complicated data, one must turn to iterative computations to get exact results.

Second, the most crucial statistical assumption underlying the applications of the binomial distribution was the assumption that the sampling of 1,000 participants from the target population was random. If the sampling was not random, then the above statistical analysis (and any inference based on it) may not be valid. Even if the sampling was random, further assumptions would be needed to make valid inferences about HIV prevalence in the sampled population, among them that the measurement technique (here, the test for HIV) used by the survey is error-free (see Chapter 29 for sensitivity analysis methods when this assumption is not viewed as being realistic).

Third, by computing P-values for many different test hypotheses, we are in effect drawing out the P-value function. Returning to the HIV example, we may continue to draw out the P-value function for the HIV prevalence based on our random-sampling model by writing a general form for the probability distributions:

$$\Pr(Y = y | R) = \binom{1,000}{y} R^y (1 - R)^{1,000 - y}.$$

The earlier distributions are special cases of this formula, with R hypothesized to equal 0.004, 0.005, 0.0048, 0.001, and 0.0011, respectively. Generically, R in this formula is referred to as a *parameter* of the distribution; each different value for R produces a different probability distribution. While R represents the true prevalence of HIV in the sampled population in the example; in other instances, R may represent risk of disease or death.

Finally, we can be even more general by letting N represent the size of our random sample; then the last equation becomes:

$$\binom{N}{y} R^y (1 - R)^{N - y}.$$

[16-3]

Given a fixed sample size N and parameter R, any probability distribution of this form is called a *binomial distribution*. Equations 16-1 and 16-2 are examples of Equation 16-3 with $N = 1,000$ and with $R = 0.004$ and 0.005, respectively.

Approximate Statistics: The Score Method

Exact distributions such as the binomial can be unwieldy to work with if N is very large. This difficulty has led to extensive development of approximations to such distributions, which allow calculation of approximate P-values and estimates. For the binomial distribution, some approximations are very accurate. Rather than display the most accurate, however, we focus on two approximate methods, the score method and the Wald method, that are simpler and are special cases of the most common methods. While we present many examples of score and Wald statistics in later chapters, we note that the reader has probably encountered other examples in past reading.

Suppose that we have a test statistic Y and formulas that give us the exact mean and variance of Y when the true parameter value is R [i.e., $E(Y|R)$ and $V(Y|R)$, respectively]. We may then construct approximate tests of the parameter by treating Y as if it were a normally distributed with mean and variance computed from the formulas. In the HIV example, Y is binomial, and the formulas for its mean and variance are NR and $NR(1-R)$. With these, we could test values of R by treating Y as if it were normal with mean NR and standard deviation $\left[NR(1-R)\right]^{\frac{1}{2}}$. This procedure implies that the *score statistic,* given by:

$$\chi_{score} = \frac{Y - NR}{\left[NR(1-R)\right]^{\frac{1}{2}}}$$

[16-4]

has a "standard" normal distribution (that is, a normal distribution with a mean of 0 and a standard deviation of 1). Thus, to find an approximate lower P-value when $Y = y$, we merely look up the probability that a standard normal variate would be less than or equal to χ_{score} with y substituted for Y. To find an approximate upper P-value, we look up the probability that a standard normal deviate would be greater than or equal to χ_{score} with y substituted for Y.

To illustrate this process, suppose that, in the HIV example, the test hypothesis is that the HIV prevalence R is 0.004. Because $N = 1,000$ subjects were observed and only $Y = 1$ was HIV positive, we get

$$\chi_{score} = \frac{1 - 1,000(0.004)}{\left[1,000(0.004)(1-0.004)\right]^{\frac{1}{2}}} = -1.503.$$

To get the lower P-value based on this statistic, we need to only use a table of the standard normal distribution to find the probability that a standard normal variate would be less than or equal to -1.503; this probability is 0.067. Note, this value is not particularly close to the exact lower P-value of 0.091 that we obtained earlier. The discrepancy is not surprising, however, considering that the accuracy of the approximation depends on both NR and $NR(1-R)$ being "large" (5 or more), and that NR is here only $1,000(0.004) = 4$. If, however, we next test $R = 0.005$, we get $NR = 5$, a score statistic of $\chi_{score} = -1.793$, and an approximate lower P-value of 0.036, practically the same as the exact lower P-value of 0.040 for $R = 0.005$. As before, to get a two-sided P-value, we would just double the smaller of the upper and lower P-values.

This example illustrates that some care is needed when using approximations such as the one given by formula 16-4. The criteria for valid approximation are usually summarized by saying that the sample size N must be "large." Unfortunately, a truly large sample is neither necessary nor sufficient for a close approximation. For example, a sample size of 10 can yield a useful approximation if $R = 0.5$, for then $NR = N(1-R) = 5$. In contrast, a sample size of 100,000 is not big enough to test approximately a hypothesized prevalence of 0.00002, since NR is only 2.

We could, if we wished, find approximate 90% confidence limits for the HIV prevalence R just as before, by trying different hypothesized prevalences R in the score statistic until we found the pair of prevalences with approximate two-sided P-values of 0.10. From a table of the standard normal distribution, we can see that this pair of prevalences must be the pair that yields score statistics (i.e., χ_{score}) of -1.645 and 1.645 because a standard normal deviate has a 5% chance of falling below -1.645 and a 5% chance of falling above 1.645. For 95% limits, we would need to find the pair of prevalences that yield score statistics of -1.96 and 1.96. From trying different values for R in formula 16-4 with $N = 1,000$, we can see that a prevalence of 0.0045 yields a score statistic χ_{score} of -1.645. Thus, 0.0045 must be the approximate (upper) 90% confidence limit based on the score statistic given above. This value is not far from the exact limit of 0.0047, which we could have anticipated from the fact that $1,000(0.0045) = 4.5$ is close to 5.

Relative to approximate confidence limits, the approximate point estimate corresponding to the score statistic is easy to find. Taking the criterion to be the value for which the approximate upper and lower P-values are equal, this can only happen when the estimated prevalence, $\hat{R}$, makes $\chi_{score} = 0$. The latter can happen only if the numerator of χ_{score} is zero, which is equivalent to the equation:

$$Y - NR = 0.$$

Solving for R yields the approximate estimator: $\hat{R} = Y/N$. Thus, we have the intuitive result that the score estimate equals the observed sample proportion. In our example, $\hat{R} = 1/1{,}000 = 0.0010$, corresponding to an estimated HIV prevalence of 0.1%. This approximate estimate is remarkably close to the median-unbiased estimate of 0.0011, considering that the informal large-sample criterion $N\hat{R}$ equals $1{,}000(0.0010) = 1$ and so is nowhere near "large."

Summarizing and generalizing the above discussion, the score method is based on taking a test statistic Y for which we can compute the exact mean and variance, $E(Y|R)$ and $V(Y|R)$ and creating from these quantities a *score statistic:*

$$\chi_{score} = \frac{Y - E(Y|R)}{V(Y|R)^{1/2}}.$$

Approximate P-values are then found by treating this score statistic as normal with a mean of 0 and a standard deviation of 1. Furthermore, an approximate point estimate may be found by solving the score equation:

$$Y - E(Y|R) = 0$$

to obtain the $\hat{R}$ that has a score statistic of 0 and, hence, a two-sided score P-value of 1 (the largest possible value).

Under the most commonly used probability models (such as those that assume the observed outcomes are independent and have a binomial, Poisson, or normal distribution), the point estimate $\hat{R}$ obtained from the score equation turns out to equal the *maximum-likelihood estimate* (see below). This equivalence arises because the numerator of the score statistic equals the derivative of the log-likelihood function produced by those models. A score statistic obtained by differentiating the log-likelihood function is sometimes called the *efficient score statistic* under the assumed probability model.[17] Some statistics books drop the word *efficient* and use the term *score statistic* to refer only to the score statistic derived from the log-likelihood function.

Approximate Statistics: The Wald Method

Although score statistics are much easier to use than exact statistics, they still require some modest computing to find confidence limits. This computational requirement arises because the standard deviation in the denominator of a score statistic changes for each test hypothesis (prevalence). A simpler approximation, called the *Wald method,* replaces the standard deviation in the score statistic (formula 16-5) by a single unchanging value, specifically the standard deviation when $R = \hat{R}$ (*i.e.*, that based on the approximate point estimate). This substitution yields the *Wald statistic* based on Y:

$$\chi_{Wald} = \frac{Y - E(Y|R)}{V(Y|R)^{1/2}}$$

[16-5]

In the HIV example, $\hat{R} = Y/N$, so

$$\chi_{\text{Wald}} = \frac{Y - NR}{\left[N\hat{R}\left(1 - \hat{R}\right)\right]^{1/2}} = \frac{Y - NR}{\left[Y\left(N - Y\right)/N\right]^{1/2}}.$$

[16-6]

If we replace χ_{Wald} by the value that a desired upper confidence limit would yield, say R_U, we could solve the resulting equation for this R_U. For example, to get the upper limit of a two-sided 90% interval, we need to find the prevalence R_U that solves:

$$\chi_{\text{Wald}} = \frac{Y - NR_U}{\left[Y\left(N - Y\right)/N\right]^{1/2}} = -1.645.$$

Solving for R_U, we get:

$$R_U = \frac{Y + 1.645\left[Y\left(N - Y\right)/N\right]^{1/2}}{N}.$$

In our HIV example, with $Y = 1$, we have:

$$R_U = \frac{1 + 1.645\left(999/1{,}000\right)^{1/2}}{1{,}000} = 0.0026.$$

Recalling that the exact upper limit was 0.0047, this Wald statistic–based upper limit of 0.0026 is clearly a poor approximation relative to that obtained from the score statistic which yielded an upper limit of 0.0045. This result should not be surprising: formulae that make increasingly greater simplifications (in this case for the variance in the denominator) should be expected to yield increasingly poor approximations.

In general, P-values and intervals from the Wald method are less accurate than those from the score method because the Wald method is itself an approximation to the score method (in the above example, it replaces the varying denominator of the score statistic χ_{score}, which depends on R, with a single standard deviation). Because the score method is also an approximation, the Wald method is an approximation to an approximation and so requires criteria that are more stringen—for binomial distributions, specifically that NR and $N(1-R)$ are large—than those required for the score method to be accurate. Nonetheless, because it is so simple, the Wald method is the most widely used approximation. Furthermore, its accuracy can be improved by applying it to a function of the proportion, such as the logit transform, instead to the proportion itself (see Chapter 17).

Likelihood Functions

Likelihood functions play a central role in modern statistical theory. Consider again the general formula 16-3 for the binomial distribution with sample size N, number of observed cases y, and probability parameter R. Substituting into this formula, the data values for N and y from our hypothetical HIV survey, we get:

$$\binom{1{,}000}{1} R^1\left(1 - R\right)^{1{,}000-1} = 1{,}000R\left(1 - R\right)^{999}.$$

[16-7]

Note carefully the following crucial point: Once we replace the data variables in the general binomial probability formula, Equation 16-3, with actual data numbers, we are left with a formula, Equation 16-8, that has only one variable, R, which is the unknown prevalence parameter that we are trying to estimate. Thus, we can view this equation as representing a simple mathematical function of the parameter R. This function is called the *likelihood function* for R and is typically denoted by $L(R)$. That is,

$$L(R) = 1{,}000R\left(1 - R\right)^{999}$$

[16-8]

is the likelihood function for R given the hypothetical data in the HIV prevalence example. This function has a number of applications in statistical analysis. First, it can be used to measure directly the relative support the data provide to various hypotheses. Second, it can supply approximate tests and estimates that have reasonable accuracy in large samples. Third, it can be used to compute Bayesian statistics.

The first two applications begin by finding the value for R, the unknown parameter, that makes the likelihood function as large as it can be. In other words, we find the value of R that brings $L(R)$ to its *maximum* value. For example, with calculus, we can show that the maximum of formula 16-9 occurs when R is $1/1{,}000 = 0.001$. This value is correspondingly referred to as the *maximum-likelihood estimate* of R. More generally, with calculus, we can show that the MLE for a binomial parameter R is equal to the observed number of cases divided by the number sampled, *i.e.*, y/N. We denote this estimate by $\hat{R}_{ml}$ to distinguish it from the median-unbiased estimate, which was 0.0011 in our example.

Next, consider the maximum value of the likelihood function:

$$L\left(\hat{R}_{ml}\right) = L(0.001) = 1{,}000(0.001)(1-0.001)^{999} = 0.3681.$$

Suppose that we are interested in testing a particular hypothesized value for R, say 0.005. One way to do so would be to take the ratio of the likelihood function at $R = 0.005$ to the likelihood function at $\hat{R}_{ml} = 0.001$. Noting that:

$$L(0.005) = 1{,}000(0.005)(1-0.005)^{999} = 0.0334,$$

this ratio is equal to $0.0334/0.3681 = 0.0908$ of the maximum value. Thus, the value of the likelihood at the hypothesized value of 0.005 is approximately 9% of the maximum value of the likelihood function (*i.e.*, much smaller). Intuitively, one can interpret this as saying that there is relatively little support in the data for the hypothesized value for R of 0.005. More generally, if we are given a hypothesized value R, then we may measure the relative support the data give R by the *likelihood ratio:*

$$LR(R) = \frac{L(R)}{L\left(\hat{R}_{ml}\right)}$$

[16-9]

or its natural logarithm $\ln[LR(R)]$. Such an approach to measuring relative support is sometimes referred to as a "pure likelihood" approach.[18,19]

Returing to the HIV prevalence example, the likelihood ratio for a test value of 0.005 is:

$$LR(0.005) = \frac{L(0.005)}{L\left(\hat{R}_{ml}\right)} = \frac{0.0334}{0.3681} = 0.0908.$$

If, on the other hand, the test value is 0.004, the likelihood ratio is:

$$LR(0.004) = \frac{L(0.004)}{L\left(\hat{R}_{ml}\right)} = \frac{0.0730}{0.3681} = 0.198.$$

Note, this is twice the likelihood ratio for 0.005. Thus, we could say from a pure likelihood perspective that a prevalence of 0.004 has twice as much relative support from the data as a prevalence of 0.005.

In likelihood theory, all support is measured relative to the MLE. Consequently, the MLE $\hat{R}_{ml}$ (0.001 in our example) always has 100% relative support because

$$LR\left(\hat{R}_{ml}\right) = \frac{L\left(\hat{R}_{ml}\right)}{L\left(\hat{R}_{ml}\right)} = 1.0.$$

Although there are no firm guidelines, one rule of thumb is to say test values for the study parameter R that have likelihood ratios below $e^{-2} = 0.135$ (*i.e.*, 13.5% or about 1/7) of the maximum are not well supported by the data.[20] In the HIV example, the upper-score 90% confidence limit of 0.0045 determined earlier has a likelihood ratio of

$$LR(0.0045) = \frac{0.0497}{0.3681} = 0.135$$

and so by the 13.5% criterion is on the boundary in terms of relative support. The value 0.0045 is thus an example of a *pure likelihood limit* at the 13.5% relative support level. It is an upper limit, as can be seen from the fact that 0.004 has more relative support and 0.005 has less.

Approximate Statistics: The Likelihood-Ratio Method

Although pure likelihood limits are not conceptually the same as confidence limits, 13.5% likelihood limits and 95% confidence limits tend to be close in value in large samples. Moreover, the two types of limits are guaranteed to be close if the confidence limits are approximate ones calculated by the likelihood-ratio method, which we now describe.

As before, suppose that R is the test value of the parameter of interest. Now consider the following statistic:

$$\chi^2_{LR} = -2 \times \ln\left[LR(R)\right]$$

[16-10]

that is, -2 times the natural log of the likelihood ratio. Using the theory of mathematical statistics, one can show that χ^2_{LR} has an approximately χ^2 distribution with one degree of freedom if (1) R is the true value of the parameter (*i.e.*, if the test hypothesis is true); (2) all the usual validity conditions hold (*i.e.*, absence of bias and the correct probability model is used to construct the likelihood function); and (3) the sample is "large" in the sense described earlier [*i.e.*, NR and $N(1-R)$ both greater than 5].[17,21] The test statistic χ^2_{LR} in formula 16-11 is called the *likelihood-ratio statistic* or *deviance statistic* for testing the hypotheses that R is the true value, and the test of R based on it is called the *likelihood-ratio test* or *deviance test*.

Unlike the score and Wald statistics, the likelihood-ratio statistic bears no resemblance to the ordinary test statistics of elementary courses. It requires some calculus (specifically, the use of a Taylor-series expansion) to show the rather remarkable fact that χ^2_{score}, the square of the test statistic given by formula 16-5, approximates χ^2_{LR}, if the sample size is large enough and the test value has reasonably high support.[17] Because the P-value from χ^2_{score} is two-sided, we can see that the P-value derived from χ^2_{LR} must also be two-sided.

How good are the likelihood-ratio statistics in our example? Because there is only one case among the 1,000 persons sampled, they appear poor relative to the exact statistics. The likelihood ratio for an HIV prevalence of 0.004 was found earlier to be 0.198, so the likelihood-ratio statistic for this prevalence is $-2 \times \ln(0.198) = 3.24$. From a one-degree-of-freedom χ^2 table, we see that this statistic yields a two-sided P-value of 0.072. Contrast this result with the corresponding two-sided exact P-value of $2 \times 0.091 = 0.18$ or the two-sided score P-value of $2 \times 0.067 = 0.13$. Only the two-sided Wald P-value looks less accurate than the likelihood-ratio result in this example. The Wald statistic is

$$\frac{1 - 1{,}000(0.004)}{\left[1{,}000(0.001)(1 - 0.001)\right]^{\frac{1}{2}}} = -3.00$$

which yields a two-sided P-value of 0.003.

In this example, the large disparities among the statistics are due chiefly to the fact that the MLE of the expected number of cases is far from the large-sample criterion: $N\hat{R}_{ml} = 1{,}000(0.001) = 1$ in this example. If each of $N\hat{R}_{ml}$, NR, $N(1 - \hat{R}_{ml})$ and $N(1-R)$ were at least 5, we would expect the likelihood-ratio statistic to be much closer to the score statistic.

Finally, likelihood-ratio confidence limits are computed by finding the two parameter values that have likelihood-ratio P-values equal to 1 minus the confidence level. This calculation is equivalent to finding the two limits that have likelihood-ratio statistics equal to the desired percentile of a one-degree-of-freedom χ^2 distribution. Thus, noting that 2.71 is the 90th percentile of a χ^2 distribution with one degree of freedom, to find 90% likelihood-ratio confidence limits, we need to find the two parameter values R_L and R_U that solve the equation:

$$-2 \times \ln\left[LR(R)\right] = 2.71.$$

[16-11]

In the HIV example, with an observed value of $Y = 1$, this equation becomes:

$$-2 \times \ln\left[\frac{1,000R(1-R)^{999}}{0.3681}\right] = 2.71.$$

The solution for the upper limit R_U is 0.0036. This limit is not close to either the exact limit of 0.0047 or the score limit of 0.0045, but it is still better than the Wald limit of 0.0030. Again, with more cases, the likelihood-ratio result would be much closer to the score result, and all the results would converge to one another. If we had desired 95% limits instead, we would solve

$$-2 \times \ln\left[LR(R)\right] = 3.84$$

[16-12]

because 3.84 is the 95th percentile of a χ^2 distribution with one degree of freedom. This equation yields an upper 95% limit for R of 0.0044, very close to the 13.5% upper pure likelihood limit found earlier. This is no coincidence. Recall that the pure-likelihood limit was the upper value for R such that $LR(R) = e^{-2}$. If we solve the confidence-limit Equation 16-13 for the likelihood ratio $LR(R)$, we get

$$LR(R) = e^{-3.84/2} = e^{-1.92} = 0.147.$$

Thus, the pure likelihood equation for 13.5% limits and the likelihood-ratio equations for 95% confidence limits are almost the same and so should yield almost the same interval estimates for R.

For more thorough discussions of the uses of likelihood functions in testing and estimation and their relation to the score and Wald methods, Clayton and Hills[22] provide a basic treatment oriented toward epidemiologic applications, while Cox and Hinkley[17] provide a classic treatment oriented toward general conceptual issues as well as mathematical details (the latter authors refer to the Wald statistic as the "maximum-likelihood test statistic").

Likelihoods in Bayesian Analysis

The third application of likelihood ratios is in computing Bayesian statistics, which may be illustrated in its simplest form by combining likelihood ratios with prior odds of hypotheses to find posterior odds of hypotheses. Returning to the HIV survey, suppose that, *before seeing the data,* we think it twice as probable that the prevalence R is 0.004 relative to 0.005. That is, perhaps because of results reported by some other study or our own preliminary results, we would bet in favor of 0.004 over 0.005 with two-to-one (2:1) odds. How should we revise these betting odds upon seeing the data? More generally, given the *prior odds* (i.e., the odds *before* seeing the data) for parameter value R_1 versus parameter value R_0, what should the *posterior odds* (i.e., the odds *after* seeing the data) be? The answer can be computed using elementary probability theory to be:

$$\text{Odds after data} = \frac{\text{Likelihood for } R_1}{\text{Likelihood for } R_0} \times \text{Odds before data},$$

or, equivalently:

$$\text{Posterior odds} = \frac{L(R_1)}{L(R_0)} \times \text{Prior odds}.$$

[16-13]

Unlike the earlier applications, the likelihood ratio in formula 16-14 does *not* involve the MLE, which is often unnecessary for a Bayesian analysis.

Returning to the example, combining the prior odds of 2:1 with $L(R_1) = L(0.004) = 0.0730$ and $L(R_0) = L(0.005) = 0.0334$, we get:

$$\text{Posterior odds} = \frac{0.0730}{0.0334} \times 2 = 4.36.$$

Thus, if we started out with 2:1 odds in favor of $R = 0.004$ over $R = 0.005$, after seeing the data, we should be in favor of 0.004 over 0.005 with 4.36:1 odds.

One must take care to note that the last answer applies only to the stated pair of hypotheses: $R_1 = 0.004$ and $R_0 = 0.005$. Even though we may favor 0.004 over 0.005 by a wide margin, it does *not* mean that 0.004 should be viewed as the most favored, not that 0.005 should be viewed as the least favored hypothesis. Moreover, one should consider *other* hypotheses, with the calculation of other posterior odds for other pairs of values for R needed to broaden the scope of the analysis.

Bayesian philosophy and elementary Bayesian methods will be covered in Chapter 23 where it is shown how Bayesian statistics can be computed from ordinary frequentist programs via the device of "prior data." More broadly, the Bayesian philosophy has led to a huge variety of methods tailored to a broad range of data scenarios. Indeed, there are now many books that give comprehensive treatments of Bayesian theory and methods for applied researchers.[23-25]

Choice of Test Statistics

So far, while we have considered a number of statistics, Y, we have given no indication of how one should go about choosing a specific statistic on which to base testing and estimation. In any analysis, there will be many possibilities. In the HIV prevalence example, we took the number of positives (cases) as our test statistic Y. If we let A stand for the number of cases, we can say we took $Y = A$. But we could have taken $Y = \ln(A)$ or $Y = \text{logit}(A/N) = \ln\left[A/(N - A)\right]$ as alternative test statistics, to name only two of many possibilities. As such, why choose Y to be the number of cases?

This is a subtle issue, and we can only outline certain aspects of it here. Statisticians have used various criteria to choose test statistics in a given problem. The primary criterion, confidence validity, requires that the chosen statistic yield approximate confidence intervals with "proper coverage." That is, for reasonably sized samples and reasonable parameter values, an approximate interval should contain (cover) the true parameter with a frequency no less than its stated (nominal) confidence level. For example, an approximate 95% confidence interval is valid if it will contain the true parameter with a frequency no less than 95% over study repetitions. To choose among valid approximate intervals, we may further impose a second criterion, which is precision. For reasonable-sized samples and reasonable parameter values, a valid and precise interval has an average width over the repetitions that is no greater than other valid intervals. Taken together, the two criteria of validity and precision are sometimes referred to as *accuracy* criteria.

Although we have stated these two criteria qualitatively, it is more practical to use them quantitatively and note the potential for a trade-off between validity and precision. For example, in a given setting, one approximate 95% confidence interval might cover 94% of the time, while another might cover 95% of the time, but if the second interval were always 30% wider than the first, we should prefer the first interval for precision, even though it is not quite as valid as the second.

A third criterion in choosing a statistic Y is the ease or availability of computational formulas for its mean and variance. For most choices of Y, including logit(A/N) in the preceding example, one must use approximate means and variances. Worse, approximate intervals that use $\ln(A)$ or logit(A/N) directly as test statistics tend to be less valid than those based on $Y = A$, with little or no precision or computation advantage. On the other hand, taking $Y = \arcsine\left[(A/N)^{\frac{1}{2}}\right]$ can produce more valid intervals than taking $Y = A$, but it also requires use of approximations to its mean and variance that become unwieldy in stratified analyses. We thus might view the choice $Y = A$, the number of cases, as representing a compromise between accuracy and simplicity. The choice $Y=A$ can also be derived from consideration of score statistics and likelihood functions.[26]

Continuity Corrections and Mid-P-Values

As we saw in earlier sections, there can be discrepancies between exact and approximate results. There are two major philosophies for dealing with these discrepancies, each with corresponding methods.

The traditional philosophy is based on the fact that only traditional exact confidence intervals are *conservatively calibrated*: If the underlying assumptions are correct, a traditional exact 90% interval is guaranteed to cover (contain) the true measure of occurrence or effect with a frequency *no less than 90%*. Parallel statements apply for other confidence levels. We emphasize the phrase "no less than 90%" because, although in some situations the actual frequency will be 90%, in others, the traditional exact 90% interval will cover the true measure with a greater frequency—as much as 100% in some extreme examples. From this, it should be clear that the traditional philosophy maintains that overcoverage (coverage frequency above the stated confidence level) is always preferable to undercoverage (coverage frequency below the confidence level). Thus, because traditional exact intervals never suffer from undercoverage, the traditional philosophy would have us adjust our approximation methods so that our approximate P-values and intervals come close to the traditional exact P-values and intervals. In other words, it would have us take traditional exact results as the "gold standard."

Perhaps the simplest way to implement this philosophy is to adopt what are known as *continuity corrections* for approximate statistics.[27] Recall that the score approximation uses a normal distribution with mean and standard deviation, $E(Y|R)$ and $V(Y|R)^{\frac{1}{2}}$. In the preceding example, the lower P-value was taken as the area under the normal curve to the left of the observed Y value. It turns out that a better approximation is obtained by taking the area under the normal curve to the left of the point *midway* between the observed Y and the next largest Y. That is, to get a better approximation to the traditional exact lower P-value, we can replace Y by $Y+\frac{1}{2}$ in the score statistic, χ_{score} given by Equation 16-5. Similarly, to get a better approximation to the traditional exact upper P-value, we should replace Y by $Y-\frac{1}{2}$ in the score statistic.

The factors $\frac{1}{2}$ for P_{lower} and $-\frac{1}{2}$ for P_{upperr} are examples of continuity corrections, and the statistics obtained when using them are said to be *continuity corrected*. In the HIV example, with $Y = 1$, the continuity-corrected score statistic for getting a lower P-value to test a prevalence of 0.004 is:

$$\frac{(1+1/2)-1,000(0.004)}{\left[1,000(0.004)(1-0.004)\right]^{\frac{1}{2}}} = -1.253.$$

This statistic yields a continuity-corrected lower P-value of 0.105, which (as desired) is closer to the traditional exact value of 0.091 than the uncorrected value of 0.067 found earlier.

The second philosophy rejects the notions that traditional exact P-values should be taken as the "gold standard" and that overcoverage is always preferable to undercoverage. Instead, it maintains that we should seek procedures that produce the narrowest confidence intervals whose coverage is (in some average sense) as close as possible to the stated confidence level. In this view, a confidence interval with a stated confidence level of 90% that sometimes covered the truth with only 88% frequency would be preferable to a much wider interval that always covered with at least 90% frequency. In other words, some risk of moderate undercoverage is acceptable if worthwhile precision gains can be obtained.

One way of implementing this alternative philosophy is to replace traditional exact P-values with *mid-P-values*.[28,29] The lower mid-P-value is defined as the probability under the test hypothesis that the test statistic Y is less than its observed value, plus half the probability that Y equals its observed value. Thus, for the HIV example with $Y = 1$, we get:

$$\text{mid-}P_{\text{lower}} = \Pr\left(Y < 1\middle| R = 0.004\right) + \Pr\left(Y = 1\middle| R = 0.004\right)/2$$

$$= \left(1 - 0.004\right)^{1,000} + \frac{1,000\left(0.004\right)\left(1 - 0.004\right)^{999}}{2}$$

$$= 0.055$$

This mid-P-value is notably less than the traditional exact P-value of 0.091. For an HIV prevalence of 0.0041, the lower mid-P-value is 0.050, so 0.0041 is the upper mid-P 90% confidence limit for the HIV prevalence. This limit is notably less than the traditional exact upper limit of 0.0047, so it more precisely bounds the HIV prevalence.

To approximate the lower mid-P-value using a normal distribution, we should take the area under the normal curve to the left of the observed Y value. It follows that, if we wish to approximate the results from mid-P-values, we should *not* use continuity corrections.[30] This conclusion is apparent in the HIV survey example, in which the mid-P-value and the uncorrected score P-value for a prevalence of 0.004 are 0.055 and 0.067, while the continuity-corrected score P-value is 0.105.

Upper mid-P-values are defined analogously to lower mid-P-values: The upper mid-P-value is the probability under the test hypothesis that the test statistic Y is greater than its observed value, plus half the probability that Y equals its observed value. The two-sided mid-P-value is then just twice the smaller of the upper and lower mid-P-values. One pleasant property of the two-sided mid-P-value is that (unlike the traditional two-sided P-value) it cannot exceed 1. To see this, note that the upper and lower mid-P-values always sum to 1:

$$\text{mid-}P_{\text{lower}} + \text{mid-}P_{\text{upper}}$$

$$= \left[\Pr\left(Y \text{ less than observed}\middle| \text{test hypothesis}\right) + \Pr\left(Y \text{ equals observed}\middle| \text{test hypothesis}\right)/2 \right]$$

$$+ \left[\Pr\left(Y \text{ greater than observed}\middle| \text{test hypothesis}\right) + \Pr\left(Y \text{ equals observed}\middle| \text{test hypothesis}\right)/2 \right]$$

$$= \Pr\left(Y \text{ less than observed}\middle| \text{test hypothesis}\right) + \Pr\left(Y \text{ equals observed}\middle| \text{test hypothesis}\right)$$

$$+ \Pr\left(Y \text{ greater than observed}\middle| \text{test hypothesis}\right) = 1.$$

This result implies that the smaller of mid-P_{lower} and mid-P_{upper} must be half or less, so twice this smaller value (the two-sided mid-P-value) cannot exceed 1. Note, the median-unbiased point estimate was earlier defined as the point for which the upper and lower traditional exact P-values are equal. This estimate is also the point for which the upper and lower mid-P-values are equal. Thus, use of mid-P-values in place of traditional exact P-values does not change the point estimate.

Mid-P-values are always smaller than traditional exact P-values. As a result, for a given confidence level, fewer points will fall inside the confidence interval produced from mid-P-values than the traditional exact interval; in other words, the mid-P interval will always be narrower than the traditional exact interval.

These advantages of mid-P-values do have a price. For example, in some situations involving small observed numbers, mid-P intervals can suffer from notable undercoverage, as can intervals based on normal approximations. Thus, mid-P intervals, like the approximate intervals, are not guaranteed to perform well when the observed numbers are very small. They do, however, perform as well as or better than approximate methods such as the score or Wald method.

Another disadvantage of mid-P-values is that they cannot be interpreted as exact probabilities. Whereas upper and lower (but not two-sided) traditional exact P-values are exact frequency probabilities of certain events, mid-P-values have no such straightforward frequency interpretation.

They do have useful Bayesian probability interpretations,[31] but these are beyond our present discussion. In any case, it can be argued that this interpretational disadvantage of mid-P-values is of no practical concern if the P-values are used only to construct confidence intervals.

In sum, one position is that traditional exact P-values are the "gold standard" because confidence intervals based on them have coverage frequencies no less than the stated (nominal) confidence level (*e.g.*, 95%). If one accepts this position, one should use continuity corrections with approximate statistics. The alternative position is that one should not ignore precision concerns but instead seek the narrowest interval that is consistent with keeping coverage close to the stated confidence level of the interval. In particular, some risk of moderate undercoverage is tolerable. If one accepts this position, one should use mid-P-values in place of traditional exact P-values and not use continuity corrections with approximate statistics.

Neither position is completely logically compelling nor is either position dominant in statistics today. It may also be argued that the choice is of little practical importance because any dataset in which the choice makes a large numerical difference must have very little information on the measure of interest. It can be shown that when the sample size is large, all the methods (traditional, mid-P, approximate with or without correction) will give similar results. The difference among them is marked only when the results are so statistically unstable that most inferences from the data are unwarranted, even in the absence of biases. For example, in the HIV survey example, the mid-P confidence limits are not close to the traditional exact limits because only one case was observed and hence the results are imprecise.

For simplicity, in the remainder of this book, we limit our discussion of approximate statistics to those without continuity corrections.

Computation and Interpretation of Two-Sided P-Values

As we have mentioned, only traditional one-tailed P-values can be interpreted as probabilities in all circumstances (this is because they are defined as probabilities). Mid-P-values and two-sided P-values do not share this property except in special circumstances. Nonetheless, if the sample numbers are large enough so that the traditional, approximate, and mid-P-values are all nearly equal, the two-sided P-values will have an approximate probability interpretation. Specifically, in this situation, the two-sided P-values will approximately equal the probability that the square of the score statistic is greater than or equal to its observed value.

For example, if Y has a binomial distribution (as we have taken to be the case in the HIV example), the square of the score statistic χ_{score} for testing R is:

$$\chi^2_{score} = \frac{(Y-NR)^2}{NR(1-R)}.$$

[16-14]

In most of the statistics literature, χ^2_{score}, rather than χ_{score}, is called the score statistic. If both NR and $N(1-R)$ are more than 5 or so, all the two-sided P-values discussed above (traditional, score, Wald, and mid-P) will approximate the probability that χ^2_{score} is greater than or equal to its observed value. In this large-sample situation, χ_{score} has approximately a normal distribution with a mean of 0 and a standard deviation of 1, and so χ^2_{score} will have approximately a χ^2 distribution with one degree of freedom. Thus, if we are interested only in the two-sided P-value, we can simply compute χ^2_{score} and look up the probability that a χ^2 variate with one degree of freedom is this large or larger. Tables and functions for this purpose are widely available in statistics books and software.

A common misinterpretation of the two-sided P-value is that it represents the probability that the point estimate would be as far or farther from the test value as was observed. This interpretation is not even approximately correct for many epidemiologic estimates, particularly risk differences, because a P-value refers to the distribution of a test statistic, not a point estimate. As an example, consider again the HIV survey, this time taking the sample proportion of HIV positives (which was 0.001) as the test statistic. Suppose our test hypothesis is that the HIV prevalence is 0.005. The distance between the observed sample proportion of 0.001 and the test value of 0.005 is 0.004. For the sample proportion to be as far or farther from the test value of 0.005 as was observed, it would have to be either less than or equal to 0.005 to 0.004 = 0.001 or greater than or equal to 0.005 + 0.004 = 0.009.

If the true prevalence is 0.005, the probability of the sample proportion being less than 0.001 or more than 0.009 is 0.11. This probability is more than the traditional two-sided P-value of 0.080 computed earlier and more than twice the size of the two-sided mid-P-value of 0.047.

Again, the preceding interpretational obstacles need not concern us if we use two-sided P-values only to find confidence limits, rather than attempting to interpret them directly. This advantage is yet another reason to focus on confidence intervals and their coverage interpretation when analyzing data.

MULTIPLE COMPARISONS

Consider the following problem: We conduct a study in which we examine every exposure-disease association among 10 exposures and 10 diseases, for a total of $10 \times 10 = 100$ exposure-disease pairs associations. To analyze each association, suppose we use a "perfect" method to set 95% confidence limits—i.e., one that produces intervals containing the true association with exactly 95% frequency. If the coverage of each interval is independent of the coverage of every other interval, how many of the 100 resulting confidence intervals should we expect to contain their respective true value? The answer to this question is simply 95% of the 100 or 95. This means that of the 100 independent confidence intervals we are to examine, we should expect five to miss their target (the corresponding true value). Of course, anywhere from 0 to 100 may actually miss their target, and five represents only an average over hypothetical repetitions of the study. But the point is that we should *expect* several of these intervals to miss their target, even if we use a perfectly valid 95% confidence interval method.

Unfortunately, because we do not know the 100 true values, we cannot identify the intervals that missed their targets. With this in mind, suppose we are uncomfortable with the idea of reporting five intervals that miss their targets completely, even if the other 95 intervals cover their targets. One alternative is to increase the confidence level of our intervals. For example, if we increase our confidence level to 99%, we can then expect only one of the 100 intervals to miss their targets. Although this will widen every interval by a considerable factor (for Wald intervals, the factor will be 2.576/1.960-1, or 31%), the widening is an inevitable price of reducing the 5% miss rate to 1%.

The trade-off we have just described, between the width and the miss rate of the confidence interval, in no way affects the P-values computed for each association; we simply choose a lower alpha level and hence a lower slice through the P-value functions to get our interval estimates. There is, however, another perspective, which leads to an entirely different P-value function from the data. It is the result of a *multiple-comparisons* analysis, also known as simultaneous testing, joint testing, or multiple inference. In this view, we do *not* treat the 100 associations as 100 separate parameters to be estimated. Instead, we treat them as composing a *single* entity with 100 components, called the joint parameter or *vector* parameter for the associations. Here we provide an example for a conceptual introduction and discuss the issues further in Chapter 19.

Suppose that the true values of the 100 associations correspond to 100 risk ratios of 3.0, 2.1, 4.2, 0.6, 1.0, 1.5, and so on (up to 100 values). Then the single vector parameter representing these 100 true values is the ordered list of the values, specifically:

$$(3.0, 2.1, 4.2, 0.6, 1.0, 1.5, \ldots),$$

where the "..." represents the remaining 94 values. Note, each number in this ordered vector is called a *component* of the list, that is, every single association is only one component of the entire list.

With this simultaneous view of the 100 associations, we can formulate a *joint hypothesis* that the entire list of true associations equals a particular list of 100 specified numbers. Most commonly, this hypothesized list is a list of null values; for risk ratios, this would comprise 100 values of 1.0:

$$(1.0, 1.0, 1.0, 1.0, 1.0, 1.0, \ldots),$$

where the "…" represents 94 more 1.0s. This null list or null vector corresponds to the *joint null hypothesis* that there is no association among all 100 exposure-disease pairs. It is also possible to test other joint hypotheses, for example, that all 100 risk ratios are equal to 2.0 or that the first 50 in the list equal 1.0 and the remaining 50 in the list equal 0.5.

For any joint hypothesis we can imagine, it is possible to construct a statistic for testing that the hypothesis is true, which yields a *P*-value and test for that hypothesis. Such a *P*-value and test are called a *joint P-value* and *joint test* (or simultaneous test) for the associations. In particular, we can perform a simultaneous test of the joint null hypothesis (that no exposure is associated with any disease). If the joint test is valid *and* the joint null hypothesis is correct—so that there really are no associations at all—there will be no more than a 5% chance that the joint *P*-value from the test will fall below 0.05.

Joint Confidence Regions

We can consider the joint *P*-values for all possible vectors of values for the 100 associations. This collection of *P*-values is the multiple-comparisons analogue of the *P*-value function. The collection of all vectors that have a joint *P*-value of at least 0.05 is called a 95% *joint confidence region* for the vector of parameter values. A 95% confidence region constructed from a valid testing method has the useful property that it will include the true parameter vector with a frequency no less than 95%, provided there is no bias and all assumptions underlying the method are satisfied.

How is this joint confidence region for the vector of 100 associations related to the 100 single-association confidence intervals that we usually compute? If the joint null hypothesis is indeed correct and single-association intervals are independent of one another, then, on average, we should expect about five of the single-association intervals to miss their target, which in every case is the null value (a risk ratio of 1.0). We should also expect a valid joint confidence region to include the null vector 95% of the time because there is at least a 95% chance that $P > .05$ when the joint null hypothesis is correct. Thus, if there are no associations, we have this apparently paradoxical result: The joint confidence region will probably contain the null vector, apparently saying that the joint null hypothesis is compatible with the data, yet it is also probable that at least a few of the single 95% confidence intervals will miss the null, apparently saying that at least a few single null hypotheses are not compatible with the data. In other words, we expect the joint confidence region to indicate that every association may be null, and the single intervals to indicate that some associations are not null. In fact, if all the null hypotheses are correct, the single-interval coverage probabilities are exactly 95%, and the intervals are independent, then the probability that at least two of the single intervals will miss the null is 1 minus the binomial probability that only none or one of the intervals misses the null.

$$1 - 0.95^{100} - 100(0.05)(0.95)^{99} = 0.96.$$

This apparent paradox has been the source of much confusion. Its resolution comes about by recognizing that the joint confidence region and the 100 single intervals are all addressing different questions and have different objectives. A single 95% interval addresses the question: "What is the value of this parameter?" where "this" refers to just one of the 100 values (*i.e.*, ignoring the other 99). Its objective is to miss the correct value of that one parameter no more than 5% of the time, *without regard to whether any of the other intervals miss or not*. Thus, each single interval addresses only one of 100 distinct single-association questions and has only one of 100 distinct objectives. In contrast, the joint confidence region addresses the question, "What is the *vector* of parameter values?"; its objective is to miss the true *vector* of all 100 associations no more than 5% of the time.

If we are indeed trying to meet the latter objective, we must recognize that some misses by the single intervals are likely to occur by chance even if no association is present. Thus, to meet the objective of joint estimation, we cannot naively combine the results from the single intervals. For example, suppose that we take as our confidence region, the set of all vectors for which the first component (*i.e.*, the first association in the list) falls within the single 95% interval for the first association, the second component falls within the single 95% interval for the second association, and so on for all 100 components. The chance that such a combined region will contain the true vector of associations is equal to the chance that *all* the single intervals will contain the corresponding components. If all the exposures and diseases are independent of one another, this probability will be 0.95^{100}, which is only 0.006! These issues are discussed further in Chapter 19.

Problems with Conventional Approaches

The preceding example illustrates how the tasks of joint testing and estimation are much more stringent than those of single one-at-a-time testing and estimation. One extreme response to this stringency is to construct the single confidence intervals to have a confidence level that guarantees the naive combination method just described will yield a valid joint confidence region. This procedure is called the *Bonferroni* method for "adjusting for multiple comparisons." If we want a 95% confidence region from overlapping the single intervals, in the preceding example, we will need a single-interval alpha level that is one-hundredth the desired joint alpha level. This value is $\alpha = 0.05/100 = 0.0005$, which corresponds to a single-interval confidence level of $(1-0.0005) \times 100 = 99.95\%$. This choice yields a 0. $0.9995^{100} = 0.95$, chance that a naïve combination of all the single 99.95% confidence intervals will produce a confidence region that includes the true vector of associations. Thus the Bonferroni method is valid, but the single intervals it produces will typically be much too wide (conservative) for use in single-association estimation. For example, Wald intervals have to be 70% wider to get a 95% joint Bonferroni region when there are 100 associations. In addition, the joint Bonferroni confidence region is typically much larger (more imprecise) than it needs to be, that is, the Bonferroni region is also unnecessarily imprecise for joint estimation purposes. For hypothesis testing, a procedure that is equivalent to the Bonferroni adjustment, and equally bad, is to use a 0.05 alpha level but multiply all the single-association *P*-values by the number of associations before comparing them to the alpha level.

A deeper problem in the multiple-comparisons literature is that joint confidence regions have been recommended in situations in which the scientific objectives of the study call for single intervals. Typically, the different associations in a study are of interest on a purely one-at-a-time basis, often to different investigators with different interests. For example, a large health survey or cohort study may collect data pertaining to many possible associations, including data on diet and cancer, on exercise and heart disease, and perhaps many other distinct topics. A researcher can legitimately deny interest in any joint hypothesis regarding all of these diverse topics, instead wanting to focus on those few (or even one) pertinent to his or her specialties. In such situations, multiple-inference procedures such as we have outlined are irrelevant, inappropriate, and wasteful of information (because they will produce improperly imprecise single intervals).[32-34]

Nevertheless, it is important to recognize that investigators frequently conduct data searches or "data dredging," for which the assessment of joint hypotheses is most appropriate.[35,36] Such searches are usually done with multiple single-inference procedures, when special multiple-inference procedures should be used instead. Classic examples of such misuse of single-inference procedures involve selecting for further analysis only those associations or interactions that are "statistically significant." This approach is commonly used in attempts to identify harmful exposures, high-risk population subgroups, or subgroups that are selectively affected by study exposures. Such attempts represent multiple-inference problems because the study question and objectives concern the vector of all the tested associations. For example, central questions that drive searches for harmful exposures may include "Which (if any) of these associations is positive?" or "Which of these associations is important in magnitude?"

Unfortunately, conventional approaches to multiple-inference questions (such as Bonferroni adjustments) are poor choices for answering such questions, in part, because they have low efficiency or poor accuracy.[37] More modern procedures, such as hierarchical (empirical-Bayes) modeling, can offer dramatic performance advantages over conventional approaches and are well suited to epidemiologic data searches.[35,38-42]

Summary

In any analysis involving testing or estimation of multiple parameters, it is important to clarify the research questions to discern whether multiple-inference procedures will be needed.

Multiple-inference procedures will be needed if and only if joint hypotheses are of interest. Even if one is interested in a joint hypothesis, conventional or classical multiple-inference procedures will usually provide poor results, and many better procedures are now available.

When in doubt about the best strategy to pursue, most audiences will find acceptable a presentation of the results of all single-inference procedures (*e.g.*, confidence intervals for all associations examined). When this is not possible and one must select associations to present based on statistical criteria, one should at least take care to note the number and nature of the associations examined and the probable effect of such selection on the final results (for example, the high probability that at least a few intervals have missed their target). Chapter 19 provides further discussion of multiple-comparisons procedures and a graphical illustration of the distinction between single- and multiple-comparison procedures.

References

1. Greenland S. Summarization, smoothing, and inference in epidemiologic analysis. 1991 Ipsen Lecture, Hindsgavl, Denmark. *Scand J Soc Med*. 1993;21:227-232.
2. Maclaughlin DS. A data validation program nucleus. *Comput Programs Biomed*. 1980;11:43-47.
3. Tukey JW. *EDA: Exploratory Data Analysis*. Reading, MA: Addison-Wesley; 1977.
4. Cochran WG. The effectiveness of adjustment by subclassification in removing bias in observational studies. *Biometrics*. 1968;24:295-313.
5. Rothman KJ, Keller AZ. The effect of joint exposure to alcohol and tobacco on risk of cancer of the mouth and pharynx. *J Chronic Dis*. 1972;25:711-716.
6. Little RJ, Rubin DB. *Statistical Analysis with Missing Data*, John Wiley & Sons; 2019.
7. Allison PD. *Missing Data*. Thousand Oaks, CA: Sage Publications; 2001.
8. Tsiatis AA. *Semiparametric Theory and Missing Data*. New York, NY: Springer; 2006.
9. Sterne JA, White IR, Carlin JB, et al. Multiple imputation for missing data in epidemiological and clinical research: potential and pitfalls. *Br Med J*. 2009;338:b2393.
10. Robins JM, Rotnitzky A, Zhao LP. Estimation of regression coefficients when some regressors are not always observed. *J Am Stat Assoc*. 1994;89:846-866.
11. Seaman SR, White IR. Review of inverse probability weighting for dealing with missing data. *Stat Methods Med Res*. 2013;22:278-295.
12. Vach W, Blettner M. Biased estimation of the odds ratio in case-control studies due to the use of ad hoc methods of correcting for missing values for confounding variables. *Am J Epidemiol*. 1991;134:895-907.
13. Greenland S, Finkle WD. A critical look at methods for handling missing covariates in epidemiologic regression analyses. *Am J Epidemiol*. 1995;142:1255-1264.
14. Greenland S. Randomization, statistics, and causal inference. *Epidemiology*. 1990;1:421-429.
15. Bishop YMM, Fienberg SE, Holland PW. *Discrete Multivariate Analysis: Theory and Practice*. Cambridge, MA: Mit Press; 1975.
16. Greenland S. Smoothing observational data: a philosophy and implementation for the health sciences. *Int Stat Rev*. 2006;74:31-46.
17. Cox DR, Hinkley DV. *Theoretical Statistics*. New York, NY: Chapman and Hall; 1974.
18. Goodman SN, Royall R. Evidence and scientific research. *Am J Public Health*. 1988;78:1568-1574.
19. Royall R. *Statistical Inference: A Likelihood Paradigm*. New York, NY: Chapman and Hall; 1997.
20. Edwards AWF. *Likelihood*. Baltimore, MD: Johns Hopkins University Press; 1992.
21. Lehmann EL. *Testing Statistical Hypotheses*. New York, NY: Wiley; 1986.
22. Clayton D, Hills M. *Statistical Models in Epidemiology*. New York, NY: Oxford University Press; 1993.
23. Gelman A, Carlin JB, Stern HS, Dunson DB, Vehtari A, Rubin DB. *Bayesian Data Analysis*. Boca Raton; London; New York: CRC press; 2013.
24. Daniels MJ, Hogan JW. *Missing Data in Longitudinal Studies: Strategies for Bayesian Modeling and Sensitivity Analysis*. Boca Raton, FL: CRC Press; 2008.
25. Wakefield J. *Bayesian and Frequentist Regression Methods*. Berlin: Springer Science & Business Media; 2013.
26. Gart JJ, Tarone RE. The relation between score tests and approximate UMPU tests in exponential models common in biometry. *Biometrics*. 1983;39:781-786.
27. Yates F. Contingency tables involving small numbers and the chi-square test. *JR Stat Soc Suppl*. 1934;1:217-235.
28. Lancaster HO. The combination of probabilities arising from data in discrete distributions. *Biometrika*. 1949;36:370-382.
29. Berry G, Armitage P. Mid-P confidence intervals: a brief review. *Statistician*. 1995;44:417-423.
30. Miettinen OS. Comment. *J Am Stat Assoc*. 1974;69:380-382.

31. Nurminen M, Mutanen P. Exact Bayesian analysis of two proportions. *Scand J Stat*. 1987;14:67-77.
32. Rothman KJ. No adjustments are needed for multiple comparisons. *Epidemiology*. 1990;1:43-46.
33. Savitz DA, Olshan AF. Multiple comparisons and related issues in the interpretation of epidemiologic data. *Am J Epidemiol*. 1995;142:904-908.
34. Mayo DG, Cox DR. Frequentist statistics as a theory of inductive inference. In: Rojo J, ed. *2nd Lehmann Symposium - Optimality. IMS Lecture Notes - Monographs Series*. Institute of Mathematical Statistics; 2006.
35. Greenland S, Robins JM. Empirical-Bayes adjustments for multiple comparisons are sometimes useful. *Epidemiology*. 1991;2:244-251.
36. Thompson JR. A response to "Describing data requires no adjustment for multiple comparisons." *Am J Epidemiol*. 1998;147:815.
37. Greenland S. Basic problems in interaction assessment. *Environ Health Perspect*. 1993;101(suppl 4):59-66.
38. Thomas DC, Greenland S. The efficiency of matching in case-control studies of risk-factor interactions. *J Chronic Dis*. 1985;38:569-574.
39. Greenland S. A semi-Bayes approach to the analysis of correlated multiple associations, with an application to an occupational cancer-mortality study. *Stat Med*. 1992;11:219-230.
40. Greenland S, Poole C. Empirical-Bayes and semi-Bayes approaches to occupational and environmental hazard surveillance. *Arch Environ Health*. 1994;49:9-16.
41. Steenland K, Bray I, Greenland S, Boffetta P. Empirical Bayes adjustments for multiple results in hypothesis-generating or surveillance studies. *Cancer Epidemiol Biomarkers Prev*. 2000;9:895-903.
42. Greenland S. When should epidemiologic regressions use random coefficients? *Biometrics*. 2000;56:915-921.

CHAPTER 17

Introduction to Categorical Statistics

Sebastien Haneuse[*]

In Chapter 16, we discussed the fundamentals of epidemiologic data analysis, focusing on methods used to estimate the proportion of a population with a disease. In this chapter, we turn to the comparison of disease proportions, odds, or rates between two populations. Toward this, we present basic statistical techniques for categorical data analysis of person-count and person-time data, focusing on methods for unstratified (crude) data. Although it is usually necessary to take into account factors beyond the exposure and the disease of interest, either through stratification or regression, it is instructive to consider methods based on crude data for a number of reasons. First, in some settings, for example, a large randomized trial that compares two treatment arms, such analyses are appropriate. Second, outside of such settings, consideration of methods for crude data provides an important foundation for understanding key concepts related to estimation and inference before working to understand why and how more complex methods are needed (*e.g.*, to control for confounding bias). Finally, simple analyses can often provide useful insight about the data and observed associations, either as a preliminary step before layering on more complexity or *post hoc* when considering the impact of introducing the additional complexity.

Following the introduction of the methods in this chapter, Chapter 18 presents extensions to settings where the data are stratified by some other variable(s), either for the purposes of controlling confounding bias or to investigate and report on heterogeneity. Chapter 18 also presents methods regarding estimation of the attributable fraction. Following that, methods for settings where the exposure and/or outcome are polytomous (*i.e.*, have more than two levels) are provided in Chapter 19, while regression-based analyses are discussed in Chapters 20 and 21.

CLASSIFICATION OF ANALYSIS METHODS

Epidemiologists often group basic types of epidemiologic studies into cohort, case-control, or cross-sectional studies (see Chapter 6). An alternative classification arises when one considers the underlying probability model that gives rise to the observed data. Suppose, for example, that the

---

[*]This chapter is based on original material by Sander Greenland and Kenneth J. Rothman.

outcome is binary and that a cohort study has been conducted. Furthermore, suppose that there is no late entry and that subjects are followed for the same time frame with no loss to follow-up. The cohort can then be viewed as a closed cohort (see Chapter 4), so that the observed data are the number of diseased individuals in relation to the size of the cohort. We refer to this as *person-count cohort* data. From such data, one can compute and report the proportion of subjects who are diseased, the *incidence proportion*, which can then serve as an estimate of *risk*.

Now suppose that the cohort is not closed; that is, late entry and loss to follow-up manifest in the data. In this setting, the subjects in the cohort contribute differing amounts of information regarding risk (*i.e.*, depending on when they enter and when they leave). Thus, it would be inappropriate to use the number of people in the cohort as a denominator when estimating risk. Instead, one can use the number of diseased individuals in relation to the total time at-risk, referred to as *person-time cohort* data, to estimate the *incidence rate* at which the outcome occurs.

Under suitable assumptions (including those discussed below), many of the statistical methods developed for cohort data can also be applied to data arising from a case-control study or a cross-sectional study.[1-8] Furthermore, as discussed in Chapter 18, only relatively minor modifications are required for basic analyses of two-stage or two-phase data.[9] Collectively, these facts greatly reduce the number of analytic methods needed in epidemiology. As explained below, however, slightly more complicated methods are needed for estimating risk ratios from case-cohort data.[10]

In studies that involve extended follow-up, some subjects may leave observation before the study disease occurs or the risk period of interest ends (*e.g.*, because of loss to follow-up or competing risks). For such studies, methods that stratify on follow-up time will be needed; these methods are discussed in Chapter 22.

FUNDAMENTAL DISTRIBUTIONS

Following the distinction between person-count and person-time cohort data, two probability distributions form the foundation for the methods presented in this chapter: the binomial distribution and the Poisson distribution.

Assumptions

As explained in the next two subsections, underpinning both the binomial and Poisson distributions are two key assumptions: (1) some form of *homogeneity* regarding the risk across subjects in the population(s) of interest; and (2) the outcomes of the study subjects are *independent*. Intuitively, independence corresponds to the notion that once you know the risk of a group, discovering the outcome status of one group member will tell you nothing about the outcome status of any other group member.

Both assumptions serve to greatly simplify the statistical theory that underpins the methods presented in this chapter. The assumption of homogeneity serves to enable borrowing of information across study subjects in order to learn about the risk or the rate of occurrence of the outcome. In the absence of some form of homogeneity (either overall or within subgroups), we would have to view each individual as having his or her own unique risk, greatly complicating any analysis.

While the details of these assumptions are given below, we note that methods that permit their relaxation are covered in Chapters 18, 20, and 24. Finally, as is usually done in presentation of introductory material, we assume no sources of bias in the study; that is, no measurement error, selection bias, follow-up bias, or confounding bias.

The Binomial Distribution

Although the binomial distribution was derived in Chapter 16, we briefly summarize it here. Suppose we consider the closed cohort setting and let N denote the total number of people in the cohort and A the number of diseased individuals or cases. Furthermore, let R denote the probability that a given subject will experience the outcome. Note, in some settings R may refer to the incidence or risk of the outcome while in others to the prevalence of the outcome (see Chapter 4). Assuming that the outcomes across the N subjects are independent, the binomial distribution characterizes the probability associated with observing $A = a$ cases out of N subjects:

$$P(A = a) = \binom{N}{a} R^a (1 - R)^{N-a} \qquad [17\text{-}1]$$

where $\binom{N}{a}$ is the binomial coefficient, read as "N choose a." Note, implicit in expression 17-1 is that the probability, R, is assumed to be the same (*i.e.*, homogeneous) across all N people in the cohort. Finally, we have that under the binomial distribution, the average or expected value of A is $E(A) = NR$ and the variance of A is $V(A) = NR(1 - R)$.

The Poisson Distribution

Now consider the setting where the cohort is not closed. Letting A again denote the number of diseased individuals or cases, let T denote the total observed person-time. Furthermore, let I denote the rate at which cases arise per unit time. Assuming that whether or not a subject is observed to have the disease during some interval of person-time is independent of how many diseased individuals there were at the start of the interval, the Poisson distribution characterizes the probability associated with observing $A = a$ cases during the T units of person-time as:

$$P(A = a) = \frac{(IT)^a \exp(-IT)}{a!} \qquad [17\text{-}2]$$

Implicit in this expression is that the rate I does not change during the time frame covered by the cohort study; that is, it is constant over time. Also implicit is the concept that a given amount of person-time, say 100 person-years, can be derived from observing many people for a short period of time or few people for a long period of time. That is, the experience of 100 persons for 1 year, 200 persons for 6 months, 50 persons for 2 years, or 1 person for 100 years are assumed to be equivalent. Finally, we have that, under the Poisson distribution, the average or expected value and variance of A are $E(A) = IT$ and $V(A) = IT$, respectively, and that the Poisson distribution can be used as an approximation to the binomial distribution when N is large and R is small.[11]

STUDIES OF SINGLE GROUPS

Epidemiologic studies are typically interested in comparing risks or rates across two or more groups. In order to do this, however, it is important to be able to quantify the risk or rate of a disease in a single group or population of interest. Indeed, such quantification may be of intrinsic scientific and public-health interest. In occupational and environmental epidemiology, for example, it is often of interest to quantify and query excess morbidity or mortality in a single workplace, community, or neighborhood. In such studies, it may also be of interest to compare incidence (*i.e.*, risk) or prevalence of the disease in this group with that of some external population. Lancaster,[12] for example, quantified the prevalence of neural tube defects among live births conceived through in vitro fertilization and subsequently compared this prevalence with that of the general population of live births.

Person-Count Cohort Data

Given observed values of N and A, expression 17-1 viewed as a function of the unknown parameter R is referred to as the *binomial likelihood*. From this, we have that the maximum likelihood estimator (MLE) of R is $\hat{R} = A/N$. See Chapter 16 for more discussion on likelihood-based estimation.

To quantify uncertainty in $\hat{R}$ as an estimate of R, a natural way forward would be to use the Wald method to construct a confidence interval. For example, a Wald-based approximate 95% confidence interval is:

$$\hat{R} \pm 1.96 \times SE\left(\hat{R}\right),$$

where $SE\left(\hat{R}\right) = \left[\hat{R}\left(1-\hat{R}\right)/N\right]^{1/2} = \left[A(N-A)/N^3\right]^{1/2}$ is the *standard error* of $\hat{R}$. A problem with this approach, however, is that there is no guarantee that the resulting lower and upper limits of the interval remain between 0 and 1. An alternative, one which is common in practice, is to use the Wald method to construct a confidence interval for an estimate of the logit of R, that is the natural logarithm of the odds:

$$\phi = \text{logit}(R) = \ln\left(\frac{R}{1-R}\right),$$

and then back-transform to obtain a confidence interval for the estimate of π using the fact that:

$$R = \text{expit}(\phi) = \frac{\exp(\phi)}{1+\exp(\phi)}.$$

Crucially, ϕ can take on any negative or positive value so that one does not have to worry about any constraints when constructing a confidence interval for a given estimator. Toward this, again using the theory likelihood-based estimation, the MLE of the logit of π can be obtained simply as the logit of the MLE of R; that is, the MLE of ϕ is $\hat{\phi} = \text{logit}\left(\hat{R}\right)$, where $\hat{R}$ is the MLE of R. Furthermore, one can show that the large-sample standard error of $\hat{\phi}$ is $SE\left(\hat{\phi}\right) = \left[1/A + 1/(N-A)\right]^{1/2}$. Thus, an approximate 95% confidence interval for $\hat{\phi}$ is:

$$\left(\hat{\phi}_L, \hat{\phi}_U\right) = \hat{\phi} \pm 1.96 \times SE\left(\hat{\phi}\right)$$

and an approximate 95% confidence interval for $\hat{\pi}$ is:

$$\left(\hat{R}_L, \hat{R}_U\right) = \left[\text{expit}\left(\hat{\phi}_L\right), \text{expit}\left(\hat{\phi}_U\right)\right].$$

In addition to R, interest may lie in estimating and reporting the *relative risk (or relative prevalence,* as appropriate*), $RR = R/R_E$, where R_E is the risk (or prevalence) in some external population. From the theory of likelihood-based estimation, we have that the MLE of RR is $\widehat{RR} = \hat{R}/R_E$; that is, one can simply substitute in the value of the MLE for R into the formula for RR. Furthermore, an approximate 95% confidence interval for $\widehat{RR}$ is $\left(\widehat{RR}_L, \widehat{RR}_U\right) = \left(\hat{R}_L/R_E, \hat{R}_U/R_E\right)$.

In the aforementioned study by Lancaster,[12] $A = 6$ infants from a cohort of $N = 1{,}694$ live births conceived through in vitro fertilization were born with neural tube defects, giving an estimated prevalence of $\hat{R} = 6/1{,}694 = 0.00354$ or 3.5 per 1,000 live births. Noting that $\left[1/A + 1/(N-A)\right]^{1/2} = 0.409$, a Wald-based approximate 95% confidence interval for the estimated prevalence is

$$\left(\hat{R}_L, \hat{R}_U\right) = \text{expit}\left[\text{logit}(0.00354) \pm 1.96 \times 0.409\right] = (0.0016, 0.0079).$$

Lancaster[12] also noted a general population prevalence of $R_G = 0.0012$, or 1.2 per 1,000. Thus, the estimated prevalence ratio for neural tube defects in live births conceived through in vitro fertilization is $\widehat{RR} = \hat{R}/R_E = 0.00354/0.0012 = 2.95$, with an approximate 95% confidence interval of $\left(\widehat{RR}_L, \widehat{RR}_U\right) = (1.33, 6.55)$. The results suggest that if the binomial model is correct, either a bias is present or there is an elevated prevalence of defects in the study cohort, but the magnitude of elevation is imprecisely estimated.

One concern with the above approximate calculations is their reliance on large-sample statistical properties of Wald-based confidence intervals. As a general rule of thumb, Wald-based limits are reasonably accurate when both $N\hat{R}_L$ and $N\left(1 - \hat{R}_U\right)$ are at least 5. In the Lancaster study, however, $N\hat{R}_L = 1,694(0.0016) = 2.7$, so that small-sample methods analogous to those described in Chapter 16 should be considered. Toward this, recall from Chapter 16 that the lower mid-P-value is defined as the probability under some hypothesized value of R that A is less than its observed value, say $A = a$, plus half the probability that A equals its observed value:

$$\text{mid-}P_{\text{lower}} = P\left(A < a \mid R\right) + \frac{1}{2}P\left(A = a \mid R\right)$$

$$= \sum_{k=0}^{a-1}\binom{N}{k}R^k\left(1 - R\right)^{N-k} + \frac{1}{2}\binom{N}{a}R^a\left(1 - R\right)^{N-a}$$

Furthermore, the upper mid-P-value, defined as the probability under some hypothesized value of R that A is greater than its observed value, say $A = a$, plus half the probability that A equals its observed value, is mid-$P_{\text{upper}} = 1 - \text{mid-}P_{\text{lower}}$. From these, the median-unbiased estimate of R is the value at which mid-$P_{\text{lower}} = \text{mid-}P_{\text{upper}} = 0.5$.[13] To get a two-sided $(1 - \alpha)$-level mid-P confidence interval, one can take the lower limit to be the value of R for which mid-$P_{\text{upper}} = \alpha/2$ and the upper limit to be the value of R for which mid-$P_{\text{lower}} = \alpha/2$.

For the Lancaster data, we have $A = 6$, $N = 1,694$, and $R_E = 0.0012$, so that substituting $R_E \times RR$ for R into the above expression we have:

$$\text{mid-}P_{\text{lower}} = \sum_{k=0}^{5}\binom{1,694}{k}\left(0.0012RR\right)^k\left(1 - 0.0012RR\right)^{1694-k}$$

$$+ \frac{1}{2}\binom{1694}{6}\left(0.0012RR\right)^6\left(1 - 0.0012RR\right)^{1688}.$$

Setting mid-$P_{\text{lower}} = 0.5$ and solving for RR yields a median-unbiased estimate of 3.03 for the prevalence ratio. Other substitutions yield 95% mid-P limits of (1.20, 6.13). Thus, despite the initial concern regarding the small number of cases, these confidence limits are similar to the large-sample limits.

Person-Time Cohort Data

Given observed values of T and A, expression 17-2 viewed as a function of the unknown parameter I is referred to as the *Poisson likelihood*. From this, the MLE of I is $\hat{I} = A/T$. Furthermore, the standard error of $\hat{I}$ is $SE\left(\hat{I}\right) = \sqrt{A/T^2}$, which can be used to construct a Wald-based confidence interval. As an example, Boice and Monson[14] reported $A = 41$ breast cancer cases out of $T = 28,010$ person-years at risk in a cohort of women treated for tuberculosis with x-ray fluoroscopy. Thus, the MLE of the rate of breast cancer in the population of such women is $\hat{I} = 41/28,010 = 0.00146$ or, equivalently, 146 cases per 100,000 person-years, with a Wald-based 95% confidence interval of (102, 191) cases per 100,000 person-years.

In addition to I, interest may lie in estimating and reporting the *rate ratio*, $IR = I/I_E$ where I_E is the rate in some external population. Again, using the theory of likelihood-based estimation, we have that the MLE of IR is $\widehat{IR} = \hat{I}/I_E$. If I_E is not be readily available but the expected number of cases given the observed person-time, say E, is, then the MLE of IR is $\widehat{IR} = A/E$. Boice and

Monson,[14] for example, report that only 23.3 cases were expected based on age-year–specific rates among women in Connecticut. Thus, the MLE of IR is $\widehat{IR} = 41/23.3 = 1.76$. To construct a Wald-based approximate confidence interval for this estimate, we first construct a confidence interval for the MLE of the natural log of IR, $\ln(\widehat{IR})$. We then use the fact that the large-sample standard error for $\ln(\widehat{IR})$ is:

$$SE\left[\ln\left(\widehat{IR}\right)\right] = \frac{1}{\sqrt{A}}.$$

From this, and exponentiating to transform back to the IR scale, a Wald-based approximate 95% confidence interval for $\widehat{IR}$ is:

$$\left(\widehat{IR}_L, \widehat{IR}_U\right) = \exp\left\{\ln\left(\widehat{IR}\right) \pm 1.96 \times SE\left[\ln\left(\widehat{IR}\right)\right]\right\}.$$

Applying this to the Boice and Monson[14] study, an approximate Wald-based 95% confidence interval is:

$$\left(\widehat{IR}_L, \widehat{IR}_U\right) = \exp\left[\ln\left(41/23.3\right) \pm 1.96 \times \left(1/\sqrt{41}\right)\right] = (1.30, 2.39)$$

These results suggest that, if the Poisson model is correct, if the variability in E is negligible, and if there is no bias, there appears to be an excess of breast cancers among fluoroscoped women relative to the Connecticut women, but the amount of that excess could readily span a wide range of values.

As with estimation and the quantification of uncertainty for RR under the binomial model, the validity of the methods presented for IR hinge on large-sample results. As a general rule of thumb, Wald-based confidence intervals can be viewed as being reasonably accurate if both $\widehat{IR}_L \times E$ and $\widehat{IR}_U \times E$ exceed 5. For settings where either of these do not hold, we can again appeal to the small-sample methods described in Chapter 16. Toward this, note that the expected value of A under a Poisson model can be written as:

$$E(A) = IT = \left(\frac{I}{E/T}\right) \times \frac{E}{T} \times T = \left(\frac{I}{I_E}\right) \times E = IR \times E.$$

We can then compute the mid-P-value functions for IR from the Poisson distribution using expression 17-2 with IT replaced with $IR \times E$:

$$
\begin{aligned}
\text{mid-}P_{\text{lower}} &= P\left(A < a|I\right) + \frac{1}{2}P\left(A = a|I\right) \\
&= \sum_{k=0}^{a-1} \frac{(IR \times E)^k \exp(-IR \times E)}{k!} + \frac{1}{2}\frac{(IR \times E)^a \exp(-IR \times E)}{a!} \\
&= 1 - mid\text{-}P_{upper}.
\end{aligned}
$$

Setting mid-$P_{\text{lower}} = 0.5$ and solving for IR yields the corresponding median-unbiased estimate. To get a two-sided $(1 - \alpha)$-level mid-P confidence interval, one can take the lower limit to be the value of IR for which mid-$P_{\text{upper}} = \alpha/2$ and the upper limit to be the value of IR for which mid-$P_{\text{lower}} = \alpha/2$.

As an example, Waxweiler et al.[15] observed $A = 7$ deaths from liver and biliary cancer in a cohort of workers who were exposed for at least 15 years to vinyl chloride. Only $E = 0.436$ deaths were expected based on general population rates. Using the above expression, the lower mid-P-value for the data is:

$$\text{mid-}P_{\text{lower}} = \sum_{k=0}^{6} \frac{\left(IR \times 0.436 \right)^{k} \exp\left(-IR \times 0.436\right)}{k!} + \frac{1}{2} \frac{\left(IR \times 0.436 \right)^{7} \exp\left(-IR \times 0.436\right)}{7!}.$$

From this, the median-unbiased estimate of IR is 16.4, while a 95% mid-P confidence interval is (6.9, 32.0). The number of cases observed is clearly far greater than we would expect under the Poisson model with $IR = 1$. Thus, unless biases are present, it appears that there is a considerably higher rate of liver and biliary cancer in this cohort relative to the general population.

Finally, for comparison, the MLE of IR using the data from the study by Waxweiler et al.[15] is $\widehat{IR} = 7/0.436 = 16.1$ while the Wald-based approximate 95% confidence interval is:

$$\left(\widehat{IR}_{L}, \widehat{IR}_{U} \right) = \exp\left\{ \ln\left(\widehat{IR}\right) \pm 1.96 \times SE\left[\ln\left(\widehat{IR}\right) \right] \right\} = (7.7, 34.0).$$

Standardization

Usually, E is calculated by applying stratum-specific incidence rates obtained from a large reference population (such as vital statistics data for a state or country) to the stratum-specific person-time experience of the study group. The process by which this is done is an example of *standardization,* which in this situation involves taking a weighted sum of the reference rates, using the stratum-specific person-time from the study group as weights (see Chapter 4). For example, if we are studying stomach cancer rates in a group consisting of persons aged 51 to 75 years divided into three age categories (ages 51-60 years, 61-70 years, 71-75 years), two sexes, and two ethnicity categories, there are a total of $3 \times 2 \times 2 = 12$ possible age-sex-ethnicity categories. Suppose that the person-times observed in each subgroup are $(T_1, T_2, \ldots, T_{12})$, and the corresponding age-sex-ethnicity–specific rates in the reference population are known to be $(I_1, I_2, \ldots, I_{12})$. Then, for a cohort that had the same age-sex-ethnicity–specific rates as the reference population and the same person-time distribution as that observed in the study group, the number of cases we should expect is:

$$E = T_1 I_1 + T_2 I_2 + \ldots + T_{12} I_{12}.$$

Note, the quantity E is generally not precisely equal to the number of cases one should expect in the study group if it had experienced the rates of the reference population.[16] This inequality arises because an alteration of the person-time rates in the study group will usually alter the distribution of person-time in the study group (see Chapters 4 and 5).

COMPARISONS OF TWO STUDY GROUPS

So far we have considered settings where the observed data came from a single group. While comparisons, in the form of relative risks and relative rates, were considered, they were done so through only conceiving of the data from the single group as being subject to statistical variation; that is, the values of R_E, I_E, and E from the external population were taken to be "known" constants. In the remainder of this chapter we consider settings where the observed data come from two groups, generically referred to as the "exposed" and "unexposed" groups. Throughout, we use the same notational conventions as those used for the single group setting but with a subscript "1" for the exposed group and a subscript "0" for the unexposed group.

Person-Count Cohort Data

In the two-group setting, person-count cohort data can be displayed in a 2×2 table of counts as illustrated in Table 17-1. The four cells of the table are the numbers of subjects classified into

Notation for a Crude Person-Count 2 × 2 Table

	Exposed	Unexposed	Total
Cases	A_1	A_0	M_1
Noncases	B_1	B_0	M_0
Total	N_1	N_0	N

each combination of presence or absence of exposure and occurrence or nonoccurrence of disease. Thus, A_0 is the number of cases among the N_0 subjects in the unexposed group (so that B_0 were not observed to experience the outcome), while A_1 is the number of cases among the N_1 subjects in the unexposed group (so that B_1 were not observed to experience the outcome).

As in the single group setting, assuming homogeneity of risk and independence of outcomes, one could use a binomial model for the observed number of cases in each of the two groups. Letting R_1 and R_0 denote the risk (*i.e.*, the probability that a given subject will experience the outcome) in the exposed and unexposed groups, respectively, the joint probability of observing $A_1 = a_1$ and $A_0 = a_0$ is the product of the two group-specific binomial probabilities:

$$P\left(A_1 = a_1, \ A_0 = a_0\right) = P\left(A = a_1\right)P\left(A_0 = a_0\right) = \binom{N_1}{a_1}R_1^{a_1}\left(1 - R_1\right)^{N_1 - a_1}\binom{N_0}{a_0}R_0^{a_0}\left(1 - R_0\right)^{N_0 - a_0}.$$

[17-3]

Note, that the joint probability can be written as the product of the two group-specific probabilities arises from the assumption that the outcomes across the groups are independent of each other. This parallels the assumption that the outcomes of subjects within the groups are independent of each other.

Given observed data in the form of (A_1, N_1, A_0, N_0), expression 17-3 viewed as a function of the two unknown parameters R_1 and R_0 is referred to as the *binomial likelihood for two groups*. Under this model, we have:

1. The MLEs of R_1 and R_0 are $\hat{R}_1 = A_1/N_1$ and $\hat{R}_0 = A_0/N_0$, respectively.
2. The MLE of the risk ratio, $RR = R_1/R_0$ is:

$$\widehat{RR} = \frac{A_1/N_1}{A_0/N_0}.$$

3. The MLE of the risk difference, $RD = R_1 - R_0$ is:

$$\widehat{RD} = \frac{A_1}{N_1} - \frac{A_0}{N_0}.$$

4. The MLE of the risk odds ratio,

$$OR = \frac{R_1/\left(1 - R_1\right)}{R_0/\left(1 - R_0\right)}$$

is the observed incidence-odds ratio:

$$\widehat{OR} = \frac{A_1/B_1}{A_0/B_0}.$$

5. If $R_1 = R_0$, that is, if there is no difference in risk between the two groups, the expected number of exposed cases, A_1, is $E = N_1M_1/N$, where M_1 is the total number of cases. Furthermore, the variance of the number of exposed cases is:

$$V = E \times \frac{M_0N_0}{N(N-1)} = \frac{M_1N_1M_0N_0}{N^2(N-1)}.$$

It follows from the last fact that a large-sample statistic for testing the null hypothesis $H_0:R_0 = R_1$, which is the same hypothesis as $RR = 1$ and $RD = 0$, is:

$$\chi_{score} = \frac{A_1 - E}{V^{1/2}},$$

which can be assessed against a standard normal distribution (that is a normal distribution with mean 0 and variance 1) to obtain a P-value.

To illustrate the various calculations, Table 17-2 presents data from a cohort study of diarrhea in breast-fed infants colonized with *Vibrio cholerae* 01, classified by level of antibody titers in their mother's breast milk.[17] A low titer is hypothesized to confer an elevated risk and so is taken to correspond to the "exposed" group (and, thus, is the first column of Table 17-2). From these data, we obtain:

$$\widehat{RR} = (12/14)/(7/16) = 1.96$$
$$\widehat{RD} = 12/14 - 7/16 = 0.42$$
$$\widehat{OR} = (12/2)/(7/9) = 7.71$$
$$E = (19 \times 14)/30 = 8.87$$
$$V = 8.87 \times (11 \times 16)/(30 \times 29) = 179$$

TABLE 17-2

Diarrhea During a 10-Day Follow-Up Period in 30 Breast-Fed Infants Colonized With *Vibrio cholerae* 01, According to Antipolysaccharide Antibody Titers in the Mother's Breast Milk

	Antibody Level		Total
	Low	High	
Diarrhea	12	7	19
No diarrhea	2	9	11
Totals	14	16	30

From Glass RI, Svennerholm AM, Stoll BJ, et al. Protection against cholera in breast-fed children by antibiotics in breast milk. *N Engl J Med.* 1983;308:1389-1392.

and

$$\chi_{\text{score}} = \frac{12 - 8.87}{(179)^{1/2}} = 2.34.$$

The latter yields an upper-tailed P-value of 0.01. Thus, a score statistic as large or larger than that observed has low probability in the absence of bias or an antibody effect.

Turning to interval estimation, an estimate of the standard error for $\widehat{RD}$ is:

$$SE\left(\widehat{RD}\right) = \left[\frac{A_1\left(N_1 - A_1\right)}{N_1^2\left(N_1 - 1\right)} + \frac{A_0\left(N_0 - A_0\right)}{N_0^2\left(N_0 - 1\right)}\right]^{1/2}.$$

Using this, one can construct a Wald-based approximate 95% confidence interval as:

$$\left(\widehat{RD}_L, \widehat{RD}_U\right) = \widehat{RD} \pm 1.96 \times SE\left(\widehat{RD}\right).$$

In data applications, this formula may produce limits that fall below -1 or above 1, especially when the cell sizes are small. To mitigate this problem, Zou and Donner[18] proposed an alternative approach to constructing interval limits for $\widehat{RD}$, specifically:

$$\left(\widehat{RD}_L, \widehat{RD}_U\right) = \left[\frac{\exp(-s) - d}{\exp(-s) + d}, \frac{\exp(s) - d}{\exp(s) + d}\right] \qquad [17\text{-}4]$$

where $s = \left[2 \times 1.96 \times SE\left(\widehat{RD}\right)\right] \Big/ \left(1 - \widehat{RD}^2\right)$ and $d = \left(1 - \widehat{RD}\right) \Big/ \left(1 + \widehat{RD}\right)$.

Approximate confidence intervals for $\widehat{RR}$ and $\widehat{OR}$ can both be obtained by first constructing confidence intervals for $\ln(\widehat{RR})$ and $\ln(\widehat{OR})$ and back-transforming by exponentiating. Toward this, standard error estimates for $\ln(\widehat{RR})$ and $\ln(\widehat{OR})$ are:

$$SE\left[\ln\left(\widehat{RR}\right)\right] = \left[\frac{1}{A_1} - \frac{1}{N_1} + \frac{1}{A_0} - \frac{1}{N_0}\right]^{1/2}$$

and

$$SE\left[\ln\left(\widehat{OR}\right)\right] = \left[\frac{1}{A_1} + \frac{1}{N_1 - A_1} + \frac{1}{A_0} + \frac{1}{N_0 - A_0}\right]^{1/2},$$

respectively. From this, Wald-based approximate 95% confidence intervals for $\widehat{RR}$ and $\widehat{OR}$ are:

$$\left(\widehat{RR}_L, \widehat{RR}_U\right) = \exp\left\{\ln\left(\widehat{RR}\right) \pm 1.96 \times SE\left[\ln\left(\widehat{RR}\right)\right]\right\}$$

and

$$\left(\widehat{OR}_L, \widehat{OR}_U\right) = \exp\left\{\ln(\widehat{OR}) \pm 1.96 \times SE\left[\ln(\widehat{OR})\right]\right\},$$

respectively.

Returning to the diarrhea data in Table 17-2, we have:

$$SE\left(\widehat{RD}\right) = \left(\frac{12 \times 2}{14^2 \times 13} + \frac{7 \times 9}{16^2 \times 15}\right)^{1/2} = 0.161,$$

$$SE\left[\ln\left(\widehat{RR}\right)\right] = \left(\frac{1}{12} - \frac{1}{14} + \frac{1}{7} - \frac{1}{16}\right)^{1/2} = 0.304,$$

$$SE\left[\ln\left(\widehat{OR}\right)\right] = \left(\frac{1}{12} + \frac{1}{2} + \frac{1}{7} + \frac{1}{9}\right)^{1/2} = 0.915.$$

From these, Wald-based approximate 95% confidence intervals are:

$$\left(\widehat{RD}_L, \widehat{RD}_U\right) = 0.42 \pm 1.96 \times 0.161 = (0.10, 0.74),$$

$$\left(\widehat{RR}_L, \widehat{RR}_U\right) = \exp\left[\ln(1.96) \pm 1.96 \times 0.304\right] = (1.08, 3.56),$$

$$\left(\widehat{OR}_L, \widehat{OR}_U\right) = \exp\left[\ln(7.71) \pm 1.96 \times 0.915\right] = (1.28, 46.3).$$

Furthermore, the 95% confidence interval for $\widehat{RD}$ based on the approach of Zou and Donner[18] is $\left(\widehat{RD}_L, \widehat{RD}_U\right) = (0.06, 0.68)$, which is slightly shifted toward the null compared with the Wald-based limits. Collectively, although the results indicate a positive association, each of the measures is imprecisely estimated, especially the odds ratio.

There are at least two cautions to consider in interpreting the statistics just given. First, infant diarrhea is usually infectious in origin, and causative agents could have been transmitted between subjects if there was contact between the infants or their mothers. This lack of independence could render the use of the binomial distribution inappropriate with a key implication that the estimates of standard errors are invalid (that is they are too small or too big relative to the true extent of uncertainty). Second, as a general rule of thumb, one may expect that a Wald-based confidence interval for $\widehat{OR}$ is reasonably accurate when all four cell expectations given the lower odds ratio limit, $\widehat{OR}_L$, and all four cell expectations given the upper odds ratio limit, $\widehat{OR}_U$, exceed 5. In the diarrhea data, however, there are only $N_1 - A_1 = 2$ low-antibody noncases, raising concern regarding the accuracy of the MLE for OR. Thus, while transformation-based approaches (such as using the natural logarithm and back-transforming) yield confidence intervals with improved characteristics, it remains important to be aware of small-sample methods. Toward this, note that the calculations for E and V, the expectation and variance of A_1 under no association between the exposure and outcome, are computed conditional on the marginal totals (M_1, M_0, N_1, N_0). That is, the calculations treat the marginal totals as fixed rather than variable. In reality, none of the designs we have described has both margins fixed. In a cohort study, the case total, M_1 in Table 17-1, is not set by design and so is free to vary; in a case-control study, while M_1 is set by design, the exposed total, N_1, is not and so is free to vary; and in a prevalence survey, all the margins may be free to vary. Nevertheless, with origins in the context of null hypothesis testing in randomized experiments,[19-22] this practice is virtually universal in epidemiologic statistics.

One useful consequence of treating (M_1, M_0, N_1, N_0) as fixed, or *conditioning* on their values, is that it greatly simplifies small-sample statistics. Consider the sharp (strong) null hypothesis (*i.e.*, that exposure has no effect on anyone) in the context of an experiment that will assign exactly N_1 out of N persons to exposure. Then, under the potential outcomes model (see Chapters 3 and 5), no causal "type 2" or preventive "type 3" persons are in the study, and the total number of cases M_1 is just the number of doomed "type 1" persons in the study. Once persons are chosen for the study, M_1 is unaffected by exposure and so, in this sense, is fixed, given the cohort. In particular, if only exposure status may vary (*e.g.*, via experimental assignment), and the number exposed N_1 is also predetermined, then under the sharp null hypothesis, the only quantities left to vary are the internal table cells. Furthermore, given one cell and the fixed margins, we can compute all the other cells by subtraction. For example, given A_1 and the fixed margins: the number of unexposed cases is $A_0 = M_1 - A_1$; the number of exposed noncases is $N_1 - A_1$; and the number of unexposed noncases is $N_0 - A_0 = N_0 - M_1 + A_1$. Finally, if exposure is assigned by simple randomization, the distribution for A_1 given the marginal totals under the null of no association is the *hypergeometric distribution* for which:

$$P\left(A_1 = a_1 \middle| M_1, M_0, N_1, N_0\right) = \frac{\dbinom{N_1}{a_1}\dbinom{N_0}{M_1 - a_1}}{\dbinom{N}{M_1}}.$$

Note, *Fisher's exact test* computes *P*-values for the null hypothesis directly from this distribution.

In the nonnull situation, the rationale for computing statistics by fixing the margins is less straightforward and applies only to inference on odds ratios. For this purpose, it has the advantage of reducing small-sample bias in estimation even if the margins are not actually fixed.[23,24] Those who remain uncomfortable with the use of fixed margins for a table in which the margins are not truly fixed may find comfort in the fact that the fixed-margins assumption makes little difference compared with statistical methods that do not assume fixed margins when the observed table cells are large enough to give precise inferences.

When treating all margins as fixed, we can compute mid-*P*-values confidence interval limits for the odds ratio using the *noncentral hypergeometric distribution* for A_1 given the marginal totals and value of *OR*, for which:

$$P\left(A_1 = a_1 \middle| M_1, M_0, N_1, N_0, OR\right) = \frac{\dbinom{N_1}{a_1}\dbinom{N_0}{M_1 - a_1}OR^{a_1}}{\sum_k \dbinom{N_1}{k}\dbinom{N_0}{M_1 - k}OR^k}.$$

[17-5]

where *k* ranges over all possible values for A_1 that are consistent with the marginal totals.[25,26] Under the null hypothesis, $OR = 1$ and this distribution reduces to the hypergeometric.

Viewing the values of (M_1, M_0, N_1, N_0) in expression 17-5 as fixed, given an observed value of A_1, only one unknown remains: the odds ratio *OR*. Thus, expression 17-5 can be viewed as a likelihood function for *OR* and is sometimes called the *conditional-likelihood* function. From this, one can obtain the *conditional maximum-likelihood estimate* (CMLE) as the value of *OR* that maximizes expression 17-5. This CMLE does *not* equal the familiar unconditional maximum-likelihood estimate, specifically $\widehat{OR} = \left[A_1/\left(N_1 - A_1\right)\right]/\left[A_0/\left(N_0 - A_0\right)\right]$; in fact, there is no closed-form, explicit formula for the CMLE of the odds ratio. Thus, it must be calculated using software.

For the data in Table 17-2 on infant diarrhea, Equation 17-5 yields the mid-*P*-value function:

$$\text{mid-}P_{\text{lower}} = P\left(Y < 12 \middle| I\right) + \frac{1}{2}P\left(A = 12 \middle| I\right) = \frac{\sum_{k=1}^{11}\dbinom{14}{k}\dbinom{16}{19-k}OR^k}{\sum_{k=1}^{14}\dbinom{14}{k}\dbinom{16}{19-k}OR^k} + \frac{1}{2}\left[\frac{\dbinom{14}{12}\dbinom{16}{7}OR^{12}}{\sum_{k=1}^{14}\dbinom{14}{k}\dbinom{16}{19-k}OR^k}\right]$$

$$= 1 - \text{mid-}P_{\text{upper}}.$$

From this the median-unbiased estimate of the odds ratio (*i.e.*, the *OR* for which mid-P_{lower} = mid-P_{upper} = 0.5) is 6.9. The conditional maximum-likelihood estimate is 7.2, whereas the unconditional (ordinary) maximum-likelihood estimate is $(12 \times 9)/(7 \times 2) = 7.7$. The mid-*P* 95% confidence limits (*i.e.*, the values of OR at which mid-P_{upper} = 0.025 and mid-P_{lower} = 0.025, respectively) are (1.3, 61.0), which can be compared with the (large-sample) Wald-based approximate 95% confidence interval of (1.3, 46.0).

Person-Time Cohort Data

With two-group comparisons based on data from a person-time cohort study, the crude (*i.e.*, unstratified) data can be displayed in the format shown in Table 17-3, with A_1 and A_0 again denoting the number of diseased cases in the exposed and unexposed groups, respectively, and with T_1 and T_0 denoting the corresponding total person-time in the two groups. Assuming independence within and across the two groups, and homogeneity with respect to the group-specific rates, I_1 and I_0, the probability of observing $A_1 = a_1$ cases in the exposed group and $A_0 = a_0$ cases in the unexposed group is the product:

$$P(A_1 = a_1, A_0 = a_0) = P(A_1 = a_1)P(A_0 = a_0) = \frac{(I_1 T_1)^{a_1} \exp(-I_1 T_1)}{a_1!} \frac{(I_0 T_0)^{a_0} \exp(-I_0 T_0)}{a_0!}. \qquad [17\text{-}6]$$

Given observed data in the form of (A_1, N_1, A_0, N_0) expression 17-6 viewed as a function of the two unknown parameters I_1 and I_0 is referred to as the *Poisson likelihood for two groups*. Under this model, we have:

1. The MLEs of I_1 and I_0 are $\hat{I}_1 = A_1/T_1$ and $\hat{I}_0 = A_0/T_0$, respectively.
2. The MLE of the rate ratio, $IR = I_1/I_0$ is:

$$\widehat{IR} = \frac{A_1/T_1}{A_0/T_0}.$$

3. The MLE of the rate difference, $ID = I_1/I_0$ is:

$$\widehat{ID} = \frac{A_1}{T_1} - \frac{A_0}{T_0}.$$

4. If $I_1 = I_0$, that is, there is no difference in rate between the two groups, the expected number of exposed cases, A_1, is $E = M_1 T_1/T$, where M_1 is the total number of cases and T is the total observed person-time. Furthermore, the variance of the number of exposed cases is:

$$V = E \times \frac{T_0}{T} = \frac{M_1 T_1 T_0}{T^2}.$$

TABLE 17-3

Format for Unstratified Data With Person-Time Denominators

	Exposed	Unexposed	Total
Cases	A_1	A_0	M_1
Person-time	T_1	T_0	T

TABLE 17-4

Breast Cancer Cases and Person-Years of Observation for Women With Tuberculosis, Who Are Repeatedly Exposed to Multiple X-ray Fluoroscopies, and Unexposed Women With Tuberculosis

	Radiation Exposure		Total
	Yes	No	
Breast cancer cases	41	15	56
Person-years	28,010	19,017	47,027

From Boice JD, Monson RR. Breast cancer in women after repeated fluoroscopic examinations of the chest. *J Natl Cancer Inst*. 1977;59:823-832.

It follows from the last fact that a large-sample statistic for testing the null hypothesis H_0: $I_0 = I_1$, which is the same hypothesis as $IR = 1$ and $ID = 0$, is:

$$\chi_{\text{score}} = \frac{A_1 - E}{V^{1/2}}.$$

which, as with the corresponding statistic for person-count cohort data, can also be compared against a standard normal distribution to obtain a P-value.

To illustrate the various calculations, Table 17-4 provides summary information on a study of the association between x-ray fluoroscopy and breast cancer among women with tuberculosis.[14] For these data, we have:

$$\widehat{IR} = (31/28,010)/(15/19,017) = 1.86$$
$$\widehat{ID} = 41/28,010 - 15/19,017 = 68 \text{ per } 100,000 \text{ person years}$$
$$E = (58 \times 28,010)/47,027 = 33.35$$
$$V = 33.35 \times 19,017/47,027 = 13.49$$

and

$$\chi_{\text{score}} = \frac{41 - 33.35}{(13.49)^{1/2}} = 2.08$$

which, from a standard normal table, corresponds to an upper-tailed P-value of 0.02 for the null of H_0: $I_0 = I_1$.

Toward constructing confidence intervals for $\widehat{IR}$, we first note that:

$$SE\left[\ln\left(\widehat{IR}\right)\right] = \left(\frac{1}{A_1} + \frac{1}{A_0}\right)^{1/2}.$$

Thus, a Wald-based approximate 95% confidence interval for $\widehat{IR}$ is:

$$\left(\widehat{IR}_L, \widehat{IR}_U\right) = \exp\left\{\ln\left(\widehat{IR}\right) \pm 1.96 \times SE\left[\ln\left(\widehat{IR}\right)\right]\right\}.$$

Furthermore, a Wald-based approximate 95% confidence interval for $\widehat{ID}$ is:

$$\left(\widehat{ID}_L, \widehat{ID}_U\right) = \exp\left[\widehat{ID} \pm 1.96 \times SE\left(\widehat{ID}\right)\right].$$

where

$$SE\left(\widehat{ID}\right) = \left(\frac{A_1}{T_1^2} + \frac{A_0}{T_0^2}\right)^{1/2}.$$

For the breast cancer data from Boice and Monson,[14] we have:

$$SE\left[\ln\left(\widehat{IR}\right)\right] = \left(\frac{1}{41} + \frac{1}{15}\right)^{1/2} = 0.302$$

and

$$SE\left(\widehat{ID}\right) = \left(\frac{41}{(28{,}101)^2} + \frac{15}{(19{,}017)^2}\right)^{1/2} = 31 \text{ per } 100{,}000 \text{ person-years.}$$

From these, an approximate 95% confidence interval for $\widehat{IR} = 1.86$ is $\left(\widehat{IR}_L, \widehat{IR}_U\right) = (1.03, 3.35)$ while an approximate 95% confidence interval for $\widehat{IR} = 68$ per 100,000 person-years is $\left(\widehat{ID}_L, \widehat{ID}_U\right) = (7.6, 128)$ per 100,000 person-years. Thus, although the results suggest a nonrandom excess of breast cancers among fluoroscoped women, they are imprecise about just how large this excess might be.

Under the two-Poisson model, a general rule of thumb regarding whether the Wald-based limits for $\widehat{IR}$ will be reasonably accurate is that both

$$\frac{M_1 T_0}{\widehat{IR}_U T_1 + T_0}$$

and

$$\frac{M_1 \widehat{IR}_L T_1}{\widehat{IR}_L T_1 + T_0}$$

should exceed 5. For the limits reported above, these quantities are 9.4 and 33.8, respectively. If the preceding criteria had not been met, however, small-sample methods are recommended. Recall that in developing small-sample methods for person-count cohort data, we conditioned on the marginal totals, (M_1, M_0, N_1, N_0) in Table 17-1. That is, they were treated as if they were fixed. For person-time cohort data, as summarized in Table 17-3, by treating the total number of cases, M_1, as fixed, we can compute mid-P limits for the incidence rate ratio IR. Specifically, consider the probability that a randomly sampled case is an exposed case. Denoting this probability by R_s, assuming independence, it may be reasonable to assume that the number of cases from among M_1 total cases that are exposed (*i.e.*, A_1 in Table 17-3), follows a binomial distribution with:

$$P\left(A_1 = a_1 | M_1\right) = \binom{M_1}{a_1} R_s^{a_1} \left(1 - R_s\right)^{M_1 - a_1}.$$

Using this, the mid-P-value functions are:

$$\text{mid-}P_{\text{lower}} = \sum_{k=0}^{a_1-1} \binom{M_1}{k} R_s^k \left(1-R_s\right)^{M_1-k} + \frac{1}{2}\binom{M_1}{y_1} R_s^{a_1} \left(1-R_s\right)^{M_1-a_1} = 1 - \text{mid-}P_{\text{upper}}.$$

Setting $\text{mid-}P_{\text{lower}} = \text{mid-}P_{\text{upper}}$ and solving for R_s yields the corresponding median-unbiased esti-mate, $\hat{R}_s$, while the lower limit of a 95% confidence interval, $\hat{R}_{s,L}$, is the value of R_s for which $\text{mid-}P_{\text{upper}} = 0.025$. Finally, the upper limit of a 95% confidence interval, $\hat{R}_{s,U}$, is the value of R_s for which $\text{mid-}P_{\text{lower}} = 0.025$.

It turns out that, under the two-Poisson model with T_1 and T_0 fixed, R_s is the ratio of the expected number of exposed cases under the expected total number of cases, which can be expressed as a function of IR and the observed person-time:

$$R_s = \frac{I_1 T_1}{I_1 T_1 + I_0 T_0} = \frac{\left(I_1/I_0\right) T_1}{\left(I_1/I_0\right) T_1 + T_0} = \frac{IR \times T_1}{IR \times T_1 + T_0}.$$

Rearranging this expression we have:

$$IR = \frac{R_s}{1-R_s} \times \frac{T_0}{T_1}.$$

which, coupled with the median-unbiased estimate and 95% confidence interval limits for R_s, can be used to compute a median-unbiased estimate of IR and corresponding 95% confidence interval.

Applying these techniques to the data in Table 17-4, we have:

$$\text{mid-}P_{\text{lower}} = \sum_{k=0}^{40} \binom{56}{k} R_s \left(1-R_s\right)^{56-k} + \frac{1}{2}\binom{56}{41} R_s^{41} \left(1-R_s\right)^{15}$$

where

$$R_s = \frac{IR \times 28{,}010}{IR \times 28{,}010 + 19{,}017}$$

so that

$$IR = \frac{R_s}{1-R_s} \times \frac{19{,}017}{28{,}010}.$$

The lower and upper 95% mid-P limits for R_s are 0.61 and 0.84, respectively, which translate to a 95% confidence interval for IR of $\left(\widehat{IR}_L, \widehat{IR}_U\right) = (1.04, 3.45)$. Because the number of cases in the study is large, these small-sample statistics are close to the large-sample statistics obtained earlier.

Case-Control Data

Assuming that the underlying source cohort is closed, the odds-ratio estimates given earlier can be applied directly to cumulative case-control data (see Chapter 8). Table 17-5 provides data from a case-control study of the association between chlordiazepoxide use in early pregnancy and con-genital heart defects. Based on these data, using the expressions given above, an estimate of the odds ratio association is:

$$\widehat{OR} = \frac{4/4}{386/1{,}250} = 3.24.$$

TABLE 17-5

History of Chlordiazepoxide Use in Early Pregnancy for Mothers of Children Born With Congenital Heart Defects and Mothers of Normal Children

	Chlordiazepoxide Use		Total
	Yes	No	
Case mothers	4	386	390
Control mothers	4	1,250	1,254
Totals	8	1,636	1,644

From Rothman KJ, Fyler DC, Goldblatt A, et al. Exogenous hormones and other drug exposures of children with congenital heart disease. *Am J Epidemiol.* 1979;109:433-439.

Furthermore, the standard error for $\ln(\widehat{OR})$ is:

$$SE\left[\ln(\widehat{OR})\right] = \left(\frac{1}{4} + \frac{1}{4} + \frac{1}{386} + \frac{1}{1,250}\right)^{1/2} = 0.710$$

which can be used to construct a Wald-based approximate 95% interval:

$$\left(\widehat{OR}_L, \widehat{OR}_U\right) = \exp\left[\ln(3.24) \pm 1.96 \times 0.710\right] = (0.81, 13.0).$$

Thus, the data exhibit a positive association but do so with little precision, indicating that, even in the absence of bias, the data are reasonably compatible with effects ranging from little or nothing up through more than a 10-fold increase in risk. Finally, for testing the null of no association, that is, $H_0: OR = 1$, we have

$$E = \frac{380 \times 8}{1,644} = 1.90$$

$$V = \frac{1.90 \times 1,254 \times 1,636}{1,644 \times 1,643} = 1.44$$

so that

$$\chi_{score} = \frac{4 - 1.90}{(1.44)^{1/2}} = 1.75$$

which yields an upper-tailed *P*-value of 0.04.

If the exposure prevalence does not change over the sampling period, these formulae can also be used to estimate rate ratios from case-control studies done with density sampling (see Chapter 8). Because controls in such studies represent person-time, individuals may be sampled more than once as controls (*i.e.*, at different times) and may be included as a case after being sampled as a control. Data from such an individual must be carefully considered in the data analysis, just as if the individual had been a different individual at each sampling time. If an individual's exposure changes over time, the data entered at each sampling time will differ. For example, in a study of smoking, it is conceivable that a single individual could first be sampled as a smoking control, then later be sampled as a nonsmoking control (if, in particular, they quit between the sampling times); if they then fell ill, he or she could be sampled a third time as a case (smoking or nonsmoking, depending on whether they resumed between the second and third sampling times).

The repeated-use rule may at first appear odd, but it is no more odd than the use of multiple person-time units from the same individual in a cohort study. One caution should be borne in mind, however: If exposure prevalence changes over the course of subject selection, and risk changes over time or subjects are matched on sampling time, one should treat sampling time as a potential confounder and thus stratify on it.[27] With fine enough time strata, no individual will appear twice in the same time stratum. Such fine stratification should also be used if one desires a small-sample (exact) analysis of density-sampled data.

Case-Cohort Data

Finally, we consider data from a case-cohort study where a *subcohort* from a closed-source cohort is initially selected at random. This subcohort, which includes some subjects who eventually go on to become cases, is then supplemented with all cases that arise during follow-up but who were not initially selected. Collectively, the data consist of all M_1 cases, M_{10} of which were observed from the subcohort and M_{11} of which were observed from outside the subcohort, together with M_0 noncases or controls. Among the M_1 cases, A_1 were observed to have been exposed while A_0 were unexposed. The total number of exposed and unexposed subjects in the data are N_1 and N_0, respectively. Thus, the subcohort contributed $B_1 = N_1 - A_1$ exposed controls and $B_0 = N_0 - A_0$ unexposed controls. Table 17-6 provides a summary of the notation.

One can estimate the risk ratio directly from the case-cohort data using large-sample formulas that generalize the risk-ratio methods for full-cohort data. To describe the maximum-likelihood estimator of the risk ratio in case-cohort data,[28] we first must define the "pseudodenominators"

$$N_1^* = \frac{A_1 M_{10}}{M_1} + B_1$$

and

$$N_0^* = \frac{A_0 M_{10}}{M_1} + B_0$$

Note, M_{10}/M_1 is the proportion of cases that arise from the subcohort. Using these, one can take

$$\widehat{RR} = \frac{A_1/N_1^*}{A_0/N_0^*} = \frac{A_1/A_0}{N_1^*/N_0^*}$$

TABLE 17-6

Notation for Crude Case-Cohort Data When All Cases in the Cohort Are Selected

	Exposed	Unexposed	Total
Cases outside of the subcohort	A_{11}	A_{01}	M_{11}
Cases from the subcohort	A_{10}	A_{00}	M_{10}
All cases	A_1	A_0	M_1
Controls from the subcohort	B_1	B_0	M_0
Total	N_1	N_0	N

as an estimate of RR. Furthermore, a large-sample estimate of the standard error of $\ln\left(\widehat{RR}\right)$ is:

$$SE\left[\ln\left(\widehat{RR}\right)\right] = \left[\frac{1}{A_1} + \frac{1}{A} + \left(\frac{M_{11} - M_{10}}{M_1}\right)\left(\frac{1}{N_1^*} + \frac{1}{N_0^*}\right) + \left(\frac{1}{A_1} + \frac{1}{A_0}\right)\left(\frac{1}{N_1^*} + \frac{1}{N_0^*}\right)^2\left(\frac{M_{11}M_{10}}{M_1^2}\right)\right]^{1/2}$$

so that a Wald-based approximate 95% confidence interval is:

$$\left(\widehat{RR}_L, \widehat{RR}_U\right) = \exp\left\{\ln\left(\widehat{RR}\right) \pm 1.96 \times SE\left[\ln\left(\widehat{RR}\right)\right]\right\}.$$

Finally, if the disease is so uncommon that no cases appear in the subcohort, then $M_{10} = 0$, $M_{11} = M_1$, $N_1^* = B_1$, and $N_0^* = B_0$, so that:

$$\widehat{RR} = \frac{A_1 B_0}{A_0 B_1} = \widehat{OR}$$

and

$$SE\left[\ln\left(\widehat{RR}\right)\right] = \left(\frac{1}{A_1} + \frac{1}{A} + \frac{1}{B_1} + \frac{1}{B_0}\right)^{1/2}.$$

Note, these are identical to the point and standard error estimates for OR based on case-control data. On the other hand, if every cohort member is selected as a control, then $M_{11} = 0$ and these formulas become identical to the risk-ratio formulas for closed cohort data.

RELATIONS AMONG EFFECT MEASURES FOR PERSON-COUNT DATA

As discussed in Chapter 5, OR is always further from the null value of 1 than RR. In a parallel fashion, $\widehat{OR}$ is always further from 1 than $\widehat{RR}$ in an unstratified study; use of $\widehat{OR}$ from a cohort study as an estimate for RR will therefore tend to produce estimates that are too far from 1. The disparity between OR and RR increases with both the size of the risks, R_1 and R_0, and the strength of the association (as measured by OR or RR). For Table 17-2, $\widehat{RR} = 2.0$ and $\widehat{OR} = 7.7$ are far apart because both observed proportions exceed 40% and the association is strong.

One often sees statements that the odds ratio approximates the risk ratio when the disease is "rare." This statement can be made more precise in a study of a closed population: If the risk odds in both the exposed individuals, that is, $R_1/(1 - R_1)$, and the unexposed individuals, that is, $R_0/(1 - R_0)$, are less than 0.10, then the disparity between OR and RR will be less than 10%.[29] In a parallel fashion, if both observed incidence odds A_1/B_1 and A_0/B_0 are less than 0.10, the disparity between $\widehat{OR}$ and $\widehat{RR}$ will be less than 10%.

The relation of either the odds ratio or risk ratio to the rate ratio, IR, is more complex. If the incidence rates change only slightly across small subintervals of the actual follow-up period (i.e., the incidence rates are nearly constant across small time strata), IR will be further from the null than RR and closer to the null than OR.[27] It follows that, given constant incidence rates over time, $\widehat{OR}$ tends to be too far from the null as an estimate of IR, and $\widehat{IR}$ as an estimate of RR tends to be too far from the null. Again, however, the disparity among the three measures will be small when the incidence is low.

References

1. Anderson JA. Separate sample logistic disrimination. *Biometrika*. 1972;59:19-35.
2. Mantel N. Synthetic retrospective studies and related topics. *Biometrics*. 1973;29:479-486.
3. Prentice RL, Breslow NE. Retrospective studies and failure-time models. *Biometrika*. 1978;65:153-158.

4. Farewell VT. Some results on the estimation of logistic models based on retrospective data. *Biometrika*. 1979;66:27-32.
5. Prentice RL, Pyke R. Logistic disease incidence models and case-control studies. *Biometrika*. 1979;66:403-411.
6. Thomas DC. General relative risk models for survival time and matched case-control analysis. *Biometrics*. 1981;37:673-686.
7. Greenland S. Multivariate estimation of exposure-specific incidence from case-control studies. *J Chronic Dis*. 1981;34:445-453.
8. Weinberg CR, Wacholder S. Prospective analysis of case-control data under general multiplicative-intercept risk models. *Biometrika*. 1993;80:461-465.
9. White JE. A two stage design for the study of the relationship between a rare exposure and a rare disease. *Am J Epidemiol*. 1982;115:119-128.
10. Prentice RL. A case-cohort design for epidemiologic studies and disease prevention trials. *Biometrika*. 1986;73:1-11.
11. Clayton D, Hills M. *Statistical Models in Epidemiology*. OUP Oxford; 2013.
12. Lancaster PA. Congenital malformations after in-vitro fertilisation. *Lancet*. 1987;2:1392-1393.
13. Birnbaum A. Median unbiased estimators. *Bull Math Stat*. 1964;11:25-34.
14. Boice JD Jr, Monson RR. Breast cancer in women after repeated fluoroscopic examinations of the chest. *J Natl Cancer Inst*. 1977;59:823-832.
15. Waxweiler RJ, Stringer W, Wagoner JK, Jones J, Falk H, Carter C. Neoplastic risk among workers exposed to vinyl chloride. *Ann NY Acad Sci*. 1976;271:40-48.
16. Keiding N, Vaeth M. Calculating expected mortality. *Stat Med*. 1986;5:327-334.
17. Glass RI, Svennerholm AM, Stoll BJ, et al. Protection against cholera in breast-fed children by antibodies in breast milk. *N Engl J Med*. 1983;308:1389-1392.
18. Zou G, Donner A. A simple alternative confidence interval for the difference between two proportions. *Control Clin Trials*. 2004;25:3-12.
19. Fisher RA. The logic of inductive inference. *J R Stat Soc Ser A*. 1935;98:39-54.
20. Cox DR, Hinkley DV. *Theoretical Statistics*. New York, NY: Chapman and Hall; 1974.
21. Little RJA. On testing equality of two independent binomial proportions. *Am Stat*. 1989;43:283-288.
22. Greenland S. On the logical justification of conditional tests for two-by-two contingency tables. *Am Stat*. 1991;45:248-251.
23. Mantel N, Hankey BF. The odds ratios of a 2 × 2 table. *Am Stat*. 1975;29:143-145.
24. Pike MC, Hill AP, Smith PG. Bias and efficiency in logistic analyses of stratified case-control studies. *Int J Epidemiol*. 1980;9:89-95.
25. Breslow NE, Day NE. *Statistical Methods in Cancer Research. Volume I: The Analysis of Case-Control Data*. Lyon: IARC; 1980.
26. Mccullagh P, Nelder JA. *Generalized Linear Models*. New York, NY: Chapman and Hall; 1989.
27. Greenland S, Thomas DC. On the need for the rare disease assumption in case-control studies. *Am J Epidemiol*. 1982;116:547-553.
28. Sato T. Estimation of a common risk ratio in stratified case-cohort studies. *Stat Med*. 1992;11:1599-1605.
29. Greenland S. Estimation of exposure-specific rates from sparse case-control data. *J Chronic Dis*. 1987;40:1087-1094.

CHAPTER 18

Stratification and Standardization

Sebastien Haneuse and Kenneth J. Rothman*

Chapter 17 presents methods for estimation and inference regarding effect measures based on "crude" data, that is, simple totals regarding the outcome and denominator measures (be they person-counts or person-time totals). Outside of randomized studies, most epidemiologic studies will require, in one form or another, consideration of factors beyond the exposure and outcome. Toward this, stratification is the mainstay of epidemiologic analyses. As with the methods presented in Chapter 17, even in studies that ultimately require more complex analyses, methods that build on data that are stratified provide an important opportunity to gain initial insight regarding the data and associations. Moreover, it provides a means for the investigator to become familiar with the distributions of key variables and with patterns in the data that may be less transparent when using methods such as regression. Additionally, several analytic concerns motivate stratification. Most prominent among these are the evaluation and control of confounding bias, and certain forms

---

*This chapter is based on material by Sander Greenland and Kenneth J. Rothman.

of selection bias such as that produced by case-control matching. Another important motivation is in the evaluation of effect-measure modification or heterogeneity of measures (as we will refer to it here). Third, stratification on follow-up time is also used in cohort studies to address problems of loss to follow-up (see Chapter 22).

This chapter presents elementary stratified-analysis methods for dealing with confounding and heterogeneity of a measure. While much of the chapter focuses on estimation of measures of effect using data from unmatched studies, we also discuss how basic stratified methods can be applied toward the analysis of data from studies that employ matching.

HETEROGENEITY VERSUS CONFOUNDING

As discussed in Chapter 5, *effect-measure modification* refers to variation in the magnitude of a measure of exposure effect across levels of another variable. This concept is often confused with biologic interaction, but it is a distinct concept (see Chapter 26). The variable across which the effect varies is called an *effect modifier.* Effect-measure modification is also known as heterogeneity of effect, nonuniformity of effect, and effect variation. Absence of effect-measure modification is also known as homogeneity of effect, uniformity of effect, and commonality of effect across strata. In most of this chapter, we will use the more general phrase *heterogeneity of a measure* to refer to variation in any measure of effect or association across strata.

Effect-measure modification differs from confounding in several important ways. The most salient difference is that, whereas confounding is a bias that the investigator hopes to prevent or remove from the effect estimate, effect-measure modification is a property of the effect under study. Thus, effect-measure modification is a finding to be reported rather than a bias to be avoided or removed. Moreover, in epidemiologic analysis, one tries to eliminate confounding, but one may be interested in describing effect-measure modification.

Confounding originates from the interrelation of the confounders, exposure, and disease in the source population from which the study subjects are selected. By changing the source population that will be studied, design strategies such as restriction can prevent a variable from acting as a confounder and thus eliminate the burden of adjusting for the variable. Unfortunately, the same design strategies may also impair the ability to study effect-measure modification by the variable. For example, restriction of subjects to a single level of a variable will prevent it from being a confounder in the study but will also prevent one from examining whether the exposure effect varies across levels of the variable.

Epidemiologists commonly use at least two different types of effect measures: ratios and differences. As discussed in Chapter 5, the degree of heterogeneity of a measure depends on the measure one uses. In particular, ratios and differences can vary in opposite directions across strata. Consider stratifying by age and suppose that the outcome measure varies both within age strata (with exposure) and across age strata (*e.g.*, the exposure-specific rates or risks vary across strata). Then at least one of (and usually both) the difference and ratio must vary across the age strata (*i.e.*, they cannot both be homogeneous over age). In contrast to this measured dependence, confounding can be defined without reference to a particular measure of effect (although its apparent severity may differ according to the chosen measure).

EXAMINATION OF STRATUM-SPECIFIC ESTIMATES

In its simplest form, stratified analysis involves computing a separate estimate from each stratum, so that the single crude estimate is replaced with a set of estimates, one per stratum. In most stratified analyses, there will be some variation in the estimates across the strata. One must then determine: (1) whether the variation in the stratum-specific estimates is of any scientific or public-health importance; and (2) the extent to which the variation is compatible with random statistical fluctuation. The answers to these questions determine what analytic methods are used and how the results are to be presented.

Consider the coronary death-rate ratio for smokers relative to nonsmokers in the data in Table 18-1. The crude mortality-rate ratio across all ages is $(630/142,247)/(101/39,220) = 1.72$, which will likely be confounded by age. Within each of the 10-year age categories, however, the confounding effect of age will likely be much reduced because of the homogenization of risk for

TABLE 18-1

Age-Specific Coronary Disease Deaths, Person-Years Observed, and Coronary Death Rates Among British Male Doctors by Cigarette Smoking

Age (y)	Cigarette Smokers			Nonsmokers			Rate Ratio
	Deaths	Years	Rate[a]	Deaths	Years	Rate[a]	
35-44	32	52,407	6.1	2	18,790	1.1	5.7
45-54	104	43,248	24.0	12	10,673	11.2	2.1
55-64	206	28,612	72.0	28	5,710	49.0	1.5
65-74	186	12,663	146.9	28	2,585	108.3	1.4
75-84	102	5,317	191.8	31	1,462	212.0	0.9
Total	630	142,247	—	101	39,220	—	—

[a]Deaths per 10,000 person-years.
From Doll R, Hill AB. Mortality of British doctors in relation to smoking; observations on coronary thrombosis. In: Haenszel W, ed. *Epidemiological Approaches to the Study of Cancer and Other Chronic Diseases*. Bethesda, MD: National Cancer Institute; 1966:205-268.

the outcome of mortality. In addition to removing most of the age confounding, stratification has revealed that the rate-ratio estimates decline with age (although the risk differences increase until the oldest category). One often sees such a decline in ratio estimates across categories of a variable as the risk of disease among the unexposed increases. This pattern is sometimes called modification by baseline risk. Finding such a pattern of variation in the estimates is a key result of the analysis.

This example illustrates the importance of examining stratum-specific estimates whenever it is feasible to do so. Unfortunately, however, it is not always feasible to do so since some variables may have too many categories to examine each separately. For example, studies may be conducted with potential confounding by family or neighborhood, for which there are too few subjects to produce stable estimates within each stratum. One can treat such variables as confounders and adjust for them when assessing effects of other factors, but one cannot easily examine how effects change across categories of family or neighborhood. When there are adequate numbers to examine stratum-specific estimates, however, it may be desirable to report findings separately for each stratum. These stratum-specific estimates may themselves be adjusted for other variables. For example, we might infer that the rate ratio differs for males and females and so report sex-specific estimates, each adjusted for age and perhaps other confounding variables.

In addition to the stratum-specific presentation of results, the investigator might choose to fit a regression model to the pattern of estimates and use the model to describe and summarize the heterogeneity. A regression model, for example, could be used to model the variation in the stratum-specific rate ratios. We discuss such models in Chapters 20 and 21. Regression methods, however, may not be as easily understood as stratum-specific results. Furthermore, a regression model can summarize a set of stratum-specific estimates parsimoniously only if each stratum can be assigned a meaningful numeric value. For example, a model for the variation of the risk difference across age strata can be greatly simplified by making use of the natural ordering of age; the same simplification is not available when examining variation across strata of race/ethnicity or other nominal scale variables.

STANDARDIZATION

As discussed in Chapters 4 and 5, standardization provides a means to summarize epidemiologic measures (*i.e.*, rates, risks, prevalences, or means) across strata by taking a weighted average of the stratum-specific measures. The weights used in computing the weighted average are referred to as the *standard*. For example, if the only stratification variable is age, a standard might be the amount of person-time or number of persons in a standard population that fall into each of the age categories.

The formula we will use for a standardized rate is:

$$I_w = \frac{\sum_i w_i I_i}{\sum_i w_i}$$

where w_i is the weight for stratum i and I_i is the rate in stratum i; w_i is usually the amount of person-time observed in stratum i of a standard population. Similarly, the standardized risk formula we will use is:

$$R_w = \frac{\sum_i w_i R_i}{\sum_i w_i}$$

where w_i is the weight for stratum i and R_i is the risk in stratum i; w_i is usually the number of persons in stratum i of a standard population. Standardized prevalences or standardized means can be constructed using the same formulae, substituting stratum-specific prevalences or means for the stratum-specific rates or risks.

The standard should be chosen to facilitate interpretation of the results. For some applications, there may be a conventional standard, such as the world age-sex distribution in a given year or a national age-sex distribution from a specific census, that facilitates comparisons with other data. For most analyses, however, the standard should be derived from the specific population for which one wants to estimate an exposure effect. As an example, if the stratum-specific incidences of a population are standardized to that population's distribution, then the standardized incidence will be equal to the crude incidence for that population. Thus, a crude incidence can be viewed as the average weighted by the distribution of the study population itself. Equivalently, a standardized incidence can be interpreted as the crude incidence in a population that has the same stratum-specific incidences as those of the observed population, but in which the distribution of the stratification variable(s) is given by the standard.

As mentioned in Chapter 5, if exposure affects the distribution used to construct the standardization weights, comparisons of standardized incidences will not properly reflect the net exposure effect on the population incidence if the same standard weights are used to construct each standardized incidence. This problem will occur, for example, when exposure alters the person-time distribution of the population, and the weights are person-times.[1] If exposure has an effect, it will alter not only the rates but also the distribution of person-time over the follow-up period.

If one wishes to estimate the total effect of exposure when exposure affects the weighting distribution, it will be necessary to use weights that change with exposure in a manner that reflects the exposure effect. Inverse-probability-of-exposure weighting provides examples of such exposure-dependent weighting. For this chapter, we will assume that exposure has negligible effects on the weights. This assumption would be satisfied in risk standardization when the standard is the baseline (starting) distribution of confounders in a cohort study, and exposure occurs only at baseline.

Standardized Differences

If I_{1i} is the rate among the exposed in stratum i and I_{0i} is the rate among the unexposed in stratum i, then the standardized rate difference is $ID_w = I_{1w} - I_{0w}$, the difference between the standardized rates for exposed and unexposed. The following algebra shows that a standardized rate difference is the weighted average of the stratum-specific rate differences, using the same standard weights:

$$ID_w = \frac{\sum_i w_i I_{1i}}{\sum_i w_i} - \frac{\sum_i w_i I_{0i}}{\sum_i w_i} = \frac{\sum_i w_i (I_{1i} - I_{0i})}{\sum_i w_i} = \frac{\sum_i w_i ID_i}{\sum_i w_i}.$$

Thus, an estimate of the standardized rate difference, $\widehat{ID}_w$, can be obtained by taking a weighted average of the estimated stratum-specific rate differences, $\widehat{ID}_i$.

Similarly, the standardized risk difference, $RD_w = R_{1w} - R_{0w}$, is the weighted average of the stratum-specific risk differences $RD_i = R_{1i} - R_{0i}$ based on the standard weights:

$$RD_w = \frac{\sum_i w_i RD_i}{\sum_i w_i}.$$

Using data from Table 18-2, suppose that we wish to estimate what the effect of tolbutamide would have been if every patient in the study (not just those randomized to tolbutamide) had received tolbutamide. To adjust for age, we should use the distribution of the entire cohort as the standard, which corresponds to weights of $106 + 120 = 226$ for the "younger than 55 years" stratum and $98 + 85 = 183$ for the "age 55+" stratum. These yield standardized risk estimates of:

$$\hat{R}_{0w} = \frac{226(5/120) + 183(16/85)}{226 + 183} = 0.107$$

$$\hat{R}_{1w} = \frac{226(8/106) + 183(22/98)}{226 + 183} = 0.142$$

which, in turn, yield a standardized risk difference estimate of $\widehat{RD}_w = 0.142 - 0.107 = 0.035$.

Returning to the British doctors' data in Table 18-1, using the age distribution of smoking subjects as the standard yields an estimated standardized coronary death rate for smoking doctors, $\hat{I}_{1w}$, that is the same as the crude rate for this group, specifically 630/142,247 years = 44.3 cases per 10^4 person-years. The corresponding standardized rate for the nonsmoking British doctors is estimated by taking a weighted average of the age-specific rates for the nonsmoking doctors using the number of person-years in each age category of the smoking doctors as the weights:

$$\hat{I}_{0w} = \frac{52,407(2/18,790) + \cdots + 5,317(31/1,462)}{52,407 + \cdots + 5,317} = \frac{444.41}{142,247} = 31.2 \text{ cases per } 10^4 \text{ person-years.}$$

The estimated standardized rate difference, $\widehat{ID}_w$, is the difference between these two standardized rate estimates, which is about 13 cases per 10^4 person-years. This value can also be obtained by taking a weighted average of the stratum-specific rate differences, weighting by the number of person-years among smoking doctors in each age category.

TABLE 18-2

Age-Specific Comparison of Deaths From all Causes for Tolbutamide and Placebo Treatment Groups, University Group Diabetes Program (1970)

	Stratum 1, Age <55 y		Stratum 2, Age 55+ y		Total (Crude)	
	Tolbutamide	Placebo	Tolbutamide	Placebo	Tolbutamide	Placebo
Dead	8	5	22	16	30	21
Surviving	98	115	76	69	174	184
Total	106	120	98	85	204	205
Average risk	0.076	0.042	0.224	0.188	0.147	0.102
RD		0.034		0.036		0.045
RR		1.81		1.19		1.44

From University Group Diabetes Program. A study of the effects of hypoglycemic agents on vascular complications in patients with adult onset diabetes. *Diabetes*. 1970;19:747-830.

Standardized Ratios

A standardized risk ratio is the ratio of two standardized risks, $RR_w = R_{1w}/R_{0w}$, which can be expressed as:

$$RR_w = \frac{\sum_i w_i R_{1i}/\sum_i w_i}{\sum_i w_i R_{0i}/\sum_i w_i} = \frac{\sum_i w_i R_{1i}}{\sum_i w_i R_{0i}} = \frac{\sum_i w_i R_{0i} RR_i}{\sum_i w_i R_{0i}}$$

where $RR_i = R_{1i}/R_{0i}$ is the stratum-specific risk ratio. From the far-right expression, we see that RR_w can be viewed as a weighted average of the stratum-specific risk ratios but with the weight corresponding to the ith stratum being the product $w_i R_{0i}$ and not just the weight from the standard (i.e., w_i).

Similarly, a standardized rate ratio is the ratio of two standardized rates, $IR_w = I_{1w}/I_{0w}$, which can be expressed as:

$$IR_w = \frac{\sum_i w_i I_{1i}/\sum_i w_i}{\sum_i w_i I_{0i}/\sum_i w_i} = \frac{\sum_i w_i I_{1i}}{\sum_i w_i I_{0i}} = \frac{\sum_i w_i I_{0i} IR_i}{\sum_i w_i I_{0i}}$$

where $IR_i = I_{1i}/I_{0i}$ is the stratum-specific rate ratio. As with RR_w, IR_w can be viewed as a weighted average of the stratum-specific rate ratios, IR_i, but with the weight corresponding to the ith stratum being the product $w_i I_{0i}$.

Returning to the tolbutamide data in Table 18-2, using the total cohort as the standard, the estimated standardized risk ratio is $\widehat{RR}_w = 0.142/0.107 = 1.33$. Similarly, we estimate a standardized rate ratio from the data in Table 18-1 by dividing the standardized rate estimate among the smokers by the standardized rate estimate among the nonsmokers. Using smokers as the standard gives $\widehat{IR}_w = 44.3/31.2 = 1.42$.

Standardized Morbidity Ratios

A standardized ratio that is standardized to the distribution of the exposed group, that is the group in the numerator of the standardized ratio, is traditionally referred to as a *standardized morbidity ratio* (SMR). Note that, conversely, a standardized ratio will not be an SMR if it does not use the exposed group as the standard. As explained in Chapter 5, if the stratum-specific ratios are heterogeneous and there is confounding across the strata, a comparison of two or more SMR estimates (say from two different studies) will remain confounded by the stratifying factors, because the SMRs are standardized to different exposure groups.

Confidence Intervals

Confidence intervals for estimates of standardized measures can be constructed using the same data and weights. Suppose that A_i cases are observed out of T_i person-time units or N_i persons in stratum i. An estimate of the variance of $\hat{I}_w$ is:

$$\widehat{Var}\left(\hat{I}_w\right) = \frac{\sum_i w_i^2 \widehat{Var}\left(\hat{I}_i\right)}{\left(\sum_i w_i\right)^2}$$

[18-1]

where $\widehat{Var}\left(\hat{I}_i\right)$, the estimated variance of the rate estimate in stratum i, depends on the probability model assumed for the number of cases A_i in each stratum. For example, given person-time cohort data and a Poisson model for the A_i:

$$\widehat{Var}\left(\hat{I}_i\right) = A_i/T_i^2 = \hat{I}_i/T_i.$$

[18-2]

For pure count data from a closed cohort and a binomial model for A_i, we use formula 18-1 to obtain $\widehat{Var}\left(\hat{R}_w\right)$, but with

$$\widehat{Var}\left(\hat{R}_i\right) = \frac{\hat{R}_i\left(1-\hat{R}_i\right)}{N_i-1} = \frac{A_i\left(N_i-A_i\right)}{N_i^2\left(N_i-1\right)}$$

in place of $\widehat{Var}\left(\hat{I}_i\right)$. As noted in Chapter 17, the Poisson and binomial models assume no contagion or other sources of dependence among outcomes. Less restrictive models lead to more generally applicable variance formulae.[2,3]

Suppose now that the data are divided into two exposure groups, distinguished by a subscript that is either 1 (for exposed) or 0 (for unexposed). Confidence intervals for a standardized rate difference and a standardized rate ratio can be constructed using the variance estimates:

$$\widehat{Var}\left(\widehat{ID}_w\right) = \widehat{Var}\left(\hat{I}_{1w}\right) + \widehat{Var}\left(\hat{I}_{0w}\right) \qquad [18\text{-}3]$$

$$\widehat{Var}\left[\ln\left(\widehat{IR}_w\right)\right] = \widehat{Var}\left(\hat{I}_{1w}\right)\big/\hat{I}_{1w}^2 + \widehat{Var}\left(\hat{I}_{0w}\right)\big/\hat{I}_{0w}^2 \qquad [18\text{-}4]$$

Note, both of these formulae assume that the standardized rate in the exposed varies independently of the standardized rate in the unexposed. Parallel formulae can be applied to estimated risk differences $\widehat{RD}_w$, risk ratios $\widehat{RR}_w$, and standard errors of $\widehat{RD}_w$ and $ln(\widehat{RR}_w)$, using $\hat{R}_{1w}$ and $\hat{R}_{0w}$ in place of $\hat{I}_{1w}$ and $\hat{I}_{0w}$, respectively. For constructing confidence intervals on the standardized risk difference, we recommend using the improved formula due to Zou and Donner[4] in Chapter 17 (specifically 17-4).

For the data in Table 18-1, taking the person-years for smokers as the stratum-specific weights, we use formulae 18-1 to 18-3 to obtain an estimate of the variance of $\widehat{ID}_w$. Intermediate calculations are given in Table 18-3; we get:

$$\widehat{Var}\left(\hat{I}_{1w}\right) = \frac{630}{142,247^2} = \frac{3.114}{\left(10^4 \text{ years}\right)^2}$$

$$\widehat{Var}\left(\hat{I}_{0w}\right) = \frac{1,997.56}{142,247^2} = \frac{9.872}{\left(10^4 \text{ years}\right)^2}$$

$$\widehat{Var}\left(\widehat{ID}_w\right) = \widehat{Var}\left(\hat{I}_{1w}\right) + \widehat{Var}\left(\hat{I}_{0w}\right) = \frac{12.9}{\left(10^4 \text{ years}\right)^2}$$

TABLE 18-3

Intermediate Calculations for Estimating the Variance of Standardized Estimates From the Data in Table 18-1

Age (y)	w_i	$w_i\hat{I}_{1i}$	$w_i\hat{I}_{0i}$	$w_i^2 Var(\hat{I}_{1i})$	$w_i^2 Var(\hat{I}_{0i})$
35-44	52,407	32	5.58	32	15.56
45-54	43,248	104	48.63	104	197.03
55-64	28,612	206	140.30	206	703.04
65-74	12,663	186	137.16	186	671.91
75-84	5,317	102	112.74	102	410.02
Total	142,247	630	444.41	630	1,997.56

Taking the square root, the estimated standard error is $\widehat{SE}\left(\widehat{ID}_w\right) = 3.6$ per 10,000 person-years. From this, a Wald-based approximate 95% confidence interval is $\left(\widehat{ID}_{w,L}, \widehat{ID}_{w,U}\right) = (5.8, 20.0)$ per 10,000 person-years.

For the standardized rate ratio, using the smokers in Table 18-1 as the standard gives the SMR. From formula 18-4, an estimate of the variance of $\ln\left(\widehat{SMR}\right)$ is:

$$\widehat{Var}\left[\ln\left(\widehat{SMR}\right)\right] = \frac{3.114\left(10^4\,y\right)^2}{\left(44.29/10^4\,y\right)^2} + \frac{9.872\left(10^4\,y\right)^2}{\left(31.24/10^4\,y\right)^2} = 0.00159 + 0.01012 = 0.0117.$$

From this the estimated standard error is $\widehat{SE}\left[\ln\left(\widehat{SMR}\right)\right] = \sqrt{0.0117} = 0.1082$, which yields a Wald-based approximate 95% confidence interval of:

$$\left(\widehat{SMR}_L, \widehat{SMR}_U\right) = \exp\left[\ln(1.42) \pm 1.96 \times 0.1082\right] = (1.15, 1.76).$$

Case-Control Data

Without external information, case-control studies do not provide stratum-specific rate or rate-difference estimates. They can, however, provide standardized rate-ratio estimates under density sampling schemes or a rare-disease assumption that can then be used to estimate the SMR. Following the notation of Chapter 8, let A_{1i} and A_{0i} be the numbers of exposed and unexposed cases in stratum i, and B_{1i} and B_{0i}, the corresponding numbers of exposed and unexposed controls. Furthermore, suppose the source population experiences T_{1i} and T_{0i} person-time units at risk during the study period. Recall from Chapter 8 that, assuming the outcome is rare and in the absence of biases, B_{1i}/B_{0i} can serve as an estimate of the ratio of exposed to unexposed person-time in the source population, T_{1i}/T_{0i}. It follows that $E_{1i} = A_{0i}/T_{0i} \times T_{1i} \approx A_{0i} \times B_{1i}/B_{0i}$ is an estimate of the number of exposed cases one should expect in stratum i of the study *if* the exposed population in that stratum experienced the unexposed rate (*i.e.*, A_{0i}/T_{0i}) and T_{1i} person-time units. Using this, an estimator of the SMR based on case-control data is $\widehat{SMR} = A_{1+}/E_{1+}$, where $A_{1+} = \sum_i A_{1i}$ and $E_{1+} = \sum_i E_{1i}$.[5]

Furthermore, under the binomial model for case-control data, an estimate of the variance of $\ln\left(\widehat{SMR}\right)$ is:

$$\widehat{Var}\left[\ln\left(\widehat{SMR}\right)\right] = \frac{1}{A_{1+}} + \frac{\sum_i E_{1+}^2 \times \left(1/A_{0i} + 1/B_{1i} + 1/B_{0i}\right)}{E_{1+}^2}$$

which can be used to construct a confidence interval for $\widehat{SMR}$.

It is also possible to estimate a standardized rate ratio from case-control data using other standards.[5] For example, in the absence of biases, $E_{0i} = A_{1i}B_{0i}/B_{1i}$ estimates the number of cases one should have expected among the unexposed in stratum i if they had experienced the exposed rate and T_{0i} person-time units; thus, an estimator of the standardized rate ratio using the unexposed population as the standard is $\widehat{SMR}_u = A_{0+}/E_{0+}$, where $A_{0+} = \sum_i A_{0i}$ and $E_{0+} = \sum_i E_{0i}$. An estimate of the variance of $\ln\left(\widehat{SMR}_u\right)$ is:

$$\widehat{Var}\left[\ln\left(\widehat{SMR}_u\right)\right] = \frac{\sum_i E_{0+}^2 \times \left(1/A_{1i} + 1/B_{1i} + 1/B_{0i}\right)}{E_{0+}^2} + \frac{1}{A_{0+}}.$$

Finally, an estimate of the standardized rate ratio using the total population as the standard is $\widehat{SMR}_t = \left(A_{1+} + E_{0+}\right)/\left(A_{0+} + E_{1+}\right)$, while an estimate of the variance of $\ln\left(\widehat{SMR}_t\right)$ is:

$$\widehat{Var}\left[\ln\left(\widehat{SMR}_t\right)\right] = \frac{A_{1+} + \sum_i E_{0+}^2 \times \left(1/A_{1i} + 1/B_{1i} + 1/B_{0i}\right)}{\left(A_{1+} + E_{0+}\right)^2} + \frac{A_{0+} + \sum_i E_{1+}^2 \times \left(1/A_{0i} + 1/B_{1i} + 1/B_{0i}\right)}{\left(A_{0+} + E_{1+}\right)^2}.$$

Note, the standardized estimators presented above assume that the expected values of the stratum-specific numbers $(A_{1i}, B_{1i}, A_{0i}, B_{0i})$ are "large" (specifically, at least 5). If the data are sparse, as is often the case in matched case-control studies, one should instead use estimators based on homogeneity assumptions or regression models. Such estimators need not assume homogeneity over all stratification variables[6-9]

ESTIMATION ASSUMING HOMOGENITY ACROSS STRATA

Rationale

Standardization provides a means to summarize measures across strata (*i.e.*, report a single value) without assuming that the measures are homogenous across those strata. Here we describe methods for estimating a single value of a given measure using data that are stratified while assuming homogeneity across the strata. Use of such methods does not require that one actually believes that the assumption holds. Their use can be viewed as a decision to simplify the analysis and the reporting of results, based on the idea that any heterogeneity that is present cannot be accurately analyzed given the study's size. This rationale is reasonable as long as the homogeneity assumption is not clearly contradicted by the data or other evidence and, thus, could be viewed as a potentially useful approximation.

Given that one can never be sure of homogeneity, how should one interpret estimates based on such an assumption? When the ratios do not vary much across strata, the homogeneous risk and rate ratio estimates discussed here appear to provide good estimates of risk and rate ratios standardized using the total population (exposed plus unexposed) as the standard.[10] This is also true of homogeneous odds ratio estimators derived from unmatched case-control studies, provided that the stratum-specific odds ratios approximate the stratum-specific risk or rate ratios. These approximations provide a straightforward interpretation of homogeneous ratio estimators and so justify their use even when some ratio heterogeneity is present (as is always the case). Nonetheless, they do not provide a rationale for failing to search for heterogeneity and report it when it appears likely to be of important magnitude.

Pooled Estimates Under the Assumption of Homogeneity

Even if the true measure is identical across strata, however, it is reasonable to expect that estimates of the measure will vary across strata because of random error. Thus, even if one assumes homogeneity across strata, one must derive an overall estimate of association or effect from stratified data. A summary estimate derived under the homogeneity assumption is sometimes called a "pooled estimate."

Pooled estimates are usually weighted averages of stratum-specific estimates. Taking a weighted average of stratum-specific estimates describes standardization as well as pooling. The difference is that with standardization, the weights are derived from a standard distribution that may be external to the data and are applied to the estimated occurrence measures (or case-control ratios) rather than to association or effect measures, and the entire process does not assume homogeneity of any measure across strata. With pooling, the weights are applied to the estimated association or effect measure, are determined solely by the data under an assumption of homogeneity, and are chosen to reduce the random variability of the summary estimate. In particular, if the measure is homogeneous across strata, its value is constant and each stratum provides an estimate of the same quantity. The analytic task is to average these stratum-specific estimates in a manner to minimize the variance of the estimate of the overall measure.

One important consequence of these differences is that a standardized estimate may assign relatively large weight to strata with little data and little weight to strata with ample data. In contrast, pooling is designed to assign weights that reflect the amount of information in each stratum. If the measure is homogeneous, one way to minimize the variance of the overall weighted average without introducing bias is to assign weights to the stratum-specific values that are inversely proportional to the estimated variance of each stratum-specific estimate. Direct pooling, or precision weighting, involves first estimating the stratum-specific variances, then inverting these to get the weights, and finally averaging the stratum-specific estimates using these weights; this is sometimes known as the Woolf method or weighted least squares.[11] To be valid, direct pooling requires large numbers within each cell in each stratum. Because many stratified analyses have sparse data, directly weighted approaches are not as broadly applicable as the alternatives we will discuss below.[12]

One alternative covered below is to find the value of the measure that maximizes the probability of the data under the homogeneity assumption. This maximum-likelihood (ML) method (Chapter 16) produces the pooled estimate without explicitly determining stratum-specific weights. ML estimates have certain desirable statistical properties, such as minimum large-sample variance among approximately unbiased estimators, and are consequently often considered the optimal large-sample estimating methods. Nonetheless, there are other relevant statistical criteria (such as mean-squared error) under which ML estimation is inferior to certain methods (such as penalized-likelihood estimation; see Chapter 21).

Another approach to estimating a homogeneous measure is the Mantel-Haenszel method, also covered below. Mantel-Haenszel estimators are easy to calculate and, in many applications, perform nearly as well as ML estimators. In the following, because likelihood computations can be complex and are invariably obtained via statistical software, we will omit formulae for ML estimates and, instead, focus on Mantel-Haenszel formulae. For a more detailed introduction to likelihood methods in epidemiologic analysis, see the works of Clayton and Hills, Newman, and Jewell.[13-15]

Maximum-Likelihood Estimation

Maximum-likelihood estimation of a homogeneous measure involves taking the data probabilities for each stratum (dictated by the choice of underlying probability distribution, such as the Poisson distribution or the binomial distribution) and multiplying them together across strata to produce a total data probability. For person-time data, the latter probability is a function of the stratum-specific rates in the exposed, I_{1i}, and in the unexposed, I_{0i}. If no constraint is imposed on these rates, the maximum-likelihood estimates (MLEs) of the stratum-specific rates under a Poisson distribution will simply be the observed rates $\hat{I}_{1i} = A_{1i}/T_{1i}$ and $\hat{I}_{0i} = A_{0i}/T_{0i}$. If, however, we assume that one of the association measures is homogeneous across the strata, either that all I_{1i}/I_{0i} equal some common value, say IR, across strata or that all $I_{1i} - I_{0i}$ equal some common value, say ID, across strata, the MLEs of the stratum-specific rates and this homogeneous measure requires iterative computation and, thus, software. Most such software assumes a Poisson probability model for the stratum-specific counts A_{1i} and A_{0i} (Chapter 17) or a Poisson regression model (Chapter 21), and that the counts are independent within and across strata. As has been mentioned, neither assumption is realistic when the disease under study is contagious, but they may be reasonable for many other diseases.

For person-count data with stratum-specific denominators N_{1i} and N_{0i}, if no constraint is imposed, the MLEs of the stratum-specific average risks under a binomial distribution are the observed incidence proportions $\hat{R}_{1i} = A_{1i}/N_{1i}$ and $\hat{R}_{0i} = A_{0i}/N_{0i}$. If, however, we constrain either the risk ratio, odds ratio, or risk difference measure to be homogeneous across the strata, then the MLEs of the stratum-specific risks and the ratio or difference measure must be found by iterative computation. Much software is available for estimating a homogeneous odds ratio, that is, assuming that the stratum-specific odds ratios:

$$OR_i = \frac{R_{1i}/(1-R_{1i})}{R_{0i}/(1-R_{0i})}$$

are the same across strata. Most such software assumes a binomial probability model for the counts A_{1i} and A_{0i} (Chapter 17) and that these counts are independent within and across strata. Assuming either that R_{1i}/R_{0i} all equal some common value RR across strata or that $R_{1i} - R_{0i}$ all equal some common value RD across strata will typically involve the use of software for fitting a binomial regression (Chapter 21).

Unconditional Versus Conditional Analysis

Chapter 17 introduced two different probability models used for analyzing rate ratios: a two-Poisson model and a single-binomial model that was based on taking the observed number of cases, M_1, as given or "fixed." It also introduced two different models for analysis of odds ratios in a 2×2 table: a two-binomial model and a single-hypergeometric model that was based on taking all the table margins (M_1, M_0, N_1, N_0) as fixed. The fixed-margin models are called conditional models, because they condition all data probabilities on the observed margins.

For the analysis of odds ratios, the hypergeometric likelihood statistics are called conditional-likelihood statistics, and the MLE of the common odds ratio derived from the hypergeometric model is called the *conditional maximum-likelihood estimate* (CMLE). In contrast, the binomial-likelihood statistics are often called unconditional likelihood statistics, and the MLE of the common odds ratio derived from the two-binomial model is often called the *unconditional MLE*. Usually, if a discussion does not specify which MLE is being considered, it is the unconditional estimate that is under discussion.

Stratified analysis of rate and odds ratios may also be conducted with or without conditioning on the stratum margins. For rate ratios, the difference is essentially only computational. For odds ratios, however, the choice of whether to model each stratum with two binomials or a single hypergeometric probability can have a profound effect on the resulting common odds ratio analysis. Only conditional-likelihood methods (based on the hypergeometric model, conditioning on all stratum margins [M_{1i}, M_{0i}, N_{1i}, N_{0i}]) and Mantel-Haenszel methods (described below) remain approximately valid in sparse data, that is, data in which the number of subjects per stratum is small. As discussed below, however, they require that the total number of subjects contributing to the estimates at each exposure-disease combination be adequate.[16-18] Unconditional likelihood methods for the odds ratio based on the two-binomial model additionally require that each binomial denominator in each stratum (that is, N_{1i} and N_{0i} in a cohort study, M_{1i} and M_{0i} in a case-control study) be "large," specifically at least 10.[19]

Only exact methods have no size requirement. Because the unconditional MLE of the odds ratio additionally requires large numbers *within* strata, whereas the conditional MLE does not, one may well ask why the unconditional MLE is used at all. There are at least two reasons: First, the conditional MLE is computationally much more demanding, and when the numbers within strata are large (N_{1i} and N_{0i} are at least 10), the two estimators will usually be almost equal and so there will be no need to use the conditional MLE. Second, only the unconditional method is theoretically justifiable for estimation of quantities other than rate ratios and odds ratios, such as risks, risk differences, and risk ratios.

Mantel-Haenszel Estimation: Person-Time Data

We consider estimation of a common rate difference, ID, and common rate ratio, IR, based on person-time data. For the first of these, the Mantel-Haenszel estimate of ID is a standardized rate difference with standard weights given by:

$$w_{MHi} = T_{1i} T_{0i} / T_{+i}$$

where $T_{+i} = T_{1i} + T_{0i}$. Coupled with the stratum-specific estimates $\hat{I}_{1i} = A_{1i}/T_{1i}$ and $\hat{I}_{0i} = A_{0i}/T_{0i}$, this weighting yields:

$$\widehat{ID}_{MH} = \frac{\sum_i w_{MHi} \left(\hat{I}_{1i} - \hat{I}_{0i} \right)}{\sum_i w_{MHi}} = \frac{\sum_i \left(A_{1i} T_{0i} - A_{0i} T_{1i} \right)/T_{+i}}{\sum_i T_{1i} T_{0i}/T_{+i}}.$$

An estimate of the variance of $\widehat{ID}_{MH}$ is:

$$\widehat{Var}\left(\widehat{ID}_{MH}\right) = \frac{\sum_i w^2_{MHi} \left(\hat{I}_{1i}/T_{1i} + \hat{I}_{0i}/T_{0i} \right)}{\left(\sum_i w_{MHi}\right)^2}$$

[18-5]

which can be used to construct valid confidence intervals even if the data are sparse.[20]

An alternative estimate of the variance of $\widehat{ID}_{MH}$ can be obtained by using $T_{1i}T_{0i}/M_{1i}$ instead of w_{MHi} in expression 18-5. While this change will often result in tighter confidence intervals, this change renders the estimator invalid for sparse data. Finally, we note that $\widehat{ID}_{MH}$ typically has a much higher variance than the corresponding MLE.[20] We therefore recommend ML for estimating a homogeneous rate difference, subject to the caution that there be at least 10 cases per stratum. If, however, there are fewer than 10 cases per stratum, the MLE of the rate difference can become excessively biased, whereas $\widehat{ID}_{MH}$ remains unbiased.

For settings where a common rate ratio is assumed, the Mantel-Haenszel estimate has the simple form given by[21,22]:

$$\widehat{IR}_{MH} = \frac{\sum_i w_{MHi} \hat{I}_{1i}}{\sum_i w_{MHi} \hat{I}_{0i}} = \frac{\sum_i A_{1i} T_{0i}/T_{+i}}{\sum_i A_{0i} T_{1i}/T_{+i}}.$$

To construct a Wald-based approximate confidence interval, we consider the following estimate of the variance of $\ln\left(\widehat{ID}_{MH}\right)$[20]:

$$\widehat{Var}\left[\ln\left(\widehat{IR}_{MH}\right)\right] = \frac{\sum_i M_{1i} T_{1i} T_{0i}/T_{+i}^2}{\left(\sum_i A_{1i} T_{0i}/T_{+i}\right)\left(\sum_i A_{0i} T_{1i}/T_{+i}\right)}.$$

Thus, letting $\widehat{SE}\left[\ln\left(\widehat{IR}_{MH}\right)\right]$ denote the square-root of the above expression, a Wald-based approximate 95% confidence interval is:

$$\left(\widehat{IR}_{MH,L}, \widehat{IR}_{MH,U}\right) = \exp\left\{\ln\left(\widehat{IR}_{MH}\right) \pm 1.96 \times \widehat{SE}\left[\ln\left(\widehat{IR}_{MH}\right)\right]\right\}.$$

Note, the above formulae are valid even if the data are sparse. Nonetheless, like the MLEs, both are "large-sample" formulae, in that their validity requires adequate numbers of subjects observed at each exposure-disease combination. As a rough guide, one should use exact limits if either:

$$\sum_i \frac{M_{1i} \widehat{IR}_{MH,L} T_{1i}}{\widehat{IR}_{MH,L} T_{1i} + T_{0i}}$$

or

$$\sum_i \frac{M_{1i} T_{0i}}{\widehat{IR}_{MH,U} T_{1i} + T_{0i}}$$

is less than 5. Finally, unlike $\widehat{ID}_{MH}$, in most situations, $\widehat{IR}_{MH}$ based on the weights w_{MHi} has a variance equal to or not much larger than that of the MLE of the common rate ratio.[20,23]

Table 18-4 gives the intermediate calculations for Mantel-Haenszel analysis of the coronary mortality data in Table 18-1. In units of deaths per 10^4 years,

$$\widehat{ID}_{MH} = \frac{13,831(6.1 - 1.1) + \cdots + 1,147(191.8 - 212.0)}{30,445^2} = 11.44$$

$$\widehat{Var}\left(\widehat{ID}_{MH}\right) = \frac{13,831^2(6.1/52,407 + 1.1/18,790) + \cdots}{30,445^2} = 9.57$$

which yield a 95% confidence interval for $\widehat{ID}_{MH}$ of $11.44 \pm 1.96 \times \sqrt{9.57} = (5.38, 17.50)$ per 10^4 person-years. If, instead, we assume a common rate ratio, we get:

$$\widehat{IR}_{MH} = 11.68/82.0 = 1.42$$

$$\widehat{Var}\left[\ln\left(\widehat{IR}_{MH}\right)\right] = \frac{110.1}{116.8(82.0)} = 0.01150$$

TABLE 18-4

Intermediate Calculations for Mantel-Haenszel Analysis of the Smoking/Coronary Mortality Data in Table 18-1

Age (y)	$T_{1i} T_{0i}/T_{+i}$	$A_{1i} T_{0i}/T_{+i}$	$A_{0i} T_{1i}/T_{+i}$	$M_{1i} T_{1i}/T_{+i}$	$M_{1i} T_{1i} T_{0i}/T_{+i}^2$
35-44	13,831	8.45	1.47	25.05	6.60
45-54	8,560	20.59	9.62	93.04	18.42
55-64	4,760	34.27	23.34	195.07	32.45
65-74	2,147	31.53	23.25	177.72	30.13
75-84	1,147	22.00	24.31	104.32	22.50
Total	30,445	116.8	82.0	595.2	110.1

which yield a Wald-based 95% confidence interval

$$\left(\widehat{IR}_{MH,L}, \widehat{IR}_{MH,U}\right) = exp\left[ln(1.42) \pm 1.96 \times \sqrt{0.01150}\right] = (1.15,\ 1.75).$$

Although details are not shown, maximum likelihood estimation yields virtually the same point estimate and confidence limits for *IR*.

Mantel-Haenszel Estimation: Pure Count Data

Now suppose that our data come from a closed cohort. Mantel-Haenszel estimates of the common risk difference, *RD*, and common risk ratio, *RR*, are equivalent to standardized estimators based on the standard weights:

$$w_{MHi} = N_{1i} N_{0i}/N_{+i}$$

where $N_{+i} = N_{1i} + N_{0i}$. Note, these weights are direct analogs of the weights for Mantel-Haenszel estimation based on person-time data. Thus, the Mantel-Haenszel estimate of the risk difference is[24]:

$$\widehat{RD}_{MH} = \frac{\sum_i (A_{1i}N_{0i} - A_{0i}N_{1i})/N_{+i}}{\sum_i N_{1i} N_{0i}/N_{+i}},$$

while the Mantel-Haenszel estimate of the risk ratio is[21]:

$$\widehat{RR}_{MH} = \frac{\sum_i A_{1i} N_{0i}/N_{+i}}{\sum_i A_{0i} N_{1i}/N_{+i}}.$$

As in the person-time situation, these Mantel-Haenszel estimators can have much higher variance than the MLEs of the homogeneous risk difference or ratio. Unlike the MLEs, however, the Mantel-Haenszel estimators remain valid in sparse data.[20] An estimate of the variance of $\widehat{RD}_{MH}$ that is valid for all types of data is given by Sato.[25] It is rather complex and so is omitted here. If N_{1i} and N_{0i} in all strata are greater than 1, then one can use the following estimate:

$$\widehat{Var}\left(\widehat{RD}_{MH}\right) = \frac{\sum_i w_{MHi}^2\left[\dfrac{A_{1i}B_{1i}}{N_{1i}^2(N_{1i}-1)} + \dfrac{A_{0i}B_{0i}}{N_{0i}^2(N_{0i}-1)}\right]}{\left(\sum_i w_{MHi}\right)^2}.$$

Unless all the cell counts are large, however, it is best to set limits using the improved approximation formula given for the crude RD in Chapter 17 (see expression 17-4).

An estimate of the variance for $\ln\left(\widehat{RR}_{MH}\right)$ is:

$$\widehat{Var}\left[\ln\left(\widehat{RR}_{MH}\right)\right] = \frac{\sum_i\left(M_{1i}N_{1i}N_{0i}//N_{+i}^2 - A_{1i}A_{0i}/N_{+i}\right)}{\left(\sum_i A_{1i}N_{0i}/N_{+i}\right)\left(\sum_i A_{0i}N_{1i}/N_{+i}\right)}. \qquad [18\text{-}6]$$

Like the MLE, $\widehat{RR}_{MH}$ and its variance estimator are "large-sample" estimators, but $\widehat{RR}_{MH}$ does not require the strata to be large.

The variance of $\widehat{RD}_{MH}$ can be greatly reduced by using $N_{1i}N_{0i}/M_{1i}$ instead of w_{MHi} as the weight. Similarly, if $M_{0i} = N_{+i} - M_{1i}$ is the total number of noncases in stratum i, the variance of $\widehat{RR}_{MH}$ can be reduced by using $N_{1i}N_{0i}/M_{0i}$ instead of w_{MHi} as the weight.[26] These modifications, however, render the estimates invalid for sparse data.

Consider again Table 18-2, comparing tolbutamide with placebo. From these data, we obtain the Mantel-Haenszel risk difference estimate of $\widehat{RD}_{MH} = 0.035$, with an estimated standard error of $\widehat{SE}\left(\widehat{RD}_{MH}\right) = 0.032$. Together, these yield a Wald-based 95% confidence interval of $\left(\widehat{RD}_{MH,L},\widehat{RD}_{MH,U}\right) = 0.035 \pm 1.96 \times 0.032 = (-0.027, 0.098)$. For comparison, the MLE of the risk difference is $\widehat{RD} = 0.034$ with an estimated standard error of $\widehat{SE}\left(\widehat{RD}\right) = 0.028$; these yield 95% confidence limits of $\left(\widehat{RD}_L,\widehat{RD}_U\right) = (-0.021, 0.089)$, somewhat narrower than the Mantel-Haenszel limits.

The Mantel-Haenszel risk-ratio estimate from Table 18-2 is $\widehat{RR}_{MH} = 1.33$, and the variance estimate for its logarithm is $\widehat{Var}\left[\ln\left(\widehat{RR}_{MH}\right)\right] = 0.0671$. Together, these yield an approximate 95% confidence interval for $\widehat{RR}_{MH}$ of:

$$\left(\widehat{RR}_{MH,L},\widehat{RR}_{MH,U}\right) = \exp\left[\ln(1.33) \pm 1.96 \times \sqrt{0.0671}\right] = (0.80, 2.21).$$

Finally, we consider estimation of the common odds ratio, OR, which may be of interest in settings where the data arise from a cohort study or from cross-sectional or case-control data. The Mantel-Haenszel estimate of OR is[27]:

$$\widehat{OR}_{MH} = \frac{\sum_i A_{1i}B_{0i}/N_{+i}}{\sum_i A_{0i}B_{1i}/N_{+i}}.$$

For values of the OR not far from 1, this estimator has a variance not much greater than the MLE and remains valid in sparse data.[12,28] Toward constructing a confidence interval, an estimate of the variance of $\ln\left(\widehat{OR}_{MH}\right)$ is:

$$\widehat{Var}\left[\ln\left(\widehat{OR}_{MH}\right)\right] = \frac{\sum_i G_i P_i}{2\left(\sum_i G_i\right)^2} + \frac{\sum_i\left(G_i Q_i + H_i P_i\right)}{2\sum_i G_i \sum_i P_i} + \frac{\sum_i H_i Q_i}{2\left(\sum_i H_i\right)^2}$$

where $G_i = A_{1i}B_{0i}/N_{+i}$, $H_i = A_{0i}B_{1i}/N_{+i}$, $P_i = (A_{1i} + B_{0i})/N_{+i}$, $Q_i = (A_{0i} + B_{1i})/N_{+i}$.[29,30]

Table 18-5 provides data from a case-control study of congenital heart disease, Down syndrome, and maternal spermicide use before conception. The Mantel-Haenszel estimate of the maternal-age stratified odds ratio relating maternal spermicide use to Down syndrome is:

$$\widehat{OR}_{MH} = \frac{(3 \times 1059)/1,175 + (1 \times 86)/95}{(104 \times 9)/1,175 + (5 \times 3)/95} = 3.78.$$

TABLE 18-5

Infants With Congenital Heart Disease and Down Syndrome, and Healthy Controls, According to Maternal Spermicide Use Before Conception and Maternal Age at Delivery

	Maternal Age <35 y, Spermicide Use			Maternal Age 35+ y, Spermicide Use		
	Yes	No	Total	Yes	No	Total
Down syndrome	3	9	12	1	3	4
Control	104	1,059	1,163	5	86	91
Total	107	1,068	1,175	6	89	95

From Rothman KJ. Spermicide use and Down syndrome. *Am J Public Health.* 1982;72:399-401.

The estimated variance from the above formula is 0.349, which yields a Wald-based 95% confidence interval of:

$$\left(\widehat{OR}_{MH,L}, \widehat{OR}_{MH,U}\right) = \exp\left[\ln(3.78) \pm 1.96 \times \sqrt{0.349}\right] = (1.19, 12.0).$$

Mantel-Haenszel Estimation: Case-Cohort Data

As for unstratified case-cohort data (Chapter 17), one can obtain a pooled estimate of the odds ratio simply by combining all cases together (whether they come from the case sample or the cohort sample) and then analyzing the data as if they were case-control data. For risk-ratio estimation, however, we must distinguish cases that are not controls (*i.e.*, not part of the cohort sample) and cases that are controls (*i.e.*, are part of the cohort sample). We will use the notation in Table 18-6 to represent a stratum in the study. Furthermore, let

$A_{1i} = A_{11i} + A_{10i} =$ exposed cases in stratum i
$A_{0i} = A_{01i} + A_{00i} =$ unexposed cases in stratum i
$M_{1i} = A_{1i} + A_{0i} =$ total cases in stratum i
$C_{1i} = A_{10i} + B_{1i} =$ exposed controls in stratum i
$C_{0i} = A_{00i} + B_{0i} =$ unexposed controls in stratum i

TABLE 18-6

Notation for a Stratum in a Case-Cohort Study

	Exposed	Unexposed	Total
Case, not control	A_{11i}	A_{01i}	M_{11i}
Case and control	A_{10i}	A_{00i}	M_{10i}
Noncase control	B_{1i}	B_{0i}	M_{0i}
Total	N_{1i}	N_{0i}	N_{+i}

A Mantel-Haenszel risk-ratio estimator for case-cohort data is[31]:

$$\widehat{RR}_{MH} = \frac{\sum_i A_{1i} C_{0i}/N_{+i}}{\sum_i A_{0i} C_{1i}/N_{+i}}$$

while an estimate of the variance of $\ln\left(\widehat{RR}_{MH}\right)$ is[32]:

$$\widehat{Var}\left[\ln\left(\widehat{RR}_{MH}\right)\right] = \frac{\sum_i\left[\left(A_{01i}+B_{0i}\right)A_{1i}C_{1i}+\left(A_{11i}+B_{1i}\right)A_{0i}C_{0i}+A_{11i}B_{0i}+A_{01i}B_{1i}\right]/N_{+i}^2}{\left(\sum_i A_{1i} C_{0i}/N_{+i}\right)\left(\sum_i A_{0i} C_{1i}/N_{+i}\right)}.$$

Like the other Mantel-Haenszel estimators, both of these estimators remain valid for sparse data but require adequate numbers of subjects contributing to the estimate at each exposure-disease combination. The variance of the risk-ratio estimator $\widehat{RR}_{MH}$ can be reduced by replacing N_i with $C_i = C_{1i} + C_{0i}$ throughout (including the variance formula), but then the estimator will no longer be valid for sparse data.

Maximum-likelihood analysis of stratified case-cohort data is also feasible,[33] but as in other designs the MLEs require iterative computation, and the MLE of the risk ratio will not be valid in sparse data.

Mantel-Haenszel Estimation: Two-Stage Data

In a two-stage (two-phase) study, the exposure and disease status of an entire study cohort is known, so a crude (unstratified) analysis can be computed for the entire cohort, but data on other variables are obtained only on subsamples from each of the four exposure-disease cells (Chapter 8). Maximum-likelihood analysis of two-stage data is possible, but rather complex.[34,35] We focus here on slightly less efficient but much simpler methods.

Let $\left(A_1^*, A_0^*, B_1^*, B_0^*\right)$ be the numbers of exposed and unexposed cases and exposed and unexposed noncases in the *entire* cohort. Suppose that simple random subsamples of size $(A_{1+}, A_{0+}, B_{1+}, B_{0+})$ are selected from the four cohort cells and we obtain covariate information only for the subjects in these subsamples. Estimates of the stratum-specific full-cohort numbers and measures are then:

$$\hat{A}_{1i}^* = A_{1i}\left(A_1^*/A_{1+}\right) \quad \hat{A}_{0i}^* = A_{0i}\left(A_0^*/A_{0+}\right)$$
$$\hat{B}_{1i}^* = B_{1i}\left(B_1^*/B_{1+}\right) \quad \hat{B}_{0i}^* = B_{0i}\left(B_0^*/B_{0+}\right)$$
$$\hat{N}_{1i}^* = \hat{A}_{1i}^* + \hat{B}_{1i}^* \quad \hat{N}_{0i}^* = \hat{A}_{0i}^* + \hat{B}_{0i}^*$$
$$\hat{R}_{1i} = \hat{A}_{1i}^*/\hat{N}_{1i}^* \quad \hat{R}_{0i} = \hat{A}_{0i}^*/\hat{N}_{0i}^*$$
$$\widehat{RD}_i = \hat{R}_{1i} - \hat{R}_{0i} \quad \widehat{RR}_i = \hat{R}_{1i}/\hat{R}_{0i}$$

and

$$\widehat{OR}_i = \hat{A}_{1i}^* \hat{B}_{0i}^*/\hat{A}_{0i}^* \hat{B}_{01}^*.$$

General variance formulae for two-stage estimators are much more complicated than those given earlier for unsampled cohort data. We will give only simple approximate formulae for estimating odds ratios under the condition that the subsample sizes are fixed by design. Let F be the crude odds ratio for the total cohort divided by the crude odds ratio for the sample:

$$F = \frac{\left(A_{0+}/A_0^*\right)\left(B_{1+}/B_1^*\right)}{\left(A_{1+}/A_1^*\right)\left(B_{0+}/B_0^*\right)} = \frac{A_1^* B_0^*}{A_0^* B_1^*}\left(\frac{A_{1+} B_{0+}}{A_{0+} B_{1+}}\right)^{-1}.$$

Then the stratum-specific odds-ratio estimator given above can be rewritten as:

$$\widehat{OR}_i = \frac{F \times A_{1i}B_{0i}}{A_{0i}B_{1i}}.$$

Similarly, the Mantel-Haenszel estimator of the homogeneous odds ratio for two-stage data is:

$$\widehat{OR}_{MH} = F \times \frac{\sum_i A_{1i}B_{0i}/N_{+i}}{\sum_i A_{0i}B_{1i}/N_{+i}}$$

where N_{+i} is the actual stratum-specific sampled number of subjects.[36] An approximate variance estimator for the two-stage $\ln\left(\widehat{OR}_{MH}\right)$ can be computed by subtracting

$$1/A_1 + 1/A_{0+} + 1/B_{1+} + 1/B_{0+} - 1/A_1^* - 1/A_0^* - 1B_1^* - 1/B_0^*$$

from the usual Mantel-Haenszel variance estimator given in formula 18-6; this variance correction was originally derived for the estimator given by Cain and Breslow.[37]

Case-Crossover and Other Case-Only Designs

Chapter 8 described several case-only designs related to case-control studies. When the exposure status of cases is known over the entire time period of a case-crossover study, and the exposure distribution of case time at risk is representative of the source population distribution, one may estimate the rate ratio from the data as if it were person-time data from a cohort study.[38] Similarly, if case exposure status is known only at certain time points, and the exposure distribution of these points is representative of the time at risk in the source population, one may estimate the rate ratio from case-crossover data as if it were matched case-control data, with the data from a single case at different time points forming a matched set.[39,40] This set comprises a "case" (the case record as of disease incidence time) and "controls" (the records from other time periods, which are used for reference).

The assumptions that permit such simple approaches to case-crossover data depend heavily on how the time points were sampled, as well as on the disease process under study, and cannot be expected to hold in general. Sampling designs and analysis methods to address these issues are discussed by Lumley and Levy,[41] Vines and Farrington,[42] Navidi and Weinhandl,[43] Janes et al.,[44] and Janes et al.[45]

Analysis of case-specular studies may be conducted by treating the case and specular as matched pairs.[40,46] See Chapter 37 and the work by Thomas[47] for discussions of the analysis of genetic case-only studies, as well as other genetic designs.

Small-Sample Methods

One can avoid approximations and conduct stratified analyses of a homogeneous measure by computing traditional exact or mid-P-values (and hence confidence limits) directly from an exact probability model for the data. These approaches are direct extensions of the small-sample methods discussed in Chapter 16. Although conceptually simple, the necessary formulae and computations become quite complex in stratified data and are limited to rate-ratio and odds-ratio analyses.[11,48] The chief advantage of such analyses is that no assumption is needed about study size. For a description of these methods, see Ref. 49 or 50.

TESTING HOMOGENEITY ACROSS STRATA

Rationale

There are no rigid criteria for deciding whether the homogeneity assumption that underpins the above methods can be used. Regardless, the first step should be to compute and inspect the stratum-specific estimates. Although one should expect some random variation in the stratum-specific estimates even when the underlying parameter is homogeneous, excessive variation (relative to that expected by chance) or obvious nonrandom patterns of variation may be evident. The investigator's judgment about heterogeneity should not be limited to the appearance of the data under analysis; if it is available, knowledge from previous studies or more general biologic insight should be integrated into the evaluation process.

For settings where outside knowledge is scant, investigators may desire a more formal statistical evaluation of the extent to which variation in the stratum-specific estimates is consistent with purely random behavior. Toward this end, a variety of statistical tests can be applied. Part of the variety derives from the fact that ratio and difference measures require separate evaluations, because homogeneity of the ratio measure usually implies heterogeneity of the difference measure and vice versa. In Chapter 15, we criticized the use of statistical tests and, especially, the concept of "statistical significance," which artificially forces a continuous measure (the P-value) into a dichotomy. The use of statistical tests is more defensible, however, when an immediate analytic decision rests on the outcome of a single statistical evaluation. Such may be the case if an investigator is attempting to decide whether the extent of variation in a set of stratum-specific estimates is consistent with probable random departures from a homogeneous measure, so that homogeneity is tenable in light of the data. In Chapter 22, we argue that this logic also applies when assessing proportional hazards in a Cox model for time-to-event outcomes.

Testing the Hypothesis

The general form of a Wald statistic for testing the hypothesis that a measure U is homogeneous across strata is:

$$\chi^2_{Wald} = \sum_i \frac{\left(\hat{U}_i - \hat{U}\right)^2}{\hat{V}_i}$$

where $\hat{U}_i$ is the stratum-specific MLE of the measure, $\hat{V}_i$ is the corresponding estimated variance, and $\hat{U}$ is the MLE of the hypothesized homogeneous (common) value of the measure. Thus, a test based on χ^2_{Wald} of the hypothesis that the measure has a "common" or constant value across the strata is based on a comparison of the stratum-specific estimates against a summary estimate that assumes homogeneity.

Under the null hypothesis that the true values of the measures, U_i, are homogeneous across the strata, this statistic will have a χ^2 distribution with degrees of freedom equal to the number of strata minus 1. Thus, a P-value for the homogeneity hypothesis can be obtained using the appropriate χ^2 distribution. Note, the stratum-specific estimates $\hat{U}_i$ may be adjusted for factors other than the modifier under study. For example, we may test homogeneity across age strata while adjusting for sex, so that i varies across age strata; $\hat{U}_i$ is then the MLE obtained by stratifying on sex within stratum i of age, and $\hat{U}$ is the overall MLE obtained by stratifying on age and sex.

One important caution in using χ^2_{Wald} is that, for ratio measures, U should be taken to be the *logarithm* of the ratio. Substitution of the logarithm of the Mantel-Haenszel estimate of the rate or odds ratio for the logarithm of the corresponding MLE, though not theoretically correct, will usually make little difference in the result. If U is a rate or risk difference or a risk ratio, however, one should *not* use the Mantel-Haenszel estimate in place of the MLE, as this would invalidate the statistic.

Consider again the tolbutamide data in Table 18-2. Applying the unstratified formulae from Chapter 17 to each age stratum yields:

$$\text{Stratum 1}: \widehat{RR}_1 = 1.81, \widehat{Var}\left[ln\left(\widehat{RR}_1\right)\right] = 0.307$$

$$\text{Stratum 2}: \widehat{RR}_2 = 1.19, \widehat{Var}\left[ln\left(\widehat{RR}_2\right)\right] = 0.0860.$$

Earlier, we mentioned that the MLE of a common RR for these data is $\widehat{RR} = 1.31$. Thus

$$\chi^2_{Wald} = \frac{\left[ln(1.81) - ln(1.31)\right]^2}{0.3072} + \frac{\left[ln(1.19) - ln(1.31)\right]^2}{0.0860} = 0.45.$$

Because there are only two strata, this statistic has $2 - 1 = 1$ degree of freedom and yields a P-value of 0.50. Thus, there is little evidence to indicate that the data are incompatible with the hypothesis of homogeneity of the risk ratio.

Repeating the process for the risk difference, we get:

$$\text{Stratum 1}: \widehat{RD}_1 = 0.034, \widehat{Var}\left(\widehat{RD}_1\right) = 0.0010$$

$$\text{Stratum 2}: \widehat{RD}_2 = 0.036, \widehat{Var}\left(\widehat{RD}_2\right) = 0.0036.$$

Because the MLE of a common RD is $\widehat{RD} = 0.034$, we get:

$$\chi^2_{Wald} = \frac{(0.034 - 0.034)^2}{0.0010} + \frac{(0.036 - 0.034)^2}{0.0036} = 0.001$$

with one degree of freedom, which yields $P = 1.00$. Thus, as is evident from the point estimates, the same data are almost perfectly compatible with the hypothesis of homogeneity of the risk difference.

As mentioned earlier, if both the exposure and the stratifying variables are risk factors, then at most either the risk ratio or risk difference can be homogeneous. Thus, if there is any stratum-specific association of tolbutamide with death, at least one of the above homogeneity hypotheses *must* be wrong. Yet the tests rejected neither hypothesis. This reflects a general problem of homogeneity testing in that it will have low power in a typical epidemiologic study; that is, even if there is heterogeneity in the true values, the probability of rejecting homogeneity will typically be small.[11,51] Moreover, studies are often designed to have "sufficient" power (*e.g.*, 80%) to detect an "overall" association of a fixed, plausible size. Tests of homogeneity, however, require that the data be divided into strata and that the stratum-specific estimates—each with its own variance estimate—are compared with one another. The power of tests of homogeneity is therefore reduced in two ways relative to the power for the overall effect: (1) the study sample is divided into strata, which increases the total variance; and (2) every stratum, some of much smaller size than the total, must be used to estimate its own measure for comparison with other strata.

When there are more than two strata, it is often possible to use more powerful tests that make use of ordering of the strata with respect to the stratifying variables. Such tests are more easily described in the context of testing product terms in regression models (Chapters 20 and 21). Even with such improved tests, however, one should always bear in mind that a high P-value from a homogeneity test does not necessarily indicate that the measure is homogeneous; it means only that heterogeneity was not detected by the test. When heterogeneity is detected, it is usually best to present and discuss stratum-specific estimates. Nonetheless, standardized summaries (as opposed to summaries that assume homogeneity) retain valid interpretations and can be used as measures of population effect.[5,52]

Consider again the coronary death and smoking data in Table 18-1. We will test the homogeneity of the rate ratio using the Mantel-Haenszel estimate. Because the variances of the stratum-specific log rate-ratio estimates are $1/A_{1i} + 1/A_{0i}$ (Chapter 17), the value of the test statistic is:

$$\chi^2_{Wald} = \sum_i \frac{\left[\ln\left(\widehat{IR}_i\right) - \ln\left(\widehat{IR}_{MH}\right)\right]^2}{1/A_{1i} + 1/A_{0i}} = \frac{\left[\ln(6.1/1.1) - \ln(1.42)\right]^2}{1/32 + 1/2} + \ldots + \frac{\left[\ln(191.8/212.0) - \ln(1.42)\right]^2}{1/102 + 1/31}$$

$$= 10.41.$$

Because there are five age strata, this statistic a has χ^2 distribution with $5 - 1 = 4$ degrees of freedom, which yields a P-value of 0.03. Thus, it appears that homogeneity of the rate ratio is not a good assumption for analyzing the data. It also appears that the declining trend in ratios seen in Table 18-1 should be accounted for in the analysis and presentation of results. For a simple trend such as that in Table 18-1, a regression analysis may provide the most parsimonious complete summary, although the estimated SMR of $\overline{SMR} = 1.43$ remains a valid (if incomplete) summary.

Most software for stratified analysis provide an approximate test of homogeneity, such as a Wald test, score test, or likelihood-ratio test; a few packages, such as StatXact[50] can supply an exact homogeneity P-value if the numbers are not too large. Tests for qualitative interaction (that is, reversal of association) have also been developed.[53]

Except for exact tests, basic homogeneity tests require the study numbers to be large within strata. It is possible to apply the study-size criteria given in Chapter 17 on a stratum-by-stratum basis to determine whether unconditional maximum-likelihood estimates and unconditional homogeneity tests can be validly applied to stratified data. For example, if every stratum is large enough for the valid estimation of the stratum-specific rate ratio, the Wald test of rate-ratio homogeneity will usually be approximately valid as well. This stratum-by-stratum criterion is probably stricter than needed for score and likelihood-ratio tests of homogeneity. Nonetheless, if the criterion is not satisfied, it is unlikely that any of the standard homogeneity tests will yield a small P-value, and thus, use of an exact test is unlikely to alter the inferences.

TESTING THE NULL HYPOTHESIS OF NO ASSOCIATION

Thus far we have considered comparisons between exposure groups through consideration of differences or ratios of either a rate or a risk measure. In any given analysis, it possible that a pooled estimate of a homogeneous rate difference shows a negative association, whereas a pooled estimate of a homogeneous rate ratio shows a positive association for the same data. Such discrepancies stem from differences in the optimal weighting schemes for the different pooled estimators and reflect the fact that at most one of the measures can be homogeneous. However, for the purposes of testing the null hypothesis of no association in any stratum, the efficient (variance-minimizing) weighting schemes are approximately equivalent for all measures. Consequently, whatever be the parameter used to measure the association, only a single hypothesis test of no association need be considered.

Hypothesis testing is generally performed with respect to the overall departure of the data from the null value of no association. Even if the chosen measure varies substantially across strata, tests of the null that assume homogeneity can often outperform tests that do not. If the stratum-specific values of the rate ratio (in person-time data) or odds ratio (in pure count data) are in fact homogeneous, the tests described below are optimal under certain restrictive criteria.[54]

If the true values of the rate ratio or odds ratio vary across strata, specialized tests can be constructed that will be more powerful than the tests of overall departure from the null value described here. Even in this situation, the tests given below are still valid. More problematic, however, is that it is possible that some stratum-specific estimates are strongly positive while others are strongly negative. In such circumstances, the pooled estimate may be near the null value as a result of the balancing of the opposing estimates in individual strata. If the underlying stratum-specific measures change direction across strata, the tests given below may have little power to detect the presence of stratum-specific associations.

Test statistics for stratified data represent a straightforward extension of the corresponding statistics for unstratified data. The score tests for stratified data retain the general form of the score tests in Chapter 17; they extend the formulas for crude data by summing stratum-specific components for the test statistics (*i.e.*, the observed number of exposed cases, the number expected under the null hypothesis, and the null variance).

Testing Based on Stratified Pure Count Data

As with unstratified data, consider the total number of exposed cases, $A_{1+} = \sum_i A_{1i}$, as the test statistic. The expectations and variances for the number of exposed cases under the test hypothesis are calculated within each stratum and are summed over the strata. Assuming that all stratum margins are fixed, the expectation and variance for the number of exposed cases under the null hypothesis, $H_0{:}OR = 1$, are:

$$E = E\left(A_{1+} \mid OR = 1\right) = \sum_i \frac{M_{1i}N_{1i}}{N_{+i}}$$

and

$$V = Var\left(A_{1+}\,\middle|\,OR=1\right) = \sum_i \frac{M_{1i}M_{0i}N_{1i}N_{0i}}{N_{+i}^2\left(N_{+i}-1\right)}.$$

Together, these can be used to form the test statistic:

$$\chi_{score} = \frac{A_{1+}-E}{V^{1/2}}$$

which was first derived by Cochran,[24] later modified by Mantel and Haenszel[27] to the above form, and is now known as the *Mantel-Haenszel statistic*. It is identical to the test statistic for unstratified person-time data, except that the three components of the test statistic are obtained by summing their stratum-specific contributions. It is valid in sparse data but requires "large" numbers overall. The precise requirements are rather complex[16] and so are not given here, but they imply that small-sample methods should be used if any of the crude totals (A_{1+}, A_{0+}, B_{1+}, B_{0+}) or their null expected values (E, $M_{1+}-E$, $N_{1+}-E$, $N_{0+}-M_{1+}+E$) are less than 5.

Consider the *P*-value for the hypothesis of no association between tolbutamide and death using the data in Table 18-2 and the Mantel-Haenszel statistic. The number of exposed cases A_{1+}, where "exposed" indicates tolbutamide therapy, equals $8 + 22 = 30$. The expected value and variance of A_{1+} under the null hypothesis are:

$$E = \frac{(106)(13)}{226} + \frac{(98)(38)}{183} = 6.10 + 20.35 = 26.45$$

$$V = \frac{(106)(120)(13)(213)}{(226)^2(225)} + \frac{(98)(85)(35)(145)}{(183)^2(182)} = 3.06 + 7.53 = 10.60,$$

respectively, so that the statistic is:

$$\chi_{score} = \frac{30-26.45}{(10.60)^{1/2}} = 1.09$$

which gives a lower-tailed *P*-value of 0.86, or a two-sided *P*-value of 0.28. (Because tolbutamide was being studied as preventive of the complications of diabetes, departures from the null value were expected to occur in the direction of preventing death. Therefore, the relevant one-sided null hypothesis is that there is no inverse association, which is tested by the lower-tailed *P*-value.)

Consider again the spermicide and Down syndrome data in Table 18-5. The Mantel-Haenszel (score) statistic is 2.41 with an upper-tailed *P*-value of 0.008, which is not close to the upper-tailed mid-*P*-value of 0.023. This discrepancy reflects the fact that the study size is too small (only four exposed cases) for the Mantel-Haenszel *P*-value to approximate the mid-*P*-value.

Testing Based on Stratified Person-Time Data

The extension of the unstratified score test for pure count data to stratified 2×2 tables is analogous to the extension of the unstratified score test for person-time data. As before, the contributions to each of the three components of the test statistic (*i.e.*, the number of exposed cases and the expectation and variance for the number of exposed cases) are derived separately for each stratum and then summed over the strata. Conditional on the total numbers of cases M_{1i} in each stratum, the expectation and variance for the number of exposed cases under the null hypothesis, $H_0 : IR = 1$, are:

$$E = E\left(A_{1+}\,\middle|\,IR=1\right) = \sum_i \frac{M_{1i}T_{1i}}{T_{+i}}$$

and

$$V = Var\left(A_{1+}\,\middle|\,IR=1\right) = \sum_i \frac{M_{1i}T_{1i}T_{0i}}{T_{+i}^2},$$

respectively, which yield the Mantel-Haenszel statistic[55]:

$$X_{score} = \frac{A_{1+} - E}{V^{1/2}}.$$

As with the person-count data counterpart, it is valid in sparse data, but it requires large total numbers. As a rough guide, small-study methods are recommended if either E or the quantity

$$\sum_i \frac{M_{1i} \widehat{IR}_{MH} T_{1i}}{\widehat{IR}_{MH} T_{1i} + T_{0i}}$$

is less than 5 or greater than $M_{1+} - 5$.

For the data in Table 18-1, the number of exposed cases, A_{1+}, equals 630, whereas the expected value and variance of A_{1+} under the null hypothesis are seen from Table 18-3 to be $E = 595.2$ and $V = 110.1$. Hence,

$$\chi_{score} = \frac{630 - 595.2}{(110.1)^{1/2}} = 3.30,$$

which corresponds to an upper-tailed P-value of 0.0005.

ANALYSIS OF DATA FROM MATCHED STUDIES

Analysis of matched data involves the same statistical methods as are used for unmatched data. Even though many textbooks present special "matched-data" techniques, these techniques are just special cases of general stratified methods for sparse data. The evenly balanced nature of matched covariates, however, can result in great simplifications of more general formulae, especially when the data are pair-matched. We will illustrate this simplification by showing how the general Mantel-Haenszel formulae introduced above reduce to simple matched-pair analysis formulae.

With modern computing resources, there is little practical need to consider other simplifications (*e.g.*, for matched data with multiple controls). Instead, a general approach to matched data as stratified data may be used. There is, however, one important guideline to follow in such an approach: Each matching category should be treated as a unique stratum, at least in the initial stages of analysis. Exceptions occur only if one can demonstrate that such detailed stratification makes no difference in the study results. For example, suppose that subjects have been matched on sex (two levels) and age in four 5-year categories of age 60 to 64 years, age 65 to 69 years, age 70 to 74 years, and age 75 to 79 years. To account fully for the matched nature of subject selection, it is necessary to stratify on at least the eight composite matching strata formed by each sex-age category combination. In particular, broader age categories are not sufficient to remove the selection bias introduced by matching.

On the other hand, any stratification that is as fine as or finer than the original matching criteria will remove the bias induced by the matching. For example, given enough data, one could use 1-year age strata with 5-year age category matching; this additional stratification will adjust for any residual age confounding within the original 5-year matching strata. One could also include unmatched variables in the stratification process. The limitation of such extensions is that many strata could end up with only a single subject and thus contribute nothing to the estimation process. For this reason, many analysts turn to "matched" modeling methods such as conditional logistic regression, which allow use of regression terms to control residual confounding (the confounding left after stratification on the matching factors). In some situations, it may instead be possible to use the matching factors as regressors in an ordinary model. This use can lead to bias, however, if the factors are continuous and treated as such instead of being categorized to reflect the matching protocol.[31,56]

Sometimes care is needed in determining what constitutes sufficient stratification by the matching factors. It is not always necessary and can be inefficient to retain the original matches made in subject selection.[57] For example, if two cases and their paired controls all have identical values for the matching factors (say, all four subjects have the same age, sex, and neighborhood), then combining these subjects into a single stratum will produce an estimator with lower variance and no less validity than that produced by an analysis in which the two pairs are kept separate. Another advantage of combining matched sets with identical matching values is that it can eliminate "double loss" of subjects. When one member of a pair has missing data, its corresponding match will be ignored by any paired analysis method that requires the missing information. If, however, the matched pair belongs to a larger stratum, the corresponding match can be retained as part of that stratum.

If a continuous variable is matched using caliper intervals rather than fixed categories, some ambiguity can arise in determining proper analysis strata, and a small amount of bias may be unavoidable, regardless of the analysis used.[58] For example, matching "age ±2 years" could yield two case-control pairs: one with case of age 65 years and matched control of age 63 years, and the other with a case of age 63 years and a matched control of age 61 years. Among these four subjects, the first control and the second case are the best age match and should be in the same stratum. Nonetheless, combining all four subjects in the same age 61 to 65 stratum will yield a 4-year age range for the stratum, twice that specified by the 2-year caliper radius. A conservative approach is to form strata no wider than the caliper radius, but this might produce strata with only one subject from a pair. A more accurate result will likely be obtained by using a slightly biased but less variable estimator based on broader categories (such as 4-year or even 5-year categories). In general, however, there is no unambiguously best way to analyze caliper-matched data, because of the inherent bias in such matching.[58] We view this ambiguity as constituting a minor but practical reason for preferring fixed-category matching over caliper matching.

To summarize, validity of the odds ratio estimate in a matched case-control study may require that one stratify on any matching factors related to exposure in at least as much detail as was used for matching. In contrast, control of matching factors is not necessary for validity of point estimates of the risk difference or risk ratio in a cohort study. Nonetheless, stratification by matched risk factors is, in principle, necessary in cohort studies because matching on risk factors affects the *variance* (and hence the confidence limits) of the risk difference and ratio estimators. This matching effect is accounted for by stratification on the matching factors.[20,59]

The remainder of this section illustrates some special formulae that apply when each stratum contains one matched pair of subjects.

Analysis of Matched-Pair Cohort Data

Suppose that stratification of a cohort yields P uniquely matched pairs of exposed and unexposed subjects. Each stratum (pair) can then be one of only four possible types.

1. Both exposed and unexposed get disease, so that $A_{1i} = A_{0i} = 1$, $B_{1i} = B_{0i} = 0$.
2. Exposed get disease but unexposed does not, so that $A_{1i} = B_{0i} = 1$, $A_{0i} = B_{1i} = 0$.
3. Unexposed get disease but exposed does not, so that $A_{1i} = B_{0i} = 0$, $A_{0i} = B_{1i} = 1$.
4. Neither exposed nor unexposed get disease, so that $A_{1i} = A_{0i} = 0$, $B_{1i} = B_{0i} = 1$.

Note that, in every stratum, $N_{1i} = N_{0i} = 1$, so $N_{+i} = N_{1i} + N_{0i} = 2$. We can summarize the four types of strata in a cohort *matched-pair table*, given in a general form in Table 18-7. In this notation, there are T, U, V, and W strata (or pairs) of types 1, 2, 3, and 4, respectively. Recall that the Mantel-Haenszel estimator of a common risk ratio based on person-count cohort data is:

$$\widehat{RR}_{MH} = \frac{\sum_i A_{1i} N_{0i} / N_{+i}}{\sum_i A_{0i} N_{1i} / N_{+i}}$$

TABLE 18-7

General Form for Uniquely Pair-Matched Cohort Data

		Unexposed Pair Member		Exposed Totals
		Disease	No Disease	
Exposed	Disease	T	U	$T + U$
Pair Member	No disease	V	W	$V + W$
	Unexposed totals	$T + V$	$U + W$	P

The T type-1 pairs and U type-2 pairs have $A_{1i} = 1$, and so have $A_{1i} N_{0i}/N_{+i} = \frac{1}{2}$, whereas the V type-3 and W type-4 pairs have $A_{1i} = 0$, and so have $A_{1i} N_{0i}/N_{+i} = 0$. Similarly, the T type-1 and V type-3 pairs have $A_{0i} = 1$, and so have $A_{0i} N_{1i}/N_{+i} = \frac{1}{2}$, whereas the U type-2 and W type-4 pairs have $A_{0i} = 0$, and so have $A_{0i} N_{1i}/N_{+i} = 0$. Hence, the Mantel-Haenszel risk ratio given above simplifies to:

$$\widehat{RR}_{MH} = \frac{(T+U)/2}{(T+V)/2} = \frac{T+U}{T+V}$$

Note that $T + U$ and $T + V$ are just the total (crude) numbers of exposed and unexposed cases. Because there are P pairs, there are exactly P exposed and P unexposed subjects total. Hence, Mantel-Haenszel risk ratio estimate is equal to the crude risk ratio. This equality illustrates how pair matching in a cohort study prevents confounding by the matching factors if no loss to follow-up occurs.

In a manner analogous to that just shown for $\widehat{RR}_{MH}$, the estimate of the variance of $\ln\left(\widehat{RR}_{MH}\right)$ simplifies to:

$$\frac{U+V}{(T+U)(T+V)} \qquad\qquad [18\text{-}7]$$

and is different from the estimate of the variance of the crude estimator:

$$\frac{1}{T+U} + \frac{1}{T+V} - \frac{2}{P} = \frac{2t+U+V}{(T+U)(T+V)} - \frac{2}{P} = \frac{2T}{(T+U)(T+V)} + \frac{U+V}{(T+U)(T+V)} - \frac{2}{P}.$$

This quantity is larger than that in formula 18-7 if the pair outcomes are positively associated (*i.e.*, if $TW > UV$), as is usually the case. In this case, the crude variance estimator is upwardly biased for the matched data, even though the crude point estimator is unbiased.

Although we forgo the details, one can similarly show that the Mantel-Haenszel risk difference for the matched pairs simplifies to the crude risk difference,

$$\frac{T+U}{P} - \frac{T+V}{P} = \frac{U-V}{P}$$

but the (correct) Mantel-Haenszel variance estimate is smaller than the crude variance estimate if $TW > UV$. The Mantel-Haenszel odds ratio reduces to an even simpler form for matched-pair cohort data: It equals U/V, the ratio of discordant pairs. We show later that the same type of simplification occurs for matched-pair case-control data.

A useful fact about the matched-cohort risk-ratio and test statistic is that they do not depend on any matched sets with no disease. This fact implies that one can estimate risk ratios from a population by using only case surveillance (population registry) data, as long as the data are naturally matched and the exposure status of cases and their matches can be ascertained. Examples of such naturally matched sets include twins, siblings, spouses, and vehicle riders. As an illustration, consider the problem of estimating the risk ratio comparing accident fatalities of motorcycle drivers and passengers. The Fatal Accident Reporting System (FARS) of the US National Highway Safety Administration attempts to register all US motor vehicle accidents that report a fatality and obtains basic data on the accidents and persons involved. Evans and Frick[60] reported from these data that among two-rider motorcycle crashes in which both driver and passenger were male and neither wore a helmet, in $T = 226$ both died, in $U = 546$ only the driver died, and in $V = 378$ only the passenger died. Because accidents without a fatality are not reported to the FARS, we do not know W = number of two-rider crashes in which neither died. Nonetheless, we can estimate the death-risk ratio for drivers versus passengers as

$$\widehat{RR}_{MH} = \left(226 + 546\right)/\left(226 + 378\right) = 1.278.$$

The logarithm of this ratio has an estimated standard error of:

$$\left\{\left(546 + 378\right)/\left[\left(226 + 546\right)\left(226 + 378\right)\right]\right\}^{1/2} = 0.0445$$

which yields a Wald-based approximate 95% confidence interval of:

$$\left(\widehat{RR}_{MH,L}, \widehat{RR}_{MH,U}\right) = \exp\left[\ln\left(1.278\right) \pm 1.96 \times 0.0445\right] = \left(1.17, 1.39\right).$$

Thus, in two-rider motorcycle crashes in the United States in which both riders are men and neither is helmeted, there is evidence to suggest that the driver is at moderately higher risk of death than the passenger.

Basic analysis of matched cohort data may proceed by stratifying on the matching factors (and by other factors, if deemed necessary) and employing appropriate stratified analysis methods. We nonetheless caution that one should examine the strata visually and use sparse-data methods (such as Mantel-Haenszel methods) if most within-stratum numerators (A_{1i} and A_{0i}) are small. If the number of exposed cases is small or the number of unexposed cases is small, small-sample ("exact") methods should be used. As a rough guide, "small" may be taken as "under five."

For person-time analyses of follow-up data, the analysis formulae do not simplify as extensively as do the formulae for count data, so we do not present them. Similar to count data, matched person-time data may be analyzed using ordinary stratified-analysis formulae.

Analysis of Matched-Pair Case-Control Data

Suppose that stratification of a case-control data set yields P uniquely matched pairs of case and control subjects. Each stratum (pair) can then be one of only four possible types:

1. Both the case and control are exposed, so that $A_{1i} = B_{1i} = 1$, $A_{0i} = B_{0i} = 0$.
2. The case is exposed, but the control is not, so that $A_{1i} = B_{0i} = 1$, $A_{0i} = B_{1i} = 0$.
3. The control is exposed, but the case is not, so that $A_{1i} = B_{0i} = 0$, $A_{0i} = B_{1i} = 1$.
4. Neither case nor control are exposed, so that $A_{1i} = B_{1i} = 0$, $A_{0i} = B_{0i} = 1$.

Note that, in every stratum, $M_{1i} = M_{0i} = 1$ and $N_{+i} = M_{1i} + M_{0i} = 2$. We can summarize the four types of strata in a case-control matched-pair table, given in general form in Table 18-8. In this notation, there are, respectively, T, U, V, and W strata (pairs) of type 1, 2, 3, and 4 listed above.

Recall that the Mantel-Haenszel estimator of a common odds ratio based on case-control data is:

$$\widehat{OR}_{MH} = \frac{\sum_i A_{1i} B_{0i}/N_{+i}}{\sum_i A_{0i} B_{1i}/N_{+i}}.$$

TABLE 18.8

General Form for Uniquely Pair-Matched Case-Control Data

		Control Pair Member		
		Exposed	Unexposed	Case Totals
Case	Exposed	T	U	$T + U$
Pair Member	Unexposed	V	W	$V + W$
	Control totals	$T + V$	$U + W$	P

The T type-1 and W type-4 pairs have $A_{1i} B_{0i}/N_{+i} = A_{0i} B_{1i}/N_{+i} = 0$ and so contribute nothing to $\widehat{OR}_{MH}$. The U type-2 pairs have $A_{1i}B_{0i}/N_{+i} = 1(1)/2 = \frac{1}{2}$ and $A_{0i} B_{1i}/N_{+i} = 0$, whereas the V type-3 pairs have $A_{1i} B_{0i}/N_{+i} = 0$ and $A_{0i} B_{1i}/N_{+i} = 1(1)/2 = \frac{1}{2}$. Hence, the Mantel-Haenszel odds ratio simplifies to:

$$\widehat{OR}_{MH} = \frac{U(1/2)}{V(1/2)} = \frac{U}{V}.$$

This formula may be recognized as the classical matched-pair odds ratio estimator,[61] which is the ratio of the two types of exposure-discordant pairs. It is also identical to the conditional maximum-likelihood estimator of the common odds ratio across strata (pairs).[11] In a similar fashion, the standard error estimate for $\ln\left(\widehat{OR}_{MH}\right)$ given above simplifies to $(1/U + 1/V)^{1/2}$ for matched-pair data. The latter expression is just the usual estimate of the standard error for $\ln(U/V)$.[11] Finally, using essentially the same derivation as given earlier for matched-pair cohort data, one can show that the Mantel-Haenszel test statistic applied to case-control pairs simplifies to the McNemar statistic $(U - V)/(U + V)^{1/2}$.

The crude counts obtained by ignoring the matching are $A_{1+} = T + U$, $A_{0+} = V + W$, $B_{1+} = T + V$, and $B_{0+} = U + W$. The crude odds ratio is thus:

$$\widehat{OR}_C = \frac{(T + U)(U + W)}{(T + V)(V + W)}.$$

Furthermore, the degree to which the case and control exposures are associated can be measured by the difference in diagonal products $TW - UV$. This quantity is positive if the case and control exposures are positively associated, and negative if these exposures are negatively associated. In general, the crude odds ratio $\widehat{OR}_C$ will be closer to 1.0 than $\widehat{OR}_{MH}$, if the case and control exposures are positively associated, and will be farther from 1.0 than $\widehat{OR}_{MH}$, if the case and control exposures are negatively associated. Typically, we expect matching to make cases and controls more alike on exposure and, thus, to induce a positive association of the case and control exposures. Thus, ordinarily we expect the crude odds ratio to be closer to the null (*i.e.*, 1.0) than the matched odds ratio. Exceptions occur, however.

As an illustration of the above points and formulae, we consider data from a matched-pair study of risk factors for adenomatous polyps of the colon.[62] In this study, both cases and controls had undergone sigmoidoscopy screening, and controls were matched to cases on time of screening (3-month categories), clinic (two clinics), age (50-54 years, 55-59 years, 60-64 years, 65-69 years, 70+ years; 76 years maximum age), and sex. Of major interest is the possible effect of low fruit and vegetable consumption; here, low consumption (exposure) is defined as two or fewer servings per day. There were $U = 45$ pairs in which the case but not the control reported low consumption, and $V = 24$ pairs in which the control but not the case reported low consumption. Thus, the

Mantel-Haenszel odds ratio is $\widehat{OR}_{MH} = 45/24 = 1.875$ while the estimated standard error of the logarithm of $\widehat{OR}_{MH}$, $\widehat{SE}\left[\ln\left(\widehat{OR}_{MH}\right)\right]$, is $(1/45 + 1/24)^{1/2} = 0.253$. These yield a Wald-based 95% confidence interval of:

$$\left(\widehat{OR}_{MH,L}, \widehat{OR}_{MH,U}\right) = exp\left[\ln(1.875) \pm 1.96 \times 0.253\right] = (1.14,\ 3.08).$$

These results can be contrasted to those obtained from the crude data. In $T = 4$ pairs, both the case and control reported low consumption, while in $W = 415$ pairs, neither reported low consumption. The crude counts are thus $A_{1+} = 4 + 45 = 49$, $A_{0+} = 24 + 415 = 439$, $B_{1+} = 4 + 24 = 28$, and $B_{0+} = 415 + 45 = 460$, which yield a crude odds ratio of $\widehat{OR}_C = 1.83$ and a Wald-based 95% confidence interval of $\left(\widehat{OR}_{C,L}, \widehat{OR}_{C,U}\right) = (1.13, 2.97)$. These are very similar to the matched results, indicating that the matching factors were not closely related to exposure (low consumption).

Many authors have noted, with some discomfort, that the matched-pair estimator U/V makes no use of the $T + W$ concordant pairs (which often compose most of the pairs). It is possible to derive odds ratio estimators that make use of the concordant pairs, and which as a result have smaller variance than U/V.[63] The cost of this variance reduction is the introduction of some bias, although the bias is often considered worth the increase in accuracy afforded by the variance reduction. Because the formulae for these estimators are not simple, we do not present them here.

For more complex matched case-control data, an analysis may proceed by stratifying on the matching factors and employing appropriate stratified analysis methods. As always, however, one should examine the strata and use sparse-data methods (such as Mantel-Haenszel or conditional maximum likelihood) if most of the within-stratum case or control counts are small. If the total numbers of exposed and unexposed cases and controls are also small, small-sample (exact) methods should be used.

ESTIMATION OF THE ATTRIBUTABLE FRACTION

Suppose that we study a closed cohort and, in the sense described in Chapter 5, an exposure that is causal. Furthermore, suppose interest lies in estimating the fraction of exposed cases that would not have occurred if exposure had not occurred, AF_e, also known as the attributable fraction among the exposed. Let RR denote the causal risk ratio, that is the proportionate increase in average risk among the exposed that is due to exposure. From Chapter 5, we have the relation:

$$AF_e = (RR - 1)/RR.$$

Now, if stratification has successfully removed all confounding and there is no bias, the SMR (that is the risk ratio standardized to the exposed) will equal RR. Thus, one can obtain an estimate and confidence limits for AF_e from any valid estimate of the SMR, say $\widehat{SMR}$, and corresponding confidence intervals, say $\left(\widehat{SMR}_L,\ \widehat{SMR}_U\right)$, via the formulae:

$$\widehat{AF}_e = \left(\widehat{SMR} - 1\right)/\widehat{SMR}$$
$$\left(\widehat{AF}_{e,L},\ \widehat{AF}_{e,U}\right) = \left[\left(\widehat{SMR}_L - 1\right)/\widehat{SMR}_U, \left(\widehat{SMR}_U - 1\right)/\widehat{SMR}_L\right]$$

Now suppose interest lies in estimating the fraction of all cases (exposed and unexposed) that would not have occurred if exposure had not occurred, AF_p, also known as the population attributable fraction. If no adjustment is needed, we have the simple relation:

$$AF_p = \frac{N_1(R_1 - R_0)}{N_1 R_1 + N_0 R_0} = \frac{p(RR - 1)}{p(RR - 1) + 1}$$

where N_1 and N_0 are the number of exposed and unexposed individuals in the cohort, respectively, and $p = N_1/(N_1 + N_0)$ is the proportion exposed. Thus, as with AF_e, if no adjustment is needed, this relation provides a means to estimating AF_p and constructing a confidence interval given results regarding the SMR.

If adjustment is needed and stratification successfully removes confounding, one can use the following relation:

$$AF_p = p_c AF_e = p_c \frac{SMR - 1}{SMR},$$

where p_c is exposure prevalence among the cases.[64] Another useful decomposition of AF_p is as a weighted average of stratum-specific population attributable fractions AF_{pi}:

$$AF_p = \sum_i p_i AF_{pi},$$

where p_i is the proportion of cases falling in stratum i.[65]

In almost all situations, p_c and the p_i will not be known and must be estimated from the data. If, however, they can be validly estimated from the study data, we can estimate AF_p via:

$$\widehat{AF}_p = \hat{p}_c \frac{\widehat{SMR} - 1}{\widehat{SMR}},$$

where $\hat{p}_c = A_{1+}/M_{1+}$ and $\widehat{SMR}$ is the estimate of the risk ratio standardized to the exposed or via:

$$\widehat{AF}_p = \sum_i \hat{p}_i \widehat{AF}_{pi}$$

where $\hat{p}_i = M_{1i}/M_{1+}$ and

$$AF_{pi} = \frac{A_{1i}}{M_{1i}} \frac{\widehat{RR}_i - 1}{\widehat{RR}_i}.$$

If the risk ratio is homogeneous across strata and the disease is uncommon, we can use:

$$AF_p = \frac{A_{1+}}{M_{1+}} \frac{\widehat{RR} - 1}{\widehat{RR}} \qquad [18\text{-}8]$$

where $\widehat{RR}$ may be a maximum-likelihood or Mantel-Haenszel estimator of a common rate ratio, IR, or a common odds ratio, OR. To construct confidence intervals, it helps to initially consider the standard error of $\hat{H} = \ln\left(1 - \widehat{AF}_p\right)$, which can be estimated by:

$$\widehat{SE}\left(\hat{H}\right) = \frac{\widehat{AF}_p}{\left(1 - \widehat{AF}_p\right)} \left[\frac{\hat{V}}{\left(\widehat{RR} - 1\right)^2} + \frac{2}{A_{1+}\left(\widehat{RR} - 1\right)} + \frac{A_{0+}}{A_{1+}M_{1+}} \right]^{1/2} \qquad [18\text{-}9]$$

where $\hat{V}$ is a variance estimator for $\ln\left(\widehat{RR}\right)$, such as one of those given in Chapter 17, as appropriate.[66] From this, 95% confidence interval limits for $\hat{H}$ formed using Equation 18-9, that is $\left(\hat{H}_L, \hat{H}_U\right) = \hat{H} \pm 1.96 \times SE\left(\hat{H}\right)$, can be back-transformed using the relation $AF_p = 1 - \exp(H)$ to construct limits for $\widehat{AF}_p$. Note, the point and interval estimators of $\widehat{AF}_p$ obtained from Equations 18-8 and 18-9 will be valid in sparse data if the RR and variance estimators used in the formulae are valid in sparse data (e.g., a Mantel-Haenszel or a CML estimator).

To estimate the fraction of coronary deaths in the British Doctors Study (Table 18-1) that could be attributable to smoking, we use the Mantel-Haenszel estimate which is $\widehat{IR}_{MH} = 1.424$ and the corresponding estimate of the variance for $\ln\left(\widehat{IR}_{MH}\right)$ which equals 0.01150. These yield:

$$\widehat{AF}_p = \frac{630}{731} \times \frac{1.424 - 1}{1.424} = 0.255$$

$$\widehat{SE}\left[\ln\left(1 - \widehat{AF}_p\right)\right] = \frac{0.255}{0.745}\left(\frac{0.01150}{0.424^2} + \frac{2}{630(0.424)} + \frac{101}{630(731)}\right)^{1/2} = 0.0916$$

which, in turn, result in a Wald-based approximate 95% confidence interval for $\hat{H} = \ln\left(1 - \widehat{AF}_p\right)$ of $\ln(1 - 0.255) \pm 1.96 \times 0.0916 = (-0.4740, -0.1148)$. Back-transforming yields a Wald-based approximate 95% confidence interval for $\widehat{AF}_p$ of (0.108, 0.377). Using the estimate of the *SMR* instead yields almost the same estimate of AF_p:

$$\widehat{AF}_p = \frac{630}{731} \times \frac{1.43 - 1}{1.43} = 0.259$$

One might be tempted to interpret these estimates as indicating that on the order of 25% fewer coronary deaths would have occurred had these doctors not smoked. Of course, this interpretation assumes that biases are absent. The interpretation also assumes that absence of smoking would not expand the person-years at risk of coronary death by removing other (competing) risks for death, such as lung cancer. This assumption cannot be exactly true, because smoking does affect the rates of many other causes of death, particularly lung cancer.

The preceding example points out that the common public health interpretation of the attributable fraction (as potential caseload reduction) assumes that removing exposure will not affect the size of the population at risk. This assumption is not always correct, and it needs to be scrutinized in any discussion of any estimate of the attributable fraction. For example, to estimate the excess of Down syndrome cases that could be attributable to spermicide exposure in the study in Table 18-5, we might use the Mantel-Haenszel estimate of the odds ratio, $\widehat{OR}_{MH} = 3.78$ as an approximate risk-ratio estimate (because Down syndrome is uncommon), to give:

$$\widehat{AF}_p = \frac{4}{16} \times \frac{3.78 - 1}{3.78} = 0.18$$

This result seems to suggest that on the order of 20% fewer cases would have occurred if no one had used spermicide. Again, this interpretation assumes that bias is absent. Even if the study were perfectly valid, however, this estimate could not be interpreted as the effect of spermicide use on the number of Down syndrome cases; such an interpretation unrealistically assumes that absence of spermicide use would not lead to more pregnancies. In reality, absence of spermicide use would probably lead to more pregnancies, thus expanding the source cohort and increasing the number of cases.

References

1. Greenland S. Absence of confounding does not correspond to collapsibility of the rate ratio or rate difference. *Epidemiology*. 1996;7:498-501.
2. Carriere KC, Roos LL. Comparing standardized rates of events. *Am J Epidemiol*. 1994;140:472-482.
3. Stukel TA, Glynn RJ, Fisher ES, Sharp SM, LU-Yao G, Wennberg JE. Standardized rates of recurrent outcomes. *Stat Med*. 1994;13:1781-1791.
4. Zou G, Donner A. A simple alternative confidence interval for the difference between two proportions. *Control Clin Trials*. 2004;25:3-12.
5. Miettinen OS. Standardization of risk ratios. *Am J Epidemiol*. 1972;96:383-388.
6. Flanders WD, Rhodes PH. Large sample confidence intervals for regression standardized risks, risk ratios, and risk differences. *J Chronic Dis*. 1987;40:697-704.

7. Greenland S. Estimating variances of standardized estimators in case-control studies and sparse data. *J Chronic Dis*. 1986;39:473-477.
8. Greenland S. Estimation of exposure-specific rates from sparse case-control data. *J Chronic Dis*. 1987;40:1087-1094.
9. Greenland S. Reducing mean squared error in the analysis of stratified epidemiologic studies. *Biometrics*. 1991;47:773-775; discussion 776.
10. Greenland S, Maldonado G. The interpretation of multiplicative-model parameters as standardized parameters. *Stat Med*. 1994;13:989-999.
11. Breslow NE, Day NE. *Statistical Methods in Cancer Research. Volume I: The Analysis of Case-Control Data*. Lyon: IARC; 1980.
12. Breslow NE. Odds ratio estimators when the data are sparse. *Biometrika*. 1981;68:73-84.
13. Clayton D, Hills M. *Statistical Models in Epidemiology*, New York, NY: Oxford University Press; 1993.
14. Newman SC. *Biostatistical Methods in Epidemiology*. New York, NY: Wiley; 2001.
15. Jewell N. *Statistics for Epidemiology*. Boca Raton: Chapman and Hall/CRC; 2004.
16. Mantel N, Fleiss JL. Minimum expected cell size requirements for the Mantel-Haenszel one-degree-of-freedom chi-square test and a related rapid procedure. *Am J Epidemiol*. 1980;112:129-134.
17. Greenland S, Schwartzbaum JA, Finkle WD. Problems due to small samples and sparse data in conditional logistic regression analysis. *Am J Epidemiol*. 2000;151:531-539.
18. Greenland S. Multiple-bias modeling for analysis of observational data (with discussion). *J R Stat Soc Ser A*. 2005;168:267-308.
19. Pike MC, Hill AP, Smith PG. Bias and efficiency in logistic analyses of stratified case-control studies. *Int J Epidemiol*. 1980;9:89-95.
20. Greenland S, Robins JM. Estimation of a common effect parameter from sparse follow-up data. *Biometrics*. 1985;41:55-68.
21. Nurminen M. Asymptotic efficiency of general noniterative estimators of common relative risk. *Biometrika*. 1981;68:525-530.
22. Rothman KJ, Boice JD. *Epidemiologic Analysis with a Programmable Calculator*, Newton, MA: Epidemiology Resources; 1982.
23. Walker AM. Small sample properties of some estimators of a common hazard ratio. *Appl Stat*. 1985;34:42-48.
24. Cochran WG. Some methods for strengthening common chi-square tests. *Biometrics*. 1954;10:417-451.
25. Sato T. On the variance estimator for the Mantel-Haenszel risk difference (letter). *Biometrics*. 1989;45:1323-1324.
26. Tarone RE. On summary estimators of relative risk. *J Chronic Dis*. 1981;34:463-468.
27. Mantel N, Haenszel W. Statistical aspects of the analysis of data from retrospective studies of disease. *J Natl Cancer Inst*. 1959;22:719-748.
28. Breslow NE, Liang KY. The variance of the Mantel-Haenszel estimator. *Biometrics*. 1982;38:943-952.
29. Robins JM, Breslow NE, Greenland S. Estimators of the Mantel-Haenszel variance consistent in both sparse-data and large-strata limiting models. *Biometrics*. 1986;42:311-323.
30. Robins J, Greenland S, Breslow NE. A general estimator for the variance of the Mantel-Haenszel odds ratio. *Am J Epidemiol*. 1986;124:719-723.
31. Greenland S . Partial and marginal matching in case-control studies. In: Moolgavkar SH, Prentice RL (eds.) *Modern Statistical Methods in Chronic Disease Epidemiology*. New York, NY: Wiley; 1986.
32. Sato T. Maximum likelihood estimation of the risk ratio in case-cohort studies. *Biometrics*. 1992;48:1215-1221.
33. Sato T. Estimation of a common risk ratio in stratified case-cohort studies. *Stat Med*. 1992;11:1599-1605.
34. Breslow NE, Holubkov R. Maximum likelihood estimation of logistic regression parameters under two-phase, outcome dependent sampling. *J R Stat Soc Ser B*. 1997;59:447-461.
35. Breslow NE, Holubkov R. Weighted likelihood, pseudo-likelihood and maximum likelihood methods for logistic regression analysis of two-stage data. *Stat Med*. 1997;16:103-116.
36. Walker AM. Anamorphic analysis: sampling and estimation for covariate effects when both exposure and disease are known. *Biometrics*. 1982;38:1025-1032.
37. Cain KC, Breslow NE. Logistic regression analysis and efficient design for two-stage studies. *Am J Epidemiol*. 1988;128:1198-1206.
38. Maclure M. The case-crossover design: a method for studying transient effects on the risk of acute events. *Am J Epidemiol*. 1991;133:144-153.
39. Mittleman MA, Maclure M, Robins JM. Control sampling strategies for case-crossover studies: an assessment of relative efficiency. *Am J Epidemiol*. 1995;142:91-98.
40. Greenland S. A unified approach to the analysis of case-distribution (case-only) studies. *Stat Med*. 1999;18;1-15.

41. Lumley T, Levy D. Bias in the case-crossover design: implications for studies of air pollution. *Environmetrics*. 2000;11:689-704.

42. Vines SK, Farrington CP. Within-subject exposure dependency in case-crossover studies. *Stat Med*. 2001;20:3039-3049.

43. Navidi W, Weinhandl E. Risk set sampling for case-crossover designs. *Epidemiology*. 2002;13:100-105.

44. Janes H, Sheppard L, Lumley T. Overlap bias in the case-crossover design, with application to air pollution exposures. *Stat Med*. 2004;24:285-300.

45. Janes H, Sheppard L, Lumley T. Case-crossover analyses of air pollution exposure data: referent selection strategies and their implications for bias. *Epidemiology*. 2005;16:717-726.

46. Zaffanella LE, Savitz DA, Greenland S, Ebi KL. The residential case-specular method to study wire codes, magnetic fields, and disease. *Epidemiology*. 1998;9:16-20.

47. Thomas DC. *Statistical Methods in Genetic Epidemiology*, New York, NY: Oxford University Press; 2004.

48. Breslow NE, Day NE. *Statistical Methods in Cancer Research. Volume II: The Design and Analysis of Cohort Studies*. Lyon: IARC; 1987.

49. Hirji K. *Exact Analysis of Discrete Data*. Boca Raton, Fl: Crc Press/Chapman and Hall; 2006.

50. Corporation C 2006. *Statexact 7*.

51. Greenland S. Tests for interaction in epidemiologic studies: a review and a study of power. *Stat Med*. 1983;2:243-251.

52. Greenland S. Interpretation and estimation of summary ratios under heterogeneity. *Stat Med*. 1982;1:217-227.

53. Gail MH, Simon R. Testing for qualitative interactions between treatment effects and patient subsets. *Biometrics*. 1985;41:361-372.

54. Gart JJ, Tarone RE. The relation between score tests and approximate UMPU tests in exponential models common in biometry. *Biometrics*. 1983;39:781-786.

55. Shore RE, Pasternack BS, Curnen MG. Relating influenza epidemics to childhood leukemia in tumor registries without a defined population base: a critique with suggestions for improved methods. *Am J Epidemiol*. 1976;103:527-535.

56. Greenland S. "Estimating relative risk functions in case-control studies using a nonparametric logistic regression". *Am J Epidemiol*. 1997;146:883-885.

57. Brookmeyer R, Day NE, Moss S. Case-control studies for estimation of the natural history of preclinical disease from screening data. *Stat Med*. 1986;5:127-138.

58. Austin H, Flanders WD, Rothman KJ. Bias arising in case-control studies from selection of controls from overlapping groups. *Int J Epidemiol*. 1989;18:713-716.

59. Weinberg CR. On pooling across strata when frequency matching has been followed in a cohort study. *Biometrics*. 1985;41:117-127.

60. Evans L, Frick MC. Helmet effectiveness of preventing motorcycle driver and passenger fatalities. *Accid Anal Prev*. 1988;20:447-458.

61. Kraus AS. Comparison of a group with a disease and a control group from the same families, in the search for possible etiologic factors. *Am J Public Health Nations Health*. 1960;50:303-311.

62. Witte JS, Longnecker MP, Bird CL, Lee ER, Frankl HD, Haile RW. Relation of vegetable, fruit, and grain consumption to colorectal adenomatous polyps. *Am J Epidemiol*. 1996;144:1015-1025.

63. Kalish LA. Reducing mean squared error in the analysis of pair-matched case-control studies. *Biometrics*. 1990;46:493-499.

64. Miettinen OS. Comment. *J Am Stat Assoc*. 1974;69:380-382.

65. Walter SD. The estimation and interpretation of attributable risk in health research. *Biometrics*. 1976;32:829-849.

66. Greenland S. Variance estimators for attributable fraction estimates consistent in both large strata and sparse data. *Stat Med*. 1987;6:701-708.

CHAPTER 19

Categorical Analysis of Polytomous Exposures and Outcomes

Sebastien Haneuse[*]

Chapters 17 and 18 focused on settings where the primary comparison being performed involved two groups, that is, a binary exposure such as "exposed" or "unexposed." Furthermore, the methods focused on a binary outcome of "diseased" or "not diseased." In this chapter, we introduce extensions of tabular analysis methods to polytomous data—data in which the exposure or outcome has more than two levels. In addition to being useful in their own right, these extensions provide a conceptual bridge between simple tabular methods and more sophisticated regression analysis. They also provide an initial approach to dose-response and trend analyses. Finally, they provide an important means of checking the results of regression analyses, specifically to see if patterns suggested by regressions can be seen in the basic counts that summarize the data.

Much of this chapter is focused on methods for analyzing an exposure with multiple levels and a binary disease outcome. In some settings, the exposure may have been categorized before the analyst receives the data. In other settings, the exposure may be available in an underlying continuous form so that the use of the methods in this chapter requires the analyst to impose his or her own categorization. We therefore begin by reviewing issues in categorization of variables.

CATEGORIZATION OF ORDERED VARIABLES

As discussed in Chapter 17, choosing categories for variables is an important step in data analysis. When the variable is measured on an ordered scale with many levels, one often sees this step disposed

[*]This chapter is based on original material by Sander Greenland.

of by using percentile category boundaries. For example, one commonly sees a variable carved into four categories formed by the quartiles, that is the 25th, 50th, and 75th percentiles, or five categories formed by the quintiles, that is the 20th, 40th, 60th, and 80th percentiles. Such automatic procedures for category formation are suboptimal in most applications and can sometimes be harmful to power, precision, and confounder control.[1-4] Percentile boundaries also make it difficult to compare associations or effects across studies, because those boundaries will correspond to different exposure values in each study.

Most important, percentile categories rarely correspond to subject-matter knowledge. Instead, they blindly lump together disparate subgroups of subjects and may thereby hide important effects. For example, vitamin C levels are high enough in most Western diets that persons with borderline or deficient intakes will constitute less than 10% of a typical study group. As a result, these people will compose fewer than half of the subjects in the lowest quarter of the distribution of vitamin C intake. If only this deficient minority suffers an elevated disease risk, this fact will be obscured by the quartile analysis. The elevated risk of the 10% minority is averaged with the normal risk of the 15% majority in the lowest quarter and then compared with the normal risk in the three higher-intake quarters. As a result, only a limited elevation of risk in the lowest quarter will arise, which itself might be difficult to detect in a categorical analysis. As another example, in many occupational and environmental studies, only a small percentage of subjects have a biologically important amount of exposure. Here again, the use of quartiles or quintiles to categorize the variable submerges these subjects among a larger mass of barely exposed (and thus unaffected) subjects, thereby reducing power and possibly inducing a biased impression of dose-response.[2,5] Finally, mixing persons of different risks in broad categories is also problematic when the categorized variable is a strong confounder. In this situation, broad categories of the confounder can result in stratum-specific estimates with substantial residual confounding.

Perhaps the most common alternative to percentiles is equally spaced boundaries. For example, vitamin C intake might be categorized in 10- or 20-mg increments of daily average intake. Such boundaries often make more subject-matter sense than percentiles, because they allow those with very low or very high intake to be put in separate categories and because the categories conform with familiar units of dose. Nonetheless, as with percentile boundaries, care is needed when using equally spaced boundaries to avoid submerging high-risk groups and in being aware of creating categories comprising small groups that may, in turn, yield poor power and precision.[2]

Ideally, categories should make sense based on external information. This guideline can be especially important and easiest to accomplish in categorization of confounders, because the prior information that led to their identification can also be used to create categories. To illustrate, consider maternal age as a potential confounder in perinatal studies. The relation of maternal age to risk can be poorly captured by either percentile or equally spaced categories, because most maternal-age effects tend to be concentrated at one or both extremes. For example, the risk of neonatal death is highest when the mother is under 18 or over 40 years of age, whereas the risk of Down syndrome is highest when the mother is over 40 years of age, with little change in the risk of either outcome during the peak reproductive ages of 20 to 35 years. Yet in typical US or European populations, quartile or quintile boundaries would fall within this homogeneous risk range, as would standard equally spaced maternal age category boundaries of, say, 20, 25, 30, and 35 years. Quartile categories, quintile categories, and these equally spaced categories would all fail to separate the heterogeneous mix of risks at the extremes of maternal age and would instead focus too much attention on the intermediate age range, with its small differences in risk.

Ideal categories would be such that any important differences in risk will exist between them but not within them. Unfortunately, this scheme may result in some categories (especially end categories) with too few subjects to obtain a reasonably precise estimate of the outcome measure in that category. One way to cope with this problem is to broaden the categories gradually until there are adequate numbers in each one, while retaining meaningful boundaries. In doing so, however, it is important to avoid defining categories based on the size of the estimates obtained from the categorizations; if category choice is based on the resulting estimates, the trend estimates and standard errors from the final categorization may be biased. For example, if we collapse together adjacent categories to maximize the appearance of a linear trend, the apparent trend in the final estimates will be biased toward a linear pattern, away from any true departures from linearity.

Open-ended categories (*e.g.*, "20+ years exposure") are particularly hazardous because they may encompass a broad range of exposure or confounder effects. We thus recommend that one makes sure the single boundary of an open-ended category is not too far from the most extreme value in the category. For example, if having more than 10 additional years of exposure could have a large effect on risk, we would try to avoid using the "20+ years exposure" category if the largest exposure value in the data is >30 years. Another drawback of open-ended categories is the practical difficulty of assigning a point to the category against which its response might be plotted.

We emphasize again that all the above problems of exposure categorization also apply to confounder categorization.[1,2,6-8] In particular, the use of automated categorization methods such as percentile boundaries can easily lead to overly broad categories in which much residual confounding remains.

BASIC TABULAR ANALYSIS

Table 19-1 displays the notation we use for stratified person-time data with $J + 1$ exposure levels and with strata indexed by i. In this table, the ellipses represent all the remaining exposure levels X_j, counts A_{ji}, and person-times T_{ji} between level X_j and level X_1. (If there are only three levels, $J = 2$ and there is no level between X_j and X_1.) We will always take the rightmost (X_0) exposure column to be the reference level of exposure, against which the J nonreference levels will be compared. Usually, X_0 is an "unexposed" or "low exposure" level when the levels X_0 to X_j correspond to increasing levels of exposure to a possibly harmful agent. Sometimes, however, X_0 is simply a commonly found level, as may be the case when X_0 to X_j are the range of an unordered variable such as religion or race. For preventive exposures, the highest exposure level is sometimes chosen for X_0.

The notation in Table 19-1 may be modified to represent person-count data by adding a row for noncase counts, $B_{ji}, \ldots B_{1i}, B_{0i}$ and then changing the person-times T_{ji} to column totals $N_{ji} = A_{ji} + B_{ji}$, as in Table 19-2. It may also be modified so that known expected values E_{ji} for the case-counts A_{ji} replace the person-times T_{ji}. The notations used in Chapter 18 are just the special cases of these notations in which $X_1 =$ "exposed" and $X_0 =$ "unexposed."

If the exposure variable is unordered or its ordering is ignored, analyses of polytomous data may proceed using computations identical in form to those given in Chapters 17 and 18. To start, we may use any and all of the binary-exposure techniques given earlier to compare any pair of exposure levels. As an example, Table 19-3 presents crude data from a study of fruit and vegetable intake in relation to colon polyps, divided into three index categories of equal width and a broad reference category. Also presented are the odds ratios and 95% confidence limits obtained from comparing each category below the highest intake level to the highest intake level and each category to the next higher category. It appears that the odds ratios decline as intake increases, with the sharpest decline occurring among the lowest intakes. Stratification of the data on the matching factors and computation of Mantel-Haenszel statistics yield virtually the same results.

The number of possible comparisons grows rapidly as the number of exposure levels increases: the number of exposure-level pairs is $(J + 1)J/2$, which equals 3 when there are three exposure levels ($J = 2$) but rises to 6 when there are four exposure levels ($J = 3$, as in Table 19-3) and 10 when there are five exposure levels ($J = 4$). Pairwise analysis of a polytomous exposure thus raises an issue of multiple comparisons, which was discussed in general terms in Chapter 16. This issue can be addressed by using either a trend test or an unordered simultaneous test statistic. Both approaches provide P-values for the joint null hypothesis that there is no association between exposure and disease across all levels of exposure.

TABLE 19-1

Notation for Stratified Person-Time Data With a Polytomous Exposure

| | Exposure Level | | | |
	X_j	...	X_1	X_0	
Cases	A_{ji}	...	A_{1i}	A_{0i}	M_{1i}
Person-time	T_{ji}	...	T_{1i}	T_{0i}	T_{+i}

TABLE 19-2

Notation for Stratified Count Data With a Polytomous Exposure

	Exposure Level				
	X_J	...	X_1	X_0	
Cases	A_{Ji}	...	A_{1i}	A_{0i}	M_{1i}
Noncases	B_{Ji}	...	B_{1i}	B_{0i}	M_{0i}
Totals	N_{Ji}	...	N_{1i}	N_{0i}	N_{+i}

Several equivalent simultaneous test statistics can be used for unstratified data. Arguably, the best-known statistic is the *Pearson χ^2 statistic*, which for unstratified person-time data has the form:

$$\chi_P^2 = \sum_j \frac{\left(A_j - E_j\right)^2}{E_j}$$

[19-1]

where the sum is from $j = 0$ to J, and $E_j = M_1 T_j / T_+$ is the expected value for A_j under the joint null hypothesis that there is no exposure-disease association. Note, the notation here is as in Table 19-1 but without the stratum subscript i. If there are no biases and the joint null hypothesis holds, χ_P^2

TABLE 19-3

Data on Fruit and Vegetable Intake (Average Number of Servings per Day) in Relation to Colon Polyps, Odds Ratios, 95% Confidence Limits, and Two-Sided *P*-Values

	Servings of Fruits and Vegetables per Day				
	≤2	>2, ≤4	>4, ≤6	>6	Totals
Cases	49	125	136	178	488
Controls	28	111	140	209	488
Total	77	236	276	387	976
Comparison to Highest (>6) Category					
Odds ratio	2.05	1.32	1.14	1.0 (Referent)	
Lower limit	1.24	0.96	0.84		
Upper limit	3.41	1.83	1.55		
P-value	0.005	0.092	0.40		
Incremental Comparisons to Next Higher Category					
Odds ratio	1.55	1.16	1.14		
Lower limit	0.91	0.82	0.84		
Upper limit	2.64	1.64	1.55		
P-value	0.10	0.41	0.40		

From Witte JS, Longnecker MP, Bird CL, et al. Relation of vegetable, fruit, and grain consumption to colorectal adenomatous polyps. *Am J Epidemiol.* 1996;144:1015-1025.

has approximately a χ^2 distribution with J degrees of freedom. For pure count data with exposure totals $N_j = A_j + B_j$ (where B_j is the observed number of noncases) and grand total $N_+ = \sum_j N_j$, the Pearson χ^2 statistic equals

$$\chi_P^2 = \sum_j \frac{\left(A_j - E_j\right)^2}{V_j}$$

[19-2]

where $E_j = M_1 N_j / N_+$ and $V_j = E_j(N_j - E_j)/N_j$ are the mean and variance of A_j under the joint null hypothesis. Equation 19-2 is equivalent to the more familiar form

$$\chi_P^2 = \sum_j \left[\frac{\left(A_j - E_j\right)^2}{E_j} + \frac{\left(B_j - F_j\right)^2}{F_j} \right]$$

[19-3]

where $F_j = M_0 N_j / N_+$ is the mean of B_j under the joint null hypothesis. For the data in Table 19-3, Equation 19-3 yields

$$\chi_P^2 = \frac{[49 - 488(77)/976]^2}{488(77)/976} + \cdots + \frac{[209 - 488(387)/976]^2}{488(387)/976} = 9.1$$

which has $J = 3$ degrees of freedom and $P = .03$. Note that this simultaneous P-value is smaller than all but one of the pairwise P-values in Table 19-3.

We use the Pearson statistic here because it is easy to compute. For unstratified data, the quantity $\chi_P^2 \times (N-1)/N$ is identical to the generalized Mantel-Haenszel statistic for testing the joint null hypothesis.[9,10] When it is extended to stratified data, the Pearson statistic requires that all stratum expected counts be "large" (usually taken to be at least five), whereas the generalized Mantel-Haenszel statistic can remain valid even if all the stratum counts are small (although the crude counts must be "large"). When stratification is needed, joint statistics can be more easily computed using software, however. We discuss unordered statistics further in the section on simultaneous analysis below.

Note that the pairwise P-values considered singly or together do *not* provide an appropriate P-value for the null hypothesis that there is no association of exposure and disease. As will be illustrated in the final section, it is possible to have all the pairwise P-values be much larger than the simultaneous P-value. Conversely, it is possible to have one or more of the pairwise P-values be much smaller than the simultaneous P-value. Thus, to evaluate a hypothesis that involves more than two exposure levels, one should compute an overall test statistic.

For stratified data, the ordinary Mantel-Haenszel estimates can be inefficient when exposure is polytomous because they do not make use of the fact that the product of the common ratios comparing level i with level j and level j with level k must equal the common ratio comparing level i with level k (the "common ratio" may be a risk, rate, or odds ratio). They can, however, be modified to use this information and so be made more efficient.[11] Efficient estimates can also be obtained from regression analyses; see Chapter 20.

DOSE-RESPONSE AND TREND ANALYSIS

If the exposure levels have a natural ordering, a serious source of inefficiency in the pairwise and unordered analyses is that the statistics take no account of this ordering. Dose-response and trend analysis concerns the use of such ordering information.

Table 19-4 presents the data used in Table 19-3 in more detail, using the finest categories with integer boundaries that yield at least four cases and four controls per category. These data will be used in the examples that follow. Note, in those examples, subjects often had fractional values of average servings per day since servings per day were calculated from questions asking the consumption frequencies of individual fruits and vegetables, such as apples and broccoli.

TABLE 19-4

Data on Fruit and Vegetable Intake and Colon Polyps, Including Mean Servings per Day, Mean Log Servings, and Case-Control Ratios in Each Category

Upper Category Boundary	Mean Servings	Mean Log Servings	No. of Cases	No. of Controls	Case-Control Ratio
1	0.68	−0.52	13	4	3.25
2	1.58	0.45	36	24	1.50
3	2.57	0.94	55	44	1.25
4	3.55	1.26	70	67	1.04
5	4.52	1.51	77	74	1.04
6	5.51	1.71	59	66	0.89
7	6.50	1.87	54	48	1.12
8	7.58	2.02	33	41	0.80
9	8.51	2.14	33	31	1.06
10	9.43	2.24	24	22	1.04
11	10.48	2.35	10	26	0.38
12	11.49	2.44	6	12	0.50
14	12.83	2.55	9	12	0.75
18	15.73	2.75	4	11	0.36
27	20.91	3.03	5	6	0.83
Totals	–	–	488	488	–

Graphing a Trend

Perhaps the simplest example of trend analyses is a plot of estimates against the exposure levels. Such occurrence plots are straightforward. For example, given population data, one may plot estimates of the average risks $R_0, R_1, \ldots, R_J$ or the incidence rates $I_0, I_1, \ldots, I_J$ against the exposure levels $X_0, X_1, \ldots, X_J$. For unmatched case-control data, the case-control ratios $A_0/B_0, A_1/B_1, \ldots, A_J/B_J$ may substitute for the risk or rate estimates.[12,13] If important confounding appears to be present, one may plot them separately for different confounder strata or plot a single set of estimates that have been appropriately standardized (Chapter 18).

The pattern exhibited by plotted estimates is called a trend. A trend is *monotonic* or *monotone* if every change in the height of the plotted points is always in the same direction. A monotone trend never reverses direction, but it may have flat segments. A trend is *strictly monotone* if it is either always increasing or always decreasing. Such a trend never reverses and has no flat segments. One commonly sees phrases such as "the data exhibited a dose-response relation" used to indicate that a plot of estimates versus exposure level was monotone. The term "dose-response," however, can refer to any pattern whatsoever, and here we use it in this general sense. That is, *dose-response* will here mean the pattern relating the outcome or effect measure to exposure, whatever it may be. The term "trend" is often used as a synonym for "dose-response," though it is more general still, as in "the trend in risk was upward but fluctuations occurred in later years." In particular, a trend may be observed over time, age, weight, or other variables for which the concept of "dose" is meaningless.

Figure 19-1 presents the case-control ratios A_j/B_j computed from Table 19-4, plotted against the category means, and connected by straight line segments. The inner dotted lines are approximate 80% confidence limits, and the fainter outer dotted lines are 99% limits. These limits are computed using the formula:

$$exp\left[ln\left(A_j/B_j \right) \pm Z_\gamma \times \widehat{SE} \right],$$

where Z_γ is the 100γ percentile of the standard normal distribution ($Z_{0.8} = 1.282$, $Z_{0.99} = 2.576$) and $\widehat{SE}$ is the estimated standard error obtained as the square root of

$$\hat{V} = \widehat{Var}\left[\ln\left(A_j/B_j\right)\right] = 1/A_j + 1/B_j.$$

The figure gives an impression of a steeper trend in the ratios at low consumption levels (less than three servings per day) than at higher levels. If no important bias or error is present, the trends in Figure 19-1 should reflect those in the underlying source-population rates.

A common approach to graphing risk or rate ratios uses a single reference level; for example, with X_0 as the reference level in rate ratios, one would plot $I_1/I_0, \ldots, I_j/I_0$ or their logarithms against the nonreference exposure levels $X_1, \ldots, X_j$. With this approach, the resulting curve is proportional to the curve obtained by plotting the rates, but it appears to be less precisely estimated.[12]

Plotting Confidence Limits

Although it is helpful to plot confidence limits along with point estimates, care must be taken to prevent the graph from visually overemphasizing imprecise points. The conventional approach of placing error bars around the points produces such overemphasis. Thus, we recommend instead that the upper and lower limits receive their own graph line, as in Figure 19-1, rather than connecting the limits to their point estimate by error bars. The resulting graphs of the lower and upper limits together form a *confidence band* for the curve being estimated.

Two serious problems arise in plotting estimated associations or effects that are derived using a shared reference level. One is that the widths of the confidence intervals at nonreference levels depend on the size of the counts in the chosen reference category; the other is that no confidence interval is generated for the curve at the reference category. If the counts in the reference category are smaller than those in other categories, the confidence limits around the estimates at the nonreference levels will be far apart and will thus make the shape of the dose-response curve appear much more imprecisely estimated than it actually is. Graphs of confidence limits for rates, risks, and case-control ratios do not suffer from these problems but are sometimes not an option (as in

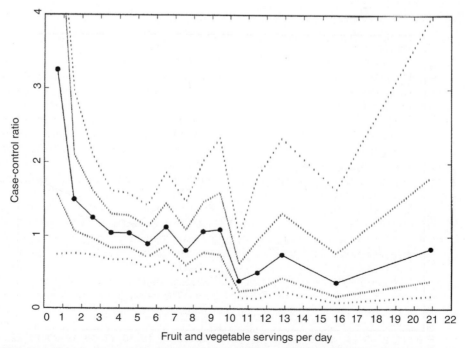

FIGURE 19-1 Plot of case-control ratios and 80% and 99% confidence limits from data in Table 19-4, using the arithmetic scale.

matched case-control studies). A more general solution, known as the *floating absolute risk*,[12,13] circumvents the problems but is designed for regression analyses and so will not be described here. To address the problems in tabular analyses of cohort or unmatched case-control data, we again recommend plotting rates, risks, case-control ratios, or their transforms, rather than rate ratios, risk ratios, or odds ratios. For matched case-control analyses, we suggest taking as the reference category the one that yields the narrowest confidence intervals, although a narrower confidence band can be obtained using the floating absolute risk method.

The limits obtained using the methods presented earlier in this book are known as pointwise limits. If no bias is present, a 90% pointwise confidence band has at least a 90% chance (over study repetitions) of containing the true rate, risk, or effect at any single observed exposure level. Nonetheless, there is a much lower chance that a conventional pointwise confidence band contains the entire true dose-response curve. That is, there will be *less* than a 90% chance that the true curve runs inside the pointwise band at every point along the graph. Construction of confidence bands that have a 90% chance of containing the true curve everywhere is best accomplished using regression methods; see Hastie et al.[14]

As a final caution, note that neither the pointwise limits nor the corresponding graphical confidence band provide an appropriate test of the overall null hypothesis of no exposure-outcome association. For example, it is possible (and not unusual) for all the 99% confidence limits for the exposure-specific associations to contain the null value, and yet the trend statistic may yield a *P*-value of less than .01 for the association between exposure and disease.

Vertical Scaling

Rates, risks, and ratio measures are often plotted on a semilogarithmic graph, in which the vertical scale is logarithmic. Semilogarithmic plotting is equivalent to plotting the log rates, log risks, or log ratios against exposure and is useful as a preliminary step to log-linear (exponential) and logistic regression. Such regressions assume linear models for the log rates, log risks, or log odds, and departures from the models are easiest to detect visually when using a logarithmic vertical scale. Figure 19-2 is a plot of the case-control ratios and confidence limits from Figure 19-1, using a logarithmic vertical scale. In this scale, the difference in trend at high and low doses appears less than in Figure 19-1.

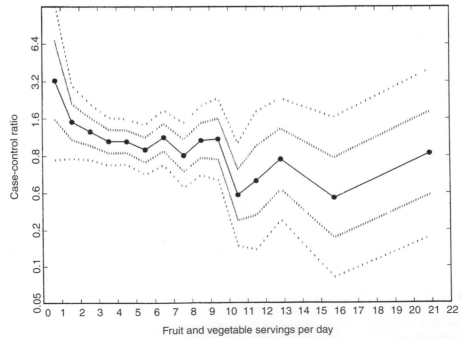

FIGURE 19-2 Plot of case-control ratios and 80% and 99% confidence limits from data in Table 19-4, using the logarithmic vertical scale.

There are various arguments for examining semilogarithmic plots,[15] but there can be subject-matter reasons for also examining plots with other scales for the vertical or horizontal axis.[16,17] In particular, the untransformed scale (that is, direct plotting of the measures) is important to examine when one wishes to convey information about absolute effects and health impacts.[18] For example, suppose the average risks at levels X_0, X_1, and X_2 of a potentially modifiable exposure follow the pattern $R_0 = 0.001$, $R_1 = 0.010$, and $R_2 = 0.050$. A plot of the risk ratios $R_0/R_0 = 1$, $R_1/R_0 = 10$, and $R_2/R_0 = 50$ against X_0, X_1, and X_2 will indicate that the proportionate risk reduction produced by moving from level X_2 to level X_1 is $(50 - 10)/50 = 0.80$. This reduction is over 80% of the maximum potential reduction of $(50 - 1)/50 = 0.98$ produced by moving from X_2 to X_0. In other words, reducing exposure from X_2 to X_1 may yield most of the total potential risk reduction. A plot of the log risk ratios at X_0, X_1, and X_2 (which are 0, 2.3, and 3.9) will not make clear the preceding point and may convey the mistaken impression that moving from X_2 to X_1 does not achieve most of the possible benefit from exposure modification.

Another approach to graphical analysis is to plot attributable and prevented fractions (relative to a common reference level) against exposure levels. Attributable fractions are plotted above the horizontal axis for exposure levels with risks higher than the reference level risk, and preventable fractions are plotted below the horizontal axis for levels with risks lower than the reference level.[17]

Incremental (Slope) Plots

The slope (direction) of a curve may be assessed directly by plotting incremental (adjacent) differences, such as $I_1 - I_0, I_2 - I_1, \ldots, I_J - I_{J-1}$, or incremental ratios, such as $I_1/I_0, I_2/I_1, \ldots, I_J/I_{J-1}$, against the category boundaries.[19] Incremental differences will be greater than zero and incremental ratios will be greater than one wherever the trend is upward; the differences will be less than zero and the ratios less than one wherever the trend is downward. Figure 19-3 displays the incremental odds ratios and their 80% and 99% confidence limits from the data in Table 19-4 plotted on a logarithmic vertical scale against the category boundaries. This graph supplements Figure 19-2 by showing that the data are fairly consistent with an unchanging slope in the logarithmic trend across consumption, which corresponds to an exponential trend on the original scale.

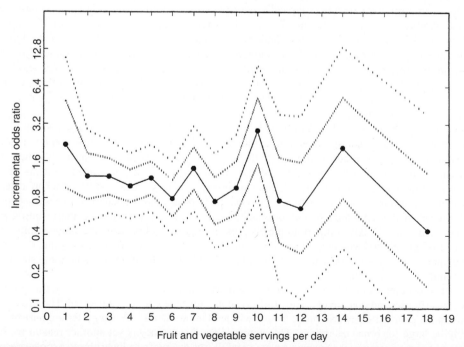

FIGURE 19-3 Plot of incremental odds ratios and 80% and 99% confidence limits from data in Table 19-4, using the logarithmic vertical scale.

Because incremental ratios are based on division by a shifting reference quantity, their pattern does not follow that of underlying rates or risks, and so they are not well suited for evaluating health impacts. They need logarithmic transformation to avoid distorted impressions produced by the shifting reference level. Suppose, for example, that average risks at X_0, X_1, and X_2 are $R_0 = 0.02$, $R_1 = 0.01$, and $R_2 = 0.02$, such as might occur if exposure was a nutrient for which both deficiency and excess are harmful. On the untransformed scale, the change in risk from X_0 to X_1 is exactly opposite the change in risk from X_1 to X_2. As a result, in going from X_0 to X_2, the exposure effects cancel out to yield identical risks at X_0 and X_2. Yet the incremental risk ratios are $R_1/R_0 = \frac{1}{2}$ and $R_2/R_1 = 2$, so that the second exposure increment will appear visually to have a larger effect than the first, if the ratios are plotted on the arithmetic scale. In contrast, on a logarithmic scale R_1/R_0 will be the same distance below zero as R_2/R_1 is above zero. This equidistance shows that the effects of the two increments cancel exactly.

Horizontal Scaling and Category Scores

One must also choose the horizontal (exposure) scale for a plot. When each exposure level X_0, $X_1,\ldots, X_J$ represents a unique exposure value, an obvious choice is to use this unique value. For example, if X_j corresponds to "j previous pregnancies," one may simply use the number of previous pregnancies as the horizontal axis. If, however, the exposure levels represent internally heterogeneous categories, such as five-year groupings of exposure time, a numeric value or score must be assigned to each category to form the horizontal scale.

Category midpoints are perhaps the simplest choice that will often yield reasonable scores. For example, this scheme would assign scores of $s_0 = 0$, $s_1 = 2.5$, $s_2 = 7$, and $s_3 = 12$ years for exposure categories of 0, 1 to 4, 5 to 9, and 10 to 14 years. Midpoints do not, however, provide scores for open-ended categories such as 15+ years.

Two slightly more involved choices that do provide scores for open-ended categories are category means and medians. Category means have an advantage that they will on average produce a straight line if there is no bias and the true dose-response curve is a line. If, however, there are categories within which exposure has large nonlinear effects (such as an exponential trend and a fivefold risk increase from the lower to the upper end of a category), no simple scoring method will provide an undistorted dose-response curve.[2] Thus, as indicated above avoidance of broad categories is advisable when strong effects may be present within such categories.

One seemingly natural and yet typically poor method of scoring categories is to assign them ordinal numbers (that is, $s_j = j$, so that 0, 1,..., J is assigned to category X_0, $X_1,\ldots, X_J$). If any category is internally heterogeneous, it will only be accidental that such ordinal scores yield a biologically meaningful horizontal axis. If the categories span unequal intervals, as in Tables 19-3 and 19-4, ordinal scores can easily yield quantitatively meaningless dose-response curves and harm the power of trend tests.[1-3] These shortcomings arise because the distance between these ordinal scores is 1, and this distance will not, in general, correspond to any difference in average exposure or effect across the categories.

In choosing the horizontal scale, it is possible to transform the exposure in any fashion that is of scientific interest. Suppose, for example, one has a carcinogenesis model that predicts that the logarithm of lung cancer rates will increase linearly with the logarithm of exposure. To check the prediction, one may plot the logarithms of the rates against the category-specific means of log exposure. Equivalently, one may plot the rates against the geometric means of the exposure categories, using logarithmic scales for both axes. (Recall that the geometric mean exposure is the antilog of the mean of the logarithms of the individual exposures.) Under the theory, the resulting plot should, on average, follow a line if no bias is present. Figure 19-4 presents the same results as in Figure 19-2 but plotted with logarithmic horizontal and vertical scales. With this scaling, the entire curve appears reasonably consistent with a straight line (especially if one considers the statistical uncertainty in the results).

In the preceding example, a different (and nonlinear) curve would result if one used the arithmetic means (the second column of Table 19-4) as scores for the exposure categories. The difference between the geometric and arithmetic means will tend to be small if the categories are narrow, but it may be large for broad categories. This potential for discrepancy is yet another reason we recommend keeping categories as narrow as practical. When examining a logarithmic exposure scale,

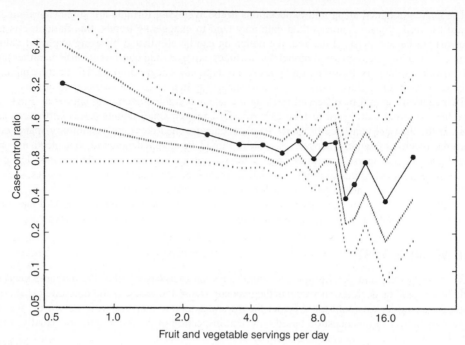

FIGURE 19-4 Plot of case-control ratios and 80% and 99% confidence limits from data in Table 19-4, using the logarithmic horizontal and vertical scales.

geometric means will provide a more meaningful analysis than will arithmetic means because the logarithm of the geometric mean is the average of the logarithms of the potentially unique individual exposure measurements, whereas the logarithm of the arithmetic mean is not.

Smoothing the Graph

Small counts may produce graphs with highly implausible fluctuations. A common approach to this problem is to add ½ to each table cell. A superior approach is to average the observed counts with expected counts (Chapter 12 of Bishop et al. and Greenland[20,21]). A simple way to do so is as follows. Suppose there are $J + 1$ exposure levels and I strata, for a total of $K = I(J + 1)$ case cells (numerators). If there is no association between the exposure *or* the stratification variables and the outcome, the expected value for A_{ji} is $E_{ji} = (M_{1+}/T_{++}) T_{ji}$ for person-time data, which is just the overall crude rate times the person-time at exposure j, stratum i. For count data, this expected value is $E_{ji} = (M_{1+}/N_{++})N_{ji}$. The smoothed case count that replaces A_{ji} in graphing rates or proportions or case-control ratios is then a weighted average of the observed cases and null expected number of cases. One such average is

$$S_{ji} = \left[M_{1+}A_{ji} + (K/2)E_{ji} \right] / (M_{1+} + K/2)$$

in which the observed counts A_{ji} are weighted by the number of cases M_{1+}, and the null expected number of cases E_{ji} are weighted by half the number of case cells K.[20] The smoothed case count S_{ji} yields a smoothed rate S_{ji}/T_{ji}, smoothed proportion S_{ji}/N_{ji}, or smoothed case-control ratio $S_{ji}/(N_{ji} - S_{ji})$. The numbers in Table 19-4 are so large that this smoothing approach produces a barely perceptible difference in the graphs in Figures 19-1 to 19-4.

There are other simple averaging schemes, each of which can greatly improve accuracy of rate or risk estimates when the observed counts A_{ji} are small. More complex schemes can do even better.[21] All operate as in the preceding equation by putting more weight on the observed (i.e., A_{ji}) value as the study size grows and by putting more weight on the expected value (i.e., E_{ji}) as the cases are spread over more cells.

The curves obtained using null expectations in the averaging formula are somewhat flattened toward the null. Because unsmoothed data may tend to exaggerate trends, this flattening is not necessarily a bad property. If desired, the flattening can be eliminated by using expected values derived from a logistic regression model that includes exposure and confounder effects rather than null expected values. If, however, one goes so far as to use a regression model for the graphical analysis, one can instead use model extensions such as splines to generate smoothed graphs.[14]

Two cautions should be observed in using the above weighted-averaging approach. First, the smoothed counts are designed to take care of only sporadic small counts (especially zeros and ones). If the data are consistently sparse (such as pair-matched data), only summary sparse-data measures (such as Mantel-Haenszel estimates) should be graphed. Second, one need not and should not compute sparse-data summaries or trend statistics from the smoothed counts. The purpose of the smoothed counts is only to stabilize estimates that depend directly on cell sizes, such as stratum-specific and standardized rates, proportions, and case-control ratios.

Finally, if the exposure measurement is continuous (or nearly so), one may instead use more sophisticated smoothing techniques. One such method, kernel smoothing, is discussed below.

THE MANTEL TEST

In examining tables and trend graphs, a natural question to ask is whether the outcome measure tends to increase or decrease in value as the exposure score increases. If the outcome measure is a rate, for example, we could ask whether the true rates tend to increase with the scores. We can suggest an answer to this question based on visual inspection of the graph, but one usually wants some formal statistical assessment as well.

The standard approach to statistical assessment of trend is to perform a regression analysis of the variation in the outcome measure with the scores. Such methods are discussed in Chapters 20 and 21. The basic qualitative question—"Does the outcome measure tend to go up or down with the exposure scores?"—can, however, be addressed by a relatively simple and popular trend test developed by Mantel.[22] Unfortunately, its simplicity and popularity have led to extensive misinterpretation of the P-value derived from the test.[19] Therefore, before we present the statistic, we explain its meaning.

Consider two hypotheses about the true outcome measures. Under the null hypothesis, these measures are not associated with the exposure scores. Under the linear hypothesis, the true measures will fall along a line when plotted against the scores. (The hypothesis is sometimes said to be log-linear if the outcome measures are logarithms of more basic measures such as rates or rate ratios.) The null hypothesis is a special case of the linear hypothesis, the one in which the line is horizontal (*i.e.*, the slope of the line is zero). The Mantel trend P-value is often misinterpreted as a P-value for the linear hypothesis; it is not, however. Rather, it is a P-value for testing the null hypothesis. If no bias is present, it provides a valid test of that hypothesis, in that the P-value will tend toward small values *only* if the null hypothesis is false; that is, for *any* alternative, including those that are linear and those that are nonlinear.

In addition to validity, we would like a statistic to have the highest power possible, so that if the null hypothesis is false, the P-value will tend toward small values. The Mantel test will be powerful when the linear hypothesis holds for the rate, risk, log rate, or log odds. That is, if any of these outcome measures has a linear relation to the scores, the Mantel test will have good power relative to the best power achievable from the study. If, however, the relation of the outcomes to the scores is nonlinear to the point of being nonmonotonic, the Mantel test may have poor power relative to the best achievable. In some extreme situations involving U-shaped relations between outcome measures and scores, the Mantel test may have little chance of detecting even a strong association.

The basic cautions in using the Mantel test may be summarized as follows: as always, a large P-value means only that the test did not detect an association; it does *not* mean that the null hypothesis is true or probably true, nor does it mean that further analyses will not reveal some violation of the null. A small P-value means only that some association was detected by the test; it does *not* mean that the association of the outcome with exposure is linear or even that it is monotone. The test is related to the linear hypothesis only in that it is much more capable of detecting linear and log-linear associations than nonmonotone associations.

With these cautions in mind, we now describe the test. The Mantel trend statistic is a type of score statistic, and it is a direct generalization of the Mantel-Haenszel statistic for binary exposures. It has the form

$$\chi_{trend} = \frac{S - E}{V^{1/2}},$$

where S is the sum of the case scores when every person is assigned the score in his or her category, and E and V are the expected value and variance of S under the null hypothesis. S and E may be computed from $S = \sum_i \sum_j A_{ji} s_j$ and $E = \sum_i M_{1i} E_i$, where s_j is the score assigned to category j and E_i is the expected case score in stratum i under the null hypothesis. For person-count data, we have $E_i = \sum_j N_{ji} s_j / N_{+i}$, while $E_i = \sum_j T_{ji} s_j / T_{+i}$ for person-time data. Furthermore, for person-count data, we have

$$V = \sum_i \left(\frac{M_{1i} M_{0i}}{N_{+i} - 1} \right) \times \left(\frac{\sum_j N_{ji} s_j^2}{N_{+i}} - E_i^2 \right)$$

while for person time data,

$$V = \sum_i E_i M_{1i} \times \left(\frac{\sum_j T_{ji} s_j^2}{T_{+i}} - E_i^2 \right).$$

Note, if there are only two exposure categories ($J = 1$), χ_{trend} simplifies to the usual Mantel-Haenszel statistic described in Chapter 18.

If no bias is present and the null hypothesis is correct, χ_{trend} will have a standard normal distribution (that is, a normal distribution with mean 0 and variance 1). Thus, its observed value can be found in a standard normal table to obtain a P-value for the null hypothesis. Special care is needed in interpreting the sign of χ_{trend} and the P-values based on it, however. A negative value for χ_{trend} may only indicate a trend that is predominantly but not consistently decreasing; similarly, a positive value may only indicate a trend that is predominantly but not consistently increasing. We emphasize again that a small P-value from this statistic means only that an association was detected, *not* that this association is linear or even monotone.

The data in Table 19-4 have only one stratum. As such, using the arithmetic category means as the scores, the formulas simplify to

$$S = \sum_j A_j s_j = 13 \times 0.68 + \ldots + 5 \times 20.91 = 2{,}694.3$$

$$E = M_1 \times \sum_j N_j s_j / N_+ = 488 \times (17 \times 0.68 + \ldots + 11 \times 20.91) = 2{,}870.8$$

and

$$V = \left(\frac{M_1 M_0}{N_+ - 1} \right) \times \left(\frac{\sum_j N_{ji} s_j^2}{N_+} - \frac{E^2}{M_1^2} \right) = \frac{488^2}{975} \left[17(0.68)^2 / 976 + \cdots + 11(20.91)^2 / 976 - 5.8828^2 \right] = 2814.6$$

From these, we have $\chi_{trend} = (2{,}694.3 - 5.8828)/2{,}814.6^{1/2} = -3.33$, which has a two-sided P-value of 0.0009. If we use the mean log servings as the scores, we instead get $\chi_{trend} = -3.69$ and $P = 0.0002$. This larger χ_{trend} and smaller P reflect the fact that the log case-control ratios appear to follow a line more closely when plotted against log servings (Figure 19-4) than when plotted against servings (Figure 19-2).

The Mantel statistic is well suited for sparse stratifications in that it remains valid even if all the counts A_{ji} are only zeros or ones, and even if there is never more than two subjects per stratum. Thus, it may be applied directly to matched data. It is, however, a large-sample statistic in that it requires (among other things) at least two of the exposure-specific case totals A_{j+} be large and (for pure count data) at least two of the exposure-specific noncase totals B_{j+} be large. When there is doubt about the adequacy of sample size for the test, one may instead use a stratified permutation (exact) test.[23]

One positive consequence of their sparse-data validity is that neither the Mantel test nor its permutation counterparts require that one collapse subjects into heterogeneous exposure categories. In particular, the Mantel statistic can be applied directly to continuous exposure data, in which each subject may have a unique exposure value. By avoiding degradation of exposure into broad categories, the power of the test can be improved.[1,3] This improvement is reflected in the preceding example, in that χ_{trend} obtained from the broad categories in Table 19-3 using mean log servings is -2.95, two-sided $P = 0.003$, whereas the χ_{trend} obtained using the individual data in Table 19-4 on log servings is -3.77, two-sided $P = 0.0002$. To compute χ_{trend} from subject-specific data, note that the formula for S, E, and V can use "categories" that contain only a single person. For example, in the data in Table 19-4, there was one person (a case) who reported eating only one serving every other week, which is 1/14 serving per day. Using subject-specific data, this person is the sole member of the first ($j = 1$) serving category, which has $A_1 = 1$, $B_1 = 0$, $N_1 = 1$, and $s_1 = \ln(1/14)$. This category contributes to the sums in S, E, and V, the amounts $A_1 s_1 = \ln(1/14)$, $M_1 N_1 s_1/N_+ = 488[\ln(1/14)]/976$, and $N_1 s_1^2/N_+ = \ln(1/14)^2/976$. By applying the above formulas to each case and control separately and summing the results over all subjects, we obtain a χ_{trend} statistic of -3.77, which yields a smaller P-value than any of the categorical (grouped) analyses.

The Mantel statistic takes on an exceptionally simple and well-known form in matched-pair case-control studies. For such studies, $M_{1i} = M_{0i} = 1$ and $N_i = 2$ in all strata. Let s_{1i} and s_{0i} be the case and control scores or exposures in pair (stratum) i. We then have $S = \sum_i s_{1i}$ as the number of exposed cases, $E_i = (s_{1i} + s_{0i})/2$ and

$$V_i = (s_{1i}^2 + s_{0i}^2)/2 - (s_{1i} + s_{0i})^2/2^2 = (s_{1i} - s_{0i})^2/4.$$

From these, we have

$$S - E = \sum_i s_{1i} - \sum_i (s_{1i} + s_{0i})/2 = \sum_i (s_{1i} - s_{0i})/2 = \sum_i d_i/2$$

and

$$V^{1/2} = \frac{1}{2}\left(\sum_i d_i^2\right)^{1/2}$$

where $d_i = s_{1i} - s_{0i}$ is the case-control exposure difference. Thus

$$\chi_{trend} = \sum_i d_i \Big/ \left(\sum_i d_i^2\right)^{1/2},$$

which may be recognized as the classical t-statistic for testing pairwise differences.[24] When exposure is dichotomous, χ_{trend} simplifies further, to the McNemar matched-pairs statistic (Chapter 18).

SPECIAL HANDLING OF THE ZERO LEVEL

When exposure is a nonnegative physical or temporal quantity (such as grams, years, or meters), some authors recommend routine deletion of the zero level (unexposed) before computation of trend estimates or statistics. Caution is needed in doing so, however. In particular, as we elaborate below, a number of context-specific factors must be evaluated to develop a rationale for retaining or deleting the unexposed.[25]

One valid rationale for deleting the unexposed arises if there is good evidence that such subjects differ to an important extent from exposed subjects on uncontrolled confounders or selection factors. This hypothesis is plausible when considering, for example, alcohol use: abstainers may differ in many health-related ways from drinkers. If such differences are present, the estimated outcome measure among the unexposed may be biased to a different extent from the estimates from other categories. This differential bias can distort the shape of the dose-response curve and bias the entire sequence of estimates. Suppose, for example, that j = years exposed, and the corresponding true risks R_j fall on a straight line with a slope of 0.010/y, with R_0 = 0.010, R_1 = 0.020, R_2 = 0.030, and R_3 = 0.040. The sequence of risks relative to the unexposed risk will then also be linear: R_1/R_0 = 2, R_2/R_0 = 3, and R_3/R_0 = 4. Suppose next that the net bias in the estimated risks is 0% (none) among the unexposed, but is −30% among the four exposed levels. The expected estimates for the R_j will then be 0.010, 0.014, 0.021, and 0.028. The resulting risk curve will no longer be a straight line (which has a constant slope throughout); instead, the slope will increase from 0.014 − 0.010 = 0.004 per year to 0.021 − 0.014 = 0.007 per year after the first year, whereas the resulting risk ratios will be 1.4, 2.1, and 2.8, all downward biased.

On the other hand, if the unexposed group is not subject to bias different from the exposed, there is no sound reason to discard them from the analysis. In such situations, deleting the unexposed will simply harm the power and precision of the study, severely so if many or most subjects are unexposed. In real data analyses, one may be unsure of the best approach. If so, it is not difficult to perform analyses both with and without the unexposed group to see if the results depend on its inclusion. If such dependence is found, this fact should be reported as part of the results.

Another problem that arises in handling the zero exposure level is that one cannot take the logarithm of zero. Thus, if one retains the zero exposed in a dose-response analysis, one cannot use the log transform of exposure, $\ln(x)$, nor can one plot exposure on a logarithmic scale. A common solution to this problem is to add a small positive number c to the exposure before taking the logarithm; the resulting transform is then $\ln(c + x)$. For example, one could use $\ln(1 + x)$, in which case subjects with zero exposure have a value of $\ln(1 + 0) = \ln(1) = 0$ on the new scale. This solution has a drawback of being arbitrary, as the transform $\ln(1 + x)$ depends entirely on the units used to measure exposure. For example, if exposure is measured in servings per day, persons who eat 0, 1, and 5 servings per day will have $\ln(1 + x)$ equal to $\ln(1) = 0$, $\ln(2) = 0.7$, and $\ln(6) = 1.8$, so that the first two people are closer together than the second two. If we instead use servings per week, the same people will have $\ln(1 + x)$ equal to 0, $\ln(1 + 7) = 2.1$, and $\ln[1 + 7(5)] = 3.6$, so that the second two people will be closer together than the first two. Likewise, use of a different added number, such as $\ln(0.1 + x)$ instead of $\ln(1 + x)$, can make a large difference in the results. Unfortunately, there is no general solution for this arbitrariness except to be aware that $\ln(c + x)$ represents a broad variety of transforms, depending on both c and the units of exposure measurement. The smaller the value of c, the more closely the transform produces a logarithmic shape, which is extremely steep near $x = 0$ and which levels off rapidly as x increases; as c is increased, the transform moves gradually toward a linear shape.

MOVING AVERAGES FOR EXPOSURES

Categorical analysis of trends involves numerous decisions including the number of categories, the category boundaries, and the category scores. A simpler alternative, with potentially better statistical properties, is to plot a *moving average* or *running mean* of the outcome variable across exposure levels. This approach may be viewed as a smoothing technique suitable for exposures measured on a fine quantitative scale. It involves moving a window (interval) across the range of exposure; one computes a rate, risk, or relative-risk estimate within the window each time one moves the window. The width of the window may be fixed, or it may be varied as the window is moved; often this variation is done to keep the same number of subjects in each window. The window radius is half its width and so is also known as its "half-width". The main choice to be made is that of this radius. Once the radius is selected, one plots the average outcome for each window against the exposure value at the center of the window. The number and spacing of window moves depend on how much detail one wants in the final graph. For example, in plotting rates against pack-years of smoking, one could have the window center move from 0 to 20 in increments of 0.5 pack-years, with a radius of 4 pack-years.

To improve statistical performance, it is customary to employ weighted averaging within a window, such that any subject at the center of the window is given maximum weight, with weight smoothly declining to zero for subjects at the ends of the window. There are a number of standard weighting functions in use, all of which tend to yield similar-looking curves in typical epidemiologic data. These weight functions are also known as *kernels;* hence, the weighted averaging process is often called *kernel smoothing,* and algorithms for carrying out the process are called *kernel smoothers.*[14]

To describe the weighted-averaging process, let x be a given exposure value and let h be the radius of the window centered at x. Let $w_u(x)$ denote the weight to give to a person whose exposure level is u when estimating the average outcome at exposure level x. The weight (kernel) function we will use is:

$$w_u(x) = \begin{cases} 1-(u-x)^2/h^2 & \text{when}\,|x-u|<h \\ 0 & \text{otherwise} \end{cases}.$$

This function reaches a maximum of 1 when $u = x$, drops toward 0 as u moves away from x, and is 0 when u is more than h units from x (for then u is outside the window centered at x). For example, consider a window centered at $x = 9$ pack-years with radius $h = 4$. The weight given a person with 9 pack-years is $w_9(9) = 1 - (9-9)^2/4^2 = 1$, whereas the weights given persons with 7, 11, 5, and 13 pack-years are

$$w_7(9) = 1 - (7-9)^2/4^2 = 0.75 = 1 - (11-9)^2/4^2 = w_{11}(9)$$

and

$$w_5(9) = 1 - (5-9)^2/4^2 = 0 = 1 - (13-9)^2/4^2 = w_{13}(9)$$

Thus, persons whose exposure level is near x are given more weight for estimating the average outcome at x than persons whose exposure level is further from x. Persons whose exposure level is outside the window centered at x are given zero weight.

When averaging rates or proportions, the statistical properties of the smoothed estimate may be further improved by multiplying the kernel weight, $w_u(x)$, by the denominator (person-time or number of persons) observed at u. When this is done, the formula for the moving weighted-average rate at x becomes

$$\hat{I}_x = \frac{\sum_u T_u w_u(x) A_u / T_u}{\sum_u T_u w_u(x)} = \frac{\sum_u w_u(x) A_u}{\sum_u w_u(x) T_u} = \frac{\left.\sum_u w_u(x) A_u \middle/ \sum_u w_u(x)\right.}{\left.\sum_u w_u(x) T_u \middle/ \sum_u w_u(x)\right.} = \frac{\overline{A}(x)}{\overline{T}(x)}$$

where A_u is the number of cases and T_u is the amount of person-time observed at exposure level u. Note that A_u/T_u is the rate observed at exposure level u. The rate estimate $\hat{I}_x$ is just the ratio of two weighted averages with weights $w_u(x)$: the weighted average number of cases observed, $\overline{A}(x)$, and the weighted average amount of person-time observed, $\overline{T}(x)$. To estimate the average risk at x, we would instead use the number of persons observed at u, N_u, in place of the person-time T_u in the preceding formula.

For case-control data, we could plot the moving weighted-average case-control ratio by using control counts B_u in place of T_u. To adjust for confounders, the smoothed rate or risk estimates or case-control ratios may be computed within strata (using the same window weights in each stratum), and then standardized (averaged) across strata, to obtain moving standardized averages.

Weighted averaging can be applied directly to uncategorized (*i.e.,* continuous) data and so does *not* require any choice of category boundaries or category scores. It is much simpler to illustrate for categorical data, however, and so we construct an example from the data in Table 19-4. To do so, we must consider the choice of the exposure scale on which we wish to construct the weights $w_u(x)$. This choice is a different issue from the choice of plotting scale considered earlier, because once we construct the moving averages, we can plot them on any axis scales we wish.

The kernel weights $w_u(x)$ depend on the distance from u to x, and so their relative magnitude as u varies will depend strongly on whether and how one transforms exposure before computing the weights. For example, one could measure distances between different numbers of servings per day on an arithmetic (untransformed) scale, in which case u and x represent servings per day. A common alternative is to measure distances on a geometric (log-transformed) scale, in which case u and x represent the logarithms of servings per day. The moving weighted averages described here tend to work better when the outcome being averaged (such as a rate or risk) varies linearly across the exposure scale used to construct the weights. Comparing Figures 19-2 and 19-4 shows that a log transform of servings per day yields a more linear plot than does an untransformed scale, and so we use weights based on log servings for our illustration.

The radius h based on log exposure has a simple interpretation on the original (untransformed) scale. If x represents a log exposure level, then only persons whose log exposure level u is between $x - h$ and $x + h$ will have nonzero weight for the average computed at x. Taking antilogs, we see that only persons whose exposure level e^u is between $e^{x-h} = e^x e^{-h}$ and $e^{x+h} = e^x e^h$ will have nonzero weight in the average computed at the exposure level e^x. For example, if we use a radius of $h = \ln(2)$ to construct the weights at 8 servings per day, only persons whose daily number of servings is between $\exp[\ln(8) - \ln(2)] = 4$ and $\exp[\ln(8) + \ln(2)] = 16$ servings will have nonzero weight in the average case-control ratio (Figures 19-5 and 19-6).

As one example, we compute the average case-control ratio for the third category in Table 19-4, using a radius on the log-servings scale of $h = \ln(2) = 0.69$. Only the logarithmic means of categories 2, 3, 4, and 5 are within a distance of 0.69 from 0.94, the logarithmic mean of category 3, so only the case-control ratios of categories 2, 3, 4, and 5 will have nonzero weights. The weights for these categories are

$$w_{0.45}(0.94) = 1 - (0.45 - 0.94)^2 / 0.69^2 = 0.50$$

$$w_{0.94}(0.94) = 1 - (0.94 - 0.94)^2 / 0.69^2 = 1.00$$

$$w_{1.26}(0.94) = 1 - (1.26 - 0.94)^2 / 0.69^2 = 0.78$$

$$w_{1.51}(0.94) = 1 - (1.51 - 0.94)^2 / 0.69^2 = 0.32$$

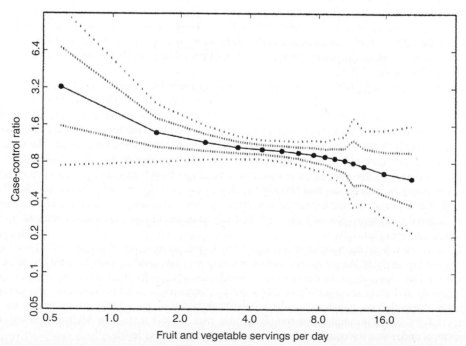

FIGURE 19-5 Plot of running weighted-average (kernel-smoothed) case-control ratios from data in Table 19-4, using the logarithmic horizontal and vertical scales and logarithmic weight (kernel) function.

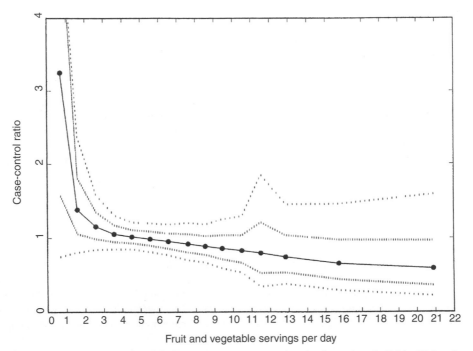

FIGURE 19-6 Plot of running weighted-average case-control ratios from data in Table 19-4, using the arithmetic scale and logarithmic weight function.

The weighted average case-control ratio for $e^{0.94} = 2.56$ servings per day is thus

$$\frac{\overline{A}(0.94)}{\overline{B}(0.94)} = \frac{0.50(36) + 1.00(55) + 0.78(70) + 0.32(77)}{0.50(24) + 1.00(44) + 0.78(67) + 0.32(74)} = \frac{152.2}{131.9} = 1.15$$

We repeat this averaging process for each category in Table 19–4 and obtain 15 smoothed case-control ratios. The solid line in Figure 19–5 provides a log-log plot of these ratios, with dotted lines for the 80% and 99% confidence bands. Because of their complexity, we omit the variance formulas used to obtain the bands; for a discussion of confidence bands for smoothed curves, see Hastie and Tibshirani, 1990.[26]

Comparing this curve with the unsmoothed curve in Figure 19–4, we see that the averaging has provided a much more stable and smooth curve. The smoothed curve is also much more in accord with what we would expect from a true dose-response curve, or even one that is biased in some simple fashion. As the final step in our graphical analysis, we replot the curve in Figure 19–5 using the original (arithmetic) scales for the coordinate axes. Figure 19–6 shows the result: The slightly nonlinear log-log curve in Figure 19–5 becomes a profoundly nonlinear curve in the original scale. Figure 19–6 suggests that most of the apparent risk reduction from fruit and vegetable consumption occurs in going from less than one serving per day to two servings per day, above which only a slight (but consistent) decline in risk occurs. Although the initial large reduction is also apparent in the original categorical plot in Figure 19–1, the gradual decline is more clearly imaged by the smoothed curve in Figure 19–6.

We have used both the transformed (Figure 19–5) and untransformed (Figure 19–6) scales in our smoothing analysis. As mentioned earlier, moving averages tend to work best (in the sense of having the least bias) when the curve being smoothed is not too far from linear; in our example, this property led us to use logarithmic exposure and outcome scales for computing the moving averages. Nevertheless, transforming the results back to the original scale can be important for interpretation; in our example, this transformation makes clear that, even after smoothing, the association under study is concentrated largely at the lowest intake levels.

VARIABLE-SPAN SMOOTHERS

Instead of being constant, the window width $2h$ can be allowed to vary with x so that there are either a fixed number of subjects or (equivalently) a fixed percentage of subjects in each window. For example, the width may be chosen so each window has as close to 100 subjects as possible. (It may not be possible to have exactly 100 subjects in some windows, because there may be subjects with identical exposure values that have to be all in or all out of any window.) The width may instead be chosen so that each window has as close to 50% of all subjects as possible. These types of windows are called (asymmetric) *nearest-neighbor* windows. The proportion of subjects in each window is called the *span* of the window.

In a person-time rate analysis or in an analysis in which the number of cases is far less than the number of noncases, the window widths can be chosen to include a fixed percentage of cases instead of subjects. There are many sophisticated methods for choosing window widths, but the basic nearest-neighbor approaches just described are adequate for exploratory analyses. The larger the span is, the smoother the curve that will be generated. As such, using different spans can provide a feel for the stability of patterns observed in the graphs.

CATEGORICAL ESTIMATES AS MOVING AVERAGES

The curves obtained from moving weighted averages tend to be biased toward flatness, especially when wide windows are used or the curve is highly nonlinear in the scales used for averaging. The latter problem is one of the reasons we used the log scale rather than the original scale when smoothing the curve in the example. Nonetheless, moving averages are generally less biased than the curves obtained using fixed categories of width that are less than the window width of the moving weighted average. The curves obtained by plotting rates or risks from fixed categories are special cases of moving averages in which only a few (usually four to six) nonoverlapping windows are used. Curves from fixed categories correspond to using a weight function $w_u(x)$ that equals 1 for all exposure levels u in the category of x and equals 0 for all u outside the category. In other words, the fixed-category curves in Figures 19–1 through 19–4 may be viewed as just very crude versions of moving-average graphs.

MORE GENERAL SMOOTHERS

One way to avoid flattening of the smoothed curve is to use a running-weighted regression curve (such as *a running weighted line*) rather than a running weighted average. Moving averages and running curves are examples of *scatterplot smoothers*.[14,26] Such techniques can be extended to include covariate adjustment and other refinements. Software that produces and graphs the results from such smoothers is becoming more widely available. We strongly recommend use of smoothers whenever one must study trends or dose-response with a continuous exposure variable, and a substantial number of subjects are spread across the range of exposure. The smoothed curves produced by these techniques can help alert one to violations of assumptions that underlie common regression models, can make more efficient use of the data than categorical methods, and can be used as presentation graphics.

BASIC ANALYSIS OF MULTIPLE OUTCOMES

So far, this chapter has focused on polytomous exposures. Here we turn our attention to polytomous outcomes, which are outcomes that classify individuals beyond the simply dichotomy of "diseased/nondiseased" or "case/control." Such data arise when disease is subclassified by subtype, or competing causes of death are studied, or multiple case or control groups are selected in a case-control study. For example, studies of cancer usually subdivide cases by cancer site; a study of cancer at a given site may subdivide cases by stage at diagnosis or by histology; and in hospital-based case-control studies, controls may be subdivided according to diagnosis.

The simplest approach to multiple-outcome analysis is to perform repeated dichotomous-outcome analyses, one for each disease rate or risk in a cohort study, or one for each case-control group combination in a case-control study. Such repeated analyses are rarely sufficient, however;

for example, in case-control studies with multiple control groups, one should also conduct a comparison of the control groups. It can also be important to examine simultaneous estimates of all effects of interest,[27] for which polytomous logistic regression provides a statistical efficient approach (see Chapter 20).

When the outcome is polytomous, we recommend that one begin with tabular analyses, cross-classifying all outcomes (including the noncases or denominators) against the exposure variable. Table 19–5 presents results on the association of male genital implants with seven distinct cancers diagnosed a year or more following the implant.[28] The estimates in the table were adjusted using 5-year age categories and 1-year categories for year of diagnosis. The first panel of the table compares the five different diagnoses chosen as control diseases, using the largest group (colon polyps) as referent. The differences observed here were judged small enough to warrant combination of the controls into one group for the main analysis in the second panel of the table. This analysis suggests an association of the implants with liver cancer and possibly bone and connective-tissue cancer as well.

As with an analysis of a polytomous exposure, analysis of multiple diseases should include examination of a simultaneous statistic that tests for all exposure-disease associations. For unstratified data, one can use the Pearson χ^2 statistic, which when applied to the numbers in the second panel of Table 19–5 has a value of 10.23 with seven degrees of freedom (the number of cancers). This statistic yields $P = 0.18$ for the joint hypothesis of no exposure–cancer association, indicating that the spread of estimates and P-values seen in the table is fairly consistent with purely random variation. This fact would not be apparent from examining only the pairwise comparisons in the table. We further discuss simultaneous analysis of multiple outcome data in the next section.

SIMULTANEOUS STATISTICS FOR TABULAR DATA

Earlier we mentioned the multiple-comparisons problem inherent in separate pairwise comparisons of multiple exposure levels. This problem is ordinarily addressed by presenting a *simultaneous* or *joint* analysis of the exposure levels. In the remainder of this chapter, we describe the principles of simultaneous analysis in more detail.

To understand better the distinction between separate and joint analyses of multiple exposure levels, consider the following $J(J + 1)/2$ questions regarding an exposure with $J + 1$ levels (one question for each pair i, j of exposure levels):

Question ij: Do exposure levels X_i and X_j have different rates of disease?

For an exposure with three levels (*i.e.* $J = 2$), this represents $2(3)/2 = 3$ different questions. Each of these questions could be addressed by conducting a Mantel-Haenszel comparison of the corresponding pair of exposure levels. We would then get three different Mantel-Haenszel statistics,

TABLE 19-5

General Data Layout for Simultaneous Analysis of Three Diseases in a Person-Time Follow-Up Study

	Exposure Level			Total
	X_J	...	X_0	
Disease		...		
D_1	A_{1J}	...	A_{10}	M_1
D_2	A_{2J}	...	A_{20}	M_2
D_3	A_{3J}	...	A_{30}	M_3
All diseases D	A_J	...	A_0	M
Person-time	T_J	...	T_0	T

χ_{MH10}, χ_{MH20}, and χ_{MH21}, which compare exposure levels X_1 to X_0, X_2 to X_0, and X_2 to X_1. In the absence of biases, χ_{MHij} would have a standard normal distribution under the single null hypothesis:

H_{0ij}: Exposure levels X_i and X_j have the same disease rate, regardless of the rates at other levels. Thus, in Table 19–3, the first P-value of 0.005 refers to the hypothesis that the ≤2 category has the same polyp rate as the >6 category, regardless of the rate in any other exposure category.

Contrast the above set of questions and hypotheses, which consider only two exposures at a time, with the following question that considers all exposure levels simultaneously:

Joint Question: Are there *any* differences among the rates of disease at different exposure levels? This question is a compound of all the separate (pairwise) questions, in that it is equivalent to asking whether there is a difference in the rates between *any* pair of exposure levels. To address this joint question statistically, we need to use a test statistic (such as the Pearson statistic χ_P^2 or the Mantel trend statistic χ_{trend}) that specifically tests the joint null hypothesis:

H_{Joint}: There is no difference among the disease rates at different exposure levels. This hypothesis asserts that the answer to the joint question is "no."

We may extend the Pearson statistic to test joint hypotheses other than the joint null. To do so, we must be able to generate expected values under non–null hypotheses. For example, if exposure has three levels indexed by $j = 0, 1, 2$, we must be able to generate expected values under the hypothesis that the rate ratios IR_1 and IR_2 comparing level 1 and 2 to level 0 are 2 and 3 (H_{Joint}: $IR_1 = 2$, $IR_2 = 3$), as well as under other hypotheses. Consider the person-time data in Table 19–1. Under the hypothesis that the true rate ratios for $X_1, \ldots, X_J$ versus X_0 are $IR_1, \ldots, IR_J$, the expectation of A_j is

$$E_j = \frac{IR_j T_j}{\sum_k IR_k T_k}.$$

[19-4]

The summation index k in the denominator ranges from 0 to J; IR_0 (the rate ratio for X_0 vs. X_0) is equal to 1 by definition. To obtain a test statistic for the hypothesis that the true rate ratios are $IR_1, \ldots, IR_J$, we need to only substitute these expected values into the Pearson χ^2 formula (Equations 19-1 or 19-2). If there is no bias and the hypothesis is correct, the resulting χ_P^2 will have approximately a χ^2 distribution with J degrees of freedom. Again, the accuracy of the approximation depends on the size of the expected values E_j.

Although the nonnull Pearson statistic can be extended to stratified data, this extension requires the expected numbers to be large in all strata, and so methods based on regression models are preferable (Chapters 20 and 21).

Joint Confidence Regions

Rarely is a particular nonnull hypothesis of special interest. The Pearson statistic based on nonnull expected values (Equation 19-4) can, however, be used to find *joint* (or simultaneous) *confidence regions*. Such a region is the generalization of a confidence interval to encompass several measures at once. To understand the concept, suppose that exposure has three levels, X_0, X_1, and X_2 and that we are interested in the log rate ratios $\ln(IR_1)$ and $\ln(IR_2)$ comparing levels X_1 and X_2 to X_0. Figure 19-7 shows an elliptical region in the plane of possible values for $\ln(IR_2)$ and $\ln(IR_1)$. Such a region is called a *C% confidence region* for $\ln(IR_1)$ and $\ln(IR_2)$ if it is constructed by a method that produces regions containing the pair of true values for $\ln(IR_1)$, $\ln(IR_2)$ with at least $C\%$ frequency.

Suppose we have an approximate statistic for testing that the pair of true values equals a particular pair of numbers, such as the simultaneous Pearson statistic X_P^2 described earlier. Then we can construct an approximate $C\%$ confidence region for the pair of true values by taking it to be the set of all points that have a P-value greater than $1 - C/100$. For example, to get an approximate 90% confidence region for IR_1, IR_2 in the preceding examples, we could take the region to be the set of all points that have $P \geq .10$ by the Pearson χ^2 test. We could also obtain a 90% confidence region for $\ln(IR_1)$, $\ln(IR_2)$ just by plotting these points for IR_1, IR_2, using logarithmic axes.

The notion of joint confidence region extends to any number of measures. For example, in studying a four-level exposure with three rate ratios, IR_1, IR_2, and IR_3, we could use the Pearson statistic to obtain a three-dimensional confidence region. Given large enough numbers, the corresponding region for $\ln(IR_1)$, $\ln(IR_2)$, and $\ln(IR_3)$ will resemble an ellipsoid.

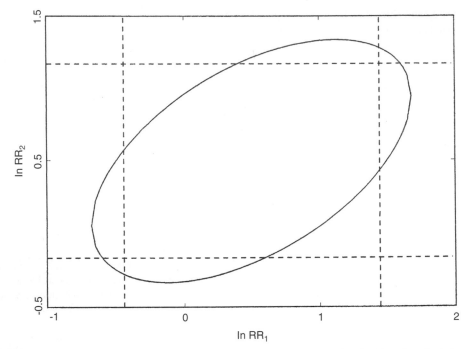

FIGURE 19-7 Graphical comparison of single 95% confidence intervals (dashed lines) and a joint 95% confidence region (ellipse).

Simultaneous Analysis of Multiple Outcomes

Table 19-5 illustrates a general data layout for simultaneous analysis of three diseases in a person-time follow-up study. There are several parameters that can be studied with these data, including:

1. the association of the combined-disease outcome D ("all diseases") with exposure,
2. the association of each disease D_h ($h = 1, 2, 3$) with exposure, and
3. the differences among the separate exposure-disease associations.

For example, we could have D = colon cancer with D_1 = ascending, D_2 = transverse, and D_3 = descending colon cancer. The associations of exposure with the combined site D and each of the separate sites D_1, D_2, and D_3 could be examined one at a time, using any of the methods described earlier for analyzing a single-disease outcome.

We also have the option of analyzing the separate sites simultaneously. To understand the distinction between separate and joint analyses, consider the following questions (one each for $h = 1, 2, 3$):

Question h: Is exposure associated with disease D_h?

For the colon cancer example, this represents three different questions, one for each of the ascending ($h = 1$), transverse ($h = 2$), and descending ($h = 3$) sites. Each of these questions could be examined separately by repeatedly applying the unordered Pearson statistic or the Mantel trend statistic described earlier in this chapter, each time using a different row for the number of cases but keeping the same denominators T_j. The unordered analyses would yield three Pearson statistics $\chi^2_{P1}, \chi^2_{P2}, \chi^2_{P3}$, one for each disease site D_h, and we might also obtain three corresponding trend statistics χ_{T1}, χ_{T2}, and χ_{T3}. In the absence of biases, the statistic χ^2_{Ph} would have approximately a χ^2 distribution with J degrees of freedom if the following null hypothesis (a "no" answer to Question h) was true:

H$_{0h}$: Exposure is unassociated with disease D_h, regardless of the exposure association with any other disease site.

Similarly, in the absence of biases, the statistic χ_{Th} would have approximately a standard normal distribution if H$_{0h}$ were true.

Contrast the three questions that consider each disease site one at a time with the following question that considers all sites simultaneously:

Joint Question: Is exposure associated with *any* of the sites D_1, D_2, or D_3?

Logically, the answer to this question is "no" if and only if the answer is "no" to all of the three preceding questions. That is, the joint null hypothesis:

$$H_{\text{Joint}}: \text{Exposure is not associated with any site}$$

is equivalent to stating that H_{0h} is true for every site D_h. A test statistic for H_{Joint} that does not require or make use of any ordering of exposure is the joint Pearson statistic:

$$\chi^2_{P+} = \sum_h E_j \left(A_{hj} - E_{hj} \right)^2 \big/ E_{hj}$$

where $E_{hj} = M_h T_j / T_+$ is the expectation of A_{hj} under the joint null hypothesis H_{Joint}. With I diseases, this statistic has approximately a χ^2 distribution with IJ degrees of freedom if there is no bias and H_{Joint} is true. Note that $\chi^2_{P+} = \sum_h \chi^2_{Ph}$. For pure count data, χ^2_{P+} is equal to $N_+/(N_+ - 1)$ times the generalized Mantel-Haenszel statistic for pure count data. The latter statistic generalizes to stratified data without an increase in degrees of freedom, but requires matrix inversion.[10] Alternatively, one may test H_{Joint} using a deviance statistic computed using a polytomous logistic regression program (see Chapter 20).

A test statistic for H_{Joint} that makes use of ordered exposure scores $s_0, s_1, \ldots, s_J$ is the joint trend statistic:

$$\chi^2_{T+} = \sum_h \left(S_h - E_h \right)^2 \big/ V_h$$

where

$$S_h = \sum_j A_{hj} s_j, \quad E_h = M_h \sum_j T_j s_j \big/ T$$

and

$$V_h = M_h \left(\sum_j T_j s_j \big/ T - E_h^2 \right)$$

χ^2_{T+} has approximately a χ^2 distribution with the number of diseases as its degrees of freedom if there are no biases and the joint null is true. For person-time data, $\chi^2_{T+} = \sum_h \chi^2_{Th}$. Like the Mantel-Haenszel statistic, the stratified version of χ^2_{T+} requires matrix inversion, but it is also easily computed using a polytomous logistic regression program. If both the disease and exposure have ordered scores, a one-degree-of-freedom statistic can be constructed for testing H_{Joint} that will usually be more powerful than χ^2_{T+}.[22]

Relation Between Simultaneous and Single Comparisons

It is an important and apparently paradoxical fact that the simple logical relations between simultaneous and single-comparison hypotheses do *not* carry over to simultaneous and single-comparison statistics. For example, the joint null hypothesis that there is no difference in disease rates across exposure levels can be false if and only if at least one of the single null hypotheses is false. Nonetheless, it is possible to have the *P*-value from the multiple-disease statistic χ^2_P much smaller than each of the *P*-values from the single-disease statistics χ^2_{Ph}. For example, suppose we had rates at three disease sites and four exposure levels ($J = 3$ with three nonreference levels), with

$\chi^2_{P1} = \chi^2_{P2} = \chi^2_{P3} = 6.3$ with $J = 3$ degrees of freedom for each disease separately. These statistics each yield $P = 0.10$, but the joint statistic is then $\chi^2_{P+} = 6.3 + 6.3 + 6.3 = 18.9$ on $3 + 3 + 3 = 9$ degrees of freedom, which yields $P = 0.03$.

Conversely, a joint null hypothesis can be true if and only if all the single null hypotheses are true. Yet it is possible for the P-value from one or more (but not all) of the single statistics to be much smaller than the P-value from the joint statistic, χ^2_P. For example, with rates at two disease sites and four exposure levels, we could get $\chi^2_{P1} = 0$ and $\chi^2_{P2} = 8.4$ with three degrees of freedom for the two sites, which yield P-values of 1.0 and 0.04. But then, $\chi^2_{P+} = 0 + 8.4 = 8.4$ with six degrees of freedom, which has a P-value of 0.20. The results in the second panel of Table 19-6 illustrate a similar phenomenon for pure count data: the liver and bone cancer associations have $P = 0.02$ and $P = 0.04$, yet the joint P-value for all seven diseases is 0.18. Similar examples can be found using other statistics, such as the simultaneous trend statistic χ^2_{T+}.

In general, simultaneous (joint hypothesis) P-values do not have a simple logical relation to the single-hypothesis P-values. This counterintuitive lack of relation also applies to confidence intervals. For example, a simultaneous 95% confidence region for two rate ratios need not contain a point contained in the two one-at-a-time 95% confidence intervals; conversely, a point in the simultaneous 95% confidence region may not be in all of the one-at-a-time confidence intervals.

TABLE 19-6

Case-Control Data on Male Genital Implants (Penile and Testicular) and Cancers Diagnosed >1 Year After Implant

	Implant		Odds Ratio	(95% Limits)	P-Value
	Yes	No			
I. Comparisons of Control Diseases					
Benign stomach tumors[a]	6	1,718	1.24	(0.48, 2.59)	0.63
Deviated septum	17	7,874	1.04	(0.61, 1.76)	0.88
Viral pneumonia	10	3,616	1.22	(0.63, 2.38)	0.55
Gallstones	49	20,986	0.91	(0.64, 1.29)	0.60
Colon polyps	94	32,707	1.00	(Reference group)	
II. Comparison of Cancers against Combined Controls					
Liver[a]	10	1,700	2.47	(1.22, 4.44)	0.02
Bone[a]	19	4,979	1.70	(1.02, 2.65)	0.04
Connective tissue[a]	8	2,119	1.54	(0.69, 2.92)	0.27
Brain	26	10,296	1.14	(0.75, 1.73)	0.53
Lymphomas	10	4,068	1.02	(0.54, 1.93)	0.95
Myelomas[a]	3	1,455	0.84	(0.20, 2.21)	0.76
Leukemias[a]	5	2,401	0.89	(0.31, 1.94)	0.79
All control diseases	176	66,901	1.00	(Reference group)	

[a]Median-unbiased estimates and mid-P statistics; remainder are Mantel-Haenszel statistics. Statistics were derived with stratification on age in 5-year intervals from 30 to 89 years of age and year of diagnosis in 1-year intervals from 1989 to 1994. P-values are two sided.
From Greenland S, Finkle WD. A case-control study of prosthetic implants and selected chronic diseases. *Ann Epidemiol.* 1996;6:530-540.

A resolution of the apparent paradox may be obtained by overlaying a simultaneous 95% confidence region for two log rate ratios with two single 95% confidence intervals, as in Figure 19-7. The single 95% confidence intervals are simply a vertical band for $\ln(RR_1)$ and a horizontal band for $\ln(RR_2)$. For a valid study design, the vertical band contains $\ln(RR_1)$ with at least 95% probability (over study repetitions) and the horizontal band contains $\ln(RR_2)$ with at least 95% probability; nonetheless, the overlap of these bands (which is the dashed square) contains the true pair $[\ln(RR_1), \ln(RR_2)]$ with as little as $0.95(0.95) \doteq 0.90$ or 90% probability. In contrast, the joint 95% confidence region is the ellipse, which contains the true pair $[\ln(RR_1) \ \ln(RR_2)]$ with at least 95% probability over study repetitions. Note that two of the square's corners are outside the ellipse; points inside these corners are inside the overlap of the single confidence intervals, but outside the joint confidence region. Conversely, there are sections inside the ellipse that are outside the square; points inside these sections are inside the joint confidence region but outside one or the other single confidence interval.

Figure 19-7 may help one visualize why a joint confidence region and the single confidence intervals have very different objectives: simultaneous methods use a single region to try to capture *all* the true associations at once at a given minimum frequency, while keeping the area (or volume) of the region as small as possible. In contrast, single methods use a single interval to capture just one true association at a given minimum frequency, while keeping this one interval as narrow as possible. Overlapping the regions produced by the single intervals will not produce joint confidence regions that are valid at the confidence level of the single intervals.

References

1. Greenland S. Avoiding power loss associated with categorization and ordinal scores in dose-response and trend analysis. *Epidemiology*. 1995;6:450-454.
2. Greenland S. Dose-response and trend analysis in epidemiology: alternatives to categorical analysis. *Epidemiology*. 1995;6:356-365.
3. Lagakos SW. Effects of mismodelling and mismeasuring explanatory variables on tests of their association with a response variable. *Stat Med*. 1988;7:257-274.
4. Zhao LP, Kolonel LN. Efficiency loss from categorizing quantitative exposures into qualitative exposures in case-control studies. *Am J Epidemiol*. 1992;136:464-474.
5. Greenland S. Problems in the average-risk interpretation of categorical dose-response analyses. *Epidemiology*. 1995;6:563-565.
6. Austin PC, Brunner LJ. Inflation of the type 1 error rate when a continuous confounding variable is categorized in logistic regression analyses. *Stat Med*. 2004;23:1159-1178.
7. Brenner H. A potential pitfall in control of covariates in epidemiologic studies. *Epidemiology*. 1998;9:68-71.
8. Brenner H, Blettner M. Controlling for continuous confounders in epidemiologic research. *Epidemiology*. 1997;8:429-434.
9. Breslow NE, Day NE. *Statistical Methods in Cancer Research. Volume I: The Analysis of Case-Control Data*. Lyon: IARC; 1980.
10. Somes GW. The generalized Mantel-Haenszel statistic. *Am Statist*. 1986;40:106-108.
11. Yanagawa T, Fujii Y, Mastuoka J. Generalized Mantel-Haenszel procedures for 2 × J tables. *Environ Health Perspect*. 1994;102(suppl 8):57-60.
12. Easton DF, Peto J, Babiker AG. Floating absolute risk: an alternative to relative risk in survival and case-control analysis avoiding an arbitrary reference group. *Stat Med*. 1991;10:1025-1035.
13. Greenland S. The relation of the probability of causation to the relative risk and the doubling dose: a methodologic error that has become a social problem. *Am J Public Health*. 1999;89:1166-1169.
14. Hastie T, Tibshirani R, Friedman J. *The Elements of Statistical Learning: Data Mining, Inference, and Prediction*. New York, NY: Springer Science & Business Media; 2009.
15. Gladen BC, Rogan WJ. On graphing rate ratios. *Am J Epidemiol*. 1983;118:905-908.
16. Devesa SS, Donaldson J, Fears T. Graphical presentation of trends in rates. *Am J Epidemiol*. 1995;141:300-304.
17. Morgenstern H, Greenland S. Graphing ratio measures of effect. *J Clin Epidemiol*. 1990;43:539-542.
18. Rothman KJ, Wise LA, Hatch EE. Should graphs of risk or rate ratios be plotted on a log scale? *Am J Epidemiology*. 2011;174:376-377.
19. Maclure M, Greenland S. Tests for trend and dose response: misinterpretations and alternatives. *Am J Epidemiol*. 1992;135:96-104.
20. Bishop YMM, Fienberg SE, Holland PW. *Discrete Multivariate Analysis: Theory and Practice*. Cambridge, MA: Mit Press; 1975.

21. Greenland S. Smoothing observational data: a philosophy and implementation for the health sciences. *Int Stat Rev*. 2006;74:31-46.
22. Mantel N. Chi-square tests with one degree of freedom: extensions of the Mantel-Haenszel procedure. *J Am Stat Assoc*. 1963;58:690-700.
23. Cytel Corporation. *Statexact 7*. Cambridge, MA: Cytel; 2006.
24. Dixon WD, Massey FJ. *Introduction to Statistical Analysis*. New York, NY: McGraw-Hill; 1969.
25. Greenland S, Poole C. Interpretation and analysis of differential exposure variability and zero-exposure categories for continuous exposures. *Epidemiology*. 1995;6:326-328.
26. Hastie T, Tibshirani R. *Generalized Additive Models*. New York, NY: Chapman and Hall; 1990.
27. Thomas DC. The problem of multiple inference in identifying point-source environmental hazards. *Environ Health Perspect*. 1985;62:407-414.
28. Greenland S, Finkle WD. A case-control study of prosthetic implants and selected chronic diseases. *Ann Epidemiol*. 1996;6:530-540.

CHAPTER 20

Regression Analysis Part I: Model Specification

Sebastien Haneuse*

Basic tabular and graphical methods, as described in Chapters 17 to 19, are an essential component of epidemiologic analysis and may be sufficient, especially when one need to consider only a few variables at a time. They are, however, limited in the number of variables that they can examine simultaneously; while one can construct a stratification based on an arbitrary number of variables, for a fixed sample size, the strata become increasingly sparse as the number of variables increases. Thus, even though sparse-strata methods (such as Mantel-Haenszel) enable analyses when there are few subjects per strata, eventually the number will fall to 0 or 1 and those methods may no longer be reasonable to apply.

Regression analysis encompasses a vast array of techniques designed to overcome the numerical limitations of simpler methods. This advantage is offset, however, by the requirement of stronger assumptions, which are typically compactly represented by a *regression model.* While such models (and hence the assumptions they represent) have some appeal in that they can be explicitly represented, care is needed since the models may not be well understood by the intended audience or even the user.

---

*This chapter is based on original material by Sander Greenland and Kenneth J. Rothman.

Regression models can and should be tailored by the analyst to suit the study question at hand; this process, sometimes called *model specification*, is part of the broader task of *regression modeling*. To ensure that the assumptions underlying a given model specification are realistic, it is essential that the modeling process be performed in collaboration with subject-matter experts involved in the research, rather than letting it be left solely to the discretion of a purely data-driven algorithm. Such active guidance requires familiarity with the variety and interpretation of models that researchers have at their disposal, as well as familiarity with the scientific context and subject matter.

A crucial point is the distinction between a *regression function* and a *regression model*. While a regression function speaks to the true relationship between a set of covariates and an outcome, a regression model is another (usually simpler) function that is chosen by the researcher to enable the conduct of the study and it is also implicitly an approximation of true regression function. This distinction is often obscured, and even unrecognized in elementary treatments of regression, which in turn has generated much misunderstanding of regression modeling. Therefore, this chapter provides separate discussions of regression functions and regression models.

Throughout this chapter, consistent with the notational convention adopted in this book, we use X to denote an exposure of interest or X when there is more than one exposure of interest. Furthermore, we use Z to denote an adjustment variable and Z when there is more than one such variable. In some instances, an example or model specification may not require consideration of a specific exposure of interest (such as may be the case if the goal is to develop a model for prediction); in these cases, we simply use Z.

Finally, we note that regression modeling is a vast topic. As such, this chapter and the next only provide outlines of key concepts and tasks; in this chapter we outline the general theory needed to understand regression analysis together with detail on various model forms and specification; in Chapter 21 we provide detail on approaches to model selection, fitting, and assessment. More detailed treatments of regression analysis can be found in many books, including Mosteller and Tukey,[1] Leamer,[2] Breslow and Day,[3] Breslow and Day,[4] McCullagh and Nelder,[5] Clayton and Hills,[6] Hosmer and Lemeshow,[7] Berk,[8] McCulloch et al.,[9] Wakefield,[10] Faraway,[11] and Agresti.[12] Leamer[2] and Berk[8] are particularly recommended for their attention to deficiencies of regression analysis in scientific applications. Of specific note, Berk[8] gives special attention to causal analysis via regression while Mosteller and Tukey[1] provide detailed connections of regression analysis to descriptive analysis.

REGRESSION FUNCTIONS

A *regression* of a variable Y on another variable, say an exposure X, is a function that describes how some feature of the distribution of Y changes across population subgroups defined by values of X. Typically, the feature is taken to be the average (mean) value of Y, often written as $E(Y|X=x)$, which should be read as "the average of Y conditional on when the variable X takes on the specific value x." Note, we restrict attention here to settings where X is a single variable and leave the generalization to multiple covariates to a later section. Furthermore, we note that the "E" part of the notation stands for "expectation," which here is just another word for "population mean."

As an example, suppose that Y stands for "height" to the nearest centimeter at some time t, X stands for "weight" to the nearest kilogram at time t, and the population of interest is that of Denmark at time t. If we subclassify the Danish population at t into categories of weight X, compute the average height in each category, and tabulate or graph these average heights against the weight categories, the result displays the regression, $E(Y|X=x)$, of height Y on weight X in Denmark at time t. Several important points should be emphasized:

1. The *concept* of regression involves no modeling. Some describe this fact by saying that the concept of regression is essentially "nonparametric." The regression of Y on X is just a property of the physical world, like the orbital path of Earth around the Sun.
2. There is nothing mathematically sophisticated about the regression function. Displayed graphically, each point on a regression curve could be computed by taking the average of Y within a subpopulation defined as having a particular value of X. In the example, the value of the regression function at $X=50$, $E(Y|X=50)$, is just average height at time t among Danes who weigh 50 kg at time t.
3. A regression function cannot be unambiguously computed until we carefully define X, Y, *and* the population over which the averages are to be taken. We will call the latter population the

target population of the regression. This population is all too often left out of regression definitions, often resulting in confusion.

4. Although we focus on $E(Y|X = x)$, as implied, other features of the distribution of Y could be chosen, including the median value of Y (sometimes referred to as median regression) or, more generally, some other quantile.

5. The concept of regression applies to variables measured on any scale: The outcome and covariate may be continuous or discrete, or even binary. For the special case where Y is binary, $E(Y|X = x)$ is equivalent to $P(Y = 1|X = x)$, that is, the average of Y when $X = x$ equals the proportion with $Y = 1$ when $X = x$. Thus, if Y is an indicator of *disease presence* at a given time, the regression of Y on X, $E(Y|X = x)$, provides the proportion *with* the disease at that time, or prevalence proportion, given $X = x$.

It is also important to accept that some degree of ambiguity will inevitably arise and is, indeed, unavoidable in practice. In our example, some ambiguity remains in that we did not specify whether t is measured to the nearest year, day, minute, or millisecond. Furthermore, it was not explicitly specified whether the "Danish population" included all citizens, all residents, or all persons present in Denmark at t. While reducing ambiguity should always be a central goal, we may decide that leaving certain questions unanswered is tolerable because varying the definitions over a modest range will not change the result to an important extent. If we left time completely out of the definition, however, the regression would become hopelessly ambiguous since we would not have a good idea of who to include or exclude from our average: Should we include people living in Denmark in prehistoric times or in the time of King Canute (the 11th century AD) or in the distant future (a thousand years from now)? The choice could strongly influence our answer, because of the large changes in height-to-weight relations that have occurred over time.

Concepts of Population

It is important to distinguish between the terms *target population* and *source population*. The target population of regression is defined without regard to our observations. For example, the regression of diastolic blood pressure on cigarette usage in China is defined whether or not we conduct a study in China (the target for this regression). The source population is the source of subjects for a particular study and is defined by the selection methods of the study. For example, a random sample survey of all residents of Beijing would have Beijing as its source population. The concepts of target and source populations connect only insofar as inferences about a regression function drawn from a study are most easily justified when the source population of the study is identical to the target population of the regression. Otherwise, issues of generalization from the source to the target have to be addressed (see Chapter 14).

In some literature, regression functions (and many other concepts) are defined in terms of averages within a "superpopulation" or a "hypothetical universe." A superpopulation is an abstraction of a target population, sometimes said to represent the distribution (with respect to all variables of interest) of all possible persons that ever were or ever could be targets of inference for the analysis at hand. Because the superpopulation approach focuses on purely hypothetical distributions, we believe it has encouraged substitution of mathematical theory for the more prosaic task of connecting study results to populations of immediate public health concern. Thus, in this chapter, we define a regression function in terms of averages within a real target population.

Regression and Causation

When considering a regression function, such as $E(Y|X = x)$, the variable Y is termed the dependent variable or the outcome variable, while the variable X is termed the independent variable, predictor, or covariate. While the "dependent/independent" terminology is most common, it is problematic because it invites confusion with unrelated probabilistic and causal concepts of dependence and independence. For example, if Y is age and X is blood pressure, then $E(Y|X = x)$ represents the average age of persons given blood pressure, X. But it is blood pressure X that causally depends on age Y, not the other way around.

More generally, for any pair of variables X and Y, we can consider either the regression of Y on X, $E(Y|X = x)$, or the regression of X on Y, $E(X|Y = y)$. Thus, the concept of regression does not imply any causal or even temporal relation between the two variables. For example, Y could be blood pressure at the start of follow-up of a cohort, and X could be blood pressure after 1 year of follow-up. Then, $E(Y|X = x)$ represents the average initial blood pressure among cohort members whose blood pressure after 1 year of follow-up is x. Below we will introduce a notation that distinguishes causation from association in regression.

Multiple Regression

The concept of multiple regression (or multivariable regression) is a simple extension of the ideas discussed above to situations in which there are multiple (*i.e.*, two or more) covariates. To illustrate, suppose that Y is an indicator of diabetes, Z_1 stands for "sex" (coded 1 for females, 0 for males), and Z_2 stands for "weight" (in kilograms). Then the regression of Y on Z_1 and Z_2, written $E(Y|Z_1 = z_1, Z_2 = z_2)$, corresponds to the average of Y among population members of a given sex, specifically z_1, and weight, specifically z_2. For example, $E(Y|Z_1 = 1, Z_2 = 70)$ is the average diabetes indicator (and, hence, the diabetes prevalence) among women who weigh 70 kg.

We can add as many covariates as we want. For example, we could add age (in years) to the last regression. Let Z_3 stand for "age." Then $E(Y|Z_1 = z_1, Z_2 = z_2, Z_3 = z_3)$ provides the diabetes prevalence among population members of a given sex, weight, and age. Since continuing to add covariates in this way will be clumsy, we use vector notion to simplify. Specifically, in the diabetes example, we let $\mathbf{Z}$ stand for the horizontal list (Z_1, Z_2, Z_3) of "sex," "weight," and "age." Similarly, we will let z without a subscript stand for the horizontal ordered list of values (z_1, z_2, z_3) for $\mathbf{Z} = (Z_1, Z_2, Z_3)$. Thus, if we write $E(Y|\mathbf{Z} = z)$, it is a shorthand for $E(Y|Z_1 = z_1, Z_2 = z_2, Z_3 = z_3)$ when there are three covariates under consideration.

More generally, if there are p covariates, say $Z_1, \ldots, Z_p$, we will write $\mathbf{Z}$ for the ordered list $(Z_1, \ldots, Z_p)$ and z for the ordered list of values $(z_1, \ldots, z_p)$. The horizontal ordered list of variables $\mathbf{Z}$ is called a *row vector* of covariates, and the horizontal ordered list of values z is called a *row vector* of values. Above, the vector $\mathbf{Z}$ is composed of the $p = 3$ items "sex," "weight," and "age"; the list z is composed of specific values for sex (0 or 1), weight (kilograms), and age (years). The number of items, p, is called the length or dimension of $\mathbf{Z}$.

Regression Measures of Effect

As discussed earlier, regression functions do not involve any assumptions of time order or causal relations. Thus, regression coefficients and quantities derived from them represent measures of association, not measures of effect. To interpret the exposure coefficients as measures of effect, the exposure variables X must be interpretable as potential intervention variables (Chapter 5) and the regression function must be modeled to provide an unconfounded representation of the effects of interest. Issues of selection bias and measurement error do not arise at this point because here, and throughout this chapter, the models are assumed to refer to population relations (*i.e.*, before selection and measurement).

To make this unconfounded representation more precise, suppose that X is either a single exposures or a vector containing multiple exposures of interest, $\mathbf{Z}$ is another vector containing the other covariates, and that the covariates in $\mathbf{Z}$ are proper confounder candidates, that is, they are unaffected by X or Y (see Chapters 3 and 12). We may then write:

$$E[Y|\text{Set}(X = x), \mathbf{Z} = z]$$

for the average value Y would have *if* everyone in the target population with $\mathbf{Z} = z$ had their X value set to x. If Y_x is the corresponding potential outcome with X set to x, then, as in Chapters 3 and 12 and elsewhere in the book, we can also write $E[Y|\text{Set}(X = x), \mathbf{Z} = z]$ as $E(Y_x|\mathbf{Z} = z)$. Note, this *average potential outcome* can be very different from the actual average $E(Y|X = x, \mathbf{Z} = z)$. The latter refers only to those population members with $X = x$ and $\mathbf{Z} = z$, whereas the former refers to *all* population members with $\mathbf{Z} = z$, including those who actually had X equal to values other than x. Thus, the average potential outcome generalizes the potential outcome concept from Chapter 3 to regressions. In terms of causal diagrams, the average potential outcome $E(Y_x|\mathbf{Z} = z)$ refers to a graph with an intervention to set $X = x$ so that there is no arrow into any member of X for the subpopulation with $Z = z$ (see Chapters 3 and 12).

As an example, suppose the target population is all persons born between 1901 and 1950 who survived to age 50 years. Let Y be an indicator of death by age 80 and X only include $X =$ pack-years of cigarettes smoked by age 50. Finally, let $Z = (Z_1, Z_2)$ where $Z_1 = 1$ if female, 0 if male and $Z_2 =$ year of birth. Then,

$$E\left[Y \mid X = 20, Z = (1, 1940)\right]$$

is the average risk of dying by age 80 years (mortality proportion) among women born in 1940 and surviving to age 50 who smoked 20 pack-years by age 50. In contrast,

$$E\left[Y_{20} \mid Z = (1, 1940)\right]$$

is the average risk of dying by age 80 among all women born in 1940 and surviving to age 50 *if* all such women had smoked 20 pack-years by age 50.

In Chapter 5, we defined effect measures as contrasts (such as differences and ratios) of occurrence in the *same* population under different conditions. In regression analysis, we may similarly define effect measures as contrasts of averages in the same population under different conditions. Because occurrence measures are averages, this definition subsumes the preceding definition. As an example, consider the average of Y in the subpopulation with $Z = z$ when X is set to x^* versus that average when X is set to x. The ratio effect measure is:

$$\frac{E\left(Y_{x^*} \mid Z = z\right)}{E\left(Y_x \mid Z = z\right)},$$

the difference effect measure is:

$$E\left(Y_{x^*} \mid Z = z\right) - E\left(Y_x \mid Z = z\right),$$

and the attributable fraction is:

$$\frac{E\left(Y_{x^*} \mid Z = z\right) - E\left(Y_x \mid Z = z\right)}{E\left(Y_{x^*} \mid Z = z\right)}.$$

Returning to the example, the ratio

$$\frac{E\left[Y_{20} \mid Z = (1, 1940)\right]}{E\left[Y_0 \mid Z = (1, 1940)\right]}$$

measures the *effect* of smoking 20 pack-years by age 50 versus no smoking on the risk of dying by age 80 among women born in 1940. On the other hand, the ratio

$$\frac{E\left[Y \mid X = 20, Z = (1, 1940)\right]}{E\left[Y \mid X = 0, Z = (1, 1940)\right]}$$

represents only the *association* of smoking 20 pack-years by age 50 versus no smoking with the risk among women born in 1940 because it contrasts two different subpopulations (one with $X = 20$ and the other with $X = 0$).

To infer that all associational measures estimated from our analysis equal their corresponding effect measures, we have to make the following assumption of no confounding given Z (which is sometimes expressed by stating that there is no residual confounding):

$$E(Y|X = x, Z = z) = E(Y_x | Z = z)$$

This assumption states that the average we observe or estimate in the subpopulation with both $X = x$ and $Z = z$ is equal to what the average in the larger subpopulation with $Z = z$ would have been if everyone had X set to x. It is important to appreciate the strength of the assumption. In the above example, the no-confounding assumption entails:

$$E\left[Y | X_1 = 20, Z = (1,1940)\right] = E\left[Y_{20} | Z = (1,1940)\right]$$

which states that the risk we will observe among women born in 1940 who smoked 20 pack-years by age 50 equals the risk we would have observed in *all* women born in 1940 if they all had smoked 20 pack-years by age 50. The social variables associated with both smoking and death should lead us to doubt that the two quantities are even approximately equal.

The plausibility, or lack thereof, of no-confounding assumptions is often the chief limitation in using epidemiologic data for causal inference. This limitation applies to both tabular and regression methods. Randomization of persons to values of X can largely overcome this limitation because it ensures that effect estimates follow an identifiable probability distribution centered around the true effect. In the absence of randomization, one must rely on a strategy of ensuring that there are enough well-measured confounders in Z so that the no-confounding assumption is at least plausible. In practice, this strategy often leads a large number of components in Z so that one may end up with few subjects at each value x of X and z of Z, which in turn leads to the sparse data problems that regression modeling attempts to address.[13]

Multivariate Regression

Multiple regression concerns averages of an outcome within levels of multiple covariates. Such an analysis is sometimes called "multivariate analysis," although it should not be confused with *multivariate regression*, a term used in advanced statistics to refer to regressions for multiple outcomes simultaneously. To illustrate multivariate regression, suppose that Y_1 is an indicator of the presence of diabetes and Y_2 is diastolic blood pressure. Let $Y = (Y_1, Y_2)$ be the vector composed of these two variables and $Z = (Z_1, Z_2, Z_3)$ the list composed of the sex indicator, weight, and age. Then the multivariate regression of diabetes and blood pressure jointly on sex, weight, and age provides the average diabetes indicator *and* average blood pressure for each specific combination of sex, weight, and age:

$$E(Y_1, Y_2 | Z_1 = z_1, Z_2 = z_2, Z_3 = z_3) = E(Y | Z = z)$$

More generally, there may be any number of outcomes in the list Y and covariates in the list Z of a multivariate regression.

BASIC REGRESSION MODELS

In any given instance, the true regression of Y on X and Z, $E(Y|X = x, Z = z)$, may be an extremely complicated function of the covariates X and Z. Thus, even if we observe this function without error, we may wish to formulate simplified pictures of reality; that is, develop and investigate *models* that approximate this regression. These models, though inevitably incorrect, can be very useful. A classic example is the representation of the distance from the earth to the sun, Y, as a function of day of the year T. To the nearest kilometer, this distance is a complex function of T because of the gravitational effects of the moon and of the other planets in the solar system. If we represent the orbit of the earth around the sun as a circle with the sun at the center, our regression model will predict the distance $E(Y|T=t)$ by a single number (about 150 million kilometers) that does not change with t. This model is adequate if we can tolerate a few percent error in our predictions. If we represent the orbit of the earth as an ellipse, our regression model will predict the earth-sun distance as smoothly and cyclically varying over the course of a year (within a range of about 147-153 million kilometers). Although it is not perfectly accurate, this second model will be more accurate than the first (*i.e.*, the one based on a circle) and will be adequate if we can tolerate a few tenths of a percent error in our predictions.

Model Specification Versus Model Fitting

Our description of the preceding models must be refined by distinguishing between the *form* of a model and a *fitted* model. "Circle" and "ellipse" refer to forms, that is, general classes of shapes. The circular model form corresponds to assuming a constant earth-sun distance over time; the elliptical model form allows this distance to vary over a temporal cycle. The process of deciding between these two forms is a simple example of *model specification*.

If we decide to use the circular form, we must also select a value for the radius (which is the Earth-Sun distance in the model). This radius specifies which circle (out of the many possible circles) to use as a representation of the Earth's orbit and is an example of a model *parameter*. The process of selecting the "best" estimate of the radius is an example of *model fitting*, and the circle that results is sometimes called the *fitted model* (although the latter term is sometimes used instead to refer to the model form).

There are two important relations between a set of data and a model fit to those data. First, there is "distance" from the fitted model to the data; second, there is "resistance" or "stability" of the fitted model, which is the degree to which the model predictions or parameter estimates change when the data themselves are changed. Chapter 21 describes approaches to evaluating distance and stability, including *delta-beta* analysis.

Depending on our accuracy requirements, we may have several simplified pictures of reality at hand and, hence, several candidate models. At best, our choice may require a trade-off between simplicity and accuracy, as in the preceding example. There is an old dictum, often referred to as *Occam razor*, that one should not introduce needless complexity for purposes of prediction or explanation. Following this dictum, if we need only 2% accuracy in predicting the earth's distance from the sun, then we should not bother with the ellipse model and instead use the constant distance derived from the circle model.

There is a more subtle benefit from this advice than avoiding needless mental exertion. Suppose that we are given two models, one (the more complex) containing the other (the more simple) as a special case, and some data with which to fit the two models. Then the more complex model will be able to fit the available data more closely than the simpler model, in the sense that the predictions from the more complex model will (on average) be closer to what is seen in the data than will the predictions from the simpler model. In the preceding example, this arises because the ellipse contains the circle as a special case. Nonetheless, there is a penalty for this closeness to the data: The predictions obtained from the more complex model tend to be less stable than those obtained from the simpler model.

Consider now the use of the two different model forms to predict events outside of the data set to which the models were fitted. One example is forecasting the Earth's distance from the Sun; another is predicting the incidence of AIDS at a time 5 years in the future. Intuitively, we might expect that if one model is both closer to the data and more stable than the other, that model will give more accurate predictions. The choice among models is rarely so clear-cut, however. Usually, one model will be closer to the data, while the other will be more stable, and it will be difficult to tell which will be more accurate. We often face this dilemma in a choice between a more complex and simpler model.

To summarize, model specification is the process of selecting a model form, whereas model fitting is the process of using data to estimate the parameters in a given model form. There are many methods of model fitting, and the topic is vast and often technical; Chapter 21 provides an overview of key concepts.

Background Example

The following epidemiologic example will be used at various points to illustrate specific models. In the 1990s, a controversy arose over whether women with no history of breast cancer but thought to be of high risk (because of family history or perhaps other factors) should be given the drug tamoxifen as a prophylactic regimen. Evidence suggested that tamoxifen might not only prevent breast cancer[14] but also cause or promote endometrial and liver cancer.

One measure of the net effect of tamoxifen prophylaxis up to a given age is the change in risk of death by that age. Suppose that the outcome Y is an indicator of death by age 70 years ($Y = 1$ for dead, 0 for alive) and X is the time of tamoxifen therapy (in years). Furthermore, let $Z = (Z_1, Z_2, Z_3, Z_4)$, where Z_1 = age (in years) at start of tamoxifen therapy, Z_2 = age at menarche, Z_3 = age at menopause, and Z_4 = parity. Suppose that the target population is American women born between 1925 and 1950 who survived to age 50 years and did not use tamoxifen before that age. If tamoxifen was not taken during follow-up, we set age at tamoxifen start (Z_1) to 70 because women who started at age 70 or later and women who never took tamoxifen have the same exposure history during the age interval under study.

In this example, the regression $E(Y \mid X = x, Z = z)$ is the average risk, or incidence proportion, of death by age 70 among women in the target population who have $X = x$ and $Z = z$. Therefore, we will write $R(x, z)$ as a shorthand for $E(Y \mid X = x, Z = z)$. We will also write R for the crude (overall) average risk $E(Y)$, $R(x)$ for the average risk $E(Y \mid X = x)$ in the subpopulation defined by having $X = x$ (without regard to the other variables), and so on.

Vacuous Models

Consider the model:

$$E(Y) = R = \alpha. \qquad [20\text{-}1]$$

There is only one regression parameter (or coefficient) in this model, specifically α, and it corresponds to the average risk in the target population. Note, model 20-1 has no implications in the sense that it imposes neither restrictions nor any constraints on the value of the regression, $E(Y)$. Moreover, it has no implications for any other regressions that may be of interest, such as $E(Y \mid X = x)$ in the subpopulation defined by having $X = x$. Put another way, all that model 20-1 is doing is speaking to the overall average and nothing else. As such, model 20-1 is said to be *vacuous*.

Two models are said to be *equivalent* if they have identical implications for the regression. Given that $R > 0$, a model that is equivalent to model 20-1 is:

$$R(X) = R = \exp(\alpha). \qquad [20\text{-}2]$$

Model 20-2 has no implication beyond forcing R to be positive. In this model, α is the natural logarithm of the overall average risk, $\alpha = \ln(R)$. Note, while models 20-1 and 20-2 are equivalent, the interpretation of the parameter α is distinct between the two models.

Given that $R > 0$ and $R < 1$, a model that is equivalent to models 20-1 and 20-2 is:

$$E(Y) = R = \operatorname{expit}(\alpha), \qquad [20\text{-}3]$$

where expit(α) is the *logistic* transform of α, defined as:

$$\operatorname{expit}(\alpha) = \frac{\exp(\alpha)}{1 + \exp(\alpha)}.$$

Model 20-3 has no implication beyond forcing R to fall between 0 and 1. Now, however, the parameter α in model 20-3 is the logit (log odds) of the overall average risk:

$$\alpha = \ln\left(\frac{R}{1-R}\right) = \text{logit}(R).$$

Finally, since models 20-2 and 20-3 are equivalent to 20-1 and that 20-1 is vacuous, we have that both 20-2 and 20-3 are also vacuous.

Constant Models

Now consider the following model:

$$E(Y|X = x) = R(x) = \alpha. \tag{20-4}$$

Superficially, 20-4 is similar to model 20-1 in the sense that the right-hand side consists of a single parameter, α. Model 20-4 is, however, much stricter since it implies a constant and common average risk, α, across all subpopulations defined by years of tamoxifen. Thus, model 20-4 is called a *constant* regression.

Note, model 20-4 is a special case of model 20-1; if all the X-specific averages equal α, as in model 20-4, then the overall average must equal α as well, as in model 20-1. More generally, consider two models, labeled model A and model B, respectively. In comparing the complexity and implications of the two models, we say that model A is more general, more flexible, or more complex than model B, or that A contains B, if all the implications of model A are also implications of model B, but not vice versa (that is, if B imposes some restrictions beyond those imposed by A). Other ways of stating this relation are that B is simpler, stronger, or stricter than A, B is contained or nested within A, or B is a special case of A.

Given that $R(x) > 0$ and $R(x) < 1$, a model that is equivalent to model 20-4 is:

$$E(x) = \exp(\alpha) \tag{20-5}$$

which can be rewritten as

$$\ln[R(x)] = \alpha.$$

Another model that is equivalent to model 20-4 is:

$$R(x) = \text{expit}(\alpha) = \frac{\exp(\alpha)}{1 + \exp(\alpha)} \tag{20-6}$$

which can be rewritten as:

$$\text{logit}[R(x)] = \alpha.$$

In model 20-5, α is the common value of the log risks, $\ln[R(x)]$, whereas α in model 20-6 is the common value of the logits, $\text{logit}[R(x)]$. Each of the models 20-4 to 20-6 is a special case of the more general models 20-1 to 20-3. In other words, models 20-4 to 20-6 are simpler, stronger, or stricter than models 20-1 to 20-3 and are contained or nested within models 20-1 to 20-3.

A constant regression is of course implausible in most situations. For example, age is related to most health outcomes. In the above example, we expect the average death risk to vary across the subgroups defined by age at start of tamoxifen use (Z_1). Moving forward, there are infinite ways to model these variations. Prior to addressing the problem of selecting a useful model from among the many choices, we first describe some of the more common choices, focusing on models for average risks (incidence proportions), incidence odds, and person-time incidence rates. The models for risks and odds can also be used to model prevalence proportions and prevalence odds.

Linear Risk Models

When considering how $E(Y|X = x)$ might vary as a function of x, that is moving beyond the constant model 20-4, one has many options. One such model is:

$$R(x) = \alpha + \beta x. \qquad [20\text{-}7]$$

This model allows the average risk to vary across subpopulations with different values for X, but only in a very specific, linear fashion. In particular, the model implies that subtracting the average risk in the subpopulation with $X = x$ from that in the subpopulation with $X = x+1$ will always yield β, *regardless* of what x is. Put another way, under model 20-7, we have:

$$R(x+1) = \alpha + \beta(x+1)$$

so that

$$R(x+1) - R(x) = \beta.$$

Thus, β_1 represents the difference in risk between the subpopulation defined by having $X = x+1$ and that defined by having $X = x$. Crucially, model 20-7 implies that this difference does not depend on the reference level x for X used for the comparison.

Model 20-7 is an example of a *linear* risk model. Just as with model 20-4, model 20-7 is stricter than model 20-1; that is, model 20-7 is a special case of model 20-1. Model 20-7 also contains model 20-4 as a special case: the latter can be seen to be a special case of the former by setting $\beta = 0$ (*i.e.*, so average risks do not vary across levels of X).

Linear risk models, such as model 20-7, are easy to understand, but when the outcome is binary they have a severe technical problem that makes them difficult to fit and/or interpret in practice: There are combinations of α and β that will produce impossible values (*i.e.*, less than 0 or greater than 1) for one or more of the risks $R(x)$. Several models partially or wholly address this problem by transforming the linear term $\alpha + \beta x$, also known as the *linear predictor*, before equating it to the risk. We will study two of these models.

Exponential Risk Models

Consider the following model:

$$R(x) = \exp(\alpha + \beta x). \qquad [20\text{-}8]$$

Since the exponential function is always positive, model 20-8 will produce positive $R(x)$ for any combination of α and β. This can be viewed as an advantage relative to the linear model given by 20-7, which may produce negative values $R(x)$ for certain combinations of α and β.

Model 20-8 is sometimes called an *exponential* risk model. It is a special case of the vacuous model 20-2; it also contains the constant model 20-5 as the special case in which $\beta = 0$. To understand the implications of the exponential risk model, we can recast it in an equivalent form by taking the natural logarithm of both sides:

$$\ln[R(x)] = \ln[\exp(\alpha + \beta x)] = \alpha + \beta x. \qquad [20\text{-}9]$$

Model 20-9 is often called a *log-linear* risk model.

The exponential and equivalent log-linear model allows risk to vary across subpopulations defined by X, but only in an exponential fashion. To interpret the coefficients, we may compare the log risks under model 20-9 for the two subpopulations defined by $X = x+1$ and $X = x$, specifically:

$$\ln\left[R(x+1)\right] = \alpha + \beta(x+1)$$

and

$$\ln\left[R(x)\right] = \alpha + \beta x.$$

Taking the difference, we have

$$\ln\left[R(x+1)\right] - \ln\left[R(x)\right] = \beta.$$

Now, because $\ln\left[R(x+1)\right] - \ln\left[R(x)\right] = \ln\left[R(x+1)/R(x)\right]$, we have

$$\ln\left[R(x+1)/R(x)\right] = \beta$$

Thus, under models 20-8 and 20-9, β represents the log risk ratio comparing the subpopulation defined by having $X = x+1$ and that defined by $X = x$, regardless of the chosen reference level x. Also, if $X = 0$, then $\ln[R(0)] = \alpha + \beta \times 0 = \alpha$; thus, α represents the log risk for the subpopulation with $X = 0$ (and so is meaningful only if X can be zero).

We can derive another equivalent interpretation of the parameters in the exponential risk model by noting that:

$$R(x+1) = \exp\left[\alpha + \beta(x+1)\right]$$

and

$$R(x) = \exp(\alpha + \beta x)$$

so that

$$R(x+1)/R(x) = \exp\left[\alpha + \beta(x+1) - (\alpha + \beta x)\right] = \exp(\beta).$$

Thus, under models 20-8 and 20-9, $\exp(\beta)$ represents the *ratio* of risks between the subpopulations defined by $X = x + 1$ and $X = x$, and this ratio does not depend on the reference level x (because x does not appear in the final expression for the risk ratio). Also, if $X = 0$, then $R(0) = \exp(\alpha + \beta \times 0) = \exp(\alpha)$; thus, $\exp(\alpha)$ represents the average risk for the subpopulation with $X = 0$.

As with linear risk models, exponential risk models have the technical problem that some combinations of α and β will yield risk values greater than 1, which are impossible. This problem will not be a practical concern, however, if all the fitted risks and their confidence limits fall well below 1.

Logistic Models

Consider the model:

$$R(x) = expit(\alpha + \beta x) = \frac{exp(\alpha + \beta x)}{1 + exp(\alpha + \beta x)} \qquad \text{[20-10]}$$

This model is called a *logistic* risk model. Because the range of the logistic function is between 0 and 1, the model will only produce risks between 0 and 1 regardless of the values for α, β, and x.

The logistic model is perhaps the most commonly used model in epidemiology, so we examine it in some detail.

To understand the implications of the logistic model, it is helpful to recast it as a model for the odds, $O(x) = R(x)/[1 - R(x)]$. Toward this, first note that under model 20-10, we have:

$$1 - R(x) = 1 - \frac{\exp(\alpha + \beta x)}{1 + \exp(\alpha + \beta x)} = \frac{1}{1 + \exp(\alpha + \beta x)}.$$

Dividing Equation 20-10 by this expression, we get:

$$O(x) = \frac{R(x)}{1 - R(x)} = \frac{\dfrac{\exp(\alpha + \beta x)}{1 + \exp(\alpha + \beta x)}}{\dfrac{1}{1 + \exp(\alpha + \beta x)}} = \exp(\alpha + \beta x). \qquad [20\text{-}11]$$

From this we see that logistic risk model is equivalent to an exponential *odds* model. Furthermore, taking logarithms of both sides of Equation 20-11, we see that the logistic model is also equivalent to the log-linear odds model:

$$\ln[O(x)] = \alpha + \beta x. \qquad [20\text{-}12]$$

Now recall that the logit of risk is defined as the log odds:

$$\operatorname{logit}[R(x)] = \ln[R(x+1)/R(x)] = \ln[O(x)]$$

Hence, from Equation 20-12, the logistic model can be rewritten in one more equivalent form, specifically:

$$\ln[O(x)] = \alpha + \beta x. \qquad [20\text{-}13]$$

This equivalent of the logistic model is often called the logit-linear risk model, or *logit model*. We can now derive two related interpretations of the logistic model parameters. First, since

$$\ln[O(x+1)] = a + \beta(x+1)$$

and

$$\ln[O(x)] = a + \beta x,$$

we have

$$\ln[O(x+1)] - \ln[O(x)] = \beta.$$

Thus, under the logistic model given by Equation 20-10, β represents the log odds ratio comparing the subpopulations with $X = x + 1$ and $X = x$. Also, if $X = 0$, then $ln[O(0)] = \alpha + \beta \times 0 = \alpha$; thus, α represents the log odds for the subpopulation with $X = 0$. Equivalently, we have:

$$O(x+1)/O(x) = \exp(\beta)$$

and

$$O(0) = \exp(\alpha)$$

so that $\exp(\beta)$ is the odds ratio comparing the subpopulations with $X = x + 1$ and $X = x$, and $\exp(\alpha)$ is the odds for the subpopulation with $X = 0$.

Other Risk and Odds Models

In addition to those given so far, several other risk models are occasionally mentioned but rarely used in epidemiology. The linear odds model is obtained by replacing the average risk by the odds in the linear risk model:

$$O(x) = \alpha + \beta x \qquad [20\text{-}14]$$

Here, β is the *odds* difference between subpopulations with $X = x + 1$ and $X = x$, and α is the odds for the subpopulation with $X = 0$. Like risk, the odds cannot be negative; unfortunately, some combinations of α and β in model 20-14 will produce negative odds. As a result, this model (like the linear risk model) may be difficult to fit and gives unsatisfactory results in some settings.

Another model replaces the logistic transform (expit) in the logistic model (Equation 20-10) by the inverse of the standard normal distribution, which also has a range between 0 and 1. The resulting model, called a *probit* model, has seen much use in bioassay studies. Its absence from epidemiologic use may stem from the fact that (unlike the logistic model) its parameters have no simple epidemiologic interpretation, and the model appears to have no advantage over the logistic in epidemiologic applications.

Several attempts have been made to use models that are mixtures of different basic models. These mixtures have various drawbacks, including difficulties in fitting the models and interpreting the parameters.[15] We thus do not describe them here.

Rate Models

Instead of modeling average risk, we may model person-time incidence rates. If we let Y denote the *rate* observed in a study subpopulation, so that Y is the observed number of cases per unit of observed person-time, the regressions $I(x) = E(Y|X = x)$ and $I(x,z) = E(Y|X = x, Z = z)$ represent the average number of cases per unit of person-time in the target subpopulation defined by $X = x$ and by $X = x$ and $Z = z$, respectively.

Most rate models are analogs of risk and odds models. For example, the model

$$I(x) = \alpha + \beta x \qquad [20\text{-}15]$$

is a linear *rate* model, analogous to but distinct from the linear risk model, given by Equation 20-7, and the linear odds models, given by Equation 20-14. This rate model implies that the difference in average rates between subpopulations with $X = x + 1$ and $X = x$ is β, regardless of x. Also, α is the average rate for the subpopulation with $X = 0$.

Model 20-15 can be problematic, however, because some combinations of α and β can produce negative rate values, which are impossible. To prevent this, most rate modeling begins with an exponential *rate* model such as:

$$I(x) = \exp(\alpha + \beta x) \qquad [20\text{-}16]$$

Crucially, because exponentiating can never result in a negative value, this model will not produce negative $I(x)$ for any α, β, or x. Note, taking the natural logarithm of both sizes, model 20-16 can be seen to be equivalent to the log-linear *rate* model:

$$\ln[I(x)] = \alpha + \beta x. \qquad [20\text{-}17]$$

Following the same approach used for the log-linear risk model 20-9, the parameter β in models 20-16 and 20-17 is the log of the rate ratio comparing the subpopulation with $X = x + 1$ to the subpopulation with $X = x$, regardless of x; hence, $\exp(\beta)$ is the corresponding rate ratio $I(x + 1)/I(x)$. Also, α is the log of the rate for the subpopulation with $X = 0$; hence, $\exp(\alpha)$ is the average rate $I(0)$ when $X = 0$.

Multiple-Regression Models

Suppose now that we wish to model the multiple regression $E(Y|X=x,Z=z)$. Each of the previous models for the single regression $E(Y|X=x)$ can be extended to handle this more general situation by replacing "βx" with:

$$\beta_x x + \beta_1 z_1 + \beta_2 z_2 + \ldots + \beta_p z_p. \qquad [20\text{-}18]$$

To illustrate, suppose that we wish to model average risk of death by age 70 years across female subpopulations defined by X = years of tamoxifen therapy; Z_1 = age at start of tamoxifen use; and, Z_2 = age at menarche. Letting $Z = (Z_1, Z_2)$, the multiple linear risk model for $R(x, z)$ is:

$$R(x,z) = \alpha + \beta_x x + \beta_1 z_1 + \beta_2 z_2,$$

while the multiple logistic risk model is

$$R(x,z) = \text{expit}(\alpha + \beta_x x + \beta_1 z_1 + \beta_2 z_2).$$

If instead we wished to model the death rate, we could use the multiple linear rate model

$$I(x,z) = \alpha + \beta_x x + \beta_1 z_1 + \beta_2 z_2$$

or a multiple exponential rate model.

$$I(x,z) = \exp(\alpha + \beta_x x + \beta_1 z_1 + \beta_2 z_2).$$

Because expression 20-18 can be clumsy to write out when there are three or more adjustment covariates (that is, $p \geq 3$), several shorthand notations are in use. Toward this, let $\boldsymbol{\beta}_z = (\beta_1, \ldots, \beta_p)$ represent the vertical list (column vector) of coefficients. Recall that $z = (z_1, \ldots, z_p)$ stands for the horizontal list (row vector) of covariate values. If we let

$$z\boldsymbol{\beta}_z = \beta_1 z_1 + \beta_2 z_2 + \ldots + \beta_p z_p,$$

we can succinctly represent the multiple linear risk model by:

$$R(x,z) = \alpha + \beta_x x + z\boldsymbol{\beta}_z, \qquad [20\text{-}19]$$

the multiple logistic model by:

$$R(x,z) = \text{expit}(\alpha + \beta_x x + z\boldsymbol{\beta}_z), \qquad [20\text{-}20]$$

the multiple exponential rate model by:

$$I(x,z) = \exp(\alpha + \beta_x x + z\boldsymbol{\beta}_z), \qquad [20\text{-}21]$$

and so on for all the models discussed earlier.

It is important to note that the multiple-regression models given by expressions 20-19 to 20-21 are not more general than the single regression models 20-7, 20-10, and 20-16, nor do they contain those models as special cases, because they refer to entirely different subclassifications of the target population. The single-regression models refer to variations in averages across subpopulations defined by levels of just one variable; the multiple-regression models, in contrast, refer to variations across the much finer subdivisions defined by the levels of several variables. For example, it is at least logically possible for $R(x)$ to follow the single-logistic model (Equation 20-10) without $R(x, z)$ following the multiple-logistic model (Equation 20-20); conversely, it is possible for $R(x, z)$ to follow the multiple-logistic model without $R(x)$ following the single-logistic model.

The preceding point is often overlooked because the single-regression models are often confused with multiple-regression models in which all covariate coefficients except one are 0. The difference, however, is analogous to the differences discussed earlier between the vacuous models 20-1 to 20-3 (which are so general as to imply nothing) and the constant regression models 20-4 to 20-6 (which are so restrictive as to be unbelievable in typical situations). To see this analogy, consider the multiple-logistic model:

$$R(x,z) = \text{expit}(\alpha + \beta_x x) \qquad [20\text{-}22]$$

The right side of this equation is the same as in the single-logistic model (Equation 20-10), but the left side is crucially different: It is the multiple-risk regression $R(x, z)$, instead of the single-regression $R(x)$. Unlike model 20-10, model 20-22 *is* a special case of the multiple-logistic model (Equation 20-20), the one in which $\beta_1 = \ldots = \beta_p = 0$. Moreover, model 20-22 asserts that risk does not vary across subpopulations defined by $X, Z_1, \ldots, Z_p$ *except* to the extent that X varies. This model is far more strict than model 20-20, which allows risk to vary with $Z_1, \ldots, Z_p$ as well as X (albeit only in a logistic fashion). It is also far more strict than model 20-10, which does not attempt to say anything about whether or how risk varies across subpopulations defined by $Z_1, \ldots, Z_p$, within specific levels of X.

We must be careful to distinguish between models that refer to different multiple regressions. For example, compare the two exponential rate models

$$I(x,z_1) = \exp(\alpha + \beta_x x + \beta_1 z_1) \qquad [20\text{-}23]$$

and

$$I(x,z_1,z_2) = \exp(\alpha + \beta_x x + \beta_1 z_1). \qquad [20\text{-}24]$$

To be clear, these are fundamentally different models. The first is a model for the regression of rates on X and Z_1 only, whereas the second is a model for the regression of rates on X, Z_1, and Z_2. The first model in no way refers to Z_2, whereas the second asserts that rates do not vary across levels of Z_2 if one looks within levels of X and Z_1. Thus, model 20-24 is the special case of

$$I(x,z_1,z_2) = \exp(\alpha + \beta_x x + \beta_1 z_1 + \beta_2 z_2)$$

in which $\beta_2 = 0$, whereas model 20-23 is not.

Many textbooks and software manuals fail to distinguish between models such as 20-23 and 20-24, which differ in what is actually being modeled (*i.e.*, the left-hand side) and instead focus only on the form/structure of the model (*i.e.*, the right-hand side). Most software fits the less restrictive model that ignores other covariates (Equation 20-23 in the preceding example) rather than the more restrictive model (Equation 20-24) when requested to fit a model with only X and Z_1 as covariates. Note that if the less restrictive model is inadequate, then the more restrictive model must also be inadequate.

Unfortunately, if the less restrictive model appears adequate, it does *not* follow that the more restrictive model is also adequate. For example, it is possible for the model form $\exp(\alpha + \beta_x x + \beta_1 z_1)$ to describe adequately the double regression $I(x, z_1)$ (which means it describes adequately the rate variation across X and Z_1 when Z_2 is ignored) and yet at the same time describe poorly the triple regression $I(x, z_1, z_2)$ (which means that it describes inadequately the rate variation across X, Z_1, and Z_2). That is, a model may describe poorly the rate variation across X, Z_1, and Z_2 even if it describes adequately the rate variation across X and Z_1 when Z_2 is ignored. The decision as to whether the model is acceptable should depend on whether the rate variation across Z_2 is relevant to the analysis objectives. For example, if the objective is to estimate the effect of changes in X on the death rate, and Z_1 and Z_2 are both potential confounders (as in the tamoxifen example), we want the model to describe adequately the rate variation across all three variables. But if Z_2 is instead affected by the study exposure X (such as when X is past estrogen exposure and Z_2 is an indicator of current uterine bleeding), we usually will not want to include Z_2 in the regression model (because we will not want to adjust our exposure-effect estimate for Z_2).

Outcome Transformations

Suppose now that Y is quantitative (*e.g.*, CD4 count or diastolic blood pressure). In some settings, it may be desirable to transform the outcome prior to modeling using some function, say $h(Y)$, defined for all possible values of Y. One may wish to do this, for example, if the distribution of Y is highly skewed in which case the mean is less useful as a summary measure than, say, the median. In such settings, using the natural logarithm, that is using $h(Y) = \ln(Y)$, can reduce the skewness so that meaningful analysis can proceed by modeling: $E\left[h(Y) \middle| X = x, Z = z\right]$. Another somewhat more technical reason for using an outcome transformation is that the accuracy of standard error estimation can be improved; in the absence of a transformation, standard error estimates may be biased (particularly in small-sample settings) when the distribution of Y is highly skewed. For this reason, transformations such as the natural logarithm are sometimes called variance-stabilizing transformations.

An important consequence of transforming the outcome prior to modeling is that the interpretation of the component coefficients is fundamentally changed. Compare, for example, model 20-7 with the model:

$$E\left[\ln(Y) \middle| X = x\right] = \alpha + \beta x. \qquad [20\text{-}25]$$

Both are linear models in the sense that the right-hand side varies linearly as a function of x_1. However, the left-hand side of model 20-7 queries the average value of Y within subpopulations defined by X while the left-hand side of model 20-25 queries the average value of $ln(Y)$ within subpopulations defined by X. Thus, the numerical values of α and β in the two models are distinct, as are their interpretations and (in that sense) the conclusions that one can draw by fitting them.

GENERALIZED LINEAR MODELS

An alternative to transforming the outcome is to transform the regression, $E(Y | X = x, Z = z)$, itself. Crucially, in doing so, one leaves the interpretation of the final model in terms of the expectation of the original Y. To see this, consider again the exponential risk and rate models,

$$R(x,z) = \exp\left(\alpha + \beta_x x + z\boldsymbol{\beta}_z\right)$$

and

$$I(x,z) = \text{expit}\left(\alpha + \beta_x x + z\boldsymbol{\beta}_z\right)$$

and the logistic risk model,

$$R(x,z) = \text{expit}\left(\alpha + \beta_x x + z\boldsymbol{\beta}_z\right).$$

Each of these models is of the general form

$$E(Y | X = x, Z = z) = f\left(\alpha + \beta_x x + z\boldsymbol{\beta}_z\right) \qquad [20\text{-}26]$$

where $f(u)$ is a function that is smooth and strictly increasing as u increases. That is, as $\alpha + \beta_x x + z\beta_z$ gets larger, $f(\alpha + \beta_x x + z\beta_z)$ gets larger, but it never jumps or bends suddenly.

For any such smooth and strictly increasing function $f(u)$, one can define the inverse function $g(v)$ that "undoes" $f(u)$ in the sense that $g[f(u)] = u$ whenever $f(u)$ is defined. Hence, a general form that is equivalent to 20-26 is:

$$g\left[E(Y | X = x, Z = z)\right] = \alpha + \beta_x x + z\boldsymbol{\beta}_z \qquad [20\text{-}27]$$

A model of the form 20-27 is called *a generalized linear model*. The function $g(v)$ is called the *link function* for the model; thus, the link function is $\ln(v)$ for the log-linear model 20-9 and $\text{logit}(v)$ for the logit-linear model 20-13. The "$\alpha + \beta_x x + z\boldsymbol{\beta}_z$" term in 20-27 is called the *linear predictor* for the model and is often abbreviated by the Greek letter η (eta); that is, $\eta = \alpha + \beta_x x + z\boldsymbol{\beta}_z$, by definition.

Almost all the models in this chapter are generalized linear models. Ordinary linear models (such as the linear risk model) are the simplest examples, in which $f(u)$ and $g(v)$ are both the identity function, that is, $f(u) = u$ and $g(v) = v$, so that:

$$E\left(Y \mid X = x, \mathbf{Z} = z\right) = \alpha + \beta_x x + z\boldsymbol{\beta}_z$$

The inverse of the exponential function $\exp(u)$ is the natural log function $\ln(v)$. Hence the generalized linear model forms of the exponential risk and rate models are the log-linear risk and rate models:

$$\ln\left[R(x,z)\right] = \alpha + \beta_x x + z\boldsymbol{\beta}_z$$

and

$$\ln\left[I(x,z)\right] = \alpha + \beta_x x + z\boldsymbol{\beta}_z$$

respectively. Similarly, the inverse of the logistic function $\text{expit}(u)$ is the logit function $\text{logit}(v)$. Hence the generalized linear form of the logistic risk model is the logit-linear risk model:

$$\text{logit}\left[R(x,z)\right] = \alpha + \beta_x x + z\boldsymbol{\beta}_z.$$

Although f is required to be smooth and strictly increasing, there are many choices for the function. In epidemiology, however, the logit link $g(v) = \text{logit}(v)$ is in common use for risks while the log link $g(v) = \ln(v)$ is in common use for rates. These link functions are almost always the default in software implementations and are sometimes the only options in software for risk and rate modeling. Some packages, however, allow selection of linear risk, rate, or odds models, and some allow users to define their own link function.

The choice of link function can have a profound effect on the interpretation of model parameters. It also has a profound effect on the shape of the trend or dose-response surface allowed by the model, especially if exposure is represented by only one or two terms. For example, if exposure is represented by a single term $\beta_x x$ in a risk model, use of the identity link results in a linear risk model and a linear trend for risk; use of the log link results in an exponential (log-linear) risk model and an exponential trend for risk; and, use of a logit link results in a logistic model and an exponential trend for the odds.

Generalized linear models differ from transformed-outcome models in that they transform the regression (conditional expectation) of Y by a link function g before imposing linearity assumptions, rather than by transforming Y itself. The generalized linear forms 20-26 and 20-27 can therefore be applied to any type of outcome, including a discrete or continuous Y. They may even be combined with a transformation $h(Y)$ of Y to create a generalized linear model for the transformed outcome:

$$g\left\{E\left[h(Y) \mid X = x, \mathbf{Z} = z\right]\right\} = \alpha + \beta_x x + z\boldsymbol{\beta}_z.$$

Because of their great flexibility, generalized linear models encompass a much broader range of forms for risks and rates than the linear, log-linear, and logistic models. One example is the complementary log-log risk model:

$$R(x,z) = 1 - \exp\left[-\exp\left(\alpha + \beta_x x + z\boldsymbol{\beta}_z\right)\right]$$

which translates to the generalized linear form:

$$\ln\left\{-\ln\left[1 - R(x, z)\right]\right\} = \alpha + \beta_x x + z\beta_z.$$

This model corresponds to the link function $\ln[-\ln(1 - v)]$ and arises naturally in certain biology experiments.

For further reading on generalized linear models, see McCulloch and Nelder,[5] Hosmer and Lemeshow,[7] McCulloch et al,[9] Wakefield,[10] Faraway,[11] and Agresti.[12]

CATEGORICAL EXPOSURES

Consider a covariate whose possible values are discrete and few, and perhaps purely nominal (that is, with no natural ordering or quantitative meaning). An example is marital status which may take on levels: never married, currently married, or formerly married. Such covariates may be entered into a multiple-regression model using *category indicator variables*. Toward this, there are many options; here we describe two.

Disjoint Category Coding

When using disjoint category coding, we first choose one level of the covariate as the *reference level* against which we want to compare risks or rates. For each of the remaining levels, we create a binary variable to indicate whether a person is at that level (1 if at the level, 0 if not). One can then enter these indicators into the regression model as individual covariates.

The entire set of indicators is called the *coding* of the original covariate. As an example, to code the marital status variable described above, assuming it is the exposure of interest, we can take "currently married" as the reference level and define:

$X_1 = 1$ if formerly married, 0 if currently or never married; and,
$X_2 = 1$ if never married, 0 if currently or formerly married (*i.e.*, ever married).

An important point is that knowing the marital status of an individual requires knowing the numerical value of *both* indicators: $(X_1, X_2) = (0, 0)$ indicates that the individual was "currently married" at the time of data collection; $(X_1, X_2) = (1, 0)$ indicates that the individual was "formerly married"; and, $(X_1, X_2) = (0, 1)$ indicates that the individual was "never married." Note, while there are $2 \times 2 = 4$ possible numerical combinations of values for X_1 and X_2, only three of them are logically possible. The combination $(X_1, X_2) = (1, 1)$ is logically impossible because an individual cannot be formerly married (*i.e.*, $X_1 = 1$) and never married (*i.e.*, $X_2 = 1$) at the same time.

More generally, we need $J - 1$ indicators to code a variable with J levels. Although these indicators will have 2^{J-1} possible numerical combinations, only J of these combinations will be logically possible. For example, we need four indicators to code a variable with five levels. These indicators have $2^4 = 16$ numerical combinations, but only 5 of the 16 combinations will be logically possible.

Interpretation of the indicator coefficients depends on the model form and the chosen coding. For example, in the logistic model

$$R(x_1, x_2) = \text{expit}(\alpha + \beta_1 x_1 + \beta_2 x_2) \tag{20-28}$$

$\exp(\beta_2)$ is the odds ratio comparing $X_2 = 1$ persons (never married) to $X_2 = 0$ persons (ever married) within levels of X_1. Because one cannot have $X_2 = 1$ (never married) and $X_1 = 1$ (formerly married), the only level of X_1 within which we can compare $X_2 = 1$ to $X_2 = 0$ is the zero level (never or currently married). Thus, $\exp(\beta_2)$ is the odds ratio comparing never married ($X_2 = 1$) with currently married ($X_2 = 0$) people among those never or currently married ($X_1 = 0$). In a similar fashion, $\exp(\beta_1)$ compares those formerly married with those currently married among those ever married.

Nested Indicator Coding

A different kind of coding is *nested indicator coding* in which levels of the covariate are grouped, and then codes are created to facilitate comparisons both within and across groups. For example, suppose we wish to compare those not currently married (never or formerly married) with those currently married, and also compare those never married with those formerly married. We can then use the indicators:

$X_1^* = 1$ if never or formerly married (*i.e.*, not currently married), 0 otherwise (currently married); and,

$X_2^* = 1$ if never married, 0 if ever married.

Note, X_2^* is the same as the X_2 used above, although X_1^* is different from X_1. The combination $X_1^* = 0$ (currently married) and $X_2^* = 1$ (never married) is impossible, while the coding $X_1^* = X_2^* = 1$ will be used for people who never married. In the logistic model

$$R\left(x_1^*, x_2^*\right) = \operatorname{expit}\left(a + \beta_1 x_1^* + \beta_2 x_2^*\right) \qquad [20\text{-}29]$$

$\exp(\beta_2)$ is now the odds ratio comparing those never married $\left(X_2^* = 1\right)$ with those ever married $\left(X_2^* = 0\right)$ among those not currently married $\left(X_1^* = 1\right)$. Similarly, $\exp(\beta_1)$ is now the odds ratio comparing those formerly married $\left(X_1^* = 1\right)$ with those currently married $\left(X_1^* = 0\right)$ among those ever married $\left(X_2^* = 0\right)$.

Choosing the Referent Category

As indicated, beyond the choices considered in models 20-28 and 20-29, there can be many options for coding category indicators. The choice among these options may be dictated by which comparisons are of most interest. As long as each level of the covariate can be uniquely represented by the indicator coding, the choice of coding will not alter the assumptions represented by the model nor the overall fit of the model (see Chapter 21). There is, however, one technical point to consider in choosing codes. The precision of the estimated coefficient for an indicator depends directly on the numbers of subjects at each indicator level. For example, suppose that in the data there are 1,000 currently married subjects, 200 formerly married subjects, and only 10 never married subjects. Then an indicator that has "never married" as one of its levels (0 or 1) has a much less precise coefficient estimate than other indicators. If "never married" is chosen as the reference level for a disjoint coding scheme, all the indicators will have that level as their zero level, and so all will have very imprecise coefficient estimates. To maximize precision, many analysts prefer to use disjoint coding in which the largest category (currently married in the preceding example) is taken as the reference level.

In choosing a coding scheme, one should not let precision concerns prevent one from making interesting comparisons. Coding schemes that distinguish among the same categories produce equivalent models. Therefore, one may fit a model repeatedly using different but equivalent coding schemes, in order to easily examine all comparisons of interest. For example, one could fit model 20-28 to compare those never or formerly married with those currently married, then fit model 20-29 to compare the never with formerly married.

CONTINUOUS EXPOSURES

Now consider a covariate that is, in principle at least, continuous. In the running tamoxifen example, Z_2, which represents the age at menarche, is such a variable. In this section we outline a number of issues related to modeling continuous covariates. Although the issues arise in all models, for simplicity we consider them in the context of the linear risk model for $E\left(Y \mid X = x\right)$ given by model 20-7 and, for convenience, is repeated here:

$$R(x) = \alpha + \beta x.$$

Recentering

Under model 20-7, the risk for the subpopulation with $X = 0$ is

$$R(0) = \alpha + \beta \times 0 = \alpha,$$

so that α can be interpreted as the risk in the subpopulation defined by "$X = 0$." Thus, if α is to have a meaningful interpretation, one must have that the population defined by "$X = 0$" be meaningful. In the tamoxifen example, $X = 0$ represents "no tamoxifen use" so that the parameter α represents the risk in that (well-defined) population. Now consider the alternative linear risk model

$$R(z_2) = \alpha + \beta_2 z_2,$$

where, as before, Z_2 is age at menarche. Because age at menarche cannot equal 0, however, α in this model has no meaningful interpretation.

One approach to mitigating this problem is to recenter the variable, that is, subtract some value, so that is $Z_2 = 0$ is rendered meaningful. For example, age 13 is a frequently observed value for age at menarche. We can redefine Z_2 to be "age at menarche minus 13 years." With this redefinition, $R(z_2) = \alpha + \beta_2 z_2$ refers to a different model, one in which $R(0) = \alpha$ represents the average risk for women who were age 13 at menarche. We will see later that such recentering is advisable when using any model, and it is especially important when product terms ("interactions") are used in a model.

Rescaling

A simple way of describing β in model 20-7 is that it is the difference in risk per unit increase in X. In this sense it is a slope parameter. Often the units used to measure X are small, relative to exposure increases of substantive interest. Suppose, for example, that X is diastolic blood pressure (DBP) measured in mm Hg; β is then the risk difference per millimeter increase in DBP. A 1-mm Hg increase, however, will be of no clinical interest; instead, we will want to consider increases of at least 5 and possibly 10 or 20 mm Hg. Under model 20-7, the difference in risk per 10 mm Hg increase is 10β. If we want to have β represent the difference in risk per 10 mm Hg, we need only redefine X as DBP divided by 10; X will then be DBP in cm Hg.

Division of a variable by a constant, as just described, is sometimes called *rescaling* of the variable. Such rescaling is advisable whenever it changes the measurement unit to a more meaningful value. It is sometimes the case that analysts rescale a variable by dividing it by its standard deviation in the sample. Unfortunately, this can sometimes make the measurement unit *less* meaningful since the sample standard deviation is an irregular unit that is unique to the study data and, as such, depends heavily on how subjects were selected into the analysis. For example, the standard deviation of DBP might be 12.7 mm Hg in one study and 15.3 mm Hg in another study. Suppose that each study divides DBP by its standard deviation before entering it in model 20-7. In the first study, β refers to the change in risk per 12.7 mm Hg increase in DBP, whereas in the second study, β refers to the change in risk per 15.3 mm Hg. Rescaling by the standard deviation thus renders the coefficients interpretable only in peculiar and different units so that they cannot be compared directly with one another or to coefficients from other studies. Correspondingly, methods that involve division by sample standard deviations (such as transformations of variables to Z-scores) should often be avoided.[16,17] Of course, simply providing the standard deviation within the sample entirely alleviates this issue. Moreover, for scales which readers are not familiar with (*e.g.*, certain psychosocial measures), rescaling by standard deviations may make the interpretation more straightforward for many readers; and, provided the standard deviation is given, results can be easily reconverted to the original scale. Similar considerations pertain to rescaling of continuous outcomes. When the relationships between a single exposure and numerous continuous outcomes are examined simultaneously, rescaling of outcomes by standard deviations can give some indication as to which outcomes are most affected by the exposure[18]; but it should again always be kept in mind that such rescaling is relative to the sample under consideration. Furthermore, noting that what is best may vary by context, we recommend that rescaling be done using simple and easily interpreted constants for the division.

Transformations

Consider again the linear risk model given by expression 20-7. If this model is correct, a plot of average risk across the subpopulations defined by X (that is, a plot of risk against X) will yield a straight line. In many instances, however, there may be no compelling reason to think that $E(Y|X = x)$ varies linearly as a function of x; that is, that model 20-7 correctly represents the trend as a function of X. We may, therefore, wish to entertain other models for the trend in risk across exposure levels. One option is to *transform* the exposure, that is, replace X in the model with some function of X.

To illustrate, suppose x on the right-hand side in model 20-7 is replaced with $\ln(x)$ to give:

$$R(x) = \alpha + \beta \ln(x). \qquad \text{[20-30]}$$

Note, the left-hand side remains unchanged in that model 20-30 remains a model for $E(Y|X = x)$. Furthermore, model 20-30 still defines a linear risk model, because a plot of average risk against the new covariate [*i.e.*, $\ln(X)$] will yield a line. It is a very different linear model from model 20-7, however, because if model 20-30 is correct, a plot of average risk against years exposed [*i.e.*, against X instead of $\ln(X)$] will yield a *logarithmic curve* rather than a line. Such a curve starts off very steep for $X < 1$ but it levels off rapidly beyond $X > 1$.

A technical problem when using the logarithmic transform is that it is not defined if X is negative or zero. If the original exposure measurement can be negative or zero, it is common practice to add a number c to X that is big enough to ensure that $X + c$ is always positive. The resulting model is:

$$R(x) = \alpha + \beta ln(x + c).$$

Unfortunately, the shape of the curve represented by this model (and hence results derived using the model) can be very sensitive to the value chosen for c, especially when the values of X may be less than 1. Frequently, c is set equal to 1, although there is usually no compelling reason for this choice.

Among other possibilities for exposure transforms are simple power curves of the form:

$$R(x) = \alpha + \beta x^p \qquad \text{[20-31]}$$

where p is some number (typically ½ or 2) chosen in advance according to some desired property. For example, with X as years exposed, use of $p = 1/2$ yields the *square root* model:

$$R(x) = \alpha + \beta x^{1/2},$$

which produces a trend curve that levels off as X increases above zero. In contrast, use of $p = 2$ yields the simple *quadratic* model:

$$R(x) = \alpha + \beta x^2$$

which produces a trend that becomes steeper as X moves away from zero.

Similar to problems with negative or zero values of X when one uses a logarithm transformation, when using the power model 20-31, one must take care if p is fractional and X can be negative. To get around this limitation, we may add some number c to X_1 that is big enough to ensure that $X+c$ is never negative, and then use $(x + c)^p$ in the model; nonetheless, as with using this approach with a logarithmic transformation, the result may be sensitive to the choice of c.

The trend implications of linear and exponential models are vastly different, and hence the implications of exposure transforms are also different. Consider again the exponential risk model (Equation 20-8) repeated here for convenience:

$$R(x) = \exp(\alpha + \beta x).$$

If this model is correct, a plot of average risk against X will yield an exponential curve rather than a line. If β is positive, this curve starts out slowly but rises more and more rapidly as X increases; it eventually rises more rapidly than does any power curve (Equation 20-31). Such rapid increase is often implausible, and we may wish to use a slower-rising curve to model risk.

One means of moderating the trend implied by an exponential model is to replace x by a fixed power, that is, x^p, with $0 < p < 1$, for example,

$$R(x) = \exp\left(\alpha + \beta x^{1/2}\right).$$

Another approach is to take the logarithm of exposure which produces the model:

$$R(x) = \exp\left[\alpha + \beta \ln(x)\right] = \exp(\alpha)\exp\left[\beta \ln(x)\right] = \exp(\alpha)\left\{\exp\left[\ln(x)\right]\right\}^{\beta} = \exp(\alpha)x^{\beta}. \quad [20\text{-}32]$$

A graph of risk against exposure under this model produces a power curve, but now (unlike model 20-31) the power is the unspecified (unknown) coefficient β instead of a prespecified value p, and the multiplier of the exposure power is $\exp(\alpha)$ (which must be positive) instead of β. Model 20-32 may thus appear to be more appropriate than model 20-31 when we want the power of X to appear as an unknown coefficient β in the model, rather than as a prespecified value p. As earlier, however, X must always be positive in order to use model 20-32; otherwise, we must add a constant c to it such that $X + c$ is always positive.

When β is negative in model 20-32, risk declines more and more gradually across increasingly exposed subpopulations. For example, if $\beta = -1$, then under model 20-32, $R(x) = R(x) = \exp(\alpha)x^{-1} = \exp(\alpha)/x$, which implies that risk declines 50% [from $\exp(\alpha)/1$ to $\exp(\alpha)/2$] when going from $X = 1$ to $X = 2$, but declines less than 10% [from $\exp(\alpha)/10$ to $\exp(\alpha)/11$] when going from $X = 10$ to $X = 11$.

The exposure transforms and implications just discussed carry over to the analogous models for odds and rates. For example, we can modify the logistic model (which is an exponential odds model) by substituting the odds $O(x)$ for the risk $R(x)$ in models 20-30 to 20-32. Similarly, we can modify the rate models by substituting the rate $I(x)$ for $R(x)$. Each model will have implications for the odds or rates analogous to those described earlier for the risk; because the risks, odds, and rates are functions of one another (Chapter 4), each model will have implications for other measures as well.

Any trend in the odds will appear more gradual when transformed into a risk trend. To see this, note that:

$$R(x) = O(x)/\left[1 + O(x)\right] < O(x)$$

and, hence, that:

$$O(x)/R(x) = 1 + O(x).$$

From this we see that the ratio of odds to risk grows as the odds (and the risks) get larger. Thus, the logistic risk model implies a less than exponential trend in the risk. Conversely, any trend in the risks will appear steeper when transformed into an odds trend. Thus, the exponential risk model implies a greater than exponential trend in the odds. When all the risks are low (say less than 10% for all possible X values), however, the risks and odds will be similar and so there will be little difference between the shape of the curves produced by analogous risk and odds models.

The relation of risk and odds trends to rate trends is, in general, more complex but in typical applications follows the simple rule that rate trends tend to fall between the less steep risk and more steep odds trends. For example, an exponential rate model typically implies a less than exponential risk trend but more than exponential odds trend. To see why these relations can be reasonable to expect, from Chapter 4 if incidence is measured over a span of time Δt in a closed population, then $R(x) < I(x)\,\Delta t < O(x)$. When the risks are uniformly low, we obtain $R(x) \approx I(x)\Delta t \approx O(x)$, and so there will be little difference in the curves produced by analogous risk, rate, and odds models.

Interpreting Models After Transformation

One drawback of models with transformed covariates is that the interpretation of the coefficients depends on the transformation. As an example, consider the model 20-32, which has $\ln(x)$ in place of x. Under this model, the risk ratio for a one-unit increase in X is:

$$R(x+1)/R(x) = \exp(\alpha)(x+1)^\beta / \exp(\alpha)x^\beta = \left[(x+1)/x\right]^\beta$$

which will depend on the value x used as the reference level: If $\beta = 1$ and x is 1, the risk ratio is 2, but if $\beta = 1$ and x is 2, the ratio is 1.5. Here, β is the power to which x is raised, and so it determines the shape of the trend. The interpretation of the intercept α is also altered by the transformation. Under model 20-32, $R(1) = \exp(\alpha)1^\beta = \exp(\alpha)$; thus, α is the log risk when $X = 1$, rather than when $X = 0$, and so is meaningful only if 1 is a possible value for X.

As a contrast, consider again the model $R(x) = \exp(\alpha + \beta x^{1/2})$. Use of $x^{1/2}$ rather than x moderates the rapid increase in the slope of the exponential dose-response curve, but it also leads to difficulties in coefficient interpretation. Under this model, the risk ratio for a 1-unit increase in X (*i.e.*, comparing $X = x + 1$ to $X = x$) is:

$$\exp\left[\alpha + \beta(x+1)^{1/2}\right] / \exp\left(\alpha + \beta x^{1/2}\right) = \exp\left\{\beta\left[(x+1)^{1/2} - x^{1/2}\right]\right\}.$$

Here, β is the log risk ratio per unit increase in the *square root* of X, which is rather obscure in meaning. Interpretation may proceed better by considering the shape of the curve implied by the model, for example, by plotting $\exp(\alpha + \beta x^{1/2})$ against possible values of X for several values of β. Note, the intercept α is less important in this model because it determines only the vertical scale of the curve rather than its shape. Such plotting is often needed to understand and compare different transforms.

Power Models

A more expansive approach to trend analysis (and confounder control) is to use multiple power terms for each covariate. Traditionally, the powers used are positive integers (*e.g.*, x, x^2, x^3), but fractional powers may also be used.[19] As an illustration, suppose that X represents the number of servings of fruits and vegetables per week. We can model trends across this covariate by using X in the model along with $X^{1/2}$, which is the square root of X, and X^2, which is the square of X, to give the following *fractional polynomial* model:

$$\ln\left[I(x)\right] = \alpha + \beta_1 x + \beta_2 x^{1/2} + \beta_3 x^2. \tag{20-33}$$

Note, we could equivalently represent model 20-33 as multiple log-linear rate regression model by setting X_1 to be the exposure of interest and then defining $X_2 = X_1^{1/2}$ and $X_3 = X_1^2$ to give:

$$\ln\left[I(x_1, x_2, x_3)\right] = \alpha + \beta_1 x_1 + \beta_2 x_2 + \beta_3 x_3.$$

While the individual coefficients in model 20-33 are difficult to interpret, one can plot fitted rates from this model using very narrow spacing to produce *a smooth curve* as an estimate of rate trends across X. As always, we may also include confounders in the model and plot model-adjusted trends. One disadvantage of power models is the potential sensitivity of estimates to *outliers*, that is, persons with unusual values or unusual *combinations* of values for the covariates. This problem can be addressed by performing model diagnostics that examine the influence of individual contributions to estimates (Chapter 21).

Categorization

While power models provide useful flexibility in modeling trends, as mentioned it is often difficult to interpret individual coefficients. While graphical representations of effect measures (such as the relative rate associated with a unit increase in X in model 20-33) can be reported, the model is not structured to enable simple and easy-to-communicate effect measures. An alternative is to categorize the covariate category indicator coding such as discussed earlier. The resulting analysis may then parallel the categorical (tabular) trend methods discussed in Chapter 19. Much of the advice given there also applies here. Specifically, to the extent allowed by background information and the sample size, the categories should represent scientifically meaningful constructs within which risk is not expected to change dramatically. Purely mathematical categorization methods such as percentiles (quantiles) can do very poorly in this regard and so are best avoided when prior risk information is available.[20,21] On the other hand, the choices of categories should *not* be dictated by the results produced; for example, manipulation of category boundaries to maximize the effect estimate will produce an estimate that is biased away from the null, whereas manipulation of boundaries to minimize a P-value will produce a downwardly biased P-value. Similarly, manipulation to minimize the estimate or maximize the P-value will produce a null-biased estimate or an upwardly biased P-value.

As a concrete example, we return to the exposure of the number of weekly servings of fruits and vegetables, and suppose the cut points of 15, 36, and 42 servings have been chosen. Taking the "15 to 35" category as the referent, one example of a disjoint category coding is to take:

X_1 = 1 if the number of servings is <15 per week, 0 otherwise;
X_2 = 1 if the number of servings is between 36 and 41 per week, 0 otherwise; and,
X_3 = 1 if the number of servings is ≥42 per week, 0 otherwise.

Using these in the log-linear rate model:

$$\ln\left[I\left(x_1, x_2, x_3\right)\right] = \alpha + \beta_1 x_1 + \beta_2 x_2 + \beta_3 x_3 \qquad [20\text{-}34]$$

we have that $\exp(\beta_1)$ is the rate ratio comparing the "<15" category with the referent "15 to 35" category, and so on, whereas $\exp(\alpha)$ is the rate in the "15 to 35" category (since this category is identified when all the X_j are 0). When model 20-34 is fit, we can plot the fitted rates on a graph as a step function. This plot provides a crude impression of the trends across (but not within) categories.

To illustrate the use of nested indicator coding, consider:

X_1^* = 1 if the number of servings is ≥ 15 per week, 0 otherwise;
X_2^* = 1 if the number of servings is ≥ 36 per week, 0 otherwise; and,
X_3^* = 1 if the number of servings is ≥ 42 per week, 0 otherwise.

Note that if $X_2^* = 1$, then $X_1^* = 1$, and if $X_3^* = 1$, then $X_1^* = 1$ and $X_2^* = 1$. Using these in the log-linear rate model:

$$\ln\left[I\left(x_1^*, x_2^*, x_3^*\right)\right] = \alpha + \beta_1 x_1^* + \beta_2 x_2^* + \beta_3 x_3^*$$

$\exp(\beta_1)$ is the rate ratio comparing the "15 to 35" category ($X_1^* = 1$ and $X_2^* = X_3^* = 0$) to the "<15" category ($X_1^* = X_2^* = X_3^* = 0$). Similarly, $\exp(\beta_2)$ is the rate ratio comparing the "36 to 42" category ($X_1^* = X_2^* = 1$ and $X_3^* = 0$) to the "15 to 35" category ($X_1^* = 1$ and $X_2^* = X_3^* = 0$). Finally, $\exp(\beta_3)$ compares the ">42" category ($X_1^* = X_2^* = X_3^* = 1$) to the "36 to 42" category ($X_1^* = X_2^* = 1$ and $X_3^* = 0$). Thus, $\exp(\beta_1)$, $\exp(\beta_2)$, and $\exp(\beta_3)$ are the incremental rate ratios across adjacent categories. Again, we may add confounders to the model and plot adjusted trends.

As a final note on categorizing variables, a common practice in epidemiology is to assign a score to each category and then enter scores into the model instead of the original variable values. The issues involved in assigning such scores were discussed in Chapter 19 under the heading, "Horizontal Scaling and Category Scores" in the "Dose-Response and Trend Analysis" section.

Briefly, using ordinal scores or codes (*e.g.*, 1, 2, 3, 4, 5 for a series of five categories) in this way should be avoided, as they can yield quantitatively meaningless dose-response curves and harm the power and precision of the results.[21-23] Category midpoints can be much less distortive but are not defined for open-ended categories; category means or medians can be even less distortive and are defined for open-ended categories. Unfortunately, if there are important nonlinear effects within categories, no simple scoring method will yield an undistorted dose-response curve, nor will it achieve the power and precision obtainable by entering the uncategorized covariates into the model.[21,23] We thus recommend that categories be kept narrow and that scores be derived from category means or medians, rather than from midpoints or ordinal scores. We further recommend that one also examine models using the covariates in their uncategorized (continuous) form whenever associations are clearly present.

Regression Splines

Finally, it is often possible to combine the advantages of categorical and power models through the use of *spline models*. Such models can be defined in a number of equivalent ways, and we present only the simplest. In all approaches, one first categorizes the covariate, as in categorical analysis (although fewer, broader categories may be sufficient in a spline model). The boundaries between these categories are called the *knots* or *join points* of the spline. Next, one chooses the *power* (or order) of the spline, according to the flexibility one desires within the categories (higher powers allow more flexibility).

Use of category indicators corresponds to a zero-power spline, in which the trend is flat within categories but may jump suddenly at the knots; thus, category indicator models are just special types of spline models. In a first-power or *linear* spline, the trend is modeled by a series of connected line segments. The trend within each category corresponds to a line segment; the slope of the trend may change only at the knots, and no sudden jump in risk (discontinuity in trend) can occur.

To illustrate how a linear spline may be represented, let X_1 again be "number of servings per week" and define:

$X_2 = X_1 - 14$ if $X_1 \geq 15$ per week, 0 otherwise; and
$X_3 = X_1 - 35$ if $X_1 \geq 36$ per week, 0 otherwise.

Using these in the log-linear rate model:

$$\ln\left[I\left(x_1, x_2, x_3\right)\right] = \alpha + \beta_1 x_1 + \beta_2 x_2 + \beta_3 x_3 \qquad [20\text{-}35]$$

produces a log rate trend that is a series of three line segments that are connected at the knots (category boundaries) of 14 and 35. To see this, note that for any value of X_1 that is less than 15 (*i.e.*, 0-14), X_2 and X_3 are both 0, so that model 20-35 simplifies to a line with slope β_1:

$$\ln\left[I\left(x_1, x_2, x_3\right)\right] = \alpha + \beta_1 x_1.$$

That is, model 20-35 over values of X_1 between 0 and 14 simplifies to one that is solely a function of which X_1 and for which the slope is β_1. When X_1 is greater than 14 but less than 36, the model simplifies from expression 20-35 to:

$$\ln\left[I\left(x_1, x_2, x_3\right)\right] = \alpha + \beta_1 x_1 + \beta_2\left(x_1 - 14\right) = \alpha - \beta_2 14 + \left(\beta_1 + \beta_2\right)x_1.$$

That is, model 20-35 over values of X_1 between 15 and 35 simplifies to one that is solely a function of which X_1 and for which the slope is $\beta_1 + \beta_2$. Finally, when X_1 is greater than 35, model 20-35 becomes:

$$\ln\left[I\left(x_1, x_2, x_3\right)\right] = \alpha + \beta_1 x_1 + \beta_2\left(x_1 - 14\right) + \beta_3\left(x_1 - 35\right) = \alpha - \beta_2 14 - \beta_3 35 + \left(\beta_1 + \beta_2 + \beta_3\right)x_1.$$

That is, model 20-35 over values of X_1 between 15 and 35 simplifies to one that is solely a function of which X_1 and for which the slope is $\beta_1 + \beta_2 + \beta_3$. Furthermore, in considering the sequence of models across the intervals defined by the categorization, we see that β_1 is the slope of the spline in the first category; β_2 is the change in slope in going from the first to the second category; and β_3 is the change in slope in going from the second to the third category.

The pattern produced by a linear spline will likely be more realistic than a categorical trend, but it has the drawback of specifying a trend where there are sudden changes in the slope at the knots. To smooth out such sudden changes, we may increase the order of the spline. Increasing the power to 2 produces a *quadratic* spline, which comprises a series of parabolic curve segments smoothly joined together at the knots. To illustrate how such a trend may be represented, let $X_1, X_2,$ and X_3 be as just defined. Then the model

$$\ln\left[I\left(x_1, x_2, x_3\right)\right] = \alpha + \beta_1 x_1 + \gamma_1 x_1^2 + \gamma_2 x_2^2 + \gamma_3 x_3^2 \qquad [20\text{-}36]$$

will produce a log rate trend that is a series of three parabolic segments smoothly connected at the knots of 14 and 35. The coefficient γ_1 corresponds to the curvature of the trend in the first category, while γ_2 and γ_3 correspond to the changes in curvature when going from the first to the second category and from the second to the third category. A still smoother curve, and often popular approach, is obtained by using a *cubic* spline.

One disadvantage of quadratic and cubic splines is that the curves in the end categories (tails) may become very unstable, especially if the category is open-ended. This instability may be reduced by *restricting* one or both of the end categories to be a line segment rather than a curve. To restrict the lower category to be linear in a quadratic spline, we need to only remove the *first* quadratic term, that is, $\gamma_1 x_1^2$, from the model. To restrict the upper category, we must subtract the *last* quadratic term from all the quadratic terms; in doing so, we must remove the last term from the model because it will be 0 after the subtraction.

To illustrate an upper category restriction, suppose we wish to restrict the above quadratic spline model for log rates 20-36 so that it is linear in the upper category only. Toward this, define:

$X_1^* = X_1$, that is the number of servings per week;
$X_2^* = X_1^2 - X_3^2$; and,
$X_3^* = X_2^2 - X_3^2$.

Using these in the log-linear rate model

$$\ln\left[I\left(x_1^*, x_2^*, x_3^*\right)\right] = \alpha + \beta_1 x_1^* + \beta_2 x_2^* + \beta_3 x_3^* \qquad [20\text{-}37]$$

will produce a log rate trend that comprises smoothly connected parabolic segments in the first two categories ("<14" and "15-35") and a line segment in the last category (">35") that is smoothly connected to the parabolic segment in the second category. (If we also wanted to force the log rate curve in the first category to follow a line, we would remove X_2^* from the model.)

To plot or tabulate the curve from a spline model, we select a set of X_1 values spaced across the range of interest, compute the set of spline terms for each X_1 value, combine these terms with the coefficients in the model to get the model-predicted outcomes, and plot these predictions. To illustrate, suppose that X_1 is servings per week and we wish to plot model 20–37 with $\alpha = -6.00$, $\beta_1 = -0.010$, $\beta_2 = -0.001$, and $\beta_3 = 0.001$ over the range 0 to 50 servings per week in 5-serving increments. We then compute $\left(X_1^*, X_2^*, X_3^*\right)$ at 0, 5, 10,..., 50 servings per week, compute the predicted rate

$$\exp\left(-6.00 - 0.010 x_1^* - 0.001 x_2^* + 0.001 x_3^*\right)$$

at each set of $\left(X_1^*, X_2^*, X_3^*\right)$ values, and, finally, plot these predictions against the corresponding X_1 values 0, 5, 10,..., 50. For example, at $X_1 = 40$, we get $X_1^* = 40$, $X_2^* = 40^2 - (40 - 35)^2 = 1{,}575$, and $X_3^* = (40 - 14)^2 - (40 - 35)^2 = 651$, for a predicted rate of

$$\exp\left[-6.00 - 0.010(40) - 0.001(1{,}575) + 0.001(651)\right] = 0.00066$$

or 6.6 per 10,000 person-years.

As with other trend models, we may obtain model-adjusted trends by adding confounder terms to our spline models. The confounder terms may be splines or any other form we prefer; spline plotting will be simplified, however, if the confounders are centered before they are entered into the analysis, for then the above plotting method may be used without modification. Further discussions of splines and their application are given by Wahba,[24] De Boor,[25] and Hastie et al.[26]

POLYTOMOUS OUTCOMES

Suppose that the outcome variable, Y, is polytomous in that it can take on one of $J+1$ mutually exclusive categories or levels, specifically, $y_0, \ldots, y_J$. The second part of Table 19-5 in Chapter 19 provides an example in which Y is a disease outcome variable, with y_0 = all control diseases as the reference category and $J = 7$ other categories corresponding to the cancer outcomes listed in the table. This outcome may be labeled as an *unordered* polytomous outcome, in the sense that there is no natural progression across the cancer types. For other polytomous outcomes, the categories $y_0, \ldots, y_J$ may be naturally ordered, such as is the case for any variable measured on a Likert scale (which takes on values of "strongly disagree," "disagree," "neither disagree or agree," "agree," or "strongly agree") or for categorical scales such as the Inpatient Multidimensional Psychiatric Scale item 79, which measures severity of schizophrenia illness, with values: 0 = "no illness," 1 = "borderline mentally ill," …, and, 7 = "among the most extremely ill". Such outcomes are often labeled as being *ordinal*.

Polytomous outcomes, as with continuous outcomes, are often analyzed by reducing them to just two categories and applying, say, a logistic model. The cancer outcomes in Table 19-5, for example, might be reduced to a dichotomous outcome of cancer versus no cancer. Alternatively, multiple categories may be created with one designated as a referent, and the other categories compared one at a time to the referent using separate logistic models for each comparison. Although they are not necessarily invalid, these approaches disregard the information contained in differences within categories, in differences between nonreference categories, and in ordering among the categories. As a result, models designed specifically for polytomous outcomes can yield far more precision and power than simple dichotomous outcome analyses.

Let $R_j(x, z)$ denote the average risk of falling in outcome category y_j $(j = 0,1,\ldots, J)$ given exposure X is x and adjustment variables Z take on values z; that is, let

$$R_j(x,z) = P\left(Y = y_j \middle| X = x, Z = z\right).$$

Several points are worth making. First, that $J+1$ risks must be specified for a single outcome represents an important departure from the material presented so far in this chapter. Second, when specifying models for the $J+1$ risks, one must take care to ensure that they each are between 0 and 1 for all levels of x and z. Otherwise, one could end up with nonsensical results where one or more of the risks are either negative or greater than 1. Finally, assuming that the $J+1$ levels correspond to the totality of all outcomes relevant to the study at hand, the sum of the $R_j(x, z)$ must add up to 1. Thus, care is needed when specifying and fitting models for polytomous outcomes to ensure that this constraint is satisfied for all values of $(X = x, Z = z)$.

Polytomous Logistic Models

One approach to ensuring that for any given value of $(X = x, Z = z)$, each of the risks is between 0 and 1 and that the total across the $J+1$ levels equals 1 is to fit a *polytomous logistic model*. Doing so involves specification of a referent outcome level and then specifying models for the remaining J levels. Generically, we take the referent level to be y_0 and note that the specific choice will need to be context specific although will often entail the notion of "no disease" or a collection of "control diseases" (as in Table 19-5). For the remaining J levels, $y_1, \ldots, y_J$, consider the following model for the risk:

$$R_j(x,z) = \frac{\exp\left(\alpha_j + \beta_{j,x}x + z\boldsymbol{\beta}_{j,z}\right)}{1 + \sum_{l=1}^{J}\exp\left(\alpha_l + \beta_{l,x}x + z\boldsymbol{\beta}_{l,z}\right)}. \qquad [20\text{-}38]$$

Note, the set of equations given by expression 20-38 involve J intercepts, specifically the α_j, and J coefficients for X, specifically the $\beta_{j,x}$, and J vectors of coefficients for Z, specifically $\boldsymbol{\beta}_{j,z} = (\beta_{j,1}, \ldots, \beta_{j,p})$. Thus, with p covariates in Z, the polytomous logistic model 20-38 involves $J \times (1 + 1 + p)$ model parameters. For example, with seven nonreference outcome levels, an exposure, and three adjustment factors, the model would involve $7 \times 5 = 35$ model parameters.

One important feature of expression 20-38 is that each of the J $R_j(x, z)$ is between 0 and 1. To see this, note that exponentiating any number yields a positive number. Thus, both the numerator and denominator of 20-38 are positive so that their ratio cannot be negative. Furthermore, since the numerator, $\exp(\alpha_j + \beta_{j,x} + z\boldsymbol{\beta}_{j,z})$, is a component of the summation in the denominator, the denominator must always be bigger than the numerator. Thus, the ratio cannot be greater than 1.

Using the J models given by expression 20-38, one can derive the induced risk for the referent category by noting that it must equal 1 minus the sum of the risks of falling in the nonreference categories. That is, we have:

$$R_0(x,z) = P(Y = y_0 | X = x, Z = z) = 1 - \sum_{j=1}^{J} P(Y = y_j | X = x, Z = z) = 1 - \sum_{j=1}^{J} \frac{\exp(\alpha_j + \beta_{j,x} + z\boldsymbol{\beta}_{j,z})}{1 + \sum_{l=1}^{J} \exp(\alpha_l + \beta_{l,x} + z\boldsymbol{\beta}_{l,z})}$$

$$= 1 - \frac{\sum_{j=1}^{J} \exp(\alpha_j + \beta_{j,x} + z\boldsymbol{\beta}_{j,z})}{1 + \sum_{l=1}^{J} \exp(\alpha_l + \beta_{l,x} + z\boldsymbol{\beta}_{l,z})} = \frac{1}{1 + \sum_{l=1}^{J} \exp(\alpha_l + \beta_{l,x} + z\boldsymbol{\beta}_{l,z})}. \qquad [20\text{-}39]$$

It is immediate, using the same arguments as those above, that $R_0(x, z)$ is between 0 and 1, and that the sum of the $R_j(x, z)$ across the $J + 1$ levels is equal to 1.

Toward interpreting the components of the model given by expression 20-38, we consider the odds of falling in outcome category y_j versus the referent category y_0, that is, $O_j(x,z) = R_j(x,z)/R_0(x,z)$. Dividing Equations 20-38 by 20-39, we arrive at the following induced model for these odds:

$$O_j(x,z) = \exp(\alpha_j + \beta_{j,x}x + z\boldsymbol{\beta}_{j,z}).$$

Thus, the polytomous logistic model given by 20-38 induces an exponential model for the odds of falling in outcome category y_j versus the referent category. A benefit of writing the model in this form is that it provides a familiar interpretation for the covariate coefficients. Specifically, suppose (x^*, z) and (x, z) are two different vectors of values for the covariates (X, Z). Then the ratio of the odds of falling in category y_j versus y_0 comparing $X = x^*$ to $X = x$ within levels z of Z is:

$$\frac{O_j(x^*,z)}{O_j(x,z)} = \frac{\exp(\alpha_j + \beta_{j,x}x^* + z\boldsymbol{\beta}_{j,z})}{\exp(\alpha_j + \beta_{j,x}x + z\boldsymbol{\beta}_{j,z})} = \exp\left[\beta_{j,x}(x^* - x)\right].$$

From this equation, we see that $\exp(\beta_{j,x})$ corresponds to the proportionate change in the odds of outcome y_j versus y_0 when the covariate X increases by 1 unit, holding Z constant. For further reading about the model, see McCulloch and Nelder[5] and Hosmer and Lemeshow[7].

Models for Ordinal Outcomes

While flexible, the polytomous regression model given by 20-38 does not acknowledge the ordering that naturally arises across the levels of an ordinal outcome. It can also be viewed as somewhat unwieldy in that the totality of the "effect" of some covariate on the outcome requires the simultaneous consideration of J sets of association parameters. Here we consider a number of models for ordinal outcomes that explicitly acknowledge the ordering, each through some simplifying assumption that yields a single, common vector of association parameters. While the plausibility any such assumption will need to be carefully considered, employing one of these models may be appealing in that: (1) it will typically result in enhanced statistical precision, relative to having to estimate J such vectors; and, (2) the reporting of results is considerably simplified since one need to only report a single set of effect measures. Note, for simplicity, we present these models for

$P(Y = y_j | X = x)$, that is, when the regression solely considers X, although the ideas extend readily (as above) when the regression is within levels of (X, Z).

The first model we consider is the *adjacent-category logistic model* which specifies an exponential model of the odds of falling into outcome category y_j versus category y_{j-1}, that is, the next lowest category, as:

$$\frac{R_j(x)}{R_{j-1}(x)} = \frac{P(Y = y_j | X = x)}{P(Y = y_{j-1} | X = x)} = \exp\left(\alpha_j^* + \beta_x^* x\right). \qquad [20\text{-}40]$$

As with the polytomous regression model, model 20-40 is only specified for $j = 1, \ldots J$; there is no "next lowest category" for the lowest level in an ordinal variable. Key to this model is that there is a common value for the β_x^* across all J pairs of adjacent categories; thus, the proportionate change in the odds of outcome y_j versus y_{j-1} when the X increases by 1 unit, $\exp(\beta_x^*)$, is the same for all pairs of adjacent categories.

Interestingly, the adjacent category logistic model can be viewed as a special case of the polytomous regression model: From 20-38, the polytomous logistic model implies that:

$$\frac{R_j(x)}{R_{j-1}(x)} = \frac{R_j(x)/R_0(x)}{R_{j-1}(x)/R_0(x)} = \frac{\exp\left(\alpha_j + \beta_{j,x} x^*\right)}{\exp\left(\alpha_{j-1} + \beta_{j-1,x} x^*\right)} = \exp\left[\left(\alpha_j - \alpha_{j-1}\right) + x\left(\beta_{j,x} - \beta_{j-1,x}\right)\right].$$

Comparing this with 20-40, the adjacent category logistic model sets $\alpha_j^* = \alpha_j - \alpha_{j-1}$ and forces the J coefficient differences, $\beta_{j,x} - \beta_{j-1,x}$ for $j = 1, \ldots, J$, to equal a common value β_x^*.

A second model that directly acknowledges the ordering of an ordinal outcome is the *cumulative odds* or *proportional odds* model which specifies the odds of falling *above* category y_j versus falling *in or below* category y_j as:

$$\frac{P(Y > y_j | X = x)}{P(Y \le y_j | X = x)} = \exp\left(\alpha_j^* + \beta_x^* x\right) \qquad [20\text{-}41]$$

Note, this model is defined for $j = 0, \ldots, J - 1$ and that it can be derived by assuming that Y was obtained by categorizing a special type of continuous variable.[5] A third option is to use an exponential model to represent the odds of falling *above* outcome category y_j versus being *in* category y_j:

$$\frac{P(Y > y_j | X = x)}{P(Y = y_j | X = x)} = \exp\left(\alpha_j^* + \beta_x^* x\right) \qquad [20\text{-}42]$$

where, as with 20-41, the model is defined for $j = 0, \ldots, J - 1$. This is called the *continuation ratio model*. Finally, the *reverse continuation ratio model* uses an exponential model to represent the odds of falling *in* category y_j versus falling *below* y_j:

$$\frac{P(Y = y_j | X = x)}{P(Y < y_j | X = x)} = \exp\left(\alpha_j^* + \beta_x^* x\right)$$

where, as with 20-40, the model is defined for $j = 1, \ldots, J$. It can also be derived by reversing the order of the levels of Y in model 20-42, but in any given application it is not equivalent to model 20-42.

Finally, all the above models can be generalized to allow variation in the coefficients β_x^* across levels of Y, as in the polytomous logistic model.[27-31] When this variation is modeled, the adjacent category model is known as the *stereotype* model.

Certain guidelines may be of use for choosing among ordinal models, although none is absolute. First, the adjacent category and cumulative odds models are *reversible*, in that only the signs of the coefficients change if the order of the Y levels is reversed. In contrast, the two continuation ratio models are not reversible. This observation suggests that the continuation ratio models may be more appropriate for modeling irreversible disease stages (*e.g.*, osteoarthritic severity), whereas the adjacent category and cumulative odds models may be more appropriate for potentially reversible outcomes (such as remission and relapse). Second, because the coefficients of adjacent category models contrast pairs of categories, the model appears best suited for discrete outcomes with few levels (*e.g.*, cell types along a normal-dysplastic-neoplastic scale). Third, because the cumulative odds model can be derived from categorizing certain special types of continuous outcomes, it is often considered most appropriate when the outcome under study is derived by categorizing a single underlying continuum (*e.g.*, blood pressure). Finally, an advantage of the continuation ratio models over the other models is that they can be fit using ordinary software without categorization of Y, even if Y is continuous.[28] The primary caution is that conditional maximum likelihood (see Chapter 17) must be used for model fitting if the observed outcomes are sparsely scattered across the levels of Y (as will be inevitable if Y is continuous).

For a more detailed comparative discussion of ordinal logistic models and guidelines for their use, see Refs. McCullagh and Nelder,[5] Greenland,[28] and Agresti.[12]

References

1. Mosteller F, Tukey JW. *Data Analysis and Regression*. Reading, MA: Addison-Wesley; 1977.
2. Leamer EE. *Specification Searches*. New York, NY: Wiley; 1978.
3. Breslow NE, Day NE. *Statistical Methods in Cancer Research. Volume I: The Analysis of Case-Control Data*. Lyon: IARC; 1980.
4. Breslow NE, Day NE. *Statistical Methods in Cancer Research. Volume II: The Design and Analysis of Cohort Studies*, Lyon: IARC; 1987.
5. McCullagh P, Nelder JA. *Generalized Linear Models*. New York, NY: Chapman and Hall; 1989.
6. Clayton D, Hills M. *Statistical Models in Epidemiology*. New York, NY: Oxford University Press; 1993.
7. Hosmer D, Lemeshow S. *Applied Logistic Regression*. New York, NY: Wiley; 2000.
8. Berk RA. *Regression Analysis: A Constructive Critique*. Newbury Park, CA: Sage; 2004.
9. McCulloch CE, Searle SR, Neuhaus JM. *Generalized, Linear, and Mixed Models*. Hoboken, NJ: Wiley; 2008:M38.
10. Wakefield J. *Bayesian and Frequentist Regression Methods*. New York, NY: Springer Science & Business Media; 2013.
11. Faraway JJ. *Linear Models with R*. Boca Raton, FL: CRC Press; 2014.
12. Agresti A. *An Introduction to Categorical Data Analysis*. Hoboken, NJ: John Wiley & Sons; 2018.
13. Robins JM, Greenland S. The role of model selection in causal inference from nonexperimental data. *Am J Epidemiol*. 1986;123:392-402.
14. Fisher B, Costantino JP, Wickerham DL, et al. Tamoxifen for prevention of breast cancer: report of the National surgical adjuvant breast and bowel project P-1 study. *J Natl Cancer Inst*. 1998;90(18):1371-1388.
15. Moolgavkar SH, Venzon DJ. General relative risk regression models for epidemiologic studies. *Am J Epidemiol*. 1987;126:949-961.
16. Greenland S, Schlesselman JJ, Criqui MH. The fallacy of employing standardized regression coefficients and correlations as measures of effect. *Am J Epidemiol*. 1986;123:203-208.
17. Greenland S, Maclure M, Schlesselman JJ, Poole C, Morgenstern H. Standardized regression coefficients: a further critique and review of some alternatives. *Epidemiology*. 1991;2:387-392.
18. Vanderweele TJ, Mathur MB, Chen Y. Outcome-wide longitudinal designs for causal inference: a new template for empirical studies. *Stat Sci*. 2020;35(3):437-466.
19. Royston P, Altman DG. Regression using fractional polynomials of continuous covariates: parsimonious parametric modeling (with discussion). *Appl Stat*. 1994;43:425-467.
20. Greenland S. Avoiding power loss associated with categorization and ordinal scores in dose-response and trend analysis. *Epidemiology*. 1995;6:450-454.
21. Greenland S. Problems in the average-risk interpretation of categorical dose-response analyses. *Epidemiology*. 1995;6:563-565.
22. Lagakos SW. Effects of mismodelling and mismeasuring explanatory variables on tests of their association with a response variable. *Stat Med*. 1988;7:257-274.
23. Greenland S. Dose-response and trend analysis in epidemiology: alternatives to categorical analysis. *Epidemiology*. 1995;6:356-365.

24. Wahba G. *Spline Models for Observational Data*. Boston, MA, Cambridge University Press; 1990.

25. De Boor C. *A Practical Guide to Splines*. New York, NY: Springer; 2001.

26. Hastie T, Tibshirani R, Friedman J. *The Elements of Statistical Learning: Data Mining, Inference, and Prediction*. New York, NY: Springer Science & Business Media; 2009.

27. Peterson B, Harrell F. Partial proportional odds models for ordered response variables. *Appl Stat*. 1990;39:205-217.

28. Greenland S. Alternative models for ordinal logistic regression. *Stat Med*. 1994;13:1665-1677.

29. Ananth CV, Kleinbaum DG. Regression models for ordinal responses: a review of methods and applications. *Int J Epidemiol*. 1997;26:1323-1333.

30. Cole SR, Ananth CV. Regression models for unconstrained, partially or fully constrained continuation odds ratios. *Int J Epidemiol*. 2001;30:1379-1382.

31. Kuss O. On the estimation of the stereotype regression model. *Comput Stat Data Anal*. 2006;50:1877-1890.

CHAPTER 21

Regression Analysis Part II: Model Fitting and Assessment

Sebastien Haneuse*

In Chapter 20, we introduced regression analysis, covering a range of topics including the distinction between a regression function and a regression model, and options for the treatment of both categorical and continuous exposures. The chapter also covered the specification of models for binary or dichotomous outcomes such as an indicator of disease presence/absence, models for continuous outcomes such as blood pressure or BMI, and models for polytomous outcomes such as disease severity quantified by some finite number of levels. For dichotomous or continuous outcomes, a general specification that encompasses nearly all models presented in Chapter 20 is given by expression 20-27 and is repeated here for convenience:

$$g\left[E\left(Y \mid X = x, Z = z\right)\right] = \alpha + \beta_x x + z\beta_z, \qquad [21\text{-}1]$$

where Y is the outcome and X is an exposure of interest and Z is a vector of adjustment variables.

In this chapter, we build on that introduction and cover topics in four areas. The first relates to the task of fitting a model, that is, obtaining estimates of $(\alpha, \beta_x, \beta_z)$, the parameters that index the model. The second relates to the task of assessing the fit of the model and performing diagnostics to determine whether there are potential problems that may compromise conclusions. The third relates to model selection, specifically how one chooses the components of X. Finally, we present methods where the broader research goal is the investigation of some specific exposure-outcome association for which the control of confounding bias is a key task.

---

*This chapter is based on original material by Sander Greenland and Kenneth J. Rothman.

While the presentation of these topics is (necessarily) ordered in this chapter, it is important to bear in mind that analysts will often have to iterate between the tasks and methods that they cover. For example, diagnostics performed following an initial model fit may indicate an apparent nonlinear association between X and the outcome, whereas only a linear association has been specified. At this point, an analyst may opt to modify the specification and then fit the new model.

As mentioned in the introduction to Chapter 20, regression analysis encompasses a vast array of methods, and there are many texts that are devoted to it. For the specific topics covered in this chapter, recommended texts that provide additional comprehensive detail are McCullagh and Nelder,[1] Clayton and Hills,[2] Hosmer and Lemeshow,[3] Agresti,[4] Dobson,[5] Hardin and Hilbe,[6] Hoffman,[7] McCulloch et al.,[8] Hastie et al.,[9] and Wakefield.[10]

MODEL FITTING

Suppose that a model has been specified and that the immediate task is to estimate the unknown parameters; in the case of model 21-1, the unknown parameters are $(\alpha, \beta_x, \beta_z)$. We take the available data to consist of observations of $Y, X,$ and Z from a sample of N study units (*e.g.*, study participants or individuals in a database); that is, we consider settings where there are no missing data. The process of model fitting involves finding the specific values of $(\alpha, \beta_x, \beta_z)$ that best fit the observed data. Practically, analysts have at their disposal many ways of achieving this result, with the key differences being the criteria used to assess "fit" and the assumptions made beyond those implicit by the specification of the regression model; expressions such as 21-1 only make statements about how the mean of the outcome, Y (or a transformation of it), varies as a function of the components of X and Z and nothing else about the distribution of Y.

Among the assumptions that can be made, the assumption of independence across study units is central to all methods for fitting models. Recall from Chapter 17 that the notions of independence and homogeneity underpin both the binomial and Poisson distribution, albeit through different mechanisms. In this chapter, independence corresponds to the notion that, conditional on (or within levels of) X and Z, the outcome of one study unit does not influence the outcome of any other study unit. Chapter 24 considers settings where such independence may not hold.

Beyond the assumption of conditional independence, analysts may approach estimation by making an assumption that the outcome is distributed according to some specific distribution, such as the binomial or the Poisson distribution if Y is a count variable or the Normal distribution if Y is continuous; or by making an assumption about the variance of the outcome (since the regression solely specifies the mean); or by making no additional assumptions. As we discuss below, implicit to the first of these options is the use of a likelihood as the criterion by which the specific values of $(\alpha, \beta_x, \beta_z)$ are chosen. Throughout, it is important to remember that different approaches to fitting a model may, and often will, lead to different estimates, so that in presenting results one should specify the method used to obtain the estimates.

Maximum Likelihood

In Chapter 16, we introduced likelihoods and maximum likelihood (ML) estimation. Briefly, for any distribution there is a corresponding unique *probability mass function* (for categorical variables) or *probability density function* (for continuous variables). From either of these, one can compute the probability of specific events regarding the variable. For example, suppose Y is an indicator of whether a patient with type 2 diabetes who undergoes bariatric surgery experiences a remission of diabetes within 12 months. Letting π denote the probability of remission, Y is said to follow a Bernoulli distribution for which the probability mass function is:

$$Pr\left(Y = y|\pi\right) = \pi^{y}(1-\pi)^{1-y}. \qquad [21\text{-}2]$$

The Bernoulli distribution is a special case of the binomial distribution from Chapter 17, with $N = 1$. From expression 21-2, given any value of π, one can compute the probability of not remitting within 12 months, that is, $Pr\left(Y = 0\right) = 1 - \pi$, or the probability of remitting within 12 months, that is, $Pr\left(Y = 1\right) = \pi$. As a second example, suppose Y is change in weight between the time of surgery and 12 months postsurgery, measured in kg. If one assumes that this continuous outcome follows a Normal distribution with mean μ and variance σ^2, then the probability density function is:

$$f\left(y\big|\mu,\sigma^2\right)=\frac{1}{\sqrt{2\pi\sigma^2}}\exp\left(-\frac{\left(y-\mu\right)^2}{2\sigma^2}\right).$$

[21-3]

From this expression one can compute the probability of having at least 20 kg of weight loss by 12 months, that is, $Pr(Y \le -20)$, using integration.

Viewed as functions of the parameters, expressions 21-2 and 21-3 are both referred to as *likelihoods* and are denoted by $L(\pi)$ and $L(\mu, \sigma^2)$, respectively. Given some value of Y (e.g., an observed data point), one can compute the value of the likelihood that corresponds to any given value of the (otherwise unknown) parameters. Intuitively, values of the parameters that yield a low likelihood can be viewed as being "incompatible" with the data, while values of the parameters that yield a high likelihood can be viewed as being "compatible" with the data. Thus, the likelihood can be used as a criterion for estimating the parameters by seeking those that yield the largest or maximum value, either via calculus or via an optimization algorithm. The result is referred to as the ML estimate.

ML estimation follows just as naturally for regression analyses, with the important provision that, in addition to the model itself, the analyst must specify the distribution of Y within levels of X and $\mathbf{Z}$. This latter distribution is sometimes referred to as the (random) error distribution or the residual distribution. Interestingly, in the case of a dichotomous outcome, there is only one choice for this distribution, specifically the Bernoulli distribution. Thus, there is only one way to form a likelihood. To illustrate this, suppose we have specified the following logistic model:

$$\pi = P\left(Y=1\big|X=x,\mathbf{Z}=z\right)=\frac{\exp\left(\alpha+\beta_x x+z\boldsymbol{\beta}_z\right)}{1+\exp\left(\alpha+\beta_x x+z\boldsymbol{\beta}_z\right)}.$$

Given a sample of size N, assuming conditional independence, the likelihood is the product of N terms, each of the same form as expression 21-2:

$$L\left(\alpha,\beta_x,\boldsymbol{\beta}_z\right)=\prod_{i=1}^{N}\pi_i^{y_i}\left(1-\pi_i\right)^{1-y_i}.$$

Note that each of the π_i is implicitly a function of the same set of unknown parameters $(\alpha, \beta_x, \boldsymbol{\beta}_z)$. Thus, the structure of the likelihood provides a means to learn about $(\alpha, \beta_x, \boldsymbol{\beta}_z)$ using the observed values of Y, X, and $\mathbf{Z}$ on all N study units. Finally, as with the simpler examples given above, one could employ calculus or any maximization algorithm to find the ML estimates of $(\alpha, \beta_x, \boldsymbol{\beta}_z)$ by maximizing $L(\alpha, \beta_x, \boldsymbol{\beta}_z)$ or, equivalently, the log-likelihood log $L(\alpha, \beta_x, \boldsymbol{\beta}_z)$.

When the outcome is anything other than a dichotomous variable, there are many (indeed infinitely many) choices that one can make for the residual distribution. If Y is a count variable, for example, common choices include the binomial and Poisson distributions as well as the beta-binomial and negative binomials.[1] If Y is a continuous outcome that can take on both negative and positive values, then the Normal distribution and the t-distribution are common choices; the gamma and Weibull distributions are common choices for an outcome that is strictly positive. Since the probability mass function or probability density function, as appropriate, is unique to each distribution, so is the form of the likelihood. As such, while the mechanics of obtaining the ML estimates are the same as outlined above, the final ML estimates will be different across different choices for the residual distribution, even if the same regression model (*i.e.*, the model for the mean of Y within levels of X and $\mathbf{Z}$) is considered.

If the choice on which the final fit is based happens to coincide with the true residual distribution, then the resulting ML estimates enjoy a number of appealing statistical guarantees, including consistency (intuitively, they are unbiased in large samples) and efficiency (intuitively, they exhibit the greatest precision among consistent estimators). If, on the other hand, the distribution that is assumed does not coincide with the true residual distribution, then some bias must be expected, even if no other source of bias is present, although the bias has been shown to be small in a broad range of settings.[11,12] More problematic, however, is that the estimated standard errors will be biased, sometimes heavily so. This, in turn, will result in confidence intervals that are invalid (either too wide or too tight). In the next two subsections, we examine this phenomenon in detail for continuous and categorical outcomes, respectively.

Least Squares Estimation

Returning to an example presented above, suppose interest lies in a linear regression model of the association between a vector of covariates, Z, and weight change at 12 months postsurgery among patients with diabetes who have undergone bariatric surgery. Furthermore, for this continuous outcome, suppose the residual distribution is taken to be a Normal with mean μ_i given by the regression model:

$$\mu_i = E\left(Y_i \middle| Z = z_i\right) = \alpha + z_i\beta,$$

for the ith study unit and with variance, sometimes referred to as the *error variance*, $V\left(Y_i \middle| Z = z_i\right) = \sigma^2$.

Taking the residual distribution to be a Normal distribution, one could proceed with estimation via ML. Specifically, one could estimate the unknown parameters, which include the error variance in addition to the regression parameters, by maximizing the likelihood:

$$L\left(\alpha, \beta, \sigma^2\right) = \prod_{i=1}^{N} \frac{1}{\sqrt{2\pi\sigma^2}} \exp\left\{-\frac{\left[y_i - \left(\alpha + z_i\beta\right)\right]^2}{2\sigma^2}\right\},$$

$$[21\text{-}4]$$

formed by the product of N terms, each of the same form as expression 21-3. Although details are omitted, the resulting ML estimates for α and β are equivalent to those obtained by minimizing:

$$\sum_{i=1}^{N}\left[y_i - \left(\alpha + z_i\beta\right)\right]^2,$$

$$[21\text{-}5]$$

that is, the sum of squared residuals. A number of points are worth making here. First, since expression 21-5 does not involve σ^2, we find that estimation of (α, β) under the assumed Normal residual distribution does not require consideration of the variance. This is in contrast to estimation for categorical outcomes where the mean-variance relationship ties estimation of (α, β) to variation in the outcome (see below). Second, expression 21-5 has the intuitive interpretation that it quantifies the total (squared) distance between the observed value of the outcome (*i.e.*, y_i) and its expected value under the model (*i.e.*, $\alpha + z_i\beta$). That is, it provides a measure of fit of a given model to the data. Third, because expression 21-5 provides a measure of fit of a given model to the observed data, it can be used as a criterion for finding the "best" values of (α, β). As such, instead of estimating (α, β) by choosing some residual distribution and then maximizing the corresponding likelihood, one can approach the task by directly minimizing 21-5. Thus, if one is willing to adopt 21-5 as a reasonable measure of fit of a given model to the data, then one can completely avoid the need to specify the residual distribution.

The estimator obtained by minimizing 21-4, or equivalently 21-5, is referred to as the *ordinary least squares* (OLS) estimator.[13] A more general class of estimators is obtained by weighting each of the contributions to the sum of squared residuals:

$$\sum_{i=1}^{N} w_i\left[y_i - \left(\alpha + z_i\beta\right)\right]^2,$$

with the result referred to as the *weighted least squares* (WLS) estimator. In theory, assuming the model for μ_i is correctly specified, the optimal weighting scheme is to set $w_i = 1/V(Y_i|Z = z_i)$, that is, the inverse of the conditional variance of the outcome; using this weight, the estimator is referred to as the *generalized least squares* (GLS) estimator and it is optimal in the sense of having the smallest variance in the class of weighted estimators.

In the above example, we assumed that $V(Y_i|Z = z_i) = \sigma^2$. If this actually holds, then the OLS estimator is optimal since the weighting implicit in 21-5 is one where each individual receives the same weight. If, however, this homogeneity assumption regarding the conditional variance does not hold, that is, $V(Y_i|Z = z_i)$ varies across levels of Z, then the standard variance estimate that is returned by most software implementations will be biased so that confidence intervals will either be too wide or too narrow. This bias, however, can be resolved through the use of a so-called sandwich estimator for the standard error.[11]

Quasi-Likelihood and Related Methods

Recall from Chapter 17 that if a variable Y follows a Poisson distribution, then the mean and the variance are the same; that is, $E(Y) = V(Y)$. There is also a direct mean-variance relationship for the binomial distribution, specifically that $V(Y) = E(Y)[N - E(Y)]/N$. Such mean-variance relationships are a common feature across many distributions for categorical variables. Underpinning these relationships are assumptions, such as the homogeneity and independence assumptions that underpin the Poisson and binomial distributions (Chapter 17). If these underpinning assumptions do not hold, however, then the actual variance of Y may be larger or smaller than the nominal variance that is suggested by the mean-variance relationship for the distribution. Of the two possibilities, the former is more common; in this case, we often say that the data are *overdispersed* relative to the nominal variance or exhibit *extra-Poisson variation* if a Poisson distribution is being considered or *extra-binomial variation* if a binomial distribution is being considered.

To illustrate overdispersion, suppose Y is the number of eyes affected by glaucoma in an individual. In a natural population, $Y = 0$ for most people and $Y = 2$ for most of the remainder. Moreover, $Y = 1$ will likely occur only infrequently since it seems reasonable that, for a given individual, if one eye is (or is not) affected by glaucoma, then the other will be (or will not be) affected. With that intuition, it seems implausible that the glaucoma status of the two eyes is independent. Suppose that one nevertheless considers a binomial distribution for Y. Under this distribution the possible values (*i.e.*, 0, 1, 2) are the same, but the probability of $Y = 1$ is higher than the probabilities of either $Y = 0$ or $Y = 2$. As such, in contrast to the observations in the population (which are largely limited to the extremes of 0 and 2), under a binomial distribution one would expect more observations in the middle (*i.e.*, values of $Y = 1$). Because of this, the variance under the binomial distribution would be smaller than the actual variance of Y; equivalently, the actual variance of Y will be larger than that expected under a binomial distribution.

In the regression context, when one couples a specification for a regression model for a categorical outcome with some specific choice for the distribution, then, because of the mean-variance relationship, one is implicitly specifying the conditional variance of the outcome within levels of Z, that is, $V(Y|Z = z)$. If, however, the actual variance of the outcome within levels of Z is larger than that suggested by the choice of distribution, then the data will be said to be overdispersed. That the assumed variance is smaller than the actual variance will generally lead to standard error estimates that are too small and, thus, confidence intervals that are too tight.

Two major approaches have been developed to cope with potential overdispersion. The first approach is to remain within the ML framework but use a residual distribution that allows a broader range of variation for Y, such as the negative binomial in place of the Poisson or the beta-binomial in place of the binomial.[1] While such distributions have been implemented in most software, the fundamental challenge remains in that if the variance under the more flexible distribution does not reflect the variance in the data, then standard error estimates may remain too small.

The second approach involves direct specification of the residual variance of Y, rather than relying on the implied variance that comes from specifying the residual distribution completely. That is, in addition to specifying a model for $E(Y|Z = z)$, one specifies a model for $V(Y|Z = z)$. While this may, at first, seem challenging, fitting methods that employ this approach are typically accompanied by methods for standard error estimation that are "robust" to misspecification of the model for $V(Y|Z = z)$; such standard error estimators are often labeled "sandwich estimators." Thus, the key advantage of this approach is that the validity of confidence intervals does not hinge on correct specification of the model for $V(Y|Z = z)$. Because of this, the model for $V(Y|Z = z)$ that is adopted is referred to as a *working model*. The drawback of using this approach, in lieu of the first, is that the estimates may be less precise (*i.e.*, have larger standard errors) than those that would be obtained through correct specification of the residual distribution. Fitting methods that employ this approach are discussed by various authors under the topics of quasi-likelihood, pseudo-likelihood, and estimating equation methods; see McCullagh and Nelder,[1] McCullagh,[14] and Diggle et al.[15] for descriptions of these methods, as well as Chapter 24.

MODEL ASSESSMENT AND DIAGNOSTICS

Following the fit of a model, it is important to assess the results against the data. The nature and extent of these checks will typically depend on what purpose we want the model to serve. At one extreme, we may only want the fitted model to provide approximately valid *summary* estimates or trends for a few key relationships. For example, we may want only to estimate the average increment in risk produced by a unit increase in exposure. At the other extreme, we may want the model to provide approximately valid *covariate-specific* predictions of outcomes, such as exposure-specific risks by age, sex, and ethnicity. The latter goal is more demanding and requires more detailed scrutiny of results, sometimes on a subject-by-subject basis.

Model diagnostics can detect discrepancies between data and a model only within the range of the data and then only when there are enough observations to provide adequate diagnostic power. For example, there has been much controversy concerning the health effects of "low-dose" radiation exposure (exposures that are only modestly in excess of natural background levels). This controversy arose because the natural incidence of key outcomes (such as leukemia) is low, and few cases had been observed in "low-dose" cohorts. As a result, several proposed dose-response models "fitted the data adequately" in the low-dose region, in that each model passed the conventional battery of diagnostic checks. Nonetheless, the health effects predicted by these models were mutually conflicting to an important extent.

More generally, one should bear in mind that a good-fitting model is not the same as a correct model. In particular, a model may appear to be correct in the central range of the data but produce grossly misleading predictions for combinations of covariate values that are poorly represented or absent in the data.

Tabular Checks

Both tabular methods, such as those presented in Chapters 17-19, and regression methods produce estimates by merging the observed data with assumptions about population structure (such as that of a common odds ratio or of an explicit regression model). When an estimate is derived using a regression model, especially one with many covariates, it may become difficult to judge the relative influence of the data versus that of the assumed population structure. To investigate this issue, we recommend that one compare model-based results with the corresponding tabular (categorical analysis) results. Careful attention should be paid to how covariates are treated in the tabular analysis. As an illustration, suppose we wish to check a logistic model in which X is the exposure under study, and four other covariates, Z_1, Z_2, Z_3, and Z_4, appear in the model. Additionally, suppose X, Z_1, and Z_2 are continuous while Z_3 and Z_4 are binary and that products among X, Z_1, and Z_3 are included in the model. Because the model is logistic and both Z_1 and Z_3 appear in products with X, they should be treated as modifiers of the X odds ratio in the corresponding tabular analysis. Furthermore, since Z_2 and Z_4 do not appear in products with X, they should be treated as pure confounders (adjustment variables) in the corresponding tabular analysis. Finally, because X, Z_1, Z_2 are continuous in the model, they must have at least three levels in the tabular analysis, so that the results can at least crudely reflect trends seen with the model.

If all three of the continuous covariates are categorized into four levels, the resulting table of disease (two levels) by all covariates will have $2 \times 4^3 \times 2^2 = 512$ cells and perhaps many zero cells depending on the size of the sample. From this table, we can attempt to compute three (for exposure X strata 1, 2, and 3 vs. 0) adjusted odds ratios (*e.g.*, using the Mantel-Haenszel summary) for each of the $4 \times 2 = 8$ combinations of X_2 and X_4, adjusting all $3 \times 8 = 24$ odds ratios for the $4 \times 2 = 8$

pure confounder levels. Some of these 24 adjusted odds ratios may be infinite or undefined as a result of small numbers, which will indicate that the corresponding regression estimates are largely model projections. Similarly, the tabular estimates may not exhibit a pattern seen in the regression estimates, which will suggest that the pattern was induced by the population structure implied by the regression model, rather than the data. For example, the regression estimates might exhibit a monotone trend with increasing exposure even if the tabular estimates did not. Interpretation of such a conflict will depend on the context: If we are certain that dose-response is monotone (*e.g.*, smoking and esophageal cancer), the monotonicity of the regression estimates will favor their use over the tabular results; in contrast, doubts about monotonicity (*e.g.*, as with alcohol and coronary heart disease) should lead us to use the tabular results or switch to a model that does not impose monotonicity.

Tests of Regression and R^2

Most software implementations of regression analyses report, in addition to the estimates themselves and standard error estimates, output from various assessments of model fit. One such assessment that is commonly supplied is a "test of regression" or "test of model," which is a test of the hypothesis that all the regression coefficients (except the intercept α) are zero. For instance, in the exponential rate model

$$I(x,z) = \exp(\alpha + \beta_x x + z\boldsymbol{\beta}_z),$$

the "test of regression" provides a P-value for the null hypothesis that all the covariate coefficients are zero, that is, $\beta_x = \beta_1 = \ldots = \beta_p = 0$. Similarly, the "test of R^2" provided by linear regression programs is just a test that all the covariate coefficients are 0. A small P-value from these tests suggests that the variation in outcome observed across covariate values appears improbably large under the hypothesis that the covariates are unrelated to the outcome. Such a result suggests that at least one of the covariates is associated with the outcome. It does *not*, however, imply that the model fits well or is adequate in any way.

To understand this crucial point, suppose that X comprises the single smoking indicator, with $X = 1$ for smokers and $X = 0$ for nonsmokers, and that the outcome Y is the 20-year risk of lung cancer. In most studies of reasonable size and validity, "test of regression" (which here is just a test of $\beta = 0$) will yield a small P-value. Nonetheless, such a model would clearly be inadequate as a means to describe variation in risk since it neglects important risk factors such as amount smoked, age at start, and sex. More generally, a small P-value from the test of regression tells us only that at least one of the covariates in the model is associated with the outcome; it does not tell us which covariate or what form to use, nor does it tell us anything about what has been left out of the model. Conversely, a large P-value from the "test of regression" does not imply that all the covariates in the model are unimportant or that the model fits well. It is always possible that transformation of those covariates will result in a small P-value or that their importance cannot be discerned given the random error in the data.

A closely related mistake is interpreting the squared multiple correlation coefficient R^2 for a regression as a goodness-of-fit measure. R^2 indicates only the proportion of Y variance that is attributable to variation in the fitted mean of Y. Although $R^2 = 1$ (the largest possible value) does correspond to a perfect fit, R^2 can also be close to 0 under a correct model if the residual variance of Y (*i.e.*, the variance of Y around the true regression curve) is always close to the total variance of Y.

The preceding limitations of R^2 apply in general. Correlational measures such as R^2 can become patently absurd measures of fit or association when the covariates and outcome are discrete or bounded.[16-19] As an example, consider Table 21-1, which shows a large association of a factor with a rare disease. The logistic model $R(x) = \text{expit}(\alpha + \beta x)$ fits these data perfectly because it uses two parameters to describe only two proportions; thus, it is a saturated model. Furthermore, $X = 1$ is associated with a 19-fold increase in risk, yet the correlation coefficient for X and Y (derived using standard formulas) is only 0.09, and the R^2 for the regression is only 0.008.

Correlation coefficients and R^2 can give even more distorted impressions when multiple covariates are present.[18,20] For this reason, we strongly recommend against their use as measures of association or effect when modeling incidence or prevalence.

TABLE 21-1

Hypothetical Cohort Data Illustrating Inappropriateness of R^2 for Binary Outcomes (See Text)

	$X_1 = 1$	$X_1 = 0$
$Y = 1$	1,900	100
Total	100,000	100,000
Risk ratio = 19, $R^2 = 0.008$		

ASSESSMENTS OF MODEL FIT

Assessments of model fit involve checking for systematic or nonrandom incompatibilities between the fitted regression model and the data. Such incompatibilities could be in the form of the model having assumed a linear association between a given exposure and the outcome when there is, in fact, a nonlinear association and also in the form of the assumed variance being incorrect (*i.e.*, the data exhibit overdispersion relative to the assumed residual distribution). With this framing, the general approach to assessing model fit involves consideration of a more elaborate model and testing whether the elaboration is necessary. For example, if the index model under consideration assumed a linear association, the more elaborate model may consider adding a quadratic term. In this sense, most assessments of model fit are *relative* assessments.

There are many approaches to performing these assessments and in the remainder of this subsection we cover some of the more common ones. Throughout, it is important to note that these tests must assume that the fitting method used was appropriate; in particular, test validity may be sensitive to assumptions about the residual distribution that was used in fitting. Furthermore, it is important to bear in mind that different elaborations may result in different conclusions regarding the adequacy of the fit of the fitted index model. For example, suppose the true trend for a given covariate is an upward but nonlinear trend and that the index model assumed linearity. An elaboration that solely includes a quadratic term may lead to the conclusion that the index model was adequate (since the true trend does not conform to the usual U-shape of a quadratic trend). However, an elaboration that includes both quadratic and cubic terms may be better equipped to detect the nonlinear upward trend and, thus, suggests that the linear association assumed by the index model is inadequate.

When models are fit by ML, a standard method for testing the fit of a simpler model against a more complex model is the *deviance test*, also known as the *likelihood ratio test*. Suppose that X represents cumulative dose of an exposure and that the index model we want to assess is the simple linear-logistic model:

$$R(x) = \text{expit}(\alpha + \beta x). \tag{21-6}$$

Let $(\widetilde{\alpha}, \widetilde{\beta})$ denote the ML estimates and $L(\widetilde{\alpha}, \widetilde{\beta})$ the value of the maximized likelihood. To assess the assumption of linearity in this model, suppose we consider the elaborations embedded in the following fractional polynomial-logistic model:

$$R(x) = \text{expit}\left(\alpha + \beta_1 x + \beta_2 x^{1/2} + \beta_3 x^2\right). \tag{21-7}$$

Note that the two models will be equivalent if both β_2 and β_3 are zero, so that a hypothesis test of the null hypothesis $\beta_2 = \beta_3 = 0$ can be used to assess whether the additional components are warranted (in lieu of the index model that assumes linearity being sufficient).

For any given model fit via ML, one can compute the *deviance*, which is twice the difference between the maximized log-likelihood under the model (*i.e.*, evaluated at the ML estimates) and the overall maximized log-likelihood under a saturated model in which there are the same number of parameters as data points. For the two model fits under consideration, the deviances are:

$$D\left(\widetilde{\alpha},\widetilde{\beta}\right) = 2\left[\log L^s - \log L\left(\widetilde{\alpha},\widetilde{\beta}\right)\right]$$

and

$$D\left(\hat{\alpha},\hat{\beta}_1,\hat{\beta}_2,\hat{\beta}_3\right) = 2\left[\log L^s - \log L\left(\hat{\alpha},\hat{\beta}_1,\hat{\beta}_2,\hat{\beta}_3\right)\right]$$

where $(\hat{\alpha},\hat{\beta}_1,\hat{\beta}_2,\hat{\beta}_3)$ is the ML estimate for model 21-7, $L(\hat{\alpha},\hat{\beta}_1,\hat{\beta}_2,\hat{\beta}_3)$ the corresponding value of the maximized likelihood, and, in both cases, L^s is the overall maximum of the likelihood under the saturated model. Intuitively, $D\left(\widetilde{\alpha},\widetilde{\beta}\right)$ and $D\left(\hat{\alpha},\hat{\beta}_1,\hat{\beta}_2,\hat{\beta}_3\right)$ can be viewed as measuring the discrepancy between the best overall fit of the data which comes from permitting each data point to serve as its own mean (and, hence, there is no structure) and the best fit of the data under the structure of the model. Taking the difference between the two yields:

$$\Delta D(\beta_2,\beta_3) = D\left(\widetilde{\alpha},\widetilde{\beta}\right) - D\left(\hat{\alpha},\hat{\beta}_1,\hat{\beta}_2,\hat{\beta}_3\right),$$

[21-8]

which provides a relative assessment of the "best" fits under the two model structures given in 21-6 and 21-7. If the linear-logistic model is correct (so that $\beta_2 = \beta_3 = 0$) and the sample is large enough, this statistic has an approximately χ^2 distribution with two degrees of freedom. Note, the degrees of freedom are obtained by calculating the difference in the number of parameters between the two models. A small *P*-value from such a test would suggest that the linear-logistic model is inadequate or fits poorly; that is, the inclusion of either or both the terms $\beta_2 x^{1/2}$ and $\beta_3 x^2$ helps capture deviations of the true regression from the linear-logistic model 21-6. A large *P*-value does *not*, however, imply that the linear-logistic model is adequate or fits well; it means only that is insufficient evidence to indicate the need for the terms $\beta_2 x^{1/2}$ and $\beta_3 x^2$. In particular, a large *P*-value from this test leaves open the possibility that $\beta_2 x^{1/2}$ and $\beta_3 x^2$ are important for describing the true regression function, but that the test failed to detect this condition. It also leaves open the possibility that some other terms that are not present in the reference model may be important. These unexamined terms may involve X_1 or other covariates. Note, because $\log L^s$ is the same in $D\left(\widetilde{\alpha},\widetilde{\beta}\right)$ and in $D\left(\hat{\alpha},\hat{\beta}_1,\hat{\beta}_2,\hat{\beta}_3\right)$, the statistic given by expression 21-8 can also be written as:

$$\Delta D(\beta_2,\beta_3) = -2\left[\log L\left(\widetilde{\alpha},\widetilde{\beta}\right) - \log L\left(\hat{\alpha},\hat{\beta}_1,\hat{\beta}_2,\hat{\beta}_3\right)\right].$$

Noting that the difference between two log-likelihoods can be expressed (after exponentiating) as the ratio of the two corresponding likelihoods, the statistic $\Delta D(\beta_2, \beta_3)$ is also referred to as the likelihood ratio test statistic, and the test itself a likelihood ratio test.

While the above was specific to comparing models 21-6 and 21-7, the ideas apply more generally. Specifically, suppose we want to assess an index model against a referent model in which it is nested; by "nested" we mean that the index model is a special case, in some way, of the referent model through setting select parameters to zero. In the case of models 21-6 and 21-7, the former is nested with the latter; setting $\beta_2 = \beta_3 = 0$ in model 21-7 gives model 21-6. Now suppose that both models are fit using ML, that $\log L_i$ and D_i are the maximized log-likelihood and deviance for the index model, respectively, and that $\log L_r$ and D_r are the maximized log-likelihood and deviance for the referent model, respectively. If the sample is large enough and the index model is correct, the deviance statistic:

$$\Delta D = D_i - D_r = -2\left(L_i - L_r\right)$$

will have an approximately χ^2 distribution with q degrees of freedom, where q is the number of parameters set to zero under the null (*i.e.*, to make the two models equivalent). Again, a small *P*-value suggests that the index model does not fit well, but a large *P*-value does *not* mean that the index model fits well, except in the very narrow sense that the test did not detect a need for the extra terms in the reference model.

Unfortunately, comparing nonnested models is a more difficult task. If the compared models have the same number of parameters, it has been suggested that (absent other considerations) one should choose the model with the highest log-likelihood.[21] In the general case, other strategies include basing comparisons on measures of fit that adjust for the number of model parameters. Examples include the *Akaike information criterion* (AIC), often defined as the model deviance plus $2p$, where p is the number of model parameters; the *Schwarz information criterion* or *Bayesian information criterion* (BIC), often defined as the model deviance plus $p \times \log N$ where N is the number of observations; and criteria based on *cross-validation*.[9] Larger values of these criteria suggest poorer out-of-sample predictive performance of the model. The definitions of these criteria vary considerably across textbooks;[20] fortunately, the differences do not typically affect the ranking of models by each criterion.

As mentioned earlier, a major problem induced by model selection strategies is that they invalidate the conventional confidence intervals and *P*-values. Nonetheless, advances in computing have led to strategies that address these selection effects via bootstrapping or related methods[9] or that finesse the selection problem by averaging over the competing models.[9,23-26]

MODEL DIAGNOSTICS

Suppose now we have found a model that has passed preliminary checks such as those for additional terms. Before adopting this model as a source of estimates, it is wise to check the model further against the basic data and assess the trustworthiness of any model-based inferences we wish to draw. Such activity is subsumed under the topic of *model diagnostics* and its subsidiary topics of residual analysis, influence analysis, and model sensitivity analysis.[27] These topics are vast, and we can only mention a few approaches here. In particular, residual analysis is not discussed here, largely because its proper use involves a number of technical complexities when dealing with the censored data and nonlinear models predominant in epidemiology.[1]

Delta-Beta Analysis

One important form of influence analysis is a *delta-beta analysis* for which the overarching goal is to assess the impact of each individual in dataset (or a group, as appropriate) on the final estimates. Suppose, for example, that the dataset consists of N individuals. Operationally, after fitting the model using the entire dataset, one refits the model N times with each of these new instances based on a dataset that removes exactly one of the individuals. Alternatively, if the dataset consists of N groups, with each containing subjects with a unique covariate pattern (*e.g.*, a particular exposure-age-sex-education combination), then the model is refit N times with each instance removing one of the groups. If the data consist of N matched sets, then one proceeds by refitting the model N times removing one set in each instance. Across all of these settings, the output is N different sets of parameter estimates (in addition to the original set of estimates based on the complete data). These sets are then examined to see if any one subject, group, or matched set influences the resulting estimates to an unusual extent.

To illustrate, suppose our objective is to estimate the rate ratio per unit increase in an exposure X, to be measured by $\exp\left(\hat{\beta}_x\right)$, where $\hat{\beta}_x$ is the estimated exposure coefficient in an exponential rate model. For each subject, the entire model (confounders included) is refit without that subject. Let $\hat{\beta}_{x(-i)}$ be the estimate of β_x obtained when subject i is excluded from the data. The difference $\hat{\beta}_{x(-i)} - \hat{\beta}_x \equiv \Delta\hat{\beta}_{x(-i)}$ is called the *delta-beta* for β_x for subject i. The influence of subject i on the results can be assessed in several ways. One way is to examine the effect on the rate ratio estimate. The proportionate change in the estimate from dropping subject i is:

$$\exp\left(\hat{\beta}_{x(-i)}\right)\Big/\exp\left(\hat{\beta}_x\right) = \exp\left(\hat{\beta}_{x(-i)} - \hat{\beta}_x\right) = \exp\left(\Delta\hat{\beta}_{x(-i)}\right),$$

for which a value of 1.30 indicates that dropping subject i increases the estimate of the rate ratio by 30%, and a value of 0.90 indicates that dropping subject i decreases the estimate by 10%. One can also assess the effect of dropping the subject on confidence limits, P-values, or any other quantity of interest.

Some software implementations report "standardized" delta-betas of the form $\Delta\hat{\beta}_{x(-i)}/\hat{s}_x$ where $\hat{s}_x$ is the estimated standard error for $\hat{\beta}_x$. By analogy with Z-statistics, any standardized delta-beta below -1.96 or above 1.96 is often interpreted as being unusual. This interpretation can be misleading, however, because $\hat{s}_x$ is not the standard deviation of the delta-beta $\Delta\hat{\beta}_{x(-i)}$, and so this type of standardized delta-beta does not have a standard Normal distribution.

It is possible that one or a few subjects or matched sets are so influential that deleting them alters the conclusions of the study, even when N is in the hundreds.[28] In such situations, comparison of the records of those subjects to others may reveal unusual combinations of covariate values among those subjects. Such unusual combinations likely correspond to previously undetected data errors, which may be resolvable. If it is not clear whether the unusual combination represents a real measurement, analysts will need to make a qualified assessment of whether the individual should remain in the dataset. For instance, it may be only mildly unusual to see a woman who reports having had a child at age 45 years or a woman who reports natural menopause at age 45 years. The combination in one subject, however, may arouse suspicion of a data error in one or both covariates, a suspicion worth the labor of further data scrutiny if that woman or her matched set disproportionately influences the results.

Delta-beta analysis must be replaced by a more complex analysis if the exposure of interest appears in multiple model terms, such as indicator terms, power terms, product terms, or spline terms. In that situation, one must focus on changes in estimates of specific effects or summaries, for example, changes in estimated risk ratios.

Model Sensitivity Analysis

A valuable diagnostic procedure, which is often a by-product of the model selection approaches described in this chapter, is model sensitivity analysis.[24,29,30] Given the variety of models available for fitting, it is inevitable that quite a few can be found that fit reasonably well by all standard tests and diagnostics. Model sensitivity analysis seeks to identify a spectrum of such acceptable models and asks whether various estimates and tests are sensitive to the choice of model used for inference. Those results that are consistent (stable) across acceptable model-based and stratified analyses can be presented using any one of the analyses. On the other hand, results that vary across analyses need to be reported with much more uncertainty than is indicated by their (unstable) confidence intervals; in particular, one should report the fact that the estimates were unstable.

MODEL SELECTION

So far, we have discussed estimation of the parameters in a model as well as post hoc assessments of fit. These activities hinge on a model having been specified, so a natural question is how do we choose a model (or possibly a set of models) that will be acceptable for the current research goal? The answer to this question depends, in part at least, on what the research goal is. Broadly, for the purpose of discussing model selection, one can categorize most research involving regression analyses as pertaining to either estimation and/or assessment of some causal effect or prediction of an outcome. The latter may correspond to estimation of some specific exposure-outcome association or to estimation of a potential moderating or mediating role that some other covariate has.

In selecting models, the key practical decisions relate to: (1) which covariates to include?; (2) how to include them, for example, via categorization or through the use of polynomial terms?; and, (3) the link function, that is, whether to adopt a linear or log-linear to logistic model for how the mean of the outcome, $E\left(Y\,|\,X=x, Z=z\right)$, depends on the covariates through the linear predictor $\alpha + \beta_x x + z\beta_z$. How one makes these decisions requires specification of criteria against which specific choices can be judged and an understanding of potential trade-offs. To this end, analysts may employ criteria based on background knowledge of the scientific context or statistical criteria in the form of some algorithm or a combination of the two. While this section discusses both types of criteria, with some specific examples, we first make a number of overarching points.

For the most part, the development of algorithms that employ statistical criteria has largely focused on prediction problems.[9] Nevertheless, analysts often use these algorithms when the goal is estimation of effects and the point of model selection is to construct a model which enables, to the extent possible with the measured data, the control of confounding bias.[31-33] Unfortunately, many algorithms that were initially designed or predicted lack a logical or statistical justification when the goal is estimation of an effect, and they perform poorly in theory, simulations, and case studies.[26,34-45]

One serious problem associated with the use of statistical criteria when the primary research goal is effect estimation, in particular, is that standard error estimates and P-values obtained from the final model (*i.e.*, after variables are selected) will be downwardly biased, often to a large degree. In particular, standard error estimates obtained from the selected model ignore the variability induced by model selection; intuitively, we have asked the data to tell us the form of the model but then post hoc act as if we knew the form from the beginning. As a result, the final models selected by the algorithms will tend to yield confidence intervals that are much too narrow (and hence fail to cover the true coefficient values with the stated frequency) and P-values that are much too small; see the citations in the preceding paragraph. Unfortunately, significance testing with no post hoc accounting for selection is the basis for most variable selection procedures in standard packaged software.

Other criteria for selecting variables, such as "change-in-point-estimate" criteria, do not necessarily perform better than significance testing (*e.g.*, see Maldonado and Greenland[46]). Viable alternatives to significance testing in model selection have emerged only gradually with advances in computing and with deeper insights into the problem of model selection. We outline the conventional approaches after first reinforcing one of the most essential and neglected starting points for good modeling: laying out existing information in a manner that can help avoid models that are in conflict with established facts.

Role of Prior Information

A critical initial step in any epidemiologic study is an assessment of the current state of the knowledge. What is known about the prevalence of the outcome? What, if any, are the any established risk factors, and what is the current evidence regarding the nature of their association with the outcome? In studies of effect estimation, what is the prevalence of the exposure or moderating/mediating factors? In all these, what is the strength of evidence? In answering these questions, epidemiologists may, to the extent possible, develop an understanding of important phenomena that may be relevant to the research goal. Consider, for example, a variable that is known to be associated with some specific treatment choice and yet there is no evidence that it predicts the outcome. One may plausibly use this knowledge to eliminate this variable from consideration. Similarly, if knowledge of the data collection scheme indicates that some factor was measured following exposure, then one can similarly exclude it from consideration (unless it is a potential mediator; see Chapter 12). In operationalizing this knowledge, causal diagrams provide a useful infrastructure and rules for making decisions such as assuming the diagram is correct and identifying a minimal set of covariates that will enable the control of confounding.[47,48] However, as discussed in Chapter 12, even if knowledge of a complete causal diagram is not available, other information concerning temporal and causal ordering can be used to make principled decisions about covariate selection based on a priori knowledge.[49]

In addition, background information on the study and data itself may be useful in making informed decisions. For example, if a variable is found to have too much missing data or is potentially subject to substantial misclassification or other measurement error, then a decision may be made to exclude it. In doing so, however, researchers must consider the impact of the exclusion on the interpretation of the results. In other instances, the design of the study may dictate whether a particular covariate is included. For example, in a matched cohort study, it is recommended that all matching factors be adjusted for even though they are, in principle, already balanced between the exposure groups.[50]

Ultimately, the dependence of regression results on the chosen model can be either an advantage or a drawback. When simple tabular analyses, as covered in Chapters 17-19, require severe simplification of the analysis variables, use of a regression model structure that is capable of reasonably approximating reality can improve the accuracy of the estimates by avoiding such simplifications. On the other hand, use of a model that is incapable of even approximating reality can decrease accuracy to less than that of tabular analysis.

This trade-off underscores the desirability of using flexible (and possibly complex) models. One should, however, take care to avoid models that are entirely unsupported by background knowledge. For example, in a cohort study of lung cancer, it is reasonable to restrict rates to increase with age, because there is enormous background literature documenting that this trend is found in all human populations. In contrast, one would want to avoid restricting cardiovascular disease (CVD) rates to increase strictly with alcohol consumption, because there is evidence suggesting that the alcohol-CVD relation is not strictly increasing.[51]

In some settings prior knowledge may be too limited to provide much guidance in model selection. A natural response might be to use models that are as flexible as possible; that is, a model can reproduce a wide variety of curves and surfaces. Unfortunately, however, flexible models are limited in that a larger sample will be needed to ensure approximately unbiased coefficient estimates. Also, after a certain point, increasing flexibility may increase variability of estimates so much that the accuracy of the estimates is decreased relative to estimates from simpler models, despite the greater faithfulness of the flexible model to reality.

Fortunately, estimates obtained from the most common epidemiologic regression models, such as exponential (log-linear) and logistic models, retain some interpretability even when the underlying (true) regression function is not particularly close to those forms.[46,52] For example, under common conditions, rate- or risk-ratio estimates obtained from those models can be interpreted as approximate estimates of standardized rate or risk ratios, using the total source population as the standard.[53] To ensure that such interpretations are reasonable, the model used should at least be able to replicate qualitative features of the underlying regression function. For example, if the underlying regression may have a reversal in the slope of the exposure-response curve, we should use a model that is capable of exhibiting such reversal (even if it cannot replicate the exact shape of the true curve).

Algorithmic Selection Strategies

Even with ample prior information, there will always be an overwhelming number of model choices, and so algorithm-based model search strategies are an important tool. Some strategies begin by specifying a minimal model form that is among the most simple and yet credible forms. Here "credible" means "compatible with available information." Thus, we start with a model of minimal computational or conceptual complexity that does not conflict with existing background information. There may be many such models; in order to help ensure that the analysis is credible to the intended audience, however, the starting model form should be one that most researchers will view as a reasonable possibility. Thus, to specify a simple yet credible model form, one needs some knowledge of the background scientific literature on the relations under study. This knowledge includes information about relations of potential confounders to the study exposures and study diseases, as well as relations of study exposures to the study diseases.[54] As a consequence, specification of a simple yet credible model can demand much more initial effort than is routinely used in model specification.

Once a minimal starting model has been specified, one can add complexities that seem necessary in light of the data. Such a search process is an *expanding* search.[55] Its chief drawback is that there are often too many possible expansions to consider within a reasonable length of time. If, however, one neglects to consider any possible expansion, one risks missing an important shortcoming of the initial model. As a general example, if our minimal model involves only first-order (linear) terms for 12 variables, we have $\binom{12}{2} = 66$ possible two-way products among these variables to consider, as well as 12 quadratic terms, for a total of 78 possible expansions with just one second-order term. An analyst may not have the time, patience, or resources to examine all the possibilities in detail; this predicament usually leads to use of automatic significance testing procedures to select additional terms, which can lead to distorted statistics.

Some strategies begin by specifying an initial model form that is flexible enough to approximate any credible model form. One advantage of this strategy is that a flexible starting point can be less demanding than a simple one in terms of the need for background information. For example, rather than concern ourselves with what the literature suggests about the shape of a dose-response curve, we can employ a starting model form that can approximate a wide range of curves. Furthermore, rather than concern ourselves with what the literature suggests about joint effects, we can employ a form that can approximate a wide range of joint effects. Subsequently, one can search for a simpler but adequate model by removing from the flexible model any complexities that appear to be unnecessary in light of the data. Such a search process, based on simplifying a complex model, is a *contracting* or simplifying search.[55]

The chief drawback of a purely contracting search is that a sufficiently flexible prior model may be too complex to fit to the available data. This drawback arises because more complex models generally involve more parameters; with more parameters in a model, more data are needed to produce trustworthy point and interval estimates. Conventional model fitting methods may yield biased estimates or may completely fail to yield any estimates (*e.g.*, not converge) if the fitted model is too complex. For example, if our flexible model for 12 variables contains all first- and second-order terms, there will be 12 first-order plus 12 quadratic plus 66 product terms, for a total of 90 coefficients. Depending on the size of the dataset, fitting this model by conventional methods may be well beyond what can be supported.

Because of potential fitting problems, contracting searches typically begin with something less than a fully flexible model. Some begin with a model as flexible as can be fitted or maximal model. As with minimal models, maximal models are not unique. In order to produce a model that can be fit with conventional methods, one may have to limit flexibility of dose-response, flexibility of joint effects, or both. It is also possible to start a model search anywhere in between the extremes of minimal and maximal models and then proceed by expanding as seems necessary and contracting as seems reasonable based on the data (although, again, resource limitations often lead to mechanical use of significance tests for this process). Unsurprisingly, such *stepwise* searches share some advantages and disadvantages with purely expanding and purely contracting searches. Like other searches, care should be taken to ensure that the starting and ending points do not conflict with prior information.

It is important to bear in mind that the results obtained following a model search can be sensitive to the choice of starting model. One can check for this problem by conducting several searches, starting at different models. Nonetheless, there are always far too many possible models to search through them all, and with many variables to consider, model search strategies always risk producing a misleading model form. Modern methods to address this problem and other modeling issues can be found in the literature on statistical learning, for example, under topics such as cross-validation, model averaging, nonparametric regression, smoothing, and boosting.[9,31,32,56,57]

There is also a large Bayesian literature on the topic of model selection.[58] Some of these methods reduce the selection problem by merging models or their results, for example, by averaging over competing models,[9,23-26] by using inferential methods that account for the selection process,[9,45,59,60] or by embedding the models in a hierarchical model that contains them all as special cases.[61] Finally, penalized fitting and other shrinkage methods also allow fitting of much larger models than feasible with conventional methods, often eliminating the need for variable selection in confounding control.[62]

MODEL-BASED STANDARDIZATION

Suppose that the main objective of modeling is to control confounding by a vector of covariates Z when examining the association of an exposure variable X with an outcome variable Y. A direct approach to this problem is to fit a model for the regression of Y on X and Z, which has been the focus of discussion so far. For example, if Y is binary, the most common direct approach fits the group-specific logistic risk model.

$$P(Y = 1 | X = x, Z = z) = \text{expit}(\alpha + \beta_x x + z\beta_z).$$

[21-9]

In this outcome model, provided that Z is sufficient for confounding control, the odds ratio association $\exp(\beta_x)$ is a Z-*conditional* measure, in that it reflects the (common) effect of X on Y within strata defined by values of Z. As described in Chapter 20, if the conditional effect varies with some component Z_k in the vector Z (*i.e.*, if Z_k modifies the association of X with Y), the model will need product terms between X and Z_k to capture that variation, and separate effect measures will need to be reported for every level of Z_k. This situation brings complexity to the modeling and reporting of the model and may result in potential instability in the estimation process (depending on the interplay between the complexity of the model and the sample size). To avoid this complexity, one may instead focus on using a regression model as a means to estimate a standardized effect measure.

It turns out that several modern statistical methods, such as marginal modeling and inverse probability weighting (IPW), can be viewed as forms of standardized effect estimation, and this view connects standardization to confounder scoring (below). To describe the general ideas, as in Chapter 18, let W be a standard distribution for the vector of potential confounders and modifiers Z. Specifically, W is a set of weights, $w(z)$, one for each value z of Z, that sum or integrate to 1, that is, $\sum_z w(z) = 1$. The regression of Y on X standardized to W is the average of $E\left(Y|X = x, Z = z\right)$ weighted by the $w(z)$:

$$E_W\left(Y|X = x\right) = \sum_z w(z) E\left(Y|X = x, Z = z\right).$$

[21-10]

As explained in Chapter 20, risk and prevalence parameters are expected proportions, and rates are expected counts per unit of person-time. They can thus be substituted into the standardization formula 21-10. For example, a standardized incidence rate is $R_W(x) = \sum_z w(z) R(x, z)$ and a standardized risk is $I_W(x) = \sum_z w(z) I(x, z)$. The latter is an example of a standardized probability, which has the general form:

$$P_W\left(Y|X = x\right) = \sum_z w(z) P\left(Y|X = x, Z = z\right).$$

The standardization methods discussed next apply with all these forms, although most of the illustrations will be in the probability form.

Standardization Using Outcome Models

Suppose that we know or can validly estimate the weights $w(z)$ for the standard. There are then several approaches to model-based standardization, depending on the type of model employed. The most straightforward is to model the conditional (X, Z)-specific outcomes $E\left(Y|X = x, Z = z\right)$ or $I(x, z)$ or $Pr\left(Y|X = x, Z = z\right)$ and then use predicted outcome values from the model fitted (*i.e.*, by substituting estimates of the parameters) in the preceding formulas.[63] For example, if we fit a model for the (X, Z)-specific incidence rates $I(x, z)$ to a cohort and obtain fitted covariate rates $\hat{I}(x, z)$, the estimated standardized rate is $\hat{I}_W(x) = \sum_z w(z) \hat{I}(x, z)$. Crucially, the model may be anything we choose and in particular may contain products between X and components of Z and may have a hierarchical (multilevel) structure. The specific estimates $\hat{I}(x, z)$ may even be from a fitted nonparametric regression, such as those produced by data-driven prediction algorithms.[9]

Details of standardization of risks, rates, ratios, and attributable fractions using parametric models are given by Lane and Nelder,[63] Bruzzi et al.,[64] Flanders and Rhodes,[65] Greenland and Holland,[66] Greenland and Drescher,[67] Joffe and Greenland,[68] and Greenland,[69] among others. Most of these articles also supply variance formulas; these formulas can be unwieldy, however, and one can instead obtain confidence limits via simulation or bootstrapping.[69] As always, the interpretation of these standardized estimates as effect estimates assumes that no uncontrolled bias is present, and in particular that Z is sufficient for confounding control and has a distribution unaffected by X. Again, the latter assumption is likely to be violated when the standard W is a person-time distribution and X and Z affect Y.[70]

Standardized Measures Versus Coefficients

To see the relation of standardization to the simpler approach of using a single exposure coefficient as the summary, suppose that the outcome model is of the additive form:

$$E(Y|X = x, \mathbf{Z} = \mathbf{z}) = \alpha + \beta_x x + \mathbf{z}\boldsymbol{\beta}_z.$$ [21-11]

Substitution of 21-11 into the standardization formula 21-10 yields:

$$
\begin{aligned}
E_W(Y|X = x+1) &= \sum_z w(z)\left[\alpha + \beta_x(x+1) + \mathbf{z}\boldsymbol{\beta}_z\right] = \sum_z w(z)(\alpha + \beta_x x + \beta_x + \mathbf{z}\boldsymbol{\beta}_z) \\
&= \sum_z w(z)\beta_x + \sum_z w(z)(\alpha + \beta_x x + \mathbf{z}\boldsymbol{\beta}_z) \\
&= \beta_x \sum_z w(z) + E_W(Y|X = x) = \beta_x + E_W(Y|X = x)
\end{aligned}
$$

where the last line follows because, by definition, $\sum_z w(z) = 1$. From these calculations we have that:

$$E_W(Y|X = x+1) - E_W(Y|X = x) = \beta_x.$$

In other words, under an additive model for the X contribution to the conditional outcome $E(Y|X = x, \mathbf{Z} = \mathbf{z})$, the standardized difference for a unit increase in X is equal to the X coefficient, regardless of the weighting W.

Next, suppose that the outcome model is of the log-additive (multiplicative) form:

$$E(Y|X = x, \mathbf{Z} = \mathbf{z}) = \exp(\alpha + \beta_x x + \mathbf{z}\boldsymbol{\beta}_z).$$ [21-12]

Substitution of this model into the standardization formula 21-10 yields:

$$
\begin{aligned}
E_W(Y|X = x+1) &= \sum_z w(z)\exp\left[\alpha + \beta_x(x+1) + \mathbf{z}\boldsymbol{\beta}_z\right] = \sum_z w(z)\exp(\beta_x)\exp(\alpha + \beta_x x + \mathbf{z}\boldsymbol{\beta}_z) \\
&= \exp(\beta_x)\sum_z w(z)\exp(\alpha + \beta_x x + \mathbf{z}\boldsymbol{\beta}_z) = \exp(\beta_x)E_W(Y|X = x)
\end{aligned}
$$

from which we have the ratio:

$$E_W(Y|X = x+1)/E_W(Y|X = x) = \exp(\beta_x).$$

In other words, under a multiplicative model for the X contribution to $E(Y|X = x, Z = z)$, the log-standardized ratio for a unit increase in X is equal to the X coefficient, regardless of the weighting W.

The preceding results show that if we are willing to make strong assumptions about homogeneity of the X association with Y across values of Z, we can bypass weighted averaging and use estimates of model coefficients as estimates of standardized measures. The problem with this usage is its strong dependence on the homogeneity assumptions. With weighted averaging, we can use products of X and $\mathbf{Z}$ components or even more complex regression models, and thus we need not depend on homogeneity assumptions. Nonetheless, if we use an additive model and nonadditivity (modification of the differences by $\mathbf{Z}$) is present, the resulting estimate of β_x can be a good estimate of the population-averaged difference with weights $w(z) = P(\mathbf{Z} = \mathbf{z})$ provided the $\mathbf{Z}$ contribution, that is, the "$z\beta_z$" term in model 21-11, is appropriate in reflecting how $E(Y|X=x,Z=z)$ varies within levels of z. In a similar fashion, if we use a multiplicative model when modification of the ratios by Z is present, the resulting estimate of $\exp(\beta_x)$ can be a good estimate of the population-averaged ratio, again provided the Z contribution, that is, the "$z\beta_z$" term in model 21-12, is appropriate in reflecting how $E(Y|X=x,Z=z)$ varies within levels of z.[53]

Unfortunately, unless risk is low at all (X, Z) combinations, the results just described do not carry over to logistic or linear odds models, reflecting the problem of noncollapsibility of odds ratios discussed in Chapter 5. In particular, when $\beta_x \neq 0$ and $\beta_z \neq 0$ in the regression model 21-9, the conditional odds ratio $\exp(\beta_x)$ will be farther from 1 than the odds ratio obtained by first standardizing the risks from the model and then combining them in an odds ratio.[71] For similar reasons, the results do not carry over to exponential and linear rate models unless X has negligible effect on person-time.[72]

SCORING METHODS

In the preceding section, the "$z\beta_z$" term in models 21-11 and 21-12 served to represent how $E(Y|X=x,Z=z)$ varies within levels of z. More generally, this term, which is simply a linear combination of the components of Z, could be replaced with any function of Z, $g(Z)$. Applying this notion to model 21-11, for example, gives:

$$E(Y|X=x,Z=z)=\alpha+\beta_x x+g(z).$$

There has been much work on defining and estimating an appropriate $g(Z)$, referred to as a *confounder score*, such that it may be included as a single term in subsequent models.

Confounder Scores and Balancing Scores

Standardization without modeling is equivalent to taking the confounder score, $g(Z)$, to be a categorical compound variable with a distinct level for every possible value of Z. For example, if Z = (sex, age), then $g(Z) = g$(sex, age) is the compound "sex-age." This two-dimensional $g(Z)$ has as possible values every sex-age combination $g(z)$, such as g(male, 60) = "male age 60 years," and the effect measure of interest might be a sex-age standardized risk ratio. This two-dimensional score will control all confounding by sex and age if the latter is measured with enough granularity.

Unfortunately, as the number of possible values for Z increases, the strata of a compound variable rapidly become too sparse for analysis. For example, if Z is composed of 8 levels for age, 4 levels for housing density, 6 levels for income, 5 levels for education, and 2 levels for sex, it will have 1920 possible levels, far too many strata to use directly in most studies. Thus, attention has focused on model-based construction of a simpler composite score that would control all confounding by Z.

Consider first a score $g(Z)$ with the property that Y and Z are independent given the exposure and the score. In other words, within levels of X and $g(Z)$, Y does not depend on the value of Z:

$$P[Y=y|X=x,Z=z,g(Z)=c]=P[Y=y|X=x,g(Z)=c].$$

If $g(Z)$ satisfies this property, Y will have a "balanced" (equal) distribution across the values of Z within strata defined by X and $g(Z)$; hence, $g(Z)$ may be called an *outcome balancing* score.

Consider next a score $g(Z)$ with the property that Z and X are independent given the score. In other words, suppose that Z does not depend on the value of X when $g(Z)$ is at a particular value c:

$$P[Z=z|X=x,g(Z)=c]=P[Z=z|g(Z)=c].$$

Such a $g(Z)$ will, on average, "balance" the distribution of Z across the levels of X. An equivalent condition is that X does not depend on the value of Z when $g(Z)$ is at a particular value c:

$$P\left[X = x \middle| Z = z, g(Z) = c\right] = P\left[X = x \middle| g(Z) = c\right].$$

If a score $g(Z)$ satisfies this condition, X will have a "balanced" (equal) distribution across the levels of Z within strata defined by $g(Z)$; hence, $g(Z)$ may be called an *exposure balancing* score.

Because of the balance they create, stratification on outcome balancing or exposure balancing scores will be sufficient for control of confounding by Z when estimating marginal (average) effects. Analyses that employ balancing scores, however, may be unnecessarily complicated and inefficient. For example, if there is no confounding by any component of Z, no score involving Z will be necessary and use of such a score will unnecessarily increase variances (and possibly introduce bias if some component of Z should not be controlled). The key issue is how to construct a score that is simultaneously simple and sufficient. Many regression approaches have been proposed for this purpose, and the following subsections review several that have been used in epidemiologic research.

Outcome Scores

Scores that are constructed to predict the outcome are called *outcome scores*. Early outcome scoring methods were based on fitting a model for the regression of the outcome Y on Z alone.[73] For a disease indicator Y, one could, for example, fit a logistic model:

$$P(Y = 1 | Z = z) = \operatorname{expit}\left(\alpha^* + z\beta_z^*\right)$$

and then use the fitted probability, that is, $\operatorname{expit}\left(\hat{\alpha}^* + z\hat{\beta}_z^*\right)$, for each subject as the values $g(z)$ of the confounder score. This fitted probability is also known as a *risk score* or *prognostic score*. Furthermore, because the fitted probability is just a one-to-one function of the fitted linear combination $z\hat{\beta}_z^*$, one can equivalently take $g(z) = z\hat{\beta}_z^*$ as the confounder score.

Analyses using risk scores obtained by regressing Y on Z alone (without X) appeared in various forms through the 1970s. Such scores, however, are *not* outcome balancing, and adjusting for them results in null-biased estimates of the Z-adjusted association of X on Y. This bias arises because the term $z\hat{\beta}_z^*$ incorporates any effect of X that is confounding the Z effect, and hence adjustment for $z\hat{\beta}_z^*$ adjusts away part of the X effect.[74,75] If the model is correct, however, the adjustment can give correct null P-values.[76-78]

To remove this bias, one may use as the confounder score the fitted value of the linear term at $X = 0$ from a model with both X and Z, such as $g(z) = z\hat{\beta}_z^*$, from fitting the risk model 21-9.[75,78] This score will be outcome balancing on average if the model is correct. Nonetheless, because the score is estimated, the resulting standard errors may be downwardly biased, leading to downwardly biased P-values and overly narrow confidence intervals. Thus, on theoretical grounds as well as labor, none of these basic outcome score approaches is clearly better than just using $\exp\left(\hat{\beta}_x\right)$ from the outcome model 21-9 as the effect estimate, nor are they better than model-based standardization.

Exposure Scores

Scores that are constructed to predict the exposure are called *exposure scores*. Miettinen[75] suggested creating an exposure score by regressing X on Y and Z and then (by analogy with risk scoring) setting $Y = 0$. In the context of cohort studies, Rosenbaum and Rubin[79] argued instead that one should model the probability of X as a function of Z only, which for a binary X could be:

$$P(X = 1 | Z = z) = e_1(z) = \operatorname{expit}(v + z\theta).$$

They called this probability of $X = 1$ the *propensity score* for X and showed that, if the fitted model is correct, $e_1(z)$ is the coarsest exposure balancing score, in that no further simplification of the score preserves its property of balancing Z across levels of X. Note, however, that simpler scores than $e_1(z)$ may be sufficient for control of confounding by $\mathbf{Z}$. For example, if Z_1 is not confounding given the remaining covariates in $\mathbf{Z}$, then there is no need to balance Z_1, and a score without Z_1 would be sufficient and simpler.

Subsequent work showed (rather counterintuitively) that if one knows the correct model for the propensity score, using the score from fitting that model has better statistical properties than using the true score $e_1(z)$.[80,81] That is, if the preceding model were correct, using fitted score $\hat{e}_1(z) = \text{expit}\left(\hat{v} + z\hat{\theta}\right)$ based on estimates of v and θ would be better than using $e_1(z) = \text{expit}(v + z\theta)$ with the true v and θ. Although this theory shows that taking $g(z) = \hat{e}_1(z)$ is a viable competitor to direct modeling of the regression of Y on X and $\mathbf{Z}$, the propensity model is unknown in observational studies and the theory leaves open how the exposure model should actually be built. Practically, studies suggest that the criteria for selection of variables to include in $\mathbf{Z}$ should be the same as those used for outcome regression.[82] These criteria can be roughly summarized by the common sense rule that important confounders should be forced into the model. Because the strength of confounding by a covariate Z_k is determined by its association with both X and Y, selection based on either association alone can easily select nonconfounders in addition to confounders.

As with analyses based on modeling Y, selection based on conventional variable selection criteria (*e.g.*, coefficient $P < .05$) can be especially harmful. For example, stepwise propensity modeling will retain a variable that is unassociated with Y if it is "significantly" associated with X, resulting in adjustment for a nonconfounder; yet it will remove a confounder whose association with X is "nonsignificant," resulting in uncontrolled confounding. On the other hand, it will retain variables that discriminate strongly between exposed and unexposed even if they have no relation to Y other than through X and so are not confounders, thus harming the efficiency of propensity score stratification by reducing overlap between the exposed and unexposed groups. For similar reasons, the ability of the propensity model to discriminate between the exposed and unexposed should not be a criterion for determining a good model: a model that discriminates perfectly will leave no exposed and unexposed subjects in the same stratum of the fitted score.

As with any modeling procedure, once the exposure model has been fitted, checks of its adequacy are advisable. A simple diagnostic is to check that the exposure and the covariates $\mathbf{Z}$ are independent given the exposure score, as they should be if the score is adequate. This check is often done by examining the covariate-exposure associations after stratifying the data on the fitted scores.

Assuming that one is able to construct a propensity score that appears adequate, it can be used to control confounding bias in a number of ways including stratification, matching, or as a covariate in regressions of Y on exposure.[83,84] The fitted propensity score $\hat{e}_1(z)$ can also be used to construct inverse probability weights for marginal modeling of the dependence of Y on X[85]: exposed individuals (*i.e.*, those with $X = 1$) receive weight $1/\hat{e}_1(z)$ and unexposed individuals (*i.e.*, those with $X = 0$) receive weight $1/\hat{e}_0(z)$, where $\hat{e}_0(z) = 1 - \hat{e}_1(z)$ is the fitted value of $P(X = 0 | \mathbf{Z} = z)$. In other words, a model for the regression of Y on X is fit in which each subject receives a weight $1/\hat{e}_x(z)$, the inverse of the probability of getting the exposure the subject actually had.

Concern has been raised that stratification, adjustment, and matching on the basis of a categorization of the fitted score may fail to completely resolve confounding bias.[85] Because stratification in this setting involves only a single summary confounder, however, one can limit residual confounding by creating fine strata and generating summary estimates using methods that work with sparse data, such as the Mantel-Haenszel estimators (see Chapter 18). Similarly, if the score is to be included in the outcome model, then bias may be mitigated by modeling the association between the score and the outcome flexibly (*e.g.*, using polynomial regression or splines). Finally, matching on the score using a tight caliper width can avoid these problems but can invalidate conventional interval estimates for the effect.[86]

In contrast, weighting requires neither categorization nor specification of the score effect on Y. It also generalizes easily to an exposure variable X with more than two levels, including time-varying exposures.[87,88] Its chief drawback is that it can lead to instabilities due to fitted probabilities near 0.[89] A related approach that does not require categorization uses a special transform of $\hat{e}_x(z)$ in a conditional outcome model and then averages over that model.[90]

Because of differences in implicit weightings, different approaches may be estimating different parameters if there is modification of the X effect measure across levels of $\mathbf{Z}$.[91-93] For example, standardization over propensity score strata corresponds to standardization by $w(z) = P(\mathbf{Z} = z)$, and use of other summaries over the strata often approximates this standardization.[53] But propensity score matching will alter the cohort distribution of $\boldsymbol{Z}$ and thus lead to a different standard than simply using everyone in the propensity score analysis. If matching is based on taking all those with $X = 1$ and using their score to select N matches with $X = 0$, the resulting cohort will, in expectation, have the $\boldsymbol{Z}$ distribution of the exposed, and so that $w(z) = P(\boldsymbol{Z} = z \mid X = 1)$ becomes the standard, which would be appropriate if the goal is to estimate the net effect that exposure had on the exposed.

In a similar fashion, weighting by $1/\hat{e}_1(z)$ and $1/\hat{e}_0(z)$ is equivalent to standardization to the distribution in the total cohort, $P(\boldsymbol{Z} = z)$.[89] To standardize to the distribution in the exposed, $P(\boldsymbol{Z} = z \mid X = 1)$, the weights must be set to $\hat{e}_1(z)/\hat{e}_1(z) = 1$ for the exposed and $\hat{e}_1(z)/\hat{e}_0(z)$ for the unexposed.[94] To standardize to the distribution in the unexposed, $P(\boldsymbol{Z} = z \mid X = 0)$, which would be appropriate if the goal is to estimate the net effect that exposure would have on the unexposed, the weights must be modified to $\hat{e}_0(z)/\hat{e}_1(z)$ for the exposed and $\hat{e}_0(z)/\hat{e}_0(z) = 1$ for the unexposed.

Propensity score and IPW methods are based on modeling the full probability of X given $\boldsymbol{Z}$, $P(X = x \mid \boldsymbol{Z} = z)$. When X is continuous, this task can be more challenging since it requires specification of the complete distribution and not just the regression of X on $\boldsymbol{Z}$, that is, $E(X = x \mid \boldsymbol{Z} = z)$. *E-estimation* and *intensity scoring* are based on adjustment using a fitted model for $E(X = x \mid \boldsymbol{Z} = z)$, subject to constraints on the conditional outcome regression $E(Y \mid X = x, \boldsymbol{Z} = z)$.[80,95] Like IPW, these methods generalize to time-varying exposures and confounders, where they are known as *g-estimation* (see Chapter 25).

Outcome Versus Exposure Modeling

There has been some controversy over the relative merits of outcome modeling and exposure modeling approaches, especially with regard to their model dependence. A few facts should be noted at the outset. First, confounding that is not captured by the measured $\boldsymbol{Z}$ (*e.g.*, because of measurement error in $\boldsymbol{Z}$ or failure to include some confounders in $\boldsymbol{Z}$) cannot be accounted for by either approach. Thus, neither approach addresses a truly intrinsic problem of observational studies—residual confounding by mismeasured or unmeasured confounders.[96,97] In a similar fashion, adjustment for inappropriate covariates, such as those affected by X or Y (*e.g.*, intermediates), will produce bias, regardless of the approach. See Chapters 3 and 12 for further discussion.

If $\boldsymbol{Z}$ is a confounder, mismodeling of either $E(Y \mid X = x, \boldsymbol{Z} = z)$ or $P(X = x \mid \boldsymbol{Z} = z)$ can leave residual confounding by $\boldsymbol{Z}$. It is, therefore, always possible that results from neither, only one, or both approaches suffer bias from mismodeling. The relative bias of the approaches may depend heavily on the modeling strategy. As a simple example, suppose that just one covariate Z_k in $\boldsymbol{Z}$ is the only confounder in a study, and that both the outcome models will be built by selecting only those covariates in $\boldsymbol{Z}$ with $P < .05$ in the fitted model. If Z_k has $P < .05$ in the outcome model but $P > .05$ in the exposure model, it will be selected into the outcome model and there will be no confounding of results from that model, but it will be left out of the exposure model, resulting in confounding of results from that model. Conversely, if Z_k has $P > .05$ in the outcome model but $P < .05$ in the exposure model, it will be left out of the outcome model, resulting in confounding of results from that model, but it will be selected into the exposure model and there will be no confounding of results from that model. The specification issue is often framed as a question of how accurately we can model the dependence of Y on X and $\boldsymbol{Z}$ versus how accurately we can model the dependence of X on $\boldsymbol{Z}$. In both approaches the final step may be to average (standardize) over the modeling results. In each approach, this averaging can reduce sensitivity to mismodeling. For example, when one standardizes model-based estimates of $E(Y \mid X = x, \boldsymbol{Z} = z)$ over a $\boldsymbol{Z}$-distribution similar to that in the data, the resulting summary estimates will be far more stable and less sensitive to misspecification than the $E(Y \mid X = x, \boldsymbol{Z} = z)$ estimates. This robustness arises from the averaging of residual errors to 0 over the data distribution of the regressors. Although this average need not be 0 within levels of X, one can check the X-specific averages: Large values indicate that X was mismodeled.

Early simulation studies reported higher specification robustness for propensity scoring,[98,99] but with only one confounder, no provision for model modification or expansion (and thus no adaptivity to context), and no explicit justification of parameter settings chosen for simulation. Use of modern modeling strategies in simulation can change comparisons dramatically, sometimes in favor of outcome modeling.[33]

The potential accuracy and difficulty of each approach also depends heavily on context as well as modeling strategy. For example, in a study of nutrient intakes and lung cancer, it is doubtful that modeling of intakes (the exposures) will be any simpler or more accurate than modeling of lung cancer risk. Exposure modeling would also be more laborious insofar as a new exposure model would have to be created for every nutrient we wish to examine. As an opposite example, in a focused study of a medical procedure or prescription drug and survival, we may have far more ability to model accurately who will receive the procedure or drug than who will survive the study period. Thus, one cannot judge whether outcome or exposure modeling is preferable without knowledge about the topic under study.

On the latter issue, it is frequently overlooked that adjustment via exposure modeling requires at least two models: the exposure model for X given $\mathbf{Z}$, and a model for adjustment of the X, Y association by the fitted exposure model. The latter model may involve only Y, X, and the fitted score and may be far simpler than the model for $E(Y|X=x, \mathbf{Z}=z)$ if $\mathbf{Z}$ is complicated or contains many variables. Nonetheless, that simplicity reflects only transference of complexity to modeling $P(X=x|\mathbf{Z}=z)$.

A parallel statistical issue is the amount of sample information available for each model. In this regard, the exposure model often has an advantage in practice.[100] To illustrate, suppose that Y is binary and X and $\mathbf{Z}$ are purely categorical. If, as often happens in cohort studies, the sample numbers with $Y=1$ at each level of X, $\mathbf{Z}$ tend to be very small, estimates of conditional risk $P(Y=1|X=x, \mathbf{Z}=z)$ may require a restrictive model or may become unstable and suffer small sample biases.[101] If at the same time the numbers at each level of X, $\mathbf{Z}$ are large, stable estimates of the exposure probabilities $P(X=x|\mathbf{Z}=z)$ can still be obtained. Note, however, that this small sample bias advantage of exposure modeling does not lead to greater precision, because the final precision of any estimate remains limited by the small numbers at $Y=1$. Note also that the advantage would switch to outcome modeling if the outcome ($Y=1$) is common but the exposure ($X=1$) is rare.

The relative precision of summary estimates from outcome and exposure modeling is difficult to evaluate because of the noncomparable models used by the two approaches. Theoretical results that assume homogeneous exposure effects and correct specification of both models[80] find precision or power advantages for outcome modeling as observed in examples and simulations.[99] This advantage is purchased by risk of downwardly biased standard errors if effects are heterogeneous. This risk can be reduced by use of $X - \mathbf{Z}$ product terms or more flexible outcome models, which in turn reduces the efficiency of outcome modeling. The same theory confirms empirical reports that inclusion of nonconfounders is less harmful to precision in exposure modeling than in outcome modeling (assuming, of course, that the nonconfounders are unaffected by exposure; see Chapters 3 and 12), although this difference may not be enough to compensate for the lower precision of exposure modeling relative to outcome modeling.[80,85]

Again, different approaches may be estimating different parameters, which can lead to disparate results even when all the models are correct.[91-93,102] As mentioned above, coefficients from outcome models and marginal models reflect an approximate total population weighting,[53] but propensity score matching can greatly alter the population and hence the weighting. Meaningful comparisons require modification of the weights to give the methods the same standard, as described earlier.

Doubly Robust Estimation

A straightforward resolution of the choice between outcome modeling and exposure modeling is to do both, and if disagreement appears, to attempt to discern the reason. Another resolution is to combine the two approaches, for example, by entering the score directly in a model for Y along with X and $\mathbf{Z}$ or by using the propensity score for matching and then regressing Y on X and $\mathbf{Z}$ in the matched sample.[103] Alternatively, one may use the inverse probability weights estimated from modeling $P(X=x|\mathbf{Z}=z)$ to fit the model for $E(Y|X=x, \mathbf{Z}=z)$ and then standardize over the fitted expected outcomes.[104] Intuitively, the idea is that if propensity scoring or IPW fails to adjust fully for $\mathbf{Z}$, the regression adjustment for $\mathbf{Z}$ may compensate, and vice versa.

This idea is formalized in the theory of *doubly robust estimation*, which shows how to combine outcome and exposure modeling in a fashion that gives a valid estimate if either model is correct.[104] The theory justifies the IPW regression approach and leads to new approaches to marginal modeling.[90] The term *doubly robust* reflects the fact that these methods have two ways to get the right answer, although this property does not necessarily improve performance when neither model is correct.[104] More recent approaches, however, minimize the bias if either of the two models is close to correctly specified.[105] Doubly robust approaches that also employ machine learning or ensemble and cross-validation approaches for model building may be especially promising,[56,57,106] although further work on determining when sample sizes are adequate for the desirable asymptotic properties of these estimators to apply would be desirable.

References

1. Mccullagh P, Nelder JA. *Generalized Linear Models*. New York, NY: Chapman and Hall; 1989.
2. Clayton D, Hills M. *Statistical Models in Epidemiology*. New York, NY: Oxford University Press; 1993.
3. Hosmer D, Lemeshow S. *Applied Logistic Regression*. New York, NY: Wiley; 2000.
4. Agresti AA. *Categorical Data Analysis*. New York, NY: John Wiley & Sons; 2002.
5. Dobson AJ. *An Introduction to Generalized Linear Models*. London: Chapman and Hall/CRC; 2001.
6. Hardin J, Hilbe J. *Generalized Linear Models and Extensions*. New York, NY: Chapman and Hall/CRC Press; 2007.
7. Hoffman JP. *Generalized Linear Models*. Boston, MA: Allyn and Bacon; 2003.
8. Mcculloch CE, Searle SR, Neuhaus JM. *Generalized, Linear, and Mixed Models*. Vol 279. Hoboken, NJ: Wiley; 2008:M38.
9. Hastie T, Tibshirani R, Friedman J. *The Elements of Statistical Learning: Data Mining, Inference, and Prediction*. New York, NY: Springer Science & Business Media; 2009.
10. Wakefield J. *Bayesian and Frequentist Regression Methods*. New York, NY: Springer Science & Business Media; 2013.
11. White H. Maximum likelihood estimation in misspecified models. *Econometrica*. 1982;50:1-9.
12. Royall RM. Model robust confidence intervals using maximum likelihood estimators. *Int Stat Rev*. 1986;54:221-226.
13. Searle SR, Gruber MH. *Linear Models*. New York, NY: John Wiley & Sons; 2016.
14. Mccullagh P. Quasi-likelihood and estimating functions. In: Hinkley DV, Reid N, Snell EJ, eds. *Statistical Theory and Modeling*. London: Chapman and Hall; 1991.
15. Diggle PJ, Heagerty P, Liang KY, Zeger SL. *Analysis of Longitudinal Data*. New York, NY: Oxford; 2002.
16. Cox DR, Wermuth N. A comment on the coefficient of determination for binary responses. *Am Stat*. 1992;46:1-4.
17. Greenland S. A lower bound for the correlation of exponentiated bivariate normal pairs. *Am Stat*. 1996;50:163-164.
18. Greenland S, Schlesselman JJ, Criqui MH. The fallacy of employing standardized regression coefficients and correlations as measures of effect. *Am J Epidemiol*. 1986;123:203-208.
19. Rosenthal RB, Rubin DR. A note on percent variance explained as a measure of importance of effects. *J Appl Soc Psychol*. 1979;9:395-396.
20. Greenland S, Maclure M, Schlesselman JJ, Poole C, Morgenstern H. Standardized regression coefficients: a further critique and review of some alternatives. *Epidemiology*. 1991;2:387-392.
21. Walker AM, Rothman KJ. Models of varying parametric form in case-referent studies. *Am J Epidemiol*. 1982;115:129-137.
22. Leonard T, Hsu JSJ. *Bayesian Methods*. Cambridge: Cambridge University Press; 1999.
23. Carlin B, Louis TA. *Bayes and Empirical-Bayes Methods of Data Analysis*. New York, NY: Chapman and Hall; 2000.
24. Draper D. Assessment and propagation of model uncertainty. *J R Stat Soc Ser B*. 1995;57:45-97.
25. Raftery AE. Bayesian model selection in social research (with discussion). *Sociol Methodol*. 1995;25:111-196.
26. Viallefont V, Raftery AE, Richardson S. Variable selection and Bayesian model averaging in case-control studies. *Stat Med*. 2001;20:3215-3230.
27. Belsley DA, Kuh E, Welsch RE. *Regression Diagnostics: Identifying Influential Data and Sources of Collinearity*. New York, NY: Wiley; 2004.
28. Pregibon D. Logistic regression diagnostics. *Ann Stat*. 1981;9:705-724.
29. Leamer EE. Sensitivity analyses would help. *Am Econ Rev*. 1985;75:308-313.
30. Saltelli A, Chan K, Scott M. *Sensitivity Analysis*. New York, NY: John and Wiley & Sons; 2000.
31. Belloni A, Chernozhukov V, Hansen C. Inference on treatment effects after selection among high-dimensional controls. *Rev Econ Stud*. 2014;81:608-650.
32. Chernozhukov V, Hansen C, Spindler M. *Valid post-selection and post-regularization Inference: An Elementary, General Approach*. Cambridge, MA: Massachusetts Institute of Technology; 2015.
33. Hill JL. Bayesian nonparametric modeling for causal inference. *J Comput Graph Stat*. 2011;20(1):217-240.

34. Sclove SL, Morris C, Radhakrishna R. Non-optimality of preliminary-test estimators for the mean of a multivariate normal distribution. *Ann Math Stat*. 1972;43:1481-1490.

35. Bancroft TW, Han CP. Inference based on conditional specification. *Int Stat Rev*. 1977;45:117-128.

36. Draper NR, Guttman I, Lapczak L. Actual rejection levels in a certain stepwise test. *Commun Stat*. 1979;A8:99-105.

37. Freedman DA. A note on screening regression equations. *Am Stat*. 1983;37:152-155.

38. Flack VF, Chang PC. Frequency of selecting noise variables in subset regression analysis: a simulation study. *Am Stat*. 1987;41:84-86.

39. Hurvich CM, Tsai CL. The impact of model selection on inference in linear regression. *Am Stat*. 1990;44:214-217.

40. Faraway JJ. On the cost of data analysis. *J Comput Graph Stat*. 1992;1:213-219.

41. Weiss RE. The influence of variable selection. *J Am Stat Assoc*. 1995;90:619-625.

42. Greenland S. Summarization, smoothing, and inference in epidemiologic analysis. 1991 Ipsen Lecture, Hindsgavl, Denmark. *Scand J Soc Med*. 1993;21:227-232.

43. Greenland S. When should epidemiologic regressions use random coefficients? *Biometrics*. 2000;56:915-921.

44. Greenland S. Putting background information about relative risks into conjugate prior distributions. *Biometrics*. 2001;57:663-670.

45. Harrell F. *Regression Modeling Strategies*. New York, NY: Springer; 2001.

46. Maldonado G, Greenland S. Simulation study of confounder-selection strategies. *Am J Epidemiol*. 1993;138:923-936.

47. Greenland S, Pearl J, Robins JM. Causal diagrams for epidemiologic research. *Epidemiology*. 1999;10:37-48.

48. Pearl J. *Causality*. 2nd ed. New York, NY: Cambridge University Press; 2009.

49. Vanderweele TJ. Principles of confounder selection. *Eur J Epidemiol*. 2019;34:211-219.

50. Sjölander A, Greenland S. Ignoring the matching variables in cohort studies–when is it valid and why? *Stat Med*. 2013;32:4696-4708.

51. Maclure M. Demonstration of deductive meta-analysis: ethanol intake and risk of myocardial infarction. *Epidemiol Rev*. 1993;15:328-351.

52. Maldonado G, Greenland S. A comparison of the performance of model-based confidence intervals when the correct model form is unknown: coverage of asymptotic means. *Epidemiology*. 1994;5:171-182.

53. Greenland S, Maldonado G. The interpretation of multiplicative-model parameters as standardized parameters. *Stat Med*. 1994;13:989-999.

54. Hernán MA, Hernández-Díaz S, Werler MM, Mitchell AA. Causal knowledge as a prerequisite for confounding evaluation: an application to birth defects epidemiology. *Am J Epidemiol*. 2002;155: 176-184.

55. Leamer EE. *Specification Searches*. New York, NY: Wiley; 1978.

56. van der Laan MJ, Rose S. *Targeted Learning: Causal Inference for Observational and Experimental Data*. New York, NY: Springer Science & Business Media; 2011.

57. van der Laan MJ, Rose S. *Targeted Learning in Data Science*. New York, NY: Springer; 2018.

58. Brown PJ, Vannucci M, Fearn T. Bayes model averaging with selection of regressors. *J R Stat Soc Ser B*. 2002;64:519-536.

59. Efron B. The estimation of prediction error: covariance penalties and cross-validation. *J Am Stat Assoc*. 2004;99:619-642.

60. Shen X, Huang H, Ye J. Inference after model selection. *J Am Stat Assoc*. 2004;99:751-762.

61. Greenland S. Multilevel modeling and model averaging. *Scand J Work Environ Health*. 1999;25(suppl 4):43-48.

62. Greenland S. Invited commentary: variable selection versus shrinkage in the control of multiple confounders. *Am J Epidemiol*. 2008;167:523-529; discussion 530-531.

63. Lane PW, Nelder JA. Analysis of covariance and standardization as instances of prediction. *Biometrics*. 1982;38:613-621.

64. Bruzzi P, Green SB, Byar DP, Brinton LA, Schairer C. Estimating the population attributable risk for multiple risk factors using case-control data. *Am J Epidemiol*. 1985;122:904-914.

65. Flanders WD, Rhodes PH. Large sample confidence intervals for regression standardized risks, risk ratios, and risk differences. *J Chronic Dis*. 1987;40:697-704.

66. Greenland S, Holland P. Estimating standardized risk differences from odds ratios. *Biometrics*. 1991;47:319-322.

67. Greenland S, Drescher K. Maximum likelihood estimation of the attributable fraction from logistic models. *Biometrics*. 1993;49:865-872.

68. Joffe MM, Greenland S. Standardized estimates from categorical regression models. *Stat Med*. 1995;14:2131-2141.

69. Greenland S. Interval estimation by simulation as an alternative to and extension of confidence intervals. *Int J Epidemiol.* 2004;33:1389-1397.
70. Greenland S. Confounding and exposure trends in case-crossover and case-time-control designs. *Epidemiology.* 1996;7:231-239.
71. Greenland S, Michels KB, Robins JM, Poole C, Willett WC. Presenting statistical uncertainty in trends and dose-response relations. *Am J Epidemiol.* 1999;149:1077-1086.
72. Greenland S. Absence of confounding does not correspond to collapsibility of the rate ratio or rate difference. *Epidemiology.* 1996;7:498-501.
73. Bunker JP, Forrest WH, Mosteller F, Vandam LD, eds. *The National Halothane Study. Report of the Subcommittee on the National Halothane Study of the Committee on Anesthesia.* Division of Medical Sciences, National Academy of Sciences-National Research Council. Washington, DC: U.S. Government Printing Office; 1969, Part IV.
74. Greenland S. Bias in methods for deriving standardized morbidity ratio and attributable fraction estimates. *Stat Med.* 1984;3:131-141.
75. Miettinen OS. Stratification by a multivariate confounder score. *Am J Epidemiol.* 1976;104:609-620.
76. Cook EF, Goldman L. Performance of tests of significance based on stratification by a multivariate confounder score or by a propensity score. *J Clin Epidemiol.* 1989;42:317-324.
77. Hansen BB. The prognostic analogue of the propensity score. *Biometrika.* 2008;95:481-488.
78. Pike MC, Anderson J, Day N. Some insights into Miettinen's multivariate confounder score approach to case-control study analysis. *Epidemiol Community Health.* 1979;33:104-106.
79. Rosenbaum PR, Rubin DB. The central role of the propensity score in observational studies for causal effects. *Biometrika.* 1983;70:41-55.
80. Robins JM, Mark SD, Newey WK. Estimating exposure effects by modelling the expectation of exposure conditional on confounders. *Biometrics.* 1992;48:479-495.
81. Rosenbaum PR. Model-based direct adjustment. *J Am Stat Assoc.* 1987;82:387-394.
82. Brookhart MA, Schneeweiss S, Rothman KJ, Glynn RJ, Avorn J, Sturmer T. Variable selection for propensity score models. *Am J Epidemiol.* 2006;163:1149-1156.
83. Rosenbaum PR. *Observational Studies.* New York, NY: Springer; 2002.
84. Rubin DB. Causal inference through potential outcomes and principal stratification: application to studies with "censoring" due to death. *Stat Sci.* 2006;21:299-309.
85. Lunceford JK, Davidian M. Stratification and weighting via the propensity score in estimation of causal treatment effects: a comparative study. *Stat Med.* 2004;23:2937-2960.
86. Abadie A, Imbens GW. On the failure of the bootstrap for matching estimators. Working Paper No. T0325. 2006;39.
87. Hernan MA, Brumback B, Robins JM. Marginal structural models to estimate the causal effect of zidovudine on the survival of HIV-positive men. *Epidemiology.* 2000;11:561-570.
88. Hernán MA, Brumback BA, Robins JM. Marginal structural models to estimate the joint causal effect of nonrandomized treatments. *J Am Stat Assoc.* 2001;96:440-448.
89. Robins JM, Hernan MA, Brumback B. Marginal structural models and causal inference in epidemiology. *Epidemiology.* 2000;11:550-560.
90. Bang H, Robins JM. Doubly robust estimation in missing data and causal inference models. *Biometrics.* 2005;61:962-973.
91. Kurth T, Walker AM, Glynn RJ, et al. Results of multivariable logistic regression, propensity matching, propensity adjustment, and propensity-based weighting under conditions of nonuniform effect. *Am J Epidemiol.* 2006;163:262-270.
92. Sturmer T, Rothman KJ, Glynn RJ. Insights into different results from different causal contrasts in the presence of effect-measure modification. *Pharmacoepidemiol Drug Saf.* 2006;15:698-709.
93. Sturmer T, Schneeweiss S, Brookhart MA, Rothman KJ, Avorn J, Glynn RJ. Analytic strategies to adjust confounding using exposure propensity scores and disease risk scores: nonsteroidal antiinflammatory drugs and short-term mortality in the elderly. *Am J Epidemiol.* 2005;161:891-898.
94. Sato T, Matsuyama Y. Marginal structural models as a tool for standardization. *Epidemiology.* 2003;14:680-686.
95. Brumback BA, Greenland S, Redman M, Kiviat N, Diehr P. The intensity-score approach to adjusting for confounding. *Biometrics.* 2003;59:274-285.
96. Joffe MM, Rosenbaum PR. Invited commentary: propensity scores. *Am J Epidemiol.* 1999;150:327-333.
97. Rubin DB. Estimating causal effects from large data sets using propensity scores. *Ann Intern Med.* 1997;127:757-763.
98. Drake C. Effects of misspecification of the propensity score on estimators of treatment effect. *Biometrics.* 1993;49:1231-1236.
99. Drake C, Fisher L. Prognostic models and the propensity score. *Int J Epidemiol.* 1995;24:183-187.
100. Cepeda MS, Boston R, Farrar JT, Strom BL. Comparison of logistic regression versus propensity score when the number of events is low and there are multiple confounders. *Am J Epidemiol.* 2003;158:280-287.

101. Greenland S, Schwartzbaum JA, Finkle WD. Problems from small samples and sparse data in conditional logistic regression analysis. *Am J Epidemiol*. 2000;151:531-539.
102. Austin PC, Grootendorst P, Normand SL, Anderson GM. Conditioning on the propensity score can result in biased estimation of common measures of treatment effect: a Monte Carlo study. *Stat Med*. 2007;26:754-768.
103. Rubin DB. *Matched Sampling for Causal Effects*. New York, NY: Cambridge University Press; 2006.
104. Kang JDY, Shafer JL. Demystifying double robustness: a comparison of alternative strategies for estimating a population mean from incomplete data (with discussion). *Stat Sci*. 2007;22:523-580.
105. Vansteelandt S, Bekaert M, Claeskens G. On model selection and model misspecification in causal inference. *Stat Methods Med Res*. 2012;21:7-30.
106. Schuler MS, Rose S. Targeted maximum likelihood estimation for causal inference in observational studies. *Am J Epidemiol*. 2017;185, 65-73.

Time-To-Event Analysis

Sebastien Haneuse

Much of epidemiologic research concerns itself with the occurrence of health events such as the diagnosis of a particular disease/condition, receipt of treatment, resolution or cure of a condition, and death. Inextricably bound to the occurrence of any such event is its timing. Indeed, beyond whether an event ever occurs, the timing of its occurrence is a central feature. In studies of disease incidence, for example, it is often of interest to understand the age at which patients are diagnosed. Furthermore, if the focus is on prognosis post diagnosis, the timing of key events including treatment and resolution or cure of the disease of interest will be critical to understand, as may be the timing of death. In such settings, the outcome of interest is referred to as a *time-to-event* outcome; when the event is mortality, we sometimes refer to the timing as a *survival* outcome. In principle, since the timing of an event is continuous random variable, one could use, say, linear regression as a modeling framework. As we will see, however, practical considerations often result in the value of the time-to-event outcome for a given study participant being incompletely observed; that is, one may not know the exact timing although we may know, for example, that it was not observed to occur within some window of follow-up. This limitation has given rise to a suite of specialized statistical tools for time-to-event outcome data analysis. In this chapter, we provide a brief overview of these tools.

CORE CONCEPTS

Time Scales

Crucial to any time-to-event outcome is the time scale on which it is measured, together with how time zero, sometimes referred to as the *origin*, is defined. In a study of cancer incidence, for example, one may take age in years as the time scale with birth as the origin. When interest lies in understanding differences in outcomes across birth cohorts, it may be natural to take calendar time as the time scale with, say, 1900 as the origin. In studies of prognosis, it may be natural to start follow-up at the occurrence of some relevant clinical event, such as the date of diagnosis or of treatment initiation, from which time is measured. Together, the time scale and origin form the basis of interpretation of the time-to-event outcome and, correspondingly, the study at-hand.

Right Censoring

Ideally, the study design that underpins the available data for a time-to-event analysis would (1) permit following a participant from the origin and (2) ensure sufficient follow-up so that the timing of the event for each study participant is observed and recorded by the research team. In many instances, however, one or both of these may not be possible. If we initially assume that all participants are followed from the origin (we return to this in the next subsection), failure of the second of these conditions means that the actual timing of event is not observed for some participants. In such settings, we say that the event time is *right censored*. The reasons for right censoring may vary. Funding restrictions, for example, may constrain follow-up of participants to a fixed period of time (*e.g.*, 1 year post treatment initiation) or to some fixed date (*e.g.*, July 1, 2025). This type of censoring is sometimes referred to as *administrative censoring,* since it is dictated by the research team. In other instances, the censoring mechanism may be under the partial but not complete control of the research team. For example, the study protocol may indicate that if the patient experiences an intermediate event, such as an adverse event or a pregnancy, then follow-up for the primary event will stop. Finally, there are instances where the censoring is completely outside of the control of the research team, such as when a participant decides to withdraw from the study or is lost to follow-up (*i.e.*, the study team is unable to contact the participant). Related to this latter set of instances, when mortality is not the primary event of interest, a participant's follow-up time is sometimes viewed as having been censored if he or she dies before the event is observed. The role that mortality plays, however, is distinct from that of censoring. Crucially, censoring is not a phenomenon that interferes with the *occurrence* of the event but, rather, is a phenomenon that interferes with the capacity of the research team to *observe* the event. Thus, in the absence of censoring, an implicit assumption is that the event will eventually occur and that it would be possible to observe it if it occurs during the study follow-up period. Clearly death does not fall within this rubric of censoring: once an individual dies, he or she cannot experience further events, so that the notion of observing an event is not even well defined. More appropriately death is a *competing risk*, a topic we return to below.

In any given study, the extent of censoring will depend on the interplay between whether or how the censoring mechanisms manifest and the rate (over time) of the event of interest. If the event is rare, for example, moderate censoring may have a larger relative impact on the observed number of events than it would if the event is common; for a rare disease, fewer of the actual event times from an already small number of events would be observed. As will become clear, this interplay has important implications for precision (*i.e.*, standard error estimation), which depends, in part, on the observed number of events.

To illustrate the effect of censoring, we use data from a placebo-controlled randomized trial, initially reported by Freireich et al., that assessed the use of 6-mercaptopurine (6-MP) among patients aged 20 years and younger who had a diagnosis of leukemia and had achieved partial or complete remission following treatment with corticosteroids.[1] The event of interest was whether the patient experienced a relapse of their leukemia. Table 22-1 provides the observed outcome data, measured in weeks, for 42 patients (21 in the 6-MP arm and 21 in the placebo arm). Attached to select values among patients in the 6-MP arm (11 in all) is a superscript "+" which indicates that the observed time was censored at that value. So, for example, there was one patient who was followed until week 6 and then censored without having experienced a relapse event. That there are no such values in the placebo arm indicates that the time to relapse was observed for each of these 21 patients. Figure 22-1 provides a graphical representation of the observed outcome information, with panels (A) and (B) representing the placebo arm and the 6-MP arm, respectively.

We will use the following notation: let T denote the time-to-event and X indicate treatment assignment; for the 6-MP trial, $X = 0$ indicates assignment to the placebo arm and $X = 1$ indicates assignment to the 6-MP arm. To summarize the information about the distribution of T within strata defined by X, a natural quantity to consider is the conditional mean, $\mu_x = E(T \mid X = x)$. Focusing on the placebo arm, one can use the data in Table 22-1 to estimate $\mu_0 = E(T \mid X = 0)$ in the usual way (*i.e.*, simply add up the values and divide by 21); the result is $\hat{\mu}_0 = 8.7$ weeks. Performing the same

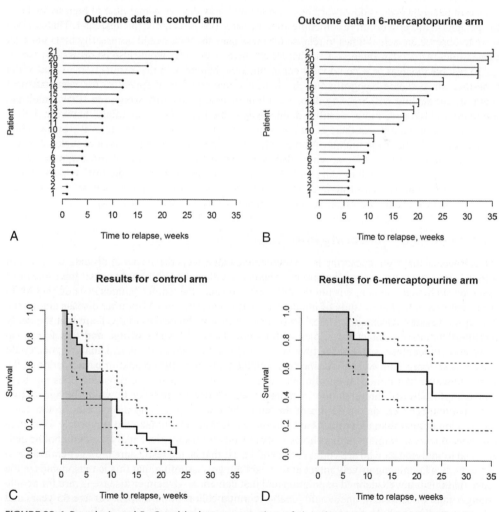

FIGURE 22-1 Panels A and B, Graphical representation of the observed outcome data for 42 patients in a placebo-randomized trial of 6-mercaptopurine for maintenance of remission following treatment for leukemia with corticosteroids, with a black dot indicating a relapse event and a square bracket indicating follow-up being censored. Panels C and D, Kaplan-Meier estimates of the survivor function (solid black line), together with 95% confidence intervals (dashed black line); the red and blue lines indicate the estimated median survival time and the 10-week survival probabilities, respectively; finally, the gray area quantifies the 10-week restricted mean survival.

TABLE 22-1

Observed Outcome Data for 42 Patients in a Placebo-Randomized Trial of 6-Mercaptopurine for Maintenance of Remission Following Treatment for Leukemia With Corticosteroids. Values Indicated With a Superscript "+" Were Right Censored

	Time to Relapse (weeks)
Placebo arm	1, 1, 2, 2, 3, 4, 4, 5, 5, 8, 8, 8, 8, 11, 11, 12, 12, 15, 17, 22, 23
6-Mercaptopurine arm	6, 6, 6, 6$^+$, 7, 9$^+$, 10, 10, 11$^+$, 13, 16, 17$^+$, 19$^+$, 20$^+$, 22, 23, 25$^+$, 32$^+$, 32$^+$, 34$^+$, 35$^+$

calculation for the 21 patients in the 6-MP arm yields an estimate of $\mu_1 = E(T|X=1)$ of 17.1 weeks. This estimate, however, is downward biased since we know that the actual time to relapse for 11 of the patients in this arm occurred sometime after the value that is recorded in Table 22-1. That is, if we were to observe the actual times to relapse for these patients, they would necessarily be larger than those values recorded in Table 22-1, so that the estimate of the mean would also be necessarily larger.

To resolve this bias, one could view censoring as a phenomenon that results in the value of the time-to-event outcome being missing. In doing so, one could then appeal to the vast statistical literature on dealing with missing data, including inverse-probability weighting (IPW), multiple imputation (MI), and, more recently, doubly-robust methods. These methods, however, fail to acknowledge or exploit that there is, in fact, partial information on the timing of the event: while we do not know the exact timing of the event, we do know that it had to have occurred at some point in time beyond the time at which they were censored. It is, therefore, more appropriate to view the observed data as providing partial or incomplete information on the timing of the event. Viewing the impact of censoring in this way, the field of time-to-event data analysis is concerned with how best to use the information that is available.

Other Forms of Censoring and Truncation

We emphasize that right censoring is a phenomenon that affects the ability to observe the event of interest and not a phenomenon that affects whether it will occur. While right censoring is the most common such phenomenon, it is not the only one. Consider the Adult Changes in Thought (ACT) study, a community-based study of incident all-cause dementia and Alzheimer disease among the elderly in western Washington state.[2] Two key features of the design of ACT are that the study recruited cognitively intact participants who were at least 65 years of age and that follow-up consisted of biennial visits. For the time scale on which to base the statistical analysis, one could use *time-on-study*, defined as time since enrollment. Outside of the context of participation in the study, however, the notion of enrollment has no meaning, so that time-on-study does not have a meaningful clinical interpretation. A more natural choice for time scale would be age, taking birth as the origin. Given the design of the study, however, there is no information in the study for people younger than 65 years. One solution to this would be to take the time scale to be *time since age 65 years*. Implicit to this choice is that results from statistical analyses could not be generalized to individuals who are younger than 65 years; that is, the results are only generalizable to individuals who are cognitively intact at 65 years of age. Assuming that this is reasonable (in the sense that this is a well-defined population and that dementia/Alzheimer disease is rare for people younger than of 65 years), one would ideally recruit a cohort of participants at age 65 years and follow them forward. As mentioned, however, this is not how ACT was designed; participants were, less stringently, only required to be at least 65 years of age. Consider, then, a participant who was enrolled at age 74 years and had three biennial visits (*i.e.*, at ages 76, 78, and 80), with the third resulting in a diagnosis of dementia. On the time scale we have chosen, their observed event time is 15 years since age 65 years. In considering their contribution to the data analysis, however, we should note that there was a 9-year period (between age 65 and 74 years) during which the research team would have had no opportunity to observe the event, had it occurred. From the perspective of the data analysis, therefore, it is not clear whether this participant can be viewed as providing the same information relative to, say, a participant who was recruited at age 65 years and followed until a diagnosis of dementia at age 80 years. When follow-up for a participant begins sometime after the origin, we say that their observed person-time in subject to *left truncation*.

A third phenomena that arises in ACT (*i.e.*, beyond right censoring and left truncation) is that while a formal diagnosis is given during one of the biennial follow-up visits, it is not clear whether the age at that visit can be taken as the exact age for their event time. Consider the aforementioned example participant who received a diagnosis during the visit when they were 80 years of age. It may have been that had they had a visit between the two biennial visits they actually had, they would have had a diagnosis at age 79 years. Given the design of the follow-up schedule, we cannot know whether this would have been the case; the most we can know is that the exact age at which the criteria for diagnosis would have been met is somewhere between the age attained at the visit during which the diagnosis was actually given and the age at the previous visit. This phenomenon, where one knows that the event occurred during some interval, but it is not known exactly when, is referred to as *interval censoring*.

Moving forward, we restrict attention to settings where the observed data are at most subject to right censoring. Although beyond the scope of this chapter, if left truncation or interval censoring is present, then they should be acknowledged and properly dealt with in the data analysis. As mentioned, by not doing so, the analysis assumes there is more information about the distribution of the time-to-event outcome than is actually available.

The Independent Censoring Assumption

In standard missing data problems, the extent to which the application of statistical methods such as IPW and MI yields valid results or conclusions hinges on the plausibility of an assumption regarding the mechanism(s) that underpin whether and why some participants have missing data and others not; that assumption is the so-called *missing-at-random* assumption.[3,4] An analogous assumption is required for statistical analyses of time-to-event data in the presence of right censoring, specifically the *independent censoring assumption*. The assumption corresponds to the notion that the censoring does not depend on the timing of the event of interest. When the censoring is purely administrative, the assumption holds; the mechanism by which person-time is censored (*e.g.*, the end of funding) is unrelated to when the event of interest occurs for any given participant. The assumption may not hold, however, if patients who are experiencing precursor symptoms to the event of interest differentially withdraw just before experiencing the actual event.

More formally, the assumption says that the timing of censoring is independent of the timing of the event of interest, conditional on any covariates that are incorporated into the analysis (including, as appropriate, an exposure or treatment of interest). Crucially, the plausibility of independence must be evaluated within levels of any such covariates. Thus, for example, even if participants in the control arm of the leukemia study were determined to be differentially withdrawing from the study (relative to those in the 6-MP arm), the assumption may be plausible for an analysis that stratifies on treatment arm. More generally, analysts must query whether there exist covariates that vary simultaneously with both censoring and the event of interest and have not been stratified or adjusted for. If there are, then the assumption of independent censoring may not be plausible and specialized methods will be needed.

PARAMETRIC ANALYSES OF TIME-TO-EVENT DATA

While statistical methods for data analysis tend to focus on estimating means, the field of time-to-event data analysis has evolved to target a range of estimands. Chief among these are the survival function and the hazard function, together with related quantities. Note that the time-to-event outcome T is a nonnegative, continuous random variable. In general, one can characterize the distribution of such a random variable in a number of ways. One could, for example, specify the *probability density function*, formally defined as:

$$f(t) = \lim_{\Delta \to 0} \frac{1}{\Delta} P(t \le T \le t + \Delta),$$

or the *survival function,* $S(t) = P(T > t)$, which is the probability that the event occurs after time t. Mathematically, these quantities are related, specifically through:

$$S(t) = 1 - P(T \le t) = 1 - F(t) = 1 - \int_0^t f(s)\,ds,$$

where $F(t)$ is the *cumulative distribution function,* sometimes referred to as the *cumulative incidence function.* Yet another characterization is via the *hazard function*:

$$\lambda(t) = \lim_{\Delta \to 0} \frac{1}{\Delta} P(t \le T \le t + \Delta \mid T \ge t),$$

which is also mathematically related to $f(t)$ and $S(t)$ via:

$$\lambda(t) = \frac{f(t)}{S(t)} = -\frac{d}{dt} \log S(t).$$

Finally, one could also characterize the distribution of T via the *cumulative hazard function*:

$$\Lambda(t) = \int_0^t \lambda(u)\,du = -\log S(t).$$

Because of its ubiquity in statistical analyses of time-to-event data, it is worth considering the precise interpretation of the hazard function, $\lambda(t)$. At the heart of the definition is $P(t \le T \le t + \Delta \mid T \ge t)$, which is the probability that the event has not occurred by time t but then does occur within the next time interval Δ; that is, it is a conditional probability of experiencing the event within the next Δ time units at time t given that the event has not occurred yet. Dividing this probability by Δ converts it into a rate, with time as the denominator. Finally, the hazard is defined by considering the limiting value of this rate as the Δ interval gets increasingly small. In the limit, therefore, the hazard function is the instantaneous rate of the event at time t, given that it has not occurred by time t.

Because of the above mathematical relationships, each of the four functions, $f(t)$, $S(t)$, $\lambda(t)$, and $\Lambda(t)$ can be used to uniquely characterize the distribution of T, albeit on different scales. Consequently, one could proceed with a data analysis by first choosing some parametric distribution and then structuring any of $f(t)$, $S(t)$, $\lambda(t)$, and $\Lambda(t)$ that correspond to that distribution to be a function of covariates. Common choices for this distribution include the exponential, Weibull, Gamma, log-normal, log-logistic, Gompertz, and generalized Gamma distributions. As with all parametric analyses, if the correct distribution is chosen and a correct specification of how the distribution depends on covariates is adopted, then one could perform valid (in the sense of obtaining consistent point estimates and valid 95% confidence intervals) and statistically efficient analyses via maximum likelihood estimation.

To illustrate this, we return to the 21 patients in the 6-MP arm of the leukemia trial. In doing so, recall that we argued that the estimate of 17.1 weeks for μ_1 was downward biased (because of the right censoring of 11 of the patients in this arm). Suppose we were willing to assume that $(T_1, \ldots, T_{21})$, the times to relapse for the 21 patients in the 6-MP arm, constitute an independent and identically distributed sample from an exponential (μ_1) distribution (*i.e.*, one with mean μ_1). In the absence of censoring (*i.e.*, we observe T for each patient), one could estimate μ_1 by maximizing the likelihood:

$$L^c(\mu_1) = \prod_{i=1}^{21} f(t_i; \mu_1) = \prod_{i=1}^{21} \frac{1}{\mu_1} \exp\left(\frac{-t_i}{\mu_1}\right),$$

where t_i is the observed time to relapse for the ith study participant in the 6-MP arm. Since t_i is not observed for each individual, however, this likelihood cannot even be evaluated. Thus, an alternative formulation for the likelihood is needed. To obtain it, we require an extended notation that permits distinguishing participants who are censored and those who are not. Toward this, let C denote the time-to-censoring, taken to be defined on the same time scale as T. Then, let Y denote the minimum of T and C; that is, Y denotes the first time at which a study participant is either censored or experiences the event. To distinguish which event the time Y corresponds to, let Δ be a binary indicator of whether the observed time is an event time. Thus, the observed outcome data for a participant who is censored is $(y_i, \delta_i) = (c_i, 0)$, whereas that for a participant who is observed to experience the event is $(y_i, \delta_i) = (t_i, 1)$.

Assuming independence across participants in the study, the new likelihood criterion will be a product of 21 contributions, as in $L^c(\mu_1)$. However, the specific contribution will depend on the nature of the observed outcome data. If the ith participant was observed to experience a relapse event, then their contribution will be $f(y_i)$ (*i.e.*, the usual contribution). If they were censored then, they cannot contribute $f(y_i)$, since we do not know the exact time at which they experienced the event. However, we can say that they survived to time y_i. Having adopted a parametric distribution for T, and assuming that independent censoring holds, this information can be encoded via the survival function evaluated at the observed time: $S(y_i)$. Jointly, these contributions can be succinctly written as:

$$L_i(\mu_1) = \begin{cases} f(y_i) & \text{if } \delta_i = 1 \\ S(y_i) & \text{if } \delta_i = 0 \end{cases}.$$

Collectively, the contributions across the 21 participants in the 6-MP arm can be expressed as:

$$L(\mu_1) = \prod_{i=1}^{21} f(y_i; \mu_1)^{\delta_i} S(y_i; \mu_1)^{1-\delta_i} = \prod_{i=1}^{21} \lambda(y_i; \mu_1)^{\delta_i} S(y_i; \mu_1)$$

$$= \prod_{i=1}^{21} \left(\frac{1}{\mu_1}\right)^{\delta_i} \exp\left(\frac{-y_i}{\mu_1}\right),$$

where the second of the above equalities comes from the relation: $\lambda(t) = f(t)/S(t)$. In comparing $L(\mu_1)$ with $L^c(\mu_1)$, while all participants (including those who are censored) contribute "$\exp(-y_i/\mu_1)$," only those participants who are observed to experience the event additionally contribute "$1/\mu_1$." Put another way, only those participants for whom the exact timing of the event is known contribute this extra information.

Due to the relative simplicity of the exponential distribution, the maximum likelihood estimate (MLE) of μ_1 can be derived analytically and is:

$$\hat{\mu}_1 = \frac{\sum_{i=1}^{21} y_i}{\sum_{i=1}^{21} \delta_i}$$

Note, the numerator of $\hat{\mu}_1$ is the sum of the observed times (be they event or censoring times), while the denominator is the number of observed events. Based on this, the MLE of the mean for the 6-MP arm is 35.9 weeks, which is more than double the naïve estimate of 17.1 weeks. Finally, if all of the observed times correspond to event times (*i.e.*, all of the $\delta_i = 1$), then the MLE under an exponential distribution is simply the sample mean. Thus, because there was no censoring in the control arm, the MLE under an exponential (μ_0) distribution for the participants in the control arm is the same as reported above, 8.7 weeks.

NONPARAMETRIC RISK ESTIMATION AND COMPARISON

The use of a likelihood based on a parametric choice for the distribution of T can easily be extended beyond estimation of a single mean. One could, for example, adopt a regression structure, as described in Chapters 19 and 20, and then estimate the parameters and perform inference in the usual way. Inherent to this is the necessity of choosing some parametric distribution for T, along with the risk that, in choosing the wrong distribution, one may end up with erroneous results and conclusions. It is therefore natural to query whether one can perform an analysis that reduces or completely removes the need to choose a specific distribution. In this subsection, we consider non-parametric estimation of the survival function, as well as methods for comparing two groups. In the following subsections, we consider regression.

Estimation of the Survival Function

As we did for the parametric analyses, it is instructive to first consider estimation of the survival function in the absence of censoring. To that end, consider the 21 patients in the control arm of the leukemia study. Since all of the observed times are actual relapse times, one could estimate the survival function at any given time t as the proportion of patients with $T > t$:

$$\hat{S}(t) = \frac{\# \text{ Participants with } T > t}{21}.$$

Thus, using the data in Table 22-1, the estimated survival at 5, 10, and 15 weeks is $12/21 = 0.571$, $8/21 = 0.381$, and $3/21 = 0.143$, respectively.

Now consider applying the same estimator to the data for the 21 participants in the 6-MP arm. At 15 weeks, one would estimate $\hat{S}(15) = 11/21 = 0.524$. The problem with this estimate, however, is that it implicitly assumes that the three participants who were censored before 15 weeks did not survive to 15 weeks. At the other extreme, one could assume that all three of these participants did survive, which would give $14/21 = 0.667$. The reality, of course, is that these values provide bounds: the actual number who survived to time 15 weeks is between 0 and 3. In principle, one could report these bounds and avoid the need to make any further assumptions (*i.e.*, about the censoring). The reporting of bounds, however, is rarely satisfactory.

One way forward would be to consider only those participants with complete data and estimate survival at 15 weeks as:

$$\hat{S}(15) = \frac{\text{Participants with } T > 15}{\text{With complete data at 15 weeks}} = \frac{11}{18} = 0.611.$$

If the independent censoring assumption holds, then this would be a reasonable strategy. It would, however, suffer from the important drawback that one throws away the partial information that the censored participants provide and, therefore, be statistically inefficient.

The *Kaplan-Meier estimator*, sometimes referred to as the *life table method*, provides a means of estimating the survival function nonparametrically by exploiting a decomposition of $S(t)$ in terms of a series of conditional probabilities. Recall that the observed data are $[(y_i, \delta_i); i = 1, \ldots, n]$. Based on this, suppose there are K unique observed event times in the sample: $t_{(1)} < t_{(2)} < \ldots < t_{(K)}$. For the 21 participants in the 6-MP arms, the $K = 7$ ordered events times are $(6, 7, 10, 13, 16, 22, 23)$. Now partition the time scale based on these times to give $K+1$ mutually exclusive intervals:

$$\left[0, t_{(1)}\right) \cup \left[t_{(1)}, t_{(2)}\right) \cup \ldots \cup \left[t_{(K-1)}, t_{(K)}\right) \cup \left[t_{(K)}, \infty\right).$$

Define the *risk set* R_k to be the set of participants who were at risk to be observed to experience the event at time $t_{(k)}$; that is, all individuals who have not experienced the event nor have been censored at the start of interval $[t_{(k)}, t_{(k+1)})$. Then, for each risk set compute: n_k, the number of participants at risk; d_k, the number of participants who experience the event at time $t_{(k)}$; and, s_k, the number of participants who do not. To illustrate these calculations, consider the fifth ordered failure time among the participants in the 6-MP arm for which $t_{(k)} = 16$, $[t_{(5)}, t_{(6)}) = [16, 22)$, $R_k = (11, 12, \ldots, 21)$, $n_k = 11$, $d_k = 1$, and $s_k = 10$. The first four columns of Table 22-2 provide a summary of these quantities across the $K = 7$ ordered event times.

TABLE 22-2

Illustration of the Calculation of the Kaplan-Meier Estimate of the Survivor Function, Using Data From the 6-Mercaptopurine Arm of the Leukemia Study

$t_{(k)}$	n_k	d_k	s_k	$\hat{P}\left(T > t_{(k)} \middle| T \geq t_{(k)}\right)$	$\hat{S}_{KM}\left(t_{(k)}\right)$
0	21	0	21	1.000	1.000
6	21	3	18	0.857	0.857
7	17	1	16	0.941	0.807
10	15	2	13	0.867	0.699
13	12	1	11	0.917	0.641
16	11	1	10	0.909	0.583
22	7	1	6	0.857	0.499
23	6	1	5	0.833	0.416

For the kth row of Table 22-1, one can estimate the conditional probability of survival past time $t_{(k)}$, given that the event had not occurred by time $t_{(k)}$ as:

$$\hat{P}\left(T > t_{(k)} \middle| T \geq t_{(k)}\right) = \frac{s_k}{n_k} = 1 - \frac{d_k}{n_k}.$$

Finally, the Kaplan-Meier estimator of $S(t)$ is the product of these conditional probability estimates across all risk sets before and including time t:

$$\hat{S}_{KM}(t) = \prod_{k:t_{(k)} \leq t} \frac{s_k}{n_k} = \prod_{k:t_{(k)} \leq t} 1 - \frac{d_k}{n_k}.$$

The right-most column of Table 22-2 provides the estimates at each of the unique event times for the 6-MP arm; panels (C) and (D) in Figure 22-1 provide a graphical representation for the control and 6-MP arms, respectively.

Two key ideas underpin the Kaplan-Meier estimator. First, it is only possible to learn about the shape of the function at times when an event occurs. Hence, as is clear in Figure 22-1, the shape has "jumps" at each of the $t_{(k)}$, the sizes of which are dictated by the relative number of events compared with the number at risk, and the estimated curve is flat between event times. Second, the product of conditional probabilities reflects the notion that in order for a participant to survive to time t without experiencing the event they must have first survived through each of the intervals before time t. Each interval leading to time t is a "step" that must be survived. For each step, the calculations address the question, "now that I have made it to this point, what is the probability that I make it to the next one?"

Summarizing Risk

In addition to a graphical representation of the estimated survival function, it may be of interest to report estimates of select measures. If, for example, some meaningful time point, say t_0, can be prespecified, then one might compute and report $\hat{S}_{KM}(t_0)$. From Figure 22-1C and D, setting $t_0 = 10$ weeks, we have $\hat{S}_{KM}(10) = 0.381$ in the control arm and $\hat{S}_{KM}(10) = 0.699$ in the 6-MP arm. Alternatively, it may be of interest to report an estimate of the mean time-to-event. In the absence of censoring, one can compute the mean estimate directly (as indicated above for the control arm). In the presence of censoring, one can estimate the mean by computing the area under the curve. For this to be a valid estimate of the mean, however, it must be that the final observed time is an event of interest (as opposed to being a censoring time). If this is the case, the Kaplan-Meier estimator descends to zero at the time of the final observed event time event, as in Figure 22-1C.

If the last observed time corresponds to a censoring event, then the Kaplan-Meier estimator plateaus at some value greater than zero, as in Figure 22-1D, and the mean cannot be estimated (unless one specifies some parametric distribution for T). In some such settings, however, one can still estimate the *median survival* time, which is the time at which 50% of the population has experienced the event. Estimating this quantity from the Kaplan-Meier estimate of $S(t)$ simply corresponds to finding the time where $\hat{S}_{KM}(t) = 0.5$. In Figure 22-1C and D, the median survival times for the control and 6-MP arms are 8 and 22 weeks, respectively; see the vertical red lines. Note, if the event rate is low and 50% of the individuals in a given sample are not observed to experience the event, then the median survival cannot be estimated either. One could, however, choose some other quantile, such as estimating the point at which 20% of the population experience the event. Finally, as a further alternative when the mean time-to-event cannot be estimated, one could estimate the *restricted mean survival time* (RMST); rather than computing the mean survival as the area under the entire curve, compute the area under the curve to some time point and interpret the quantity as the average time-to-event to that time.[5] The shaded areas in Figure 22-1C and D graphically represent the 10-week RMST. To calculate the RMST up to time t_0, one can use the following formula:

$$\text{RMST}(t_0) = \sum_{k:t_{(k)} < t_0} \hat{S}_{KM}\left(t_{(k-1)}\right) \times \left(t_{(k)} - t_{(k-1)}\right) + \hat{S}_{KM}\left(t_{(k)}\right) \times \left(t_0 - t_{(k)}\right)$$

with $t_{(0)} = 0$ and $\hat{S}_{KM}\left(t_{(0)}\right) = 1.0$. Using the values provided in Table 22-2, we have:

$$\widehat{\text{RMST}}_1(10) = 1.000 \times (6-0) + 0.857 \times (7-6) + 0.807 \times (10-7) = 9.3 \text{ weeks}$$

in the 6-MP arm. Performing the same calculation in the control arm yields $\widehat{\text{RMST}}_0(10) = 6.6$ weeks. Consequently, the results from this study suggest that patients who undergo treatment with 6-MP are estimated to experience 2.7 more relapse-free weeks, on average, during the first 10 weeks following initiation of treatment.

Quantification of Uncertainty

In addition to presenting an estimate of the survival function, or an estimate of some summary measure, it will often be of interest to present some quantification of uncertainty. Usually, this is in the form of a 95% confidence interval for which an estimate of the variance of the Kaplan-Meier estimator is needed. One such estimator is *Greenwood formula*:

$$\hat{V}_G\left[\hat{S}_{KM}(t_0)\right] = \left[\hat{S}_{KM}(t_0)\right]^2 \sum_{k:t_{(k)} \le t_0} \frac{d_k}{n_k s_k}.$$

If we let $\widehat{SE}_G(t_0)$ denote the square-root of this quantity, one can construct an approximate 95% confidence interval as:

$$\left[\hat{S}_{KM}(t_0) - 1.96\widehat{SE}_G(t_0), \hat{S}_{KM}(t_0) - 1.96\widehat{SE}_G(t_0)\right].$$

One potential problem with this interval is that there is no guarantee that it will respect the fact that $S(t_0)$ must be between 0 and 1. One solution to this problem is to construct a 95% confidence interval for $\log\left[-\log\hat{S}_{KM}(t_0)\right]$ and then back-transform onto the $S(t_0)$ scale. Toward this, an application of the delta method gives an estimate of the variance of $\log\left[-\log\hat{S}_{KM}(t_0)\right]$ as:

$$\hat{V}\left\{\log\left[-\log\hat{S}_{KM}(t_0)\right]\right\} = \left[\frac{1}{-\log\hat{S}_{KM}(t_0)}\right]^2 \sum_{k:t_{(k)} < t_0} \frac{d_k}{n_k s_k}.$$

Letting $\widehat{SE}_{ll}(t_0)$ denote the square-root of this quantity, a 95% confidence interval for $\hat{S}_{KM}(t_0)$ that respects the bounds that the underlying true value of $S(t_0)$ is:

$$\left[\hat{S}_{KM}(t_0)^{\exp\left[1.96\widehat{SE}_{ll}(t_0)\right]}, \hat{S}_{KM}(t_0)^{\exp\left[-1.96\widehat{SE}_{ll}(t_0)\right]} \right].$$

The gray dashed lines in Figure 22-1C and D provide these (pointwise) 95% confidence intervals for the two arms in the leukemia study. Beyond the log-log transformation, other options include using an arcsine transformation or a logit transformation. A final solution is to construct a 95% interval by using results for the proportion of a binomial distribution with proportion p and sample size N but with $\hat{p}$ replaced by $\hat{S}_{KM}(t_0)$ and N replaced by N^*, termed the "effective sample size," which is obtained by equating the Greenwood variance with an estimate of the variance that follows by directly applying a binomial distribution: $\hat{V}\left[\hat{S}_{KM}(t_0)\right] = \hat{S}_{KM}(t_0)\left[1 - \hat{S}_{KM}(t_0)\right]/N^*$.[6,7] All of these methods ensure admissible values of the interval limits, with results from Anderson et al. indicating that the bounds proposed by Rothman are preferred in small-sample settings.

Comparisons Between Groups

Finally, we consider settings where it is of interest to compare the survival experience of two groups. Toward this, let $S_0(t)$ denote the survival function for group 0 (e.g., the control arm in the leukemia data) and $S_1(t)$ is the survival function for group 1 (e.g., the 6-MP arm in the leukemia data). If, as considered above, some meaningful time point, say t_0, can be prespecified, one could estimate the $S_0(t_0) - S_1(t_0)$ with $\hat{S}_{1,KM}(t_0) - \hat{S}_{0,KM}(t_0)$, and construct a 95% confidence interval based on the following estimate of the standard error of the estimated difference: $\sqrt{\hat{V}\left[\hat{S}_{1,KM}(t_0)\right] + \hat{V}\left[\hat{S}_{0,KM}(t_0)\right]}$. One problem with this form of comparison, however, is that there may not be a single, clinically meaningful time point. Furthermore, even if one can be identified, focusing on a single time point effectively precludes insight into differences between the two groups that manifest at other times. As such, it is often the case that interest lies in comparing the survival experience between two groups across the entire (observed) follow-up period. This can be performed via a *log-rank test*. While the overarching philosophy of this book is to discourage the use of statistical hypothesis testing (see Chapter 2), such tests are commonplace in two-arm randomized trials. Toward this, let $t_{(1)} < t_{(2)} < \ldots < t_{(K)}$ now denote the unique ordered event times after pooling across the two groups. Then, at each such event time, consider the 2×2 table that categorizes all patients at risk to be observed to experience the event at time $t_{(k)}$ by whether they experience the event and by group membership; see Table 22-3. Under the null hypothesis of no difference in the survival functions between the two groups, that is $S_0(t) = S_1(t)$ for all t, conditional on the risk set at time $t_{(k)}$, the number of events in group 1, D_{1k}, has a hypergeometric (n_k, n_{1k}, d_k) distribution. From this, the expected number of events is $E(D_{1k}) = n_{1k}d_k/n_k$. Now let $U_k = D_{1k} - E(D_{1k})$ be the difference between the observed and expected number of events in group 1. Under the null hypothesis, it can be shown that $E(U_k) = 0$ and that,

$$V(U_k) = \frac{n_{1k}n_{0k}(n_k - d_k)d_k}{n_k^2(n_k - 1)}.$$

Using these results, one can perform a test on the basis of the log-rank test statistic:

$$T_{LR} = \frac{\left(\sum_{k=1}^{K} U_k\right)^2}{\sum_{k=1}^{K} V(U_k)},$$

which, in large samples, has a χ^2 distribution with one degree of freedom.

It may be instructive to note that the log-rank test based on T_{LR} is equivalent to the Cochran-Mantel-Haenzel test as applied to the sequence of 2×2 tables formed by stratification on time (specifically, at the K unique event times across the two groups); see Chapter 18. Viewed in this way,

TABLE 22-3

2x2 Table Associated With the *k*th Pooled Event Time, $t_{(k)}$, in a Log-Rank Test of the Difference in the Time-to-Event Experience Between Two Groups

	Event		
	No	**Yes**	
Group 0	$n_{0k} - d_{1k}$	d_{0k}	n_{0k}
Group 1	$n_{1k} - d_{1k}$	d_{1k}	n_{1k}
	$n_k - d_k$	d_k	n_k

a key feature of the log-rank test is that, while the entire quantity is standardized by the sum of the variances in the denominator, the K U_k components contribute equally; the numerator is obtained by simply adding up the contributions. This may be surprising, however, since risk sets that are formed later in the time scale are necessarily smaller because individuals who experience the event and/or are censored are subsequently removed from consideration. A consequence of this is that the magnitude of T_{LR} may be sensitive to contributions from risk sets that are formed later in the time scale. Because of this, one may wish to down-weight those contributions in a manner that reflects the notion that they are providing less "information" or, equivalently, up-weight the contributions from the risk sets that are formed early on in the time scale. One way of doing this is to perform a test on the basis of the Gehan-Breslow test statistic, which uses the size of the risk set as a weight:

$$T_{GB} = \frac{\left(\sum_{k=1}^{K} n_k U_k \right)^2}{\sum_{k=1}^{K} n_k^2 V(U_k)}.$$

As with the standard log-rank test, under the null hypothesis of no difference between the survival functions between the two groups, and in large samples, T_{GB} has a χ^2 distribution with one degree of freedom.

THE COX MODEL

For studies based on observational data, some form of statistical adjustment for potential confounding will typically be required. In the absence of censoring, since T is a continuous outcome, a natural way forward would be to consider performing a linear regression analysis. That is, one could fit a model for the conditional mean of T as a function of some set of covariates. See Chapters 20 and 21. In the presence of censoring, one could estimate the unknown regression parameters using IPW or MI although, as mentioned earlier, these approaches do not directly exploit the partial information on the outcome that the censored data provide. Another drawback of performing a linear regression analysis is the exclusive focus on the mean as a summary of the distribution of T. Moreover, it will often be of interest to learn as much as possible about the entire shape of the distribution of T since doing so provides critical, complimentary information on the prognosis of patients. Panels (C) and (D) in Figure 22-1 highlight this by providing estimates of the proportion of patients who relapse by a given time point, at multiple time points as well as the point in time at which 50% have experienced a relapse (*i.e.*, the median survival).

Modeling the Hazard Function

Suppose interest lies in learning how T depends on X, an exposure of interest, adjusting for a set of covariates given by $\mathbf{Z} = (Z_1, \ldots, Z_p)$. Recalling that the hazard function fully characterizes the distribution of T, one could proceed by specifying a model for $\lambda(t)$. One such model is the Cox model,[8] which structures the hazard function as:

$$\lambda(t \mid X, \mathbf{Z}) = \lambda_0(t) \exp\left(\beta_x X + \beta_1 Z_1 + \ldots + \beta_p Z_p \right). \qquad [22\text{-}1]$$

In this model, $\lambda_0(t)$ is referred to as the *baseline hazard* and corresponds to the hazard function for the population for which $X = Z_1 = \ldots = Z_p = 0$. In this sense, it serves a role that is analogous to the intercept in a standard regression model. Exponentiating a given regression coefficient, one can interpret the result as a *hazard ratio*. For example, suppose X is a binary indicator of whether a participant was in the 6-MP arm in the leukemia data, and consider the (unadjusted) Cox model $\lambda(t|X) = \lambda_0(t)\exp(\beta_x X)$. A simple calculation gives:

$$\frac{\lambda(t|X_1 = 1)}{\lambda(t|X_1 = 0)} = \frac{\lambda_0(t)\exp(\beta_x)}{\lambda_0(t)} = \exp(\beta_x).$$

Thus, $\exp(\beta_x)$ is the ratio of the hazard functions and, correspondingly, β_x is the log-hazard ratio. More generally, as with any regression model, if there were other covariates in the model, then one could interpret $\exp(\beta_x)$ as an *adjusted hazard ratio* for X, adjusted in the sense of holding all other covariates constant when performing the comparison. Furthermore, if X was not binary, then $\exp(\beta_x)$ would be the hazard ratio that corresponds to a one-unit increase in X.

Two features of the model given by expression 22-1, which we refer to as the "standard" Cox model, are worth noting. First, implicit to the specification is that X and the components of Z do not vary as a function of time. Consequently, in order for the model to have a meaningful interpretation across the entire time scale, X and Z must be defined and measured at or before the origin. Second, the multiplicative effect of a given covariate in the model, as represented by the corresponding hazard ratio, is constant as a function of time. This condition is often referred to as *proportional hazards*. We return to both of these features below.

Parametric Estimation

Just as in estimation of the mean survival time, one could approach estimation of the Cox model via a parametric likelihood:

$$L\left[\lambda_0(t), \beta\right] = \prod_{i=1}^{n} \lambda\left(y_i | X = x_i, Z = z_i\right)^{\delta_i} S\left(y_i | X = x_i, Z = z_i\right)$$

where $\beta = (\beta_x, \beta_1, \ldots, \beta_p)$, and $S\left(y_i | X = x_i, Z = z_i\right)$ is the survival function that corresponds to the specification of the Cox model based on the mathematical relations described above. In contrast to semiparametric analyses based on the partial likelihood (described below), this likelihood is explicitly a function of the baseline hazard which must, therefore, be specified. This specification could be achieved by assuming some parametric distribution, such as the Gompertz distribution, which would correspond to specifying:

$$\lambda_0(t) = \alpha_1 \alpha_2^t$$

or the Weibull distribution, which would correspond to specifying:

$$\lambda_0(t) = \alpha_1 \alpha_2^{\alpha_1} t^{\alpha_1 - 1}$$

Any such choice would result in a finite set of unknown parameters, generically denoted here by α, which would be estimated simultaneously with β. As a final alternative, one could specify $\lambda_0(t)$ as a function of time using a spline model (see Chapter 20 and additional references). The appeal of doing so is that one can typically achieve great flexibility with only a small number of unknown parameters. The drawback, however, is that the calculation of $S\left(y_i | X = x_i, Z = z_i\right)$ in the likelihood is less straightforward than it would be if some parametric distribution had been chosen.

Semiparametric Estimation

More typically, estimation of the parameters of a Cox model typically proceeds via the *partial likelihood*. Remaining within the setting where X and Z are defined at baseline, the observed data for the *ith* individual in the study sample are $(y_i, \delta_i, x_i, z_i)$. Letting $(t_{(1)} < t_{(2)} < \ldots < t_{(K)})$ again denote the ordered unique event times across all individuals in the sample, suppose (initially) that only a single individual was observed to experience the event of interest at any given $t_{(k)}$; that is, $d_k = 1$. Let (k) denote the index of the individual who experienced the event, $x_{[k]}$, their specific value of exposure of interest, and $z_{[k]}$, their value of Z. The partial likelihood is:

$$
\begin{aligned}
L_p(\boldsymbol{\beta}) &= \prod_{k=1}^{K} \frac{\lambda\left(t \mid X = x_{(k)}, \boldsymbol{Z} = z_{(k)}\right)}{\sum_{i \in R_k} \lambda\left(t \mid X = x_i, \boldsymbol{Z} = z_i\right)} \\
&= \prod_{k=1}^{K} \frac{\lambda_0(t)\exp\left(\beta_x x_{(k)} + \beta_1 z_{(k),1} + \ldots + \beta_p z_{(k),p}\right)}{\sum_{i \in R_k} \lambda_0(t)\exp\left(\beta_x x_i + \beta_1 z_{i,1} + \ldots + \beta_p z_{i,p}\right)} \\
&= \prod_{k=1}^{K} \frac{\exp\left(\beta_x x_{(k)} + \beta_1 z_{(k),1} + \ldots + \beta_p z_{(k),p}\right)}{\sum_{i \in R_k} \exp\left(\beta_x x_i + \beta_1 z_{i,1} + \ldots + \beta_p z_{i,p}\right)}
\end{aligned}
$$

Several aspects of $L_p(\boldsymbol{\beta})$ are worth noting. First, and perhaps central to the broad use of the Cox model, is that the partial likelihood is solely a function of the regression parameters, and, moreover, is not a function of the unknown baseline hazard function, $\lambda_0(t)$. As a result, one can estimate $\boldsymbol{\beta}$ without having to specify or estimate $\lambda_0(t)$. In this sense, the analysis is referred to as a semiparametric statistical procedure; part of the model is structured via some finite set of parameters (*i.e.*, the linear combination of the covariates), while the remainder of the model is left unspecified (*i.e.*, the baseline hazard function). This feature has substantial appeal because it means that one does not have to adopt or even consider some specific form of $\lambda_0(t)$ as function of time (which may be complex), nor does one have to assess the sensitivity of the results across alternative choices. Second, practically, one can obtain the partial likelihood estimator of $\boldsymbol{\beta}$ by solving the system of $p+1$ partial likelihood score equations given by $U_p(\boldsymbol{\beta}) = 0$, where $U_p(\boldsymbol{\beta}) = \dfrac{\partial}{\partial \boldsymbol{\beta}} \log L_p(\boldsymbol{\beta})$ is the partial likelihood score function. In this system, the first equation corresponds to β_x and is given by:

$$
\sum_{k=1}^{K} \left[x_{(k)} - \frac{\sum_{i \in R_k} x_i \exp\left(\beta_x x_i + \beta_1 z_{i,1} + \ldots + \beta_p z_{i,p}\right)}{\sum_{i \in R_k} \exp\left(\beta_x x_i + \beta_1 z_{i,1} + \ldots + \beta_p z_{i,p}\right)} \right] = 0.
$$

Subsequent equations correspond to the coefficients for Z. So, for example, the equation corresponding to the coefficient for the jth component of Z, β_j, will be:

$$
\sum_{k=1}^{K} \left[z_{(k),j} - \frac{\sum_{i \in R_k} z_{i,j} \exp\left(\beta_x x_i + \beta_1 z_{i,1} + \ldots + \beta_p z_{i,p}\right)}{\sum_{i \in R_k} \exp\left(\beta_x x_i + \beta_1 z_{i,1} + \ldots + \beta_p z_{i,p}\right)} \right] = 0.
$$

In considering the terms in the above expressions, we see that the first component in each is the covariate of the individual who actually experienced the event (*i.e.*, $x_{(k)}$ or $z_{(k),j}$), while the second is a weighted average of the same covariate among all individuals who could have experienced the event [*i.e.*, all those in risk set R_k, which includes individual (k)], with the weights jointly dictated by the totality of the covariate vectors in the risk set as well as the value of $\boldsymbol{\beta}$. Thus, in a sense, the partial likelihood encodes information about $\boldsymbol{\beta}$ by performing a comparison of the covariates of the individual who actually experienced the event to those of all individuals who could have experienced it. Put another way, the partial likelihood is asking for each risk set: why was it that, among all of the individuals who could have experienced the event at time $t_{(k)}$, individual (k) was the one to experience it? Finally, the partial likelihood only depends on the observed event times through their relative ordering; that is, how the K risk sets are ordered in the product.

Given the partial likelihood estimate of $\boldsymbol{\beta}$, one can obtain an estimate of the cumulative baseline hazard function using the so-called *Breslow estimator*[9]:

$$
\hat{\Lambda}_0(t) = \sum_{t_k \leq t} \frac{1}{\sum_{i \in R_k} \exp\left(\hat{\beta}_x x_i + \hat{\beta}_1 z_{i,1} + \ldots + \hat{\beta}_p z_{i,p}\right)}.
$$

Key to this is that, although $\lambda_0(t)$ is not explicitly specified in the analysis, one can nevertheless use this estimate of the cumulative baseline hazard to estimate the survivor function for a patient with a given covariate profile. Thus, in addition to quantifying relative risk (via the hazard ratio), one can quantify absolute risk without having to make any parametric assumptions about the underlying distribution of T.

Ties in the Observed Event Times

As indicated, the way in which the partial likelihood informs the value of β is through a series of comparisons of the covariates of the individual who experienced the event in each risk set with the collection of covariates among all those who could have experienced the event. This implicitly relies on there being a single individual who experienced the event within a risk set (*i.e.*, for the numerator in each of the K contributions). Put another way, it assumes that there are no ties in the observed event times. In the leukemia study data, however, numerous instances of tied event times are observed. From Table 22-1, two participants in the control arm were observed to relapse at week 1 and three participants in the 6-MP arm were observed to relapse at week 6. In principle, if a sufficiently granular measurement of time is adopted, there should be no ties. In the 6-MP data, this could be achieved by measuring relapse in days or perhaps hours, as necessary. In the absence of this level of granularity, if there are ties, then the partial likelihood (as given above) cannot be used since there will be at least one risk set where it is unclear which individual should be represented in the numerator. In this setting, the appropriate way forward is to consider all possible orderings of the event times within each risk set for which there are ties and then average the contributions. Thus, one would need to calculate all $3! = 6$ possible orderings of the event times for the first risk set in 6-MP arm of the leukemia study (since there are $d_k = 3$ relapses observed at $t_{(k)} = 6$ weeks).

In small datasets, the additional computation involved in considering all possible orderings may be manageable. In large datasets with many ties, however, the computational burden may be prohibitive; a risk set with 10 individuals having experienced the same event time would result in 3,628,800 possible orderings. To resolve this dilemma, a number of approximations have been developed to reduce the time taken for results to be obtained, with the best known being two proposed by Breslow[9] and Efron.[10] Among the various options, when there are many ties, while the Breslow method is often the default in software implementations, the Efron approximation tends to provide results that are closer to what one would obtain in going through all of the calculations.[11]

Time-Varying Covariates

As noted, one key feature of the standard Cox model is that it implicitly takes the covariates included to be constant over the time frame; that is, they are *time-invariant*. In many instances, this will be perfectly reasonable. For example, by definition, age at enrollment in the leukemia study will not change over time nor will the staging of the disease at the time of diagnosis. In other instances, a covariate may change over time and yet reasonably be specified as being time-invariant in the model. In the leukemia study, for example, even though a patient's treatment status may change over time (*e.g.*, they discontinue due to some adverse event), an intent-to-treat analysis would correspond to X being an indicator of the treatment arm to which the participant was randomized (*i.e.*, the value of treatment at the origin) and, thus, be time-invariant.

On the other hand, it may be that a key covariate varies over time, and the fact that it does so may be of intrinsic interest. In the context of the ACT study, for example, an investigation of the association between physical frailty and risk of Alzheimer disease may wish to acknowledge the fact that frailty changes over time. Letting $X(t)$ denote the value of a measure of physical frailty at time t, the (unadjusted) Cox model for the hazard is:

$$\lambda(t|X) = \lambda_0(t)\exp[\beta_x X(t)]$$

As with the standard form, $\lambda_0(t)$ is the baseline hazard function although it now corresponds to a population for which $X(t) = 0$ at all time points. Furthermore, following the simple calculation given for the standard Cox model, we have for each t:

$$\frac{\lambda\left[t \mid X(t)=1\right]}{\lambda\left[t \mid X(t)=0\right]} = \frac{\lambda_0(t)\exp(\beta_x)}{\lambda_0(t)} = \exp(\beta_x).$$

Thus, the hazard ratio, $\exp(\beta_x)$, is again constant as a function of time so that, even though the covariate is permitted to change over time, the model can be referred to as being a proportional hazards model.

Now consider the somewhat more general Cox model with a time-varying covariate:

$$\lambda\left[t \mid X(t), \mathbf{Z}\right] = \lambda_0(t)\exp\left[\beta_x X(t) + \beta_1 Z_1 + \ldots + \beta_p Z_p\right].$$

Estimation for this model can again proceed using the partial likelihood, with the only modification being that covariate values in each of the K contributions must reflect their values at the time the risk set is formed:

$$L_p(\beta) = \prod_{k=1}^{K} \frac{\exp\left[\beta_x x_{(k)}(t_{(k)}) + \beta_1 z_{(k),1} + \ldots + \beta_p z_{(k),p}\right]}{\sum_{i \in R_k} \exp\left[\beta_x x_i(t_{(k)}) + \beta_1 z_{i,1} + \ldots + \beta_p z_{i,p}\right]}$$

where $x_i(t_{(k)})$ is the value of covariate vector for the ith individual at time $t_{(k)}$. Operationally, one can use any software implementation for the standard Cox model to fit a model with time-varying covariates by splitting an individual's record in the dataset into a series of intervals during which the covariate values are constant. For example, although this was not the case, suppose some participants in the 6-MP arm of the leukemia study were observed to stop treatment and that interest lies in performing an as-treated analysis based on fitting a Cox model of the form: $\lambda(t \mid X) = \lambda_0(t)\exp\left[\beta_x X(t)\right]$, where $X(t)$ is an indicator of treatment ($0/1 = $ control/6-MP). Furthermore, for concreteness, suppose the participant in the 6-MP arm who was observed to relapse at week 23 (see Table 22-1) actually stopped treatment during week 20; thus, $X(t) = 1$ for $t \leq 20$ and $X(t) = 0$ for $t > 20$. Operationally, one could acknowledge this in the analysis dataset by constructing two records (*i.e.*, rows) for this individual: the first record would indicate that the interval starts at the origin (*i.e.*, $t = 0$) with $X = 1$ and has the observed outcome $(y, \delta) = (20, 0)$; the second record would indicate that the interval starts at $t = 21$ with $X = 0$ and has the outcome $(y, \delta) = (23, 1)$. Thus, the participant's record while on treatment is censored at time $t = 20$ and then viewed as being subject to left truncation at $t = 21$ when they stop treatment. Note, since the two intervals are mutually exclusive and jointly represent no more or less information than the participant's complete data, no adjustment to the standard errors need to be made to account for the fact that there are now two records in the dataset.

Further complications can arise, however, when not only the exposure is time-varying but the potential confounders are as well. If time-varying confounders of the exposure are themselves affected by prior levels of the exposure, then fitting a time-varying Cox model will not suffice to obtain estimates of causal effects of exposure trajectories.[12,13] More complex causal models for time-varying exposures are then needed. See Chapter 25 for further discussion.

Beyond Proportional Hazards

The second noted feature of the standard Cox model is that the hazard ratio that is used to represent the association between a given exposure and the outcome [*i.e.*, $\exp(\beta_x)$ for X] is constant as a function of time, and that this is referred to as "proportional hazards." Intuitively, proportional hazards corresponds to there being no effect-measure modification of the covariate effect by time on the hazard ratio scale. It is often the case that proportional hazards is viewed as an assumption. Here, we do not take this position. Instead, we view proportional hazards as a modeling choice that is made in much the same way that an analyst may choose to represent the effect of a covariate in a linear regression solely using main effects (*i.e.*, without any interactions). Such decisions are commonplace even if it is plausible that the effect of a given exposure is modified by some other covariate; models are often specified with main effects alone on the basis of parsimony, study size or power considerations, and interpretability. Furthermore, by referring to proportional hazards as an assumption, there is an implication that the analyst believes that the true association between the exposures does not vary over time. In general, however, it is implausible that this will be the case except, perhaps, in settings where the time frame under consideration is relatively short. That is, it is implausible that relative differences in risk (as represented by the hazard) that manifest in the short-term following exposure will remain at constant levels over the long run. That this is the case, however, clearly does not preclude analysts from making a decision to model a given exposure with main effects only. In the context of a Cox model, one could then interpret the estimated hazard ratio as an average over time of the time-varying hazard ratio. This average is specific to the follow-up period in the study; the average over, say, a 5-year window will differ from the average over a 10-year window.

While proportional hazards is not viewed here as an assumption, it is may still be important and of scientific interest to assess it as a modeling choice. Consequently, all of the methods that have been developed for empirically assessing the "proportional hazards assumption" are still useful. Practically, these methods fall into two broad classes. The first of these consists of graphical assessments based on fitting an initial proportional hazards model and plotting the residuals (or functions of them) against time (or some function of time).[14] Common among these approaches is to plot the *Schoenfeld residual* for each covariate against t.[15] For example, toward assessing proportional hazards for X in model $\lambda(t|X,Z) = \lambda_0(t)\exp(\beta_x X + \beta_1 Z + ... + \beta_p Z_p)$, the Schoenfeld residual is:

$$\text{resid}(t) = X_{ev}(t) - \bar{X}(t,\hat{\boldsymbol{\beta}})$$

where $X_{ev}(t)$ is the mean of X across the individual(s) who experienced the event at time t, while $\bar{X}(t,\hat{\boldsymbol{\beta}})$ is a weighted average of the covariates among those at risk at time t, weighted by the fitted linear predictor from the Cox model:

$$\bar{X}(t,\hat{\boldsymbol{\beta}}) = \frac{\sum_{t_i \leq t} x_j \exp(\hat{\beta}_x x_i + \hat{\beta}_1 z_{i,1} + ... + \hat{\beta}_p z_{i,p})}{\sum_{t_i \leq t} \exp(\hat{\beta}_x x_i + \hat{\beta}_1 z_{i,1} + ... + \hat{\beta}_p z_{i,p})}.$$

Key to the use of the Schoenfeld residual is that if proportional hazards holds for X, then resid(t) will have mean zero. Thus, any time trends in resid(t) will be indicative of nonproportional hazards.

The second class of methods is based on having the analyst specify some form of a deviation from proportional hazards and assessing the evidence in favor of that deviation. To illustrate this, consider again the leukemia trial and let X denote treatment assignment (*i.e.*, 0/1 = control/6-MP) with relapse taken to be the event of interest. In its most general form, the corresponding nonproportional hazards Cox model is:

$$\lambda(t|X) = \lambda_0(t)\exp[\beta_x(t)X],$$

with the hazard ratio, $\exp[\beta_x(t)]$, explicitly a function of time. Now consider the model:

$$\lambda(t|X_1) = \lambda_0(t)\exp(\beta_x X + \beta_{xt} Xt), \qquad \text{[22-2]}$$

where Xt is the product of X and linear term for time (*i.e.*, an interaction term). From this, the hazard ratio for X is $\exp[\beta_1(t)] = \exp(\beta_x + \beta_{xt}t)$, so that β_x can be interpreted as the immediate effect of treatment with 6-MP (*i.e.*, when $t = 0$). Now suppose $\beta_x < 0$ so that $\exp(\beta_x) < 1.0$ and the immediate effect is one of benefit since it corresponds to a reduction in the hazard for relapse. If, in addition, $\beta_{1t} < 0$ then $\beta_x + \beta_{xt}t$ will become an increasingly large negative number as time progresses. Thus, the corresponding hazard ratio will deviate further and further from 1.0, indicating that the magnitude of the benefit increases with time. If, in addition to $\beta_x < 0$, $\beta_{xt} > 0$, then $\beta_x + \beta_{xt}t$

will eventually equal zero as time progresses and beyond that be increasingly positive. Thus, the immediate benefit of 6-MP [as represented by $\exp(\beta_x)$] will wane and eventually become detrimental.

In principle, model 22-2 can be easily fit by noting that the interaction term can be viewed as a time-varying covariate and then using the methods described in the previous subsection. Then, after having fit the model, one could quantify evidence of nonproportionality by examining the estimate and confidence interval for β_{xt}. Finally, this general strategy need not be restricted to the model given by expression 22-2. One could, for example, consider other forms of nonproportionality by using alternative functions of time such as:

$$\lambda(t|X) = \lambda_0(t)\exp\left[\beta_x X + \beta_{xt} X \log(t)\right],$$

for which the hazard ratio for X is $\exp\left[\beta_x(t)\right] = \exp(\beta_x)t^{\beta_{xt}}$. As with the first model, when $\beta_{xt} = 0$, this model reduces to a proportional hazards model. More generally, the specific choice of how $\beta_x(t)$ is structured within this strategy may be guided by what the research team believes a priori to be a plausible manner in which nonproportional hazards manifests.

It is important to note that for many practical settings, these approaches may not provide a clear path forward: graphical-based approaches are inherently subjective, while testing-based approaches require specification of the deviation away from proportional hazards, and will often be underpowered since study sizes are typically determined on the basis of estimating main effects. As such, it will be important to balance what one learns from employing these methods with the goals of the analysis and the role that the specific covariate plays. If the covariate in question is the exposure of interest, then parsimony and simplicity of interpretation may lead to the decision to retain a proportional hazards characterization of its association with the outcome. On the other hand, it may be that understanding and quantifying the extent to which the effect of an exposure wanes over time may be of central interest, in which case a model that balances this parsimony against clearer interpretability should be pursued. To this end, one could adopt either of the above interaction models and report the results for β_x and β_{xt} simultaneously or flexibly specify $\beta_x(t)$ with a spline and report the results graphically; see Fisher et al. for an example of the latter.[16]

Finally, if the covariate in question is an adjustment variable, then quantification of its association with the outcome may not be paramount, relative to, say, ensuring thorough adjustment. If this is the case and the covariate is discrete (*e.g.*, study site), then one may opt to represent the association via stratification of the baseline hazard function. Specifically, suppose X is the exposure of interest and Z is a discrete adjustment variable taking values in $1,\dots,S$. The corresponding stratified Cox model is:

$$\lambda(t|X_1) = \lambda_{0z}(t)\exp(X\beta_x),$$

where $\lambda_{0z}(t)$ is a stratum-specific baseline hazard function, one for each of the S levels of Z. From this, the hazard ratio for Z comparing stratum z with stratum 1, holding X constant, is $\lambda_{0z}(t)/\lambda_{01}(t)$, which is some unspecified function of time. Estimation for this model can then proceed based on a modification of the partial likelihood that considers the ordered event times and, hence, risk sets within each of the S strata of Z:

$$L_p(\beta_1) = \prod_{z=1}^{S}\prod_{k=1}^{K_s}\frac{\exp\left(x_{[s,(k)]}\beta_x\right)}{\sum_{i\in R_{s,k}}\exp\left(x_{(s,i)}\beta_x\right)}.$$

Crucially, as with the partial likelihood for the standard Cox model, it is immediately clear that estimation of β_x can proceed without the analyst having to specify any of the S baseline hazard functions. Consequently, estimation of β_x based on this model will be robust to whatever the true association between Z and the outcome is. An important drawback of this strategy, however, is that while one could estimate the S stratum-specific baseline hazard functions, there is no single simple summary measure of the association between Z and the outcome. If, as indicated, Z is solely an adjustment factor and interpretability is not a priority, then analysts may find this a reasonable price to pay for not having to commit to a specific form of the relationship between Z and the outcome.

BEYOND THE COX MODEL

So far, we have focused exclusively on the Cox model, in various forms, as a means to performing regression analysis of time-to-event data. That the Cox model is ubiquitous in clinical and public health research is, in large part, due to the appeal of not having to specify the baseline hazard function if estimation proceeds using the partial likelihood. Another reason is that the hazard ratio is interpretable as an incidence rate ratio or short-term risk ratio (see Chapter 5) or, loosely, a relative risk. Nevertheless, the Cox model has limitations, including that covariate effects are restricted to act multiplicatively on the hazard. Additionally, recent work has questioned the interpretability of a hazard ratio or an incidence rate ratio as a measure of association, specifically as to whether it can be viewed as having a causal interpretation.[17,18] As such it is important to be aware of other regression frameworks that might be adopted. Here we provide a brief overview, focusing on model specification and interpretation, of two choices, both of which can be viewed as linear regression-type analyses of time-to-event outcome data. Throughout, while these approaches are often framed as "alternatives" to the Cox mode, they are, in fact, complimentary in that they represent distinct approaches to characterizing associations.

Additive Hazard Models

The first framework is the *additive hazards model* framework, which can intuitively be thought of as a linear regression for the hazard function.[19,20] Arguably, the simplest reasonable additive hazard model is of the form:

$$\lambda(t \mid X) = \beta_0(t) + \beta_x X + \beta_1 Z_1 + \ldots + \beta_p Z_p,$$

[22-3]

with $\beta_0(t)$ interpreted as the baseline hazard function in the same way that $\lambda_0(t)$ is in the Cox model. Covariate effects, however, are not taken to affect the hazard multiplicatively but, rather, additively. Thus, instead of reporting an estimate of $\exp(\beta_x)$ as a relative change in the hazard associated with the exposure X, one would report β_x as an absolute change in the hazard, just as one interprets the coefficient in a linear regression model as the absolute change in the mean outcome for a one-unit change in the exposure.

In the additive hazards model given by 22-3, the effects of each of the covariates do not vary over time. As with the standard Cox model, this choice could be interpreted as targeting a true common effect over time or as an average of a time-varying effect. Naturally, as appropriate to the analysis, one could choose to adopt a more flexible model for which select components have effects that do vary over time. For example, the following model permits the effect of X to vary over time while modeling the components of Z as being time-invariant:

$$\lambda(t \mid X) = \beta_0(t) + \beta_x(t)X + \beta_1 Z_1 + \ldots + \beta_p Z_p.$$

Finally, as with the Cox model, one can semiparametrically estimate components of an additive hazards model that pertain to the associations between covariates and the outcome without having to prespecify the baseline hazard function; see Martinussen and Peng[21] for details.

Accelerated Failure Time Models

Beyond models that structure the hazard function, another common regression framework for time-to-event data is the accelerated failure time (AFT) modeling framework. Before presenting this framework, consider a linear regression analysis of the association between X, a covariate of interest, and a continuous outcome Y, adjusting for a set of confounders $Z=(Z_1,\ldots,Z_p)$. One way of specifying a linear regression is to adopt the structure:

$$Y = \beta_0 + \beta_x X + \beta_1 Z_1 + \ldots + \beta_p Z_p + \varepsilon,$$

along with assumptions regarding the mean, the variance, and (sometimes) the distribution of the residual or error term, ε. Building on this, consider the following regression structure for a time-to-event outcome:

$$\log(T) = \beta_x X + \beta_1 Z_1 + \ldots + \beta_p Z_p + \varepsilon,$$

where the log transformation of T is adopted to acknowledge that the outcome must be positive. Coupled with a distributional assumption regarding the residual terms, specifically for e^ε (because of the log transformation), the above model is referred to as an *accelerated failure time model*. In considering the distribution of e^ε, which may initially seem unintuitive, it is helpful to note that it corresponds to the distribution of T when all of the components of X and $\mathbf{Z}$ equal 0. Thus, it can loosely be interpreted as a "baseline distribution" for the model specification. Since this distribution characterizes variation in T across time, an intercept in the model would be superfluous and is, therefore, not needed in the specification.

The central appeal of the AFT model is that the regression parameters have an intuitive interpretation in terms of the impact that covariates have on the quantiles of the distribution of T. To see this, consider the leukemia trial data with X consisting of a single binary covariate that denotes treatment assignment (*i.e.*, $X = 0$ for the placebo arm and $X = 1$ for the 6-MP arm). Mathematically, the AFT model for the time to relapse:

$$\log(T) = \beta_x X + \varepsilon,$$

can be equivalently represented in terms of the survivor function for the distribution of T, specifically:

$$S(t \mid X) = S_0\left[t \times \exp(-\beta_x X)\right]$$

where $S_0(t)$ is the "baseline" survivor function (*i.e.*, the survivor function for the placebo group), that corresponds to the choice of the baseline distribution of T in the linear regression-type specification given above. Now suppose that $\beta_x = -0.69$ so that $\exp(-\beta_x) = 2$. From the above, we have that the survivor function for the 6-MP group is given by $S(t; X = 1) = S_0(t \times 2)$. Moreover, we can write.

$$S(t \mid X = x) = \begin{cases} S_0(t) & \text{if } x = 0 \\ S_0(t \times 2) & \text{if } x = 1. \end{cases}$$

From this, we can see that the AFT model structures differences in the survival experience of the two groups through a doubling of the timings at which quantiles of T arise. For example, if the median time to relapse in the placebo group is 10 weeks, then the median time to relapse in the 6-MP will be 20 weeks. Put another way, if the 10-week mark is the point in time at which 50% of patients taking placebo will relapse, the corresponding point in time for patients in the 6-MP arm is 20 weeks. Thus, the effect of treatment is to decelerate (or push back in time) events on the time scale. If $\beta_x = 0.69$ so that $\exp(-\beta_x) = 0.5$, the median time to relapse in the 6-MP arm would be half of the median time to relapse. Thus, the effect of treatment would be to accelerate (or bring forward) events on the time scale.

That the interpretation of covariate effects in an AFT model is through an effect on the actual timing of the events (as opposed to an effect on the hazard function) may provide an intuitively appealing alternative or compliment to both the Cox model and the additive hazards model. Interestingly, for select choices of the baseline distribution, the AFT model can be rerepresented in a form that is structurally the same as the Cox model, albeit with some specific form for the baseline hazard function that is dictated by the choice of distribution. Suppose, for example, that the baseline distribution of T is taken to be a Weibull distribution with shape parameter $\alpha > 0$ and scale parameter $\kappa > 0$, so that the baseline survivor function is $S_0(t) = \exp(-\kappa t^\alpha)$. The corresponding baseline hazard function is $\lambda_0(t) = \kappa \alpha t^{\alpha-1}$ with the induced model for the hazard as a function of X:

$$\lambda(t \mid X) = \kappa \alpha \left[t \times \exp(\beta_x X)\right]^{\alpha-1} \exp(\beta_x X).$$

This, in turn, can be succinctly written as:

$$\lambda(t|X) = \lambda_0(t)\exp(\beta_x^* X),$$

where $\beta_x^* = -\alpha \times \beta_x$. That is, the induced model for the hazard that arises from combining the AFT model $log(T) = \beta_x X + \varepsilon$ with a Weibull distribution has the same form as the standard Cox model with proportional hazards for the (multiplicative) effect of X.

Given an AFT model specification, an analysis can proceed by specifying a parametric baseline distribution and performing maximum likelihood-based estimation and inference. Alternatively, one may wish to proceed with a semiparametric analysis that leaves the baseline distribution unspecified. For this case, methods for estimation and inference within the frequentist framework have been developed that exploit the connection between an AFT model and its induced hazard function.[21] These methods can be unstable, however, and an alternative is to perform estimation and inference within the Bayesian paradigm for which there is a rich literature.[22]

COMPETING RISKS

Key Cause-Specific Quantities

As indicated, censoring is a phenomenon that affects the ability of the research team to observe the event of interest. Implicit to this is that the participant continues to be at risk to experience the event. In some settings, however, phenomena may arise that preclude the occurrence of the event of interest altogether. Such phenomena are referred to as *competing risks*. Possibly the most common competing risk scenario is where the primary event of interest is death due to some specific cause, with death due to other causes constituting competing risks.

Another scenario is where interest lies in some nonmortality event, the occurrence of which is subject to whether the study participant is alive. In the leukemia study, for example, mortality (either overall or in a cause-specific manner) is a competing risk for the primary outcome of time to relapse. A second example of this scenario is that of the study of preeclampsia, a condition characterized by elevated blood pressure during pregnancy. Since preeclampsia is a condition that is specific to pregnancy, delivery of the baby precludes a diagnosis and is, therefore, a competing risk.

In considering methods for competing risks, it is helpful to bear in mind the two most important (and complementary) quantities in time-to-event data analysis: (1) the rate at which events occur in time (*i.e.*, the hazard function) and (2) the probability of an event occurring at a given time (*i.e.*, the survival function). In the absence of meaningful competing risks, either because overall mortality is of primary interest or because mortality due to any cause is rare, there is a direct correspondence between learning about the hazard and learning about the survival function. In particular, because of the mathematical relationship between $\lambda(t)$ and $S(t)$, in learning that a risk factor is associated with a reduction in the rate at which events occur, one can also conclude that it will be associated with a reduction in the probability of the event occurring. Unfortunately, this does not hold when competing risks are present. To see this, suppose there are $K \geq 2$ event types. As an analogue to the cumulative incidence function, $F(t) = 1 - S(t)$, define the *cumulative incidence function* for the kth event type as:

$$CIF_k(t) = P(T \leq t, D = k),$$

where D is a random variable that indicates the event type. This quantity can be interpreted as the probability of experiencing an event by time t and that the event experienced is of type k. Note, since:

$$\sum_{k=1}^{K} P(T \leq t, D = k) = P(T \leq t) = F(t),$$

there is some intuitive appeal in reporting the K cause-specific $CIF_k(t)$ since their total is equal to the overall probability of having experienced any event by that time point.

Additionally, as an analogue to $\lambda(t)$, define the *cause-specific hazard function* for the kth event type as:

$$\lambda_k^{cs}(t) = \lim_{\Delta \to 0} \frac{1}{\Delta} P(t \leq T \leq t + \Delta, D = k | T \geq t),$$

To interpret $\lambda_k^{cs}(t)$, recall that the standard hazard function, $\lambda(t)$, is the instantaneous rate of the event at time t given that it has not occurred by time t. Analogously, $\lambda_k^{cs}(t)$ is the instantaneous rate associated with the occurrence of event type k at time t given that no event of any type has occurred by time t. Thus, $\lambda_k^{cs}(t)$ is sometimes interpreted as the rate at which event type k occurs in the presence of competing risks. Finally, as with the K cause-specific $CIF_k(t)$, it is straightforward to show that the sum of the K cause-specific $\lambda_k^{cs}(t)$ equals the overall hazard rate of experiencing any of the events at time t.

As with $\lambda(t)$ and $S(t)$, there is a mathematical relationship between the cause-specific hazards and the cause-specific cumulative incidence functions. Specifically, one can show that:

$$CIF_k(t) = \int_0^t \lambda_k^{cs}(u)P(T \geq u)du = \int_0^t \lambda_k^{cs}(u)\exp\left[-\sum_{j=1}^K \Lambda_j^{cs}(u)\right]du,$$

where $\Lambda_j^{cs}(t) = \int_0^t \lambda_j^{cs}(u)du$ is the cause-specific cumulative hazard function. From this, we see the crucial result that $CIF_k(t)$ is a function of all K cause-specific hazards. Because of this, we make two important comments. First, in contrast to the setting in which there are no competing risks, there is no guarantee of a one-to-one relationship between the rate at which an event occurs, as characterized by the cause-specific hazard $\lambda_k^{cs}(t)$, and the probability of the event having occurred, as characterized by the cause-specific cumulative incidence function, $CIF_k(t)$. Consequently, if a regression analyses for $\lambda_k^{cs}(t)$ suggests that a given risk factor is protective for cause K in that it reduces the rate at which it occurs at time t, it may nevertheless be the case that the risk factor is detrimental in terms of incidence by time t. Second, notwithstanding the above relation, it may be tempting to forge ahead with estimation of $CIF_k(t)$ via an analysis that effectively ignores any competing events. One could, for example, use the usual Kaplan-Meier estimator by censoring the person-time for any participant that experiences an event of a type other than type k. Doing so, however, effectively assumes the absence of competing risks in the population; that is, the interpretation pertains to a hypothetical population in which one can only die from cause k. Beyond being of questionable relevance to the real world, one can also show that the Kaplan-Meier estimator in the presence of competing risks is upward-biased since participants who have experienced some other event are nevertheless presumed to still be at risk. Another option would be to use a Breslow-type estimator of $CIF_k(t)$ based solely on using, say, a model for $\lambda_k^{cs}(t)$. While a model for $\lambda_k^{cs}(t)$ can be fit without assumptions regarding the dependence among the competing risks (see below), the corresponding Breslow-type estimator of $CIF_k(t)$ requires the competing risks to be independent. This assumption, however, cannot be empirically verified.[23] Moreover, in many biomedical applications where comorbidities such as hypertension and diabetes have an influence on a range of causes of death, independent competing risks may not be plausible.

Motivated by these issues, Fine and Gray proposed that analysts consider the *subdistribution hazard function*, defined as:

$$\lambda_k^{sd}(t) = -\frac{d}{dt}\left[1 - CIF_k(t)\right],$$

for the kth cause or, equivalently, through the relation:

$$CIF_k(t) = 1 - \exp\left[-\int_0^t \lambda_k^{sd}(u)du\right].$$

In contrast to $\lambda_k^{cs}(t)$, which speaks to the rate at which event k occurs at time t among those who have not experienced any event, by its construction (*i.e.*, through the above definition), $\lambda_k^{sd}(t)$ can be interpreted as the instantaneous rate at which event k occurs at time t among those individuals who have not experienced event k at that time. Because of the direct one-to-one correspondence between the cause-specific subdistribution function and the cause-specific cumulative incidence function, unintuitive discrepancies (such as when a risk factor is protective when one considers the rate but detrimental when one considers incidence) will not arise. Of course, though, it is important to stress that while the direction of the two associations will be the same, the magnitude of the effect of a risk factor on $\lambda_k^{sd}(t)$ will not be the same as the magnitude of the effect of a risk factor on $CIF_k(t)$.

Analyses

Although application of the usual Kaplan-Meier estimator will result in bias unless independent competing risks holds, a consistent estimator of $CIF_k(t)$ that does not rely on this assumption is the Nelson-Aalen estimator:

$$\widehat{\text{CIF}}_k(t) = \sum_{t_i < t} \hat{S}_{KM}(t_i - 1) d\hat{\Lambda}_k(t_i)$$

where $\hat{S}_{KM}(t)$ is the Kaplan-Meier estimator for the overall survivor and $\hat{\Lambda}_k(t)$ is the Nelson-Aalen estimator for $\Lambda_k^{cs}(t)$, the cause-specific cumulative hazard function defined above.

For regression analyses, one could proceed with modeling the K cause-specific $\lambda_k^{cs}(t)$ or the K cause-specific $\lambda_k^{sd}(t)$ as functions of covariates using the same approaches that one might model $\lambda(t)$ in the standard time-to-event setting. So, for example, we could adopt a multiplicative Cox-type specification for the cause-specific hazard functions of the form:

$$\lambda_k^{cs}(t|X,Z) = \lambda_{0k}^{cs}(t)\exp\left(\beta_{xk}^{cs}X + \beta_{1k}^{cs}Z_1 + \ldots + \beta_{pk}^{cs}Z_p\right).$$

As with the standard Cox model, exponentiating a given regression parameter provides a hazard ratio contrast, albeit with the precise interpretation specific to the fact that $\lambda_k^{cs}(t)$ speaks to the rate at which event k occurs at time t among those individuals who have not experienced any event at that time. Practically, estimation of this regression model is straightforward since it follows by using the same partial likelihood-based approach for the standard Cox regression model, with the only modification being that participants who experience an event of some type other than type k are treated as having been censored. Thus, with a small modification to the analysis dataset, any software for the standard Cox model can be used. Note, no assumption regarding the dependence structure across the competing risks is needed for estimation of $\lambda_k^{cs}(t)$.

Similarly, one could proceed with modeling the K cause-specific subdistribution hazard functions:

$$\lambda_k^{sd}(t|X) = \lambda_{0k}^{sd}(t)\exp\left(\beta_{xk}^{sd}X + \beta_{1k}^{sd}Z_1 + \ldots + \beta_{pk}^{sd}Z_p\right),$$

with the interpretation of an exponentiated regression parameter again speaking to a hazard ratio, with the precise interpretation specific to the fact that $\lambda_k^{sd}(t)$ speaks to the rate at which event k occurs at time t among those individuals who have not experienced event k at that time. Practically, estimation again proceeds as in the standard Cox model with the key difference being that one ignores if or when a participant experiences an event that is not of type k. That is, the participant is retained in all future risk sets; she has not been censored nor experienced event k. This may be counterintuitive. However, in retaining participants in future risk sets, an implicit constraint is imposed on estimation of $\lambda_k^{sd}(t)$ that can be interpreted as providing a "placeholder" for the proportion of the population that cannot experience event k.

Although details are not given here, as with the standard Cox model, there is substantial scope for building on the above models to permit consideration of time-dependent effects as well as time-varying effects and for building models that target additive, rather than multiplicative, associations.[24-27]

We conclude this subsection with a note on the substantial debate regarding whether one should report results based on modeling of the cause-specific hazard functions or the subdistribution hazard functions. In particular, some have argued that cause-specific hazard functions may be best-suited to the study of etiology since they correspond to the instantaneous rate at which events occur among those who are event free. Furthermore, because of the direct correspondence with the cause-specific cumulative incidence function, subdistribution hazards may be best-suited to the studies where the interest lies in risk prediction and the development of risk scoring systems.[28] Others have argued, however, that the distinction between the two frameworks should be viewed as a positive in that they provide complementary information about how a given risk factor has an effect on a set of competing risks endpoints. As such, Latouche et al. recommend that both frameworks should be considered and provide practical guidance on how to perform analyses and present results.[29]

SEMICOMPETING RISKS

The Distinction With Competing Risks

The standard setting for competing risks analysis is that primary interest lies with mortality as the outcome, coupled with the recognition that there are multiple causes of death. Central to the challenge of analyzing such data is that death due to any given cause is *terminal* for all other causes in the sense that once an individual dies due to some specific cause they cannot experience further outcomes; indeed, subsequent outcomes are not even well defined.

A distinct setting is one where interest lies in some *nonterminal* event, the occurrence of which is subject to a terminal event. In the ACT study, for example, primary scientific interest lies in incident Alzheimer disease. Although mortality is not the primary focus, it is clearly a competing risk for Alzheimer disease (especially among the elderly). Of course, the reverse is not the case: once an individual is diagnosed with Alzheimer disease, they remain at risk for death. In this sense, Alzheimer disease can be viewed as a nonterminal event.

More generally, settings where primary interest lies with some nonterminal event for which the occurrence is subject to a terminal event are referred to as *semicompeting risks*.[30-32] Although less familiar than competing risks, semicompeting risks are ubiquitous in clinical and public health research. Examples include: the study of cancer recurrence, following successful treatment of an initial tumor; the study of acute graft-versus-host disease among patients undergoing hematopoietic stem cell transplantation for leukemia; the assessment of palliative measures to improve quality of end-of-life among patients with a terminal diagnosis; the study of end-stage renal disease among individuals with chronic kidney disease; and, the study of clinical and behavioral outcomes among preterm infants admitted to a neonatal intensive care unit. In each of these examples, death is the competing risks although this need not always be the case. As mentioned above, preeclampsia is only diagnosed during pregnancy so that delivery of the baby constitutes a terminal event. Thus, studies of risk factors and prophylactic strategies for preeclampsia fall within the rubric of semicompeting risks.

A critical feature of semicompeting risks data is that one will observe the timing of both events on at least some study participants. This is in contrast to competing risks where one can only observe the timing of at most one event (*i.e.*, that associated with the observed cause of death for the individual). Figure 22-2 provides a graphical representation of this important difference. A consequence of being able to observe both events on individual study units is that the data provide at least partial

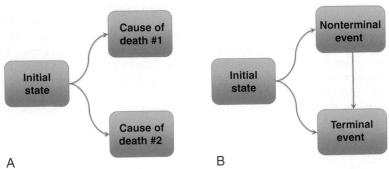

FIGURE 22-2 Graphical representation of the distinction between competing risks (A) and semicompeting risks (B).

information on the dependence between the nonterminal and terminal events. This, in turn, provides two key benefits. First, it provides analysts with an opportunity to acknowledge this dependence in the analysis, an important consideration when dealing with multiple outcomes within a study participant (see also Chapter 24). Second, one can view the two events as a bivariate outcome and model them simultaneously in a single joint model. This, in turn, permits a broader range of scientific questions to be addressed, including the extent to which risk factors affect how the two events covary.

Naïve Methods

Before outlining statistical approaches that have been developed for the analysis of semicompeting risks data, it is worth considering various naïve analysis strategies that are commonly used. Among these, one approach is to perform an analysis of the nonterminal event using standard univariate methods in time-to-event analysis, such as the Kaplan-Meier estimator of the survival function or a Cox model, treating the terminal event as a censoring mechanism (*i.e.*, in addition to other censoring mechanisms, such as loss-to-follow-up or the end of the study). Problematic with this strategy is that the meaning and interpretation of the independent censoring assumption, critical to the validity of these methods, is unclear. To see this, note that, intuitively, the independent censoring assumption can be thought of saying that, conditional upon covariates included in the analysis, the experience with respect to the event of interest among those individuals who are censored would have been the same as those who were not been censored. This, however, clearly cannot be applied to individuals who die since there is no subsequent "experience." Thus, prior to consideration of the plausibility of the independent censoring assumption, there is a strong argument that one should not view death as a censoring mechanism. Indeed, this notion has led to some authors to refer to its occurrence by saying that person-time was "truncated by death."[33]

Another way forward would be to construct and analyze a composite endpoint. That is, a new outcome that represents the time of the first instance of either event. This is a strategy often used in oncology studies where progression-free survival, which corresponds to the first of disease progression or death, is commonly used as an outcome. Benefits of adopting this approach are that one can use standard univariate methods in time-to-event analysis and that the larger number of "events" (since we are counting two types) will typically lead to an increase in statistical power. An important drawback of this strategy, however, is that the mixing of two distinct outcomes results in a fundamental change in the scientific question.[31] That is, the focus of the analysis has shifted away from one in which the nonterminal event is of primary interest. Thus, in using a composite endpoint, one sacrifices the ability to investigate risk factors for the nonterminal event unless it is plausible that the set of risk factors that are predictive of the two events are the same and that the magnitude and directions of the associations are the same.

Beyond these naïve strategies, there is a small but rich literature on methods for the analysis of semicompeting risks data in which three major threads have emerged.

The Survivor Averaged Causal Effect

The first major thread embeds the analysis within the causal counterfactual paradigm (see Chapter 3). Focusing on settings where interest lies in comparing the relative impact of two (or more) treatment options on the risk of the nonterminal event, the overarching strategy has been to define some causal contrast together with the assumptions under which the contrast is identified. One such contrast is the *survivor averaged causal effect* (SACE) which considers the impact of treatment choice among "always survivors," that is the principal stratum or subpopulation of patients who would survive under either treatment and, as such, for whom the nonterminal event is always well-defined.[33-36] Because this stratum of individuals who would have survived under either treatment is unknown, SACE is not fully identified from the data. However, a variety of methods use bounds or sensitivity analysis to draw inferences about this particular estimand.[37-41]

Copula-Based Methods

A second general approach builds on methods for standard bivariate time-to-event analyses (*i.e.*, where neither event is terminal for the other). Briefly, let T_1 and T_2 denote the times to the nonterminal and terminal events, respectively, and consider modeling the joint survivor function: $P(T_1 > t_1, T_2 > t_2)$. One approach to modeling this function is to first specify models for the marginal survivor functions of T_1 and T_2, that is $S_1(t_1) = P(T_1 > t_1)$ and $S_2(t_2) = P(T_2 > t_2)$, respectively. Then these quantities can then be "linked" to form a model for the joint survivor function, specifically $P(T_1 > t_1, T_2 > t_2) = C_\theta[S_1(t_1), S_2(t_2)]$, where $C_\theta(\cdot, \cdot)$ is a *copula* (essentially a mathematical function) that is indexed by an unknown parameter θ that must be estimated. One well-known copula was proposed by Clayton[42] and is motivated through consideration of a latent patient-specific frailty or random effect. This frailty is then assumed to impact the risk of both events, thus representing a form of dependence between the two outcomes; see Chapter 24 for more on how random effects can be used to account for dependence between outcomes. Moreover, if the frailties arise from a Gamma distribution with mean 1.0 and variance θ, then the Clayton copula is of the form:

$$C_\theta\left[S_1(t_1),\ S_2(t_2)\right] = \left[S_1(t_1)^{1-\theta} + S_2(t_2)^{1-\theta} - 1\right]^{1/(1-\theta)}.$$

In applying this idea from bivariate time-to-event analysis to the semicompeting risks setting, one can only use a copula to define a joint model on the upper wedge of the (T_1, T_2) plane, that is where $T_1 < T_2$ since one cannot observe the nonterminal event after the terminal event.[30] Then, using the copula, one may use the data to simultaneously estimate $S_1(t_1)$ and $S_2(t_2)$ and θ, possibly putting regression structure on $S_1(t_1)$ and $S_2(t_2)$.[43,44] One limitation of copula-based methods, however, is that $S_1(t_1)$ in $C_\theta[S_1(t_1), S_2(t_2)]$ is not the same as the marginal distribution of T_1, even though it is sometimes interpreted as such. Furthermore, as mathematical devices, copulas can only encompass a narrow range of dependence structures. The Clayton copula, for example, only permits positive dependence between T_1 and T_2. Consequently, copula-based strategies may be limited if interest lies (in part, at least) on how T_1 and T_2 covary.

The Illness-Death Model

A third general framework views semicompeting risks data as arising from an *illness-death* model, a special form of a multistate model.[45] Briefly, the illness-death model posits that, at any given point in time, the study participant is in one of the three "states": (1) an initial state, prior to experiencing either event; (2) a state of having experienced the nonterminal event, necessarily prior to experiencing the terminal event; and, (3) an absorbing state of having experienced the terminal event. Figure 22-2B provides a graphical representation of these states. With this infrastructure, one can then proceed with modeling by placing structure on the three hazard functions that dictate the rates at which individuals transition between the states:

$$\text{I} \rightarrow \text{II}: \quad \lambda_1(t_1) = \lim_{\Delta \to 0} \frac{1}{\Delta} P\left(t_1 \leq T_1 \leq t_1 + \Delta \mid T_1 \geq t_1, T_2 \geq t_1\right),$$

$$\text{I} \rightarrow \text{III}: \quad \lambda_2(t_2) = \lim_{\Delta \to 0} \frac{1}{\Delta} P\left(t_2 \leq T_2 \leq t_2 + \Delta \mid T_1 \geq t_2, T_2 \geq t_2\right),$$

$$\text{II} \rightarrow \text{III}: \quad \lambda_3(t_2 \mid t_1) = \lim_{\Delta \to 0} \frac{1}{\Delta} P\left(t_2 \leq T_2 \leq t_2 + \Delta \mid T_1 = t_1, T_2 \geq t_2\right),$$

Such models can be the form of a set of Cox models[46,47] or a set of AFT models.[48] As part of these specifications, one may additionally choose to include a patient-specific frailty as a means to structure any residual dependence between T_1 and T_2 (as was used to motivate the Clayton copula).

In an illness-death model, dependence between T_1 and T_2 is jointly structured via the interplay between $\lambda_2(t_2)$ and $\lambda_3(t_2 \mid t_1)$, and the magnitude of the variance of the frailties.[31] One representation of the former is the *explanatory hazard ratio*, $\text{EHR}(t_2, t_1) = \lambda_3(t_2 \mid t_1) / \lambda_2(t_2)$, defined for $t_2 > t_1$. Intuitively, $EHR(t_2, t_1)$ provides a summary of the relative influence of experiencing the nonterminal event at time t_1 on subsequent risk of the terminal event. Moreover, depending on how $\lambda_2(t_2)$ and $\lambda_3(t_2 \mid t_1)$ are specified, one can summarize the impact of covariates on how having experienced the nonterminal event influences subsequent risk of the terminal event. Thus, through this interplay, a much broader class of dependence structures can be captured than can, say, via copula-based methods.

STUDY DESIGNS IN TIME-TO-EVENT ANALYSES

So far, the presentation of methods for time-to-event data analysis has focused on settings where, although the outcome may be censored, complete data on all relevant covariates are available. In practice, however, the latter may not readily apply; data on a particular covariate may not be routinely collected (*e.g.*, race or smoking status in an EHR-based study) or may be too expensive to obtain for all participants (*e.g.*, the level of some biomarker measured from a biologic specimen). In such settings, a cost-effective strategy may be to collect the otherwise-unavailable information on a subsample of the study population. Furthermore, if information on the outcome is available, then it can be used to inform a statistically efficient outcome-dependent sampling design for selecting the subsample. Here, we present two classes of such designs.

Basic Design Options

Arguably, the best-known outcome-dependent sampling design is the case-control study design for binary outcomes, with analyses typically performed with respect to a logistic regression model (see Chapter 8). When the outcome of interest is a time-to-event outcome, the two most common outcome-dependent sampling designs are the nested case-control design and the case-cohort design, both of which are described in the context of a binary outcome in Chapter 8.

Arguably, the simplest nested case-control design proceeds as follows: for each case, consider the risk set that is formed at the time of the event and use simple random sampling to select $m-1$ "controls" who did not experience the event; then ascertain the otherwise-unknown covariate information on the m selected individuals given by the case and controls.[49] Throughout, it is assumed that the sampling of controls is independent in the sense that, at any given point in time, knowledge of which individuals have been previously selected as controls or who have been censored (1) does not influence selection in subsequent risks sets and (2) provides no information about the risk of experiencing the event beyond that time. This assumption may be violated if, for example, an individual who is selected as a control early on in the study changes her behavior in a way that modifies her risk for the event thereafter. Crucially, under the assumption of independent sampling, any given individual may serve as a control for multiple cases during follow-up. Furthermore, an individual who eventually becomes a case may serve as a control for other cases before the point in time that they experience the event themselves.

As proposed by Prentice,[50] the original case-cohort design proceeds by first selecting a subcohort from the initial study population via simple random sampling. The subcohort is then supplemented with all individuals who go on to experience the event of interest during follow-up but were not initially selected. Collectively, therefore, the individuals on whom the otherwise unavailable covariates are ascertained consist of all cases and a random sample of the noncases.

Analogous to the nested case-control design, the case-cohort design assumes that selection into the subcohort does not influence an individual's behavior in such a way that would change their future risk of the event of interest. In contrast to the nested case-control design, however, where the selection of controls is on a person-by-person basis and is not influenced by prior selection as a control, under the case-cohort design all cases share the same pool of controls (subject to their being at risk at the time the case experiences the event). This, as we elaborate upon below, has important consequences for the statistical analysis of data from a case-cohort design.

Estimation for the Cox Model and of Absolute Risk

Given data from a nested case-control study, the standard approach to estimation of the regression parameters from a Cox model is to maximize a modified version of the partial likelihood, specifically:

$$L_{ncc}(\boldsymbol{\beta}) = \prod_{k=1}^{K} \frac{\exp\left(\beta_x x_{(k)} + \beta_1 z_{(k),1} + \ldots + \beta_p z_{(k),p}\right)}{\sum_{i \in \tilde{R}_k} \exp\left(\beta_x x_i + \beta_1 z_{i,1} + \ldots + \beta_p z_{i,p}\right)},$$

where $\tilde{R}_k \subseteq R_k$ is a modified risk set that only includes the kth case and the $m-1$ controls. As such, analogous to logistic regression analysis of data from a case-control study for a binary outcome, one can estimate the regression parameters in a Cox model without regard to the fact that the data arise from an outcome-dependent sampling design. Moreover, one can employ any software for fitting the Cox model directly to the subsample selected by the design to obtain point estimates. Finally, the estimated standard errors from such a fit can be used to construct valid confidence intervals for the regression parameters and, hence, hazard ratios.[51]

One limitation of basing estimation on $L_{ncc}(\beta)$ is that the information on the cases is only used at the point in time when their corresponding risk set is formed. Consider a nested case-control study in which all relevant covariates (including those to be ascertained via the design) are time-invariant. Furthermore, suppose that two of the cases experience the event of interest at the 6-month mark and at the 12-month mark, respectively, and that second of these cases had not been selected as a control for the first. An analysis based on the above modified partial likelihood would not use information on the second case at the 6-month mark (*i.e.*, they would not contribute to the corresponding risk set in the denominator), despite the analyst having complete covariate information and knowing that they had not experienced the event at 6 months. Motivated by a desire to recover this "lost" information, it has been proposed that the matching be ignored or broken at the analysis stage, therefore treating the data as if it arose from a case-cohort design albeit with a nonstandard approach to selecting the subcohort. To ensure unbiased estimation, analysts can use either IPW or multiple imputation.[52,53]

Given data from a case-cohort study, one can estimate the regression parameters from a Cox model by maximizing the following pseudo-likelihood:

$$L_{caco}(\beta) = \prod_{k=1}^{K} \frac{\exp\left(\beta_x x_{(k)} + \beta_1 z_{(k),1} + \ldots + \beta_p z_{(k),p}\right)}{\sum_{i \in \tilde{S}_k} \exp\left(\beta_x x_i + \beta_1 z_{i,1} + \ldots + \beta_p z_{i,p}\right)},$$

where $\tilde{S}_k \subseteq R_k$ is the set of all individuals in the kth risk set who were selected by the design (*i.e.*, the subcohort together all remaining cases). Because the form of $L_{caco}(\beta)$ resembles that of the usual partial likelihood, as well as $L_{ncc}(\beta)$, one can use any standard software for obtaining point estimates. Unlike the nested case-control design, however, one cannot use the standard errors returned from such a fit to construct valid confidence intervals; since the same pool of controls is used for each case (subject to their being at risk at the time of the event), a form of statistical dependence is induced across the K contributions in $L_{caco}(\beta)$ which has to be accounted for to ensure valid estimation of standard errors.[54]

As with the nested case-control design, developments in statistical methodology since the case-control design was originally proposed have given analysts a range of tools to make use of all of the available information (*i.e.*, not just that provided by the subcohort). The framing for these methods is to reorient the analysis around the entire initial sample and then view those not selected by the design as having missing data. With this framing, one can use all of the tools that have been developed for efficient analyses of missing data, including IPW as well as multiple imputation.[53,55]

Finally, in addition to estimation of the regression coefficients, methods for both designs have been developed to permit estimation of absolute risk in the context, say, of a risk prediction study. Given data from a nested case-control study, for example, one can combine estimates of the regression parameters with a weighted version of the Breslow estimator of the cumulative baseline hazard function (as applied to those individuals selected by the design):

$$\hat{\Lambda}_0(t) = \sum_{t_k \leq t} \frac{1}{\sum_{i \in \tilde{R}_k} w_i(t_k) \exp\left(\beta_x x_i + \beta_1 z_{i,1} + \ldots + \beta_p z_{i,p}\right)}$$

where $w_i(t_k)$ depends on the sampling scheme for the controls. A similar approach can be used to estimate the cumulative baseline hazard function based on data from a case-cohort study.

Stratified Designs

Beyond simple random sampling for the selection of controls, a stratified version of the nested case-control design has been proposed. Referred to as *counter-matching,* the design uses covariate information that is readily available on all members of the initial cohort to form a stratification with S levels.[56] The counter-matched design then proceeds via risk-set sampling (as in the standard design) but with a prespecified number of individuals selected from each of the S strata within the risk set. As an example, suppose a design is prespecified such that m_s is to be selected from stratum s, for $s = 1,...,S$. For the specific stratum that the case belongs to, additional $m_s - 1$ controls are selected at random from that stratum. For each of the other strata, m_s controls are selected at random. As a special case, suppose the exposure of interest is binary and consider a 1:1 nested case-control design that counter-matches solely on the exposure. For this setup, a single control would be selected at random from among those that have the opposite exposure status to the case in the risk set. Thus, each of case-control dyad would have exactly one exposed individual and one unexposed individual. The central benefit of having gone through this process is that it facilitates the avoidance of matched sets for which there is no exposure variation; these sets would drop out from $L_{ncc}(\beta)$ and, thus, provide no information. More generally, the design ensures maximal variation in the representation of the levels of S (in a sense providing a balanced design across S) which will increase statistical efficiency for the variables that define S. Given data from a counter-matched nested case-control design, an analysis can proceed for the Cox model based on a weighted version of the modified partial likelihood, $L_{ncc}(\beta)$, with the weights calculated on the basis of the prespecified m_s and the number of individuals within each stratum within each risk set.

One can also use information that is readily available on all individuals in the initial cohort to construct a stratified sampling frame for the subcohort that may yield gains in efficiency. Suppose, for example, that the exposure of interest is rare but known on all individuals and that the purpose of the subsampling is to collect information one or more otherwise-unavailable confounders. In using simple random sampling to select the subcohort one could, by chance, have few controls who are exposed, thereby limiting statistical precision. Since the exposure is known, one could stratify the selection of the subcohort and increase precision for estimation of the association between the exposure and the time-to-event outcome. Practically, estimation can proceed with a relatively simple modification to $L_{caco}(\beta)$, specifically with the introduction of weights that reflect the sampling of the controls.[55]

Relative Merits of the Designs

The key structural distinction between the two classes of designs rests with selection of controls: in nested case-control studies, the selection is performed, in part at least, by matching on time; in case-cohort studies, there is no such matching, so that the subcohort can be viewed as being directly representative (on average at least) of the population from which the initial cohort was selected. This difference results in a number of downstream consequences, through which the relative merits of the designs can be compared.[57,58] Broadly, these merits can be characterized into two groups: those that are scientific/statistical in nature and those that are practical/logistical in nature.

A central goal of epidemiologic study design is to provide the means to address a given scientific question in as cost-efficient manner as possible. With this in mind, much of the initial work on investigating the relative merits of the designs focused on comparing their statistical efficiency in regard to estimation of the log-hazard ratios from a Cox model.[59-61] On the whole, the two designs appear to have comparable performance when the total number of individuals selected to have complete data (*i.e.*, the otherwise-unknown covariates are ascertained) is the same. One setting where nested case-control studies enjoy an advantage, however, is when there is substantial late entry into the study or if there is substantial right censoring.

Beyond statistical efficiency, early comparisons also considered the extent to which the subsample selected to have complete data could be used to analyze secondary outcomes (*i.e.*, outcomes other than the primary one that was as the basis for the design). Consider, for example, a hypothetical study of the association between some novel biomarker and the risk of recurrence following treatment among individuals diagnosed with prostate cancer. Furthermore, suppose the study is to be conducted in the context of an established cohort for which biological specimens have been collected. If a case-cohort study was conducted, the biomarker would be evaluated on all individuals in the random subcohort as well as among all remaining individuals who experience a recurrence during follow-up. After the completion of the study, the data from the subcohort could readily be used to investigate the association between the biomarker and a secondary outcome of, say, mortality. From an analysis perspective, since the subcohort was obtained via random sampling, no adjustment would be needed to account for the fact that the data were originally collected via a case-cohort design for recurrence. In contrast, because of the matching on time, where controls are matched to cases as they experience the primary event of interest, one cannot directly perform an analysis of some secondary outcome given data from a nested case-control study. Recent statistical developments, however, provide researchers with the tools to reuse the controls from a nested case-control study to conduct studies for secondary outcomes.[52,62] As such, it is no longer the case that the case-cohort design enjoys this particular advantage.

From a practical/logistical perspective, if the sampling is to be performed prospectively, then the case-cohort has the advantage of identifying all controls at the outset, with the burden of identifying additional individuals to be selected restricted to the cases. In contrast, before the selection of any controls in a nested case-control design, one must identify all individuals in the risk set formed as each case experiences the primary event. This will likely require greater administrative real-time coordination, specifically to acknowledge censoring and since some individuals may move between satisfying eligibility criteria and not, as well as result in a less predictable workflow.

One setting where the nested case-control design has a distinct advantage is when one or more of the otherwise unknown covariates is time dependent (*e.g.*, smoking history or history of exposure to some pharmacotherapy). In particular, controls selected in a case-cohort design will only have this information ascertained at the outset (*i.e.*, when the subcohort is identified) so that their information will not be up-to-date when they are used as comparators in the denominator of $L_{caco}(\beta)$. For controls selected in a nested case-control design, however, this information will be collected at the time they are selected (*i.e.*, when the case is identified) which coincides with the point in time at which they contribute to the denominator of $L_{ncc}(\beta)$.

ADDITIONAL TOPICS

The field of time-to-event analysis is huge and continuously evolving. While this chapter provides an overview of key concepts and topics, there are many that could not be covered including estimation in the presence of left truncation and/or interval censoring, the control of time-dependent confounding, the analysis of recurrent events, and Bayesian methods. Fortunately, are there numerous excellent texts that are specifically devoted to the analysis of time-to-event outcomes, ranging from those that are more theoretical[63,64] to those that emphasize practical issues as well as software.[14,65-68]

References

1. Freireich EJ, Gehan E, FREI E III, et al. The effect of 6-mercaptopurine on the duration of steroid-induced remissions in acute leukemia: a model for evaluation of other potentially useful therapy. *Blood*. 1963;21:699-716.
2. Kukull WA, Higdon R, Bowen JD, et al. Dementia and Alzheimer disease incidence: a prospective cohort study. *Arch Neurol*. 2002;59:1737-1746.
3. Little RJ, Rubin DB. *Statistical Analysis with Missing Data*. Hoboken, NJ: John Wiley & Sons; 2019.
4. Seaman S, Galati J, Jackson D, Carlin J. What is meant by "missing at random"? *Stat Sci*. 2013;28(2):257-268.
5. Royston P, Parmar MK. The use of restricted mean survival time to estimate the treatment effect in randomized clinical trials when the proportional hazards assumption is in doubt. *Stat Med*. 2011;30:2409-2421.
6. Rothman KJ. Estimation of confidence limits for the cumulative probability of survival in life table analysis. *J Chronic Dis*. 1978;31:557-560.
7. Anderson J, Bernstein L, Pike M. Approximate confidence intervals for probabilities of survival and quantiles in life-table analysis. *Biometrics*. 1982;38(2):407-416.
8. Cox DR. Regression models and life-tables. *J R Stat Soc Ser B (Methodological)*. 1972;34(2):187-220.
9. Breslow N. Covariance analysis of censored survival data. *Biometrics*. 1974;30(1):89-99.
10. Efron B. The efficiency of Cox's likelihood function for censored data. *J Am Stat Assoc*. 1977;72:557-565.
11. Farewell V, Prentice RL. The approximation of partial likelihood with emphasis on case-control studies. *Biometrika*. 1980;67:273-278.
12. Robins JM. *Marginal structural models versus structural nested models as tools for causal inference*. In: *Statistical Models in Epidemiology, the Environment, and Clinical Trials*. Springer; 2000.
13. Hernan MA, Brumback B, Robins JM. Marginal structural models to estimate the causal effect of zidovudine on the survival of HIV-positive men. *Epidemiology*. 2000;11:561-570.
14. Therneau TM, Grambsch PM. *Modeling Survival Data: Extending the Cox Model*. Springer Science & Business Media; 2000.

15. Schoenfeld D. Partial residuals for the proportional hazards regression model. *Biometrika*. 1982;69:239-241.

16. Fisher DP, Johnson E, Haneuse S, et al. Association between bariatric surgery and macrovascular disease outcomes in patients with type 2 diabetes and severe obesity. *J Am Med Assoc*. 2018;320:1570-1582.

17. Hernán MA. The hazards of hazard ratios. *Epidemiology*. 2010;21:13.

18. Uno H, Claggett B, Tian L, et al. Moving beyond the hazard ratio in quantifying the between-group difference in survival analysis. *J Clin Oncol*. 2014;32:2380.

19. Martinussen T, Scheike TH. A flexible additive multiplicative hazard model. *Biometrika*. 2002;89:283-298.

20. Rod NH, Lange T, Andersen I, Marott JL, Diderichsen F. Additive interaction in survival analysis: use of the additive hazards model. *Epidemiology*. 2012;23:733-737.

21. Martinussen T, Peng L. Alternatives to the Cox model. In: Klein J, VAN Houwelingen H, Ibrahim J, Scheike T, eds. *Handook of Survival Analysis*. 2013.

22. Ibrahim JG, Chen MH, Sinha D. *Bayesian Survival Analysis*. Wiley; 2014.

23. Tsiatis A. A nonidentifiability aspect of the problem of competing risks. *Proc Natl Acad Sci*. 1975;72:20-22.

24. Pintilie M. *Competing Risks: A Practical Perspective*. John Wiley & Sons; 2006.

25. Beyersmann J, Allignol A, Schumacher M. *Competing Risks and Multistate Models with R*. Springer Science & Business Media; 2011.

26. Crowder MJ. *Multivariate Survival Analysis and Competing Risks*. CRC Press; 2012.

27. Geskus RB. *Data Analysis with Competing Risks and Intermediate States*. CRC Press; 2015.

28. Austin PC, Lee DS, Fine JP. Introduction to the analysis of survival data in the presence of competing risks. *Circulation*. 2016;133:601-609.

29. Latouche A, Allignol A, Beyersmann J, Labopin M, Fine JP. A competing risks analysis should report results on all cause-specific hazards and cumulative incidence functions. *J Clin Epidemiol*. 2013;66:648-653.

30. Fine JP, Jiang H, Chappell R. On semi-competing risks data. *Biometrika*. 2001;88:907-919.

31. Jazić I, Schrag D, Sargent DJ, Haneuse S. Beyond composite endpoints analysis: semicompeting risks as an underutilized framework for cancer research. *J Natl Cancer Inst*. 2016;108.

32. Haneuse S, Lee KH. Semi-competing risks data analysis: accounting for death as a competing risk when the outcome of interest is nonterminal. *Circ Cardiovasc Qual Outcomes*. 2016;9:322-331.

33. Zhang JL, Rubin DB. Estimation of causal effects via principal stratification when some outcomes are truncated by "death". *J Educ Behav Stat*. 2003;28:353-368.

34. Robins JM. A new approach to causal inference in mortality studies with a sustained exposure period-application to control of the healthy worker survivor effect. *Math Model*. 1986;7:1393-1512.

35. Frangakis CE, Rubin DB. Principal stratification in causal inference. *Biometrics*. 2002;58:21-29.

36. Tchetgen Tchetgen EJ. Identification and estimation of survivor average causal effects. *Stat Med*. 2014;33:3601-3628.

37. Mattei A, Mealli F. Application of the principal stratification approach to the Faenza randomized experiment on breast self-examination. *Biometrics*. 2007;63:437-446.

38. Hayden D, Pauler DK, Schoenfeld D. An estimator for treatment comparisons among survivors in randomized trials. *Biometrics*. 2005;61:305-310.

39. Jemiai Y, Rotnitzky A, Shepherd BE, Gilbert PB. Semiparametric estimation of treatment effects given base-line covariates on an outcome measured after a post-randomization event occurs. *J R Stat Soc Ser B (Statistical Methodology)*. 2007;69:879-901.

40. Egleston BL, Scharfstein DO, Freeman EE, West SK. Causal inference for non-mortality outcomes in the presence of death. *Biostatistics*. 2007;8:526-545.

41. Chiba Y, Vanderweele TJ. A simple method for principal strata effects when the outcome has been truncated due to death. *Am Journal Epidemiology*. 2011;173:745-751.

42. Clayton DG. A model for association in bivariate life tables and its application in epidemiological studies of familial tendency in chronic disease incidence. *Biometrika*. 1978;65:141-151.

43. Peng L, Fine JP. Regression modeling of semicompeting risks data. *Biometrics*. 2007;63:96-108.

44. Hsieh JJ, Wang W, ADAM Ding A. Regression analysis based on semicompeting risks data. *J R Stat Soc Ser B (Statistical Methodology)*. 2008;70:3-20.

45. Putter H, Fiocco M, Geskus RB. Tutorial in biostatistics: competing risks and multi-state models. *Stat Medicine*. 2007;26:2389-2430.

46. Xu J, Kalbfleisch JD, Tai B. Statistical analysis of illness–death processes and semicompeting risks data. *Biometrics*. 2010;66(3):716-725.

47. Lee KH, Haneuse S, Schrag D, Dominici F. Bayesian semi-parametric analysis of semi-competing risks data: Investigating hospital readmission after a pancreatic cancer diagnosis. *J R Stat Soc Ser C Appl Stat*. 2015;64(2):253.

48. Lee KH, Rondeau V, Haneuse S. Accelerated failure time models for semi-competing risks data in the presence of complex censoring. *Biometrics*. 2017;73(4):1401-1412.

49. Thomas DC. Addendum to Methods of cohort analysis: appraisal by application to asbestos mining. By FDK Liddell, JC McDonald and DC Thomas. *J R Stat Soc Ser A*. 1977;140:469-491.

50. Prentice R. A case-cohort design for epidemiologic cohort studies and disease prevention trials. *Biometrika*. 1986;73:1-11.

51. Goldstein L, Langholz B. Asymptotic theory for nested case-control sampling in the Cox regression model. *Ann Stat*. 1992;20(4):1903-1928.

52. Samuelsen SO. A pseudolikelihood approach to analysis of nested case-control studies. *Biometrika*. 1997;84:379-394.

53. Keogh RH, White IR. Using full-cohort data in nested case–control and case–cohort studies by multiple imputation. *Stat Med*. 2013;32:4021-4043.

54. Onland-Moret NC, van der Schouw YT, Buschers W, et al. Analysis of case-cohort data: a comparison of different methods. *J Clin Epidemiol*. 2007;60:350-355.

55. Borgan O, Langholz B, Samuelsen SO, Goldstein L, Pogoda J. Exposure stratified case-cohort designs. *Lifetime Data Anal*. 2000;6:39-58.

56. Langholz B, Borgan O. Counter-matching: a stratified nested case-control sampling method. *Biometrika*. 1995;82:69-79.

57. Wacholder S. Practical considerations in choosing between the case-cohort and nested case-control designs. *Epidemiology*. 1991;2:155-158.

58. Borgan O, Samuelsen SO. Nested case-control and case-cohort studies. In: Klein J, Van Houwelingen H, Ibrahim J, Scheike T, eds. *Handbook of Survival Analysis*. Boca Raton, FL: CRC Press; 2013.

59. Langholz B, Thomas DC. Nested case-control and case-cohort methods of sampling from a cohort: a critical comparison. *Am J Epidemiol*. 1990;131:169-176.

60. Langholz B, Thomas DC. Efficiency of cohort sampling designs: some surprising results. *Biometrics*. 1991;47(4):1563-1571.

61. Barlow WE, Ichikawa L, Rosner D, Izumi S. Analysis of case-cohort designs. *J Clin Epidemiol*. 1999;52:1165-1172.

62. Saarela O, Kulathinal S, Arjas E, Läärä E. Nested case–control data utilized for multiple outcomes: a likelihood approach and alternatives. *Stat Med*. 2008;27:5991-6008.

63. Kalbfleisch JD, Prentice RL. *The Statistical Analysis of Failure Time Data*. John Wiley & Sons; 2011.

64. Andersen PK, Borgan O, Gill RD, Keiding N. *Statistical Models Based on Counting Processes*. Springer Science & Business Media; 2012.

65. Hosmer D, Lemeshow S, May S. *Applied Survival Analysis: Regression Modeling of Time-To-Event Data*. Wiley-Interscience; 2008.

66. Allison PD. *Survival Analysis Using SAS: A Practical Guide*. SAS Institute; 2010.

67. Royston P, Lambert PC. *Flexible Parametric Survival Analysis Using STATA: Beyond the Cox Model*. STATA Press; 2011.

68. Collett D. *Modelling Survival Data in Medical Research*. CRC Press; 2015.

CHAPTER 23

Introduction to Bayesian Statistics

Sander Greenland

Earlier chapters briefly introduced the central concepts of Bayesian statistics. Beginning with Laplace in the 18th century, these methods were used freely alongside other methods. In the 1920s, however, several influential statisticians (*e.g.*, R. A. Fisher, J. Neyman, and E. Pearson) developed bodies of frequentist techniques intended to supplant entirely all others, based on notions of objective probability represented by relative frequencies in hypothetical infinite sequences of randomized experiments or random samplings. For the rest of the 20th century, these methods dominated statistical research and became the sole body of methods taught to most students. Chapters 16-22 describe the fundamentals of these frequentist methods for epidemiologic studies.

In the context of randomized trials and random-sample surveys in which they were developed, these frequentist techniques appear to be highly effective tools. As the use of the methods spread from designed surveys and experiments to observational studies, however, an increasing number of statisticians questioned the objectivity and realism of the hypothetical infinite sequences invoked by frequentist methods.[1-8] They argued that a subjective Bayesian approach better represented situations in which the mechanisms generating study samples and exposure status were heavily

---

This chapter has been reprinted without revision from the Third Edition.

nonrandom and poorly understood. In those settings, which typify most epidemiologic research, the personal judgments of the investigators play an unavoidable and crucial role in making inferences and often override technical considerations that dominate statistical analyses (as perhaps they should; cf. Susser[9]).

In the wake of such arguments, Bayesian methods have become common in advanced training and research in statistics,[10-13] even in the randomized trial literature for which frequentist methods were developed.[14,15] Elementary training appears to have lagged, however, despite arguments for reform.[16] This chapter illustrates how conventional frequentist methods can be used to generate Bayesian analyses. In particular, it shows how basic epidemiologic analyses can be conducted with a hand calculator or ordinary software packages for stratified analysis.[17] The same computational devices can also be used to conduct Bayesian regression analyses with ordinary regression software.[18] Thus, as far as computation is concerned, it is a small matter to extend current training and practice to encompass Bayesian methods.

The chapter begins with a philosophical section that criticizes standard objections to Bayesian approaches, and that delineates key parallels and differences between frequentist and Bayesian methods. It does not address distinctions within frequentist and Bayesian traditions. See Goodman for a review of the profound divergence between Fisherian and Neyman-Pearsonian frequentism.[19] This chapter argues that observational researchers (not just statisticians) need training in subjective Bayesianism[1,2,20] to serve as a counterweight to the alleged objectivity of frequentist methods. For this purpose, neither "objective" Bayesian methods[21] nor "pure likelihood" methods[22] will do, because they largely replicate the pretense of objectivity that renders frequentist methods so misleading in observational research.

Much of the modern Bayesian literature focuses on a level of precision in specifying a prior and analytic computation that is far beyond anything required of frequentist methods or by the messy problems of observational data analysis. Many of these computing methods obscure important parallels between traditional frequentist methods and Bayesian methods. High precision is unnecessary given the imprecision of the data and the goals of everyday epidemiology. Furthermore, subjective Bayesian methods are distinguished by their use of informative prior distributions; hence their proper use requires a sound understanding of the meaning and limitations of those distributions, not a false sense of precision. In observational studies, neither Bayesian nor other methods require extremely precise computation, especially in light of the huge uncertainties about the processes generating observational data (represented by the likelihood function), as well as uncertainty about prior information.

After an introduction to the philosophy of Bayesian methods, the chapter focuses on basic Bayesian approaches that display prior distributions as prior estimates or prior data, and that employ the same approximate formulas used by frequentist methods.[5,17,18,23-29] Even for those who prefer other computing methods, the representation of prior distributions as prior data is helpful in understanding the strength of the prior judgments.

FREQUENTISM VERSUS SUBJECTIVE BAYESIANISM

There are several objections that frequentists have raised against Bayesian methods. Some of these are legitimate but apply in parallel to frequentist methods (and indeed to all of statistics) in observational studies. Most important, perhaps, is that the assumptions or models employed are at best subjective judgments. Others are propaganda—*e.g.*, that adopting a Bayesian approach introduces arbitrariness that is not already present. In reality, the Bayesian approach makes explicit those subjective and arbitrary elements that are shared by all statistical inferences. Because these elements are hidden by frequentist conventions, Bayesian methods are left open to criticisms that make it appear only they are using those elements.

Subjective Probabilities Should Not Be Arbitrary

In subjective (personalist) Bayesian theory, a prior for a parameter is a probability distribution Pr(parameters) that shows how a particular person would bet about parameters if she disregarded the data under analysis. This prior need not originate from evidence preceding the study; rather, it represents information apart from the data being analyzed. When the only parameter is a risk ratio, RR, the 50th percentile (median) of her prior Pr(RR) is a number RR_{median} for which she would give even odds that RR < RR$_{median}$ versus RR > RR$_{median}$, *i.e.*, she would assign Pr(RR < RR$_{median}$) = Pr(RR > RR$_{median}$) if she disregarded the analysis data. Similarly, her 95% prior limits are a pair of numbers RR$_{lower}$ and RR$_{upper}$ such that she would give 95:5 = 19:1 odds that the true risk ratio is between these numbers, *i.e.*, Pr(RR$_{lower}$ < RR < RR$_{upper}$) = 0.95 if she disregarded the analysis data.

Prior limits may vary considerably across individuals; mine may be very different from yours. This variability does not mean, however, that the limits are arbitrary. When betting on a race with the goal of minimizing losses, no one would regard it reasonable to bet everything on a randomly drawn contestant; rather, a person would place different bets on different contestants, based on their previous performance (but taking account of differences in the past conditions from the present). Similarly, in order for a Bayesian analysis to seem reasonable or credible to others, a prior should reflect results from previous studies or reviews. This reflection should allow for possible biases and lack of generalizability among studies, so that prior limits might be farther apart than frequentist meta-analytic confidence limits (even if the latter incorporated random effects).

The prior Pr(parameters) is one of the two major inputs to a Bayesian analysis. The other input is a function Pr(data|parameters) that shows the probability the analyst would assign the observed data for any given set of parameter values, usually called the *likelihood function*. In subjective-Bayesian analysis, this function is another set of bets: The model for Pr(data|parameters) summarizes how one would bet on the study outcome (the data) if one knew the parameters (*e.g.*, the exposure-covariate specific risks). Any such model should meet the same credibility requirements as the prior. This requirement parallels the frequentist concern that the model should be able to approximate reality. In fact, any competent Bayesian has the same concern, albeit perhaps with more explicit doubts about whether that can be achieved with standard models.

The same need for credibility motivates authors to discuss other literature when writing their research reports. Credible authors pay attention to past literature in their analyses by adjusting for known or suspected confounders, by not adjusting for factors affected by exposure, and by using a dose-response model that can capture previously observed patterns (*e.g.*, the J-shaped relation of alcohol use to cardiovascular mortality). They may even vary their models to accommodate different views on what adjustments should be done. In a similar manner, Bayesian analyses need not be limited to using a single prior or likelihood function. Acceptability of an analysis is often enhanced by presenting results from different priors to reflect different opinions about the parameter, by presenting results using a prior that is broad enough to assign relatively high probability to each discussant's opinion (a "consensus" prior), and by presenting results from different degrees of regression adjustment (which involves varying the likelihood function).

The Posterior Distribution

Upon seeing the outcome of a race on which a person had bet, she would want to update her bets regarding the outcome of another race involving the same contestants. In this spirit, Bayesian analysis produces a model for the posterior distribution Pr(parameters|data), a probability distribution that shows how she should bet about the parameters *after* examining the analysis data. As a minimal criterion of reasonable betting, suppose she would never want to place her bets in a manner that allows an opponent betting against her to guarantee a loss. This criterion implies that her bets should obey the laws of probability, including Bayes' theorem,

$$\Pr\left(\text{parameters}|\text{data}\right) = \Pr\left(\text{data}|\text{parameters}\right)\Pr\left(\text{parameters}\right)/\Pr\left(\text{data}\right)$$

where the portion Pr(data) is computed from the likelihood function and the prior.[30] The 50th percentile (median) of her posterior about a risk ratio RR is a number RR$_{median}$ for which Pr(RR < RR$_{median}$|data) = Pr(RR > RR$_{median}$|data), where "|data" indicates that this bet is formulated in light of the analysis data. Similarly, her 95% posterior limits are a pair of numbers RR$_{lower}$ and RR$_{upper}$ such that after analyzing the data she would give 95:5 = 19:1 odds that the true relative risk is between these numbers, *i.e.*, Pr(RR$_{lower}$ < RR < RR$_{upper}$|data) = 0.95.

As with priors, posterior distributions may vary considerably across individuals, not only because they may use different priors Pr(parameters) but also because they may use different models for the data probabilities Pr(data|parameters). This variation is only to be expected given disagreement among observers about the implications of past study results and the present study's design. Bayesian analyses can help pinpoint sources of disagreement, especially in that they distinguish sources in the priors from sources in the data models.

Frequentist-Bayesian Parallels

It is often said (incorrectly) that "parameters are treated as fixed by the frequentist but as random by the Bayesian." For frequentists and Bayesians alike, the value of a parameter may have been fixed from the start, or it may have been generated from a physically random mechanism. In either case, both suppose that it has taken on some fixed value that we would like to know. The Bayesian uses probability models to express personal uncertainty about that value. In other words, the "randomness" in these models represents personal uncertainty; it is *not* a property of the parameter, although it should accurately reflect properties of the mechanisms that produced the parameter.

A crucial parallel between frequentist and Bayesian methods is their dependence on the model chosen for the data probability Pr(data|parameters). Statistical results are as sensitive to this choice as they are to choice of priors. The choice should thus ideally reflect the best available knowledge about forces that influence the data, including effects of unmeasured variables, biased selection, and measurement errors (such as misclassification). Instead, the choice is almost always a default built into statistical software, based on assumptions of random sampling or random treatment assignment (which are rarely credible in observational epidemiology), plus additivity assumptions. Worse, the data models are often selected by mechanical algorithms that are oblivious to background information and, as a result, often conflict with contextual information. These problems afflict the majority of epidemiologic analyses today, in the form of models (such as the logistic, Poisson, and proportional-hazards models) that make interaction and dose-response assumptions that are rarely if ever justified. These models are never known to be correct and in fact cannot hold exactly, especially when one considers possible study biases.[31,32]

Acceptance of results derived from these models (whether the results are frequentist or Bayesian) thus requires the doubtful assumption that existing violations have no important effect on results. The model for Pr(data|parameters) is thus a weak link in the chain of reasoning leading from data to inference, shared by both frequentist and Bayesian methods. In practice, the two approaches often use the same model for Pr(data|parameters), whence divergent outputs from the methods must arise elsewhere. A major source of divergence is the explicit prior Pr(parameters) used in Bayesian reasoning. The methods described in this chapter will show the mechanics of this divergence and provide a sense of when it will be important.

Empirical Priors

The addition of the prior Pr(parameter) raises the point that the validity of the Bayesian answer will depend on the validity of the prior model as well as the validity of the data model. If the prior should not just be some arbitrary opinion, however, what should it be?

One answer arises from frequentist shrinkage-estimation methods (also known as Stein estimation, empirical Bayes, penalized estimation, and random-coefficient or ridge regression) to improve repeated-sampling accuracy of estimates. These methods use numerical devices that translate directly into priors[4,5,33] and thus leave unanswered the same question asked of subjective Bayesians: Where should these devices come from? Empirical-Bayes and random-coefficient methods assume explicitly that the parameters as well as the data would vary randomly across repetitions according to an actual frequency distribution Pr(parameters) that can be estimated from available data. As in Bayesian analyses, these methods compute posterior coefficient distributions using Bayes' theorem. Given the randomness of the coefficients, however, the resulting posterior intervals are also frequentist confidence intervals in the sense of containing the true (if varying) parameter values in the stated percentage of repetitions.[11]

Those who wish to extend Bayes-frequentist parallels into practice are thus led to the following empirical principle: When true frequency distributions exist and are known for the data or the parameter distribution (as in multilevel random sampling[34]), they should be used as the distributions in Bayesian analysis. This principle reflects the idea of placing odds on race contestants based on their past frequencies of winning and corresponds to common notions of induction.[35] Such frequency-based priors are more accurately termed "empirical" rather than "subjective," although the decision to accept the empirical evidence remains a subjective judgment (and subject to error). Empirical priors are mandated in much of Bayesian philosophy, such as the "principal principle,"[36] which states that when frequency probabilities exist and are known (as in games of chance and in quantum physics), one should use them as personal probabilities. More generally, an often-obeyed (if implicit) inductive principle is that the prior should be found by fitting to available empirical frequencies, as is often done in frequentist hierarchical regression.[5,24,37,38] The fitted prior is thus no more arbitrary than (and may even be functionally identical to) a fitted second-stage frequentist model. With empirical priors, the resulting frequentist and Bayesian interval estimates may be numerically identical.

Frequentist-Bayesian Divergences

Even when a frequentist and a Bayesian arrive at the same interval estimate for a parameter, the interpretations remain quite different. Frequentist methods pretend that the models are laws of chance in the real world (indeed, much of the theoretical literature encourages this illusion by calling distributions "laws"). In contrast, subjective-Bayesian methods interpret the models as nothing more than summaries of tentative personal bets about how the data and the parameters would appear, rather than as models of a real random mechanism. The prior model *should* be based on observed frequencies when those are available, but the resulting model for the posterior Pr(parameters|model) is a summary of personal bets after seeing the data, not a frequency distribution (although if the parameters are physically random, it will also represent a personal estimate of their distribution).

It is important to recognize that the subjective-Bayesian interpretation is much less ambitious (and less confident) than the frequentist interpretation, insofar as it treats the models and the analysis results as systems of personal judgments, possibly poor ones, rather than as some sort of objective reality. Probabilities are nothing more than expressions of opinions, as in common phrasings such as "It will probably rain tomorrow." Reasonable opinions are based heavily on frequencies in past experience, but they are never as precise as results from statistical computations.

Frequentist Fantasy Versus Observational Reality

For Bayesian methods, there seems no dispute that the results should be presented with reference to the priors as well as to the data models and the data. For example, a posterior interval should be presented as "*Given these priors, models, and data*, we would be 95% certain that the parameter is in this interval."

A parallel directive should be applied to frequentist presentations. For example, 95% confidence intervals are usually presented as if they account for random error, without regard for what that random error is supposed to represent. For observational research, one of many problems with frequentist ("repeated-sampling") interpretations is that it is not clear what is "random" when no random sampling or randomization has been done. Although "random variation" may be present even when it has not been introduced by the investigator, in observational studies there is seldom a sound rationale for claiming it follows the distributions that frequentist methods assume, or any known distribution.[31] At best, those distributions refer only to thought experiments in which one asks, "*If* data were repeatedly produced by the *assumed* random-sampling process, the statistics would have their stated properties (*e.g.*, 95% coverage) across those repetitions." They do not refer to what happens under the distributions actually operating, for the latter are unknown. Thus, what they do say is extremely hypothetical, so much so that to understand them fully is to doubt their relevance for observational research.[4]

Frequentist results are hypothetical whenever one cannot be certain that the assumed data model holds, as when uncontrolled sources of bias (such as confounding, selection bias, and measurement error) are present. In light of such problems, claims that frequentist methods are "objective" in an observational setting seem like propaganda or self-delusion.[4-6,30,32] At best, frequentist methods in epidemiology represent a dubious social convention that mandates treating observational data as if they arose from a fantasy of a tightly designed and controlled randomized experiment on a random sample (that is, as if a thought experiment were reality). Like many entrenched conventions, they provoke defenses that claim utility[13,39] without any *comparative* empirical evidence that the conventions serve observational research better than would alternatives. Other defenses treat the frequentist thought experiments as if they were real—an example of what has been called the mind-projection fallacy.[40]

Were we to apply the same truth-in-packaging standard to frequentists as to Bayesians, a "statistically significant" frequentist result would be riddled with caveats such as "*If* these data had been generated from a randomized trial with no drop-out or measurement error, these results would be very improbable were the null true; but because they were not so generated we can say little of their actual statistical significance." Such brutal honesty is of course rare in presentations of observational epidemiologic results because emphasizing frequentist premises undermines the force of the presentation.

Summary

A criticism of Bayesian methods is that the priors must be arbitrary, or subjective in a pernicious or special way. In observational studies, however, the prior needs to be no more arbitrary than the largely arbitrary data models that are routinely applied to data and can often be given a scientific foundation as or more firm than that of frequentist data models. Like any analysis element, prior models should be scrutinized critically (and rejected as warranted), just as should frequentist models. When relevant and valid external frequency data are available, they should be used to build the prior model (which may lead to inclusion of those data as part of the likelihood function, so that the external and current data become pooled).

When prior frequency data are absent or invalid, however, other sources of priors will enter, and must be judged critically. Later sections will show how simple log relative-risk priors can be translated into "informationally equivalent" prior frequency data, which aids in this judgment, and which also allows easy extension of Bayesian methods to regression analysis and non-normal priors.[18,28]

SIMPLE APPROXIMATE BAYESIAN METHODS

Exact Bayesian analysis proceeds by computing the posterior distribution via Bayes' theorem, which requires Pr(data). The latter can be difficult to evaluate (usually requiring multiple integration over the parameters), which seems to have fostered the misimpression that practical Bayesian analyses are inherently more complex computationally than frequentist analyses. But this impression is based on an unfair comparison of *exact* Bayesian methods to *approximate* frequentist methods.

Frequentist teaching evolved during an era of limited computing, so they focused on simple, large-sample approximate methods for categorical data. In contrast, the Bayesian resurgence occurred during the introduction of powerful personal computers and advanced Monte Carlo algorithms, hence much Bayesian teaching focuses on exact methods, often presented as if simple approximations are inadequate. But Bayesian approximations suitable for categorical data have a long history,[23,24] are as accurate as frequentist approximations, and are accurate enough for epidemiologic studies. The approximations also provide insights into the meaning of both Bayesian and frequentist methods and hence are the focus of the remainder of this chapter.

In the examples that follow, the outcome is very rare, so we may ignore distinctions among risk, rate, and odds ratios, which will be generically described as "relative risks" (RR). Because a normal distribution has equal mode, median, and mean, we may also ignore distinctions among these measures of location when discussing a normal ln(RR). When we take the antilog $e^{\ln(RR)} = RR$, however, we obtain a log-normal distribution, for which mode < median and geometric mean < arithmetic mean. Only the median transforms directly: median RR $= e^{\text{median ln(RR)}}$.

INFORMATION-WEIGHTED AVERAGING

Information (or precision) is here defined as the inverse of the variance.[10] Weighting by information shows how simple Bayesian methods parallel frequentist summary estimation based on inverse-variance weighting. It assumes that both the prior model and the data model are adequately approximated by normal distributions. This assumption requires that the sample sizes (both actual and prior) are large enough for the approximation to be adequate. As with the approximate frequentist methods on which they are based, there is no hard-and-fast rule on what size is adequate, in part because of disagreement

TABLE 23-1

Case-Control Data on Residential Magnetic Fields ($X = 1$ is >3 mG Average Exposure, $X = 0$ is ≤3 mG) and Childhood Leukemia[42] and Frequentist Results

	$X = 1$	$X = 0$	
Cases	3	33	Table odds ratio = RR estimate = 3.51
Controls	5	193	95% confidence limits = 0.80, 15.4

$\ln(OR) = \ln(RR)$ estimate = $\ln(3.51)$, estimated variance = 0.569

From Savitz DA, Wachtel H, Barnes FA, John EM, Tvrdik JG. Case-control study of childhood cancer and exposure to 60-Hz magnetic fields. *Am J Epidemiol.* 1988;128(1):21-38.

about how much inaccuracy is tolerable (which depends on context). The same approximations in frequentist categorical statistics are arguably adequate down to cell sizes of 4 or 5.[41]

A Single Two-Way Table

Table 23-1 shows case-control data from the first widely publicized study to report a positive association between residential magnetic fields and childhood leukemia.[42] Although previous studies had reported positive associations between household wiring and leukemia, strong field effects seemed unlikely at the time, and very strong effects seemed very unlikely. Suppose we model these *a priori* ideas by placing 2:1 odds on a relative risk (RR) between ½ and 2 and 95% probability on RR between ¼ and 4 when comparing children above and below a 3 milligauss (mG) cut point for fields. These bets would follow from a normal prior for the log relative risk $\ln(RR)$ that satisfies

exp(prior mean − 1.96·prior standard deviation) = ¼
exp(prior mean + 1.96·prior standard deviation) = 4.

Solving this pair of equations, we get

$$\text{Prior mean of } \ln(RR) = \text{average of the limits} = \frac{\ln(¼) + \ln(4)}{2} = 0$$

$$\text{Prior standard deviation of } \ln(RR) = \frac{\text{width of interval in } \ln(RR) \text{ units}}{\text{width of interval in standard deviation units}}$$

$$= \frac{\ln(4) - \ln(¼)}{2(1.96)} = 0.707$$

$$\text{Prior variance of } \ln(RR) = 0.707^2 = 0.500 = ½.$$

Thus, the normal prior distribution that would produce the stated bets has mean zero and variance ½.

Three of 36 cases and 5 of 198 controls had estimated average fields above 3 milligauss (mG). These data yield the following frequentist RR estimates:

Estimated RR = sample odds ratio = 3(193)/5(33) = 3.51
Estimated variance of log odds ratio = 1/3 + 1/33 + 1/5 + 1/193 = 0.569
95% confidence limits = exp[ln(3.51) ± 1.96 × 0.569$^{1/2}$] = 0.80, 15.4

Assuming there is no prior information about the prevalence of exposure, an approximate posterior mean for $\ln(RR)$ is just the average of the prior mean $\ln(RR)$ of 0 and the data estimate $\ln(3.51)$, weighted by the information (inverse variance) of $1/(½)$ and $1/0.569$, respectively:

Posterior mean for $\ln(RR)$ = expected $\ln(RR)$ given data

$$\approx \left[0/(½) + \ln(3.51)/0.569\right] / \left[1/(½) + 1/0.569\right] = 0.587$$

The approximate posterior variance of ln(RR) is the inverse of the total information:

Posterior variance for $\ln(RR) \approx 1/[1/(\frac{1}{2}) + 1/0.569] = 0.266$

Together, this mean and variance produce

Posterior median for $RR \approx \exp(0.587) = 1.80$
95% posterior limits for $RR \approx \exp(0.587 \pm 1.96 \times 0.266^{1/2}) = 0.65, 4.94$

The posterior RR of 1.80 is close to a simple geometric averaging of the prior RR (of 1) with the frequentist estimate (of 3.51), because the data information is $1/0.569 = 1.76$, whereas the prior information is $1/(\frac{1}{2}) = 2$, giving almost equal weight to the two. This equal weighting arises because both the study (with only three exposed cases and five exposed controls) and the prior are weak. Note too that the posterior RR of 1.80 is much closer to the frequentist odds ratios from other studies, which average around 1.7.[32]

Bayesian Interpretation of Frequentist Results

The weighted-averaging formula shows that the frequentist results arise from the Bayesian calculation when the prior information is made negligibly small relative to the data information. In this sense, frequentist results are just extreme Bayesian results, ones in which the prior information is zero, asserting that absolutely nothing is known about the RR outside of the study. Some promote such priors as "letting the data speak for themselves." In reality, the data say nothing by themselves: The frequentist results are computed using probability models that assume complete absence of bias, and so filter the data through false assumptions.

A Bayesian analysis that uses these frequentist data models is subject to the same criticism. Even with no bias, however, assuming absence of prior information is empirically absurd. Prior information of zero implies that a relative risk of (say) 10^{100} is as plausible as a value of 1 or 2. Suppose the relative risk was truly 10^{100}; then every child exposed above 3 mG would have contracted leukemia, making exposure a sufficient cause. The resulting epidemic would have come to everyone's attention long before the above study was done because the leukemia rate would have reflected the prevalence of high exposure, which is about 5% in the United States. The actual rate of leukemia is 4 cases per 100,000 person-years, which implies that the relative risk cannot be extremely high. Thus there are ample background data to rule out such extreme relative risks.

So-called objective-Bayes methods[21] differ from frequentist methods only in that they make these unrealistic "noninformative" priors explicit. The resulting posterior intervals represent inferences that no thoughtful person could make, because they reflect nothing of the subject under study or even the meaning of the variable names. Genuine prior bets are more precise. Even exceptionally "strong" relations in noninfectious disease epidemiology (such as smoking and lung cancer) involve RR of the order of 10 or 1/10, and few noninfectious study exposures are even that far from the null. This situation reflects the fact that, for a factor to reach the level of formal epidemiologic study, its effects must be small enough to have gone undetected by clinical practice or by surveillance systems. There is almost always some surveillance (if only informal, through the healthcare system) that implies limits on the effect size. If these limits are huge, frequentist results serve as a rough approximation to a Bayesian analysis that uses an empirically based prior for the RR; otherwise the frequentist results may be very misleading.

Adjustment

To adjust for measured confounders without using explicit priors for their confounding effects, one need only to set a prior for the adjusted RR and then combine the prior ln(RR) with the adjusted frequentist estimate by inverse-variance averaging. For example, in a pooled analysis of 14 studies of magnetic fields (>3 mG vs. less) and childhood leukemia,[32] the only important measured confounder was the source of the data (*i.e.*, the variable coding "study"), and thus stratification by study was crucial. The maximum-likelihood odds-ratio estimate of the common odds ratio across the studies was 1.69, with 95% confidence limits of 1.28, 2.23; thus the log odds ratio was $\ln(1.69) = 0.525$ with variance estimate $[\ln(2.23/1.28)/3.92]^2 = 0.0201$. Combining this study-adjusted frequentist result with a normal$(0, \frac{1}{2})$ prior yields

$$\text{Posterior mean for } \ln(RR) \approx \left[0/(\tfrac{1}{2}) + \ln(1.69)/0.0201\right] / \left[1/(\tfrac{1}{2}) + 1/0.0201\right] = 0.504$$

$$\text{Posterior variance for } \ln(RR) \approx 1/\left[1/(\tfrac{1}{2}) + 1/.0201\right] = 0.0193$$

$$\text{Posterior median for } RR \approx \exp(0.504) = 1.66$$

$$95\% \text{ posterior limits for } RR \approx \exp\left(0.504 \pm 1.96 \cdot 0.0193^{1/2}\right) = 1.26, 2.17$$

This posterior hardly differs from the frequentist results, reflecting that the data information is $1/0.0201 = 50$, or 25 times the prior information of $1/(\frac{1}{2}) = 2$. In other words, the data information dominates the prior information.

One can also make adjustments based on priors for confounding, which may include effects of unmeasured variables.[32,43-45]

Varying the Prior

Many authors have expressed skepticism over the existence of an actual magnetic field effect, so much so that they have misinterpreted positive findings as null because they were not "statistically significant."[46] The Bayesian framework allows this sort of prejudice to be displayed explicitly in the prior, rather than forcing it into misinterpretation of the data.[47] Suppose that the extreme skepticism about the effect is expressed as a normal prior for $\ln(RR)$ with mean zero and 95% prior limits for RR of 0.91 and 1.1.[48] The prior standard deviation is then $[\ln(1.1) - \ln(0.91)]/3.92 = 0.0484$. Averaging this prior with the frequentist summary of $\ln(1.69)$ yields 95% posterior RR limits of 0.97, 1.16. Here, the prior weight is $1/0.0484^2 = 427$, more than 8 times the data information of 50, and so the prior dominates the final result.

It can be instructive to examine how the results change as the prior changes.[4,15,32,49] Using a normal$(0, v)$ prior, a simple approach examines the outputs as the variance v ranges over values that different researchers hold. For example, when examining a relative risk (RR), prior variances of $\frac{1}{8}, \frac{1}{2}, 2, 4$ for $\ln(RR)$ correspond to 95% prior intervals for RR of $(\frac{1}{2}, 2)$, $(\frac{1}{4}, 4)$, $(1/16, 16)$, $(1/50, 50)$. The frequentist results represent another (gullible) extreme prior based on two false assumptions: first, that the likelihood (data) model is correct (which is falsified by biases); and second, that nothing is known about any explicit parameter, corresponding to infinite v and hence no prior upper limit on RR (which is falsified by surveillance data). At the other extreme, assertions of skeptics often correspond to priors with $v < \frac{1}{8}$ and hence a 95% prior interval within $(\frac{1}{2}, 2)$.

Bayes Versus Semi-Bayes

The preceding example analyses are *semi*-Bayes in that they do not introduce an explicit prior for all the free parameters in the problem. For example, they do not use a prior for the population exposure prevalence $\Pr(X = 1)$ or for the relation of adjustment factors to exposure or the outcome. Semi-Bayes analyses are equivalent to Bayesian analyses in which those parameters are given noninformative priors and correspond to frequentist mixed models (in which some but not all coefficients are random). As with frequentist analyses, the cost of using no prior for a parameter is that the results fall short of the accuracy that could be achieved if a realistic prior were used. The benefit is largely one of simplicity in not having to specify priors for many parameters. Good provides a general discussion of cost-benefit trade-offs of analysis complexity,[5] under the heading of "Type-II rationality." Good[5] (1983) and Greenland[38] also describe how multilevel (hierarchical) modeling subsumes frequentist, semi-Bayes, and Bayes methods, as well as shrinkage (empirical-Bayes) methods.

TABLE 23-2

General Notation for 2 × 2 Prior-Data Layout

	$X = 1$	$X = 0$		
Cases	A_1	A_0	Table RR = RR_{prior}	$= (A_1/N_1)/(A_0/N_0)$
Total	N_1	N_0		$= (A_1/A_0)/(N_1/N_0)$

PRIOR DATA: FREQUENTIST INTERPRETATION OF PRIORS

Having expressed one's prior bets as intervals about the target parameter, it is valuable to ask what sort of data would have generated those bets as confidence intervals. In the previous examples, we could ask: What would constitute data "equivalent" to the prior? That is, what experiment would convey the same information as the normal (0, ½) prior for ln(RR)? Answers to such Bayesian questions can be found by frequentist thought experiments,[47] which show how Bayesian methods parallel frequentist methods for pooled analysis of multiple studies.

Suppose we were given the results of a trial with N_1 children randomized to exposure ($X = 1$) and N_0 to no exposure (a trial that would be infeasible and unethical in reality but, as yet, allowed in the mind), as in Table 23-2. With equal allocation, $N_1=N_0=N$. The frequentist RR estimate then equals the ratio of the number of treated cases A_1 to the number of untreated cases A_0:

$$\text{Estimated RR} = \left(A_1/N\right)/\left(A_0/N\right) = A_1/A_0$$

Given the rarity of leukemia, N would be very large relative to A_1 and A_0. Hence $1/N \approx 0$, and

$$\text{Estimated variance for ln(RR)} = 1/A_1 + 1/A_0 - 1/N - 1/N \approx 1/A_1 + 1/A_0$$

To yield our prior for RR, these estimates must satisfy

$$\text{Estimated RR} = A_1/A_0 = 1$$

So $A_1 = A_0 = A$, and

$$\text{Estimated variance of ln(RR) estimate} \approx 1/A_1 + 1/A_0 = 1/A + 1/A = 2/A = \text{½}$$

So $A_1 = A_0 = A = 4$. Thus, data roughly equivalent to a normal(0, ½) prior would comprise four cases in each of the treated and the untreated groups in a very large randomized trial with equal allocation, yielding a prior estimate RR_{prior} of 1 and a ln(RR) variance of ½. The value of N would not matter, provided it was large enough so that $1/N$ was negligible relative to $1/A$. Table 23-3 shows an example.

Expressing the prior as equivalent data leads to a general method for doing Bayesian and semi-Bayes analyses with frequentist software:

1. Construct data equivalent to the prior.
2. Add those prior data to the actual study data as a distinct (prior) stratum.

The resulting point estimate and C% confidence limits from the frequentist analysis of the augmented (actual + prior) data provide an approximate posterior median and C% posterior interval for the parameter.

In the example, this method leads to a frequentist analysis of two strata: one stratum for the actual study data (Table 23-1) and one stratum for the prior-equivalent data (Table 23-3). Using information weighting (which assumes both the prior and the likelihood are approximately normal), these strata produce a point estimate of 1.80 and 95% limits of 0.65, 4.94, as above. A better

TABLE 23-3

Example of Bayesian Analysis via Frequentist Methods: Data Approximating a Log-Normal Prior, Reflecting 2:1 Certainty That RR is Between ½ and 2, 95% Certainty That RR is Between ¼ and 4, and Result of Combination With Data From Table 23-1. ($X = 1$ is >3 mG Average Exposure, $X = 0$ is ≤3 mG.)

	$X = 1$	$X = 0$	
Cases	4	4	Table RR = RR_{prior} = 1
Total	100,000	100,000	Approximate 95% prior limits = 0.25, 4.00

$\ln(RR_{prior}) = 0$, approximate variance = ¼ + ¼ = ½

Approximate posterior median and 95% limits from stratified analyses combining prior with Table 18-1:

From information (inverse-variance) weighting of RR estimates: 1.80, 95% limits 0.65, 4.94

From maximum-likelihood (ML) estimation: 1.76, 95% limits 0.59, 5.23

---

approximation is supplied by using maximum likelihood (ML) to combine the strata, which here yields a point estimate of 1.76 and 95% limits of 0.59, 5.23. This approximation assumes only that the posterior distribution is approximately normal.

With other stratification factors in the analysis, the prior remains just an extra stratum, as above. For example, in the pooled analysis there were 14 strata, one for each study (Table 23-1).[32] Adding the prior data used above with $A = 4$ and $N = 100,000$ as if it were a 15th study, and applying ML, the approximate posterior median RR and 95% limits are 1.66 and 1.26, 2.17, the same as from information weighting.

After translating the prior to equivalent data, one might see the size of the hypothetical study and decide that the original prior was overconfident, implying a prior trial larger than seemed justified. For a childhood leukemia incidence of $4/10^5$ years, eight cases would require 200,000 child-years of follow-up, which is quite a bit larger than any real randomized trial of childhood leukemia. If one were not prepared to defend the amount of one's prior information as being this ample, one should make the trial smaller. In other settings, one might decide that the prior trial should be larger.

Reverse-Bayes Analysis

Several authors describe how to apply Bayes' theorem in reverse (inverse-Bayes analysis) by starting with hypothetical posterior results and asking what sort of prior would have led to those results, given the actual data and data models used.[5,50] One hypothetical posterior result of interest has the null as one of the 95% limits. In the above pooled analysis, this posterior leads to the question: How many prior cases per group (A) would be needed to make the lower end of the 95% posterior interval equal 1?

Repeating the ordinary Bayes analysis with different A and N until the lower posterior limit equals 1, we find that $A = 275$ prior leukemia cases per group (550 total) forces the lower end of the 95% posterior interval to 1.00. That number is more than twice the number of exposed cases seen in all epidemiologic studies through 2008. At a rate of about 4 cases/10^5 person-years, a randomized trial capable of producing $2A = 550$ leukemia cases under the null would require roughly 550/$(4/10^5) > 13$ million child-years of follow-up. The corresponding prior variance is $2/275 = 0.00727$, for a 95% prior interval of

$$\exp\left(0 \pm 1.96 \cdot 0.00727^{1/2}\right) = 0.85, 1.18$$

Although this is an extremely skeptical prior, it is not as skeptical as many of the opinions written about the relation.[48] Upon seeing this calculation, we might fairly ask of skeptics, "Do you actually have evidence for the null that is equivalent to such an impossibly large, perfect randomized trial?" Without such evidence, the calculation shows that any reasonable posterior skepticism about the association must arise from methodologic shortcomings of the studies. These shortcomings correspond to shortcomings of standard frequentist data models (see Ref. 32 and Chapter 29).

Priors With Non-Null Center

Suppose we shift the prior estimate RR_{prior} for RR to 2, with 95% prior limits of ½ and 8. This shift corresponds to $\ln(RR_{prior}) = \ln(2)$ with a prior variance of ½. Combining this prior with the Savitz data[42] by information weighting yields

$$\text{Posterior variance} \approx 1/\left[1/(\tfrac{1}{2}) + 1/0.569\right] = 0.266 \quad \text{(as before)}$$

$$\text{Posterior } \ln(RR) \text{ median} \approx \left[\ln(2)/(\tfrac{1}{2}) + \ln(351)/0.569\right]/\left[1/(\tfrac{1}{2}) + 1/0.569\right] = 0.956$$

$$\text{Posterior RR median} \approx \exp(0.956) = 2.60$$

$$95\% \text{ posterior RR limits} \approx \exp\left(0.956 \pm 1.96 \cdot 0.266^{1/2}\right) = 0.95, 7.15$$

One can accomplish the same by augmenting the observed data set with a stratum of prior data. To preserve approximate normality, we keep $A_1 = A_0$ (so $A_1/A_0 = 1$) and adjust the denominator quotient N_1/N_0 to obtain the desired $RR_{prior} = (A_1/A_0)/(N_1/N_0) = 1/(N_1/N_0) = N_0/N_1$. In the preceding example, this change means keeping $A_1 = A_0 = 4$ and $N_1 = 100,000$, but making $N_0 = 200,000$, so that

$$RR_{prior} = (4/100,000)/(4/200,000) = 200,000/100,000 = 2$$

The approximate prior variance of $\ln(RR)$ remains $\frac{1}{4} + \frac{1}{4} = \frac{1}{2}$. Thus, data equivalent to the upshifted prior would be the observation of four cases in each of the treated and the untreated groups in a randomized trial with a 1:2 allocation to $X = 1$ and $X = 0$.

Choosing the Sizes of the Prior Denominators

The absolute size of N_1 and N_0 used will matter little, provided both $N_1 > 100 \cdot A_1$ and $N_0 > 100 \cdot A_0$. Thus, if we enlarge A_1 and A_0, we enlarge N_1 and N_0 proportionally to maintain disease rarity in the prior data. Although it may seem paradoxical, this rarity is simply a numerical device that can be used even with common diseases. This procedure works because standard frequentist RR estimators do not combine baseline risks across strata. By placing the prior data in a separate stratum, the baseline risk in the prior data may take on any small value, without affecting either the baseline risk estimates for the actual data or the posterior RR estimates. N_1 and N_0 are used only to move the prior estimate RR_{prior} to the desired value: When they are very large, they cease to influence the prior variance and only their ratio, N_1/N_0, matters in setting the prior.

For the thought experiment used to set N_1 and N_0, one envisions an experimental group that responds to treatment (X) with the relative risk one expects, but in which the baseline risk is so low that the distinctions among odds, risk, and rate ratios become unimportant. The estimator applied to the total (augmented) data will determine what is estimated. An odds-ratio estimator will produce an odds-ratio estimate, a risk-ratio estimator will produce a risk-ratio estimate, and a rate-ratio estimator will produce a rate-ratio estimate. For rate-ratio analyses, N_1 and N_0 represent person-time rather than persons.

Non-Normal Priors

The addition of prior data shown above (with very large N_1, N_0) corresponds to using an F distribution with $2A_1$, $2A_0$ degrees of freedom as the RR prior.[28,51] With $A_1 = A_0 = A$ the above lognormal approximation to this prior appears adequate down to about $A = 4$; for example, at $A = 4$, the approximate 95% RR interval of (¼, 4) has 93.3% exact prior probability from an F (8, 8) distribution; at $A = 3$ the approximate 95% interval is (1/5, 5) and has 92.8% exact probability from an $F(6, 6)$. These are minor discrepancies compared to other sources of error, and the resulting discrepancies for the posterior percentiles are smaller still. As with the accuracy of maximum likelihood, the accuracy of the posterior approximation depends on the total information across strata (prior + data). Nonetheless, if we want to introduce prior data that represent even less information or that represent non-normal ln(RR) priors, we can employ prior data with $A_1 \neq A_0$ to induce ln(RR)-skewness, and with $A_1, A_0 < 3$ to induce heavier tails than the normal distribution. Generalizations beyond the F distribution are also available.[27,28]

Further Extensions

Prior-data methods extend easily to multivariable modeling and to settings in which some or all variables (including the outcome) have multiple levels. For example, one may add a prior stratum for each regression coefficient in a model; coefficients for continuous variables can be represented as trials comparing two levels of the variable (*e.g.*, 800 vs. 0 µg/d folic acid supplementation); and prior correlations can be induced using a hierarchical prior-data structure.[18,45]

CHECKING THE PRIOR

A standard recommendation is to check homogeneity of measures before summarizing them across strata. An analogous recommendation is to check the compatibility of the data and the prior,[52] which is subsumed under the more general topic of Bayesian model checking.[12,15,53] For normal priors, one simple approximate check examines the P-value from the "standardized" difference,

(Frequentist estimate − prior estimate) × (frequentist variance + prior variance)$^{1/2}$

which is the analog of the frequentist two-stratum homogeneity statistic. Like frequentist homogeneity tests, this check is neither sensitive nor specific, and it assumes that the prior is normal and the observed counts are "large" (>4). A small P-value does indicate, however, that the prior and the frequentist results are too incompatible to average by information weighting.

For the pooled magnetic field data with a normal(0, ½) prior ($A_1 = A_0 = 4 \ll N_1 = N_0$), the check is $[\ln(1.69) - 0]/(0.0201 + ½)^{1/2} = 0.72$, $P = .47$. Thus, by this check the prior and the frequentist result appear to be compatible, largely because the prior is compatible with such a broad range of results. Despite this compatibility, their average may still be misleading (*e.g.*, as a result of study biases). In contrast, with the skeptical normal (0, 0.0484^2) prior ($A_1 = A_0 = 854 \ll N_1 = N_0$), the check is $[\ln(1.69) - 0]/(0.0201 + 0.0484^2)^{1/2} = 3.50$, $P = .0005$, which indicates extreme incompatibility of the prior and the frequentist result, and which suggests that the average would be misleading because at least one of the prior and the frequentist result is misleading (and perhaps both are).

The P-value for the exposure-disease (X-Y) association in the actual data equals the homogeneity P-value from comparing the frequentist result to a dogmatic normal(0, 0) prior concentrated entirely at the null with zero variance (equivalent to overwhelming prior data, *e.g.*, $A = 10^{100}$ and $N = 10^{100,000}$). For the pooled-data example, this P-value is 0.0002, corresponding to the usual interpretation that a small P-value is indicative of a conflict between the null and the data. The P-value comparing the prior mean to the frequentist estimate can be viewed as a generalization of the usual P-value to allow testing of nondogmatic ("fuzzy") hypotheses in which the true parameter is specified only up to a distribution, rather than asserted to equal a single number.

DISCUSSION

Data Alone Say Nothing at All

It is sometimes recommended that the prior should be given up if it appears to be in conflict with the "actual data."[54] The conflict, however, is between the prior and the frequentist result from the data *model*; without a model for the data-generating mechanism, the data alone can conflict with nothing.[55]

If we truly believed the frequentist results were from perfect data from a randomized trial conducted on a random sample from the target population, we would no doubt afford them precedence over a prior composed from mere impressions of other evidence. Indeed, a key inferential property of randomized studies is that, if they are precise enough, they force agreement among those who believe that the randomization was carried out properly and not undermined by subsequent events. Observational studies stray from this ideal, however, and do so to an unknown extent. A conflict between a prior and a frequentist result can arise from an invalid data model (resulting from study biases or an incorrect analytic method), as opposed to an incorrect prior. Thus, an apparent conflict only calls attention to a discrepancy in need of explanation. This situation is starkly illustrated by the magnetic field controversy, in which many scientists still postulate that the frequentist result (rather than their skeptical prior) is in error.

Although (as is often said) frequentist statistics better reflect the data than do Bayesian statistics, those data should not be regarded as sacrosanct when making inferences beyond the observations. Even rough but contextually well-informed priors can provide information as reliable as or more reliable than current observations. To put it negatively, one may be justifiably afraid of the unreliability of subjective priors, but this fear does not license exclusive reliance on unreliable data. Frequentist statistics and their "objective" Bayesian analogs indeed stay closer to the observations, but this closeness will harm inference when those observations are riddled with error and better external information is available. Conversely, for the goal of data description (as opposed to inference), neither Bayesian nor frequentist modeling results are an adequate substitute for tabular and graphical data summaries.

Data Priors as a General Diagnostic Device

The data representation of priors is far more important and general than is realized by most of the statistics community. For teaching, data priors provide both a Bayesian interpretation of frequentist statistics (as Bayesian statistics with no prior data) and a frequentist interpretation of Bayesian statistics (as frequentist statistics based in part on external data). For analysis, data priors provide a critical perspective on a proposed prior and can lead to refinements to better match the level of prior information one wishes to assume. Other prior representations are also conceptually helpful; for example, the penalized-likelihood approach illustrates how Bayesian statistics can be viewed as frequentist statistics with probabilistic constraints on parameters.[26,56] These interpretations show that entering and deleting variables in a regression are extremes along a continuum in which the variable may enter partially, to the extent allowed by the constraint.[4,57,58]

Data representations are not limited to conjugate priors (priors that have the same functional form as the likelihood function). Any prior that can be viewed as a product of likelihood functions can be translated into data, namely, the data arising from the statistical studies represented by the functions. These functions may be of varying forms, and those forms may differ from that of the actual-data likelihood (*i.e.*, they may be nonconjugate). The translation clarifies the evidential claims that the prior is making. Conversely, to say that a given prior cannot be viewed as augmenting data means that one could not envision a series of studies that would lead to the prior (let alone point to actual studies that produce the prior). Such a prior is arguably nonempirical in principle and hence scientifically meaningless (in the same sense that a theory that is empirically untestable in principle is scientifically meaningless). Translation between forms for a prior is thus a scientific (as opposed to statistical) diagnostic for priors.

The Role of Markov Chain Monte Carlo

Translation of the prior into various forms does not dictate the manner of posterior computation. One could, for example, translate for diagnostic purposes and then sample from the posterior distribution using a Markov chain Monte Carlo (MCMC) program such as WinBUGS. Nonetheless, MCMC is subject to technical problems that are not always easily detected. MCMC also does not display the parallels between frequentist and Bayesian analyses. Hence it is arguably inadequate alone or as a starting point for Bayesian instruction, and analytic methods are valuable for starting and checking MCMC analyses.

One can question, however, whether MCMC analyses are necessary once approximate results are in hand. Given perfectly correct models, and if allowed to run long enough, MCMC can produce more accurate results than the methods described above. Nonetheless, upon considering all the poorly understood sources of bias that plague observational research, our models are always highly inaccurate, and MCMC refinements may only add a false sense of precision to inaccurate results.

Connections to Sensitivity Analysis

There is a close and complementary connection between Bayesian methods and sensitivity analyses (see Chapter 29), in which parameters fixed at defaults by frequentist methods are varied to see their effect on statistics. Simple sensitivity analyses will reveal unlimited sensitivities to certain variations and hence convey no information unless coupled with contextual information to determine what variations are meaningful.[59] That contextual information is none other than prior information, which can be formalized in a prior distribution for use in Bayesian or analogous prior-sampling methods for risk and decision analysis[32,45,60,61] (see Chapter 29). In this format, one can also conduct Bayesian sensitivity analysis by seeing how results vary as the prior is varied. For this process, data representations can help one judge which priors are credible enough to examine.

Some Cautions on Use of Priors

Many have argued for integrating the Bayesian perspective into the teaching of basic methods (*e.g.*, see Ref. 16 and the ensuing discussion). The prior data approach facilitates this goal because it requires no new statistical formulas or software. Standard frequentist methods for stratified and regression analysis become Bayesian by adding just a few data records and covariates.

With this new capacity, however, comes risk of abuse. Although Bayesian methods are now widely accepted as a way to improve inferences using prior information,[11,12] one cannot expect improvement over ordinary methods using just any prior. Worsening could occur from using a badly misinformed prior (a prior that assigns relatively low probability to values near the truth), which suggests being generous in setting the spread of the prior. If the resulting prior remains highly influential, subject-matter justification will be especially important, as will statistical checks of the compatibility of priors with the likelihood. Among basic diagnostics are visual comparisons of prior and likelihood summaries or graphs, *e.g.*, comparing the prior mode and limits to the maximum-likelihood (ML) estimate and confidence limits, or comparing entire graphs. Another simple check is the *P*-value for comparing the actual and prior data as if the latter were an actual data stratum, as described above. Although a large *P*-value means only that the check detected no problem, a small *P*-value indicates incompatibility of the prior with the model for the actual data, which could arise from faulty prior information, faulty actual data (resulting from, *e.g.*, study defects), a faulty model for the data (*i.e.*, a faulty likelihood model), or some combination.

Concerns about background information argue for retaining frequentist results to compare with Bayesian results whenever the former are sensible to apply, and for using vaguely informative and relatively simple priors. "Vaguely informative" is a context-dependent notion, however, in which the percentiles of the prior distribution would be viewed as at least reasonable if not liberally inclusive by all those working in the research topic. With 95% limits of ¼, 4 and 2:1 (67%) limits of ½, 2, the normal(0, 0.5) prior for ln(RR) may often seem reasonable when the RR is expected to be in the "weak" (½, 2) range and there is no strong directional information. But in some contexts (*e.g.*, environmental and occupational research), only adverse health effects are of serious concern, and the use of more directional priors may then be justifiable.

Vaguely informative should not be construed as noninformative. Noninformative priors correspond to using values of A_1 and A_0 of zero, which give back the ML estimate and confidence interval as the posterior mode and interval. So-called reference priors[21] correspond to using very small values and thus give similar results. Such "objective Bayesian" methods confer none of the predictive benefits obtainable from well-informed priors, rarely make sense on subject-matter grounds,[17,35] and (like frequentist methods) break down in the face of nonidentification.[32] In essence, they discard prior information, the key source of Bayesian strengths as well as weaknesses. Thus, like frequentism, objective Bayesianism leads to mechanical procedures that software or a robot could apply to data. Such decontextualized algorithmic statistics form the bulk of current statistical training. Epidemiologic inference requires contextual input, however, and prior specification is one crucial aspect that should not be automatic.

CONCLUSIONS

Bayesian and frequentist methods address different questions. Bayesian methods address questions of the form "Having seen the data, what betting odds should I place on this hypothesis versus another?" and seek to use contextual information to improve the bet. The methods focus on the observed data, rather than on counterfactual data as might arise under a hypothetical long run. In contrast, frequentist methods address questions of the form "If I applied this method to a hypothetical long run of studies like this one, how would it behave over that long run?" and seek methods with desirable long-run properties, such as correct confidence-interval coverage rates. Frequentist methods do not provide odds of hypotheses, nor do they address whether the particular inference they produce from the observed data is better than other inferences one could make from those data, without reference to a long run.

Despite their focus on actual data, Bayesian methods exhibit desirable frequentist (long-run) properties when both they and the evaluation are well informed by the scientific context.[62] Thus, even for a frequentist, Bayesian thinking is necessary as part of a broad and well-rounded approach. Bayesian and related methods become particularly worthwhile when conventional frequentist statistics become questionable and priors matter, as when confronting sparse data, multiple comparisons, collinearity, or nonidentification.[18,26,32,38,45,56,62-65] Frequentist interval estimates inevitably get interpreted as if they were Bayesian, without appreciating that the priors implicit in those interpretations are rarely if ever contextually plausible. Because this appreciation seems essential for proper interpretation of frequentist as well as Bayesian methods in observational settings,[4,17,32,45,66] the inclusion of Bayesian perspectives in teaching would be helpful even if frequentist results remained the norm for presentation.

A major flaw shared by conventional statistical methods (be they frequentist, likelihoodist, or Bayesian), however, is that they pretend the data came from an ideal study in which all important influences on the data (including those of the investigators and the subjects) can be approximated by a known model. In observational epidemiology, this assumption can be drastically flawed, resulting in far too much certainty placed on statistical results. Chapter 29 discusses how statistics can approach this problem in a contextually informed manner by using bias models with explicit priors for unknown bias parameters.

In summary, Bayesian analysis can be performed easily by information weighting of prior estimates with frequentist estimates (as if doing a meta-analysis of prior studies and the current study). More generally, it can be done by representing prior information as hypothetical study data to be added to the analysis as new strata (as if doing a pooled analysis of prior studies and the current study). This data-prior approach provides a diagnostic for contextual strength and relevance of the prior, and also facilitates Bayesian regression analysis.[18,28] Both approaches allow one to produce Bayesian analyses from formulas and software for frequentist analyses, and both facilitate introduction of Bayesian ideas into introductory statistics training alongside the corresponding frequentist approaches.

References

1. Lindley DV. *Introduction to Probability and Statistics from a Bayesian Viewpoint*. Cambridge: Cambridge University Press; 1965.
2. DeFinetti B. *The Theory of Probability*. Vol 1. New York, NY: Wiley; 1974.
3. Cornfield J. Recent methodological contributions to clinical trials. *Am J Epidemiol*. 1976;104(4):408-421.
4. Leamer EE. *Specification Searches*. New York, NY: Wiley; 1978.
5. Good IJ. *Good Thinking*. Minneapolis, MN: University of Minnesota Press; 1983.
6. Berger JO, Berry DA. Statistical analysis and the illusion of objectivity. *Am Scientist*. 1988;76:159-165.
7. Berk RA, Western B, Weiss RE. Statistical inference for apparent populations. *Sociol Methodol*. 1995;25:421-458.
8. Greenland S. On sample-size and power calculations for studies using confidence intervals. *Am J Epidemiol*. 1988;128(1):231-237.
9. Susser M. Judgement and causal inference: criteria in epidemiologic studies. *Am J Epidemiol*. 1977;105(1):1-15.
10. Leonard T, Hsu JSJ. *Bayesian Methods*. Cambridge: Cambridge University Press; 1999.
11. Carlin B, Louis TA. *Bayes and Empirical-Bayes Methods of Data Analysis*. 2nd ed. New York, NY: Chapman and Hall; 2000.

12. Gelman A, Carlin JB, Stern HS, Rubin DB. *Bayesian Data Analysis*. 2nd ed. New York, NY: Chapman and Hall/CRC; 2003.

13. Efron B. Bayesians, frequentists, and scientists. *J Am Stat Assoc*. 2005;100:1-5.

14. Spiegelhalter DJ. Bayesian methods for cluster randomized trials with continuous responses. *Stat Med*. 2001;20(3):435-452.

15. Spiegelhalter David J, Abrams KR, Myles JP. *Bayesian Approaches to Clinical Trials and Health-Care Evaluation*. New York, NY: Wiley; 2004.

16. Berry DA. Teaching elementary Bayesian statistics with real applications in science (with discussion). *Am Stat*. 1997;51:241-271.

17. Greenland S. Bayesian perspectives for epidemiological research: I. Foundations and basic methods. *Int J Epidemiol*. 2006;35(3):765-775.

18. Greenland S. Bayesian perspectives for epidemiological research. II. Regression analysis. *Int J Epidemiol*. 2007;36(1):195-202.

19. Goodman SN. p values, hypothesis tests, and likelihood: implications for epidemiology of a neglected historical debate. *Am J Epidemiol* 1993;137(5):485-496; discussion 497-501.

20. Goldstein M. Subjective Bayesian Analysis: Principles and Practice. *Bayesian Anal*. 2006;1(3):403-420.

21. Berger JO. The case for objective Bayesian analysis. *Int Soc Bayesian Anal*. 2004;1:1-17.

22. Royall R. *Statistical Inference: A Likelihood Paradigm*. New York, NY: Chapman and Hall; 1997.

23. Lindley DV. The Bayesian analysis of contingency tables. *Ann Math Stat*. 1964;35:1622-1643.

24. Good IJ. *The Estimation of Probabilities*. Boston, MA: MIT Press; 1965.

25. Bedrick EJ, Christensen R, Johnson W. A new perspective on generalized linear models. *J Am Stat Assoc*. 1996;91:1450-1460.

26. Greenland S. Putting background information about relative risks into conjugate prior distributions. *Biometrics*. 2001;57(3):663-670.

27. Greenland S. Generalized conjugate priors for Bayesian analysis of risk and survival regressions. *Biometrics*. 2003;59(1):92-99.

28. Greenland S. Prior data for non-normal priors. *Stat Med*. 2007;26(19):3578-3590.

29. Greenland S, Christensen R. Data augmentation priors for Bayesian and semi-Bayes analyses of conditional-logistic and proportional-hazards regression. *Stat Med*. 2001;20(16):2421-2428.

30. Greenland S. Induction versus Popper: substance versus semantics. *Int J Epidemiol*. 1998;27(4):543-548.

31. Greenland S. Randomization, statistics, and causal inference. *Epidemiology*. 1990;1(6):421-429.

32. Greenland S. Multiple-bias modeling for analysis of observational data (with discussion). *J R Stat Soc Ser A*. 2005;168:267-308.

33. Titterington DM. Common structure of smoothing techniques in statistics. *Int Stat Rev*. 1985;53:141-170.

34. Goldstein H. *Multilevel Statistical Models*. 3rd ed. London: Arnold; 2003.

35. Greenland S. Probability logic and probabilistic induction. *Epidemiology*. 1998;9(3):322-332.

36. Lewis DK. A subjectivist's guide to objective chance. In: Jeffrey RC, ed. *Studies in Inductive Logic and Probability*. Berkeley: University of California Press; 1981;263-293.

37. Good IJ. Hierarchical Bayesian and empirical Bayesian methods (letter). *Am Stat*. 1987;41:92.

38. Greenland S. Principles of multilevel modelling. *Int J Epidemiol*. 2000;29(1):158-167.

39. Zeger SL. Statistical reasoning in epidemiology. *Am J Epidemiol*. 1991;134(10):1062-1066.

40. Jaynes ET, Bretthorst GL. *Probability Theory: The Logic of Science*. New York, NY: Cambridge University Press; 2003.

41. Agresti AA. *Categorical Data Analysis*. 2nd ed. New York, NY: John Wiley & Sons; 2002.

42. Savitz DA, Wachtel H, Barnes FA, John EM, Tvrdik JG. Case-control study of childhood cancer and exposure to 60-Hz magnetic fields. *Am J Epidemiol*. 1988;128(1):21-38.

43. Leamer EE. False models and post-data model construction. *J Am Stat Assoc*. 1974;69:122-131.

44. Graham P. Bayesian inference for a generalized population attributable fraction: the impact of early vitamin A levels on chronic lung disease in very low birthweight infants. *Stat Med*. 2000;19(7):937-956.

45. Greenland S. The impact of prior distributions for uncontrolled confounding and response bias: a case study of the relation of wire codes and magnetic fields to childhood leukemia. *J Am Stat Assoc*. 2003;98:47-54.

46. Exposure to power-frequency magnetic fields and the risk of childhood cancer. UK Childhood Cancer Study Investigators. *Lancet*. 1999;354(9194):1925-1931.

47. Higgins JP, Spiegelhalter DJ. Being sceptical about meta-analyses: a Bayesian perspective on magnesium trials in myocardial infarction. *Int J Epidemiol*. 2002;31(1):96-104.

48. Taubes G. Fields of fear. *Atlantic*. 1994;274:94-100.

49. Spiegelhalter DJ, Freedman LS, Parmar MKB. Bayesian approaches to randomized trials (with discussion). *J R Stat Soc Ser A*. 1994;156:357-416.

50. Matthews RAJ. Methods for assessing the credibility of clinical trial outcomes. *Drug Inf J*. 2001;35:1469-1478.

51. Jones MC. Families of distributions arising from distributions of order statistics. *Test*. 2004;13:1-44.

52. Box GEP. Sampling and Bayes inference in scientific modeling and robustness. *J R Stat Soc Ser A*. 1980;143:383-430.

53. Geweke J. Simulation methods for model criticism and robustness analysis. In: Bernardo JM, Berger JO, Dawid AP, Smith AFM, eds. *Bayesian Statistics 6*. New York, NY: Oxford University Press; 1998.

54. Robins JM, Greenland S. The role of model selection in causal inference from nonexperimental data. *Am J Epidemiol*. 1986;123(3):392-402.

55. Robins JM. Data, design, and background knowledge in etiologic inference. *Epidemiology*. 2001;12(3):313-320.

56. Greenland S. When should epidemiologic regressions use random coefficients? *Biometrics*. 2000;56(3):915-921.

57. Greenland S. Multilevel modeling and model averaging. *Scand J Work Environ Health*. 1999;25(suppl 4):43-48.

58. Greenland S. Causal analysis in the health sciences. *J Am Stat Assoc*. 2000;95:286-289.

59. Greenland S. *The sensitivity of a sensitivity analysis (invited paper)*. In: *1997 Proceedings of the Biometrics Section*. Alexandria, VA: American Statistical Association; 1998:19-21.

60. Eddy DM, Hasselblad V, Schachter R. *Meta-analysis by the Confidence Profile Method*. New York, NY: Academic Press; 1992.

61. Greenland S. Sensitivity analysis, Monte Carlo risk analysis, and Bayesian uncertainty assessment. *Risk Anal*. 2001;21(4):579-583.

62. Gustafson P, Greenland S. The performance of random coefficient regression in accounting for residual confounding. *Biometrics*. 2006;62(3):760-768.

63. Greenland S. Basic problems in interaction assessment. *Environ Health Perspect*. 1993;101(suppl 4): 59-66.

64. Greenland S. Small-sample bias and corrections for conditional maximum-likelihood odds-ratio estimators. *Biostatistics*. 2000;1(1):113-122.

65. Greenland S, Schwartzbaum JA, Finkle WD. Problems due to small samples and sparse data in conditional logistic regression analysis. *Am J Epidemiol*. 2000;151(5):531-539.

66. Rubin DB. Practical implications of modes of statistical inference for causal effects and the critical role of the assignment mechanism. *Biometrics*. 1991;47(4):1213-1234.

Longitudinal and Cluster-Correlated Data Analysis

Sebastien Haneuse

In Chapter 17, we introduced the notion of independence as an assumption that underpins the binomial distribution and the Poisson distribution for count random variables. The assumption of independence also arose in the discussion of likelihood-based estimation in Chapters 17, 18, 21, and 22. Intuitively, assuming independence implies that knowing the outcome of one study unit tells us nothing about the outcome of some other study unit. In the regression context where, for example, X is an exposure of interest and Z is a collection of adjustment factors, the assumption is typically considered within levels of (X, Z). In many instances, however, the assumption of independence for the outcomes across study units may not be plausible. Consider, for example, a study of patient-specific risk factors for hospital-acquired sepsis based on information from multiple hospitals. While knowing the outcome of a patient in a given hospital may not tell us much about the outcomes of patients at other hospitals, it may give some information about the outcomes of other patients at the same hospital; shared resources and standards of care may render the risk of sepsis among patients at the same hospital more similar to each other than to patients admitted to a different hospital. Similarly, consider a longitudinal study of risk factors for stunted growth in the 6 months following birth, where repeated weight measurements are obtained, say, monthly. For this study, the individual observations are the monthly weight measurements; that is, the "study units" are the infant/month-specific weight measurements. In considering an infant's growth trajectory, it seems reasonable that knowing the weight measurements at months 1, 2, and 3 for a given infant will tell us something about the distribution of their weight measurements at month 4. It also seems reasonable that this information might not tell us anything about the weight at month 4 of a different infant. As such, the infant/month-specific weight measurements may plausibly be independent between infants (unless, perhaps, if they are related) but not within an infant.

If independence across the outcomes does not hold, what are the consequences of naïvely applying the methods for estimation and inference that have been described in Chapters 16 to 22? That is, what are the consequences of naïvely treating the study units in the data set as if they were all independent of each other when they, in fact, exhibit dependence? Statistically, the primary consequence of using the methods described in Chapters 16 to 22 is that inference will be invalid. Specifically, estimates of standard errors will be wrong, either too small or too big depending on the data and the analysis/model, with downstream consequences being that 95% confidence intervals and P-values will be invalid. Much of this chapter, therefore, is devoted to describing methods that seek to ensure valid standard error estimation and, hence, inference.

Beyond statistical considerations, another important consequence of naïvely applying methods developed for independent data is that doing so will likely unnecessarily limit the scope of scientific inquiry. Moreover, longitudinal and cluster-correlated data provide both *within-* and *between-*cluster information (by "cluster" we mean the hospital in the first example above and the infant in the second example) that can be used to address a range of scientific questions that could not be addressed if all one had was purely independent data (*e.g.*, a single patient at each hospital). This point is elaborated upon in the first subsection of this chapter.

Because of the need to acknowledge how study units are dependent, the analysis of longitudinal and cluster-correlated data is typically more complex than the analysis of independent data. This complexity is both conceptual, in that careful consideration must be paid to both the mean and the dependence structure, and practical, in that there are many choices that one can make regarding the model that one fits and the methods used for estimation and inference. Unfortunately, one cannot be prescriptive in how to approach the analysis of dependent data since there is no single method/approach that can be viewed as universally "most" appropriate. As such, decisions in any given analysis will require simultaneous consideration of the scientific goals, the assumptions that one is willing to make, and an understanding of the analytic tools that one has at one's disposal.

The methodologic focus in this chapter is on the two most common regression-based analysis approaches for longitudinal and cluster-correlated data: (1) marginal models, with estimation and inference via generalized estimating equations (GEE), and (2) mixed effects models, with estimation and inference via maximum likelihood. However, these are by no means the only approaches for regression-based analysis of longitudinal and cluster-correlated data; the broader field is extensive and continuously evolving, and there are many textbooks that have been devoted to the topic. One text that provides a balance between theoretical and practical considerations is Fitzmaurice et al.[1] For readers interested in technical and statistical details, comprehensive treatments are given by Diggle et al.,[2] Fitzmaurice et al.,[3] and McCulloch et al.[4]

CORE CONCEPTS

The Nature of Dependence

Key to all statistical methods for dependent data is how dependence across outcomes is structured, either implicitly or explicitly, within the analysis. As will become clear, different methods approach this task in different ways, each corresponding to different assumptions and, thus, having different robustness properties. Before considering how one might approach the analysis of dependent data, therefore, it is worth considering how dependence arises and manifests. To that end, consider the data presented in Figure 24-1. Shown are longitudinal measurements, at ages 8, 10, 12, and 14 years, of the length (mm) from the pituitary gland to the pterygomaxillary fissure among 11 girls and 15 boys, collected at the University of North Carolina Dental School.[5] Thus, the study units are the child's age-specific length measurements.

Let Y be the vector of $N = 26 \times 4 = 104$ measurements, with the first four values corresponding to those at ages 8, 10, 12, and 14 years for the first child, the next four corresponding to those at ages 8, 10, 12, and 14 years for the second child, and so on. In considering these data, the assumption of independence would imply that the correlation between all pairs of measurements in Y is zero; that is, $\mathrm{Cor}(Y_i, Y_j) = 0$ for all (i, j) pairs, regardless of whether the observations are from the same child or from different children. This clearly represents a strong, and likely implausible,

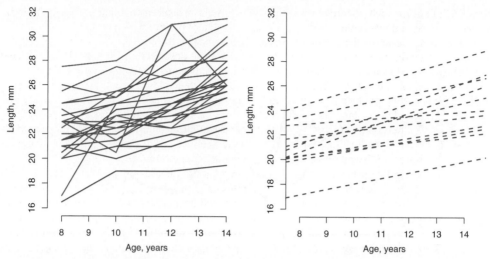

FIGURE 24-1 Longitudinal data on the length (mm) from the pituitary gland to the pterygomaxillary fissure among 11 girls and 15 boys, collected at the University of North Carolina Dental School. In the left-hand side plot are the raw data, with black lines for the boys and red lines for the girls. In the right-hand side plot are the fitted values from individual linear regressions for each of the 11 girls.

assumption for the data in Figure 24-1. At the other extreme, one could adopt a completely agnostic position and permit the possibility that there is dependence between all pairs of measurements in Y. For example, one could consider the possibility that $\mathrm{Cor}(Y_i, Y_j)$ is nonzero for all (i, j) pairs. While this has the appeal of being flexible, such an analysis implicitly introduces $N(N - 1)/2$ additional dependence parameters [*i.e.*, one new correlation parameter for each unique (i, j) pair] that would need to be estimated. For the dental length data, this would mean estimating $104 \times 103/2 = 5{,}356$ additional parameters even though there are only $N = 104$ data points! Moreover, adopting this position is likely overly flexible since it is plausible that the measurements of two unrelated children in two different households are indeed independent.

Since neither extreme will be satisfactory in most studies, consideration of dependence typically results in some middle ground, specifically by assuming independence for certain pairs of observations while permitting dependence between other pairs. The key practical tasks, therefore, are to:

1. specify which pairs are taken to be independent; and,
2. structure the dependence between those that are not.

To guide these tasks, it may be helpful to think of dependence as arising through some phenomenon (or phenomena) that, informally, "connects" the outcomes of study units such that their values covary or depend on each other in some way. Conceptually, one might think of these connections as arising due to one or more shared characteristics. For the dental length data, each subset of four measurements represented by one of the 26 lines in Figure 24-1 shares the "characteristic" of having been obtained from the same child. More generally, we might say that the characteristics that underpin the connections can be summarized through the notion that the N study units are *clustered* in some way. For the dental length data, one natural clustering is at the level of the child; the first four measurements in Y are clustered within the first child, while the next four are clustered within the second child and so on. Based on this, one could approach the first practical task by positing that the measurements are independent between children but that the observations within a child are not. In doing so, the number of correlations would be reduced from 5,356 to $26 \times 6 = 156$ [since there are 26 children and $(4 \times 3)/2 = 6$ unique pairs of measurements within each child]. While this is a substantial reduction, there are still more parameters than data points. To mitigate this, one could assume that the dependence between the measurements at age 8 years and at age 10 years is the same for all 26 children, and so on for all pairs of ages. This is one choice

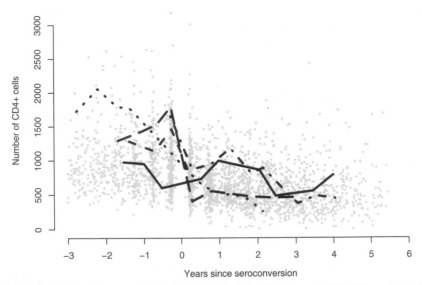

FIGURE 24-2 CD4+ cell measurements on 369 men from the Multicenter AIDS Cohort Study who seroconverted during follow-up. Also shown are the longitudinal trajectories for five randomly selected men.

for structuring dependence (*i.e.*, the second practical task above), for which only six additional dependence parameters would need to be estimated. Other choices are, of course, possible; the sections on marginal models and mixed effects models below provide detail on how each framework approaches this task.

The data in Figure 24-1 are *longitudinal* in that the timing of the measurements defines a natural ordering, one that is of intrinsic scientific interest and will, therefore, likely require consideration in the analysis. A second example of this type of data is given in Figure 24-2, which presents $N = 2,376$ CD4+ cell measurements on 369 men from the Multicenter AIDS Cohort Study (MACS) who seroconverted during follow-up.[6,7] For these data, CD4+ cell count measurements are clustered according to which study participant they were obtained from; Figure 24-2 highlights this by presenting the observed trajectories for 5 randomly selected men. One important difference between these data and those in Figure 24-1 is that the number of measurements varies across the 369 men, specifically between 1 and 12, as does the timing of when the measurements were obtained (relative to seroconversion). This, as will become clear, has important implications for statistical analyses.

Not all dependent data are longitudinal in nature. Li et al.,[8] for example, examine the association between exposure to gestational diabetes in utero and the risk of obesity in childhood using data from the Growing Up Today Study (GUTS). This is an ongoing prospective cohort study, the participants of which are the offspring of women enrolled in the Nurses' Health Study II. That participants in the GUTS could potentially be siblings raises the possibility of dependence in their outcomes due to the shared environment of their family. Beyond family structures, such as GUTS, another example of dependent data that is not longitudinal when individual subjects are clustered by some geographic schema, such as a city or county or state. Such data are common in spatial epidemiology, including studies of air pollution.[9] For both of these settings, we label the data as being *cluster-correlated*.

That we make the distinction between longitudinal and cluster-correlated data is important because doing so may help make decisions regarding how to structure both the mean model and the dependence structure within clusters (*i.e.*, the second practical task above). In a longitudinal study, for example, one might include time as a covariate in a regression analysis. Furthermore, one might make use of information on timing to adopt a dependence structure that permits measurements that are close to each other in time to exhibit greater dependence than measurements that are far apart in time. In the absence of a natural ordering of time, such structure in the regression model or the dependence may be irrelevant and thus does not need consideration. However, the distinction does not necessarily imply a particular analysis method; indeed, both the marginal model and mixed effects model frameworks described below can be used to analyze either type of data.

Multilevel Data

It will often be the case that multiple ways of clustering the data can be conceived. In the dental length data, for example, it may be that some of the children were related, perhaps as siblings or as cousins. If this was the case, then it may be reasonable to presuppose that shared genetic characteristics among children within a family could induce dependence between measurements; if two of the children in the data happened to be twins, for example, one would not expect their measurements at any given age to be independent. Such a scenario may be labeled as the data being *multilevel*: the dental length measurements are clustered within children who are clustered within families. Conventionally, the labeling of levels is according to the granularity within which the population of study units is clustered. Thus, in the clustering just described for the dental length data, the first level is the family, the second level is the child, and the third level is the dental length measurement.

Another feature of the family/child/measurement multilevel clustering is that it is *nested*. By this we mean that there is hierarchical structure such that all length measurements within a child only belong to a single family. An example where the data may be *nonnested* is given in Figure 24-3, which reports on data from Medicare on $N = 121,557$ patients aged 65 years or older who were diagnosed with pancreatic cancer during a hospitalization and subsequently discharged alive, between 2000 to 2009. Specifically, Figure 24-3A provides the ordered 90-day readmission rates across 1,031 hospitals at which there were at least 50 such diagnoses during the study time period, while Figure 24-3B presents the ordered percentage of non-White patients across the 1,031 hospitals. Note, the ordering in the two subfigures is not the same. Implicit in both subfigures is that the patients (who are the "study units") are clustered within the hospitals. While this seems reasonable, one could also conceive of the patients as being additionally clustered on the basis

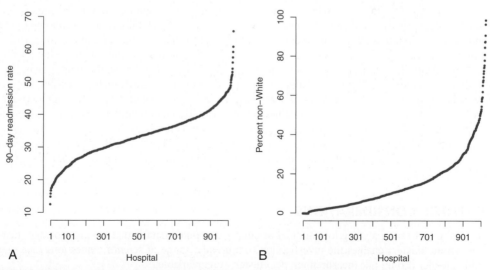

A   Hospital

B   Hospital

FIGURE 24-3 Hospital-specific 90-day readmission rates (right-hand side plot; **A**) and percent non-White (left-hand side plot; **B**) based on $N = 121,557$ Medicare patients aged 65 years or older who were diagnosed pancreatic cancer during a hospitalization and subsequently discharged alive, between 2000-2009, at one of 1,031 hospitals at which there were at least 50 such diagnoses during the study time period. In both plots, the values have been ordered but the ordering is not the same between the plots; that is, the hospital with the lowest 90-day readmission rate (*i.e.*, #1 in the right-hand side plot; **A**) is not the same as the hospital with the lowest percent non-White (*i.e.*, #1 in the left-hand side plot; **B**).

of who the attending physician was during the initial hospitalization in which they received their diagnosis, or by the state in which the hospital is located. Adopting the latter would result in a nested multilevel clustering; all patients within a hospital would belong to the same cluster defined by "state." In adopting the former, however, we may find that some physicians work at multiple hospitals. Suppose, for example, that Dr Snow was the attending physician for 35 patients in the data. Furthermore, suppose Dr Snow splits their time between two hospitals, and that 20 of their patients in the data were admitted to hospital A with the other 15 admitted to hospital B. While all 35 patients share the characteristic of having been attended by Dr Snow, they do not all belong to the same cluster defined by "hospital." In this sense, there is no nesting of the patients treated by Dr Snow within a single hospital.

In the remainder of this chapter, we present methods in the context of a single level of clustering. Nevertheless, everything that is covered translates readily to nested and nonnested multilevel settings. For example, just as naïvely assuming independence when there is dependence can lead to invalid inference, if the true underlying dependence structure is multilevel, ignoring one level may also result in invalid inference. Furthermore, the approaches used within the marginal model and mixed effects model frameworks to structuring dependence when there is only a single level translate in a straightforward, albeit somewhat more involved, way to settings where there are multiple levels.[4,10,11]

Notation

A central feature of dependent data is that there are multiple measurements within clusters. We therefore need a notation that distinguishes between study units that belong to the same cluster and those that belong to different clusters. To that end, we let K denote the number of clusters. For the dental length data in Figure 24-1, we have $K = 26$, while $K = 369$ and $K = 1,031$ for the MACS data and Medicare data in Figures 24-2 and 24-3, respectively. Let n_k denote the number of study units in the kth cluster. In the dental length data, $n_k = 4$ for all $K = 26$ children, while it varies from 51 to 1,035 for the hospital-specific number of patients in the Medicare data. Collectively, the total number of study units across all K clusters is $N = \sum_{k=1}^{K} n_k$.

Toward the specification of regression models, let $\boldsymbol{Y}_k = \left(Y_{k1}, \ldots, Y_{kn_k} \right)$ denote the vector of n_k responses for the kth cluster. Furthermore, associated with the ith response from the kth cluster is a vector of p covariates or risk factors, denoted by $\boldsymbol{Z}_{ki} = \left(Z_{ki,1}, \ldots, Z_{ki,p} \right)$. Finally, as appropriate to the context, let X_{ki} denote the exposure or covariate of interest for the ith study unit in the kth cluster.

Some covariates in $\boldsymbol{Z}_{ki}$ or X_{ki} may take on the same value across all study units within a cluster. In the dental length data, if X_{ki} is sex, then $X_{k1} = X_{k2} = X_{k3} = X_{k4}$; that is, the four age-specific length measurements have the same value of X. Depending on the context, such a covariate may be referred to as being *cluster-specific* or *between-subject* or *time-invariant*. In contrast, other covariates in $\boldsymbol{Z}_{ki}$ or X_{ki} may take on different values across the study units within a cluster. In the dental length data, the age at which any given measurement was taken is such a variable, while non-White race/ethnicity is such a variable in the Medicare data (Figure 24-3B). Depending, again, on the context, such a covariate may be referred to as being *subject-specific* or *within-cluster* or *time-dependent*.

SCIENTIFIC CONSIDERATIONS

A central benefit of analyzing longitudinal or cluster-correlated data is that having repeated measures within clusters enables the investigation of a broader range of scientific questions than one could consider if only one measurement per cluster were available.

Benefits of Analyzing Longitudinal Data

If the data are longitudinal in nature, one can investigate trajectories of an outcome over time, as well as how those trajectories differ between treatment or exposure groups. Arterburn et al.,[12] for example, report on a study of long-term weight outcomes following bariatric surgery. They find that patients who undergo bariatric surgery tend, on average, to lose substantial weight during the first year following surgery (up to 30%), but then reach a nadir and slowly regain weight, albeit not back to the original value. In the absence of longitudinal data, that is with only a single weight measurement, one could not characterize this trend.

For longitudinal studies where the time scale is age, one can take advantage of the repeated measures to examine different effects of age. To illustrate this, consider the MACS data of Figure 24-2 and suppose interest lies in understanding the association between age and CD4+ cell counts at and around the time of seroconversion. Because longitudinal data are available, the data in Figure 24-2 could be used to simultaneously investigate potential cohort effects, such as that younger men have higher CD4+ cell counts at the time of seroconversion, as well as longitudinal effects, such as that the postseroconversion CD4+ cell count trajectory is steeper for older men.

Finally, longitudinal data can be used to investigate how a change in some exposure or risk factor is associated with the outcome or changes in the outcome. Consider, for example, a study of the association between CES-D (Center for Epidemiologic Studies Depression Scale), a measure of depression, and CD4+ cell count around the time of seroconversion. Let $X_{k'}$ denote the CES-D score just before seroconversion and $Y_{k'}$ the corresponding CD4+ cell count. Ignoring, for simplicity, any other covariates that one might consider (for example, for the purposes of adjustment), consider the following linear regression model for the mean of the CD4+ cell count at the ith observation for the kth man in the MACS data, as a function of the longitudinally measured CES-D measurements:

$$E\left(Y_{ki}\big|X_{k1},\ldots,X_{kn_k}\right) = \beta_0 + \beta_C X_{k'} + \beta_L\left(X_{ki} - X_{k'}\right). \qquad [24\text{-}1]$$

Note, in contrast to the presentation of regression models in previous chapters, in this chapter we use β_0 to denote the intercept. From model 24-1, we have that:

$$E\left(Y_{k'}\big|X_{k1},\ldots,X_{kn_k}\right) = \beta_0 + \beta_C X_{k'}$$

so that β_C can be seen to represent the association between CES-D and CD4+ cell count at the time of seroconversion. Formally, β_C is the change in expected CD4+ cell count at the time of seroconversion that is associated with a unit increase in CES-D. Because the interpretation is specific to the time of seroconversion, one could label β_C as being a *cross-sectional contrast*.

With a little algebra, we also have from model 24-1 that:

$$E\left(Y_{ki} - Y_{k'}\big|X_{k1},\ldots,X_{kn_k}\right) = \beta_L\left(X_{ki} - X_{k'}\right).$$

Thus, β_L speaks to how changes in CES-D over time are associated with changes in CD4+ cell count over time. Formally, among subjects with the same CD4+ cell count just before seroconversion, if the change in CES-D from just before seroconversion to the ith measurement were one unit larger, the expected change in CD4+ cell count from just before seroconversion to the ith measurement would be β_L units larger. Because the changes in both the exposure and outcome are occurring over time, one might label β_L as being a *longitudinal contrast*.

To emphasize the distinction between the two types of association, suppose we hypothesize that the true values of β_C and β_L are negative. The first of these corresponds to a hypothesis that men with more severe symptoms of depression at seroconversion tend to have lower CD4+ cell counts at that time, while the second corresponds to the hypothesis that men who experience increases in depressive symptoms (*i.e.*, their depression gets worse) around the time of seroconversion tend to experience greater decreases in CD4+ cell count over time. Crucially, in the absence of repeated measures, one could not distinguish between these hypotheses. If only a single measurement were available and it was at the time of seroconversion for all men in the data set, then one could estimate β_C (assuming the absence or appropriate adjustment for potential sources of bias). If, however, only a single measurement was obtained but at different points relative to seroconversion, then one could not estimate either β_C or β_L unless they were assumed to be the same.

Benefits of Analyzing Cluster-Correlated Data

Analogously distinct effects can also be investigated with cluster-correlated (as opposed to longitudinal) data. Returning to the Medicare data, Figure 24-3B highlights that there is substantial variation in the racial composition of the pancreatic cancer patients across the $K = 1,031$ hospitals represented in the data set; the percent non-White varies from 0.0% to 98.6%. It may be of interest, then, to distinguish between the effect of an individual's race on their outcome from the effect on their outcome of the racial composition across all patients treated at the hospital. Such effects are sometimes referred to as *contextual effects*.[13] Toward this, let X_{ki} be a binary indicator of non-White race ($0 =$ no, $1 =$ yes), and consider the following logistic model for the probability of readmission within 90 days for the ith patient in the kth hospital:

$$\text{logit Pr}\left(Y_{ki} = 1 \middle| X_{k1}, \ldots, X_{kn_k}\right) = \beta_0 + \beta_1 X_{ki} + \beta_2 \bar{X}_k^* + \beta_3 X_{ki} \bar{X}_k^* \qquad [24\text{-}2]$$

where $\bar{X}_k^* = \left(\bar{X}_k - 0.5\right) \times 10$, with $\bar{X}_k$ the mean of X_{ki} (*i.e.*, the proportion non-White in the kth hospital). Note, by standardizing $\bar{X}_k^*$ in this way one can interpret: (1) $\bar{X}_k^* = 0$ as representing the setting where the percent non-White in the hospital is 50%; and, (2) a unit increase in $\bar{X}_k^*$ as representing an increase of 10% in the percent non-White.

From model 24-2, one can loosely interpret the slope parameters as addressing the following questions:

$\exp(\beta_1)$: Is there a difference in the odds of a readmission within 90 days between non-White and White patients at a hospital that serves 50% non-White patients?

$\exp(\beta_2)$: Is there a difference in the odds of a readmission within 90 days between White patients served at hospitals that differ in the racial composition of the populations they serve (specifically by 10% in the percent non-White)?

$\exp(\beta_3)$: If there is a difference between non-White and White patients, does this difference vary between hospitals that differ in the racial composition of the populations they serve?

Note, if each hospital only had one study unit, then the value of $\bar{X}_k$ would be the same as X_{k1}, that is, the race of the first (and only) patient. Consequently, in the absence of repeated measures within the hospitals one could not estimate β_3 nor could one distinguish between β_1 and β_2.

STATISTICAL CONSIDERATIONS

Ensuring Valid Inference

The primary statistical pitfall that one faces when analyzing longitudinal or cluster-correlated data is the impact of ignoring or inappropriately accounting for the dependence on the data, specifically in regard to the validity of standard error estimates. By this we mean that the standard error estimates will not properly reflect the actual uncertainty that the estimates of the regression parameters exhibit. As a consequence, Wald-based 95% confidence intervals (see Chapter 17) will be either too wide or too tight, depending on whether the standard error estimates are overestimated or underestimated. Furthermore, P-values computed using naïve standard errors will be incorrect so that the validity of hypothesis tests based on the Wald statistics is compromised. Unfortunately, general rules of thumb regarding whether the standard error estimates are too small or too large do not exist, in part because the extent of underestimation or overestimation depends on the interplay between the nature of the dependence structure that is ignored by the naïve analysis and the nature of the naïve analysis itself.

Study Size

A second statistical consideration is the notion that there are two distinct "study sizes": the number of clusters, K; and, the cluster-specific number of study units, n_k. Distinguishing between these is important because of the differential impact of increasing one or the other on precision of estimated regression coefficients. To illustrate, suppose primary interest lies in the association between educational attainment in early life and cognitive decline in later life, with the latter assessed longitudinally. Intuitively, precision of an estimate of the association between educational attainment and cognitive decline will be enhanced by observing a wider range of educational attainment values (that is, increasing the variation in the education attainment covariate). Since educational attainment in the context of this study is likely a between-cluster or time-invariant covariate, precision will be enhanced with a larger number of clusters in the study (*i.e.*, individuals). In contrast, if interest lies in characterizing the association between physical fitness later life, a time-varying covariate, and cognitive function in later life, then precision may also be enhanced with a larger number of observations per individual. Moreover, this distinction is critical when conducting assessments of statistical power during the design phase of a longitudinal or cluster-correlated observational study,[14] or of a cluster-randomized trial.[15] In particular, the requirements regarding K and n_k will differ dramatically depending on whether the exposure of interest or intervention is at the level of the cluster or at the level of the individual study unit.

Distinguishing between the two types of study size is also important when one considers the settings under which a given statistical analysis procedure can provide valid results. Below, for example, we discuss how the usual standard error estimates for an analysis based on GEE require K to be at least 40, and that for K less than 40 some adjustment is required.

The Role of the Regression Model

Third, we note that dependence in the regression context is *residual* in the sense that it is beyond what has already been accounted for in the regression model for the mean. To see this, note that one way of interpreting any regression model is that it provides a way to structure variation in the outcome as a function of the covariates included; as more of this variation is structured through the mean (for example, by including additional, relevant covariates or through flexible modeling such as the use of polynomial terms; see Chapter 20), less unexplained or residual variation remains. Similarly, the extent and nature of dependence in a regression context will depend on the regression model for the mean that is under consideration. Returning to the dental length data in Figure 24-1, let $Z_{ki,1}$ denote the age at which the ith measurement on the kth child was obtained, and let $Z_{ki,2}$ denote the sex (0 = female, 1 = male) of the kth child at the ith measurement. Consider the following two linear regression models for the mean dental length:

$$E\left(Y_{ki}|Z_{ki}\right) = \beta_0 + \beta_1 Z_{ki,1}$$

[24-3]

and

$$E\left(Y_{ki}|Z_{ki}\right) = \beta_0 + \beta_1 Z_{ki,1} + \beta_2 Z_{ki,2} + \beta_3 Z_{ki,1} Z_{ki,2}.$$

[24-4]

Assuming the true values of either (or both) of β_2 and β_3 are nonzero, model 24-4 will explain more of the variation in the outcome than model 24-3. As such, the residual variance that remains, that is the variance of:

$$R_{ki} = Y_{ki} - E\left(Y_{ki}|Z_{ki}\right)$$

will be lower under model 24-4 than under model 24-3. Similarly, the residual dependence between observations within a cluster will be smaller. Returning to the intuition provided above, the lack of $Z_{ki,2}$ in model 24-3 means that sex remains an unaccounted-for phenomenon that connects the measurements within a child and, therefore, induces dependence. By including $Z_{ki,2}$ in model 24-4, the influence that sex exerts as a "connection" between measurements within a child will be diminished, so that the magnitude of dependence will be lower. In the limit, if one were able to identify and include into the model a set of covariates that represented all phenomena that connects the study units, then the residual dependence would go to zero. That is, the data could be viewed as being independent.

Time-Varying Exposures

Finally, we emphasize that special consideration must be given in longitudinal studies in which the goal is to estimate causal effects in regard to an exposure that is time-varying. Moreover, if the time-varying exposure is affected by previous outcome levels or previous values of a time-varying confounder, then standard regression techniques, including those described in this chapter, will generally fail to estimate causal effects without bias. In these settings, techniques based on counterfactuals must be used; these are covered in Chapter 25. If the time-varying exposure is independent of the outcome over time, perhaps conditionally on a set of time-invariant confounders, then the methods presented here would be appropriate. Examples of such exposures include an individual's age, as in the dental growth data, or a time-varying exposure that is completely external to the individual such as may be the case with ambient air pollution levels. Furthermore, the methods presented here are appropriate for estimating causal effects of time-invariant or point exposures, such as receipt of bariatric surgery in Arterburn et al.[12]

EXPLORATORY DATA ANALYSIS

Throughout Part III of this book we have emphasized that, while the final analysis of a given study may rely on a relatively complex technique, such as regression, an initial exploratory data analysis (EDA) based on crude statistics can be invaluable in helping avoid certain problems and pitfalls, and in aiding subsequent decisions. As with all EDA, there can be no prescription for how one proceeds, although an often useful first step is to investigate potentially unusual observations. For example, the graphical representation of the data in Figure 24-1 reveals that there are several instances where length measurement decreases from one time point to the next. While initially unintuitive, a plausible explanation for this may lie with understanding that the measurement is the length between two points in a child's head and that the rate of growth may not be the same for the two points. Thus, while it would nevertheless be wise to check the validity of the measurement, the decrease may accurately reflect a real physiological phenomenon.

Another useful EDA technique is to perform an initial exploration of the mean structure. While this is something that can be done for all studies in which regression will be used, it can be particularly useful in the dependent data setting where the association between a given covariate and the outcome can manifest in several ways; see the example regarding CES-D and CD4+ cell counts above. Toward illustrating such an initial exploration, Table 24-1 reports on the mean length for the data in Figure 24-1 stratified by sex and age, as well as the difference in mean length between the males and females. From the table there appears to be preliminary evidence for: *trends over time*, in that the average length increases with age for both males and females; *cross-sectional differences*, in that males have larger average lengths at each age; and *longitudinal differences*, in that the increase in average length over time is greater for males than females. Knowing this could be helpful in making future decisions regarding the structure of a regression model.

TABLE 24-1

Numerical Summaries of the Dental Length Data Shown in Figure 24-1

	Age, years			
	8	10	12	14
Mean length (mm)				
Males	22.9	24.0	25.9	27.6
Females	21.2	22.2	23.1	24.1
Difference (mm)	1.7	1.8	2.8	3.5

To accompany a crude analysis as in Table 24-1, one could perform initial unadjusted regression analyses of each cluster. The right-hand side image in Figure 24-1, for example, provides the fitted lines from a series of simple linear regressions of length against age for each of the 11 girls. From the figure, there appears to be preliminary evidence for: *trend*, in that the length is increasing with age for all females; *tracking*, in that females with large lengths at younger ages tend to have large dental lengths at older ages; and *comparable variation over time*, in that the variation across females is (roughly) similar across the four ages at which measurements were taken.

A final component of EDA that is particularly useful in the context of this chapter is an exploration of the dependence structure. Since dependence is residual (see above), any exploration in an EDA requires specification of a model for the mean. With that in mind, suppose a mean model has been fit and consider the standard deviation and correlation matrix of the residuals for the kth cluster:

$$S = \begin{pmatrix} \sigma_1 & & & \\ \rho_{12} & \sigma_2 & & \\ \vdots & \vdots & \ddots & \\ \rho_{1n_k} & \rho_{2n_k} & \cdots & \sigma_{n_k} \end{pmatrix}$$

where $\sigma_i = \sqrt{V(R_{ki})}$ is the standard deviation for the residual of the ith study unit and $\rho_{ij} = \mathrm{Cov}(R_{ki}, R_{kj}) / \sqrt{V(R_{ki})V(R_{kj})}$ is the correlation between residuals for the ith and jth study units. Calculating this matrix for the dental length data for the 11 females in Figure 24-1 with a mean model that solely includes a linear term for age, yields:

$$\hat{S} = \begin{pmatrix} 2.12 & & & \\ 0.83 & 1.90 & & \\ 0.86 & 0.90 & 2.36 & \\ 0.84 & 0.88 & 0.95 & 2.44 \end{pmatrix}.$$

From the diagonal of $\hat{S}$, there is a suggestion of *heteroskedasticity* since the standard deviation in the residuals increases with age. Furthermore, from the off-diagonals there is evidence of very strong correlation between measurements within the children (at least 0.83 for all pairs), and that the magnitude of the correlation is fairly constant across all pairs. As elaborated upon below, the latter observation may lead one to adopt an exchangeable correlation structure or use a random intercepts model.

The use of S as an exploratory tool for the MACS data in Figure 24-2 requires additional work since, in contrast to the dental length data, the measurements across the $K = 369$ men were not obtained at a common set of times. In particular, the use of S requires categorizing time and binning measurements accordingly. To that end, the following $\hat{S}$ was obtained by: (1) fitting a flexible polynomial linear regression model for the mean CD4+ count as a function of time relative to seroconversion; and, (2) categorizing time relative to seroconversion into 7 intervals using cut-offs $(-1.5, -0.5, 0.5, 1.5, 2.5, 3.5)$:

$$\hat{S} = \begin{pmatrix} 379 & & & & & & \\ 0.70 & 397 & & & & & \\ 0.61 & 0.58 & 349 & & & & \\ 0.47 & 0.55 & 0.59 & 264 & & & \\ 0.30 & 0.46 & 0.51 & 0.75 & 301 & & \\ 0.50 & 0.56 & 0.46 & 0.67 & 0.81 & 296 & \\ 0.89 & 0.47 & 0.49 & 0.59 & 0.73 & 0.83 & 323 \end{pmatrix}.$$

From this, there is again some evidence of heteroskedasticity in that the standard deviations of the residuals increase as one moves away from the time of seroconversion (the fourth row/column). Furthermore, there is some evidence that correlation between pairs of residuals decays as the distance between them (in time) increases. Finally, when there is a lack of balance in the timing of the measurements, it will be important to characterize how many data points one has to estimate the various components of S. For example, the estimate of 0.89 for the correlation between residuals at the two extremes of the time scale is only based on nine pairs of such observations (since there are only nine men in the data set that contribute data at the two extremes). This estimate is therefore subject to substantially more uncertainty than other estimates in $\hat{S}$ and, thus, should be taken with a grain of salt.

MARGINAL MODELS

Chapter 20 introduced generalized linear models as a class that encompasses many regression models that are commonly fit in epidemiologic studies. Building on that, one general specification for the regression model of the mean outcome of the ith study unit in the kth cluster is:

$$g\left[E\left(Y_{ki} \mid X_k = x_k, Z_k = z_k\right)\right] = \beta_0 + f_x\left(x_k, \boldsymbol{\beta}_x\right) + f_z\left(z_k, \boldsymbol{\beta}_z\right) \qquad [24\text{-}5]$$

where g is the link function, with specific choices of the identity link resulting in a linear regression specification, the log link resulting in a log-linear specification, and the logit link resulting in a logistic specification (see Chapter 20).

From the left-hand side of model 24-5, we see that the regression is specifying the mean of the outcome for the ith study unit conditional on the totality of exposures and adjustment variables across all study units in the cluster, X_k and Z_k, respectively. This is so that the specification can encompass models where exposure (or covariate) information on other study units is relevant for modeling the mean of the ith study unit, such as those given by models 24-1 and 24-2. From the right-hand side of model 24-5, the way in which the mean of the outcome depends on X_k is left general, through the function f_x, again to encompass a broad range of ways in which the mean for the ith study unit depends on the totality of exposures in the kth cluster. Similarly, the way in which the mean of the outcome depends on Z_k is left general through the function f_z.

To further illustrate possibilities within the class of models defined by model 24-5, suppose the data are longitudinal and consider the model:

$$g\left[E\left(Y_{ki} \mid X_k = x_k, Z_{ki} = z_{ki}\right)\right] = \beta_0 + \beta_{x,1} x_{ki} + \beta_{x,2} x_{k(i-1)} + z_{ki} \boldsymbol{\beta}_z. \qquad [24\text{-}6]$$

This model states that the way in which the mean for the outcome at the ith time point for the kth cluster depends on the totality of exposure information is through the current exposure (*i.e.*, X_{ki}) and the exposure at the previous time point (*i.e.*, $X_{k(i-1)}$). Such a model, referred to as a *distributed lag mean model*, is commonly used in air pollution studies to capture persistent effects of exposure.[16-18] Another common model is the *cross-sectional mean model*:

$$g\left[E\left(Y_{ki} \mid X_{ki} = x_{ki}, Z_{ki} = z_{ki}\right)\right] = \beta_0 + \beta_x x_{ki} + z_{ki} \boldsymbol{\beta}_z \qquad [24\text{-}7]$$

which solely specifies how the mean of the outcome for the ith study unit in the kth cluster depends on the exposure and covariates for that study unit.

Focusing on model 24-7, β_x can be interpreted as a contrast in the mean response between two populations of study units that differ in their value of X_{ki} by one unit but have the same value of Z_{ki}. Note, this interpretation does not require direct consideration of cluster membership; again, the interpretation is one that compares two populations of study units that are defined solely in terms of the values of X_{ki} and Z_{ki}. Because of this, one can think of β_x as representing an "average" association between X and Y, adjusted for Z, where the averaging is over the population of clusters. In this sense we say that β_x is a *population-averaged* parameter, as are all the other parameters in the model. Furthermore, these arguments can be applied to the distributed lag model given by model

24-6 and the more general specification given by model 24-5, to conclude that their component parameters are also population-averaged.

An important feature of models 24-5 to 24-7 is that each solely structures the mean of the outcome, within levels of X and Z. Moreover, they do not imply any assumptions about the dependence between the outcomes of two study units within a cluster. This is in contrast to mixed effects models (see below). To distinguish between models that do and do not imply assumptions about the dependence structure, the latter are referred to as *marginal models*; those models that do imply an assumption about the dependence structure are referred to as *conditional models*.

Generalized Estimating Equations

Suppose a marginal model has been specified and let β denote the collection of unknown regression parameters. In model 24-7, for example, $\beta = (\beta_0, \beta_x, \beta_z)$. The primary statistical tasks are then to obtain valid estimates of the unknown regression parameters and their standard errors. If there is choice in how one achieves these tasks, it is also desirable to obtain statistically efficient estimates (*i.e.*, those with the smallest standard errors). One framework for achieving both of these is the *generalized estimating equations* framework which involves estimating β by solving:

$$\sum_{k=1}^{K} D_k^T W_k (Y_k - \mu_k) = 0, \qquad [24\text{-}8]$$

where $\mu_k = (\mu_{k1}, \mu_{k2}, \ldots, \mu_{kn_k})$, with $\mu_{ki} = E(Y_{ki} | X_k, Z_{ki})$, is the vector of study unit-specific means in the kth cluster under the specified marginal model. Furthermore, D_k is an $n_k \times (p + 2)$ matrix of partial derivatives with the ith row equal to $\partial \mu_{ki}/\partial \beta$ and W_k an $n_k \times n_k$ symmetric matrix of weights. Note, model 24-8 is a system of $(p + 2)$ equations, one for each of the unknown parameters in β.

From the form of model 24-8, we see that, in a sense, the estimating equation is adding up contributions across the K clusters. This form arises because of the assumption that outcomes across clusters are taken to be independent. We also see from model 24-8 that the way in which we learn about β from the data is through a comparison of the observed outcomes, Y_k, and the expected outcomes under the model, μ_k, across the K clusters. Intuitively, we find the "best" values of β by minimizing the distance between the observed and expected outcomes. In principle, we could achieve this without D_k or W_k, that is by solving: $\sum_{k=1}^{K} (Y_k - \mu_k) = 0$. So, what are the roles of D_k and W_k? For the former, the reason is somewhat technical, but it essentially serves to rescale the system of equations to help find the estimator more quickly. Since these are completely determined by the specification of the marginal model, one need not be too concerned with their role.

The role of the weight matrix W_k is important to consider, however, particularly because it must be specified by the analyst. Setting aside exactly how one specifies W_k, which is discussed below, a crucial property of GEE is that if the marginal model for $E(Y_{ki} | X_{ki} = x, Z_{ki} = z)$ is correctly specified, then solving 24-8 will, in general, result in consistent estimates of β *regardless* of the choice of W_k. In addition, regardless of the choice of W_k, valid standard errors for $\hat{\beta}$ can be obtained using the robust sandwich variance estimator, the formula for which can be written as:

$$\widehat{\text{Cov}}(\hat{\beta}) = A^{-1}(\hat{\beta}) B(\hat{\beta}) A^{-1}(\hat{\beta}) \qquad [24\text{-}9]$$

where

$$A(\beta) = \sum_{k=1}^{K} D_k^T W_k D_k$$

and

$$B(\beta) = \sum_{k=1}^{K} D_k^T W_k (Y_k - \mu_k)(Y_k - \mu_k)^T W_k D_k$$

Note, the term "sandwich" comes from the form of 24-9; the two A^{-1} components form two pieces of "bread," while the B is the "cheese" between them. Because of the two critical properties just noted, estimation and inference are said to be *robust* to specification of the weight matrix W_k.

Given the robustness property, it is natural to ask: are some choices of W_k better than others? And, if so, how do we go about making good choices? It turns out that, while the choice of W_k does not affect validity, it does affect the statistical precision of the resulting estimate. Furthermore, the choice that leads to the minimum variance of the estimate is to use the inverse of the covariance matrix of the response vector, Y_k, as a weight, such that $W_k = \text{Cov}(Y_k)^{-1}$. With this choice, we say that the resulting estimator is *efficient* in the class of estimators defined by model 24-8. Informally, taking the inverse of $\text{Cov}(Y_k)$ will downweight study units in the kth cluster that have high variance and upweight study units that have low variance; that is, study units which have less variability in the outcomes will contribute more "information." At the same time, adopting $\text{Cov}(Y_k)^{-1}$ as a weighting structure directly acknowledges (and exploits) the fact that the study units are dependent (*i.e.*, W_k has nonzero values in the off-diagonals), which then translates into efficiency gains. Finally, we note that if we were able to use $\text{Cov}(Y_k)^{-1}$ as a weighting scheme, then a valid estimate of the covariance of the resulting point estimate of β is $\widehat{\text{Cov}}(\hat{\beta}) = A^{-1}(\hat{\beta})$.

In most settings we do not know the exact form of $\text{Cov}(Y_k)$. Because of the robustness properties, however, as one makes some choice for W_k, the only potential loss incurred is that the resulting estimator is less efficient (*i.e.*, one for which standard error estimates will, typically, be larger) than the one we would have obtained had we set $W_k = \text{Cov}(Y_k)^{-1}$. If that choice of W_k is reasonably close to $\text{Cov}(Y_k)^{-1}$, however, then we might not expect the loss to be substantial. This, in turn, suggests a strategy where one first develops as good a working understanding of $\text{Cov}(Y_k)$ as possible, and then uses that working understanding as an inverse weight. That is, one can thoughtfully develop a *working dependence structure*, say $\widetilde{\text{Cov}}(Y_k)$, and then use $W_k = \widetilde{\text{Cov}}(Y_k)^{-1}$. Crucially, because the working dependence structure need not be the exact true dependence structure, one should not say that we "assume" that it is correct. Indicating that $\widetilde{\text{Cov}}(Y_k)$ is the assumed structure implies that it is necessary for this specification to be correct in order to ensure valid estimation and inference. Since this is not the case, one should say that a given working dependence structure is "adopted." For example, one might adopt independence between study units as a working structure and still obtain valid inference, even when the study units are not actually independent and it would be inappropriate to "assume" so.

In the next subsection, we discuss how one can approach the task of specifying $\widetilde{\text{Cov}}(Y_k)$. Before doing so, we note an important exception to the robustness properties of GEE that arises when interest lies in the cross-sectional mean, $E(Y_{ki} | X_{ki} = x_{ki}, Z_{ki} = z_{ki})$, a model for which is given by model 24-7, in settings where X or any components of Z vary across study units within a cluster. In this case, in addition to the model for the cross-sectional mean being correctly specified, one must also assume that it equals the full conditional mean, as represented by expression 24-5. That is, one must have that:

$$E(Y_{ki} | X_k = x_k, Z_k = z_k) = E(Y_{ki} | X_{ki} = x_{ki}, Z_{ki} = z_{ki}).$$

If the assumption does not hold, then using model 24-8 to estimate β in the cross-sectional mean model will result in bias unless W_k is an $n_k \times n_k$ identity matrix (*i.e.*, a matrix of 1's on the diagonal and 0's on the off-diagonals).[19] That is, valid estimation and inference (using the sandwich estimator) can still be achieved but only if working independence is adopted for the dependence structure. Of course, even though adopting a working independence structure seems antithetical to the notion that the outcomes in a cluster are dependent, we are still able to perform valid inference using the sandwich estimator given by expression 24-9.

Structuring the Working Dependence Structure

To illustrate how one might approach the task of specifying the working dependence structure, we return to the dental length data in Figure 24-1. For these data, since $n_k = 4$ for each child, we have that the true $\text{Cov}(Y_k)$ for the kth child is a symmetric 4×4 matrix given by:

$$\text{Cov}(Y_k) = \begin{bmatrix} \text{Var}(Y_{k1}) & \text{Cov}(Y_{k1}, Y_{k2}) & \text{Cov}(Y_{k1}, Y_{k3}) & \text{Cov}(Y_{k1}, Y_{k4}) \\ \text{Cov}(Y_{k1}, Y_{k2}) & \text{Var}(Y_{k2}) & \text{Cov}(Y_{k2}, Y_{k3}) & \text{Cov}(Y_{k2}, Y_{k4}) \\ \text{Cov}(Y_{k1}, Y_{k3}) & \text{Cov}(Y_{k2}, Y_{k3}) & \text{Var}(Y_{k3}) & \text{Cov}(Y_{k3}, Y_{k4}) \\ \text{Cov}(Y_{k1}, Y_{k4}) & \text{Cov}(Y_{k2}, Y_{k4}) & \text{Cov}(Y_{k3}, Y_{k4}) & \text{Var}(Y_{k4}) \end{bmatrix}.$$

Consider, now, the following working dependence structure:

$$\widetilde{\text{Cov}}(Y_k) = \sigma^2 \begin{pmatrix} 1 & \rho & \rho & \rho \\ \rho & 1 & \rho & \rho \\ \rho & \rho & 1 & \rho \\ \rho & \rho & \rho & 1 \end{pmatrix}.$$

[24-10]

This specification adopts three simplifications regarding $\text{Cov}(Y_k)$. First, because the right-hand side does not depend on k, the specification amounts to adopting a dependence structure that is the same for all K clusters. Second, the working variances of each of the age-specific measurements are taken to be the same: $\widetilde{\text{Var}}(Y_{k1}) = \widetilde{\text{Var}}(Y_{k3}) = \widetilde{\text{Var}}(Y_{k3}) = \widetilde{\text{Var}}(Y_{k4}) = \sigma^2$. Finally, it takes the correlation between pairs of observations to be constant across all pairs; that is, $\text{Corr}(Y_{ki}, Y_{kj}) = \rho$ for all $i \neq j$, a structure that is sometimes referred as an *exchangeable* correlation structure.

Two appealing features of model 24-10 are that the structure is simple and easy to communicate, and that only two dependence parameters need be estimated (*i.e.*, σ^2 and ρ). The simplifications adopted, however, are severe and may result in $\widetilde{\text{Cov}}(Y_k)$ being far from the true $\text{Cov}(Y_k)$. If this is the case, then making the simplifications less severe may yield benefits in terms of statistical efficiency. One approach to doing this would be to adopt a working dependence structure that is exchangeable as in model 24-10 but allow the dependence parameters to vary across the levels of some cluster-specific covariate. In the dental length data, for example, rather than assuming that the dependence parameters are the same for all children, one could specify separate exchangeable structures for the boys and the girls. That is, have separate values of σ^2 and ρ for the two sexes. Another option would be explicitly acknowledging the longitudinal nature of the data and adopting a working dependence structure in which the dependence between two study units is determined by how far apart in time they are. For the dental growth data, since the measurements are all 2 years apart, one could adopt the following *banded* correlation structure:

$$\widetilde{\text{Cov}}(Y_k) = \sigma^2 \begin{pmatrix} 1 & \rho_1 & \rho_2 & \rho_3 \\ \rho_1 & 1 & \rho_1 & \rho_2 \\ \rho_2 & \rho_1 & 1 & \rho_1 \\ \rho_3 & \rho_2 & \rho_1 & 1 \end{pmatrix},$$

[24-11]

where ρ_1 is the common correlation between all pairs of measurements that are 2 years apart, ρ_2 is the common correlation between all pairs of measurements that are 4 years apart, and ρ_3 is the common correlation between all pairs of measurements that are 6 years apart. For the dental growth data, this may be a reasonable choice because it only results in two additional parameters beyond model 24-10. As n_k increases, however, this may result in a large number of parameters that require estimation. One compromise between models 24-10 and 24-11 is a structure that decays as function of time such as an *autoregressive* correlation structure:

$$\widetilde{\text{Cov}}(\boldsymbol{Y}_k) = \sigma^2 \begin{pmatrix} 1 & \rho & \rho^2 & \rho^3 \\ \rho & 1 & \rho & \rho^2 \\ \rho^2 & \rho & 1 & \rho \\ \rho^3 & \rho^2 & \rho & 1 \end{pmatrix}.$$

[24-12]

In this structure, ρ is the common correlation between all pairs of measurements that are 2 years apart, while squaring it gives the common correlation between all pairs that are 4 years apart and cubing it gives the common correlation between all pairs that are 6 years part. Crucially, model 24-12 offers a very different structure from that encoded in model 24-10 while having the same total number of dependence parameters. Furthermore, as with model 24-10, one could permit σ^2 and ρ in model 24-12 to depend on cluster-specific covariates.

Finally, we note that while it is possible to quantify uncertainty in estimates of the parameters that index the working dependence structure in a GEE analysis, doing so requires making additional assumptions that may be difficult to specify and justify.[20] Furthermore, related to this is that formal testing of the dependence structure in the marginal model framework is less straightforward than it is in the mixed model framework (see below).

Adjustments in Small-Sample Settings

The validity of the robust sandwich estimator given by expression 24-9 requires the number of clusters to be large, with some rules of thumb suggesting that K be at least 40.[21,22] For settings where K is smaller than 40, the sandwich estimator tends to underestimate the standard error; thus, 95% confidence intervals and P-values will be too small. To resolve this, a number of corrections have been proposed. Perhaps the simplest is a degrees of freedom correction that involves multiplying the usual variance estimate by a factor of $K/(K-p)$. Since this will always be greater than 1.0, the impact is an increase in the estimates for all parameters. When there is substantial variation in the cluster sizes, however, this rather crude adjustment, which does not take cluster size into account, has been shown to exhibit poor performance.[23]

Of the remaining strategies, most follow an approach that involves modifying the sandwich estimator in some way, specifically through $\boldsymbol{B}$.[21,24,25] Based on a number of simulation studies, however, it seems that no method can be taken to be universally superior, suggesting that the relative performance of the corrections depends on a number of factors including the type of outcome, the degree of the variability in cluster sizes, and the model of interest.[23,26,27]

MIXED EFFECTS MODELS

Intuitively, marginal models such as 24-5, 24-6, and 24-7 can be viewed as permitting the analysis to "borrow information" across the clusters via the estimation of a set of parameters that is common to all clusters. Doing so, however, fails to acknowledge the potential for heterogeneity across clusters. This problem motivates fitting separate regression models to each cluster. For example, consider the following modification of model 24-7:

$$g\left[E\left(Y_{ki} | X_{ki} = x_{ki}, \boldsymbol{Z}_{ki} = \boldsymbol{z}_{ki}\right)\right] = \beta_{0,k} + \beta_{x,k} x_{ki} + \boldsymbol{z}_{ki} \boldsymbol{\beta}_{z,k}$$

[24-13]

In this model, while $\beta_{x,k}$ is interpreted as a contrast between two populations of study units, the comparison is specific to the kth cluster. In this sense $\beta_{x,k}$ is a *cluster-specific* parameter, as are all other parameters in the model.

To help illustrate and distinguish between models 24-7 and 24-13, Figure 24-4 presents their application to the dental length data. In the figure, the two solid lines correspond to the fitted lines from a linear marginal regression model with sex and age (as a linear term), and their interaction:

$$E\left(Y_{ki} | \text{Age}_{ki} = a, \text{Sex}_{ki} = s\right) = \beta_0 + \beta_a a + \beta_s s + \beta_{as} as,$$

[24-14]

with the red line depicting to the fitted line for the females and the black line depicting the fitted line for the males. Note, these lines could also have been obtained by fitting two separate linear regression models of dental length against age, stratified by sex. Also shown in the figure are $K = 26$ separate regressions of dental length outcome against age of the form:

$$E\left(Y_{ki}\big|\mathrm{Age}_{ki} = a\right) = \beta_{0,k} + \beta_{a,k}a \qquad [24\text{-}15]$$

for the kth child. In the figure, the pink dashed lines correspond to the 11 females while the gray dashed lines correspond to the 15 males.

It is clear from Figure 24-4 that there is substantial heterogeneity in the intercepts (*i.e.*, the fitted lines at age 8 years) and in the slopes. In this sense, model 24-13 provides a measure of insight that is not obtained when one only considers the results from the marginal model (*i.e.*, the solid lines). One important limitation of the separate regressions specification 24-13, however, is that it does not provide a direct means of quantifying the association between a cluster-specific or time-invariant covariate and the outcome; in Figure 24-4 one would need to obtain a summary of the 26 dashed lines in order to quantify the association between sex and dental length. This motivates consideration of models that permit heterogeneity in select parameters but not others. As an example, a model that is intermediate between models 24-7 and 24-13 is:

$$g\left[E\left(Y_{ki}\big|X_{ki} = x_{ki}, \mathbf{Z}_{ki} = \mathbf{z}_{ki}\right)\right] = \beta_{0,k} + \beta_x x_{ki} + \mathbf{z}_{ki}\boldsymbol{\beta}_z \qquad [24\text{-}16]$$

In this model β_x and $\boldsymbol{\beta}_z$ are common regression parameters across all clusters while the intercept is permitted to vary. Such a model might be reasonable if one wanted to acknowledge variation in baseline risk while estimating a common association for some exposure of interest, and if a common adjustment parameter (*i.e.*, $\boldsymbol{\beta}_z$) across clusters is sufficient for the control of confounding bias. Despite being common across clusters, however, the interpretation of β_x remains cluster-specific. This is because isolating the two study unit populations that form the contrast (*i.e.*, that differ in X by one unit) requires "holding constant" not just $\mathbf{Z}_{ki}$ but also the intercept, $\beta_{0,k}$. That is, the comparison is not just within levels of $\mathbf{Z}_{ki}$ but also within cluster.

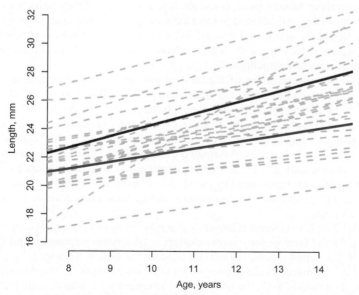

FIGURE 24-4 Fitted lines from two sets of regression analysis of the dental length data shown in Figure 24-1. The solid lines present population-averaged results from a marginal model with an interaction between age (represented as a linear term) and sex (black for boys and red for girls). The dashed lines present 26 child-specific regressions of the mean length as a linear function of age.

Models such as 24-16 provide a compromise between being able to quantify and estimate associations for between-cluster covariates and acknowledging heterogeneity. Nevertheless, they require estimating a relatively large number of parameters. Fitting model 24-16, for example, would require estimating $K + 2$ parameters. While this is fewer than $3 \times K$ parameters in model 24-13, the extent to which reliable estimates can be obtained will depend on the interplay between the number of clusters and the cluster-specific study sizes. In the extreme, if each cluster only has $n_k = 2$ study units, so that $N = 2K$, then the number of unknown parameters is more than half of the study size. Moreover, there are relatively little data to inform the magnitude of each of the $\beta_{0,k}$. To mitigate this problem one can incorporate additional structure across the $\beta_{0,k}$. One approach to this is given by the following model:

$$g\left[E\left(Y_{ki}\middle|X_{ki}=x_{ki},\mathbf{Z}_{ki}=z_{ki},\gamma_{0,k}\right)\right]=\left(\beta_0+\gamma_{0,k}\right)+\beta_x x_{ki}+z_{ki}\boldsymbol{\beta}_z, \qquad [24\text{-}17]$$

which replaces "$\beta_{0,k}$" model in 24-16 with "$\beta_0 + \gamma_{0,k}$." Comparing this model to model 24-16, we see that model 24-17 reconceptualizes heterogeneity in the intercepts across the clusters through a set of cluster-specific deviations, specifically the $\gamma_{0,k}$, that are centered around an overall intercept, β_0. One can then build on this by assuming that the cluster-specific deviations arise from some underlying distribution such as a Normal distribution with mean zero and variance, say, σ_γ^2. Whatever choice is made, it is important that the distribution has mean zero; this ensures that β_0 can be interpreted as the intercept that corresponds to the "average" cluster. Finally, since the cluster-specific $\gamma_{0,k}$ are conceived as arising from some distribution, they are often referred to as *random effects*. Correspondingly, the regression parameters, $\boldsymbol{\beta} = (\beta_0, \beta_x, \boldsymbol{\beta}_z)$ often referred as *fixed effects*, with the overall model referred to as a *mixed effects model*.

Some additional points are worth noting. First, recall that one approach to intuiting how dependence arises is through the notion that there are characteristics that are specific to the cluster that "connect" the responses of study units within the cluster. With this in mind, one interpretation of $\gamma_{0,k}$ is as a latent factor that, in some sense, summarizes the collective impact of these characteristics on the outcome of the ith study unit in the kth cluster. The factor is "latent" in the sense that it is not a quantity that we can directly measure. Nevertheless, because the same value is "shared" across all study units within the kth cluster, it serves as a useful statistical device to connect their outcomes and, consequently, dependence. Study units in a cluster with a large positive value of $\gamma_{0,k}$ will all tend to have higher risk for the outcome, so that their observed outcomes will tend to be similar and thus exhibit dependence. Similarly, study units in a cluster with a large negative value of $\gamma_{0,k}$ will all tend to have lower risk, so that their outcomes will also be similar and, thus, exhibit dependence.

Second, with this interpretation of the random effects, the variance component σ_γ^2 can be interpreted as a measure of the extent of dependence. To see this, suppose σ_γ^2 is equal to zero. That is, there is no heterogeneity in the intercepts across the clusters so that each of the $\gamma_{(0,k)}$ must equal zero. Intuitively, within the confines of the model structure, this tells us that there is nothing special about being in one cluster or another; there are no specific "connections" among the study units in a given cluster, so their outcomes can be viewed as being independent. As σ_γ^2 increases, the heterogeneity across the clusters increases, as does the influence of their cluster-specific characteristics (as represented by the random effects) so that the outcomes of study units within a cluster will exhibit greater dependence among themselves relative to that with study units in other clusters.

Third, model 24-17, sometimes referred to as a *random intercepts model*, can be extended to acknowledge potential heterogeneity across clusters in association parameters. In Figure 24-4, for example, the 26 fitted child-specific regressions indicate that there is heterogeneity in dental length at age 8 years (*i.e.*, the intercept) and heterogeneity in the trajectories (*i.e.*, the slopes corresponding to age). Building on model 24-17, the latter type of heterogeneity can be directly incorporated into a mixed effects model as follows:

$$g\left[E\left(Y_{ki}\middle|X_{ki}=x,\mathbf{Z}_{ki}=z,\boldsymbol{\gamma}_k\right)\right]=\left(\beta_0+\gamma_{0,k}\right)+\left(\beta_x+\gamma_{x,k}\right)x+z\boldsymbol{\beta}_z. \qquad [24\text{-}18]$$

Thus, each cluster has two random effects, $\gamma_k = (\gamma_{0,k}, \gamma_{x,k})$, with $\gamma_{0,k}$ a random intercept that quantifies the deviation around the common intercept, β_0, and $\gamma_{x,k}$ a random slope that quantifies the deviation around the common slope parameter, β_x. More generally, a mixed effects model may also have random effects for the components of Z_{ki}. To complete the specification, one would need to specify the distribution of the random effects which must have mean zero in each component. While many choices are possible, one common choice is a bivariate Normal distribution in which the components may be correlated. This would permit the random intercept to be correlated with the random slope, which may be relevant if, for example, individuals with higher starting values tend to have steeper trajectories over time.

Fourth, viewing the introduction of the random effects as a means to structure dependence, we see an important distinction between marginal models and mixed effects models. Specifically, recall that specification of a marginal mean model says nothing about the dependence structure (which must be specified separately). In contrast, when one specifies a mixed effects model, assumptions regarding the dependence structure are being implicitly made. Consider, for example, fitting the linear mixed effects model:

$$E\left(Y_{ki} \mid X_{ki} = x_{ki}, Z_{ki} = z_{ki}, \gamma_{0,k}\right) = \left(\beta_0 + \gamma_{0,k}\right) + \beta_x x_{ki} + z_{ki}\beta_z \qquad [24\text{-}19]$$

with the assumption that $\gamma_{0,k}$ follows a Normal distribution with mean zero and variance σ_γ^2. Furthermore, assume the residuals in this linear model follow a Normal distribution with mean zero and variance σ_ε^2. Then the induced dependence structure for the response vector (conditional on X and Z) is an exchangeable structure as in model 24-10. In more general settings, such as when the model being fit is a logistic model and/or when random slopes are included, it may not be possible to derive the induced dependence structure mathematically. As such, approaching the task of deciding which random effects to include and how may best be done through attempting to characterize heterogeneity across clusters rather than dependence within clusters.

Likelihood-Based Estimation

Analyses for marginal models via GEE can be referred to as being *semiparametric* because they rely only on the correct specification of the mean model. Moreover, as discussed, validity does not hinge on correct specification of the dependence structure nor the full distribution of the data. In contrast, analyses for mixed effects models are *parametric* because one is required to specify the full distribution of the data; in addition to the model for the mean (as in models 24-17 to 24-19) and the distribution of the random effects, one must specify the underlying conditional distribution of the outcome (*i.e.*, conditional on the covariates included in the model and the random effects). In describing model 24-19, for example, the distribution of the response was specified via the assumed normal distribution for the residuals. While one can only take the distribution of the outcome to be Bernoulli when it is binary, there are many choices, when the outcome is a count variable, with the binomial and Poisson distributions being well-known examples (see Chapter 17). Collectively, therefore, there up to four sets of unknown quantities in a mixed effects model:

1. the fixed effects, denoted by β;
2. the K cluster-specific random effects, denoted by γ_k;
3. the variance components of the random effects distribution, denoted by Σ_γ; and,
4. any additional parameters that index the distribution of the response, denoted by ϕ.

Note, in models 24-17 and 24-19, Σ_γ is a single variance component, that is the variance of $\gamma_{0,k}$, while in model 24-18, Σ_γ denotes the three parameters that index the 2×2 variance matrix of $(\gamma_{0,k}, \gamma_{x,k})$: the variance of $\gamma_{0,k}$, the variance of $\gamma_{1,k}$, and the correlation between $\gamma_{0,k}$ and $\gamma_{1,k}$. Furthermore, in the specification of model 24-19, ϕ is the variance of the residuals (*i.e.*, σ_ε^2 in the specified normal); if the outcome was binary, then no additional parameters need be estimated (since the mean fully specifies the Bernoulli distribution).

Given specification of the full data distribution, the usual approach to estimating β is to use maximum likelihood (see Chapters 16 and 21). In the context of a mixed effects model, there are a number of distinct likelihoods that one could use. One choice is the *conditional likelihood*:

$$L\left(\beta,\gamma_1,\ldots\gamma_K,\phi\right) = \prod_{k=1}^{K} L_k\left(\beta,\gamma_k,\phi\right)$$

which, although details are not given, is constructed by combining the assumption of independence across clusters (hence the product), with the mixed effects regression specification and the assumption regarding the underlying conditional distribution of the outcome. One problem with using this likelihood, however, is that the number of unknown quantities increases as the number of clusters increase; as K increases, so does the number of cluster-specific random effects that must be estimated. This poses special challenges when statistical theory is used to establish the properties of the resulting estimator, challenges that are not usually of central interest in an epidemiologic study. To resolve this, estimation for a mixed effects model is usually performed by integrating out the random effects to form what is known as the *marginal likelihood*:

$$L\left(\beta,\Sigma_\gamma,\phi\right) = \prod_{k=1}^{K} L_k\left(\beta,\Sigma_\gamma,\phi\right) = \prod_{k=1}^{K} \int L_k\left(\beta,\gamma_k,\phi\right) f\left(\gamma_k|\Sigma_\gamma\right) \partial\gamma_k. \qquad [24\text{-}20]$$

Intuitively, we use structure that comes from the assumption that the random effects arise from some specified distribution, encoded by $f\left(\gamma_k|\Sigma_\gamma\right)$, to eliminate the task of estimating each of the γ_k. In their place, we are required to estimate the variance components, Σ_γ, but the number of such parameters will typically be small. Thus, although some component of β, typically β_x, may be of primary interest, the analysis proceeds by simultaneously estimating β, Σ_γ, and (as necessary) ϕ via maximization of 24-20.

Inference for the Mean Model and the Dependence Structure

An important benefit of basing an analysis on the marginal likelihood 24-20 is that inference for β follows from standard statistical theory. Thus, standard errors for the estimate of β, and consequently confidence intervals, as well as P-values from a likelihood ratio test (see Chapter 21) are straightforward to obtain (although must be coded up in software).

Another important benefit of using a likelihood-based analysis is that one can use hypothesis testing to formally investigate heterogeneity across the clusters. For example, if one views the variance component in a random intercepts model, σ_γ^2, as a measure of dependence, one can formally assess whether there is any evidence in the data to indicate a lack of independence by performing a likelihood ratio test of the null hypothesis that $\sigma_\gamma^2 = 0$.[28] Similarly, one could formally assess whether the random intercepts in model 24-18 contribute to the fit of the model by testing the null hypothesis that the variance of the $\gamma_{x,k}$ random slopes is equal to zero. On a technical note, care is needed when computing P-values for the likelihood ratio test statistic since the sampling distribution is not a χ^2 distribution but, rather, a mixture of χ^2 distributions, with the mixture depending on the models being considered.

That one can perform formal hypothesis testing for the variance components is important for a number of reasons. First, as we elaborate upon below, the validity of a mixed effects model-based analysis hinges on correct specification of the distribution of the random effects (in addition to correct specification of the other components). Because dependence is typically more challenging to conceive of than the mean, it may not be clear how to proceed, and hypothesis testing can provide insight directly from the data that may be helpful. Although this book generally downplays the use of hypothesis testing, for settings where primary interest lies in estimating the association between some exposure and the outcome (*i.e.*, β_x), the dependence structure will be of secondary interest (if at all), so that the use of hypothesis use may be justifiable as a means to selecting the variance components.

A second reason why being able to perform hypothesis testing for the variance components is important is because doing so may be appropriate to answer the question of interest. In studies of hospital variation in quality of care, for example, mixed effects models are used as a means to analyze patient outcomes across hospitals.[29] Consider, for example, a study of hospital variation in 90-day readmission among Medicare patients diagnosed with pancreatic cancer using the data summarized in Figure 24-3. For such a study, it will be important to adjust for differences in case-mix across the hospitals, such as differences in the sex and age distribution of the patients.[30] One approach to the achieving this is to fit the following logistic mixed effects model:

$$\text{logit}\left[E\left(Y_{ki}\middle|\boldsymbol{Z}_{ki}=z_{ki},\gamma_{0,k}\right)\right]=\left(\beta_0+\gamma_{0,k}\right)+z_{ki}\boldsymbol{\beta}_z,$$

where $\boldsymbol{Z}_{ki}$ is a vector of patient-specific characteristics and $\gamma_{0,k}$ is a hospital-specific random effect that, intuitively, summarizes all aspects of the hospital that contribute to high or low quality of care. Using this model, one could formally assess whether there is variation in readmission rates across hospitals by testing the variance component for $\gamma_{0,k}$.

Estimation of Random Effects

In the event that the null hypothesis is rejected, one may conclude that interventions or policies that improve the quality of low-performing hospitals should be developed, implemented, and assessed. This, in turn, requires identifying the low-performing hospitals although the use of the marginal likelihood model 24-20 as a basis for the analysis eliminated the random effects from the analysis. To resolve this, following the fit of a mixed effects model, one can posthoc estimate the random effects using empirical Bayes methods.[31,32]

Robustness

An important caveat for likelihood-based analyses of mixed effects models is that if the assumed distribution of the random effects is incorrect, that is, it is misspecified, then there are no guarantees that estimation and inference using 24-20 will be valid. In particular, if the random effects are misspecified (*e.g.*, a random slope should have been included, as in model 24-18, but it was not) or if the assumed distribution of the random effects is misspecified (*e.g.*, the true distribution is skewed but a symmetric Normal distribution was adopted), then the maximum likelihood estimates for β may be biased even if the mean model is correctly specified. Furthermore, standard error estimates may also be biased. Thus, it is important that the task of specifying structure, via the random effects, in heterogeneity across clusters is approached with care. This is in contrast to the specification of the working dependence structure in a GEE-based analysis, where the only consequence of misspecification is a loss of statistical efficiency.

While important to be aware of, in practice this issue seems to be primarily a theoretical one. Moreover, theoretical calculations as well as extensive simulation studies indicate that for a broad range of mixed effects models, estimation and inference for β is generally robust to misspecification of the distribution of the random effects; see McCulloch and Neuhaus[33] for a summary. Nevertheless, numerous methods have been developed to mitigate potential bias due to misspecification, including methods based on estimating/specifying the random effects distribution nonparametrically or smoothly[34-36]; methods based on flexible families of parametric distributions[37-39]; and, Bayesian nonparametric methods.[40,41]

COMPARING THE PARAMETERS FROM MARGINAL AND MIXED EFFECTS MODELS

The two previous sections provide an overview of marginal models, with estimation and inference via GEE, and mixed effects models, with estimation and inference via maximum likelihood. From these overviews, we find that the frameworks differ in numerous ways, including how they seek to account for dependence in the outcomes within a cluster; their approaches to estimation and inference; their robustness properties; and, in whether/how inference can be performed for the dependence structure. Another important distinction is in the precise interpretation of the parameters. To see this, compare the marginal linear model:

$$E\left(Y_{ki} \mid X_{ki} = x_{ki}\right) = \beta_0^m + \beta_x^m x_{ki} \qquad\qquad [24\text{-}21]$$

to the corresponding conditional, random intercepts model:

$$E\left(Y_{ki} \mid X_{ki} = x_{ki}, \gamma_k\right) = \beta_0^c + \beta_x^c x_{ki} + \gamma_k. \qquad\qquad [24\text{-}22]$$

To emphasize the distinction between the two models, superscripts "m" and "c" have been added to the notation for the intercept and slope parameters. Just as with models 24-5 through 24-7, β_x^m, the slope parameter that characterizes how the mean of Y varies as a function of X in model 24-21 has a population-averaged interpretation. Furthermore, just as with models 24-13, 24-15, and 24-16, the interpretation of β_x^c in model 24-22 is cluster-specific. Thus, the marginal model is speaking to the association between X and Y averaging *across* clusters while the mixed effects model is speaking to the association *within* clusters.

Now consider the interpretations of β_x^m and β_x^c in the specific context of the dental length data, with X taken to be the sex of the child coded as 0 = female and 1 = male. β_x^m is the difference in expected dental length between two populations of measurements; one taken from females and one from males. While the interpretation of β_x^c also corresponds to a difference in the average of length measurements, it must be within-child. It is unclear, however, whether one can attribute any meaning to a contrast between females and males that is within-child. More generally, the interpretation of any cluster-specific covariate coefficient in a mixed effects model will suffer from this seemingly unsettling problem.

Setting aside this important conceptual issue regarding mixed effects models, since both β_x^m and β_x^c are seeking to quantify the association between X and Y, are they the same numerically? For linear models such as 24-21 and 24-22, the answer is yes: even though they have fundamentally different interpretations, they are numerically the same. As an analogy, consider the mean and median of a symmetric distribution (such as is the case for a Normal distribution). Clearly, the definitions (and thereby interpretations) of the mean and median are distinct and yet they will be numerically equivalent for a symmetric distribution. As such, for a symmetric distribution, one can learn about the mean of a population with knowledge about the median. Thus, returning to the regression context, even if one were to fit a linear mixed effects model, it may be reasonable to interpret the results as pertaining to population-averaged contrasts. Outside of linear mixed models, however, the values of β_x^m and β_x^c will, in general, not be the same numerically. That this is the case is closely linked to the notion of noncollapsibility (see Chapter 5). Nevertheless, they will often be similar unless the variance of the random effects is large.

ADDITIONAL TOPICS

As mentioned in the introduction, the field of repeated measures data analysis is huge, and we have only covered select topics. Additional topics that readers may encounter in their own analyses include alternative tools for EDA, such as the sample variogram and semivariogram; spatial and spatiotemporal data analysis; time series data analysis; the joint analysis of longitudinal and time-to-event data; outcome-dependent sampling in the repeated measures context; methods for twin studies; missing data; informative clustering; Bayesian methods for mixed effects models; cluster-randomized trials and step-wedge designs; transition regression models; and marginalized models. Each of these topics could be addressed with their own distinct sections or, indeed, their own chapters. Most of these topics are covered in some capacity in the texts mentioned in the introduction.

References

1. Fitzmaurice GM, Laird NM, Ware JH. *Applied Longitudinal Analysis*. New York, NY: John Wiley & Sons; 2012.
2. Diggle PJ, Heagerty P, Liang KY, Zeger SL. *Analysis of Longitudinal Data*. New York, NY: Oxford; 2002.
3. Fitzmaurice G, Davidian M, Verbeke G, Molenberghs G. *Longitudinal Data Analysis*. Hoboken, NJ: CRC Press; 2008.
4. Mcculloch CE, Searle SR, Neuhaus JM. *Generalized, Linear, and Mixed Models*. Hoboken, NJ: Wiley; 2008:M38.
5. Potthoff RF, Roy S. A generalized multivariate analysis of variance model useful especially for growth curve problems. *Biometrika*. 1964;51:313-326.
6. Kaslow RA, Ostrow DG, Detels R, Phair JP, Polk BF, Rinaldo CR Jr. The Multicenter AIDS Cohort Study: rationale, organization, and selected characteristics of the participants. *Am J Epidemiol*. 1987;126:310-318.
7. Zeger SL, Diggle PJ. Semiparametric models for longitudinal data with application to CD4 cell numbers in HIV seroconverters. *Biometrics*. 1994;50(3):689-699.
8. Li S, Zhu Y, Yeung E, et al. Offspring risk of obesity in childhood, adolescence and adulthood in relation to gestational diabetes mellitus: a sex-specific association. *Int J Epidemiol*. 2017;46:1533-1541.
9. Elliot P, Wakefield JC, Best NG, Briggs DJ. *Spatial Epidemiology: Methods and Applications*. Oxford, UK: Oxford University Press; 2000.
10. Miglioretti DL, Heagerty PJ. Marginal modeling of nonnested multilevel data using standard software. *Am J Epidemiology*. 2007;165:453-463.
11. Luke DA. *Multilevel Modeling*. Los Angeles: SAGE Publications Inc.; 2019.
12. Arterburn DE, Johnson E, Coleman KJ, et al. Weight outcomes of sleeve gastrectomy and gastric bypass compared to nonsurgical treatment [published online ahead of print September 28, 2020]. *Ann Surg*. 2020.
13. Diez-Roux AV. A glossary for multilevel analysis. *J Epidemiol Community Health*. 2002;56(8):588-594.
14. Snijders TA. Power and sample size in multilevel linear models. In: Everitt BS, Howell DC, eds. *Encyclopedia of Statistics in Behavioral Science*. Hoboken, NJ: Wiley; 2005.
15. Rutterford C, Copas A, Eldridge S. Methods for sample size determination in cluster randomized trials. *Int J Epidemiol*. 2015;44:1051-1067.
16. Schwartz J. The distributed lag between air pollution and daily deaths. *Epidemiology*. 2000;11:320-326.
17. Samet JM, Zeger SL, Dominici F, et al. The national morbidity, mortality, and air pollution study. Part II: morbidity and mortality from air pollution in the United States. *Res Rep Health Eff Inst*. 2000;94:5-79.
18. Welty LJ, Zeger SL. Are the acute effects of particulate matter on mortality in the National Morbidity, Mortality, and Air Pollution Study the result of inadequate control for weather and season? A sensitivity analysis using flexible distributed lag models. *Am J Epidemiol*. 2005;162:80-88.
19. Pepe M, Anderson GL. A cautionary note on inference for marginal regression models with longitudinal data and general correlated response data. *Commun Stat Simul Comput*. 1994;23:939-951.
20. Prentice RL, Zhao LP. Estimating equations for parameters in means and covariances of multivariate discrete and continuous responses. *Biometrics*. 1991;47(3):825-839.
21. Mancl LA, Derouen TA. A covariance estimator for GEE with improved small-sample properties. *Biometrics*. 2001;57:126-134.
22. Pan W, Wall MM. Small-sample adjustments in using the sandwich variance estimator in generalized estimating equations. *Stat Med*. 2002;21:1429-1441.
23. Li P, Redden DT. Small sample performance of bias-corrected sandwich estimators for cluster-randomized trials with binary outcomes. *Stat Med*. 2015;34:281-296.
24. Kauermann G, Carroll RJ. A note on the efficiency of sandwich covariance matrix estimation. *J Am Stat Assoc*. 2001;96:1387-1396.
25. Fay MP, Graubard BI. Small-sample adjustments for Wald-type tests using sandwich estimators. *Biometrics*. 2001;57:1198-1206.
26. Lu B, Preisser JS, Qaqish BF, Suchindran C, Bangdiwala SI, Wolfson M. A comparison of two bias-corrected covariance estimators for generalized estimating equations. *Biometrics*. 2007;63:935-941.
27. Fan C, Zhang D, Zhang CH. A comparison of bias-corrected covariance estimators for generalized estimating equations. *J Biopharm Stat*. 2013;23:1172-1187.
28. Self SG, Liang KY. Asymptotic properties of maximum likelihood estimators and likelihood ratio tests under nonstandard conditions. *J Am Stat Assoc*. 1987;82:605-610.
29. Haneuse S, Dominici F, Normand SL, Schrag D. Assessment of between-hospital variation in readmission and mortality after cancer surgical procedures. *JAMA Netw Open*. 2018;1(6):e183038.
30. Normand SLT, Ash AS, Fienberg SE, Stukel TA, Utts J, Louis TA. League tables for hospital comparisons. *Annu Rev Stat Appl*. 2016;3:21-50.
31. Casella G. An introduction to empirical Bayes data analysis. *Am Stat*. 1985;39:83-87.
32. Ten Have TR, Localio AR. Empirical Bayes estimation of random effects parameters in mixed effects logistic regression models. *Biometrics*. 1999;55:1022-1029.

33. Mcculloch CE, Neuhaus JM. Misspecifying the shape of a random effects distribution: why getting it wrong may not matter. *Stat Sci.* 2011;26(3):388-402.

34. Laird N. Nonparametric maximum likelihood estimation of a mixing distribution. *J Am Stat Assoc.* 1978;73:805-811.

35. Zhang D, Davidian M. Linear mixed models with flexible distributions of random effects for longitudinal data. *Biometrics.* 2001;57:795-802.

36. Agresti A, Caffo B, Ohman-Strickland P. Examples in which misspecification of a random effects distribution reduces efficiency, and possible remedies. *Comput Stat Data Anal.* 2004;47:639-653.

37. Magder LS, Zeger SL. A smooth nonparametric estimate of a mixing distribution using mixtures of Gaussians. *J Am Stat Assoc.* 1996;91:1141-1151.

38. Piepho HP, Mcculloch CE. Transformations in mixed models: application to risk analysis for a multienvironment trial. *J Agric Biol Environ Stat.* 2004;9:123-137.

39. Caffo B, An MW, Rohde C. Flexible random intercept models for binary outcomes using mixtures of normals. *Comput Stat Data Anal.* 2007;51(11):5220-5235.

40. Dey DD, Müiler P, Sinha D. *Practical Nonparametric and Semiparametric Bayesian Statistics.* New York, NY: Springer Science & Business Media; 2012.

41. Antonelli J, Trippa L, Haneuse S. Mitigating bias in generalized linear mixed models: the case for Bayesian nonparametrics. *Stat Sci.* 2016;31:80.

CHAPTER 25

Causal Inference With Time-Varying Exposures

Tyler J. VanderWeele

INTRODUCTION

This chapter will provide an introduction to the methodology concerning causal inference for longitudinal data with exposures that may vary over time. Causal inference from observational data poses challenges, but these are compounded when what is being studied is an exposure that can change over time.[1-6] Central to the complexities involved is the potential for feedback, that is to say, the possibility that the outcome under study, or something related to it, itself affects subsequent values of the exposure, in addition to the exposure affecting the outcome. When causal influence in both directions is possible, it becomes even more difficult to assess causality and causal effects.

As an example of the complications that can arise, we will discuss research on the relationship between religious service attendance and depression. Dozens of studies have found that service attendance is correlated with lower rates of depression.[7] This is sometimes interpreted as that service attendance itself protects against depression. The majority of such studies, however, have been carried out with cross-sectional data[7] with all variables measured at the same period of time. Recent work, moreover, suggests that those who become depressed tend to be more likely to stop attending religious services.[8] If this is so, the inverse association between religious service attendance and depression could potentially arise not because attendance protects against depression but simply because those who are depressed stop attending services.[8,9] Cross-sectional data cannot distinguish the direction of the causal relation. For that, we need longitudinal data and multiple measurements of both service attendance and depression over time.

In the example of attendance and depression, it is also possible that effects are present in both directions, that is to say, that there is feedback.[9-11] Again the only way to assess this issue is with multiple measurements over time of both depression and attendance. These questions illustrate the challenges in studying the effect of exposures that vary over time. The present chapter will discuss methodology appropriate to the setting of such time-varying exposures when interest lies in assessing causal effects. We will discuss some of the analytic challenges of assessing causal effects for time-varying exposures and will discuss what is and is not possible with standard regression techniques when assessing causal effects.[4,12] We will further discuss classes of causal models—marginal structural models, structural nested models, and parametric g-formula approaches—that can address a broader range of causal effects with time-varying exposures.[4,5,13]

TIME-VARYING EXPOSURES AND CAUSAL INFERENCE

Suppose we have some exposure X (*e.g.*, religious service attendance) and some outcome of interest Y (*e.g.*, depressive symptoms) measured at the end of follow-up. Let Z denote a set of covariates measured at baseline. Suppose we have repeated measurements of the exposure over time; let X_k denote the exposure at follow-up time k. Suppose that other variables L might confound the relationship between the exposure and the outcome and that these too can change over time. Let L_k denote values of these potential time-varying confounders at follow-up time k. The relationships among the variables are depicted in Figure 25-1. Note that the figure here does not depict a linear structural equation model but instead simply illustrates the structural relationships among the variables.

The time-varying confounders L might also include intermediate values of our outcome (*e.g.*, intermediate values of depressive symptoms before the end of follow-up). We can then see from the figure the potential for feedback. For example, service attendance X_1 at time 1 may affect depressive symptoms at time 2, L_2, which may in turn subsequently affect service attendance at time 3, X_3, etc. Such feedback complicates the assessment of causal effects. The difficulties arise when an intermediate variable is on the pathway from prior exposure to the outcome and also confounds the effect of subsequent exposure on the outcome. Depressive symptoms at time 2 could be such a variable. For example, depressive symptoms at follow-up 2 (denoted by L_2) are potentially on the pathway from attendance at follow-up 1 (denoted by X_1) to final depressive symptoms at the end of follow-up (denoted by Y). But depressive symptoms at follow-up 2 (L_2) may also confound the relationship between attendance at follow-up 3 (denoted by X_3) and final depressive symptoms, Y.

In this setting, problems arise if we are trying to assess the joint effects of attendance at follow-up visits 1, 2, and 3 and we try to apply standard regression techniques. If the joint effect of attendance at follow-up visits 1, 2, and 3 is of interest, then we must consider whether to make adjustment for intermediate depressive symptoms at time 2. If an adjustment is made for depressive symptoms at follow-up 2, that adjustment will block some of the effect of attendance at follow-up 1 on final depressive symptoms Y because depressive symptoms at time 2 are on the causal pathway. But if adjustment is not made for depressive symptoms at follow-up 2, then the effect of attendance at follow-up 3 on final depressive symptoms Y will be biased because depressive symptoms at follow-up 2 may confound the relationship between attendance at follow-up 3 and final depressive symptoms Y. The regression analysis would thus be biased, regardless of whether adjustment is made for depressive symptoms at time 2. This problem will arise whenever there is a time-varying variable that is on the pathway from prior exposure to the outcome and also confounds the relationship between subsequent exposure and the outcome.[4] The issue is sometimes referred to as "time-dependent confounding," because one of the confounders is temporally subsequent to, and on the pathway from, the exposure. The problem is common whenever we are studying exposures that vary over time. It is one of the issues that make assessing causal effect of time-varying exposures challenging.

Although standard regression techniques generally fail when we attempt to examine the joint effects of an exposure over time, some causal questions can be assessed with a time-varying exposure using standard regression techniques. We will discuss these in the next section. Later in the chapter, we will also consider causal models, including marginal structural models and others, that allow for estimating broader classes of causal effects.

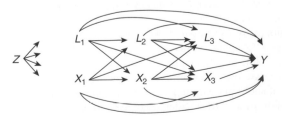

FIGURE 25-1 Causal diagram illustrating effects of time-varying exposures (X_1, X_2, X_3) on outcome Y with time-dependent confounders (L_1, L_2, L_3) and time-fixed confounder Z.

STANDARD REGRESSION APPROACHES AND CAUSAL INFERENCE WITH TIME-VARYING EXPOSURES

In the previous section, we discussed how standard regression techniques would fail if we were interested in studying the joint effects of an exposure that changes over time. However, if instead we are interested simply in assessing the extent to which the exposure measured at one time affects the outcome, this relation can be assessed with standard regression techniques. Suppose that we are interested in the effect of X_2 on Y, and suppose again that our exposure (*e.g.*, service attendance) changes over time. Also, suppose that we focus our inquiry on the extent to which the exposure at follow-up 2, X_2, affects outcome Y. In this case, from the rules governing (see Chapter 3),[14] we would see that if we controlled for prior attendance, X_1, prior depressive symptoms, L_1, and the baseline covariates Z, then these steps would suffice to control for confounding of the effect of X_2 on Y. We could then assess the effect of exposure at follow-up 2, X_2, on outcome Y using standard regression-based methods. Thus, some causal effects are accessible to standard regression analysis even when exposures do vary over time. It is only when we are interested in the joint effects of a time-varying exposure over time that the complexities discussed in the previous section arise.

However, with a time-varying exposure, even if we are only interested in assessing the effect of an exposure at one particular time, we still must be careful in thinking about covariate control. We noted above that to control for confounding of the effect of exposure at time 2 on the depressive symptoms outcome Y, we needed also to control for the depressive symptoms at the previous time, L_1. Otherwise, prior depressive symptoms L_1 could induce bias as this affect both the exposure at time 2 and later depressive symptom outcomes. In other words, if we did not control for the outcome (*e.g.*, depressive symptoms) at time 1, association between exposure at time 2 and outcome Y could be confounded by the earlier depressive symptoms, due to "reverse causation." In the context of the service attendance example, an association between attendance X_2 and depression Y could be explained entirely or in part because prior depression (L_1) leads people to cease attending (X_2) and also results in subsequent depression (Y). Thus, in the context of assessing causal effects, even when studying the effect of an exposure at a single point in time, it is important to control for the prior values of the outcome to try to rule out reverse causation. Exceptions can arise when there is considerable measurement error,[15] and if the effect of prior outcome on subsequent exposure is weak, but generally control for prior outcome will be important if it has a strong effect on subsequent exposure.

We also noted above that to assess the effect of exposure X_2 on outcome Y in Figure 25-1, control should also be made for the prior value of the exposure, X_1. This is because if prior exposure X_1 affects subsequent exposure X_2, and also independently affects the outcome Y not through X_2, then prior exposure X_1 itself confounds the effect of subsequent exposure X_1 on outcome Y. Intuitively, if we are interested in assessing only the effect of exposure at time 2 on outcome Y and we do not control for the exposure at time 1, then the associations between X_2 and Y will reflect not only the potential effect of X_2 on Y, but also some of the independent effect of X_1 on Y that is captured by X_2 serving as a proxy for X_1. When control is made for prior exposure, it is sometimes said that one assesses the effects of "incident exposure" or current exposure rather than "prevalent exposure" (see Danaei et al.[16] and Hernán[17]). Because of the potential for reverse causation, and other issues, "prevalent exposure" analyses are often subject to a broader range of biases than "incident exposure" analyses. See Danaei et al.[16] and Hernán[17] for further discussion.

A few additional comments merit attention. First, the need to control for prior exposure is only relevant if that prior exposure affects the outcome independently of current exposure. For example, if only the most recent exposure affected subsequent depressive symptoms so that there were arrows from X_1 to L_2, but no direct arrows from X_1 to L_3 or Y, as in Figure 25-2, then control for X_1 would not be necessary. In Figure 25-2, control for L_1 and Z alone and also L_2 would suffice to control for confounding for the effect of X_2 on Y. Note, however, that even here we must still control for L_2 in addition to L_1 to control for confounding. However, control for prior exposure is only absolutely needed when the prior exposure can affect the outcome through pathways independent of subsequent exposure and the confounders.

We have discussed the need, when using regression analyses to assess the effect of an exposure at a given time, of controlling for prior outcome and prior exposure. But how far back does this extend? If the exposure and outcome are varying over time, do we also need to control for the

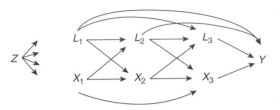

FIGURE 25-2 Causal diagram illustrating effects of time-varying exposures (X_1, X_2, X_3) on outcome Y with time-dependent confounders (L_1, L_2, L_3) and time-fixed confounder Z, with only most recent exposure X_t affecting subsequent time-dependent confounder L_{t+1}.

outcome two periods back? The answer to this question depends upon how far back the outcome affects subsequent exposure independent of other intervening intermediate outcome measures and how far back the exposure affects the subsequent outcome independent of the intervening exposure measures. Suppose we were interested in assessing the effect of exposure X_3 on the outcome Y. In Figure 25-1, if all of the arrows present on the diagram did indeed reflect direct effects that were present, then to estimate the magnitude of the effect of X_3 on Y, we would indeed need to control for not just prior exposure and outcome X_2 and L_2, but for the exposure and outcome the period before that, *i.e.*, for X_1 and L_1. For example, if control was not made for L_1, and if L_1 had an effect on X_3, independent of L_2 and X_2, and also had an effect on Y independent of L_2, X_2, L_3, and X_3, then it would confound the relationship between X_3 and Y. If, however, as in Figure 25-2, L_1 does not affect X_3 independent of X_2 and L_2, then control for X_1 and L_1 here would not be necessary. To estimate the effect of X_3 on Y, control for baseline covariates Z and X_2 and L_2 alone would be sufficient. Thus, the extent to which we must use earlier data depends on how far back we must go to control adequately for confounding of the effect of current exposure. That in turn depends on how strong the effect of the prior exposure is on subsequent outcome, and the effect of the prior outcome is on subsequent exposure, independent of intervening exposures and outcomes. Unless we expect these independent lagged effects (*i.e.*, effects of past exposure not through more recent exposure) to be substantial, control for the immediately prior exposure and prior outcome should suffice, but it may in practice be good to assess this assumption by comparing results with and without inclusion of the additional lagged exposures and outcomes. In any case, control for the immediately prior exposure and outcome will usually be important in the control for confounding of the effect of an exposure at a single period of time.

The considerations above apply to regression analyses with a single outcome at the end of follow-up, but they apply also to various repeated outcome analyses and to time-to-event analyses as well. Sometimes, in these settings, if time-varying exposures are measured, covariate values are updated over time as well. As discussed above and elsewhere,[4,5] using updated values of the covariates can be problematic in the study of causal effects if these covariate values are themselves affected by prior exposure. However, if what is in view is just the effect of current exposure on the outcome, then updating the covariates over time and also controlling for time-updated prior exposure and outcome can still yield valid estimates of the effect of current exposure on the outcome. Thus, for example, a proportional hazards model that controls for time-updated covariates and also prior exposure and outcome can give valid estimates of a causal hazard ratio relating current exposure to the outcome. See Koegh et al.[12] for further discussion. It is only when the joint effects of a time-varying exposure over time are of interest that standard regression methods cannot be used and the causal models described below are necessary. As emphasized in this section, however, when standard regression models are used to assess the effects, in many situations it will be important to control for prior outcome and exposure.

HIERARCHY OF ROBUSTNESS TO CONFOUNDING ACROSS STUDY DESIGNS

A hierarchy of robustness to confounding from different study designs for assessing causality might thus be formulated. In general, cross-sectional designs and analyses will be least robust to confounding unless a clear argument can be made for the temporal ordering of the exposure preceding the outcome and control can be made for confounding variables that likewise temporally precede the exposure and outcome. Second, designs in which the exposure clearly precedes the outcome and in which control can be made for a rich set of baseline covariates that potentially confound the relationship between the exposure and the outcome may be somewhat more robust. Third, if control can also be made for prior measures of the outcome, it strengthens the evidence further as prior levels of the outcome may often be the strongest confounders for the relationship between the current exposure and subsequent outcome. Fourth, if control can also be made for prior exposure, it strengthens the evidence yet further. Fifth, as we will discuss in the next section of the chapter, designs in which both the exposure and the outcome are assessed repeatedly and for which analyses assess the effects of the time-varying exposures contribute yet further evidence. Sixth, a randomized trial of the exposure generally provides, at least in the absence of complications such as noncompliance and drop-out, the greatest robustness to potential uncontrolled confounding.

There are of course some ambiguities across levels. Even in a cross-sectional design, as perhaps obtained in a survey, if the exposure of interest is assessed retrospectively in childhood and the outcomes are assessed at the time the survey is taken, the temporal ordering between exposure and outcome may be clear, and if confounding variables are likewise assessed in childhood, then such a design approximates what we have described as the second level. Furthermore, analyses of the exposure at a single point in time that control for multiple values of past outcome and past exposure are similar in the evidence that they contribute toward establishing causality as those which explicitly model the joint effects of time-varying exposures controlling for the entire past, creating ambiguity between levels 4 and 5 above. Finally, although randomized trials are often considered the "gold standard" for assessing causality, in practice, investigators often face issues of noncompliance and drop-out, in which case the results from a trial may not be an improvement over the evidence that is available from observational data. These subtleties must all be taken into account in assessing evidence for robustness to confounding. Moreover, evidence for a causal relationship depends, of course, not only on robustness to confounding but also on the details of the design, the size of the study, the magnitude of the effect estimate, the richness of the covariate data, and the possibility of other biases such as measurement error and selection bias. Furthermore, sensitivity analysis to assess how strong unmeasured confounding, or measurement error, or selection bias must be to explain away the effect estimate is also important in assessing the strength of evidence (see Chapters 12 and 29).[18-20] Nevertheless, questions of temporality in study design and controlling for prior values of outcome and exposure ought also be given considerable weight in assessing evidence for causality. Keeping this hierarchy with regard to robustness to confounding in mind can be helpful in assessing one aspect of the evidence for causality and in thinking about design and analysis choices.

INTRODUCTION TO MARGINAL STRUCTURAL MODELS

Although standard regression methods can be used to assess some causal effects in the presence of a time-varying exposure, they cannot be used to address all such effects. If we are interested in the joint effects of X_1, X_2, and X_3 on the outcome Y, then standard regression methods can fail, as noted above. Likewise, if we are interested in studying whether exposure X_2 has an independent effect on Y not through subsequent exposure X_3, this too is a question for which standard regression methods often do not suffice.

One class of models that has gained considerable popularity in epidemiology and to some extent in the social sciences, due to its ability to assess joint effects of time-varying exposures and due to its relative ease of use, is marginal structural models, introduced by Robins.[3,4] Marginal structural models are models for the counterfactual outcome[13,21,22] under hypothetical interventions on the exposure. For example, consider the effects of hypothetical interventions on exposure at follow-up visits 1, 2, and 3 on the final outcome Y. The models predict the expected outcomes, possibly conditional on baseline covariates Z, had there been interventions on the exposure at follow-up visits 1, 2, and 3 to fix these values. The model on a linear scale would then take the form:

$$E\left[Y_{x_1 x_2 x_3} \mid Z = z\right] = \mu + \gamma z + \beta_1 x_1 + \beta_2 x_2 + \beta_3 x_3$$

where $Y_{x_1 x_2 x_3}$ is the outcome at the end of follow-up for an individual that would have resulted under hypothetical joint interventions to set exposure at follow-up visits 1, 2, and 3 to levels x_1, x_2, and x_3, respectively, and where Z denotes one or more covariates at baseline. The variable $Y_{x_1 x_2 x_3}$

is sometimes referred to as a "counterfactual outcome" (see Chapter 3), as it is the outcome that would have resulted had the exposure at follow-up visits 1, 2, and 3, been set, possibly contrary to fact, to x_1, x_2, and x_3. In the model, the effects on the outcome of joint interventions on the exposure at follow-up visits 1, 2, and 3 are β_1, β_2, and β_3 respectively. The coefficient β_2 is the effect of X_2 on Y not through X_3, and the coefficient β_1 is the effect of X_1 on Y not through X_2 or X_3.

For a causal interpretation of estimates, marginal structural models, like traditional regression analyses or growth curve models or structural equation models, make certain "no unmeasured confounding" assumptions. These assumptions essentially state that the groups receiving different exposure levels are, within strata of the past measured variables, comparable with one another in all ways related to the outcome. For regression analyses using an exposure at a single period of time and a single outcome at the end of follow-up, the assumption is straightforward, but can of course be challenging to satisfy in practice. It would hold if the exposure were randomized. In an observational study, control is made for covariates thought to affect both the exposure and the outcome (see Chapter 12). In the context of assessing causal effects of a time-varying exposure, the assumption of no unmeasured confounding needs to be made repeatedly over time. Specifically, one must assume that at each period k, the baseline covariates and the history of the time-varying covariates and exposures up through time $k-1$ suffice to control for confounding of the effect of the exposure, at time k, on the final outcome. This condition would hold under the causal diagram in Figure 25-1. It would also hold if there were an underlying latent variable U in Figure 25-1 that affected all the time-varying variables L_1, L_2, and L_3, even if no control was made for U. It would fail, however, if that unmeasured variable U also affected any of the exposures X_1, X_2, and X_3; in such a case, the effects of the exposures would not be unconfounded unless one also controlled for U.

Even if we make the confounding assumptions above, traditional regression methods do not permit the assessment of the joint effects of a time-varying exposure, but, under the no unmeasured confounding assumptions above, one can assess the joint effects by fitting a marginal structural model using a weighting technique. The weighting method is to weight observations by the inverse of the probability of exposure. Doing so controls effectively for confounding, not through regression adjustment but by reweighting of the data to negate the confounding that is present. This weighting approach has been used in survey sampling for decades[23] but was more recently extended to the context of longitudinal data and time-varying exposures.[4] The weighting technique is analogous to the dynamic use of propensity scores (see Chapter 21).[24] The weights are calculated as the inverse of the probability of having the exposure level that was in fact present, conditional on past covariate history. The overall weight for each subject is computed by taking the product of the weights at each period in time. Thus, the final weight for an individual i at the end of follow-up T is given by:

$$W = \prod_{k=1}^{T} \frac{1}{\Pr\left(X_k = x_k^i \mid X_1 = x_1^i, \ldots, X_{k-1} = x_{k-1}^i, Z = z^i, L_1 = l_1^i, \ldots, L_{k-1} = l_{k-1}^i\right)}$$

where x_k^i is the actual exposure for an individual i at time k, z^i is the actual baseline covariate values for the individual i, and l_k^i are the actual time-varying covariate values for the individual i at time k. For binary exposures, each of the probabilities

$$\Pr\left(X_k = x_k^i \mid X_1 = x_1^i, \ldots, X_{k-1} = x_{k-1}^i, Z = z^i, L_1 = l_1^i, \ldots, L_{k-1} = l_{k-1}^i\right)$$

is generally obtained by logistic regression and then, to obtain the weight for an individual, one obtains from the logistic regression predicted probabilities for each individual using their covariate and exposure values. Importantly, by using a different weight for each time, the task of confounding control can be achieved for each point in time for which different measurements are available. Thus for the weight for X_3, one can adjust for L_2, whereas for the weight for the exposure X_1, one does not adjust for L_2, thereby circumventing the problems with regression-based approaches. For continuous exposures, the probabilities are replaced by probability density functions. See also Robins et al.[4] for further details.

The marginal structural model for the expected counterfactual outcomes conditional on baseline covariates is then fit by regressing the observed outcome on the exposures at each time period, in a model where each subject is weighted by the inverse-probability-of-treatment weights described above. The weighting controls for the confounding by balancing the time-varying covariates at each time point. Robust variance estimation is used for standard errors to account for sampling error in the estimation of the weights.[4] This weighting technique will give consistent estimates of the parameters of the marginal structural model provided control has been made, at each exposure period, for confounding given the past exposure and covariates. Whether the weighting successfully balances the time-varying covariates across levels of exposure can also be examined empirically.[25] If the outcome is binary, a similar logistic marginal structural model can be fit. All steps described above are the same, except that the final weighted linear regression model is replaced by a weighted logistic regression model.

Weighting techniques can lead to imprecise estimates; one can improve the precision of estimates by reducing the variability of weights using what are sometimes referred to as "stabilized weights."[4] Stabilized weights are given by:

$$W = \prod_{k=1}^{T} \frac{\Pr\left(X_k = x_k^i \middle| X_1 = x_1^i, \ldots, X_{k-1} = x_{k-1}^i, Z = z^i\right)}{\Pr\left(X_k = x_k^i \middle| X_1 = x_1^i, \ldots, X_{k-1} = x_{k-1}^i, Z = z^i, L_1 = l_1^i, \ldots, L_{k-1} = l_{k-1}^i\right)}$$

where the denominator of the weight is the same as before but the numerator of the weight is the probability that individuals had the exposure that they in fact did have, conditional on their past exposure history and their baseline covariates (but not their past time-varying covariate history). The numerator probabilities can likewise be obtained by logistic regression. The use of such stabilized weights tends to perform better in practice. It is especially important in the context of continuous exposures.[4] Extreme weights are sometimes also trimmed at the 1st and 99th percentile of the weight distribution say (cf. Cole and Hernán[26]) to make estimates of the causal effects more stable.

Marginal structural models can also be used to assess moderation by baseline covariates of the effects of the exposures on the outcome. They can also be fit to nonlinear models.[4] They can be used to assess possible interaction between the effects of exposure at different times and to assess the extent to which the exposure, *e.g.*, at time 2, has an effect on the final outcome Y, independent of exposure at time 3 or subsequent times.

Marginal structural models can also be extended to settings with effects on repeated outcome measurements over time[27] or to settings with time-to-event outcomes.[28] They can also be used to address issues of censoring and loss to follow-up over time. The marginal structural model approach tends to work better when exposures are binary or categorical and is less stable when exposures are continuous. Other types of causal models, such as structural mean models, which are considered below, are generally preferable when exposures are continuous. Other discussions are also given elsewhere.[5,27,28]

FURTHER EXTENSIONS TO MARGINAL STRUCTURAL MODELS

With repeated outcome measurements, the marginal structural model approach can be extended to fit a repeated measures marginal structural model. We will consider a simple example here of a repeated measures marginal structural model using outcomes at two different follow-up periods, *e.g.*, follow-up 3 and 4. The repeated measures marginal structural model[27] effectively combines analyses in which the effect of exposure at follow-up visits 2 and 3 on the outcome at follow-up 4 is simultaneously assessed with the effect of the exposure at follow-up visits 1 and 2 on the outcome at follow-up 3. In this model, it is assumed that the outcome depends only on the values of the exposure at the previous two periods. The model takes the form:

$$E\left[Y_{x_{t-1}x_{t-2}}(t)\middle| Z = z\right] = \mu + \lambda t + \gamma z + \beta_1 x_{t-1} + \beta_2 x_{t-2}$$

for $t = 3$ and $t = 4$, where $Y_{x_{t-1}x_{t-2}}(t)$ is the outcome at follow-up t for an individual that would have resulted under hypothetical joint interventions to set the exposure at follow-up visits $t-1$ and $t-2$ to levels x_{t-1} and x_{t-2}, respectively, and where Z denotes baseline covariates. In the model, the effects of the outcome at time t of joint interventions on the exposure at follow-up visits $t-1$ and $t-2$ are β_1 and β_2, respectively, for a one point change in the exposure.

The parameters of the model can be estimated by fitting a weighted conditional repeated measures model (see Chapter 24) with time-varying weights. The conditional repeated measures model is:

$$E\left[Y(t)|Z = z, X_{t-1} = x_{t-1}, X_{t-2} = x_{t-2}\right] = \mu + \lambda t + \gamma z + \beta_1 x_{t-1} + \beta_2 x_{t-2}$$

where $Y(t)$ is the observed depressive symptoms at follow-up visit t. The weights for visit t are given by the stabilized weights[27]:

$$W(t) = \prod_{k=1}^{t} \frac{\Pr\left(X_k = x_k^i \middle| X_1 = x_1^i, \ldots, X_{k-1} = x_{k-1}^i, Z = z^i\right)}{\Pr\left(X_k = x_k^i \middle| X_1 = x_1^i, \ldots, X_{k-1} = x_{k-1}^i, Z = z^i, L_1 = l_1^i, \ldots, L_{k-1} = l_{k-1}^i\right)}$$

where Z denotes the baseline values of the covariates and $L_1, \ldots, L_{k-1}$ denote the history of the time-varying covariates up through follow-up visit $k-1$. The distributions, $\Pr(x_k | x_1, \ldots, x_{k-1}, z)$ and $\Pr(x_k | x_1, \ldots, x_{k-1}, z, l_1, \ldots, l_{k-1})$, are often modeled using logistic regression if the exposures are binary or using multinomial regression if they are categorical. For continuous exposures, the density function must be modeled.[4] In general, however, marginal structural models and weighting techniques are often less stable with continuous exposures. In the next section, we describe an alternative class of causal models that often perform better with continuous exposures.

The estimates obtained from the weighting procedure described above will have a causal interpretation as the parameters of the marginal structural model under the assumption that the effect of the exposure at each follow-up visit k on the outcome at subsequent times is unconfounded, conditional on the baseline covariates, the history of the time-varying covariates up through follow-up visit $k-1$, and the history of the exposure up through follow-up visit $k-1$. See Hernán et al.[27] for further details on the repeated measures of marginal structural model. The marginal structural model approach can also be extended to time-to-event outcomes. See Hernán et al.[28] for details.

Analyses can also take into account censoring and missingness using an inverse-probability-of-censoring technique. At each time-point, indicators for censoring and missingness are regressed on baseline covariates and on prior history of each of the time-varying covariates. Adjustment for missingness and censoring is made by weighting each subject by the inverse-probability-of-censoring weight[4] defined as the product at each time of the probabilities of being uncensored at that time, conditional on baseline covariates, past exposure history, and past time-varying covariate history. The weight given to each subject in the final marginal structural model analysis is then the product of the inverse-probability-of-treatment-weight and the inverse-probability-of-censoring weight. The adjustment for missingness/censoring assumes that conditional on the baseline covariates and past exposure and time-varying covariates, missingness is not predictive of what an individual's outcome would have been under interventions on the exposure. Under this assumption and assuming that at each time period, the baseline covariates and the prior history of the time-varying covariates suffice to control for confounding of the effect of the exposure at each period on the final outcome, this inverse-probability-of-treatment-and-censoring weighting technique will give consistent estimates of the parameters of the marginal structural model.[4,27]

Some of the modeling described here could potentially also be attempted using a structural equation model. While possible, the modeling and confounding assumptions required to address these questions with a structural equation model are considerably stronger than for a marginal structural model. For example, to address the joint effects of the exposures over time on the outcome with structural equation models requires modeling each of the time-varying variables at each point in time, each of the exposures, and the outcome, as a function of the past. In contrast, the marginal structural model technique described above only requires modeling the exposure at follow-ups 1, 2, and 3 and the outcome at follow-up 4. Thus distributional and functional form assumptions (e.g., normality and linearity) are made for far fewer variables in the marginal structural model approach as contrasted with the structural equation model approach (cf. VanderWeele and VanderWeele et al.)[29,30] Other more subtle biases to which simple regression adjustment and structural equation modeling techniques are subject can also be addressed with marginal structural models.[31,32]

STRUCTURAL MEAN MODELS

In this section, we will briefly describe an alternative analytic approach and model for assessing the joint causal effects of a time-varying exposure, sometimes referred to as structural nested models, a special subclass of which is structural mean models. These models have been used extensively with time-to-event data. Unfortunately, the model fitting procedures are more complex with these models than with marginal structural models. See Hernán and Robins[5] and Vansteelandt and Sjolander[33] for recent overviews. Here we will consider one relatively straightforward approach that can be employed when estimating the joint effects of the exposure on the outcome over just two time periods, X_1 and X_2.

The confounding assumptions here will be the same as considered above. Specifically, it is assumed that at each period k, the baseline covariates and the history of the time-varying exposure and covariates up through time $k-1$ suffice to control for confounding of the effect of the exposure, at time k, on the final outcome. In the context of evaluating the effect of exposure at just two time periods, X_1 and X_2, we assume that conditional on baseline covariates Z, the effect of X_1 on Y, is unconfounded and that conditional on Z, X_1, and L_1, the effect of X_2 on Y, is unconfounded.

Consider a model for the counterfactual outcomes, in which, if desired, we allow for potential interaction between X_1 and X_2:

$$E\left(Y_{x_1 x_2} \middle| Z = z\right) = \beta_0 + \beta_1 x_1 + \beta_2 x_2 + \beta_3 x_1 x_2 + \beta_4' z$$

This model can then be fit, instead of by weighting, by using a two-stage regression approach.[34] In the first stage, we fit a regular linear regression model of Y on X_1, X_2, Z, and L_1, allowing for potential interaction between X_1 and X_2:

$$E\left(Y \middle| x_1, x_2, z, l\right) = \gamma_0 + \gamma_1 x_1 + \gamma_2 x_2 + \gamma_3 x_1 x_2 + \gamma_4' z + \gamma_5' l$$

We then use coefficient estimates of this regression model in two ways. First, we take the estimate of regression coefficient for the exposure X_2, γ_2, and the coefficient for the interaction, γ_3, as the estimates for β_2 and β_3 in the counterfactual mean model. Second, we take the coefficient estimates of γ_2 and γ_3, call them $\hat{\gamma}_2$ and $\hat{\gamma}_3$, and for each individual i, we calculate the following outcome residuals:

$$\hat{Y} = Y - \hat{\gamma}_2 x_2 - \hat{\gamma}_3 x_1 x_2$$

We then regress these residuals on the exposure X_1 and covariates Z:

$$E\left(\hat{Y} \middle| x_1, z\right) = \mu_0 + \mu_1 x_1 + \mu_2' z$$

We then take the estimate of μ_1 from this regression as our estimate of β_1 in the counterfactual mean model. Provided the confounding assumptions described above hold, this approach will provide consistent estimates for the parameters of the structural mean model.[34] Standard errors can be obtained by bootstrapping. Although the procedure is somewhat involved, it can be carried out using standard software and it tends to be more stable if the exposures under study are continuous rather than binary or categorical.

G-FORMULA AND PARAMETRIC G-FORMULA

The approaches described above using marginal structural models and structural mean models have come to be routinely used methods for assessing the effects of time-varying exposures. The marginal structural model approach, due to its relative straightforward implementation, has become especially popular. However, these tools were developed somewhat after the original theory for causal inference with time-varying exposures appeared. The initial theory of causal inference for time-varying exposures[1] instead gave formulas for the causal effects based on a generalization of standardization. This generalization is often referred to as the g-formula. Robins[1] showed that if, at each period k, the baseline covariates and the history of the time-varying covariates and exposures up through time $k-1$ suffice to control for confounding of the effect of the exposure, at time k, on the final outcome, then one could estimate the causal effects comparing two different exposure trajectories. Specifically, the effect comparing two exposure trajectories $(x_1,\ldots,x_T)$ and $(x'_1,\ldots,x'_T)$ (for example, for a binary exposure we might take $(x_1 = 1,\ldots,x_T = 1)$ and $(x'_1 = 0,\ldots,x'_T = 0)$) is then given by:

$$\sum_{l,z} E\left(Y\middle|x_1,\ldots,x_T,z,l_1,\ldots,l_T\right)\prod_{k=1}^{T}\Pr\left(l_k\middle|x_1,\ldots,x_{k-1},z,l_1,\ldots,l_{k-1}\right)\Pr(z)-$$

$$\sum_{l,z} E\left(Y\middle|x'_1,\ldots,x'_T,z,l_1,\ldots,l_T\right)\prod_{k=1}^{T}\Pr\left(l_k\middle|x'_1,\ldots,x'_{k-1},z,l_1,\ldots,l_{k-1}\right)\Pr(z)$$

These formulas are standardizations of the conditional expectation of the final outcome Y conditional on exposure history, baseline covariates, and time-varying covariate history, standardized by the probability of the time-varying and baseline covariates, conditional on the past values of these covariates and the past values of the exposure history. In the absence of time-varying covariates, the formula above simplifies to

$$\sum_{z} E\left(Y\middle|x_1,z\right)\Pr(z)-\sum_{z} E\left(Y\middle|x'_1,z\right)\Pr(z)$$

which is just the standardization discussed for causal effects for an exposure at a single point in time in Chapters 3 and 5. The g-formula is the generalization of this standardization for time-varying exposures.

In principle, with very large amounts of data, one could estimate each of the conditional expectations $E\left(Y\middle|x_1,\ldots,x_T,z,l_1,\ldots,l_T\right)$ and each of the probabilities $\Pr\left(l_k\middle|x_1,\ldots,x_{k-1},z,l_1,\ldots,l_{k-1}\right)$ by just taking sample averages. However, with a relatively lengthy covariate or exposure history, this approach would require a very large sample size to do accurately. An alternative strategy would be to use parametric models for the conditional expectation and for the covariate probabilities. The approach of using parametric models for the expectations and probabilities is sometimes referred to as the parametric g-formula. After fitting the parametric models with the data and using the g-formula to obtain estimates of causal effects, one can use bootstrapping to obtain standard errors and confidence intervals. While being intuitively attractive, the parametric g-formula approach was shown to suffer from certain theoretical problems. In particular, it can be shown that under certain specifications of the parametric models, when some of the variables are binary and some are continuous, it can be possible that the models are specified in such a way that it is impossible for the parametric g-formula to obtain an effect of zero when in fact the null of no effect is true. This problem is sometimes referred to as the g-null paradox. See Robins and Wasserman[35] and Robins and Hernán[5] for further discussion of this problem. For this reason, for some time, the use of parametric g-formula approaches had been avoided in the literature and it was in part this problem that motivated some of the developments described above concerning marginal structural models and structural mean models, which do not suffer from these problems.

More recently, the use of parametric g-formula approach has been re-evaluated. While the problem of the g-null paradox is relevant in theory, it has been suggested that the bias that results in practice may often be very small. Even if one cannot obtain an exact numerical estimate of zero under the null, one might get very close. Moreover, the problems of the g-null paradox may be attenuated further by using flexible parametric models for the conditional expectations and probabilities such as splines. The magnitude of bias implied by the g-null paradox may not be as substantial as was thought and, depending on the setting, may be large or small. For some further consideration of the g-null paradox using numerical examples, see Young and Tchetgen Tchetgen.[36] As a result of these considerations, the parametric g-formula approach has been used somewhat more frequently in recent years than in the past and macros have been developed for its implementation.[37,38]

EXAMPLES OF EFFECTS IN BOTH DIRECTIONS

In this section, we will illustrate the marginal structure model methodology for time-varying exposures using the example of religious service attendance and discussion that was mentioned in the Introduction section. Again, numerous studies have reported that service attendance is associated with lower depression. However, the majority of these studies have used cross-sectional data. Koenig et al.[7] report that of the studies on the association published since 2000, the cross-sectional studies outnumber those using longitudinal data by a ratio of 6:1. As noted in the Introduction section, using cross-sectional data to study this relation is problematic, because there is evidence also that depression leads to lower rates of service attendance.[8] Thus, even if there were no effect of service attendance on depression, one would find an inverse association with cross-sectional data simply because those who are depressed stop attending services.

There have, however, been studies of the association of service attendance and depression using longitudinal data, and some of these have also controlled for baseline depression.[39-42] These studies also have found association between service attendance and subsequent depression, even after controlling for baseline depression and various potential confounding variables. Such studies provide stronger evidence for a causal relationship. One study has controlled for prior exposure and has in fact used a marginal structural model analysis to assess the time-varying effects of religious service attendance on subsequent depression and also the effect of depression on subsequent service attendance.[10,11] We briefly present these results here to illustrate the methodology.

Li et al.[10] used data on 48,984 nurses from the Nurses' Health Study with repeated measures of service attendance and depression, beginning in 1992 and measured every 4 years. For the purpose of the analysis, depression was defined as self-reported or clinically diagnosed depression, or use of antidepressant medications, or depressive symptoms with a CESD-10 measure of above 10. They assessed the effects of service attendance in 1996 and 2000 on depression in 2004. Extensive health, demographic, and socioeconomic covariates at baseline in 1992 were controlled, as well as baseline depression in 1992 and baseline service attendance in 1992. Specifically, control was made for sociodemographic, social, lifestyle factors, smoking status, alcohol consumption, postmenopausal hormone use, and health/medical conditions and physical/functional limitations or disability. Covariate information was updated during the follow-up and controlled for as time-varying confounders. A marginal structural model was fit, using the techniques described above to assess the effects of service attendance in 1996 and 2000 on depression in 2004. Thus for the effect of exposure in 1996, adjustment was made for covariates in 1992, and for the effect of the exposure in 2000, adjustment was made for covariates in 1996. See Li et al.[10,11] for further details. Service attendance in 2000 more than once per week had an effect estimate odds ratio of 0.71 (95% CI: 0.62, 0.82) for depression in 2004 compared with those never attending and those attending weekly had an effect estimate odds ratio of 0.75 (95% CI: 0.67, 0.84). However, service attendance in 1996 did not seem to affect depression in 2004 above and beyond service attendance in 2000. It seemed as though only most recent service attendance was relevant.

Li et al. also examined the effects of depression on service attendance using a marginal structural model for the effects of depression in 1996 and 2000 on service attendance in 2004, controlling for baseline covariates in 1992 and updated in the marginal structural model. Those who were depressed in 2000 had an odds ratio 0.74 (95% CI: 0.68, 0.80) of attending services once per week or more in 2004 compared to those who were not depressed in 2000. Here, however, there was also evidence for an independent effect of depression in 1996 on service attendance in 2004 above and beyond that effect of depression in 2000 on attendance. Specifically, the direct effect of depression in 1996 on attendance in 2004, independent of depression in 2000, was to lower the odds of attendance by 0.91-fold (95% CI: 0.83, 1.00).

Using the marginal structural model analysis, there appeared to be evidence for an effect in both directions, of service attendance on subsequent depression and of depression on subsequent service attendance. In the case of the effect of depression on subsequent service attendance, it appeared that not only recent depression was relevant but also depression even 8 years earlier. It is this capacity to assess such joint effects and the direct effect of past exposure above and beyond present exposures that is one of the chief advantages of marginal structural models. As discussed above, regression-based methods are not adequate for such purposes because of the issue of time-dependent confounding. Marginal structural models get around this issue of time-dependent confounding and take into account potential feedback by carrying out confounding control through the weighting techniques described above. Such models can give considerable insight into the dynamics when feedback and effects in both directions are present.

With the depression example, the presence of effects in both direction means that cross-sectional data are essentially useless for assessing causation concerning effects of attendance on depression. However, the seemingly protective associations did hold up even in longitudinal analysis. This will not, however, always be the case. For example, using the same Nurses' Health study data but taking cross-sectional associations between religious service attendance and cardiovascular disease with all variables measured in 1992, there is a strong association with those attending more than once per week, at 0.61 (95% CI: 0.42-0.98) times lower odds for cardiovascular disease. With control of age, body mass index, smoking, alcohol, physical activity, diet quality, and social support, the association persists with an odds ratio of 0.64 (95% CI: 0.42-0.98). However, when using longitudinal data and controlling also for baseline cardiovascular disease and for baseline attendance, the association is greatly reduced (0.88, 95% CI: 0.74-1.03) (cf. Li et al.).[11] Likewise with a large cohort study and longitudinal study design, Schnall et al.[43] report essentially no association between attendance and incidence of cardiovascular disease. Thus, although numerous cross-sectional studies suggest an association between attendance and cardiovascular disease,[7] here, unlike in the depression example, the associations do not seem to hold up under more rigorous analyses for causal inference. One cannot generally assess causality using cross-sectional data unless a case can be made for temporal and causal ordering on other grounds or if exposures are recalled retrospective or do not change with time. Without actually carrying out the longitudinal analysis, it is impossible to distinguish between the scenario that characterized the depression example, when associations are robust to more rigorous designs, and the cardiovascular disease example, where associations were not robust.

CONCLUSION

In this chapter, we have reviewed some of the advances over the past 3 decades relating to causal inference with time-varying exposures. This is an area in which epidemiologic methods have expanded considerably and in which major contributions to the field have occurred, owing principally to the work of Robins and colleagues. While we can address certain questions about causal inference from time-varying exposures using traditional regression methods, there are many other questions for which these more modern methods are needed. This chapter has provided an introduction to these questions and the methods that apply. The literature on structural nested models and structural mean models is large and many more methods are available than have been considered here. Unfortunately, many of these methods are still difficult to implement with standard software, but some progress has been made. See Vansteelandt and Sjolander[33] for a recent overview. Likewise, the statistical methodology for marginal structural models has improved with so-called doubly robust and targeted maximum likelihood estimators of marginal structural model parameters now available. These estimators are more robust to model misspecification and more efficient.[44,45] Coverage of these approaches is beyond the scope of this chapter, but their application has become easier with newer software.[46] The statistical tools and conceptual frameworks now available to assess causal effects of time-varying exposures are now dramatically different and improved from the release of the first edition of this text in 1986, which was also the year that the seminal paper of Robins on the topic was published. The field has been transformed by this work. It is one of the central methodological achievements of modern epidemiology.

References

1. Robins JM. A new approach to causal inference in mortality studies with sustained exposure period–application to control of the healthy worker survivor effect. *Math Model*. 1986;7:1393-1512.
2. Robins JM. Addendum to a new approach to causal inference in mortality studies with sustained exposure period - application to control of the healthy worker survivor effect. *Comput Math Appl*. 1987;14:923-945.
3. Robins JM. Association, causation, and marginal structural models. *Synthese*. 1999;121:151-179.
4. Robins JM, Hernán MA, Brumback B. Marginal structural models and causal inference in epidemiology. *Epidemiology*. 2000;11:550-560.

5. Robins JM, Hernán MA. In: *Estimation of the Causal Effects of Time-Varying Exposures*. Fitzmaurice G, Davidian M, Verbeke G, Molenberghs G, eds. New York, NY: Chapman and Hall/CRC Press; 2009.
6. Robins JM. Marginal structural models versus structural nested models as tools for causal inference. In Halloran ME, Berry D, eds. *Statistical Models in Epidemiology: The Environment and Clinical Trials*. New York, NY: Springer-Verlag; 1999:95-134.
7. Koenig HG, King DE, Carson VB. *Handbook of Religion and Health*. 2nd ed. Oxford, New York: Oxford University Press; 2012.
8. Maselko J, Hayward RD, Hanlon A, Buka S, Meador K. Religious service attendance and major depression: a case of reverse causality? *Am J Epidemiol*. 2012;175(6):576-583.
9. VanderWeele TJ. "Religious service attendance and major depression: a case of reverse causality?" *Am J Epidemiol*. 2013;177(3):275-276.
10. Li S, Okereke OI, Chang SC, Kawachi I, VanderWeele TJ. Religious service attendance and lower depression among women–a prospective cohort study. *Ann Behav Med*. 2016;50(6):876-884.
11. Li S, Stamfer M, Williams DR, VanderWeele TJ. Association between religious service attendance and mortality among women. *JAMA Intern Med*. 2016;176(6):777-785.
12. Keogh RH, Daniel RM, VanderWeele TJ, Vansteelandt S. Analysis of longitudinal studies with repeated outcome measures: adjusting for time-dependent confounding using conventional methods. *Am J Epidemiol*. 2018;187(5):1085-1092.
13. Hernán MA, Robins JM. *Causal Inference*. Boca Raton: Chapman & Hall; 2021, forthcoming.
14. Pearl J. *Causality: Models, Reasoning, and Inference*. 2nd ed. Cambridge: Cambridge University Press; 2009.
15. Glymour MM, Weuve J, Berkman LF, Kawachi I, Robins JM. When is baseline adjustment useful in analyses of change? An example with education and cognitive change. *Am J Epidemiol*. 2005;162(3):267-278.
16. Danaei G, Tavakkoli M, Hernán MA. Bias in observational studies of prevalent users: lessons for comparative effectiveness research from a meta-analysis of statins. *Am J Epidemiol*. 2012;175(4):250-262.
17. Hernán MA. Epidemiology to guide decision-making: moving away from practice-free research. *Am J Epidemiol*. 2015;182(10):834-839.
18. Rosenbaum PR. *Observational Studies*. New York, NY: Springer-Verlag; 2002.
19. Lash TL, Fox MP, Fink AK. *Applying Quantitative Bias Analysis to Epidemiologic Data*. New York, NY: Springer; 2009.
20. Ding P, VanderWeele TJ. Sensitivity analysis without assumptions. *Epidemiology*. 2016;27(3):368-377.
21. Imbens G, Rubin DB. *Causal Inference in Statistics, Social, and Biomedical Sciences: An Introduction*. New York, NY: Cambridge University Press; 2015.
22. Morgan SL, Winship C. *Counterfactuals and Causal Inference*. 2nd ed. Cambridge, United Kingdom: Cambridge University Press; 2014.
23. Horvitz DG, Thompson DJ. A generalization of sampling without replacement from a finite universe. *J Am Stast Assoc*. 1952;47:663-685.
24. Rosenbaum PR, Rubin DB. The central role of the propensity score in observational studies for causal effects. *Biometrika*. 1983;70:41-55.
25. Jackson JW. Diagnostics for confounding of time-varying and other joint exposures. *Epidemiology*. 2016;27(6):859-869.
26. Cole SR, Hernán MA. Constructing inverse probability weights for marginal structural models. *Am J Epidemiol*. 2008;168:656-664.
27. Hernán MA, Brumback B, Robins JM. Estimating the causal effect of zidovudine on CD4 count with a marginal structural model for repeated measures. *Stat Med*. 2002;21:1689-1709.
28. VanderWeele TJ. Structural equation modeling in epidemiologic analysis. *Am J Epidemiol*. 2012;176:608-612.
29. Hernán MA, Brumback B, Robins JM. Marginal structural models to estimate the causal effect of zidovudine on the survival of HIV-positive men. *Epidemiology*. 2000;11:561-570.
30. VanderWeele TJ, Hawkley LC, Cacioppo JT. On the reciprocal relationship between loneliness and subjective well-being. *Am J Epidemiol*. 2012;176:777-784.
31. Barber JS, Murphy SA, Verbitsky N. Adjusting for time-varying confounding in survival analysis. *Sociol Methodol*. 2004;34:163-192.
32. Bray BC, Almirall D, Zimmerman RS, Lynam D, Murphy SA. Assessing the total effect of time-varying predictors in prevention research. *Prev Sci*. 2006;7:1-17.
33. Vansteelandt S, Sjolander A. Revisiting g-estimation of the effect of a time-varying exposure subject to time-varying confounding. *Epidemiologic Methods*. 2016;5(1):37-56.
34. Vansteelandt S. Estimating direct effects in cohort and case-control studies. *Epidemiology*. 2009;20:851-860.
35. Robins JM, Wasserman L. *Estimation of effects of sequential treatments by reparameterizing directed acyclic graphs*. In: *Proceedings of the Thirteenth Conference on Uncertainty in Artificial Intelligence*. San Francisco, CA: Morgan Kaufmann Publishers Inc.; 1997:409-420.

36. Young JG, Tchetgen Tchetgen EJ. Simulation from a known Cox MSM using standard parametric models for the g-formula. *Stat Med.* 2014;33(6):1001-1014.

37. Daniel RM, De Stavola BL, Cousens SN. Gformula: estimating causal effects in the presence of time-varying confounding or mediation using the g-computation formula. *Stata J.* 2011;11 (4):479-517.

38. HSPH. *Causal Inference Program.* 2020. Available at https://www.hsph.harvard.edu/causal/software/.

39. Strawbridge WJ, Shema SJ, Cohen RD, Kaplan GA. "Religious attendance increases survival by improving and maintaining good health behaviors, mental health, and social relationships." *Ann Behav Med.* 2001;23(1):68-74.

40. Van Voorhees BW, Paunesku D, Kuwabara SA, et al. Protective and vulnerability factors predicting new-onset depressive episode in a representative of U.S. adolescents. *J Adolesc Health.* 2008;42(6):605-616.

41. Norton MC, Singh A, Skoog I, et al. Church attendance and new episodes of major depression in a community study of older adults: the Cache County Study. *J Gerontol B Psychol Sci Soc Sci.* 2008;63(3):P129-P137.

42. Balbuena L, Baetz M, Bowen R. Religious attendance, spirituality, and major depression in Canada: a 14-year follow-up study. *Can J Psychiatry.* 2013;58:225-232.

43. Schnall E, Wassertheil-Smoller S, Swencionis C, et al. The relationship between religion and cardiovascular outcomes and all-cause mortality in the Women's Health Initiative Observational Study. *Psychol Health.* 2010;25(2):249-263.

44. Rosenblum M, van der Laan MJ. Targeted maximum likelihood estimation of the parameter of a marginal structural model. *Int J Biostat.* 2010;6(2):1557-4679. doi:10.2202/1557-4679.1238.

45. van der Laan MJ, Rose S. *Targeted Learning: Causal Inference for Observational and Experimental Data.* San Francisco, CA: Springer Science & Business Media; 2011.

46. Gruber S, van der Laan MJ. Tmle: an R package for targeted maximum likelihood estimation. *J Stat Softw.* 2012;51(13):1-35.

CHAPTER 26

Analysis of Interaction

Tyler J. VanderWeele, Timothy L. Lash, and Kenneth J. Rothman

$\mathbf{I}$t is common for the effect of one exposure on an outcome to depend in some way on the presence or absence of another exposure. When this is the case, we say that there is interaction between the two exposures. Recent years have seen increasing interest in interaction between genetic and environmental exposures, where environmental exposures are usually widely defined as anything outside the genome or its related biology. Interaction can also occur between two or more environmental or behavioral exposures or between two different genetic exposures or between other types of exposures. Drug-drug interactions, for example, are of growing interest in the topic area of pharmacovigilance, as are gene-drug interactions in the topic area of pharmacogenetics. Interactions between pollutants, between pollution and the built environment, or between lifestyle behaviors and the built environment are receiving substantial attention from environmental epidemiologists. In social epidemiology, research has recently emphasized intersectionality theory, which was originally developed to address the nonadditivity of effects of sex or gender with race or ethnicity,[1] and which has been extended to many other social domains.[2-5] The processes giving rise to illness, health, and a variety of other outcomes are often inherently complex. Interaction between exposures, from whatever categories of types of exposures, is one manifestation of this complexity. In this chapter, we present an overview of concepts and methods for assessing interaction, including some of the motivations for studying interaction.

MOTIVATIONS FOR ASSESSING INTERACTION

There are a number of practical and theoretical considerations that motivate the study of interaction. One of the most prominent is that, in a number of settings, resources to implement interventions may be limited. It may not be possible to intervene on or treat an entire population. Resources may only be sufficient to address a small fraction of the target population. If this is the case, then it may be important to identify the subgroups in which the intervention or treatment is likely to have the largest effect. As will be discussed below, methods for assessing additive interaction can help to determine which subgroups would benefit most from an intervention or treatment. Other methods can help to identify groups of individuals, based on a large number of covariates, who would or would not benefit, or who would benefit to the greatest extent, from an intervention or treatment. Even in settings in which resources are not limited and it is possible to intervene on everyone, it may be the case that a particular intervention is beneficial for some individuals and harmful for others. In such cases, it is very important to identify those groups for which the intervention or treatment may be harmful and refrain from the intervention for such persons. Techniques for assessing such so-called "qualitative" or "cross-over" interactions are discussed below.

Another reason sometimes given for assessing interaction is that it may shed insight on the mechanisms for the outcome. We will describe below how it is possible to sometimes detect individuals for whom an outcome would occur if both exposures are present but would not occur if just one or the other were present. We will see that this more mechanistic notion of interaction is quite distinct from more statistically based notions of interaction. In some cases, we can gain insight into whether there might be a mechanism requiring two or more specific causes to operate and we will discuss the limits of such reasoning.

As noted above, one of the motivations for studying interaction is to identify which subgroups would benefit most from intervention when resources are limited. However, in some settings, it may not be possible to intervene directly on the primary exposure of interest, and one might instead be interested in which other covariates could be intervened upon to eliminate much or most of the effect of the primary exposure of interest in the target population. In these cases, methods for attributing effects to interactions, discussed in the latter part of this chapter, can be useful for assessing and identifying the most relevant covariates for intervention. Finally, sometimes interactions are modeled not with any specific scientific or policy goal in mind concerning interactions per se, but simply because a statistical model fits the data better when the model includes the additional flexibility allowed by an interaction term. Sometimes, such considerations may give insights into potential generalizability of effect estimates. These various motivations for studying interaction are distinct so, as we will see throughout, when studying interaction, it is important to clearly state the goal of an analysis or assessment of interaction.

MEASURES OF INTERACTION AND SCALE OF INTERACTION

As a motivating example, consider data presented in Hilt et al.[6] concerning the effect of smoking on lung cancer and how this varied by self-reported history of occupational exposure to asbestos. The projected 10-year risk of lung cancer comparing current and ex-smokers with never-smokers varied by self-reported history of occupational asbestos exposure, as shown in Table 26-1. Lung cancer risk is much higher when both smoking and asbestos exposure are present together. This is an example of an interaction.

Let Y denote a binary outcome. Let G and X denote two binary exposures of interest. These might be a genetic factor and an environmental factor, respectively, but our discussion will not be restricted to gene-environment interaction and G and X could represent any two factors. Later in the chapter, we will also explicitly discuss interaction when the factors are not binary, but much of the discussion here generalizes in a straightforward manner to polytomous or continuous exposures. Let $p_{gx} = P(Y = 1|G = g, X = x)$ be the risk of the outcome when G is value g and

TABLE 26-1

Ten-Year Projected Risk of Lung Cancer by Smoking and Asbestos Status

	No Asbestos	Asbestos
Never-smoker	0.0011	0.0067
Ever smoker	0.0095	0.0450

X is value x. A natural way to assess interaction is to measure the extent to which the effect of the two factors together exceeds the effect of each considered individually (cf. Refs. 7, 8). This could be measured by:

$$(p_{11} - p_{00}) - [(p_{10} - p_{00}) + (p_{01} - p_{00})] \qquad [26\text{-}1]$$

Here $(p_{11} - p_{00})$ would be interpreted as the effect of both factors together compared with the reference category of both factors absent. For now, we will assume that the probabilities of the outcome under different exposure combinations correspond to the actual effects of the exposures on the outcome; we will consider issues of confounding and covariate adjustment in interaction analyses further below. The expressions $(p_{10} - p_{00})$ and $(p_{01} - p_{00})$ would be the effects of the first factor alone and the second factor alone, respectively. We would then consider the contrast between the effects of both factors together versus the sum of each considered separately. If this difference is nonzero, we say that there is interaction on the difference scale.

The measure in 26-1 is called the interaction contrast, or IC, and is a measure of interaction on the additive scale, or equivalently, a measure of departure from additive effects. The measure in 26-1 can be simplified as:

$$p_{11} - p_{10} - p_{01} + p_{00} \qquad [26\text{-}2]$$

If $p_{11} - p_{10} - p_{01} + p_{00} > 0$, the interaction is said to be positive or "super-additive," which suggests that persons exposed to both factors have a higher risk (p_{11}) than can be explained by subtracting the effect of the first factor alone $(p_{10} - p_{00})$, the effect of the second factor alone $(p_{01} - p_{00})$, and the baseline risk of disease in those exposed to neither factor (p_{00}). For the data in Table 26-1, we have:

$$p_{11} - p_{10} - p_{01} + p_{00} = 0.0450 - 0.0095 - 0.00670 + 0.0011 = 0.0299 > 0.$$

We would have evidence here of positive or "super-additive" interaction, meaning that the risk of lung cancer over 10 years is projected to be higher in ever smokers with history of occupational exposure than can be explained by the effects of smoking alone, occupational exposure to asbestos alone, and the risk of lung cancer in those exposed to neither. If $p_{11} - p_{10} - p_{01} + p_{00} < 0$, the interaction is said to be negative or "subadditive."

The measure can also be written as the difference in risk differences for X across strata of G, $(p_{11} - p_{10}) - (p_{01} - p_{00})$ and can likewise be written as the difference in risk differences for G across strata of X, $(p_{11} - p_{01}) - (p_{10} - p_{00})$, which are both just rearrangements of Equation 26-2.

Sometimes, instead of using risk differences to measure effects, one might use risk ratios or other relative measures of association. For example, we could define the risk ratio effect measures as:

$$RR_{10} = p_{10}/p_{00}$$
$$RR_{01} = p_{01}/p_{00}$$
$$RR_{11} = p_{11}/p_{00}$$

These estimates can be used to estimate departure from additive effects by dividing all terms in Equation 26-2 by p_{00}. The resulting estimate of departure from additive effects equals,

$$RERI_{RR} = RR_{11} - RR_{10} - RR_{01} + 1. \qquad [26\text{-}3]$$

This quantity is referred to as the "relative excess risk due to interaction" or RERI.[7] It is also sometimes referred to as the "interaction contrast ratio" or ICR. This gives us something similar to additive interaction but using risk ratios rather than risks. Subsequently, we will refer to this quantity in 26-3 as $RERI_{RR}$. $RERI_{RR} > 0$ if and only if for the additive interaction in 26-2,

$IC = p_{11} - p_{10} - p_{01} + p_{00} > 0$; likewise $RERI_{RR} < 0$ if and only if $IC = p_{11} - p_{10} - p_{01} + p_{00} < 0$; and $RERI_{RR} = 0$ if and only if $IC = p_{11} - p_{10} - p_{01} + p_{00} = 0$. Thus, we can assess whether additive interaction is positive, negative, or zero using risk ratios and $RERI_{RR}$. It should be noted that although $RERI_{RR}$ gives the direction (positive, negative, zero) of the additive interaction, we cannot in general use $RERI_{RR}$ to make statements about the relative magnitude of the underlying additive interaction for risks, $p_{11} - p_{10} - p_{01} + p_{00}$, unless we know p_{00}. If the magnitude (rather than just the sign) of $RERI_{RR}$ is going to be interpreted, then it must be kept in mind that this magnitude is on the excess relative risk scale, and this does not necessarily correspond to the relative magnitude of additive interaction for risks. This is because the baseline risks may differ across groups.

However, only the direction, rather than the magnitude, of $RERI_{RR}$ is needed to draw conclusions about the public health relevance of interaction. Essentially, if we are trying to decide which subgroup of G to target for an intervention when resources are limited, $RERI_{RR} > 0$ implies the public health consequences of an intervention on X would be larger in the $G = 1$ group, while $RERI_{RR} < 0$ implies the public health consequences of an intervention on X would be larger in the $G = 0$ group. In the example from Table 26-1:

$$RR_{10} = p_{10}/p_{00} = 0.0095/0.0011 = 8.64$$
$$RR_{01} = p_{01}/p_{00} = 0.0067/0.0011 = 6.09$$
$$RR_{11} = p_{11}/p_{00} = 0.0450/0.0011 = 40.9$$

The ICR therefore equals $40.9 - 8.64 - 6.09 + 1 = 27.17 = IC/p_{00} = 0.0299/0.0011$. Because ICR is greater than zero, the effects of smoking and occupational asbestos exposure on 10-year lung cancer risk are super-additive. A tobacco intervention program would be more productively targeted at persons with occupational history of asbestos exposure than at persons without an occupational history of asbestos exposure. Note that this evaluation of "productive targeting" an intervention pays no attention to the prevalence of occupational history of asbestos exposure. If this history is rare (as it was in most industrialized nations), or largely restricted to one demographic group (occupational exposure to asbestos affected primarily men in most industrialized nations), or if there are competing risks associated with tobacco use or occupational history of asbestos exposure (as there are), then these considerations would also weigh into an evaluation of productive targeting of the tobacco cessation intervention.

In this case, IC can be estimated directly because the 10-year risks of lung cancer are available for all four exposure combinations. However, in some case-control studies, only ratio estimates of effect are available, so the RERI formulation is useful to estimate departure from additive effects in studies of that design. As discussed in Chapter 8, case-control odds ratios will validly estimate risk ratios (even when the outcome is common) in case-control designs when the controls are selected from the entirety of the underlying population rather than just from the noncases (see Ref. 9, for further review and discussion of this point). In cumulative case-control and cross-sectional study designs, only the disease odds ratio can be estimated, and thus effect measures and interaction measures are evaluated on an odds ratio scale. The effects for each of the exposures considered separately and both considered together on the odds ratio scale are defined, respectively, by:

$$OR_{10} = \left[p_{10}/(1 - p_{10}) \right]/\left[p_{00}/(1 - p_{00}) \right]$$
$$OR_{01} = \left[p_{01}/(1 - p_{01}) \right]/\left[p_{00}/(1 - p_{00}) \right]$$
$$OR_{11} = \left[p_{11}/(1 - p_{11}) \right]/\left[p_{00}/(1 - p_{00}) \right].$$

A measure of interaction potentially relevant to the additive scale for odds ratio might then be taken as:

$$RERI_{OR} = OR_{11} - OR_{10} - OR_{01} + 1 \qquad\qquad [26\text{-}4]$$

This quantity measures the extent to which, on the odds ratio scale, the effect of both exposures together exceeds the additive effects of the two exposures considered separately. In general, measures of interaction on the odds ratio and risk ratio scales will be close to one another whenever the outcome is rare. When the outcome is rare, both $(1 - p_{gx})$ and $(1 - p_{00})$ will be close to 1, and thus the odds ratios approximate risk ratios, since $OR_{gx} = \left[p_{gx}/(1-p_{gx}) \right]/\left[p_{00}/(1-p_{00}) \right] \approx p_{gx}/p_{00} = RR_{gx}$ (see also Chapters 4 and 5). For example, using the data in Table 26-1, an estimate of RERI using disease odds instead of disease risk would be obtained from:

$$OR_{10} = \left[0.0095/(1-0.0095) \right]/\left[0.0011/(1-0.0011) \right] = 8.71 \approx 8.64$$
$$OR_{01} = \left[0.0067/(1-0.0067) \right]/\left[0.0011/(1-0.0011) \right] = 6.13 \approx 6.09$$
$$OR_{11} = \left[0.0450/(1-0.0450) \right]/\left[0.0011/(1-0.0011) \right] = 42.8 \approx 40.9$$

The $RERI_{OR}$ estimated with these odds ratios equals $42.8 - 8.71 - 6.13 + 1 = 28.95$, which approximately equals the $RERI_{RR}$ of 27.17 estimated from the risk data.

One might also be interested in the departure from multiplicative effects. Both departure from additive effects and departure from multiplicative effects can be estimated while also reporting difference or ratio estimates of association. It is important, therefore, to avoid connecting the study's design or analysis plan to the choice of the scale (departure from additive or multiplicative effects) by which interaction will be evaluated. A measure of interaction on the multiplicative scale for risk ratios would be:

$$\left[(RR_{11})/(RR_{10}RR_{01}) \right] = \left[(p_{11}p_{00})/(p_{10}p_{01}) \right] \qquad \text{[26-5]}$$

This quantity measures the extent to which, on the risk ratio scale, the effect of both exposures together exceeds the product of the effects of the two exposures considered separately. We compare the measure $RR_{11}/(RR_{10}RR_{01})$ to 1 rather than to 0 here since $RR_{11}/(RR_{10}RR_{01})$ is a ratio. If the ratio is 1, then the effect of both exposures together is equal to the product of the effect of the two exposures considered separately, that is, there is no interaction on the multiplicative scale for risk ratios and, equivalently, no departure from multiplicative effects. If $RR_{11}/(RR_{10}RR_{01}) > 1$, the multiplicative interaction is said to be positive or supermultiplicative. If $RR_{11}/(RR_{10}RR_{01}) < 1$, the multiplicative interaction is said to be negative or submultiplicative. This measure of multiplicative interaction can be rewritten as $RR_{11}/(RR_{10}RR_{01}) = (p_{11}/p_{01})/(p_{10}/p_{00})$, i.e., as the ratio of (1) the relative risk for G when $X = 1$ versus (2) the relative risk for G when $X = 0$. Likewise, it can be written as $RR_{11}/(RR_{10}RR_{01}) = (p_{11}/p_{10})/(p_{01}/p_{00})$, i.e., as the ratio of (1) the relative risk for X when $G = 1$ versus (2) the relative risk for X when $G = 0$.

Using the data in Table 26-1, we have that the measure of multiplicative interaction is given by:

$$\left[(RR_{11})/(RR_{10}RR_{01}) \right]$$
$$= \left\{ (0.0450/0.0011)/\left[(0.0095/0.0011) \times (0.0067/0.0011) \right] \right\}$$
$$= \left[(40.9)/(8.64 \times 6.09) \right] = 0.78.$$

We would have evidence here of negative multiplicative interaction. In other words, the risk ratio comparing ever smokers with a history of occupational exposure to asbestos to those without exposure to smoking or asbestos (40.9) is less than the product of the risk ratio comparing ever smokers to those without exposure to smoking or asbestos (8.64) and the risk ratio comparing those with a history of occupational exposure to asbestos to those without exposure to smoking or asbestos (6.09). We can also use odds ratios to estimate departure from multiplicativity. If $OR_{11}/(OR_{10}OR_{01}) > 1$, the multiplicative interaction is said to be positive. If $OR_{11}/(OR_{10}OR_{01}) < 1$, the multiplicative interaction is said to be negative. As also discussed above, case-control odds ratios provide valid estimates of the risk ratios when controls are selected from the population that gave rise to the cases and not from noncases at the end of follow-up. For cumulative case-control designs and cross-sectional designs, the odds ratios provide reasonable estimates of the risk ratio if the disease is rare in strata defined by all combinations of G and X. For the data in Table 26-1, we have:

$$OR_{11}/(OR_{10}OR_{01}) = 42.8/(8.71 \times 6.13) = 0.80$$

The measure of multiplicative interaction on the odds ratio scale indicates negative interaction and is close to what was obtained for the estimate of multiplicative interaction on the risk ratio scale (0.78).

Table 26-1 example demonstrates that whether an interaction is positive or negative may depend on whether effects are estimated by differences or ratios. In this example, there is a positive interaction when effects are measured by risk differences, sometimes referred to as interaction on the additive scale, but there is a negative interaction when effects are measured by risk ratios, sometimes referred to as interaction on the multiplicative scale. Said another way, the estimated effect of both exposures together on the risk difference scale exceeds the sum of the estimated effects on the risk difference scale of each considered separately, while it is also the case that the estimated effect of both exposures together on the risk ratio scale is less than the product of the estimated effects on the risk ratio scale of each considered separately.

Likewise, interaction may be present on one scale but absent on another. Consider the synthetic data in Table 26-2.

Here there is no additive interaction since $p_{11} - p_{10} - p_{01} + p_{00} = 0.10 - 0.07 - 0.05 + 0.02 = 0$, but there is a negative multiplicative interaction since

$$RR_{11}/(RR_{10}RR_{01}) = (0.10/0.02)/[(0.07/0.02)(0.05/0.02)] = 5/(3.5 \times 2.5) = 0.57 < 1.$$

In other settings, we might have additive interaction but no multiplicative interaction. Consider the synthetic data in Table 26-3.

Here the additive interaction is positive since $p_{11} - p_{10} - p_{01} + p_{00} = 0.10 - 0.04 - 0.05 + 0.02 = 0.03 > 0$, but there is no multiplicative interaction since $RR_{11}/(RR_{10}RR_{01}) = (0.10/0.02)/[(0.04/0.02)(0.05/0.02)] = 5/(2 \times 2.5) = 1$. In fact, if both of the exposures have an effect on the outcome, then the absence of interaction on the additive scale implies the presence of multiplicative interaction for relative risks and likewise, the absence of multiplicative interaction for relative risks implies the presence of additive interaction. In other words, if both of the exposures have an effect on the outcome, then there must be interaction on at least one scale or both. This makes clear that just to say that there is an interaction on some scale is relatively uninteresting; all it implies is that both exposures have some effect on the outcome. It also raises the question of why interaction is of interest, and which scale is to be preferred. When undertaking interaction analyses, it is important to clearly state the goal or the motivation for the analysis and to choose a measure of interaction accordingly. In a subsequent section, we will turn to the arguments for and interpretation of additive versus multiplicative interaction.

One reason why additive interaction is important to assess (rather than only relying on multiplicative interaction measures) is that it is the more relevant public health measure.[10-13] Consider again the outcome probabilities in Table 26-3. Suppose that the outcome probabilities represent the

TABLE 26-2

Risk of Outcome by Cross-Classified Exposure Status

	$X = 0$	$X = 1$
$G = 0$	0.02	0.05
$G = 1$	0.07	0.10

TABLE 26-3

Risk of Outcome by Cross-Classified Exposure Status

	$X = 0$	$X = 1$
$G = 0$	0.02	0.05
$G = 1$	0.04	0.10

probability of a disease being cured for a drug (X) stratified by genotype status (G). The effect of X on the risk difference scale among those with $G = 0$ is $0.05 - 0.02 = 0.03$; while the effect of X among those with $G = 1$ is $0.10 - 0.04 = 0.06$. If we had only 100 doses of the drug and we had to decide which group to treat, we could cure three additional persons if we used all of the drug supply among those with $G = 0$, but we could cure six additional persons if we used all of the drug supply among those with $G = 1$. All other things being equal, we would clearly want to give the drug supply to those with $G = 1$. The additive interaction measure, $p_{11} - p_{10} - p_{01} + p_{00} = 0.03 > 0$, allows us to see this. The multiplicative interaction measure, $RR_{11}/(RR_{10}RR_{01}) = 1$, does not.

In fact, the multiplicative scale can indicate the wrong subgroup to treat. Suppose in Table 26-3 we replace the probability of cure in $G = 1$, $X = 1$ of 0.10 with 0.09. Then the effect on the difference scale of X among those with $G = 0$ is $0.05 - 0.02 = 0.03$; the effect of X among those with $G = 1$ is $0.09 - 0.04 = 0.05$. Thus, on the difference scale, the effect size is larger for the $G = 1$ subgroup, indicating this is the subgroup we would like to treat if resources are limited. However, on the risk ratio scale, the effect for those with $G = 0$ is $0.05/0.02 = 2.5$ and for those with $G = 1$ it is $0.09/0.04 = 2.25$; the risk ratio effect size is larger for the $G = 0$ subgroup; however, this is not the subgroup to which we would want to allocate limited resources. If we had only 100 doses of the drug, we could cure three additional persons if we used the drug supply among those with $G = 0$, but we could cure five additional persons if we used the drug supply among those with $G = 1$. All other things being equal, we would clearly want to give the drug supply to those with $G = 1$. The issue with the multiplicative scale is that the baseline risk is different in the two subgroups, and thus the risk ratio is operating on different baseline risks.

The possibility of positive additive interaction, but negative or null multiplicative interaction is not simply a theoretical possibility. This situation is in accordance with the lung cancer data in Table 26-1, where we had a positive additive interaction but a negative multiplicative interaction. It was likewise the case in analyses of the joint effects of *Helicobacter pylori* and use of nonsteroidal anti-inflammatory drugs (NSAIDs) in causing peptic ulcer[14] with slightly positive additive interaction but negative multiplicative interaction. Similarly, in analyses of interaction between factor V Leiden mutation and oral contraceptive use in causing venous thrombosis, the multiplicative interaction was found to be close to null, but there was a positive additive interaction.[15] Using the multiplicative interaction results in any of these cases to determine which subgroups to prioritize intervention would have given the wrong conclusion. For example, from the data in Table 26-1, more lives would be saved by removing asbestos from homes of smokers first; the risk ratios suggest the opposite conclusion. Indeed dismissing the importance of one factor in assessing the effects of another because of the absence of multiplicative interaction can be quite dangerous: the null multiplicative interaction between factor V Leiden mutation and oral contraceptive use may lead to false reassurances that "it does not matter" whether one carries the mutation or not for the decision to start using oral contraceptives; whereas, in fact, because those with the factor V Leiden mutation have a roughly seven times higher baseline risk than those without the mutation,[15] the "constant risk ratio" for oral contraceptive use results in a much higher increase in absolute risk for those with the factor V Leiden mutation than those without.

More generally, $p_{11} - p_{10} - p_{01} + p_{00} > 0$ implies the public-health consequence of an intervention on X to address this particular outcome would be larger in the $G = 1$ group, while $p_{11} - p_{10} - p_{01} + p_{00} < 0$ implies the public-health consequence of an intervention on X would be larger in the $G = 0$ group. Thus, while it may be of interest to assess multiplicative interaction and it may be viewed as simpler to assess multiplicative interaction in the inherently multiplicative regression models used to analyze many epidemiologic data sets, additive interaction should also always be examined, if for no other reason than to assess public-health importance.

A few other measures of additive interaction using data from risk ratios or odds ratios are sometimes employed. The synergy index[7] is defined as:

$$S = (RR_{11} - 1)/[(RR_{10} - 1) + (RR_{01} - 1)].$$

It measures the extent to which the risk ratio for both exposures together exceeds 1, and whether this is greater than the sum of the extent to which each of the risk ratios considered separately each exceed 1. Suppose the denominator of S is positive, then if $S > 1$ we will have $RERI_{RR} > 0$ and thus $p_{11} - p_{10} - p_{01} + p_{00} > 0$. If $S < 1$, then we will have $RERI_{RR} < 0$ and thus $p_{11} - p_{10} - p_{01} + p_{00} < 0$. Thus, the synergy index can be used to assess departure from additive effects. As with $RERI_{RR}$, the risk ratios in the synergy index are often replaced and, approximated, by odds ratios when it is used with estimates from case-control designs. The interpretation of the synergy index becomes difficult in settings in which one or both exposures are preventive rather than causative so that the denominator of S is negative.[16] When one or both of the exposures is preventive, rather than causative (*i.e.*, $RR_{10} < 1$ and/or $RR_{01} < 1$), such that the denominator of S, $(RR_{10} - 1) + (RR_{01} - 1)$, is less than 0, then with an inequality like $S > 1$, multiplying both sides of this inequality by $(RR_{10} - 1) + (RR_{01} - 1)$, which is negative, will reverse the sign of the inequality, because of multiplication by a negative number, to give $RR_{11} - 1 < (RR_{10} - 1) + (RR_{01} - 1)$ or $RERI_{RR} < 0$; and thus when the denominator of S is negative, $S < 1$ becomes the condition for positive additive interaction, which can be confusing. In general it is thus best not to report S unless the denominator, $(RR_{10} - 1) + (RR_{01} - 1)$, is positive. This issue does not arise with $RERI_{RR}$ because the denominator of $RERI_{RR}$ is never negative. The issue can be resolved with the synergy index S by recoding the exposures so that neither is preventive in the absence of the other.[16] Another measure of additive interaction that is sometimes used is called the attributable proportion and is defined as:

$$AP = (RR_{11} - RR_{10} - RR_{01} + 1)/RR_{11}$$

and essentially measures the proportion of the risk in the doubly exposed group that is due to the interaction. The attributable proportion is a derivative measure of the relative excess risk due to interaction: $AP > 0$ if and only if $RERI_{RR} > 0$; and $AP < 0$ if and only if $RERI_{RR} < 0$. A variant on the attributable proportion may also be potentially of interest. The attributable proportion measure above measures the proportion of risk in the doubly exposed group that is due to interaction.

$$AP = RERI_{RR}/RR_{11} = (RR_{11} - RR_{10} - RR_{01} + 1)/RR_{11} = (p_{11} - p_{10} - p_{01} + p_{00})/p_{11}$$

Alternatively, we might consider the proportion of the joint effects of both exposures together that is due to interaction.[7,17] This measure is given by:

$$AP^* = RERI_{RR}/(RR_{11} - 1) = (RR_{11} - RR_{10} - RR_{01} + 1)/(RR_{11} - 1)$$
$$= (p_{11} - p_{10} - p_{01} + p_{00})/(p_{11} - p_{00}).$$

This is different from $AP = RERI_{RR}/RR_{11}$, which captures the proportion of the *disease* in the doubly exposed group that is due to the interaction. The alternative measure, $AP^* = RERI_{RR}/(RR_{11} - 1)$, captures the proportion of the *effect* of both exposures on the additive scale that is due to interaction. Whereas most of the literature has focused on the former measure, $AP = RERI_{RR}/RR_{11}$, both measures may be of interest, although they capture different things. With the measure $AP = RERI_{RR}/RR_{11}$, even if all of the joint effect were due to interaction so that the effects of G alone and X alone were both risk ratios of 1, *i.e.*, $RR_{10} = 1$ and $RR_{01} = 1$, we would nevertheless have an attributable proportion measure for disease in the doubly exposed less than 1:

$$AP = RERI_{RR}/RR_{11} = (RR_{11} - RR_{10} - RR_{01} + 1)/RR_{11}$$
$$= (RR_{11} - 1 - 1 + 1)/RR_{11} = (RR_{11} - 1)/RR_{11} < 1$$

TABLE 26-4

Odds Ratios for Breast Cancer by Strata of Alcohol Consumption and XRCC3-T241 M

	No Alcohol	Alcohol
T/T or T/M	1	1.12
M/M	1.21	2.09

That is, even if the entirety of the joint effect of both exposures was due to interaction, the attributable proportion $AP = RERI_{RR}/RR_{11}$ measure would be less than 100%. This result arises because some of the disease risk in the doubly exposed group (p_{11}) is attributed to causes other than G or X (p_{00}). By subtracting $p_{00}/p_{00} = 1$ from RR_{11} in the denominator, the measure $RERI/(RR_{11} - 1)$ would equal 100% when the main effects of G alone and X alone are both risk ratios of 1 and the entirety of the joint effect is due to interaction.

All of these measures can be used in both cohort studies and case-control studies. To estimate the measures that would be obtained using risk data from a cohort study, a case-control odds ratio would have to be estimated using case-cohort design or, if estimated by cumulative case-control design, the disease would have to be rare in every stratum of combined G and X categories. These expectations of unbiased estimation of these measures using case-control design follow directly from principles explained in Chapter 8.

As an example, Figueiredo et al.[18] studied the effects of XRCC3-T241 M polymorphisms and alcohol consumption on breast cancer risk using a case-control design. The genetic risk factor was considered the M/M genotype versus a reference of the T/T or T/M genotype. They obtained the odds ratios in Table 26-4 from their case-control study.

Although we cannot assess additive interaction directly using risks, $p_{11} - p_{10} - p_{01} + p_{00}$, from the odds ratios in Table 26-4, we can still estimate:

$$RERI_{OR} = OR_{11} - OR_{10} - OR_{01} + 1 = 2.09 - 1.21 - 1.12 + 1 = 0.76 > 0$$

so we have evidence of positive additive interaction $(IC > 0)$. Breast cancer is a relatively rare outcome, and so odds ratios will closely approximate risk ratios in this study. Likewise, we could calculate the synergy index $S = (RR_{11} - 1)/[(RR_{10} - 1) + (RR_{01} - 1)] \approx 3.30 > 1$, again indicating positive additive interaction. And we can calculate the proportion of risk in the doubly exposed group attributable to interaction, $AP = [(RR_{11} - RR_{10} - RR_{01} + 1)/(RR_{11})] \approx 36.4\%$ or the proportion of the joint effects of both exposures attributable to interaction, $AP^* = [(RR_{11} - RR_{10} - RR_{01} + 1)/(RR_{11} - 1)] \approx 69.7\%$.

STATISTICAL INTERACTIONS AND REGRESSION MODELS

In practice, interactions are often estimated by using statistical models by including a product term for the two exposures in the model. A statistical model on the linear scale accommodating interaction might take the form:

$$P(Y = 1 | G = g, X = x) = \alpha_0 + \alpha_1 g + \alpha_2 x + \alpha_3 xg. \qquad [26\text{-}6]$$

It is easy to verify under this model that $\alpha_0 = p_{00}$ estimates the risk in the doubly unexposed group, $\alpha_1 = p_{10} - p_{00}$ estimates the effect of g as a risk difference, $\alpha_2 = p_{01} - p_{00}$ estimates the effect of x as a risk difference, and $\alpha_3 = p_{11} - p_{10} - p_{01} + p_{00}$ estimates IC. The coefficient α_3 is thus equal to our measure of additive interaction based on risks; for this reason, α_3 is sometimes referred to as a statistical interaction on the additive scale.

Similarly, one might use a log-linear model for risk ratios, including a product term:

$$\log[P(Y = 1 | G = g, X = x)] = \beta_0 + \beta_1 g + \beta_2 x + \beta_3 xg. \qquad [26\text{-}7]$$

Here we have that $\exp(\beta_0) = p_{00}$ estimates the risk in the doubly unexposed group, $\exp(\beta_1) = RR_{10}$ estimates the effect of g as a risk ratio, $\exp(\beta_2) = RR_{01}$ estimates the effect of x as a risk ratio, and $\exp(\beta_3) = RR_{11}/(RR_{10}RR_{01})$ estimates the departure from multiplicative effects. The so called "main effects" β_1 and β_2, when exponentiated, simply give the risk ratios for each of the two exposures when each is considered alone. The coefficient β_3, when exponentiated, gives our measure for multiplicative interaction for risk ratios, $RR_{11}/(RR_{10}RR_{01})$. The coefficient β_3 is thus often referred to as a statistical interaction for a log-linear model. Likewise, one might use a logistic model for odds ratios, including a product term:

$$\operatorname{logit}\left[P\left(Y = 1 \middle| G = g, X = x\right)\right] = \gamma_0 + \gamma_1 g + \gamma_2 x + \gamma_3 xg. \qquad [26\text{-}8]$$

Here we have that $\exp(\gamma_0) = p_{00}/(1 - p_{00})$ estimates the disease odds in the doubly unexposed group, $\exp(\gamma_1) = OR_{10}$ estimates the effect of g as a disease odds ratio, $\exp(\gamma_2) = OR_{01}$ estimates the effect of x as a disease odds ratio, and $\exp(\gamma_3) = OR_{11}/(OR_{10}OR_{01})$ estimates the departure from multiplicative effects as a function of disease odds ratios. The main effects, γ_1 and γ_2, when exponentiated, give the odds ratios for each of the two exposures. The coefficient γ_3, when exponentiated, gives our measure for multiplicative interaction for odds ratios, $OR_{11}/(OR_{10}OR_{01})$. Thus, γ_3 is referred to as a statistical interaction for a logistic model. The equality $\exp(\gamma_0) = p_{00}/(1 - p_{00})$ will only hold with cohort data. However, all the other equalities, $\exp(\gamma_1) = OR_{10}$, $\exp(\gamma_2) = OR_{01}$, and $\exp(\gamma_3) = OR_{11}/(OR_{10}OR_{01})$, will hold for both cohort data and case-control data, subject to the principles described in Chapter 8. We can thus assess both main effects of the exposures and the multiplicative interaction between the exposures on an odds ratio scale using case-control data.

When the outcome and both exposures are binary and no further covariates are included, it is straightforward to fit these models to the data using standard software. The estimate and confidence interval obtained by maximum likelihood estimation and given by such software for α_3 will constitute an estimate and confidence interval for the additive interaction $p_{11} - p_{10} - p_{01} + p_{00}$. The estimates and confidence intervals obtained by maximum likelihood estimation and given by such software for β_3 and γ_3, when exponentiated, will constitute an estimate and confidence interval for the multiplicative interaction on the risk ratio and odds ratio scales, respectively.

Often we may want to control for other covariates in models 26-6 to 26-8. For example, we may want to fit the following analogous models, which include an additional vector of covariates Z:

$$P\left(Y = 1 \middle| G = g, X = x, Z = z\right) = \alpha_0 + \alpha_1 g + \alpha_2 x + \alpha_3 xg + \alpha_4' z$$

$$\log\left[P\left(Y = 1 \middle| G = g, X = x, Z = z\right)\right] = \beta_0 + \beta_1 g + \beta_2 x + \beta_3 xg + \beta_4' z .$$

$$\operatorname{logit}\left[P\left(Y = 1 \middle| G = g, X = x, Z = z\right)\right] = \gamma_0 + \gamma_1 g + \gamma_2 x + \gamma_3 xg + \gamma_4' z$$

Unfortunately, the linear and log-linear models, when fit to data, will often encounter convergence problems in the maximum likelihood algorithms used to fit the models, especially when there are continuous covariates in Z. The models do not ensure that the predicted risks satisfy the constraint of lying between 0 and 1. The logistic model with covariates does not suffer from this problem. For this reason, a common approach to assessing interaction in practice has become fitting the logistic model with covariates and assessing the estimate and confidence interval for the product term coefficient, γ. This approach is also popular because it can be implemented in a straightforward way with case-control data as well. However, as discussed throughout this chapter, it is also recommended that investigators assess additive interaction as well. This can be more challenging when covariates are in the model. Additional strategies to fit linear and log-linear models with covariates using data from cohort studies have been described elsewhere (cf., Refs. 19, 20 for overviews of several different methods). In the next section, we will describe what has become a standard approach[21] to estimating additive interaction, with covariate control, which consists of using a logistic regression with additional covariates and transforming the parameter estimates to obtain estimates and confidence intervals for the relative excess (RERI).

ADDITIVE INTERACTION AND REGRESSION MODELS

Suppose the following model is fit to the data:

$$\text{logit}\left[P\left(Y = 1 | G = g, X = x, Z = z\right)\right] = \gamma_0 + \gamma_1 g + \gamma_2 x + \gamma_3 xg + \gamma_4' z. \qquad [26\text{-}9]$$

We then have that:

$$\text{RERI}_{OR} = OR_{11} - OR_{10} - OR_{01} + 1 = \exp\left(\gamma_1 + \gamma_2 + \gamma_3\right) - \exp\left(\gamma_1\right) - \exp\left(\gamma_2\right) + 1.$$

Thus, we can estimate a measure of additive interaction, RERI_{OR}, using the parameters of a logistic regression. This approach has the advantage that the logistic regression in 26-9 can more easily be fit to data when there are continuous covariates than the corresponding linear or log-linear models for binary outcomes given in the previous section. This approach with logistic regression also has the advantage that it can be employed even with case-control data. Even with cohort data—if the outcome is rare in all strata of all combinations of g, x, and z—this approach to additive interaction using RERI_{OR} can often be helpful because the logistic regression model often fits data quite well and has fewer convergence issues than a linear or log-linear model for risk. The logistic regression model has the interesting implication that if the model is correctly specified so that the log odds are linear in the covariates Z, then the RERI_{RR} measure will also be constant across strata of the covariates. This approach to RERI_{RR}, as other modeling approaches, presupposes that the statistical model is correctly specified. We discuss below other modeling approaches for additive interaction that make different modeling assumptions.

Standard errors for RERI_{RR}, as estimated above, can be obtained using the delta method.[21] Software options are now available to estimate these standard errors (*e.g.*, Refs. 22-26). To estimate standard errors for RERI_{OR} using logistic regression, in addition to the delta method described by Hosmer and Lemeshow,[21] one may also use bootstrapping, which can have more accurate standard errors when the sample size is small[27]; other resampling-based approaches are available when some of the outcome counts for particular exposure combinations are low.[28] Bayesian approaches to RERI_{OR} are also now available.[29] When sample sizes are relatively large, the approaches to estimating RERI_{OR} will give fairly comparable confidence intervals; when sample sizes are small the resampling-based approach may be more accurate. However, in general, fairly large sample sizes are required to obtain even moderately precise estimates of interaction; thus, for the most part, in those very settings in which it is possible and reasonable to evaluate interaction, the various approaches to estimate RERI_{OR} are likely to give comparable estimates and standard errors. Easy-to-implement software[30,31] is also available for estimating RERI_{OR} using so-called linear odds models.[32] This approach, however, can have difficulty handling continuous covariates Z. Such covariates can be handled in linear odds models by using a weighting approach for covariate control,[33] and this approach can be employed with case-control data as well.

The approach described above works well if the outcome is rare so that RERI_{OR} approximates RERI_{RR}. If the outcome is common, RERI_{OR} may not be an adequate measure of additive interaction. In such cases, for cohort data, one could estimate RERI_{RR} by replacing the logistic model in 26-9 with a log-linear model, though such log-linear models with continuous covariates Z may not always converge. An approach for risk ratios using modified Poisson, rather than logistic regression, has also been proposed that can be used with a common outcome.[34] Alternatively, with cohort data with a common outcome, one may use a weighting approach to estimating additive interaction.[35] This approach models the relationship between the exposures and the covariates, rather than between the outcome and the covariates.

Our discussion thus far has focused on binary exposures. A similar approach can be used with categorical, ordinal, or continuous exposures. The logistic regression model above in 26-9 could be fit to the data if the two exposures G and X were ordinal or continuous. However, when additive interaction is carried out for ordinal or continuous exposures using this approach based on logistic regression, two things must be kept in mind, one analytical and one interpretative. First analytically, for ordinal and continuous exposures, it is important to consider the magnitude of the change in the exposures for which one is examining interaction. If one is considering a change for the value of G from g_0 to g_1 and a value of X from x_0 to x_1, then instead of using $\exp(\gamma_1 + \gamma_2 + \gamma_3)$-$\exp(\gamma_1) - \exp(\gamma_2) + 1$ as an estimate of RERI_{OR}, one uses:

$$
\begin{aligned}
\text{RERI}_{OR} = {} & \exp\left[\left(g_1 - g_0 \right)\gamma_1 + \left(x_1 - x_0 \right)\gamma_2 + \left(g_1 x_1 - g_0 x_0 \right)\gamma_3 \right] \\
& - \exp\left[\left(g_1 - g_0 \right)\gamma_1 + \left(g_1 - g_0 \right)x_0\gamma_3 \right] \\
& - \exp\left[\left(x_1 - x_0 \right)\gamma_2 + \left(x_1 - x_0 \right)g_0\gamma_3 \right] + 1.
\end{aligned}
$$

This needs to be taken into account when using software so that estimates and covariance matrices are multiplied by the appropriate factors. Software implementation is described in more detail in the appendix of VanderWeele and Knol.[26] Similar expressions could be given using categorical exposures: under any specific statistical model and for any two levels of each of the two exposures, one simply calculates the three relative risks comparing the various exposure combinations to the reference group and one subtracts from the risk ratio of the doubly exposed group, the two risk ratios for each of the singly exposed groups and adds 1. The second, more interpretative point, when ordinal, continuous, or categorical exposures are being employed, is that it is important to keep in mind that the RERI_{OR} measure (or the analogous RERI_{RR} measure) does vary according to the levels being compared and can vary in sign as well. The additive interaction measure for a change in X from 10 to 20 and in G from 0 to 1 may be different than the additive interaction measure for a change in X from 20 to 30 and in G from 0 to 1; the sign of the additive interaction measure may even be different. But if this is so, then this can have important public health implications; it would indicate that if a change in X from 20 to 30 is being considered, then it might be best to target one group, whereas if a change in X from 10 to 20 is being considered, it might be best to target the other. See also Knol et al.,[36] for further discussion.

INTERPRETING ADDITIVE VERSUS MULTIPLICATIVE INTERACTION

The fact that interaction can be assessed on different scales and that inferences from interaction analyses are scale-dependent raises the question on which scale interaction should be assessed: additive or multiplicative or some other. Our view is that it is almost always best to present both additive and multiplicative measures of interaction.[26,37-39] In practice, measures of multiplicative interaction, using logistic regression, are most frequently reported. This preference very likely arises because of convenience, rather than because careful thought has been given to which measure is to be preferred. Standard software using logistic regression will automatically give an estimate and confidence interval for multiplicative interaction. As noted in the previous section, additional work is required in most current software packages to obtain measures of additive interaction, and for this reason, it is not often done. In a review of a random sample of 25 cohort and 50 case-control studies from five highly ranked epidemiological journals, Knol et al.[40] noted that although 61% of the studies included at least as secondary analyses an assessment of effect modification or interaction, only one reported a measure of additive interaction. It is in general a mistake not to report additive interaction. As noted above and as discussed further below, additive interaction is always relevant for assessing the public health significance of an interaction. Although both additive and multiplicative interaction should in general be reported, we nonetheless review some of the reasons that have been put forward for using one scale versus the other.

Departure from additive effects is useful for assessing the public health importance of interventions and the public health significance of interaction.[10-13] As noted above, if the effect of an intervention is larger on the difference scale in one subgroup versus another, then this indicates that there would be larger numbers for whom the disease would be prevented or cured in giving a hundred individuals in the first subgroup treatment versus giving a hundred individuals in the second subgroup treatment. Such information is useful for targeting subpopulations for which the intervention is most effective. This will be relevant whenever resources are constrained and thus relevant also for cost-effectiveness.[41] As discussed above, the additive, not the multiplicative, scale gives this information. Other metrics related to the additive scale for assessing public-health impact can also be employed.[42] A second reason sometimes given for using additive interaction is that it more closely corresponds to tests for mechanistic interaction, rather than merely statistical interaction.[11,43-45] As discussed further below, evaluations of additive interaction can sometimes be used to detect synergism in Rothman's[46] sufficient cause framework. Conceived of another way, assessing additive interaction can sometimes be used to assess whether there are persons for whom the outcome would occur if both exposures were present but not if only one or the other of the exposures were present. As discussed below, this ends up being a different and, in many cases, stronger notion of interaction than merely a statistical interaction.

Several reasons are also often put forward for using the multiplicative scale. First, as noted above, it is easier to fit multiplicative models (such as logistic regression), and the multiplicative scale is the most natural scale on which to assess interaction for such models; moreover, when using such models, measures of multiplicative interaction are readily obtained from standard software. Second, it is sometimes claimed that there is in general less heterogeneity on the multiplicative scale. Studies of meta-analyses have suggested that in terms of statistical significance, the risk ratio and odds ratio are less heterogeneous than the risk difference.[47-49] Engels et al.[48] found that for 107 of 125 meta-analyses (86%), the P-value for heterogeneity for risk differences was less than that for the odds ratios. With a P-value cutoff of 0.10, they found that 59 (47%) meta-analyses were heterogeneous for the risk difference and 44 (35%) were heterogeneous for the odds ratio. Deeks and Altman[47] likewise report that the risk difference was more heterogenous than the odds ratio or risk ratio using 1889 meta-analyses. Sterne and Egger[50] reviewed 78 meta-analyses and found that the P-value for heterogeneity was less than 0.05 in 29%, 27%, and 35% of these meta-analyses, for the odds ratio, risk ratio, and risk difference, respectively. If this is so, it may have implications for the generalizability of ratio effect estimates to other settings.

However, it is not entirely clear the extent to which the supposed evidence proposed is simply due to difference in power across the different scales or whether there is genuinely less heterogeneity.[51] More convincing evidence would come from large studies suggesting goodness of fit of the multiplicative model.[51,52] Nevertheless, if it is indeed the case that the multiplicative scales (odds ratio or risk ratio) are "less heterogeneous" and this indicates something about the underlying biology as to how effects typically operate (see comments on the "Limits of Biologic Inference" below), then detecting an interaction on a multiplicative scale may be of greater import than detecting interaction on the additive scale. A third reason sometimes given for using the multiplicative scale for overall effects (but also potentially applicable to interaction), stated in some epidemiology textbooks, is that the relative effect measures are better suited to "assessing causality." According to Poole,[53] this notion can be traced back to a paper by Cornfield et al.[54] showing that smoking was strongly related to lung cancer but not to other diseases on a relative risk scale, while smoking seemed similarly related to lung cancer and also to other diseases on an absolute risk scale. Because specificity of effect was seen as a criterion of causality,[55] the relative risk scale was seen as superior over the absolute risk scale in assessing causality. As noted by Poole,[53] whether the relative or absolute measure is more useful for "assessing causality" will, however, vary by setting. In some cases, such as that considered by Cornfield et al.,[54] the multiplicative scale may indeed prove to be more useful, and it might be thought that this general argument then is also relevant to interaction.

Arguments can be given in favor of each of the two scales. However, it would seem that the primary reasons for assessing and interpreting multiplicative interactions are software convenience and perhaps overstated evidence that ratio estimates of association are less heterogeneous than difference estimates of heterogeneity. Neither is compelling from the point of view of interpretation, whereas the primary arguments for assessing and interpreting additive interactions are based on either mechanism or public-health issues. Moreover, nothing prohibits investigators from reporting measures of interaction on both additive and multiplicative scales, and, in most settings, we think this approach is best because both can be informative.[37-39] Results from this maximally informative approach are straightforward to report. In fact, with knowledge of interaction on both scales, it is also possible to place the form of interaction along a range of 11 distinct ordered states,[56] which, for two exposures that are each causative at least in the absence of the other, may be described as positive-multiplicative positive-additive, no-multiplicative positive-additive, negative-multiplicative positive-additive, negative-multiplicative zero-additive, negative-multiplicative negative-additive, single-pure interaction, single-qualitative interaction, single-qualitative single-pure interaction, double-qualitative interaction, perfect antagonism (where the risk of the outcome in the doubly exposed group is the same as in the doubly unexposed group), and inverted interaction (where the risk of the outcome in the doubly exposed group is less than that in the doubly unexposed group). Analogous orderings can be obtained when both exposures are preventive or when one is causative and the other preventive.[56]

The presence or absence of interaction on either scale may be of interest and as noted above, provided both exposures have an effect on the outcome, there will always be interaction on at least one scale. The only way there can be no interaction on any scale is for at least one of the two exposures to have no effect on the outcome at all. This brings us back to the point that was made at the beginning of the chapter, that, when studying interaction, it is important to clearly understand what the goal of the analysis is: What is it that we are trying to learn? What scientific or policy question are we trying to answer and how does an interaction analysis help us? We have seen above already that interaction on the additive scale gives insight into which subgroups are best to treat. We will see below that interaction on the additive scale can also sometimes give insight into more mechanistic forms of interaction. As also discussed below, the absence of interaction on either the additive or multiplicative scale may also give some clues (though rarely definitive evidence) as to the underlying biology; likewise we will see that the presence of positive-multiplicative interaction may give some clues as to mechanisms. But it is always important to clarify what the goal of the analysis is and what we are trying to learn. Again, the fact that there is interaction *on some scale* is otherwise nothing more than acknowledging that both exposures have some effect.

CONFOUNDING AND THE INTERPRETATION OF INTERACTION

Thus far, we have considered measures of interaction using risk differences, risk ratios, and odds ratios. In general, however, we want to know whether our effect estimates correspond to causal effects rather than mere associations. In observational studies, we thus attempt to control for confounding. Analytically, this is often done through regression adjustment for other covariates. In interaction analyses, we have two exposures and thus potentially two sets of confounding factors to consider. The causal interpretation of interaction measures depends on whether control has been made for one or both sets of confounding factors or neither.

Suppose we have controlled for one set of confounding factors, those for the relationship between our primary exposure of interest and the outcome, but that we have possibly not controlled for confounding of the relationship between the secondary factor and the outcome. We would in this case still be able to obtain valid estimates of the effect of the primary exposure within strata defined by our secondary factor. For example, suppose we found substantial interaction between a drug and hair color when examining some health outcome. If we had controlled for the confounding factors for the drug-outcome relationship, or if the drug were randomized, we could interpret our interaction measure as a measure of heterogeneity concerning how the actual causal effect of the drug varied across subgroups defined by hair color. If we found that the effect of our primary exposure varied by strata defined by the secondary factor in this way, then we might call this "effect heterogeneity" or "effect modification." This might be useful, for example, in decisions about which subpopulations to target to maximize the effect of interventions. Provided we have controlled for confounding of the relationship between the primary exposure and the outcome, these estimates of effect modification or effect heterogeneity could be useful even if we have not controlled for confounding of the relationship between the secondary factor and the outcome. What we would not know, however, is whether the effect heterogeneity was due to the secondary factor itself or something else associated with it. If we have not controlled for confounding for the secondary factor, the secondary factor itself may simply be serving as a proxy for something that is causally relevant for the outcome.[44] For example, if we found that the effect of the drug varied by strata defined by hair color, this may simply be because hair color is associated with genotype and it is this genotype that is causally relevant for modifying the effect of the drug on the outcome. If we were simply to dye someone's hair, this intervention would not change the effect of the drug.

If we are interested principally in assessing the effect of the primary exposure within subgroups defined by a secondary factor, then simply controlling for confounding for the relationship between the primary exposure and the outcome is sufficient. However, if we want to intervene on the secondary factor to change the effect of the primary exposure, then we need to control for confounding of the relationships of both factors with the outcome. When we control for confounding for both factors, we might refer to this as "causal interaction" in distinction from mere "effect heterogeneity" mentioned above.[57]

As another example, VanderWeele and Knol[58] consider a randomized trial for a housing intervention program for homeless adults to reduce the number of hospitalizations. Suppose that the effect of the housing program were examined within strata defined by whether the participants had at least part time employment. Here, the housing program is randomized, but employment status is not. If it were found that the housing intervention had a larger effect for those with part-time employment than for those without, this could be used as a valid estimate for the effect of the intervention within these different subgroups and could be useful in subsequently targeting the intervention toward the subgroups for which it would be most effective. By randomization, we have controlled for confounding of the housing intervention, but we have not necessarily controlled for confounding of employment status. Thus, while we could get valid estimates of effects of the housing intervention within strata defined by employment status, we could not draw conclusions on what would happen if we intervened on employment status as well to try to improve the effect of the intervention. Again, employment status has not been randomized. Employment status may, for instance, be serving as a proxy for mental health, and it may be that mental health is in fact what is relevant in altering the effects of the intervention. It is possible that if we intervened on employment status, without changing mental health, then this would not alter at all the effect of the housing intervention. We would only be able to assess what the effect of interventions on employment status in altering the effect of the housing intervention would be if we had controlled for confounding of the relationship between the factor defining subgroups, namely employment status, and the outcome.

In summary, if we are interested in identifying which subpopulations it is best to target with a particular intervention, then assessing effect heterogeneity is fine and only the confounding factors of the relation between the primary exposure and outcome need be considered (though even here it is sometimes argued control for other factors can help with external validity and extrapolation to other settings). If we are interested in potentially intervening on the secondary factor to change the effects of the primary intervention (or if we are interested in assessing mechanistic interaction, described below), then we want measures of causal interaction and we would need to control for confounding for the relationships between both factors and the outcome.

In practice, typically a regression model is simply fit to the data, regressing the outcome on the two exposures, a product term, and possibly other covariates. However, whether the regression coefficient for the product term can be interpreted as a measure of effect heterogeneity or causal interaction or both or neither depends on what confounding factors have been controlled. For effect heterogeneity, we only have one set of confounding factors to consider, just those for the relationship between the primary exposure and the outcome. For causal interaction, we have two sets of confounding factors to consider, those for the primary exposure and the outcome and those for the secondary factor and the outcome. Epidemiologists are careful to control for confounding and think carefully about confounding in observational studies for overall causal effects. However, too often issues of confounding have been neglected in interaction analyses. Careful thought needs to be given to interaction analyses in interpreting associations as causal and in distinguishing between whether an attempt is being made to control for one or both sets of confounding factors; and which of "effect heterogeneity" (also sometimes called "effect modification") or "causal interaction" is of interest will depend upon the context. Additional subtleties also arise in distinguishing between causal interaction and effect heterogeneity. For example, VanderWeele[57] showed that there can be cases in which effect heterogeneity is present but not causal interaction or when causal interaction is present but not effect heterogeneity. Likewise, there are also cases in which effect heterogeneity measures are identified from the data, but casual interaction measures are not; there are more subtle cases in which casual interaction measures are identified from the data but effect heterogeneity measures are not.

The terms "interaction" and "effect modification" in practice are often used interchangeably. In some sense, what we have called "effect modification" or "effect heterogeneity" is still a type of interaction analysis and what we have called "causal interaction" could almost be viewed as "effect modification" by intervening on a secondary variable.[57,59] There is some ambiguity in terminology, and it would be difficult to insist on a set of rules for terminology. However, even if the terms themselves are used interchangeably, it is important to keep in mind that there are still two distinct concepts. The distinction has to do with whether one or two potential interventions are in view. Failure to take the distinction into account could lead to incorrect policy recommendations. In writing papers, researchers can make clear which of the two concepts is in view (without having to adopt a strict terminological stance) by clarifying, in a Methods section, whether confounding control is intended for one or both exposures and by commenting, in a Discussion section, whether interventions on one or both exposures are being considered when interpreting the implications of the results.

PRESENTING INTERACTION ANALYSES

Very often when interaction or effect modification is of interest, effect measures are presented for each stratum separately using separate reference groups. Suppose for example, we had data as in Table 26-1 and that effect measures were computed on the risk ratio scale. We let $X = 1$ denote asbestos exposure and $X = 0$ the absence of asbestos exposure, and we let $G = 1$ denote smoking and $G = 0$ nonsmoking. It is not uncommon for papers to present, *e.g.*, the (adjusted) risk ratio effect measures for say the exposure X separately across strata of the other factor G. For example, the effect measures might be presented as in Table 26-5.

While it may be useful to see that the risk ratio in the nonsmoking ($G = 0$) stratum is larger than the risk ratio in the smoking ($G = 1$) stratum, and for calculating multiplicative interaction: $4.74/6.09 = 0.78$ as above, there are several other comparisons for which Table 26-5 is uninformative. For example, by presenting the analyses with separate reference groups for each of the $G = 0$ and $G = 1$ strata, we will not know from such a presentation whether the ($G = 0, X = 1$) subgroup or the ($G = 1, X = 0$) subgroup is at higher risk for the outcome. In fact, simply from the information in Table 26-5, we would not know whether the ($G = 1, X = 1$) subgroup or the ($G = 0, X = 1$) subgroup is at higher risk for the outcome, or whether the ($G = 1, X = 0$) subgroup or the ($G = 0, X = 0$) subgroup is at higher risk for the outcome. Nor do we know from Table 26-5 what the sign is for measures of additive interaction. For these reasons, current guidelines[38,39] recommend that interaction and effect modification analyses be presented with a single common reference group, say the ($G = 0, X = 0$) subgroup, or that the original data be presented,[37] or both. If risk ratios with a common reference group were used for the data in Table 26-1, the risk ratio estimates could then be presented as in Table 26-6.

From the information presented in Table 26-6, which uses a single common reference group, we would know that the increasing order of risk across $G \times X$ subgroups was ($G = 0, X = 0$), then ($G = 0, X = 1$), then ($G = 1, X = 0$), and then ($G = 1, X = 1$). We could still calculate the individual risk ratios for X in the different strata of G as: $6.09/1 = 6.09$ for $G = 0$ and $40.9/8.64 = 4.74$ for $G = 1$ (and we could also add these to the table if desired). We could thus also estimate measures of multiplicative interaction. We could moreover estimate the risk ratios for G across strata of X: *e.g.*, $8.64/1 = 8.64$ for $X = 0$ and $40.9/6.09 = 6.72$ for $X = 1$ (and we could present these in the table if desired). And we could moreover estimate measures of additive interaction from the information in Table 26-6: $\text{RERI}_{RR} = 40.9 - 8.64 - 6.09 + 1 = 27.2 > 0$. The presentation of interaction analyses in Table 26-6 thus gives the reader far more information (using a single common reference category) than the presentation in Table 26-5 (using multiple reference categories). Presenting interaction analyses using a single common reference category such as the presentation in Table 26-6 is thus to be preferred. If the study is a cohort study, then it may be even further preferable to present the actual risks, as in Table 26-1, in the cells of the table, rather than the risk ratios.[37,38]

TABLE 26-5

Risk Ratios With Separate Reference Groups (Less Informative Presentation)

	No Asbestos ($X = 0$)	Asbestos ($X = 1$)
Nonsmoker ($G = 0$)	1 (Reference)	RR = 6.09
Smoker ($G = 1$)	1 (Reference)	RR = 4.74

TABLE 26-6

Risk Ratios With a Common Reference Group (More Informative Presentation)

	No Asbestos ($X = 0$)	Asbestos ($X = 1$)
Nonsmoker ($G = 0$)	1 (Reference)	6.09
Smoker ($G = 1$)	8.64	40.9

Knol and VanderWeele[38] suggest that when interaction and effect modification analyses are presented, the following items all be given in Table 26-1: (1) risk differences or risk ratios (or odds ratios if risk differences or relative risks cannot be calculated) for each (G, E) stratum with a single reference category (possibly taken as the stratum with the lowest risk of the outcome); (2) risk differences, risk ratios, or odds ratios for G within strata of X, and for X within strata of G; (3) interaction measures on additive and multiplicative scales, along with confidence intervals and P-values for these; (4) the exposure-outcome confounders for which adjustment has been made either for one of the exposures (for effect modification/heterogeneity analyses) or for both of the exposures (for interaction analyses) with clear indication of whether attempt is being made to control for one or two sets of confounding factors. Knol and VanderWeele[38] also consider different layout options for this information and how to further extend such presentations when one or both exposures has more than two levels. If multiple different interaction analyses are conducted in the same paper and presented in the same table, it may be desirable to put all of these items on a single line of a table so that multiple interactions analyses can be presented in the same table.

QUALITATIVE INTERACTION

In some cases, we might think that an exposure has a positive effect for one subgroup and a negative effect for a different subgroup. Such instances are sometimes referred as "qualitative interactions" or "crossover interactions."[60,61] The term "quantitative interaction" is sometimes used exclusively for interactions which are not qualitative interactions.[61] However, others use the term "quantitative interaction" to describe a statistical interaction on any scale and prefer using "noncrossover interaction" for the presence of interaction which is not a "qualitative interaction."[60] Unlike statistical interactions, qualitative interactions do not depend on the scale that is being used.[62] If there is a qualitative interaction on the difference scale, there will also be a qualitative interaction on the ratio scale, and vice versa.

As an example of such qualitative interaction, Gail and Simon[60] consider data from a trial of two therapies for breast cancer, one of which does and the other of which does not involve tamoxifen. For patients younger than 50 years with low progesterone receptor levels, the treatment without tamoxifen led to higher proportions who were disease-free after 3 years. However, for all other groups (who were either older or had higher progesterone receptor levels, or both), the treatment with tamoxifen led to higher proportions who were disease-free after 3 years. Here we would likely want to give young patients with low progesterone receptor levels the treatment without tamoxifen, and others the treatment with tamoxifen.

In an example like this, we see then that qualitative interaction is very important in decision-making. We discussed above that in settings in which the intervention is beneficial for everyone, but the magnitude of the benefit varies across subgroups, additive interaction can be useful in assessing whether it would be better to target the intervention to some subgroups rather than others if resources are limited. However, in such settings, if resources are not limited and the intervention is beneficial for everyone we may well want to treat all subgroups. Qualitative interaction, in contrast, has implications for treatment or interventions decisions even if resources are unlimited. In the presence of qualitative interaction, we do not want to treat all subgroups, because the treatment is in fact harmful in some subgroups. If qualitative interaction is present, it is thus important to be able to detect it. Often, in a randomized trial, if a particular treatment or drug is known to be detrimental in some subgroups, such subgroups are typically then excluded from the trial when choosing participants. If this is so, qualitative interaction would then not be apparent because the groups for which the treatment has harmful effects are excluded in advance.

Several statistical approaches have been developed to evaluate such qualitative interaction (*e.g.*, Refs. 60, 63-66). The details of these various approaches and their power properties do vary, but they all essentially coincide when one is simply testing for qualitative interaction between two subgroups. The approaches differ when examining qualitative interaction across three or more subgroups. Pan and Wolfe[64] describe a fairly straightforward way to carry out this evaluation. Their approach allows for multiple subgroups and allows estimation of qualitative interaction of at least a certain magnitude (rather than simply whether one of the effects is larger, and the other smaller, than 0). It requires constructing confidence intervals of various sizes depending on the number of subgroups. Their approach is equivalent to that described by Piantadosi and Gail,[65] sometimes referred to as the "range test," but the implementation described by Pan and Wolfe[64] is easier to carry out. An alternative approach was proposed by Gail and Simon[60] that involves not simply constructing confidence intervals for the effects in each subgroup but rather constructing a confidence interval for the sum of the positive versus negative standardized effects across subgroups.

The approach of Gail and Simon[60] tends to perform better when there are several subgroups with effects that are positive and several also with effects that are negative. The approaches of Piantadosi and Gail[65] and Pan and Wolfe[64] tend to perform better if the effects in most of the subgroups are in one direction and there are only one or very few subgroups for which the effect is in the opposite direction. The motivation for these various approaches involving several subgroups is often having a continuous covariate or multiple covariates of interest, which might define subgroups for which a qualitative interaction is thought to be present. However, with continuous covariates or multiple covariates, an approach described below for detecting effect heterogeneity based on a vector of covariate values, and determining for which individuals the treatment effects are positive versus negative, may ultimately prove to be more useful.

A special case or limit case of qualitative interaction is what is sometimes called a pure interaction, in which the exposure has no effect whatsoever in one subgroup but does have an effect in a different subgroup. Like qualitative interactions, pure interactions do not depend on the scale being used. As an example of such a "pure" interaction, certain genetic variants on chromosome 15q25.1, which seem to only affect lung cancer for individuals who smoke, and otherwise appear to have no effect for those who do not smoke.[67] We will consider this example further below.

SYNERGISM AND MECHANISTIC INTERACTIONS

Thus far, we have been considering different notions of statistical interaction and their interpretation. We noted above that such notions of statistical interaction were scale dependent. In this section, we will consider drawing conclusions about more mechanistic forms of interaction. We might say that a "sufficient cause interaction" is present if there are individuals for whom the outcome would occur if both exposures were present but would not occur if just one or the other exposure were present.[43,45] If we let Y_{gx} denote the counterfactual outcome (the outcome that would have occurred) for each subject if, possibly contrary to fact, G had been set to g and X had been set to x, then a sufficient cause interaction is present if for some individual $Y_{11} = 1$ but $Y_{10} = Y_{01} = 0$. This is in some sense a "mechanistic interaction" insofar as when both exposures are present, the outcome is turned "on," but when only one or the other exposure is present, the outcome is turned "off." It can furthermore be shown that if such a sufficient cause interaction is present, then within the sufficient cause framework (see Chapter 3),[46] there must be a sufficient cause for Y that has both G and X as components.[43,45] This is thus sometimes called "synergism" between G and X in the sufficient cause framework. Note that a sufficient cause interaction does require some individual with $Y_{11} = 1$ but $Y_{10} = Y_{01} = 0$, but does not require $Y_{00} = 0$ for this individual. Below we will also consider an even stronger notion of "mechanistic interaction," which requires some individual for whom $Y_{11} = 1$ and $Y_{10} = Y_{01} = Y_{00} = 0$. However, we will begin our discussion of mechanistic interaction with the slightly weaker notion of a sufficient cause interaction, as this is all that is required for synergism between G and X within the sufficient cause framework. Patterns of this sort are sometimes referred to as "response types" and have been discussed extensively elsewhere.[58,68-70]

Additive interaction is sometimes used to evaluate such mechanistic or sufficient cause interaction. However, having positive additive interaction only implies such sufficient cause interaction under additional assumptions. If it can be assumed that both exposures are never preventive for any individual (formally, if Y_{gx} is nondecreasing in g and x for all individuals), then provided control is also made for confounding of both exposures, positive-additive interaction, $p_{11} - p_{10} - p_{01} + p_{00} > 0$, suffices for sufficient cause interaction.[11,43] The assumption that neither exposure can ever be preventive for any individual is sometimes referred to as a positive "monotonicity" assumption; it is a strong assumption. In some contexts, it might be plausible. For example, we would probably never think that smoking is protective for lung cancer for any individual. There may be some persons for whom smoking causes lung cancer, there may be others for whom smoking is neutral, but we would never think that smoking prevents lung cancer for anyone (*i.e.*, that they would not have lung cancer if they smoked, but that they would have lung cancer if they did not smoke). Thus the positive monotonicity assumption for the effect of smoking on lung cancer may be plausible. But, in other cases, the assumption may be less plausible. For example, if we were to consider the effect of alcohol consumption on stroke, alcohol may be protective for stroke in some persons but causative for others; the monotonicity assumption would not be plausible here. Positive monotonicity requires that the effect is never preventive for the outcome for any person in the population. Importantly, to assess sufficient cause interaction simply by examining whether additive interaction is positive requires that the effects of both exposures on the outcome be monotonic. This will in many contexts be a strong assumption, and it is an assumption that is not possible to verify empirically; it must be argued for on substantive grounds.

Fortunately, it is also possible to assess sufficient cause interaction even without such monotonicity assumptions, but the standard approaches no longer suffice. VanderWeele and Robins[43,45] showed that if the effect of the two exposures were unconfounded, then,

$$p_{11} - p_{10} - p_{01} > 0$$

would imply the presence of a sufficient cause interaction. This is a stronger condition than regular positive-additive interaction, which only requires $p_{11} - p_{10} - p_{01} + p_{00} > 0$ because, with the condition $p_{11} - p_{10} - p_{01} > 0$, we are no longer adding back in the outcome probability p_{00} for the doubly unexposed group. This condition for a sufficient cause interaction, without making monotonicity assumptions, thus does not correspond to, and is stronger than, the regular test for additive interaction, or than simply examining whether interaction is positive in a statistical model.[71] In these various cases, the magnitude of the contrast $p_{11} - p_{10} - p_{01} + p_{00}$ with monotonicity or $p_{11} - p_{10} - p_{01}$ without monotonicity in fact gives a lower bound on the prevalence of individuals manifesting sufficient cause interaction patterns.[72]

If data are only available on the ratio scale, then if both exposures have positive monotonic effects on the outcomes, we can also test for sufficient cause interaction by the condition $RERI_{RR} > 0$. Likewise, the condition $p_{11} - p_{10} - p_{01} > 0$ without imposing monotonicity assumptions can expressed as $RERI_{RR} > 1$; again this is stronger than simply the ordinary condition for positive additive interaction $RERI_{RR} > 0$. However $RERI_{RR}$ can still be used in a straightforward way to test for such sufficient cause interaction by testing whether $RERI_{RR} > 1$ rather than simply $RERI_{RR} > 0$.

Note that when the empirical conditions above are satisfied, the conclusion is that there are some individuals for whom $Y_{11} = 1$ and $Y_{10} = Y_{01} = 0$; the conclusion is not that all individuals or even all diseased cases have this response pattern. Note also that these conditions are sufficient but not necessary for sufficient cause interaction, *i.e.*, if these conditions are satisfied, then a sufficient cause interaction must be present, but if the conditions are not satisfied, then there may or may not be a sufficient cause interaction—one simply cannot determine this from the data. The conditions given here are the weakest possible empirical conditions to test for sufficient cause interaction without making further assumptions.[73]

VanderWeele[35,74] discussed empirical tests for an even stronger notion of interaction. We might say that there is a "singular" or "epistatic" interaction if there are individuals in the population who will have the outcome if and only if both exposures are present; in counterfactual notation, that is, there are individuals for whom $Y_{11} = 1$ but $Y_{10} = Y_{01} = Y_{00} = 0$. In the genetics literature, when gene-gene interactions are considered, such response patterns are sometimes called instances of "compositional epistasis"[75,76] and constitute settings in which the effect of one genetic factor is masked unless the other is present. VanderWeele[35,74] showed that if the effects of the two exposures on the outcome were unconfounded then,

$$p_{11} - p_{10} - p_{01} - p_{00} > 0$$

would imply the presence of such an "epistatic interaction." Again, this is an even stronger notion of interaction; in this condition for "epistatic interaction," we are now subtracting p_{00}. The condition $p_{11} - p_{10} - p_{01} - p_{00} > 0$ expressed in terms of $RERI_{RR}$ is equivalent to $RERI_{RR} > 2$. For epistatic interactions, if the effect of at least one of the exposures is positive monotonic (Y_{gx} is nondecreasing in at least one of g or x), then $p_{11} - p_{10} - p_{01} > 0$ suffices for an epistatic interaction and tests for $RERI_{RR} > 1$ could be used; if the effect of both exposures are positive and monotonic, then $p_{11} - p_{10} - p_{01} + p_{00} > 0$ suffices and tests for $RERI_{RR} > 0$ could be used to test for an epistatic interaction.[35,74] These conditions are likewise sufficient but not necessary for an epistatic interaction; if these conditions are satisfied, then an epistatic interaction must be present, but if the conditions are not satisfied, then an epistatic interaction may or may not be present. Note also that when the empirical conditions above are satisfied, the conclusion is that there are some individuals for whom $Y_{11} = 1$ but $Y_{10} = Y_{01} = Y_{00} = 0$; the conclusion is not that all individuals or all diseased cases have this response pattern. The various results are summarized in Table 26-7.

The sufficient conditions given here for mechanistic interaction require that control has been made for confounding of the effects of both exposures. The sufficient conditions for $RERI_{RR}$ for mechanistic interaction in Table 26-7 still apply when adjustment is made for confounders (*e.g.*, when the relative excess risk due to interaction is calculated using logistic regression as described above adjusting for a sufficient set of confounders). When statistical models are used to adjust for confounding, this requires correct model specification. Within the sufficient cause framework, such statistical models can impose constraints on the sufficient causes, which are sometimes thought undesirable.[72] In such cases, alternative modeling approaches using weighting or semiparametric methods can help relax these modeling assumptions[33,72,77,78] but are beyond the scope of this chapter.

In assessing additive interaction using $RERI_{RR}$, it thus is useful to examine not only whether the estimate and confidence interval for $RERI_{RR}$ are greater than 0 (*i.e.*, whether there is additive interaction) but also whether the estimate and confidence interval for $RERI_{RR}$ are all greater than 1 or are all greater than 2. This examination is useful because $RERI_{RR}$ of this magnitude would provide evidence for mechanistic interaction (sufficient cause or epistatic interaction) without the need for additional assumptions. The $RERI_{RR}$ scale is the natural scale on which to assess mechanistic interaction and has the thresholds of 0, 1, and 2 for varying degrees of evidence (according to the strength of the assumptions needed for the conclusion). We noted above that $RERI_{RR}$ cannot be used to assess the magnitude of the underlying additive interaction for risks, but we see here that although its magnitude does not necessarily correspond to the magnitude of the additive interaction for risks, the magnitude of $RERI_{RR}$ does give differing degrees of evidence for mechanistic interaction.

As an example, Bhavnani et al.,[79] using age-standardized measures, report risk ratios for diarrheal disease across groups infected with rotavirus and/or Giardia. With the doubly uninfected group as the reference category, the risk ratio for rotavirus (in the absence of Giardia) is 2.63, the

TABLE 26-7

Relations Between the Additive Relative Excess Risk due to Interaction (RERI) and Forms of Mechanistic Interaction Under Different Monotonicity Assumptions
("S" Indicates the Presence of a Sufficient Cause Interaction; "E" Indicates an Epistatic Interaction)

Monotonicity Assumption	$RERI_{RR} > 0$	$RERI_{RR} > 1$	$RERI_{RR} > 2$
No assumptions about monotonicity	-	S	S, E
One of G or X have positive monotonic effects	-	S, E	S, E
Both G and X have positive monotonic effects	S, E	S ,E	S, E

risk ratio for Giardia (in the absence of rotavirus) is 1.13, and the risk ratio when both rotavirus and Giardia are present as 10.72. This gives $\text{RERI}_{RR} = 10.72 - 2.63 - 1.13 + 1 = 7.96$ (95% CI: 3.13, 18.92). The value of RERI_{RR} and its entire 95% confidence interval exceed the value 2, suggesting strong evidence for mechanistic interaction (both "sufficient cause" and "epistatic" interaction) even in the absence of any monotonicity assumptions.

Evaluation of sufficient cause or epistatic interaction can also be done simply by using the interaction parameter of a log-linear model (or logistic model if odds ratios approximate risk ratios) directly. The log-linear model for risk ratios that includes a product term takes the form:

$$\log\left[P\left(Y = 1 \middle| G = g, X = x\right)\right] = \beta_0 + \beta_1 g + \beta_2 x + \beta_3 xg.$$

Here, if both G and X have positive monotonic effects on Y, then the condition $\beta_3 > 0$ implies both a sufficient cause interaction and an epistatic interaction.[71,74] If at least one of G or X has positive monotonic effects on Y, then, provided both the main effect of G and X on Y are nonnegative (i.e., $\beta_1 \geq 0$ and $\beta_2 \geq 0$), the condition $\beta_3 > \log(2)$ implies both a sufficient cause interaction and an epistatic interaction.[71,74] Since $\exp(\beta_3) = \text{RR}_{11}/(\text{RR}_{10}\text{RR}_{01})$, this simplifies to the condition for the multiplicative risk ratio interaction $\text{RR}_{11}/(\text{RR}_{10}\text{RR}_{01}) > 2$. If neither G nor X have positive monotonic effects on Y, then, provided both the main effect of G and X on Y are nonnegative (i.e., $\beta_1 \geq 0$ and $\beta_2 \geq 0$), the condition $\beta_3 > \log(2)$ implies a sufficient cause interaction and the condition $\beta_3 > \log(3)$ implies an epistatic interaction.[71,74] Thus, once again, without monotonicity assumptions a positive statistical multiplicative interaction, $\beta_3 > 0$, alone does not suffice and we need strong conditions, e.g., $\beta_3 > \log(2)$ or $\beta_3 > \log(3)$. However, if we can estimate the parameters of the multiplicative model $\beta_1, \beta_2, \beta_3$ then, as described above, we can calculate the relative excess risk due to interaction by $\text{RERI}_{RR} = \exp(\beta_1 + \beta_2 + \beta_3) - \exp(\beta_1) - \exp(\beta_2) + 1$ and we would be better off testing for sufficient cause synergism using the conditions $\text{RERI}_{RR} > 0$ or $\text{RERI}_{RR} > 1$ or $\text{RERI}_{RR} > 2$, respectively, as these conditions are more often satisfied than those for the multiplicative interaction [$\beta_3 > 0$, $\beta_3 > \log(2)$, and $\beta_3 > \log(2)$]. The comments here for statistical interaction for risk ratios in a log-linear model pertain also approximately to statistical interaction for disease odds ratios in a logistic regression model when the outcome is rare.

Although it is beyond the scope of the current chapter, extensions of these ideas are available for exposures with more than two levels[74,80] and for multiway interactions between three or more exposures[45,73] as well as for settings with causal antagonism in which the presence of one exposure may block the operation of the other.[81] In the next section, we will discuss how even these so-called mechanistic interactions (sufficient cause or epistatic interactions) give limited information about the underlying biology.

LIMITS OF INFERENCE CONCERNING BIOLOGY

Although evaluations of sufficient cause interaction, like those considered in the previous section, can shed light on whether there are individuals for whom the outcome would occur if both exposures are present but not if just one or the other is present, even such "mechanistic interaction" does not imply that the two exposures are physically interacting in any biologic sense.[43,75,76,82,83] To see this, suppose that G_1 and G_2 are two genetic factors. Suppose that when $G_1 = 1$ protein 1 is not produced and that when $G_2 = 1$ protein 2 is not produced. Suppose that the outcome Y occurs if and only if neither protein 1 nor protein 2 is present. We then have an epistatic interaction because the outcome occurs if and only if $G_1 = 1$ and $G_2 = 1$, but we do not have physical interaction here. It is the absence of the proteins that gives rise to the outcome; there simply is nothing to interact biologically.

We should thus distinguish between (1) statistical interaction on the one hand and (2) mechanistic interaction (e.g., the outcome occurs if both exposures are present but not if just one or the other is present), on the other, and finally, (3) "biological" or "functional" interaction in which the two exposures physically interact to bring about the outcome.[35,75,76,84] In the example just given, we have mechanistic interaction but not "functional" or biological interaction. Thus, although we can sometimes empirically draw conclusions about mechanistic interaction from data, empirical tests will not generally inform conclusions about functional or biological interaction between exposures, and it is important to understand the limits of the conclusions being drawn about these alternative forms of interaction.

Other examples of the limitation of biologic inference concerning interaction were given by Siemiatycki and Thomas.[82] Consider, for example, a setting in which for the outcome to occur, two stages of disease development must take place. Suppose that the two exposures of interest, G_1 and G_2, affect different stages: G_1 acts on stage 1 and G_2 acts on stage 2. Suppose also in this example that stage 1 and stage 2 are completely independent of each other. Assume that the baseline probability of stage 1 occurring is 1% and the baseline probability of stage 2 occurring is also 1%, so that the baseline risk of disease is 0.01%. Suppose that G_1 increases the probability of stage 1 occurring from 1% to 2% and G_2 increases the probability of stage 2 occurring from 1% to 5%. Suppose, however, that the presence of G_2 in no way alters the effect of G_1's increasing the probability of stage 1 occurring from 1% to 2%; i.e., the probability of stage 2 is 1% if $G_1 = 0$ and 2% if $G_1 = 1$, irrespective of whether G_2 is present or absent. Suppose, similarly, that the presence of G_1 in no way alters the effect of G_2's increasing the probability of stage 2 occurring from 1% to 5%. Here then we seem to have no interaction between G_1 and G_2 at the biologic level. As noted above, if neither exposure ($G_1 = 0$ and $G_2 = 0$) is present, then the risk of stage 1 and stage 2 are both 1% and the overall risk of the outcome is $1\% \times 1\% = 0.01\%$. If just G_1 is present ($G_1 = 1$ and $G_2 = 0$) then the risk of stage 1 is 2% and the risk of stage 2 is 1% and the overall risk of the outcome is $2\% \times 1\% = 0.02\%$. If $G_1 = 0$ and $G_2 = 1$, then the risk of stage 1 is 1% and the risk of stage 2 is 5% and the overall risk of the outcome is $1\% \times 5\% = 0.05\%$. If $G_1 = 1$ and $G_2 = 1$, then the risk of stage 1 is 2% and the risk of stage 2 is 5% and the overall risk of the outcome is $2\% \times 5\% = 0.10\%$. In this example our measure of multiplicative interaction is:

$$\left(p_{11}p_{00}\right)/\left(p_{10}p_{01}\right) = \left[0.10\%\left(0.01\%\right)\right]/\left[0.02\%\left(0.05\%\right)\right] = 1$$

However, our measure of additive interaction is:

$$p_{11} - p_{10} - p_{01} + p_{00} = 0.10\% - 0.02\% - 0.05\% + 0.01\% = 0.04\% > 0.$$

We have positive-additive interaction but no biologic interaction in this example. Here our conditions for sufficient cause interaction are satisfied since:

$$p_{11} - p_{10} - p_{01} = 0.10\% - 0.02\% - 0.05\% = 0.03\% > 0$$

and even our conditions for "epistatic" or "singular" interaction are satisfied:

$$p_{11} - p_{10} - p_{01} - p_{00} = 0.10\% - 0.02\% - 0.05\% - 0.01\% = 0.02\% > 0$$

But we stipulated there was no functional interaction between G_1 and G_2 at the biologic level. How are we to make sense of this? What we can conclude from the condition for a epistatic or singular interaction is that there are some individuals who would have the outcome if both exposures were present but who would not if just one or the other or neither exposure were present. But we see here that not even this necessarily indicates interaction at some functional biologic level. We have this form of "singular" or "sufficient cause" interaction because, if both exposures are present, 0.10% have the outcome and this cannot be accounted by those individuals whose outcome only required the first exposure (0.02%) or only the second (0.05%) or who required neither (0.01%). Even if these three groups were mutually exclusive, they would not account for the risk of 0.10% that occurs if both exposures are present $[0.10\% - (0.02\% + 0.05\% + 0.01\%) = 0.02\% > 0]$. There must be some individuals for whom the outcome occurs if and only if both exposures are present. But again, this does not, as this example shows, indicate interaction in any functional biologic sense.

On the basis of these and other similar examples, Thompson[83] suggested that if an outcome required stages and one exposure affected the first stage and another exposure affected the second stage (a "multistage model") then if there were no biologic interaction, we would expect a multiplicative model. He likewise suggested that if the occurrence of a single adverse event was sufficient for the development of the disease (a "single-hit model"), then in the absence of biologic interaction, we would expect an additive model. Finally, he suggested that if the outcome occurred if an individual failed to experience any of one or more occurrences of a beneficial event (a "no-hit model" cf. Ref. 85), then the model should again be multiplicative. While such heuristics may be of some use, if we do find that an additive model fits well it is not necessarily the case that we have a "single-hit model" with no biologic interaction; it could equally be the case that we have a "multistage model" in which the factors operate antagonistically. Or if we were to find that the multiplicative model fit well, this fit does not necessarily indicate a "multistage model" with no biologic interaction, but could also be a "single-hit model" in which there was biologic interaction. We cannot in general draw conclusions about the type of biologic model and the presence or absence of biologic interaction simply from the statistical models we use. If we find positive multiplicative interaction, this could be a "multistage model" or a "no-hit" model with biologic interaction, or it could be a "single-hit model" with biologic interaction, or it could be a more complicated model with no biologic interaction whatsoever. We cannot tell from the data alone. Our inferences about biology are limited.

We can assess statistical interaction (on any scale we choose), we can assess additive interaction to determine how best to allocate interventions, and we can assess "sufficient cause" or "epistatic/singular" interaction to determine whether there are individuals who would have the outcome if both exposures were present but not if only one or the other were present. All of these may provide some insight into the underlying biology, but we have no way of going from any of these forms of interaction, which we can assess with data, directly to the underlying biology itself.

In some earlier literature, sufficient cause synergism was sometimes referred to as "biologic interaction" (*e.g.*, Ref. 86), and sometimes additive interaction was referred to as "biologic interaction" (*e.g.*, Ref. 23). However, as we have seen in the examples above, neither statistical additive interaction nor even sufficient cause interaction or epistatic interaction necessarily tells us anything about physical or functional interactions. Statistical analyses can only tell us limited information about the underlying biology.[82-84,87] Because of this, there has been a suggestion to move away from the use of "biologic interaction" for sufficient cause interaction or synergism in the sufficient cause framework (cf. Refs. 84, 88). It may be more appropriate to refer to these sufficient cause or epistatic interactions as "mechanistic interactions"; these are still cases in which both exposures together turn the outcome "on" and the removal of one turns the outcome "off" and thus the "mechanistic" description seems appropriate. If even this is thought to be language that is too strong (if "mechanistic" is still thought to indicate biology rather than indicating "on" and "off"), then simply using the terms "sufficient cause interaction" may be best.

ATTRIBUTING EFFECTS TO INTERACTIONS

At the beginning of the chapter, we discussed different measures concerning the proportion of risk or effect attributable to interaction. In fact, we can decompose the joint effects of the two exposures, G and X, into three components: (1) the effect due to G alone, (2) the effect due to X alone, and (3) the effect due to their interaction. On the risk difference scale, this decomposition is:

$$p_{11} - p_{00} = \left(p_{10} - p_{00}\right) + \left(p_{01} - p_{00}\right) + \left(p_{11} - p_{10} - p_{01} + p_{00}\right)$$

where the first component, $(p_{10} - p_{00})$, is the effect due to G alone, the second component, $(p_{01} - p_{00})$, is the effect due to X alone, and the final component, $(p_{11} - p_{10} - p_{01} + p_{00})$, is the standard additive interaction. We could then also compute the proportion of the joint effect due to G alone, $(p_{10} - p_{00})/(p_{11} - p_{00})$, due to X alone, $(p_{01} - p_{00})/(p_{11} - p_{00})$, and due to their interaction, $(p_{11} - p_{10} - p_{01} + p_{00})/(p_{11} - p_{00})$. We can also carry out a similar decomposition with ratio measures using excess relative risks. We can decompose the excess relative risk for both exposures, $RR_{11} - 1$, into the excess relative risk for G alone, for X alone, and the excess relative risk due to interaction, RERI. Specifically, we have[89]:

$$RR_{11} - 1 = \left(RR_{10} - 1\right) + \left(RR_{01} - 1\right) + RERI_{RR}.$$

We could then likewise compute the proportion of the effect due to G alone, $(RR_{10} - 1)/(RR_{11} - 1)$, due to X alone, $(RR_{01} - 1)/(RR_{11} - 1)$, and due to their interaction $RERI_{RR}/(RR_{11} - 1)$.

As noted earlier, Rothman[7] proposed an attributable proportion defined as $AP = RERI_{RR}/RR_{11}$, which captures the proportion of the disease in the doubly exposed group that is due to the interaction. However, the measure in the decomposition above, $RERI_{RR}/(RR_{11} - 1)$, is the proportion of the joint effect due to interaction.[17]

Under the logistic regression model:

$$\operatorname{logit}\left[P\left(Y = 1 \mid G = g, X = x, Z = z\right)\right] = \gamma_0 + \gamma_1 g + \gamma_2 x + \gamma_3 xg + \gamma_4' z.$$

for an outcome that is rare, the joint effect attributable to G alone, X alone, and to their interaction is given approximately by:

$$\left(RR_{10} - 1\right)/\left(RR_{11} - 1\right) \approx \left[\exp(\gamma_1) - 1\right]/\left[\exp(\gamma_1 + \gamma_2 + \gamma_3) - 1\right]$$
$$\left(RR_{01} - 1\right)/\left(RR_{11} - 1\right) \approx \left[\exp(\gamma_2) - 1\right]/\left[\exp(\gamma_1 + \gamma_2 + \gamma_3) - 1\right]$$
$$RERI_{RR}/\left(RR_{11} - 1\right) \approx \left[\exp(\gamma_1 + \gamma_2 + \gamma_3) - \exp(\gamma_1) - \exp(\gamma_2) + 1\right]/\left[\exp(\gamma_1 + \gamma_2 + \gamma_3) - 1\right]$$

The expressions can be used even when control is made for covariates in the logistic regression. VanderWeele and Tchetgen Tchetgen[89] provide software to do this automatically and to calculate standard errors and confidence intervals for the proportions and also discuss extensions to exposures that are not binary. Note that to interpret the effects above causally, one would have to control for confounding of the relationships of both exposures with the outcome. For these measures to make sense as proportions, RR_{11}, RR_{10}, and RR_{01} must all be greater than or equal to 1.

We illustrate the various decompositions with an example from genetic epidemiology presented by VanderWeele and Tchetgen Tchetgen[89] using data from a case-control study of 1,836 cases of lung cancer at Massachusetts General Hospital and 1,452 controls.[90] The study included information on smoking and genotype information on locus 15q25.1. For simplicity, we will code the exposure as binary so that smoking is ever versus never and the genetic variant is a comparison of 0 versus 1/2 T alleles at rs8034191. Analyses were restricted to Caucasians and covariate data include age (continuous), gender, and educational history (college degree or more, yes/no). The regression yielded $\gamma_1 = 0.04$, $\gamma_2 = 1.33$, and $\gamma_3 = 0.49$. If we proceed with the decomposition of the joint effect, then the proportions attributable to G alone, X alone, and to their interaction are:

$$\left(RR_{10} - 1\right)/\left(RR_{11} - 1\right) = \left[\exp(0.04) - 1\right]/\left[\exp(0.04 + 1.33 + 0.49) - 1\right]$$
$$\approx 0.8\% \left(95\% \text{ CI}: -6.2\%, 7.7\%\right)$$
$$\left(RR_{01} - 1\right)/RR_{11} - 1 = \left[\exp(1.33) - 1\right]/\left[\exp(0.04 + 1.33 + 0.49) - 1\right]$$
$$\approx 51.4\% \left(95\% \text{ CI}: 33.4\%, 69.4\%\right)$$
$$RERI/\left(RR_{11} - 1\right) = \left[\begin{array}{c}\exp(0.04 + 1.33 + 0.49) \\ -\exp(0.04) - \exp(1.33) + 1\end{array}\right]/\left[\exp(0.04 + 1.33 + 0.49) - 1\right]$$
$$\approx 47.8\% \left(95\% \text{ CI}: 33.3\%, 62.3\%\right)$$

Almost none ($\sim$0.8%) of the joint effect (comparing both G and X present to both absent) is due to the effect of G in the absence of X, about 51% is due to X in the absence of G, and about 48% is due to the interaction between G and X.

We will now consider a somewhat different decomposition that involves decomposing a total effect, rather than joint effects, into the component due to interaction. If the two exposures G and X are independent (*i.e.*, uncorrelated) in the population, then we can also decompose the total effect of one of the exposures (*e.g.*, total effect of X) into two components[89]:

$$\left(p_{x=1} - p_{x=0}\right) = \left(p_{01} - p_{00}\right) + \left(p_{11} - p_{10} - p_{01} + p_{00}\right)P\left(G=1\right).$$

This decomposes the overall effect of X on Y into two pieces: the first piece is the conditional effect of X on Y when $G = 0$, the second piece is the standard additive interaction, $(p_{11} - p_{10} - p_{01} + p_{00})$, multiplied by the probability that $P(G = 1)$. We can then attribute the total effect of X on Y to the part that would be present still if G were 0 (this is $p_{01} - p_{00}$), and to a part that has to do with the interaction between G and X [this is $(p_{11} - p_{10} - p_{01} + p_{00})P(G=1)$]. If we could remove the genetic exposure, *i.e.*, set it to 0, we would remove the part that is due to the interaction and be left with only $p_{01} - p_{00}$. Since we can do this decomposition, we can define a quantity $\text{pAI}_{G=0}(X)$ as the proportion of the overall effect of X that is attributable to interaction, with a reference category for the genetic exposure of $G = 0$, as:

$$\text{pAI}_{G=0}\left(X\right) := \left[\left(p_{11} - p_{10} - p_{01} + p_{00}\right)P\left(G=1\right)\right]\Big/\left(p_{x=1} - p_{x=0}\right)$$

The remaining portion $(p_{01} - p_{00})/(p_{x=1} - p_{x=0})$ is the proportion of the effect of X that would remain if G were fixed to 0. VanderWeele and Tchetgen Tchetgen[89] provide SAS and Stata code to do this automatically and handle more general cases and models. Note that the three-way decomposition above for joint effects did not require that the exposures be independent of one another. However, the two-way decomposition for a total effect given here does require that the exposures are independent. VanderWeele and Tchetgen Tchetgen[89] and VanderWeele[91] also discuss similar, but more complex, decompositions when the two exposures, G and X, are correlated.

As already discussed earlier in this chapter, one of the motivations for studying interaction is to identify which subgroups would benefit most from intervention when resources are limited. In settings in which it is not possible to intervene directly on the primary exposure of interest, one might instead be interested in which other covariates could be intervened upon to eliminate much or most of the effect of the primary exposure of interest. The methods here for attributing effects to interactions can be useful in assessing this and identifying the most relevant covariates for intervention.

CASE-ONLY DESIGNS

In some settings, especially within genetic contexts, it is sometimes possible to obtain estimates of multiplicative interaction with only a sample of cases. Consider the statistical interaction β_3 in the log-linear model:

$$\log\left[P\left(Y = 1\middle|G = g, X = x\right)\right] = \beta_0 + \beta_1 g + \beta_2 x + \beta_3 xg.$$

Suppose now also that the distribution of the two exposures, G and X, are independent in the population. This assumption may be plausible in many gene-environment interaction studies. Suppose further that data are only collected on the cases ($Y = 1$). It can be shown that under this independence assumption, the odds ratio relating G and X among the cases is equal to the interaction measure on the multiplicative scale β_3[92,93]:

$$\left[P\left(G = 1\middle|X = 1, Y = 1\right)\Big/P\left(G = 0\middle|X = 1, Y = 1\right)\right]\Big/\left[P\left(G = 1\middle|X = 0, Y = 1\right)\Big/P\left(G = 0\middle|X = 0, Y = 1\right)\right]$$

$$= \left[\left(RR_{11}\right)\Big/\left(RR_{10}RR_{01}\right)\right] = \beta_3$$

Somewhat surprisingly, to get measures of multiplicative interaction, all that is needed is data on G and X among the cases. The use of the odds ratio relating G and X among the cases is referred to as the "case-only" estimator of interaction. With the case-only estimator, we can estimate the interaction parameter β_3, but we cannot estimate the main effects of the log-linear regression, β_1 and β_2.

The case-only estimator depends critically on the assumption that the distribution of the two exposures are independent in the population and can be biased if this assumption is violated.[94] However, under this assumption of independence in distribution, the case-only estimator is in fact more efficient than using the standard estimate from a log-linear regression.[95]

The same result holds for statistical interaction in logistic regression.

$$\operatorname{logit}\left[P\big(Y=1\big|G=\mathrm{g},X=\mathrm{x}\big)\right]=\gamma_0+\gamma_1\mathrm{g}+\gamma_2\mathrm{x}+\gamma_3\mathrm{gx}$$

under the assumption that the outcome is rare.[93] The result for log-linear models does not require a rare outcome. Sometimes, for logistic regression, the independence assumption is articulated as one of independence of G and X among the noncases. For a rare outcome, this is approximately equivalent to independence in the population.

The result also holds for log-linear or logistic regression if we control for covariates. The conditional independence assumption is then that the distributions of G and X are independent conditional on Z. Estimates and confidence intervals for the case-only estimator can be obtained by running a logistic regression of G on X and Z among the cases:

$$\operatorname{logit}\left[P\big(G=1\big|X=\mathrm{x},Z=\mathrm{z},Y=1\big)\right]=\theta_0+\theta_1\mathrm{x}+\theta_2'\mathrm{z}.$$

The coefficient and confidence interval for θ_1 in this regression on the cases will equal that of the product term coefficient β_3 in the log-linear model provided the distributions of G and X are independent conditional on Z in the population and will equal that of γ_3 in the logistic model, provided, in addition, that the outcome is rare.

Note that in all cases, to interpret the multiplicative interaction parameter estimate from the statistical model as causal interaction on a multiplicative scale, it would be necessary to assume that the effects of both exposures on the outcome are unconfounded (conditional on covariates Z). To interpret the parameter estimate as a measure of effect heterogeneity on the multiplicative scale, it would be necessary to assume that the effect of one of the exposures on the outcome is unconfounded (conditional on covariates Z). In a case-only study, simply assuming that the effect of one exposure on the other exposure is unconfounded does not suffice to give a causal interpretation for the effects of either or both exposures on the outcome Y.

As an example, Bennet et al.,[96] use data on nonsmoking lung cancer cases and report exposure status for GSTM1 genotype and passive smoking as in Table 26-8.

Using data only on the cases, the estimate of multiplicative interaction is:

$$\mathrm{RR}_{11}/\big(\mathrm{RR}_{10}\mathrm{RR}_{01}\big)$$

$$=\left[P\!\left(\begin{array}{c}G=1\\X=1,Y=1\end{array}\right)\!\Big/P\!\left(\begin{array}{c}G=0\\X=1,Y=1\end{array}\right)\right]\!\Big/\!\left[P\!\left(\begin{array}{c}G=1\\X=0,Y=1\end{array}\right)\!\Big/P\!\left(\begin{array}{c}G=0\\X=0,Y=1\end{array}\right)\right]$$

$$=\big(37/14\big)/\big(27/28\big)=2.74$$

When adjusted also for age, radon exposure, saturated fat intake, and vegetable intake using logistic regression, the case-only estimate of multiplicative interaction is 2.6 (95% CI: 1.1, 6.1). There is evidence here for multiplicative interaction between passive smoking and the absence of GSTM1 on lung cancer.

TABLE 26-8

Number of Cases by Genotype and Smoking Status

	No Smoking	Smoking
GSTM1 present, $G = 0$	28	14
GSTM1 absent, $G = 1$	27	37

From Bennett WP, Alavanja MCR, Blomeke B, et al. Environmental tobacco smoke, genetic susceptibility, and risk of lung cancer in never-smoking women. *J. Natl. Cancer Inst.* 1999;91:2009-2014.

VanderWeele et al.[72] discuss using the case-only estimator to assess mechanistic interaction and show that if the main effects of both exposures are nonnegative (which cannot be assessed directly in a case-only study, but could be evaluated on substantive grounds), then a sufficient cause interaction is present if $\theta_1 > \log(2)$ without any individual level monotonicity assumptions, or if $\theta_1 > 0$ when it can be assumed that both exposures have positive monotonic effects on the outcome. They also note that if the main effects of both exposures are nonnegative, then an epistatic interaction is present if $\theta_1 > \log(3)$ without any individual-level monotonicity assumptions or if $\theta_1 > \log(2)$ and at least one of the two exposures has a positive monotonic effect or if $\theta_1 > 0$ and both exposures have positive monotonic effects.

INTERACTIONS FOR CONTINUOUS OUTCOMES

When continuous outcomes are the focus of study, linear and log-linear regression can still be used to estimate measures of additive and multiplicative interaction, respectively. For additive interaction, a linear regression model for the continuous outcomes could be used:

$$E\left(Y|G = g, X = x, Z = z\right) = \alpha_0 + \alpha_1 g + \alpha_2 x + \alpha_3 xg + \alpha_4' z$$

and α_3 can be taken as a measure of additive interaction. This parameter is equal to the additive interaction measure:

$$\alpha_3 = E\left(Y|G = 1, X = 1, Z = z\right) - E\left(Y|G = 1, X = 0, Z = z\right)$$
$$- E\left(Y|G = 0, X = 1, Z = z\right) + E\left(Y|G = 0, X = 0, Z = z\right).$$

For multiplicative interaction, a log-linear regression model for the continuous outcomes could be used:

$$\log\left[E\left(Y|G = g, X = x, Z = z\right)\right] = \beta_0 + \beta_1 g + \beta_2 x + \beta_3 xg + \beta_4' z$$

and β_3 can be taken as a measure of multiplicative interaction. This parameter, when exponentiated, is equal to the multiplicative interaction measure:

$$\exp(\beta_3) = \left[E\left(\begin{matrix}Y|G = 1, \\ X = 1, Z = z\end{matrix}\right) \middle/ E\left(\begin{matrix}Y|G = 1, \\ X = 0, Z = z\end{matrix}\right)\right] \middle/ \left[E\left(\begin{matrix}Y|G = 0, \\ X = 1, Z = z\end{matrix}\right) \middle/ E\left(\begin{matrix}Y|G = 0, \\ X = 0, Z = z\end{matrix}\right)\right].$$

Note that with a continuous outcome, most of the arguments for preferring one scale to another are no longer applicable. With a continuous outcome, we generally no longer run into convergence problems for the additive scale. But the argument for the public health significance of the additive scale is not as applicable for a continuous outcome because we are no longer analyzing discrete events. Moreover, with a continuous outcome, it is not clear that the additive scale gives any insight into mechanistic interaction. Whether additive or multiplicative scales are to be preferred for a continuous outcome will generally depend on the distribution of the outcome data.

IDENTIFYING SUBGROUPS TO TARGET TREATMENT USING MULTIPLE COVARIATES

Thus far our focus has been on estimating and interpreting interactions; we have focused on binary exposures but have also briefly considered ordinal or continuous exposures. As we had noted above, one motivation for examining interaction is determining whether a particular intervention might be more effective for one subgroup than another. It was noted that assessing interaction on the additive scale was most important for this purpose. This motivation does, however, raise the question as to how to choose the variable or variables that are to define subgroups. Most of our discussion has presupposed that we have a particular secondary variable in mind that will define subgroups and for which we will examine whether there is effect heterogeneity across subgroups. In some settings, data on many such variables that could potentially define subgroups may be available. One option would then be to use each of these and see if any of them are such that there is evidence for substantial effect heterogeneity. A downside of this approach is that by evaluating effect heterogeneity across many variables, we may find spurious results suggesting effect heterogeneity by chance. An approach that is often advocated in the literature is to decide in advance, based on substantive knowledge, which factor or factors are thought most likely to show evidence for effect heterogeneity and evaluate only these.

An additional complication arises when the variable that is going to define subgroups is continuous. One might then have to decide what cutoffs of the continuous variable are to be used to define categories. One might also be interested in whether there is an optimal set of category boundaries such that whenever the variable is above some level, it is best to treat. Methods to address this type of question are now available for a single continuous variable.[97-99]

However, further complications arise when one is interested in using multiple continuous or categorical variables simultaneously. An even more general approach involves forming anticipated "effect scores" for every person in a sample or population based on many baseline covariates and then targeting treatment to those above a certain "effect score" threshold. One approach to forming such effect scores is to fit a regression model for the outcome on all or several covariates for the treated or exposed subjects and then to fit a separate model for the untreated or unexposed subjects. For each person in the sample, one can then use the two models, once they are fit to the data, to obtain a predicted outcome (or probability of the outcome) under exposure or treatment and a predicted outcome (or probability of the outcome) under the unexposed or untreated condition. The difference between these two predicted outcomes would then be the individual's estimated "effect score." One might then consider targeting treatment only to those above a certain threshold. This approach has the advantage of being able to incorporate information from many different covariates in defining subgroups to try to optimize the population-level effect of treatment. It would even be possible to compare different models for the outcome under the exposed and unexposed conditions or different sets of covariates, in these models, to see which has the "effect scores" that best allows one to predict the outcome and target subpopulations.[100]

The approach is appealing and intuitive. Several complications arise, however, in trying to make inferences in this manner, though methods have been developing to address these. One complication is "overfitting": if the same data are used to fit the models and to evaluate which of the effect scores, and models, and covariates, have the best predictive properties in forming subgroups, then the performance in a different sample might not be very good. Because of the potential for overfitting, the evaluation of the effect scores and models and covariates may be misleading because the model parameters were specifically estimated to fit the available data as well as possible and if the same parameters were used to get predicted outcomes in a different sample drawn from the same population, its performance would not be as good. Zhao et al.[100] have proposed a cross-validation procedure which involves splitting the sample into a training dataset (which is used to fit the models) and an evaluation dataset (which is used to evaluate and compare effects scores and models and covariates) to address this problem. Based on simulations they recommend using 4/5 of the data to fit the models and 1/5 to evaluate the models. Another complication that can arise with this effect-score approach is that if the models to get predicted outcomes are not correctly specified, then the inferences about the effects for different subgroups defined by the effect score may be misleading. Cai et al.[101] have proposed a two-stage approach which helps address this issue. They recommend fitting parametric regression model for the treated and control subjects to form the effect scores and then to use nonparametric regression to estimate the effects of the treatment on the outcome across subgroups defined by these effect scores. They describe procedures to carry out inference and form confidence intervals for the effects across subgroups defined by the effect scores. These procedures are applicable even if the parametric models initially used to form the effect scores are not correctly specified.

More recent work has developed cross-validated targeted minimum loss-based approach to estimate the optimal treatment rule and the outcomes under it.[102-105] These approaches have a number of desirable theoretical properties, but work remains to be done in assessing the sample sizes that are needed for these techniques to be useful and how the various methods that have been proposed in the literature compare to one another in actual practice. Sample sizes larger than what is currently typically available in many randomized trials will often be needed.[106]

These approaches using multiple covariates to identify subgroups for which to target treatment are appealing and potentially powerful. Each of these approaches to optimal selection of subgroups for treatment using many covariates suggests a move away from examining two-way interactions one by one and also a move away from using "prognostic scores" (*i.e.*, stratifying by the predicted risk of the outcome among the unexposed) as such practices are suboptimal.[105] More methodological development remains to be done so that these are easy to implement and to optimally choose cutoffs, and to evaluate sample sizes needed to carry out this work in practice, but as these methods develop, it is likely they will be very useful in observational and experimental research.

ROBUSTNESS OF INTERACTION TO UNMEASURED CONFOUNDING AND SENSITIVITY ANALYSIS

As noted earlier, if we are interested in estimates of causal interaction, *e.g.*, assessing what the effects on the outcome would be if we were to intervene on both exposures, then we must control for confounding for both the exposures. If we have failed to control for confounding, then our interaction estimates may be biased. There are, however, cases in which unmeasured confounding will lead to unbiased estimates of interaction. Specifically suppose we had an unmeasured confounder U of one of the exposures, say X, then if G and X are independent, and if U does not interact with G on the additive scale, then estimates of additive interaction will be unbiased even if control is not made for U[107] and even though the main effect for X is thus biased. Likewise, if G and X are independent, and if U does not interact with G on the multiplicative scale, then estimates of multiplicative interaction will be unbiased even if control is not made for U.[107] Analogous results hold if the unmeasured confounder affects G rather than X and analogous results also hold in some cases in which there are unmeasured confounders of G and of X[107]; the independence assumption can also be somewhat relaxed.[108] Finally, if these assumptions of independence and no interaction between U and G or X fail, then sensitivity analysis techniques for interaction on the additive or multiplicative scale[107] can be employed to assess how robust one's conclusions about interaction are to unmeasured confounding. Note also that, as discussed above, if only one of the two exposures is subject to confounding then (even without controlling for such confounding), interaction estimates can sometimes still be interpreted as measures of effect heterogeneity (*i.e.*, how interventions on the effect of one exposure vary across strata defined by the second exposure, where we do not intervene on the second exposure).

FURTHER READING

There are a number of issues that we have not been able to touch upon in this chapter. We have focused here on binary outcomes. Similar issues concerning additive versus multiplicative interaction are also relevant for time-to-event outcomes: Li and Chambless[109] discuss additive interaction for the proportional hazard models; VanderWeele[110] and Strensrud et al.[111] discuss mechanistic interpretation of such additive interactions in time-to-event models; Rod et al.[112] discuss interaction analysis in additive hazard models. A number of papers have considered power and sample size calculations for interaction including settings of multiplicative interaction using logistic regression,[113-118] case-only estimators of interaction,[95,119] additive interaction,[120] and for multiplicative interaction using matched case-control data.[121]

Another important topic on analysis of interaction concerns methods to robustly estimate interaction even if models for the main effects are misspecified.[77,78,122,123] Another group of papers has examined methods to better exploit the conditional independence assumption of the case-only estimator when data are also available on controls[124-126] or methods that exploit the conditional independence assumption while still being at least partially protected against possible violations of this assumption.[127,128] Methods are also available to jointly test a main effect and an interaction[129-131] so as to leverage potential interaction to be able to more powerfully detect genetic associations.

Other work has examined methods to estimate interaction in family-based genetic studies design.[132-135] Recently there has also been considerable interest in the challenges of assessing interaction in genome-wide-association studies when multiple comparison problems are present.[136-141] In some settings, exposures may vary over time and new methods have been developing to assess effect modification by time-varying covariates and/or exposures.[72,142-144] Further literature has noted that in many settings, interaction may be robust to measurement error[145-152] even when such sources of bias render estimates of main effect invalid. We have not been able to describe all of these methods and developments in this chapter, but the interested reader can consult the relevant literature.

HISTORICAL NOTES

We provide here a brief summary of the theoretical and technical advances in terms of the evolution of the concepts, methods, and measures of interaction in epidemiology and biostatistics. There is a substantial literature on the concept of interaction from other disciplines (*e.g.*, genetics) or on empirical descriptions of interaction[153] which is not the focus of the present summary.

Concerning concepts of interaction, the conceptualization of interaction in terms of sufficient causes was put forward in epidemiology by Rothman.[46] The use of additive interaction measures for determining the public-health importance of interactions was explicitly made by Hammond et al.,[154] though awareness of the point seems present much earlier including discussion in the bioassay literature of the 1920s and 1930s (cf. Refs. 155, 156). A series of letters on the topic of the scale of interaction and the public health importance of interaction, concluding with a short commentary[12] is widely regarded as having "settled" the issue of the additive scale being the scale of relevance for public health, though the point is still often neglected in practice. In 1990, Ottman and Susser characterized types of two-way interactions. The distinction between interaction and effect heterogeneity was first made by VanderWeele,[57] though there were perhaps hints in prior literature that two distinct concepts were present.

Concerning measures and statistical approaches to interaction, although the paper on Simpson's paradox is often cited in connection to confounding, it was in fact originally a discussion about interaction.[157] Simpson showed that discarding the interaction terms in a regression could impact the estimation of the pooled effect even when the stratum-specific effects were homogeneous.[157] Explicit reference to the scale-dependence of interaction is given in Mantel et al.[158]

The synergy index was proposed by Rothman.[159] The attributable proportion was proposed by Walker.[160] The relative excess risk due to interaction (RERI) or ICR was proposed by Rothman.[7] Delta-method standard errors for these measures were given by Hosmer and Lemeshow.[21]

Early tests for qualitative interaction were given by Peto[61] and Gail and Simon.[60] In 1984, Smith and Day proposed methods to compute the statistical power of a study to assess interactions. The case-only estimator for multiplicative interaction was first given by Piegorsch et al.[93]

Testing for sufficient cause interaction under monotonicity assumptions using the condition of positive additive interaction was proposed by Koopman.[161] The second edition of this text[86] provided the first analytic proof of the result. Excepting Rothman and Greenland,[86] there was often lack of awareness that the monotonicity assumptions were needed for the use of this condition of positive additive interaction. Tests for sufficient cause interaction without requiring monotonicity were first proposed by VanderWeele and Robins.[43,45]

References

1. Bauer GR. Incorporating intersectionality theory into population health research methodology: challenges and the potential to advance health equity. *Soc Sci Med.* 2014;110:10-17.
2. Coley SL, Nichols TR. Race, age, and neighborhood socioeconomic status in low birth weight disparities among adolescent mothers: an intersectional inquiry. *J Health Dispar Res Pract.* 2016;9(4):1-16.
3. Jackson JW, Williams DR, VanderWeele TJ. Disparities at the intersection of marginalized groups. *Soc Psychiatry Psychiatr Epidemiol.* 2016;51(10):1349-1359.
4. Pachankis JE, Hatzenbuehler ML, Berg RC, et al. Anti-LGBT and anti-immigrant structural stigma: an intersectional analysis of sexual minority men's HIV risk when migrating to or within Europe. *J Acquir Immune Defic Syndr.* 2017;76(4):356-366.
5. Vives-Cases C, Eriksson M, Goicolea I, Öhman A. Gender and health inequalities: intersections with other relevant axes of oppression. *Glob Health Action.* 2015;8(1):30292.
6. Hilt B, Langård S, Lund-Larsen PG, Lien JT. Previous asbestos exposure and smoking habits in the county of Telemark, Norway: a cross-sectional population study. *Scand J Work Environ Health.* 1986;12:561-566.
7. Rothman KJ. *Modern Epidemiology.* 1st ed. Boston, MA: Little, Brown and Company; 1986.
8. Szklo M, Nieto FJ. *Epidemiology: Beyond the Basics.* 2nd ed.. Boston, MA: Jones and Bartlee Publishers; 2007.
9. Knol MJ, Vandenbroucke JP, Scott P, Egger M. What do case-control studies estimate? Survey of methods and assumptions in published case-control research. *Am J Epidemiol.* 2008;168:1073-1081.
10. Blot WJ, Day NE. Synergism and interaction: are they equivalent? *Am J Epidemiol.* 1979;110:99-100.
11. Greenland S, Lash TL, Rothman KJ. Concepts of interaction. In: Rothman KJ, Greenland S, Lash TL, eds. *Modern Epidemiology.* 3rd ed. Philadelphia: Lippincott Williams and Wilkins; 2008:chap 5.
12. Rothman KJ, Greenland S, Walker AM. Concepts of interaction. *Am J Epidemiol.* 1980;112:467-470.
13. Saracci R. Interaction and synergism. *Am J Epidemiol.* 1980;112:465-466.
14. Kuyvenhoven JP, Veenendaal RA, Vandenbroucke JP. Peptic ulcer bleeding: interaction between non-steroidal anti-inflammatory drugs, Helicobacter pylori infection, and the ABO blood group system. *Scand J Gastroenterol.* 1999;34:1082-1086.
15. Vandenbroucke JP, Koster T, Briët E, Reitsma PH, Bertina RM, Rosendaal FR. Increased risk of venous thrombosis in oral-contraceptive users who are carriers of factor V Leiden mutation. *Lancet.* 1994;344:1453-1457.
16. Knol MJ, VanderWeele TJ, Groenwold RHH, Klungel OH, Rovers MM, Grobbee DE. Estimating measures of interaction on an additive scale for preventive exposures. *Eur J Epidemiol.* 2011;26:433-438.
17. VanderWeele TJ. Reconsidering the denominator of the attributable proportion for additive interaction. *Eur J Epidemiol.* 2013;28:779-784.
18. Figueiredo JC, Knight JA, Briollais L, Andrulis IL, Ozcelik H. Polymorphisms XRCC1-R399Q and XRCC3-T241M and the risk of breast cancer at the Ontario site of the Breast Cancer Family Registry. *Cancer Epidemiol Biomarkers Prev.* 2004;13:583-591.
19. Knol MJ, le Cessie S, Algra A, Vandenbroucke JP, Groenwold RHH. Overestimation of risk ratios by odds ratios in trials and cohort studies: alternatives to logistic regression. *Can Med Assoc J.* 2012;184:895-899.
20. Yelland LN, Salter AB, Ryan P. Relative risk estimation in randomized controlled trials: a comparison of methods for independent observations. *Int J Biostat.* 2011;7(1):5.
21. Hosmer DW, Lemeshow S. Confidence interval estimation of interaction. *Epidemiology.* 1992;3:452-456.
22. Ai C, Norton EC. Interaction terms in logit and probit models. *Econ Lett.* 2003;80:123-129.
23. Andersson T, Alfredsson L, Kallberg H, Zdravkovic S, Ahlbom A. Calculating measures of biological interaction. *Eur J Epidemiol.* 2005;20:575-579.
24. Lundberg M, Fredlund P, Hallqvist J, Diderichsen F. A SAS program calculating three measures of interaction with confidence intervals. *Epidemiology.* 1996;7:655-656.
25. Norton EC, Wang H, Ai C. Computing interaction effects and standard errors in logit and probit models. *Stata J.* 2004;4:154-167.
26. VanderWeele TJ, Knol MJ. A tutorial on interaction. *Epidemiol Methods.* 2014;3:33-72.
27. Assmann SF, Hosmer DW, Lemeshow S, Mundt KA. Confidence intervals for measures of interaction. *Epidemiology.* 1996;7:286-290.
28. Nie L, Chu H, Li F, Cole SR. Relative excess risk due to interaction: resampling-based confidence intervals. *Epidemiology.* 2010;21:552-556.
29. Chu H, Nie L, Cole SR. Estimating the relative excess risk due to interaction: a Bayesian approach. *Epidemiology.* 2011;22:242-248.
30. Kuss O, Schmidt-Pokrzywniak A, Stang A. Confidence intervals for the interaction contrast ratio. *Epidemiology.* 2010;21:273-274.
31. Richardson DB, Kaufman JS. Estimation of the relative excess risk due to interaction and associated confidence bounds. *Am J Epidemiol.* 2009;169:756-760.
32. Skrondal A. Interaction as departure from additivity in case-control studies: a cautionary note. *Am J Epidemiol.* 2003;158(3):251-258.

33. VanderWeele TJ, Vansteelandt S. A weighting approach to causal effects and additive interaction in case-control studies: marginal structural linear odds models. *Am J Epidemiol*. 2011;174:1197-1203.

34. Zou GY. On the estimation of additive interaction by use of the four-by-two table and beyond. *Am J Epidemiol*. 2008;168:212-224.

35. VanderWeele TJ. Empirical tests for compositional epistasis. *Nat Rev Genet*. 2010;11:166.

36. Knol MJ, van der Tweel I, Grobbee DE, Numans ME, Geerlings MI. Estimating interaction on an additive scale between continuous determinants in a logistic regression model. *Int J Epidemiol*. 2007;36:1111-1118.

37. Botto LD, Khoury MJ. Facing the challenge of gene-environment interaction: the two-by-four table and beyond. *Am J Epidemiol*. 2001;153:1016-1020.

38. Knol MJ, VanderWeele TJ. Guidelines for presenting analyses of effect modification and interaction. *Int J Epidemiol*. 2012;41:514-520.

39. Vandenbroucke JP, von Elm E, Altman DG, et al. Strengthening the reporting of observational studies in epidemiology (STROBE): explanation and elaboration. *Epidemiology*. 2007;18:805-835.

40. Knol MJ, Egger M, Scott P, Geerlings MI, Vandenbroucke JP. When one depends on the other: reporting of interaction in case-control and cohort studies. *Epidemiology*. 2009;20:161-166.

41. Greenland S. Interactions in epidemiology: relevance, identification and estimation. *Epidemiology*. 2009;20:14-17.

42. Spiegelman D, Khudyakov P, Wang M, VanderWeele TJ. Evaluating public health interventions: 7. Let the subject matter choose the effect measure. Ratio, difference or something else entirely. *Am J Public Health*. 2018;108:73-76.

43. VanderWeele TJ, Robins JM. The identification of synergism in the SCC framework. *Epidemiology*. 2007;18:329-339.

44. VanderWeele TJ, Robins JM. Four types of effect modification—a classification based on directed acyclic graphs. *Epidemiology*. 2007;18:561-568.

45. VanderWeele TJ, Robins JM. Empirical and counterfactual conditions for sufficient cause interactions. *Biometrika*. 2008;95:49-61.

46. Rothman KJ. Causes. *Am J Epidemiol*. 1976;104:587-592.

47. Deeks JJ, Altman DG. Effect measures for met-analysis of trials with binary outcomes. In: Egger M, Davey Smith G, Altman DG, eds. *Systematic Reviews in Health Care: Meta-Analysis in Context*. London: BMJ Publishing Group; 2003:313-335.

48. Engels EA, Schmid CH, Terrin N, et al. Heterogeneity and statistical significance in meta-analysis: an empirical study of 125 meta-analyses. *Stat Med*. 2000;19:1707-1728.

49. Sterne JA, Egger M. Funnel plots for detecting bias in meta-analysis: guidelines on choice of axis. *J Clin Epidemiol*. 2001;54:1046-1055.

50. Sterne JA, Egger M. Funnel plots for detecting bias in meta-analysis: guidelines on choice of axis. *J Clin Epidemiol*. 2001;54:1046-1055.

51. Poole C, Shrier I, VanderWeele TJ. Is the risk difference really a more heterogeneous measure? *Epidemiology*. 2015;26(5):714-718.

52. Spiegelman D, VanderWeele TJ. Evaluating public health interventions: 6. Ratios or differences? Let the data tell us. *Am J Public Health*. 2017;107:1087-1091.

53. Poole C. On the origin of risk relativism. *Epidemiology*. 2010;21:3-9.

54. Cornfield J, Haenszel W, Hammond EC, Lilienfeld AM, Shimkin MB, Wynder LL. Smoking and lung cancer: recent evidence and a discussion of some questions. *J Natl Cancer Inst*. 1959;22:173-203.

55. Hill AB. The environment and disease: association or causation? *Proc R Soc Med*. 1965;58:295-300.

56. VanderWeele TJ. The interaction continuum. *Epidemiology*. 2019;30:648-658.

57. VanderWeele TJ. On the distinction between interaction and effect modification. *Epidemiology*. 2009;20:863-871.

58. VanderWeele TJ, Knol MJ. The interpretation of subgroup analyses in randomized trials: heterogeneity versus secondary interventions. *Ann Intern Med*. 2011;154:680-683.

59. VanderWeele TJ. Response to "On the definition of effect modification," by E. Shahar and D.J. Shahar. *Epidemiology*. 2010;21:587-588.

60. Gail M, Simon R. Testing for qualitative interactions between treatment effects and patient subsets. *Biometrics*. 1985;41:361-372.

61. Peto R. Statistical aspects of cancer trials. In: Halnan KE, ed. *Treatment of Cancer*. London: Chapman and Hall;1982:867-871.

62. de González AB, Cox DR. Interpretation of interaction: a review. *Ann Appl Stat*. 2007;1:371-385.

63. Li J, Chan IS. Detecting qualitative interactions in clinical trials: an extension of range test. *J Biopharm Stat*. 2006;16:831-841.

64. Pan G, Wolfe DA. Test for qualitative interaction of clinical significance. *Stat Med*. 1997;16:1645-1652.

65. Piantadosi S, Gail MH. A comparison of the power of two tests for qualitative interactions. *Stat Med*. 1993;12:1239-1248.

66. Silvapulle MJ. Tests against qualitative interaction: exact critical values and robust tests. *Biometrics*. 2001;57:1157-1165.

67. Li Y, Sheu C-C, Ye Y, et al. Genetic variants and risk of lung cancer in never smokers: a genome-wide association study. *Lancet Oncol*. 2010;11:321-330.

68. Miettinen OS. Causal and preventive interdependence: elementary principles. *Scand J Work Environ Health*. 1982;8:159-168.

69. Greenland S, Poole C. Invariants and noninvariants in the concept of interdependent effects. *Scand J Work Environ Health*. 1988;14:125-129.

70. Greenland S, Brumback B. An overview of relations among causal modelling methods. *Int J Epidemiol*. 2002;31(5):1030-1037.

71. VanderWeele TJ. Sufficient cause interactions and statistical interactions. *Epidemiology*. 2009;20:6-13.

72. VanderWeele TJ, Vansteelandt S, Robins JM. Marginal structural models for sufficient cause interactions. *Am J Epidemiol*. 2010;171:506-514.

73. VanderWeele TJ, Richardson TS. General theory for interactions in sufficient cause models with dichotomous exposures. *Ann Stat*. 2012;40(4):2128-2161.

74. VanderWeele TJ. Epistatic interactions. *Stat Appl Genet Mol Biol*. 2010;9(Article 1):1-22.

75. Cordell HJ. Detecting gene-gene interaction that underlie human diseases. *Nat Rev Genet*. 2009;10:392-404.

76. Phillips PC. Epistasis—the essential role of gene interactions in the structure and evolution of genetic systems. *Nat Rev Genet*. 2008;9:855-867.

77. Vansteelandt S, VanderWeele TJ, Tchetgen EJ, Robins JM. Multiply robust inference for statistical interactions. *J Am Stat Assoc*. 2008;103:1693-1704.

78. Vansteelandt S, VanderWeele TJ, Robins JM. Semiparametric inference for sufficient cause interactions. *J R Stat Soc Ser B*. 2012;74:223-244.

79. Bhavnani D, Goldstick JE, Cevallos W, Trueba G, Eisenberg JNS. Synergistic effects between rotavirus and coinfecting pathogens on diarrheal disease: evidence from a community-based study in northwestern Ecuador. *Am J Epidemiol*. 2012;176:387-395.

80. VanderWeele TJ. Sufficient cause interactions for categorical and ordinal exposures with three levels. *Biometrika*. 2010;97:647-659.

81. VanderWeele TJ, Knol MJ. Remarks on antagonism. *Am J Epidemiol*. 2011;173:1140-1147.

82. Siemiatycki J, Thomas DC. Biological models and statistical interactions: an example from multistage carcinogenesis. *Int J Epidemiol*. 1981;10:383-387.

83. Thomas W. Effect modification and the limits of biological inference from epidemiologic data. *J Clin Epidemiol*. 1991;44:221-232.

84. VanderWeele TJ. A word and that to which it once referred: assessing "biologic" interaction. *Epidemiology*. 2011;22:612-613.

85. Walter SD, Holford TR. Additive, multiplicative, and other models for disease risks. *Am J Epidemiol*. 1978;108(5):341-346.

86. Rothman KJ, Greenland S, eds. *Modern Epidemiology*. 2nd ed. Philadelphia: Lippincott; 1998.

87. Cordell HJ. Epistasis: what it means, what it doesn't mean, and statistical methods to detect it in humans. *Hum Mol Genet*. 2002;11(20):2463-2468.

88. Lawlor DA. Biological interaction: time to drop the term? *Epidemiology*. 2011;22:148-150.

89. VanderWeele TJ, Tchetgen Tchetgen EJ. Attributing effects to interactions. *Epidemiology*. 2014;25(5):711-722.

90. Miller DP, Liu G, De Vivo I, et al. Combinations of the variant genotypes of GSTP1, GSTM1, and p53 are associated with an increased lung cancer risk. *Cancer Res*. 2002;62:2819-2823.

91. VanderWeele TJ. A unification of mediation and interaction: a four-way decomposition. *Epidemiology*. 2014;25(5):749-761.

92. Yang Q, Khoury MJ, Sun F, Flanders WD. Case-only design to measure gene-gene interaction. *Epidemiology*. 1999;10:167-170.

93. Piegorsch WW, Weinberg CR, Taylor JA. Non-hierarchical logistic models and case-only designs for assessing susceptibility in population-based case—control studies. *Stat Med*. 1994;13:153-162.

94. Albert PS, Ratnasinghe D, Tangrea J, Wacholder S. Limitations of the case-only design for identifying gene-environment interactions. *Am J Epidemiol*. 2001;154:687-693.

95. Yang Q, Khoury MJ, Flanders WD. Sample size requirements in case-only designs to detect gene-environment interaction. *Am J Epidemiol*. 1997;146:713-719.

96. Bennett WP, Alavanja MCR, Blomeke B, et al. Environmental tobacco smoke, genetic susceptibility, and risk of lung cancer in never-smoking women. *J Natl Cancer Inst*. 1999;91:2009-2014.

97. Bonetti M, Gelber RD. A graphical method to assess treatment-covariate interactions using the cox model on subsets of the data. *Stat Med*. 2000;19:2595-2609.

98. Bonetti M, Gelber RD. Patterns of treatment effects in subsets of patients in clinical trials. *Biostatistics*. 2005;5:465-481.

99. Song X, Pepe MS. Evaluating markers for selecting a patient's treatment. *Biometrics*. 2004;60:874-883.
100. Zhao L, Tian L, Cai T, Claggett B, Wei LJ. Effectively selecting a target population for a future comparative study. *J Am Stat Assoc*. 2013;108:527-539.
101. Cai T, Tian L, Wong PH, Wei LJ. Analysis of randomized comparative clinical trial data for personalized treatment selections. *Biostatistics*. 2011;12:270-282.
102. Luedtke AR, van der Laan MJ. Targeted learning of the mean outcome under an optimal dynamic treatment rule. *J Causal Inference*. 2015;3:61-95.
103. Luedtke AR, van der Laan MJ. Statistical inference for the mean outcome under a possibly non-unique optimal treatment strategy. *Ann Stat*. 2016;44:713-742.
104. Luedtke AR, van der Laan MJ. Optimal dynamic treatments in resource limited settings. *Int J Biostat*. 2016;12:283-303.
105. VanderWeele TJ, Luedtke AR, van der Laan MJ, Kessler RC. Selecting optimal subgroups for treatment using many covariates. *Epidemiology*. 2019;30:334-341.
106. Luedtke A, Sadikova E, Kessler RC. Sample size requirements for multivariate models to predict between-patient differences in best treatments of major depressive disorder. *Clin Psychol Sci*. 2019;7(3):445-461.
107. VanderWeele TJ, Mukherjee B, Chen J. Sensitivity analysis for interactions under unmeasured confounding. *Stat Med*. 2012;31:2552-2564.
108. Tchetgen Tchetgen EJ, VanderWeele TJ. Robustness of Measures of Interaction to Unmeasured Confounding. COBRA Preprint. Available at http://biostats.bepress.com/cobra/art89.
109. Li R, Chambless L. Test for additive interaction in proportional hazards models. *Ann Epidemiol*. 2007;17:227-236.
110. VanderWeele TJ. Causal interactions in the proportional hazards model. *Epidemiology*. 2011;22:713-717.
111. Stensrud MJ, Ryalen PC, Røysland K. Sufficient cause interaction for time-to-event outcomes. *Epidemiology*. 2019;30(2):189-196.
112. Rod NH, Lange T, Andersen I, Marott JL, Diderichsen F. Additive interaction in survival analysis: use of the additive hazards model. *Epidemiology*. 2012;23:733-737.
113. Demidenko E. Sample size and optimal design for logistic regression with binary interaction. *Stat Med*. 2008;27:36-46.
114. Foppa I, Spiegelman D. Power and sample size calculations for case-control studies of gene-environment interactions with a polytomous exposure variable. *Am J Epidemiol*. 1997;146:596-604.
115. Garcia-Closas M, Lubin JH. Power and sample size calculations in case-control studies of gene-environment interactions: comments on different approaches. *Am J Epidemiol*. 1999;149:689-692.
116. Gauderman WJ. Sample size requirements for association studies of gene-gene interaction. *Am J Epidemiol*. 2002;155:478-484.
117. Greenland S. Tests for interaction in epidemiologic studies: a review and study of power. *Stat Med*. 1983;2:243-251.
118. Hwang S-J, Beaty TH, Liang K-Y, Coresh J, Khoury MJ. Minimum sample size esitimation to detect gene-environment interaction in case-control designs. *Am J Epidemiol*. 1994;140:1029-1037.
119. VanderWeele TJ. Sample size and power calculations for case-only interaction studies: formulas for common test statistics. *Epidemiology*. 2011;22:873-874.
120. VanderWeele TJ. Sample size and power calculations for additive interactions. *Epidemiologic Methods*. 2012;1:159-188.
121. Gauderman WJ. Sample size requirements for matched case-control studies of gene-environment interaction. *Stat Med*. 2002;21:35-50.
122. Tchetgen Tchetgen EJ. On the interpretation, robustness, and power of varieties of case-only tests of gene-environment interaction. *Am J Epidemiol*. 2010;172:1335-1338.
123. Tchetgen Tchetgen EJ, Robins JM. The semi-parametric case-only estimator. *Biometrics*. 2010;66:1138-1144.
124. Chatterjee N, Carroll RJ. Semiparametric maximum likelihood estimation exploiting gene-environment independence in case-control studies. *Biometrika*. 2005;92:399-418.
125. Han SS, Rosenberg PS, Garcia-Closas M, et al. Likelihood ratio test for detecting gene (G)-environment (X) interactions under an additive risk model exploiting G-E independence for case-control data. *Am J Epidemiol*. 2012;176(11):1060-1067.
126. Mukherjee B, Zhang L, Ghosh M, Sinha S. Semiparametric Bayesian analysis of case-control data under conditional gene-environment independence. *Biometrics*. 2007;63:834-844.
127. Dai J, Logsdon B, Huang Y, et al. Simultaneous testing for marginal genetic association and gene-environment interaction in genome-wide association studies. *Am J Epidemiol*. 2012;176:164-173.
128. Mukherjee B, Chatterjee N. Exploiting gene-environment independence for analysis of case-control studies: an empirical-Bayes type shrinkage estimator to trade off between bias and efficiency. *Biometrics*. 2008;64:685-694.
129. Chatterjee N, Kalaylioglu Z, Moleshi R, Peters U, Wacholder S. Powerful multilocus tests of genetic association in the presence of gene-gene and gene-environment interactions. *Am J Hum Genet*. 2006;79:1002-1016.

130. Kraft P, Yen YC, Stram DO, Morrison J, Gauderman WJ. Exploiting gene-environment interaction to detect disease susceptibility loci. *Hum Hered.* 2007;63:111-119.

131. Maity A, Carroll RJ, Mammen E, Chatterjee N. Testing in semiparametric models with interaction, with applications to gene-environment interactions. *J R Stat Soc Ser B.* 2009;71:75-96.

132. Hoffmann TJ, Lange C, Vansteelandt S, Laird NM. Gene-environment interaction tests for dichotomous traits in trios and sibships. *Genet Epidemiol.* 2009;33:691-699.

133. Lake S, Laird N. Tests of gene-environment interaction for case-parent triads with general environmental exposures. *Ann Hum Genet.* 2004;68:55-64.

134. Umbach D, Weinberg C. The use of case-parent triads to study joint effects of genotype and exposure. *Am J Hum Genet.* 2000;66:251-261.

135. Weinberg CR, Shi M, Umbach DM. A sibling-augmented case-only approach for assessing multiplicative gene-environment interactions. *Am J Epidemiol.* 2011;174:1183-1189.

136. Gayan J, González-Pérez A, Bermudo F, et al. A method for detecting epistasis in genome-wide studies using case--control multi-locus association analysis. *BMC Genomics.* 2008;9:360.

137. Khoury MJ, Wacholder S. From Genome-wide association studies to gene-environment-wide interaction studies - challenges and opportunities. *Am J Epidemiol.* 2009;169:227-230.

138. Kraft P. Multiple comparisons in studies of gene x gene and gene x environment interaction. *Am J Hum Genet.* 2004;74:582-585.

139. Murcray CE, Lewinger JP, Gauderman WJ. Gene-environment interaction in genome-wide association studies. *Am J Epidemiol.* 2009;169:219-226.

140. Pierce BL, Ahsan H. Case-only genome-wide interaction study of disease risk, prognosis and treatment. *Genet Epidemiol.* 2010;34:7-15.

141. Thomas D. Gene-environment-wide association studies: emerging approaches. *Nat Rev Genet.* 2010;11:259-272.

142. Almirall D, Ten Have T, Murphy SA. Structural nested mean models for assessing time-varying effect moderation. *Biometrics.* 2010;66:131-139.

143. Petersen ML, Deeks SG, Martin JN, van der Laan MJ. History-adjusted marginal structural models for estimating time-varying effect modification. *Am J Epidemiol.* 2007;166:985-993.

144. Robins JM, Hernán MA, Rotnitzky A. Effect modification by time-varying covariates. *Am J Epidemiol.* 2007;166:994-1002.

145. Cheng KF, Lin WJ. The effects of misclassification in studies of gene-environment interactions. *Hum Hered.* 2009;67:77-87.

146. Garcia-Closas M, Thompson WD, Robins JM. Differential misclassifcation and the assessment of gene-enviornment interactions. *Am J Epidemiol.* 1998;147:426-433.

147. Jiang Z, VanderWeele TJ. Additive interaction in the presence of a mismeasured outcome. *Am J Epidemiol.* 2015;181:81-82.

148. Lindström S, Yen Y-C, Spiegelman D, Kraft P. The impact of gene-environment dependence and misclassification in genetic association studies incorporating gene-environment interactions. *Hum Hered.* 2009;68:171-181.

149. Tchetgen Tchetgen EJ, Kraft P. On the robustness of tests of genetic associations incorporating gene-environment interaction when the environmental exposure is misspecified. *Epidemiology.* 2011;22:257-261.

150. VanderWeele TJ. Interaction tests under exposure misclassification. *Biometrika.* 2012;99:502-508.

151. VanderWeele TJ. Multiplicative interactions under differential outcome measurement error with perfect specificity. *Epidemiology.* 2019;30(3):e15-e16.

152. Zhang L, Mukherjee B, Ghosh M, Gruber S, Moreno V. Accounting for error due to misclassification of exposures in case-control studies of gene-environment interaction. *Stat Med.* 2008;27:2756-2783.

153. Morabia A. Interaction–epidemiology's brinkmanship: discussion of a tutorial on interaction, by Tyler VanderWeele and Mirjam Knol. *Epidemiol Method.* 2014;3(1):73-77.

154. Hammond EC, Selikoff IJ, Seidman H. Asbestos exposure, cigarette smoking and death rates. *Ann NY Acad Sci.* 1979;330:473-490.

155. Ashford JR, Cobby JM. A system of models for the action of drugs applied singly or jointly to biological organisms. *Biometrics.* 1974;30:11-31.

156. Weinberg CR. Applicability of the simple independent action model to epidemiologic studies involving two factors and a dichotomous outcome. *Am J Epidemiol.* 1986;123:162-173.

157. Simpson EH. The interpretation of interaction in contingency tables. *J R Stat Soc Series B (Methodol).* 1951;13(2):238-241.

158. Mantel N, Brown C, Byar DP. Tests for homogeneity of effect in an epidemiologic investigation. *Am J Epidemiol.* 1977;106:125-129.

159. Rothman KJ. Synergy and antagonism in cause-effect relationships. *Am J Epidemiol.* 1974;99:385-388.

160. Walker AM. Proportion of disease attributable to the combined effect of two factors. *Int J Epidemiol.* 1981;10:81-85.

161. Koopman JS. Interaction between discrete causes. *Am J Epidemiol.* 1981;113:716-724.

Mediation Analysis

Tyler J. VanderWeele

Mediation analysis concerns the set of principles and analytic techniques to identify and quantify how much of the effect of an exposure on an outcome operates through one or more different causal pathways. Such techniques can be useful in epidemiology to evaluate the presence and importance of different mechanisms in understanding how the effect of exposures on different health outcomes is brought about. Methodology for mediation has expanded dramatically over the past decade. The topic of methodology for mediation has traditionally been more the provenance of social scientists and psychologists; training and education on methodological approaches for mediation has been less common in epidemiology and public health. Many of the recent methodologic advances have, however, come out of the causal inference and epidemiologic research communities. This chapter will walk the reader through what some of those advances have been, with an eye toward methods that are likely most useful in the practice of epidemiology and public health research. The topic is broad and a full book–length overview of these topics is now available.[1] This chapter will provide a succinct overview of methodology for mediation, describe when and in what contexts traditional approaches are valid and in what settings other analytic approaches need to be sought out, and point to relevant articles and relevant sections of the book-length overview for further reading.

Questions of mediation concern settings in which a particular mediator may be responsible for some of, or most of, the effect of an exposure on an outcome. The methods for mediation attempt to assess what portion of the effect of the exposure on the outcome is in fact operating through that particular mediator and what portion might be through other mechanisms or pathways. The effect of the cause on the outcome that operates through the mediator of interest is sometimes referred to as an indirect effect or mediated effect. The effect of the cause on the outcome that is not through the mediator of interest is sometimes referred to as the direct effect or unmediated effect. It is important, however, to keep in mind that such effects are direct only relative to the mediator of interest; there will likely be other mediators or mechanisms that account for other aspects of the effect of the cause on the outcome. The phenomenon whereby a cause affects a mediator and the change in the mediator goes on to affect the outcome is what is generally referred to as "mediation," and the techniques by which a researcher assesses the relative magnitude of these direct and indirect effects is sometimes referred to as "mediation analysis."

In this chapter, attention will be given to the confounding assumptions required for a causal interpretation of direct and indirect effect estimates. Methods from the causal inference literature to conduct mediation in the presence of exposure-mediator interactions, binary outcomes, binary mediators, and case-control study designs will be presented. Sensitivity analysis techniques for unmeasured confounding and measurement error will be introduced. Discussion will be given to extensions to time-to-event outcomes and multiple mediators. Further flexible modeling strategies arising from the precise counterfactual definitions of direct and indirect effects will also be described.

MOTIVATIONS FOR ASSESSING MEDIATION

Methods for mediation help us understand the mechanisms, and pathways, and mediators whereby a cause affects an outcome. There are a number of motivations for wanting to understand the phenomenon of mediation. In some instances, the motivation may principally be explanation and understanding. For example, genetic variants on chromosome 15 were found to be associated with both smoking behavior and lung cancer. A question that arose in this context was whether the variants affected lung cancer only because they affected smoking, which causes lung cancer, or whether the variants affected lung cancer through pathways other than through smoking.[2] Methods for mediation can give insight into the pathways and mechanisms by which causal effects arise. Empirically studying mediation can also help confirm and refute theory. As another example, it has been repeatedly found that low socioeconomic status (SES) during childhood is associated with adverse health outcomes later in life. However, there remains debate as to whether this relation exists principally because low SES during childhood affects adult SES, which in turn affects adult health (a "social trajectory" model), or whether childhood SES affects adult health through pathways other than through adult SES (a "latent effects/sensitive period" model), or both. Understanding the role of adult SES in the association between childhood SES and health outcomes can provide empirical evidence in settling which of these theoretical models is better supported.[3] Empirical methods for mediation can be used to evaluate the evidence for these different theories.

Another motivation sometimes given for the empirical study of mediation is to refine interventions. We may be in a setting in which we have established through a randomized trial that an intervention has a beneficial effect on average for the study population. We might be interested in further refining the intervention so as to increase the magnitude of the effect. This might be done by altering or improving components of the intervention that target a particular mechanism for the outcome. However, before proceeding with such refinements, it might be thought desirable to know whether, and the extent to which, the mechanism targeted is an important pathway from the intervention to the outcome. If the mechanism targeted explains a large portion of the effect, then refining the intervention further to target this mechanism may be desirable. However, if the mechanism is found not to be important, then it may be best to redirect efforts at refining the intervention elsewhere. Methods for mediation can help to assess the relative importance of various mechanisms.

Likewise, if an intervention has an effect on an outcome, then knowing something about the mechanisms and pathways by which these effects arise may allow for the discarding of components of an intervention which perhaps are not ultimately important for the outcome. For example, a randomized trial of a cognitive therapy intervention[4] was found to have a beneficial effect on depressive symptoms. However, it was also noted that the intervention had an effect on the use of antidepressants: those in the cognitive behavioral therapy arm were more likely to use antidepressants during follow-up. This led to questions concerning whether the cognitive behavioral therapy intervention had a beneficial effect on depressive symptoms simply because it led to higher antidepressant use, or whether the intervention affected depressive symptoms through other pathways, *e.g.*, by changing the thought and behavioral patterns of the participants. If the intervention was only beneficial because of higher use of antidepressant, then the cognitive-behavioral aspects of the intervention could perhaps be abandoned without much loss, and a more cost-effective intervention just focusing on antidepressant adherence could be developed. Alternatively, it may have been that the intervention was effective both because of increased antidepressant use and because of cognitive-behavioral changes. Methods for assessing mediation can again be useful in assessing the relative contribution of these various pathways.

Methods for mediation might also be of interest in settings in which an intervention is found not to have an effect on an outcome. By considering various possible mechanisms and mediators, it may be possible to assess whether the intervention did not affect the outcome because it failed to affect the mediator, or whether the intervention did in fact affect the mediator but rather the mediator under consideration failed to change the outcome. Such knowledge may be useful in determining whether an intervention needs to be refined by better targeting a particular mechanism or mediator, or whether the mechanism or mediator that was targeted was in fact the wrong one because it had little effect on the outcome. It is also possible that an intervention might affect the outcome positively through one mechanism and negatively through a different mechanism, leading to an overall null effect. Assessing mediation can also help identify such settings.

We might also be interested in empirically assessing mediation because in some settings in which we may not be able to intervene on the primary exposure or cause of the outcome directly, we might be interested in whether we can eliminate a detrimental effect of an exposure by intervening instead on some particular mechanism or mediator. For example, in the context of the aforementioned genetic epidemiology example, we cannot intervene directly on the genetic variants, but we might be interested in how much of the effect of the genetic variants on lung cancer we could block if we could intervene to eliminate smoking. As we will see in a later section, the portion of the effect that operates through a particular mechanism (*e.g.*, by changing smoking) and the portion of the effect that could be eliminated if we intervened on a mechanism (*e.g.*, completely eliminated smoking) may be very different from one another, and different methods and different measures of effect are useful in these different contexts. These two measures to assess the portion of the effect that operates through a particular mechanism (*e.g.*, by changing smoking) and the portion of the effect that could be eliminated if we intervened on a mechanism will diverge when both mediation and interaction are simultaneously present so that the exposure both affects and interacts with the mediator. Similar motivations concerning the effects of interventions on a mechanism when we cannot intervene directly on the exposure itself likewise arise in health disparities research. We may, for example, find differences in a health outcome across racial groups. We cannot intervene on race, but we might be interested in the extent to which the health disparities across racial groups might be reduced or eliminated if we could intervene to equalize educational school quality across racial groups; such ideas can likewise be formalized within a causal framework of mediation.[5,6]

TRADITIONAL APPROACHES TO MEDIATION ANALYSIS

There have been two traditional approaches to mediation analysis: sometimes referred to as the difference method and the product method (or product-of-coefficients method). We will consider each in turn.

The Difference Method

The difference method has been employed frequently in epidemiology and the biomedical sciences. It consists of fitting two regression models. Let X denote an exposure of interest, M a potential mediator, Y an outcome, and Z a set of baseline covariates. The first regression model for the difference method is a regression of the outcome Y on the exposure X and covariates Z:

$$E(Y|x,z) = \phi_0 + \phi_1 x + \phi_2' z$$

The coefficient, ϕ_1, is often interpreted as the total effect of the exposure X on the outcome Y. The second regression is similar but includes the mediator as a variable in the regression as well:

$$E(Y|x,m,z) = \theta_0 + \theta_1 x + \theta_2 m + \theta_4' z$$

If the exposure coefficient of the first regression, ϕ_1, without the mediator, goes down considerably when comparing it to the exposure coefficient in the second regression, θ_1, when adding the mediator, then it is thought that this gives evidence for mediation, since it seems as though the mediator explains some of the effect of the exposure on the outcome. The difference between these two coefficients is sometimes interpreted as a mediated or indirect effect (IE):

$$\mathrm{IE} = \phi_1 - \theta_1$$

The exposure coefficient itself, θ_1, in the model that includes the mediator is then generally taken as a measure of the direct effect (DE) as this is seemingly the effect on the outcome that remains even when control has been made for the mediator:

$$\mathrm{DE} = \theta_1$$

We will return in the next section to the assumptions under which the interpretation of these estimates as direct and indirect effects is valid.

The Product Method

A slightly different method, sometimes called the product method or the product-of-coefficients method, is used with frequency in the social sciences. The approach was made popular in part by an article by Baron and Kenny,[7] though it had been proposed earlier.[8-11] With the product method, two regressions are again employed. We once again regress the outcome on the exposure, the mediator and the covariates:

$$E(Y|x,m,z) = \theta_0 + \theta_1 x + \theta_2 m + \theta_4' z$$

We then regress the mediator itself on the exposure and the covariates:

$$E(M|x,z) = \beta_0 + \beta_1 x + \beta_2' z$$

The direct effect is once again taken as θ_1, the exposure coefficient in the outcome regression model that includes the mediator. The indirect effect, however, is taken as the product of β_1 and θ_2, i.e., the exposure coefficient in the mediator model times the mediator coefficient in the outcome model. The product $\beta_1 \theta_2$, taken as a measure of the indirect effect, has a seemingly intuitive interpretation as the effect of the exposure on the mediator times the effect of the mediator on the outcome.

With these two methods, the product method and difference method, the question naturally arises how they compare. Fortunately, for a continuous outcome and mediator with linear regression models fit by ordinary least squares, the two approaches coincide. It can be shown that we will always have for our mediated effect that $\beta_1 \theta_2 = \phi_1 - \theta_1$.[12] However, this is not the case with logistic regression models. With logistic regression with a binary outcome, the product and difference methods can diverge; they do not give numerically identical results. We will return to this question of which, if either, of these methods for logistic regression is valid in a subsequent section.

CONFOUNDING ASSUMPTIONS FOR MEDIATION ANALYSIS

Fairly strong assumptions are needed for the estimates of direct and indirect effects described previously to be interpreted causally. First, as in ordinary observational studies, control must be made for exposure-outcome confounding (Assumption A1). Second, because with direct and indirect effects, we are also drawing conclusions about the effects of the mediator on the outcome, control must be made for mediator-outcome confounding (Assumption A2). Third, because mediation analysis is essentially about the exposure changing the mediator (and that change in the mediator affecting the outcome), control must also be made for exposure-mediator confounding (Assumption A3). Finally, for standard estimates, as mentioned earlier, to be interpreted as direct and indirect effects, there should be no mediator-outcome confounder that is itself affected by the exposure (Assumption A4). We will now consider each of these confounding assumptions in more detail.

Graphically, one might picture these first three assumptions as in Figure 27-1. These three assumptions—control for exposure-outcome, mediator-outcome, and exposure-mediator confounding—essentially amount to controlling for the vectors of variables Z_1, Z_2, and Z_3 in Figure 27-1, corresponding to exposure-outcome confounders, mediator-outcome confounders, and exposure-mediator confounders, respectively. In practice, some of the covariates might affect all of the exposure, mediator, and outcome; and the covariates may affect each other. None of this is problematic and the covariates groups Z_1, Z_2, and Z_3 need not be distinguished from one another. What is important is that the covariates included in the regression models mentioned earlier suffice to control for exposure-outcome, mediator-outcome, and exposure-mediator confounding (Assumptions A1-A3). These are of course strong assumptions; in a later section, we will consider sensitivity analyses that will allow us to assess how robust our direct and indirect effect estimates are to violations of these assumptions and how substantial a violation in the assumptions would have to be in order to considerably alter our inferences about direct and indirect effects.

We have thus far considered the first three of the assumptions described earlier. The fourth assumption is that none of the mediator-outcome confounders is affected by the exposure. Diagrammatically, in Figure 27-1, this assumption essentially corresponds to there being no arrow from the exposure X to the mediator-outcome confounders Z_2. If the exposure did affect a mediator-outcome confounder Z_2, then this would be problematic for the estimation of direct and indirect effects, because the variable Z_2 would then itself also be a mediator for the effect of the exposure X on the outcome Y and one that itself also confounded the effect of the mediator of interest, M, on the outcome Y. The fourth assumption would thus be violated in a setting like that depicted in Figure 27-2 by the variable L. Addressing scenarios like this (when another variable is both a mediator and a confounder for our mediator of interest, M) is more complicated. We will consider this setting again in a later section in which we discuss concepts and methods for handling multiple mediators. For the next several sections, however, we will assume that this fourth assumption of no mediator-outcome confounders affected by the exposure also holds. Another way to think about the fourth assumption is that there should be relatively little time between the exposure and the mediator. If there is a substantial gap, then the fourth assumption requires that nothing on the pathway from the exposure to the mediator itself also independently affects the outcome. This assumption will often become less and less plausible the more time that elapses between the exposure and mediator.

The confounding assumptions for mediation analysis are extremely important. Violations of these assumptions can give rise to very misleading results. Assumptions A1 (control for exposure-outcome confounding) and A3 (control for exposure-mediator confounding) correspond to assumptions typically made in observational studies for total effects. What distinguishes the assumptions required in the mediation context is that control must also be made for mediator-outcome confounding (Assumption A2). This assumption is not necessary for analysis of total effects, but it is needed for the analysis of direct and indirect effects. For the estimation of direct and indirect effects, this assumption is moreover needed even if the exposure has been randomized. In a randomized trial, although the exposure has been randomized, the mediator has not been, and once we start reasoning about direct and indirect effects, we are considering the effects of not only the exposure but also of the mediator as well. Failure to control for mediator-outcome confounding in a randomized trial can substantially bias estimates of direct and indirect effects.

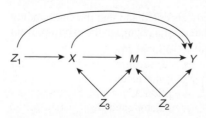

FIGURE 27-1 Relations between exposure X, mediator M, and outcome Y, and confounders of the exposure-outcome relationship (Z_1), the mediator-outcome relationship (Z_2), and the exposure-outcome relationship (Z_3).

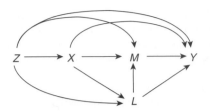

FIGURE 27-2 A mediator-outcome confounder L that is itself affected by the exposure *X*.

As an example of such bias, Strong et al.,[4] as noted earlier, consider the effects of a randomized cognitive behavioral therapy intervention on depressive symptoms at 3 months follow-up, and found there to be a beneficial effect: those who had received the therapy had lower depressive symptoms in follow-up. It was also noted, however, that those in the therapy arm had, at 3 months follow-up, higher rates of antidepressant use. This led to questions with regard to whether the cognitive behavioral therapy intervention had a beneficial effect on depressive symptoms only because it resulted in higher antidepressant use, or whether the intervention affected depressive symptoms through other pathways by changing thought and behavioral patterns. To address this question, if we apply the traditional approaches to mediation analysis mentioned earlier to the Strong et al.[4] data and regress depressive symptoms on antidepressant use and therapy, then the coefficient for antidepressant use in this regression is positive. With the naïve analysis, it looks like antidepressants increase depression! The effect mediated by antidepressant use thus looks harmful; and the direct effect is larger than the total effect. Essentially, we get nonsense from the traditional approach if we ignore mediator-outcome confounding. What is almost certainly occurring here is that those using antidepressants are likely also those in more difficult contexts, *e.g.*, those who are having relationship troubles or who have lost loved ones. The confounding between antidepressant use and depressive symptoms (*i.e.*, mediator-outcome confounding) is so severe that we even get the direction of the regression coefficient for antidepressant use wrong. See Section 3.4 of Ref. 1 for further discussion of this example and reanalysis of the data.

This example highlights the fact that if we are interested in mediation analysis we must control mediator-outcome confounders. This point applies to the traditional approaches to mediation analysis described previously as well as to more recent methods described later. With either the traditional approaches or the more recent approaches, for direct and indirect effect estimates to have a causal interpretation, we need assumptions (A1)-(A4). In a subsequent section, we will consider sensitivity analysis for such mediator-outcome confounding.

ALLOWING FOR EXPOSURE-MEDIATOR INTERACTION

In addition to clarifying the confounding assumptions required for the estimation of direct and indirect effects, the causal inference literature on mediation has also clarified how mediation analysis can be conducted, and how a total effect can be decomposed into direct and indirect effects even when the exposure and the mediator interact in their effects on the outcome. Suppose, for example, that our model for the outcome included an exposure-mediator:

$$E(Y|x,m,z) = \theta_0 + \theta_1 x + \theta_2 m + \theta_2 xm + \theta_4' z$$

and that we fit a linear regression model for the mediator as was the case with the product method:

$$E(M|x,z) = \beta_0 + \beta_1 x + \beta_2' z$$

It has been shown that provided that the models are correctly specified and that the confounding assumptions (A1)-(A4) hold, direct and indirect effect estimates, for a change in the exposure from level x^* to x (*e.g.*, for a binary exposure $x = 1, x^* = 0$), are given by[13]:

$$DE = \left[\theta_1 + \theta_3 \left(\beta_0 + \beta_1 x^* + \beta_2' z \right) \right] \left(x - x^* \right)$$

$$IE = \left(\beta_1 \theta_2 + \beta_1 \theta_3 x \right) \left(x - x^* \right)$$

Standard errors for these expressions are also available,[13] and software to compute these effects and their standard errors and confidence intervals is available.[14] The total effect is the sum of the direct and indirect effects, and sometimes a proportion-mediated measure is used, obtained by dividing the indirect effect by the total effect; see Section 2.13 of Ref. 1 for further discussion of the measure and its properties.

Note that when there is no exposure-mediator interaction (*i.e.*, when $\theta_3 = 0$), these expressions just given simply reduce to θ_1 for the direct effect and $\beta_1\theta_2$ for the indirect effect, which are the same estimates as those of the product method described earlier (which also, with linear regression, coincides with the difference method). The other terms in the formulas for direct and indirect effects account for the presence of exposure-mediator interaction.

BINARY OUTCOMES AND LOGISTIC REGRESSION

A similar approach can be applied with a binary outcome and logistic regression. Suppose we have a binary outcome and a normally distributed continuous mediator and we fit a logistic regression model for the outcome, possibly allowing for exposure-mediator interaction:

$$logit\left[P\left(Y=1|x,m,z\right)\right]=\theta_0+\theta_1 x+\theta_2 m+\theta_2 xm+\theta_4' z$$

and that we fit a linear regression model for the mediator:

$$E\left(M|x,z\right)=\beta_0+\beta_1 x+\beta_2' z$$

Provided that the outcome is relatively rare (a point to which we will return), that confounding assumptions (A1)-(A4) hold, and that the models are correctly specified, direct and indirect effect estimates on an odds ratio scale are given approximately by[15]:

$$OR^{DE}=\exp\left\{\left[\theta_1+\theta_3\left(\beta_0+\beta_1 x^*+\beta_2' z+\theta_2\sigma^2\right)\right]\left(x-x^*\right)+0.5\theta_3^2\sigma^2\left(x^2-x^{*2}\right)\right\}$$

$$OR^{IE}=\exp\left[\left(\beta_1\theta_2+\beta_1\theta_3 x\right)\left(x-x^*\right)\right]$$

where σ^2 is the variance of the error term in the regression for the mediator. Standard errors for these expressions are available,[15] as is software to compute these effects, their standard errors, and confidence intervals.[14] For a rare outcome, a proportion-mediated measure on the risk difference scale can be obtained from the direct and indirect effect odds ratios by the formula: $OR^{DE}(OR^{IE}-1)/(OR^{DE}OR^{IE}-1)$.

If there is no exposure-mediator interaction (*i.e.*, if $\theta_3 = 0$), these expressions simply reduce to $\exp(\theta_1)$ for the direct effect and $\exp(\beta_1\theta_2)$ for the indirect effect, equivalent to the product method-type expressions. We had noted earlier that the product method and the difference method do not necessarily coincide for logistic regression. However, it can be shown that if the outcome is rare (and there is no interaction in the model) then the product method and difference method do at least approximately coincide.[15]

If the outcome is not rare, however (10% is often used a cutoff), then the product method and the difference method can and do diverge and, in fact, neither approach nor the expressions given earlier are valid for the direct and indirect effects. We will return to this issue shortly. However, one way around the problem if the outcome is common is to replace the logistic regression model with a log-binomial model. If we use a log-binomial model for the outcome, then the aforementioned expressions are valid for the direct and indirect effects on a risk ratio scale and, in the absence of interaction, the product and difference methods will coincide. Software for estimating direct and indirect effects with log-binomial models is available.[14]

The problem with logistic regression with binary outcomes that are not rare has to do with the fact that logistic regression uses the odds ratio, which is a measure that is "noncollapsible,"[16] and thus marginal and conditional odds ratios are not directly comparable. With a common outcome, the odds ratios with the mediator in the model versus without the mediator in the model are thus not directly comparable, and this lack of comparability leads to a problem with the difference method. The problem arises because as we add covariates to the logistic regression model (even if these are not confounders), the coefficients in logistic regression tend to increase in magnitude.[17] Viewed intuitively, when the outcome is common, the odds ratio does not approximate the risk ratio, and the extent of this lack of approximation can vary with the other covariates in the models. If we add the mediator to the logistic regression outcome model, then the coefficient of the exposure in the logistic regression may go down because of mediation but go up because of the additional variable in the model. It might then look like the coefficient of the exposure does not change at all even though there is in fact mediation. We would then draw the wrong conclusion from the difference method. In fact, because of this noncollapsibility of odds ratios, it can be shown that, with logistic regression, the difference method is conservative for mediation. That is to say, if one uses the difference method and the confounding assumptions hold, the difference method will in general underestimate the indirect effect when used with logistic regression.[18] Thus, if the difference method with logistic regression indicates the presence of a mediated effect, and the no-confounding assumptions hold, then there is in fact evidence for a mediated effect. However, if the difference method suggests a null estimate of the indirect effect, this does not necessarily indicate that there is no mediation. There may still be mediation; the difference method does not allow one to draw conclusions in this case because the difference method is conservative.

When the outcome is rare, odds ratios approximate risk ratios and these problems diminish and may be ignorable. When the outcome is common, we can get around these issues by fitting a log-linear model rather than a logistic model. Further discussion is given in Chapter 2 of Ref. 1.

One final point is worth noting when studying a binary outcome. Our discussion so far is relevant for estimating direct and indirect effects with cohort data or randomized trials. Often in epidemiologic studies, data are available from a case-control study. With a case-control study design in which sampling is done based on the outcome Y, the estimates from the logistic regression model for that outcome can be used in the analysis. However, the regression model for the mediator needs to be modified to take into account the sampling design. One can do this using a weighting technique,[15] or, if the outcome is rare, a much simpler approach is to fit the mediator model only among the controls. With a rare outcome, the distribution of the mediator among the controls will be a very close approximation to the distribution of the mediator in the underlying population, and so the direct and indirect effect estimates with the mediator model fit only among the controls will give a very close approximation to the direct and indirect effects. Software for estimating direct and indirect effects for a case-control design is available.[14] With a matched case-control study, a similar approach of fitting the mediator regression only among the controls can be employed but then the direct and indirect effect estimates pertain to a subpopulation with a covariate distribution that corresponds to those of the cases.[19]

BINARY MEDIATORS

If the mediator is binary, a similar regression-based approach to estimating direct and indirect effects is also applicable. Suppose that the mediator is binary and the outcome is continuous and that the following models are correctly specified, which potentially allows for exposure-mediator interaction:

$$E(Y|x,m,z) = \theta_0 + \theta_1 x + \theta_2 m + \theta_3 xm + \theta_4' z$$
$$logit[P(M = 1|x,z)] = \beta_0 + \beta_1 x + \beta_2' z$$

If the models are correctly specified and the confounding assumptions (A1)-(A4) hold, then direct and indirect effect estimates can again be given by a simple combination of the regression coefficients of the two regression models (see Ref. 14 or Ref. 1 for the explicit formulas). Likewise, if both the mediator and the outcome are binary and we fit two logistic regression models:

$$logit\left[P\left(Y = 1|x,m,z\right)\right] = \theta_0 + \theta_1 x + \theta_2 m + \theta_2 xm + \theta_4' z$$

$$logit\left[P\left(M = 1|x,z\right)\right] = \beta_0 + \beta_1 x + \beta_2' z$$

Again if the models are correctly specified and the confounding assumptions (A1)-(A4) hold, then direct and indirect effect estimates are again given by a combination of the coefficients of the two models.[1,14] Software to estimate direct and indirect effects with binary mediators is also available.[14]

SENSITIVITY ANALYSIS FOR UNMEASURED CONFOUNDING

We have emphasized earlier the assumptions that are needed to draw conclusions about direct and indirect effects. Assumptions (A1)-(A4) are strong and may often not be met. It is therefore important to assess how robust one's conclusions are about direct and indirect effects when there are violations of the assumptions being made. Sensitivity analysis techniques help one assess, for example, how strong an unmeasured confounder would have to be related to both the mediator and to the outcome to substantially change conclusions being drawn about the direct and indirect effects. Several sensitivity analysis techniques for mediation have been proposed in the literature.[20-25] See Chapter 3 of Ref. 1 for an overview of many of these methods.

Here we will focus on one recent sensitivity analysis technique[20,23] that, at least for a binary outcome, has broad applicability, makes relatively few assumptions, and is thus of potential use in a wide range of potential applications. The technique will make use of two sensitivity analysis parameters. It will assume control has been made for exposure-outcome confounding (Assumption A1) and exposure-mediator confounding (Assumption A3), but that there might be unmeasured mediator-outcome confounders (*i.e.*, Assumption A2 is violated), though it is assumed none of these is affected by the exposure (*i.e.*, assumption A4 is satisfied). In other words, we will consider a causal structure like that in Figure 27-3. Consider a binary outcome Y. Let U be an unmeasured mediator-outcome confounder and let:

$$\gamma = max_m \frac{max_u P(Y = 1 \mid x = 1,m,z,u)}{min_u P(Y = 1 \mid x = 1,m,z,u)}$$

denote the maximum risk ratio relating U and the outcome Y among the exposed across strata of the mediator, conditional on covariates. This parameter will be the maximum ratio by which U can increase the likelihood of the outcome Y. Second, let

$$\lambda = max_{m,u} \frac{P(u \mid x = 1,m,z)}{P(u \mid x = 0,m,z)}$$

denote the maximum risk ratio relating U and the exposure *conditional across different levels of M*. It is the maximum of these associations that we are specifying so both parameters should always be specified as being greater than or equal to 1. This second parameter, however, is more difficult to interpret. If both X and U affect M, then conditional on M, there will be an association between X and U even if neither affects the other (see Chapter 3 on causal diagrams). Some intuition for this parameter can be gained by noting that over many scenarios,[23,26] the association between X and U within strata of M will generally be smaller than the association between X and M, and also smaller than that between U and M, so these can be helpful in specifying possible values of the second sensitivity analysis parameter λ.

It can be shown[20] that under the scenario in Figure 27-3, the maximum ratio that such an unmeasured confounder can decrease the direct effect or increase the indirect effect is given by:

$$B = \frac{\gamma\lambda}{\gamma + \lambda - 1}$$

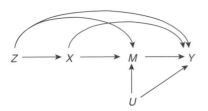

FIGURE 27-3 An unmeasured confounder U of the mediator-outcome relationship.

Thus to get a "bias-adjusted estimate" (understood as the most that such an unmeasured confounder can alter the direct and indirect effects), we can take our direct and indirect effects estimates and their confidence intervals from the observed data and divide the direct effect ratio estimate and both limits of its confidence interval by the bias factor B. For the indirect effect, we multiply the ratio estimate and both limits of its confidence interval by the bias factor B to obtain such bias-adjusted estimates. Thus the mechanics of this technique are fairly simple in practice. Moreover, the technique holds under only the single assumption that Figure 27-3 is the correct causal structure, *i.e.*, we have only unmeasured mediator-outcome confounding, and that our other confounding assumptions (A1, A2, and A4) hold.

We of course do not know what the sensitivity analysis parameters, γ and λ, are, but we can vary them and see how large they must be before estimates change in meaningful ways or are reduced to the null. In practice, reporting an entire table of bias-adjusted direct and indirect effect estimates across a whole range of sensitivity analysis parameters can be helpful. This table can be arranged by putting increasingly large values of one sensitivity analysis parameter, λ, on the rows, and the other, γ, on the columns and reporting the bias-adjusted estimates and confidence intervals for each of these settings. This array gives the reader considerable information on how sensitive, or not, estimates are to violations in the assumptions. At the very least, however, it is good practice to report how much unmeasured confounding would be required to reduce the direct effect estimate to the null; and also how much confounding would be required to reduce to confidence interval to include the null. This can be done in a manner exactly analogous to the E-value calculations[27] described in Chapter 12 on confounding. See Smith and VanderWeele[23] for a straightforward description for mediation. Likewise, at a minimum, it is good to report how much unmeasured confounding would be required to reduce the indirect effect estimate to the null; and also how much confounding would be required to reduce to confidence interval to include the null. This can all be done in a relatively straightforward manner.

The aforementioned technique applies for an unmeasured confounder that increases both the mediator and the outcome. If an unmeasured confounder decreases the probability of the outcome, one defines γ as the inverse of the aforementioned definition, calculates the bias factor B using the same formula as mentioned earlier, but then one multiplies the direct effect estimate and both limits of its confidence interval by B; and one divides the indirect effect estimate and both limits of its confidence interval by B (rather than vice versa) to obtain bias-adjusted estimates. The technique we have described here is relevant for binary outcomes. However, similar techniques can be used for continuous, count, and time-to-event outcomes and can also be applied on a difference rather than a ratio scale. Further discussion of these techniques is given elsewhere.[20,23]

MEASUREMENT ERROR AND MISCLASSIFICATION

There has also been some recent work on the impact of measurement error and misclassification on direct and indirect effect estimates. Several bias adjustment methods are now available for nondifferential measurement error[28-33] that employ regression calibration techniques, SIMEX methods, methods of moments estimators, weighting approaches, and the EM (expectation-maximization) algorithm. See also Chapter 13 for more discussion concerning misclassification and measurement error for total effects. Some work has also considered differential measurement error of the mediator.[30] Some of these various techniques have software available for implementation, but the software resources are still currently limited. The reader is referred to the relevant articles cited above for further information, or to Section 3.5 of Ref. 1. Here we will focus on some intuitive results concerning the direction of the bias subject to nondifferential measurement error of the mediator, exposure, or outcome.

We will begin with potential measurement error or misclassification of the mediator. If either the mediator is binary, or if both the mediator and outcome are continuous, and there is no exposure-mediator interaction, then it can be shown[33,34] that the indirect effect will be biased toward the null and the direct effect will be biased away from the null. The intuition here is that measurement error or misclassification of the mediator will weaken the association between the mediator and the outcome and as the indirect effect can often be thought of as the product of the effect of the exposure on the mediator and that of the mediator on the outcome, this indirect effect will be biased downward by the measurement error, weakening the association between the mediator and the outcome. Because the indirect effect is biased toward the null, the direct effect will be biased away from the null. This intuition always holds if either the mediator is binary, or if both the mediator and outcome are continuous, and there is no exposure-mediator interaction. It will often hold in other scenarios (*e.g.*, if the mediator has three or more levels, or is continuous with exposure-mediator interaction), but it will not always hold in these other scenarios. Bias-adjustment techniques[31,35] can still be used in these other scenarios if it is unclear whether the intuition applies.

Other work has considered the biases of direct and indirect effect estimators in the presence of nondifferential measurement error of the exposure or the outcome.[28,29] For nondifferential measurement error of the outcome, both direct and indirect effects are unbiased for continuous outcomes, and both are biased toward the null for dichotomous outcomes.[28] Drawing intuitive conclusions about the direction of the bias of direct and indirect effects is thus relatively straightforward in the context of measurement error of the outcome.

For nondifferential measurement error of the exposure, in the absence of exposure-mediator interaction, the natural direct effect is biased toward the null, but the indirect effect can be biased in either direction.[29] The intuition for the indirect effect is that measurement error of the exposure will tend to weaken the exposure-mediator association, but will strengthen the mediator-outcome association. Which of these two consequences is more substantial will determine whether the indirect effect is biased toward or away from the null. Correction methods for direct and indirect effects estimators in the presence of nondifferential measurement error of the exposure and outcome are also available.[29]

TIME-TO-EVENT OUTCOMES

A similar approach to mediation analysis can be used with time-to-event outcomes as well. Fuller discussion is given elsewhere,[1] but one can once again specify, for example, either a proportional hazard model or an accelerated failure time model for a time-to-event outcome, and either a linear or logistic regression for a continuous or binary mediator, respectively. The coefficients can again be combined to get estimates of direct and indirect effects. As was the case with logistic regression, so also with proportional hazards models, the product and the difference methods require a rare outcome assumption (*e.g.*, less than 10% cumulative risk in every combination of exposure, covariates, and mediators by the end of follow-up) to be applicable.[36] The use of accelerated failure time models does not require this rare outcome assumption. Software to implement these approaches is available.[32] For a proportional hazards model with a common outcome, a weighting approach can be used.[37] Methods for mediation with time-to-event outcomes have also been developed using additive hazard models.[37] Sensitivity analysis techniques are also available.[38] Further discussion of mediation with time-to-event outcomes can be found in Chapter 4 of Ref. 1.

MULTIPLE MEDIATORS

Our discussion thus far has concerned only a single mediator. Methods are also available for multiple mediators. Sometimes an informal approach is used for multiple mediators by assessing mediation one mediator at a time and then summing up the proportion mediated across mediators. If the mediators affect one another, then this approach fails. Even if the mediators do not affect one another, this approach will still fail if there are interactions between the effects of the various mediators on the outcome. A regression-based approach, similar to that described previously, for assessing the extent to which the effect of an exposure is mediated by an entire set of mediators can be used to address these settings in which the mediators might affect one another.[39] These methods can be used even if the ordering of the mediators is unknown. A weighting-based approach can be used for even greater flexibility.[39] More information and the precise assumptions and methodology required are given in Chapter 5 of Ref. 1.

A more challenging setting is assessing the effect mediated through one mediator when there are other mediators that precede and affect the mediator of interest such as in Figure 27-2. In this context, direct and indirect effects are not in general identified even if one has data on all the variables[1,40] unless one makes further strong modeling assumptions about linearity of the models and the absence of certain interactions,[41-44] as is done in a linear structural equation model. Some progress can be made in this context using sensitivity analysis.[42-44] One can in this context still, however, assess the effects mediated by a particular mediator of interest together with all those preceding it. Certain path-specific effects can also be estimated[1,40,45] and, as described in the next section, yet further progress with multiple mediators can be made by slightly altering the formal definitions of the direct and indirect effects.[46,47]

PRECISE COUNTERFACTUAL INTERPRETATION

The recent progress that has been made in methods for mediation analysis has come about by approaching the question of mediation through a counterfactual-based perspective on causal inference (See Chapter 3). We will briefly describe here the counterfactual definitions of direct and indirect effects that have allowed this progress. Let Y_x denote a subject's outcome if exposure X were set, possibly contrary to fact, to x. Let M_x denote a subject's counterfactual value of the mediator M if exposure X were set to the value x. Finally, let Y_{xm} denote a subject's counterfactual value for Y if X were set to x and M were set to m. Robins and Greenland[48] and Pearl[49] gave the following definitions for controlled direct effects and natural direct and indirect effects based on interventions on the mediator M.

The controlled direct effect of exposure X on outcome Y comparing $X = x$ with $X = x^*$ and setting M to m is defined by $\text{CDE}(m) = Y_{xm} - Y_{x^*m}$ and measures the effect of X on Y not mediated through M—that is, the effect of X on Y after intervening to fix the mediator to some value m. As discussed further below, the controlled direct effect is useful for assessing whether there are pathways from the exposure to the outcome not through the mediator; these effects can also be useful for assessing how much of an effect of an exposure on an outcome could be eliminated by intervening on a mediator. However, for the purposes of effect decomposition, *i.e.*, assessing how much of an effect is operating through a mediator versus through other pathways, a different formal set of definitions and effects is employed—sometimes referred to as a natural direct (NDE) and a natural indirect effect (NIE)—and it is this set of effects that has formed the foundation of the methods and approaches in this chapter, and to which we now turn.

In contrast to controlled direct effects, natural direct effects fix the mediator variable for each individual to the level it naturally would have been under—for example, the absence of exposure. The natural direct effect of exposure X on outcome Y comparing $X = x$ with $X = x^*$ intervening to set M to what it would have been if exposure had been $X = x^*$ is formally defined by $Y_{xM_{x^*}} - Y_{x^*M_{x^*}}$. Corresponding to a natural direct effect is a natural indirect effect formally defined by $Y_{xM_x} - Y_{xM_{x^*}}$. The natural indirect effect assumes that exposure is set to some level $X = x$ and then compares what would have happened if the mediator were set to what it would have been if exposure had been x versus what would have happened if the mediator were set to what it would have been if exposure had been x^*. Under the technical assumptions of consistency and composition (see Chapter 3; cf. Refs. 13, 49), we also have that the total effect (TE) decomposes into the sum of a natural direct and indirect effect: TE = NIE + NDE. In counterfactual notation, this is

$$(Y_x - Y_{x^*}) = (Y_{xM_x} - Y_{xM_{x^*}}) + \left(Y_{xM_{x^*}} - Y_{x^*M_{x^*}}\right).$$

Under the no confounding assumptions (A1)-(A4), these effects are identified on average for a population by the methods and expressions mentioned earlier. The controlled direct effects require only assumptions (A1) and (A2). Controlled direct effects can also be estimated even when there are mediator-outcome confounders affected by the exposure as in Figure 27-2, though special methods such as marginal structural models and structural nested models are then needed[50-52] as the aforementioned regression methods will no longer suffice. In the absence of exposure-mediator interaction in the models mentioned earlier, the controlled direct effects are equal to the natural direct effects. Controlled direct effects cannot otherwise be used for effect decomposition or to assess the relevance of a particular pathway (there is not in general a "controlled indirect effect"). However, as described in the next section, controlled direct effects are often considered to be of greater policy relevance as they consider the effect of the exposure that would remain under an intervention on the mediator to fix it to a specific value.

The interpretation of assumption (A4), in particular, has been the subject of some controversy. It is sometimes referred to as a "cross-world independence assumption" as its formalization requires the independence of two different counterfactuals. Such independence does follow from certain causal diagrams interpreted as nonparametric structural equation models,[49] but does not follow under other interpretations of causal diagrams.[53] See Robins and Richardson[54] and Sections 2.3 and 7.3 of Ref. 1 for further discussion of the assumption (A4), its interpretation, and some of the controversies concerning this interpretation.

Some of these controversies can be avoided by slightly altering the definition of the direct and indirect effects so that, for the direct effect, for example, when comparing the effect of being exposed versus unexposed, instead of fixing, for each individual, the level of the mediator to what it would have been in the absence of exposure, one fixes, for each individual, the mediator to a random draw from the distribution of the mediator among the unexposed.[6,45,55,56] Such effects are sometimes referred to as "interventional direct and indirect effects" or "randomized interventional analogues of direct and indirect effects." Identification of such interventional direct and indirect effects can be made under weaker assumptions. Using such interventional direct and indirect effects can also facilitate further progress with settings of multiple mediators,[45,47] path-specific effects,[32] and mediation analysis with time-varying exposures and mediators.[56-58] While the definition of the effects is thereby slightly altered, within the context of health disparities research, these interventional direct and indirect effects are arguably what is in fact most relevant.[5,6]

PROPORTION ELIMINATED VERSUS PROPORTION MEDIATED

Although natural direct and indirect effects are useful in assessing the importance of particular pathways, they do not correspond to any particular intervention that we could typically carry out in actual practice. This is because they require, for example, for each individual, fixing the mediator to the level it would have been in the absence of exposure, whereas we do not in general know what those values are for those persons actually exposed. Natural direct and indirect effects, although potentially helpful for assessing the impact of different pathways, are thus of more limited interest from a policy perspective.

An alternative proportion measure may be of more interest in policy settings. The controlled direct effect fixing the mediator to level $M = m$, CDE(m), captures the effect of the exposure on the outcome if the mediator were set, possibly contrary to fact, to level m. This is an intervention we might hope to be able to carry out in practice. We might hope that by intervening on the mediator we could block a substantial part of the effect of the exposure on the outcome.[1,48] A proportion measure that could then be used, and that would be of policy relevance, would be the proportion of the effect of the exposure on the outcome that could be eliminated by intervening to set the mediator to some fixed level m. We might call this measure the proportion eliminated and denote it by PE(m). On a difference scale, this would be:

$$PE(m) = \left[TE - CDE(m) \right] / TE$$

That is, the difference between the total effect and the controlled direct effect fixing the mediator level to m (which measures the extent of the effect that is eliminated by fixing the mediator to level m) divided by the total effect itself, to obtain a proportion. If this "proportion eliminated" (PE) were large and we wanted to prevent the effect of the exposure on the outcome, we might try to implement policies to intervene on the mediator. Whereas the proportion mediated essentially captures what would happen to the effect of the exposure if we were to somehow disable the pathway from the exposure to the mediator (setting it to its natural value), the proportion eliminated captures what would happen to the effect of the exposure on the outcome if we were to fix the mediator to the same fixed value $M = m$ for all persons.

Importantly, the "proportion eliminated" measure will not always equal the proportion mediated. Suppose that the exposure and the mediator interacted but that the exposure had no effect on changing the mediator itself. In this case the indirect effect of the exposure on the outcome through the mediator would be 0 (because the exposure does not change the mediator) and we would have a proportion mediated of $PM = NIE/TE = 0/TE = 0\%$. However, if, with interaction, the effect of the exposure were large with the mediator but small without the mediator, then the "proportion eliminated" by fixing the mediator to 0 might be substantial. If we were to fix the mediator to 0 for everyone, the exposure may not have much of an effect on the outcome, $i.e.$, $CDE(m = 0)$ might be quite small, and the proportion eliminated $PE(m = 0) = [TE - CDE(m = 0)]/TE$ might be close to 100%. In the extreme case in which there is a "pure interaction" (so that the exposure has no effect on the outcome unless the mediator is present) but if it is also the case that the exposure has no effect on the mediator itself, then the proportion mediated is 0%, but the proportion eliminated by fixing $m = 0$ is 100%.

More generally the proportion mediated measure $PM = NIE/TE$ and the proportion eliminated measure $PE(m) = [TE - CDE(m)]/TE$ may differ because, in the presence of an interaction between the exposure and the mediator, we may have a different proportion eliminated measure for every value of m. Because the total effect decomposes into a natural direct effect and natural indirect effect ($TE = NIE + NDE$), we can reexpress the proportion mediated as $PM = (TE - NDE)/TE$. In the technical language of the causal inference literature, the proportion eliminated and the proportion mediated may differ because the controlled direct effect may not equal the natural direct effect; the natural direct effect essentially averages over the various controlled direct effects. The two measures will coincide when there is no interaction between the exposure and the mediator [either at the individual level[1] or at the expected population level under no confounding assumptions (A1)-(A4)[13]].

An example where the proportion mediated and proportion eliminated measures do diverge is in the example from genetic epidemiology mentioned earlier for the effects of chromosome 15q25 genetic variants on lung cancer with cigarettes smoked per day as an mediator: each variant allele on 15q25 increases the risk of lung cancer by about 1.3 fold. A small proportion (perhaps no more than 5%-10%) of this effect is mediated by increasing cigarettes per day.[2] However, there is strong interaction between these variants and cigarettes per day in their effects on lung cancer and there may in fact be a "pure" interaction such that the variants have no effect on lung cancer for those who do not smoke. The variants may operate by increasing the nicotine and toxins extracted per cigarettes smoked. In this case, the controlled direct effect if we were able to fix cigarettes per day to 0 for everyone would be $CDE(m = 0) = 0$ and thus the proportion of the effect eliminated would be $PE(m = 0) = [TE - CDE(m = 0)]/TE = [TE - 0]/TE = 100\%$. By eliminating smoking, we eliminate all of the effect of the variants. The proportion mediated (by cigarettes per day) is small because the variants do not increase cigarettes per day all that substantially (only by about 1 cigarette per day); but the proportion eliminated by fixing cigarettes per day to 0 is large because the variants do not seem to affect lung cancer without smoking.

The two measures, proportion eliminated and proportion mediated, have differing interpretations. The proportion eliminated is in general the more relevant policy measure. It captures how much of the effect of the exposure on the outcome we could eliminate by intervening on the supposed mediator variable. The proportion mediated captures how much of the effect of the exposure on the outcome is because of the effect of the exposure on the mediator. It gives insight into the role of different pathways but not necessarily on what would happen if we were to intervene on particular mediators. The proportion eliminated measure is attractive because it concerns the effect of actual potential policy intervention and because it requires only the estimation of controlled direct effects, which, as we have seen, can be identified under somewhat weaker assumptions than natural direct and indirect effects. If effect decomposition and evaluation of the operation of various pathways are of interest, natural direct and indirect effects and the proportion mediated measure may still be of interest. But for policy purposes, the proportion eliminated is often the more relevant measure.

STUDY DESIGN AND MEDIATION ANALYSIS

We discussed previously four assumptions about confounding that were important in giving causal interpretations to the direct and indirect effect estimates. Our assumptions were that control had been made for (A1) exposure-outcome, (A2) mediator-outcome, and (A3) exposure-mediator confounding and that (A4) none of the mediator-outcome confounders was itself affected by the exposure. These assumptions also effectively require an assumption about temporality: that the exposure preceded the mediator and that the mediator preceded the outcome. If such temporality did not hold, then associations between the exposure, mediator, and outcome would not reflect causal effects, implying violations of the confounding assumptions.

Several important implications follow from this temporality requirement that relate to study design. First, these issues of temporality and confounding have important implications for the timing and measurement of variables. Studies should be designed and data collected in such a way that it is ensured, to the greatest extent possible, that the exposure precedes the mediator and that the mediator precedes the outcome. This will often require that data are collected on at least two, and often even three, different time points. It will also often rule out the use of cross-sectional designs. The trouble with cross-sectional designs is that it will often be difficult to know the direction of causality. If the exposure and mediator are associated in a cross-sectional design, it will be difficult to know if this is because the exposure affects the mediator, or if the mediator affects the exposure, or if both are the case. In other words, with cross-sectional data, it will be difficult to rule out feedback and reverse causation. For example, if cognitive behavioral therapy were taken as the exposure, antidepressant use as the mediator and depressive symptom scores as the outcome, but cross-sectional data are used, then it will be difficult to know if an association between therapy and antidepressant use exists because therapy encourages patients to comply with antidepressants, or whether those who take antidepressant medications are more functional and therefore more likely to attend therapy sessions. We cannot distinguish between these two explanations for associations with cross-sectional data or assess their relative contributions. Likewise, if we found the supposed mediator, antidepressant use, were associated with the outcome, depressive symptom scores, then, with cross-sectional data, we would not know to what extent such associations reflected an actual effect of the antidepressant on depressive symptoms, and to what extent the associations resulted from, or were muted by, those with more severe depression being more motivated to use an antidepressant. Again, with cross-sectional data, we cannot determine the direction of causality or, in the case of feedback, the relative magnitudes of the two possible directions causality may operate.

To assess causality, and thus mediation, we need designs that capture data at different points in time. If, because of the design of the study, and the timing of the measurements, we know that the exposures precede the mediator and that the mediator precedes the outcome, then these issues of reverse causation will be of less concern. The most straightforward way to design a study to ensure temporality is to measure the exposure, the mediator, and the outcome used in the analysis at three different times. However, even with data collected at a single point in time, it is at least sometimes possible to have the temporal ordering clear. For example, in the genetic epidemiology example mentioned earlier concerning lung cancer, a case-control study was employed: the exposure was a genetic variant; the mediator, cigarettes per day; and the outcome, lung cancer. Even if the data were collected at a single point in time, it is clear that the genetic variant precedes the mediator and the outcome (since the genetic variant is fixed at conception) and likewise, if the cigarettes per day measure is an average measure of cigarettes per day during the time preceding the assessment of lung cancer status, then it will also be clear that the mediator precedes the outcome. Thus, in some cases, it will be possible to establish the temporal ordering of variables even if all the actual data collection takes place at a single point in time. However, in general, with cross-sectional data in which temporal ordering is not clear and in which causality may occur in both directions, we cannot reliably draw conclusions about mediation.

Conceived of in another way, we might say that, with cross-sectional data, we cannot in general distinguish between mediation and confounding. If the variable X precedes M and M affects Y, then M may be a mediator of the effect of X on Y; but if M precedes X and M affects Y, then M may be a confounder of the effect of X on Y. No statistical techniques will distinguish between these two possibilities if we do not know the temporal ordering or something further about causal relationships between these variables. Establishing whether a variable potentially plays the role of a mediator or a confounder can only be done with substantive knowledge about the nature of the variables, the design of the study, and the timing of measurements.

Of course, in some cases, a variable may be both a mediator and a confounder. Therapy may affect subsequent antidepressant use (and thus antidepressant use may mediate some of the effect of therapy on the outcome), but it may also be the case that antidepressant use may affect whether a patient shows up for subsequent therapy (and thus prior antidepressant use might be a confounder for the effect of subsequent therapy). Once again, with cross-sectional data, it is not possible to tease apart these issues and distinguish between mediation and confounding when there is such feedback. Methods for mediation that handle feedback between variables in the context of time-varying exposures, mediators, and confounders are now available.[56] However, the possibility of feedback is relevant even when we have a single exposure, a single mediator, and a single outcome. This is because, even if we have measured an exposure at time t, a mediator at time $t + 1$, and an outcome at time $t + 2$, and thus know the temporal ordering of these variables, it is possible that the prior values of the exposure, the mediator, and the outcome could in fact serve as the most important confounding variables. The prior value of the mediator at time $t - 1$, say, may affect both the exposure at time t and the outcome at time $t + 2$ and thus serve as a confounder. Because of this potential for feedback and reverse causation, the strongest study designs for providing evidence for mediation will be those in which the exposure precedes the mediator, which precedes the outcome, and in which previous values of the exposure, mediator, and outcome can also be included in the set of potential baseline confounders (*i.e.*, the values of the exposure, mediator, and outcome, measured before the exposure measurement used as the actual exposure in the analysis, are included in the set of confounders Z). Control for prior values of the exposure, mediator, and outcome helps to ensure that the confounding assumptions, required for a causal interpretation of the direct and indirect effects, are more likely to be plausible.

In some settings, prior values of a particular exposure (or mediator, or outcome) do not exist and such considerations are then rendered irrelevant. For example, in the genetics example considered earlier, the exposure was a genetic variant and this is fixed at conception and has no prior value (though, even here, controlling for the genotype of the parents can help control for confounding). Likewise, in some examples, mortality might be the outcome and, assuming everyone is alive at study entry, there is no "prior outcome" to control. Similarly, if the exposure is an intervention that no one has previously received, there will be no "prior exposure" to control; control effectively is made for it automatically since no one previously had the exposure. However, in general, when the exposure, mediator, or outcome varies over time, control for prior values of these variables as confounders will render the confounding assumptions more plausible and help rule out the possibility of reverse causation.

These issues are mitigated somewhat if the exposure itself is randomized. In that case, there will be no exposure-outcome confounding and no exposure-mediator confounding. However, as we have already noted, even if the exposure is randomized, there may still be mediator-outcome confounding (since the mediator has not been randomized) and thus, in such circumstances, controlling for past values of the mediator and the outcome (values before the exposure's randomization) can help control for mediator-outcome confounding. Even previous values of the exposure (if defined before randomization) may help control for such mediator-outcome confounding if such prerandomization values of the exposure are thought to likewise affect the postrandomization values of both the mediator and the outcome.

In summary, if we have a single exposure, mediator, and outcome used in the analysis and employ the methods described earlier in this chapter, then the no confounding assumptions (A1)-(A4) will often be more plausible if we can control for prior values of the exposure, mediator, and outcome (*i.e.*, values measured before the measurement of the exposure variable used in the analysis). The importance of study design is often emphasized in trying to draw causal inferences from observational data. Within the context of assessing mediation and direct and indirect effects, issues of temporality and study design are even more complex and subtle as the effects of multiple variables are in view.

MORE FLEXIBLE MODELS

In this chapter, we have considered various parametric models to undertake mediation analysis. However, the causal inference approach to mediation is very flexible and can be pursued under any model. The difficulty is that each time the model is changed, new expressions for the effects have to be derived. The SAS, Stata, and SPSS macros mentioned earlier[14] consider different scenarios. However, if greater flexibility is desired, a simulation-based approach has been developed by Imai et al.[22] that allows investigators to specify much more flexible models for the outcome and the mediator and then estimate the direct and indirect effects by simulation. The approach effectively makes the same no confounding assumptions (A1)-(A4) described earlier but allows for more modeling flexibility. Software is available in both R and Stata.[59,60] See Imai et al.,[22] Tingley et al.,[67] and Sections 2.17 and 2.18 of Ref. 1 for further discussion.

Additional flexibility in modeling can also be achieved in weighting approaches that allow one to model the exposure and the mediator, or the exposure and the outcome, rather than mediator and the outcome.[24,61-66] Other approaches make use of target maximum likelihood techniques to allow for more flexible modeling.[67] Recent work has compared statistical power of these various approaches under a range of scenarios.[68] Power and sample size calculation have traditionally relied on approximations from simulations using tables,[69] but Rudolph et al.[68] now provide tools to carry out such calculations for a range of more recent methods.

CONCLUSION

Mediation analysis has expanded rapidly over the past decade. Numerous other methods have been developed[12,24,57,58,61,62,66,67,70-72] beyond what we have covered here. Several of these are discussed in a book-length treatment of the topic.[1] Methods have begun to be developed for handling questions of mediation for time-varying exposure and mediators,[56,57] and there have been further developments with time-to-event outcomes with repeatedly measured mediators.[58,73-75]

Concepts and methods are now also available to assess mediation and interaction simultaneously. A total effect can be decomposed into not just two, but into four distinct components: that due to just mediation, that due to just interaction, that due to both mediation and interaction, and that due to neither.[76] This new methodology considers how much of the direct effect described earlier is or is not due to interaction, and how much of the indirect effect described earlier is or is not due to interaction. The approach provides maximum insight into the phenomena of mediation and interaction simultaneously. Software to implement this type of analysis is also available.[76] See Ref. 76 and Chapter 14 of Ref. 1 for further discussion.

The methods for mediation discussed in this chapter can be useful for a number of purposes. Some potential uses of these ideas and methods include trying to understand etiology, providing evidence to confirm and refute theory, assessing the impact of intervening on a mediator when it is not possible to alter an exposure, and in trying to understand why an intervention succeeded or failed. The application of these techniques makes some strong assumptions, and should thus always be accompanied by sensitivity analysis, but in some instances at least, these approaches can give considerable insight into pathways.

HISTORICAL NOTES

Modern approaches to quantifying the extent of mediation are often traced back to the work of Wright[77-79] using path analysis, effectively giving rise to the "product" or "product-of-coefficients" method, with formulas for indirect effects also given explicitly by Hyman[9] and Alwin and Hauser.[8] Sobel[11] gave an explicit formula for the standard error of the indirect effect via the product method.

Kendall and Lazarsfeld[80] and Lazarsfeld[81] gave early descriptions of the difference method for mediation of adding the mediator to a regression model of the outcome on the exposure to assess mediation. The difference method approach was described in the epidemiologic methods textbook of Susser.[82] Although the method was subsequently frequently employed in epidemiology and the biomedical sciences, formal exposition of the approach remained minimal within epidemiology. Prentice[83] proposed using the approach for evaluating the relevance of a surrogate endpoint. The equivalence of the product and difference method for linear regression was shown analytically by MacKinnon et al.[84]

Judd and Kenny[10] explicitly noted that control needed to be made for mediator-outcome confounders in conducting analyses of mediation. Baron and Kenny[7] distinguished a mediator from a moderator (or what is often called in epidemiology an "effect modifier"); the distinction drew attention to their article and subsequently their discussion of mediators became the canonical reference for mediation analysis, especially within psychology. Unfortunately, unlike Judd and Kenny,[10] the Baron and Kenny[7] article did not note that control needed to be made for mediator-outcome confounding, and thus this central assumption was subsequently ignored in much of the applied and methodological literature, and is still often ignored in psychology today. Statistical methodology for mediation, much of it coming from the psychology literature, expanded rapidly during the 1990s and subsequently.

With regard to the counterfactual approach to causal inference, Holland[85] provided counterfactual definitions for controlled direct effects. Robins and Greenland[48] gave counterfactual definitions for natural direct and indirect effects. Pearl[49] described a sufficient set of confounding assumptions on causal diagrams, interpreted as nonparametric structural equation models, that would identify average natural direct and indirect effects for a population. The work of Robins and Greenland[48] and Pearl[49] made clear more formally the importance of control for mediator-outcome confounders. Regression methods employing natural direct and indirect effects were described by Petersen et al.[86]; explicit analytic formulae using natural direct and indirect effects allowing for exposure-mediator interaction were given by VanderWeele and Vansteelandt[13,15] and Imai et al.[22] and relating these to the product and difference methods. After the first decade of the 21st century, the methodological literature on mediation from a causal inference perspective expanded very rapidly.

References

1. VanderWeele TJ. *Explanation in Causal Inference: Methods for Mediation and Interaction*. New York: Oxford University Press; 2015.
2. VanderWeele TJ, Asomaning K, Tchetgen Tchetgen EJ, et al. Genetic variants on 15q25.1, smoking and lung cancer: an assessment of mediation and interaction. *Am J Epidemiol*. 2012;175:1013-1020.
3. Nandi A, Glymour MM, Kawachi I, VanderWeele TJ. Using marginal structural models to estimate the direct effect of adverse childhood social conditions on onset of heart disease, diabetes and stroke. *Epidemiology*. 2012;23:223-232.
4. Strong V, Waters R, Hibberd C, et al. Management of depression for people with cancer (SMaRT oncology 1): a randomised trial. *Lancet*. 2008;372:40-48.
5. Jackson JW, VanderWeele TJ. Decomposition analysis to identify intervention targets for reducing disparities. *Epidemiology*. 2018;29(6):825-835.
6. VanderWeele TJ, Robinson W. On the causal interpretation of race in regressions adjusting for confounding and mediating variables. *Epidemiology*. 2014;25:473-484.
7. Baron RM, Kenny DA. The moderator-mediator variable distinction in social psychological research: conceptual, strategic, and statistical considerations. *J Pers Soc Psychol*. 1986;51:1173-1182.
8. Alwin DF, Hauser RM. The decomposition of effects in path analysis. *Am Sociol Rev*. 1975;40:37-47.
9. Hyman HH. *Survey Design and Analysis: Principles, Cases and Procedures*. Glencoe, IL: Free Press; 1955.
10. Judd CM, Kenny DA. Process analysis: estimating mediation in treatment evaluations. *Eval Rev*. 1981;5:602-619.
11. Sobel ME. Asymptotic confidence intervals for indirect effects in structural equations models. In: *Sociological Methodology*. Leinhart S, ed. San Francisco: Jossey-Bass; 1982:290-312.
12. MacKinnon DP. *Introduction to Statistical Mediation Analysis*. New York: Erlbaum; 2008.
13. VanderWeele TJ, Vansteelandt S. Conceptual issues concerning mediation, interventions and composition. *Stat Interf*. 2009;2:457-468.
14. Valeri L, VanderWeele TJ. Mediation analysis allowing for exposure-mediator interactions and causal interpretation: theoretical assumptions and implementation with SAS and SPSS macros. *Psychol Methods*. 2013;18:137-150.
15. VanderWeele TJ, Vansteelandt S. Odds ratios for mediation analysis for a dichotomous outcome. *Am J Epidemiol*. 2010;172:1339-1348.
16. Greenland S, Robins JM, Pearl J. Confounding and collapsibility in causal inference. *Stat Sci*. 1999;14:29-46.
17. Robinson L, Jewell NP. Some surprising results about covariate adjustment in logistic regression models. *Int Stat Rev*. 1991;59:227-240.

18. Jiang Z, VanderWeele TJ. When is the difference method conservative for mediation? *Am J Epidemiol.* 2015;182(2):105-108.

19. VanderWeele TJ, Tchetgen Tchetgen EJ. Mediation analysis with matched case-control designs. *Am J Epidemiol.* 2016;183:869-870.

20. Ding P, VanderWeele TJ. Sharp sensitivity bounds for mediation under unmeasured mediator-outcome confounding. *Biometrika.* 2016;103:483-490.

21. Hafeman DM. Confounding of indirect effects: a sensitivity analysis exploring the range of bias due to a cause common to both the mediator and the outcome. *Am J Epidemiol.* 2011;174:710-717.

22. Imai K, Keele L, Tingley D. A general approach to causal mediation analysis. *Psychol Methods.* 2010;15:309-334.

23. Smith LH, VanderWeele TJ. Mediational E-values: approximate sensitivity analysis for unmeasured mediator–outcome confounding. *Epidemiology.* 2019;30(6):835-837.

24. Tchetgen Tchetgen EJ, Shpitser I. Semiparametric theory for causal mediation analysis: efficiency bounds, multiple robustness, and sensitivity analysis. *Ann Stat.* 2012;40:1816-1845.

25. VanderWeele TJ. Bias formulas for sensitivity analysis for direct and indirect effects. *Epidemiology.* 2010;21:540-551.

26. Greenland S. Quantifying biases in causal models: classical confounding vs collider-stratification bias. *Epidemiology.* 2003;14:300-306.

27. VanderWeele TJ, Ding P. Sensitivity analysis in observational research: introducing the E-value. *Ann Intern Med.* 2017;167:268-274.

28. Jiang Z, VanderWeele TJ. Causal mediation analysis in the presence of a mismeasured outcome. *Epidemiology.* 2015;26:e8-e9.

29. Jiang Z, VanderWeele TJ. Causal mediation analysis in the presence of a misclassified binary exposure. *Epidemiologic Methods.* 2019;8(1).

30. le Cessie S, Debeij J, Rosendaal FR, Cannegieter SC, Vandenbroucke J. Quantification of bias in direct effects estimates due to different types of measurement error in the mediator. *Epidemiology.* 2012;23:551-560.

31. Valeri L, Lin X, VanderWeele TJ. Mediation analysis when a continuous mediator is measured with error and the outcome follows a generalized linear model. *Stat Med.* 2014;33:4875-4890.

32. Valeri L, VanderWeele TJ. SAS macro for causal mediation analysis with survival data. *Epidemiology.* 2015;26:e23-24.

33. VanderWeele TJ, Valeri L, Ogburn EL. The role of misclassification and measurement error in mediation analyses. *Epidemiology.* 2012;23:561-564.

34. Ogburn EL, VanderWeele TJ. Analytic results on the bias due to nondifferential misclassification of a binary mediator. *Am J Epidemiol.* 2012;176:555-561.

35. Valeri L, VanderWeele TJ. The estimation of direct and indirect causal effects in the presence of a misclassified binary mediator. *Biostatistics.* 2014;15:498-512.

36. VanderWeele TJ. Causal mediation analysis with survival data. *Epidemiology.* 2011;22:575-581.

37. Lange T, Hansen JV. Direct and indirect effects in a survival context. *Epidemiology.* 2011;22:575-581.

38. VanderWeele TJ. Unmeasured confounding and hazard scales: sensitivity analysis for total, direct and indirect effects. *Eur J Epidemiol.* 2013;28:113-117.

39. VanderWeele TJ, Vansteelandt S. Mediation analysis with multiple mediators. *Epidemiol Methods.* 2013;2:95-115.

40. Avin C, Shpitser I, Pearl J. Identifiability of path-specific effects. In: *Proceedings of International Joint Conferences on Artificial Intelligence.* Edinburgh, Scotland, UK; 2005:357-363.

41. Daniel RM, De Stavola BL, Cousens SN, Vansteelandt S. Causal mediation analysis with multiple mediators. *Biometrics.* 2015;71:1-14.

42. Imai K, Yamamoto T. Identification and sensitivity analysis for multiple causal mechanisms: revisiting evidence from framing experiments. *Polit Anal.* 2012;21:141-171.

43. Tchetgen Tchetgen EJ, VanderWeele TJ. On identification of natural direct effects when a confounder of the mediator is directly affected by exposure. *Epidemiology.* 2014;25:282-291.

44. Vansteelandt S, VanderWeele TJ. Natural direct and indirect effects on the exposed: effect decomposition under weaker assumptions. *Biometrics.* 2012;68:1019-1027.

45. VanderWeele TJ, Vansteelandt S, Robins JM. Methods for effect decomposition in the presence of an exposure-induced mediator-outcome confounder. *Epidemiology.* 2014;25:300-306.

46. Lin S-H, VanderWeele TJ. Interventional approach for path-specific effects. *J Causal Inference.* 2017;5(1):1-10.

47. Vansteelandt S, Daniel RM. Interventional effects for mediation analysis with multiple mediators. *Epidemiology.* 2017;28(2):258-265.

48. Robins JM, Greenland S. Identifiability and exchangeability for direct and indirect effects. *Epidemiology.* 1992;3:143-155.

49. Pearl J. *Direct and indirect effects.* In: *Proc. Seventeenth Conference Uncertainy in Artificial Intelligence.* San Francisco, CA: Morgan Kaufmann; 2001:411-420.

50. Robins JM, Hernan MA, Brumback B. Marginal structural models and causal inference in epidemiology. *Epidemiology*. 2000;11:550-560.

51. Vansteelandt S. Estimating direct effects in cohort and case–control studies. *Epidemiology*. 2009;20(6):851-860.

52. VanderWeele TJ. Marginal structural models for the estimation of direct and indirect effects. *Epidemiology*. 2009;20:18-26.

53. Richardson TS, Robins JM. Single world intervention graphs (SWIGs): a unification of the counterfactual and graphical approaches to causality. Center for the Statistics and the Social Sciences, University of Washington Series. Working Paper 128. 2013.

54. Robins JM, Richardson TS. Alternative graphical causal models and the identification of direct effects. In: Shrout P, ed. *Causality and Psychopathology: Finding the Determinants of Disorders and Their Cures.* UK: Oxford University Press; 2010

55. Didelez V, Dawid AP, Geneletti S. Direct and indirect effects of sequential treatments. In: *Proceedings of the Twenty-Second Conference on Uncertainty in Artificial Intelligence.* Cambridge, MA, USA; 2006.

56. VanderWeele TJ, Tchetgen Tchetgen EJ. Mediation analysis with time-varying exposures and mediators. *J R Stat Soc Ser B*. 2017;79:917-938.

57. Lin S-H, Young J, Logan R, Tchetgen Tchetgen EJ, VanderWeele TJ. Parametric mediational g-formula approach to mediation analysis with time-varying exposures, mediators, and confounders: an application for smoking, weight, and blood pressure. *Epidemiology*. 2017;28:266-274.

58. Lin S-H, Young J, Logan R, VanderWeele TJ. Mediation analysis for a survival outcome with time-varying exposures, mediators, and confounders. *Stat Med*. 2017;20:4153-4166.

59. Daniel RM, De Stavola BL, Cousens SN. gformula: estimating causal effects in the presence of time-varying confounding or mediation using the g-computation formula. *Stata J*. 2011;11:479-517.

60. Tingley D, Yamamoto T, Hirose K, Keele L, Imai K. Mediation: R package for causal mediation analysis. *J Stat Softw*. 2014;59:1-38.

61. Albert JM. Distribution-free mediation analysis for nonlinear models with confounding. *Epidemiology*. 2012;23:879-888.

62. Hong G, Nomi T. Weighting methods for assessing policy effects mediated by peer change. *J Res Educ Eff*. 2012;5(3):261-289.

63. Lange T, Vansteelandt S, Bekaert M. A simple unified approach for estimating natural direct and indirect effects. *Am J Epidemiol*. 2012;176:190-195.

64. Nguyen QC, Osypuk TL, Schmidt NM, et al. Practical guidance for conducting mediation analysis with multiple mediators using inverse odds ratio weighting. *Am J Epidemiol*. 2015;181(5):349-356.

65. Steen J, Loeys T, Moerkerke B, Vansteelandt S. Medflex: an R package for flexible mediation analysis using natural effect models. *J Stat Softw*. 2017;76(11):1-46.

66. Tchetgen Tchetgen EJ. Inverse odds ratio-weighted estimation for causal mediation analysis. *Stat Med*. 2013;32(26):4567-4580.

67. Zheng W, van der Laan MJ. Targeted maximum likelihood estimation of natural direct effects. *Int J Biostat*. 2012;8:1-40.

68. Rudolph KE, Goin DE, Stuart EA. The peril of power: a tutorial on using simulation to better understand when and how we can estimate mediating effects. *Am J Epidemiol*. 2020 (in press). doi:10.1093/aje/kwaa083.

69. Fritz MS, MacKinnon DP. Required sample size to detect the mediated effect. *Psychol Sci*. 2007;18(3):233-239.

70. Albert JM, Nelson S. Generalized causal mediation analysis. *Biometrics*. 2011;67:1028-1038.

71. Goetgeluk S, Vansteelandt S, Goetghebeur E. Estimation of controlled direct effects. *J R Stat Soc Ser B Stat Methodol*. 2008;70:1049-1066.

72. Martinussen T, Vansteelandt S, Gerster M, von Bornemann Hjelmborg J. Estimation of direct effects for survival data by using the Aalen additive hazards model. *J R Stat Soc Ser B Stat Methodol*. 2011;73:773-788.

73. Aalen OO, Stensrud MJ, Didelez V, Daniel R, Røysland K, Strohmaier S. Time-dependent mediators in survival analysis: modeling direct and indirect effects with the additive hazards model. *Biometrical J*. 2019;62(3):532-549.

74. Didelez V. Defining causal mediation with a longitudinal mediator and a survival outcome. *Lifetime Data Anal*. 2019;25(4):593-610.

75. Vansteelandt S, Linder M, Vandenberghe S, Steen J, Madsen J. Mediation analysis of time-to-event endpoints accounting for repeatedly measured mediators subject to time-varying confounding. *Stat Med*. 2019;38(24):4828-4840.

76. VanderWeele TJ. A unification of mediation and interaction: a four-way decomposition. *Epidemiology*. 2014;25:749-761.

77. Wright S. The relative importance of heredity and environment in determining the piebald pattern of guinea-pigs. *Proc Natl Acad Sci USA*. 1920;6:320-332.
78. Wright S. Correlation and causation. *J Agric Res*. 1921;20:557-585.
79. Wright S. The theory of path coefficients: a reply to Niles's criticism. *Genetics*. 1923;8:239-255.
80. Kendall PL, Lazarsfeld PF. Problems of survey analysis. In: Merton RK and Lazarsfeld PF, eds. *Continuities in Social Research: Studies in the Scope and Method of the "The American Solider"*. Gencoe, IL: Free Press; 1950:133-196.
81. Lazarsfeld PF. Interpretation of statistical relations as a research operation. In: Lazarsfeld PF, Rosenberg M, eds. *The Language of Social Research: A Resader in the Methodology of Social Research*. Glencoe, IL: Free Press; 1955:115-125.
82. Susser M. *Causal Thinking in the Health Sciences: Concepts and Strategies of Epidemiology*. New York: Oxford University Press; 1973.
83. Prentice RL. Surrogate endpoints in clinical trials: definition and operational criteria. *Stat Med*. 1989;8:431-440.
84. MacKinnon DP, Warsi G, Dwyer JH. A simulation study of mediated effect measures. *Multivariate Behav Res*. 1995;30:41-62.
85. Holland PW. Causal inference, path analysis, and recursive structural equations models. In: Clogg CC, ed. *Sociological Methodology*. Washington, DC: American Sociological Association; 1988:449-484.
86. Petersen ML, Sinisi SE, van der Laan MJ. Estimation of direct causal effects. *Epidemiology*. 2006;17:276-284.

CHAPTER 28

Instrumental Variables and Quasi-Experimental Approaches

M. Maria Glymour and Sonja A. Swanson

THE EPIDEMIOLOGIST'S DREAM: EVALUATING CAUSATION DESPITE CONFOUNDING

In this chapter, we consider a group of methods that share a common feature: they can be used to evaluate causal effects of an exposure or treatment on an outcome even when there is unmeasured confounding of the exposure-outcome relationship. All of these designs depend on the availability of an effectively random source of variation in the exposure (and we will provide a precise definition of what constitutes "effectively random" below). In this chapter, we introduce study designs based on quasi-experiments and the closely related concept of an instrumental variable (IV). These methods have a long history in economics, epidemiology, and related fields. The emergence of Mendelian randomization (MR) designs, which leverage genetic information with IV methods, has sparked renewed attention and elaboration of methods. We review the assumptions under which quasi-experiments allow us to test certain causal null hypotheses and identify various causal estimands, and we describe common analytic approaches. In most cases, the interpretation of these types of analyses rests on very strong assumptions, and we review approaches to evaluating these assumptions. This is an area of rapid methodological development, and we mention a handful of important extensions. Randomization in a double-blind placebo-controlled trial is a special case of an IV that is familiar to most epidemiologists, as we explain further below. We therefore use comparisons to randomized controlled trials (RCTs) as a framework to understand quasi-experiments and IV analyses.

Quasi-experiments are defined inconsistently by different researchers (even between different chapters of the previous edition of *Modern Epidemiology*)[7,8] and some but not all definitions invoke IVs. The IV approach was published a century ago[2,9] and has been developed across multiple disciplines.[10] An influential paper in the mid-1990s launched an outpouring of studies using IV methods to circumvent confounding.[3,11] In this chapter, we refer to a quasi-experiment as a setting in which (i) there is an effectively random source of variation in the exposure of interest, or probability of being exposed, such that (ii) that source of variation is unrelated to the counterfactual value of the outcome under any particular value of exposure. In other words, a quasi-experiment occurs if there is a factor that influences whether an individual is likely to be exposed but has no other reason to be associated with the outcome. These assumptions can be formalized with counterfactuals or with directed acyclic graphs (DAGs). For the counterfactual-IV criteria, we say G serves as an IV or instrument for estimating the effect of X on Y if both counterfactual-IV condition 1 (specifying that G is associated with X) and counterfactual-IV condition 2 (specifying that G is unrelated to potential outcomes of Y under different values of X) are met:

$$\text{CF-IV 1. } G \not\perp\!\!\!\perp X \qquad\qquad\qquad [28\text{-}1]$$

$$\text{CF-IV 2. } G \perp\!\!\!\perp Y_X \qquad\qquad\qquad [28\text{-}2]$$

These assumptions often seem plausible only after conditioning on some set of covariates, and we return to that setting below. Note that counterfactual-IV 2 is implied by two separate assumptions, which readers may find more intuitive. These assumptions specify that G is unrelated to the potential outcome Y would take once the actual values of G and X are set (counterfactual-IV 2a, thereby ruling out shared causes of G and Y) and that the potential outcome of Y once the value of X is set does not depend on the value of G (counterfactual-IV 2b, ruling out effects of G on Y that are not mediated by X):

$$\text{CF-IV 2a. } G \perp\!\!\!\perp Y_{G=g,X=x} \qquad\qquad\qquad [28\text{-}3]$$

$$\text{CF-IV 2b. } Y_{G=g,X=x} = Y_{G=g',X=x} \qquad\qquad\qquad [28\text{-}4]$$

If we imagine a double-blind, placebo-controlled RCT, which assesses a point intervention and achieves complete follow-up, we would expect that the randomization indicator G would satisfy these conditions. Most RCTs have imperfect adherence, in which case, as discussed in Chapter 6, the intent-to-treat (ITT) association between G and Y does not correspond to the effect of X on Y. What we will shortly see is that, by satisfying the IV conditions, we can learn something about the effect of X on Y, despite the nonadherence. In the prior discussion of randomization, it was noted that strategies to account for nonadherence by comparing study participants based on their actual treatment received ("as treated" analysis) or restricting to participants who adhered to their randomly assigned treatment ("per-protocol" analysis) break randomization and are informative only if common causes of adherence and the outcome are measured. IV methods permit insights even if the common causes of adherence and the outcome are unknown. Although the IV conditions may be reasonable in many well-conducted RCTs beyond the idealized one described here, we focus on a simple setting for clarity, though we will consider more complex settings later.

Typically, when the source of variability G is not under the control of a researcher evaluating the effect of X, the situation is called a quasi-experiment and we refer to G as a *proposed* instrument. The line between an RCT and a quasi-experiment is not crisp, with some disagreement about whether certain studies should be called quasi-experiments or experiments. For example, important exposures such as military draft and subsidized housing are often assigned by lottery[12,13]; studies that leverage such lotteries to evaluate the effects of military service or housing on health fall into a gray area between RCTs and quasi-experiments. The key issue when evaluating either an RCT or a quasi-experiment is whether the IV conditions are met; informally, people tend to refer to the design as quasi-experimental when there is greater uncertainty about the assumptions or when the source of G (randomization) was not a research study.

One can use an IV to evaluate the sharp causal null hypothesis that there is no effect of X on Y for any individual in the study (as with nearly any study, it is not possible to prove the null, merely to disprove it). Testing the sharp null is as simple as evaluating the association of G with Y, that is, in the language of an RCT, evaluating the ITT effect. In Chapter 6, it was noted that this advantage of RCTs extends far beyond calculating the probability of the observed association under the null hypothesis: with randomization to treatment, we can compute the probability of the observed association under various hypotheses about how treatment assignment affects the outcome and thereby estimate the size of the effect of random assignment. When adherence is imperfect, we need additional assumptions (detailed below) to estimate the magnitude of the effect of X on Y using IV analyses. To the extent the IV conditions are violated, the IV effect estimate does not correspond with an effect of X on Y. Even in an RCT, if the IV conditions are not met, the interpretation of the ITT estimate also changes, and it can no longer be considered a test of the null hypothesis that X does not affect Y or used to evaluate the effect of X on Y.[14,15]

The conditions we described in counterfactual-IV 1 and counterfactual-IV 2 can also be conveniently represented graphically, following the rules of causal DAGs.[10] In the causal DAGs in Figure 28-1A, G fulfills the IV conditions above with respect to X and Y. When expressing the assumptions graphically, it is more common to list three conditions:

DAG-IV 1. G is associated with X (because, say, G influences X or G shares a common cause with X).
DAG-IV 2. There are no back-door paths linking G and Y, for example, no shared causes of G and Y.
DAG-IV 3. There are no paths via which G influences Y that do not pass through X.

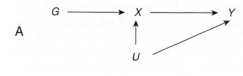

A

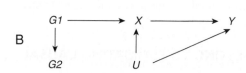

B

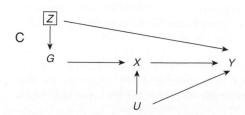

C

FIGURE 28-1 Directed acyclic graphs showing causal assumptions under which G **(A)** or $G1$ or $G2$ **(B)** are valid instrumental variables for the effect of X on Y, despite the presence of an unmeasured confounder (U) of the X-Y association. In **C**, G is a valid instrument for the effect of X on Y only conditional on Z. Z is shown with a box around it to indicate that analyses must condition on Z.

The graphical assumptions are nearly equivalent to the counterfactual assumptions, and as with the counterfactual assumptions can be modified to accommodate settings in which they are fulfilled only when conditioning on a set of covariates. Researchers can typically adopt either the counterfactual or the graphical criteria, whichever they find most illuminating. For example, the DAG-based assumptions may be more easily evaluated using subject matter expertise in applied settings.[16,17] These assumptions are all that is needed to evaluate the sharp null hypothesis that X does not affect Y for any individual in the sample; a DAG helps us see why the sharp null implies G is d-separated from and therefore independent of Y. If the association of G and Y is not null, then either the sharp null that there is no effect of X on Y does not hold or the DAG-IV conditions are violated. This sharp null assessment can be conducted even if X is unmeasured since it only requires information on G and Y. This has powerful implications: even in situations when X is not measured at all, it may be possible to evaluate the sharp null hypothesis that X has no effect on Y for any individual in the population. In fact, this is even true for certain sharp null hypotheses when the exposure is time varying.[15]

Applying the d-separation rules reveals some helpful extensions of conventional IV. First, considering Figure 28-1B, it is clear that either $G1$ or $G2$ provides an IV for the effect of X on Y: $G2$ is d-connected to Y if and only if X influences Y; $G2$ is sometimes referred to as a noncausal IV.[18] Another important extension is to incorporate covariates. The IV conditions may be true only conditional on a set of covariates. If so, we can assess the association between G and Y conditioning on the covariate set to test the null hypothesis that X has no effect on Y for any individual. For example, if there is one shared cause of G and Y (say, Z) but we have measured and controlled for that factor, G may then be a conditionally valid IV (Figure 28-1C). Similarly, if there is one path via which G affects Y not mediated by X, we might be able to control for a variable to block that path and still use G as an IV. In both cases, we must evaluate whether the proposed covariate control introduces collider bias such that G would be d-connected to Y even if X did not influence Y. This idea is also easily expressed as a set of counterfactual assumptions:

$$\text{Conditional CF} - \text{IV1. } G \not\!\perp\!\!\!\perp X \mid Z$$

$$\text{Conditional CF} - \text{IV2. } G \perp\!\!\!\perp Y_{X=x} \mid Z$$

The need to incorporate covariate control may seem disappointing if a primary goal of IV analyses is to circumvent the no-unmeasured-confounding assumption. However, the no-unmeasured-confounding assumption in conventional analyses applies to the X-Y association, whereas for IV, it applies to the G-Y association. In some situations, the no-unmeasured-confounding assumption may be more plausible for G-Y than for X-Y. Even if both assumptions are controversial in a given setting, if the no-confounding assumption for G-Y is unrelated to the no-confounding assumption for X-Y, finding a similar result with the IV analysis and a conventional analysis can strengthen the evidence that X has a causal effect. New evidence based on the IV conditions may be far more convincing than multiple replications based on designs that rely on the assumption of no unmeasured X-Y confounding.[19]

MOVING BEYOND NULL HYPOTHESIS TESTING TO ESTIMATING CAUSAL EFFECTS

As emphasized throughout this textbook, it is typically desirable to go beyond evaluating the sharp null hypothesis and quantify the causal effect of the exposure, that is, derive a point estimate for the effect of X on Y. Many different possible causal estimands may be of interest to a researcher, and for convenience, we note several of relevance for this chapter, along with the corresponding counterfactual contrast for each, in Table 28-1.

Consider again an RCT with nonadherence. Nonadherence to the randomly assigned treatment could occur for many reasons: individuals are assigned to treatments they prefer not to take, the assigned treatment is belatedly deemed to be medically inappropriate for some individuals

TABLE 28-1

Causal Estimands Referred to in This Chapter

Estimand	Description	Counterfactual Expression
Population Average Treatment Effect (PATE)	Effect of X on Y, in the full population	$E(Y_{X=1} - Y_{X=0})$
Sample Average Treatment Effect (SATE)	Effect of X on Y in the sample	$E(Y_{X=1} - Y_{X=0}|S = 1)$
Intent-to-Treat Effect (ITT) and its quasi-experiment analogue	Effect of different values of an instrumental variable on Y	$E(Y_{G=1} - Y_{G=0})$
Local Average Treatment Effect (LATE)	Effect of X on Y among the subgroup in which the IV affects exposure	$E(Y_{X=1} - Y_{X=0}|X_{G=1} = 1, X_{G=0} = 0)$
Effect of Treatment among the Treated (ETT)	Effect of X on Y among those who were actually exposed to X	$E(Y_{X=1} - Y_{X=0}|X = 1)$

The above specifies causal estimands for dichotomous exposures, but all can be extended to settings with continuous exposures. We do not further discuss the distinction between the SATE and the PATE, because the issues do not differ in the context of quasi-experimental designs compared to conventional observational studies.

(for example see Brott et al.[20]), or there is insufficient availability of the treatment for everyone assigned to receive it. As a result, the ITT effect estimate does not equal the effect of treatment received. IV analyses account for nonadherence to randomly assigned treatment and can be used to estimate a per-protocol effect of treatment received (*i.e.*, the effect if everyone had adhered to assigned treatment, which should equal the sample average treatment effect, SATE).[21] The difference between the ITT effect estimate and the effect of actually receiving a treatment generally grows larger as nonadherence to randomly assigned treatment increases. Quasi-experimental sources of variation in exposure often change the average exposure only a bit—much less than random assignment in most RCTs—so the divergence between the analogue of an ITT effect and the analogue of a per-protocol effect is even greater in quasi-experiments than most RCTs. Thus, in quasi-experimental settings, IV analyses to estimate the effect of receiving treatment are especially important.

However, in order for results from an IV analysis to be interpreted as a causal effect estimate derived from the IV analysis, more assumptions beyond the core IV conditions listed above are needed—the interpretation of the causal effect estimate depends on which assumption is invoked. Indeed, results from IV analyses are often interpreted as an effect estimate for a specific subgroup of the population.[16] Before discussing alternatives for additional assumptions and what parameter may be estimated under each alternative, we discuss specific approaches to IV effect estimation.

ESTIMATORS USED IN INSTRUMENTAL VARIABLE ANALYSES

Given that the IV conditions are fulfilled, how do we conduct an IV analysis to estimate the effect of treatment? We consider three statistical methods to derive an IV estimate. We will first discuss the estimators that are typically employed and in the next section, we will consider the assumptions that are required to interpret these estimators as corresponding to one or more of the causal estimands given in Table 28-1.

The first, sometimes called a Wald estimator, is rarely used directly in practice but provides a useful intuition. The Wald estimator's most frequently presented form is for a binary IV (*e.g.*, random assignment to experimental vs. placebo group) and a binary treatment X with a continuous or binary Y. In this setting, the Wald estimator is the ratio of the association between the instrument (G) and the outcome (Y) (the numerator) and the association between the instrument and the treatment (X) (the denominator):

$$\frac{E(Y|G=1)-E(Y|G=0)}{E(X|G=1)-E(X|G=0)} \qquad [28\text{-}5]$$

In an RCT, this is a ratio of the ITT effect estimate to the estimate of adherence. If everyone adheres to random assignment, then the denominator of this ratio is 1, and the Wald estimate equals the ITT estimate. With nonadherence, the IV estimate will typically be farther from the null than the ITT estimate. This makes sense: the lower the adherence, the more we will need to "correct" the ITT to estimate the effect of treatment received. The Wald estimator is usually presented expressing the numerator and denominator as risk differences, but one can also use covariances or extend to continuous IVs by conceptualizing the denominator as a difference in propensity score at contrasting levels of the IV.[22,23]

The Wald estimator also helps give the intuition behind *why* IV methods can help us learn about the effect of X on Y. Returning to Figure 28-1A, we see that the effect of G on Y is unconfounded, and the effect of G on X is unconfounded. Informally, it seems that with these two pieces of information—if we can estimate the G-Y and G-X effects—we can somehow disentangle the effect of X on Y. The Wald estimator indeed is simply the ratio of these two components. Note this logic extends to noncausal instruments such as $G2$ in Figure 28-1B.

Two-stage least squares (2SLS) regression is an alternative to the Wald approach that conveniently incorporates covariates, handles multiple proposed IVs for the same treatment, and evaluates treatments with continuous distributions.[11,24] The first stage of a 2SLS model uses the treatment as the dependent variable and predicts treatment as a function of the instrument and any covariates of interest (denoted by the vector Z in the model below) where the estimates of the regression coefficients are denoted with "hats" such as $\widehat{\beta_0}$. The estimated regression coefficients are then used to calculate the predicted value of the treatment $(\tilde{X})$, which is used to predict the outcome Y:

$$\tilde{X} = \widehat{\alpha_0} + \widehat{\alpha_1}G + \widehat{\alpha_k}Z_k \qquad [28\text{-}6]$$

$$Y = \widehat{\beta_0} + \widehat{\beta_1}\tilde{X} + \widehat{\beta_k}Z_k + \varepsilon \qquad [28\text{-}7]$$

Why does this work? This predicted value from the first-stage model $(\tilde{X})$ can be thought of as a rescaled value of the IV. Considering the DAG in Figure 28-1A, the predicted value of X from equation 28-2 varies only in response to the IV and measured covariates, but is unaffected by U. Thus, the second stage is assessing the difference in Y in response to the difference in X that is attributable specifically to G.

The third approach we mention is g-estimation of structural nested models (SNMs) under the IV conditions. Readers familiar with g-estimation of SNMs may recognize this as one of the so-called "g-methods" for estimating causal effects, typically used under some no-unmeasured-confounding assumption.[25,26] However, the parameters in an SNM could also be estimated under the IV conditions in tandem with additional assumptions described below.[27] Intuitively, the SNM specifies that the observed outcome for each individual i could be decomposed into, first, that person's potential outcome had they never been exposed (*i.e.*, $Y_{i,X=0}$, which we will refer to as U_i) and second, the effect of person i's actual exposure on the outcome. Although we do not observe the values of U_i (except for those individuals who are in fact not exposed) the IV conditions imply that U_i is independent of G. If we know each individual's actual exposure level, we can then calculate the effect of exposure which would fulfill the assumption that U_i is independent of G. This is straightforward, for example, if the effect is specified as a linear model with a single exposure time period. If we assume the causal model is:

$$Y_i = U_i + \beta_1 X_i \qquad [28\text{-}8]$$

For any proposed value of β_1, we can calculate the U_i for each individual implied by that β_1:

$$U_i = Y_i - \beta_1 X_i \qquad [28\text{-}9]$$

We can then test whether, assuming the proposed β_1 is correct, the values of U_i calculated this way are independent of the randomly assigned treatment group G. If the calculated U_is are associated with G, this implies the proposed β_1 is not correct. This approach allows one to go beyond the point intervention X considered in most of this chapter and also consider effects of time-varying exposures: as long as each individual's sequence of exposures is known, any proposed effect estimate can be used to "back out" the exposure effect and calculate U_i, providing a test for the proposed effect estimate. Note that with a single binary IV, although we can accommodate time-varying exposure, we cannot estimate time-varying effect estimates. We must express the effect of exposure at any time point with a single parameter. A more typical application, for example, is based on accelerated failure-time models, in which the effect estimate is expressed as the percent change in survival time due to each period of exposure.[28,29] Although g-estimation of SNMs is not used nearly as frequently as 2SLS or other approaches, it has the appeal of a more general framework for extensions involving time-varying IVs and/or exposures, failure-time outcomes, and some alternative model specifications.[27,30-32]

IV estimation can sometimes be conducted even when there is no data set that includes measures of the instrument, the exposure, and the outcome concurrently.[33,34] If we have two data sets, one that includes information on the proposed IV and the exposure and another that includes information on the proposed IV and the outcome, then we can nonetheless estimate a causal effect. The intuition for why this works can be seen via considering the separate stages of 2SLS, or considering the numerator and denominator of the Wald estimator separately. Doing such a two-sample IV analysis, not surprisingly, requires that the effect of G on X (conditional on any covariates used in the analyses) is the same in the two populations. Separate-sample or two-sample applications have proven especially valuable for MR studies in which genetic information is used as the IV.[34]

We do not discuss variance calculations for the above estimators except to note that they are often not straightforward but are built into standard software packages. When considering an IV approach or interpreting IV estimates, it is important to recognize that IV methods nearly always have less statistical power than conventional analyses using the same sample size to estimate the same effect (*i.e.*, the effect of X on Y). No matter how large the analytic sample may be, the information about the treatment effect in an IV analysis derives only from those individuals whose exposure was influenced by the IV. Just as the effective sample size in an RCT declines in proportion to the adherence to randomization, the effective sample size of an IV analysis declines in proportion to the association of the proposed IV with the exposure.

INTERPRETING AN EFFECT ESTIMATE FROM AN IV ANALYSIS

To interpret the effect estimate derived from any of these types of estimators as a causal effect of X on Y, one must adopt one or more assumptions beyond the core conditions described earlier. Researchers have some choices among additional assumptions, and the choice influences the interpretation of the effect estimate obtained from an IV analysis. In this section, we describe options for this additional assumption (which we refer to as point-identifying assumptions because they are needed to derive a point estimate for the causal effect of X on Y) and what interpretation can be given to the IV estimate when adopting each such assumption. Because much of the literature discussing these interpretations and assumptions addresses settings with a binary IV G that influences the exposure, a binary exposure X, and continuous or binary outcome Y, we tackle this setting here unless otherwise indicated.

Homogeneity

A simple option for a point-identifying assumption is that the effect of the treatment on the outcome (effect of X on Y) is the same for all people, that is, a "constant treatment effect" or the strongest version of a "homogeneity" assumption. In this case, the IV methods estimate therefore the average treatment effect $\left[E\left(Y_{X=1} - Y_{X=0}\right) \right]$. However, this assumption is unreasonable in many epidemiologic settings. If counterfactuals are conceptualized as deterministic, it would be mathematically illogical for binary outcomes. For example, if counterfactuals are deterministic and exposure caused the outcome to occur for one individual in the population so that $Y_{i,X=1} - Y_{i,X=0} = 1$, the constant treatment effect assumption implies that exposure would cause the outcome to occur for *every* individual, precluding the existence of any other causes of Y besides X. Because such a strong homogeneity assumption is often implausible, it is not commonly invoked.

One could instead adopt a slightly weaker version of a homogeneity assumption to estimate a different causal effect. Assuming no additive effect modification by the IV among the treated:

$$E\left(Y_{X=1} - Y_{X=0} \middle| X = 1, G = 1\right) = E\left(Y_{X=1} - Y_{X=0} \middle| X = 1, G = 0\right) \qquad [28\text{-}10]$$

allows for estimation of the average treatment effect among the treated $\left[E\left(Y_{X=1} - Y_{X=0} \middle| X = 1\right) \right]$. Assuming instead no *multiplicative* effect modification by the IV among the treated also allows for the same effect to be estimated, albeit with a different estimator.[18,35] Making the additional assumption that no such effect modification occurs among the untreated ($X = 0$) allows for estimation of the average treatment effect. We would generally expect this version of a homogeneity assumption to be fulfilled only if there were no unmeasured factors that modified the effect of the IV on treatment and also modified the effect of treatment on the outcome.[36]

Altogether, these types of homogeneity assumptions have received criticism for being implausible in many research settings. Existing and ongoing research addresses alternative assumptions beyond those reviewed here that would permit identification of causal effects with IV analyses. By far the most common choice for this additional assumption, however, is called the monotonicity assumption.

Monotonicity

The monotonicity assumption is that the IV does not have opposite effects on the exposure for any two individuals in the population.[11] In other words, if the IV increases the average value of X for some individuals, it must not decrease the average value of X for other individuals. More formally:

$$X_{i,G=1} \geq X_{i,G=0} \text{ for all individuals in the population, or}$$
$$X_{i,G=1} \leq X_{i,G=0} \text{ for all individuals in the population}$$

In contrast to the homogeneity assumptions described previously, which relate to the effect of X on Y, the monotonicity assumption relates to the effect of G on X and does not require that the magnitude of the effect of G on X be identical for all individuals. The monotonicity assumption refers to counterfactuals and cannot be proven, although it can be disproven in some circumstances.[18,37]

Although the monotonicity assumption is seen as more plausible than the homogeneity assumptions described above, invoking it changes the interpretation of the effect estimated via IV analysis. Rather than estimating the effect in the full study population, or among the treated, it estimates the effect among those individuals whose treatment status would have been changed by the IV. More formally, for example, this effect is written as follows:

$$E\left(Y_{X=1} - Y_{X=0} \middle| X_{G=1} = 1, X_{G=0} = 0\right) \qquad [28\text{-}11]$$

and is referred to as a local average treatment effect (LATE) or complier average causal effect in the literature.[38-40] The LATE expression conditions on counterfactuals, highlighting the fact that we cannot directly observe which individuals' effects are included in the group whose treatment status would have been changed by the IV. Therefore, although the LATE tells us the causal effect for some people, we do not know precisely which people those are.

The LATE nomenclature and the significance of this subgroup are most clearly understood in the context of a randomized trial. The LATE draws on the ideas of principal stratification, in that we conceptualize the trial population as having four mutually exclusive types of individuals: people who would have adhered to random assignment, regardless of whether assigned to treatment or placebo (referred to as "compliers"); people who would have been treated regardless of random assignment ("always-takers"); people who would not have taken treatment, regardless of random assignment ("never-takers"); and people who would have done the opposite of what they were assigned, that is, take treatment if assigned to control and take control if assigned to treatment ("defiers"). The monotonicity assumption amounts to claiming that there are no "defiers" in a population and thereby allows us to estimate the effect in the "compliers." We emphasize that monotonicity does not require that the effect of G on X is identical for everyone in the population, or even that G influences X for everyone in the population; it merely requires that there not be people for whom G influences X in opposite directions. It is generally impossible to identify these compliance types based on the observed data alone: a person randomized to treatment who took treatment may be a "complier" or an "always-taker" (because $X_{G=1} = 1$ for both groups) and it would be impossible to know which based on this information alone. If we assume there are no "defiers," we can, however, estimate the fraction of the whole population which are "compliers": this is the difference in the fraction treated among people randomized to $G = 1$ compared to those randomized to $G = 0$. Knowing this fraction can be useful because if most people are "compliers," this suggests that the LATE could be a close approximation of the SATE and, setting aside sampling differences, the PATE.

Although the terminology of compliance types makes less sense outside of the randomized trial context, the counterfactual definition of who is a "complier" or what it means to assume there are no "defiers" can still be applied to other causal IVs. The reference to the four compliance types breaks down with a continuous instrument or treatment, but the intuition for the interpretation is the same: it is a weighted average of the effect of changes in the treatment that were induced by the value of the IV, now with unidentifiable weights.[11] Just as it is impossible to identify which individuals are "compliers" in the case of binary IV and treatments, it is similarly impossible to know the weight for each individual in a setting with continuous IV or treatment. The idea of these compliance types and monotonicity also presumes that the IV causes the exposure, rather than simply being associated with exposure like the noncausal IV $G2$ in Figure 28-1B. For noncausal IVs, monotonicity and the LATE are defined with respect to the underlying causal IV ($G1$ in Figure 28-1B) rather than the measured noncausal IV.[41]

Another option is to assume that the effect of G on X for any individual is unrelated to the effect of X on Y. This implies that the average effect of X on Y is the same for "compliers" as for "defiers." In this case, the LATE and the PATE are identical to each other and the IV estimate is consistent for the PATE. Although this assumption seems unlikely to be strictly true in most settings, plausible violations may be too small to substantively impact conclusions in some cases (see further discussion below regarding the impact of "defiers" on the IV effect estimate).

CONTROVERSIES ABOUT THE MONOTONICITY ASSUMPTION AND THE LOCAL AVERAGE TREATMENT EFFECT

The monotonicity assumption was introduced in the classic paper providing a causal interpretation for IV-based effect estimates[11] and widely adopted in subsequent IV analyses. There are two general concerns raised about using monotonicity to estimate the LATE, and we discuss the merits of each claim in more detail below: (1) the monotonicity assumption is not plausible in many applied settings and (2) the LATE is not of substantive interest.

The plausibility of monotonicity depends on the setting, and we consider it in the examples discussed below. Like any assumption underlying any causal inference, this will need to be considered on a case-by-case basis. An important question is the extent to which IV estimators are biased from the LATE under modest monotonicity violations, for example, if a small fraction of the sample is "defiers." This will depend on the magnitude of the difference in the effect of X on Y among the "compliers" compared to the "defiers" as well as the fraction of the sample who are "defiers" versus "compliers."[38] If the effect of X on Y is smaller in the "defiers" than in the "compliers," the IV estimate may counter-intuitively be *larger* than the LATE. Likewise, if the effect of X on Y is larger in the "defiers" than in the "compliers," the IV estimate may counter-intuitively be *smaller* than the LATE. Conceptually, this occurs because the IV estimate is a weighted average of the effect of X on Y in the "compliers" and the "defiers," but the "defiers" receive a negative weight (because the IV discourages them from being treated). If the effect of X on Y is the same for "compliers" and "defiers," the IV analysis estimates this effect.

The substantive relevance of the LATE has been questioned on the grounds that it is impossible to identify the individuals within the sample who are "compliers."[37] Further, there is no guarantee that the "compliers" in one IV analysis will be the same types of individuals who are "compliers" in another study or in a large-scale implementation of the treatment being evaluated. For example, consider an RCT of an experimental medication with substantial nonadherence. If the same individuals who refuse to take the experimental medication in the trial also refuse to take it when prescribed in clinical practice, then the LATE would be a better estimate than the ITT for the effects of using the medication in practice. However, the compliers in clinical practice may systematically differ from the compliers in the RCT. For example, if the RCT results indicate that the medication is extremely effective, subsequent take-up of the medication might be much higher than in the trial. Note that this possibility—that the medication effects for future users may be substantially different from the effects in people induced to take the medication in the RCT—would similarly reduce the relevance of ITT and per-protocol estimates derived from the RCT data. If subsequent take-up approached 100%, although the per-protocol estimand would be of interest,[37] any valid estimate of it would depend on a heroic, usually implausible, homogeneity condition as described above.

The LATE is likely of greater interest than the PATE when the population studied includes some people who are certain to be treated or certain not to be treated, but it is not easy to identify those "definitely treat" or "definitely do not treat" individuals in advance or based on data collected. Good RCT design would ideally specify eligibility criteria such that people for whom the best treatment strategy is already known are not enrolled, but this may not be possible in some cases, especially with natural experiments. For example, if two judges disagree about whether to incarcerate a defendant for a crime of moderate severity, it would be useful to know how incarceration likely affects the long-term outcomes of such a defendant, that is, the LATE. If the crimes were so severe that all judges agree the defendant must be incarcerated, it is of less interest to know whether the incarceration harms the long-term outcomes of the criminal, because this information is unlikely to affect the decision about whether to incarcerate this individual. Thus, the PATE, which averages the effects of the incarceration across all defendants, including those who committed trivial, moderate, or severe crimes, is of less interest. The usefulness of the LATE of course depends on whether future judges can identify the moderate cases for whom the effect estimate is applicable—that is, that the definition of a "complier" would map onto information available to future judges.

When the IV does not directly cause exposure (*i.e.*, as in $G2$ in Figure 28-1), then assuming monotonicity and targeting the LATE has even more challenges. In these settings, the LATE that is estimated refers to the underlying, unmeasured causal IV—and any bias due to violations of monotonicity must be considered with respect to that unmeasured causal IV.[18] This implies that, for proposed IVs that are unlikely to directly cause exposure (*e.g.*, provider's preference as approximated by previous patient treatment decisions in pharmacoepidemiologic studies[42]), we have even less information about the "compliers" than with a causal IV and the LATE may be of less interest.

In summary, in some cases, the LATE might map closely to the effect of most substantive interest and indeed could more closely align to it than the PATE. In other settings, it is undesirable that we cannot access the PATE, and we care about the IV effect estimate only because we think it gives us insight into the likely sign and magnitude of the PATE. The relevance of the LATE can at least be partially improved by reporting further information about the proportion of the population who are "compliers" and their measured characteristics.[18,38,41,43]

Bounding Causal Effects

In situations when none of the above point-identifying assumptions—which would permit a specific causal interpretation of the IV estimate—are plausible, it is still possible to estimate bounds (*i.e.*, the largest and smallest mathematically possible values) on the average causal effect. The IV conditions alone imply mathematical constraints on the size and direction of the average causal effect.[44-46] There is also the possibility of combining the IV conditions with additional assumptions that are not strong enough to lead to point identification but can provide narrower bounds than the IV assumptions alone.[47] For example, by making assumptions about the counterfactual outcome under treatment among the "never-takers" (*i.e.*, a counterfactual about which we have no information in the observed data but for which we may have strong prior beliefs), much narrower bounds are implied.[47-49]

Bounds on the average causal effect have been described more broadly for nonbinary IVs as well. In the setting in which the outcome is continuous, bounds could also be generated if one is willing to assume an upper and lower possible limit on what the continuous outcome can be.[50] IV-based bounds can also be applied in less standard study designs, such as case-control studies and for two-sample IV studies.

COMPARISON WITH OTHER APPROACHES TO CAUSAL INFERENCE

IV-based methods, including experiments and quasi-experiments, can be contrasted with more conventional methods of observational epidemiology.[51] Typical approaches for causal inferences in observational epidemiology rely on the assumption that all factors which influence both exposure and outcome can be accounted for so fully that, within covariate strata, the treatment an individual receives is unrelated to that individual's potential outcome under that treatment:

$$X \perp\!\!\!\perp Y_{X=x} \mid Z \qquad\qquad [28\text{-}12]$$

This entails no unmeasured confounders of X and Y and is a key part of what is sometimes called the back-door criterion, that is (assuming no variable in Z is a descent of X), Z fulfills the back-door criterion with respect to the effect of X on Y.[52] Fulfilling this "no-unmeasured-confounding" assumption may be implausible for many exposure-outcome associations and is nearly always questionable. In settings where accounting for all shared causes of exposure and outcome seems difficult or impossible, quasi-experimental study designs accompanied by IV analyses can be invaluable.

As noted earlier, weighing the assumptions for the IV effect estimate in comparison to the assumptions for conventional observational analyses should be done on a case-by-case basis. Combining IV and conventional methods can help triangulate causal effects because the two approaches rely on substantively different assumptions.[19,51] Evaluating a research question repeatedly using designs that rely on identical assumptions provides little new information; evaluating the same question with a design that relies on entirely different assumptions can be much more enlightening.

Although epidemiologists often hope that observational studies will lay the groundwork for an RCT, for many important research questions, ideal RCTs are unlikely to ever be fielded. In the domain of social epidemiology, this is obvious: we are unlikely to randomize children to drop out of high school versus to complete their degree; we foresee no RCTs of many exposures of importance in social epidemiology, such as an incarceration or divorce. Nevertheless, the challenge of fielding classical RCTs prevails in many settings beyond social epidemiology. A major effort to field an RCT evaluating the health effects of alcohol consumption foundered in part due to ethical concerns.[53] RCTs of medications already established as effective in a population overall cannot be ethically repeated, even if there are important uncertainties about effects within subgroups (*e.g.*, HIV preexposure prophylaxis [PrEP]).[54] Despite these ethical challenges to RCTs, the chance that an individual will be exposed to each of these exposures is subject to numerous random (or plausibly random) influences that are otherwise unrelated to health outcomes. Educational attainment and alcohol consumption are influenced by state and local policies or by happenstance of geographic proximity.[55] Incarceration chances are influenced by the mercy of the randomly assigned district attorney and judge.[56] Changes in divorce laws influence the likelihood of marriage dissolution.[57] After the initial RCT evidence, numerous PrEP programs were rolled out across the world; the likelihood that a person at risk of HIV infection uses PrEP is influenced by the local programs, access rules, and marketing strategies.[58] In each of these cases, quasi-experimental approaches can provide insights available from no other methods.

Contrasting covariate control and IV-based methods requires recognizing trade-offs. IV analyses, when applied to settings with intentional or accidental randomization, can deliver a scientifically important effect estimate, albeit with some additional assumptions.[14] This causal effect estimate can be obtained even when there is intractable confounding of exposure and outcome, including due to nonadherence in an RCT. Despite these advantages, due to the limitations of IV-based methods discussed throughout the chapter, IV methods are not a panacea. The IV assumptions are very strong and in many cases, it is difficult to identify a plausibly valid IV for the research question. Adopting the monotonicity assumption for point-identification implies that the IV effect estimates may not be generalizable beyond the mysterious "compliers." Using IVs versus covariate-control methods can sometimes also entail a trade-off between statistical precision and potential bias. When combining both sources of error in an effect estimate, one might in some settings prefer a slightly biased but precise estimate.[59]

The contrast we make here—between designs that rely on fulfilling the "no-unmeasured-confounding" assumption with respect to exposure and outcome versus designs that rely on the existence of an IV—emphasizes the connection between study designs often taught as separate quasi-experimental designs: regression discontinuity, difference-in-difference, interrupted time series approaches, and the recently popularized MR approach. We now briefly consider some common sources of IVs and then show how IV methods and concepts overlap with these classic quasi-experimental approaches, before we dive into a small group of illustrative examples in a bit more detail.

COMMONLY PROPOSED IVs

IV analyses are often conducted in observational data. These settings fall on a spectrum from situations in which the IV conditions seem very plausible to situations in which the IV conditions are questionable (but might hold or approximately hold with appropriate covariate control). A major practical challenge for would-be IV analysts is recognizing a potential IV. For that purpose, examples of common types of IVs can be enlightening. Table 28-2 lists some of the many sources of IVs. Below we discuss a few examples to provide more specificity.

First, let us consider an example that seems very similar to an RCT but randomization was applied for purposes unrelated to research: allocation of housing subsidies by lottery. Many families in the United States are eligible for a government subsidy for rental housing. There is not

TABLE 28-2

Sources of Seemingly Random Variation in Exposure, Potentially Applicable as Instrumental Variables in Health Research

- Lotteries randomly allocating limited resources
- The timing of a policy change in a particular location or setting
- Policy changes implemented at different times in different places
- Policy changes affecting only some subgroups of otherwise similar individuals
- Arbitrary thresholds for eligibility for a resource or enrollment in a study
- Arbitrarily assigned judges, interviewers, providers, classmates, or roommates
- Providers or interviewers selected for reasons unrelated to the potential outcome ("as-good-as-random")
- Distance to a resource
- Genetic variants influencing exposure to a phenotype (*i.e.*, Mendelian randomization studies)
- Study design randomly assigning interviewers or interventionists who have varying success at delivering a treatment
- Study design randomly assigning exposure

sufficient funding provided to subsidize all eligible families, and so this subsidy is often allocated by random assignment across a list of eligible families. This random assignment is intended to provide a fair mechanism to distribute a limited resource, and it thereby creates a potential IV to evaluate the effect of receipt of housing subsidies on social and health outcomes.[13] Note that this IV is valid only among individuals who were eligible and signed up for the lottery. It is not a valid IV when considered in the whole US population, because individuals who did not sign up for the lottery could not possibly have been awarded a housing subsidy. Just as with a trial, researchers using this type of proposed IV need to carefully consider whether lottery assignment might affect the social and health outcomes via mechanisms unrelated to exposure of interest (*i.e.*, in Figure 28-1A, the existence of a path from G to Y not passing through X). For example, although the lottery influenced the financial burden related to housing costs, it could not be used as an IV specifically for the exposure of housing-related financial burden. This is because being randomized to receive a housing subsidy also likely implies a move to a new residence; an interruption of ties to current neighbors after moving to new housing; as well as possibly a change in schools for children. A comparison of those who were and were not randomized to receive the subsidy would correspond with the potential effects of this bundle of changes.

Randomly assigned judges are an example of an IV that seems more distant from an RCT.[56] Many resources, such as eligibility for social security disability benefits, are determined by an essentially randomly assigned case reviewer. The reviewer has discretion to award disability payments or deny payments based on the application information. However, reviewers vary substantially in their propensity to award payments. Some reviewers are much more inclined to award benefits than other reviewers. Since the assignment of the reviewer has nothing to do with the merits of the case, the reviewer's decision pattern offers a possible IV to estimate the effect of receiving social security disability benefits on outcomes.[60] A similar idea has been proposed in pharmacoepidemiology, in which it has been argued that (a) physicians have a preference or tendency to prescribe one medication over another, but (b) which physician a patient sees is effectively random.[36,42] Under these assumptions, the physicians' prescribing tendencies may offer an IV for the effect of particular medications. Of course, if the assignment is not actually random, it is possible that the IV conditions would not hold. For example, if certain physicians tend to see more severe patients (*e.g.*, because they are specialists or have a reputation for handling specific case types), then the proposed IV would not be valid.

A large body of IV work draws on how policy changes occur across time or space. For example, in 1947, England increased mandatory schooling so children were required to remain in school for an additional year (to age 15). Children born before 1933 were not affected and could leave school at age 14. Banks and Mazzonna compared late-life cognitive outcomes for individuals born in England before and after 1933, in order to evaluate the effect of additional education on cognitive outcomes.[61] Individuals born in 1933 having markedly better cognition than individuals born in 1932 indicates the additional education likely had a benefit.

IVs can also be built into study designs. For example, behavioral change interventions premised on one-on-one counseling might randomly assign the counselor, recognizing that some counselors will likely be more effective than others at eliciting behavioral change among trial participants. This creates an IV for the effect of behavior change. Even for researchers who never plan to use a quasi-experiment, recognizing the power of IV methods can lead to improvements in conventional study designs. In studies with prospective participant enrollment, randomly assigning recruitment representatives could allow for rigorous estimation of selection bias if some representatives achieve much higher enrollment rates than others.[62,63]

In interventions with multiple possible mediators, randomly assigning interventionists can offer an additional opportunity to disentangle multiple mediating pathways, without resorting to implausible assumptions of no confounding. For example, consider an intervention aiming to improve poststroke quality of life via two mechanisms, say (1) improvements in environmental accommodations to promote independence (*e.g.*, bathroom grab bars) and (2) improvements in communication with close friends and family about how to most effectively provide emotional or practical support. Some interventionists might be much better at identifying opportunities for environmental accommodations, whereas other interventionists might be better at facilitating intimate conversations among social network members. These two mechanisms can be conceptualized as exposures themselves, and if interventionists are assigned at random, the identity of the interventionist can be used as an IV to estimate the effect of each mechanism.

LINKING IV METHODS WITH QUASI-EXPERIMENTAL DESIGNS

Quasi-experimental studies have a long history in health research, but linking quasi-experimental methods with IV analyses vastly extends the usefulness of quasi-experiments. The IVs we discussed above are often used in a set of research designs referred to with special names such as interrupted time series, regression discontinuity, difference-in-difference, or MR designs. When linking these designs with IV methods, we distinguish between two types of research questions. Consider Figure 28-1A. We have focused on situations in which the question of interest addresses the effect of X on Y and noted that we can use the effect of G on Y to learn about the effect of X on Y. In such a research question, G is simply a convenient tool, not of interest in and of itself. However, one can imagine settings in which a question of interest is limited to the effect of G on Y per se, that is, settings in which the ITT analogue is of intrinsic interest. To distinguish between these two types of questions, consider a situation in which G is a policy change that increases taxes on cigarettes. A policymaker considering implementing a similar tax policy in a new but generally similar location might care most about the overall effects of that precise policy on cardiovascular disease (CVD) incidence. On the other hand, an *individual* considering whether to stop smoking would not care much about the effect of the tax policy but would instead want to know the cardiovascular effects of smoking cessation, which might be estimated by using the tax policy implementation as an IV. Further, policymakers in the new location may find other policy strategies known to reduce smoking—for example, indoor smoking bans—more politically feasible than the tax. If so, the policymaker would not care about the effect of taxation per se, but rather the effect of reducing smoking on CVD incidence. By combining information on the effect of smoking on CVD (derived from using tax policy as an IV) with information on the effect of the indoor smoking ban on smoking, the policymaker could try to anticipate the CVD benefits of the proposed indoor smoking ban. In short, different audiences may find either the effect of the policy or the IV estimate of the effect of smoking cessation of greater relevance.[51] Keeping these interests and motivations in mind helps us navigate the world of quasi-experimental methods because the assumptions required to answer the two types of questions differ.[51]

Sharp and Fuzzy Regression Discontinuity Approaches

Regression discontinuity methods apply when there is a threshold for a measured variable around which the probability of being treated changes very rapidly.[7,64] Such a threshold might be an eligibility criterion for a specific resource for example. Examples of this include rules that specify eligibility criteria for randomized trials of medications[65] or programs that guarantee college admissions[66] or provide financial subsidies to every student in a particular community with standardized test scores above a certain threshold. We expect people just above and just below the test score threshold to be otherwise similar or exchangeable. We can compare these groups to estimate the effects of receiving the subsidy and, assuming the subsidy increases the chances of attending college, apply an IV analysis such as 2SLS to estimate the effects of attending college. In this example, the test score is referred to as the forcing or running variable. This threshold might be used, for example, to estimate the effects of receiving the financial subsidy (which is equivalent to scoring above the threshold) on mental health outcomes 5 years later. Because we may think that individuals with higher test scores would average different mental health even if they did not receive a subsidy, we must account for the continuous, incremental association of test scores with mental health. This design creates a sharp regression discontinuity occurring exactly at the threshold above which individuals receive the subsidy (where we use the notation: I(test score > threshold) to represent an indicator variable for whether the test score is above the threshold):

$$Mental\ Health = \alpha_0 + \alpha_1 I \left(test\ score > threshold \right)$$
$$+ \alpha_2 test\ score + \varepsilon \qquad [28\text{-}13]$$

If we had extremely large samples immediately above and immediately below the threshold, we could just compare individuals in this very narrow range. In typical finite data sets though, we need to extend the range around the threshold and the model for the running

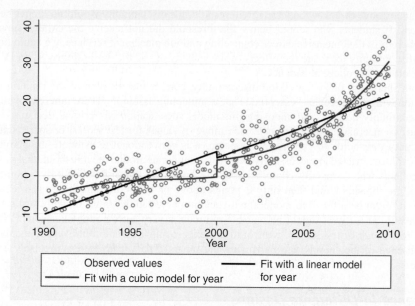

FIGURE 28-2 Misspecification of the running variable in a regression discontinuity or related design. Assuming the event causing a discontinuity occurred in the year 2000, alternative specifications of the underlying time-trend lead to very different estimates of the discontinuity at the time the policy was introduced. A linear model for year (solid black line) would suggest a small negative discontinuity in 2000. If year is modeled with linear, quadratic, and cubic polynomials (solid red line), the estimated discontinuity is instead positive.

variable will be very important. The coefficient of interest, α_1, will in general be very sensitive to correct specification of the relationship between the running variable and the outcome. If, for example, the association between test score and mental health in the absence of a subsidy would be nonlinear, but we specify it as linear, the misspecification will alter the estimated coefficient for the threshold (see an example of egregious misspecification in Figure 28-2).

This approach can be modified to estimate the effect of college attendance on mental health, using performance above the threshold (and therefore receipt of a subsidy) as an IV. In this setting, it is considered a fuzzy regression discontinuity because the value of the running variable does not perfectly determine the exposure variable. Some people with below-threshold test scores nonetheless attend college, whereas some people with above-threshold scores do not. To account for this fuzziness, we might use an IV analysis, with the threshold as the IV, college attendance (CA) as the exposure, and mental health as the outcome:

$$\widetilde{CA} = \widehat{\gamma_0} + \widehat{\gamma_1} I\left(test\ score > threshold\right) + \widehat{\gamma_2}\left(test\ score\right) \qquad [28\text{-}14]$$

$$Mental\ Health = \widehat{\beta_0} + \widehat{\beta_1}\widetilde{CA} + \widehat{\beta_2} test\ score + \varepsilon \qquad [28\text{-}15]$$

Contrasting the sharp and fuzzy regression discontinuity, note the variable that is the IV in the fuzzy regression discontinuity is instead identical to the exposure of interest in the sharp regression discontinuity. There is thus no need to apply an IV analysis to identify the effect of this variable in the sharp regression discontinuity study. Many of the factors that would violate the IV assumptions necessary to identify the causal effect of interest in the fuzzy regression discontinuity would also violate the assumptions necessary to identify the effect of interest in the sharp regression discontinuity case. For example, if some other resources besides the college subsidy were tied to performance above or below the test score threshold, the discontinuity would no longer be a valid instrument. If students who scored below the threshold did not receive the college subsidy but instead were provided intensive career counseling and job placement services, we could no longer use the discontinuity to isolate the effects of the subsidy or use the discontinuity as an IV to estimate the effects of college attendance.

In both sharp and fuzzy regression discontinuity, correct specification of the running variable association with the outcome is essential. That is, modeling assumptions are inherent in all regression discontinuity designs, and choosing this model specification is a critical decision.[67] This is particularly concerning when there is a wide range of values for test scores, or sparse data at the discontinuity threshold. To explore this concern, it is conventional to estimate the above model using a sample restricted to successively narrower boundaries around the threshold, that is, restricting to students who score only 10 points above or below the threshold, then only 5 points above or below the threshold, and then only 2 points above or below the threshold. The idea is that although it might be difficult to model the association between the entire range of test scores and mental health correctly, it should be feasible to model a very narrow range correctly. Within the very narrow range of test scores, we would not expect much variation in average mental health in the absence of the subsidy, but narrowing the range of data leads to less precisely estimated coefficients.

Difference-in-Difference Designs

Difference-in-difference designs build upon regression discontinuity designs by incorporating comparison groups that were not treated to help model the counterfactual values for individuals who were treated. For example, a difference-in-difference approach with the test score example might involve a comparison group of test-takers who were not eligible for the subsidy regardless of their test, for example, students from a neighboring community, and we would estimate:

$$
\begin{aligned}
Mental\ Health = \widehat{\beta_0} + \widehat{\beta_1}I\left(test\ score > threshold\right) + \widehat{\beta_2}test\ score \\
+ \widehat{\beta_3}I\left(lives\ in\ eligible\ community\right) \\
+ \widehat{\beta_4}I\left(\begin{matrix} test\ score > threshold\ and \\ lives\ in\ eligible\ community \end{matrix}\right) + \varepsilon
\end{aligned}
\qquad [28\text{-}16]
$$

In this difference-in-difference model, the estimate for β_1 refers to the discontinuity at the test score threshold for students in the comparison (reference) community, who are not eligible for a subsidy. For these students, there should be no difference in mental health if we have correctly modeled the running variable (test score). The coefficient β_3 refers to the difference between people in the eligible community with below-threshold test scores and people in the comparison community with below-threshold test scores. We are interested specifically in the coefficient β_4, which describes the differential discontinuity at the test score threshold for those students who live in the community eligible for the subsidy versus students who live in comparison communities. This model is unbiased even if the eligible community and the comparison community differ overall with respect to average mental health, provided those differences are the same regardless of test score; such differences are accounted for by adjusting for the indicator for community. In essence, difference-in-difference models use trends in a comparison group to account for possible sources of deviation in trends among the treated.

Just as with regression discontinuity and interrupted time series, we can apply an IV-based analysis to a difference-in-difference setting to identify the effect of a resource or exposure influenced but not perfectly determined by the test score threshold. The analysis is the same as the other IV analyses discussed here, but the interaction between test score threshold and living in an eligible community is considered the IV; both the first and second stages of the IV analysis include control for the continuous test score as well as indicators for being above the test score threshold and for living in an eligible community, whereas the interaction term is included in the first stage but omitted from the second stage.

A very common setting for this design leverages implementation of a policy at different times in different places as an IV for the effect of the resource or treatment influenced by that policy. For example, consider using a policy which delivers resource X and was implemented at different times in multiple communities to estimate the effect of X on Y. With data on individuals in communities, one might use an indicator for whether the policy had yet been implemented in a specific community j at year t, controlling for either a continuous or a segmented time trend and a vector of indicators for each community of k communities (Z_j):

$$\widetilde{X_{t,j}} = \widehat{\alpha_0} + \widehat{\alpha_1}I\left(policy\ in\ force\ in\ community\right)_{t,j} + \widehat{\alpha_2}time_t + \sum_{j=3}^{k+2} \widehat{\alpha_j}Z_j \qquad [28\text{-}17]$$

$$Y_{t,j} = \widehat{\beta_0} + \widehat{\beta_1}\widetilde{X_{t,j}} + \widehat{\beta_2}time_t + \sum_{j=3}^{k+2} \widehat{\beta_j}Z_j + \varepsilon_{t,j} \qquad [28\text{-}18]$$

In Equation 28-17, the indicator for whether the policy is in force in the community is only 1 for observations that refer to a community which adopted the policy and only for those years after the policy was already in force. In other words, it is parallel to the indicator variable in Equation 28-16 for whether the test score is above the threshold and the individual lives in an eligible community. Correctly modeling the running variable, in this case time, is very important in this model, as in the regression discontinuity model. We return to special consideration when time is the running variable below for interrupted time series and time series modeling.

Versions of the above difference-in-difference model could be estimated with grouped data for each community and at multiple time points before and after policy implementation or with multilevel data on individuals within each community across multiple time points (either the same or different individuals across multiple time points). If individual-level data are available, it permits additional covariate control to account for potential differences in the composition of the community or address other possible mechanisms via which the policy may have influenced Y.

Improvements in strategies to derive an optimal comparison group or other approaches to modeling the counterfactual values of the treated are an active area of research. The use of synthetic comparison groups based on averages of multiple locations is growing in popularity.[68] Other work uses matching to select the comparison groups that would offer the most statistical power.[69]

Interrupted Time Series Designs and Modeling Time Series

Interrupted time series approaches can be thought of as regression discontinuity studies in which time is the running variable. The discontinuity occurs, for example, at the date when a new policy is implemented or expected to take effect. Interrupted time series studies face essentially identical challenges as other regression discontinuity designs with respect to correct modeling of the running variable (time). With interrupted time series approaches, we must anticipate the temporal trends in the outcome that would have occurred in the absence of the event causing the discontinuity. When time is the running variable, the most plausible threats relate to other events that occurred simultaneously, besides the policy or event of interest. As with regression discontinuity, we can analyze interrupted time series to evaluate the effect of something perfectly determined at the time of the interruption (*e.g.*, the effect of the policy as implemented) or to evaluate the effect of a resource or exposure that was influenced at the time of the interruption, but not perfectly determined. In the latter case, we use an IV analysis to estimate first the effect of the interruption on the exposure of interest and then how that change in exposure due to the interruption influenced the outcome of interest.

Interrupted time series designs draw on a large set of methods for modeling time series data. These methods are generally equally relevant to those difference-in-difference designs in which time is the source of one of the differences. Many important data streams provide repeated measures on contextual variables (such as daily high temperature) or grouped variables (such as daily mortality rate) over a long period of time for a particular location or set of locations. Some time series research aims merely to describe the structure of a time series, that is, how past values of the series predict future values, and we refer readers to time series textbooks for more details on these methods.[70] Similar considerations are applicable to settings in which researchers evaluate the association between two time series to offer insight into causal processes, for example, whether values of an exposure at time t (X_t) influence future values of an outcome Y.

Ecological variables that appear in time series data are often used as IVs to reveal causal effects of another variable. For example, time series data on alcohol sales and motor vehicle fatality rates have been used to evaluate the effects of population level alcohol consumption on motor vehicle fatalities.[71] Motor vehicle fatality time series data, combined with information on the timing of policy campaigns to deter drunk driving, were used to evaluate the success of these campaigns.[71] Historical time series on famine exposure and birth-cohort-specific mortality rates have been used to test the hypothesis that nutritional deprivation in utero has enduring effects on mortality rate.[72] In this case, we can conceptualize the famine time series data as providing IVs for an individual level exposure (in utero nutrition) that was not measured. Even with no directly measured data on in utero nutrition, we can potentially evaluate whether this exposure influences later mortality risk. Rainfall time series data have been used as IVs for a surprising and sometimes controversial array of exposures,[73,74] but also used as direct measures of drought exposure to evaluate how drought influences child health outcomes.[75] Many policy datasets used as IVs can be described as time series data. For example, data on state schooling policies for the 20th century, frequently used as IVs for the effects of education, are a time series for each state.[14,54] In a slight variation on classic IV methods, time series on regulatory actions, air pollution, and mortality have been combined to identify locations for which regulatory action improved air quality and then, within those locations, estimate the effect of the regulatory action on mortality.[76]

Many aspects of using time series data for causal research largely overlap with design and analysis considerations for typical individual level or multilevel data, but several aspects of time series data merit special consideration. Some time series methods that are typical in descriptive or predictive work may be inappropriate in causal research. The relevance of one time series for another may be lagged, so X_t may influence Y_{t+1} or Y_{t+2} or even Y_{t+30}; standard analytic approaches can identify statistically optimal lags, but this choice should also reflect substantive knowledge. Choosing the wrong lag period can deliver entirely incorrect results. To see this, consider the lag between population smoking rates and lung cancer mortality.[77] Smoking rates have declined dramatically in many countries in recent decades, but lung cancer mortality lags smoking by decades. Estimating a model in which lung cancer mortality was predicted by contemporaneous smoking rates could incorrectly indicate that declines in smoking lead to increases in lung cancer mortality. This is critical to note in chronic disease research because the pathologic processes may take years to culminate in illness. When the exposure of interest is the introduction of a policy at time k, the independent variable time series might be conceptualized $X_t = 0$ if $t < k$ and $X_t = 1$ if $t \geq k$, consistent with equation 28-13 replacing "test score > threshold" with "time period $\geq k$." If the policy is expected to have small initial effects that accumulate until the policy is in full force, this might require the estimation of two terms, to capture the rate of accumulation and another to capture the maximum effect. Alternatively, some policies might be expected to have large initial effects that subsequently attenuate. The choice among possible specifications should reflect substantive knowledge and consistency with the data.

Transformations may be necessary for a time series to be rendered "stationary," that is, with similar variance and autocorrelation regardless of when one examines the time series. Repeated measures of the same variable in the same location are typically correlated (autocorrelation), which may invalidate conventional standard error (SE) calculations. First differencing (e.g., instead of using X_t as the independent variable, use $X_t - X_{t-1}$ and instead of using Y_t as the dependent variable, use $Y_t - Y_{t-1}$) is a common technique because it sometimes eliminates autocorrelation and improves stationarity. First differencing can also induce spurious inverse correlation in some cases however, and this transformation changes the meaning of the exposure and imposes strong assumptions about the timing of the causal process.

Periodicity is common in time series data, for example, due to seasonal fluctuations. In regression models of time series data, periodicity may be addressed by incorporating concise functional forms (e.g., cosine functions of time), indicator variables for the cycle clock (e.g., indicators for each calendar month), or flexible models such as splines to allow for periodicity that evolves over time. The goal is to choose a specification that removes the periodicity, so that conditional on the control variables for periods, the residual values of the outcome series do not show cycles.

Addressing the periodicity is important because such cycles often affect both the exposure and outcome time series and therefore create spurious associations. For example, both flu rates and prevalence of wearing mittens increase during winter. Removing periodicity can therefore be considered a strategy to address confounders.[78] Similarly, many time series show long-term trends, such as increasing educational attainment or declining cardiovascular mortality, over the past century. Time series regression models must account for such trends, recognizing that some of the similarity in trends over time might be due to unrelated factors but others may be attributable to a causal effect of one variable on the other. Usually, disentangling these relies on some smoothing assumptions about how temporal trends would evolve in the absence of the causal factor of interest.

Even when both exposure and outcome time series refer to place-level variables, interest in health research is often about a process that influences individual health outcomes. Many time series analyses are strictly ecological, using grouped or ecological data for both exposure and outcome. Merging time series exposure data onto individual level data on outcomes and covariates, that is, evaluating multilevel data, can help address bias due to shared time trends.

Methods specific for time series analysis are well developed in other disciplines, and the language used is often inconsistent with terminology adopted in modern epidemiology. For example, the phrase Granger causality is used to describe a setting in which current values of one time series variable (X_t) predict future values of another time series variable (Y_{t+1}), even when conditioning on current values of the outcome variable (Y_t). Granger causality can be a useful assessment, but it does not imply causality as defined in this textbook, because the conditional association may reflect uncontrolled confounding or collider bias.[10,79]

Mendelian Randomization

MR applications—which use genetic polymorphisms as IVs to estimate the effects of a phenotype influenced by those genetic variants—have blossomed since a series of influential articles in 2004.[71,80,81] Although not originally presented as a version of IV, Didelez and others noted that MR approaches were a special case of IV.[82] This recognition helped link extensive prior scholarship on IV to MR applications.

The original conceptualization of MR used information on a single genetic variant as an IV to estimate the effect of a phenotype directly influenced by that variant on a downstream health outcome. For example, genetic variants that influence alcohol consumption have been used to evaluate the effects of alcohol on CVDs, cancers, and other health outcomes.[83,84] As genetic data have increased, recent MR analyses tend to combine information on several genetic variants as proposed IVs individually or jointly.[85,86]

In fact, the special features of the genetic data now available to the scientific community have driven innovation in MR methods. Specifically, we now pool many large data sets to field Genome-Wide Association Studies (GWAS), which identify numerous genetic variants, each of which has a small correlation with the phenotype of interest measured in those data sets. The genetic polymorphisms (*i.e.*, places in the genetic code where differences between humans are common) typically identified with GWAS have very small associations with the phenotype and are generally not thought to be causal variants: the GWAS method is premised on the idea that variation across the genome is clustered because segments of chromosomes are inherited together. As a result, a polymorphism at one location on the genome is highly correlated with nearby genetic variation. The magnitude of association between individual polymorphisms and phenotypes of interest is often very small; major investments in GWAS have allowed datasets of hundreds of thousands of individuals, supporting identification of genetic variants with tiny effect sizes.

In many cases, the datasets used to field GWAS for a specific phenotype are not the same data sets in which the health outcome of interest has been measured. For example, in research on the effects of BMI on mental health, many datasets may include genetic information and BMI data, or genetic information and mental health data, but not all three variables necessary for a classic IV analysis: genetic information, BMI, and mental health data. These problems in combination have driven IV analysis methods that leverage polygenic risk scores, novel approaches for evaluating IV validity (discussed more below), and two-sample IV approaches.

For MR, potential threats to the core IV assumptions follow the same structure as for any IV, but correspond with particular biological phenomena and thus sometimes come with their own nomenclature.[87-89] Population stratification refers to the clustering of particular genetic variants within subpopulations with shared ancestry, who may also have shared social experiences. These variants may predict health outcomes only because of their different prevalence within the group and thus correlation with the distinctive social experiences of that group. For this reason, MR analyses nearly always control for detailed measures of genetic ancestry. MR studies may also be biased by the influences of parental genetics on the health of their offspring. Many genetic variants may have numerous pathways via which they influence a health outcome; such so-called "pleiotropic pathways" can lead to spurious MR results. A final commonly invoked threat is canalization, processes such that the early developmental effects of a genetic polymorphism are offset by changes over the life-course elicited in response to the immediate consequences of the gene.

When there are multiple genetic variants that might be used as candidate IVs, the estimates based on each of the genetic variants may differ. Such inconsistency may indicate a violation of the IV assumptions or may reflect true differences in the individuals who are "compliers" with different genetic variants. Inconsistent estimates across multiple genetic variants may also indicate heterogeneity in the phenotype of interest. For example, although there are genetic variants confirmed to predict BMI, BMI is a heterogeneous exposure and may not meet the consistency assumption for causal inference.[90] Different genetic variants may identify effects of different facets of BMI (*e.g.*, abdominal adiposity vs. peripheral adiposity). Although this is a problem in interpreting IV estimates of effects of BMI, the problem in the context of IV is very similar to the problem when using BMI as an exposure in conventional analyses. In some settings, then, the IV approach can help identify the consistency violation and even potentially disentangle effects of different components of BMI, effects that may be impossible to evaluate with conventional approaches.[91-93]

The growth of genetic studies of social and behavioral phenotypes,[94] such as education,[95] has prompted interest in the possibility of MR studies for evaluation of the causal effects of social factors. Given the tragic misuses invoking genetic explanations for social stratification, these applications merit special caution. It is often unclear for which causal structures such analyses might provide evidence. In some cases, the proposed IV seems as strongly linked to potential confounders as to the exposure of interest. For example, Nguyen evaluated whether genetic variants linked to education could provide a valid IV to estimate the effect of education on dementia. She found that genetic variants predicted dementia risk more strongly than they predicted education and concluded that they were unlikely to be valid IVs.[96] Further, the health effects of social factors are of great interest because there are numerous policies and individual decisions that can influence the social factors, many of which have been used in prior IV studies.[80,81] The very modifiability of social factors—the feature which accounts for their substantive importance in public health—may also define plausible IVs. IV analyses leveraging genetic variants would not necessarily provide evidence on the likely effect of changes in social factors achieved via policy strategies.

EVALUATING THE VALIDITY OF AN IV ANALYSIS

The validity of a proposed IV should always be considered with respect to a specific exposure and outcome; an IV that is valid to estimate the effect of an exposure on one outcome may not be valid for another outcome. To guide interpretation, we need to provide evidence on the core IV conditions (CF-IV 1 and CF-IV 2 or DAG-IV 1, DAG-IV 2, and DAG-IV 3) plus any point-identifying assumption invoked, for example, monotonicity. There are several available approaches for trying to falsify each of these assumptions and to understand the robustness of the IV estimate to plausible violations of each assumption.

We noted above that many of the other quasi-experimental approaches can be viewed as based on having an IV or making IV-type assumptions, even when an IV analysis is not applied. As such, many of the strategies for evaluating the validity of an IV analysis can also be adapted for regression discontinuity, interrupted time series, and difference-in-difference designs. For ease of presentation, we focus specifically on techniques for evaluating traditional IV analyses here.

Is the IV Associated with Exposure?

If condition DAG-IV 1, that a proposed IV is associated with the exposure of interest, is not met, then we do not expect the proposed IV to predict Y even if X influences Y. In this case, the proposed

IV is at best useless because a null IV estimate would tell us nothing. The proposed IV may be worse than useless, however, because of "weak-instruments bias." Weak-instruments bias occurs in finite samples when there are multiple potential IVs, which have no or very weak associations with the exposure. In this case, the 2SLS estimator is biased in the direction of the ordinary least squares (OLS) estimate, so if the OLS estimate is biased away from the causal effect, in situations where X has no true effect on Y, the 2SLS estimate will also be so biased.[97,98] Weak-instruments bias attenuates with larger sample size; is exacerbated by more IVs; and if X has no effect on Y, is largely ameliorated by separate sample approaches.

The association between a proposed IV and the exposure of interest is easily demonstrated, and this association should always be reported. Traditionally, minimum F-tests have been used as a criterion for a "weak instrument," so it is conventional to report the F-statistic for the IV-exposure association as evidence of the "strength" of the instrument.[97] The F-statistic will depend on sample size, which is appropriate because weak instruments bias also depends on sample size. The F-statistic also decreases with additional IVs; this is a major concern in MR methods because there are often many genetic variants each with small effects and has motivated the approach of combining variants into a single polygenic score.[99] Conceptually, weak instruments bias can be thought of as due to overfitting the first stage of the 2SLS model, so that the predicted value of the treatment variable is slightly correlated with the unmeasured confounders. This will happen by chance in any regression model with multiple predictor variables in a finite sample; it becomes worse with additional predictors (*i.e.*, multiple IVs) or smaller samples.

It is also useful to report other metrics describing the strength of the association between the IV and the exposure, such as the correlation coefficient (or denominator of the Wald estimator). If it is necessary to include covariates in the analysis, it is the partial correlation between the IV and the exposure—conditional on other covariates—that is relevant. In a single-sample analysis, this assessment is straightforward. In two sample analyses, the strength of the IV may differ in the two samples, and the *measured* strength of the IV will almost certainly differ because of finite sample variation, different sample sizes, and imperfect harmonization of the measurements available in the two samples. In general, if X has no effect on Y, two sample approaches avoid the above-described version of weak-IV bias, so the lack of power (*i.e.*, information about the effect of X on Y) will be clear from the wide confidence intervals. If X does affect Y, but G does not affect X, the denominator of the IV estimator converges to 0, so the IV estimator will be extremely variable. In contrast, in single sample analyses, extremely weak IVs may nonetheless lead to spuriously precise effect estimates biased toward the confounded observational estimate of the exposure-outcome association.[97]

Even if the condition DAG IV-1 is technically fulfilled, the strength of the association between the IV and exposure is important because it is inversely proportional to the variance of the IV estimate and the bias that would be introduced by any violation of the other IV conditions. If the effect of G on X is very small, the IV estimate will be very imprecise and is unlikely to be informative. The LATE estimate provides an intuition for this: the effect is based only on the small fraction of people for whom G influenced X. Because of this, evaluating the confidence interval for an IV estimate is essential: wide CIs often reveal that little has been learned from the IV analysis. The potential for bias magnification with a weak proposed IV is more insidious than the impact on variance. If there is a direct effect of a proposed IV on the outcome not mediated by the exposure, the bias in a 2SLS IV effect estimate equals the magnitude of the direct effect divided by the correlation between the proposed IV and the exposure. The smaller the first-stage association, the larger the bias. Unlike the weak-instruments bias discussed above, this bias is *not* attenuated with larger sample sizes or separate samples.

Using Substantively Informed Tests to Evaluate the Validity of IVs

The plausibility of assumptions DAG-IV 2 and DAG-IV 3 should be considered separately based on subject matter knowledge, but the empirical approaches to evaluating these assumptions are often identical. Just as it is not possible to prove the standard no-confounding assumption in analyses based on confounder control, it is in general not possible to prove that either DAG-IV 2 or DAG-IV 3 assumption is true. It is possible to provide supportive evidence for DAG-IV 2 or DAG-IV 3, however, or to disprove these assumptions.[91] These methods can be summarized as substantively informed tests based on the implications of the IV assumptions; tests that take advantage of the availability of multiple proposed IVs to triangulate evidence; and tests that evaluate mathematical implications of the IV assumptions.

Substantively informed tests may draw on any of the following:

1. Balance of measured potential confounders: In conventional analyses, it is useful to evaluate the balance of measured covariates across levels of treatment. In IV analyses, it is useful to evaluate the balance of measured covariates across levels of the proposed IV. Because small confounding biases due to unbalanced confounders are inflated in IV analyses, as described above, we recommend evaluating such bias after applying a scaling factor proportional to the proposed IV-exposure association.[36,100] In other words, when illustrating the balance of a potential confounder C by level of the proposed IV, one should consider the scaled difference in the confounder by levels of the IV: $\left[E\left(C|G=1\right)-E\left(C|G=0\right)\right]/\left[\Pr\left(X=1|G=1\right)-\Pr\left(X=1|G=0\right)\right]$. If the confounder imbalance is assessed without accounting for this scaling factor (the effect of the proposed IV on exposure), it is tempting to dismiss small differences although they might be important in the IV analysis.

2. Negative control outcomes, which are likely to be subject to the same (if any) biasing pathways as the main outcome of interest, but which are not thought to be affected by the exposure: if the IV predicts negative control outcomes, this implicates biasing pathways. Note that such a test should not condition on the exposure.

3. Populations for which the IV is known not to influence the exposure: in such populations, a valid IV should be unrelated to the outcome, but a biased IV might nonetheless predict the outcome. For example, analyses using a genetic variant related to alcohol consumption *(ALDH2)* to evaluate the effects of alcohol use on stroke took advantage of the fact that in their research setting, alcohol use was extremely rare among women, regardless of genetic background. The genetic IV was associated with stroke among men (for whom it also predicted alcohol use) but not among women (for whom the genetic variant was unrelated to alcohol use). This finding was interpreted as supporting the validity of the genetic variant as an IV for the effect of alcohol, because pleiotropic pathways would presumably have operated similarly for men and women.[84]

4. Sensitivity or bias analysis to evaluate whether effects are robust to plausible violations of the IV conditions: for example, the IV conditions entail that the instrument G has no direct effect on Y, but we might posit some range of direct effects in violation of this condition. We can then derive the range of estimates for the effect of X on Y consistent with the specified magnitude of the violating pathway.[87,101] Calculations of the e-value, that is, the strength of a confounder that would be sufficient to fully explain the observed association assuming the confounder had equal magnitude of effect on G and Y, have been proposed for MR and are equally applicable for any IV method.[102]

Developing substantively informed tests relies on understanding of the process by which the IV is thought to operate, for example, in order to identify subgroups that should *not* be affected. These are valuable complements to IV analyses of data from quasi-experiments.

Taking Advantage of Multiple Proposed IVs to Search for Assumption Violations

Tests that leverage the availability of multiple proposed IVs are widely used in economics and are referred to as over-identification tests. The basic idea is to test whether IV effect estimates derived from one proposed IV are statistically consistent with effect estimates derived from other proposed IVs. The caveat to this is that all proposed IVs may be similarly biased, in which case over-identification tests would fail to flag the problem.

If over-identification tests *do* indicate that effect estimates from different proposed IVs are inconsistent with one another, there are several possible explanations. First, one or more of the proposed IVs may be biased (but the over-identification test gives you no insight into which one is the problem). Alternatively, heterogeneity in the effect of treatment may explain the discrepancy. The "compliers" in the LATE for different IVs may be different subgroups, and the effect of X on Y for the "compliers" to the first IV may differ from the effect of X on Y for the "compliers" to the second IV.

A related complication with interpreting over-identification tests occurs for exposures that violate the consistency assumption (see Chapter 3 for discussion of consistency), that is, the assumption that each individual's potential outcome setting exposure to a particular value equals that person's actual outcome if they have that value of the exposure $\left[\left(Y_{i,X=x} \middle| X = x \right) = \left(Y_i \middle| X = x \right) \right]$. For example, some compulsory schooling laws regulate the age at which children must begin school, whereas other policies regulate the age at which children may leave school. It is very possible that even though both types of policies lead to additional schooling on a population basis, the effects of starting school when younger differ from the effects of finishing when older. In population studies, educational attainment is nearly always characterized as years or credentials completed, without regard to the ages at which the individual attended school. The evidence that children's brains are particularly plastic during rapid developmental periods in early childhood would suggest that education so measured violates the consistency assumption. Distinguishing the effects of these two educational experiences (an extra year of schooling in early childhood vs. an extra year in adolescence) is an important scientific opportunity provided by an IV. This type of heterogeneity could be discovered with an IV analysis using different types of policies as IVs even in data sets for which the timing of education was never recorded. However, an adequately powered over-identification test would show that effect estimates from the different types of compulsory schooling laws were different, suggesting invalid IVs. Given this possibility, over-identification tests must be interpreted carefully, with consideration for whether a failed test indicates heterogeneous treatment effects, consistency violations, or invalid IVs.

Over-identification tests can be applied when there are multiple proposed IVs or when it is feasible to evaluate interactions between prerandomization variables and a single proposed IV. This extremely powerful idea makes over-identification tests much more broadly applicable. For example, in a multisite individually randomized trial, one could use the interaction between site and random assignment to implement over-identification tests. This boils down to evaluating whether the IV-estimated effect of treatment in some sites is statistically different from that in other sites. If so, this suggests there may be a violation of the IV assumptions in some sites. Note that this comparison of IV effect estimates is much more informative than a comparison of ITT effect estimates across sites, because ITT estimates may differ simply due to differences in adherence. However, for the IV effect estimates to be comparable, some type of homogeneity assumption is implicit—otherwise, the estimates may differ because each estimate is for a different LATE and not because one or more of the proposed IVs are invalid per se.

Tests That Evaluate Mathematical Implications of the IV Assumptions

Above, we described how the IV model implies certain mathematical constraints that allow us to compute bounds on the causal effect. These same mathematical constraints can provide a test of the IV assumptions. Consider an example with a binary IV G, binary exposure X, and binary outcome Y, so the possible effects of X on Y for any individual (β_i) are defined by the two counterfactuals, and we can consider four types of people (where β_i refers to the effect of X on Y for individual i) labeled below assuming Y is an undesirable outcome:

a. $Y_{X=1} = 1, Y_{X=0} = 1: \beta_i = 0$ (doomed: no effect of treatment)
b. $Y_{X=1} = 0, Y_{X=0} = 1: \beta_i = -1$ (helped: treatment prevents the outcome)
c. $Y_{X=1} = 1, Y_{X=0} = 0: \beta_i = 1$ (harmed: treatment causes the outcome)
d. $Y_{X=1} = 0, Y_{X=0} = 0: \beta_i = 0$ (immune: no effect of treatment)

Consider that every individual in the sample can also be defined based on the effect of the IV on their treatment (as described above: "always-taker," "never-taker," "complier," and "defier") and the effect of exposure on the outcome (types doomed, helped, harmed, or immune), for a total of 16 types of people. Summing the prevalence of any subset of those 16 types must always total less than or equal to 100% of the sample. The IV bounds leverage this point by summing the probability of various combinations of the 16 types.[103] The bounds derive from the following inequality, which must be true for any value of X or Y under the IV conditions:

$$\Pr\left(X = x, Y = y \middle| G = 1 \right) + \Pr\left(X = x, Y = 1 - y \middle| G = 0 \right) \leq 1 \qquad [28\text{-}19]$$

To see the intuition, consider the case where $X = 1$ and $Y = 0$:

$$\Pr\left(X = 1, Y = 0 \middle| G = 1\right) + \Pr\left(X = 1, Y = 1 \middle| G = 0\right) \leq 1 \qquad \text{[28-20]}$$

Note that the first term includes only "compliers" and "always-takers" (we know this because $G = 1$ and $X = 1$) who either are helped by the treatment or are immune to the outcome (types b and d, because $Y_{X=1} = 0$). The second term includes only "defiers" and "always-takers" (because $G = 0$, but $X = 1$) who are either doomed or harmed by the treatment (types a and b because $Y_{X=1} = 1$). In other words, the two terms refer to mutually exclusive subgroups and the sum captures at most 8 of the 16 possible types. Therefore, it must sum to less than or equal to 100% of the sample. If it is more than 100%, the IV assumptions cannot be true. Thus, this provides a falsification test of the structural IV assumptions. A similar falsification test is possible if we apply the inequality with $X = 0$ and $Y = 1$. In general, the inequalities can be expanded for multiple values of G and must fulfill the following:

$$max_X \left\{ \sum_Y max_G \left[\Pr\left(X, Y \middle| G\right) \right] \right\} \leq 1$$

where $max_G()$ refers to the maximum value of the quantity in parentheses across all possible values of G.

If this is violated, it is evidence against our IV conditions. Stronger constraints than these have been derived,[104] and it has been proven that such constraints exist beyond the all-binary case as long as the exposure is not continuous. Because these inequalities can be applied for any proposed IV, they can also be applied to sets of proposed IVs jointly and separately to assess each one's validity.[105] This allows for a parallel to the "over-identification" tests described above without needing to assume homogeneity.

METHODS TO ACCOMMODATE VIOLATIONS OF THE STRUCTURAL ASSUMPTIONS

MR analyses have stimulated new insights into how to evaluate the validity of the IV assumptions and methods that are robust to violations—that is, how we can conduct an IV-based analysis when one or more proposed instruments may not actually be instruments. This is an area of rapid development, so we discuss only illustrative examples of new approaches. Most of these approaches now leverage the availability of multiple possible IVs and trade-off between alternative assumptions, offering strategies that may be more appealing in some settings.

MR analyses commonly use numerous genetic variants as IVs. Egger regression uses each potential IV as a single observation and regresses the effect of the instrument on the outcome on the effect of the instrument on the exposure.[106] The slope of this regression line equals a summary IV effect estimate. This can be easily visualized graphically, plotting the effect of the instrument on the outcome on the Y-axis against the effect of the instrument on the exposure on the X-axis.

The appeal of Egger regression is that it can deliver a valid causal effect even if assumptions DAG-IV-2 and 3 are violated. Egger regression requires instead a different assumption, called the instrument strength independent of direct effect (InSIDE) assumption. InSIDE requires that the magnitude of any biasing pathways linking the proposed IVs and the outcome is unrelated to the magnitude of the effects of the proposed IVs on the exposure. In other words, knowing that a particular IV strongly increases probability of exposure tells us nothing about the direction or magnitude of the biasing pathway linking it to the outcome. Under the InSIDE assumption plus monotonicity, not only is the slope of the Egger regression a valid causal effect, but also the intercept of the Egger regression is the average magnitude of the biasing paths. A major limitation of Egger regression is that it has very low statistical power. Also, the InSIDE assumption may seem plausible if the primary threat to the IV conditions is pleiotropic pathways from the genetic variant to the outcome, but it does not seem plausible if the threat is due to sources such as population stratification or collider bias.

Other approaches also take advantage of having numerous proposed genetic IVs and assume that some IV estimates might be biased up and others down, but the distribution of or majority of IV estimates using different proposed IVs are centered on the true causal effect. With this assumption, the median or mode of the estimates from different proposed IVs is adopted.

WHEN ARE POTENTIALLY BIASED "INSTRUMENTS" INFORMATIVE?

In the context of natural experiments, the structural assumptions for IV may be controversial. Even if there is uncertainty about these assumptions, the natural experiment or IV methods may be valuable. For example, precisely estimated null IV results are unlikely to reflect violations of the structural assumptions, as this would only occur if the structural violation was of the same magnitude but opposite direction of the causal effect estimated by the IV. If the IV strongly predicts the exposure but does not predict the outcome, the most likely explanation is that the exposure does not affect the outcome, or at least, variations in the exposure induced by the IV do not influence the outcome.

The most plausible sources of bias in an IV can also guide interpretation of an IV effect estimate, since the estimate reflects a combination of any true causal effect and biasing pathways. If the plausible bias is of an opposite sign as the IV effect estimate, we might at least infer a direction for the causal effect. If the plausible bias is of the same sign as the IV effect estimate—for example, both the estimate and the likely bias are positive—the IV estimate is not informative. Any bias is inflated by the IV analyses, so even if the likely direct effect is small, the IV estimate can be extremely biased. This discussion suggests the likely value of quantitative bias analysis in IV methods.

In some cases, problems with IV analyses point to problems with conventional analyses that might otherwise be overlooked. For example, consistency violations that may be unrecognized in typical data can be observed in IV analyses.

EXAMPLE 1: RANDOMIZED CONTROLLED TRIAL OF A POINT IN TIME TREATMENT

The Norwegian Colorectal Cancer Prevention trial was a randomized trial involving nearly 100,000 Norwegians who had no history of colorectal cancer and were of ages 55 to 64 years in 1998 or 50 to 54 years in 2000.[107] Those randomized to the screening arm were invited for a one-time colorectal cancer screening via a mailed invitation, while those assigned to the control arm were not offered any screening (and the particular screening was not available outside the context of the study). Primary study endpoints included colorectal cancer incidence and mortality, with outcomes measured through national registries. The ITT 10-year risk difference estimate for colorectal cancer risk was −0.2% (95% confidence interval −0.4% to −0.1%). However, while by design there was perfect adherence in the control arm, only about two-thirds of those randomized to the screening arm were actually screened. As such, it was of interest to also estimate a per-protocol effect: what was the effect of screening, rather than the effect of being randomized to screening?

This is in many ways a textbook case for IV analysis, with randomization proposed as an IV. The first condition, that randomization is associated with screening, is met. The second condition is expected by design (of note, there was also minimal loss to follow-up). The third condition, that randomization did not affect outcomes except through screening, is not guaranteed here but there is no obvious plausible way in which it would be substantially violated. Even monotonicity is guaranteed by design here: since nobody in the control arm received screening, there are no "defiers" (and no "always-takers," though this is not required for monotonicity).

Under these conditions, the researchers could estimate the effect of screening in the "compliers" subgroup: −0.4% (95% confidence interval −0.7% to −0.2%).[107] Moreover, because there was perfect adherence in the control arm, we can actually describe the "compliers" as being simply those individuals who were screened in the screening arm. However, it may also be interesting to know something about the effect in the full study population and not just the "compliers." Without making a homogeneity assumption, that effect estimate from an IV analysis would not extend to the whole study, however. Bounds estimated under the IV conditions alone suggest that screening may, on average, be much more beneficial than this point estimate suggests, but the bounds are also consistent with smaller benefits and do not rule out the possibility of harm.[49] However, the bounds are this wide specifically because we have no information, by definition, on what would have happened to the "never-takers" had they been screened. If we make some reasonable assumptions about that group's unobserved risk (*e.g.*, that at most 10% of them would have developed colorectal cancer), then the resulting bounds are substantially narrower.

EXAMPLE 2: NATURAL EXPERIMENT

Educational attainment is associated with a wide range of health outcomes, but in most cases, the association is plausibly confounded by numerous unmeasured confounders, such as parental social advantage, intelligence, personality characteristics, or community economic resources. Conventional RCTs for education are rarely feasible or ethical, so IV-based approaches have emerged as a popular strategy to identify the social and health consequences of increases in education. De Neve et al.[108] took advantage of a major expansion in access to 10th grade in Botswana to estimate the effect of an additional year of schooling on the risk of HIV infection. In 1996, Botswana reclassified the 10th grade from upper secondary school to lower secondary school. Because there were many more lower secondary schools available, and there were substantial incentives to complete lower secondary school, children who completed 9th grade in 1996 or later were much more likely to complete 10th grade than children from earlier cohorts. In fact, children born in cohorts affected by the reform averaged nearly 0.8 additional years of schooling compared to children from cohorts prior to the reform. The authors applied a 2SLS analysis and estimated that completing an additional year of schooling reduced HIV infection risk by 8.1 percentage points (SE = 3.1) overall, 11.6 percentage points (SE = 5.8) for women and 5.0 percentage points (SE = 2.9) for men.

Because the model relied on a policy discontinuity across cohorts of schoolchildren who completed 9th grade in 1996 or later, the authors were especially concerned about potential bias due to misspecification of temporal trends in HIV incidence. To address this, their primary model specification included a linear term for year of birth. They also confirmed that results were not substantially changed when including quadratic terms for year of birth, when restricting to a narrower set of birth cohorts, or when allowing the slope across birth cohorts to change before and after the cohorts affected by the policy implementation. In additional validity checks, they confirmed that the birth cohort after the policy discontinuity was not associated with changes in HIV infection among individuals who completed 9 or fewer grades of schooling, that is, those whose schooling was not affected by the policy change.

De Neve et al. interpreted their coefficient as a local average treatment effect and noted that it was a larger effect than derived using conventional covariate adjusted regression models to estimate the effect of an additional year of schooling on HIV risk. In their OLS analysis, each additional year of schooling above 9 years was associated with a 3.7 percentage point (SE = 0.4) lower risk of HIV infection. When IV-based estimates are larger than OLS estimates, there are several possible explanations. First, the LATE may differ from the PATE estimated by OLS. De Neve noted that this was possible in the Botswana study because the effects of completing 10th grade may differ from the effects of completing other grades (there was likely a nonmonotonic relationship between education and HIV risk). The children who completed 10th grade due to the policy change may benefit more from the extra schooling than other children might benefit. Children who complete additional schooling because of a policy change may, for example, be unusually talented but socially disadvantaged. Alternatively, the OLS estimate may be biased downwards due to model misspecification or confounding. De Neve and colleagues hypothesize that unobserved factors, such as personal charisma, may increase both education and HIV risk, which would introduce a downward bias into the OLS coefficient. Finally, it is also possible that the IV is biased, although their numerous robustness checks increase confidence in the results.

EXAMPLE 3: MENDELIAN RANDOMIZATION

Evaluations of the role of C-reactive protein (CRP) in CVD provide a valuable illustration of an MR study, using genetic variation as a proposed IV to estimate the effects of a phenotype (CRP level) on subsequent health outcomes. CRP is well established as a predictor of CVD and the strong association made it a possible candidate for a potential therapeutic target in drug development.[109] However, there was uncertainty about whether CRP causally influenced CVD, perhaps via an inflammatory mechanism, or merely reflected a physiologic response to the processes that culminated in CVD. Similar questions relate to many biomarkers of disease: is this biomarker predictive because it is a physiologic mechanism or just a marker of incipient disease? Established genetic variants strongly predict CRP level, and these variants were proposed as IVs to estimate the effect of CRP on CVD. In fact, variants that increase CRP level have little or no relationship to CVD,[110] and this evidence indicates CRP is unlikely to be on the causal pathway and should not be considered an intervention target.

The example of CRP is a relatively ideal MR study because the genetic variants are closely genetically linked to CRP (*i.e.*, CRP is the protein directly coded by the genes). This is a case in which the null finding was very informative, because there had been prior non-MR estimates in favor of the existence of a causal effect. MR studies are often criticized because of uncertainty about whether the genetic variants fulfill the core IV condition of no direct effects of the IV on the outcome. However, a violation of this assumption would need to perfectly offset the causal effect to explain a null finding. Thus, well-powered MR studies with narrow confidence intervals around a null effect estimate, as was the case with CRP, may be substantively more informative than MR results that suggest causal effects.[87]

In general, IV assumptions are more plausible if the phenotype (exposure) of interest is closely biologically connected to the genetic variants proposed as IVs. For example, consider a situation in which the exposure of interest is the RNA product of a genetic variant; in this case, biasing paths from the genetic variant to health outcomes of interest that do not pass through the RNA product are very unlikely. If the exposure of interest is the primary protein encoded by the genetic variant, this also seems promising, although we must consider how alternative splicing might create pleiotropic pathways. IV methods for complex biological phenotypes such as BMI are challenging because any of the numerous steps linking the genetic variant and the phenotype may have pleiotropic consequences. Canalization may also be likely: individuals with genetic variants that increase their body weight from early in life may develop buffering physiologic characteristics that reduce, for example, adverse cardiovascular consequences of the extra body weight.

PROBLEMS QUASI-EXPERIMENTAL METHODS DO NOT SOLVE

Given epidemiologists' increased interest in and application of quasi-experimental designs, it is worth noting some problems which these methods do not overcome. First, IVs are used to address causal questions, so they are not relevant for problems in which the goal is strictly description or optimal prediction. In general, selection bias due to collider stratification is not solved.[89] For example, if the exposure influences a collider, the IV also influences that collider (via the exposure) and therefore is subject to the same collider bias (Figure 28-3). Similarly, bias due to differential mismeasurement of the outcome is generally not resolved. For example, if the exposure is associated with a disease merely because exposed individuals with the disease are more likely to be diagnosed than unexposed individuals with the disease, the IV analysis will be affected by the same diagnostic bias (Figure 28-4).

Generally, all the quasi-experimental approaches reviewed here are developed for time-fixed or point interventions, and extensions to studying the effects of sustained interventions to date have been limited. For example, IV applications for time-varying treatments are complicated because

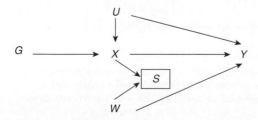

FIGURE 28-3 Directed acyclic graph showing how collider stratification bias due to selection on *S* that affects the *X-Y* association will also bias the instrumental variable association.

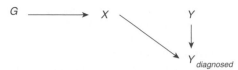

FIGURE 28-4 Directed acyclic graph showing how bias due to effects of exposure on diagnosis of outcome Y ($Y_{\text{diagnosed}}$) will also bias the instrumental variable estimate because even under the null that X has no effect on Y, G, and $Y_{\text{diagnosed}}$ are d-connected. Unmeasured common causes of X and Y are omitted for simplicity.

an IV (even in an RCT) that increases exposure at one point in time may have no effect or even decrease exposure probability at a subsequent time period.[111] Thus, IVs have seen limited applications that explicitly model time-varying exposures. As discussed above, in theory, IVs can be integrated in SNMs and used to estimate time-varying treatment effects or effects of complex treatment regimes. To take advantage of such an approach, it would be necessary to identify an IV that influences treatment across time and to make detailed modeling assumptions about how treatment over time affects the outcome.[18,27,32,112] While these challenges with implementing more elaborate IV models for time-varying exposures are notable, ignoring the true time-varying nature of an exposure and using a single measure in order to fit conventional IV models lead to incorrect effect estimates. To see this, consider the setting in Figure 28-5, where G is an instrument for the whole history of an exposure considered jointly but not for exposure at any single time point. In this case, using any IV estimator to estimate the effect of the exposure as measured at a single time point on the outcome will be biased. Moreover, it will generally be a biased estimate of the effect of the full exposure history too.[87,88,113,114] These challenges may preclude point estimation of effects in settings with inherently time-varying exposures but either incomplete measures of the exposure history or uncertainty about how to conceptualize the exposure history; testing a sharp null that exposure at any time point has no effect on the outcome may nonetheless be feasible. This concern is particularly salient with MR studies, in which genetic variants may influence phenotype across the life course and age-specific effects of the phenotype on subsequent health outcomes are likely.[15,87]

CONCLUSION: HOW SHOULD IV AND OTHER QUASI-EXPERIMENTAL METHODS BE ADOPTED IN EPIDEMIOLOGY?

IV analyses are often a useful complement to ITT analyses of RCTs. When it is feasible to calculate an IV effect estimate, it should typically be presented alongside ITT estimates, along with clear delineation of the assumptions for interpreting the IV estimate. Quasi-experiments and IV analyses are mainstay methods in some disciplines.[43] These approaches can frequently be valuable tools in epidemiology as alternatives or complements to causal identification methods based on the back-door criterion. In most cases, epidemiologists consider the back-door criterion difficult to fulfill, which is why RCTs are often placed at the pinnacle of the hierarchy of evidence for causal inference. No matter how long the list of confounders that have been measured, one can imagine some that were not measured. Even if there is a measured variable blocking every back-door path between X and Y, it is difficult to imagine that each of those has been measured perfectly. Moreover, even if the researchers have obtained a perfect measurement of at least one variable on

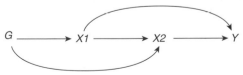

FIGURE 28-5 Directed acyclic graph showing a variable (G) which is a valid instrument for the joint effect of exposure at time 1 ($X1$) and exposure at time 2 ($X2$) but not a valid instrument to isolate the effect of $X1$ or $X2$ alone. Unmeasured common causes of $X1$, $X2$, and Y are omitted for simplicity.

every back-door path, have they selected a correct model to account for the confounders? These are strong assumptions to fulfill the back-door criterion and may be entirely implausible, in which case IV-based methods may offer the most credible approach to causal identification. However, IV methods also rely on strong assumptions, so there is no obvious reason to always prefer IV approaches over back-door criterion-based approaches. In many cases, the assumptions for IV-based causal inference may seem at least as controversial as the back-door criterion, but IV-based methods can provide complementary evidence to buttress inferences. We emphasize the importance of considering the context when evaluating the plausibility of either the IV or the back-door criterion assumptions.

Other valuable applications for IV-based methods arise when an estimand such as the LATE is of more interest than the ITT or even the PATE. IV-based approaches should also be considered when the exposure of interest is not measured or is not measured well in the same data set as the outcome. IVs can be used to test the sharp null of no effect even if the exposure is unmeasured by estimating the ITT effect or its analogue. Exposure measurement is expensive or infeasible in some data sets, and IVs with two-sample methods can be used to derive effect estimates even if the exposure and outcome are not available on the same individuals. Although we did not discuss it in this chapter, IV analyses have wide applications to addressing measurement error in a treatment or exposure. With a valid IV and a few more assumptions, one can estimate the effect of X on Y even if X is measured with noise. This is often applied in settings such as nutritional and environmental epidemiology, when exposure measurement is especially challenging, but likely has wider relevance in other fields.[115]

Recognizing the potential power of IVs can also inform study design. Opportunities for IVs can be created by careful study designs, for example, by randomizing interviewers in a data collection initiative or randomly selecting units for staggered rollout of a new clinical protocol or randomly assigning "encouragements" for alternative treatment protocols. Quasi-experimental methods are invaluable in program evaluation, implementation science, and related work.[116] Building in such likely IVs may be a nearly costless strategy to allow for more rigorous assessment of causal questions.

When considering whether to pursue quasi-experimental or IV-based approaches, epidemiologists must consider the strong assumptions and evaluate whether these assumptions are plausible. Finding credible possible IVs is difficult, but often there are multiple potential sources of IVs for the same or closely related exposure-outcome effects. Because good instruments are often recognized by careful understanding of the processes that lead some individuals to be exposed while others are unexposed, the same thinking that helps find IVs is also relevant for accounting for confounding in conventional back-door-based approaches. Even if perfect fulfillment of the assumptions is unlikely, an IV analysis may offer insights. Imperfect IV analyses may be useful if the likely assumptions are well understood or if the results can rule out at least some causal explanations that cannot be evaluated with methods based on the back-door criterion. New data sources offer new potential quasi-experiments and IVs, so these methods are likely to be of growing relevance in the future of epidemiology.

References

1. Greenland S. An introduction to instrumental variables for epidemiologists. *Int J Epidemiol.* 2000;29:722-729.
2. Stock JH, Trebbi F. Retrospectives – who invented instrumental variable regression? *J Econ Perspect.* 2003;17:177-194.
3. Angrist JD, Krueger AB. Instrumental variables and the search for identification: from supply and demand to natural experiments. *J Econ Perspect.* 2001;15:69-85.
4. Irwig L, Groeneveld H, Becklake M. Relationship of lung-function loss to level of initial function – correcting for measurement error using the reliability coefficient. *J Epidemiol Community Health.* 1988;42:383-389.
5. Karvonen M. Epidemiology in the context of occupational health. In: Karvonen M, Mikheev MI, eds. *Epidemiology of Occupational Health.* Copenhagen: World Health Organization; 1986:1-15.
6. Cook TD, Campbell DT. *Quasi-Experimentation: Design & Analysis Issues for Field Settings.* Boston, MA: Houghton Mifflin Company; 1979.
7. Cook TD, Campbell DT, Shadish W. *Experimental and Quasi-Experimental Designs for Generalized Causal Inference.* Boston, MA: Houghton Mifflin; 2006.

8. Rothman KJ, Greenland S, Lash TL. *Modern Epidemiology*. Philadelphia, PA: Lippincott Williams & Wilkins; 2008.
9. Wright PG. *Tariff on Animal and Vegetable Oils*. New York, NY: Macmillan Company; 1928.
10. Pearl J. *Causality: models, reasoning and inference*. Cambridge: Cambridge University Press; 2000.
11. Angrist JD, Imbens GW. 2-stage least-squares estimation of average causal effects in models with variable treatment intensity. *J Am Stat Assoc*. 1995;90:431-442.
12. Angrist JD. Lifetime earnings and the Vietnam era draft lottery: evidence from social security administrative records. *Am Econ Rev*. 1990;80:313-336.
13. Jacob BA, Ludwig J, Miller DL. The effects of housing and neighborhood conditions on child mortality. *J Health Econ*. 2013;32:195-206.
14. Hernán MA, Hernández-Díaz S. Beyond the intention-to-treat in comparative effectiveness research. *Clin Trials*. 2012;9:48-55.
15. Swanson SA, Labrecque J, Hernán MA. Causal null hypotheses of sustained treatment strategies: what can be tested with an instrumental variable? *Eur J Epidemiol*. 2018;33:723-728.
16. Swanson SA, Hernán MA. Commentary: how to report instrumental variable analyses (suggestions welcome). *Epidemiology*. 2013;24:370-374.
17. Swanson SA. Communicating causality. *Eur J Epidemiol*. 2015;30:1073-1075.
18. Hernán MA, Robins JM. Instruments for causal inference – an epidemiologist's dream? *Epidemiology*. 2006;17:360-372.
19. Lawlor DA, Tilling K, Davey SG. Triangulation in aetiological epidemiology. *Int J Epidemiol*. 2017;45(6):1866-1886.
20. Brott TG, Hobson RW II, Howard G, et al; CREST Investigators. Stenting versus endarterectomy for treatment of carotid-artery stenosis. *N Engl J Med*. 2010;363:11-23.
21. Hernán MA, Robins JM. Per-protocol analyses of pragmatic trials. *N Engl J Med*. 2017;377:1391-1398.
22. Tan Z. Regression and weighting methods for causal inference using instrumental variables. *J Am Stat Assoc*. 2006;101:1607-1618.
23. Wooldridge JM. *Introductory Econometrics: A Modern Approach*. Mason, Ohio: Thomson Southwestern; 2003.
24. Angrist JD, Krueger AB. Does compulsory school attendance affect schooling and earnings? *Q J Econ*. 1991;106:979-1014.
25. Robins JM. A new approach to causal inference in mortality studies with sustained exposure periods – application to control of the healthy worker survivor effect. *Math Model*. 1986;7:1393-1512.
26. Tilling K, Sterne JA, Szklo M. Estimating the effect of cardiovascular risk factors on all-cause mortality and incidence of coronary heart disease using G-estimation: the atherosclerosis risk in communities study. *Am J Epidemiol*. 2002;155:710-718.
27. Robins JM. The analysis of randomized and non-randomized AIDS treatment trials using a new approach to causal inference in longitudinal studies. In: Sechrest L, Freeman H, Mulley A, eds. *Health Service Research Methodology: A Focus on AIDS*. Washington, DC: U.S. Public Health Service, National Center for Health Services Research; 1989:113-159.
28. Mark SD, Robins JM. A method for the analysis of randomized trials with compliance information – an application to the multiple risk factor intervention trial. *Control Clin Trials*. 1993;14:79-97.
29. Mark SD, Robins JM. Estimating the causal effect of smoking cessation in the presence of confounding factors using a rank preserving structural failure time model. *Stat Med*. 1993;12:1605-1628.
30. Vansteelandt S, Joffe M. Structural nested models and G-estimation: the partially realized promise. *Stat Sci*. 2014;29:707-731.
31. Robins JM, Blevins D, Ritter G, Wulfsohn M. G-estimation of the effect of prophylaxis therapy for *Pneumocystis carinii* pneumonia on the survival of AIDS patients. *Epidemiology*. 1992;3:319-336.
32. Robins JM. Correcting for non-compliance in randomized trials using structural nested mean models. *Commun Stat Theory Methods*. 1994;23:2379-2412.
33. Angrist JD, Krueger AB. Split sample instrumental variables. *Natl Bur Econ Res Tech Pap*. 1994;150.
34. Pierce BL, Burgess S. Efficient design for Mendelian randomization studies: subsample and 2-sample instrumental variable estimators. *Am J Epidemiol*. 2013;178:1177-1184.
35. Hernán M, Robins J. Instruments for causal inference: an epidemiologist's dream? Erratum. *Epidemiology*. 2014;25:164.
36. Brookhart MA, Rassen JA, Schneeweiss S. Instrumental variable methods in comparative safety and effectiveness research. *Pharmacoepidemiol Drug Saf*. 2010;19:537-554.
37. Robins JM, Greenland S. Identification of causal effects using instrumental variables: comment. *J Am Stat Assoc*. 1996;91:456-458.
38. Angrist JD, Imbens GW, Rubin DB. Identification of causal effects using instrumental variables. *J Am Stat Assoc*. 1996;91:444-455.
39. Imbens GW, Angrist JD. Identification and estimation of local average treatment effects. *Econometrica*. 1994;62:467-475.

40. Baker SG, Lindeman KS. The paired availability design: a proposal for evaluating epidural analgesia during labor. *Stat Med*. 1994;13:2269-2278.

41. Swanson SA, Hernán MA. The challenging interpretation of instrumental variable estimates under monotonicity. *Int J Epidemiol*. 2017;47:1289-1297.

42. Brookhart MA, Wang PS, Solomon DH, Schneeweiss S. Evaluating short-term drug effects using a physician-specific prescribing preference as an instrumental variable. *Epidemiology*. 2006;17:268-275.

43. Angrist JD, Pischke JS. *Mostly Harmless Econometrics: An Empiricist's Companion*. Princeton: Princeton University Press; 2009.

44. Balke A, Pearl J. Bounds on treatment effects from studies with imperfect compliance. *J Am Stat Assoc*. 1997;92:1171-1176.

45. Manski CF. Nonparametric bounds on treatment effects. *Am Econ Rev*. 1990;80:319-323.

46. Richardson TS, Robins JM. ACE bounds; SEMs with equilibrium conditions. *Stat Sci*. 2014;29:363-366.

47. Swanson SA, Hernán MA, Miller M, Robins JM, Richardson TS. Partial identification of the average treatment effect using instrumental variables: review of methods for binary instruments, treatments, and outcomes. *J Am Stat Assoc*. 2018;113:933-947.

48. Richardson T, Robins JM. Analysis of the binary instrumental variable model. In: Dechter R, Geffner H, Halpern JY, eds. *Heuristics Probability and Causality: A Tribute to Judea Pearl*. London, United Kingdom: College Publications; 2010:415-444.

49. Swanson SA, Holme Ø, Løberg M, et al. Bounding the per-protocol effect in randomized trials: an application to colorectal cancer screening. *Trials*. 2015;16:541.

50. Manski CF, Pepper J. Monotone instrumental variables: with an application to the returns to schooling. *Econometrica*. 2000;68:997-2010.

51. Matthay EC, Hagan E, Gottlieb LM, et al. Alternative causal inference methods in population health research: evaluating tradeoffs and triangulating evidence. *SSM Popul Health*. 2020;10:100526.

52. Pearl J. *Causality: Models, Reasoning, and Inference*. Cambridge: Cambridge University Press; 2009.

53. US Department of Health & Human Services. *NIH to End Funding for Moderate Alcohol and Cardiovascular Health Trial*. Bethesda, MD: National Institutes of Health (NIH); 2018. Available at https://www.nih.gov/news-events/news-releases/nih-end-funding-moderate-alcohol-cardiovascular-health-trial.

54. Grant RM, Lama JR, Anderson PL, et al. Preexposure chemoprophylaxis for HIV prevention in men who have sex with men. *N Engl J Med*. 2010;363:2587-2599.

55. Lleras-Muney A. Were compulsory attendance and child labor laws effective? An analysis from 1915 to 1939. *J Law Econ*. 2002;45:401-435.

56. Aizer A, Doyle JJ Jr. Juvenile incarceration, human capital, and future crime: evidence from randomly assigned judges. *Q J Econ*. 2015;130:759-803.

57. Stevenson B, Wolfers J. Bargaining in the shadow of the law: divorce laws and family distress. *Q J Econ*. 2006;121:267-288.

58. Amico KR, Bekker LG. Global PrEP roll-out: recommendations for programmatic success. *Lancet HIV*. 2019;6:e137-e140.

59. Boef AG, Dekkers OM, Vandenbroucke JP, le Cessie S. Sample size importantly limits the usefulness of instrumental variable methods, depending on instrument strength and level of confounding. *J Clin Epidemiol*. 2014;67:1258-1264.

60. Maestas N, Mullen KJ, Strand A. Does disability insurance receipt discourage work? Using examiner assignment to estimate causal effects of SSDI receipt. *Am Econ Rev*. 2013;103:1797-1829.

61. Banks J, Mazzonna F. The effect of education on old age cognitive abilities: evidence from a regression discontinuity design. *Econ J*. 2012;122:418-448.

62. Tchetgen Tchetgen EJ, Wirth KE. A general instrumental variable framework for regression analysis with outcome missing not at random. *Biometrics*. 2017;73:1123-1131.

63. Marden JR, Wang L, Tchetgen Tchetgen EJ, Walter S, Glymour MM, Wirth KE. Implementation of instrumental variable bounds for data missing not at random. *Epidemiology*. 2018;29:364-368.

64. Oldenburg CE, Moscoe E, Bärnighausen T. Regression discontinuity for causal effect estimation in epidemiology. *Curr Epidemiol Rep*. 2016;3:233-241.

65. Oldenburg CE, Venkatesh Prajna N, Krishnan T, et al. Regression discontinuity and randomized controlled trial estimates: an application to the Mycotic Ulcer Treatment Trials. *Ophthalmic Epidemiol*. 2018;25:315-322.

66. Goodman J, Hurwitz M, Smith J. Access to 4-year public colleges and degree completion. *J Labor Econ*. 2017;35:829-867.

67. Gelman A, Imbens G. Why high-order polynomials should not be used in regression discontinuity designs. *J Bus Econ Stat*. 2019;37:447-456.

68. Abadie A, Diamond A, Hainmueller J. Synthetic control methods for comparative case studies: estimating the effect of California's tobacco control program. *J Am Stat Assoc*. 2010;105:493-505.

69. Baiocchi M, Small DS, Yang L, Polsky D, Groeneveld PW. Near/far matching: a study design approach to instrumental variables. *Health Serv Outcomes Res Methodol*. 2012;12:237-253.

70. Shumway RH, Stoffer DS. *Time Series Analysis and its Applications: With R Examples*. New York, NY: Springer International Publishing; 2017.

71. Jiang H, Livingston M, Room R. Alcohol consumption and fatal injuries in Australia before and after major traffic safety initiatives: a time series analysis. *Alcohol Clin Exp Res*. 2015;39:175-183.

72. Catalano R, Gemmill A, Bruckner T. A test of famine-induced developmental programming in utero. *J Dev Orig Health Dis*. 2019;10:368-375.

73. Miguel E, Satyanath S, Sergenti E. Economic shocks and civil conflict: an instrumental variables approach. *J Polit Econ*. 2004;112:725-753.

74. Lind JT. Rainy day politics. An instrumental variables approach to the effect of parties on political outcomes. *Eur J Polit Econ*. 2020;61:101821.

75. Epstein A, Benmarhnia T, Weiser SD. Drought and illness among young children in Uganda, 2009-2012. *Am J Trop Med Hyg*. 2020;102:644-648.

76. Zigler CM, Choirat C, Dominici F. Impact of national ambient air quality standards nonattainment designations on particulate pollution and health. *Epidemiology*. 2018;29:165.

77. Shibuya K, Inoue M, Lopez AD. Statistical modeling and projections of lung cancer mortality in 4 industrialized countries. *Int J Cancer*. 2005;117:476-485.

78. Catalano R, Serxner S. Time series designs of potential interest to epidemiologists. *Am J Epidemiol*. 1987;126:724-731.

79. Maziarz M. A review of the Granger-causality fallacy. *J Philos Econ*. 2015;8:86-105.

80. Davey Smith G, Ebrahim S. 'Mendelian randomization': can genetic epidemiology contribute to understanding environmental determinants of disease? *Int J Epidemiol*. 2003;32:1-22.

81. Davey Smith G, Ebrahim S. Mendelian randomization: prospects, potentials, and limitations. *Int J Epidemiol*. 2004;33:30-42.

82. Didelez V, Sheehan N. Mendelian randomization as an instrumental variable approach to causal inference. *Stat Methods Med Res*. 2007;16:309-330.

83. Boccia S, Hashibe M, Gallì P, et al. Aldehyde dehydrogenase 2 and head and neck cancer: a meta-analysis implementing a Mendelian randomization approach. *Cancer Epidemiol Biomarkers Prev*. 2009;18:248.

84. Millwood IY, Walters RG, Mei XW, et al. Conventional and genetic evidence on alcohol and vascular disease aetiology: a prospective study of 500 000 men and women in China. *Lancet*. 2019;393:1831-1842.

85. Burgess S, Smith GD, Davies NM, et al. Guidelines for performing Mendelian randomization investigations. *Wellcome Open Res*. 2019;4:186.

86. Burgess S, Foley CN, Allara E, Staley JR, Howson JM. A robust and efficient method for Mendelian randomization with hundreds of genetic variants. *Nat Commun*. 2020;11:1-11.

87. VanderWeele TJ, Tchetgen Tchetgen EJ, Cornelis M, Kraft P. Methodological challenges in Mendelian randomization. *Epidemiology*. 2014;25:427-435.

88. Swanson SA, Tiemeier H, Ikram MA, Hernán MA. Nature as a trialist? Deconstructing the analogy between Mendelian Randomization and randomized trials. *Epidemiology*. 2017;28:653-659.

89. Swanson SA. A practical guide to selection bias in instrumental variable analyses. *Epidemiology*. 2019;30:345-349.

90. Hernán MA, Taubman SL. Does obesity shorten life? The importance of well-defined interventions to answer causal questions. *Int J Obes*. 2008;32:S8-S14.

91. Glymour MM, Tchetgen EJT, Robins JM. Credible Mendelian Randomization studies: approaches for evaluating the instrumental variable assumptions. *Am J Epidemiol*. 2012;175:332-339.

92. Glymour MM, Walter S, Tchetgen EJT. Natural experiments and instrumental variables analyses in social epidemiology. In: Oakes JM, Kaufman JS, eds. *Methods in Social Epidemiology*. San Francisco: Jossey-Bass; 2017:493-537.

93. Shen L, Walter S, Melles RB, Glymour MM, Jorgenson E. Diabetes pathology and risk of primary open-angle glaucoma: evaluating causal mechanisms by using genetic information. *Am J Epidemiol*. 2016;183:147-155.

94. Benjamin DJ, Cesarini D, Chabris CF, et al. The promises and pitfalls of genoeconomics. *Annu Rev Econom*. 2012;4:627-662.

95. Lee JJ, Wedow R, Okbay A, et al. Gene discovery and polygenic prediction from a 1.1-million-person GWAS of educational attainment. *Nat Genet*. 2018;50:1112.

96. Nguyen TT, Tchetgen EJT, Kawachi I, et al. Instrumental variable approaches to identifying the causal effect of educational attainment on dementia risk. *Ann Epidemiol*. 2016;26:71-76.e1-e3.

97. Bound J, Jaeger DA, Baker RM. Problems with instrumental variables estimation when the correlation between the instruments and the endogenous explanatory variable is weak. *J Am Stat Assoc*. 1995;90:443-450.

98. Staiger D. Instrumental Variables with weak instruments. *Econometrics*. 1997;65:557-586.

99. Pierce BL, Ahsan H, VanderWeele TJ. Power and instrument strength requirements for Mendelian randomization studies using multiple genetic variants. *Int J Epidemiol*. 2011;40:740-752.

100. Jackson JW, Swanson SA. Toward a clearer portrayal of confounding bias in instrumental variable applications. *Epidemiology*. 2015;26:498-504.

101. Conley TG, Hansen CB, Rossi PE. Plausibly exogenous. *Rev Econ Stat*. 2010;94:260-272.

102. Swanson SA, VanderWeele TJ. E-values for mendelian randomization. *Epidemiology*. 2020;31:e23.

103. Wang L, Robins JM, Richardson TS. On falsification of the binary instrumental variable model. *Biometrika*. 2017;104:229-236.

104. Bonet B. *Instrumentality Tests Revisited*. San Francisco, CA: Morgan Kaufmann; 2001:48-55.

105. Diemer EW, Labrecque J, Tiemeier H, Swanson SA. Application of the instrumental inequalities to a Mendelian randomization study with multiple proposed instruments. *Epidemiology*. 2020;31(1):65-74.

106. Bowden J, Davey Smith G, Burgess S. Mendelian randomization with invalid instruments: effect estimation and bias detection through Egger regression. *Int J Epidemiol*. 2015;44:512-525.

107. Holme Ø, Løberg M, Kalager M, et al. Effect of flexible sigmoidoscopy screening on colorectal cancer incidence and mortality: a randomized clinical trial. *J Am Med Assoc*. 2014;312:606-615.

108. De Neve JW, Fink G, Subramanian SV, Moyo S, Bor J. Length of secondary schooling and risk of HIV infection in Botswana: evidence from a natural experiment. *Lancet Glob Health*. 2015;3:e470-e477.

109. Ridker PM. A test in context: high-sensitivity C-reactive protein. *J Am Coll Cardiol*. 2016;67:712-723.

110. Prins BP, Abbasi A, Wong A, et al. Investigating the causal relationship of C-reactive protein with 32 complex somatic and psychiatric outcomes: a large-scale cross-consortium Mendelian randomization study. *PLoS Med*. 2016;13:e1001976.

111. Sternberg CN, Hawkins RE, Wagstaff J, et al. A randomised, double-blind phase III study of pazopanib in patients with advanced and/or metastatic renal cell carcinoma: final overall survival results and safety update. *Eur J Cancer*. 2013;49:1287-1296.

112. Robins JM, Rotnitzky A, Zhao LP. Estimation of regression coefficients when some regressors are not always observed. *J Am Stat Assoc*. 1994;89:846-866.

113. Labrecque JA, Swanson SA. Interpretation and potential biases of Mendelian randomization estimates with time-varying exposures. *Am J Epidemiol*. 2019;188(1):231-238.

114. Labrecque JA, Swanson SA. Mendelian randomization with multiple exposures: the importance of thinking about time. *Int J Epidemiol*. 2019. doi:10.1093/ije/dyz234.

115. Fraser GE. A search for truth in dietary epidemiology. *Am J Clin Nutr*. 2003;78:521S-525S.

116. Handley MA, Lyles CR, McCulloch C, Cattamanchi A. Selecting and improving quasi-experimental designs in effectiveness and implementation research. *Annu Rev Public Health*. 2018;39:5-25.

Bias Analysis

Timothy L. Lash

INTRODUCTION

This chapter introduces quantitative methods for evaluating potential biases (systematic errors) in individual studies. Earlier chapters covered basic methods to assess sensitivity of results to confounding by an unmeasured variable, misclassification, and selection bias. These methods quantify systematic errors by means of *bias parameters,* which in a bias analysis are fixed at initial values and then in a sensitivity analysis of the bias analysis varied to see how the results change with the changes to the values assigned to the parameters. These basic methods are reviewed again here, applied by way of example to a single research result that carries throughout the chapter.

This chapter then extends these basic bias-sensitivity analyses by assigning a prior probability distribution to the bias parameters (probabilistic bias modeling) to produce *distributions* of results as output. The methods are typically implemented via simulation, and their outputs have a natural interpretation as semi-Bayesian posterior distributions (Chapter 23) for exposure effects. They are "semi-" Bayesian because they use prior distributions for the bias parameters but not for the effect under study. We focus on the special case in which the observed data can be represented in a 2×2 table of an exposure indicator X (coded 1 = present, 0 = absent) and a disease indicator D. Many of the basic principles and difficulties of bias analysis can be illustrated with this simple case, because the 2×2 table can be thought of as a stratum from a larger data set. After describing simulation methods, we discuss empirical and Bayesian bias analysis methods.

Most statistical methods also assume specific models for the form of effects (of exposure, modifiers, and confounders) and of random errors. Use of erroneous model forms is sometimes called *specification error* and can lead to systematic errors known as *specification biases*. *Model-sensitivity analysis* addresses these biases by seeing how the results change as the model form is changed.[1-3] We do not cover model-sensitivity analysis, because it involves technical issues of model selection beyond the scope of this chapter.

We also do not address general *missing-data bias* (bias due to nonrandomly incomplete data)[4,5] or *informative* or *nonignorable missing data*.[6] All the problems we discuss can be viewed as extreme cases of missing-data bias[7]: uncontrolled confounding is due to missing data on a confounder; misclassification is due to missing measurements of the gold standard variables; and selection bias is due to nonrandomly missing members or follow-up of the source population.

All analysis methods, whether conventional methods or those described here, consider the data as given; that is, they assume that we have the data and that the data have not been corrupted by miscodings, programming errors, forged responses, etc. Thus, the methods assume that there is no misclassification due to data processing errors, participants' malintent, or investigator fraud. Such problems arise from isolated events that may affect many records, and their correction depends entirely on detection by logic checks, data examination, and comparison of data sources. Thus, we do not see such problems as falling within the sphere of bias analysis amenable to quantitative bias-adjustments.

The Need for Bias Analyses

Aside from simple bias analysis methods described in earlier chapters, our discussion of statistical methods has so far focused on accounting for measured confounders and random errors in the data-generating process. Randomization of exposure assignment is the conventional assumption of statistical methods for causal inference within a study cohort, for it makes confounding a chance phenomenon.[8] Random sampling forms the analogous conventional assumption of statistical methods for inference from the sample to a larger population (*e.g.*, in descriptive epidemiology or from the controls in a case-control study to a source population), for it makes sampling error a chance phenomenon. Most methods assume that measurement error is absent, but those that account for errors assume that the errors are random.[9] Upon stratification, these assumptions (that confounding, sampling errors, and measurement errors are random) are made within the levels of the stratifying variables. We will call methods based on these randomness assumptions *conventional methods*.

By assuming that all errors are random and that any modeling assumptions (such as homogeneity of effect estimates across strata of control variables) are correct, all uncertainty about the effect of errors on estimates is subsumed within conventional standard deviations for the estimates (standard errors), such as those given in earlier chapters (which assume no measurement error), and any discrepancy between an observed association and the target effect may be attributed to chance alone. When the assumptions are incorrect, however, the logical foundation for conventional statistical methods is absent, and those methods may yield highly misleading inferences. Epidemiologists recognize the possibility of incorrect assumptions in conventional analyses when they talk of uncontrolled confounding (from nonrandom exposure assignment), selection bias (from nonrandom subject selection or follow-up), and information bias (from imperfect measurement). These biases rarely receive quantitative analysis,[7,10,11] a situation that is understandable given that the analysis requires specifying values (such as the amount of selection bias) for which little or no data may be available.[10,12] An unfortunate consequence of this lack of quantification is the statistical reification of those aspects of error that are more readily quantified,[13] namely, the random components.

Systematic errors can be and often are larger than random errors, and failure to appreciate their impact may yield highly misleading research results and inferences based on them. This concern is magnified by qualitative treatments of systematic errors, in which investigators acknowledge concerns about systematic errors as study limitations and then dismiss or marginalize these concerns without any quantitative treatment. The problem is further magnified in large studies and pooling projects, because in those studies, the large size reduces the amount of random error, and as a result the random error may be only a small component of total error. In such studies, a focus on "statistical significance" or even on the location of confidence limits[14] may amount to nothing more than a decision to focus on artifacts of systematic error as if they reflect a real causal effect.

Addressing concerns about systematic errors in a constructive fashion is not easy, but is nonetheless essential if the results of a study are to be used to inform decisions in a rational fashion.[10] We shall call the process of addressing bias quantitatively *bias analysis.* As described in a number of books,[15-18] the basic ideas have existed for decades under the topic of *sensitivity analysis* and the more general topics of *uncertainty analysis, risk assessment,* and *risk analysis.* These topics address more sources of uncertainty than we shall address, such as model misspecification and informatively missing data. Here we focus only on the effects of basic validity problems.

A discomforting aspect of these analyses is that they reveal the highly tentative and subjective nature of inference from observational data, a problem that is concealed by conventional statistical analysis. Bias analysis often requires educated guesses about the likely sizes of systematic errors, guesses that may vary considerably across observers. The conventional approach is to make the guess qualitatively by describing the study's limitations. An assessment of the extent of bias, compared with the extent of exposure effects, therefore becomes an exercise in intuitive reasoning under uncertainty.

The ability to reason under uncertainty has been studied by cognitive psychologists and sociologists, who have found it susceptible to many predictable patterns of mistakes.[19-21] This literature, where it deals with situations analogous to epidemiologic inference, indicates that the qualitative approach tends to favor exposure effects over systematic errors as an explanation for observed associations.[22] Unfortunately, students of sciences, including epidemiology, seldom receive training in the heuristics and cognitive biases that influence their evaluation and inferences from the evidence they generate or gather.[13] Quantitative methods such as those described in this chapter offer a potential safeguard against these failures, by providing insight into the importance of various sources of error and by helping to assess the uncertainty of study results. For example, such assessments may argue persuasively that certain sources of bias cannot by themselves plausibly explain a study result, or that a bias explanation cannot be ruled out, conditional on the accuracy of the bias model. As discussed in Chapters 2 and 23, and later in this section, the primary caution is that what appears "plausible" may vary considerably across persons and time.

There are several reasons why quantitative methods that take account of uncontrolled biases have traditionally seen much less development than methods for addressing random error. First, until recently, randomized experiments supplied much of the impetus for statistical developments. These experiments were concentrated in agriculture, manufacturing, and clinical medicine and often could be designed so that systematic errors played little apparent role in the results. A second reason is that most uncontrolled biases cannot be analyzed by conventional methods (*i.e.*, without explicit priors for bias parameters) unless additional "validation" data are available. Such data are usually absent or limited, possibly because investigators are incentivized to allocate study resources toward increasing the number of participants or duration of follow-up rather than toward conducting a validation substudy.[23] Furthermore, validation studies may themselves be subject to systematic errors beyond those present in the main study, such as potentially biased selection of participants for validation (*e.g.*, if validation requires further subject consent and participation). As a result, investigators must resort to less satisfactory partial analyses or quantify only the uncertainty due to random error.

Reviewers, editors, and funders in the health sciences seldom call on authors of submitted manuscripts or investigators of submitted research proposals to quantitatively assess systematic errors.[24] Because of the labor and expertise required for a bias analysis, and the limited importance of single studies for policy issues, it makes little sense to require such an analysis of every study.[10] For example, studies whose conventional 95% confidence limits exclude no reasonable possibility should be viewed as inconclusive regardless of any further analysis. It can be argued that the best use of effort and journal space for single-study reports is to focus on a thorough description of the study design, methods, and data to facilitate later use of the study data in reviews, meta-analyses, and pooling projects.[25]

On the other hand, any report with policy implications may damage public health if the claimed implications are wrong. Thus, it is justifiable to demand quantitative bias analysis in such studies.[10,26] Going further, it is arguably an ethical duty of granting agencies and editors to require a thorough quantitative assessment of relevant literature and of systematic errors to support claimed implications for public policy or medical practice. Without the endorsement of these gatekeepers of funding and publication, there is little motivation to collect validation data or to undertake quantitative assessments of bias.[24]

Caveats About Bias Analysis

As noted above, results of a bias analysis are derived from inputs specified by the analyst, a point that should be emphasized in any presentation of the methods or their results. These inputs are constructed from judgments, opinions, or inferences about the likely magnitude of bias sources or parameters.[13] Consequently, bias analyses do not establish the existence or absence of causal effects any more than do conventional analyses. Rather, they show how the analysts developed their output judgments (inferences) from their input judgments.

An advantage of bias analysis over a qualitative discussion of study limitations is that it allows mathematics to replace unsound intuitions and heuristics at many points in judgment formation. For example, stakeholders who draw different inferences based on the same evidence base can evaluate whether their differences emanate from differences in the inputs they assign to inform the strength of bias. For example, one stakeholder may view an epidemiology study as strongly suggesting a causal effect, whereas a second stakeholder may view the nonnull association as likely emanating from differential misclassification of the outcome. Bias analysis would allow them to evaluate whether differences in their credible inputs for outcome misclassification are in fact consistent with their differences in inference. If so, then these differences could presumably be resolved by improving measurement of the outcome, including designing a study unlikely to have differential misclassification of the outcome. In this way, bias analysis can guide the productive allocation of rare research resources to resolve stakeholder differences.[27]

Nonetheless, the mathematics should not entice researchers to phrase judgments in objective terms that mask their subjective origin. For example, a claim that "our analysis indicates the conventional results are biased away from the null" would be misleading. A better description would say "our analysis indicates that, *under the assumed bias model and the values we chose for the bias parameters,* the conventional results *would be* biased away from the null." The latter description acknowledges the fact that the results are sensitive to judgmental inputs, some of which may be speculative. The more advanced methods of this chapter require input distributions (rather than sets of values) for bias parameters, but the same caveat holds: the results of the bias analysis, and inferences resting on the results, apply only under those chosen distributions. The analysis will be more convincing if the analyst provides evidence that the chosen distributions assign high probability to reasonable combinations of the parameters, and especially that the values chosen for the bias parameters cover the range of reasonable combinations of those parameters. These and other good practices for presentation and interpretation of quantitative bias analyses have been more completely explained elsewhere.[10]

To some extent, criticisms similar to the above apply to conventional frequentist and Bayesian analyses (Chapters 16-24), insofar as those analyses require many choices and judgments from the investigators.[13] Examples include choice of methods used to handle missing data, choice of category boundaries for quantitative variables, choice of methods for variable selection, and choice of priors assigned to effects under study. As the term "conventional" connotes, many choices have default answers (*e.g.*, a binomial model for the distribution of dichotomous outcomes). Although the scientific basis for these defaults is often doubtful or lacking (*e.g.*, missing-data indicators; percentile boundaries for continuous variables; stepwise variable selection; noninformative priors for effects), and the underlying assumptions are almost never explicitly stated or evaluated, deviations from the defaults may prompt requests for explanations from referees and readers.

Bias analysis requires more input specifications than do conventional analyses, and as yet, there is no accepted convention regarding these specifications. As a result, input judgments are left entirely to the analyst, opening avenues for manipulation to produce a desired output.[13] Thus, when examining a bias analysis, a reader must bear in mind that other reasonable inputs might produce quite different results. This input sensitivity is why we emphasize that bias analysis is a collection of methods for explaining and refining subjective judgments in the light of data (like the subjective Bayesian methods of Chapter 23), rather than a method for detecting nonrandom data patterns. In fact, a bias analysis can sometimes be made to produce virtually any estimate for the study effect without altering the data or imposing an objectionable prior on that effect. Such outcome-driven analyses, however, may require assignment of values or distributions to bias parameters that have doubtful credibility. Therefore, it is crucial that the inputs used for a bias analysis be described in detail so that those inputs can be examined critically by the reader. It is also good practice to provide the statistical computing code or applications used to perform a quantitative bias analysis, along with the data required to perform it, so that stakeholders can check for coding errors, verify results, and evaluate different assumption sets for themselves.[10]

Terminology

Bias analyses modify a conventional estimate of diseases or exposure frequency (for descriptive epidemiology) or of the effect an exposure contrast has on a health outcome (for etiologic epidemiology) to account for bias introduced by systematic error. Bias analysis therefore combines the data used for the conventional estimate with equations that adjust the conventional estimate for the estimated impact of the systematic error. The equations linking the conventional estimate to the bias-adjusted estimate are called the *bias model*. These equations have parameters, called *bias parameters*. For example, imagine a case-control study in which not all eligible participants agree to participate. The bias model linking the conventional estimate to a bias-adjusted estimate would use the proportions of all eligible subjects who participated in the study as the bias parameters. These proportions would be within strata of persons with and without the outcome and within categories of the exposure variable. If the exposure variable is dichotomous, then there would be four bias parameters: the proportion participating among exposed cases, the proportion participating among unexposed cases, the proportion participating among exposed controls, and the proportion participating among unexposed controls. The values assigned to these parameters would determine the direction and magnitude of selection bias, assuming a valid bias model. When presenting and interpreting bias analyses, it is crucial to keep this assumption of a valid bias model in mind. This assumption encompasses both an assumption that the equations of the bias model adequately represent the influence of the systematic error on the conventional estimate and that the values assigned to the bias parameters are valid.

Realize, however, that the values assigned to the bias parameter cannot be known for certain, so cannot be known to be valid.[10,12] If they were known for certain, so were identifiable, there would be no bias. To know the participation proportions within exposure categories of a case-control study, exposure and disease status of every member of the source population would have to be known, which can only be realized when everyone participates in the study population, hence there could be no selection bias. Likewise, to know the sensitivity and specificity of exposure classification with certainty, one would have to measure the gold standard in every member of the study population, in which case there would be no information bias because the gold standard measure of exposure and not the misclassified measure would be used in the analysis. To know the strength of association of an unmeasured confounder with the exposure and the outcome with certainty, it would have to be measured in the study population, and it would no longer be an uncontrolled confounder. The very nature of bias analysis requires that the values of the bias parameters are uncertain, an assumption critical to proper interpretation of the bias analysis results.

ANALYSIS OF UNMEASURED CONFOUNDERS

Sensitivity analysis and external adjustment for confounding by dichotomous variables appeared in the study of Cornfield et al. (1959)[28] and were further elaborated by Bross,[29,30] Yanagawa,[31] Axelson and Steenland,[32] and Gail et al.[33] Extensions of these approaches to multiple-level confounders are available.[34-37] Although most of these methods assume that the odds ratios (ORs) or risk ratios are constant across strata, it is possible to base external adjustment on other assumptions.[31,33] Practical extensions to multiple regression analyses typically involve modeling the unmeasured confounders as latent (unobserved) variables.[12,38-40]

External Adjustment

Suppose that we have conducted an analysis of an exposure X and a disease D, adjusting for the recorded confounders, but we know of an unmeasured potential confounder and want to assess the possible effect of failing to adjust for this confounder. For example, in a case-control study of occupational exposure to resin systems (resins) and lung cancer mortality among male workers at a transformer-assembly plant,[41] the authors could adjust for age and year of death, but they had no data on smoking. Upon adjustment for age and year at death, a positive association was observed for resins exposure and lung cancer mortality ($OR = 1.77$, 95% confidence limits = 1.18, 2.64). A limitation of the study was incomplete control for potential confounding by history of tobacco smoking. A conventional approach to this concern would be to describe the lack of control for potential confounding by history of tobacco smoking as a limitation of the study and then to conjecture that this limitation is unlikely to account for the entire observed association. The authors might even cite earlier papers that showed the effects of not controlling for smoking are rather modest, unless the smoking habits of the study population are quite extreme.[32] A quantitative bias analysis takes a more direct approach, seeking to answer to what extent did confounding by smoking affect the observation?

For simplicity, suppose that resins exposure and smoking are treated as dichotomous: $X = 1$ for resin-exposed, 0 otherwise and $Z = 1$ for smoker, 0 otherwise. We might wish to know how large the resins-smoking association has to be so that adjustment for smoking removes the resins-lung cancer association. The answer to this question depends on a number of parameters, among which are (a) the resins-specific associations (*i.e.*, the associations within levels of resins exposure) of smoking with lung cancer, (b) the resins-specific prevalences of smoking among the controls, and (c) the prevalence of resins exposure among the controls. Resins prevalence is observed, but the second two quantities are unobserved, and therefore must be informed by external information, including other research and educated guessing by the analyst.

It is this process of assigning values to the bias parameters of the bias models that forms the basis for quantitative bias analysis. We will assume various plausible combinations of values for the smoking-lung cancer association and resins-specific smoking prevalences, and then see what values we get for the smoking-adjusted resins-lung cancer association. If all the latter values are substantially elevated, we have a basis for doubting that the unadjusted resins-lung cancer association is due entirely to confounding by smoking. Otherwise, confounding by smoking is a plausible explanation for the observed resins-lung cancer association.

We will use the crude data in Table 29-1 for illustration. There is no evidence of important confounding by age or year in these data, probably because the controls were selected from other chronic-disease deaths. For example, the crude OR is 1.76 versus an age-year adjusted OR of 1.77. The corresponding 95% confidence limits are 1.20 and 2.58 for the crude OR and 1.18 and 2.64 for the age-year adjusted OR. If it is necessary to stratify on age, year, or both, we could repeat the computations given below for each stratum and then summarize the results across strata, or we could use regression-based adjustments.[12]

TABLE 29-1

Crude Data for Case-Control Study of Occupational Resins Exposure (*X*) and Lung Cancer Mortality (Greenland et al., 1994[41]); Controls Are Selected Noncancer Causes of Death

	X = 1	*X* = 0	Total
Cases (*D* = 1)	$A_{1+} = 45$	$A_{0+} = 94$	$M_{1+} = 139$
Controls (*D* = 0)	$B_{1+} = 257$	$B_{0+} = 945$	$M_{0+} = 1202$

Odds ratio after adjustment for age and death year: 1.77.
Age-year adjusted conventional 95% confidence limits for OR_{DX}: 1.18, 2.64.
From Greenland S, Salvan A, Wegman DH, Hallock MF, Smith TJ. A case-control study of cancer mortality at a transformer-assembly facility. *Int Arch Occup Environ Health*. 1994;66(1):49-54.

TABLE 29-2

General Layout (Expected Data) for Bias Analysis and External Adjustment for a Dichotomous Confounder Z

	Z = 1			Z = 0		
	X = 1	X = 0	Total	X = 1	X = 0	Total
Cases	A_{11}	A_{01}	M_{11}	$A_{1+} - A_{11}$	$A_{0+} - A_{01}$	$M_{1+} - M_{11}$
Controls	B_{11}	B_{01}	M_{01}	$B_{1+} - B_{11}$	$B_{0+} - B_{01}$	$M_{0+} - M_{01}$

Consider the general notation for the expected stratified data given in Table 29-2. We will use hypothesized values for the stratum-specific prevalences to fill in this table and solve for an assumed common OR relating exposure to disease within levels of Z.

$$OR_{DX} = \frac{A_{11}B_{01}}{A_{01}B_{11}} = \frac{(A_{1+} - A_{11})(B_{0+} - B_{01})}{(A_{0+} - A_{01})(B_{1+} - B_{11})}$$

Suppose that the smoking prevalences among the exposed and unexposed populations are estimated or assumed to be P_{Z1} and P_{Z0}, and the OR relating the confounder and disease within levels of exposure is OR_{DZ} (i.e., we assume OR homogeneity, although heterogeneity can be incorporated with only a slightly more complicated bias model[31,33]). Assuming that the control group is representative of the source population, we set $B_{11} = P_{Z1}B_{1+}$ and $B_{01} = P_{Z0}B_{0+}$. Next, to find A_{11} and A_{01}, we solve the following pair of equations:

$$OR_{DZ} = \frac{A_{11}(B_{1+} - B_{11})}{(A_{1+} - A_{11})B_{11}}$$

and

$$OR_{DZ} = \frac{A_{01}(B_{0+} - B_{01})}{(A_{0+} - A_{01})B_{01}}$$

These have solutions:

$$A_{11} = OR_{DZ}A_{1+}B_{11}/(OR_{DZ}B_{11} + B_{1+} - B_{11}) \qquad [29\text{-}1]$$

and

$$A_{01} = OR_{DZ}A_{0+}B_{01}/(OR_{DZ}B_{01} + B_{0+} - B_{01}) \qquad [29\text{-}2]$$

Having obtained data counts corresponding to A_{11}, A_{01}, B_{11}, and B_{01}, we can put these numbers into Table 29-2 and compute directly a Z-adjusted estimate of the exposure-disease odds ratios OR_{DX}. The answers from each smoking stratum should agree.

The preceding estimate of OR_{DX} is sometimes said to be "indirectly adjusted" for Z, because it is the estimate of OR_{DX} that one would obtain if one had data on the confounder Z and disease D that displayed the assumed prevalences and confounder odds ratio OR_{DZ}. More precise terms for the resulting estimate of OR_{DX} are "externally adjusted" or "bias-adjusted," because the estimate makes use of an estimate of OR_{DZ} obtained from sources external to the study data. The smoking prevalences must also be obtained externally; occasionally (and preferably), they may be obtained from a survey of the underlying source population from which the subjects were selected. (Because we assumed that the ORs are constant across strata, the result does not depend on the exposure prevalence.)

To illustrate external adjustment with the data in Table 29-1, suppose that the smoking prevalences among the resins exposed and unexposed are 70% and 50%. Then,

$$B_{11} = P_{Z1}B_{1+} = 0.70(257) = 179.9$$

and

$$B_{01} = P_{Z0}B_{0+} = 0.50(945) = 472.5$$

Taking $OR_{DZ} = 5$ for the resins-specific smoking-lung cancer OR, Equations 29-1 and 29-2 yield

$$A_{11} = 5(45)179.9/[5(179.9) + 257 - 179.9] = 41.45$$

and

$$A_{01} = 5(94)472.5/[5(472.5) + 945 - 472.5] = 78.33$$

Putting these results into Table 29-2, we obtain the stratum-specific resins-lung cancer ORs.

$$OR_{DX} \frac{41.45(472.5)}{179.9(78.33)} = 1.39$$

and

$$OR_{DX} \frac{(45 - 41.45)(945 - 472.5)}{(257 - 179.9)(94 - 78.33)} = 1.39$$

which agree (as they should). We see that confounding by smoking could account for much of the excess of the crude resins OR above 1, if there were a much higher smoking prevalence among the resin exposed relative to the unexposed.

In a sensitivity analysis of the bias analysis, we repeat the above external adjustment process using other plausible values for the prevalences and the confounder effect, as implemented also in other examples.[42-44] Table 29-3 presents a summary of results using other values for the resins-specific smoking prevalences and the smoking OR. The table also gives the smoking-resins OR.

$$OR_{XZ} = O_{Z1}/O_{Z0} = P_{Z1}(1 - P_{Z0})/(1 - P_{Z1})P_{Z0}$$

TABLE 29-3

Sensitivity of Externally Adjusted Resins-Cancer Odds Ratio OR_{DX} to Choice of P_{Z1} and P_{Z0} (Smoking Prevalences Among Exposed and Unexposed) and OR_{DZ} (Resins-specific Smoking-Cancer Odds Ratio)

| | | | OR_{DZ} | | |
| | | | 5 | 10 | 15 |
P_{Z1}	P_{Z0}	OR_{XZ}			
0.40	0.30	1.56	$OR_{DX} = 1.49$	$OR_{DX} = 1.42$	$OR_{DX} = 1.39$
0.55	0.45	1.49	1.54	1.49	1.48
0.70	0.60	1.56	1.57	1.54	1.53
0.45	0.25	2.45	1.26	1.13	1.09
0.60	0.40	2.25	1.35	1.27	1.24
0.75	0.55	2.45	1.41	1.35	1.33

where $O_{zj} = P_{zj}/(1 - P_{zj})$ is the odds of $Z = 1$ versus $Z = 0$ when $X = j$. There must be a substantial exposure-smoking association to remove most of the exposure-cancer association. Because there was no reason to expect an exposure-smoking association at all, Table 29-3 supports the notion that the observed resins-cancer association is probably not due entirely to confounding by the dichotomous smoking variable used here, assuming a valid bias model. We would have to consider a polytomous smoking variable to further address confounding by smoking.

Relation of Unadjusted to Adjusted ORs

An equivalent approach to that just given computes the ratio of the unadjusted to Z-adjusted ORs as a measure of the strength of uncontrolled confounding,[31] assuming a valid bias model. For example, one could compute:

$$
\begin{aligned}
\frac{OR_{DX \text{ unadjusted}}}{OR_{DX \text{ adjusted}}} &= \frac{(OR_{DZ}O_{Z1}+1)(O_{Z0}+1)}{(OR_{DZ}O_{Z0}+1)(O_{Z1}+1)} \\
&= \frac{(OR_{DZ}OR_{XZ}O_{Z0}+1)(O_{Z0}+1)}{(OR_{DZ}O_{Z0}+1)(OR_{XZ}O_{Z0}+1)} \\
&= \frac{OR_{DZ}OR_{XZ}O_{Z0}+1-P_{Z0}}{(OR_{DZ}P_{Z0}+1-P_{Z0})(OR_{XZ}P_{Z0}+1-P_{Z0})} \\
&= \frac{OR_{DZ}P_{Z1}+1-P_{Z1}}{OR_{DZ}P_{Z0}+1-P_{Z0}}
\end{aligned}
$$

[29-3]

Assuming that Z is the sole uncontrolled confounder, this ratio can be interpreted as the degree of bias due to failure to adjust for Z. This series of equations shows that when Z is not associated with the disease ($OR_{DZ} = 1$) or is not associated with exposure ($OR_{XZ} = 1$), the ratio of the unadjusted and adjusted ORs is 1, implying that there is no confounding by Z. In other words, under this bias model, a confounder must be associated with the exposure and the disease in the source population (see Chapters 5 and 12). Recall, however, that these associations are not sufficient for Z to be a confounder, because a confounder must also satisfy certain causal relations (e.g., it must not be affected by exposure or disease; see Chapters 3, 5, and 12). Equation 29-3 also shows that the ratio of unadjusted to adjusted ORs depends on the prevalence of $Z = 1$; that is, the degree of confounding depends not only on the magnitude of the associations but also on the confounder distribution.

In many circumstances, we may have information about only one or two of the three parameters that determine the unadjusted/adjusted ratio. Nonetheless, it can be seen from Equation 29-3 that the ratio cannot be further from 1 than are $OR_{DZ}/(OR_{DZ}P_{Z0}+1-P_{Z0})$, $OR_{XZ}/(OR_{XZ}P_{Z0}+1-P_{Z0})$, $1/(OR_{DZ}P_{Z0}+1-P_{Z0})$, or $1/(OR_{XZ}P_{Z0}+1-P_{Z0})$; the ratio is thus bounded by these quantities. Furthermore, because the bound $OR_{DZ}/(OR_{DZ}P_{Z0}+1-P_{Z0})$ cannot be further from 1 than OR_{DZ}, the ratio cannot be further from 1 than OR_{DZ}, and similarly cannot be further from 1 than OR_{XZ}.[28,30] Thus, the OR bias from failure to adjust Z cannot exceed the OR relating Z to D or to X.

These methods readily extend to cohort studies. For data with person-time denominators T_{ji}, we use the T_{ji} in place of the control counts B_{ji} in the previous equations to obtain an externally adjusted rate ratio. For data with count denominators N_{ji}, we use the N_{ji} in place of the B_{ji} to obtain an externally adjusted risk ratio.[36] Bounds analogous to those above can be derived for risk differences.[45]

Improved bounds can be derived under deterministic causal models relating X to D in the presence of uncontrolled confounding.[46] There is also a large literature on bounding causal risk differences from randomized trials when uncontrolled confounding due to noncompliance may be present (see Chapter 8 of Pearl, 2000[47]).

A slightly different bounding approach is to plot isopleths of combinations of values assigned to the parameters of the bias model that yield strengths of bias equal to the observed association.[48] One then evaluates the plausibility of these values to reach a judgment about whether uncontrolled confounding is likely to fully explain the observed association. Winkelstein used this approach to evaluate whether uncontrolled confounding by an infectious agent might explain the association between smoking and cervical cancer.[48] One can reduce the isopleths to the common minimum point for the factors to obtain a less complicated index than the full isopleths.[48] Vanderweele and Ding call this point the E-value,[49-52] which is described more completely in Chapter 12. Similar approaches are available for measurement error and selection bias.[53,54]

Combination With Adjustment for Measured Confounders

The preceding equations relate the unadjusted OR to the OR adjusted only for the unmeasured confounder (Z) and thus ignore the control of any other confounders. If adjustment for measured confounders has an important effect, the equations must be applied using bias parameters conditioned on those measured confounders. To illustrate, suppose that age adjustment was essential in the previous example. We should then have adjusted for confounding by smoking in the age-adjusted or age-specific ORs. Application of the previous equations to these ORs will require age-specific parameters, for example, P_{Z0} will be the age-specific smoking prevalence among unexposed noncases, OR_{DZ} will be the age-specific association of smoking with lung cancer among the unexposed, and OR_{XZ} will be the age-specific association of smoking with resins exposure among noncases.

Although most estimates of confounder-disease associations are adjusted for major risk factors such as age, information adjusted for other parameters is often unavailable. Use of unadjusted parameters in the preceding equations may be misleading if they are not close to the adjusted parameters (*e.g.*, if the unadjusted and age-adjusted ORs associating smoking with exposure are far apart). For example, if age is associated with smoking and exposure, adjustment for age could partially adjust for confounding by smoking, and the association of smoking with exposure will change upon age adjustment. Use of the age-unadjusted smoking-exposure odds ratio (OR_{XZ}) in the preceding equations will then give a biased estimate of the residual confounding by smoking after age adjustment. More generally, proper external adjustment in combination with adjustments for measured confounders requires information about the unmeasured variables that is conditional on the measured confounders. This information is often difficult to obtain, and use of the more readily available unconditional information is likely to overestimate the bias due to uncontrolled confounding. One alternative, described in more detail below, is to model the strength of confounding directly and then to account quantitatively for the possibility that the strength of uncontrolled confounding is less than what has been directly estimated.[55]

ANALYSIS OF MISCLASSIFICATION

As noted in Chapter 14, nearly all epidemiologic studies suffer from some degree of measurement error, which is usually referred to as classification error or *misclassification* when the variables are discrete. The effect of even modest amounts of error can be profound, yet rarely is the error quantified.[11] Chapter 13 presents simple bias models to address misclassification using basic algebra. We revisit these basic methods below and apply them to the resins and lung cancer example as a foundation for the more advanced methods later in this chapter. See Chapter 13 for a complete discussion of misclassification and simple bias analyses to address it.

Exposure Misclassification

Consider first the estimation of exposure prevalence from a single observed category of subjects, such as the control group in a case-control study. Define the following quantities in this category:

X = 1 if exposed, 0 if not

X^* = 1 if *classified* as exposed, 0 if not

PVP = probability that someone classified as exposed is truly exposed

= predictive value of an exposure "positive" = $Pr(X = 1|X^* = 1)$, or positive predictive value

PVN = probability that someone classified as unexposed is truly unexposed

= predictive value of an exposure "negative" = $Pr(X = 0|X^* = 0)$, or negative predictive value

B_1^* = number classified as exposed (with $X^* = 1$)

B_0^* = number classified as unexposed (with $X^* = 0$)

B_1 = number truly exposed (with $X = 1$)

B_0 = number truly unexposed (with $X = 0$)

If estimates of the predictive values are available, they can be used directly to estimate the numbers truly exposed (B_1) and truly unexposed (B_0) from the misclassified counts $B_1{}^*$ and $B_0{}^*$ via the expected relations.

$$B_1 = PVP\left(B_1{}^*\right) + \left(1 - PVN\right)B_0{}^*$$
$$B_0 = PVN\left(B_0{}^*\right) + \left(1 - PVP\right)B_1{}^* \qquad [29\text{-}4]$$

Note that the total M_0 is not changed by exposure misclassification:

$$
\begin{aligned}
M_0 &= B_1 + B_0 \\
&= PVP\left(B_1{}^*\right) + \left(1 - PVN\right)B_0{}^* + PVN\left(B_0{}^*\right) + \left(1 - PVP\right)B_1{}^* \\
&= \left(PVP + 1 - PVP\right)B_1{}^* + \left(PVN + 1 - PVN\right)B_0{}^* \\
&= B_1{}^* + B_0{}^*
\end{aligned}
$$

Thus, once we have estimated B_1, we can estimate B_0 from $B_0 = M_0 - B_1$. From the preceding equations, we can estimate the true exposure prevalence as $P_{e0} = B_1/M_0$. Parallel equations for cases or person-time follow by substituting A_1, A_0, $A_1{}^*$, and $A_0{}^*$ or T_1, T_0, $T_1{}^*$, and $T_0{}^*$ for B_1, B_0, $B_1{}^*$, and $B_0{}^*$ in Equation 29-4. The bias-adjusted counts obtained by applying the equation to actual data are only estimates derived under the assumption that the true predictive values are PVP and PVN and there is no other error in the observed counts (*e.g.*, no random error). To make this clearer, one can denote the solutions in Equation 29-4 by $\hat{B}_1$ and $\hat{B}_0$ instead of B_1 and B_0; for notational simplicity, we have not done so here.

Unfortunately, valid measures of predictive values are seldom available. For example, when predictive values are measured in an internal validation study requiring extra respondent burden, the highly cooperative study participants who agree to participate may have different patterns of exposure and measurement accuracy than other study participants. When valid measures of predictive values are available, they ordinarily apply only to the study population in which they were measured because they depend directly on exposure prevalence, which varies across target populations (see Equations 29-9 and 29-10). Owing to variations in exposure prevalence across target populations and time, predictive values from a different study are unlikely to apply to a second study. Even when one can reliably estimate predictive values for a study, these estimates should be allowed to vary with disease and confounder levels, because exposure prevalence will vary across these levels.

These problems in applying predictive values lead to alternative adjustment methods, which use classification parameters that do not depend on true exposure prevalence. The following four probabilities are common examples of such parameters:

Se = probability that someone exposed is classified as exposed
    = sensitivity = $\Pr(X^* = 1 | X = 1)$

Fn = probability that someone exposed is classified as unexposed
    = false-negative probability = $\Pr(X^* = 0 | X = 1) = 1 - \text{Se}$

Sp = probability that someone unexposed is classified as unexposed
    = specificity = $\Pr(X^* = 0 | X = 0)$

Fp = probability that someone unexposed is classified as exposed
    = false-positive probability = $\Pr(X^* = 1 | X = 0) = 1 - \text{Sp}$

The following equations then relate the expected misclassified counts to the true counts:

$$B_1{}^* = \text{expected number of subjects classified as exposed}$$
$$= \text{Se } B_1 + \text{Fp } B_0 \qquad [29\text{-}5]$$

and

$B_0{}^*$ = expected number of subjects classified as unexposed

$$= \mathrm{Fn}\, B_1 + \mathrm{Sp}\, B_0 \qquad\qquad [29\text{-}6]$$

Note that Se + Fn = Sp + Fp = 1, showing again that the total is unchanged by the exposure misclassification:

$$
\begin{aligned}
M_0 &= B_1 + B_0 \\
&= (\mathrm{Se} + \mathrm{Fn})B_1 + (\mathrm{Sp} + \mathrm{Fp})B_0 \\
&= \mathrm{Se}B_1 + \mathrm{Fp}B_0 + \mathrm{Fn}B_1 + \mathrm{Sp}B_0 \\
&= B_1{}^* + B_0{}^*
\end{aligned}
$$

In most studies, one observes only the misclassified counts $B_1{}^*$ and $B_0{}^*$. If we assume that the sensitivity and specificity are equal to Se and Sp (with Fn = 1 − Se and Fp = 1 − Sp), we can estimate B_1 and B_0 by solving Equations 29-5 and 29-6. From Equation 29-6.

$$B_0 = \left(B_0{}^* - \mathrm{Fn}B_1\right)\big/\mathrm{Sp}$$

We can substitute the right side of this equation for B_0 in Equation 29-5, which yields

$$B_1{}^* = \mathrm{Se}B_1 + \mathrm{Fp}\left(B_0{}^* - \mathrm{Fn}B_1\right)\big/\mathrm{Sp}$$

We then solve for B_1 and compute B_0

$$
\begin{aligned}
B_1 &= \left(\mathrm{Sp}B_1{}^* - \mathrm{Fp}B_0{}^*\right)\big/\left(\mathrm{SeSp} - \mathrm{FnFp}\right) \\
&= \left(B_1{}^* - \mathrm{Fp}M_0\right)\big/\left(\mathrm{Se} + \mathrm{Sp} - 1\right) \\
B_0 &= M_0 - B_1 = \left(B_0{}^* - \mathrm{Fn}M_0\right)\big/\left(\mathrm{Se} + \mathrm{Sp} - 1\right) \qquad [29\text{-}7]
\end{aligned}
$$

From these equations we can also estimate the true exposure prevalence as $P_{e0} = B_1/M_0$. Again, the B_1 and B_0 obtained by applying Equation 29-7 to actual data are only estimates derived under the assumption that the true sensitivity and specificity are Se and Sp. To estimate a bias-adjusted measure of association, we must also apply analogous equations to estimate A_1 and A_0 from the observed (misclassified) case counts $A_1{}^*$ and $A_0{}^*$:

$$A_1 = \left(A_1{}^* - \mathrm{Fp}M_1\right)\big/\left(\mathrm{Se} + \mathrm{Sp} - 1\right) \qquad\qquad [29\text{-}8]$$

from which $A_0 = M_1 - A_1$, where M_1 is the observed case total. These equations may be applied to case-control, closed-cohort, or prevalence-survey data. For person-time follow-up data, Equation 29-7 can be modified by substituting T_1, T_0, $T_1{}^*$, and $T_0{}^*$ for B_1, B_0, $B_1{}^*$, and $B_0{}^*$.

The equations may be applied within strata of confounders as well. After application of the equations, we may compute bias-adjusted, stratum-specific, and summary effect estimates from the estimates of the true counts. Finally, we tabulate the bias-adjusted estimates obtained by using different combinations of estimates for Se and Sp and thus obtain a picture of how sensitive the bias analysis results are to various degrees of misclassification. See Chapter 13 for further discussion of assigning values to Se and Sp.

Valid variances for adjusted estimates cannot be calculated from the adjusted counts using conventional equations (such as those in Chapters 16 and 17), even if we assume that sensitivity and specificity are known or are unbiased estimates from a validation study. This problem arises because conventional equations do not take account of the data transformations and random errors in the adjustments. Equations that do so are available.[56-61] Probabilistic bias analysis, which is described below, can also account for these technical issues and for other sources of uncertainty as well.

Nondifferentiality

In the preceding description, we assumed nondifferential exposure misclassification, that is, the same values of Se and Sp of exposure classification applied to both the cases (Equation 29-8) and the noncases (Equation 29-7). To say that a classification method is nondifferential with respect to disease means that it has identical operating characteristics among cases and noncases, so that sensitivity and specificity of exposure classification do not vary with disease status. We expect this property to hold when the mechanisms that determine the classification are identical among cases and noncases. This expectation is reasonable when the mechanisms that determine exposure classification precede the disease occurrence and are not affected by uncontrolled risk factors, as in many cohort studies, although even then it is not guaranteed to hold. Thus, to say that there is nondifferential exposure misclassification (such as when exposure data are collected from records that predate the outcome) means that neither disease nor uncontrolled risk factors result in different accuracy of response for cases compared to noncases.

Nondifferential misclassification is even then an expectation about how the classification mechanisms are thought to influence the observed result. One can never verify from the result that the observed data were misclassified nondifferentially. Such a verification would require a comparison of the sensitivity of exposure classification in all cases with the sensitivity in all noncases and a comparison of the specificity of exposure classification in all cases with the specificity in all noncases. As noted above, these complete data sensitivities and specificities are never available; if they were, the study would have a gold-standard measurement of exposure classification in all participants, obviating the need to use the misclassified measurement. Thus, labels of misclassification as nondifferential or differential apply only to the expectation of how the information bias is thought to have operated, without any guarantee of how closely the particular study result adhered to the expectation.[62] As usual, large deviations from expectations are less likely as sample size increases. See Chapter 13 for further discussion.

When differential misclassification is a reasonable possibility, we can extend the bias analysis by using different sensitivities and specificities for cases and noncases. Letting Fp_1, Fp_0 be the case and noncase false-positive probabilities, and Fn_1, Fn_0 the case and noncase false-negative probabilities, the bias-adjusted OR for a single 2×2 table simplifies to

$$\frac{\left(A_1{}^* - Fp_1 M_1\right)\left(B_0{}^* - Fn_0 M_0\right)}{\left(A_0{}^* - Fp_1 M_1\right)\left(B_1{}^* - Fn_0 M_0\right)}$$

This equation is sensible, however, only if all four parenthetical terms in the ratio are positive.

Application to the Resins-Lung Cancer Example

As an example, we bias-adjust the resins-lung cancer data in Table 29-1 under the assumption that the sensitivity and specificity of exposure ascertainment among cases are 0.9 and 0.8, and the sensitivity and specificity of exposure ascertainment among controls are 0.8 and 0.8. This assumption means that exposure detection is somewhat better for cases. (Because this study is record based with deaths from other diseases as controls, it seems unlikely that the actual study would have had such differential misclassification.) From Equations 29-7 and 29-8, we obtain

$$B_1 = \left[257 - 0.2(1,202)\right]/(0.8 + 0.8 - 1) = 27.67$$
$$B_0 = 1,202 - 27.67 = 1,174.33$$
$$A_1 = \left[45 - 0.2(139)\right]/(0.8 + 0.9 - 1) = 24.57$$
$$A_0 = 139 - 24.57 = 114.43$$

These yield a bias-adjusted OR of 24.57(1,174.33)/114.43(27.67) = 9.1. This value is much higher than the conventional OR of 1.76, despite the fact that exposure detection is better for cases. This better exposure detection in the cases might have suggested that the original estimate was biased away from the null, so that the bias-analysis would have been expected to yield a bias-adjusted

TABLE 29-4

Bias-Adjusted Resins-Lung Cancer Mortality Odds Ratios Under Various Assumptions About the Resins Exposure Sensitivity (Se) and Specificity (Sp) Among Cases and Controls

Cases		Controls			
		Se: 0.90	0.80	0.90	0.80
Se	*Sp*	*Sp*: 0.90	0.90	0.80	0.80
0.90	0.90	2.34[a]	2.00	19.3	16.5
0.80	0.90	2.83	2.42[a]	23.3	19.9
0.90	0.80	1.29	1.11	10.7[a]	9.1
0.80	0.80	1.57	1.34	12.9	11.0[a]

[a]Nondifferential misclassification.

estimate nearer the null. The difference between the bias-adjusted estimate we obtained and the expected direction of the bias illustrates the utility of using quantitative bias-analysis to overcome faulty intuitions.

By repeating the preceding bias analysis, we obtain a resins-misclassification sensitivity analysis for the data in Table 29-1. Table 29-4 provides a summary of the results of this sensitivity analysis. As can be seen, under the nondifferential misclassification scenarios along the descending diagonal, the bias-adjusted OR estimates (2.34, 2.42, 10.7, and 11.0) are always further from the null than the conventional estimate computed directly from the data (1.76, which corresponds to the estimate assuming $Se = Sp = 1$, no misclassification). This result reflects the fact that, if the exposure is dichotomous and the misclassified measurement of exposure is better than random labeling, nondifferential, and independent of other errors (whether systematic or random), the bias produced by the exposure misclassification is toward the null. We caution, however, that this rule does not extend automatically to other situations, such as those involving a polytomous exposure (see Chapter 13).

In one form of recall bias, cases remember true exposure more than do controls, that is, there is higher sensitivity among cases (see Chapter 13). Table 29-4 shows that even if we assume that this form of recall bias is present, bias-adjustment may move the estimate away from the null; in fact, three bias-adjusted estimates (2.00, 16.5, and 9.1) are further from the null than the conventional estimate (1.76). These results show that the association can be considerably diminished by misclassification, even in the presence of recall bias. To understand this apparently counterintuitive phenomenon, one may think of the classification procedure as having two components: a nondifferential component shared by both cases and controls and a differential component reflecting the recall bias. In many plausible scenarios, the bias toward the null produced by the nondifferential component overwhelms the bias away from the null produced by the differential component.[63]

Table 29-4 also shows that the specificity has a more powerful effect on the observed OR than does the sensitivity in this example (*e.g.*, with $Se = 0.8$ and $Sp = 0.9$, the bias-adjusted estimate is 2.42, whereas with Se = 0.9 and Sp = 0.8, the bias-adjusted estimate is 10.7), because the exposure prevalence is low. In general, when the exposure prevalence is low, the OR estimate is more sensitive to false-positive error than to false-negative error, because false positives arise from a larger group and thus can easily overwhelm true positives. See Chapter 13 for further discussion.

Finally, the example shows that the uncertainty in results due to the uncertainty about the classification probabilities can be much greater than the uncertainty conveyed by conventional confidence intervals. The conventional 95% confidence interval in the example extends from 1.2 to 2.6, whereas the misclassification-adjusted ORs range above 10 if we allow specificities of 0.8, even if we assume that the misclassification is nondifferential, and to as low as 1.1 if we allow differential misclassification. Note that this large range of uncertainty does not incorporate random error, which is the only source of error reflected in the conventional confidence interval.

Relation of Predictive Values to Sensitivity and Specificity

Arguments are often made that the sensitivity and specificity of an instrument will be roughly stable across similar populations, at least within levels of disease and covariates such as age, sex, and socio-economic status. Nonetheless, as mentioned earlier, variations in sensitivity and specificity can occur under many conditions—for example, when the measure is an interview response and responses are interviewer dependent.[64] These variations in sensitivity and specificity will also produce variations in predictive values, which can be seen from equations that relate the predictive values to sensitivity and specificity. To illustrate the relations, again consider exposure classification among noncases, where $M_0 = B_1 + B_0 = B_1* + B_0*$ is the noncase total, and let $P_{e0} = B_1/M_0$ be the true exposure prevalence among noncases. Then, in expectation, the positive predictive value among noncases is

$$PVP_0 = \left(\text{number of correctly classified subjects in } B_1*\right)\big/B_1*$$
$$= \text{Se } B_1\big/\left(\text{Se } B_1 + \text{Fp } B_0\right)$$
$$= \text{Se}\left(B_1/M_0\right)\big/\left[\text{Se}\left(B_1/M_0\right) + \text{Fp}\left(B_0/M_0\right)\right]$$
$$= \text{Se}P_{e0}\big/\left[\text{Se}P_{e0} + \text{Fp}\left(1 - P_{e0}\right)\right] \tag{29-9}$$

Similarly, in expectation, the negative predictive value among noncases is

$$PVN_0 = \text{Sp}\left(1 - P_{e0}\right)\big/\left[\text{Fn}P_{e0} + \text{Sp}\left(1 - P_{e0}\right)\right] \tag{29-10}$$

Equations 29-9 and 29-10 show that predictive values are a function of the sensitivity, specificity, *and* the unknown true exposure prevalence in the population to which they apply. When bias-adjustments to address misclassification are based on internal validation data and those data are a random sample of the study population, or can be reweighted to the entire study population, there is no issue of generalization across populations. In such situations, the predictive-value approach to bias-adjustment to address misclassification is simple and efficient.[65,66] We again emphasize, however, that validation studies may be afflicted by selection bias, thus violating the generalizability assumption used by this approach.

Disease Misclassification

Most equations and concerns for exposure misclassification also apply to disease misclassification. For example, Equations 29-4 and 29-7 can be modified to adjust for disease misclassification. For disease misclassification in a closed-cohort study or a prevalence survey, *PVP* and *PVN* will refer to the predictive values for disease, and *A*, *B*, and *N* will replace B_1, B_0, and M_0. For the adjustments using sensitivity and specificity, consider first the estimation of the incidence proportion from a closed cohort or of prevalence from a cross-sectional sample. The preceding equations can then be adapted directly by redefining Se, Fn, Sp, and Fp to refer to disease. Let

D = 1 if diseased, 0 if not

$D*$ = 1 if classified as diseased, 0 if not

Se = probability someone diseased is classified as diseased

    = disease sensitivity = $\Pr(D* = 1|D = 1)$

Fn = false-negative probability = $1 - \text{Se}$

Sp = probability someone nondiseased is classified as nondiseased

    = disease specificity = $\Pr(D* = 0|D = 0)$

Fp = false-positive probability = $1 - Sp$

Suppose that *A* and *B* are the true numbers of diseased and nondiseased subjects, and *A** and *B** are the numbers classified as diseased and nondiseased. Then Equations 29-5 to 29-7 give the expected relations between A, B and A^*, B^*, with A, B replacing B_1, B_0; A^*, B^* replacing B_1^*, B_0^*; and $N = A + B = A^* + B^*$ replacing M_0. With these changes, Equation 29-7 becomes

$$A = \left(A^* - \text{Fp}N\right)\big/\left(\text{Se} + \text{Sp} - 1\right) \qquad\qquad [29\text{-}11]$$

and $B = N - A$. These equations can be applied separately to different exposure groups and within strata, and bias-adjusted summary estimates can then be computed from the bias-adjusted counts. Results of repeated application of this process for different pairs of Se, Sp can be tabulated to provide a sensitivity analysis. Also, the pair Se, Sp can either be kept the same across exposure groups (nondifferential disease misclassification) or allowed to vary across groups (differential misclassification). As noted earlier, however, special variance equations are required to estimate intervals or other statistics for the bias-adjusted results.[56-60]

The situation differs slightly for person-time follow-up data. Here, one must replace the specificity Sp and false-positive probability Fp with a different concept, that of the *false-positive rate,* Fr:

Fr = number of false-positive diagnoses (noncases diagnosed as cases) per unit person-time. We then have

$$A^* = \text{Se }A + Fr\,T \qquad\qquad [29\text{-}12]$$

where T is the true person-time at risk. Also, false negatives (of which there are FnA) will inflate the observed person-time T^*; how much depends on how long the false negatives are followed. Unless the disease is very common, however, the false negatives will add relatively little person-time and we can take T to be approximately T^*. Upon doing so, we need to only solve Equation 29-12 for A:

$$A = \left(A^* - FrT^*\right)\big/\text{Se} \qquad\qquad [29\text{-}13]$$

and get a bias-adjusted rate A/T^*. Sensitivity analysis then proceeds (similarly to before) by applying Equation 29-13 to the different exposure groups, computing bias-adjusted summary measures and repeating this process for various combinations of Se and Fr (which may vary across subcohorts).

The preceding analysis of follow-up data is simplistic, in that it does not account for possible effects if exposure lengthens or shortens the time from incidence to diagnosis. These effects have generally not been correctly analyzed in the medical literature[67,68] (see the discussion of standardization in Chapter 18). In these cases, one should treat the time of disease onset as the outcome variable and bias-adjust for errors in measuring this outcome using methods for continuous variables.[9]

Often studies make special efforts to verify case diagnoses, so that the number of false positives within the study will be negligible. If such verification is successful, we can assume that Fp = 0, Sp = 1, and Equations 29-11 and 29-13 then simplify to $A = A^*/Se$. If we examine a risk ratio RR under these conditions, then, assuming nondifferential misclassification, the observed RR^* will be

$$RR^* = \frac{A_1^*/N_1}{A_0^*/N_0} = \frac{\text{Se}A_1/N_1}{\text{Se}A_0/N_0} = \frac{A_1/N_1}{A_0/N_0} = RR$$

In other words, with perfect specificity, nondifferential sensitivity of disease misclassification will not bias the risk ratio. Assuming that the misclassification negligibly alters person-time, the same will be true for the rate ratio[69] and will also be true for the OR when the disease is uncommon. The preceding fact allows extension of the result to case-control studies in which cases are carefully screened to remove false positives.[70]

Suppose now that the cases cannot be screened, so that in a case-control study there may be many false cases (false positives). It would be a severe mistake to apply the disease-misclassification adjustment Equation 29-11 to case-control data if (as is almost always true) Se and Sp are determined from other than the study data themselves,[71] because the use of different sampling probabilities for cases and controls alters the sensitivity and specificity within the study relative to the source population.[72] To see the problem, suppose that all apparent cases A_1^*, A_0^* but only a fraction f of apparent noncases B_1^*, B_0^* are randomly sampled from a closed cohort in which disease has been classified with sensitivity Se and specificity Sp. The expected numbers of apparent cases and controls selected at exposure level j are then

$$A_j^* = \text{Se } A_j + \text{Fp } B_j$$

and

$$f B_j^* = f\left(\text{Fn } A_j + \text{Sp } B_j\right)$$

The numbers of true cases and noncases at exposure level j in the case-control study are

$$\text{Se } A_j + f \text{ Fn } A_j = \left(\text{Se} + f \text{ FN}\right)A_j$$

and

$$\text{Fp } B_j + f \text{ Sp } B_j = \left(\text{Fp} + f \text{ Sp}\right)B_j$$

whereas the numbers of correctly classified cases and noncases in the study are SeA_j and $fSpB_j$. The sensitivity and specificity in the study are thus

$$\text{Se } A_j / \left(\text{Se} + f \text{ Fn}\right)A_j = \text{Se}/\left(\text{Se} + f \text{ Fn}\right)$$

and

$$f \text{ Sp } B_j / \left(\text{Fp} + f \text{ Sp}\right)B_j = f \text{ Sp}/\left(\text{Fp} + f \text{ Sp}\right)$$

The study specificity can be far from the population specificity. For example, if $Se = Sp = 0.90$, all apparent cases are selected, and controls are 1% of the population at risk, the study specificity will be $0.01(0.90)/[0.1 + 0.01(0.90)] = 0.08$. Use of the population specificity 0.90 instead of the study specificity 0.08 in a bias analysis could produce extremely distorted results.

Confounder Misclassification

The effects of dichotomous confounder misclassification lead to residual and possibly differential residual confounding.[73] These effects can be explored using the methods discussed previously for dichotomous exposure misclassification.[74-76] One may apply Equations 29-7 and 29-8 to the confounder within strata of the exposure (rather than to the exposure within strata of the confounder) and then compute a summary exposure-disease association from the bias-adjusted data. The utility of this approach is limited, however, because most confounder adjustments involve more than two strata. We discuss a more general (matrix) approach below.

Misclassification of Multiple Variables

So far, our analyses have assumed that only one variable requires bias-adjustment. In many situations, age and sex (which tend to have negligible error) are the only important confounders, the cases are carefully screened, and only exposure remains seriously misclassified. There are, however, many other situations in which not only exposure but also major confounders are misclassified. Disease misclassification may also coexist with these other problems, especially when studying disease subtypes.

In examining misclassification of multiple variables, it is commonly assumed that the classification errors for each variable are independent of *errors* in other variables. This assumption is different from that of nondifferentiality, which asserts that errors for each variable are independent of the *true values* of the other variables. Neither, either one, or both assumptions may hold, and all have different implications for bias. As mentioned in Chapter 13, the generalization that "nondifferential misclassification of exposure always produces bias toward the null" is false if the errors are dependent or if exposure has multiple levels.

If all the classification errors are independent across variables, we can apply the bias-adjustment equations in sequence for each misclassified variable, one at a time. For example, in a prevalence survey, we may first obtain counts bias-adjusted for exposure misclassification from Equations 29-7 and 29-8 and then further bias-adjust these counts for disease misclassification using Equation 29-11. If, however, the classification errors are dependent across variables, we must turn to more complex bias-adjustment methods such as those based on matrix adjustment of counts.[56-58,71] Dependent errors most easily arise when the same method, such as an interview or medical record review, is used to ascertain more than one variable involved in the analysis.[77] Matrix methods are also useful for adjustments of polytomous (multilevel) variables. In some cases, one can reason about the direction, but not the magnitude, of the bias from more than one misclassified variable using signed graphs.[78]

A Matrix Adjustment Method

We now briefly outline one simple matrix approach that is the natural generalization of the equations given earlier[58,71,79,80] and can be applied under any misclassification setting, including dependent and differential misclassification of polytomous variables. Imagine that we have a multiway table of data classified by disease, one or more exposures, and one or more stratification variables (all of which may have multiple levels). Suppose that this table has K cells. We can list these cells in any order and index them by a subscript $k = 1,...,K$. Suppose that C_k^* subjects are classified into cell k, whereas C_k subjects truly belong in that cell. Next, define

p_{mk} = probability of being classified into cell m when the true cell is k.

Then, in expectation,

$$C_m^* = \sum_{k=1}^{K} p_{mk} C_k \qquad [29\text{-}14]$$

This equation is a generalization of Equations 29-5 and 29-6.

If we write C^* and C for the vectors of C_m^* and C_k and P for the matrix of p_{mk}, then Equation 29-14 reduces to $C^* = PC$. The adjusted counts, assuming that P contains the true classification probabilities, can then be found from the observed (misclassified) counts C^* by inverting P, to get $C = P^{-1}C^*$. The practical utility of this equation will of course depend on the information available to specify plausible values for the p_{mk} in each application.

Use of Validation Data

In the previous bias-adjustment equations, we assumed that Se and Sp were educated guesses, perhaps suggested by or estimated from external literature. Suppose instead that classification probabilities can be estimated directly from an internal validation subsample of the study subjects, that the latter subsample is itself free of bias, and that the sampling is random within levels of exposure, disease, and any adjustment covariates. Several statistically efficient ways of using these data are then available, beginning with the predictive-value approaches described earlier, but also including two-stage and missing-data analysis methods. From such methods, correctly classified counts may be estimated using maximum-likelihood or related techniques, and full statistics (including confidence intervals) can be obtained for the resulting effect estimates.[6,56-59,65,81-85] Regression methods may also be used to adjust for errors in continuous measurements.[9,86-89] Robins et al.[4] and Carroll et al.[9] review and compare a number of methods and their relation to missing-data techniques and discuss general methods for continuous as well as discrete variables.

A general bias-adjustment equation for the predictive-value approach follows if we have estimates of q_{km} = probability of truly belonging to cell k when classified into cell m. We can then obtain estimates of the true counts from the equation

$$C_k = \sum_{m=1}^{M} q_{km} C_m *$$

[29-15]

which is a generalization of Equation 29-4. In the matrix algebra formulation, we can write this equation as $C = QC^*$, where Q is the matrix of q_{km}. Bias-adjustment methods more efficient and more general than the preceding approach can be obtained using likelihood-based techniques; see Carroll et al.[9] for a model-based treatment.

An important caution in interpreting the results from formal bias-adjustment methods is that most methods assume that the validation standard is measured without error. If, however, the validation measurement taken as the truth is itself subject to error, then the bias-adjusted estimate will also be biased, possibly severely so.[90] Many studies labeled as validation studies actually substitute one imperfect measure of a variable for another. They are thus measures of agreement, not validity. For binary exposures, the bias in the bias-adjusted estimate can be kept below that of the unadjusted estimate if the validation measurement has higher sensitivity and specificity than the original measurement, and the bias-adjustment method does not assume nondifferentiality.[91] More generally, by introducing assumptions (models) for the joint relation of the available measurements to each other and to the true values, as well as assumptions about randomness of validation sampling, further adjustments can be made to account for errors in the validation measurements.[85,87,88,92,93] These assumptions may then be subjected to sensitivity analyses of the impact of assumption violations.

We have underscored the random-sampling assumptions in validation methods because of the high potential for selection bias in many validation studies. Validation studies often require an additional respondent burden (*e.g.*, to complete a diet diary for validation of a food frequency questionnaire or to submit a biospecimen for validation of a self-reported estimate of exposure), leading to questions about the representativeness of those who volunteer to participate. Even when no burden is imposed, selection bias may occur. For example, studies that validate self-reported history by record review sometimes treat those who refuse permission to review their records as if they were no different from those who permit review. Nonetheless, one reason to refuse permission may be to avoid detection of an inaccurate self-report. If this type of refusal is common enough, extrapolation of the results from those who permit review to the larger study group will exaggerate the validity of self-reported history. Bias analysis of selection bias (discussed next) can be used to assess such problems.

In summary, when the validation study is itself subject to systematic error and bias, sensitivity analysis remains an important adjunct to more formal bias-adjustment methods.

SELECTION BIAS

Selection bias (including response and follow-up bias) is perhaps the simplest to deal with mathematically and yet is often the hardest to address convincingly, although attempts have been made.[94-97] The chief obstacle is lack of sufficient information to perform a quantitative bias analysis because, by definition, the information required for a bias analysis is missing among nonparticipants or those lost to follow-up.

Some early writings mistakenly implied that selection bias, like confounding, can always be controlled if one obtains data on factors affecting selection. Although some forms of selection bias can be controlled like confounding, other forms can be impossible to control without external information. An example of controllable selection bias is that induced by matching in case-control studies. As discussed in Chapter 8, one needs only to control the matching factors to remove the selection bias introduced by the matching. Other examples include two-stage studies, which employ biased selection with known selection probabilities and then use those probabilities to adjust for the selection bias.[98-102] Examples of ordinarily uncontrollable bias occur when controls are matched to cases on factors affected by exposure or disease and for which the population distribution is unknown, such as intermediate causal factors or disease symptoms.[103]

Selection bias is controllable when the factors that affect selection are measured on all study subjects, and either (a) these factors are antecedents of both exposure and disease, and so can be controlled like confounders (see Chapter 12), or (b) one knows the joint distribution of these factors (including exposure and disease, if they jointly affect selection) in the entire source population, and so can adjust for the bias using methods such as shown in Equation 29-3 or the one given below. A condition equivalent to (b) is that one knows the selection probabilities for each level of the factors affecting selection. Unfortunately, this situation is rare. It usually occurs only when the study incorporates features of a population survey, as in two-stage designs[98,99] and randomized recruitment.[104]

There is a well-known decomposition for the OR that can be used for bias analysis of selection bias.[80,98] Suppose that S_{Aj} and S_{Bj} are the probabilities of case and noncase selection at exposure level j. For a dichotomous exposure, $j = 1$ for the exposed and 0 for the unexposed. In a density-sampled case-control study, let S_{Bj} be the person-time rate of control selection at exposure level j. Then the population case counts can be estimated by A_j/S_{Aj} and the population noncase counts (or person-times) can be estimated by B_j/S_{Bj}. Therefore, the bias-adjusted OR or rate-ratio estimate comparing exposure level j to level 0 is

$$\frac{\left(A_j/S_{Aj}\right)\left(B_0/S_{B0}\right)}{\left(A_0/S_{A0}\right)\left(B_j/S_{Bj}\right)} = \frac{A_j B_0}{A_0 B_j}\left(\frac{S_{Aj} S_{B0}}{S_{A0} S_{Bj}}\right)^{-1} \qquad [29\text{-}16]$$

In words, an adjusted estimate can be obtained by dividing the sample OR by a selection bias factor $S_{Aj}S_{B0}/S_{A0}S_{Bj}$. Equation 29-16 can be applied within strata of confounders, and the selection bias factor can vary across the strata. Generalizations of this equation to regression settings are also available.[95,105] It can also be applied repeatedly to account for independent sources of selection bias. We have presented an extension to an equivalent reweighting approach and an example application of both approaches, in Chapter 14. We will illustrate its application to the resins and lung cancer example in the section on probabilistic bias analysis.

The obstacle to any application is estimating values to assign to the selection probabilities S_{Aj} and S_{Bj}. Again, these usually can be estimated only if the study in question incorporates survey elements to determine the true population frequencies. Otherwise, a sensitivity of a bias analysis based on Equation 29-16 may have to encompass a broad range of possibilities. Equation 29-16 does provide one minor insight: no bias occurs if the selection bias factor is 1. One way the latter will occur is if disease and exposure affect selection independently, in the sense that $S_{Aj} = t_A u_j$ and $S_{Bj} = t_B u_j$, where t_A and t_B are the marginal selection probabilities for cases and noncases, and u_j is the marginal selection probability at exposure level j (in density studies, t_B will be the marginal rate of control selection). Occasionally one may reason that such independence will hold, or independence can be forced to hold through careful sampling. Nonetheless, when refusal is common and subjects know their own exposure and disease status, there may be good reasons to doubt the assumption.[106]

Now suppose that the selection bias is a consequence of having a covariate Z affected by exposure X that influenced selection (e.g., as when Z is an intermediate or is affected by exposure X and the study disease D). Recall that Equation 29-3 gives the ratio of the unadjusted OR_{DX} to the Z-adjusted OR_{DX} in terms of the prevalence P_{Z0} of $Z = 1$ among unexposed noncases, the OR_{DZ} relating Z to D given X, and the OR_{XZ} relating Z to X given D. Our present situation is the reverse of when Z is an unmeasured confounder: we now have the Z-stratified OR_{DX} but want the unadjusted OR_{DX}. The inverses of the expressions in Equation 29-3 are equal to the ratio of the adjusted and unadjusted DX odds ratios and thus equal to the selection bias produced by stratifying on Z, assuming that the Z-specific DX odds ratio (OR_{DX}) is constant across Z levels.[107] If the OR for the association of Z with selection does not vary with D or X, we can estimate OR_{DX}, OR_{DZ}, and OR_{XZ} from the data and then do a bias analysis of selection bias as a function of O_{Z0}, which equals the sample odds of $Z = 1$ versus $Z = 0$ divided by the ratio of selection probabilities when $Z = 1$ versus $Z = 0$.

MULTIPLE-BIAS ANALYSES

Quantitative bias analyses for different biases may be combined into a multiple-bias analysis. This combination, however, requires proper ordering of the bias-adjustments because order can make a difference. As a general rule, bias-adjustments should be made in the *reverse* of the order in which the problems occurred during the data-generation process.[12,108] In particular, because differential misclassification bias as a function of sensitivity and specificity does not reduce to a simple multiplicative bias factor in the OR, the result of the combined bias-adjustment will depend on the order in which misclassification bias-adjustment is made.

Confounding originates in population causal relations (see Chapter 12) so is usually the first problem to occur, but selection from the source population may occur before or after classification. As an example, suppose that we wish to make bias-adjustments for uncontrolled smoking confounding and exposure misclassification, and we have external data indicating a likely joint distribution for smoking and exposure. Suppose also that these external data are themselves based on exposure measurements misclassified in a manner like the study data (as would be the case if the data came from the same cohort as the study data). The bias-adjustment for uncontrolled confounding by smoking will then yield a hypothetical smoking-stratified table of *misclassified* exposure by disease, which then must be bias-adjusted for exposure misclassification. In other words, the smoking stratification should precede the misclassification bias-adjustment. On the other hand, if the joint distribution of smoking and exposure used for external adjustment was a purely hypothetical one referring to the *true* exposure, the misclassification bias-adjustment should precede the construction of the hypothetical smoking-stratified table.

To complicate matters further, the ordering of classification may differ for different variables; for example, in a case-control study, exposure classification typically occurs after selection, but disease classification typically occurs before. Sometimes even the ordering of classification steps for a single variable is mixed; for example, in the resins example, job information came from records that preceded the study, but exposure classification based on the jobs came from hygienist evaluations made after selection. An optimal analysis would make separate bias-adjustments for each source of exposure misclassification, with misclassification adjustments occurring both before and after selection-bias-adjustments.

Another problem in multiple-bias analysis is the complexity of examining and presenting results from multiple bias-adjustments. The minimum number of parameters for a realistic analysis of an effect is arguably three confounding parameters, four classification probabilities, and four selection probabilities. Yet if we assigned only five values to each of these $3 + 4 + 4 = 11$ bias parameters and eliminated half the combinations from each of the three parameter groups based on symmetry considerations, we would still have $5^{11}/2^3$ or more than 6 million combinations to consider. This problem has led to the development of simulation methods for summarizing over these combinations, which we address next.

PROBABILISTIC BIAS ANALYSIS

The methods in the preceding sections describe simple bias analyses that provide a quantitative assessment of one bias at a time, or as ordered adjustments. The bias parameters (*e.g.*, associations of an unmeasured confounder with the exposure and outcome; false-positive and false-negative classification probabilities; selection probabilities) are assigned one value or a limited number of values. Although these methods yield an estimate of the direction and magnitude of bias, they treat the bias parameters as if they were perfectly measured themselves (one assigned value) or as if they can only take on a limited combination of values (as in Tables 29-3 and 29-4). Neither treatment is likely correct. In addition, when a set of bias-adjustments arises from different combinations of bias parameters, these simple methods provide no sense of which adjustment is most plausible and which adjustment is least plausible. All combinations are treated as if they are equally likely, and presentation of multiple combinations is both cumbersome and difficult to interpret.[109]

The simple methods we have presented do not combine the adjustment for systematic error with the random error reflected in the conventional confidence interval. The effect of bias-adjustments on the *P*-value and confidence interval can be nonintuitive. For example, although a bias-adjustment for nondifferential misclassification of a binary exposure can easily move a small unadjusted association far from the null (see Table 29-4), the same bias-adjustment will either have no effect on the *P*-value or, through an overwhelming increase in variance, will make the *P*-value larger than it was before bias-adjustment. Therefore, the bias-adjustment does not yield stronger evidence against the null hypothesis, even though it yields an estimate of association that is farther from the null.[61]

As we have mentioned, a major problem with conventional statistical analysis is its exclusive focus on random error as the only source of uncertainty. Early attempts to integrate bias analysis with random-error analysis applied sensitivity analyses to *P*-values and confidence limits,[37,110] for example, by repeatedly applying conventional equations to the adjusted data obtained from multiple scenarios. Such approaches, however, may convey an unduly pessimistic or conservative picture of the uncertainty surrounding results. For example, the lowest lower 95% limit and highest upper 95% limit from a broad-ranging analysis will contain a very wide interval that could have a coverage rate much greater than 95%. This problem occurs in part because these analyses treat all scenarios equally, regardless of plausibility. More recent attempts have calibrated a study's *P*-value or confidence interval to account for its expected result given empirical evidence about the influence of systematic and random errors in similar studies.[111,112] Theoretical and practical concerns about this approach have also been raised.[113-115] Probabilistic bias analysis provides a more coherent approach by integrating the results using explicit prior distributions for the bias parameters, so this approach is the focus of the remainder of the chapter.

We will illustrate probabilistic bias analysis in perhaps its simplest and most common form, Monte-Carlo sensitivity analysis (MCSA). After outlining this approach, we apply it to adjustments for an unmeasured confounder, misclassification, and selection bias, following the outline and example used above for simple sensitivity analysis. We conclude with a brief description of Bayesian bias analysis, which provides a more general approach to probabilistic bias analysis based on the same models and distributions. Both approaches can be thought of as supplying a posterior distribution for the target parameter (*e.g.*, an effect measure), in the sense of a Bayesian analysis.[116] The chief limitation of MCSA (which it shares with conventional frequentist methods) is that it implicitly assumes we have no prior information about the target parameter and certain other parameters. In contrast, the Bayesian approach can use prior information on all the parameters of the models.

Introduction to the Method

Probabilistic bias analysis extends simple bias analysis by assigning probability distributions to the bias parameters,[12,95,117-122] rather than using a few fixed values for the parameters. Assuming that the data under analysis provide no information about the bias parameters, these distributions must be developed based on information outside the data, such as experiences in other studies. The distributions for the bias parameters are then Bayesian prior distributions.[116,123,124]

At each iteration of a probabilistic bias analysis, values for the bias parameters are randomly selected from their assigned probability distributions and then used in the bias-analysis equations given earlier to produce a single bias-adjusted estimate. There may be adjustments for multiple biases as well as for random error. Repeating this random selection-and-adjustment process, we generate a frequency distribution of bias-adjusted estimates of the target parameter. This distribution can be summarized using percentiles, such as the median (the 50th percentile), and using intervals between percentiles. For example, the 2.5th and 97.5th percentiles of the distribution are the limits of an interval that contains 95% of the simulated estimates.

Percentiles and intervals from this distribution depict in a compact and accessible way the frequency of estimates obtained from repeated bias-adjustment for systematic errors (or both systematic and random errors) based on the priors. To distinguish them from confidence intervals, we will call them *simulation intervals*. Conventional confidence intervals implicitly assume absence of uncontrolled systematic error, and they usually cover the true value with much less than their stated frequency when this assumption is not approximately correct. In the latter case, if the priors used in probabilistic bias analysis assign high relative probability to the actual values of the bias parameters, the resulting simulation interval typically has better coverage of the true value than the corresponding conventional confidence interval.[125]

Suppose that our overall model of bias and random error is a good approximation to the actual data-generating process, that we have negligible background information about the target parameter, and that our distributions for the bias parameters fairly reflect our best information about the biases. The probabilistic bias analysis then provides a reasonable sense of where the target parameter is "most likely" to be, where "most likely" is meant in a Bayesian (betting) sense.[116] The final probabilistic bias analysis distribution incorporates biases judged potentially important and random error. It provides a sense of the total uncertainty about the target parameter that is warranted under the assumed models and distributions, given the data. This more complete sense of uncertainty stems from using a model that makes fewer assumptions than are used by conventional statistical methods, which neglect sources of bias, except possibly control for measured confounders.

Analysis of Uncontrolled Confounding

We will illustrate a probabilistic bias analysis of confounding by smoking, an unmeasured potential confounder, in the study of the association between occupational resins exposure and lung cancer mortality (Table 29-1). Multiple combinations of the bias parameters yielded the 18 adjusted estimates in Table 29-3. Our probabilistic bias analysis begins by assigning prior probability distributions to each of the bias parameters, which are the prevalence of smoking in those exposed to resins (P_{Z1}), the prevalence of smoking in those unexposed to resins (P_{Z0}), and the OR associating smoking with lung cancer mortality (OR_{DZ}).

As an initial simple illustration, we give P_{Z0} and P_{Z1} independent prior distributions that are uniform between 0.40 and 0.70. These bounds reflect that we know smoking prevalence among men in the United States was high (over 50%) during the time under study,[126] but we do not know how the study population differed from the general population, nor do we know how smoking was associated with exposure, if at all. To draw a uniform random number P between 0.40, 0.70, one can use a uniform random-number generator (available in most statistical software) to obtain a number u between 0 and 1 and then transform u to $p = 0.40 + (0.70 - 0.40)u = 0.4 + 0.3u$.

We emphasize that our use of independent uniform distributions is unrealistic. One problem is that the uniform distribution imposes sharp boundaries on supported (allowed) values, where in fact no sharp boundary exists, and makes the probabilities jump from 0 to a maximum value at those boundaries. Another problem is that the uniform distribution makes all supported values equally probable, when in fact there will be differences in plausibility among these values. We will describe later how to obtain more realistic distributions for proportions and how to deal with dependencies.

Our prior distribution for OR_{DZ} is log-normal with 95% limits of 5 and 15. To simulate from this distribution, at iteration i we draw $\ln(OR_{DZ,i})$ from a normal distribution with 95% limits of $\ln(5)$ and $\ln(15)$, reflecting our high certainty that the OR_{DZ} for the smoking indicator Z is between 5 and 15. The solid curve in Figure 29-1A shows the density of this distribution. The limits imply that the mean of this symmetrical distribution is $[\ln(15) + \ln(5)]/2 = 2.159$. Because the number of standard deviations between the upper and lower 95% limits is $2(1.96) = 3.92$, the standard deviation (SD) of this distribution is $[\ln(15) - \ln(5)]/3.92 = 0.280$. To draw a normal random number w with mean = 2.159 and SD = 0.280, one can use a standard (mean = 0, SD = 1) normal random-number generator (available in most software) to obtain a random standard normal deviate z and then transform z to $w = $ mean $+ z \cdot$ SD $= 2.159 + z(0.280)$. Finally, we use w as our draw of $\ln(OR_{DZ})$ and hence e^w as our draw of OR_{DZ}.

To generate a large number (K) of adjusted estimates based on the chosen distributions, we proceed as follows. At iteration i (where i goes from 1 to K), we execute the following steps:

1. For each bias parameter, draw a random value from its prior distribution: $P_{Z0,i}$ from a uniform (0.40, 0.70), $P_{Z1,i}$ from a uniform (0.40, 0.70), and $\ln(OR_{DZ,i})$ from a normal with mean = 2.159 and SD = 0.280.
2. Using the bias parameter values drawn in step 1, solve Equations 29-1 or 29-3 to obtain the corresponding $OR_{DX,i}$ bias-adjusted for smoking. Record this value.

Repeating steps 1 and 2 K times generates a frequency distribution of K bias-adjusted $OR_{DX,i}$. Ideally, K is chosen so that the simulated percentiles of most interest (such as the median OR_{DX}) are accurate to the number of digits used for presentation (e.g., three digits). This criterion may require far more iterations than needed to obtain sufficient accuracy for practical purposes, however.

In this example, after one simulation run of $K = 20,000$ iterations, the median $OR_{DX,i}$ equaled 1.77 with 95% simulation limits of 1.25 and 2.50, which have a ratio of 2.50/1.25 = 2.00. We use the ratio of limits to measure the width of the interval because the measure of association being simulated is itself a ratio measure. Note that this ratio of limits will vary with the chosen interval percentage. The limits and their ratio reflect only our uncertainty about the values assigned to the bias parameters, as modeled by their prior distributions. They can be contrasted with the conventional 95% confidence limits for OR_{DX} of 1.18 and 2.64, which have a ratio of 2.64/1.18 = 2.24. The similar ratios of limits reflect the fact that our priors induce uncertainty about confounding that is of a magnitude comparable with that for our uncertainty about random error.

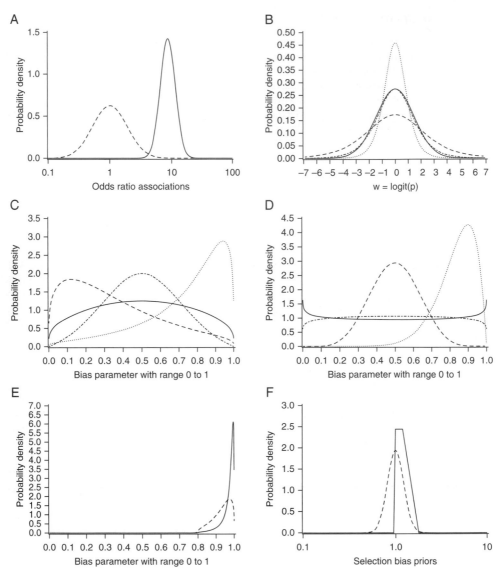

FIGURE 29-1 Probability densities for distributions discussed in text. **A,** Densities for unmeasured-confounding example (semilogarithmic plot): solid curve (——), normal prior for ln(OR_{DZ}) with mean [ln(15) + ln(5)]/2 = 2.159 and standard deviation 0.280; dashed curve (— —), normal prior for ln(OR_{XZ}) with mean 0 and standard deviation 0.639. **B,** Densities for logistic distributions of unbounded w with location m and scale factor s, where w = logit(P) and P is a proportion: solid curve (——), normal density $m = 0$ and standard deviation = $\sigma = s = 1.45$; dashed curve (– – –), logistic density with $m = 0$, $s = 0.8$, $\sigma = 0.8\pi/\sqrt{3} = 1.45$; mixed dashed curve (– – – ·), logistic density with $m = 0$ and $s = 0.5$; dotted curve (····), logistic density with $m = 0$ and $s = 0.3$. **C,** Densities for a proportion P with location m and scale factor s: solid curve (——), logit-logistic density with $m = 0$ and $s = 0.8$; dashed curve (– – –), logit-logistic density with m = logit(0.3) and $s = 0.8$; mixed dashed curve (– – – ·), logit-logistic density with $m = 0$ and $s = 0.5$; dotted curve (····), logit-logistic density with m = logit(0.8) and $s = 0.8$. **D,** Densities for a proportion P: solid curve (——), beta distribution with $\alpha = 0.9$ and $\beta = 0.9$; dashed curve (– – –), beta distribution with $\alpha = 7$ and $\beta = 7$; mixed dashed curve (– – – ·), beta distribution with $\alpha = 1.1$ and $\beta = 1.1$; dotted curve (····), beta distribution with $\alpha = 10$ and $\beta = 2$. **E,** Densities for misclassification example: solid curve (——), prior for sensitivity Se_i of resin exposure classification, where $Se_i = 0.8 + 0.2 \cdot \text{expit}(w)$ and w has a logistic distribution with m = logit(0.9) and $s = 0.8$; dashed curve (– – –), prior for specificity Sp_i of resin exposure classification, where $Sp_i = 0.8 + 0.2 \cdot \text{expit}(w)$ and w has a logistic distribution with m = logit(0.7) and $s = 0.8$. **F,** Densities for selection-bias example (semilogarithmic plot): dashed curve (– – –), normal prior for log selection-bias factor with mean ln(1) = 0 and standard deviation 0.207; solid curve (——), trapezoidal prior density for log selection-bias factor with b_l = –ln(0.95), b_u = –ln(1.8), m_l = –ln(1) = 0, m_u = –ln(1.2).

Incorporating Adjustment for Random Error

We next generate a distribution for OR_{DX} that incorporates two sources of uncertainty: confounding and random error. We take each adjusted $\ln(OR_{DX,i})$ and subtract from it a random error generated from a normal distribution with a standard deviation equal to the conventional standard deviation estimate for the log OR. From the equation in Chapter 17, that estimated standard deviation

is $SD = \sqrt{\dfrac{1}{45} + \dfrac{1}{94} + \dfrac{1}{257} + \dfrac{1}{945}} = 0.1944$. Thus, to incorporate independent random error into the

above simulation, we add a third step to each iteration:

1. Draw a number z_i from a standard normal distribution. Then construct a smoking and random error bias-adjusted OR

$$OR_{DX,i}^* = e^{\ln\left(OR_{DX,i}\right) - z_i \widehat{SD}} \qquad [29\text{-}17]$$

If we apply step 3 without steps 1 and 2, the resulting frequency distribution will adjust for random error only and its 2.5th and 97.5th percentiles will approach the conventional confidence limits (Figure 29-2A) as K grows large. As described above, repeating steps 1 and 2 without step 3 generates a distribution of $OR_{DX,i}$ that is bias-adjusted for smoking only. Repeating all three steps together generates a distribution of $OR_{DX,i}^*$ that is bias-adjusted for smoking and incorporates random error. After one simulation run of $K = 20,000$ iterations, the median $OR_{DX,i}^*$ equals 1.77 with 95% simulation limits 1.04 and 3.03, which have a ratio of 3.03/1.04 = 2.91. In contrast, the conventional 95% confidence limits for OR_{DX} have a ratio of 2.24, which is only 2.24/2.91 ≈ 77% that of the new ratio. The larger ratio of upper to lower limits from the three-step simulation reflects the fact that our priors allow for some uncertainty about a source of uncontrolled confounding. The simulation returns the conventional interval if in step 1 of our simulation we make $P_{Z1,i} = P_{Z0,i}$, for then smoking and exposure are unassociated in every iteration, and there is no confounding by smoking. In other words, the conventional interval is equivalent to a simulation interval that assumes that there is no uncontrolled confounding.

Step 3 as given above uses the same normal approximation to random error on the log OR scale as used in conventional statistics (see Chapters 16-18). An alternative that is sometimes easier to employ (particularly with the record-level adjustments described later) is *resampling*. At each iteration, before making the bias-adjustment in step 2, a new data set of the same size as the original is sampled with replacement from the original data set (separately for cases and controls in a case-control study, to maintain the original case and control numbers). The distribution of estimates obtained with this added step simultaneously bias-adjusts for the unmeasured confounder and incorporates random error, whereas the distribution of estimates from the original data bias-adjusts only for the unmeasured confounder. Rather than using the resampled data directly, more sophisticated *bootstrap* approaches use the resampled data to make adjustments for statistical biases as well as for random error.[127-129]

Building More Realistic Prior Distributions

The uniform distributions assigned to the prevalences P_{Z1} and P_{Z0} of smoking in exposed and unexposed assign the same probability to every possible pair of values for these prevalences. Thus, a 70% smoking prevalence in the exposed and 40% prevalence in the unexposed are assigned the same probability as a 50% prevalence for both. We have no basis for expecting that any difference actually existed, and we think that small differences are more likely than large ones. If we knew the smoking prevalence in one group, it would lead us to expect a similar prevalence in the other. Assignment of independent and uniform distributions to the prevalence of smoking bias parameters therefore corresponds poorly to our prior beliefs. As a result of placing overly high probabilities on large differences, the preceding simulation may exaggerate the uncertainty due to confounding. It may also understate uncertainty by excluding improbable—but possible—large values for the differences. One way to give higher probabilities to pairs with smaller differences, and thus more accurately reflect our uncertainty, is to generate the pairs so that the two prevalences are correlated. We will discuss generation of correlated pairs under misclassification.

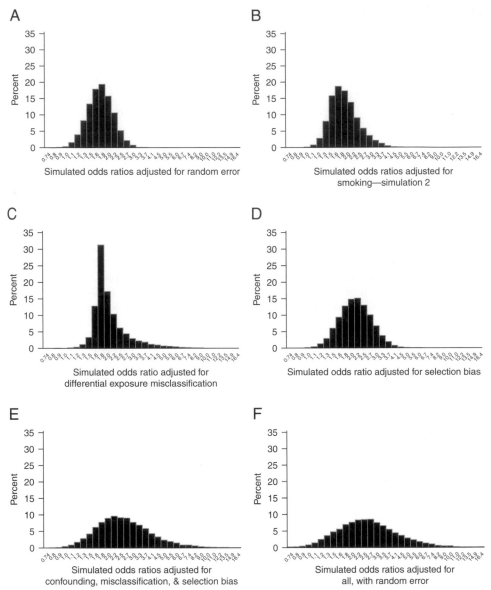

FIGURE 29-2 Histograms of simulation results ($K = 20,000$) from probabilistic bias analyses applied to the resins-lung cancer example. **A,** Adjustment for random error only: median = 1.77, 95% simulation limits = 1.18, 2.64 (equal to the conventional 95% confidence limits), ratio of limits = 2.24. **B,** Bias-adjustment for unmeasured confounding by smoking, without random error: median = 1.77, 95% simulation limits = 1.26, 3.06, ratio of limits = 2.43. **C,** Bias-adjustment for misclassification of resin exposure, without random error: median = 1.92, 95% simulation limits = 1.46, 4.90, ratio of limits = 3.36. **D,** Bias-adjustment for selection biases, without random error: median = 2.14, 95% simulation limits = 1.32, 3.57, ratio of limits = 2.70. **E,** Bias-adjustment for uncontrolled confounding by smoking, misclassification of resin exposure, and selection biases, without random error: median = 2.52, 95% simulation limits = 1.21, 7.54, ratio of limits = 6.23. **F,** Bias-adjustment for uncontrolled confounding by smoking, misclassification of resin exposure, and selection biases, with random error: median = 2.54, 95% simulation limits = 1.10, 7.82, ratio of limits = 7.11.

Another way to better represent our prior beliefs is to switch to a bias model in which it is reasonable to treat the bias parameters as independent.[120] Equation 29-3 is an example. Using this bias model, instead of sampling from a distribution for P_{Z1}, we sample from a distribution for OR_{XZ}, the exposure-confounder OR. Unlike with P_{Z1}, knowing OR_{XZ} will have little if any influence on our expectation for P_{Z0}, so giving OR_{XZ} and P_{Z0} independent priors is not unreasonable.

The sharp bounds of the uniform prior distributions assigned to P_{Z1} and P_{Z0} likewise impose sharp bounds on OR_{XZ}, excluding as impossible values those that are less than $(1 - 0.7)0.4/0.7(1 - 0.4) = 2/7$ or more than $0.7(1 - 0.4)/(1 - 0.7)0.4 = 7/2 = 3.5$. Because we do not know for certain that OR_{XZ} is within these bounds, we can better reflect our uncertainty by using a distribution that allows some chance of falling outside these bounds, which is a second advantage to a bias model that involves OR_{XZ} instead of both P_{Z1} and P_{Z0}. For illustration, suppose that we assign $\ln(OR_{XZ})$ a normal distribution with 95% prior limits at the extreme values from the uniform distributions for P_{Z1} and P_{Z0}, which are $\pm \ln[0.7(1 - 0.4)/(1 - 0.7)0.4] = \pm\ln(3.5)$. The mean of this normal distribution is 0, and the width of the 95% prior interval is $2\cdot\ln(3.5)$, so the SD is $2\cdot\ln(3.5)/3.92 = 0.639$. The dashed curve in Figure 29-1A shows the density of this distribution. We then replace step 1 above with 1′. For each bias parameter, draw a random value from its prior distribution: $P_{Z0,i}$ from a uniform distribution (0.40, 0.70), $\ln(OR_{XZ,i})$ from a normal distribution with mean = 0 and SD = 0.639, and $\ln(OR_{DZ,i})$ from a normal distribution with mean = 2.16 and SD = 0.280.

Repeating steps 1′ through 3 K times generates a new frequency distribution of K bias-adjusted $OR_{DX,i}$ (Figure 29-2B) and also a frequency distribution of K bias-adjusted $OR_{DX,i}$* that incorporate random errors as well. After one simulation run of $K = 20,000$ iterations, the median $OR_{DX,i}$* equaled 1.77 with 95% simulation limits 1.05 and 3.47, which have a ratio of $3.47/1.05 = 3.30$. The conventional 95% confidence limits for OR_{DX} have a ratio of $2.64/1.18 = 2.24$, which is only $2.24/3.30 \approx 2/3$ that of the new ratio. The earlier simulation limits based on unrealistic independent priors have a ratio of $3.03/1.04 = 2.91$, which is only $2.91/3.30 = 88\%$ that of the new ratio.

Analysis of Uncontrolled Confounding via Direct Bias Simulation

Confounding analyses are sometimes conducted by placing a prior directly on the amount of confounding in the conventional estimate.[55,130,131] For example, if earlier studies of the same association measured the confounder in question and reported both the unadjusted and adjusted estimates, the adjusted could be divided into the unadjusted to provide an estimate of the bias due to failing to adjust for the confounder[132]; one can also construct confidence intervals for this ratio.[133] These results and other considerations can be used as a basis for a prior on the size of the bias factor in a study that fails to adjust for the confounder.

Some Easily Generated Distributions

As mentioned earlier, the uniform is a rigid and unrealistic distribution. Although prior distributions are usually little more than educated guesses or bets about the parameters (hopefully reflecting relevant external data), flexible alternatives are needed to capture the rough distinctions that can be made (*e.g.*, among "likely," "probable," "reasonable," and "implausible" values). One alternative we have illustrated for log ORs is the normal distribution. This choice can be adequate if our uncertainty about the parameter can be approximated by a symmetric, unbounded, and peaked distribution. Often, however, our uncertainty is better represented by a distribution with asymmetries, boundaries, or broad areas of equally probable values. Although normal random numbers can be transformed to capture these properties, other distributions better suited for this purpose can be derived from uniform random numbers.

Logistic Distributions

Consider a number u generated from the uniform distribution between 0 and 1. Let m and s be any fixed numbers with $s > 0$, and let

$$w = m + s \bullet logit(u) \, where \, logit(u) = \ln(u) - \ln(1-u) \qquad [29\text{-}18]$$

The new random number w has what is known as a *logistic distribution* recentered at m and rescaled by s. It has mean, median, and mode at m, and scale s. Like a normal distribution, it is symmetric with an unbounded range, but it has heavier tails, reflected in the fact that the standard deviation of a logistic distribution is $\sigma = \dfrac{\pi}{\sqrt{3}}s \approx 1.81s$, or 81% larger than the scale factor s. In contrast, for a normal distribution, the standard deviation σ and the scale factor s are equal ($\sigma = s$), which is why elementary statistics books rarely distinguish the scale factor from the standard deviation. Figure 29-1B shows densities of logistic distributions for various choices of s, along with the density of a normal distribution with $\sigma = 1.81(0.8) \approx 1.45$ for comparison (solid curve). Relative to the normal, the logistic spreads mass from the center hump into the tails. Thus, a logistic prior can be used as an alternative to a normal prior when extreme values are not considered more probable than a normal prior makes them appear.

The logistic prior can be generalized further into recentered and rescaled log-F distributions (also known as generalized-conjugate distributions). These distributions can generate a large variety of shapes, including skew distributions, and can be extended further to encompass multiple correlated parameters.[134-136]

Transformation to Proportions and Bounded Variables

Now let $p = \text{expit}(w) = \dfrac{e^w}{1+e^w}$ where w has an unbounded distribution with median m, such as a normal, logistic, or log-F distribution. The new random number P has a distribution from 0 to 1 with median $\text{expit}(m)$. Consider first the special case in which w has a logistic distribution with $m = 0$. The distribution of P is then symmetric about 0.5 and is uniform if, in addition, $s = 1$. If $s < 1$, however, the distribution of P will give more probability to the middle values (near 0.5) than to extreme values (near 0 and 1), and if $s > 1$ it will give more probability to the extremes (near 0 and 1) than to the middle. For $s = 0.9$, the distribution of P is largely flat from 0.1 to 0.9, and then falls off, and for $s = 0.8$, the distribution of P is a rounded hill or semicircle between 0 and 1. As s gets smaller, the hill becomes less rounded and more peaked; for $s = 0.3$, the density of P becomes a bell curve between 0 and 1. Figure 29-1B shows the density of P for various choices of s when w is logistic and $m = 0$. We caution that for logistic distributions with $s > 1$ or normal distributions with $\sigma > 1.6$, the resulting density for P is bimodal.

With nonzero m, the distribution of P becomes skewed even if the starting distribution of $w = \text{logit}(P)$ is symmetric. Suppose that we start with a symmetric distribution for w that is determined by its median m and scale factor s, such as a normal or a logistic distribution. To skew the distribution of P to a median of, say, 0.3, we shift w by $m = \text{logit}(0.3)$, so that $w = m + s \cdot logit(u)$, where u is again uniform. Thus, starting from a uniform u, we get

$$ p = expit(w) = expit\big[\, m + s \cdot logit(u) \,\big] $$

Figure 29-1C shows the density of the distribution of P for $m = \text{logit}(0.3)$ with $s = 0.8$. If we take the logit of P, we get back the logistic or normal distribution that we started with. Therefore, by analogy with the term "log-normal" for a variable whose log has a normal distribution, we say that the distribution of $P = \text{expit}(w)$ is *logit-logistic* if w is logistic and *logit-normal* if w is normal.[137]

We can also shift and rescale the range of P to get yet another random number q that falls between a desired minimum (lower boundary) b_l and maximum (upper boundary) b_u, by setting $q = b_l + (b_u - b_l)p$. If $w - \text{logit}(P)$ has a distribution determined by its median m and scale factor s, four parameters specify the distribution of q: m, s, and the boundaries b_l and b_u. The median of q is then $b_l + (b_u - b_l)\text{expit}(m)$.

Trapezoidal Distributions

A *trapezoidal distribution* has as parameters a minimum (lower boundary) b_l, a maximum (upper boundary) b_u, a lower mode m_l, and an upper mode m_u. The minimum and maximum set the range of values allowed (supported) by the distribution, and the lower and upper modes set a zone of indifference in which all values are considered equally probable. The density of the distribution has a lower triangular tail sloping upward between b_l and m_l, a flat table between m_l and m_u, and an upper triangular tail sloping downward between m_u and b_u. The density is symmetric if $b_u - m_u = m_l - b_l$ and becomes more peaked as m_u and m_l become closer. In the extreme case with $m_l = m_u$, the density becomes triangular with a sharp peak at the modes. At the other extreme, at which the lower mode equals the minimum ($m_l = b_l$) and the upper mode equals the maximum ($m_u = b_u$), the density becomes uniform.

A trapezoidal random number t can be obtained from a random uniform $(0, 1)$ number u as follows:

Let $v = \sqrt{b_u + m_l + u(b_u + m_u - b_l - m_l)}$. Then

$$\text{(i)} \quad \text{If } m_l \leq v \leq m_u, \text{then } t = v$$

$$\text{(ii)} \quad \text{If } v < m_l, \text{then } t = b_l + \sqrt{(m_l - b_l)(2v - m_l - b_l)}$$

$$\text{(iii)} \quad \text{If } v > m_u, \text{then } t = b_u - \sqrt{2(b_u - m_u)(v - m_u)} \qquad [29\text{-}19]$$

The trapezoidal distribution is a useful candidate prior for logically bounded quantities such as proportions and for other quantities when one is comfortable with placing sharp lower and upper bounds on the possible values. Uncertainty about the bounds to use can be accommodated by setting those bounds very wide to accommodate all remotely reasonable possibilities, thus making the tails long (*i.e.*, making $m_1 - b_1$ and $b_u - m_u$ large relative to $m_u - m_1$).

Beta Distributions

The beta distribution provides a second probability density function that takes on a wide range of shapes. It is especially well suited for assignment to proportions—such as sensitivity, specificity, or predictive values—because it is constrained to the interval $(0,1)$. The beta distribution is parameterized by two positive shape parameters, often denoted as α and β. The expected value of a random variable X drawn from a beta distribution and its variance are:

$$E(X) = \frac{\alpha}{\alpha + \beta}$$

$$Var(X) = \frac{\alpha\beta}{(\alpha + \beta)^2 (\alpha + \beta + 1)} \qquad [29\text{-}20]$$

With α and β both set equal to 1.1, the beta distribution yields a near uniform density, but without the sharp boundaries of the uniform distribution. With α and β both set equal to 7, the beta distribution yields a symmetric density like the normal distribution. With α and β set to different values, the beta distribution yields asymmetric densities centered on different means. In general, if α and β are both less than 1, then the density distribution will be u-shaped, giving more weight to values at the tails than values at the center. If α and β are both greater than 1, then the density distribution will be unimodal, giving more weight to values at the center than values at the tails. Figure 29-1D illustrates the wide variety of shapes that can be generated using the beta distribution.

The beta distribution addresses many of the shortcomings of some of the other distributions. Unlike the uniform and trapezoidal distributions, the beta distribution does not yield sharp boundaries (except at 0 and 1). Unlike the normal distribution, the beta distribution does not yield values outside of an allowed range (such as proportions less than zero or greater than one). A shortcoming of the beta distribution is that the connection between the desired density shape and the values assigned to α and β are not always directly apparent, except for proportions informed by observed counts. In general, for a classification parameter (sensitivity, specificity, positive predictive value, or negative predictive value), one can use the observed counts from a validation study to assign values to the beta distribution parameters. For example, to parameterize the sensitivity of classification, one can set α equal to the number of test positives and β equal to the number of test negatives. This method adopts the results of the validation study to parameterize directly the beta distribution, and therefore, it should be implemented only after consideration of the direct applicability of the validation study results to the classification problem at hand. For example, if a validation substudy of resin exposure in our example found that among workers truly exposed to resin, 15 were correctly categorized as resin exposed and 2 were incorrectly classified as resin unexposed, the sensitivity would be 15/17 ~ 88% with Wald 95% CI: 73% to 100%. If we used these data to directly inform a beta distribution, it would be of the form: $sens \sim beta(\alpha = 15, \beta = 2)$. Using Equation 29-20 for mean and variance, we find this distribution has a mean of 15/(15 + 2) = 0.88

and a standard deviation of 0.08 resulting in a Wald 95% interval of 0.73, 1.00. The beta specification matches our initial results well.

When one wishes to parameterize the beta distribution less directly, an approximate guide for choosing values for α and β is to specify a range of likely values with minimum = a, maximum = b, and mean = x. The minimum and maximum values can be substituted for confidence limits to solve for the standard deviation. Continuing with the example, we could specify $a = 0.73$ and $b = 1.00$ along with $x = 0.88$, so $sd = \dfrac{1.00 - 0.73}{3.92} = 0.07$. Given the estimated mean (x) and standard deviation (sd), we can solve for α and β with the following equations:

$$\alpha = x\left[\frac{x(1-x)}{sd^2} - 1\right]$$

$$\beta = (1-x)\left[\frac{x(1-x)}{sd^2} - 1\right]$$

Using these equations with this example yields $\alpha = 18.7$ and $\beta = 2.5$, which are close to the actual shape parameters ($\alpha = 15$, $\beta = 2$).

Generating Dependent Variables

So far, we have discussed only use of independent distributions for the different bias parameters. For realism, however, it is sometimes essential to build dependence into these distributions. Earlier we noted that the prevalences of smoking in those exposed to resins (P_{Z1}) and in those unexposed to resins (P_{Z0}) were likely similar, although both may have been in a wide range (we used 0.4-0.7). More generally, when considering analogous classification or selection probabilities across different subgroups (*e.g.*, cases and controls, men and women), it is often unrealistic to consider the probabilities to be equal (nondifferential) across the subgroups, but it is usually even more unrealistic to pretend that they are completely unrelated, for we often expect these probabilities to be similar across the subgroups. Even if we think that they are not necessarily close together, finding evidence that a probability of misclassification (or of refusal) is high in one subgroup will lead us to think that it is high in other subgroups. In other words, we usually expect analogous bias parameters to be positively associated across subgroups.

If we can translate the degree of association we expect between two unknown parameters π and τ into a correlation coefficient r, there is a simple way to generate pairs of random draws of π and τ that have that correlation. At each iteration, we first generate three (instead of two) independent random numbers, labeled h_1, h_2, and h_3. These three numbers need not come from the same distribution; all that matters is that they are drawn independently and have the same variance. Then the pair of random numbers

$$g_1 = h_1\sqrt{r} + h_2\sqrt{1-r}$$
$$g_2 = h_1\sqrt{r} + h_3\sqrt{1-r} \qquad\qquad [29\text{-}21]$$

will have correlation r across the iterations. Now g_1 and g_2 may not have the location, spread, or shape desired for the π and the τ distributions (*i.e.*, they might not have the desired mean and standard deviation, or the desired bounds, or desired modes). If, however, the h_k are all drawn from distributions with mean 0 and variance 1, then g_1 and g_2 will also have mean 0 and variance 1; in that case, to get different means μ_1, μ_2 and variances σ_1^2, σ_2^2 for the pair members, we use instead $\mu_1 + \sigma_1 g_1$, $\mu_2 + \sigma_2 g_2$, which will still have correlation r. For this reason, it is often easiest to start with distributions for h_k that have means of 0 and variances of 1 and then transform the output pair to have the desired means and variances. This approach can be generalized to create multiple correlated parameters via hierarchical modeling.[12,95]

Use of Equation 29-20 will be illustrated in application to differential misclassification adjustment in the probabilistic bias analysis example. If the inputs h_k are normal, the output pair g_1 and g_2

will also be normal. If the inputs h_k have the same distribution (*e.g.*, all logistic or all trapezoidal), the distributions of the outputs g_1 and g_2 will tend to have a more normal shape than the inputs. When using Equation 29-21 with nonnormal inputs, one should create histograms of the final generated variables to check that they have distributions that match well enough the expected shape of the assigned density distribution, which is good practice for draws from distributions assigned to any parameter of a bias model.[10] If we require nonnormality of one or both of the final pair members, we can transform g_1 or g_2 or both in a nonlinear fashion. For example, starting with normal g_1 and g_2, we could use $\exp(g_1)$ and $\text{expit}(g_2)$ to obtain a final pair with $\exp(g_1)$ a positive log-normal number and $\text{expit}(g_2)$ a logit-normal number between 0 and 1. Nonlinear transforms sometimes have little effect on the final pair correlation if r is positive, but they can be changed dramatically by certain transformations.[138] Hence, if nonlinear transforms are used, one should check the actual correlation as well as means and variances of the final pairs generated.

Analysis of Misclassification

Consider again Table 29-4, which shows the results of our initial sensitivity analysis of the bias analysis of resin exposure misclassification. The four bias parameters that govern these results are the sensitivities and specificities of exposure classification among cases and controls. For a probabilistic bias analysis of misclassification paralleling Table 29-4, one needs to assign prior distributions to the four bias parameters. A simple way to use the simulation draws from these distributions is as follows: at each iteration, the misclassification-adjusted counts B_{1i}, B_{0i}, A_{1i}, and A_{0i} are derived from Se_i and Sp_i using Equations 29-7 and 29-8. The misclassification-adjusted OR estimate from iteration i is then $OR_{DX,i} = A_{1i} B_{0i}/A_{0i} B_{1i}$. Finally, Equations 29-7 and 29-8 are applied iteratively using draws from these distributions.

Nondifferential Misclassification

To continue the resins-lung cancer example assuming nondifferential misclassification, at each iteration we draw two independent uniform random numbers u_1, u_2 and transform them to logistic draws $g_1 = \text{logit}(0.9) + 0.8 \cdot \text{logit}(u_1)$ and $g_2 = \text{logit}(0.7) + 0.8 \cdot \text{logit}(u_2)$. We then set

$$Se_i = 0.8 + 0.2\,expit\!\left(g_1\right) \quad \text{and}$$
$$Sp_i = 0.8 + 0.2\,expit\!\left(g_2\right)$$

which force Se_i and Sp_i to lie between 0.8 and 1, with a median of $0.8 + 0.2(0.9) = 0.98$ for Se_i and a median of $0.8 + 0.2(0.7) = 0.94$ for Sp_i. Figure 29-1E shows the resulting densities for Se_i and Sp_i. After one simulation run of $K = 20{,}000$ iterations, the median $OR_{DX,i}$ adjusted for nondifferential misclassification is 2.01, and the 95% simulation limits are 1.78 and 4.71, which have a ratio of 2.65. This ratio is 18% greater than the ratio of the conventional confidence limits. As in the confounding examples, one can also account for random error by applying Equation 29-17 (step 3) to generate $OR^*_{DX,i}$ from the $OR_{DX,i}$. With random error added, the median $OR^*_{DX,i}$ is 2.10 and the 95% simulation limits are 1.32 and 4.99, which have a ratio of 3.78. These limits are shifted upward relative to the conventional limits of 1.18 and 2.64, and have a ratio about 70% greater than that of the conventional limits. This shift arises because the assumed exposure misclassification is nondifferential, and other, downward sources of bias are not included in the bias-adjustment model.

Treatment of Negative Cell Frequencies Yielded by Bias-Adjustment

To avoid negative bias-adjusted cell frequencies, the prior distributions for sensitivity and specificity must be bounded by $Se \geq B_1^*/M_0$ and $Sp \geq B_0^*/M_0$ among noncases and by $Se \geq A_1^*/M_1$ and $Sp \geq A_0^*/M_1$ among cases. If a distribution is used that extends into the region of negative adjustment (*i.e.*, if it allows draws that violate any of these inequalities), there are several options. If one regards the region as a reasonable possibility and regards the prior distribution as fair, one may set the negative counts to 0 and then tally the resulting 0 or infinite ORs in the final simulation percentiles. On the other hand, if one does not regard the region as realistic, one can either revise the prior distribution to fall above the region or let the simulation do this revision automatically by having it discard draws that fall in the region.

If draws are discarded, the result is the same as using a distribution that is truncated at the point where the region of negative adjustments begins. One should thus check whether the resulting truncated distribution still appears satisfactory by plotting the histogram of draws against the density assigned to the bias parameter. As an example, Fox et al. (2005) used trapezoidal prior distributions for the parameters in the resins-lung cancer example.[139] For nondifferential misclassification scenarios, at iteration i, Fox et al. independently drew a sensitivity Se_i and a specificity Sp_i from a trapezoidal distribution with $b_1 = 75\%$, $b_u = 100\%$, $m_1 = 85\%$, and $m_u = 95\%$. This distribution results in negative adjusted counts when $Sp_i \leq B_0^*/M_0 = 945/1{,}202 = 0.786$. Discarding these draws (as Fox et al. did) truncates the distribution at 0.786, so that the actual simulation distribution is no longer trapezoidal. Instead, the probability of $Sp < 0.786$ is 0. The resulting prior density jumps from 0 to about $(0.786-0.75)/(0.85-0.75) \approx 40\%$ of its maximum at 0.786 and continues upward, paralleling the original trapezoidal density.

Using this truncated prior, the median bias-adjusted OR obtained by Fox et al. was 2.5, with 95% simulation limits of 1.7 and 14 before accounting for random error and limits of 1.4 and 15 (ratio $15/1.7 \approx 9$) after accounting for random error. The distribution assigned to sensitivity and specificity was meant to parallel the fixed values used in Table 29-4, rather than to reflect actual prior beliefs about the values that ought to be assigned to the sensitivities and specificities. As a consequence, all of the bias-adjusted ORs from the earlier sensitivity analysis of the bias analysis that assumed nondifferential misclassification (the descending diagonal of Table 29-4) fall within the 95% simulation limits.

Record-Level Adjustment

To obtain their results, Fox et al. (2005) used a simulation procedure more complex but approximately equivalent to the one based on Equations 29-7 and 29-8.[139] At each iteration, the adjusted counts $A_{1,i}$ and $B_{1,i}$ derived from Se_i and Sp_i are used to compute the prevalences among cases and controls, and then predictive values are estimated from Equations 29-9 and 29-10. For each data record, these predictive values are used to impute the "true" value of exposure from the observed misclassified value. The resulting bias-adjusted data set at iteration i is then used to compute a bias-adjusted OR. The advantage of this procedure is that it retains the same form even if further adjustments are needed (*e.g.*, for age, sex, and other confounders recorded in the data). It also parallels multiple imputation for measurement-error adjustment based on validation data,[140] and so it is easily combined with imputations for missing data. The disadvantage is that it can be computationally demanding,[141] because it requires construction of a new data set at each iteration.

Differential Misclassification

To allow for differential misclassification, we must generate separate sensitivities $Se_{1,i}$, $Se_{0,i}$ and separate specificities $Sp_{1,i}$, $Sp_{0,i}$ for cases and controls. In doing so, however, we must note that case sensitivities are not a priori independent of the control sensitivities, nor are the case specificities a priori independent of the control specificities, and take these facts into account in the simulations. For example, if we found out the sensitivity and specificity for the controls, the information would definitely influence the distributions we would assign to the case sensitivity and specificity. One way to address this dependence in the resins-lung cancer example is as follows. At each iteration i, we:

1. Draw three independent uniform random numbers u_1, u_2, and u_3, transform them to logistic numbers $h_k = \text{logit}(0.9) + 0.8 \cdot \text{logit}(u_k)$, and use Equation 29-21 to generate pairs of numbers g_1 and g_2 from the h_k, with correlation $r = 0.8$. We then set

$$Se_{1,i} = 0.8 + 0.2expit(g_1) \quad \text{and}$$
$$Se_{0,1} = 0.8 + 0.2expit(g_2)$$

2. Draw three more independent uniform random numbers u_4, u_5, and u_6, transform them to logistic numbers $h_k = \text{logit}(0.7) + 0.8 \cdot \text{logit}(u_k)$, and use Equation 29-21 to generate pairs of numbers g_3 and g_4 from the h_k, with correlation $r = 0.8$. We then set

$$Sp_{1,i} = 0.8 + 0.2expit(g_3) \quad \text{and}$$
$$Sp_{0,1} = 0.8 + 0.2expit(g_4)$$

$Se_{1,i}$, $Sp_{1,i}$ are then used to bias-adjust the case counts via Equation 29-8, and $Se_{0,i}$, $Sp_{0,i}$ are used to bias-adjust the control counts via Equation 29-7.

After one simulation run of $K = 20,000$ iterations, the correlation of $Se_{1,i}$ and $Se_{0,i}$ was 0.76 and the correlation of $Sp_{1,i}$ and $Sp_{0,i}$ was 0.78. The median $OR_{DX,i}$ was 1.92 and the 95% simulation limits were 1.46 and 4.90, which have a ratio of 3.36 (Figure 29-2C). This ratio is $3.36/2.24 \approx 1.5$ times larger than the ratio of the conventional limits and is $3.36/2.65 \approx 1.27$ times larger than the ratio of the limits from the nondifferential simulations. Upon adding random error using Equation 29-17, the median $OR^*_{DX,i}$ is 2.01 and the 95% simulation limits are 1.20 and 5.13, which have a ratio of 4.28. This ratio is $4.28/3.36 \approx 1.27$ times larger than that without random error.

We use the same classification priors for cases and controls, because in this study we have no basis for presuming that any difference exists. By generating separately the parameters for cases and controls with a correlation less than 1, however, we produce a limited and random degree of differentiality at each draw. The distribution of differentiality is partially controlled by the correlation parameter r, with less differentiality expected as r approaches 1. With the same priors for cases and controls, a correlation of 1 corresponds to nondifferentiality, because it would make $g_1 = g_2$ and $g_3 = g_4$ and thus yield the same sensitivity and specificity for cases and controls at every iteration. The distribution of differentiality is also controlled by the final transformation to sensitivity and specificity, with less differentiality expected as the bounds become narrower. Equality of the distributions for cases and controls simply reflects our ignorance about how differentiality might have occurred, if it occurred.

Had the exposure histories been based on subject recall rather than on records, we would have made the case sensitivity distribution higher and the case specificity distribution lower relative to the control distributions, to reflect in our priors some expectation of recall bias. A more-detailed model for the underlying continuous exposure measurement could also lead to a difference in the case and control distributions for sensitivity and specificity, even if the continuous error distribution was the same for both cases and controls.[142]

The sensitivity distribution is set higher than the specificity distribution because the dichotomy into exposed versus unexposed corresponds to positive exposure versus no exposure in the original quantitative exposure evaluation. It thus favors sensitivity over specificity. If a very high cutpoint is used, the sensitivity distribution might be set lower than the specificity distribution.

Both the differential and nondifferential results are more compatible with larger ORs than the conventional result. One should bear in mind that disagreements are due entirely to the different priors underlying the analyses. The conventional result assumes perfect classification and gives a result equivalent to a simulation in which the prior probability that Se = Sp = 1 is 100%. In contrast, our simulations allow for the possibility that both false-positive and false-negative exposure misclassification might be common. One's preferences should depend on which priors better reflect one's own judgment about the mechanisms of exposure classification that generated Table 29-1.

In all the preceding simulations, sensitivities were generated independently of specificities. An assumption of independence might be justified if there were forces that move the correlation of sensitivity with specificity in the positive direction, other forces that moved the correlation in the negative direction, and we do not know the relative strength of these forces.[12] As an upward force on the correlation, the association of the original quantitative exposure assessment with true exposure level is unknown: If it is high, then both sensitivity and specificity will be high, and if it is low, then both sensitivity and specificity will be low. As a downward force, sensitivity will decline and specificity will increase as the cutpoint chosen for dichotomization is increased. An ideal analysis would attempt to model the relative contribution of these forces to the final correlation. In the present example, however, the cutpoint is known and is at its minimum; hence, arguably the downward force is eliminated and sensitivity and specificity should have been given a positive correlation.

Analysis of Selection Bias

As noted earlier, when the factors affecting selection are measured on all study subjects and are not affected by exposure or disease, the selection bias produced by the factors can be controlled by adjusting for the factors. Thus, if such a factor Z is unmeasured but we can assign prior distributions to its prevalence and its associations with exposure and disease, we can conduct a probabilistic bias analysis of selection bias using the equations presented earlier for analysis of confounding. When selection bias arises because exposure X affects Z and Z influences selection, the inverse of

Equation 29-3 gives the selection bias produced by stratifying on Z. If Z is measured, the quantities OR_{DZ} and OR_{XZ} can be estimated from the data, and the simulation requires only a prior on the prevalence of $Z = 1$ within one of the exposure-disease combinations, for example, prevalence odds O_{Z0} among the unexposed noncases. If Z is unmeasured, however, priors on OR_{DZ} and OR_{XZ} will be needed as well.

If data are available that indicate the size of the selection bias factor $S_{Aj}S_{B0}/S_{A0}S_{Bj}$ in Equation 29-16, they can be used to create a prior directly for this factor. Draws from this prior are then divided into the OR estimate to provide a selection-bias-adjusted estimate from that iteration. This approach generalizes easily to regression-model coefficients.[95]

Consider again the resins-lung cancer example. In this study, 71 of 210 (34%) lung cancer cases and 787 of 1,989 (40%) control deaths were omitted from the analysis because of lack of adequate job records for exposure reconstruction, due mostly to routine record disposal during the history of the facility under study.[41] If lack of records was strongly related to both resin exposure and cause of death, considerable selection bias could result. The magnitude could be bounded by the (absurd) extremes in which either all 71 missing cases were exposed and all 787 missing controls were unexposed, which yields a bias factor of $45(945)/[(45 + 71)(945 + 787)] = 0.21$, or all 71 missing cases were unexposed and all 787 missing controls were exposed, which yields a bias factor of $[(94 + 71)(257 + 787)]/94(257) = 7.1$.

Because we see only a small association between lack of records and cause of death, we expect the bias (if any) from lack of records to be small; hence, these bounds are of no help. Instead, we assign a normal prior to the component of bias in the log OR due to missing records with mean 0 (no bias) and standard deviation 0.207 (Figure 29-1F, dashed curve), which yields 95% prior probability of the bias factor falling between $e^{\pm1.96 \cdot 0.207} = 0.67$ and 1.5, and 2:1 odds of the factor falling between $e^{\pm0.97 \cdot 0.207} = 0.82$ and 1.22. Draws z from a standard normal distribution are thus used to bias-adjust the resin-lung cancer OR by dividing $e^{z \cdot 0.207}$ into the OR. A more thorough analysis would attempt to relate lack of records to dates of employment, trends in resin use, and trends in mortality from lung cancer and the control diseases (lack of records was far more frequent among earlier employees than later employees and was modestly associated with the cause of death).

Other sources of selection bias include use of lung cancer deaths as a substitute for incident cases and use of other deaths as controls. To build a prior distribution for these sources, assume for the moment that lack of records is not a source of bias. Given the relative socioeconomic homogeneity of the underlying occupational cohort, we expect similar survival rates among the exposed and unexposed, making it plausible that the use of deaths for cases produced little bias. Thus, we neglect case-selection bias, that is, we assume that $S_{A1} \approx S_{A0}$. On the other hand, use of other deaths as controls is suspect. For example, if resins exposure is positively associated with death from these control causes of deaths, controls will exhibit too much exposure relative to the source population (i.e., $S_{B1} > S_{B0}$), leading to $S_{B0}/S_{B1} \approx S_{A1}S_{B0}/S_{A0}S_{B1} < 1$ if $S_{A1} \approx S_{A0}$. Furthermore, if resin association with control deaths were the sole source of selection bias, the inverse of this bias factor, S_{B1}/S_{B0}, would equal the rate ratio for that association (for related discussion, see "Number of Control Groups" in Chapter 8). Thus, a prior for the control selection bias in this example is approximated by a prior for the inverse of the OR relating resin exposure to the control causes of death. Equivalently, a prior for the log selection-bias factor is approximated by the negative of the prior for the log OR relating exposure to control deaths.

The control deaths were primarily from cardiovascular causes, which were chosen based on a prior that assigned low probability to an association with the study exposures. Even if there were an association, occupational factors for cardiovascular deaths usually have small ratios (less than smoking-cardiovascular disease rate ratios, which are typically on the order of 2), as one would expect owing to the high frequency and heterogeneity of cardiovascular deaths. To approximately capture these ideas, we assign a trapezoidal prior to the log selection-bias factor for control selection bias, with $b_1 = -\ln(.95)$, $b_u = -\ln(1.8)$, $m_1 = -\ln(1) = 0$, and $m_u = -\ln(1.2)$ (Figure 29-1F, solid). Draws w from this distribution are then used to adjust the resin-lung cancer OR by dividing e^w into the OR.

Combining the two selection-bias-adjustments under the assumption of independence of the sources, at each iteration we draw a standard normal z and a trapezoidal w and then divide the resin-lung cancer OR by $e^{z \cdot 0.207 + w}$. After one simulation run with $K = 20,000$ iterations, the median $OR_{DX,i}$ is 2.14 and the 95% simulation limits are 1.32 and 3.57, which have a ratio of 2.70 (Figure 29-2D).

This ratio is $2.70/2.24 \approx 1.21$ times larger than the ratio of the conventional limits. After accounting for random error using Equation 29-17, the median $OR^*_{DX,i}$ is 2.15 and the 95% simulation limits are 1.14 and 4.14, which have a ratio 3.63, which is $3.63/2.24 \approx 1.62$ times larger than the ratio of the conventional limits. The conventional limits are obtained from a simulation in which the priors for both selection-bias factors assign 100% probability to 1 (no bias).

Comparative and Combined Analyses

Table 29-5 summarizes the results of the probabilistic bias analyses given here. With the example prior distributions, it appears that random error, confounding, and selection bias make similar contributions to uncertainty about the resins-lung cancer OR, whereas exposure classification errors are a somewhat larger source of uncertainty.

Extension of these methods to multiple probabilistic bias analyses is straightforward if the parameters from each source of bias (confounding, exposure misclassification, disease misclassification, confounder misclassification, selection bias) can be treated as if they are independent. An important caution is that, even if the parameters from each source are independent, the order of adjustment can still matter if misclassification adjustment is made. As discussed earlier, adjustments should be made in reverse order of their occurrence. Thus, some misclassification adjustments may come before selection-bias-adjustments, whereas others may come after.

If all the tabular data counts are large and random error is independent of the bias parameters, the order in which random error is added will usually not matter much, especially when (as in the present example) random error turns out to be small compared with systematic errors. Nonetheless, the sensitivity of random-error adjustment to order can be investigated by comparing results from resampling the data first, versus adding random error last as in Equation 29-17. No ordering is universally justified, however, because random variation can occur at any stage of the data-generating process. Exposure and disease occurrence have random components (which lead to random components in confounding), and selection and classification errors have random components. An ideal analysis would also model these sources separately, although again, given large enough data counts, their combination into one step may have little effect.

In the resins-lung cancer example, we assume that the study problems occurred in the order of confounding, selection bias, and misclassification. Thus, at each iteration of our multiple-bias analysis, we

1. Draw sensitivities and specificities to bias-adjust the OR for misclassification.
2. Draw the selection-bias factors to bias-adjust this misclassification-adjusted OR.
3. Draw the independent confounding parameters P_{Z0}, OR_{DZ}, and OR_{XZ}, to create a confounding factor to bias-adjust the OR bias-adjusted for misclassification and selection.

We use the priors illustrated earlier, allowing differential misclassification. After one simulation run of $K = 20,000$ iterations, the resulting median $OR_{DX,i}$ is 2.52 and the 95% simulation limits are 1.21 and 7.54, which have a ratio of 6.23 (Figure 29-2E). This ratio is $6.23/2.24 \approx 2.8$ times larger than the ratio of conventional limits, demonstrating that random error is of far less importance than total bias uncertainty under our priors. Adding random error using Equation 29-17 gives a median $OR^*_{DX,i}$ of 2.54 and 95% simulation limits of 1.10 and 7.82, which have a ratio of 7.11 (Figure 29-2F). This ratio is $7.11/2.24 \approx 3.2$ times larger than the ratio of conventional limits, demonstrating that the conventional limits grossly understate the uncertainty one should have if one accepts our priors.

Figures 29-2A to D display the separate sources of uncertainty that contributed to the final bias assessment in Figure 29-2F. Other sets of priors could give very different results. Nonetheless, we expect that any set of priors that is reasonably consistent with the limited study design (a record-based mortality case-control study in an occupational cohort) will also yield a combined simulation interval that is much wider than the conventional confidence interval, because the simulation interval will incorporate uncertainty about biases as well as random error.

The priors we chose did lead to a point of agreement with the conventional analysis: both analyses suggest that workplace exposure to resins is positively associated with lung cancer in the underlying cohort. In our final combined assessment, the proportion of simulations in which the adjusted OR estimate fell below 1 was 0.014; the analogous conventional statistic is the upper-tailed P-value

TABLE 29-5

Summary of Results From Monte-Carlo Analyses of Biases in the Study of Occupational Resins Exposure (*X*) and Lung Cancer Mortality (Table 29-1)

Bias Model	Without Incorporating Random Error			With Random Error Incorporated		
	Median	2.5th and 97.5th Percentiles	Ratio of Limits	Median	2.5th and 97.5th Percentiles	Ratio of Limits
1. None (conventional)	1.77	1.77, 1.77	1.00	1.77	1.18, 2.64	2.24
2. P_{Z0} and $P_{Z1} \sim$ uniform (0.4, 0.7); $\ln(OR_{DZ}) \sim$ normal(2.159, 0.280)	1.77	1.25, 2.50	2.00	1.77	1.04, 3.03	2.91
3. $P_{Z0} \sim$ uniform (0.4, 0.7); $\ln(OR_{XZ}) \sim$ normal(0, 0.639); $\ln(OR_{DZ}) \sim$ normal(2.159, 0.280)	1.77	1.26, 3.06	2.43	1.80	1.05, 3.47	3.30
4. $Se = 0.8 + 0.2 \cdot \text{expit}(g_1)$ and $Sp = 0.8 + 0.2 \cdot \text{expit}(g_2)$, where $g_1 = \text{logit}(0.9) + 0.8 \cdot \text{logit}(u_1)$ and $g_2 = \text{logit}(0.7) + 0.8 \cdot \text{logit}(u_2)$ and u_1 and $u_2 \sim$ uniform(0, 1)	2.01	1.78, 4.71	2.65	2.10	1.32, 4.99	3.78
5. $Se_1 = 0.8 + 0.2 \cdot \text{expit}(g_1)$ and $Se_0 = 0.8 + 0.2 \cdot \text{expit}(g_2)$, where g_1 and $g_2 = \text{logit}(0.9) + 0.8 \cdot \text{logit}(u_k)$ with $r = 0.8$; $Sp_1 = 0.8 + 0.2 \cdot \text{expit}(g_3)$ and $Sp_0 = 0.8 + 0.2 \cdot \text{expit}(g_4)$, where g_3 and $g_4 = \text{logit}(0.7) + 0.8 \cdot \text{logit}(u_k)$ with $r = 0.8$, and $u_k \sim$ uniform(0, 1)	1.92	1.46, 4.90	3.36	2.01	1.20, 5.13	4.28
6. $\ln(S_{A0}S_{B0}/S_{A0}S_{B1}) \sim 0.207z +$ trapezoidal with $b_1 = -\ln(0.95)$, $b_u = -\ln(1.8)$, $m_1 = -\ln(1)$ and $m_u = -\ln(1.2)$	2.14	1.32, 3.57	2.70	2.15	1.14, 4.14	3.63
7. Combined in order 5, then 6, and then 3	2.52	1.21, 7.54	6.23	2.54	1.10, 7.82	7.11

for testing $OR_{DX} \leq 1$, which from Table 29-1 is 0.002. We emphasize, however, that this degree of agreement with the conventional result might not arise from bias analyses with other defensible sets of priors.

Our assessment assumed independence among the different sources of uncertainty (random error, confounding, misclassification, and selection bias). Parameter dependencies within and between the different steps (1-3) can be accommodated by inducing correlations using Equation 29-20. Our ability to specify such correlations knowledgeably is often limited. Nonetheless, information about the mechanisms responsible for the correlations is often available; for example, vitamin intakes estimated from food-intake data have substantially correlated errors owing to the errors in capturing food and supplement consumption. Hierarchical models can be used to capture available information about such correlations.[12,95]

Bayesian and Semi-Bayesian Analysis

Bayesian approaches to bias analysis begin with a bias model as used in a sensitivity analysis, then add prior distributions for the bias parameters. Thus, they involve the same initial work, inputs, and assumptions as probabilistic bias analysis. They may also employ prior distributions for other parameters in the analysis, such as one for the effect under study. If all parameters are given an explicit prior, the analysis is fully Bayesian; otherwise, it is semi-Bayesian. To describe these methods, we will use the term *distribution* to refer to what is technically known as a probability density or mass function.

If only the bias parameters are given explicit priors, the only difference between semi-Bayesian analysis and probabilistic bias analysis is in the ensuing computations. To outline the differences, suppose that:

- Y represents the observed data under analysis; above, Y represents the four counts in Table 29-1.
- β represents all the bias parameters; above, β would contain the parameters involving an unmeasured confounder, sensitivities, and specificities, and selection-bias factors.
- α represents all other parameters in the problem; above, α would contain the effect of interest (the log OR adjusted for all bias and random error) and the true exposure prevalence.
- $P(\beta)$ represents the joint prior distribution of the bias parameters; if, as above, parameters for different bias sources are given independent priors, $P(\beta)$ is just the product of all the bias-prior distributions.
- $P(\varepsilon)$ represents the assumed distribution of random errors; above, $P(\varepsilon)$ was approximated by a normal distribution on the log OR scale.

A probabilistic bias analysis iterates through draws of the bias parameters β from their prior $P(\beta)$, along with draws of random errors ε from $P(\varepsilon)$, then plots or tabulates the adjusted results, as in Table 29-5. It is thus a simple extension of classical bias and sensitivity analysis using priors to choose the possible bias-parameter values and adding random-error adjustment.

In contrast, a Monte-Carlo Bayesian analysis iterates through draws of all parameters from the joint *posterior distribution* $P(\alpha,\beta|Y)$ for both α and β. From Bayes's theorem, the posterior $P(\alpha,\beta|Y)$ is proportional to $P(Y|\alpha,\beta)P(\alpha,\beta)$, where $P(\alpha,\beta)$ is the joint prior distribution for α and β and $P(Y|\alpha,\beta)$ is the probability of seeing the data Y given the parameters α and β. The latter data probability is a function of α, β, and the random-error distribution $P(\varepsilon)$. In a semi-Bayesian bias analysis, all values of α are taken to have equal prior probability, in that $P(\alpha,\beta)$ is assumed to equal $P(\beta)$; that is, a "noninformative" prior for α is assumed. The semi-Bayesian posterior distribution is thus proportional to $P(Y|\alpha,\beta)P(\beta)$.

Posterior sampling can be computationally demanding and technically subtle, especially when the data contain no direct information about certain parameters, as in the bias models used earlier.[60,143-145] Computational details can be largely handled by free Internet software such as WinBUGS and R, however. There are also analytic approximations to Bayesian analyses that are easy to implement using ordinary commercial software, such as the prior-data approach[135,146,147] or missing data methods,[148] and that can be adapted to bias analysis and combined with Monte-Carlo methods.[149]

Under the models for bias discussed earlier in this chapter, probabilistic bias analysis with random error included tends to give results similar to semi-Bayesian bias analysis, provided the priors do not lead to impossible outputs (*e.g.*, negative adjusted counts) in the analysis.[12,116] For example, in an analysis of smoking as an unmeasured confounder in an occupational cohort study of silica exposure and lung cancer, Steenland and Greenland obtained conventional 95% confidence limits of 1.31 and 1.93. In contrast, the 95% probabilistic bias analysis simulation limits (including random error) were 1.15 and 1.78, while the Bayesian posterior simulation limits using the same confounding prior and a noninformative prior for the silica effect were 1.13 and 1.84.[150] In general, we expect the PSA and semi-Bayesian results to be similar when, under the assumed model and prior, the data provide no information about the bias parameters, that is, when the posterior distribution $P(\beta|Y)$ equals the prior $P(\beta)$.[12,116] The confounding and selection models used earlier are examples. Gustafson provides a general discussion of conditions for the latter equality.[145]

Although they are less transparent computationally than probabilistic bias analysis, Bayesian approaches have advantages in interpretation and flexibility. First, unlike with probabilistic bias analysis, the Bayesian output distribution is guaranteed to be a genuine posterior probability distribution. This guarantee means, for example, that the 95% Bayesian interval is a fair betting interval under the assumed prior and data model. Second, Bayesian analysis has no difficulty accommodating priors that would sometimes yield impossible outputs in a bias analysis. Recall that an impossible bias-analysis output might reflect a problem with the data (*e.g.*, large random error) rather than the prior; hence, such an output is not a sufficient reason to reject or modify the prior. Third, Bayesian analyses can reveal counterintuitive phenomena in uncertainty assessments that are not apparent in probabilistic bias analysis.[151]

Fourth and perhaps most important, the Bayesian formulation facilitates use of prior information about any parameter in the analysis, not just those in the bias models. For example, in addition to bias priors, one can use priors for effects of measured confounders[125,152] or for the effect under study.[120,149] The "noninformative" effect priors implicit in conventional methods, in probabilistic bias analysis, and in semi-Bayesian analysis are always contextually absurd, in that they treat effects that are enormous and effects that are small as if they were equally probable,[146] despite years of epidemiologic research experience to show that enormous and very small effects are extraordinarily rare. The consequence of this treatment is unnecessary imprecision and greater susceptibility to false-positive results. Nonetheless, probabilistic bias analysis provides an easily implemented bridge between simple bias analysis and Bayesian analysis and will often be sufficient for bias analysis, especially when random error is a small component of total uncertainty.

CONCLUSION

Bias analysis is a quantitative extension of the qualitative speculations that characterize good discussions of study results. In this regard, it can be viewed as an attempt to move beyond conventional statistics, which are based on implausible randomization and random-error assumptions,[8,12,14] and the more informed but informal inferences that recognize the importance of biases, but do not attempt to estimate their magnitude.

No analysis should be expected to address every conceivable source of uncertainty.[10] There will be many sources that will be of minor importance in a given context, and preliminary considerations will often identify just a few sources of concern. At one extreme, conventional results may show that the random error in a study is potentially so large that no important inference could be drawn under any reasonable scenario (as in studies with few exposed cases). In that case, bias analysis will be a superfluous exercise. Bias analysis may also be justifiably avoided if the author is content with a descriptive approach to the study report and can refrain from making inferences or recommendations.[25]

Nonetheless, bias analysis will often be essential to obtain an accurate picture of the net uncertainty one should have in light of study data and a given set of prior judgments. The results quantify the degree to which a study should seem informative under those priors, rather than classifying the study into crude and often misleading categories of "valid" versus "invalid" or "high quality" versus "low quality" based on qualitative assessments. This quantification can be most important for large studies, pooled analyses, and meta-analyses claiming to have clear findings. It can even become essential to the public interest when results are likely to be used for public policy or medical practice recommendations. In these settings, conventional results can become an impediment to sound recommendations if they appear to provide conclusive inferences and are not tempered by formal bias analysis.

As mentioned in the introduction, a danger of quantitative bias analyses is the potential for analysts to exaggerate or obscure reported associations by manipulating bias parameters or priors until they obtain favored results. As various controversies have revealed, however, there is ample opportunity for investigators to inject their own biases (or those of their sponsors) by manipulating study protocols, study data, and conventional analyses.[153] Thus, as with all methods, the potential for abuse is not an argument against honest use, nor does it argue for the superiority of conventional approaches.

Honest use of quantitative bias analyses and Bayesian analyses involves attempts to base priors and models on empirical evidence, uninfluenced by the consequences (both analytically and politically). As emphasized in the introduction, however, it also requires presentation of results as judgments based on the chosen models and priors, rather than as data analyses or as objective study findings. Because conventional results are themselves based on doubtful models and implicit priors of no bias, they would be presented as nothing more than ill-founded judgments if they were subject to the same truth-in-packaging requirement.[12]

An advantage of formal bias analyses over narrative evaluations of conventional results is that opinions and prejudices about parameter values are made explicit in the priors, thus opening the assumptions underpinning any inferences to public scrutiny and criticism. Readers can evaluate the reasonableness of the analysis in light of their own priors and background information. When controversy arises, alternative analyses will be needed.

Once a bias analysis is programmed, however, alternative bias models and priors can be examined with little extra effort. Comparisons of alternative formulations can be viewed as a sensitivity analysis of the bias analysis.[109] Such comparisons allow observers to isolate more easily sources of disagreement and identify formulations that best reflect their own judgment, thereby helping move debates beyond qualitative assertions and counterassertions, and possibly guiding the most productive avenue for further research investment.[27]

References

1. Leamer EE. Sensitivity analyses would help. *Am Econ Rev*. 1985;75:308-313.
2. Draper D. Assessment and propagation of model uncertainty. *J R Stat Soc Ser B*. 1995;57:45-97.
3. Saltelli A, Chan K, Scott EM. *Sensitivity Analysis*. New York, NY: Wiley; 2000.
4. Robins JM, Rotnitzky A, Zhao LP. Estimation of regression coefficients when some regressors are not always observed. *J Am Stat Assoc*. 1994;89:846-866.
5. Little RJA, Rubin DB. *Statistical Analysis with Missing Data*. 2nd ed. New York, NY: Wiley; 2002.
6. Lyles RH, Allen AS. Estimating crude or common odds ratios in case-control studies with informatively missing exposure data. *Am J Epidemiol*. 2002;155(3):274-281.
7. Howe CJ, Cain LE, Hogan JW. Are all biases missing data problems? *Curr Epidemiol Rep*. 2015;2(3):162-171.
8. Greenland S. Randomization, statistics, and causal inference. *Epidemiology*. 1990;1(6):421-429.
9. Carroll RJ, Ruppert D, Stefanski LA, Crainiceanu C. *Measurement Error in Nonlinear Models*. Boca Raton, FL: Chapman and Hall; 2006.
10. Lash TL, Fox MP, MacLehose RF, Maldonado G, McCandless LC, Greenland S. Good practices for quantitative bias analysis. *Int J Epidemiol*. 2014;43(6):1969-1985.
11. Jurek AM, Maldonado G, Greenland S, Church TR. Exposure-measurement error is frequently ignored when interpreting epidemiologic study results. *Eur J Epidemiol*. 2006;21(12):871-876.
12. Greenland S. Multiple-bias modeling for analysis of observational data (with discussion). *J R Stat Soc Ser A*. 2005;168:267-308.
13. Greenland S. Invited commentary: the need for cognitive science in methodology. *Am J Epidemiol*. 2017;186(6):639-645.
14. Greenland S, Senn SJ, Rothman KJ, et al. Statistical tests, P values, confidence intervals, and power: a guide to misinterpretations. *Eur J Epidemiol*. 2016;31(4):337-350.
15. Eddy DM, Hasselblad V, Schachter R. *Meta-analysis by the Confidence Profile Method*. New York, NY: Academic Press; 1992.
16. National Research Council Committee on Risk Assessment of Hazardous Air Pollutants. *Science and Judgment in Risk Assessment*. Washington, DC: National Academy Press; 1994.

17. Vose D. *Risk Analysis*. New York, NY: John Wiley and Sons; 2000.
18. Lash TL, Fox MP, Fink AK. *Applying Quantitative Bias Analysis to Epidemiologic Data*. Statistics for biology and health. New York, NY: Springer; 2009.
19. Kahneman D, Slovic P, Tversky A. *Judgment under Uncertainty: Heuristics and Biases*. New York, NY: Cambridge University Press; 1982.
20. Gilovich T, Griffin D, Kahneman D. *Heuristics and Biases: The Psychology of Intuitive Judgment*. New York, NY: Cambridge University Press; 2002.
21. Gilovich T. *How We Know What Isn't So*. New York, NY: Free Press; 1993.
22. Lash TL. Heuristic thinking and inference from observational epidemiology. *Epidemiology*. 2007;18(1):67-72.
23. Greenland S. Statistical uncertainty due to misclassification: implications for validation substudies. *J Clin Epidemiol*. 1988;41(12):1167-1174.
24. Fox MP, Lash TL. On the need for quantitative bias analysis in the Peer-review process. *Am J Epidemiol*. 2017;185(10):865-868.
25. Greenland S, Gago-Dominguez M, Castelao JE. The value of risk-factor ("black-box") epidemiology. *Epidemiology*. 2004;15(5):529-535.
26. Lash TL, Fox MP, Cooney D, Lu Y, Forshee RA. Quantitative bias analysis in regulatory settings. *Am J Public Health*. 2016;106(7):1227-1230.
27. Lash TL, Ahern TP. Bias analysis to guide new data collection. *Int J Biostat*. 2012;8(2).
28. Cornfield J, Haenszel W, Hammond EC, Lilienfeld AM, Shimkin MB, Wynder EL. Smoking and lung cancer: recent evidence and a discussion of some questions. *J Natl Cancer Inst*. 1959;22(1):173-203.
29. Bross ID. Spurious effects from an extraneous variable. *J Chronic Dis*. 1966;19(6):637-647.
30. Bross ID. Pertinency of an extraneous variable. *J Chronic Dis*. 1967;20(7):487-495.
31. Yanagawa T. Case-control studies: assessing the effect of a confounding factor. *Biometrika*. 1984;71:191-194.
32. Axelson O, Steenland K. Indirect methods of assessing the effects of tobacco use in occupational studies. *Am J Ind Med*. 1988;13(1):105-118.
33. Gail MH, Wacholder S, Lubin JH. Indirect corrections for confounding under multiplicative and additive risk models. *Am J Ind Med*. 1988;13(1):119-130.
34. Schlesselman JJ. Assessing effects of confounding variables. *Am J Epidemiol*. 1978;108(1):3-8.
35. Simon R. "Assessing effects of confounding variables". *Am J Epidemiol*. 1980;111(1):127-129.
36. Flanders WD, Khoury MJ. Indirect assessment of confounding: graphic description and limits on effect of adjusting for covariates. *Epidemiology*. 1990;1(3):239-246.
37. Rosenbaum PR. *Observational Studies*. 2nd ed. New York, NY: Springer; 2002.
38. Lin DY, Psaty BM, Kronmal RA. Assessing the sensitivity of regression results to unmeasured confounders in observational studies. *Biometrics*. 1998;54(3):948-963.
39. Robins JM, Rotnitzky A, Scharfstein DO. Sensitivity analysis for selection bias and unmeasured confounding in missing data and causal inference models. In: Halloran ME, Berry DA, eds. *Statistical Models in Epidemiology*. New York, NY: Springer-Verlag; 1999:1-92.
40. McCandless LC, Gustafson P, Levy A. Bayesian sensitivity analysis for unmeasured confounding in observational studies. *Stat Med*. 2007;26(11):2331-2347.
41. Greenland S, Salvan A, Wegman DH, Hallock MF, Smith TJ. A case-control study of cancer mortality at a transformer-assembly facility. *Int Arch Occup Environ Health*. 1994;66(1):49-54.
42. Sundararajan V, Mitra N, Jacobson JS, Grann VR, Heitjan DF, Neugut AI. Survival associated with 5-fluorouracil-based adjuvant chemotherapy among elderly patients with node-positive colon cancer. *Ann Intern Med*. 2002;136(5):349-357.
43. Marshall SW, Mueller FO, Kirby DP, Yang J. Evaluation of safety balls and faceguards for prevention of injuries in youth baseball. *J Am Med Assoc*. 2003;289(5):568-574.
44. Maldonado G, Delzell E, Tyl RW, Sever LE. Occupational exposure to glycol ethers and human congenital malformations. *Int Arch Occup Environ Health*. 2003;76(6):405-423.
45. Kitagawa EM. Components of a difference between two rates. *J Am Stat Assoc*. 1955;50:1168-1194.
46. Maclehose RL, Kaufman S, Kaufman JS, Poole C. Bounding causal effects under uncontrolled confounding using counterfactuals. *Epidemiology*. 2005;16:548-555.
47. Pearl J. *Causality: Models, Reasoning and Inference*. Cambridge, United Kingdom: Cambridge University Press; 2000.
48. Ding P, VanderWeele TJ. Sensitivity analysis without assumptions. *Epidemiology*. 2016;27(3):368-377.
49. VanderWeele TJ, Ding P. Sensitivity analysis in observational research: introducing the E-value. *Ann Intern Med*. 2017;167(4):268-274.
50. Haneuse S, VanderWeele TJ, Arterburn D. Using the E-value to assess the potential effect of unmeasured confounding in observational studies. *J Am Med Assoc*. 2019;321(6):602-603.
51. Ioannidis JPA, Tan YJ, Blum MR. Limitations and misinterpretations of E-values for sensitivity analyses of observational studies. *Ann Intern Med*. 2019;170(2):108-111.

52. VanderWeele TJ, Mathur MB, Ding P. Correcting misinterpretations of the E-value. *Ann Intern Med.* 2019;170(2):131-132.

53. VanderWeele TJ, Li Y. Simple sensitivity analysis for differential measurement error. *Am J Epidemiol.* 2019;188(10):1823-1829.

54. Smith LH, VanderWeele TJ. Bounding bias due to selection. *Epidemiology.* 2019;30(4):509-516.

55. Lash TL, Schmidt M, Jensen AO, Engebjerg MC. Methods to apply probabilistic bias analysis to summary estimates of association. *Pharmacoepidemiol Drug Saf.* 2010;19(6):638-644.

56. Selén J. Adjusting for errors in classification and measurement in the analysis of partly and purely categorical data. *J Am Stat Assoc.* 1986;81:75-81.

57. Espeland MA, Hui SL. A general approach to analyzing epidemiologic data that contain misclassification errors. *Biometrics.* 1987;43(4):1001-1012.

58. Greenland S. Variance estimation for epidemiologic effect estimates under misclassification. *Stat Med.* 1988;7(7):745-757.

59. Greenland S. Maximum-likelihood and closed-form estimators of epidemiologic measures under misclassification. *J Stat Plan Inference.* 2007;138:528-538.

60. Gustafson P. *Measurement Error and Misclassification in Statistics and Epidemiology.* Boca Raton, FL: Chapman and Hall; 2003.

61. Greenland S, Gustafson P. Adjustment for independent nondifferential misclassification does not increase certainty that an observed association is in the correct direction. *Am J Epidemiol.* 2006;164:63-68.

62. Jurek AM, Greenland S, Maldonado G, Church TR. Proper interpretation of non-differential misclassification effects: expectations vs observations. *Int J Epidemiol.* 2005;34(3):680-687.

63. Drews CD, Greeland S. The impact of differential recall on the results of case-control studies. *Int J Epidemiol.* 1990;19(4):1107-1112.

64. Begg CB. Biases in the assessment of diagnostic tests. *Stat Med.* 1987;6(4):411-423.

65. Marshall RJ. Validation study methods for estimating exposure proportions and odds ratios with misclassified data. *J Clin Epidemiol.* 1990;43(9):941-947.

66. Brenner H, Gefeller O. Use of the positive predictive value to correct for disease misclassification in epidemiologic studies. *Am J Epidemiol.* 1993;138(11):1007-1015.

67. Greenland S. A mathematic analysis of the "epidemiologic necropsy". *Ann Epidemiol.* 1991;1(6):551-558.

68. Greenland S. The relation of the probability of causation to the relative risk and the doubling dose: a methodologic error that has become a social problem. *Am J Public Health.* 1999;89:1166-1169.

69. Poole C. Exceptions to the rule about nondifferential misclassification (abstract). *Am J Epidemiol.* 1985;122:508.

70. Brenner H, Savitz DA. The effects of sensitivity and specificity of case selection on validity, sample size, precision, and power in hospital-based case-control studies. *Am J Epidemiol.* 1990;132(1):181-192.

71. Greenland S, Kleinbaum DG. Correcting for misclassification in two-way tables and matched-pair studies. *Int J Epidemiol.* 1983;12(1):93-97.

72. Jurek AM, Maldonado G, Greenland S. Adjusting for outcome misclassification: the importance of accounting for case-control sampling and other forms of outcome-related selection. *Ann Epidemiol.* 2013;23(3):129-135.

73. Greenland S. The effect of misclassification in the presence of covariates. *Am J Epidemiol.* 1980;112(4):564-569.

74. Savitz DA, Baron AE. Estimating and correcting for confounder misclassification. *Am J Epidemiol.* 1989;129(5):1062-1071.

75. Marshall JR, Hastrup JL. Mismeasurement and the resonance of strong confounders: uncorrelated errors. *Am J Epidemiol.* 1996;143(10):1069-1078.

76. Marshall JR, Hastrup JL, Ross JS. Mismeasurement and the resonance of strong confounders: correlated errors. *Am J Epidemiol.* 1999;150(1):88-96.

77. Lash TL, Fink AK. "Neighborhood environment and loss of physical function in older adults: evidence from the Alameda County Study". *Am J Epidemiol.* 2003;157(5):472-473.

78. VanderWeele TJ, Hernan MA. Results on differential and dependent measurement error of the exposure and the outcome using signed directed acyclic graphs. *Am J Epidemiol.* 2012;175(12):1303-1310.

79. Barron BA. The effects of misclassification on the estimation of relative risk. *Biometrics.* 1977;33(2):414-418.

80. Kleinbaum DG, Kupper LL, Morgenstern H. *Epidemiologic Research: Principles and Quantitative Methods.* New York, NY: Van Nostrand Reinhold; 1982.

81. Tennenbein A. A double sampling scheme for estimating from binomial data with misclassification. *J Am Stat Assoc.* 1970;65:1350-1361.

82. Lyles RH, Tang L, Superak HM, et al. Validation data-based adjustments for outcome misclassification in logistic regression: an illustration. *Epidemiology.* 2011;22(4):589-597.

83. Edwards JK, Cole SR, Troester MA, Richardson DB. Accounting for misclassified outcomes in binary regression models using multiple imputation with internal validation data. *Am J Epidemiol.* 2013;177(9):904-912.

84. Tang L, Lyles RH, Ye Y, Lo Y, King CC. Extended matrix and inverse matrix methods utilizing internal validation data when both disease and exposure status are misclassified. *Epidemiol Methods.* 2013;2(1):49-66.

85. Spiegelman D, Rosner B, Logan R. Estimation and inference for logistic regression with covariate misclassification and measurement error in main study/validation study designs. *J Am Stat Assoc.* 2000;95:51-61.

86. Rosner B, Willett WC, Spiegelman D. Correction of logistic regression relative risk estimates and confidence intervals for systematic within-person measurement error. *Stat Med.* 1989;8(9):1051-1069; discussion 1071-3.

87. Spiegelman D, Carroll RJ, Kipnis V. Efficient regression calibration for logistic regression in main study/internal validation study designs with an imperfect reference instrument. *Stat Med.* 2001;20(1):139-160.

88. Spiegelman D, Zhao B, Kim J. Correlated errors in biased surrogates: study designs and methods for measurement error correction. *Stat Med.* 2005;24(11):1657-1682.

89. Freedman LS, Fainberg V, Kipnis V, Midthune D, Carroll RJ. A new method for dealing with measurement error in explanatory variables of regression models. *Biometrics.* 2004;60(1):172-181.

90. Wacholder S, Armstrong B, Hartge P. Validation studies using an alloyed gold standard. *Am J Epidemiol.* 1993;137(11):1251-1258.

91. Brenner H. Correcting for exposure misclassification using an alloyed gold standard. *Epidemiology.* 1996;7(4):406-410.

92. Spiegelman D, McDermott A, Rosner B. Regression calibration method for correcting measurement-error bias in nutritional epidemiology. *Am J Clin Nutr.* 1997;65(4 Suppl):1179S-1186S.

93. Spiegelman D, Schneeweiss S, McDermott A. Measurement error correction for logistic regression models with an "alloyed gold standard". *Am J Epidemiol.* 1997;145(2):184-196.

94. Tang MC, Weiss NS, Malone KE. Induced abortion in relation to breast cancer among parous women: a birth certificate registry study. *Epidemiology.* 2000;11:177-180.

95. Greenland S. The impact of prior distributions for uncontrolled confounding and response bias: a case study of the relation of wire codes and magnetic fields to childhood leukemia. *J Am Stat Assoc.* 2003;98:47-54.

96. Lash TL, Fink AK. Null association between pregnancy termination and breast cancer in a registry-based study of parous women. *Int J Cancer.* 2004;110(3):443-448.

97. Stang A, Schmidt-Pokrzywniak A, Lash TL, et al. Mobile phone use and risk of uveal melanoma: results of the risk factors for uveal melanoma case-control study. *J Natl Cancer Inst.* 2009;101(2):120-123.

98. Walker AM. Anamorphic analysis: sampling and estimation for covariate effects when both exposure and disease are known. *Biometrics.* 1982;38(4):1025-1032.

99. White JE. A two stage design for the study of the relationship between a rare exposure and a rare disease. *Am J Epidemiol.* 1982;115(1):119-128.

100. Breslow N, Cain K. Logistic regression for two-stage case-control data. *Biometrika.* 1988;75:11-20.

101. Flanders WD, Greenland S. Analytic methods for two-stage case-control studies and other stratified designs. *Stat Med.* 1991;10(5):739-747.

102. Weinberg CR, Wacholder S. The design and analysis of case-control studies with biased sampling. *Biometrics.* 1990;46(4):963-975.

103. Greenland S, Neutra R. An analysis of detection bias and proposed corrections in the study of estrogens and endometrial cancer. *J Chronic Dis.* 1981;34(9-10):433-438.

104. Weinberg CR, Sandler DP. Randomized recruitment in case-control studies. *Am J Epidemiol.* 1991;134(4):421-432.

105. Scharfstein DO, Rotnitsky A, Robins JM. Adjusting for nonignorable drop-out using semiparametric nonresponse models. *J Am Stat Assoc.* 1999;94:1096-1120.

106. Criqui MH, Austin M, Barrett-Connor E. The effect of non-response on risk ratios in a cardiovascular disease study. *J Chronic Dis.* 1979;32(9-10):633-638.

107. Greenland S. Quantifying biases in causal models: classical confounding vs collider-stratification bias. *Epidemiology.* 2003;14(3):300-306.

108. Greenland S. Basic methods for sensitivity analysis of biases. *Int J Epidemiol.* 1996;25(6):1107-1116.

109. Greenland S. *The sensitivity of a sensitivity analysis (invited paper).* In: *1997 Proceedings of the Biometrics Section.* Alexandria, VA: American Statistical Association; 1998:19-21.

110. Greenland S, Robins JM. Confounding and misclassification. *Am J Epidemiol.* 1985;122(3):495-506.

111. Schuemie MJ, Ryan PB, DuMouchel W, Suchard MA, Madigan D. Interpreting observational studies: why empirical calibration is needed to correct p-values. *Stat Med.* 2014;33(2):209-218.

112. Schuemie MJ, Hripcsak G, Ryan PB, Madigan D, Suchard MA. Empirical confidence interval calibration for population-level effect estimation studies in observational healthcare data. *Proc Natl Acad Sci U S A*. 2018;115(11):2571-2577.

113. Gruber S, Tchetgen Tchetgen E. Limitations of empirical calibration of p-values using observational data. *Stat Med*. 2016;35(22):3869-3882.

114. Franklin JM. P-values and decision-making: discussion of 'Limitations of empirical calibration of p-values using observational data'. *Stat Med* 2016;35(22):3889-3891.

115. Schuemie MJ, Hripcsak G, Ryan PB, Madigan D, Suchard MA. Robust empirical calibration of p-values using observational data. *Stat Med*. 2016;35(22):3883-3888.

116. MacLehose RF, Gustafson P. Is probabilistic bias analysis approximately Bayesian? *Epidemiology*. 2012;23(1):151-158.

117. Hoffman FO, Hammonds JS. Propagation of uncertainty in risk assessments: the need to distinguish between uncertainty due to lack of knowledge and uncertainty due to variability. *Risk Anal*. 1994;14(5):707-712.

118. Shlyakhter A, Mirny L, Vlasov A, Wilson R. Monte Carlo modeling of epidemiological studies. *Hum Ecol Risk Assess Int J*. 1996;2(4):920-938.

119. Lash TL, Silliman RA, Guadagnoli E, Mor V. The effect of less than definitive care on breast carcinoma recurrence and mortality. *Cancer*. 2000;89(8):1739-1747.

120. Greenland S. Sensitivity analysis, Monte Carlo risk analysis, and Bayesian uncertainty assessment. *Risk Anal*. 2001;21(4):579-583.

121. Lash TL, Fink AK. Semi-automated sensitivity analysis to assess systematic errors in observational data. *Epidemiology*. 2003;14(4):451-458.

122. Phillips CV. Quantifying and reporting uncertainty from systematic errors. *Epidemiology*. 2003;14(4):459-466.

123. MacLehose RF, Olshan AF, Herring AH, et al. Bayesian methods for correcting misclassification: an example from birth defects epidemiology. *Epidemiology*. 2009;20(1):27-35.

124. MacLehose RF, Bodnar LM, Meyer CS, Chu H, Lash TL. Hierarchical semi-Bayes methods for misclassification in Perinatal epidemiology. *Epidemiology*. 2018;29(2):183-190.

125. Gustafson P, Greenland S. The performance of random coefficient regression in accounting for residual confounding. *Biometrics*. 2006;62(3):760-768.

126. National Centre for Chronic Disease Prevention and Health Promotion Office on Smoking and Health. *Patterns of Tobacco Use Among U.S. Youth, Young Adults, and Adults*. Atlanta, GA: Centers for Disease Control and Prevention (US); 2014.

127. Efron B, Tibshirani RJ. *An Introduction to the Bootstrap*. New York, NY: Chapman and Hall; 1994.

128. Davison AC, Hinkley DV. *Bootstrap Methods and Their Application*. New York, NY: Cambridge; 1997.

129. Carpenter J, Bithell J. Bootstrap confidence intervals: when, which, what? A practical guide for medical statisticians. *Stat Med*. 2000;19(9):1141-1164.

130. Robins JM, Greenland S, Hu F. Estimation of the causal effect of a time-varying exposure on the marginal mean of a repeated binary outcome (with discussion). *J Am Stat Assoc*. 1999;94:687-712.

131. Bodnar LM, Tang G, Ness RB, Harger G, Roberts JM. Periconceptional multivitamin use reduces the risk of preeclampsia. *Am J Epidemiol*. 2006;164(5):470-477.

132. Miettinen OS, Cook EF. Confounding: essence and detection. *Am J Epidemiol*. 1981;114(4):593-603.

133. Greenland S, Mickey RM. Closed-form and dually consistent methods for $2 \times 2 \times K$ and $I \times J \times K$ tables. *Appl Stat*. 1988;37:335-343.

134. Greenland S. Generalized conjugate priors for Bayesian analysis of risk and survival regressions. *Biometrics*. 2003;59(1):92-99.

135. Greenland S. Prior data for non-normal priors. *Stat Med*. 2007;26(19):3578-3590.

136. Jones MC. Families of distributions arising from distributions of order statistics. *Test*. 2004;13:1-44.

137. Lesaffre E, Rizopoulos D, Tsonaka R. The logistic transform for bounded outcome scores. *Biostatistics*. 2007;8(1):72-85.

138. Greenland S. A lower bound for the correlation of exponentiated bivariate normal pairs. *Am Statist*. 1996;50:163-164.

139. Fox MP, Lash TL, Greenland S. A method to automate probabilistic sensitivity analyses of misclassified binary variables. *Int J Epidemiol*. 2005;34(6):1370-1376.

140. Cole SR, Chu H, Greenland S. Multiple-imputation for measurement-error correction. *Int J Epidemiol*. 2006;35(4):1074-1081.

141. Lash TL, Abrams B, Bodnar LM. Comparison of bias analysis strategies applied to a large data set. *Epidemiology*. 2014;25(4):576-582.

142. Flegal KM, Keyl PM, Nieto FJ. Differential misclassification arising from nondifferential errors in exposure measurement. *Am J Epidemiol*. 1991;134(10):1233-1244.

143. Carlin B, Louis TA. *Bayes and Empirical-Bayes Methods of Data Analysis*. 2nd ed. New York, NY: Chapman and Hall; 2000.

144. Gelman A, Carlin JB, Stern HS, Rubin DB. *Bayesian Data Analysis*. 2nd ed. New York, NY: Chapman and Hall/CRC; 2003.

145. Gustafson P. On model expansion, model contraction, identifiability, and prior information (with discussion). *Stat Sci*. 2005;20:111-140.

146. Greenland S. Bayesian perspectives for epidemiological research: I. Foundations and basic methods. *Int J Epidemiol*. 2006;35(3):765-775.

147. Greenland S. Bayesian perspectives for epidemiological research. II. Regression analysis. *Int J Epidemiol*. 2007;36(1):195-202.

148. Greenland S. Bayesian perspectives for epidemiologic research: III. Bias analysis via missing-data methods. *Int J Epidemiol*. 2009;38(6):1662-1673.

149. Greenland S, Kheifets L. Leukemia attributable to residential magnetic fields: results from analyses allowing for study biases. *Risk Anal*. 2006;26:471-482.

150. Steenland K, Greenland S. Monte Carlo sensitivity analysis and Bayesian analysis of smoking as an unmeasured confounder in a study of silica and lung cancer. *Am J Epidemiol*. 2004;160(4):384-392.

151. Gustafson P, Greenland S. Curious phenomena in Bayesian adjustment for exposure misclassification. *Stat Med*. 2006;25(1):87-103.

152. Greenland S. When should epidemiologic regressions use random coefficients? *Biometrics*. 2000;56(3):915-921.

153. Curfman GD, Morrissey S, Drazen JM. Expression of concern reaffirmed. *N Engl J Med*. 2006;354(11):1193.

CHAPTER 30

Ecologic Studies and Analysis

Hal Morgenstern and Jon Wakefield

An ecologic or aggregate study focuses on the comparison of groups, rather than individuals. The underlying reason for this focus is that individual-level data are missing on the joint distribution of at least two and perhaps all variables within each group; in this sense, an ecologic study is an "incomplete" design.[1] Ecologic studies have been conducted by social scientists for more than a century[2] and have been used extensively by epidemiologists in many research areas. Nevertheless, the distinction between individual-level and group-level (ecologic) studies and the inferential implications are far more complicated and subtle than they first appear. Before 1980, ecologic studies were usually presented in the first part of epidemiology textbooks as simple "descriptive" analyses in which disease rates are stratified by place or time to preliminarily test hypotheses; little attention was given to statistical methods or inference; for example, see MacMahon and Pugh.[3] In the past few decades, the methods and conduct of ecologic studies have expanded considerably, and a dominant part of this field is now often labeled "spatial epidemiology"[4-7] or "spatiotemporal epidemiology."[8,9] The purpose of this chapter is to provide a methodologic overview of ecologic studies that emphasizes study design, statistical analysis, sources of bias, and causal inference. Although ecologic studies are easily and inexpensively conducted, the results are often misinterpreted.

CONCEPTS AND RATIONALE

Before discussing the design and interpretation of ecologic studies, we must first define the concepts of ecologic measurement, analysis, and inference.

Levels of Measurement

The sources of data used in epidemiologic studies typically involve direct observations of individuals; or they may also involve observations of groups, organizations, or places. These observations are then organized to measure specific variables in the study population: individual-level variables are properties of individuals (*e.g.*, age and blood-pressure level); and ecologic (macro-level) variables are properties of groups, organizations, or places (*e.g.*, degree of social organization and air-pollution level). To be more specific, ecologic measures may be classified into three types:

1. *Aggregate measures* are summaries (*e.g.*, means or proportions) of observations derived from individuals in each group (*e.g.*, the proportion of smokers and median family income).
2. *Environmental measures* are physical characteristics of the place in which members of each group live or work (*e.g.*, air-pollution level, hours of sunlight, and rurality). Note that each environmental measure has an analogue at the individual level, and these individual exposures (or doses) usually vary among members of each group (though they may remain unmeasured).
3. *Global measures* are attributes of groups, organizations, or places for which there is no distinct analogue at the individual level, unlike aggregate and environmental measures (*e.g.*, population density of each residential area, level of social disorganization, the existence of a specific law, and type of healthcare system).

Levels of Analysis

The unit of analysis is the common level for which the data on all variables are reduced and analyzed. In an *individual-level analysis,* a value for each variable is assigned to every subject in the study. It is possible, even common in environmental epidemiology, for one or more predictor variables to be ecologic measures. For example, the measured air-pollution level of a county might be assigned to every subject who is a resident of that county.

In a *completely ecologic analysis,* all variables (exposure, disease, and covariates) are ecologic measures so that the unit of analysis is the group (*e.g.*, region, worksite, school, healthcare facility, demographic stratum, or time interval). Thus, within each group, we do not know the joint distribution of any combination of variables at the individual level (*e.g.*, the frequencies of exposed cases, unexposed cases, exposed noncases, and unexposed noncases); all we know is the marginal distribution of each variable (*e.g.*, the proportion exposed and the disease rate), *i.e.*, the T frequencies in each group as illustrated in Figure 30-1.

In a *partially ecologic analysis* of three or more variables, we have additional information on certain joint distributions (the M, N, or A/B frequencies in Figure 30-1); but we still do not know the full joint distribution of all variables within each group (*i.e.*, the ? cells in Figure 30-1 are missing). For example, in an ecologic study of cancer incidence by county, the joint distribution of age (a covariate) and disease status within each county (the M frequencies in Figure 30-1) might be obtained from the census and a population tumor registry. From these sources, the investigator would be able to estimate age-specific cancer rates for each county. Because different sources are often used to obtain exposure and disease data, additional information might be obtained on the joint distribution of age and the exposure status (the N frequencies in Figure 30-1).

FIGURE 30-1 Joint distribution of exposure status ($x = 1$ vs. 0), disease status ($y = 1$ vs. 0), and covariate status ($z = 1$ vs. 0) in each group of a simple ecologic analysis: T frequencies are the only data available in a completely ecologic analysis of all three variables; M frequencies require additional data on the joint distribution of z and y within each group; N frequencies require additional data on the joint distribution of x and z within each group; A and B frequencies require additional data on the joint distribution of x and y within each group; and ? cells are always missing in an ecologic analysis.

In a *semi-ecologic analysis*, all data are collected at the individual level, except for one variable—either the exposure, disease, or covariate—which is measured ecologically. This type of analysis is frequently used to measure an environmental exposure, where the outcome and covariates are measured at the individual level.[10,11] For example, in a study of possible air-pollution effects in a state, air-pollution levels might be collected from monitors located throughout the state and used to obtain pollution levels for each county. Then, in the analysis, every person living in a given county would be assigned the pollution level for that county. This type of analysis, even when a continuous exposure level is dichotomized, cannot be fully illustrated in Figure 30-1, though the M frequencies would be known in each group.

Multilevel analysis is a modeling technique that combines data collected at two or more levels.[12-19] For example, in an educational context, one may be interested in test scores collected on students within classrooms, that are nested within schools, which are themselves nested within school districts. A multilevel approach would estimate the contributions from each of these levels, within one model. This approach is described in a later section.

Levels of Inference

The underlying goal of a given epidemiologic study or analysis may be to make *biologic* (or biobehavioral) *inferences* about effects on individual *risks* or to make *ecologic inferences* about effects on group *rates*.[20] The target level of causal inference, however, does not always match the level of analysis. For example, the explicit or implicit objective of an ecologic analysis may be to make a biologic inference about the effect of a specific exposure on individual disease risk. As discussed later in this chapter, such *cross-level inferences*[21] are particularly vulnerable to bias.

If the objective of a study is to estimate the *biologic (individual-level) effect* of wearing a motorcycle helmet on the risk of motorcycle-related mortality among motorcycle riders, the target level of causal inference is biologic. On the other hand, if the objective is to estimate the *ecologic effect* of helmet-use laws on the motorcycle-related mortality rate of riders in different states, the target level of causal inference is ecologic. Note that the magnitude of this ecologic effect depends not only on the biologic effect of helmet use, but also on the degree and pattern of compliance with the law in each state. Furthermore, the validity of the ecologic-effect estimate depends on our ability to control for differences among states in the joint distribution of confounders, including individual-level variables such as age and the time spent riding a motorcycle in the previous year.

We might also be interested in estimating the *contextual effect* of an ecologic exposure on individual risk, which is also a form of biologic inference.[11,22-24] If the ecologic exposure is an aggregate measure, we would generally want to separate its effect from the effect of its individual-level analogue, *e.g.*, when studying social factors or immunity. For instance, we might estimate the contextual effect of living in a poor area on the risk of disease, controlling for individual poverty level.[25] Contextual effects can be profound in infectious-disease epidemiology, where the risk of disease depends on the prevalence of the disease in others with whom the individual has contact.[26-28]

In evaluating motorcycle-helmet laws in the United States, we would probably not expect a contextual *effect* of living in a state that mandates helmet use on the risk of motorcycle-related mortality in riders, controlling for individual helmet use. If a rider's helmet use does not change after the helmet law takes effect, we would not expect his or her risk of motorcycle-related mortality to change. Nevertheless, we might expect to observe an *association* between the same variables after the law because of differential compliance with the law within states and possible confounding. Thus, the risk of motorcycle-related mortality among riders who do not wear helmets may be higher in states with the helmet law than in states without the law (an apparent contextual effect).

In clinical studies of a possible treatment effect on patient outcome, a contextual effect among treatment facilities may be due to unmeasured differences in the quality of care. Such contextual effects should be distinguished, however, from *compositional effects* due to differences in treatment practice among facilities, *i.e.*, a biologic effect of the treatment itself.[29,30] The better clinical outcomes in patients in certain facilities may simply reflect the greater use of the more effective treatment in those facilities. In ecologic studies, contextual and compositional effects are confounded with each other.

Rationale for Ecologic Studies

There are several reasons for the widespread use of ecologic studies in epidemiology, despite frequent cautions about their methodologic limitations:

1. *Low cost and convenience.* Ecologic studies are inexpensive and take little time because various secondary data sources, each involving different information needed for the analysis, can easily be linked at the aggregate level.[20] For example, data obtained from population registries, vital records, large surveys, and the census are often linked at the state, county, or census-tract level. Beyond more traditional sources of data, there has been an explosion in the availability of data from the web and social media sources. When the groups are defined geographically, the widespread availability of geographical information systems (GIS) allows the effective storage and combination of datasets from different sources with differing geographies.

2. *Measurement limitations of individual-level studies.* In environmental epidemiology and other research areas, we often cannot accurately measure relevant exposures or doses at the individual level for large numbers of subjects—at least not with available time and resources. Thus, the only practical way to measure the exposure may be ecologically.[20,31] This advantage is especially true when investigating apparent clusters of disease in small areas.[32] Sometimes individual-level exposures, such as dietary factors, cannot be measured accurately because of substantial within-person variability; yet ecologic measures might accurately reflect group averages.[33,34]

3. *Design limitations of individual-level studies.* Exposures must vary to study their effects. Individual-level studies may not be practical for estimating exposure effects if the exposure varies little within the study area. Ecologic studies covering a much wider area, however, might be able to achieve substantial variation in mean exposure across groups.[35-37]

4. *Limitations of confounding control in individual-level studies.* In nonrandomized studies of treatment effects, confounding tends to occur when the indication for being treated—good or poor prognosis—is a predictor of the outcome. This confounding may be challenging to control by covariate adjustment. Under certain conditions, conducting an ecologic or semi-ecologic analysis with treatment status defined ecologically (*e.g.*, the proportion treated in each facility) may control for the *confounding by indication.* This approach for reducing the bias, which is related to instrumental-variable analysis, will be discussed in a later section.

5. *Interest in ecologic effects.* As noted previously, the stated purpose of a study may be to assess an ecologic effect; *i.e.*, the target level of inference may be ecologic rather than biologic—to understand differences in disease rates among populations.[35,38] Ecologic effects are particularly relevant when evaluating the impacts of social processes or population interventions such as new programs, policies, or legislation. As discussed later in this chapter, however, an interest in ecologic effects does not necessarily obviate the need for individual-level data.[24,39]

6. *Simplicity of analysis and presentation.* In large complex studies conducted at the individual level, it may be conceptually and statistically simpler to perform ecologic analyses and to present ecologic results than to do individual-level analyses. For example, data from large periodic surveys, such as the National Health Interview Survey, are often analyzed ecologically by treating some combination of year, region, and demographic group as the unit of analysis. As discussed later in this chapter, however, such simplicity of analysis and presentation often conceals methodologic problems.

STUDY DESIGNS

In an ecologic study design, the planned unit of analysis is the group. Ecologic designs may be classified on two dimensions: the method of exposure measurement and the method of grouping.[1,20] Regarding the first dimension, an ecologic design is called *exploratory* if there is no specific exposure of interest or the exposure of potential interest is not measured, and it is called *etiologic* if the primary exposure variable is measured and included in the analysis. In practice, this dimension is a continuum, since most ecologic studies are not conducted to test a single hypothesis. Regarding the second dimension, the groups of an ecologic study may be identified by place (multiple-group design), by time (time-trend design), or by a combination of place and time (mixed design).

Multiple-Group Designs

Exploratory Study

In an exploratory multiple-group study, we compare the rate of disease among many regions during the same period. The purpose is often to search for spatial patterns that might suggest an environmental etiology or more specific etiologic hypotheses. For example, the National Cancer Institute (NCI) mapped age-adjusted cancer mortality rates in the United States by county for the period 1950 to 1969.[40] For oral cancers, they found a striking difference in geographic patterns by sex: among men, the mortality rates were greatest in the urban Northeast; but among women, the rates were greatest in the Southeast. These findings led to the hypothesis that snuff dipping, which was common among rural southern women, is a risk factor for oral cancers.[41] The results of a subsequent case-control study supported this hypothesis.[42]

Exploratory ecologic studies may also involve the comparison of rates between migrants and their offspring and residents of their countries of emigration and immigration.[3,33] If the rates differ appreciably between the countries of emigration and immigration, migrant studies often yield results suggesting the influence of certain types of risk factors for the disease under study. For example, if US immigrants from Japan have rates of a disease similar to US Whites but much lower than Japanese residents, the difference may be due to environmental or behavioral risk factors operating during adulthood. On the other hand, if US immigrants from Japan and their offspring have rates much lower than US Whites but similar to Japanese residents, the difference may be due to genetic risk factors. Such interpretations, however, especially in the first instance, are often limited by differences between countries in the classification and detection of disease or cause of death.

In mapping studies, such as the NCI investigation, a simple comparison of rates across regions is often complicated by two statistical problems. First, regions with smaller numbers of observed cases show greater variability in the estimated rate; thus, the most extreme rates tend to be observed for those regions with the fewest cases. Second, nearby regions tend to have more similar rates than do distant regions (*i.e.*, spatial dependence) because unmeasured risk factors tend to exhibit spatial structure. Statistical methods for dealing with both problems have been developed by fitting Bayesian hierarchical models, in which spatial dependence of the residuals is explicitly modeled, usually through some form of conditional autoregressive model.[7,43] Fully Bayesian computation is now relatively straightforward using the integrated nested Laplace approximation (INLA) technique.[44]

When exposures and covariates are added to the model, spatial dependence may create another serious problem, *confounding by location*, where associations with the outcome can be dramatically different in models that include or exclude error terms that allow for spatial dependence.[43,45] Furthermore, if the study objective is to predict area-specific outcomes rather than to estimate effects, some of the problems discussed here are not relevant. For example, the addition of covariates to the model may improve estimation.[46] We also note that the inferential issues encountered with exploratory multiple-group designs are closely related to the change of support problem[47,48] and the modifiable areal-unit problem.[49]

Etiologic Study

In an etiologic multiple-group study, we assess the ecologic association between the average exposure level or prevalence and the rate of disease among many groups. This is the most common ecologic design; typically, the unit of analysis is a geopolitical region. For example, Hatch and Susser examined the association between background gamma radiation and the incidence of childhood cancers between 1975 and 1985 in the region surrounding a nuclear plant.[50] Average radiation levels for each of 69 tracts in the region were estimated from a 1976 aerial survey. The authors found positive associations between radiation level and the incidence of leukemia (an expected finding) as well as solid tumors (an unexpected finding). The Small Area Health Statistics Unit in the United Kingdom has carried out a large number of such ecologic studies around point sources of pollution.

Data analysis in this type of multiple-group study usually involves fitting a mathematical model to the data. Ordinary least-squares procedures, however, will generally be inadequate because the fundamental assumption of uncorrelated error terms with constant variance will be violated. The variance of the error terms will not in general be constant but will rather depend on the mean. Further, as discussed previously, there will be spatial dependence, with error terms from areas close together tending to be more similar. To address these concerns, Pocock et al.[51] proposed a linear model in which the unexplained variation is treated as random effects. Model parameters were estimated by an iteratively reweighted least-squares procedure. A similar procedure was used by Breslow[52] to fit loglinear models. Prentice and Sheppard[53] proposed a linear relative rate model, which leads readily to the estimation of rate ratios (assuming the model is properly specified). Prentice and Thomas[54] considered an exponential relative rate model, which they argue may be more parsimonious than the linear-form model for specifying covariates. These methods can be applied to data aggregated by place and/or time (to be discussed later). Fortunately, it is now straightforward to model count data using Poisson and binomial likelihoods with random effects to reflect overdispersion (excess variation), perhaps with spatial and/or temporal structure.[43,55]

Newer statistical developments in the analysis of multiple-group ecologic data emphasize the inclusion of supplementary data and/or prior information to improve effect estimation.[18,56,57] Use of ecologic modeling to estimate exposure effects (rate ratios and differences) is described in the section "Effect Estimation." Approaches for reducing bias in ecologic studies by combining ecologic data with individual-level data are described by Haneuse and Wakefield[58,59] and Wakefield and Haneuse[60] and are discussed in the section "Multilevel Analyses and Designs."

Time-Trend Designs

Exploratory Study

An exploratory time-trend or time-series study involves a comparison of the disease rates over time in one geographically defined population. In addition to providing graphical displays of temporal trends, time-series data can also be used to forecast future rates and trends. This latter application, which is more common in the social sciences than in epidemiology, usually involves fitting autoregressive integrated moving average (ARIMA) models to the outcome data.[61-65] The autoregressive component of this model accounts for the correlation among repeated outcomes over time in the population by allowing the outcome observed at one time to depend on past outcomes. The net result is that the correlation between observations decays with increasing lag between observations. The moving-average component allows for the outcome observed at one time to depend on random disturbances in the outcome at previous times. This process allows the correlation between observations to be large for a given lag and then drop to zero for larger lags. The integrated (nonstationary) component of the model allows for long-term trends in the outcome. ARIMA modeling can also be extended to evaluate the impact of a population intervention,[63,66] to estimate associations between two or more time-series variables,[62,64,67] and to estimate associations in a mixed ecologic design[65,68] (see also later discussion). Alternative time series models, such as dynamic structures, exist, which are hidden Markov models in which latent parameters are given temporal structure.[69]

A special type of exploratory time-trend analysis often used by epidemiologists is age-period-cohort analysis (or simply, cohort analysis). This approach typically involves the collection of retrospective data from a large population over a period of 20 or more years. Through graphical or tabular displays[70,71] or formal modeling techniques,[72,73] the objective is to estimate the separate effects of three time-related variables on the rate of disease: age, period (calendar time), and birth cohort (year of birth). By describing the occurrence of disease in this way, the investigator attempts to gain insight about temporal trends, which might lead to new hypotheses.

Lee et al.[74] conducted an age-period-cohort analysis of melanoma mortality among White males in the United States between 1951 and 1975. They concluded that the apparent increase in the melanoma mortality rate was due primarily to a cohort effect. That is, persons born in more recent years experienced throughout their lives a higher rate than did persons born earlier. In a subsequent paper, Lee[75] speculated that this cohort effect might reflect increases in sunlight exposure or sunburn during youth, which he hypothesized is a risk factor for melanoma.

From a purely statistical perspective, there is an inherent problem in making inferences from the results of age-period-cohort analyses because of the linear dependency among the three time-related variables.[55,71,73,76-81] Thus, we cannot allow the value of one variable to change when the values of the other two variables are held constant. As a result of this "identifiability" problem, each data set has alternative model fits (and hence interpretations) with respect to the combination of age, period, and cohort effects; there is no unique set of effect parameters when all three variables are considered simultaneously. This phenomenon is subtle, however, since certain second-order trends are identifiable. The only way to decide which interpretation should be accepted is to consider the findings in light of prior knowledge and, possibly, to constrain the model by ignoring one effect. The latter strategy may be aided by the inclusion of relevant covariates.

Etiologic Study

In an etiologic time-trend study, we assess the ecologic association between change in average exposure level or prevalence and change in disease rate in one geographically defined population. As with exploratory designs, this type of assessment can be done by simple graphical displays or by time-series regression modeling.[62,64,65]

In their etiologic time-trend study, Darby and Doll[82] examined the associations between average annual absorbed dose of radiation fallout from weapons testing and the incidence rate of childhood leukemia in three European countries between 1945 and 1985. Although the leukemia rate varied over time in each country, they found no convincing evidence that these changes were attributable to changes in fallout radiation.

Causal inference from time-trend studies is often complicated by two problems. First, changes in disease classification and diagnostic criteria can produce distorted trends in the observed rate of disease, which can lead to substantial bias in estimating exposure effects. Second, there may be an appreciable induction/latent period between first exposure to a risk factor and disease detection. To deal with the latter issue in an ecologic time-trend study, the investigator can lag observations between average exposure and disease rate by a duration assumed to reflect the average induction/latent period of exposure-induced cases. There are two approaches for selecting the lag: (1) an *a priori* method based on knowledge of the disease; and (2) empirical methods that maximize the observed association of interest or optimize the fit of the model that includes a lag parameter. Unfortunately, the first method is often problematic because adequate prior knowledge is lacking, and the second method can produce results that are biologically meaningless and very misleading.[83] Furthermore, confounding by location discussed previously may also distort the estimation of temporal outcome trends due to temporal dependence in the residuals. A flexible temporal model for dealing with this problem has been proposed by Kelsall et al.[84]

Mixed Designs

Exploratory Study

The exploratory mixed design combines the basic features of the exploratory multiple-group study and the exploratory time-trend study. Time-series (ARIMA) modeling or age-period-cohort analysis can be used to describe or predict trends in the disease rate for multiple populations. For example, to test the hypothesis of Lee[75] that changes in sunlight exposure during youth can explain the observed increase in melanoma mortality in the United States, we might conduct an age-period-cohort analysis, stratifying on region according to approximate sunlight exposure (without measuring the exposure). Assuming the amount of sunlight in the regions have not changed differentially over the study period, we might expect the cohort effect described earlier to be stronger for sunnier regions. Riebler et al.[85] described age-period-cohort models over space from which certain relative-risk contrasts are identifiable if one is willing to make assumptions regarding at least one common time effect across regions.

Etiologic Study

In an etiologic mixed design, we assess the association between change in average exposure level or prevalence and change in disease rate among many groups. Thus, the interpretation of estimated effects is enhanced because two types of comparisons are made simultaneously: change over time within groups and differences among groups. For example, Crawford et al.[86] evaluated the hypothesis that hard drinking water (*i.e.*, water with a high concentration of calcium and magnesium) is a protective risk factor for cardiovascular disease (CVD). They compared the absolute change in CVD mortality rate between 1948 and 1964 in 83 British towns, by water-hardness change, age, and sex. In all sex-age groups, especially for men, the authors found an inverse association between trends in water hardness and CVD mortality. In middle-aged men, for example, the increase in CVD mortality was less in towns that made their water harder than in towns that made their water softer.

EFFECT ESTIMATION

A major quantitative objective of most epidemiologic studies is to estimate the effect of one or more exposures on disease occurrence in a well-defined population at risk. A measure of effect in this context is not just any measure of association such as a correlation coefficient; rather, it reflects a particular causal parameter, *i.e.*, a counterfactual contrast in disease occurrence.[31,39,87-92] In studies conducted at the individual level, effects are usually estimated by comparing the rate or risk of disease, in the form of a ratio or difference, for exposed and unexposed populations (see Chapter 5). In multiple-group ecologic studies, however, we cannot estimate effects directly in this way because of the missing information on the joint distribution within groups. Instead, we regress the group-specific disease rates (Y) on the group-specific exposure prevalences (X). Note, throughout this chapter, uppercase letters are used to represent ecologic variables and their estimated regression coefficients; lowercase letters are used to represent individual-level variables and their estimated regression coefficients.

The most common model form for analyzing ecologic data is the linear model. Ordinary least-squares methods can be used to yield the following prediction model: $E(Y|X) = B_0 + B_1 X$, where B_0 and B_1 are the estimated intercept and slope. An estimate of the biologic effect of the exposure (at the individual level) can be derived from the regression results.[93,94] The predicted disease rate in a group that is entirely exposed is $E(Y|X=1) = B_0 + B_1(1) = B_0 + B_1$, and the predicted rate in a group that is entirely unexposed is $E(Y|X=0) = B_0 + B_1(0) = B_0$. Therefore, the estimated rate difference is $E(Y|X=1) - E(Y|X=0) = B_0 + B_1 - B_0 = B_1$, and the estimated rate ratio is $(B_0 + B_1)/B_0 = 1 + B_1/B_0$.

Alternatively, fitting a loglinear model to the data yields: $E(Y|X) = \exp(B_0 + B_1 X)$. Applying the same method used previously for linear models, the estimated rate ratio is $E(Y|X=1)/E(Y|X=0) = \exp(B_1)$.

As an illustration of rate-ratio estimation in an ecologic study, consider Durkheim's examination of religion and suicide in four groups of Prussian provinces between 1883 and 1890 (Figure 30-2).[95] The groups were formed by ranking 13 provinces according to the proportion (X) of the population that was Protestant. Using ordinary least-squares linear regression, we estimate the suicide rate $\left[E(Y|X) \right]$ in each group to be 3.66 + 24.0X. Therefore, the estimated rate ratio, comparing Protestants with other religions, is 1 + (24.0/3.66) = 7.6. Note in Figure 30-2 that the fit of the linear model appears excellent ($R^2 = 0.97$). In general, however, measures of fit for ecologic models can be misleading about the underlying model at the individual level that generated the ecologic data.[96]

The ecologic method of effect estimation requires rate predictions be extrapolated to both extreme values of the exposure variable (*i.e.*, $X = 0$ and 1), which are likely to lie well beyond the observed range of the data. It is not surprising, therefore, that different model forms (*e.g.*, loglinear vs. linear) can lead to very different estimates of effect.[97] Fitting a linear model, in fact, may lead to negative, and thus meaningless, estimates of the rate ratio. And as already mentioned, a linear model and analysis using ordinary least squares is problematic due to the implicit assumption of uncorrelated errors with constant variance. Other statistical methods for estimating exposure effects in ecologic studies are discussed by Chambers and Steel,[56] Gelman et al.,[98] and Wakefield.[11,43]

Confounders and Effect Modifiers

There are two methods used to control for confounders in multiple-group ecologic analyses. The first is to treat ecologic measures of the confounders as covariates (Z) in the model, *e.g.*, percentage of males and percentage of Whites in each group. If the individual-level effects of the exposure and covariates are additive (*i.e.*, if the disease rates follow a linear model), then the ecologic regression of Y on X and Z will also be linear with the same coefficients.[39,97,99] That is, the estimated coefficient

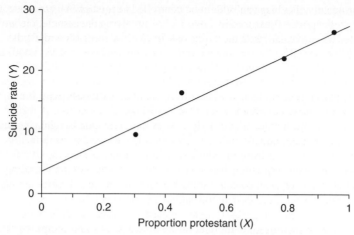

FIGURE 30-2 Suicide rate (Y, per 10^5/y) by proportion Protestant (X) for four groups of Prussian provinces, 1883-1890. The four observed points (X, Y) are (0.30, 9.56), (0.45, 16.36), (0.785, 22.00), and (0.95, 26.46); the fitted line is based on unweighted least-squares regression. (Adapted from Durkheim E. *Suicide: a Study in Sociology*. New York: Free Press; 1951.)[95]

for the exposure variable in a linear model can be interpreted as the rate difference adjusted for the covariates, provided the effects are truly additive and there are no other sources of bias. To estimate the adjusted rate ratio for the exposure effect, we must first specify values for all covariates (**Z**) in the model, because the effects of X and **Z** are assumed to be additive—not multiplicative. Thus, the estimated rate ratio, conditional on covariate levels (**Z**), is the predicted rate in a group that is entirely exposed $\left[E(Y|X=1, \mathbf{Z}) \right]$ divided by the predicted rate in a group that is entirely unexposed $\left[E(Y|X=0, \mathbf{Z}) \right]$.

Fitting a loglinear model to the ecologic data yields an estimate of the adjusted rate ratio that is independent of covariates; *i.e.*, $E(Y|X=1, \mathbf{Z})/E(Y/X=0, \mathbf{Z}) = \exp(B_1)$, where B_1 is the estimated coefficient for the exposure. (For ease of notation, parameters and their estimates are not distinguished, with the difference being clear from the context.) Thus, the effects of X and **Z** are assumed to be multiplicative. Unfortunately, this ecologic estimate is a biased estimate of the individual-level rate ratio, even if the effects are multiplicative at the individual level and no other source of bias is present.[96,100]

The second method used to control for confounders in ecologic analyses is rate standardization for these confounders (see Chapters 4 and 5), followed by regression of the standardized rates as the outcome variable. Note that this method requires additional data on the joint distribution of the covariate and disease within each group (*i.e.*, the M frequencies in Figure 30-1). Nevertheless, it cannot be expected to reduce bias unless all predictors in the model (X and **Z**) are also mutually standardized for the same confounders, using the same standard population.[97,101,102] Standardization of the exposure prevalences, for example, requires data on the joint distribution of the covariate and exposure within groups (*i.e.*, the N frequencies in Figure 30-1); unfortunately, this information is not usually available in ecologic studies.

As in individual-level analyses, product terms (*e.g.*, XZ) are often used in ecologic analyses to model interaction effects, *i.e.*, to assess effect modification. In ecologic analyses, however, the product of X and Z (both group averages) is not, in general, equal to the average product of the exposure (x) and covariate (z) at the individual level within groups. Assuming a linear model, XZ will be equal to the mean xz in each group only if x and z are uncorrelated within groups.[97] Thus, as pointed out in "Problems of Confounder Control," nonadditive interaction effects at the individual level complicate the interpretation of ecologic results.

Confounding by Indication

As mentioned earlier, in nonrandomized clinical studies of treatment effects, confounding tends to occur when the indication for being treated—good or poor prognosis—is a predictor of the outcome. Unfortunately, that bias can seldom be controlled adequately by covariate adjustment.[103] Confounding by indication is illustrated in Table 30-1A, involving the association between a binary treatment (treated vs. untreated) and mortality risk in two facilities (A and B). As shown in the table, the risk difference (RD) for treatment stratified by prognosis (poor vs. good) and facility is −0.10 (the effect parameter of interest). However, poor prognosis is positively association with both treatment status and mortality risk in each facility. Thus, the crude RD in each facility is 0.02, which is strongly biased beyond the null. If data from the two facilities are combined, the crude RD is −0.01, still strongly biased toward the null (Table 30-1A).

Now suppose we conduct an ecologic analysis with the same data by ignoring prognosis (confounder) and excluding (individual-level) data on mortality risk within each facility. As shown in Table 30-1B, the RD, obtained from the slope (B_1) in the linear model, is −0.10, *i.e.*, unbiased. While this result may seem surprising, Wen and Kramer[104] argued that confounding by indication would be less likely to occur in an ecologic study because treatment decisions among facilities are influenced by "practice style," rather than the patient's prognosis.

The ecologic analysis in Table 30-1B is not biased because, in Table 30-1A, mortality risk does not differ between facilities, conditional on treatment status and prognosis. No bias occurs because this particular ecologic analysis is equivalent to an *instrumental-variable analysis*[105] (see Chapter 28), where the instrumental variable is the treatment facility. More specifically, the data in Table 30-1A satisfy two key assumptions of a valid instrumental-variable analysis: (1) facility affects mortality risk only through (individual-level) treatment status and (2) the effect of facility on mortality risk is not confounded.[106] Note that these assumptions depend on information that is not available in an ecologic analysis; moreover, they are not likely to hold in practice.

Recognizing the methodologic limitations of ecologic analysis with Wen and Kramer's method, Johnston[107] proposed a semi-ecologic analysis, which he called a "two-level" analysis, in which the outcome and covariates are measured at the individual level, but treatment status is measured at the group level (*e.g.*, proportion treated in each facility). Using simulations, they found that their method yielded less biased estimates of the treatment effect than did a conventional analysis using the patient's treatment status.[108] In a recent application of semi-ecologic analysis in patients hospitalized with acute myocardial infarction, Pack et al.[109] found little difference in inpatient mortality risk comparing hospitals with the highest versus the lowest proportion of those patients receiving echocardiography.

METHODOLOGIC PROBLEMS

Despite the many practical advantages of ecologic studies mentioned previously, there are several methodologic problems, beyond those already discussed, that may severely limit causal inference, especially biologic inference.

Ecologic Bias

The major limitation of ecologic analysis for making causal inferences is ecologic bias, which is usually interpreted as the failure of ecologic associations to reflect the biologic effect at the individual level.[11,18,20,93,96,100,102,110] More generally, *cross-level bias* (or "cross-level fallacy") can be interpreted as the failure of associations seen at one level of grouping to correspond to effect measures at the grouping level of interest.[21,30,111] For example, relations seen in county-level data may poorly track relations that exist at the individual level (no grouping) or at the neighborhood level (neighborhood grouping), and so would be biased if individual-level or neighborhood-level relations were of interest.[24,112] This failure to capture desired effects applies also to estimating confounder effects at the level of interest, and hence threatens validity both directly and by undermining control of confounding.[24]

In addition to the usual sources of bias that threaten individual-level analyses (see Chapters 12-14), the underlying problem of ecologic analyses for estimating biologic effects is heterogeneity of exposure level and covariate levels within groups. As noted earlier, this heterogeneity is not fully captured with ecologic data because of missing information on joint distributions (Figure 30-1). Robinson[113] was the first to describe mathematically how ecologic associations could differ from the corresponding associations at the individual level within groups of the same population.[113]

TABLE 30-1A

Number (*N*) of Patients and Mortality Risk (*R*), by Facility, Treatment Status, and Patient Prognosis: Hypothetical Example of Individual-Level Analysis Showing the Risk Difference (RD) for the Protective Effect of Treatment on Mortality Risk, by Facility and Prognosis

Treatment Status	Facility A				Facility B			
	Poor Prognosis		Good Prognosis		Poor Prognosis		Good Prognosis	
	N	*R*	*N*	*R*	*N*	*R*	*N*	*R*
Treated	400	0.40	100	0.10	900	0.40	600	0.10
Untreated	600	0.50	900	0.20	100	0.50	400	0.20
Total	1,000	0.46	1,000	0.19	1,000	0.41	1,000	0.14
RD	−0.10		−0.10		−0.10		−0.10	
Crude RD[a]	0.02				0.02			
Overall RD[b]	−0.01							

[a]Ignoring prognosis within each facility.
[b]Ignoring prognosis and facility.

He expressed this relation in terms of correlation coefficients, which was later extended by Duncan et al.[114] to regression coefficients in a linear model. The phenomenon became widely known as the *ecologic(al) fallacy*,[115] *i.e.*, making incorrect inferences about biologic effects on the basis of ecologic associations. As this concept became widely recognized, researchers discovered that the magnitude of the ecologic bias may be severe in practice.[100,116-119]

As an illustration of ecologic bias, consider again Durkheim's data on religion and suicide (Figure 30-2).[95] The estimated rate ratio of 7.6 in the ecologic analysis may not mean that the suicide rate was nearly eight times greater in Protestants than in non-Protestants. Rather, since none of the regions was entirely Protestant or non-Protestant, it may have been non-Protestants (primarily Catholics) who were committing suicide in predominantly Protestant provinces. It is certainly plausible that members of a religious minority might have been more likely to take their own lives than were members of the majority. The implication of this alternative explanation is that living in a predominantly Protestant area has a contextual effect on suicide risk among non-Protestants; specifically, there is an interaction effect at the individual level between religion and religious composition of one's area of residence.

TABLE 30-1B

Number (*N*) of Patients and Mortality Risk (*R*), by Facility and Treatment Status: Hypothetical Example of an Ecologic Analysis Based on Data From Table 30-1A With Data Missing on Prognosis and the Joint Distribution of Treatment Status and Mortality Risk Within Facilities

Treatment Status	Facility A		Facility B		Total	
	N	*R*	*N*	*R*	*N*	*R*
Treated	500	?	1,500	?	2,000	?
Untreated	1,500	?	5,00	?	2,000	?
Total	2,000	0.325	2,000	0.275	4,000	0.300

$$RD^a = B_1 = \frac{Change\ in\ risk}{Change\ in\ \%\ treated} = \frac{0.325-0.275}{0.25-0.75} = -0.10$$

[a]The slope (*B*₁) of the linear regression model can be calculated algebraically since there are only two groups (facilities) in the ecologic analysis.

Interestingly, Durkheim[95] compared the suicide rates (at the individual level) for Protestants, Catholics, and Jews living in Prussia; and from his data, we find that the rate was about twice as great in Protestants as in other religious groups. Thus, there appears to be substantial ecologic bias (*i.e.*, comparing rate-ratio estimates of about 2 vs. 8). Durkheim,[95] however, failed to notice this quantitative difference because he did not actually estimate the magnitude of the effect in either analysis.

Greenland and Morgenstern[102] showed that ecologic bias can arise from three sources when using simple linear regression to estimate the crude exposure effect: the first may operate in any type of study; the latter two are unique to ecologic studies (*i.e.*, cross-level bias) but are defined in terms of individual-level parameters.

1. *Within-group bias.* Ecologic bias may result from bias within groups due to confounding, selection methods, or misclassification, even though within-group effects are not estimated. Thus, for example, if there is positive confounding of the crude effect parameter in every group, we would expect the crude ecologic estimate to be biased as well (an exception was described in the previous section).
2. *Confounding by group.* Ecologic bias may result if the background rate of disease in the unexposed population varies across groups. More specifically, bias results if there is a nonzero ecologic correlation between mean exposure level and the background rate.
3. *Effect modification by group (on an additive scale).* Ecologic bias may also result if the rate difference for the exposure effect at the individual level varies across groups.

Confounding and effect modification by group (the sources of cross-level bias) can arise in three ways: (1) extraneous risk factors (confounders or modifiers) are differentially distributed across groups; (2) the ecologic exposure variable has a contextual effect on risk separate from the biologic effect of its individual-level analogue, *e.g.*, living in a predominantly Protestant area versus being Protestant (in the suicide example)[110]; or (3) disease risk depends on the prevalence of that disease in other members of the group, which is true of many infectious diseases.[27] For nonlinear models, *pure specification bias* is another problem that is discussed in the next section.

To appreciate the sources of cross-level bias, it is helpful to consider simple numerical illustrations involving both individual-level and ecologic analyses with the same population (as in Figure 30-1). The hypothetical example in Table 30-2 involves a dichotomous exposure (x) and three groups. At the individual level, both the rate difference and rate ratio vary somewhat across the groups, but the effect is positive in all groups; the crude and group-standardized rate ratio is 2.0. Fitting a linear model to the ecologic data, however, we find that the slope for the exposure variable (X) is negative and the rate ratio is 0.50, suggesting a protective effect. The reason for such large ecologic bias is heterogeneity of the rate difference across groups (effect modification by group). In this example, there is no confounding by group because the unexposed rate is the same in all three groups, *i.e.*, 100 cases per 10^5 person-years, or more formally, 100 per 10^5/y (rates have units of inverse time; see Chapter 4).

The example in Table 30-3 illustrates the conditions for no cross-level bias. First, group is not a modifier of the exposure effect at the individual level because the rate difference (100 per 10^5/y) is uniform across groups (even though the rate ratio varies). Second, group is not a confounder of the exposure effect because there is no ecologic correlation between the percentage of exposed ($100X$) and the unexposed rate. Thus, the individual-level and ecologic estimates of the rate ratio are the same (1.8) and unbiased, even though the R^2 for the fitted model is very low ($R^2 = 0.029$).

Unfortunately, the two conditions that produce cross-level bias cannot be checked with ecologic data because those conditions are defined in terms of individual-level associations. This inability to check the validity of ecologic results seriously limits biologic inference. Furthermore, the fit of the ecologic regression model, in general, gives no indication of the presence, direction, or magnitude of ecologic bias. Thus, a model with excellent fit may yield substantial bias, and one model with a better fit than another model may yield more bias. For example, there was substantial bias when fitting a linear model to Durkheim's suicide data in Figure 30-2,[95] despite an excellent fitting model ($R^2 = 0.97$). Recall that the estimated rate ratio was 7.6, compared with a "true" rate ratio of approximately 2. If we fit a loglinear model to the same data, we get $E(Y|X) = \exp(1.974 + 1.418X)$ and $R^2 = 0.91$; therefore, the estimated rate ratio is $\exp(1.418) = 4.1$. Thus, the loglinear model produces less bias even though it has a smaller R^2 than does the linear model. In general, we cannot expect to reduce bias by using better fitting models in ecologic analysis.

TABLE 30-2

Number of New Cases, Person-Years (P-Y) of Follow-up, and Disease Rate (Y, per 100,000/Y), by Group and Exposure Status (x) (Top); Summary Parameters for Each Group (Middle); and Results of Individual-Level and Ecologic Analyses (Bottom): Hypothetical Example of Ecologic Bias due to Effect Modification by Group

Exposure Status (x)	Group 1			Group 2			Group 3		
	Cases	P-Y	Rate	Cases	P-Y	Rate	Cases	P-Y	Rate
Exposed (1)	20	7,000	286	20	10,000	200	20	13,000	154
Unexposed (0)	13	13,000	100	10	10,000	100	7	7,000	100
Total	33	20,000	165	30	20,000	150	27	20,000	135
Percentage of exposed (100X)			35			50			65
Rate difference (per 10^5/y)			286			100			54
Rate ratio			2.9			2.0			1.5

Individual-level analysis

Crude rate ratio[a] = 2.0

Adjusted rate ratio (SMR)[b] = 2.0

Ecologic analysis: linear model

$E(Y) = 200 - 100X$ $(R^2 = 1)$

Rate ratio = 0.50

[a] Rate ratio for the total population, unadjusted for group.
[b] Rate ratio standardized for group, using the exposed population as the standard.

TABLE 30-3

Number of New Cases, Person-Years (P-Y) of Follow-up, and Disease Rate (Y, per 100,000/Y), by Group and Exposure Status (x) (Top); Summary Parameters for Each Group (Middle); and Results of Individual-Level and Ecologic Analyses (Bottom): Hypothetical Example of No Ecologic Bias

Exposure Status (x)	Group 1			Group 2			Group 3		
	Cases	P-Y	Rate	Cases	P-Y	Rate	Cases	P-Y	Rate
Exposed (1)	16	8,000	200	30	10,000	300	24	12,000	200
Unexposed (0)	12	12,000	100	20	10,000	200	8	8,000	100
Total	28	20,000	140	50	20,000	250	32	20,000	160
Percentage of exposed (100X)			40			50			60
Rate difference (per 10^5/y)			100			100			100
Rate ratio			2.0			1.5			2.0

Individual-level analysis

Crude rate ratio[a] = 1.8

Adjusted rate ratio (SMR)[b] = 1.8

Ecologic analysis: linear model

$E(Y) = 133 + 100X$ ($R^2 = 0.029$)

Rate ratio = 1.8

[a] Rate ratio for the total population, unadjusted for group.
[b] Rate ratio standardized for group, using the exposed population as the standard.

A potential strategy for reducing ecologic bias is to use smaller units in an ecologic study (*e.g.*, counties instead of states) in order to make the groups more homogeneous with respect to the exposure. On the other hand, this strategy might not be feasible due to the lack of available covariate data aggregated at the same level, and it can lead to another problem: greater migration between groups[20,120] (see also "Other Problems"). From a more practical perspective, Arsenault et al.[121] proposed nine criteria for choosing the geographic unit of analysis, such as biologic relevance, communicability of results, and ease of data access. Unfortunately, the geographic areas for which data are available are typically administrative units such as census tracts or counties, which may not correspond to target areas of interest (*e.g.*, neighborhoods or hospital service areas).

Other methods for reducing ecologic bias rely on statistical modeling techniques that incorporate external information, *i.e.*, supplementary data on individuals or prior information.[4,11,19,57-60,97,122-124] For example, Best et al.[125] used a Bayesian hierarchical modeling approach to estimate the effect of environmental exposure to benzene on the incidence of childhood leukemia in Greater London. These investigators employed three units of analysis: local authority districts, census wards, and 1-km^2 grid squares. Although they found consistent positive associations between benzene exposure and childhood leukemia, the authors acknowledged several methodologic problems that limited their ability to make causal inferences. For studies investigating the health effects of air pollution, it has become common to use modeled exposure surfaces, but this practice can produce challenges in accounting for the uncertainty in the surface.[126]

A widely cited method for eliminating ecologic bias without the use of external information was proposed by King.[127] His approach combined the linear-regression method described previously[93] and the method of "bounds," proposed by Duncan and Davis.[128] Early critics of King's method maintained that it does not provide accurate estimates of individual effects in certain datasets and that the diagnostics provided by King are not sensitive to the errors.[129] One key problem of King's model, in its original form, is that it assumes no contextual effects.[57] These claims have been debated in the literature,[130,131] and the method remains controversial.[57,132,133] One critic has concluded that King's method is unlikely to reduce ecologic bias relative to simpler models.[133] As with all methods for making ecologic inference, King's approach is based on strong assumptions that are untestable with ecologic data.

Pure Specification Bias

The source of ecologic bias in Table 30-2, heterogeneity of the rate difference across groups in a linear model, extends more generally to nonlinear models. Pure specification bias, as described by Greenland,[97] also referred to as "model specification bias,"[134] arises because in general a nonlinear risk model changes its form under aggregation. In this section, we show subscripts for y and x denoting individual j within area i, for $i = 1,...,m$ areas and $j = 1,...,n(i)$ individuals within area i. To illustrate pure specification bias, we first assume the linear individual-level model with this notation:

$$E\left(y_{ij}\middle|x_{ij}\right) = b_0 + b_1 x_{ij}$$

[30-1]

The aggregate (ecologic) data are assumed to correspond to the average risk Y_i and average exposure X_i in the ith area. On aggregation (averaging) of 30-1 we obtain:

$$E\left(Y_i\middle|X_i\right) = B_0 + B_1 X_i$$

[30-2]

Thus, a linear individual risk model retains its form under aggregation, and we retain the individual-level parameters from 30-1, where $b_0 = B_0$ and $b_1 = B_1$.

When the risk is nonlinear, however, aggregation does not generally recover the same form, as we now illustrate with the loglinear individual risk model:

$$E\left(y_{ij}\middle|x_{ij}\right) = \exp\left(b_0 + b_1 x_{ij}\right)$$

[30-3]

In this model, $\exp(b_0)$ is the risk associated with $x = 0$ (baseline risk), and $\exp(b_1)$ is the relative risk corresponding to an increase in x of one unit. If we aggregate this model, we obtain the average of the individual risks:

$$E\left[Y_i \big| x_{ij}, j = 1,...,n(i)\right] = \tfrac{1}{n(i)}\sum_{i=1}^{n(i)} \exp\left(b_0 + b_1 x_{ij}\right)$$

[30-4]

A naive ecologic model, applying the same form as 30-3, would assume:

$$E\left(Y_i \big| X_i\right) = \exp\left(B_0 + B_1 X_i\right)$$

[30-5]

where the ecologic parameters are again denoted B_0, B_1 and are distinguished from the individual-level parameters in 30-4. If one tries to interpret model 30-5 at the individual level, then it would imply that there is a *contextual effect* operating since risk depends on the proportion of exposed individuals in the area. Interpreting $\exp(B_1)$ as an individual association would therefore correspond to a belief that it is average exposure that is causative and that individual exposure is irrelevant.

The difference between 30-4 and 30-5 is clear: While the former averages the risks across all exposure levels, the latter is the risk corresponding to the average exposure. Without further assumptions on the moments (in particular, the variance) of the within-area exposure distributions, we can guarantee no ecologic bias, *i.e.*, $\exp(B_1) = \exp(b_1)$, only when there is no within-area variability in exposure so that $x_{ij} = X_i$ for all individuals in area i and for all areas.

In general, there is no pure specification bias if the disease model is linear in x, as assumed in the previous section, or if all the moments of the within-area distribution of exposure are independent of the mean. If b_1 is close to zero, this form of pure specification bias is also likely to be small (since then the exponential model will be approximately a linear model for which there is no bias), though in this case confounding is likely to be a serious concern. Unfortunately, the mean-variance relation is impossible to assess without individual-level data on the exposure. If the exposure is heterogeneous within areas, we need information on the variability within each area to control the bias. Such information may come from a sample of individuals within each area. Detailed discussion of ecologic modeling with a loglinear model can be found elsewhere.[37,100,123,135]

Problems of Confounder Control

As indicated in a previous section, covariates are included in ecologic analyses to control for confounding, but the conditions for a covariate being a confounder are different at the ecologic and individual levels.[24,96,102,136] At the individual level, a risk factor must be associated with the exposure to be a confounder. In a multiple-group ecologic study, in contrast, a risk factor may produce ecologic bias (*e.g.*, it may be an ecologic confounder) even if it is unassociated with the exposure in every group, especially if the risk factor is ecologically associated with the exposure across groups.[97,102] Conversely, a risk factor that is a confounder within groups may not produce ecologic bias if it is ecologically unassociated with the exposure across groups. For example, as noted previously, there is some evidence that confounding by indication in the estimation of intended treatment effects is less severe in ecologic or semi-ecologic studies than in observational studies conducted at the individual level.[104,107]

In general, however, control for confounders is far more problematic in ecologic analyses than in individual-level analyses,[24,39,96,97,102] since rarely are data on variables required for confounder control available. Even when all variables are accurately measured for all groups, adjustment for extraneous risk factors may not reduce the ecologic bias produced by these risk factors. In fact, it is possible for such ecologic adjustment to increase bias.[96,102]

It follows from the principles presented in the previous section that there will be no ecologic bias in a multiple-linear-regression analysis if all the following conditions are met:

1. There is no residual within-group bias in exposure effect in any group due to confounding by unmeasured risk factors, selection methods, or misclassification.

2. There is no ecologic correlation between the mean value of each predictor (exposure and covariate) and the background rate of disease in the joint reference (unexposed) level of all predictors (so that group does not confound the predictor effects).
3. The rate difference for each predictor is uniform across levels of the other predictors within groups (*i.e.*, the effects are additive).
4. The rate difference for each predictor, conditional on other predictors in the model, is uniform across groups (*i.e.*, group does not modify the effect of each predictor on the additive scale at the individual level).

These conditions are sufficient, but not necessary, for the ecologic estimate to be unbiased; *i.e.*, there might be little or no bias even if none of these conditions is met (*e.g.*, see "Confounding by Indication"). On the other hand, minor deviations from the latter three conditions can produce substantial cross-level bias.[97] Since the sufficient conditions for no cross-level bias cannot be checked with ecologic data alone, the unpredictable and potentially severe nature of such bias makes biologic inference from ecologic analyses particularly problematic.

The conditions for no cross-level bias with covariate adjustment are illustrated in the hypothetical example in Table 30-4. Both the exposure (x) and covariate (z) are dichotomous variables, and there are three groups. At the individual level, the covariate is not a confounder of the exposure effect because there is no exposure-covariate association (in person-years) within any of the groups. Thus, the crude and adjusted estimates of the rate ratio are nearly the same (1.3). In the ecologic analysis, however, the covariate is a confounder because there is an inverse association between the exposure (X) and the covariate (Z) across groups. Thus, although the crude ecologic estimate of the rate ratio (0.32) is severely biased, the adjusted estimate (1.3) is unbiased. The reasons for no cross-level bias with covariate adjustment are (1) the rate (100 per 10^5/y) in the joint reference group ($x = z = 0$) does not vary across groups, *i.e.*, the second condition is met and (2) the rate difference (100 per 10^5/y) is uniform within groups and across groups—*i.e.*, the third and fourth conditions are met.

The example in Table 30-5 illustrates cross-level bias when the null hypothesis is true. At the individual level, the covariate (z) is a strong confounder because it is a predictor of the disease in the unexposed population and it is associated with exposure status (x) within groups. Thus, the crude rate ratio (2.1) is biased. At the ecologic level, however, there is no association between the exposure (X) and the covariate (Z), so that the covariate is not an ecologic confounder. Nevertheless, both the crude and adjusted rate ratios (8.6) are strongly biased because the rate in the joint reference category ($x = z = 0$) is ecologically associated with both the exposure (X) and the covariate (Z)—*i.e.*, the second condition is not met.

Lack of additivity at the individual level (refer to the third condition) is common in epidemiology, but unmeasured modifiers do not bias results at the individual level if they are unrelated to the exposure.[90] Furthermore, statistical interactions may be readily assessed at the individual level by including product terms as predictors in the model (*e.g.*, xz). In ecologic analyses, however, lack of additivity within groups is a source of ecologic bias, and this bias cannot be eliminated by the inclusion of product terms (*e.g.*, XZ) unless the effects are exactly multiplicative and the two variables are uncorrelated within groups.[137] If x and z are correlated within groups, additional data on the x-z associations (the N frequencies in Figure 30-1) can be used to improve the ecologic estimate of each predictor effect controlling for the other.[5,11,19,34,37,122,123,138,139]

Another source of ecologic bias is misspecification of confounders.[96] Although this problem can also arise in individual-level analyses, it is more difficult to avoid in ecologic analyses because the relevant confounder may be the distribution of covariate histories for all individuals within each group. In ecologic studies, therefore, adjustment for covariates derived from available data (*e.g.*, proportion of current smokers) may be inadequate to control confounding (by smoking). It is preferable, whenever possible, to control for more than a single summary measure of the covariate distribution (*e.g.*, the proportions of the group in each of several nonreference smoking categories). In addition, since it is usually necessary to control for several confounders (among which the effects may not be linear and additive), the best approach for reducing bias in an ecologic analysis is to include covariates for categories of their joint distribution within groups. For example, to control ecologically for race and sex, the investigator might adjust for the proportions of White women, non-White men, and non-White women (treating White men as the referent), rather than the conventional approach of adjusting for the proportions of men (or women) and Whites (or non-Whites).

TABLE 30-4

Number of New Cases, Person-Years (P-Y) of Follow-up, and Disease Rate (Y, per 100,000/Y), by Group, Covariate Status (z), and Exposure Status (x) (Top); Summary Parameters for Each Group (Middle); and Results of Individual-Level and Ecologic Analyses (Bottom): Hypothetical Example of No Ecologic Bias; Covariate is an Ecologic Confounder but not a Within-Group Confounder

Covariate Status (z)	Exposure Status (x)	Group 1			Group 2			Group 3		
		Cases	P-Y	Rate	Cases	P-Y	Rate	Cases	P-Y	Rate
1	Exposed (1)	18	3,000	600	24	4,000	600	24	4,000	600
	Unexposed (0)	60	12,000	500	40	8,000	500	30	6,000	500
	Total	78	15,000	520	64	12,000	533	54	10,000	540
0	Exposed (1)	4	2,000	200	8	4,000	200	12	6,000	200
	Unexposed (0)	8	8,000	100	8	8,000	100	9	9,000	100
	Total	12	10,000	120	16	12,000	133	21	15,000	140
Total	Exposed (1)	22	5,000	440	32	8,000	400	36	10,000	360
	Unexposed (0)	68	20,000	340	48	16,000	300	39	15,000	260
	Total	90	25,000	360	80	24,000	333	75	25,000	300
Percentage exposed (100X)				20			33			40
Percentage with z = 1 (100Z)				60			50			40

Individual-level analysis

Crude rate ratio[a] = 1.3

Adjusted rate ratio (SMR)[b] = 1.3

Ecologic analysis: linear models

Crude: $E(Y) = 420 - 286X$ ($R^2 = 0.94$); rate ratio = 0.32

Adjusted: $E(Y) = 100 + 100X + 400Z$ ($R^2 = 1$); rate ratio[c] = 1.3

[a] Rate ratio for the total population, unadjusted for group or the covariate.
[b] Rate ratio standardized for group and the covariate, using the exposed population as the standard.
[c] Setting $Z = 0.50$ (the mean for all three groups).

TABLE 30-5

Number of New Cases, Person-Years (P-Y) of Follow-up, and Disease Rate (Y, per 100,000/Y), by Group, Covariate Status (z), and Exposure Status (x) (Top); Summary Parameters for Each Group (Middle); and Results of Individual-Level and Ecologic Analyses (Bottom): Hypothetical Example of Ecologic Bias due to Confounding by Group; Covariate is a Within-Group Confounder but Not an Ecologic Confounder

Covariate Status (z)	Exposure Status (x)	Group 1			Group 2			Group 3		
		Cases	P-Y	Rate	Cases	P-Y	Rate	Cases	P-Y	Rate
1	Exposed (1)	40	8,000	500	195	13,000	1,500	140	14,000	1,000
	Unexposed (0)	60	12,000	500	180	12,000	1,500	60	6,000	1,000
	Total	100	20,000	500	375	25,000	1,500	200	20,000	1,000
0	Exposed (1)	2	2,000	100	6	2,000	300	12	6,000	200
	Unexposed (0)	28	28,000	100	69	23,000	300	48	24,000	200
	Total	30	30,000	100	75	25,000	300	60	30,000	200
Total	Exposed (1)	42	10,000	420	201	15,000	1,340	152	20,000	760
	Unexposed (0)	88	40,000	220	249	35,000	711	108	30,000	360
	Total	130	50,000	260	450	50,000	900	260	50,000	520
Percentage exposed (100X)		20			30			40		
Percentage with z = 1 (100Z)		40			50			40		

Individual-level analysis

Crude rate ratio[a] = 2.1

Adjusted rate ratio (SMR)[b] = 1.0

Ecologic analysis: linear models

Crude: $E(Y) = 170 + 1,300X$ ($R^2 = 0.16$); rate ratio = 8.6

Adjusted: $E(Y) = -2,040 + 1,300X + 5,100Z$ ($R^2 = 1$); rate ratio[c] = 8.6

[a] Rate ratio for the total population, unadjusted for group or the covariate.
[b] Rate ratio standardized for group and the covariate, using the exposed population as the standard; also the common rate ratio within each group.
[c] Setting Z = 0.433 (the mean for all three groups).

Within-Group Misclassification

The principles of misclassification bias with which epidemiologists are familiar when interpreting the results of analyses conducted at the individual level do not apply to ecologic analyses. At the individual level, for example, nondifferential independent misclassification of a dichotomous exposure biases the effect estimate toward the null (see Chapter 13). In multiple-group ecologic studies, however, this principle does not hold when the exposure variable is an aggregate measure. Brenner et al.[140] have shown that nondifferential misclassification of a dichotomous exposure within groups usually leads to bias away from the null and that the bias may be severe.

As an illustration of this distinct feature of ecologic analysis, consider the two-group example in Table 30-6, which contrasts analyses with correctly classified and misclassified exposure data at both the individual and ecologic levels. The sensitivity and specificity of exposure classification are assumed to be 0.9 for both cases and noncases in the population. The correct rate ratio at the individual level is 5.0. With nondifferential exposure misclassification, the observed rate ratio would be 3.4, which is biased toward the null. Although an ecologic analysis of the correctly classified data yields an unbiased estimate of the rate ratio (5.0), an analysis with misclassified data would yield an observed rate ratio of 11.0, which is strongly biased away from the null. To appreciate the direction of the misclassification bias in this ecologic analysis, notice that the difference in the percentage exposed ($100X$) between the two groups decreases from $40 - 20 = 20\%$ to $42 - 26 = 16\%$ when the exposure is misclassified (Table 30-5). Thus, the slope in the misclassified analysis increases from 200 to 250 per 10^5/y. In addition, the intercept decreases from 50 to 25 per 10^5/y. Each of these changes causes the observed rate ratio with the misclassified data to increase (away from the null).

It is possible to correct for nondifferential misclassification of a dichotomous exposure or disease in ecologic analyses, based on prior specifications of sensitivity and specificity.[140,141] Suppose, for example, we wish to correct for nondifferential exposure misclassification when using simple linear regression (no covariates) to estimate the exposure effect. The corrected estimator of the rate ratio derived from the model results is $(B_0 + B_1 Se)/[B_0 + B_1(1 - Sp)]$, where B_0 and B_1 are the estimated intercept and slope from the misclassified data, Se is the sensitivity of exposure classification, and Sp is the specificity. Substituting B_0 and B_1 from the misclassified ecologic analysis in Table 30-6 into this expression for the corrected rate ratio, we get $[25 + 250(0.9)]/[25 + 250(1 - 0.9)] = 5.0$, the correct value. Greenland and Brenner[141] also derived a corrected estimator for the variance of the estimated rate ratio.

In studies conducted at the individual level, misclassification of a covariate, if nondifferential with respect to both exposure and disease, will usually reduce our ability to control for that confounder.[142,143] That is, adjustment will not completely eliminate the bias due to the confounder. In ecologic studies, however, nondifferential misclassification of a dichotomous confounder within groups does not affect our ability to control for that confounder, provided there is no cross-level bias.[144] More generally, however, misclassification of confounders will reduce control of confounding at the ecologic level as well as the individual level.

Other Problems

Lack of Adequate Data

Certain types of data, such as medical histories, may not be available in aggregate form; or available data may be too crude, incomplete, or unreliable, such as sales data for measuring behaviors.[20,120] In addition, secondary sources of data from different administrative areas or from different periods may not be comparable. For example, disease rates may vary across countries because of differences in disease classification or case detection. Furthermore, since many ecologic analyses are based on mortality rather than incidence data, causal inference may be further limited because mortality reflects the course of disease as well as its occurrence.[1]

Temporal Ambiguity

In a well-designed cohort study of disease incidence, we can usually be confident that disease occurrence did not precede the exposure. In ecologic studies, however, use of incidence data provides no such assurance against this temporal ambiguity.[20] The problem is most troublesome when

TABLE 30-6

Number of New Cases, Person-Years (P-Y) of Follow-up, and Disease Rate (Y, per 100,000/Y), by Group, Type of Exposure Classification (Correct vs. Misclassified[a]), and Exposure Status (Top); Percentage of Exposed by Group (Middle); and Results of Individual-Level and Ecologic Analyses (Bottom): Hypothetical Example of Ecologic Bias Away From the Null due to Nondifferential Exposure Misclassification Within Groups

Exposure Classification	Exposure Status (x or x')	Group 1			Group 2		
		Cases	P-Y	Rate	Cases	P-Y	Rate
Correctly classified	Exposed ($x = 1$)	50	20,000	250	100	40,000	250
	Unexposed ($x = 0$)	40	80,000	50	30	60,000	50
	Total	90	100,000	90	130	100,00	130
Misclassified[a]	Exposed ($x' = 1$)	49	26,000	188	93	42,000	221
	Unexposed ($x' = 0$)	41	74,000	55	37	58,000	64
	Total	90	100,000	90	130	100,000	130
Percentage exposed, correctly classified ($100X$)		20			40		
Percentage exposed, misclassified ($100X'$)		26			42		

Individual-level analysis Ecologic analysis: linear models

Correct: rate ratio[b] = 5.0 Correct: $E(Y) = 50 + 200X$; rate ratio = 5.0

Misclassified: rate ratio[c] = 3.4 Misclassified: $E(Y) = 25 + 250X'$; rate ratio = 11.0

[a]Sensitivity = specificity = 0.9 for both cases and noncases (nondifferential misclassification).
[b]Common rate ratio within each group.
[c]Common rate ratio, using the Mantel-Haenszel method.

the disease can influence exposure status in individuals (reverse causation) or when the disease rate can influence the mean exposure in groups (through the impact of population interventions designed to change exposure levels in areas with high disease rates).

The problem of temporal ambiguity in ecologic studies (especially time-trend studies) is further complicated by an unknown or variable induction and latent periods between exposure and disease detection.[83,120] The investigator can only attempt to deal with this problem in the analysis by examining associations for which there is a specified lag between observations of average exposure and disease rate. Unfortunately, there may be little prior information about induction and latency on which to base the lag, the induction/latency may vary appreciably among individual cases, or appropriate data may not be available to accommodate the desired lag.

Collinearity

Another problem with ecologic analyses is that certain predictors, such as sociodemographic and environmental factors, tend to be more highly correlated with each other than they are at the individual level.[116,117] The implication of such collinearities is that it is very difficult to separate the effects of these variables statistically; analyses yield model coefficients with very large variances so that effect estimates may be highly unstable. In general, collinearity is most problematic in multiple-group ecologic analyses involving a small number of large, heterogeneous regions.[22,114]

Migration Across Groups

Migration of individuals into or out of the source population can produce selection bias in a study conducted at the individual level because migrants and nonmigrants may differ on both exposure prevalence and disease risk. Although it is clear that migration can also cause ecologic bias,[145,146] little is known about the magnitude of this bias or how it can be reduced in ecologic studies.[31] Using simulations based on "dynamic systems," Ocaña-Riola et al.[147] found that mortality rates can be overestimated by nearly 20% in areas with high uncontrolled immigration, but they did not apply their findings to ecologic analysis. With recent technological advances for tracking and mapping individuals, new spatiotemporal methods offer opportunities for studying migration and mobility patterns in an ecologic context.[8] For example, Zagheni et al.[148] used Twitter data to examine migration patterns across and within countries.

Interpreting Ecologic Associations

Knowing the severe methodologic limitations of ecologic analysis for making biologic inferences, many epidemiologists who report ecologic results argue that there can be no cross-level bias when their primary objective is to estimate an ecologic effect.[149-151] For example, we might want to estimate the ecologic effect (effectiveness) of state laws requiring smoke detectors by comparing the fire-related mortality rate in those states with the law versus other states without the law.[20] Although this is a reasonable objective, the interpretation of observed ecologic effects is complicated by several issues.

First, outcome events (disease or death) occur in individuals; thus, the disease or mortality rate in a population is an aggregate, not a global, measure. Consequently, biologic inference may be implicit to the objectives of an ecologic study unless the underlying biologic and contextual effects are already known from previous research. Can smoke detectors placed appropriately in homes reduce the risk of fire-related mortality in those homes by providing an early warning of smoke? Does living in an area where most homes are properly equipped with smoke detectors reduce the risk of fire-related mortality in homes with or without smoke detectors? The first question refers to a possible biologic effect; the second question refers to a possible contextual effect. The ecologic effect of smoke-detector laws depends on these biologic and contextual effects as well as other factors, *e.g.*, the level of enforcement, the quality of smoke-detector design and construction, the cost and availability of smoke detectors, and their proper placement, installation, operation, and maintenance. In an ecologic study without additional information, the ecologic effect completely confounds biologic and contextual effects.[39,110]

Another complicating issue in interpreting observed ecologic effects as contextual effects is that there may be a need to control for confounders measured at the individual level.[24] Even if the exposure is a global measure, such as a law, groups are seldom completely homogeneous or comparable with respect to confounders. To make a valid comparison between states with and without smoke-detector laws, for example, we would need to control for differences among states in the joint distribution of extraneous risk factors, such as socioeconomic status of residents, firefighter availability and access, building design, and construction.

When contextual effects are of interest, rarely are the available ecologic data grouped in a way closely relevant to the effect of interest. Typical vital statistics data on disease occurrence are aggregated by a convenient geopolitical unit, which may be far too coarse to allow valid estimation of small-area effects, *e.g.*, at the neighborhood level. Unfortunately, ecologic associations can be extremely sensitive to the grouping level, making claims about relations seen at one level dubious when applied to another level of interest.[24,113,121]

MULTILEVEL ANALYSES AND DESIGNS

One solution to the problem of separating individual and contextual effects is to incorporate both individual-level and ecologic measures in the same analysis. This approach might include different measures of the same factor; *e.g.*, each subject would be characterized by his or her own exposure level as well as the average exposure level for all members of the group to which he or she belongs (aggregate measure). Not only would this approach help to clarify the sources and magnitude of ecologic and cross-level bias, but it would also allow us to separate biologic, contextual, and ecologic effects. It is especially appropriate in social epidemiology, infectious-disease epidemiology, and the evaluation of population interventions.

There are various statistical methods for including both individual-level and ecologic measures in the same analysis. One method, called *contextual analysis* in the social sciences, is a simple extension of conventional (generalized linear) modeling such as multiple linear regression and logistic regression.[23,152] The model, which is fit to the data at the individual level, includes both individual-level and ecologic predictors. For example, suppose we wanted to estimate the effect of "herd immunity" on the risk of an infectious disease. The risk (y) of disease might be modeled as a function of the following linear component: $b_0 + b_1x + b_2X + b_3xX$, where x is the individual's immunity status and X is the prevalence of immunity in the group to which that individual belongs.[26] Therefore, b_2 represents the contextual effect of herd immunity, and b_3 represents the interaction effect, which allows the herd-immunity effect to depend on the individual's immune status. The interaction term is needed in this application since we would expect no herd-immunity effect among immune individuals. Note, however, that the interpretation of the interaction effect depends on the form of the model (see Chapter 20).

An important limitation of contextual analysis is that outcomes of individuals within groups are treated as independent. In practice, however, the outcomes of two individuals are more likely to be similar if they come from the same group (region) than if they come from different groups, because individuals in the same group tend to share risk factors for the outcome. Ignoring such within-group dependence ("clustering") generally results in estimated variances of contextual effects that are biased downward, making confidence intervals too narrow. To handle this problem of within-group dependence, we can add random effects to the conventional (contextual) model described previously; this approach is called *mixed-effects modeling, multilevel modeling,* or *hierarchical regression.*[7,11-19,57,60,124,138,139]

Multilevel modeling is a powerful technique with many potential applications and statistical benefits.[153-155] It can be used to estimate contextual and ecologic effects and to derive improved (empirical or full Bayes) estimates of individual-level effects. It can also be used to determine how much of the difference in outcome rates across groups (ecologic effect) can be explained by differences in the distribution of individual-level risk factors (biologic effects). For example, a two-level analysis is often used to examine individual-level and ecologic predictors. At the first level of analysis, we might predict individual risk or health status within each group as a function of several individual-level variables. At the second (ecologic) level, we predict the estimated regression parameters (*e.g.*, the intercept and slopes) from the first level as a function of several ecologic variables. The underlying assumption is that the group-specific regression parameters can be viewed as random samples from a population of such parameters. By combining results from both levels, we can predict individual-level outcome as a function of individual-level predictors, ecologic (contextual) predictors, and their interaction terms.

For example, Humphreys and Carr-Hill[25] used multilevel modeling to estimate the contextual effect of living in a poor area (electoral ward) on several health outcomes, controlling for the individual's income and other covariates. In a conventional ecologic analysis, the effects of living in a poor area and personal income would be confounded, and ecologic estimates of effect would be susceptible to cross-level bias. Similar findings for the effects of "neighborhood" socioeconomic status have been reported by several other investigators.[139,156]

Despite many new insights generated by multilevel analysis about the social determinants of disease and health, this approach for analyzing observational data also poses new challenges. First, because there are many selection factors influencing the distribution of people among neighborhoods, it is difficult to control for these factors by covariate adjustment at the individual level. Thus, estimated effects of neighborhood (ecologic) factors, especially aggregate measures, may be confounded by unmeasured risk factors.[157] Second, it is often difficult to distinguish *a priori* whether a given individual-level risk factor affects the ecologic exposure of interest and is therefore a confounder that should be controlled, or whether the risk factor is an intermediate variable (mediator) in the hypothesized causal pathway between the ecologic exposure and disease occurrence and therefore should not be controlled.[158,159] Third, estimated ecologic and contextual effects may be severely distorted when population interventions (aimed at changing the ecologic factor) are implemented in those groups with high outcome rates (reverse causation). Fourth, the ecologic units used in most multilevel analysis are administrative areas (*e.g.*, census tracks), which may not correspond to relevant social contexts for estimating neighborhood effects.[24,158] Fifth, an assumption of most multilevel analyses, based on individual surveys, is that exposure and covariate distributions are stable over time, and this assumption will be suspect when important trends are known to exist.[24] Sixth, to the extent that neighborhood characteristics (context) are determined (endogenously) by aggregating characteristics of individuals within neighborhoods, and not by global (exogenous) interventions, causal (counterfactual) interpretations of contextual and individual effects are problematic (especially when the neighborhoods are small), because we cannot change an individual's exposure status, holding constant the mean exposure status (context) of the neighborhood in which that individual resides, *i.e.*, individual and contextual effects are not completely identifiable.[39,157]

Multilevel analysis can be extended to more than two levels. For example, we might want to predict certain health outcomes in nursing-home residents as a function of characteristics of the residents (*e.g.*, age and health status), their physicians (*e.g.*, type of specialty and country of medical training), and the nursing homes (*e.g.*, size and doctor-to-patient ratio). In this type of analysis, residents are grouped by their physician, who might provide care to many residents in one home, and by their nursing home affiliation.

The simplest design for generating multilevel analyses is a single survey of a population that is large and diverse enough so that multiple groups (*e.g.*, administrative areas or ethnic groups) can be defined for ecologic measurement and analysis. In addition to environmental and global variables for regions or organizations, ecologic measures are derived by aggregating all subjects in each group. An alternative, more efficient, approach is a *multilevel* or *hybrid design* in which a two-stage sampling scheme is used first to select groups (stage 1), followed by the selection of individuals within groups (stage 2).[18,19,25,57,60,124,138,160] A hybrid design might involve conducting a conventional multiple-group ecologic study by linking different data sources, then obtaining supplemental data from individuals randomly sampled from each group. For example, by estimating the exposure-covariate association in each subsample, this approach can be used to improve the control of confounders in an ecologic analysis.[11,34,37,53,57,122,123,160] A variation of this hybrid design might involve a case-control study as the second stage, where cases and controls are identified from each group in the first (ecologic) stage, possibly matching controls to cases on known risk factors as well as group affiliation.[124]

Thus, multilevel models provide an appealing framework to apportion variation between different levels, using crossed and nested effects for example, but ultimately the ability to extract useful information in ecologic studies is critically dependent on the availability of data.

CONCLUSION

There are several practical advantages of ecologic studies that make them especially appealing for doing various types of epidemiologic research. Despite these advantages, however, ecologic analysis poses major problems of interpretation when making statistical or causal inferences and especially when making biologic inferences (due to ecologic bias, etc.). From a methodologic perspective, it is best to have individual-level data on as many relevant nonglobal measures as possible. Just because the exposure variable is measured ecologically, for example, does not mean that other variables should be as well. The validity of effect estimates from ecologic studies can often be improved by obtaining additional data on the within-group associations between covariates, between the exposure and covariates, or between the disease and covariates, and by incorporating prior information. To understand the implications of the use of ecologic data in any setting, it is useful to write down the individual-level model that would be fitted if individual-level data were available. Aggregation of an individual-level model allows the characterization of ecologic bias and reveals the individual-level data that would reduce the chance of ecologic bias. Ecologic bias can be safely removed only by combining ecologic- and individual-level data.

Several epidemiologists have called for greater emphasis on understanding differences in health status between populations—a return to a public-health orientation, in contrast to the individual (reductionist) orientation of modern epidemiology.[35,38,161-165] This recommendation represents an important challenge for the future of epidemiology, but it cannot be met simply by conducting ecologic studies. Multiple levels of measurement and analysis are needed, and additional methodologic and conceptual issues must be addressed.[24] Even when the purpose of the study is to estimate ecologic effects, individual-level information is often essential for drawing valid inferences about these effects. Thus, to address the underlying research questions, we typically would want to estimate and control for biologic and contextual effects, preferably using multilevel analysis. In contemporary epidemiology, the "ecologic fallacy" reflects the failure of the investigator to recognize the need for biologic inference and thus for individual-level data. This need arises even when the primary exposure of interest is an ecologic measure and the outcome of interest is the health status of entire populations.

References

1. Kleinbaum DG, Kupper LL, Morgenstern H. *Epidemiologic Research: Principles and Quantitative Methods*. New York: Van Nostrand Reinhold; 1982.
2. Dogan M, Rokkan S. Introduction. In: Dogan M, Rokkan S, eds. *Social Ecology*. Cambridge, MA: MIT Press; 1969:1-15.
3. MacMahon B, Pugh TF. *Epidemiology: Principles and Methods*. Boston: Little, Brown; 1970.
4. Elliott P, Wakefield JC, Best NG, Briggs DJ, eds. *Spatial Epidemiology: Methods and Applications*. New York: Oxford; 2000.
5. Lawson AB. *Statistical Methods in Spatial Epidemiology*. Chichester: Wiley; 2001.
6. Waller LA, Gotway CA. *Applied Spatial Statistics for Public Health Data*. 1st ed. Hoboken, NJ: Wiley-Interscience; 2004.
7. Banerjee S, Carllin BP, Gelfand AE. Hierarchical Modeling and Analysis for Spatial Data. 2nd ed. Boca Raton: CRC Press; 2015.
8. Meliker JR, Sloan CD. Spatio-temporal epidemiology: principles and opportunities. *Spat Spatiotemporal Epidemiol*. 2011;2(1):1-9.
9. Cressie N, Wikle CK. *Statistics for Spatio-Temporal Data*. New York: Wiley; 2011.
10. Kunzli N, Tager IB. The semi-individual study in air pollution epidemiology: a valid design as compared to ecologic studies. *Environ Health Perspect*. 1997;105(10):1078-1083.
11. Wakefield J. Ecologic studies revisited. *Annu Rev Public Health*. 2008;29:75-90.
12. Wong GY, Mason WM. The hierarchical logistic regression model for multilevel analysis. *J Am Stat Assoc*. 1985;80:513-524.
13. Wong GY, Mason WM. Contextually specific effects and other generalizations for the hierarchical linear model for comparative analysis. *J Am Stat Assoc*. 1991;86:487-503.
14. Bryk AS, Raudenbush SW. *Hierarchical Linear Models: Applications and Data Analysis Methods*. Thousand Oaks, CA: Sage; 1992.
15. Goldstein H. *Multilevel Statistical Models*. 3rd ed. London: Edward Arnold; 2003.
16. Kreft I, de Leeuw J. *Introducing Multilevel Modeling*. London: Sage; 1998.
17. Diez Roux AV. Multilevel analysis in public health research. *Annu Rev Public Health*. 2000;21:171-192.
18. Wakefield J. Multi-level modelling, the ecologic fallacy, and hybrid study designs (edit). *Int J Epidemiol*. 2009;38:330-336.
19. Haneuse S, Bartell S. Designs for the combination of group- and individual-level data. *Epidemiology*. 2011;22(3):382-389.

20. Morgenstern H. Uses of ecologic analysis in epidemiologic research. *Am J Public Health*. 1982;72(12):1336-1344.

21. Achen CH, Shively WP. *Cross-Level Inference*. Chicago: University of Chicago Press; 1995.

22. Valkonen T. Individual and structural effects in ecological research. In: Dogan M, Rokkan S, eds. *Social Ecology*. Cambridge, MA: MIT Press; 1969:53-68.

23. Boyd LHJ, Iversen GR. *Contextual Analysis: Concepts and Statistical Techniques*. Belmont, CA: Wadsworth; 1979.

24. Greenland S. Ecologic versus individual-level sources of bias in ecologic estimates of contextual health effects. *Int J Epidemiol*. 2001;30(6):1343-1350.

25. Humphreys K, Carr-Hill R. Area variations in health outcomes: artefact or ecology. *Int J Epidemiol*. 1991;20(1):251-258.

26. Von Korff M, Koepsell T, Curry S, Diehr P. Multi-level analysis in epidemiologic research on health behaviors and outcomes. *Am J Epidemiol*. 1992;135(10):1077-1082.

27. Koopman JS, Longini IM Jr. The ecological effects of individual exposures and nonlinear disease dynamics in populations. *Am J Public Health*. 1994;84(5):836-842.

28. Fisher LH, Wakefield J. Ecological inference for infectious disease data, with application to vaccination strategies. *Stat Med*. 2020;39(3):220-238.

29. Duncan C, Jones K, Moon G. Context, composition and heterogeneity: using multilevel models in health research. *Soc Sci Med*. 1998;46(1):97-117.

30. Diez Roux AV. A glossary for multilevel analysis. *J Epidemiol Community Health*. 2002;56(8):588-594.

31. Morgenstern H, Thomas D. Principles of study design in environmental epidemiology. *Environ Health Perspect*. 1993;101(suppl 4):23-38.

32. Walter SD. The ecologic method in the study of environmental health. I: Overview of the method. *Environ Health Perspect*. 1991;94:61-65.

33. Hiller JE, McMichael AJ. Ecological studies. In: Margetts BM, Nelson M, eds. *Design Concepts in Nutritional Epidemiology*. Oxford: Oxford University Press; 1991:323-353.

34. Prentice RL, Sheppard L. Aggregate data studies of disease risk factors. *Biometrika*. 1995;82:113-125.

35. Rose G. Sick individuals and sick populations. *Int J Epidemiol*. 1985;14(1):32-38.

36. Prentice RL, Kakar F, Hursting S, Sheppard L, Klein R, Kushi LH. Aspects of the rationale for the women's health trial. *J Natl Cancer Inst*. 1988;80(11):802-814.

37. Plummer M, Clayton D. Estimation of population exposure in ecological studies. *J R Stat Soc Ser B*. 1996;58:113-126.

38. McMichael AJ. The health of persons, populations, and planets: epidemiology comes full circle. *Epidemiology*. 1995;6(6):633-636.

39. Greenland S. A review of multilevel theory for ecologic analyses. *Stat Med*. 2002;21(3):389-395.

40. Mason TJ, McKay FW, Hoover R, Blot WJ, Fraumeni JF Jr. *Atlas of Cancer Mortality for US Counties: 1950-1969*. DHEW Publ No (NIH) 75-780. Washington, DC: US Government Printing Office; 1975:36-37.

41. Blot WJ, Fraumeni JF Jr. Geographic patterns of oral cancer in the United States: etiologic implications. *J Chronic Dis*. 1977;30(11):745-757.

42. Winn DM, Blot WJ, Shy CM, Pickle LW, Toledo A, Fraumeni JF Jr. Snuff dipping and oral cancer among women in the southern United States. *N Engl J Med*. 1981;304(13):745-749.

43. Wakefield J. Disease mapping and spatial regression with count data. *Biostatistics*. 2007;8:158-183.

44. Blangiardo M, Cameletti M. *Spatial and Spatio-Temporal Bayesian Models with R-INLA*. New York: Wiley; 2015.

45. Clayton DG, Bernardinelli L, Montomoli C. Spatial correlation in ecological analysis. *Int J Epidemiol*. 1993;22(6):1193-1202.

46. Rao JNK, Molina I. *Small Area Estimation*. 2nd ed. Hoboken, NJ: John Wiley & Sons; 2015.

47. Gotway CA, Young LJ. Combining incompatible spatial data. *J Am Stat Assoc*. 2002;97(458):632-648.

48. Bradley JR, Wikle CK, Holan SH. Bayesian spatial change of support for count-valued survey data with application to the American community survey. *J Am Stat Assoc*. 2016;111(514):472-487.

49. Wong D. The modifiable areal unit problem (MAUP). In: Fotheringham AS, Rogerson PA, eds. *The SAGE Handbook of Spatial Analysis*. London: Sage Publications; 2009:105-123.

50. Hatch M, Susser M. Background gamma radiation and childhood cancers within ten miles of a US nuclear plant. *Int J Epidemiol*. 1990;19(3):546-552.

51. Pocock SJ, Cook DG, Beresford SA. Regression of area mortality rates on explanatory variables: what weighting is appropriate?. *J R Stat Soc Ser C Appl Stat*. 1981;30(3):286-295.

52. Breslow NE. Extra-Poisson variation in log-linear models. *Appl Stat*. 1984;33:38-44.

53. Prentice RL, Sheppard L. Validity of international, time trend, and migrant studies of dietary factors and disease risk. *Prev Med*. 1989;18(2):167-179.

54. Prentice RL, Thomas D. Methodologic research needs in environmental epidemiology: data analysis. *Environ Health Perspect*. 1993;101(suppl 4):39-48.

55. Smith TR, Wakefield J. A review and comparison of age-period-cohort models for cancer incidence. *Statist Sci*. 2016;31(4):591-610.
56. Chambers RL, Steel DG. Simple methods for ecological inference in 2 × 2 tables. *J R Stat Soc Ser A*. 2001;164(1):175-192.
57. Wakefield J. Ecological inference for 2 × 2 tables. *J R Stat Soc Ser A*. 2004;167(2):385-445.
58. Haneuse SJ, Wakefield JC. Hierarchical models for combining ecological and case-control data. *Biometrics*. 2007;63(1):128-136.
59. Haneuse SJ, Wakefield JC. The combination of ecological and case-control data. *J R Stat Soc Ser B Stat Methodol*. 2008;70(1):73-93.
60. Wakefield J, Haneuse SJ-PA. Overcoming ecologic bias using the two-phase study design. *Am J Epidemiol*. 2008;167(8):908-916.
61. Box G, Jenkins G. *Time Series Analysis, Forecasting and Control*. San Francisco: Holden Day; 1976.
62. Ostrom CWJ. *Time Series Analysis: Regression Techniques*. 2nd ed. Newbury Park, CA: Sage Foundation; 1990.
63. Helfenstein U. The use of transfer function models, intervention analysis and related time series methods in epidemiology. *Int J Epidemiol*. 1991;20(3):808-815.
64. Chatfield C. *Time-series Forecasting*. Boca Raton: Chapman & Hall/CRC; 2001.
65. Zeger SL, Irizarry R, Peng RD. On time series analysis of public health and biomedical data. *Annu Rev Public Health*. 2006;27:57-79.
66. McDowall D, McCleary R, Meidinger EE, Hay RA Jr. *Interrupted Time Series Analysis*. Beverly Hills, CA: Sage Foundation; 1980.
67. Catalano R, Serxner S. Time series designs of potential interest to epidemiologists. *Am J Epidemiol*. 1987;126(4):724-731.
68. Sayrs LW. *Pooled Time Series Analysis*. Newbury Park, CA: Sage Foundation; 1989.
69. Prado R, West M. *Time Series: Modeling, Computation, and Inference*. 1 ed. Boca Raton: Chapman and Hall/CRC; 2010.
70. Frost WH. The age selection of mortality from tuberculosis in successive decades. *Am J Epidemiol* 1939;30-SectionA(3):91-96.
71. Glenn ND. *Cohort Analysis*, Series/No. 07-005. Thousand Oaks, CA: Sage; 1977.
72. Mason KO, Mason W, Winsborough HH, Poole WK. Some methodological issues in the cohort analysis of archival data. *Am Sociol Rev*. 1973;38:242-258.
73. Holford TR. Understanding the effects of age, period, and cohort on incidence and mortality rates. *Annu Rev Public Health*. 1991;12:425-457.
74. Lee JA, Petersen GR, Stevens RG, Vesanen K. The influence of age, year of birth, and date on mortality from malignant melanoma in the populations of England and Wales, Canada, and the white population of the United States. *Am J Epidemiol*. 1979;110(6):734-739.
75. Lee JA. Melanoma and exposure to sunlight. *Epidemiol Rev*. 1982;4:110-136.
76. Goldstein H. Age, period and cohort effects-a confounded confusion. *J Appl. Stat*. 1979;6:19-24.
77. Clayton D, Schifflers E. Models for temporal variation in cancer rates. I: age-period and age-cohort models. *Stat Med*. 1987;6(4):449-467.
78. Clayton D, Schifflers E. Models for temporal variation in cancer rates. II: age-period-cohort models. *Stat Med*. 1987;6(4):469-481.
79. Carstensen B. Age-period-cohort models for the Lexis diagram. *Stat Med*. 2007;26(15):3018-3045.
80. Kuang D, Nielsen B, Nielsen JP. Forecasting with the age-period-cohort model and the extended chain-ladder model. *Biometrika*. 2008;95(4):987-991.
81. Kuang D, Nielsen B, Nielsen JP. Identification of the age-period-cohort model and the extended chain-ladder model. *Biometrika*. 2008;95(4):979-986.
82. Darby SC, Doll R. Fallout, radiation doses near Dounreay, and childhood leukaemia. *Br Med J (Clin Res Ed*. 1987;294(6572):603-607.
83. Gruchow HW, Rimm AA, Hoffmann RG. Alcohol consumption and ischemic heart disease mortality: are time-series correlations meaningful? *Am J Epidemiol*. 1983;118(5):641-650.
84. Kelsall JE, Zeger SL, Samet JM. Frequency domain log-linear models; air pollution and mortality. *J R Stat Soc Ser C (Appl Stat)*. 1999;48(3):331-344.
85. Riebler A, Held L, Rue H. Estimation and extrapolation of time trends in registry data–borrowing strength from related populations. *Ann Appl Stat*. 2012;6:304-333.
86. Crawford MD, Gardner MJ, Morris JN. Changes in water hardness and local death-rates. *Lancet*. 1971;2(7720):327-329.
87. Rubin DB. Bayesian inference for causal effects: the role of randomization. *Ann Stat*. 1978;6:4-58.
88. Rubin DB. Comment: Neyman (1923) and causal inference in experiments and observational studies. *Stat Sci*. 1990;5:472-480.
89. Greenland S, Schlesselman JJ, Criqui MH. The fallacy of employing standardized regression coefficients and correlations as measures of effect. *Am J Epidemiol*. 1986;123:203-208.

90. Greenland S. Interpretation and choice of effect measures in epidemiologic analyses. *Am J Epidemiol.* 1987;125(5):761-768.
91. Greenland S, Maclure M, Schlesselman JJ, Poole C, Morgenstern H. Standardized regression coefficients: a further critique and review of some alternatives. *Epidemiology.* 1991;2(5):387-392.
92. Maldonado G, Greenland S. Estimating causal effects. *Int J Epidemiol.* 2002;31(2):422-429.
93. Goodman LA. Some alternatives to ecological correlation. *Am J Social.* 1959;64:610-625.
94. Beral V, Chilvers C, Fraser P. On the estimation of relative risk from vital statistical data. *J Epidemiol Community Health.* 1979;33(2):159-162.
95. Durkheim E. *Suicide: A Study in Sociology.* New York: Free Press; 1951:153-154.
96. Greenland S, Robins J. Invited commentary: ecologic studies—biases, misconceptions, and counterexamples. *Am J Epidemiol.* 1994;139(8):747-760.
97. Greenland S. Divergent biases in ecologic and individual-level studies. *Stat Med.* 1992;11(9):1209-1223.
98. Gelman A, Park DK, Ansolabehere S, Price PN, Minnite LC. Models, assumptions and model checking in ecological regressions. *J R Stat Soc Ser A.* 2001;164(1):101-118.
99. Langbein LI, Lichtman AJ. *Ecological Inference.* Thousand Oaks, CA: Sage Foundation; 1978.
100. Richardson S, Stucker I, Hemon D. Comparison of relative risks obtained in ecological and individual studies: some methodological considerations. *Int J Epidemiol.* 1987;16(1):111-120.
101. Rosenbaum PR, Rubin DB. Difficulties with regression analyses of age-adjusted rates. *Biometrics.* 1984;40(2):437-443.
102. Greenland S, Morgenstern H. Ecological bias, confounding, and effect modification. *Int J Epidemiol.* 1989;18(1):269-274.
103. Miettinen OS. The need for randomization in the study of intended effects. *Stat Med.* 1983;2(2):267-271.
104. Wen SW, Kramer MS. Uses of ecologic studies in the assessment of intended treatment effects. *J Clin Epidemiol.* 1999;52(1):7-12.
105. Rassen JA, Brookhart MA, Glynn RJ, Mittleman MA, Schneeweiss S. Instrumental variables I: instrumental variables exploit natural variation in nonexperimental data to estimate causal relationships. *J Clin Epidemiol.* 2009;62(12):1226-1232.
106. Hernan MA, Robins JM. Instruments for causal inference: an epidemiologist's dream? *Epidemiology.* 2006;17(4):360-372.
107. Johnston SC. Combining ecological and individual variables to reduce confounding by indication: case study—subarachnoid hemorrhage treatment. *J Clin Epidemiol.* 2000;53(12):1236-1241.
108. Johnston SC, Henneman T, McCulloch CE, van der Laan M. Modeling treatment effects on binary outcomes with grouped-treatment variables and individual covariates. *Am J Epidemiol.* 2002;156(8):753-760.
109. Pack QR, Priya A, Lagu T, et al. Association between inpatient echocardiography use and outcomes in adult patients with acute myocardial infarction. *JAMA Intern Med.* 2019;179(9):1176-1185.
110. Firebaugh G. A rule for inferring individual-level relationships from aggregate data. *Am Sociol Rev.* 1978;43:557-572.
111. Subramanian SV, Jones K, Kaddour A, Krieger N. Revisiting Robinson: the perils of individualistic and ecologic fallacy. *Int J Epidemiol.* 2009;38(2):342-360; author reply 370-3.
112. Openshaw S, Taylor PH. The modifiable area unit problem. In: Wrigley N, Bennett RJ, eds. *Quantitative Geography: A British View.* London: Routledge & Kegan Paul; 1981:chap 9.
113. Robinson WS. Ecological correlations and the behavior of individuals. *Am Sociol Rev.* 1950;15:351-357.
114. Duncan OD, Cuzzort RP, Duncan B. *Statistical Geography: Problems in Analyzing Areal Data.* Westport, CT: Greenwood Press; 1961:64-67.
115. Selvin HC. Durkheim's "Suicide" and problems of empirical research. *Am J Sociol.* 1958;63:607-619.
116. Stavraky KM. The role of ecologic analysis in studies of the etiology of disease: a discussion with reference to large bowel cancer. *J Chronic Dis.* 1976;29(7):435-444.
117. Connor MJ, Gillings D. An empiric study of ecological inference. *Am J Public Health.* 1984;74(6):555-559.
118. Feinleib M, Leaverton PE. Ecological fallacies in epidemiology. In: Leaverton PE, Masse L, eds. *Health Information Systems.* New York: Praeger; 1984:33-61.
119. Stidley CA, Samet JM. Assessment of ecologic regression in the study of lung cancer and indoor radon. *Am J Epidemiol.* 1994;139(3):312-322.
120. Walter SD. The ecologic method in the study of environmental health. II. Methodologic issues and feasibility. *Environ Health Perspect.* 1991;94:67-73.
121. Arsenault J, Michel P, Berke O, Ravel A, Gosselin P. How to choose geographical units in ecological studies: proposal and application to campylobacteriosis. *Spat Spatiotemporal Epidemiol.* 2013;7:11-24.
122. Guthrie KA, Sheppard L. Overcoming biases and misconceptions in ecological studies. *J R Stat Soc Ser A.* 2001;164(1):141-154.
123. Wakefield J, Salway R. A statistical framework for ecological and aggregate studies. *J R Stat Soc Ser A.* 2001;164(1):119-137.
124. Wakefield J, Haneuse S, Dobra A, Teeple E. Bayes computation for ecological inference. *Stat Med.* 2011;30(12):1381-1396.

125. Best N, Cockings S, Bennett J, Wakefield J, Elliott P. Ecological regression analyses of environmental benzene exposure and childhood leukemia: sensitivity to data inaccuracies, geographical scale and ecological bias. *J R Stat Soc A*. 2001;164(1):155-174.

126. Wakefield J, Shaddick G. Health-exposure modeling and the ecological fallacy. *Biostatistics*. 2006;7(3):438-455.

127. King G. *A Solution to the Ecological Inference Problem: Reconstructing Individual Behavior from Aggregate Data*. Princeton, NJ: Princeton University Press; 1997.

128. Duncan OD, Davis B. An alternative to ecological correlation. *Am Sociol Rev*. 1953;18:665-666.

129. Freedman DA, Klein SP, Ostland M, Roberts MR. Review of A Solution to the ecological inference problem (by G. King). *J Am Stat Assoc*. 1998;93:1518-1522.

130. King G. The future of ecological inference research: a comment on Freedman et al. *J Am Stat Assoc*. 1999;94:352-355.

131. Freedman DA, Ostland M, Roberts MR, Klein SP. Reply to G. King. *J Am Stat Assoc*. 1999;94:355-357.

132. Cho WKT. Iff the assumption fits . . .: a comment on the King ecological inference solution. *Polit Anal*. 1998;7:143-163.

133. McCue KF. The statistical foundations of the EI method. *Am Stat*. 2001;55:106-110.

134. Sheppard L. Insights on bias and information in group-level studies. *Biostatistics*. 2003;4(2):265-278.

135. Salway R, Wakefield J. Sources of bias in ecological studies of non-rare events. *Environ Ecol Stat*. 2005;12:321-347.

136. Darby S, Deo H, Doll R, Whitley E. A parallel analysis of individual and ecological data on residential radon and lung cancer in south-west England. *J R Stat Soc Ser A*. 2001;164(1):193-203.

137. Richardson S, Hémon D. Ecological bias and confounding. *Int J Epidemiol*. 1990;19(3):764-767.

138. Jackson C, Best N, Richardson S. Improving ecological inference using individual-level data. *Stat Med*. 2006;25(12):2136-2159.

139. Jackson C, Best N., Richardson S. Hierarchical related regression for combining aggregate and individual data in studies of socio-economic disease risk factors. *J R Stat Soc Ser A (Statistics Society)*. 2008;171(1):159-178.

140. Brenner H, Savitz DA, Jockel KH, Greenland S. Effects of nondifferential exposure misclassification in ecologic studies. *Am J Epidemiol*. 1992;135(1):85-95.

141. Greenland S, Brenner H. Correcting for non-differential misclassification in ecologic analyses. *Appl Stat*. 1993;42:117-126.

142. Greenland S. The effect of misclassification in the presence of covariates. *Am J Epidemiol*. 1980;112(4):564-569.

143. Savitz DA, Baron AE. Estimating and correcting for confounder misclassification. *Am J Epidemiol*. 1989;129(5):1062-1071.

144. Brenner H, Greenland S, Savitz DA. The effects of nondifferential confounder misclassification in ecologic studies. *Epidemiology*. 1992;3(5):456-459.

145. Polissar L. The effect of migration on comparison of disease rates in geographic studies in the United States. *Am J Epidemiol*. 1980;111(2):175-182.

146. Kliewer EV. Influence of migrants on regional variations of stomach and colon cancer mortality in the Western United States. *Int J Epidemiol*. 1992;21(3):442-449.

147. Ocana-Riola R, Fernandez-Ajuria A, Mayoral-Cortes JM, Toro-Cardenas S, Sanchez-Cantalejo C. Uncontrolled migrations as a cause of inequality in health and mortality in small-area studies. *Epidemiology*. 2009;20(3):411-418.

148. Zagheni E, Garimella V, Weber I, State B. Inferring international and internal migration patterns from twitter data. In: *Proceedings of the 23rd International Conference on World Wide Web Seoul*. Korea: Association for Computing Machinery; 2014.

149. Centerwall BS. Exposure to television as a risk factor for violence. *Am J Epidemiol*. 1989;129(4): 643-652.

150. Casper M, Wing S, Strogatz D, Davis CE, Tyroler HA. Antihypertensive treatment and US trends in stroke mortality, 1962 to 1980. *Am J Public Health*. 1992;82(12):1600-1606.

151. Stewart AW, Kuulasmaa K, Beaglehole R. Ecological analysis of the association between mortality and major risk factors of cardiovascular disease. *Int J Epidemiol*. 1994;23:505-516.

152. Iversen GR. *Contextual Analysis*. Thousand Oaks, CA: Sage Foundation; 1991.

153. Greenland S. Causal analysis in the health sciences. *J Am Statist Assoc*. 2000;95:286-289.

154. Witte JS, Greenland S, Kim LL, Arab L. Multilevel modeling in epidemiology with GLIMMIX. *Epidemiology*. 2000;11(6):684-688.

155. Snijders TAB, Bosker RJ. *Multilevel Analysis*. 2nd ed. Thousand Oaks, CA: Sage Publications; 2012.

156. Pickett KE, Pearl M. Multilevel analyses of neighbourhood socioeconomic context and health outcomes: a critical review. *J Epidemiol Community Health*. 2001;55(2):111-122.

157. Oakes JM. The (mis)estimation of neighborhood effects: causal inference for a practicable social epidemiology. *Soc Sci Med*. 2004;58(10):1929-1952.

158. Diez-Roux AV. Bringing context back into epidemiology: variables and fallacies in multilevel analysis. *Am J Public Health.* 1998;88(2):216-222.

159. Diez Roux AV. Estimating neighborhood health effects: the challenges of causal inference in a complex world. *Soc Sci Med.* 2004;58(10):1953-1960.

160. Navidi W, Thomas D, Stram D, Peters J. Design and analysis of multilevel analytic studies with applications to a study of air pollution. *Environ Health Perspect.* 1994;102(suppl 8):25-32.

161. Krieger N. Epidemiology and the web of causation: has anyone seen the spider? *Soc Sci Med.* 1994;39(7):887-903.

162. Link BG, Phelan J. Social conditions as fundamental causes of disease. *J Health Soc Behav.* 1995;35(Extra Issue):80-94.

163. Pearce N. Traditional epidemiology, modern epidemiology, and public health. *Am J Public Health.* 1996;86(5):678-683.

164. Susser M, Susser E. Choosing a future for epidemiology: II. From black box to Chinese boxes and eco-epidemiology. *Am J Public Health.* 1996;86(5):674-677.

165. Schwartz S, Carpenter KM. The right answer for the wrong question: consequences of type III error for public health research. *Am J Public Health.* 1999;89(8):1175-1180.

CHAPTER 31

Agent-Based Modeling

Brandon D.L. Marshall

INTRODUCTION

Agent-based models (ABMs), also known as individual-based models, are a subset of microscale computational models for simulating the actions of multiple "agents" in an attempt to reproduce, characterize, and understand complex population phenomena.[1] In most epidemiological applications of ABMs, agents represent people who interact with each other to form an artificial society, thus simulating a hypothetical population of interest. Rather than a "top-down" method (in which model outputs are a direct function of group-based rules or equations governing the system-level behavior), agent-based modeling is a "bottom-up" approach, in which outcomes are generated from microscale interactions. ABMs are useful because the representation and reproduction of complex population phenomena from individual-level behaviors can lead to critical insights into novel causal mechanisms and interventions to improve health.

One of the earliest known ABMs was a model published in 1969 and 1971, which demonstrated that neighborhood racial segregation can arise as a product of small preferences for neighbors of the same race.[2,3] Although developed without a computer, the Schelling segregation model embodies the core characteristics of an ABM: the actions of individual agents, interacting in a shared simulated environment, produce an emergent, aggregate outcome (*i.e.*, in this case, racial segregation). Since this foundational work, ABMs have been used to recreate and explain complex phenomena across a variety of disciplines, including economics,[4] ecology,[5] and social psychology.[6]

While first applied to the study of infectious disease transmission,[7] agent-based modeling can now be found across the many subdisciplines of epidemiology. Examples of ABMs are ubiquitous throughout the infectious disease literature,[8] and ABMs are increasingly employed to explore the etiology and prevention of noncommunicable diseases,[9] social determinants of health such as incarceration,[10] and the effects of place on health.[11,12] The ability to incorporate information from disparate data sources, promote interdisciplinary collaboration, and bridge scientific disciplines[13] has also contributed to the growth of agent-based modeling in public health generally, in which integrative approaches are recognized as paramount for addressing our most pressing health challenges.[14] Specific examples of their successful implementation include attempts to study the most vexing and intractable problems in public health, including the rise and persistence of obesity (Zhang et al.[15]), eradication of human immunodeficiency virus (HIV) transmission,[16] and mitigation of pervasive racial/ethnic health disparities in the United States.[17]

The purpose of this chapter is to provide an introduction to the key concepts, methods, and common applications of agent-based modeling in epidemiology. Readers interested in gaining a more in-depth appreciation for the design, construction, and validation of ABMs are referred to several excellent texts on the subject.[18,19] Finally, although ABMs are but one of the many systems science methods used in public health,[20] the chapter focuses on agent-based modeling, as the approach has become one of the more commonly employed microsimulation approaches in epidemiology.[9] The chapter begins with an introduction to ABMs and offers rationale for their use and application in epidemiology. Next, I describe the design and implementation of ABMs, including their construction, parameterization, calibration, verification and validation, and interpretation. Finally, the chapter concludes with a discussion of the distinctive characteristics and features of ABMs that make them particularly well suited as a method of epidemiological inquiry.

What Are ABMs?

ABMs simulate the behaviors and interactions of autonomous agents, which may represent individuals or collective entities (such as hospitals, schools, and governments). Agents are encoded with heterogeneous characteristics, which can include endogenous traits (*i.e.*, biological functions), sociodemographic characteristics, spatial positioning, and various exposure and disease states.[21] In many ABMs, agents interact with each other in one or more shared simulated environments, which can affect both the nature of agent interactions and individual agent behavior. ABMs are implemented, calibrated, and validated using prepackaged or custom-built computer software. The software is then used to test how changes in agent characteristics and behaviors, or manipulations to the simulated environment(s), affect model outputs. These outputs are viewed as emergent, population-level properties that arise as a function of individual-level (*i.e.*, microscale) agent behaviors and interactions. Most ABMs implemented for epidemiological applications seek to reproduce population-level disease outcomes, such as incidence, prevalence, and mortality rates. For example, an agent-based modeling study published in 2015 sought to compare the relative effectiveness of structural and psychosocial interventions on the prevalence of violence-related posttraumatic stress disorder (PTSD) in New York City.[22] Population PTSD prevalence "emerged" from the model as a result of individual agents witnessing, experiencing, and perpetrating violence.

The evolution of an ABM is determined by preprogrammed agent characteristics and by rules that regulate how agents behave, relate with each other, and interact with the simulated environments.[20] As observed in the Schelling segregation model, even simple rules governing agent behavior can result in complex, unanticipated population phenomena.[23] By comparing model outputs under different rule sets, counterfactual scenarios—representing different risk factor distributions, causal structures, public health interventions, or policies—can be simulated. Interventions that change agents' underlying characteristics or behaviors, alter contact networks (through which risk factors or diseases are transmitted), and/or modify environments can all be interrogated. Thus, ABMs provide an opportunity to evaluate the hypothetical impact of a wide variety of interventions across multiple populations and various contexts.

In this capacity, ABMs function as an in silico laboratory in which the researcher defines a set of agent characteristics, specifies initial conditions, applies rules for agent-agent interactions, and programs static or transitory exposure and disease states. By running the simulation many times and observing outcomes under different input parameters (collectively referred to as a "treatment"), the investigator can compare outcomes obtained from any number of hypothetical scenarios. Given that all agents in the population receive the treatment under various scenarios specified by the researcher, the results obtained from an ABM are analogous to *potential outcomes* as defined in the classical epidemiologic literature.[24] In this manner, agent-based modeling shares the same counterfactual understanding of disease causation as traditional epidemiological investigations.[25]

Rationale for ABMs

Agent-based modeling offers an alternative, complementary approach to the empirical study of causal effects and intervention impacts in the presence of *complexity*.[26] Disease causes can be said to exhibit complexity if some or all of the following characteristics are observed: sensitivity to initial conditions (*e.g.*, disease prevalence); adaptivity, in that individual behavior can evolve based on past history; feedback loops, such that causal effects are magnified (*i.e.*, positive feedback) or dampened (*i.e.*, negative feedback) as disease processes progress; contextual effects, such that health outcomes are shaped by specific social, economic, and political contexts; and finally, a high degree of interacting and interdependent causes, as well as structurally nonlinear relationships between causes and outcomes.[27,28] Highly interdependent causal pathways, fundamental characteristics of complex systems,[29] are integral to many of the challenges that public health now faces. To this end, the application of agent-based modeling to understand how complex disease processes affect population health has gained traction and currency.[30]

Empirical methods have been developed to address complex phenomena in epidemiology (*e.g.*, time-dependent confounding, interference) and are discussed elsewhere in this text. Agent-based modeling should thus be viewed as complementary to these modes of inquiry. In addition, agent-based modeling is a useful method to confirm or repudiate previously observed causal mechanisms. For example, an ABM that simulates friendship formation has been used to examine the causal effect of social influence on adolescent obesity.[31] In observational studies, this relationship is known to be confounded by homophily (*i.e.*, the tendency for individuals to select friends who are similar to themselves) and shared environmental influences.[32] The agent-based modeling study found evidence for social influence on adolescent body mass index and obesity-related behaviors, even after accounting for both shared environmental factors and multiple sources of homophily in friendship selection.[31] Finally, ABMs represent an efficient method to evaluate the hypothetical effects of interventions for which their evaluation using traditional approaches (*e.g.*, randomized controlled trials, RCTs) would be burdensome, unethical, or impractical.

Another important rationale for agent-based modeling arises from the fact that agent-level outcomes are, by definition, nonindependent. In agent-based modeling, an agent's state is directly influenced by the status or behavior of other agents through explicit simulation of agent-agent interactions. For example, in a study testing the effectiveness of influenza vaccine choice on viral transmission in the Washington, DC, metropolitan area, an agent's risk of acquiring influenza was dependent on his or her interactions with infected agents in various environments, including households, schools, and workplaces.[33] The authors found that increasing the type of influenza vaccines made available significantly reduced the number of influenza cases in an epidemic year.

The phenomenon of nonindependence between individuals is known generally as *interference*.[34] Interference may be present whenever the exposure or treatment assignment of one individual is influenced by the outcome(s) of others in the population.[35] Applying methods that do not account for interference can result in misleading or incorrect inference; in extreme circumstances, an exposure or treatment may appear beneficial, even when it is universally harmful.[36]

Rather than a nuisance factor such as confounding, interference is often of intrinsic interest. Investigators may wish to estimate the degree to which herd immunity protects unvaccinated individuals in a vaccine trial, for example.[37] Several methods have been developed to quantify the effect of interference in epidemiological studies.[36,38] For example, one can estimate causal effects that are conditional on contact with an exposed individual, such that the potential outcome is a two-stage counterfactual statement, dependent on both coming into contact with an exposed person (due to interference) and treatment assignment.[35] More recent work has also focused on developing inverse probability weighting estimators to obtain causal estimands of interest in the presence of interference.[39]

Agent-based modeling offers an alternative and useful method to evaluate interference. In fact, given that ABMs explicitly simulate interactions between people, elucidating the effects of interference should be a primary motivator for the adoption of agent-based modeling methods in epidemiology.[25] In addition, ABMs can be used to evaluate the potential effectiveness of network-based interventions, or interventions that target individuals based on their network location, size, or connectedness. For example, one agent-based simulation compared the effectiveness of targeting antiobesity interventions to the most highly connected nodes in social networks, versus targeting individuals at random.[40] Despite empirical evidence that an individuals' social network influences his or her risk of obesity,[41] the modeling study found no evidence that policies targeting well-connected individuals would reduce obesity prevalence more so than general population-based interventions.

Finally, ABMs can simulate the formation, dissolution, and reconstitution of relationships between agents, resulting in dynamic network structures that change over time. The modeling of dynamic networks can more accurately represent contact patterns, spatial clustering, and other social processes of interest (*e.g.*, the diffusion of health information) than many other mathematical modeling approaches.[42] For this reason, ABMs are well suited to modeling the transmission of HIV and other sexually transmitted infections, since they are able to capture heterogeneity of individual sexual behavior and the highly dynamic nature of sexual networks, both of which play important roles in determining disease incidence over time.[43]

MODEL DESIGN AND IMPLEMENTATION

Like all mathematical models, the validity of ABMs depends on the assumptions made during the model development process and the availability of accurate data with which to parameterize the model. There are a number of published frameworks for constructing, calibrating, and validating an ABM.[44-46] Guidelines for reporting ABMs in the peer-reviewed literature are also available.[47,48] Regardless of the model development framework used, agent-based modeling rests on the fundamental assumption that, for any given research question, people and their relevant health states, interactions, and environments can be credibly modeled at a reasonable level of abstraction.[49] Meeting this assumption carries at least two important challenges. First, the researcher must decide which minimal set of rules is acceptable for defining agent behavior, their relationships, and their environments, such that meaningful inferences can be made from model output. Second, data and/or prior knowledge must exist to inform the specific structure and parameterization of the model processes. In the sections that follow, I summarize the most commonly employed methods to help ensure that an ABM has internal validity and that the model's results have relevance to solving real-world epidemiological problems.

Notation and Terminology

General terminology and ABM notation are summarized in this section, with the understanding that many ABMs are developed somewhat idiosyncratically to represent the specific characteristics and mechanisms of a population health system of interest. As a first step, the modeler defines an agent population, consisting of $N > 1$ agents. Next, we must specify the universe of *agent behaviors*, which are defined as anything an agent does during a simulation, which may include making a decision, acquiring or dissolving relationships with other agents, moving environments, or changing an internal status (*e.g.*, aging). For each agent $i = 1,\dots,N$, a set of $m = 1,\dots,M$ internal characteristics (also known as traits) are described, such that the agent population at a time step $t = 0,\dots,T$ can be represented by an N-by-M matrix $\mathbf{S}^t$:

$$\mathbf{S}^t = \begin{bmatrix} s_{1,1}^t & s_{1,2}^t & \cdots & s_{1,M}^t \\ s_{2,1}^t & s_{2,2}^t & \cdots & s_{2,M}^t \\ \vdots & \vdots & \ddots & \vdots \\ s_{N,1}^t & s_{N,1}^t & \cdots & s_{N,M}^t \end{bmatrix}$$

where each row describes the values for the set of agent i's M internal traits at time t. Traits are defined broadly and can represent sociodemographic characteristics such as age and race, genetic predisposition to certain diseases, exposure states, propensity to engage in a certain health behavior, and social influence in a community. In the trait matrix $\mathbf{S}^t$, traits can be stored as any real number (*e.g.*, if the mth trait is sex at birth, $m = 1$ may represent a female agent, while $m = 2$ may represent a male agent).

As described earlier in this chapter, the purpose of agent-based modeling is to generate emergent population outcomes from agent-level interactions. At each time step t ($t = 1,...,T$), each agent i interacts with a subset of the population ($1,...,i$-1, i+1$,...,N$), described by an agent-agent interaction matrix $\mathbf{K}^t$. That is, each element $k_{i,j}^t$ of $\mathbf{K}^t$ indicates whether agent i interacts with agent j during time step t, where i and $j = 1,...,N$. Note that $\mathbf{K}^t$ is not necessarily symmetric; for example, agent i may know j but not vice versa, or information (*e.g.*, disease transmission) may be unidirectional and "flow" one way. The agent-agent interaction matrix can be dichotomous, where each element $k_{i,j}^t \in \{0,1\}$ defines an unweighted contact network [*i.e.*, agents i and j are either connected (1) or not connected (0)], or take on other values, in which case the matrix represents a weighted network structure. It is possible to construct an ABM such that there are no agent-agent interactions. In this circumstance, $\mathbf{K}^t$ is an identity matrix (ones down the diagonal and zeros everywhere else), which is analogous to the assumption of noninterference (*i.e.*, one agent's exposure does not affect the outcome of others).

In addition to the interaction network, agents can also be placed in different environments, represented by a matrix $\mathbf{E}^t$, where each agent is located within one of $P = 1,...,P$ possible environmental states at time t:

$$\mathbf{E}^t = \begin{bmatrix} e_{1,1}^t & e_{1,2}^t & \cdots & e_{1,P}^t \\ e_{2,1}^t & e_{2,2}^t & \cdots & e_{2,P}^t \\ \vdots & \vdots & \ddots & \vdots \\ e_{N,1}^t & e_{N,1}^t & \cdots & e_{N,P}^t \end{bmatrix}$$

An ABM is initialized by populating the "baseline" (*i.e.*, $t = 0$) agent trait matrix $\mathbf{S}^0$, environmental state matrix $\mathbf{E}^0$, and the interaction matrix $\mathbf{K}^0$, with values drawn from probability distributions. A model replication is defined as one execution of the model (sometimes called a model run), with a specific set of initial conditions usually set by a random number generator.

The simulation proceeds by defining a set of rules $\mathbf{Z}$. Rules govern how agents update their internal states (called agent rules), interact with other agents (agent-agent interaction rules), and move between or interact with environmental states (called an agent-environment rule). If we assume that the rules are stable and independent of agent behavior and interactions, the evolution of the model can be described by the following general functions:

$$s_{i,m}^t = f\left(\mathbf{S}^{t-1},\mathbf{K}^t,\mathbf{E}^{t-1},\varepsilon_{i,m,t}\right)$$

$$k_{i,j}^t = g\left(\mathbf{S}^{t-1},\mathbf{K}^{t-1},\mathbf{E}^{t-1},\xi_{i,j,t}\right)$$

$$e_{i,p}^t = h\left(\mathbf{S}^{t-1},\mathbf{K}^t,\mathbf{E}^{t-1},\zeta_{i,p,t}\right)$$

for all agents $i,j = 1,...,N$, $m = 1,...,M$, $P = 1,...,P$, and $t = 1,...,T$. The functions $f()$, $g()$, and $h()$, which include random error terms (ε, ξ, ζ), are responsible for updating values stored in each matrix at time $t - 1$ to values representing time t. Thus, the rules $\mathbf{Z}$ are coded in the model by defining functions $f()$, $g()$, and $h()$ and by specifying the distribution of the random error terms. In other words, at each discrete time step, the microsimulation updates the agent trait matrix, interaction matrix, and environmental state matrix, based on previous values and rules set by the modeler.

For a given replication r (where $r = 1,...,R$), after an arbitrary number of time steps T, outcome(s) of interest can be evaluated in the agent population. The simulation can produce multiple outputs (*e.g.*, disease incidence, prevalence, and mortality rates). The vector of O outcomes for run r at time T is denoted as $Y_r^T = \left(y_{r,1}^T \ y_{r,2}^T \cdots y_{r,o}^T\right)$, which can include functions and/or combinations of agent traits, interactions, or environmental locations, but are most often specific elements of interest from the R trait matrices $\mathbf{S}^T$ (*e.g.*, agent disease status, and therefore population disease prevalence, at time T across the R replications).

In most agent-based modeling studies in epidemiology, we wish to compare model outputs (*i.e.*, hypothetical disease outcomes) under various counterfactual scenarios, which might represent different exposure distributions, policy or programmatic options, changes in the agents' interaction processes, or alterations to the agent environment. We define an agent-based counterfactual treatment as a uniquely specified set of rules Z, internal traits $S^{t=0}$, interaction matrices $K^{t=0}$, and environments $E^{t=0}$. After running R replications, we often wish to compare the disease outcomes, at time T, of the agent population subjected to counterfactual scenario A $\left[\text{denoted as } \left(Z_A, S_A^T, K_A^T, E_A^T \right) \right]$ versus counterfactual scenario B $\left[\text{denoted as } \left(Z_B, S_B^T, K_B^T, E_B^T \right) \right]$.

In many instances, a Monte Carlo simulation is used to obtain outcomes from replications $r = 1, \ldots, R$ at time T, for counterfactual scenarios A and B, respectively. Specifically, by executing the model R times, we define $\hat{\mu}_{o,A}^{T,R}$ and $\hat{\mu}_{o,B}^{T,R}$ for counterfactual scenarios A and B, respectively, and outcome o ($o = 1, \ldots, O$) as:

$$\hat{\mu}_{o,A}^{T,R} = \frac{\sum_{r=1}^{R} y_{r,o,A}^{T}}{R}$$

$$\hat{\mu}_{o,B}^{T,R} = \frac{\sum_{r=1}^{R} y_{r,o,B}^{T}}{R}$$

where $\hat{\mu}_{o,A}^{T,R}$ and $\hat{\mu}_{o,B}^{T,R}$ represent point estimators for the expected value of the outcome of interest derived from R replications under hypothetical scenarios A and B, at time step T, respectively.

As an example, consider an ABM constructed to examine the effects of different policies on unhealthy eating behaviors.[50] The study found that interventions emphasizing healthful eating norms (*e.g.*, mass media campaigns) were more effective than directly targeting food prices (*e.g.*, fast-food taxation) on fruits and vegetable consumption. In this example, the outcome of interest was the mean probability of consuming ≥2 servings of fruits and vegetables per day, which was a function of individuals' taste preferences and health beliefs, in turn influenced by habits of their friends and the food marketing strategies used in the broader environment. The counterfactual scenarios of interest represented various hypothetical policy experiments, which were parameterized to affect agent behavior, agent-agent interactions, and the simulated food environment. This example demonstrates the breadth and flexibility of counterfactual treatments that can be evaluated in the agent-based modeling environment.

Theory Development

For an ABM to run, the model developer must identify, define, and program agent behaviors, agent-agent interactions, and the relationship between agents and their environments. The first step in this process is to specify a "target"—the phenomena and population the model is intended to represent, reproduce, and simulate.[18] Since no model can capture all possible characteristics, behaviors, and environments that may influence a health outcome of interest, building a model for the target requires a theoretically motivated and conceptually grounded process of abstraction.[44] We should not aim to construct an all-encompassing representation of reality, but a highly simplified depiction that nonetheless provides valid insights into real-world phenomena and improves scientific understanding.[51] In other words, the goal is to identify the most parsimonious model to approximate reality: the model should only be as complex as it needs to be.

Commonly employed conceptual frameworks in population health, including the social-ecological model of health behavior and the syndemic theory of disease production,[52,53] can be helpful in identifying the core components of an ABM as employed in epidemiology. Behavioral change theories and other models from behavioral and cognitive psychology can also be helpful to inform agent behavior processes. Given that simplification is a necessary step in all models used in epidemiology, existing tools, including causal diagramming,[54] may also be helpful in determining the key processes to be modeled in an ABM (see Figure 31-1).

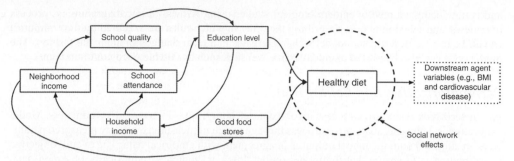

FIGURE 31-1 Causal diagram of an agent-based model representing macrosocial drivers of disparities in obesity. Note: Smoking and physical activity behaviors (at the agent level) were left out of the diagram for simplicity. (Reproduced from Orr MG, Galea S, Riddle M, Kaplan GA. Reducing racial disparities in obesity: simulating the effects of improved education and social network influence on diet behavior. *Ann Epidemiol.* 2014;24(8):563-569 with permission.)

Model Construction

ABMs require a set of code and a computational engine to be executed. Many ABMs are designed from scratch using all-purpose programming languages such as Python™, Java™, and C++. A number of modeling services (with preloaded libraries of commonly employed routines and functions) are also available. Among the most common programs are NetLogo (https://ccl.northwestern.edu/netlogo) and Repast (http://repast.sourceforge.net); other software has been reviewed elsewhere.[49] Once the model has been developed, the simulation is run by having agents repeatedly execute their behaviors and interactions according to preprogrammed rules. Most ABMs proceed in either discrete or activity-based time steps.

In an ABM, agents are endowed with static or dynamic behaviors that can depend on everything from simple "if-then" rules to complex adaptive processes. The modeler must also define which agents are (or could be) connected to whom and the dynamics of these interactions. The way in which agents are connected to each other is referred to as the model *topology*. Common topologies include a spatial grid, a more complicated spatial geography (*e.g.*, agents can only interact with other agents who are nearby), or a social network. The topology of an ABM can also evolve over time. For example, in one study that used an ABM to evaluate policies to reduce influenza transmission in the workplace, agents were assigned to and moved between specific geographic locations representing schools or workplaces.[55] During each simulated day, agents could only interact with other agents who shared the same social activity location.

The agent environment may represent a set of geographic characteristics (*e.g.*, pollutants, crime, or other aspects of the physical or built environment), venues (*e.g.*, homes, bars, workplaces), or institutions (*e.g.*, hospitals, prisons). An agent's location in the simulated landscape is usually recorded as a dynamic attribute—encoded in the environmental state matrix $\mathbf{E}^t$—as it moves in space. Different types of environments may promote, facilitate, or constrain agent behaviors. For example, in one ABM that simulated walking behaviors within a city, the agent environment was composed of 400 equal-sized neighborhoods, each with two properties: safety and esthetics.[56] A walking index (representing each person's walking experience) was a function of both individual agents' characteristics (*e.g.*, age, walking ability) and the safety and esthetic quality of all neighborhoods along a walking route. Each agent's walking index in turn affected how much she/he would walk in the subsequent day.

Summarizing the lengthy and often complicated set of model characteristics, algorithms, and rules that govern ABM processes can be challenging for the researcher. Descriptions of ABMs in the peer-reviewed literature are often incomplete or difficult to follow, which makes replicating their results difficult, if not impossible.[19] Modelers have attempted to address this issue by standardizing the reporting of ABMs using frameworks such as the "Overview, Design concepts, and Details" (ODD) protocol.[45,48] The purpose of frameworks such as the ODD protocol is to ensure that the reporting of ABMs is complete, comprehensive, and organized in a consistent fashion. The ODD protocol has been used in the ecological and social science literature for some time and is now being adopted in epidemiological studies using ABMs.[57] Flow diagramming, process overviews, and scheduling (*i.e.*, describing the order in which rules are executed by the computer) can all be used to describe the model's characteristics in a clear and comprehensible fashion. The model code can also be posted on open-source websites such as GitHub (https://github.com/).

Parameterization and Calibration

Parameterization refers to the process involved in selecting values for a model's parameters. Model calibration is defined as an iterative process through which unmeasured or poorly measured parameters are adjusted until the model output is in agreement with empirical data. The overall objective of calibration is to ensure that the model output "fits" or "matches" empirically observed data. Demonstrating that the model can reproduce real-world phenomena improves the model's overall credibility and is an important—but not the only— aspect of establishing model validity.

Calibration can be conceptualized as a two-step procedure. First, the modeler must decide on the set of targets they wish to calibrate to, and the criteria for determining when the model is sufficiently well calibrated. In epidemiology, ABMs are often calibrated to disease outcome measures of interest, such as incidence, prevalence, and mortality rates. It is important to note that biases present in observational studies impact the accuracy of calibration targets, which in turn influences the validity of a calibrated ABM. Although RCTs may be viewed as the gold standard for obtaining model calibration targets, they are often conducted with a highly selected subset of the desired target population. In addition, RCTs may not have evaluated the full set of interventions that the modeler wishes to test; in fact, agent-based modeling is often used precisely because an RCT is unethical, infeasible, or impractical to evaluate the effect of a treatment on the target population. One recent study demonstrated that modern causal inference techniques, including the *g*-formula, can be used to obtain a range of calibration targets for ABMs when observational data (on treatments, outcomes, and confounders) are available in a population of interest.[58] Additional research is needed to determine the methods, circumstances, and assumptions that result in valid ABM calibration targets from observational data.

Once the calibration targets have been selected, the modeler then aims to reproduce these targets in the simulated population. ABMs often involve a large number of rules, algorithms, and parameter sets; as such, calibration should focus on "fine-tuning" a small subset of its total parameters.[19] Calibrating a large number of parameters can lead to an overfitting problem, in which the model can reproduce a small number of output observations artificially precisely. As a general framework, modelers should seek to calibrate parameters with the most uncertainty and those that have the strongest effect on model output. Uncertain parameters include those whose true value is unknown (or has a large range of possible values) and those for which empirical data are not available. Parameters that are particularly important (*i.e.*, substantially influence model outcomes) can usually be recognized a priori, or identified in sensitivity analyses. Parameters that are highly uncertain but have little impact on model results should not be subject to calibration procedures.[19] Finally, modelers should avoid calibrating parameters that are nonorthogonal or have similar effects on agent behavior and model output. For example, in an HIV transmission ABM, if the likelihood of a transmission event is directly proportional to both the total number of sex acts and the proportion of acts in which condoms are used, only one of these parameters should be calibrated. It may seem counterintuitive to calibrate an ABM by fine-tuning only a small subset of parameters and leaving others constant. However, since the number of parameters often greatly exceeds the number of calibration targets, the risk of overfitting is significant. In addition, modelers who wish to evaluate the effect of adjusting parameters not subject to calibration can easily do so. For example, their values can be varied in sensitivity analyses to evaluate the robustness of the model to alternative model initialization specifications.

There is an extensive literature on methods for calibrating microsimulation models,[59-61] including ABMs[46,62]; a detailed description of various calibration methods is beyond the scope of this chapter. Most procedures are a variation on best-fit calibration methods, in which parameter values are chosen such that model output provides a best-fit to the observed data. As an example, an iterative hyperparameter grid search algorithm can be implemented to fit model output to target empirical data using scalar modifiers as fitting parameter inputs. This method is executed by exhaustively searching through a selected range of parameters and their predefined space and evaluating model output performance by calculating an R^2 for each calibration target as a measure of fit. If multiple calibration targets are of interest, the result that produces the least absolute Manhattan distance from the initial parameterized input variables (that is, the smallest linear combination of R^2 and absolute value of scaling parameter change from 1) can be sought. More efficient methods, such as approximate Bayesian computation, can also be implemented. The most common Bayesian method used to calibrate ABMs is called an approximate Bayesian computation rejection algorithm, which involves running models a large number of times, with parameters drawn randomly from prior distributions, rejecting unsuitable model parameterizations, and retaining only those simulations in which model output is within a predefined "tolerance" from the observed data, measured using the Euclidean distance.[63] The final result of the rejection algorithm is a posterior distribution of parameter values, which can then be sampled during model replications.[64] Calibrating an ABM to a time series can be more complicated and involves deciding from a number of possible calibration criteria (*e.g.*, minimizing maximum errors or mean squared errors and setting a number of points in the time series that are acceptably close to the observations).[19]

Verification and Validation

Model verification and validation are essential components of the ABM design process. Model verification asks the question, "Does the ABM work as intended?," whereas model validation seeks to determine whether the model accurately reproduces the target phenomena. Although there is no universal approach or consensus on how to conduct verification and validation in agent-based modeling, a number of principles and overall techniques have been previously published.[65-67]

The goal of verification is to determine whether the programming implementation of the conceptual model is correct. This process includes debugging, verification of all model calculations, and determining whether equations in the model are solved correctly. Some common verification methods include debugging procedures, code "walk-throughs" (a form of software peer review), and boundary testing (*i.e.*, determining whether the model performs as expected at the parameter boundaries).

Broadly, model validation is a process through which the research team assesses the extent to which the model is a credible representation of the real-world phenomena the model seeks to represent. Several techniques are available to demonstrate a model's validity. For example, a model is said to have *face validity* if content experts believe that the model behaves reasonably well by making subjective judgments about its performance. Most ABMs also go through a procedure known as *empirical validation*. Here, the developer determines whether the model is a good representation of the target by comparing whether the model output is consistent with observed data. A number of different approaches to conduct empirical validation have been developed and are described elsewhere.[46] Finally, a variety of statistical tests can be used to determine if the model's behavior has an acceptable level of consistency with observed data.[68]

Although a comprehensive discussion of ABM validation procedures is beyond the scope of this chapter, and is the topic of other previously published reports,[46] we note that detailed sensitivity analyses are essential to establish model validity. In addition to examining how results depend on sensitivity to initial conditions and across-run variability (arising from stochastic elements in the model), current recommendations include investigating model robustness against changes in model rules as well as timing and updating mechanisms.[46] Methodological standards and a minimally acceptable set of protocols for ABM construction, analysis, and validation[69] should be adhered to whenever feasible.

Interpreting ABMs

Interpreting the output of an ABM has distinct challenges from other mathematical modeling approaches. First, isolating the causal mechanisms and effects of one parameter can be difficult in models with a high degree of agent heterogeneity and many interdependent processes. For this reason, conducting parameter sweeps over multiple variables (*i.e.*, running replications with different combinations of input parameter values) to understand model behavior is recommended. Second, ABMs can be highly sensitive to initial conditions. In complex and chaotic systems, even small perturbations in initial conditions can lead to large differences in model output.[70] Third, precise prediction of real-world phenomena under different inputs can be problematic when many assumptions are made regarding agent behavior and interactions. Given the complexity of many ABMs, the objective should not necessarily be to predict specific population outcomes under different scenarios per se, but to conduct a robust policy analysis, such that recommendations consist of an ensemble of policy options, which perform well under plausible model specifications and are robust to model assumptions.

ABM MODEL CHARACTERISTICS

Given that many ABMs are constructed de novo, with algorithms and rule sets created to answer a particular research question and coded in a variety of different software languages, the characteristics and features of ABMs can vary substantially across models. Nonetheless, there are core characteristics and concepts that differentiate ABMs from other types of models, which are the focus of this section. Readers interested in a more in-depth discussion are referred to several excellent texts on the subjects.[1,19]

Emergence

By definition, all population health outcomes (e.g., disease incidence, prevalence, mortality rates) are an aggregation of individual health states. Each person's health status is in turn a function of their own biological characteristics, their interactions with other people in the population, and the influence of their environments. Put another way, population health outcomes *emerge* from the behaviors and characteristics of autonomous units (i.e., people) and their local interactions between each other and their environments.[71]

The concept of *emergence* is a defining characteristic of ABMs. The goal of agent-based modeling is to simulate the emergence of population-level outcomes from the local behaviors and interactions of individual agents and their environments.[1] For example, a recent agent-based modeling study simulated *Clostridium difficile* transmission in a 200-bed hospital.[72] The incidence of hospital-acquired *C. difficile* "emerged" from a series of ten possible agent-agent and agent-environment interactions that could lead to disease transmission. The inclusion of four distinct agent types (patients, visitors, nurses, and physicians) allowed the researchers to evaluate a variety of hospital- and patient-centered infection control interventions. The study, which was the first to compare patient- and hospital-focused infection control strategies, found that bundling just two interventions (e.g., daily cleaning with disinfectant and *C. difficile* screening at admission) could reduce hospital-onset infections by over 80%.[72]

The ability to simulate *emergence*—defined formally as the appearance of population-level patterns, trends, and regularities from interactions among smaller or simpler entities that themselves do not exhibit such properties—is an important strength of agent-based modeling.[73] Emergent behavior is said to occur whenever the interactions of individual entities jointly contribute to the system-level behavior that is not easily predicted from summative or aggregate properties of the individual units; in other words, the whole is greater and more complex than the sum of its parts.[74] Emergent behavior is observed throughout the physical and social sciences—the flocking behavior of birds is one example of how animals organize themselves in a complex, collective manner.[75]

In epidemiology, the unique contributions of ABMs and other "bottom-up" simulation approaches stem from their capacity to reproduce (and thus better understand) the mechanisms through which group-level phenomena are generated. It is for this reason that ABMs are employed in epidemiological practice to elucidate the origins and determinants of population-level protective factors (e.g., herd immunity) and the unintended consequences of individual behaviors in human populations.[76-78] For example, one agent-based modeling study found that the dramatic racial disparities in incarceration rates between Blacks and Whites in the United States can be reproduced from systemic biases in sentencing lengths, combined with a "social contagion" effect, in which the risk of incarceration is dependent on the prevalence of incarceration in neighborhoods and social networks.[10] Simulations without a contagion effect (i.e., in which the risk of incarceration is independent of any relationship with currently incarcerated agents) could not reproduce observed racial disparities in incarceration rates (see Figure 31-2), even with significantly increased initial prevalence and risk of incarceration among African Americans.[10]

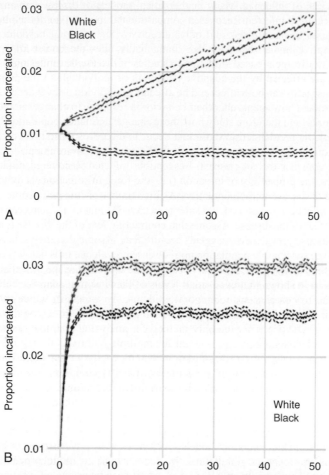

FIGURE 31-2 An example of *emergence* in an agent-based model: Biases in sentencing lengths and "transmission" of incarceration through social networks explain racial disparities in incarceration rates in the United States. **Panel A,** Prevalence of incarceration (by race) estimated from an agent-based model in which the median sentence length is 10 months for Whites and 12 months for Blacks, and in which the risk of incarceration is proportional to the number of incarcerated individuals in an agent's network. **Panel B,** Proportion of people incarcerated (by race) estimated from an agent-based model with no "contagiousness" of incarceration. Note: *x*-axis refers to a time scale in years. (Reproduced from Lum K, Swarup S, Eubank S, Hawdon J. The contagious nature of imprisonment: an agent-based model to explain racial disparities in incarceration rates. *J R Soc Interface.* 2014;11:20140409 with permission.)

Understanding the *emergent properties* of a population system (in this case, the emergence of stark racial disparities in incarceration) provides important insights into the root causes of public health problems. Agent-based modeling studies can also inform new avenues for intervention: in this case, reforms to the US criminal justice system including policies to ameliorate existing inequities in sentencing lengths, in addition to interventions that reduce the "transmission" of incarceration through social networks (*e.g.*, community-based reintegration programs), were recommended by the authors.[10]

Adaptivity

Individuals are not passive actors in their exposure to disease risks. As an everyday example, consider how members of a household might change their behavior after a relative acquires influenza (*e.g.*, increased hand washing and social distancing). These behavioral adaptions in turn decrease an individual's own risk of influenza. Many mathematical models of disease transmission (including the common Susceptible-Infected-Recovered compartmental models) do not explicitly incorporate behavioral responses to disease risk and other incentives for changing behavior, despite studies showing that adaptive human behavior can dramatically alter the course of epidemics.[79,80] An important reason to use agent-based modeling in studies of disease transmission is to simulate how model outcomes are affected by the adaptive behaviors of individuals in the population. In other words, since disease risks can both affect and be affected by individual-level decisions, ABMs allow the researcher to model how agents alter their behavior in response to changes in their environments and contact networks, and therefore study how these changes influence population health outcomes.

Adaptive behaviors are defined as those that occur in direct response to a current or past state, the influence of other agents, or due to stimuli in the modeled environment.[19] As an example of these principles, consider that in classical Susceptible-Infected-Recovered models of infectious disease epidemics, the probability of infection (*i.e.*, the force of infection) is directly proportional to the prevalence of disease in the population. As the number of infected people increases, so too does the force of infection. In contrast, consider now an ABM in which agents can contract both the disease itself *and* fear of the disease. Assume that contracting fear of the disease is also directly proportional to the disease prevalence. As agents acquire fear, assume that they self-isolate, removing themselves from the susceptible population until disease prevalence falls below a certain threshold. Self-isolation is thus an *adaptive behavior* based on the current disease prevalence. Agent-based modeling studies have shown that even small levels of fear-inspired adaptive behavior (*e.g.*, self-isolation) can lead to complex spatiotemporal epidemic dynamics, in which reoccurring waves of infection occur due to the premature return of self-isolated individuals to the susceptible population.[81] Note that ABMs are not the only method for analyzing adaptive phenomena: coupled, nonlinear dynamical systems can also account for multiple outbreaks during the same episode.[82] Nonetheless, ABMs can accommodate substantial heterogeneity within and evolution of adaptive behaviors, which may be important for modeling particularly complex transmission networks for disease processes such as obesity and sexually transmitted infections.

Stochasticity

In contrast to deterministic epidemic models (such as models governed by ordinary differential equations), ABMs are stochastic simulations. We define stochastic model processes as those based on random functions or events. In an ABM, stochasticity can be produced in a number of different ways: random number generators to produce variability in initial conditions; statistical distributions from which parameter values and agent characteristics are drawn; or rule sets that have random components (*e.g.*, a coin flip). Stochastic elements in an ABM result in variability in the model output. For this reason, an ABM often needs to be run many times, which results in a distribution of outcomes. The degree of variability across model replications depends on the nature and number of stochastic processes in the model: some ABMs may produce nearly the same result, while the output of other replications will vary widely.

In general, variability in an ABM can arise from two sources. First, at model initialization, random number generators are used to define the model's initial conditions, distributing the traits, interactions, and environmental state values randomly in the agent population, conditional on the input parameter functions and probability distributions. For example, in an ABM simulating transmission of a sexually transmitted infection, the number of sexual partners each agent is connected to may be drawn from known sexual partnership degree distributions, such as negative binomial distributions.[83] Since agents are assigned initial characteristics and interactions using random number generators, each replication will have a distinct population set using what is known as a random *seed*, even if the mean input parameter values are the same. For example, an ABM may be initialized with 12% baseline disease prevalence, yet across model replications, agent-level instances of disease may be distributed in very different ways. Therefore, even models with no other stochastic element beyond a random seed can produce variability in model output. However, for each replication, the exact sequence and distribution of random numbers (*i.e.*, its random seed) can be stored and regenerated. Setting the generator's seed can be used to eliminate the randomness at model initialization as a source of variability among the model runs.[19] The advantage is to preclude randomness as an explanation for different preliminary modeling results.

Stochastic elements in the rule sets governing agent behaviors, agent-agent interactions, and interactions with their environments are a second important source of variability in model output. For example, in an ABM that simulates HIV epidemic dynamics,[16] the overall risk of HIV transmission between an uninfected and infected agent (β_p) was determined by a binomial process:

$$\beta_p \sim Bin(n, \beta_a) = \frac{\beta_p!}{(\beta_p - n)!n!} \beta_a^{\beta_p} (1 - \beta_a)^{n - \beta_p}, \quad \beta_p \in \{1, \cdots, n\}$$

where β_a is the per-act probability of HIV transmission (specific to the behaviors engaged in between serodiscordant agents, such as condomless insertive and receptive anal intercourse). The number of trials, n, is defined as the number of sex acts between the two agents, which in turn could be dependent on other random or deterministic functions. The combination of random seeds and stochastic model processes produces a model output that varies over time and across model replications. For example, an adaptation of this HIV transmission model was used to estimate the proportion of all HIV transmission events that occur during acute HIV infection,[84] defined as the 3 to 6 month period after seroconversion.[85] Due to the rare nature of these acute transmission events, a large agent population of 100,000 was initialized and 500 model replications were conducted. As shown in Figure 31-3, the proportion of all transmission due to acute HIV infection varied over the 10-year model runs, and also across the model replications (10th and 90th simulation intervals are shown).

It is important to note that random variability observed between model replications does not represent the true degree of uncertainty present in an ABM. Uncertainty and possible biases in model structure, input parameters, and calibration procedures are important to consider; therefore, variability in model output across replications should not be used as a measure of model reliability or validity.[19] Additional procedures and analyses should be used to test the model's robustness and the extent to which the model accurately reproduces real-world phenomena (see the *Model Design and Implementation* section above). Nonetheless, model replication is important for generating

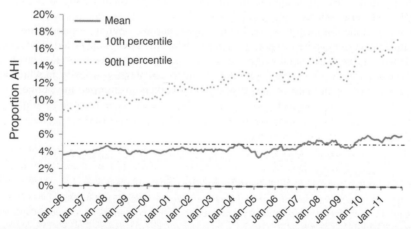

FIGURE 31-3 The estimated proportion of all HIV transmission events from acute HIV infection (AHI) among people who inject drugs in New York City, 1996 to 2011. Note: Agent population of 100,000 was used to represent the entire New York City adult population, with 1.6% prevalence of injection drug use in 1996. Results shown above are from 500 model replications. Note: The dash-dot black line represents the cumulative estimate (4.9%) for the entire 16-year period. The values for the dashed series (10th percentile) are 0 for the majority of data points due to the rarity of acute transmission events in a small population over the course of a single month; that is, the probability of observing an acute transmission event in the lowest decile of model runs for a given month is near 0. (Reproduced from Escudero DJ, Lurie MN, Mayer KH, et al. Acute HIV infection transmission among people who inject drugs in a mature epidemic setting. *AIDS*. 2016;30:2537-2544 with permission.)

random error in model output, particularly in instances in which the agent population is smaller than the target population. Moreover, replications are helpful for comparing different versions of an ABM. When we compare counterfactual scenarios by changing model inputs and assumptions, we must run the model enough times to differentiate meaningful differences from "noise" generated by stochastic elements of the model.

CONCLUSION

Epidemiology is, at its heart, a pragmatic discipline that identifies opportunities to control and prevent disease.[86] Agent-based modeling represents one method to synthesize prior knowledge of a population—and the causal structures that act on this population—to understand how an intervention could affect the public's health. In this manner, agent-based modeling is a science of evidence synthesis. Specifically, ABMs (and other simulation approaches) represent a platform for the integration of diverse evidence sources, including inconsistent or inconclusive scientific information, to support decision-making for complex public health problems. Formalized methods and frameworks for the integration of diverse data streams into simulation models (and their implications for evidence-based policy analysis) have recently been proposed for population health sciences.[87,88] Continued adoption of these methods is warranted.

I do not wish to imply that agent-based modeling is the only (or superior) method by which dynamically complex processes can be explored in epidemiology. Rather, agent-based modeling is one of many recently developed approaches that seek to account for complex phenomena in population health. These include the parametric g-formula[89,90] as well as novel approaches that assess interference using potential outcomes frameworks.[39] Additional research is required to determine under what conditions ABMs provide similar or novel insights into the causes of disease, compared to traditional epidemiologic approaches and other modern methods. Very few comparative investigations have been conducted to directly interrogate an epidemiologic question with different types of causal inference models, including those that are agent based. One recently published study found that the g-formula and an ABM consistently estimated mortality and causal effects when all inputs were from the same target population, but the latter produced biased effects when inputs were extrapolated from another population.[91] Conducting additional cross-model type comparisons will aid in the determination of the circumstances in which ABMs are likely to produce reliable results and valid causal inference.

I wish to conclude this chapter by noting that agent-based modeling of population health systems and the impact of hypothetical policy changes on health outcomes have led to novel scientific insights. However, the actual uptake of programs and policies informed by ABMs has largely yet to be evaluated in real-world settings. A multidisciplinary and iterative science, in which modelers work collaboratively with interventionists and policy makers to improve the public's health, is necessary.

References

1. Epstein JM. *Generative Social Science: Studies in Agent-Based Computational Modeling*. Princeton, NJ: Princeton University Press; 2006.
2. Schelling TC. Models of segregation. *Am Econ Rev*. 1969;59(2):488-493.
3. Schelling TC. Dynamic models of segregation. *J Math Sociol*. 1971;1(2):143-186.
4. Tesfatsion L. Agent-based computational economics: modeling economies as complex adaptive systems. *Inf Sci*. 2003;149(4):263-269.
5. Judson OP. The rise of the individual-based model in ecology. *Trends Ecol Evol*. 1994;9(1):9-14.
6. Smith ER, Conrey FR. Agent-based modeling: a new approach for theory building in social psychology. *Pers Soc Psychol Rev*. 2007;11(1):87-104.
7. Koopman JS, Longini IM Jr. The ecological effects of individual exposures and nonlinear disease dynamics in populations. *Am J Public Health*. 1994;84(5):836-842.
8. Willem L, Verelst F, Bilcke J, Hens N, Beutels P. Lessons from a decade of individual-based models for infectious disease transmission: a systematic review (2006-2015). *BMC Infect Dis*. 2017;17(1):612.
9. Nianogo RA, Arah OA. Agent-based modeling of noncommunicable diseases: a systematic review. *Am J Public Health*. 2015;105(3):e20-e31.
10. Lum K, Swarup S, Eubank S, Hawdon J. The contagious nature of imprisonment: an agent-based model to explain racial disparities in incarceration rates. *J R Soc Interface*. 2014;11(98):20140409.

11. Auchincloss AH, Riolo RL, Brown DG, Cook J, Diez Roux AV. An agent-based model of income inequalities in diet in the context of residential segregation. *Am J Prev Med*. 2011;40(3):303-311.

12. Blok DJ, de Vlas SJ, Bakker R, van Lenthe FJ. Reducing income inequalities in food consumption: explorations with an agent-based model. *Am J Prev Med*. 2015;49(4):605-613.

13. Axelrod R. Agent-based modeling as a bridge between disciplines. In: Tesfatsion L, Judd KL, eds. *Handbook of Computational Economics*. Vol 2. Amsterdam: North-Holland; 2006:1565-1584.

14. Maglio PP, Mabry PL. Agent-based models and systems science approaches to public health. *Am J Prev Med*. 2011;40(3):392-394.

15. Zhang J, Tong L, Lamberson PJ, Durazo-Arvizu RA, Luke A, Shoham DA. Leveraging social influence to address overweight and obesity using agent-based models: the role of adolescent social networks. *Soc Sci Med*. 2015;125:203-213.

16. Marshall BDL, Friedman SR, Monteiro JF, et al. Prevention and treatment produced large decreases in HIV incidence in a model of people who inject drugs. *Health Aff (Millwood)*. 2014;33(3):401-409.

17. Cerdá M, Tracy M, Ahern J, Galea S. Addressing population health and health inequalities: the role of fundamental causes. *Am J Public Health*. 2014;104(suppl 4):S609-S619.

18. Gilbert N. *Agent-Based Models*. Thousand Oaks, CA: SAGE Publications; 2008.

19. Railsback SF, Grimm V. *Agent-based and Individual-Based Modeling: A Practical Introduction*. Princetown, NJ: Princetown University Press; 2012.

20. Luke DA, Stamatakis KA. Systems science methods in public health: dynamics, networks, and agents. *Annu Rev Public Health*. 2012;33:357-376.

21. Auchincloss AH, Diez Roux AV. A new tool for epidemiology: the usefulness of dynamic-agent models in understanding place effects on health. *Am J Epidemiol*. 2008;168(1):1-8.

22. Cerdá M, Tracy M, Keyes KM, Galea S. To treat or to prevent?: reducing the population burden of violence-related post-traumatic stress disorder. *Epidemiology*. 2015;26(5):681-689.

23. Bonabeau E. Agent-based modeling: methods and techniques for simulating human systems. *Proc Natl Acad Sci USA*. 2002;99(suppl 3):7280-7287.

24. Little RJ, Rubin DB. Causal effects in clinical and epidemiological studies via potential outcomes: concepts and analytical approaches. *Annu Rev Public Health*. 2000;21:121-145.

25. Marshall BDL, Galea S. Formalizing the role of agent-based modeling in causal inference and epidemiology. *Am J Epidemiol*. 2015;181(2):92-99.

26. Naimi AI. Commentary: integrating complex systems thinking into epidemiologic research. *Epidemiology*. 2016;27(6):843-847.

27. Miller JH, Page SE. On emergence. In Levin SA & Strogatz SH eds. *Complex Adaptive Systems: An Introduction to Computational Models of Social Life*. Princeton studies in complexity. Princeton, NJ: Princeton University Press; 2007:44-53.

28. Philippe P, Mansi O. Nonlinearity in the epidemiology of complex health and disease processes. *Theor Med Bioeth*. 1998;19(6):591-607.

29. Aral SO, Leichliter JS, Blanchard JF. Overview: the role of emergent properties of complex systems in the epidemiology and prevention of sexually transmitted infections including HIV infection. *Sex Transm Infect*. 2010;86(suppl 3):iii1-iii3.

30. Pearce N, Merletti F. Complexity, simplicity, and epidemiology. *Int J Epidemiol*. 2006;35(3):515-519.

31. Shoham DA, Tong L, Lamberson PJ, et al. An actor-based model of social network influence on adolescent body size, screen time, and playing sports. *PLoS One*. 2012;7(6):e39795.

32. Cohen-Cole E, Fletcher JM. Is obesity contagious? Social networks vs. environmental factors in the obesity epidemic. *J Health Econ*. 2008;27(5):1382-1387.

33. DePasse JV, Smith KJ, Raviotta JM, et al. Does choice of influenza vaccine type change disease burden and cost-effectiveness in the United States? An agent-based modeling study. *Am J Epidemiol*. 2017;185(9):822-831.

34. Hudgens MG, Halloran ME. Toward causal inference with interference. *J Am Stat Assoc*. 2008;103(482):832-842.

35. Halloran ME, Struchiner CJ. Causal inference in infectious diseases. *Epidemiology*. 1995;6(2):142-151.

36. Sobel ME. What do randomized studies of housing mobility demonstrate?: causal inference in the face of interference. *J Am Stat Assoc*. 2006;101(476):1398-1407.

37. VanderWeele TJ, Tchetgen Tchetgen EJ, Halloran ME. Components of the indirect effect in vaccine trials: identification of contagion and infectiousness effects. *Epidemiology*. 2012;23(5):751-761.

38. Oakes JM. The (mis)estimation of neighborhood effects: causal inference for a practicable social epidemiology. *Soc Sci Med*. 2004;58(10):1929-1952.

39. Tchetgen Tchetgen EJ, VanderWeele TJ. On causal inference in the presence of interference. *Stat Methods Med Res*. 2012;21(1):55-75.

40. El-Sayed AM, Seemann L, Scarborough P, Galea S. Are network-based interventions a useful antiobesity strategy? An application of simulation models for causal inference in epidemiology. *Am J Epidemiol*. 2013;178(2):287-295.

41. Christakis NA, Fowler JH. The spread of obesity in a large social network over 32 years. *N Engl J Med.* 2007;357(4):370-379.

42. Rahmandad H, Sterman J. Heterogeneity and network structure in the dynamics of diffusion: comparing agent-based and differential equation models. *Manag Sci.* 2008;54(5):998-1014.

43. Doherty IA, Padian NS, Marlow C, Aral SO. Determinants and consequences of sexual networks as they affect the spread of sexually transmitted infections. *J Infect Dis.* 2005;191(suppl 1):S42-S54.

44. Gilbert N, Terna P. How to build and use agent-based models in social science. *Mind Soc.* 2000;1(1):57-72.

45. Grimm V, Berger U, DeAngelis DL, Polhill JG, Giske J, Railsback SF. The ODD protocol: a review and first update. *Ecol Model.* 2010;221(23):2760-2768.

46. Windrum P, Fagiolo G, Moneta A. Empirical validation of agent-based models: alternatives and prospects. *J Artif Soc Soc Simul.* 2007;10(2):8.

47. Abuelezam NN, Rough K, Seage GR III. Individual-based simulation models of HIV Transmission: reporting quality and recommendations. *PLoS One.* 2013;8(9):e75624.

48. Grimm V, Berger U, Bastiansen F, et al. A standard protocol for describing individual-based and agent-based models. *Ecol Model.* 2006;198(1-2):115-126.

49. Macal CM, North MJ. Tutorial on agent-based modelling and simulation. *J Simulation.* 2010;4:151-162.

50. Zhang D, Giabbanelli PJ, Arah OA, Zimmerman FJ. Impact of different policies on unhealthy dietary behaviors in an urban adult population: an agent-based simulation model. *Am J Public Health.* 2014;104(7):1217-1222.

51. Heesterbeek H, Anderson RM, Andreasen V, et al; Isaac Newton Institute IDD Collaboration. Modeling infectious disease dynamics in the complex landscape of global health. *Science.* 2015;347(6227):aaa4339.

52. Sallis JF, Owen N, Fisher EB. Ecological models of health behavior. In: Glanz K, Rimer BK, Viswanath K, eds. *Health Behavior and Health Education: Theory, Research, and Practice.* 4th ed. San Francisco, CA: John Wiley & Sons, Inc; 2008:465-486.

53. Singer M, Clair S. Syndemics and public health: reconceptualizing disease in bio-social context. *Med Anthropol Q.* 2003;17(4):423-441.

54. Greenland S, Pearl J, Robins JM. Causal diagrams for epidemiologic research. *Epidemiology.* 1999;10(1):37-48.

55. Kumar S, Grefenstette JJ, Galloway D, Albert SM, Burke DS. Policies to reduce influenza in the workplace: impact assessments using an agent-based model. *Am J Public Health.* 2013;103(8):1406-1411.

56. Yang Y, Diez Roux AV, Auchincloss AH, Rodriguez DA, Brown DG. A spatial agent-based model for the simulation of adults' daily walking within a city. *Am J Prev Med.* 2011;40(3):353-361.

57. Cerdá M, Tracy M, Keyes KM. Reducing urban violence: a contrast of public health and criminal justice approaches. *Epidemiology.* 2018;29(1):142-150.

58. Murray EJ, Robins JM, Seage GR, III, et al. Using Observational Data to Calibrate Simulation Models. *Med Decis Making.* 2018;38(2):212-224. doi:10.1177/272989X17738753.

59. Dowling R, Skabardonis A, Halkias J, McHale G, Zammit G. *Guidelines for calibration of microsimulation models - framework and applications.* In: *Calibration and Validation of Simulation Models.* Washington, DC: Transportation Research Board; 2004:1-9.

60. Hansen LP, Heckman JJ. The empirical foundations of calibration. *J Econ Perspect.* 1996;10(1):87-104.

61. Rutter CM, Miglioretti DL, Savarino JE. Bayesian calibration of microsimulation models. *J Am Stat Assoc.* 2009;104(488):1338-1350.

62. Thiele JC, Kurth W, Grimm V. Facilitating parameter estimation and sensitivity analysis of agent-based models: a cookbook using net logo and R. *J Artif Soc Soc Simul.* 2014;17(3):11.

63. van der Vaart E, Beaumont MA, Johnston ASA, Sibly RM. Calibration and evaluation of individual-based models using approximate Bayesian computation. *Ecol Model.* 2015;312:182-190.

64. Sunnåker M, Busetto AG, Numminen E, Corander J, Foll M, Dessimoz C. Approximate bayesian computation. *PLoS Comput Biol.* 2013;9(1):e1002803.

65. Helbing D. *Social Self-Organization: Agent-Based Simulations and Experiments to Study Emergent Social Behavior (Understanding Complex Systems).* Zurich: Springer-Verlag Berlin Heidelberg; 2012.

66. Khattak AS, Khiyal MSH, Rizvi SS. Verification and validation of agent-based model using E-VOMAS approach. *Int J Comput Sci Netw Secur.* 2015;15(3):29-35.

67. Ormerod P, Rosewell B. Validation and verification of agent-based models in the social sciences. In: Squazzoni F, ed. *Epistemological Aspects of Computer Simulation in the Social Sciences.* New York, NY: Springer Berlin Heidelberg; 2010:130-140.

68. Xiang X, Kennedy R, Madey G, Cabaniss S. *Verification and validation of agent-based scientific simulation models. Paper Presented at the Proceedings of the 2005 Agent-Directed Simulation Symposium.* 2005.

69. Richiardi M, Leombruni R, Saam N, Sonnessa M. A common protocol for agent-based social simulation. *J Artif Soc Soc Simul.* 2006;9(1):15.

70. Resnicow K, Page SE. Embracing chaos and complexity: a quantum change for public health. *Am J Public Health*. 2008;98(8):1382-1389.

71. Reidpath DD. Population health. More than the sum of the parts? *J Epidemiol Community Health*. 2005;59(10):877-880.

72. Barker AK, Alagoz O, Safdar N. Interventions to reduce the incidence of hospital-onset Clostridium difficile infection: an agent-based modeling approach to evaluate clinical effectiveness in adult acute care hospitals. *Clin Infect Dis*. 2018;66(8):1192-1203.

73. Oakes JM. Invited commentary: rescuing robinson crusoe. *Am J Epidemiol*. 2008;168(1):9-12.

74. Rickles D, Hawe P, Shiell A. A simple guide to chaos and complexity. *J Epidemiol Community Health*. 2007;61(11):933-937.

75. Paina L, Peters DH. Understanding pathways for scaling up health services through the lens of complex adaptive systems. *Health Policy Plan*. 2012;27(5):365-373.

76. El-Sayed AM, Scarborough P, Seemann L, Galea S. Social network analysis and agent-based modeling in social epidemiology. *Epidemiol Perspect Innov*. 2012;9(1):1.

77. Galea S, Riddle M, Kaplan GA. Causal thinking and complex system approaches in epidemiology. *Int J Epidemiol*. 2010;39(1):97-106.

78. Liu F, Enanoria WT, Zipprich J, et al. The role of vaccination coverage, individual behaviors, and the public health response in the control of measles epidemics: an agent-based simulation for California. *BMC Public Health*. 2015;15:447.

79. Ceddia MG, Bardsley NO, Goodwin R, Holloway GJ, Nocella G, Stasi A. A complex system perspective on the emergence and spread of infectious diseases: integrating economic and ecological aspects. *Ecol Econ*. 2013;90:124-131.

80. Fenichel EP, Castillo-Chavez C, Ceddia MG, et al. Adaptive human behavior in epidemiological models. *Proc Natl Acad Sci USA*. 2011;108(15):6306-6311.

81. Epstein JM, Parker J, Cummings D, Hammond RA. Coupled contagion dynamics of fear and disease: mathematical and computational explorations. *PLoS One*. 2008;3(12):e3955.

82. Poletti P, Caprile B, Ajelli M, Pugliese A, Merler S. Spontaneous behavioural changes in response to epidemics. *J Theor Biol*. 2009;260(1):31-40.

83. Kault D. The shape of the distribution of the number of sexual partners. *Stat Med*. 1996;15(2):221-230.

84. Escudero DJ, Lurie MN, Mayer KH, et al. Acute HIV infection transmission among people who inject drugs in a mature epidemic setting. *AIDS*. 2016;30(16):2537-2544. doi:10.1097/QAD.0000000000001218.

85. Cohen MS, Shaw GM, McMichael AJ, Haynes BF. Acute HIV-1 infection. *N Engl J Med*. 2011;364(20):1943-1954.

86. Susser M. What is a cause and how do we know one? A grammar for pragmatic epidemiology. *Am J Epidemiol*. 1991;133(7):635-648.

87. Atkinson JA, Page A, Wells R, Milat A, Wilson A. A modelling tool for policy analysis to support the design of efficient and effective policy responses for complex public health problems. *Implement Sci*. 2015;10:26.

88. Baguelin M, Flasche S, Camacho A, Demiris N, Miller E, Edmunds WJ. Assessing optimal target populations for influenza vaccination programmes: an evidence synthesis and modelling study. *PLoS Med*. 2013;10(10):e1001527.

89. Westreich D, Cole SR, Young JG, et al. The parametric g-formula to estimate the effect of highly active antiretroviral therapy on incident AIDS or death. *Stat Med*. 2012;31(18):2000-2009.

90. Young JG, Cain LE, Robins JM, O'Reilly EJ, Hernan MA. Comparative effectiveness of dynamic treatment regimes: an application of the parametric g-formula. *Stat Biosci*. 2011;3(1):119-143.

91. Murray EJ, Robins JM, Seage GR, Freedberg KA, Hernan MA. A comparison of agent-based models and the parametric G-formula for causal inference. *Am J Epidemiol*. 2017;186(2):131-142.

PART **IV**

Special Topics

CHAPTER 32

Infectious Disease Epidemiology

Matthew P. Fox and Emily W. Gower

INTRODUCTION

Humans have been experiencing and reacting to the extraordinary morbidity and mortality impacts of infectious diseases like measles and tuberculosis for millennia. Thus, it is not surprising that early attempts to understand the causes of disease were deeply rooted in understanding infectious diseases. Indeed, many with no epidemiologic training quickly make the connection between the word *epidemiology* and the study of epidemics, and much of the history of the methods we use in all areas of epidemiology is to be found here. Infectious diseases motivated many of the early developments in epidemiologic methods, and some of the earliest attempts to wrestle with how to understand and identify causation were inspired by infectious diseases and infectious disease outbreaks. One of the best-known attempts at establishing causation was developed by Robert Koch in the late 1800s to enable determination of whether an infectious pathogen was responsible for causing a disease. He developed four postulates for establishing causation that led the way to identifying the causes of tuberculosis and cholera and paved the way for later well-known attempts to evaluate causation, such as the Bradford Hill guidelines.[1] A less well-known example is the contribution made to epidemiologic methods in the late 1800s motivated by the study of diphtheria,[2] in which Nobel Prize winner Johannes Fibiger used a randomized methodology to test the effectiveness of serum treatment by giving it to patients on alternate days.[3]

The study of infectious diseases has changed dramatically since 1900. As the demographic transition led to an epidemiologic shift from mortality patterns driven by infectious diseases to increasing rates of chronic diseases, countries have been forced to grapple with an increasing burden of chronic conditions that have accompanied rising life-expectancy globally. At the same time, infectious diseases like pneumonia, diarrheal diseases, malaria, tuberculosis, and HIV continue to be major sources of morbidity and mortality, especially in low-income settings, and particularly among children. Diarrheal, lower respiratory, and other common infectious diseases accounted for almost 10% of all deaths globally in 2015 as can be seen in Table 32-1. There was an impressive decrease in under-five mortality risks worldwide between 2000 and 2016, dropping from 69.4 to 38.4 per 1,000 live births,[4] and major reductions in mortality from HIV, tuberculosis, and diarrheal diseases at older ages worldwide. Still, the Global Burden of Diseases study estimates that

TABLE 32-1

Global Distribution of Communicable Diseases in Relation to All-Cause Mortality From 2005 to 2015

	All Age Deaths (Thousands)		Age-Standardized Mortality Rate (per 100,000)	
	2005	**2015**	**2005**	**2015**
All causes	53,618.5	55,792.9	1,024.0	850.1
Communicable, maternal, neonatal, and nutritional diseases	14,023.9	11,263.6	226.2	159.3
Nutritional deficiencies	*460.8*	*405.7*	*7.8*	*5.9*
Diarrhea, lower respiratory, and other common infectious diseases	*5,773.1*	*4,959.8*	*99.3*	*73.2*
Neglected tropical diseases and malaria	*1,298.5*	*843.1*	*19.5*	*11.5*
Maternal disorders	*350.8*	*275.3*	*5.1*	*3.6*
Neonatal disorders	*2,653.5*	*2,163.2*	*37.3*	*28.8*
Other communicable, maternal, neonatal, and nutritional diseases	*347.7*	*311.3*	*5.6*	*4.4*
HIV/AIDS and tuberculosis	*3139.5*	*2305.2*	*51.6*	*31.9*
Noncommunicable diseases	34,835.6	39,804.2	719.1	624.7
Injuries	4,759.0	4,725.1	78.6	66.2

Adapted from Table 5 of GBD 2015 Mortality and Causes of Death Collaborators. Global, regional, and national life expectancy, all-cause mortality, and cause-specific mortality for 249 causes of death, 1980-2015: a systematic analysis for the Global Burden of Disease Study 2015. *Lancet.* 2016;388:1459-1544.

infectious diseases (along with maternal, neonatal, and nutritional disorders) continue to contribute just under 19% of the total estimated age-standardized mortality rate at 159.3 per 100,000 in 2015, down from 226.2 in 2005 (Table 32-1)[5]. In addition, while it would be nice to think that our long history of studying and fighting infectious diseases means we have little work left to do, tuberculosis remains the most common cause of infectious disease deaths worldwide, despite almost two centuries of combating it. Moreover, outbreaks of diseases like Ebola, Zika, SARS-CoV-2, methicillin-resistant *Staphylococcus aureus* (MRSA), dengue, and West Nile remind us that studying infectious diseases will continue to occupy us for a long time to come. Furthermore, understanding how to control these new pathogens will require not only knowledge of biology, virology, pathology, and immunology, but also the larger role of societal and environmental changes. This can already be seen with the development of sophisticated system dynamics models like agent-based models used for disease forecasting to describe the interaction of people, environment, and pathogens.[6]

Despite great advances in our ability to both prevent and treat infectious diseases, we continue to seek new tools to diagnose, treat, and prevent them, as new challenges arise, including new and emerging infectious diseases, antibiotic and antiviral resistance, suboptimal immunization rates, and overcrowding from increased urbanization. The approaches range from behavioral interventions like handwashing campaigns[7] to biological approaches such as the development of new antiviral drugs and vaccines. They also include traditional approaches to vector control like spraying with insecticides and novel attempts like genetically altering mosquitos to make them resistant to infectious agents like malaria.[8,9]

Two examples of our need to continue to grapple with infectious diseases have appeared in recent years. The first comes from the 2014 to 2016 Ebola virus outbreak in Guinea, Sierra Leone, and Liberia, which was the largest in history, responsible for over 11,000 deaths.[10,11] Poor public health infrastructure, traditional cultural practices for tending the sick and the dead, and increased globalization and access to international and intercontinental travel allowed the disease to spread rapidly across borders and raised fears that global outbreaks are increasingly likely. This outbreak underscores the importance of ensuring that public health systems are ready to combat and contain emerging threats and that we continue to push forward with the development of novel approaches to prevent and treat infectious diseases. Unfortunately, experience with such a large Ebola outbreak did not lead to adequate preparedness to prevent future large outbreaks. In December of 2019, a novel coronavirus, SARS-CoV-2, appeared in Wuhan, China, leading to the illness COVID-19. Initial estimates of case fatality rates over 10 times higher than those of seasonal flu[12] were documented, leading governments worldwide to enact social distancing measures and lockdowns designed to slow the spread of transmission. Because many of those who experienced severe illness required hospitalization and use of ventilators and because no vaccine or effective treatment existed early on in the pandemic, the global slogan of "bend the curve" began, meaning to slow the spread of transmission enough to prevent healthcare systems from being overwhelmed. While many in high-income countries had limited experience with severe epidemics, the world was again acquainted with concepts like asymptomatic transmission, incubation periods, mathematical models of transmission, and the basics of handwashing, distancing, testing and tracing, and using masks to prevent infectious disease transmission. Thus, infectious diseases are not a thing of the past.

While the world continues to urbanize, with over 50% of the world's population now living in urban areas,[13] humans are also moving into locations we have previously not inhabited, putting us in close contact with vectors and pathogens that were previously unknown or poorly described, such as Lyme disease caused by *Borrelia burgdorferi* spread by deer ticks in the late 1970s.[14] Rising global temperatures have shifted the geographic range in which pathogens and their vectors can thrive, as demonstrated by the increase in global distribution of dengue[15] and chikungunya fever.[16] Rising sea temperatures have led to increased cholera outbreaks, and rising sea levels and natural disasters have impacted water and sanitation systems,[17] which can lead to pathogens emerging in places where outbreaks had been uncommon, as happened with a cholera outbreak in Haiti after the massive 2010 earthquake.[18] Urbanization and crowding in areas where animals are kept in large numbers has allowed for facilitation of disease strains making the jump to humans, causing outbreaks like the SARS epidemic in 2003.[19]

Each of these challenges underscores the fact that, as the planet we inhabit further urbanizes, warms, and industrializes and our ways of interacting with our environments and technological advances further progress, the challenges of studying the natural history of and interventions targeted at infectious diseases remain as important as ever. In this context, epidemiology plays a critical role in identifying and preventing new diseases and outbreaks, understanding factors that contribute to the spread of those diseases, developing novel approaches to reducing risk and harm, and providing rigorous evidence of the effectiveness of interventions designed to prevent or cure those diseases. At the same time, neglected infectious diseases that continue to cause significant suffering but lack the resources necessary to bring them to elimination as a public health problem require clever solutions to advance progress toward their control.

MAJOR HISTORICAL CONTRIBUTIONS OF INFECTIOUS DISEASE EPIDEMIOLOGY

The history of infectious disease epidemiology is too long to fully cover in this chapter in a meaningful way. Here, we focus on the key contributions that shaped the field and that laid the groundwork for modern infectious disease research. We refer those wishing to gain a thorough understanding of the major events in the history of infectious disease epidemiology to some key resources on the subject.[20-22]

London's Cholera Outbreak

No history of epidemiology would be complete without mention of John Snow's famous investigation of a cholera outbreak in England in 1854, which killed hundreds in London's Golden Square neighborhood. Snow had already hypothesized that cholera was transmitted by the fecal-oral route when the Broad Street outbreak began, but the pathogen itself was not yet known. Snow used careful scientific inquiry to map where cholera cases were occurring.[23] He then analyzed the maps to determine that the source of the outbreak was the Broad Street water pump and ultimately removed the pump handle. While reports of Snow's influence on removing the pump handle and ending the outbreak are common lore, in fact, the epidemic had largely subsided by the time Snow intervened. In addition, Snow's investigation of the cholera outbreak near Broad Street was not the only investigation.[24] Foreshadowing the role of changing climate, England's Board of Health plotted the outbreak as a function of temperature, wind, air pressure, and humidity. This same investigation likely also identified the index case, a case that Snow was not even aware had occurred.[25]

Still, Snow's investigation is one of the earliest outbreak investigations and is notable since the source of the outbreak was correctly determined even before the infectious pathogen, *Vibrio cholerae*, was known. His work demonstrated that even when the causes of disease are not fully understood, progress in prevention can still be made. His work also demonstrated the value of careful and detailed epidemiologic investigation, including careful consideration of comparability of populations,[26] though controversy continues as to whether or not his maps of the outbreak preceded his conclusions.[25] What may be less commonly known is that Snow pioneered the use of Voronoi diagrams that divide geographic areas into sections that are closest to a set of points on a map.[27,28] In his case, Snow used the locations of the city's water pumps as centroids of the map segments to show that the majority of the cases of cholera were located in map segments closest to the pump. The use of this method demonstrates the critical intermingling of mathematics and the study of infectious diseases and foreshadows the development of more complex models of infectious disease transmission and geographic information systems that have become an important part of research in infectious disease epidemiology.

Puerperal Fever

Another important development in infectious disease epidemiology was the identification of hand washing as a means for preventing puerperal fever in the mid-1800s in Vienna. While recognition that puerperal fever transmitted from person to person was likely discovered much earlier and its contagiousness was well documented by Oliver Wendall Holmes, exactly how it was transmitted, what the agent was, and how to prevent the spread were unknown in the mid-1800s.[29] Upon identifying a large number of deaths due to puerperal fever in maternity wards, Ignaz Semmelweis noted that the rates of the disease differed strongly by ward. Specifically, he noted rates were higher in the ward where students were taught to deliver babies and lower in the ward where midwives delivered babies.[30] This descriptive epidemiology led him to theorize that the spread of disease might be related to the autopsies performed by the students who were also delivering babies. Like Snow's cholera example, while the mechanism of disease transmission was not yet known, he was able to test his theory by getting the students to wash their hands and instruments using a solution of chlorinated lime after autopsies. This action led to a reduction from over 10% to below 2% in the incidence of fatal puerperal fever[31] as shown in Figure 32-1. The design used was far different from the approach we might take today (his looking more like an interrupted time series), but this early intervention study provided strong evidence of an effect of handwashing on reduced incidence despite a limited understanding of the true cause of the disease. Though his discovery was not well received at that time, today this is widely seen as one of the greatest discoveries in the history of infectious diseases, and handwashing and sterilization have proven to be effective in preventing the transmission of many other infectious agents. At the same time, suboptimal hand hygiene in hospitals continues to lead to nosocomial and iatrogenic infections even today.[32-35]

Smallpox

One further historical triumph in infectious disease epidemiology relates to Edward Jenner's demonstration of the effectiveness of cowpox inoculation to prevent smallpox in the late 1700s. Jenner used data on milkmaids to support his theory by noting that milkmaids exposed to cowpox were unlikely to contract smallpox.[36] From there, Jenner hypothesized that exposing a healthy person to the pus from a person infected with cowpox could prevent infection with the more severe smallpox. He tested his theory by taking a specimen from the pustule of an infected milkmaid and inoculating an 8-year old boy. He then exposed the boy to smallpox, and the boy did not contract the more severe infection. While our methods have evolved from Jenner's day to prevent experimentation on human subjects without ethical oversight, informed consent, and demonstration of balance of benefits and harms (equipoise), Jenner's work paved the way for the development of vaccines for many infectious agents, like measles and polio, that were once seen as inevitable aspects of life. As one might expect, Jenner's discovery did not come from observation alone, but built on folk knowledge and the work of many others before him who had previously discovered the effects of inoculation.[36] Indeed, General George Washington ordered the a crude form of

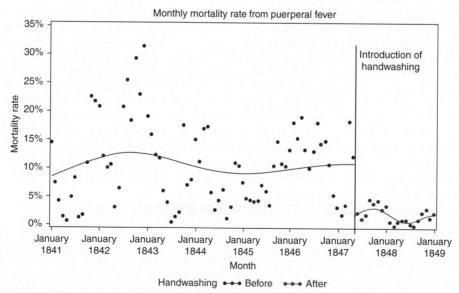

FIGURE 32-1 Change in mortality rate from puerperal fever in relation to institution of handwashing by Ignaz Semmelweis. (Reproduced from La Rochelle P, Julien AS. How dramatic were the effects of handwashing on maternal mortality observed by Ignaz Semmelweis? *J R Soc Med.* 2013;106(11):459-460.)

vaccination of his Continental army against smallpox before Jenner's work had even been done[37] and others may have already developed vaccination by the time of Jenner's work.[38] Further as recounted by Huth,[39] James Jurin published statistical analyses of the effectiveness of variolation with smallpox in the early 1700s. Smallpox eventually became the first disease to be eradicated by vaccination, as described in more detail later in this chapter.

Other Key Milestones in Infectious Disease Epidemiology

Numerous other significant milestones have led to dramatic changes in infectious disease transmission rates. These include the identification and mitigation of poor sanitation and overcrowding as a driver of transmission, the discovery and development of antibiotics to treat bacterial infections, the early vaccine trials of Sabin and Salk to prevent polio, and the development of the first antiviral drugs. While the list of significant milestones is too great to enumerate, and strongly overlaps with discoveries in infectious disease medicine and public health, these and many other advances in the prevention and treatment of infectious diseases have led to a sharp reduction in transmission in high-income countries, dramatically reducing epidemics of once common infectious diseases like tuberculosis, measles, polio, *Streptococcus pneumoniae*, *Haemophilus influenzae B*, yellow fever, typhoid, and others. Amazingly, as was found with many of the discoveries by some of the pioneers of infectious disease epidemiology described above, these reductions occurred before the discovery of the underlying infectious agent and often predate antibiotics. Instead, changes in sanitation, crowding, behavior, and diet have had a much stronger influence on the changing epidemiology of infectious diseases globally. Progress continues to be made in reducing infectious diseases, and this has strong knock on effects in reducing infant and child mortality. Indeed, in low-income countries, infant mortality rates recently have fallen sharply following strong reductions in major childhood infectious diseases like malaria[40] and diarrhea.[41]

The epidemiologic study of infectious diseases also has a history of direct experimentation to prove causation. In the mid-1980s, Barry Marshall proved his theory that peptic ulcers were caused by *Helicobacter pylori* by experimenting on himself. After demonstrating that he was ulcer free, he then ingested a culture of the bacterium. After drinking the culture, Marshall developed peptic ulcers and then subsequently cured himself by taking antibiotics.[42] This use of Koch's postulates was a strong, if not extreme, way to demonstrate causation, an act that earned him the Nobel Prize in 2005. Marshall only experimented on himself, but unfortunately, direct experimentation on humans with limited evidence to justify such experimentation and disregard for ethics is common in history. For example, initially pellagra was thought to be caused by an infectious disease, but later was proven to be caused by a lack of dietary niacin. This was determined through experimentation on prisoners in the early 1900s, in which Joseph Goldberger intentionally fed them a diet devoid of fresh fruits and vegetables,[43] and therefore with little niacin content. Other deeply concerning studies with disregard for ethics, include the infamous Tuskegee experiments conducted in the 1930s by the United States Public Health Service in which practitioners intentionally did not treat African Americans in Alabama who had syphilis in order to study the natural history of the disease. This occurred despite the fact that effective treatment was identified while the study was being conducted, and patients were told they were receiving treatment.[44] These studies, and others like them, were highly unethical. Although they provided evidence for and against competing theories of causation for these particular diseases, their larger impact is the influence they and others have had on ethical norms for the conduct of human subjects research on infectious diseases.

MAJOR OBJECTIVES OF INFECTIOUS DISEASE EPIDEMIOLOGY

The field of infectious disease epidemiology is diverse, and within it, we study many of the same things that are studied in other epidemiologic disciplines like description of the natural history and identification of risk factors. However, due to the nature of the transmission of infectious diseases from person to person or from vector to person, many aspects of infectious disease epidemiology differ from other epidemiologic disciplines. Infectious disease epidemiology covers everything from studying the natural history of infectious diseases and their distribution within populations to identifying new methods for treating infected patients and preventing the spread of disease. We investigate modes of transmission (*e.g.*, air borne, blood borne, fecal-oral, vector borne) and risk factors that increase the probability of infection or transmission, such as the role of malnutrition and immunosuppression in contracting measles. We also seek to identify and test new interventions to reduce transmission, from simple behavioral interventions such as handwashing to complex biomedical approaches such as developing vaccines to prevent the transmission of viruses and novel antibiotics to reduce morbidity and mortality. We also conduct surveillance to attempt to identify and prevent outbreaks (*e.g.*, mosquito surveillance to provide early warning for West Nile virus) and the unexpected adverse effects resulting from epidemiologic interventions. For example, through continual surveillance of the use of a particular rotavirus vaccine, we learned that in rare cases, vaccination may cause intussusception, a condition in which the intestine folds in upon itself.[45]

Infectious disease epidemiologists work on the cutting edge of developing and testing new technologies. At the same time, we also work on identifying better ways to implement proven approaches and the development of simplified tools that are focused on strengthening health systems to prevent and treat diseases in low-technology and rural settings. For example, epidemiologists developed and tested the implementation of the World Health Organization's (WHO) Integrated Management of Childhood Illness strategy that largely relies on signs and symptoms to diagnose and treat infectious diseases in settings with limited diagnostic tools.[46]

The novel SARS-CoV-2 outbreak that began in late 2019 demonstrates the extent of infectious diseases epidemiology in a very short period of time because the need for such information for action was so urgent. As of the time of writing this in August of 2020, the following has already occurred. Tracking of cases as of April 25, 2020, is shown in Figure 32-2.

When cases of SARS-CoV-2 began circulating in China, initial efforts to understand the epidemiology were focused on possible sources of transmission and whether or not human-to-human transmission was possible, as was later established.[47] As more cases were reported the world learned quickly that cases of this novel infectious disease increase exponentially, not linearly as we are used to with many other diseases. Next, there was a need to identify the route of transmission (fomites, infected objects and surfaces, large droplets from coughing and sneezing, or smaller, possibly aerosolized droplets that can last a long time in the air) and rule out others as major sources of transmission (*e.g.*, sexual, fecal-oral, etc.). Researchers worked to characterize the natural history of the disease, demonstrating that the disease was associated with symptoms that had some overlap with seasonal influenza, but in severe cases tended to be associated with a dry cough, fever and pneumonia.[48] Characterization of the demographic distribution of cases led to identification that children, although able to transmit the disease, have very low risk of severe illness, while those over the age of 65 suffer the highest rates of mortality.[12] Researchers also identified the incubation period (time from exposure to symptoms) of up to roughly two weeks (median of about 5 days),[49] which provided vital information on how long those who are exposed should quarantine. Further,

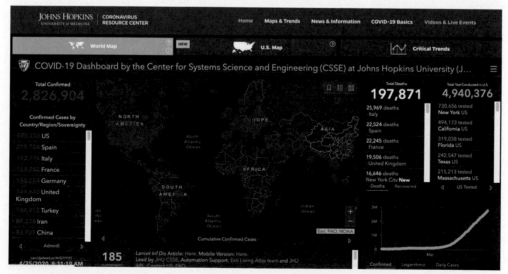

FIGURE 32-2 Screenshot of the John Hopkins COVID-19 dashboard as of April 25, 2020.

researchers identified that transmission could occur in the presymptomatic phase,[50] making it more difficult to isolate those who are infectious before they can transmit to others. Epidemiologists also identified that many people who get infected remain asymptomatic or show only mild symptoms, but have the potential to transmit the disease, making it even more challenging to determine the best approach to stopping transmission. leading to speculation about whether herd immunity (described in detail later in the chapter) could be achieved. Moreover, research was conducted on how long the virus could live on surfaces in order to identify risks from touching contaminated surfaces.[51] Indeed, the descriptive epidemiology in the early outbreak helped save lives.

Critical in all of this was the development of tests to identify infection with the novel virus. Due to our experiences with other coronaviruses (including previous SARS and MERS outbreaks), developing polymerase chain reaction tests for the virus was done in a matter of weeks after the virus was identified. This test development allowed some countries to develop testing that could be implemented at drive through facilities, allowing for rapid diagnosis and isolation. Many countries implemented physical distancing measures and travel bans designed to reduce the contact rate and the number of cases to allow burdened healthcare systems time to ramp up capacity and care for the sickest and to reduce the case fatality rate. Some countries implemented extensive contact tracing programs to identify those who may have been exposed to an infectious person so they could quarantine.[52] Some developed smart phone apps and used cell phone data to characterize travel patterns of those infected to identify potential sources of outbreaks.

As all of this was occurring, teams of researchers sought out a vaccine to prevent new cases and therapeutics to treat severe illness. As of the time of writing, a vaccine is estimated to be 6 to 12 months away, but several therapeutics are being tested in clinical trials. Convalescent plasma, taking blood of those who were infected, and then recovered and transfusing those who were experiencing severe illness, is being tested as a means to reduce morbidity and mortality, but to date, evidence is limited.[53] Antibody tests are also being developed to attempt to identify those who have already been infected and who may not be able to be infected again for some period of time.

Another critical aspect of responding to the COVID-19 outbreak has been the development of mathematical models for infectious disease (described in detail below). For many in the general public, this pandemic was the first time they had ever heard of infectious disease models. The modelers used what was known about the disease and how diseases move from person to person to project the likely progression of the pandemic and to model the effect of various interventions.[54,55] These models were used to guide decisions around community-wide shutdowns and implementation of sometimes severe physical distancing strategies to attempt to slow the spread of transmission.[56] The models also gave us a sense of the likely impact of various strategies to reduce transmission, such as wearing masks, contact tracing, and travel bans. They allowed us to make public health decisions, but they also have limitations that are difficult for the general public and even policy makers to understand,[57] exposing the need for better scientific communication on the part of epidemiologists.

This pandemic also made it clear that epidemiologists need to work with those in other fields and disciplines for epidemic control. Doctors and nurses are central to caring for the sickest patients, while laboratories are critical for ensuring the ability to identify those who are infected. Critical infrastructure and supply chains are essential to ensuring that food is still available during community-wide lockdowns. Manufacturing is critical to ensure that production of personal protective equipment can be ramped up to meet the fast increasing need. The impact of the outbreak on global economies was tremendous only months in, requiring the skills of economists to assess the economic impact and aid in developing recovery strategies. Moreover, even though epidemiologists were central to advising on how to control transmission, policy makers and those trained in policy evaluation were critical to weighing the various choices about how to confront a global pandemic. The media is critical in getting messages out to the public, requiring good science communication, and civil society organizations are needed to support communities who are suffering the most. Some media and social media also led to a need to combat misinformation. Each of these sectors is critical to combating such a massive challenge.

As of the time of writing, the COVID-19 outbreak is still continuing to expand and it is not yet clear how long it will continue and what the final impact will be. As you read this, so much more will have been learned and so many more advances will have been made. But, there will also be long-lasting impacts of this pandemic and a need to reinvest in public health infrastructure to prevent or better manage such an outbreak in the future.

CONCEPTS UNIQUE TO INFECTIOUS DISEASE EPIDEMIOLOGY

Progression of Infection

Much of what infectious disease epidemiologists study relates to understanding the ways in which pathogens lead to infection, how those infections then transmit through populations, how to interrupt transmission, and what factors influence disease severity. Although routes of transmission differ across pathogens, most, follow a standard series of stages of infection, *i.e.*, the steps necessary for a pathogen to cause infection. These include existing in a host or reservoir, a susceptible host encountering the pathogen, the pathogen entering the new host and replicating, and finally the pathogen exiting the host to infect a new person.

Each pathogen has its own characteristics, such as how effective it is at invading the host, and how it will affect the human host. Hosts also have characteristics such as how successfully the host can contain the infection. We can also describe the environment in which the pathogen and host interact (*e.g.*, frequency and degree of contact between hosts and the conditions of the environment in which the contact is made). These factors together determine how the pathogen is likely to spread within a population and with what severity illness is likely to occur. These factors influence disease incidence, severity, and transmissibility.

Although infections can occur in non-humans, we focus here on infections that occur to human hosts. For infection to occur, a human host must be susceptible to the infection and must come into contact with the pathogen, through the environment (*e.g.*, contaminated water exposure to *Giardia lamblia*), through contact with animals or insects who carry the pathogen (*e.g.*, ticks infected with *Rickettsia rickettsii*, the bacteria which causes Rocky Mountain Spotted fever), or through contact with other humans who are infectious (*e.g.*, transmission of influenza through exposure to the droplets expressed by an infectious person who is coughing or sneezing). The major determinants of whether the host will become infected are the dose of the pathogen to which the host is exposed and the route of infection.

The transmission cycle typically begins with colonization of the host, in which the pathogen (*e.g.*, a virus, bacteria, prion, etc.) exists on the host, but has yet to invade tissues and cause disease. Colonization occurs when a susceptible host encounters the pathogen. Next, infection occurs when a pathogen enters the tissue of a susceptible host and begins to replicate. For some pathogens, infection occurs without colonization, such as when an infected tick bites a human or when pathogens enter the host through contaminated water or food. In other instances, a host may be colonized without ever becoming infected. For example, *Streptococcus pneumoniae*, the cause of many severe cases of bacterial pneumonia, is often found in the nasopharynx of healthy hosts but rarely leads to infection that develops into pneumonia. The presence of commensal organisms, like *Streptococcus pneumonia*, on epithelial surfaces can make determining the cause of an infection difficult, because both the commensal organisms and the pathogen will be present in samples collected for culture, making it difficult to identify the organism responsible for infection.

Sometimes infection does not lead to clinical disease. **Subclinical infection** occurs when the host is infected but has no symptoms. Some hosts may become infected without experiencing any detrimental effects of the infection for some time, if at all. In other cases, hosts may become **colonized carriers** of disease and are able to pass on the infection to others despite never experiencing the typical symptoms of the infection. A famous example of an asymptomatic carrier comes from the early 1900s, when a cook who was infected with typhoid spread the pathogen to people she cooked for without experiencing illness herself.[58] After infection occurs, a host becomes infectious, meaning it can pass on the infectious agent to another host or to a vector to begin a new cycle of transmission. If much of the infectious period occurs before the host experiences clinical symptoms (presymptomatic) or if the host never experiences symptoms (asymptomatic), identifying infectious hosts for effective intervention is difficult or impossible. For example, when an individual with HIV becomes infectious, they may experience a short period of symptoms that are not likely recognized as being associated with HIV. The individual may then go several years without any symptoms, despite being infectious. When the asymptomatic phase is long, strategies like isolation of those infected and quarantining those exposed, treating symptomatic patients, or vaccinating contacts of symptomatic patients will have limited impact on reducing transmission, and routine testing strategies may be more effective. If, however, most of the infectious period occurs after symptoms occur, then these strategies can be highly effective. For example, the most infectious period for rubella

TABLE 32-2

Common Terms and Measures Associated With Stages of Infectious Disease Transmission

Measure	Definition
Colonization	A pathogen exists on or enters the host but has not invaded the tissue to cause infection
Infection	A pathogen enters the tissue of a susceptible host and replicates
Carrier	A host able to transmit infection even if experiencing no symptoms
Infectivity	A measure of how likely an infectious agent is to cause infection
Infectiousness	A measure of how likely an infected host is to transmit the infectious agent
Pathogenicity	A measure of the ability of an infectious agent to cause clinical disease in the host
Immunogenicity	A measure of the ability of an infectious agent to invoke an immune response in the host
Virulence	A measure of the severity of illness the infectious agent causes in the host

virus is after rash occurs, allowing for case identification before significant onward transmission occurs. Quarantine of exposed individuals and isolation of rubella cases can be highly effective.[59] On the contrary, SARS-CoV-2 is caused by a pathogen for which transmission can occur both before and after symptoms occur,[50] making it difficult to isolate all infectious persons before significant transmission occurs. During the 2020 outbreak, the lack of ability to rapidly and accurately test large segments of the population for infection led to the need for widespread community stay-at-home orders even for individuals who were thought to be healthy, in order to reduce the rate of transmission until testing and mitigation strategies could be developed.

Key measures of infectious disease transmission are defined in Table 32-2. We describe how effective a pathogen is at infecting a host in terms of its *infectivity*, which relates to how much of the agent (*i.e.*, dose) is needed to cause infection. The primary measure of incidence is the attack rate, defined as the number of new cases divided by the population at risk. For infections that spread from person to person, we can summarize the transmissibility of the pathogen using the *secondary attack rate*, which is measured as the proportion of susceptible individuals who become infected after being exposed to an infected index case. Secondary attack rates are most easily measured when exposure is known, such as in a point-source foodborne disease outbreak where both a single source of exposure and the exposed population are well defined, because the number of contacts has to be known to calculate the secondary attack rate. Infectious diseases such as measles, pertussis, and polio have high secondary attack rates, with over 80% of those exposed and susceptible becoming infected.[60]

We also characterize pathogens by their *incubation period* which is the time between exposure and clinical disease. For example, the incubation period for diphtheria is 2-5 days while the incubation period for measles is 10-14 days.[60] Other diseases, like Creutzfeldt-Jakob disease (related to bovine spongiform encephalopathy), have an incubation period of years.[61] Estimation of the incubation period can guide interventions to control the spread of the disease. For example, during the SARS-CoV-2 pandemic in 2020, those who were exposed were counseled to self-quarantine for 14 days, the estimated maximum incubation period.[47,49]

Once the pathogen enters the host, there can be a period before the host becomes infectious (and in fact, some infected persons may never become infectious) and therefore capable of transmitting the infection to a new susceptible host (or passing it on through an intermediate vector such as the bite of a mosquito). The time at which a person becomes infectious often does not coincide with clinical illness, making it difficult to measure. Because of this, we use the *serial interval* as a proxy measure. The serial interval is defined as the time between the onset of clinical disease of successive generations of infected persons. Although this interval does not measure the period of infectiousness directly, it does give us a sense for how infectious the pathogen is, with shorter serial intervals corresponding to more infectious pathogens. For example, the serial interval in an influenza outbreak in South Africa was measured to be about 2.3 days.[62]

The rate at which infected hosts become infectious and the duration of infectiousness strongly impact how quickly transmission will spread through a population of susceptible hosts and how many new cases each infected case will produce. For some pathogens, treatment can impact both the rate of becoming infectious and the duration of infectiousness. One powerful example of the impact of intervening to reduce infectiousness is the use of highly active antiretroviral therapy for individuals with HIV to prevent replication of the virus within the host. When successful, this practice can nearly eliminate the chance of transmission.[63]

The impact that an infectious agent has on the host in terms of its ability to cause illness and the severity of the illness that it causes are also important. We define the **pathogenicity** of the agent as its ability to cause disease, **virulence** in terms of how severe the illness is, (though some use this term as a synonym of pathogenicity), and **immunogenicity** as the ability of the agent to cause an immunologic response in the host. In some cases, a pathogen that is easily transmitted may have limited ability to cause severe illness. For example, polio, which can lead to acute flaccid paralysis, tends to be asymptomatic in over 70% of children infected and leads to paralysis in only about 1% of those infected.[60]

In extreme cases, where the pathogen can result in death of the host, we can summarize an infectious agent's virulence using the **case fatality rate**. This is defined as the proportion of those with the disease who die. Creutzfeldt-Jakob disease, rabies infection and Eastern Equine Encephalitis all have a very high case fatality rate.[60] However, not all infections that can have severe consequences have high case fatality rates. For example, Zika virus has a very low case fatality rate, despite the fact that children born to women who become infected while pregnant can develop microcephaly.[64] Highly virulent agents that lead to death, debilitation, or loss of quality of life are often considered a high priority for intervention (*e.g.*, hemorrhagic fevers such as Ebola, Marburg, etc.). At the same time, in some cases the virulence of pathogens that quickly kill their host can limit the period of infectiousness and prevent large-scale outbreaks. As with infectiousness, virulence and pathogenicity can be influenced by treatment, with some medications preventing the most severe effects of illness. Pathogenicity and virulence influence how important communities consider the infection and what actions should be taken to intervene to prevent further transmission. For example, in Ebola outbreaks involving more than 100 diagnosed cases, the case fatality rate has ranged from 25% to 90%.[65]

For several reasons, parameters like those described above can be difficult to determine accurately during an outbreak. First, these measures can vary across populations and demographics. Second, data from early in an outbreak often suffer from various biases including misclassification from imperfect tests, testing only the most severe cases (often those seeking medical care), delays in reporting information, and the relatively long period of time from infection to final outcome. As an example of this, in the 2020 SARS-CoV-2 outbreak, early estimates of the case fatality rate were nearly 3%, since only those individuals with symptoms severe enough to seek medical care were tested, resulting in a significant underestimate of the number of cases in the population. As testing became more widely available, the reported case fatality rate dropped. In addition, there could be a period of weeks to months from the time of symptoms at which one would seek a test and the time of death. When cases are increasing exponentially, using the current number of cases as the denominator and the current number of deaths as the numerator leads to a misaligned ratio that is likely biased. Models must be used to try to adjust for these biases[12] until final estimates can be generated.

Measures of Disease Control: Eradication Versus Elimination

Disease control can be accomplished in a variety of ways, and the ultimate targets for control are dictated by the feasibility of controlling the disease at the population level. The strongest control of an infectious agent is *extinction*, in which an infectious agent is completely eliminated, and no remaining samples of the organism exist. To date, no human pathogen has reached extinction.

Eradication is defined as a global, permanent reduction of the number of new cases of a disease to zero, which means that no human or other living organism can be infected with that disease again. In such cases, the only viable samples of the organism are located in tightly controlled laboratories. Achieving eradication is quite challenging. While political and social factors play a critical role in the success of eradication efforts, eradication ultimately requires several factors. First, an infectious agent cannot have a non-human reservoir. If an animal serves as a reservoir of infection, even if all humans are vaccinated to protect against transmission, the organism could still circulate in animal hosts and have the potential to reemerge. Eradication also requires effective interventions to interrupt transmission and that diagnostic tools that can detect disease at low levels in the host organism are readily available.[66] To date, only one disease of humans, smallpox, has been eradicated (rinderpest, a disease of cattle, has also been eradicated). Two other diseases currently targeted for eradication are dracunculiasis (guinea worm disease) and poliomyelitis, and great strides have been made to control both. In 2018, guinea worm was nearing eradication, with only 19 cases reported across three countries worldwide.[67] Concerted efforts to eradicate poliomyelitis began in 1988, and since then the incidence of new wild poliovirus cases have dropped by more than 99%. Four of the six WHO regions have been declared polio-free. However, polio remains endemic in a few countries.[68] As cases become more rare, the costs of case identification and efforts to reach elimination increase substantially. In 2019, a group of organizations pledged $2.6 billion to eliminate polio, despite only 33 reported cases globally in 2018, underscoring the massive efforts needed to reach eradication. Efforts are also underway to eradicate yaws, a chronic bacterial infection that affects skin, bones and cartilage.

Elimination of a disease typically refers to reducing the number of new infections to zero in a defined geographic area through deliberate interventions. Throughout history, many diseases have been eliminated from specific geographic areas while they remain endemic in others. A key challenge of maintaining elimination targets is trying to prevent re-emergence of the disease within an area that has been declared free of the disease. Malaria was once endemic in the United States but has since been eliminated. Measles also has been eliminated from specific geographic regions. However, in recent years, clusters of cases have been reported in previously disease-free areas, most likely due to reduced vaccination rates in those areas (see section on Modeling for more details), resulting in declarations of public health emergencies. This re-emergence highlights the challenges with elimination versus eradication.

Elimination as a public health problem is a disease control approach primarily targeting neglected tropical diseases. To reach elimination as a public health problem, countries must reach disease reduction targets defined by a group of WHO partners, with targets varying based on the disease. The underlying rationale is that if the disease burden is reduced to a low enough level within a community, the disease will no longer be a public health problem because isolated episodes of infection at the individual level will not be sufficient for community members to experience the long-term sequelae of the disease. Trachoma, lymphatic filariasis, and human African trypanosomiasis are three neglected tropical diseases that currently have targets for global elimination as a public health problem.

Trachoma's elimination targets are based both on markers of infection and presence of long-term sequelae, namely trichiasis, a condition characterized by inturned eyelashes that scratch the eye and can lead to blindness. Monitoring the presence of infection in large low- and middle-income countries (LMICs) is challenging due to limited infrastructure for diagnostic tests and lack of resources to fund such testing. To overcome these challenges, trachoma experts have identified clinical signs of current or recent infection with *Chlamydia trachomatis* that lay individuals can easily identify. Trachomatous follicles are white lymphoid follicles of the upper tarsal conjunctiva that typically are indicative of current or recent ocular chlamydial infection. In order to reach elimination targets, the prevalence of trachomatous follicles must be below 5% in children aged <10 years. Trichiasis experts believe that if the prevalence of signs of infection can be reduced to <5% in young children, community infection will be insufficient to reemerge and will not lead to long-term sequelae. Using this clinical sign allows for approximation of the burden of infection without the need for expensive diagnostic testing, enabling broader monitoring of the disease in these communities. To ensure that long-term sequelae are also well managed, the WHO also requires that the prevalence of unmanaged trichiasis is below 1 per thousand population in order for a country to declare elimination. For all diseases reaching elimination as a public health problem, ongoing surveillance efforts are required to ensure that disease does not re-emerge to a level sufficient to pose a public health problem.

Neglected Tropical Diseases

Many infectious diseases, such as influenza, are found consistently throughout the world, but others tend to be concentrated in or isolated to specific areas or to specific population subsets. Neglected tropical diseases (NTDs) are a group of communicable diseases found commonly in LMICs, primarily in tropical and subtropical climates. Currently, NTDs affect more than one billion individuals in nearly 150 countries, particularly in areas with extreme poverty and inadequate sanitation. This cluster of diseases is called neglected because they historically have not received the same attention or funding directed at their control as other infectious diseases. Many NTDs can lead to debilitating chronic conditions, which have a lasting negative impact on quality of life. In 2007, the WHO convened a partnership to target elimination of NTDs globally. This initiative has led to significant investment in NTDs, which in turn has paved the way for funding to support research on how best to manage them. At present, the WHO considers 13 diseases to be NTDs. This list evolves over time, and the most up-to-date list can be found on the WHO website.

The WHO has targeted five NTDs for eradication or global elimination as a public health problem by 2020. These include dracunculiasis (guinea worm), leprosy, lymphatic filariasis, human African trypanosomiasis, and trachoma. Multipronged efforts targeting the different stages of disease are required to reach elimination, and determining the best approaches requires extensive epidemiologic research. For example, research is required to determine how to reduce the spread of infection. In areas with low literacy, health education is clearly an important aspect of disease management, but approaches to improving health literacy may differ by country or by disease. For example, Guinea worm is a disease in which an individual ingests copepods (water fleas) that harbor dracunculiasis larvae by drinking contaminated water. The larvae mature inside the person, and when the worm is ready to reproduce, it burrows to the surface, often through the person's leg. The pain associated with this process is often alleviated by cooling one's leg in a river or lake, which then triggers the release of larvae. These larvae are consumed by water fleas, thus continuing the cycle. Efforts to reduce infection by improving water sources and health education on the need to filter water before drinking have been highly effective. However, in recent years, eradication efforts have been hampered by infections identified in multiple, previously unknown intermediate hosts, including wild dogs and frogs.[69] These issues highlight some of the challenges faced by eradication programs as they come closer to their targets.

METHODOLOGIES

Study Designs That Work Well for Infectious Diseases

Conventional Epidemiologic Study Designs

The study designs most commonly used in other fields of epidemiology are also regularly used to investigate infectious diseases. These include case-series, cross-sectional, case-control, cohort studies, and clinical trials. Often multiple types of studies are required to ultimately answer an infectious disease question. A famous case series of a cluster of rare, opportunistic infections among men who have sex with men in the early 1980s led to the identification of a new infectious disease that was eventually identified as HIV/AIDS.[70] Cross-sectional surveys led to the development of the hypothesis that male circumcision could reduce the risk of acquiring HIV infection, and this has ultimately been confirmed in randomized trials.[71-73] Cohort studies are commonly used for identifying factors that are associated with infectivity, pathogenicity, and virulence. Clinical trials are common for investigating both disease prevention through testing vaccines and disease treatment through investigating new drugs, including antibiotics and antivirals. They are also used for testing the effectiveness of strategies for infectious disease control such as clinical trials of face washing to prevent the spread of ocular chlamydial infection.[74,75] Some specific ways in which these study designs are used in infectious disease epidemiology as well as ways they have been altered or innovated upon are presented below.

Outbreak Investigations

Perhaps the most well-known design for studying infectious diseases is the outbreak investigation. Outbreak investigations attempt to identify the root cause of a particular outbreak and provide guidance for direct public health actions. An outbreak is defined as a greater than expected number of cases of a particular infection[76], often rapidly increasing, over a defined time period. Outbreak investigations may make use of several epidemiologic study designs, including case series and case-control studies. Case series are used to identify an outbreak. Once a cluster of cases is identified, investigators will often implement a case-control study to determine the source of the outbreak. In this setting, cases are often easily identifiable, and depending on the type of outbreak, the population that gave rise to the cases may also be reasonably well defined.

After initial investigations, hypotheses are refined and further investigation is often done until the source of the outbreak is identified and verified, and when possible, controlled. For example, in a 2018 outbreak of *Escherichia coli* infection, investigators first determined that romaine lettuce was the source of the outbreak, but it took nearly 3 months to determine the source of the contaminated lettuce.[77] In outbreaks of new diseases, determining the source of the infection and responsible pathogen can be particularly challenging, but is crucial to control the spread of disease. This was true of the initial cases of AIDS noted above, in which the cases were initially identified as a cluster of cases of pneumocystis pneumonia[78] and Kaposi sarcoma,[70,79] prior to determining that HIV was the primary cause of the outbreak of these secondary opportunistic infections. Methods had to be developed to identify the causal agent at the same time that the mode of transmission needed to be identified in order to prevent further transmission.

In other cases, the pathogen itself is well known and can be identified quickly, but identifying the route of transmission, which is of critical importance for control, can be challenging. For example, in 2007, a multistate outbreak of acanthamoeba, an amoeba that is commonly found in water sources and can cause blindness, was first identified from an ophthalmology listserv[80] (similar to novel surveillance approaches now being developed to mine previously untapped data sources, though using less technology). Once the outbreak was identified, careful investigation through a case-control study found that use of a particular contact lens solution believed to have insufficient ability to kill the amoebae was associated with a 15-fold increased odds of developing acanthamoeba keratitis from the infection.[81]

In an outbreak investigation, time is usually of the essence to reduce the impact of the outbreak. Outbreak investigations also differ from some other epidemiologic research in that the results typically lead to direct public health intervention and, therefore, the standards for when to ascribe causation may be loosened. In part because of the time pressure, but also because the strength of the effect of the exposure is typically quite large, some validity is often sacrificed for expediency. For example, controls are often sampled from a convenience sample of those who did not develop the outcome rather than seeking to enroll a sample representative of the study base that gave rise to the cases (even though the outcome can be common in some cases). A famous outbreak investigation that led to large changes in public health policies around food preparation occurred in 1993, when over 600 cases of food poisoning (including four deaths) related to a strain of *E. coli* bacteria (O157:H7) were linked to undercooked beef served at a fast food chain.[82] In a case-control study of 25 of the cases, those who ate at the chain in San Diego were 13 times more likely to develop *E. coli*–related food poisoning [95% CI (confidence interval): 1.7-99] compared to age- and sex-matched controls.[82] This outbreak led to large changes in the food industry to prevent future outbreaks, including changes in the minimum internal cooking temperatures of beef and the addition of warning labels on food products regarding the potential harms of undercooked meat.

Surveillance

An important aspect of epidemiologic study of infectious diseases is surveillance for outbreaks of diseases (see Chapter 9), and perhaps some of the most innovative work on infectious diseases in recent years has occurred in this area. For example, methods for syndromic surveillance[83]—in which symptom reports are monitored in real time to identify disease outbreaks earlier than they often would have been identified through conventional surveillance approaches—have accelerated over the past decades as concerns over terrorist use of infectious agents have increased. See, for example, the 2001 use of anthrax in mailings[84] and the systems set up for bioterrorism detection following the 9/11 terrorist attacks in New York City.[83-85] Hospital admission systems can be designed to mine clinical records and flag when cases of an infectious disease or symptoms that might be indicative of an infection rise above predicted levels within any given period. These data can be aggregated across the healthcare system to provide an early warning system for outbreak detection.

Furthermore, outbreaks of infectious diseases often capture the attention of the public, leading to new ways to study outbreaks. Novel methods for studying outbreaks, such as mapping news reports (http://www.healthmap.org/en/ and shown in Figure 32-3), following search term trends, or tracing changes in medication prescriptions associated with the symptoms,[86,87] may improve our ability to detect outbreaks in real time.

Surveillance approaches are not limited to medical data but instead can use novel datasets to identify and predict where disease outbreaks are or will occur. For example, pharmacy purchases of over-the-counter cold medicines can be monitored to provide an early warning of influenza outbreaks. In Iceland, call detail records were linked with data on influenza-like illness to identify Keflavik International Airport as the source of introduction of the 2009 H1N1 outbreak into the country.[88] Absenteeism data from large companies or school systems also can be used.[89] In Atlanta, school sign-out logs have been shown to give early warning of influenza activity.[90] More recently, machine-learning algorithms have been developed to monitor internet-based resources for outbreak signal detection.[87] The challenge with these methods is that it is often difficult to distinguish signal from noise, particularly when the outbreak is disseminated and no single data source is able to distinguish the outbreak from the background rate. In such instances, false positives and false negatives may be common. Future refinement of such methods to allow for more specific signals may be able to provide faster response times to control outbreaks.

Big data methods and social network data are now being developed and utilized to attempt to identify outbreaks of infectious diseases,[91] and this is particularly useful in areas where infrastructure may be poor. Such big data sources are also being interrogated to provide a better understanding of transmission dynamics themselves to allow for prediction of outbreaks much like weather forecasting, though such methods are in their infancy.[92] Mobile phone data are also allowing for better understanding of the travel and social contact patterns that drive outbreaks.[88,93] With a growing number of data sources being generated that can be analyzed in real time, the increase in attention to big data methods in infectious disease epidemiology is likely to continue. Such approaches are not without their limitations, however, and concerns about bias, model overfitting, and false signals remain[94] and will have to be addressed in much the same way as they are addressed in conventional epidemiologic studies.

Surveillance for infectious diseases can be challenging in areas where limited resources are available to detect cases, especially for diseases that are uncommon. This challenge has impeded polio surveillance, for example, where well-functioning healthcare systems may not exist in the

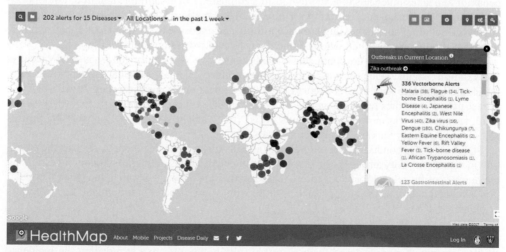

FIGURE 32-3 Healthmap data on reports of Zika outbreaks over a 1-week period (http://www.healthmap.org/en/).

areas where transmission is most likely. In such cases, methods to identify the success of the surveillance system itself can prove to be highly informative in determining whether control efforts are successful. In the case of polio, monitoring rates of acute flaccid paralysis is useful in determining how strong the polio surveillance system is, since acute flaccid paralysis can be associated with polio, but it occurs at a rate of roughly 1 per 100,000 when polio transmission is absent. Thus, in areas where fewer than 1 per 100,000 cases of acute flaccid paralysis are being detected, the surveillance system is likely poor and actions can be taken to attempt to improve the system.[95]

Vaccine Efficacy Studies

Vaccine efficacy studies are designed to evaluate how well vaccination against a specific pathogen reduces the risk of becoming infected with that pathogen. Numerous study designs are used to evaluate vaccine efficacy. While surveillance studies can be used to describe a reduction in rates of disease, such population-level ecologic studies are subject to secular trends and individual-level residual confounding, which makes it difficult to infer causation.[96] For example, analyses of surveillance data can show that the number of pneumococcal meningitis cases is inversely correlated with the proportion of persons vaccinated with pneumococcal conjugate vaccine[96]; however, such data would not include specific information linking individuals with their vaccine status.

Cohort studies and clinical trials provide more convincing evidence of a vaccine effect. Vaccine effectiveness is expressed as [(ARU − ARV)/ARU] × 100% (where ARV = attack rate in the vaccinated and ARU = attack rate in the unvaccinated) or [(1 − RR) × 100%] (where RR can be any estimate of the risk ratio). If the vaccine is protective, the resulting measure is between 0% and 100% and indicates the percent reduction in incidence among those vaccinated. Cohort and randomized clinical trial vaccine efficacy studies are challenging in that they require substantial effort and large populations to estimate the parameter of interest.

Test-negative study designs offer an alternative approach to examining vaccine efficacy.[97-99] In this design, individuals who seek hospital care for a suspected illness are tested for the condition. The approach is a variation of the case-control design in which researchers identify the vaccine status of all those who are suspected to have had the condition. Those who test negative serve as controls for those who test positive. This design has become an increasingly common approach to assess the efficacy of seasonal influenza vaccine, since there is not sufficient time to conduct randomized trials, and vaccine trials at each influenza season would probably be unethical. Instead, patients presenting to a clinic or hospital for influenza-like illness can be tested to confirm patients who have and who do not have influenza.[100] As noted, those who test negative are then used as controls and those who test positive are used as cases, and assessment of seasonal influenza vaccination is done for all participants. Case-control analysis can then be used to generate a measure of vaccine effectiveness. The strength of the design is that it can reduce confounding by care-seeking behavior and takes much less time to yield results compared to a prospective cohort or randomized trial design. The design does require some important assumptions to be met in order to be valid,[101] however, including no confounding by susceptibility and exposure to the infectious agent, assumptions that should be considered when planning a test-negative design study.[102,103]

Vaccine efficacy studies are conducted not only for new vaccines, but also for seasonal vaccines. For example, annual studies are used to assess the effectiveness of seasonal influenza vaccines, which are known to vary in effectiveness from year to year and across subtypes. A meta-analysis of test-negative studies reporting annual influenza vaccine efficacy found that between 2004 and 2015, vaccination was most effective against H1N1 (61%) and least effective against H3N2 viruses (33%), with efficacy varying widely across years.[104]

Studies are also conducted to measure other aspects of vaccine effectiveness, such as the reduction in disease severity among those who become infected. This is often measured by investigating the number of flu-related hospitalizations. These studies are conducted both at the general population level and in targeted subgroups such as those with type 2 diabetes or individuals aged 70 years or older.

Vaccine Safety Studies

While vaccines that are licensed for use are typically highly effective at reducing the incidence of infectious diseases, some vaccines may be associated with rare, serious adverse events that typically cannot be detected in preapproval clinical trials due to the limited study size of the trials for ascertaining the occurrence of these rare events. For example, an association between seasonal influenza vaccination and muscle weakness caused by Guillain-Barre syndrome has been reported to occur in about 1 person per 100,000 of the vaccinated population.[105] Because vaccination is typically done in healthy individuals, rare adverse events that are highly publicized may lead to a reduction in vaccine uptake. Thus, it is important to have accurate measures of the risk of these events. In order to identify causal relationships between vaccination and these rare, serious adverse effects, vaccination usually must be given to a very large group of individuals in the general population. Studies to identify increases in rates of these rare events typically require very large sample sizes, tight control of confounding by design and analysis, and attention to other sources of bias to obtain valid and precise effect estimates.

Variants of the case-crossover method, in which individuals who either got the vaccine or experienced the adverse event of concern are compared to themselves at a different time point, have been also employed in such situations. Such methods take advantage of the fact that the risk window for adverse events in relation to vaccination is often short, and therefore, rare outcomes can be studied by using subjects as their own controls. Two such self-controlled designs are the self-controlled case series (SCCS)[106] and the self-controlled risk interval design (SCRI),[106] also called the vaccinee only risk interval (VORI) design.[107] In the SCRI design, person-time at risk for an adverse event can be partitioned into a period shortly after vaccination (a period considered exposed) and periods before or substantially after vaccination (a period considered unexposed). By comparing periods considered to be exposed and unexposed within the same individuals, control of time-fixed confounding is achieved, strengthening the validity of the effect estimates. The SCCS design uses only those who experienced the adverse event and focuses on whether or not vaccination occurred in close proximity to the adverse event. People experiencing the adverse event have their person-time portioned into exposed and unexposed person-time (in relation to vaccination). Such designs are important to consider for vaccine adverse-event surveillance because they can be conducted in large, existing datasets like health insurance databases and can control confounding by factors that do not change over time because they use the same persons for the exposed and unexposed groups. However, while time-fixed confounding is controlled by design, time-varying confounding is not, and methods for time-varying confounding control should be implemented if it is suspected.

An example of this approach was used in the study of rotavirus vaccine, a vaccine that was shown to be effective in reducing the incidence of a common cause of diarrheal disease, particularly among children. In 2014, a VORI design showed a small increase in the absolute risk of intussusception, a severe intestinal condition in which the intestine folds in on itself, in the first 21 days after vaccination, compared to 22 to 42 days after vaccination (risk difference of 1.5 cases per 100,000 recipients of at least one dose, 95% CI: 0.2-3.2).[45] Although this approach had somewhat lower power than an equivalent cohort study, it had the benefit of strong control of confounding for time invariant factors, which is crucial in cases where the outcome is rare and the anticipated effects are small.

Community-Level Intervention Studies

For some diseases and public health measures, intervening at the community level may have a larger impact than intervening at the individual level. This is particularly true for infectious diseases where community behavioral modification is more likely to have an impact. For example, research has shown that providing bed nets at the community level has a greater impact on reducing malaria incidence than providing them to individuals. If a large proportion of a community at risk for malaria uses bed nets, even those who do not use them may accrue benefits. This community protection can occur if bed nets lead to an overall reduction in exposure to mosquitoes carrying the malaria parasite in the area, which ultimately would impact the community's immunity, not just those who used the bed nets. In the case of malaria, it has been estimated that a very large proportion of the population would actually need to be using bed nets for such a community benefit to occur,[108] but for other infectious diseases, herd immunity (discussed in detail in the section on modeling) can convey an important component of the protection obtained from a public health intervention.

Mass drug administration (MDA) is a community-level approach used to provide chemotherapy to an entire population or selected high-risk groups within a community to treat a specific infection, regardless of whether those individuals are infected. The approach is designed to reduce the community-level burden of infection to a threshold that is so low that the disease cannot spread effectively in the community. This approach is used for multiple NTDs, including schistosomiasis, onchocerciasis, lymphatic filariasis,[109] and trachoma.[110,111] More recently, use of MDA for malaria control has been tested, with some early short-term success.[112]

In designing studies to evaluate the effectiveness of MDA, factors to consider include determining required coverage rates, identifying which individuals need to be treated, and evaluating what frequency of treatment provides the most effective rate of decline. Trachoma, a chronic ocular infection with *Chlamydia trachomatis*, provides an excellent example of factors that must be considered in determining MDA protocols. The prevalence of infection is highest in children aged 1 to 9 years old, ranging from 5% to 50% in highly endemic countries. Years of repeated infection can lead to the blinding sequelae of the disease, trichiasis, a condition in which in-turned eyelashes rub the eye and can lead to blindness. Women are at increased risk of the long-term sequelae and blindness, but it is unclear whether this is a result of increased exposure to infected children or other factors. The disease is targeted for elimination as public health problem, and the WHO recommends annual provision of azithromycin to entire trachoma-endemic communities until the prevalence of signs of active trachoma is reduced to below 5% in children aged <10 years. To reach this global policy decision, community-level randomized controlled trials were conducted to assess how often to treat (annually, twice annually, etc.[111,113]), who should be treated (only children, the whole community), and what level of coverage (70%, 80%, etc.) is required to reduce disease below elimination thresholds. As some countries faced challenges in reaching the elimination targets after a few rounds of MDA, additional work was conducted to determine whether the treatment policy should be amended. One example of the community-based trials that were conducted to address this question is the Partnership for the Rapid Elimination of Trachoma (PRET).[114] PRET was conducted in three countries with varying levels of endemicity: The Gambia[115] (low endemicity), Niger[110] (moderate endemicity), and Tanzania[116] (high endemicity). Each country investigated different questions related to the frequency of treatment and the population who should be treated. Ultimately, none of the studies demonstrated a substantial benefit in changing from the existing WHO guideline of 80% coverage of the entire community.

Two clinical trials of trachoma MDA conducted in Ethiopia provide an interesting view into the importance of looking at long-term effects of MDA treatments. The first trial investigated the impact on the burden of trachoma infection of treating communities twice annually versus once annually for 2 years. The study showed that biannual treatment was more effective at reducing infection prevalence.[113] However, a longer study conducted by the same group and investigating annual versus biannual treatment over 42 months showed no difference between groups.[111] This finding highlights the importance of considering study duration and critical time points, because MDA treatments are time-consuming and costly. For trachoma, treating annually instead of twice yearly will result in substantial cost-savings over many years with similar disease outcomes.

MDA studies in trachoma also highlight the potential for important ancillary benefits and harms of MDA. In many trachoma MDA studies, community members reported better health through reduced respiratory infections. One study found a lower rate of mortality in children living in communities receiving MDA.[117] This finding led to a multinational study to investigate the potential for reducing mortality in non-trachoma endemic countries by treating all children on an annual basis with a single dose of azithromycin. That study showed a benefit of treating young children, with the majority of the benefit seen in Niger.[118]

When community-level designs are used, they come with trade-offs. For example, randomization of communities may be less likely to lead to exchangeable populations than individual randomization, particularly when few communities are randomized. In addition, statistical adjustments to variance estimates must be made to account for the clustering of information that occurs when individuals within a cluster are more similar with respect to their outcomes than those between clusters. Such adjustments may reduce the precision of estimates and as such, cluster randomized trials often require larger sample sizes than individually randomized trials. Still, when the intervention is logically delivered at a community level and when benefits to those not receiving the intervention are expected to be part of the benefit of the intervention assessed, such clustered approaches should be considered. When they are used, statistical models like generalized estimating equations can be used to account for the statistical clustering by inflating standard errors and resulting confidence intervals to have appropriate coverage properties.

Rapid Assessment Studies

In some settings, highly sophisticated epidemiologic studies using the approaches described above are not necessary to answer the most pertinent epidemiologic questions. Often, communities simply need to determine whether or not a particular disease is an important public health problem. This knowledge allows the community to begin planning resource allocation to make key services available to reduce transmission or treat the condition. Rapid assessment study designs allow for quick identification of the presence of a disease, at a significantly reduced cost. This allows for prioritizing affected regions, identifying high-risk groups within a specific geographic area, and developing targeted interventions to help those in need.[119]

Rapid assessments differ from many epidemiologic study designs in that they typically have simplified sampling strategies, are of short duration, have easy to use protocols that can easily be followed by local personnel, and employ straight forward analytic methods. Multiple approaches to sampling for rapid assessments have been described. Some of the earliest rapid assessments were conducted to determine immunization coverage. In those rapid assessments, a sampling approach developed for the WHO's Expanded Program on Immunization (EPI) (and therefore called EPI sampling) was used. This involves using census data to define clusters and then selecting a random sample of clusters for evaluation. Within each cluster, the interviewer selects a random starting household, and on arriving at that household, spins a bottle. The interviewer travels along the path from that household in the direction the bottle is facing to reach the next household. However, this "random walk" approach is vulnerable to biases, given that it is easy for the interviewer to preferentially select an easy path to follow, and even if the methodology is strictly followed, the approach may under-sample those living in more remote areas. Additionally, in low-resource areas where census estimates often are outdated and do not represent the current population, such sampling methods may not accurately depict the population. As a result, newer sampling methods, including compact segment sampling, have been developed. In compact segment sampling, geographic clusters are selected with probability of selection proportional to the size of the cluster. Clusters are then mapped to identify households and divide them into subgroups of equal size. A random set of subgroups is then selected and all individuals living within the subgroup are examined or interviewed.

Lot Quality Assurance Sampling Surveys

Rapid assessments are commonly used to establish treatment programs for NTDs, including trachoma and onchocerciasis. For both diseases, rapid assessments have been used to identify target areas for initiating treatment interventions to reach elimination targets. Once elimination programs are established, however, the use of another approach, lot quality assurance sampling surveys, is often used to assess the impact of treatment coverage on disease burden. The approach was originally developed to assess manufacturing outputs, in which the quality assessor would sample a specific number (N) of the item from a batch, with a predetermined cutoff for poor quality, X. If the assessor reached X defective items, the batch ("Lot") was deemed defective. However, if the inspector reached the target sample size N without finding a defective one, then the batch was considered acceptable. Applying this approach to public health problems is relatively straightforward. The assessor takes a small, random sample of a community to determine whether there is a reasonable likelihood that the number of individuals with the condition in a population is above a certain threshold. This estimate is useful for determining whether specific interventions need to be continued. For example, as we noted earlier, with many NTDs, annual MDA is used to reduce the burden of infection within the community. MDA must continue until the community reaches and maintains a defined elimination threshold (such as the 5% active disease target for trachoma, described above). Lot quality assessment surveys allow for a relatively low-cost approach to making an initial assessment of whether the threshold has been reached. If the lot quality assessment suggests that the threshold has not been reached, the community continues MDA. If it indicates that the threshold has been reached, more expensive, methodologically rigorous surveys are undertaken to determine a more accurate and precise measure of the level of disease in the community.

Lot quality sampling can also be used to assess whether planned intervention coverage has been reached. This approach is effective for monitoring vaccine delivery. In this setting, supervisors divide the vaccine target area into segments. They randomly select and visit segments, where they interview individuals who should have been vaccinated. Once they reach either a specified number of "no" responses or the target sample size, they determine whether the planned vaccination occurred at the planned level.[120]

Analytic Methods for Infectious Diseases

Models for Infectious Diseases

Because infectious diseases require both a susceptible host and a chain of transmission from one susceptible host to another (or from a vector to a host), the parameters we previously used to described infectious disease (such as the attack rate and secondary attack rate) can be summarized in models that allow prediction of how an infectious disease will transmit through a population. Such models are built to reflect the characteristics of the disease itself (infectiousness, pathogenicity, etc.) and also the ways that hosts interact with each other in the population of interest and with their environment. Mathematical models have been developed for many infectious diseases to describe the transmission dynamics within a population, predict where and how the infection will spread, and model the potential impact of efforts to control the infection. These models blend the evidence from traditional epidemiologic study designs, such as randomized trials and cohort studies, with assumptions about the population, the environment, and the pathogen to forecast future events.

Depending on the question being asked, the models can either be deterministic or stochastic. Deterministic compartmental models can be described using a series of differential equations. Stochastic models comprise either individual or agent-based modeling, or population-based models that simulate the number of events that will occur among a population of individuals. While a detailed description is beyond the scope of this text, we refer readers to the work of Kermack and McKendrick,[121] to Anderson and May's[122] textbook *Infectious Disease of Humans,* as well as to an introduction to the field in the textbook *Infectious Disease Epidemiology* by Nelson and Williams.[20]

Many modes of transmission dynamics can be captured using compartmental models. The term *compartmental model* refers to the fact that within such models, analysts place hosts into compartments that describe their current state in relation to the disease transmission process.[123] We can also model the rate at which hosts move between compartments, taking into account the population dynamics (interactions between hosts) and factors related to the host itself. Such models are then summarized using a series of equations that describe how hosts move between compartments over time. Modeling the dynamics of transmission allows a prediction of how an infectious disease will transmit within a fully susceptible population and allows for modeling the impact of a potential intervention. When combined with cost information, such models can aid public health decision-making.

The simplest of these models describes the different states that a person can be in with respect to many infectious diseases and categorizes hosts into one of three states, labeled S, I, and R (which leads to them being called *SIR models*). In such a model, S refers to a susceptible host, I refers to an infectious (or infected) host, and R refers to a recovered host. This model might describe measles, for which a person starts in the susceptible compartment at birth and can remain there if they are never infected and are never vaccinated. Hosts move to the infectious compartment once they become infected. Finally, they recover from the illness and develop immunity to future measles infection, in which case they are no longer susceptible or infectious. Arrows between each compartment define the ways (*i.e.*, directions) that people can move between the compartments, as well as the ways they can enter the population or be permanently removed from the population (*e.g.*, through birth and through death either related to the illness itself or independent of the infection, and possibly through migration into or out of the population). Other examples of diseases that follow an SIR model are vaccine preventable diseases like mumps and rubella. The key feature of these infectious agents is that once a person has been infected and recovered, they are no longer susceptible and do not return to the S compartment.

Finally, we can parameterize the arrows between compartments with information that describes the probability that any host within a compartment moves to another compartment within a defined time period. These parameters specify the rates at which hosts move in and out of each compartment and relate to the infectious agent, the host, and population dynamics. The parameters will describe the infectious agent (*e.g.*, how effective the pathogen is at colonizing and infecting susceptible hosts), the interaction between the host and the environment (*e.g.*, contact with other hosts, contact with vectors, etc.), and the host (*e.g.*, immune function and resistance to the pathogen). Thus, the probability of a contact being infectious and the probability of transmission occurring per contact, determine the rate at which hosts move from the S compartment to the I compartment. Host factors, which include how quickly those who are infected become noninfectious, govern movement from the I compartment to the R compartment. Population factors also determine how quickly susceptibles are replaced (as a function of the birth rate) and movement out of each of the compartments (as a function of age specific mortality rates and potentially disease specific mortality). The dynamics of the movement of the infectious agent through the population and the occurrence of clinical disease will be a function of the rate at which hosts move from one compartment to the next.

Modeling the dynamics of infectious diseases within a population can lead to important insights into transmission patterns, as shown in a very simple SIR model in Figure 32-4. The model allows susceptible hosts to become infected as a function of the contact rate between hosts and the probability of transmission per contact. Movement from S to I is a function of the size of the population in each stage of the model (S, I, and R) along with the contact rate and probability of transmission per contact. This dynamic process is typically referred to as the "force of infection" or λ. Infectious hosts move to the recovered compartment as a function of the recovery rate, defined as the inverse of the average period of infectiousness. The model can be summarized with a series of simple differential equations that define the number of subjects in each compartment at any time t. Assuming a closed population with no births, deaths, and in or out migration, these equations are as follows:

$$\frac{dS}{dt} = \frac{-cpSI}{N}$$

$$\frac{dI}{dt} = \frac{cpSI}{N} - rI$$

$$\frac{dR}{dt} = rI$$

where S, I, and R are the number of susceptible, infected, and recovered hosts, N is the total population size (S + I + R), c is the contact rate, p is the probability of transmission per contact, and r is the rate of recovery. The parameter $c*p$ is often summarized as β. The average duration of infectiousness can be summarized as $1/r$.

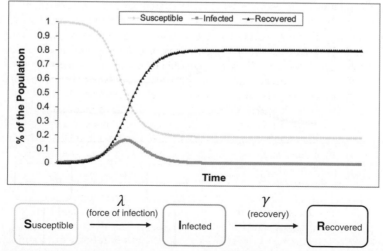

FIGURE 32-4 A simple SIR model of disease transmission in a closed population.

The model assumes we start with a completely susceptible population and one infected person and the implications are plotted in Figure 32-4. Such a model is a simplification of the reality for many infectious diseases, and the values used for c, p, and r are not meant to replicate any specific or even realistic disease or population but rather to show a general pattern. What we learn from this simple model is still important. We see that epidemics tend to follow a similar pattern. When a new infectious host enters a susceptible population, the rate of infection begins to increase rapidly. How quickly the infected proportion of the population increases is a function of the contact rate, the probability of transmission per contact, the proportion of the population infected, and how quickly infected hosts are removed from the I compartment through recovery (again assuming a closed population with no births or deaths and no migration). The infected proportion begins to level off and decline at some point without infecting everyone in the population because the number of susceptibles left in the population declines to a point that transmission cannot be sustained. Note this model is deterministic and does not account for the stochastic nature of transmission.

Without making any further assumptions about replacement of susceptibles (*e.g.*, through birth or in-migration), the infection will eventually stop as the average number of new people being infected by each person infected falls below 1 (a concept known as the reproductive rate, discussed below). In reality, replacement of susceptibles tends to occur at least through birth leading to a set point where the proportion of the population that is infected remains stable over time, as shown in Figure 32-5.

Compartmental models have been helpful in understanding the potential of various interventions to reduce HIV transmission and have been particularly influential in global HIV policy. When first rolled out globally, HIV treatment was reserved for those with compromised immune systems, defined by some value of their CD4 count. For example, initially when large-scale access to HIV treatment became available in sub-Saharan Africa (around 2004), only those with a CD4 count <200 cells/mm^3 (or those with some condition indicating severe illness) were offered treatment. This threshold was slowly increased over time (to 350 cells/mm^3 then to 500 cells/mm^3). More recently, a test-and-treat intervention was proposed, in which providers would test the entire population for HIV routinely (*e.g.*, yearly) and then would treat everyone found to be infected, regardless of their CD4 count. Under the assumption that those who take and adhere to HIV treatment are highly unlikely to transmit the virus to uninfected partners, models—like that shown in Figure 32-6 —were used to predict that such an approach could lead to dramatic reductions in HIV incidence (as shown in Figure 32-7).[124] The model contains only S and I compartments (plus a D compartment, denoting AIDS-related deaths, reported separate from μ which is the background mortality),

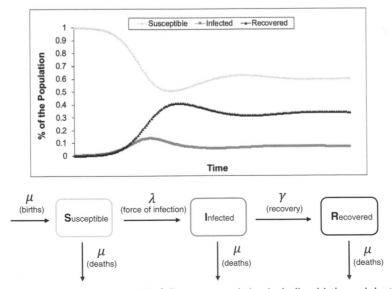

FIGURE 32-5 A simple SIR model of disease transmission including births and deaths.

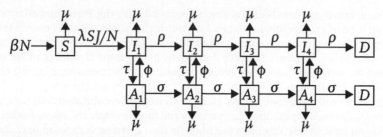

FIGURE 32-6 SIR model to describe the transmission dynamics of HIV in South Africa by Granich et al. Greek letters represent the different parameters by which people move from one compartment to another. (From Granich RM, Gilks CF, Dye C, De Cock KM, Williams BG. Universal voluntary HIV testing with immediate antiretroviral therapy as a strategy for elimination of HIV transmission: a mathematical model. *Lancet*. 2009;373:48-57.)

as currently there is no cure for HIV that would lead to a recovered state. The model also includes compartments denoted as A to represent those taking HIV treatment (antiretroviral therapy) and the reduction in infectiousness associated with treatment. The A compartments are essential in this model, as this reduction in infectiousness of people in the A boxes and the large number of people moving from I to A will reduce the overall force of infection (λ), or the rate at which new people will become infected.

While still being only a theoretical finding, this model and other similar ones[125] were given greater credibility and renewed interest by the results of the landmark HPTN052 trial, which showed a 97% reduction in HIV transmission from an infected partner if the infected partner began antiretroviral therapy at a higher CD4 count rather than waiting until the CD4 count declined.[63] The trial demonstrated that HIV treatment could be used as a prevention measure, as those taking treatment who suppressed the virus to levels undetectable in the blood almost never transmitted

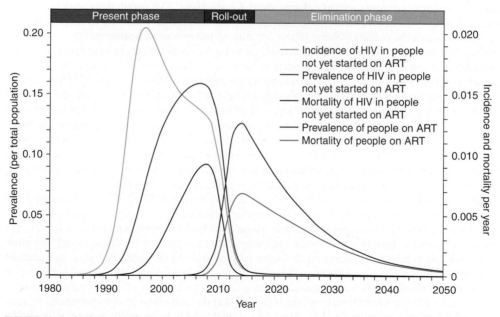

FIGURE 32-7 The impact of a test-and-treat approach to HIV management on incidence, prevalence, and mortality in South Africa using the model in Figure 6 by Granich et al. (From Granich RM, Gilks CF, Dye C, De Cock KM, Williams BG. Universal voluntary HIV testing with immediate antiretroviral therapy as a strategy for elimination of HIV transmission: a mathematical model. *Lancet*. 2009;373:48-57.)

the virus to uninfected partners. Still it is now recommended by the WHO that all those who test positive for HIV be offered treatment, and many countries have adopted this policy. Observational data have shown that as treatment coverage has increased (along with other preventive measures like male circumcision), incidence has been decreasing, giving some credibility to the approach.[126] Unfortunately, recent trials of such an approach have been mixed, demonstrating the challenge of turning predictions into reality.[127-130]

The simple SIR model explained above is not sufficient to describe all infectious diseases, but can be adapted to account for the specific dynamics and modes of transmission of other infectious agents. For example, a disease that has a lag from the time a person is exposed until they become infectious might add a compartment to create an SEIR model (as has been done for Ebola), with E describing an exposed but not yet infectious period.[131] More parameters are then needed to describe the population dynamics and the duration of the exposed period, as the modeler must specify the rate at which a host moves from susceptible to exposed and from exposed to infectious. The length of time spent in these different states will impact the rate at which an infectious agent moves through the population, and the model can be used to make inferences as to which interventions are likely to be most effective for this infectious disease compared to one with a shorter period from exposure to infectiousness. Again, this affects the force of infection and can limit the rate at which susceptible individuals become infected.

SIR and SEIR models were used to model the SARS-CoV-2 outbreak in 2020. Such models were used to estimate the number of deaths expected globally,[56] the impact of various strategies like contact tracing[55] and physical distancing,[56] the impact of second additional waves of transmission,[132] and to predict the number of hospital beds needed for planning purposes.[56] These models were used in real time to attempt to make fast decisions to improve the overall outlook. When this happens, models quickly become out of date because changes in behavior (*e.g.*, lockdowns preventing people from going outside except for essential services) reduce the contact rate, which changes the projections from the model. The further into the future we model, the less confident we should be in the predictions. As such, it is important for such models to present accompanying uncertainty intervals that express the distribution of possible results given our assumptions and the starting conditions.

For other infectious agents, an SI model with persons moving from S to I and then back to S might be more appropriate. An example of this is tuberculosis, where infection does not lead to lifelong immunity, so hosts move back into the S compartment. The populations in these models can also be divided into subpopulations that are important to the transmission dynamics, such as age- and sex-specific cohorts (where contact and mixing patterns as well as mortality rates may be different) or cohorts of high-risk populations that may be central to the spread of the infection (*e.g.*, immunocompromised persons). This concept is demonstrated in Figure 32-6, where the infectious period is divided into multiple compartments which represent different states of infectiousness corresponding to the way the host controls infection (*i.e.*, an early highly-infectious state, a period of low-level infectiousness, and finally a period of higher infectiousness as illness progresses). Models can further be adapted to account for diseases in which one or more intermediate hosts, vectors, or reservoirs are required for transmission to occur (*e.g.*, schistosomiasis in which snails act as the reservoir). For such diseases, interactions between the host and the vector or the host and the environment will have a strong influence on transmission and careful epidemiologic studies are needed to measure these interactions to get accurate predictions from models.

More recently, agent-based models have become popular for modeling infectious diseases[133,134] (see Chapter 31). These models differ from compartmental models in that they explicitly model the actual individuals within the population and interactions between them rather than modeling the expected number of people in each of the compartments at any given time. These models are more computationally intensive (taking much longer to run) and require more complex and detailed computer coding to develop. However, they permit the user to model specific contacts that occur between individuals within a population, allowing them to give a more accurate representation of reality than a compartmental model might if data exist at the individual level to parameterize such a model. They are also more flexible, allowing for stochasticity to be easily accounted for in the probability of contact and the likelihood of transmissions within any contact. The implications of this stochasticity can then be observed through multiple runs of the model and looking at the average of these runs as well as the distribution of outcomes.

Insights From Infectious Disease Models

Infectious disease models can be used to understand what to expect when a host enters a completely susceptible population or what will happen in a population that already has ongoing transmission. We can summarize the transmission dynamics for an infectious agent using the parameter R_0, the basic reproductive number. R_0 is defined as the average number of new infections created by a single infected host when entering a completely susceptible population. The higher the value of R_0, the harder it is to intervene to stop transmission of the infectious agent as the number of secondary cases is high. For example, measles has been estimated to have an R_0 value around 12, implying that each case produces about 12 new cases, which makes it hard to interrupt transmission. R_0 relates back to our model above, as it can be estimated as β/r. A pathogen like polio has an R_0 value of approximately 5, making it relatively easier to interrupt transmission.[122] As an infectious disease is transmitted through a population, the average number of new cases created by each infected case before ceasing to be infectious decreases. This pattern occurs because susceptible hosts are removed from the population, leaving fewer susceptible people for each new infectious case to contact and infect. We can summarize the average number of new infections created by each infectious host at any point in time with the parameter $R(t)$, the effective reproduction number at time t. If $R(t)$ falls below 1, sustained transmission will eventually stop, because fewer new infections are created than are removed from the infectious population. As more susceptibles are introduced into the population (*e.g.*, through birth, loss of immunity, in-migration), $R(t)$ may increase and transmission may begin again. The goal of infectious disease control programs is to push $R(t)$ below 1, in order to end transmission by intervening on one of the parameters that determines movement between compartments. For example, reducing the contact rate (through isolation of infectious hosts) and reducing the infectiousness (through treatment) are approaches to slowing or stopping movement from the S to the I compartment.

Such models can also help identify which of multiple possible interventions might have the biggest impact and how intense the intervention needs to be to be effective. For example, vaccination programs that seek to end transmission take advantage of herd immunity, the idea that with high coverage, vaccination has the potential to protect not just the individual vaccinated, but also those not vaccinated, by reducing their exposure to the infectious agent. In such cases, if vaccine coverage is high, the chances of any susceptible, unvaccinated person encountering an infectious person is low, and even if they are infected, the chances they pass on the infection to someone else is also low, reducing the chance of sustained onward chains of transmission.

Herd immunity is a critical component of any vaccine strategy as it is difficult to vaccinate 100% of the population both for practical reasons (it can be hard to reach everyone in the population with vaccines and some may refuse vaccination) and for medical reasons (some members of the population may have contraindications to vaccination, for example, those who are immunosuppressed and very young infants cannot be vaccinated). Because herd immunity can protect some of those unvaccinated, the proportion of the population needed to end transmission is not 100%, but rather a function of R_0. When a vaccine exists for a disease, the approximate proportion of the population that needs to be effectively vaccinated (*i.e.*, immune) to stop transmission is given by the formula $1 - (1/R_0)$. This implies that those pathogens that have higher R_0 values require more of the population to be vaccinated in order to end transmission than those with lower R_0 values. For a highly infectious pathogen with an R_0 of 12 (*e.g.*, measles), roughly 92% of the population (1-1/12) would need to be vaccinated (assuming perfect immunity following vaccination). In practice, a greater percentage would have to be vaccinated to achieve herd immunity given the fact that vaccines do not elicit an immune response 100% of the time. Polio, with an R_0 of around 5, would only require 80% of the population be vaccinated to end transmission. Figure 32-8 shows the relationship between R_0 and the proportion of the population that needs to be vaccinated for $R(t)$ to drop to 1. Such calculations assume a random mixing pattern within a population, such that any person is equally likely to encounter any other. This assumption is not likely realistic in many cases, because those who are unvaccinated may be more likely to be in contact with other unvaccinated people since they may, for example, share similar beliefs about vaccination. As such, the actual proportion of the population that needs to be vaccinated may be different from what is estimated from the simple model above.

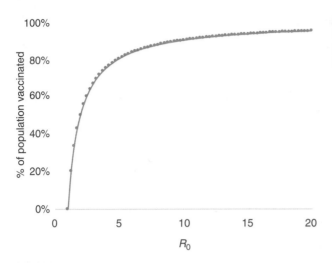

FIGURE 32-8 Relationship between R_0 and the proportion of the population needed to be vaccinated to drive *R(t)* below 1.

Transmission models can also alert us to potential problems with a proposed intervention strategy. For example, while vaccination programs generally reduce morbidity and mortality associated with the infection, they can have unintended consequences. As vaccination coverage increases for illnesses that commonly occur in unvaccinated populations in childhood, transmission of those diseases will be reduced because there are fewer susceptible hosts. While this means that fewer people will become infected, it also means that unless transmission is ended, the average age at which a susceptible host encounters an infectious person will go up, because there are fewer susceptible young people. While in many cases this creates little problem, some infections have greater consequences in adults than in children. Rubella, typically a childhood infection in unvaccinated populations, has a low rate of severe illness.[59] However, if rubella is passed from a mother to a child in utero, it can lead to congenital rubella syndrome in the offspring, a condition that can include deafness, eye abnormalities, and heart disease. If vaccination at intermediate levels of coverage does not end transmission but drives up the average age at infection, the population will experience fewer cases of rubella overall but an increase in the average age at infection. This will lead to more pregnant women being infected and more cases of congenital rubella syndrome. Thus, programs where vaccine coverage is not expected to be high may choose not to vaccinate for rubella or may choose to focus vaccination on women of childbearing age to reduce the risk of severe consequences.

CHALLENGES FOR STUDYING INFECTIOUS DISEASES

Confounding

Infectious disease epidemiology is subject to many of the same challenges as other fields of epidemiology, including confounding and effect measure modification. As described in Chapters 5 and 12, confounding variables influence both the exposure and the outcome variables and may lead to inaccurate interpretation of study results. An excellent example of unanticipated confounding is described in a trial investigating the impact of mass drug administration on the community burden of trachoma. In all but one village, MDA reduced the prevalence of trachoma. In the remaining community, the prevalence spiked following one of the treatments. Upon further investigation, the study team discovered that most of the members of the village had traveled to a village in an adjacent country for a religious celebration. Trachoma is a disease that is spread person-to-person, and the risk of infection increases when uninfected individuals stay in close quarters with infected individuals. In this study, travel resulting in exposure to an untreated community confounded the relationship between treatment and trachoma prevalence.[135] This study highlights the importance of fully examining study results and investigating when results seem improbable (*e.g.*, why would treatment increase the prevalence of disease?).

Sampling Issues—Need for Different Approaches Internationally

Many of the world's most burdensome infectious diseases are concentrated in low-income countries. In high-income settings, researchers have access to most if not all of the tools they need to produce reasonably accurate study results. Most high-income countries have detailed, updated census data readily available to provide risk and rate denominators, as well as technology that can be used to facilitate sample selection and random sampling. For example, telephone surveys can be conducted to determine public opinion with a 2 to 3% confidence interval on the accuracy of results. These surveys use computer-based algorithms to ensure that the sample population is representative of the target population with regard to age, gender, and race distribution. Keeping track of multiple characteristics of a sampled population in a low-income country is very challenging, making complex sampling strategies infeasible. In these settings, it is critical to consider the most important study aspects and to focus on those. This often will require simpler sampling schemes, such as the lot quality assurance methods described above. However, in simplifying the study design, the researchers must ensure that they do not compromise the quality of the research that they are conducting. Further, they must be mindful of the available resources and design the study that best fits the country's needs.

Symptom-Based Diagnosis Versus Laboratory-Based Diagnosis

Obtaining valid estimates of the effect of exposures on infectious disease or the effects of infectious disease on outcomes (such as the effect of herpes simplex virus on dementia) can be complicated by the fact that it can be difficult to diagnose many infectious diseases, and new laboratory methods are often needed to detect them with reasonable sensitivity and specificity. Famously, in the beginning of the HIV/AIDS epidemic, the causative agent could not be identified because there was no way to detect the virus, and such methods had to be developed before a reliable test for the virus could be created. Early tests for HIV relied on the detection of antibodies to the HIV virus, but these were complicated by the fact that antibodies did not develop immediately after infection, leaving a period when infection could be missed. Polymerase chain reaction, which detects the actual virus rather than the host's response to the virus, is now commonly used to detect the virus and is a much more accurate way to detect disease. Thus, when novel pathogens appear, it can take time for the methods to catch up to the needs of both the public health and research communities.

For infectious diseases that are typically mild among the majority of the infected, such as respiratory diseases like rhinovirus and influenza, laboratory tests typically are only used to diagnose severe cases, such as when someone is hospitalized. Otherwise, clinical diagnoses are often made based on signs and symptoms and can easily be misclassified. Thus, epidemiologic research relying on clinical datasets often identify only the most severe cases, making it difficult for valid conclusions to be drawn about the role of various exposures in facilitating transmission. Even in cases where prospective cohorts are specifically developed to study infectious diseases, tests for some infections are poor. This can be due to limitations in the test, as happens with Lyme disease, or because the infection can be cleared by the host making the infection more difficult to detect. In such cases, epidemiologists will often develop a working clinical case definition in which those suspected of having the illness are classified as *suspected, probable,* or *confirmed* cases based on what information is available. Those with few of the symptoms of the disease would be considered suspected cases, those with symptoms and some diagnostic criteria would be considered as probable cases, and those with laboratory confirmation would be considered as confirmed cases.

One striking example of the impact that misclassification of infectious diseases can have is in the detection of the causal relationship between human papillomavirus (HPV) and the development of cervical cancer. As the development of better and more accurate methods to detect HPV became available, the odds ratios relating HPV to cervical cancer increased from roughly 2.0 in the mid 1980s to over 500 in the early 2000s (Figure 32-9).[136] This change demonstrates the danger in relying on the adage that nondifferential misclassification biases toward the null, therefore estimates of effect generated from data with nondifferential exposure misclassification will be conservative. Even ignoring the many exceptions to this rule (some of which are discussed

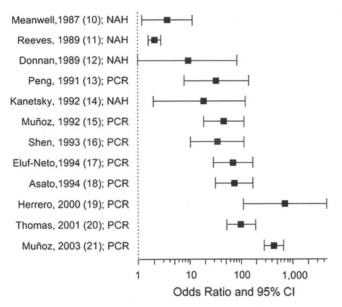

FIGURE 32-9 Increasing strength of the odds ratio relating human papillomavirus (HPV) to cervical cancer as better methods were developed to detect HPV. (From Franco EL, Tota J. Invited commentary: human papillomavirus infection and risk of cervical precancer—using the right methods to answer the right questions. *Am J Epidemiol.* 2010;171:164-168.)

in Chapter 14) and the fact that the definition of "conservative" is unclear in this case, what matters is not only the expected direction of this bias, but also the magnitude. Given that the role an epidemiologist plays is not only to determine *if* an exposure causes an outcome, but *how much* increase in incidence is occurring due to the exposure, then how much bias toward the null is occurring can change our perception of the results. The difference between an odds ratio of 2 and an odds ratio of 500 could be the difference between increased concern that requires action and a public health emergency that requires immediate attention and marshalling of resources.[137]

In cases where the infection is the outcome, it can still be difficult to accurately measure exposures. These exposures often rely on recall, such as what someone ate (in an outbreak investigation) or exposure to environmental factors that can be hard to identify (such as exposure to areas where vectors like ticks might be present). In the case of outbreaks, effect sizes are often so high as to be forgiving of exposure misclassification. In foodborne outbreaks, strong odds ratios relating an exposure to a particular food can often still be seen even in the presence of a reasonable amount of nondifferential misclassified recall of the food of interest. One has to be careful about the type of misclassification, however, as foodborne outbreaks often rely on recall and those who become sick may be more likely to remember or report what they ate than those who did not get sick. Such recall bias, a form of differential exposure misclassification, can sometimes make foods appear to be associated with the pathogen even if they arc not causally related. Outside of outbreak situations, the effects of exposures on outcomes might be far smaller, allowing nondifferential exposure misclassification to obscure true causes.

Difficulty in Patient Tracking and Contact in Low-Income Countries

As with any field of study, adequate sampling of the population is critical for calculating rates of disease, and in longitudinal studies, high follow-up rates also are needed to achieve valid estimates of disease occurrence. In areas where community infrastructure is limited, identifying and tracking patients can be quite challenging. This is particularly true in rural areas of low-income countries where some families may not own a mobile phone and traditional addresses are not used, in part because roads may not exist.

To overcome these issues, population-based studies often begin by conducting a census of each village involved in the study. In recent years, global positioning system (GPS) data have become popular for pinpointing the location of individuals[138-140] during the census. These data facilitate mapping that can be used both for planning intervention strategies and to return to the same location for follow-up visits. As an added benefit, GPS data are now commonly used to plot the burden of disease using programs like ArcGIS. These plots allow for a visual display that can be used to identify pockets of disease and, in some cases, the probable source of infection.[141] As use of GPS data expands, so do the applications of these data. For example, friction maps are now available to characterize how difficult it is to travel between two places. These maps rely on satellite imagery to determine the terrain and road infrastructure.[142] They then use complex algorithms to estimate the travel time between the two points. Overlaying these data with existing data from other sources can be used to address a wide variety of epidemiologic questions, and such applications are likely to become increasingly common with the increased use of open source software packages such as R.

Independence Assumptions

Studying infectious diseases also poses challenges in that there is not always independence between individuals or clusters in a study, an assumption made by many statistical models and, therefore, necessary for valid inference.[143] With infectious diseases, treating one person may prevent infection in another, and statistical models need to account for this. For some noninfectious conditions, this may not be the case, such that treating one person has no effect on others and standard methods would be valid. However, while it is often asserted that infectious diseases are more likely to suffer from this problem of violation of the independence assumption than other disciplines within epidemiology, there is mounting evidence for social transmission of exposures (*e.g.*, exercise, diet, behaviors, etc.) and noninfectious conditions and as such, other conditions also need to tackle this problem.[144] Infectious diseases, which have had to account for herd immunity for some time, were forced to confront this problem early, such that it is seen as critical for the field, while others may only now be wrestling with this problem and may benefit from the experience of infectious disease epidemiology.

Other Challenges

Infectious disease epidemiologists also face challenges in how to study interventions to reduce transmission. As the mode of transmission for some infectious agents involves intermediate hosts, the vector might be a better target for intervention than humans and yet the effect still best measured in humans (*e.g.*, reducing the risk for schistosomiasis by reducing the population of snails). Surveillance for such diseases can also involve sampling the vector rather than humans, as is done when mosquitos are sampled and evaluated for carrying pathogens like the arbovirus West Nile virus (a disease that rarely causes serious morbidity) and Eastern Equine Encephalitis virus (a disease which, while uncommon, can lead to encephalitis associated with a roughly 33% mortality among those infected).[145]

Infections as a Cause of Chronic Disease

Our understanding of the overlap in and relationship between infectious and chronic diseases has, in recent decades, evolved substantially. In addition to our improved understanding of the clinical effects of infectious diseases, we have begun to understand the effects that viruses and bacteria can have in both causing and exacerbating the effects of chronic diseases. We have also begun to understand the role that chronic conditions have in increasing susceptibility to and exacerbating the effects of infectious diseases. In addition, medications to treat infectious diseases, especially those that need to be taken long term, can cause chronic conditions such as metabolic syndrome, hypertension, lipodystrophy, and cancers. AIDS, a condition with an infectious disease causal agent (*i.e.*, the HIV virus) acts like a chronic disease requiring lifelong antiretroviral treatment that, if effectively managed, can turn a disease that was once a death sentence into a chronic condition with a near standard life expectancy.[146] Treatment for HIV can be associated with increased risk of hypercholesterolemia and metabolic conditions. The discovery that human papilloma virus was the major cause of cervical cancer has demonstrated the role that viruses can play in causing cancer. Since then it has been discovered that HPV infection is related to increased risk of multiple cancers, and Hepatitis B and C, Epstein-Barr, human herpes virus 8, and human T-lymphotropic virus-1, among others, can lead to various cancers as well. The HIV virus leads to a depletion of the immune system that can protect against cancers, putting those with HIV at increased risk. Treatment for chronic conditions can often be immunosuppressive, acting as a strong risk factor for development of infectious conditions including reactivation or latent tuberculosis.

Infections and the Microbiome

In recent years, science has significantly advanced the understanding of the microbiome and its role in health. The microbiome refers to the broad array of microorganisms that inhabit the human body. Multiple factors influence the biodiversity of an individual's microbiome, including genetics, food consumption, and antibiotic use, among other factors. The balance of microorganisms can play a key role in an individual's susceptibility to infection, with the microbiota playing a key role in regulating colonization of pathogenic organisms. When the balance of microorganisms changes, it can alter the body's immune responses, which ultimately can change the body's ability to fight infection, leading to both chronic conditions like celiac diseases and irritable bowel syndrome and increased susceptibility to infectious conditions like viral pneumonia and HIV.[147] Investigation of the role of the microbiome in preventing infectious disease remains an exciting area of research.

ETHICAL, LEGAL, POLICY, AND SOCIAL ISSUES

Perhaps, one of the biggest ethical and legal issues surrounding infectious diseases stems from the fact that many infectious diseases are most prevalent in low-income countries, making this an obvious place to research interventions to treat these conditions. However, when trials demonstrate the effectiveness, of, say a new drug that is very expensive, it is not clear that patients in settings where the drugs are tested will be able to afford or access such treatments. This problem was common in the early 2000s when the HIV epidemic was at its worst in sub-Saharan Africa but access to treatment was limited. While trials in Africa may have been desirable from the standpoint of having sufficient patients to enroll into studies of new treatments, was it ethical to do so if patients in the region would not be able to immediately access the treatments that might be proven to be effective? And further, would there not be an ethical imperative to ensure that those who were started on effective treatment as part of a trial were provided with the medication for the rest of their lives if effective? These questions were largely resolved when large-scale access to HIV treatment became available in 2004, but it is likely that such questions will resurface as new diseases that threaten people in both low- and high-income counties emerge (for example, in the event of a global Ebola outbreak as vaccine development ramps up[148] or as an effective vaccine is developed for SARS-CoV-2, which, at the time of writing, has yet to be demonstrated.).

Stigma

Another important ethical issue that arises in the study of infectious diseases comes from the fact that many infectious diseases have been and continue to be stigmatized. Leprosy, a condition caused by a bacterial infection that leads to severe disfigurement, has historically been a highly stigmatized disease in which those infected were ostracized from their communities or forced into quarantine. Sexually transmitted diseases such as chlamydia, syphilis, and gonorrhea also have long been stigmatized, which prevents many infected people from wanting to participate in research studies that might associate them with the condition. Issues of stigma go beyond research and impact service delivery for these diseases. For example, the HIV epidemic has caused massive changes in the delivery of health care in low-income settings where, due to the substantial disease burden, HIV is often treated in vertical programs located in standalone HIV clinics, or within primary healthcare settings, but in a separate part of the clinic or on a separate day. Presenting to those care facilities and standing in the HIV queue can easily identify a patient as having a stigmatized disease. While HIV is no longer as stigmatized, stigmatization continues, and disclosure of HIV status can result in physical abuse and loss of social standing. Reports of patients seeking HIV care at clinics far from their homes have been noted since early in the roll-out of treatment worldwide, as patients seek the anonymity of a clinic not in their own community. For research studies, this creates a very strong need to keep patient information confidential, since participating in research studies may make their status more easily identifiable.

It is not only the infectious conditions themselves that lead to stigmatization. In some cases, treatment for those conditions can lead to unintentional disclosure that researchers need to consider when designing studies. For example, some of the earlier medications to treat HIV were associated with redistribution of fat cells around the body (lipodystrophy and lipoatrophy), which could identify a person with the condition. In other instances, patients have noted that simply having to take their HIV treatment so frequently has meant they could not conceal their infection from family members, partners, friends, and coworkers. While disclosure of HIV status to close friends and relatives appears to increase the probability of seeking and staying on treatment, it also puts the infected person at risk for the stigmatizing aspects of the condition, and in some cases at risk for physical and emotional abuse.[149]

It is not only sexually transmitted diseases that face the issue of stigma. Other infectious diseases that are associated with poverty have also been highly stigmatized, such as tuberculosis. Further, conditions that are believed to have causes related to local beliefs about the impacts of a person's behavior or spiritual relationships can also be stigmatized within communities. Infectious conditions that lead to disfigurement like leprosy, trachoma, and lymphatic filariasis (leading to elephantiasis) have long been stigmatized. For any condition researchers are interested in studying, careful protocols are essential for reducing the impact that stigma may have in preventing patients from enrolling in the study.

Fear Associated With Infectious Diseases

Infectious diseases deal with the unknown. When people see dramatic increases in the number of cases of severe and sometimes new diseases, many develop a fear that other people may pose a risk to them. Such fear among susceptible populations often requires urgent political and social action. The 2014 to 2016 Ebola outbreak in Sierra Leone, Liberia, and Guinea led to dramatic responses in countries far away from West Africa and strong concerns over the risk of an outbreak in locations that were likely dramatically different from the true risk. In circumstances like this, research being conducted in infectious diseases can sometimes be under substantial pressure to obtain results quickly and under intense scrutiny and put pressure on relaxation of ethical standards.

Low-Income Versus High-Income Settings

Another challenge faced in infectious disease research has to do with the interaction between researchers from high- and low-income settings. Studies that are conducted by researchers from wealthy institutions must get ethical approval from their home institutions as well as local ethical approval for the work before research begins. In such cases, ethics boards at institutions in high-income countries often lack the local context and understanding of local ethical issues to make appropriate assessments about the study. Practices that may seem unethical in one culture may be deemed essential in others (*e.g.*, the practice of requiring consent of a local chief or elder for people within a community to participate in a research study). The reviews of the local ethics board may be in conflict with that of the international ethics board, and harmonizing the two can be substantial work. It is not always clear where ethics boards can compromise or defer to each other, but open communication and understanding of local customs and norms is essential to facilitating ethical research. Further, as attention shifts from infectious diseases to chronic conditions in low-income countries, it will be critical for researchers focused on chronic conditions to learn the lessons from those working on infectious diseases.

Antivaccination Beliefs

Vaccination is an integral part of infectious disease control. However, misinformation provided at the community level has led to fear of vaccination among some subgroups. Further, while the efficacy of many childhood vaccines has been well established, high vaccine coverage has led to a revision in the risk-benefit calculation for some considering vaccination for themselves or their children for which the risk of rare, but sometimes severe, adverse events related to vaccines is seen as greater than the risk of contracting the disease itself. This is likely to be especially true when vaccine coverage is high and few in the population have experienced or observed the negative consequences of the disease.

Concern over the risks of vaccination can lead some not to vaccinate their children, which ultimately can lead to outbreaks of disease in areas where vaccine coverage is too low to ensure herd immunity.[150,151] Furthering the trend toward reduced vaccine coverage is the scientific fraud that related the measles mumps rubella (MMR) vaccine to a form of autism, as published in the *Lancet* by Dr. Andrew Wakefield in 1998.[152] While not perfectly correlated, after publication of this fraudulent research, rates of MMR vaccination dropped[153] in England and Wales and measles outbreaks increased. In 2010, after an investigation failed to identify many of the cases or corroborate the data used for the original paper, the paper was retracted.[154,155] Yet this paper is seen as a catalyst for the antivaccination movement. As vaccination rates have declined in many areas, outbreaks like the 2015 Disneyland outbreak[156] and many others like it in areas that had not seen measles in decades have become more common.

Ironically, when outbreaks of vaccine preventable diseases occur in areas with high vaccine coverage rates, there are often more cases among the people who have been vaccinated than have not been vaccinated, leading to a general fear that the vaccine is not effective. However, even when a vaccine is highly effective, such a pattern is predictable. Because no vaccine is 100% effective, in highly vaccinated populations like the United States, a small proportion of the vaccinated population will remain at risk even after receiving a full set of vaccine doses. Introducing groups who cannot or choose not to be vaccinated makes it more likely that those who were vaccinated but remained unprotected will encounter someone who is infectious. If an outbreak does occur, there will be more vaccinated but unprotected individuals than completely unvaccinated individuals and, therefore, the number of cases will often be greater among the vaccinated.

To illustrate this phenomenon, imagine a population of 100,000 people in which 95% were vaccinated against a disease with a vaccine that was 95% effective. In this population, 5,000 people would be at risk in the unvaccinated group (5% of 100,000) while 4,750 would be at risk in the vaccinated group (5% of the 95,000 vaccinated) leaving roughly the same number of people at risk in both populations. If an outbreak occurs, we might expect similar numbers of cases in each group. An example of this occurred in a well-cited case of a measles outbreak in Texarkana in 1970.[157] While Texarkana straddled the Texas and Arkansas border, vaccination rates were estimated to be above 99% on the Arkansas side but only around 57% on the Texas side. Because the vaccination rate was so high on the Arkansas side, when an outbreak occurred, almost all the cases in Arkansas were among the vaccinated, leading to concerns among the public that the vaccine was ineffective. When proper epidemiologic studies were done comparing the risks of disease in those vaccinated to those unvaccinated, the vaccine efficacy was estimated to be above 95%. Still, with so many cases occurring among the vaccinated, such an outbreak can lead to a reduced faith in vaccination, which in turn can reduce vaccination rates and lead to new outbreaks. For more on the Texarkana example, see the excellent case study developed by the CDC using data from the outbreak at https://www.cdc.gov/eis/casestudies/Xtexark.711-903.student.pdf.

ANTICIPATED FUTURE DIRECTIONS

Big Data Mining

Epidemiologists' access to large data sets has increased significantly in recent years with healthcare systems having shifted to electronic claims data and medical records. However, many nontraditional sources of data such as pharmacy records, cell phones, social media, wearables, GPS trackers, weather data, and others are already providing a wealth of information for detecting and predicting patterns of disease transmission. These data sources likely will become an increasingly important part of infectious disease epidemiology in the future. Increased data access, increased computing power, and the development of methods for machine learning, natural language processing, artificial intelligence, and complex systems dynamics modeling are already leading to substantial advances in this field and likely will lead to the development of novel analytic and monitoring approaches in the coming years. Furthermore, wearable devices provide new opportunities to track movements of individuals and their interactions with others.

As noted above, the number of large databases that have or are soon to become available for research is likely to lead to dramatic increases in the ability to forecast disease outbreaks. As these methods are developed, they will inevitably have to grapple with the interface between modeling and public health action. As these models become more available, it will be important to link with decision makers to ensure that models that detect outbreaks early in settings where traditional surveillance systems are poor, and that yield actionable modeling results before large outbreaks occur, receive adequate public attention. However, it will be important to balance false-positive signals, where public health resources are mobilized when no outbreak is occurring against missing early outbreak detection in order to ensure that the public does not lose confidence in the approach. Careful consideration of how to deal with these problems will need to be an active area of research as these methods continue to become more popular.

mHealth Initiatives

Mobile phones have become nearly ubiquitous globally. While in very remote villages in low-income countries they are rare, often one or two individuals have a mobile phone. This increased connectivity has had a substantial impact on the way that epidemiologic studies are conducted. Project managers can inform village leaders when their study team will be traveling to the village, thereby increasing the chances that study participants will be available when they arrive. mHealth is the term used to generally describe the use of mobile technology as it is applied for health care. In many settings, mobile phones are used as education tools to teach patients and study participants about health issues. However, their application extends to other activities, like reminding patients to take medications on a regular schedule and to acting as a tool for disease surveillance. Mobile phones are now regularly used to collect study data in remote settings. Their use enables the addition of GPS data to the dataset, which facilitates tracking participants for follow-up, and utilizing the data to create maps that inform the study team about things like the distribution of disease or the distance between health centers. As technology continues to advance, it is likely that mHealth initiatives will continue to expand.

New and Emerging Diseases

Future efforts at infectious disease research will inevitably have to deal with new and emerging infectious diseases. As we discussed in the beginning of this chapter, the 2019 novel coronavirus outbreak has made this all too apparent. Because of the fear that is often associated with conditions that have severe negative health consequences and those with which the public has limited experience, the call for public health action is typically strong. The recent emergence of Zika virus in the western hemisphere has mobilized substantial resources for researching the condition, both to better understand the natural history and to identify effective methods for treatment and prevention. However, with new diseases come new challenges. The novel coronavirus has made us acutely aware that better planning is needed to combat outbreaks before they become pandemics.

As the climate warms, pathogens formerly limited to warmer climates are likely to move into previously temperate regions, increasing disease incidence and providing renewed impetus for research and action. Additionally, as new infectious diseases are identified, new treatments and strategies for control will need to be developed, tested, and implemented. Resistance to treatments (*e.g.*, antibiotic resistance) will further push us to develop novel treatments that need to be evaluated for safety and effectiveness. Just as the identification of AIDS pushed the development of lab methods to detect new viruses that could then be used for other infectious agents, new infectious diseases are likely to push us to develop novel technologies that can be used for both clinical care and research.

CONCLUSIONS

Infectious diseases have had a significant impact on the development of current epidemiologic methods and practices. In particular, early efforts at assessing cause and effect were focused on studying infectious diseases. While a shift in the global burden of disease shows a reduction in infectious diseases and an increase in chronic conditions, infectious diseases continue to have a substantial impact on global morbidity and mortality. Accordingly, epidemiologic research into infectious diseases will need to evolve in the coming decades to deal with the health problems of a changing world, an aging population, and the interaction between infectious diseases and the environment. New study designs and methods to best utilize the vast amounts of data becoming available to predict disease outbreaks are likely to be the focus of the field in coming years. However, tried and true methods for determining the causes of outbreaks, for identifying new treatments and prevention of infectious diseases will continue to be critical to advancing our understating of infectious diseases.

References

1. Hill AB. The environment and disease: association or causation? *Proc R Soc Med*. 1965;58:295-300.
2. Opinel A, Tröhler U, Gluud C, et al. Commentary: the evolution of methods to assess the effects of treatments, illustrated by the development of treatments for diphtheria, 1825-1918. *Int J Epidemiol*. 2013;42:662-676.
3. Hróbjartsson A, Gøtzsche PC, Gluud C. The controlled clinical trial turns 100 years: Fibiger's trial of serum treatment of diphtheria. *Br Med J*. 1998;317:1243-1245.
4. Wang H, Alemu Abajobir A, Hassen Abate K, et al. Global, regional, and national under-5 mortality, adult mortality, age-specific mortality, and life expectancy, 1970-2016: a systematic analysis for the Global Burden of Disease Study 2016. *Lancet*. 2017;390:1084-1150.
5. GBD 2015 Mortality and Causes of Death Collaborators. Global, regional, and national life expectancy, all-cause mortality, and cause-specific mortality for 249 causes of death, 1980-2015: a systematic analysis for the Global Burden of Disease Study 2015. *Lancet*. 2016;388:1459-1544.
6. Venkatramanan S, Lewis B, Chen J, Higdon D, Vullikanti A, Marathe M. Using data-driven agent-based models for forecasting emerging infectious diseases. *Epidemics*. 2018;22:43-49.
7. Luby SP, Agboatwalla M, Feikin DR, et al. Effect of handwashing on child health: a randomised controlled trial. *Lancet*. 2005;366:225-233.
8. Gantz VM, Jasinskiene N, Tatarenkova O, et al. Highly efficient Cas9-mediated gene drive for population modification of the malaria vector mosquito *Anopheles stephensi*. *Proc Natl Acad Sci U S A*. 2015;112:E6736-E6743.
9. Hammond A, Galizi R, Kyrou K, et al. A CRISPR-Cas9 gene drive system targeting female reproduction in the malaria mosquito vector *Anopheles gambiae*. *Nat Biotechnol*. 2016;34:78-83.
10. WHO Ebola Response Team, Aylward B, Barboza P, et al. Ebola virus disease in West Africa—the first 9 months of the epidemic and forward projections. *N Engl J Med*. 2014;371:1481-1495.
11. CDC. *2014 Ebola Outbreak in West Africa - Case Counts | Ebola Hemorrhagic Fever*. CDC; 2015. Available at https://www.cdc.gov/vhf/ebola/history/2014-2016-outbreak/case-counts.html.
12. Verity R, Okell LC, Dorigatti I, et al. Estimates of the severity of coronavirus disease 2019: a model-based analysis. *Lancet Infect Dis*. 2020;20(6):669-677. doi:10.1016/s1473-3099(20)30243-7.
13. United Nations Department of Economic and Social Affairs Population Department. *World Urbanization Prospects*. New York. 2018. Available at https://population.un.org/wup/Publications/Files/WUP2018-KeyFacts.pdf.
14. Connecticut State Department of Health. *Circular Letter #12-32*. Connecticut: Hartford; 1976. Available at https://portal.ct.gov/-/media/Departments-and-Agencies/DPH/dph/infectious_diseases/lyme/1976 circularletterpdf.pdf?la=en.
15. Butterworth MK, Morin CW, Comrie AC. An analysis of the potential impact of climate change on dengue transmission in the Southeastern United States. *Environ Health Perspect*. 2016;125:579-585.
16. Mordecai EA, Cohen JM, Evans MV, et al. Detecting the impact of temperature on transmission of Zika, dengue, and chikungunya using mechanistic models. *PLos Negl Trop Dis*. 2017;11:e0005568.
17. Moore SM, Azman AS, Zaitchik BF, et al. El Niño and the shifting geography of cholera in Africa. *Proc Natl Acad Sci U S A*. 2017;114:4436-4441.
18. Chin C-S, Sorenson J, Harris JB, et al. The origin of the Haitian cholera outbreak strain. *N Engl J Med*. 2011;364:33-42.
19. Peiris JSM, Yuen KY, Osterhaus ADME, Stöhr K. The severe acute respiratory syndrome. *N Engl J Med*. 2003;349:2431-2441.
20. Nelson KE, Williams CM. *Infectious Disease Epidemiology*. 3rd ed. Burlington, MA: Jones & Bartlett Publishers, Inc; 2013.
21. Thomas JC, Weber DJ. *Epidemiologic Methods for the Study of Infectious Diseases*. New York, NY: Oxford University Press; 2001.
22. Giesecke J. *Modern Infectious Disease Epidemiology*. 3rd ed. Boca Raton, FL: CRC Press, Taylor & Francis; 2017.

23. Snow J. *On the Mode of Communication of Cholera*. 2nd ed. London: John Churchill; 1855.

24. Paneth N, Vinten-Johansen P, Brody H, Rip M. A rivalry of foulness: official and unofficial investigations of the London cholera epidemic of 1854. *Am J Public Health*. 1998;88:1545-1553.

25. Brody H, Rip MR, Vinten-Johansen P, Paneth N, Rachman S. Map-making and myth-making in broad Street: the London cholera epidemic, 1854. *Lancet*. 2000;356:64-68.

26. Morabia A. History of the modern epidemiological concept of confounding. *J Epidemiol Community Health*. 2011;65:297-300.

27. Okabe A, Boots B, Sugihara K. *Spatial Tessellations: Concepts and Applications of Voronoi Diagrams*. 2nd ed. Toronto: John Wiley and Sons; 1999.

28. Senechal M. Spatial tessellations: concepts and applications of Voronoi diagrams. *Science*. 1993;260:1170.

29. Hallett C. The attempt to understand puerperal fever in the eighteenth and early nineteenth centuries: the influence of inflammation theory. *Med Hist*. 2005;49:1-28.

30. Loudon I. Ignaz Phillip Semmelweis' studies of death in childbirth. *J R Soc Med*. 2013;106:461-463.

31. La Rochelle P, Julien A-S. How dramatic were the effects of handwashing on maternal mortality observed by Ignaz Semmelweis? *J R Soc Med*. 2013;106:459-460.

32. Pittet D, Boyce JM. Hand hygiene and patient care: pursuing the Semmelweis legacy. *Lancet Infect Dis*. 2001;1:9-20.

33. Vincent J-L. Nosocomial infections in adult intensive-care units. *Lancet*. 2003;361:2068-2077.

34. Sickbert-Bennett EE, DiBiase LM, Willis TMS, Wolak ES, Weber DJ, Rutala WA. Reduction of healthcare-associated infections by exceeding high compliance with hand hygiene practices. *Emerg Infect Dis*. 2016;22:1628-1630.

35. Liu S, Wang M, Wang G, Wu X, Guan W, Ren J. Microbial characteristics of nosocomial infections and their association with the utilization of hand hygiene products: a hospital-wide analysis of 78,344 cases. *Surg Infect (Larchmt)*. 2017;18:676-683.

36. Richardson R. Jenner's cowskin. *Lancet*. 2000;356:1858.

37. Becker QH. George Washington and variolation; Edward Jenner and vaccination. *J Am Med Assoc*. 1986;255:1881.

38. Horton R. Myths in medicine. *Br Med J*. 1995;310:62.

39. Huth E. Quantitative evidence for judgments on the efficacy of inoculation for the prevention of small-pox: England and New England in the 1700s. *J R Soc Med*. 2006;99:262-266.

40. World Health Organization (WHO). *World Malaria Report 2015*. Geneva, Switerland: World Health Organization; 2015.

41. Fischer Walker CL, Perin J, Aryee MJ, Boschi-Pinto C, Black RE. Diarrhea incidence in low- and middle-income countries in 1990 and 2010: a systematic review. *BMC Public Health*. 2012;12:220.

42. Marshall BJ, Armstrong JA, McGechie DB, Glancy RJ. Attempt to fulfil Koch's postulates for pyloric Campylobacter. *Med J Aust*. 1985;142:436-439.

43. Goldberger J. *Goldberger on Pellagra*. Baton Rouge, LA: Louisiana State University Press; 1964.

44. Jones J. *Bad Blood the Tuskegee Syphillis Experiment: A Tragedy of Race and Medicine*. New York, NY: The Free Press; 1981.

45. Yih WK, Lieu TA, Kulldorff M, et al. Intussusception risk after rotavirus vaccination in U.S. Infants. *N Engl J Med*. 2014;370:503-512.

46. Gera T, Shah D, Garner P, Richardson M, Sachdev HS. Integrated management of childhood illness (IMCI) strategy for children under five. *Cochrane Database Syst Rev*. 2016;(6):CD010123.

47. Li Q, Guan X, Wu P, et al. Early transmission dynamics in Wuhan, China, of novel coronavirus-infected pneumonia. *N Engl J Med*. 2020;382:1199-1207.

48. Gaythorpe K, Imai N, Cuomo-dannenburg G, et al. *Symptom Progression of COVID-19*. Imperial College London (11-03-2020). doi:10.25561/77344.

49. Lauer SA, Grantz KH, Bi Q, et al. The incubation period of coronavirus disease 2019 (COVID-19) from publicly reported confirmed cases: estimation and application. *Ann Intern Med*. 2020;172(9):577-582. doi:10.7326/m20-0504.

50. Wei WE, Li Z, Chiew CJ, Yong SE, Toh MP, Lee VJ. Presymptomatic transmission of SARS-CoV-2 — Singapore, January 23–March 16, 2020. *MMWR Morb Mortal Wkly Rep*. 2020;69:411-415. doi:10.15585/mmwr.mm6914e1external icon.

51. van Doremalen N, Bushmaker T, Morris DH, et al. Aerosol and surface stability of SARS-CoV-2 as compared with SARS-CoV-1. *N Engl J Med*. 2020;382(16):1564-1567. doi:10.1056/nejmc2004973.

52. Ng Y, Li Z, Chua YX, et al. Evaluation of the effectiveness of surveillance and containment measures for the first 100 patients with COVID-19 in Singapore—January 2-February 29, 2020. *MMWR Morb Mortal Wkly Rep*. 2020;69:307-311. doi:10.15585/mmwr.mm6911e1external icon.

53. Duan K, Liu B, Li C, et al. Effectiveness of convalescent plasma therapy in severe COVID-19 patients. *Proc Natl Acad Sci U S A*. 2020;117(17):9490-9496. doi:10.1073/pnas.2004168117.

54. Hellewell J, Abbott S, Gimma A, et al. Feasibility of controlling COVID-19 outbreaks by isolation of cases and contacts. *Lancet Glob Heal*. 2020;8:e488-e496.

55. Ferretti L, Wymant C, Kendall M, et al. Quantifying SARS-CoV-2 transmission suggests epidemic control with digital contact tracing. *Science*. 2020;368(6491):eabb6936.

56. Walker PGT, Whittaker C, Watson O, et al. *The Global Impact of COVID-19 and Strategies for Mitigation and Suppression*. Imperial College London.2020. doi:10.25561/77735.

57. Jewell NP, Lewnard JA, Jewell BL. Predictive mathematical models of the COVID-19 pandemic. *J Am Med Assoc*. 2020;323(19):1893-1894. doi:10.1001/jama.2020.6585.

58. Soper GA. The work of a chronic typhoid germ distributor. *J Am Med Assoc*. 1907;48:2019.

59. Centers for Disease Control and Prevention. Rubella virus. In: Hamborsky J, Kroger A, Wolfe S, eds. *Epidemiology and Prevention of Vaccine-Preventable Diseases*. 13th ed. Washington D.C.: Public Health Foundation; 2015.

60. Hamborsky J, Kroger A, Wolfe S, eds. *Centers for Disease Control and Prevention. Epidemiology and Prevention of Vaccine-Preventable Diseases*. 13th ed. Washington, DC: Public Health Foundation; 2015.

61. WHO. *Variant Creutzfeldt-Jakob Disease*. WHO; 2016. Available at https://www.who.int/zoonoses/diseases/variantcjd/en/.

62. Archer BN, Tempia S, White LF, Pagano M, Cohen C. Reproductive number and serial interval of the first wave of influenza A(H1N1)pdm09 virus in South Africa. *PLoS One*. 2012;7:e49482.

63. Cohen MS, Chen YQ, McCauley M, et al. Prevention of HIV-1 infection with early antiretroviral therapy. *N Engl J Med*. 2011;365:493-505.

64. Center for Disease Control and Prevention. *Clinical Evaluation & Disease | Zika Virus | CDC*. CDC. 2016.

65. World Health Organization (WHO). *WHO | Ebola Virus Disease*. WHO; 2017. Available at https://www.who.int/health-topics/ebola#tab=tab_1.

66. Dowdle WR. The principles of disease elimination and eradication. *MMWR Morb Mortal Wkly Rep*. 1999;48:23-27.

67. https://www.cartercenter.org/health/guinea_worm/case-totals.html.

68. Polio Global Eradication Initiative. Polio Now. Available at http://polioeradication.org/polio-today/polio-now/.Accessed January 19, 2020.

69. The Lancet. Guinea worm disease eradication: a moving target. *Lancet*. 2019;393:1261.

70. Centers for Disease Control (CDC). Kaposi's sarcoma and Pneumocystis pneumonia among homosexual men--New York City and California. *MMWR Morb Mortal Wkly Rep*. 1981;30:305-308.

71. Auvert B, Taljaard D, Lagarde E, Sobngwi-Tambekou J, Sitta R, Puren A. Randomized, controlled intervention trial of male circumcision for reduction of HIV infection risk: the ANRS 1265 Trial. *Plos Med*. 2005;2:e298.

72. Gray RH, Kigozi G, Serwadda D, et al. Male circumcision for HIV prevention in men in Rakai, Uganda: a randomised trial. *Lancet*. 2007;369:657-666.

73. Bailey RC, Moses S, Parker CB, et al. Male circumcision for HIV prevention in young men in Kisumu, Kenya: a randomised controlled trial. *Lancet*. 2007;369:643-656.

74. Stocks ME, Ogden S, Haddad D, Addiss DG, McGuire C, Freeman MC. Effect of water, sanitation, and hygiene on the prevention of trachoma: a systematic review and meta-analysis. *Plos Med*. 2014;11:e1001605.

75. West S, Muñoz B, Lynch M, et al. Impact of face-washing on trachoma in Kongwa, Tanzania. *Lancet*. 1995;345:155-158.

76. World Health Organization. *WHO | Disease Outbreaks*. WHO; 2013. Available at https://www.who.int/csr/don/archive/year/2013/en/.

77. Centers for Disease Control and Prevention (CDC). *Outbreak of E. coli Infections Linked to Romaine Lettuce*. 2019. Available at https://www.cdc.gov/ecoli/2018/o157h7-11-18/index.html.

78. Centers for Disease Control. Pneumocystis pneumonia — Los Angeles. *MMWR Morb Mortal Wkly Rep*. 1981;30:250-252.

79. Centers for Disease Control and Prevention (CDC). A cluster of Kaposi's sarcoma and pneumocystis carinii pneumonia among homosexual male residents of Los Angeles and Orange counties, California. *MMWR Morb Mortal Wkly Rep*. 1982;31:305-307.

80. Centers for Disease Control and Prevention (CDC). Acanthamoeba keratitis multiple states, 2005-2007. *MMWR Morb Mortal Wkly Rep*. 2007;56:532-534.

81. Verani JR, Lorick SA, Yoder JS, et al. National outbreak of Acanthamoeba keratitis associated with use of a contact lens solution, United States. *Emerg Infect Dis*. 2009;15:1236-1242.

82. Centers for Disease Control and Prevention. Update: multistate outbreak of Escherichia coli O157:H7 infections from hamburgers—Western United States, 1992-1993. *MMWR Morb Mortal Wkly Rep*. 1993;42:258-263.

83. Henning KJ. Overview of syndromic surveillance: what is syndromic surveillance? *MMWR Morb Mortal Wkly Rep*. 2004;53:1-9.

84. Jernigan JA, Stephens DS, Ashford DA, et al. Bioterrorism-related inhalational anthrax: the first 10 cases reported in the United States. *Emerg Infect Dis.* 2001;7:933-944.

85. Moran GJ, Talan DA. Syndromic surveillance for bioterrorism following the attacks on the world trade center—New York city, 2001. *Ann Emerg Med.* 2003;41:414-418.

86. Johnson AK, Mehta SD. A comparison of internet search trends and sexually transmitted infection rates using google trends. *Sex Transm Dis.* 2014;41:61-63.

87. Brownstein JS, Freifeld CC, Reis BY, Mandl KD. Surveillance sans Frontières: internet-based emerging infectious disease intelligence and the HealthMap project. *PLos Med.* 2008;5:1019-1024.

88. Kishore N, Mitchell R, Lash TL, et al. Flying, phones and flu: anonymized call records suggest that Keflavik International Airport introduced pandemic H1N1 into Iceland in 2009. *Influenza Other Respi Viruses.* 2020;14:37-45.

89. Besculides M, Heffernan R, Mostashari F, Weiss D. Evaluation of school absenteeism data for early outbreak detection, New York City. *BMC Public Health.* 2005;5:105.

90. Weiss Z. Detecting the onset of infectious disease outbreaks using school sign-out logs. *Epidemiology.* 2019;30:e18-e19.

91. Ginsberg J, Mohebbi MH, Patel RS, Brammer L, Smolinski MS, Brilliant L. Detecting influenza epidemics using search engine query data. *Nature.* 2009;457:1012-1014.

92. Moran KR, Fairchild G, Generous N, et al. Epidemic forecasting is messier than weather forecasting: the role of human behavior and internet data streams in epidemic forecast. *J Infect Dis.* 2016;214:S404-S408.

93. Wesolowski A, Buckee CO, Engø-Monsen K, Metcalf CJE. Connecting mobility to infectious diseases: the Promise and limits of mobile phone data. *J Infect Dis.* 2016;214:S414-S420.

94. Bansal S, Chowell G, Simonsen L, Vespignani A, Viboud C. Big data for infectious disease surveillance and modeling. *J Infect Dis.* 2016;214:S375-S379.

95. Global Polio Eradication Initiative. Surveillance Indicators – GPEI. http://polioeradication.org/polio-today/polio-now/surveillance-indicators/. Accessed June 3, 2018.

96. Hsu HE, Shutt KA, Moore MR, et al. Effect of pneumococcal conjugate vaccine on pneumococcal meningitis. *N Engl J Med.* 2009;360:244-256.

97. Broome CV, Facklam RR, Fraser DW. Pneumococcal disease after pneumococcal vaccination. *N Engl J Med.* 1980;303:549-552.

98. Jackson ML, Nelson JC. The test-negative design for estimating influenza vaccine effectiveness. *Vaccine.* 2013;31:2165-2168.

99. Suzuki M, Dhoubhadel BG, Ishifuji T, et al. Serotype-specific effectiveness of 23-valent pneumococcal polysaccharide vaccine against pneumococcal pneumonia in adults aged 65 years or older: a multicentre, prospective, test-negative design study. *Lancet Infect Dis.* 2017;17:313-321.

100. Sullivan SG, Feng S, Cowling BJ. Potential of the test-negative design for measuring influenza vaccine effectiveness: a systematic review. *Expert Rev Vaccin.* 2014;13:1571-1591.

101. Sullivan SG, Tchetgen Tchetgen EJ, Cowling BJ. Theoretical basis of the test-negative study design for assessment of influenza vaccine effectiveness. *Am J Epidemiol.* 2016;184:345-353.

102. Lewnard JA, Tedijanto C, Cowling BJ, Lipsitch M. Measurement of vaccine direct effects under the test-negative design. *Am J Epidemiol.* 2018;187:2686-2697.

103. Feng S, Cowling BJ, Kelly H, Sullivan SG. Estimating influenza vaccine effectiveness with the test-negative design using alternative control groups: a systematic review and meta-analysis. *Am J Epidemiol.* 2018;187:389-397.

104. Belongia EA, Simpson MD, King JP, et al. Variable influenza vaccine effectiveness by subtype: a systematic review and meta-analysis of test-negative design studies. *Lancet Infect Dis.* 2016;16:942-951.

105. National Institutes of Neurological Disorders and Stroke. Guillain-Barré Syndrome Fact Sheet. https://www.ninds.nih.gov/Disorders/Patient-Caregiver-Education/Fact-Sheets/Guillain-Barré-Syndrome-Fact-Sheet. Accessed January 17, 2020.

106. Whitaker HJ, Farrington CP, Spiessens B, Musonda P. Tutorial in Biostatistics: the self-controlled case series method. *Stat Med.* 2006;25:1768-1797.

107. Baker MA, Lieu TA, Li L, et al. A vaccine study design selection framework for the postlicensure rapid immunization safety monitoring program. *Am J Epidemiol.* 2015;181:608-618.

108. Teklehaimanot A, Sachs JD, Curtis C. Malaria control needs mass distribution of insecticidal bednets. *Lancet.* 2007;369:2143-2146.

109. Bockarie MJ, Alexander NDE, Hyun P, et al. Randomised community-based trial of annual single-dose diethylcarbamazine with or without ivermectin against Wuchereria bancrofti infection in human beings and mosquitoes. *Lancet.* 1998;351:162-168.

110. Amza A, Kadri B, Nassirou B, et al. A cluster-randomized trial to assess the efficacy of targeting trachoma treatment to children. *Clin Infect Dis.* 2016;64:ciw810.

111. Gebre T, Ayele B, Zerihun M, et al. Comparison of annual versus twice-yearly mass azithromycin treatment for hyperendemic trachoma in Ethiopia: a cluster-randomised trial. *Lancet.* 2012;379:143-151.

112. von Seidlein L, Peto TJ, Landier J, et al. The impact of targeted malaria elimination with mass drug administrations on falciparum malaria in southeast Asia: a cluster randomised trial. *PLos Med.* 2019;16:e1002745. DOI:10.1371/journal.pmed.1002745.

113. Melese M, Alemayehu W, Lakew T, et al. Comparison of annual and biannual mass antibiotic administration for elimination of infectious trachoma. *J Am Med Assoc.* 2008;299:778-784.

114. Stare D, Harding-Esch E, Munoz B, et al. Design and baseline data of a randomized trial to evaluate coverage and frequency of mass treatment with azithromycin: the partnership for rapid elimination of trachoma (PRET) in Tanzania and the Gambia. *Ophthalmic Epidemiol.* 2011;18:20-29.

115. Harding-Esch EM, Sillah A, Edwards T, et al. Mass treatment with azithromycin for trachoma: when is one round enough? Results from the PRET trial in the Gambia. *PLos Negl Trop Dis.* 2013;7:e2115. doi:10.1371/journal.pntd.0002115.

116. West SK, Bailey R, Munoz B, et al. A randomized trial of two coverage targets for mass treatment with azithromycin for trachoma. *PLos Negl Trop Dis.* 2013;7:e2415. doi:10.1371/journal.pntd.0002415.

117. O'Brien K, Cotter S, Amza A, et al. Childhood mortality after mass distribution of azithromycin: a secondary analysis of the PRET cluster-randomized trial in Niger. *Pediatr Infect Dis J.* 2018;37:1082-1086.

118. Keenan J, Bailey R, West S, et al. Azithromycin to reduce childhood mortality in sub-Saharan Africa. *N Engl J Med.* 2018;378:1583-1592.

119. Marmamula S, Keeffe JE, Rao GN. Rapid assessment methods in eye care: an overview. *Indian J Ophthalmol.* 2012;60:416-422.

120. Olives C, Valadez JJ, Pagano M. Estimation after classification using lot quality assurance sampling: Corrections for curtailed sampling with application to evaluating polio vaccination campaigns. *Trop Med Int Heal.* 2014;19:321-330.

121. Kermack W, McKendrick A. A contribution to the mathematical theory of epidemics. *Proc R Soc Lond Ser A.* 1927;115:700-721.

122. Anderson RM, May RM. *Infectious Diseases of Humans: Dynamics and Control.* New York, NY: Oxford University Press; 1992.

123. Blackwood JC, Childs LM. An introduction to compartmental modeling for the budding infectious disease modeler. *Lett Biomath.* 2018;5:195-221.

124. Granich RM, Gilks CF, Dye C, De Cock KM, Williams BG. Universal voluntary HIV testing with immediate antiretroviral therapy as a strategy for elimination of HIV transmission: a mathematical model. *Lancet.* 2009;373:48-57.

125. Wagner BG, Blower S. Universal access to HIV treatment versus universal 'test and treat': transmission, drug resistance and treatment costs. *PLoS One.* 2012;7:e41212.

126. Grabowski MK, Serwadda DM, Gray RH, et al. HIV prevention efforts and incidence of HIV in Uganda. *N Engl J Med.* 2017;377:2154-2166.

127. Iwuji CC, Orne-Gliemann J, Larmarange J, et al. Universal test and treat and the HIV epidemic in rural South Africa: a phase 4, open-label, community cluster randomised trial. *Lancet HIV.* 2018;5:e116-e125.

128. Havlir DV, Balzer LB, Charlebois ED, et al. HIV testing and treatment with the use of a community health approach in rural Africa. *N Engl J Med.* 2019;381:219-229.

129. Makhema J, Wirth KE, Pretorius Holme M, et al. Universal testing, expanded treatment, and incidence of HIV infection in Botswana. *N Engl J Med.* 2019;381:230-242.

130. Hayes RJ, Donnell D, Floyd S, et al. Effect of universal testing and treatment on HIV incidence - HPTN 071 (PopART). *N Engl J Med.* 2019;381:207-218.

131. Althaus CL. Estimating the reproduction number of Ebola virus (EBOV) during the 2014 outbreak in West Africa. *PLos Curr.* 2014. doi:10.1371/currents.outbreaks.91afb5e0f2.79e7f29e7056095255b288.

132. Kissler SM, Tedijanto C, Goldstein E, Grad YH, Lipsitch M. Projecting the transmission dynamics of SARS-CoV-2 through the postpandemic period. *Science.* 2020;368(6493):860-868.

133. Willem L, Stijven S, Tijskens E, Beutels P, Hens N, Broeckhove J. Optimizing agent-based transmission models for infectious diseases. *BMC Bioinformatics.* 2015;16:183.

134. Willem L, Verelst F, Bilcke J, Hens N, Beutels P. Lessons from a decade of individual-based models for infectious disease transmission: a systematic review (2006-2015). *BMC Infect Dis.* 2017;17:612.

135. Burton MJ, Holland MJ, Makalo P, et al. Re-emergence of Chlamydia trachomatis infection after mass antibiotic treatment of a trachoma-endemic Gambian community: a longitudinal study. *Lancet.* 2005;365:1321-1328.

136. Franco EL, Tota J. Invited commentary: human papillomavirus infection and risk of cervical precancer—using the right methods to answer the right questions. *Am J Epidemiol.* 2010;171:164-168.

137. Tota J, Mahmud SM, Ferenczy A, Coutlée F, Franco EL. Promising strategies for cervical cancer screening in the post-human papillomavirus vaccination era. *Sex Health.* 2010;7:376-382.

138. García GA, Hergott DEB, Phiri WP, et al. Mapping and enumerating houses and households to support malaria control interventions on Bioko Island. *Malar J.* 2019;18:283.

139. Fornace KM, Surendra H, Abidin TR, et al. Use of mobile technology-based participatory mapping approaches to geolocate health facility attendees for disease surveillance in low resource settings. *Int J Health Geogr*. 2018;17:21.

140. Mosomtai G, Evander M, Mundia C, et al. Datasets for mapping pastoralist movement patterns and risk zones of Rift Valley fever occurrence. *Data Br*. 2018;16:762-770.

141. Iravatham CC, Kumar Neela VS, Valluri VL. Identifying and mapping TB hot spots in an urban slum by integrating geographic positioning system and the local postman—a pilot study. *Indian J Tuberc*. 2019;66:203-208.

142. Weiss DJ, Nelson A, Gibson HS, et al. A global map of travel time to cities to assess inequalities in accessibility in 2015. *Nature*. 2018;553:333-336.

143. Benjamin-Chung J, Abedin J, Berger D, et al. Spillover effects on health outcomes in low-and middle-income countries: a systematic review. *Int J Epidemiol*. 2017;46:1251-1276.

144. Buyukkececi Z, Leopold T, van Gaalen R, Engelhardt H. Family, firms, and fertility: a study of social interaction effects. *Demography*. 2020;57(1):243-266. doi:10.1007/s13524-019-00841-y.

145. Eastern Equine Encephalitis | CDC. https://www.cdc.gov/easternequineencephalitis/index.html. Accessed January 19, 2020.

146. Bor J, Herbst AJ, Newell M-L, Bärnighausen T. Increases in adult life expectancy in rural South Africa: valuing the scale-up of HIV treatment. *Science*. 2013;339:961-965.

147. Libertucci J, Young VB. The role of the microbiota in infectious diseases. *Nat Microbiol*. 2019;4:35-45.

148. Kennedy SB, Bolay F, Kieh M, et al. Phase 2 Placebo-controlled trial of two vaccines to prevent Ebola in Liberia. *N Engl J Med*. 2017;377:1438-1447.

149. Murray LK, Semrau K, McCurley E, et al. Barriers to acceptance and adherence of antiretroviral therapy in urban Zambian women: a qualitative study. *AIDS Care*. 2009;21:78-86.

150. Majumder MS, Cohn EL, Mekaru SR, Huston JE, Brownstein JS. Substandard vaccination compliance and the 2015 measles outbreak. *JAMA Pediatr*. 2015;169:494.

151. Halsey NA, Salmon DA. Measles at disneyland, a problem for all ages. *Ann Intern Med*. 2015;162:655-656.

152. Wakefield A, Murch S, Anthony A, et al. Retracted: Ileal-lymphoid-nodular hyperplasia, non-specific colitis, and pervasive developmental disorder in children. *Lancet*. 1998;351:637-641.

153. Public Health England. Completed Primary Courses at Two Years of Age: England and Wales, 1966-1977, England only 1978 onwards. http://webarchive.nationalarchives.gov.uk/20140714111349/http://www.hpa.org.uk/web/HPAweb&HPAwebStandard/HPAweb_C/1195733819251. Accessed January 19, 2020.

154. Deer B. How the case against the MMR vaccine was fixed. *Br Med J*. 2011; 342: c5347.

155. Dyer C. Lancet retracts MMR paper after GMC finds Andrew Wakefield guilty of dishonesty. *Br Med J*. 2010;340:281.

156. Zipprich J, Winter K, Hacker J, et al. Measles outbreak—California, December 2014-February 2015. *MMWR Morb Mortal Wkly Rep*. 2015;64:153-154.

157. Landrigan PJ. Epidemic measles in a divided city. *J Am Med Assoc*. 1972;221:567-570.

CHAPTER 33

Reproductive Epidemiology

Clarice R. Weinberg, Allen J. Wilcox, and Anne Marie Jukic

GENERAL CONSIDERATIONS

Reproductive epidemiology addresses the reproductive life course, including embryonic development, fetal development of reproductive systems, conception and pregnancy, delivery and health of the offspring, and reproductive senescence. The epidemiology of reproduction is complicated by irksome and intriguing methodologic problems. We begin by introducing some of the practical and conceptual issues.

1. <u>Occult health conditions</u>. Reproductive function can be abnormal without overt signs of dysfunction. Subtle changes such as alterations in menstrual function may go unrecognized. Infertile couples may have no related symptoms and may not discover their infertility until they attempt to conceive. Bias in ascertainment of infertile cases can arise from self-selection related to personal decisions about whether or when to have children and about whether or when to seek medical help. Such selection bias can produce spurious associations between infertility and the factors that lead couples to seek infertility treatment.

2. <u>Heterogeneity</u>. As in other areas of epidemiology, the tendency to dichotomize health outcomes often oversimplifies and mischaracterizes what is a continuum of risk. While heterogeneity of risk across individuals is common in other areas of epidemiology, it is especially important in reproduction because outcomes can occur repeatedly. An example

is recurrent pregnancy loss. Recurrent loss is sometimes regarded clinically as a distinct diagnosis, when it is in fact an imperfect biomarker for those at the extreme high end of the range of miscarriage risk.[1]

3. Selective attrition. Heterogeneity in risk among couples can lead to deceptive population sorting. For example, among couples who are trying to conceive, those who have relied on unreliable methods of contraception (such as spermicide) and attempt conception will as a group have lower fecundability than couples who have relied on a highly effective method of birth control (such as oral contraception). This result occurs because, among those who have used spermicides, many of the more fertile couples would have reached their desired family size through unplanned pregnancies and thus be removed from the group planning to conceive. If one ignores this differential attrition, one could wrongly conclude that spermicide use adversely affects fertility.[2]

4. Competition among outcomes. Reproductive end points are often not independent from each other and may compete directly. For example, approximately 25% of human chorionic gonadotropin (hCG)-producing pregnancies are lost before clinical recognition.[3] An exposure that increases the risk of very early loss might do so by accelerating the death of conceptuses that otherwise would have ended later as clinically recognized miscarriages. As a result, a study of recognized miscarriages might spuriously conclude that the exposure is protective. Similarly, an exposure that causes a malformed fetus to be stillborn rather than surviving to live birth might appear protective in studies of birth defects because malformations among stillbirths are less likely to be recognized and recorded. Shifts in the timing of death could also distort a dose-response pattern, producing a paradoxical decline in birth defects at higher levels of exposure.[4]

5. Cohorts work well. While case-control studies are broadly used in other areas of epidemiology, many reproductive problems are better addressed through cohort studies. Outcomes that are relatively common but incompletely ascertained in routine clinical care (like miscarriage or pregnancy complications) can be better suited for cohort studies. For longer-term outcomes related to exposures during pregnancy, cohort studies assess exposures prospectively and thereby avoid recall bias. For example, major cohort studies of pregnancy complications and later outcomes have proved fruitful.[5-7]

6. Pairs matter. For many reproductive end points, the proper unit of study is the couple. Distinguishing the effects of maternal and paternal exposures is complicated by the fact that the exposures are often correlated. Consideration of family genetics introduces further complexities. During gestation, the genomes of mother and fetus can jointly influence outcomes and influence the effects of exposures on those outcomes and may require special analytic approaches. (See the comments on genetic studies below.)

7. Time confounding. Pregnancy is, to varying degrees, under the control of the couple. When decisions to become pregnant are affected by previous pregnancy outcomes, this dependency can produce highly nonstandard forms of confounding by time. For example, women with miscarriages are likely to become pregnant again relatively soon, while women with successful pregnancies may wait several years before another pregnancy. This tendency of women to replace failed pregnancies will lead to a time bias in which the more recently occurring pregnancies will be more likely to have ended in miscarriage. If a cross-sectional study is carried out to assess the effects of an exposure on miscarriage risk and the exposure has also varied over time, spurious associations can arise.[8] Pregnancy interval can distort interpretations in other ways. A longer interval between pregnancies can be associated with changes in residence or other environmental conditions and change in the male partner. Failure to consider all those possibilities can lead to mistaken causal inferences.[9,10]

8. Obscure denominators. Denominators are easily miscounted or even unmeasurable in reproductive studies. For example, it is not possible to estimate the full extent of pregnancy loss because present techniques cannot identify all cycles in which an oocyte was fertilized. A more feasible goal is to identify all conceptions that survive long enough to produce measurable levels of the pregnancy hormone, hCG, although even this design is logistically complex.[11-13]

Similar issues afflict studies based on self-recognition of pregnancy. The detection of miscarriage is strongly affected by the stage at which pregnancy is recognized. Time of recognition should ideally be accounted for analytically. An exposure that reduces fertility prolongs the attempt time, which in turn may heighten attention to the early signs of pregnancy and motivate earlier tests for pregnancy. Earlier detection increases the *detection* of loss, even in the absence of increased *occurrence* of loss.

9. Reverse causation. Reproductive studies are particularly vulnerable to problems of reverse causality largely because events can occur closely together in time. For example, women with pregnancy complications may schedule more prenatal obstetric visits because of heightened concern, producing an association between prenatal care and bad outcomes. As another example, women who have not had a successful pregnancy are more likely to remain in the workforce and may consequently accumulate more occupational exposure than women who stay home with young children. This infertile worker effect (or reproductively unhealthy worker effect) can lead to spurious associations between occupational exposures and adverse reproductive outcomes.[14]

10. Recurrence risk and research opportunities. The availability of repeated outcomes for a woman or couple (or a family over multiple generations) offers design opportunities not seen in many other areas of epidemiology. One of the strongest risk factors for adverse reproductive outcomes is a previous occurrence of the same outcome. For example, it may be possible to explore the relative contributions of environmental and genetic causes by looking for changes in recurrence risk among women who change partners between pregnancies or who keep the same partner but change some crucial environmental exposure.[15] Another opportunity involves interventions among women with a previous occurrence of the outcome of interest. Clinical trials of women who had earlier delivered a baby with a neural tube defect provided efficient proof of the benefit of folic acid in preventing this defect.[16] Recurrence risk also presents analytic traps. Some investigators have adjusted for prior outcomes in assessing etiologic associations. This adjustment itself can produce bias if the exposures under study influenced both current and past risk.[17]

11. Collider stratification bias. Stratifying on colliders in general can open "back-door" causal pathways, leading to biased inference.[18] In particular, gestational age and birth weight, which are commonly adjusted for in reproductive epidemiology, are themselves strongly influenced by factors that also influence the outcome and thus can create strong bias.[19-22] Adjustments for either variable should be avoided in most settings.

12. Seasonal effects. Seasonal patterns in pregnancy outcomes can reflect potentially modifiable risk factors related to environment or lifestyle. However, because of widespread access to birth control, the time of conception is subject to planning. Timing is related to whether the pregnancy was intended and to fecundability, making seasonality vulnerable to confounding.[23,24] The risk set (denominator) is also important to specify properly when assessing seasonality; the characteristics of that set can vary with season. For example, the risk set for preterm birth is fetuses within a particular range of gestational age and not live births. Even among the fetuses who are at risk, the age structure of the population of fetuses will vary with season and must be taken into account.[25]

13. Mediation analysis pitfalls. Preterm birth may seem like a natural mediator when studying the effect of exposures on outcomes such as neonatal mortality. However, preterm delivery is not only a determinant of immaturity at birth but also a biomarker of prenatal distress. Directed acyclic graphs do not do a good job of capturing such subtleties. Even though early delivery is generally associated with higher neonatal mortality, preterm delivery might actually improve survival for a particular fetus under intrauterine duress (for example, in the presence of infection) compared to a counterfactual where the stressed fetus is forced to stay in an inhospitable uterine environment. We seldom fully understand the underlying biological causes for a preterm birth, and consequently standard mediation analysis can mislead us about the proportion of deaths preventable by delay of delivery.

With these general conceptual and methodologic problems in mind, we turn to specific reproductive end points.

THE REPRODUCTIVE LIFE COURSE

The reproductive life of women is bracketed by the milestones of puberty and menopause. These events are themselves topics of study. For example, the onset of puberty can be accelerated by hormonally active chemicals or retarded by inadequate nutrition.[26] Menopause can be accelerated by exposures that are toxic to the ovary[27] or by conditions that make hysterectomy advisable.

Both milestones present the investigator with definitional problems. Puberty for girls involves a series of hormonal and physical changes for which the onset of menstruation provides a convenient, though only partially relevant, marker. The timing of puberty for boys is more difficult to pinpoint. Both transitions can be studied by categorizing children according to Tanner stages,[28-30] which provide physical benchmarks for successive levels of sexual maturation.

The Menstrual Cycle

Starting at menarche, women undergo cyclic changes of their reproductive system, under neuroendocrine control. About once a month, a mature egg (or sometimes more) is released from the ovary and picked up by the oviduct for transport to the uterus. The ovum dies if not rapidly fertilized by a sperm, and menstruation begins roughly 2 weeks later. Pituitary and ovarian hormones coordinate the recruitment, selection, and maturation of the follicle and the preparation of the uterus, all under the direction of the hypothalamus.

The menstrual cycle is defined as the interval from the onset of one menstrual bleed to the onset of the next. The menstrual cycle is often described as lasting 28 days, with ovulation on day 14, but there is considerable variability in both cycle length and the timing of ovulation.[31] The variability in cycle length was well demonstrated in the extraordinary longitudinal study launched by Alan Treloar, who collected menstrual diaries from a cohort of several thousand women throughout their reproductive life.[32]

Certain exposures and physiologic states (such as intense physical training or emaciation) can cause anovulation (failure to ovulate) as an adaptive response. Less extreme forms of the same conditions would also be expected to produce measurable changes in the menstrual cycle, perhaps lengthening it or increasing its variability. The menstrual cycle can be studied noninvasively and prospectively, and menstrual-cycle characteristics are informative as markers of female reproductive function[33,34] and as key health indicators in adolescent girls.[35] Characteristics of interest include cycle length, variability in cycle length, ovulation frequency and timing, pain (dysmenorrhea), duration of menses, and amount of bleeding.[36]

The biological variability of menses (as captured, for example, in prospective menstrual diaries) presents statistical challenges. One can apply longitudinal methods to the study of cycle length based on the occurrence or nonoccurrence of abnormally long cycles.[33] Differences among women in their menstrual-cycle patterns create complex dependencies in the data. More methodologic work is needed to take full advantage of longitudinal cycle–length data for comparing exposed with unexposed women.[37,38]

If an exposure lengthens or increases the variability of menstrual cycles, studying the effect might necessitate daily biologic samples. Metabolites of luteinizing hormone (LH) (a pituitary hormone) and the ovarian hormones estrogen and progesterone can be assayed in first-morning urine specimens to describe reproductive hormonal patterns.[31,39] Alternatively, saliva carries transudates of serum hormones,[40] and current techniques also allow one to use saliva or urine to collect DNA for genetic assays.[41]

Menopause

Menopause is medically defined as the time when a woman stops menstruating. Menopause can occur naturally, with no medical intervention, or be secondary to uterine ablation, hysterectomy, or oophorectomy. While the definition is clear, the event and the age at which it occurs can be hard to pinpoint. The usual confirmation of menopause requires one nonpregnant, nonlactating year without a menstrual period, but menstruation can sometimes resume after a year. Also, this defini-tion leaves women who experience natural and permanent menopause unclassifiable for a full year. There can be awkward issues related to classifying events. For example, should a woman who dies of a heart attack 11 months after her last period be coded as premenopausal at the time of death? The most straightforward definitional remedy is probably to code the time of menopause as a year after the final period for everyone.

Another complication is that women who premenopausally have a hysterectomy with retention of one or both ovaries are menopausal in the sense that they no longer menstruate but may hor-monally cycle (and ovulate) for some unknown duration after the hysterectomy. Such uncertainties should be recognized and ideally analytically taken into account, *e.g.*, via multiple imputation of the time of hormonal menopause, in the analysis.

When the estimated age distribution of a life event is based only on those who have already experienced the event, the estimate will be biased by an overrepresentation of early events. This is a persistent problem in estimating the average age at menopause. For example, in a cross-sectional study, women who are past the mean age at menopause but still premenopausal will not contribute to the estimate, which biases the average menopausal age downward. Age at menopause for pre-menopausal women needs to be treated as censored at their observed age. Censoring of age at nat-ural menopause can also apply to hysterectomy, a competing risk. A premenopausal woman who has a hysterectomy at age 50 years has been at risk of natural menopause up to age 50 years but not after. Information for women who are premenopausal or who were premenopausal at the time of hysterectomy needs to be included through survival-analytic methods. With careful methods of analysis and certain assumptions, one can estimate the age distribution for natural menopause based on either cross-sectional data[27,42] or prospective data.[43]

FERTILITY

The most direct indicator of reproductive health is the production of a healthy baby. The word *fertility* can be confusing, as it is used in different ways by clinicians, demographers, and epide-miologists. Demographers and health statisticians refer to "fertility" as the production of children. "Fertility" for clinicians and the general public means the biologic capacity to reproduce, with "infertility" and "subfertility" referring to the involuntary impairment of that capacity. It is in this latter sense that epidemiologists approach the study of fertility.

Reduced fertility as an end point aggregates many possible reproductive impairments. Problems in gametogenesis, sperm transport, tubal patency, hormonal preparation of the uterine lining, implantation, immune response, and viability of the conceptus can all interfere with achieving a successful pregnancy. A couple in the United States is usually considered to be clinically infertile after at least 1 year without contraception and without pregnancy. For women older than 35 years, a 6-month interval may be enough to warrant clinical workup. *Primary* infertility refers to infertility in a couple with no previous live birth, while *secondary* infertility is infertility in a couple who has previously had a live birth.

The case-control design has been widely used for the study of rare, well-defined diseases, but is less well suited to the study of infertility.[44] Case-control studies often rely on infertility clinics for case identification, and many infertile couples do not seek medical help.[45] That self-selection and other socioeconomic factors produce a strong potential for ascertainment bias in identifying "cases" through the medical system, particularly when studying lifestyle factors. Some couples may fatalistically accept childlessness without seeking medical help. Others may be willing to seek help but are unable to afford it. The availability of comprehensive health insurance presumably reduces such selection.

One advantage of studying clinic-identified infertility is that additional data may be available for the proximal medical causes, such as poor sperm quality in the man or ovulatory dysfunction in the woman. Clinically distinct categories may also be etiologically distinct, and aggregating into a single "infertile" category might obscure disparate etiologies. In practice, however, medical eval-uations are often incomplete, and the categories of pathology can be provisional and overlapping. Male and female factors can both contribute. An ongoing medical workup can often be cut short by the occurrence of pregnancy.

There are also issues with diagnostic validity. The clinical dichotomy of fertile and infertile is an oversimplification. If clinically infertile "cases" are defined only by waiting time, with no requirement of documented physiologic dysfunction, there can be considerable misclassification. Couples who are normal but unlucky may be diagnosed as infertile, while others with low fertility but better luck are miscategorized as normal. Spontaneous "cures" are common: Most couples who go for a year without conceiving will eventually achieve pregnancy even without medical intervention (*Textbook of Clinical Embryology,* Cambridge University Press).

Time to Pregnancy

Another approach to the study of infertility is to regard fertility as a continuum. Biologically, there is a wide range of reproductive capacity, even among couples who achieve pregnancy. The proportion of couples conceiving in a given cycle is referred to here as the conception rate. Each noncontracepting, sexually active couple has a certain average probability of conception per menstrual cycle. This probability is called their *fecundability* and varies from zero (completely sterile) up to some limit that could be close to one. Among couples who discontinue contraception in order to become pregnant, about one-quarter conceive a clinical pregnancy in their first menstrual cycle at risk. This represents the mean fecundability of the whole group. Among those remaining at risk in the second menstrual cycle, the proportion conceiving is lower, and the conception rate continues to decline in successive cycles.[46] This declining pattern is seen even if couples who do not eventually conceive are removed from the denominators.[47,48] The declining conception rate is not a true time effect, but rather evidence of selective attrition in a heterogeneous population. The most highly fertile couples conceive early and are absent from subsequent risk sets. In this way, the successive cohorts remaining at risk are increasingly dominated by relatively subfertile couples, and the conception rate among those remaining at risk declines.

The heterogeneity in fecundability among couples suggests the possibility of modifiable factors that either promote or impair fertility. Such factors may be identified by studying time-to-pregnancy among exposed versus unexposed couples. Studies of time-to-pregnancy[49] have proved fruitful in identifying male and female exposures with adverse effects on fertility. Such studies make use of detailed time information beyond the usual clinical dichotomy of 6 or 12 months. Because each menstrual cycle provides a single ovulatory opportunity for conception, time-to-pregnancy is inherently discrete (taking only integer values), with the menstrual cycle serving as the natural scale for counting time. In a prospective study, menstrual cycles are enumerated directly through diary records. Ideally, the method for diagnosing pregnancy would be objective and standardized (*e.g.*, by use of a commercially available home test kit and a well-defined protocol).

Prospective Cohort Study Designs

An "incident cohort" study of fecundability enrolls women who discontinue their birth control in order to become pregnant. Exposures are ascertained and then participants are followed from the time they discontinue contraception until they become pregnant, resume contraception, or reach a certain maximum follow-up time without pregnancy. Survival-analytic methods allow all these women to contribute information appropriately. Web-based prospective designs can be both cost-effective and informative, as demonstrated by the Snart Forældre and PRESTO Studies.[50] A "prevalent cohort" study would enroll not only women who are about to discontinue contraception but also those who are currently trying to conceive. The analytic time-to-event model then must properly account for delayed entry into a cycle-specific risk set. This requires accurate information about the number of cycles women were at risk of conception just before enrollment—information that is not always easy to obtain retrospectively. Male exposures can also be studied in the context of time-to-pregnancy studies. For example, effects of male sleep duration on fecundability have been reported.[50]

Urine can also be used to measure metabolites of the ovarian hormones estrogen and progesterone and the pituitary hormone LH. These hormone measurements can enable the investigator to identify day of ovulation—the key reference point of the menstrual cycle.[31,39,51] Hormone assays may also provide clues about the fertile potential of each menstrual cycle. If women also record days with unprotected intercourse, the timing of intercourse in relation to ovulation can be taken into account in assessing fecundability.[52-55] Fertility can be modeled in an even more detailed way to capture specific mechanisms of effect, such as reduction in sperm survival time or uterine receptivity.

The real-time detection of ovulation and the fertile window is an area of rapidly expanding innovation. Menstrual cycle tracking apps, wearables, and at-home hormone testing are all available to the consumer with data collection and storage within phone apps. Tracking apps allow women to record menstrual cycle events, basal body temperatures, self-assessments of cervical mucus, and a breadth of health conditions. Wearable technology can detect changes in core body temperature and other markers that signal menstrual cycle stages. At-home hormone testing allows women to test their urine for changes in luteinizing hormone or estrogen, which could enable prediction of her fertile window and improve conception probability. These resources are likely to create databases for research on menstrual cycles, ovulation, fertility, and pregnancy with unprecedented sample sizes. While great potential exists for these new technologies, the epidemiologic characteristics, biases, strengths, and limitations of these data are just beginning to be explored.[56]

Retrospective Study Designs

A retrospective design requires women (or their partners) to reconstruct time-to-pregnancy retrospectively, usually for a current or recent pregnancy. In this approach, both the exposures and the time to an intended pregnancy are based on recall. (Unintended pregnancies provide little useful information on fecundability.) Certain biases, such as *post hoc* difficulties in establishing what was "intended" and differential persistence in trying, can be a problem,[57] but much has been learned from such studies. Women are able to recall these durations with surprising accuracy even many years later.[57,58] Men can provide usable data for the most recent pregnancy.[59] When the exposure of interest is rare or the available population is fixed (as in an occupational study), the number of women actively trying to conceive may be too small to be informative. In such a setting, a retrospective time-to-pregnancy study that oversamples exposed women could be more informative.

In a prevalent or incident cohort time-to-pregnancy study, the sampling unit is the attempt at pregnancy, while in the retrospective time-to-pregnancy study, the sampling unit is typically the pregnancy itself. If every attempt at pregnancy ended in pregnancy, the two designs would generate roughly comparable data. In fact, of course, couples who are unknowingly sterile will be present in cohort studies but not in retrospective studies. An exposure that causes complete sterility in a subpopulation—but with no effect on the remainder—would be missed by the retrospective time-to-pregnancy design. This is more of a problem in theory than in practice; most reproductive toxicants can be expected to cause subfertility among the exposed who have not been rendered sterile. If it is important to include sterile couples retrospectively, this could be done by sampling reproductive aged couples rather than pregnancies, and ascertaining for each couple the length of the most recent interval during which they were having unprotected intercourse, regardless of whether pregnancy occurred.[60]

In a retrospective time-to-pregnancy study, the wording of questions can strongly affect the data. It is not sufficient to ask women how many menstrual cycles they took to conceive. Some who conceived in their first cycle answer that they took "zero" cycles, while others say "one."[61] This reporting inconsistency can be avoided by asking women whether the pregnancy occurred in the very first menstrual cycle after discontinuing contraception, and if not, whether it occurred in the second or third. For times longer than three cycles, one can ascertain the calendar time between when contraception was discontinued up to the last menstrual period preceding conception. One then must divide this interval by the usual cycle length and add 1, to allow for the cycle when conception actually occurred. Women can give credible answers[51] to a short series of questions about their time to the most recent pregnancy, and retrospective data agree reasonably well with data on the same pregnancies that have been gathered prospectively in a cohort study many years before.[61]

Current Duration Study Design

Another possible design is the "current duration approach"[48,62,63] in which couples who are currently sexually active but not contracepting are asked how long ago they discontinued birth control. Such ongoing durations are subject to length bias in that attempt times that are long are at proportionally increased probability of being sampled. Those durations can be used to study relative fecundability across risk factors, provided (1) any time-varying risk factors can be accurately assessed retrospectively and (2) length-biased sampling is properly accounted for.

Data Analysis

It would take many attempts and many pregnancies to determine the exact fecundability of a given couple. However, the maximum likelihood estimate for a couple is the inverse of the number of cycles it took them to conceive. The distribution of fecundabilities across couples can be modeled parametrically.[48,64]

If we assume simple random sampling, the fraction of couples who conceive in the first cycle after discontinuing contraception provides an unbiased estimate of the pregnancy planner population's mean fecundability. This assumes that the discontinued method of contraception has no residual effect, which is not true for oral contraceptives. With information on prior contraception, this effect can be taken into account in the analysis. The very simplest comparative fecundability study would estimate the fractions of exposed and unexposed couples who conceive in their first cycle of trying and compute a *fecundability ratio* (dividing one fraction by the other). A fecundability ratio is simply a risk ratio, although the word *risk* is unnatural in this setting, where conception is a desired outcome.

Extending this approach, one can use all cycles by stratifying on each cycle number (not just cycle 1) and assuming a fixed ratio (or odds ratio) of fecundabilities across strata of cycle time. This is a discrete analog of the Cox proportional hazards model,[65] which now models the cycle-specific probability of conception and assumes an exposure imposes a fixed multiplier on fecundability. For example, a fecundability ratio of 0.3 means that the exposed are only 30% as likely as the unexposed to conceive in each menstrual cycle at risk. Such a model can easily incorporate adjustments for potential confounders. An alternative is to make the very different assumption that the odds ratio is constant across cycles and use a logistic model instead of a log-risk model to estimate the fecundability odds ratio. (See the Appendix at the end of this chapter for technical details.)

Sources of Bias

Couples vary in their fecundability. At each successive menstrual cycle during an attempt at conception, this variation implies the selective removal of the couples with highest fecundability from the couples still trying to conceive. The three study designs described above (prospective, retrospective, current duration) are subject to different degrees of bias in estimating relative fecundability for a reproductively toxic exposure, even if the effect is proportional for each couple.[66,67]

Practical issues arise in collection and analysis of time-to-pregnancy data, even if one assumes that the reporting of ongoing attempt times is accurate. For example, a couple who has been trying for three cycles before recruitment into a prospective, prevalent cohort study must be recorded as contributing data beginning at cycle 4 (not cycle 1) to avoid immortal time bias. This is analogous to the usual survival analyses, where those who enter late contribute "left-truncated" data to the analysis. This issue is particularly important if the timing of study entry is related to exposure, for example, if exposed persons who have been trying to conceive for a long time are more likely to join the study than similar unexposed persons. One might want to restrict enrollment to those who have been trying at most for six cycles, both to enroll the most informative couples and to ensure good data quality for their prior attempt time.

A second practical problem is to account for possible effects of medical interventions, which could be differential by exposure. In a prospective cohort study, one can ascertain at what point a couple seeks medical help and simply censor their data as of that cycle. Lacking such detailed information in retrospective data, analysis could be truncated at about a year because medical interventions typically begin after a year (or 6 months among older women).

A prospective study of couples attempting pregnancy allows collection of exposure data specific to the month or day. Such time-varying exposures can be used directly in fecundability modeling. In a retrospective time-to-pregnancy study, such precision is seldom possible. Exposures can be ascertained with reference to a single point in time, but one must choose this reference date carefully. If one asks about exposures around the time that pregnancy was achieved, there could be bias from behavioral changes caused by perceived difficulty in conceiving. For example, a woman who has been trying to conceive for a long time might be motivated to give up smoking to improve her chances of success. This bias could affect the results for any modifiable factor that women regard as unhealthy. One solution is to choose a reference date for exposures around the time when contraception was first discontinued.

Even if an exposure is ascertained as of the time when the attempt began, a subtle problem can occur if the prevalence of an exposure or confounder has trended over calendar time. Consider a retrospective study of female dental assistants, in which the use of latex gloves was found to enhance fertility.[8] This puzzling finding was presumably an artifact of the trend for increased use of latex gloves over time. Women with long times to pregnancy tended to have begun their attempt at a time when gloves were seldom used; those with short times to pregnancy began their attempt more recently, when glove use was common because of the AIDS epidemic. There is not an easy solution. Adjustment for calendar time at the beginning of the attempt does not solve the problem. Similarly, it is not enough to regard the exposure as time-dependent because the opportunity for exposure remains correlated with the outcome. Certain ad hoc remedies can be employed if external data are available on exposure prevalence over time.[8] Otherwise, one must rely on quantitative bias analyses to estimate the extent of possible bias from changes in exposure prevalence over calendar time.

Other subtle sources of bias in fertility studies can be equally damaging.[68-70] For example, smokers as a group have more accidental pregnancies than nonsmokers.[71] If one compares the fertility of smokers and nonsmokers, smokers can appear to be less fertile because relatively more of the highly fertile smokers have achieved their desired family size via unintended pregnancies. In this way, exposed women who are highly fertile can consequently be underrepresented in the cohort of women having planned pregnancies. This bias can afflict both retrospective and prospective studies of time-to-pregnancy,[2] and there is no secure protection against it. Some reassurance can be gained in a retrospective study by ascertaining exposure information from women whose most recent pregnancy was unintended. Similarly, in a prospective cohort study, one can ask about past unintended pregnancies (or infer it from a history of induced abortions). If the exposed and unexposed women have similar histories of unintended pregnancies and induced abortions, then this bias may not be important.

Yet another source of bias involves the definition of a birth control failure in a retrospective study. In retrospective studies, analysis is necessarily restricted to nonaccidental pregnancies. There can be systematic differences in how couples interpret a birth control failure after the fact. Conceptions that some couples report as occurring in the first menstrual cycle at risk may be reported by other couples as accidental. If accidents are differentially misclassified by exposed versus unexposed as "intentional" cycle-one conceptions, there can be bias in either direction. A useful sensitivity analysis would reanalyze the data after omitting all cycle-one data (*i.e.*, beginning the analysis at cycle 2). If results are similar to those with the entire data set, this "definitional bias" can probably be neglected.[68,69]

Finally, an "unhealthy worker" effect is possible in reproductive epidemiology. Women who are reproductively healthy are more likely to have children, to take repeated maternity leaves, and, in some populations, to leave the salaried workforce. Assessments of reproductive end points that compare employed with unemployed women may need to account for such phenomena. Even within a working population, this selective process could link job seniority and cumulative exposure to poor reproductive capacity due to reverse causality. (If gender bias in the workplace declines and the needs of women with children are better accommodated, these selective pressures will presumably be reduced.) Further difficulties may arise if work status and seniority are indirectly affected by the exposure via effects on fertility, as in the complex causal pathways with feedback discussed by Robins.[72]

In summary, time-to-pregnancy studies can identify factors that affect human fertility, but with many unique sources of bias that must be taken into account.

Making Use of Assisted Reproductive Technology Protocols

Many couples having difficulty conceiving seek medical assistance and ultimately use assisted reproductive technologies or ARTs. The woman is treated with drugs that cause her to hyperovulate, and then multiple ova are "harvested" surgically. Fertilization is achieved either by combining sperm and ova in a laboratory dish (in vitro fertilization or IVF) or through injection of single sperm directly into each ovum (intracytoplasmic sperm injection or ICSI). The use of ART is increasing. An estimated 1.7% of babies born in the United States are via ART (https://www.cdc.gov/art/artdata/index.html. Accessed September 17, 2018).

ART protocols provide an opportunity for clinical reproductive epidemiology. Although ART couples are self-selected, they provide a unique population for studying the effects of various exposures on the complex steps of fertility. The sequence of reproductive processes is under clinical observation and decomposed into its successive components. Specific effects of fertility-related factors can therefore be discovered. For example, oocyte number, quality, and fertilizability have been reported to be reduced in women who consume sweetened drinks,[73] and similar effects were seen in women with elevated urinary markers of phthalates.[74] Effects of male exposures on the functional quality of the sperm can also be explored under these protocols. For example, organophosphate flame retardant metabolites in the man's urine may be associated with reduced fertilization rates in IVF.[75]

Semen Quality

Male fertility is accessible for study in a way that female fertility is not. Women provide no ready access to their gametes, while male gametes are available and abundant. Semen quality can be assessed by automated methods that quantify sperm number, density, swimming ability, morphology, and other characteristics. Such semen characteristics are in turn related to a man's fecundability.[76,77] However, there are obstacles to both the interpretation and the collection of semen data. Certain extraneous factors (such as abstinence time and season) can have a strong influence on the results. Also, there can be difficulties in persuading men to produce a specimen for research, and recruitment rates are typically low,[78] with strong potential for selection bias. Exposures that are toxic to sperm can produce azoospermia and frank sterility,[79] while more subtle effects on sperm parameters have less certain effects on fertility.

Paternal Exposures

Effects via the father are biologically plausible and have been reported.[80] Exposures can occur via contaminated clothes or through substances that might mutate sperm or contaminate seminal fluid. Epigenetics offers a new kind of mechanism by which paternal exposures might influence pregnancy through the sperm epigenome, with effects that may persist across generations.[81] While this mechanism of effect is supported by experimental animal models, the corresponding research in humans is preliminary. Modifications in the sperm epigenome have been reported in fathers who were obese or overweight[82] or were smokers.[83] Changes have also been reported to be associated with urinary phthalate metabolites.[84] Information on paternal exposures should be collected when possible.

FETAL AND PREGNANCY COMPLICATIONS

The epidemiology of pregnancy complications and impaired fetal development is fraught with pitfalls. Fetal pathologies are seldom apparent until after delivery. By then, hidden competing risks may have distorted causal inference through selection bias. These conditions create a rich set of challenges for the collection and analysis of reproductive data.

Every healthy baby has survived a complex mix of biological processes that are only partially observable. These processes can cause extensive damage, including pregnancy loss. Death of the fertilized egg before implantation is unknowable by any current technology, but in principle attrition could be as high as 60%. The earliest stage at which pregnancy can be detected is at implantation, about 9 days after fertilization.[85] Starting from this point, a third of pregnancies are lost by natural attrition and another portion by induced abortion. Many of those losses are due to lethal genetic aberrations or developmental errors. Placental pathologies impose further stresses on the fetus, all within a maternal system that is experiencing extreme (if temporary) alterations in physiologic function.

Like infertility, pregnancy loss is not a rare event. About 25% of implanted embryos are lost without women knowing they are pregnant,[3] and an additional 10% to 15% of recognized pregnancies end in miscarriage.[86] This extensive prenatal winnowing is presumably an important selective mechanism for conserving the maternal resources spent on reproduction, ensuring that the mother invests in only the most highly fit embryos.[87]

Early Pregnancy Loss

The earliest known biomarker of pregnancy is the hormone hCG. hCG becomes detectable in mother's blood and urine around the time the developing conceptus invades the uterine wall, 6 to 12 days following ovulation.[85] In an idealized 28-day menstrual cycle with ovulation on day 14, this window of implantation would correspond to days 20 to 26, several days before the next period is expected. Given that pregnancies are typically not symptomatic at this early stage, such pregnancies can be lost without being recognized. Early loss usually occurs around the time of the expected menstrual period, with vaginal bleeding that is indistinguishable from normal menses[88] (Figure 33-1).

An early loss prolongs the time to conceive a recognized pregnancy. Time-to-pregnancy studies, however, are not a sensitive way to detect the effect of an exposure that increases the risk of unmeasured early loss. For example, an exposure that increases that risk by 50% (from 25%-38%) would reduce a couple's apparent fecundability by just 17% [relative fecundability = (1-0.38)/(1-0.25) = (0.62)/(0.75) = 0.83].

Direct studies of early pregnancy loss, via an incident cohort study, are difficult. At any given time, a relatively small proportion of women are planning to become pregnant. Even fewer are willing to participate in an intensive study that requires collection of daily urine specimens.

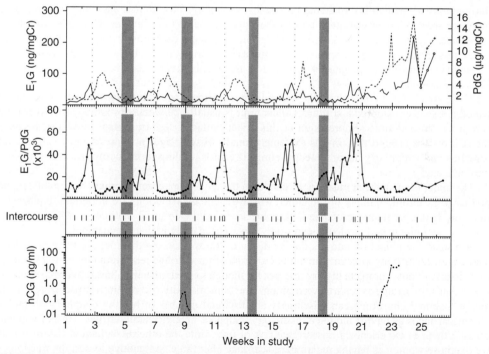

FIGURE 33-1 Hormonal data for a woman who participated in the Early Pregnancy Study for 25 weeks. The vertical shaded bars correspond to menses. The solid curve in the first panel shows the levels of a major estrogen metabolite, whereas the broken curve shows levels of a progesterone metabolite, both corrected for creatinine excretion to control for urinary diluteness. The day of ovulation was estimated by an algorithm that captures the rapid descent in the ratio of the two metabolites that accompanies luteinization of the ovarian follicle around the time of ovulation.[39] The estimated days of ovulation are shown as vertical broken lines through each menstrual cycle. The pregnancy hormone, hCG, evinces the occurrence of an early loss (week 9) followed by a clinical pregnancy (week 22).

Enrolling women before or at the time they discontinue their birth control is optimum in ensuring that the most fertile couples are not lost. Later enrollment produces a lower yield of pregnancies per observed cycle but can enrich the study through oversampling rare exposures that reduce fecundability or oversampling couples susceptible to effects of an exposure of interest. Since early pregnancy studies are also time-to-pregnancy studies, it is useful to determine accurately the number of cycles the couple had been trying before enrolling in the study.

In an effort to improve sensitivity, investigators may be tempted to define the hCG criteria for early loss with a specificity less than 1.0. Imperfect specificity can seriously bias the findings because early loss is relatively uncommon. There are far more cycles without implantation than with implantation, and even a small drop in specificity can lead to many false positives. If an exposed group of women is subfertile, they will contribute more nonimplantation cycles, with correspondingly more possibilities for false-positive early losses. This phenomenon can lead to a higher proportion of apparent early loss in the exposed, even with no difference in risk of loss between the groups. This "fertility bias" can be substantial.[11] Optimum specificity can be established by including a control group of women who cannot conceive, such as women with tubal ligation. Any criterion for early loss should be one that produces few or no false positives in those controls.

Miscarriage

Pregnancies that end spontaneously, between the time pregnancy symptoms begin and the time when a fetus is viable outside the uterus, are referred to variously as miscarriages, spontaneous abortions, or early fetal losses. Since pregnancy loss is greatest in the earliest weeks of gestation, the perceived amount of loss varies according to when a woman recognizes she is pregnant. With the widespread availability of home pregnancy tests, early detection is easy and losses can be more apparent. Women who have a history of miscarriage or infertility, or who have worrisome exposures, may test themselves earlier and thus identify more early miscarriages. One option is to define miscarriage as a loss after 6 weeks from last menstrual period (LMP). Alternatively, if data are available on time of pregnancy recognition, this can be treated as a left-truncation point for survival analysis.

There are also difficulties with the upper-limit gestational age boundary for miscarriage (after which a loss is considered a stillbirth). This limit is usually 20 weeks, but this varies over time and across jurisdictions. Imprecision at this upper bound is less important, however, because the risk of loss around this time is extremely small. Miscarriages are rarely registered in vital statistics and irregularly documented in clinical records, adding to the complications of epidemiologic study.

The underlying cause of miscarriage can lie in the fetus (*e.g.*, chromosomal abnormalities), the mother (*e.g.*, thrombophilia), or the father, whose genetic contributions are important to placental function. If the pregnancy outcome is the object of study, then usual methods can be applied to evaluate the influence of particular exposures experienced early in that pregnancy.

If instead the object of study is the condition of the woman (or the couple), there are added challenges. Identifying women who are at high risk of miscarriage requires a complete reproductive history. Even a complete history may not be enough to separate normal and abnormal couples, given that miscarriage is relatively common. The clinical entity of "recurrent miscarriage" (formerly "habitual abortion") can misclassify a substantial number of healthy couples with multiple miscarriages as having a clinical pathology.[1] Suppose an abnormality afflicts 10% of women, causing them to experience a miscarriage risk of 0.2, while the other 90% have a risk of 0.1. If we diagnose women as having recurrent miscarriage after three consecutive losses, the fraction of diagnosed women who in fact have the abnormality can be shown algebraically to be less than half. Most of the women diagnosed with recurrent miscarriage would be normal but suffering from bad luck. In other words, the number of observed miscarriages for a given couple has poor positive predictive value for underlying pathology when the majority of miscarriages occur for other reasons. Case-control approaches raise an additional problem with regard to case definition and sampling. If one compares hospitalized cases of miscarriage with hospitalized live births, one must recognize that many women with miscarriage are not hospitalized, whereas most women delivering an infant are, creating selection bias.

Induced abortions complicate the estimation of miscarriage risk in retrospective studies or studies that depend on clinical records. In such settings, the miscarriage risk is often calculated as the number of miscarriages divided by the sum of miscarriages and births. Where they are illegal, induced abortions may be reported as miscarriages. Where they are legal, induced abortions serve as a competing risk—that is, women who have an induced abortion were at risk of miscarriage up to the time of their abortion, but not after. One can in principle account for this competing risk with accurate data on the occurrence and gestational age of induced abortions. However, the confidentiality surrounding induced abortion can make such information hard to obtain, and timing may not be recalled accurately. In the absence of such information, miscarriage rates will be biased.[89] When information is available on the number of induced abortions but not their gestational age, a rough adjustment was proposed in 1983 to add a number equal to half of the induced abortions to the denominator.[90] When there is information about the gestational age distribution of induced abortions, better methods can be employed.[91] In settings where induced abortions are performed relatively early in pregnancy, the competing risk may be small enough not to warrant major concern.

An alternative retrospective design of miscarriage risk ascertains the outcome of the most recent pregnancy and relates this outcome to exposures at that time. This approach is particularly convenient for studies of a rare exposure or of a small fixed population (such as an occupational cohort) in which few women will be currently pregnant. A problem with this design is that an intended pregnancy that ends in loss is likely to be quickly followed by an additional pregnancy to achieve the desired outcome.[68,69] A successful pregnancy, in contrast, is followed by a longer interval to the next pregnancy. This selective masking of miscarriages by replacement pregnancies can produce the appearance of a change in risk over time (see point 7 "General Considerations"). The interval of time between conception and interview can act as a reverse-causation confounder and must be taken into account when studying an exposure that has changed over time.

A case-cohort approach to the study of miscarriage can be used with a cohort of pregnancies identified at the time of pregnancy diagnosis (for example, through a health maintenance organization). This requires special analysis methods (Chapters 17 and 18). The primary time scale is gestational time, not calendar time. Pregnancies that end in miscarriage can be identified as cases, and the cohort (or a random sample of the cohort) serves as the risk set. In principle, the stage of pregnancy at which loss occurs may provide further etiologic clues to the cause of the loss. Chromosomal abnormalities may be more common among early miscarriages than later, for example.[92] If exposure information is not available from prospectively recorded records (e.g., medical records), the information must be ascertained retrospectively.[93] The prospective cohort study allows pregnancies that end in induced abortion to contribute information from the time of recognition to the time of induced abortion. Women contemplating an induced abortion would tend to be reluctant to sign up for a prospective study, so there will likely be sampling bias. Exposure information can be collected repeatedly, allowing exposure effects to be targeted to the corresponding stage of gestation. Finally, exposures can be ascertained before the outcomes, avoiding potential for differential recall.

High gravidity (total number of pregnancies) is associated with higher risk of miscarriage, and it may seem natural to include gravidity as a potential confounder. However, women with one or more miscarriages require additional pregnancies to reach their desired family size, which plausibly explains the observed association. Adjustment or stratification on gravidity can introduce serious distortions.[1,94] Another subtle bias can occur because women who have a miscarriage are at increased risk of recurrence (a consequence of population heterogeneity of risk). Exposure studies may attempt to adjust for women's inherent level of miscarriage risk by controlling for prior loss. Such adjustment can distort the estimated risk ratio for current pregnancy if the earlier miscarriage was also affected by the exposure under study.[17] Causal diagrams are useful in this context[95-97] (see Chapter 3).

Statistical dependence is an issue with miscarriage risk, as with other pregnancy outcomes. Women may contribute several pregnancies in a study, and these events are not statistically independent. This problem can be addressed in the analysis using "random effects" logistic regression models or generalized estimating equation (GEE) logistic regression, which explicitly allows dependent outcomes within each woman's history. However, GEE becomes invalid if the cluster size is "informative,"[98] for example, if women with a higher risk of loss have more pregnancies in order to achieve their desired family size. In this setting, more complicated analytic methods are required. One approach is to sample one pregnancy from each woman, fit a risk model, e.g., using logistic regression, save the estimated coefficients and standard errors, and then repeat the same sampling and analysis many times.[98] This resampling approach is robust to informative cluster size and allows for complex dependencies among the outcomes. A weighted GEE approach[99] is equivalent to that resampling approach asymptotically and may work better when the study is small.

Hierarchical mixed-model methods can also be used to address dependencies among reproductive outcomes.[100] This approach might be appropriate if one has access to reproductive and exposure history data that can be linked, and one wants to estimate odds ratios in a way that uses all the pregnancies but does not assume independence among pregnancies within the same woman. This approach has been criticized, however, because reproductive decisions that couples (and their physicians) make are highly dependent on their experiences, implying that the within-couple dependency structure can be history-dependent and may not be adequately captured by a mixed model.[101] It may be preferable to focus instead on a single pregnancy, *e.g.*, a woman's first pregnancy.

Stillbirth

Stillbirth is defined as the death of a fetus after reaching a gestational age at which survival out of the womb is considered possible but before delivery. While gestational age of viability may seem like a logical line dividing miscarriages and stillbirths, it is neither fixed nor precise. For many years, viability was defined as 28 completed weeks of gestation. As medical interventions have lowered the limits of viability to 24 weeks and even earlier, the legal definition for the registration of stillbirth has also lowered. This definition varies widely across jurisdictions (*e.g.*, 20, 22, 24, 28 weeks), and sometimes includes a birth weight criterion.[102-104] Gestational age itself is hard to measure, and population differences in the methods for estimating gestational age (for example, last menstrual period vs. early ultrasound examination) add further imprecision to the definition of stillbirth.

It is not only the lower gestational age limit of stillbirth mortality that presents complications to the epidemiologist. There is also the matter of distinguishing stillbirth from live birth. The line between a death a few minutes before delivery and a few minutes after can be thin. Signs of life in the newborn may be uncertain. Given this gray area, regional or cultural differences in distinguishing fetal and neonatal death can be important. In the Soviet Union, some babies were not counted as live births until they had survived 1 week after delivery (increasing stillbirth and reducing infant mortality).[105] Valid comparisons of stillbirth rates (and neonatal mortality rates) across populations require close attention to possible differences in classification.

The question of defining stillbirth mortality at a given gestational age has provoked important methodological controversies. For many years, the standard definition of stillbirth mortality was the number of stillbirths divided by the total number of live births plus stillbirths at a given gestational week of pregnancy. However, live births are not at risk of fetal death. The proper risk set for fetal death is all fetuses alive at that gestational age. Yudkin and colleagues discussed this problem in 1987,[106] but analytic practice has been slow to change. The use of this more correct definition of stillbirth risk can radically change etiologic interpretations.[107]

Another problem in gestational age–specific stillbirth mortality is that death can occur weeks before delivery but not be detected until delivery. Without accurate information on the date of a fetal death, the next best alternative is to use the date of delivery (number of stillborn infants at a given week of pregnancy divided by the number of ongoing pregnancies at that time).

Fetal Growth

Given the role of birth weight as a marker of prenatal influences, fetal growth itself is a potentially useful indicator of prenatal effects. Before the advent of ultrasound, there was little opportunity to assess fetal growth except at delivery. As ultrasound technology has advanced, the ability to describe fetal growth has expanded dramatically. The first image of an in utero fetus was published in 1958.[108] Within a decade, biparietal diameter (skull width) had been proposed as a way to estimate fetal age.[109] In 1985, an equation for estimating fetal weight with several fetal measures (crown-rump length, biparietal diameter, head circumference, and abdominal circumference) was proposed and is still in use today.[110]

To measure fetal growth, one needs both a measure of fetal size and an accurate estimate of fetal age. One complication is that the fetal ultrasound measure most widely available is also the one used routinely to infer gestational age. Such a circular system cannot measure fetal growth. If one wishes to use a single ultrasound measure to assess fetal growth, it is essential to ascertain gestational age through a mechanism independent of fetal size (*e.g.*, by LMP or ovulation date).

With measures of fetal size at two time points, it becomes possible to assess growth, and, with an outside reference, one can also identify pathological changes in growth. Such a determination requires a "normal" standard against which fetal growth can be judged. It remains unresolved as to whether one growth standard can serve all populations or whether standards need to be tailored to a given population. If a single standard is used (as has been proposed by some),[111,112] the proportion of "growth restricted" fetuses can vary across otherwise healthy populations.[113] Variability can be reduced by instead stratifying fetal growth standards by maternal race/ethnicity.[114]

Whatever standard is chosen, it can be used to define categorical outcomes (fetal growth restriction or overgrowth, also called macrosomia) and to assign z-scores or percentiles to rates of growth. This makes it possible to determine whether a given fetus is maintaining its size relative to other fetuses of a comparable age. Toward this end, a z-score for fetal size has been proposed.[115] This approach can incorporate covariates expected to influence fetal size (for example, maternal body mass index, paternal height, maternal age, fetal sex). If measurements are available for multiple time points, appropriate random effects can also be included. The flexibility of this modeling scheme allows it to be applied to numerous types of fetal growth measures.

Disproportionate fetal growth is another characteristic that may indicate suboptimal fetal growth. Disproportionality has been suggested as a way to distinguish constitutionally small fetuses from those affected by pathological factors. A creative array of ratio measures has been proposed to detect pathological deviations in growth (head-to-abdominal circumference[116]; ponderal index[117,118]; head circumference to birth weight[119]; birth weight to placental weight[120]; and cerebral artery to umbilical artery pulsatility ratio[121]). The predictive usefulness of these ratios remains to be thoroughly tested.

NEONATAL OUTCOMES

For the baby, birth is a risky transition. The life supports of intrauterine existence are removed, and the baby must breathe and digest on its own. Not surprisingly, the mortality experienced by a baby in the hours and days after birth is higher than at any other time in life.[122, p 166] This mortality, as well as subsequent morbidity among survivors, is strongly predicted by the gestational age and weight of the baby at birth.

Neonatal Mortality

Neonatal mortality is a straightforward concept, defined as any death in the first 28 days (or sometimes 7 days) after live birth. The risk of neonatal mortality among live births climbs sharply with preterm delivery, and the mortality of preterm infants is a frequent topic of study.

The conventional definition of neonatal mortality among preterm babies is the risk observed among all live births at a given gestational age. Some authors have argued instead that the approach for stillbirths should be extended to neonatal deaths—that neonatal mortality at a given gestational age should be defined as a proportion of all fetuses alive at the gestational age at which the neonates who died were born.[123] However, neither denominator (ongoing fetuses or live births at a given gestational age) provides an estimate of neonatal mortality that is interpretable for etiologic analysis. Neonatal deaths are a mix of deaths that arise from two distinct risk sets.[13] Some neonatal deaths result from problems experienced by the fetus (such as birth defects) and for which fetuses may be the correct denominator. Other neonatal deaths are due to causes that occur only during or after delivery (for example, complications due to immaturity or hospital-acquired infection). For these deaths, live births are the correct denominator. Unfortunately, these two general sources of neonatal mortality cannot be cleanly differentiated, and some deaths are due to a combination of factors (for example, in a preterm baby with a major birth defect). As a result, it is not possible to assign a correct denominator to preterm neonatal deaths. For etiologic studies of neonatal death among babies born preterm, either denominator generates distorted results.[13] Any etiologic analysis that stratifies, conditions on, or adjusts for gestational age is subject to this caution. Estimates of gestational age–specific neonatal mortality based on live births are still valid for prediction.

Perinatal mortality is the combination of stillbirth and neonatal mortality. Perinatal mortality is a frequently used outcome and resolves the difficulties of misclassification (and competing risk) between fetal and neonatal death. Perinatal mortality does not, however, escape the difficulties of stratifying by gestational age, given that neonatal deaths are a substantial component of perinatal deaths. The same cautions regarding conditioning on gestational age in the analysis of neonatal mortality apply to the analysis of perinatal mortality.

Gestational Length

Preterm delivery is one of the most common pregnancy complications of pregnancy, occurring in 10% of US pregnancies.[124] This adverse outcome is usually defined as delivery before 37 completed weeks of gestation, measured from the start of the LMP. The risk set for gestational week–specific risk of preterm delivery is ongoing pregnancies (*i.e.*, fetuses).

One design (usually the most costly) for studying preterm delivery is prospective. Survival-analytic methods allow all pregnancies to be fully used in the analysis (see Chapter 22), where survival refers to the continuation of the pregnancy, and the primary time scale is gestational age. Pregnancies should be analyzed as left truncated at the time that a delivery could have been identified as an event in the study. One can then censor the analysis at a prespecified time point, *e.g.*, 37 completed weeks, after which (by definition) fetuses are no longer at risk of preterm delivery. Dividing preterm births into specific clinical subsets such as preterm premature rupture of membranes may clarify etiologic studies. Clinical interventions such as induction of labor and planned caesarian section should be treated as right-censoring events (events that terminate follow-up). Nevertheless, this censoring may distort the analysis if the interventions are in response to fetal distress (as is often the case), which may itself have soon caused spontaneous preterm delivery. In this case, the assumption of noninformative censoring is violated. More complex methods could be employed.[125]

A related problem arises when specific pathologic mechanisms leading to prematurity are under study. If preterm deliveries without membrane rupture are treated as independent censoring events, this implicitly assumes that the pregnancies ending in preterm delivery without membrane rupture would have had the same risk of premature membrane rupture as the pregnancies that continued in utero, had they not been delivered early. This implicit assumption is not necessarily true.

Although prematurity is not a rare outcome, one can potentially improve study efficiency by sampling all preterm deliveries in some defined population of pregnancies and comparing exposures in these pregnancies with exposures in a random subcohort of pregnancies. This design would be straightforward, for example, in a health maintenance organization. Case-cohort methods of analysis are then needed to analyze the gestational survival of the pregnancy up to a cutoff at 37 weeks, analogous to the proposed approach for miscarriage.[93] Such survival methods allow the investigator to model gestational time–specific exposure effects.

Assessment of exposures specific to the stage of pregnancy (gestational time) can be important. If exposure is crudely classified only as occurring at some time during pregnancy, this can lead to de facto exposure misclassification and bias.[4] One problem is that pregnancies that last longer have a greater opportunity for exposure than pregnancies that end early. This propensity bias can be avoided by treating exposure as time-dependent in a survival analysis, so that current hazard is not permitted to depend in any way on future exposures. A more detailed treatment of issues related to the study of pregnancy complications is provided by Olsen.[126]

While fetuses are the obvious risk set for the occurrence of preterm delivery, the risk set for postnatal outcomes among babies born preterm is not so easily defined. As is true for neonatal mortality, morbidity among preterm babies can be caused by a combination of events occurring in utero and events occurring after delivery. The same difficulties discussed above for studies of neonatal mortality also apply to studies of other outcomes after preterm birth. No single denominator adequately captures the relevant risk set. As a consequence, etiologic studies of preterm babies are subject to serious distortions in their results.[13,21,22]

Birth Weight and Fetal Origins of Adult Disease

A newborn's weight is a strong predictor of its survival, independent of gestational age.[127] Birth weight is easily measured and routinely recorded and is commonly used in perinatal research. Low birth weight (LBW, defined as births less than 2500 g) has been a frequent surrogate for perinatal health, especially when gestational age data are hard to obtain. The risk of neonatal mortality among LBW babies is typically 25-fold higher than for babies of higher weight.[128] This high mortality was mistakenly attributed for many years to premature delivery. As better data on gestational age accumulated, it became clear that half or more of LBW babies are not preterm, and that small babies are at high risk even if they are not preterm. Without prematurity to explain their mortality, a diagnosis of "growth retardation" was created. The study of LBWs shifted to a study of "intra-uterine growth retardation" or "fetal growth restriction,"[129] usually defined as the smallest 10% of babies delivered at each gestational age (SGA).

Small size is often assumed to be on the causal pathway to its associated morbidity and mortality, leading to policies and interventions intended to promote heavier babies. For example, the World Health Organization established a goal of a 30% reduction in LBW by 2025 (http://www.who.int/nutrition/publications/globaltargets2025_policybrief_lbw/en/; Accessed September 17, 2018). Maternal nutrition has been a major focus of perinatal epidemiology in part because of the expectation that better nutrition should produce heavier (and, consequently, healthier) babies.

It remains a question as to whether birth weight is a health outcome in itself. There are no clear clinical criteria that distinguish (for example) babies at the 8th percentile and those at the 12th percentile. Also, changes in birth weight do not necessarily have the predicted consequence. The great secular declines in infant mortality have occurred with little change in birth weight.[122, p 216] Conversely, babies born at high altitudes are smaller without having increased mortality.[130] But the most important challenge to a causal role for birth weight is in what is known as the LBW paradox.

A paradox emerges when stratifying by birth weight in the analysis of neonatal outcomes. An exposure (such as maternal smoking) associated with higher neonatal mortality overall may be associated with lower mortality among LBW babies[130] (Figure 33-2). In 2006, two papers suggested that this paradox could be explained by unmeasured factors that cause both severe growth restriction and high mortality.[19,131] Subsequent papers have expanded this idea[132] and seen it as an example of collider bias.[133] The pattern seen with many exposures associated with LBW (smoking, infant sex, high altitude, race, twinning) is revealing. The mortality curve shifts toward lower weights to the same extent that the birth weight distribution shifts—as if the change in birth weights is an epiphenomenon, rather than an example of causal mediation.[134,135] An upward shift in the mortality curve can occur at the same time, but that association appears to be independent of, and therefore not mediated through, the effect on birth weight.

Prenatal factors impairing the subsequent health of the child also frequently restrict the growth of the fetus. From a public health perspective, it is not possible to assess what benefits—if any—might come with interventions to produce larger babies. When considering causal associations between an exposure and a neonatal outcome, there is no justification for adjustment or stratification by birth weight. Birth weight remains useful as a biomarker, and categories such as LBW and SGA can be predictors of health outcomes.

Experiences and exposures in prenatal life can have long-lasting effects on later health. The extensive effects of fetal exposure to DES are a good example.[136] Barker promoted the idea of developmental origins of disease by focusing on the association of LBW with cardiovascular disease.[137] Barker's observations raised the perceived importance of reproductive epidemiology and provided justification for national pregnancy cohort studies with long-term follow-up (e.g., Olsen et al., 2001[138]; Magnus et al., 2016[7].)

While birth weight is a powerful predictor of long-term health, there are mechanisms that could confound those associations (as discussed above). The cautions raised above with regard to analysis of birth weight or gestational age in the context of neonatal outcomes also apply to the analysis of later health outcomes. Any analysis that treats birth weight (or preterm delivery) as a direct causal agent or as a mediator of adult risk may introduce bias. Moreover, when adjusting for adult characteristics (such body weight) that are associated with birth weight, artificial associations can be induced between birth weight and health outcomes such as blood pressure.[139] Directed acyclic graphs are an essential tool in the analysis of relationships between prenatal and long-term health.

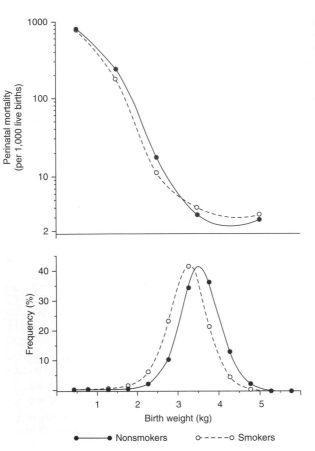

FIGURE 33-2 Frequency distributions of birth weight and weight-specific perinatal mortality rates for infants exposed and unexposed to mothers' smoking: Missouri, 1980-1984. (Reproduced with permission from Wilcox A. Birthweight and perinatal mortality: the effect of maternal smoking. *Am J Epidemiol.* 1993;137:1098-1104.)

Birth Defects

Our understanding of the etiology of birth defects has undergone radical transformation over the past century. In the first decades of the 1900s, medical dogma held that the fetus is perfectly shielded by the placenta from adverse outside influences. In 1941, Gregg[140] linked an outbreak of rubella to a rare eye defect in newborn infants, which led to the discovery of the spectrum of birth defects associated with rubella infection during pregnancy. This revelation shook the obstetrics world. Clearly the placenta was not a perfect shield.

The notion persisted that an exposure must make the mother ill in order to injure her fetus. In 1961, this dogma too fell when thalidomide (a sedative prescribed to pregnant women) was discovered to be a cause of limb-reduction defects. In this case, fetal damage was done by an exposure benign (and indeed therapeutic) to the mother.[141] Perhaps most disturbing of all was the recognition in 1971 that diethylstilbestrol (DES)—a synthetic estrogen prescribed to women during pregnancy—is a transplacental carcinogen, leading to a rare cancer in adulthood.[142] This finding demonstrated the possibility of harmful effects on the fetus that might not become apparent for decades. These discoveries led to a new era of concern about fetal vulnerability, particularly with regard to pharmacologic agents or environmental toxicants. Many of the large national birth registries in place today were launched in the 1960s with the aim of detecting new teratogens introduced into the population. Despite the subsequent expansion of epidemiologic research related to birth defects, most defects have obscure origins. Methodologic difficulties persistently frustrate research in this area.

One obstacle is accurate ascertainment of malformations at birth. The skill of the examiner and the thoroughness of examination can play a large role in the birth prevalence of defects. Even clinically obvious defects, such as facial clefts so severe as to require surgery, are underascertained in birth records.[143] Furthermore, not all birth defects are detectable at birth. Many heart defects are not manifest until after initial discharge from hospital, and some may go undiagnosed until adulthood. With careful examination, 3% of babies have major malformations identifiable at birth, and another 3% carry defects identified later.[144,145] Minor defects are at least as common. Population registries based on routine examination of newborns find overall birth prevalence in the range of 2% to 3%.

Birth defects comprise a wide spectrum of defects, and specific types are rare. Even the most common types of birth defects are found in only 1 to 4 per 1,000 babies. This scarcity may tempt an investigator to lump all defects in etiologic studies. This is as unwise as grouping all cancers—the individual categories of defects are heterogeneous in their origins, and causal associations that are strong for a given birth defect can be undetectable when looking at total defects. Even narrowly defined defects can have diverse origins, and a single teratogen may cause only a small fraction of the observed cases.[146]

A major obstacle to studies of birth defects is that incidence cannot be validly estimated. Birth defects typically originate in the earliest stages of pregnancy, when direct observation is not possible. The prevalence of any defect at birth is thus a function of incidence and intrauterine survival, with defective fetuses experiencing increased rates of embryonic and fetal loss. Survival to birth may be impaired by the defects themselves and by maternal mechanisms that screen out faulty fetuses.[87] This selective loss of defective fetuses could influence etiologic studies. For example, an exposure could in principle decrease the survival of malformed fetuses and cause the loss to occur as a miscarriage rather than as a recorded birth. Such a mechanism could lead to an association of the exposure with decreased prevalence of birth defects.

In addition, diagnostic screening and elective abortion are used to terminate pregnancies with malformed fetuses.[147] Since aborted defects are often not captured by birth defects registries, selection by induced abortion can introduce bias in etiologic studies where prenatal diagnosis (and the response to it) is nonrandom. Despite these limitations, the study of birth defects remains an important public health enterprise. Most epidemiologic studies are based on population registries or on clinic data (usually case-control studies). Registries have played a central role in our growing understanding of birth defects epidemiology, even though registries have not (yet) fulfilled their original purpose of uncovering new teratogens entering the environment.

For case-control designs, one methodologic question is whether a couple with a defective infant will be influenced by guilt or anxiety to report their adverse exposures differently than a couple with a normal infant.[148-151] A controversial remedy for this potential recall bias is to select babies with other birth defects as controls. There is a practical advantage to this approach: Parents of babies with birth defects are easier to recruit than parents of normal infants. Controls with defects can often be sampled from the same clinic or birth defect registry as the cases. A problem with such controls is that the effect measure will be biased toward the null if the defect in the controls shares etiologies with the cases.[152] But such "case-case" designs may be unnecessary—the problem of recall bias with unaffected controls may be less than feared. A comparison of odds ratios using the two types of control groups provided no evidence that differential recall of exposure is an important concern in such studies.[153] Other studies that account for potential misclassification through simulations showed little to no changes in effect estimates[154,155] although these changes varied across exposures and context. The extent of bias could be related to the type of exposure, changes in the prevalence and social acceptability of that exposure over time, and the cultural norms of the study population.

Case-control studies of birth defects (as with other pregnancy outcomes) can take advantage of short latencies between exposure and outcome. The relevant window of exposure for most defects is within the first trimester of pregnancy, so the time from exposure to diagnosis can be less than a year. The specific timing of exposure during embryonic and fetal development can provide further useful information. Teratogens often act only during a brief stage of organogenesis. For example, the structures of the heart are complete by the ninth obstetric week (counting from last menstrual period), and so an effect by a later exposure seems unlikely.

Amid this uncertainty over etiology, we know that both genetic and environmental factors play a role in most defects, presumably in interaction with each other. Concordance rates in monozygotic twins are elevated compared with dizygotic twins, as are recurrence risks in families that have already had a child with a birth defect.[15,156] Thus far, allelic variants linked to birth defects have explained little.

Sex Ratio

PubMed lists many more scientific publications on sex ratio than on preterm delivery. This is not because the ratio of boys to girls at birth is an important public health problem, but rather because it is so easily studied—and because the topic is a perennial crowd pleaser. These two features make studies of sex ratio subject to a treacherous set of pitfalls. Data on sex ratio are easily collected, easily presented, and available in enormous quantities. Things can go wrong in at least two ways. One is that easy access to data permits anyone to examine the outcome many times in many contexts. This leads to an abundance of dramatic (but unreproducible) results.[157] The second problem is that the availability of huge numbers allows the detection of (possibly) true differences that are so slight that their biological importance is nugatory.

That the sex ratio should be of popular interest is obvious: the first question asked about any new baby is whether the baby is a boy or a girl. Couples with a preference for one or the other are eager for advice that would tip the scales. Much advice has been offered (for example, on timing intercourse relative to ovulation), but the bottom line is that all timing-based methods of sex selection are successful half the time. A popular category of sex ratio studies is the study of social conditions or exposures that might shift the ratio. False-positive results have led to popular myths about changes in sex ratio after wars or during conditions of extreme stress.[158,159] As intriguing as these are, such effects have not been consistently replicated. In more recent times, environmental contaminants have been claimed to alter the sex ratio, although such differences are often miniscule (*e.g.*, a decline of the male excess from 51.5% to 51.3%[160]). The biological mechanisms that might underlie such subtle shifts remain obscure. One factor that incontrovertibly can alter the sex ratio is selective abortion. Although the practice is illegal in most countries, its effects are evident in the skewed sex distributions in certain countries with a strong cultural preference for sons.[161]

FAMILY STUDIES

Recurrence Risk in Pregnancies

Pathologies of pregnancy, including preeclampsia and preterm delivery, have a high relative risk of recurrence.[162,163] This is true also for adverse outcomes among the neonates, such as birth defects or developmental problems.[164,165] The study of pregnancy-related recurrence risks within women helps to control for both genetic and environmental confounding factors. A further advantage is that a woman's pregnancies typically occur within a relatively limited time. Factors that alter recurrence risk (such as a change in male partner) can provide clues about the underlying etiology of risk.

Patterns of recurrence can also lead to unexpected traps, as demonstrated by the example of preeclampsia. Preeclampsia is more common in first pregnancies and in pregnancies with a new male partner. These observations led to the hypothesis that women become immunologically tolerant of antigens from their male partner and that a new partner raises preeclampsia risk by introducing new antigens.[166] The new-partner observation, however, is confounded by pregnancy interval. Preeclampsia risk (for reasons still not clear) increases directly with time since previous pregnancy. Women who change partners also tend to have longer intervals between their pregnancies—and when interval is taken into account, the association of preeclampsia risk with new male partner disappears.[9,10]

Family Designs

The close biological and social connections of the nuclear family provide rich opportunities for etiologic research designs tailored to the family setting, particularly for conditions with onset that is prenatal or diagnosed fairly early in life. For example, studies of pregnancy outcomes within women show high recurrence rates for specific problems of pregnancy, as well as for poor outcomes among offspring. Sibling studies can exploit the various combinations of genetic and shared intrauterine conditions that are possible among families while implicitly adjusting for early life factors that can confound exposure effects. Fathers' exposures may affect intrauterine development. In genetic studies of offspring disease, the laws of Mendelian transmission from parents provide a natural randomization against which one can estimate effects of genetic variants on risk.

Sibling Comparisons

Twin studies comparing phenotype concordance rates in monozygotic (MZ) and dizygotic (DZ) twins are useful for assessing heritability. There are two approaches to calculate disease concordance for twins: the pairwise concordance rate and the proband-wise concordance rate.[167] Both are based on counting the excess of co-occurrences in MZ versus DZ twin pairs. (Dizygotic twins share one uterus but are genetically no more similar than any two nontwin siblings.) Pairwise concordance rates estimate the probability that both twins have the condition, conditional on at least one twin having it. Proband-wise concordance rates estimate the probability that one twin develops the disease given that the other has it. These may seem to be nearly the same, but in practice, the pairwise concordance rate can be much smaller than the proband-wise concordance rate.[167] More important, the proband-wise concordance rate corresponds to the recurrence risk in families, which makes it more clinically relevant. Also, proband-wise rates are not vulnerable to effects of incomplete ascertainment (in contrast with pairwise rates). Both rates can be influenced by changes in case definition or by the age of the population from which the twins are sampled. When prenatal risk factors are the topic of interest, it may be useful to compare dizygotic twins (who shared a uterus) with non-twin siblings (who inhabited the same uterus but at different times). The proband-wise concordance rate can be compared for the two types of sibling pairs, with a higher concordance rate in dizygotic twins suggesting prenatal influences.

A family-based approach could also be taken, based on conditional logistic analysis of data from mothers who experienced different exposures and different outcomes during her pregnancies. An example would be women who smoke in one pregnancy but not another.[168] Informative mothers would be those with offspring who varied in their outcomes and also their pregnancy exposures.

Another useful comparison involves half-siblings. One can compare pairs of half-siblings who share a mother but not a father with pairs who share a father but not a mother. Recurrence risk may be higher for maternal half-siblings if there are maternally mediated genetic effects or effects of the prenatal environment. This kind of asymmetry has been observed for the birth defect, cryptorchidism.[169] Such studies are usually set within population registries, which provide large study size for identifying these various family structures. All sibling studies are vulnerable to misclassification of paternity, although that issue is much less important for comparisons of monozygotic versus dizygotic twin pairs. While extremely useful, sibling analyses can be subject to subtle problems of interpretation. For example, if siblings are less similar with regard to confounders than with regard to the exposure under study, the within-pair estimate could be more biased than an ordinary unpaired estimate.[170-172]

Genetic Factors in Reproductive Epidemiology

The mother's genome contributes not only to the genome of her fetus but to the perinatal environment.[173] For example, the mother's genotype may confer reduced ability to metabolize toxicants during pregnancy. Thus, when exploring the genetic contributions to risk, the unit of interest is the maternal-fetal pair. A study of only the baby's genotype, or only the mother's genotype, is vulnerable to confounding because of the high correlation between the two. A carefully designed genetic study of perinatal risk should include at least the mother and child, and, if possible, the father as well.

Case-control studies are one approach to genetic studies. An alternative design (case-parent triads) can be particularly useful when studying pregnancy complications and conditions with onset early in the child's life. In this design, affected offspring and their two parents are genotyped.[174] Alleles associated with the outcome of interest will be found in affected offspring more often than Mendelian transmission would predict (see also Chapter 37). Geneticists have made use of this apparent distortion by comparing the total number of transmissions from heterozygous parents to affected offspring with a binomial (probability 1/2) distribution, in a procedure called the transmission disequilibrium test (TDT).[175]

The same data can be analyzed in family-based approach based on the autosomal genotypes of the mother, father, and child. For a simple biallelic gene (with three options AA, Aa, and aa for each family member), each family is categorized into 1 of 15 possible cells in a contingency table. The resulting multinomial counts can be analyzed by stratified log-linear regression,[174] which yields estimates of the relative-risk parameters associated with two copies or one copy, respectively, of the variant allele inherited by the affected offspring, treating the 0-copy offspring as the referent category. Statistical power for this approach often exceeds that of the TDT.[174]

Methods based on parents also avoid biases related to control selection because the biologic parents are inherently well-matched controls for genetic effects. On the other hand, one must assume not only Mendelian assortment for the gametes, but also that survival of affected offspring to the point of study does not depend on genotype, conditional on the parents' genotypes.

What if there are maternal genes that affect the mother's phenotype during gestation and thereby affect the fetus? This causal mechanism will produce asymmetry between the parents, in which mothers of affected offspring carry more copies of the susceptibility allele than fathers. There would be no distortion in transmissions to affected offspring. A simple extension of the same log-linear model accommodates such maternally mediated effects and allows them to be distinguished from direct effects due to the child's inherited genotype.[176] Families in which the genotype for a parent is missing (*e.g.*, due to nonparticipation or due to misidentified paternity) can also be fully used.[177,178]

The case-parent approach has several advantages over a case-control design. First, it requires only affected families, who are usually more willing than unaffected families to volunteer for study. By obviating the need for an independent control group, this approach also avoids some of the most problematic aspects of genetic case-control studies, basically because the untransmitted parental alleles are effectively serving as well-matched controls for the case offspring. Consequently, the case-parent approach is relatively robust against bias due to self-selection of controls. Also, the approach avoids bias due to genetic "population stratification" (when subgroups differ in both the prevalence of the allele and the baseline risk of disease), provided the analysis is conditional on parental genotypes. (Some investigators suggest that genetic stratification is not an important source of bias in diverse populations.[179]) Despite the absence of controls, the case-parent approach is similar in power to that of a case-control study with the same number of cases and an equal-size control group.[180]

One can also extend the model to look at effects due to *imprinting,* which occurs when a copy of the variant allele can be expressed differently depending on whether it came from the mother or the father.[177,178] Evidence is mounting, for example, that imprinting plays a role in autism.[181] Finally, statistical missing-data methods can be used to make full use of the data from incomplete triads,[177,178] even if the missing-data mechanism depends on the missing genotype.[182,183]

Regarding the maternal-fetal pair as the unit at risk leads naturally to questions about the potential for synergistic effects of the fetal and maternal genotypes, for example, Rh factor incompatibility. The log-linear model has been extended to detect such interactive causal mechanisms.[184] Incompatible maternal-fetal genotypes may also be related to risk of schizophrenia in the offspring.[185] Thus, the case-parent design combines opportunities to study maternal effects, parent-of-origin effects, and fetal-maternal interactions in one study—effects that would be difficult to elucidate with a classical case-control design.

The case-parent design does not permit the study of main effects of exposures unless controls are added. However, an extension of the log-linear model allows the exploration of gene-by-environment interaction,[186] the main effects of the fetal-maternal genotypes, and any departures from multiplicative joint effects between genotypes and categorical exposures. Either the mother, or the fetus/offspring, or both may be exposed to the relevant factor. Note that the design is retrospective, and the exposure obviously does not influence the transmission of alleles from parents to affected offspring. However, if a variant allele synergizes the effect of an exposure, then cases with the exposure will be relatively more likely to have inherited that allele from a heterozygous parent than will cases without the exposure.

Interactions between genotypes and continuous exposures, such as number of cigarettes smoked, can be studied in a closely related framework by looking for apparent "effects" of the offspring exposure on the patterns of allele transmission from parents to affected offspring,[187] assessed by polytomous logistic regression (see Chapter 20).

A third alternative in genetic family-based studies is a hybrid design, which exploits the best features of the case-parents approach and the population-based case-control approach. One recruits cases and their parents and also unrelated controls and their parents. The parents of controls are genotyped, but not the controls themselves, who provide only nongenetic information to the study.[188] Under the assumption that the disease is rare and that Mendelian transmission rates apply in the general population, this design permits efficient estimation of all risk-related parameters of interest under a multiplicative formulation. It is, however, susceptible to bias due to population stratification.

Quantitative traits such as birth weight can also be studied in place of dichotomous outcomes by using the same polytomous logistic regression described for assessing gene-by-exposure interaction but with the trait in place of the exposure. In such analysis, the outcome is the number of copies carried by the offspring, conditional on the parental genotypes, in relation to the value of the trait.[189-191] A convenient feature of this approach is that one need not assume Mendelian inheritance under the null, and thus one gains robustness against potential effects of the gene (and any genetic correlates) on gestational survival. The inference is based on whether the distribution of offspring genotypes, conditional on parental genotypes, varies across levels of the quantitative trait. Extensions also allow for the incorporation of trait data from multiple offspring from the same family.[189,190] (A more detailed account of family-based approaches is provided elsewhere).[192]

The availability of tools for genotyping will no doubt lead to still other options for the design of epidemiologic studies. Nevertheless, the original burst of optimism that came with the breaking of the human genetic code has largely dissipated. It has become clear that "agnostic" assessments of effects of single genetic variants will not succeed in fully explaining the heritability of traits and diseases. As new biologic hypotheses are framed, opportunities will expand for analysis of the interplay of genetic and environmental factors. Epigenetics and gene-by-gene interactions are also emerging as important players, and new methods will be needed to elucidate those complex mechanisms. This expanded research may have implications for the way we understand not just birth defects but many other problems of reproduction, pregnancy, and development.

APPENDIX

Formally, the proportional probabilities model for analysis of retrospective (pregnancy-based or attempt-based) or prospective (cohort study-based) time-to-pregnancy data is based on outcomes at each woman-cycle of observation:

$$\ln\left(\text{conception rate at cycle } i, \text{ given } E, X_1, X_2, \ldots, X_P\right) = c_i + \beta E + \beta_1 X_1 + \beta_2 X_2 + \beta_P X_P$$

where ln denotes the natural logarithm; the conception rate is the cycle-specific probability of pregnancy, given the couple is still at risk; E is the exposure of interest; and $X_1, X_2, \ldots, X_P$ denote P potential confounders. The parameter c_i denotes the baseline conception rate for the ith cycle; in effect, we establish a set of baseline stratum parameters to allow for the above-described decline in conception rate with attempt cycle. The fecundability ratio is estimated by exponentiating the estimated β from this model. Confidence intervals can be obtained by exponentiating the upper and lower confidence limits based on the estimated coefficient and its estimated standard error.

Because this is a generalized linear model (see Chapter 20), it can be fitted using standard software (GLIM, or SAS using the GENMOD procedure); however, one must force extra iterations to ensure that convergence has been achieved. One annoying feature of this model is that it can sometimes result in fitted probabilities that exceed 1.0 for individual couples, which occurs whenever their fitted linear predictor (the right-hand side of the above equation) exceeds 0. Although this is an undesirable feature in a model and can interfere with estimation of parameters, such invalid excursions seem to be rare in practice, unless the model is overparameterized or there are covariate outliers.

Other models can be used. The discrete-time model proposed by Cox[65] uses as the link function the log odds of the conception rate instead of its logarithm. Otherwise, the preceding formulation is unchanged. This alternative formulation is a logistic model and can be fitted using standard software, provided attempt cycle is entered as an unordered categorical (in SAS a *class*) variable. It is important, however, to be aware that when this Cox discrete-time model is used, the parameter being estimated by exponentiating β is now the fecundability-odds ratio, not the fecundability ratio. The fecundability ratio will always be closer to 1.0 than the fecundability-odds ratio, just as the risk ratio is closer than the odds ratio to 1.0. Because the outcome here is not rare, the two parameters may be quite different. The assumption that the fecundability ratio or, alternatively, the fecundability-odds ratio, is constant across time can be checked by examining in the respective model the coefficient for a product of the exposure and time (cycle number).

References

1. Gladen BC. On the role of "habitual aborters" in the analysis of spontaneous abortion. *Stat Med.* 1986;5:557-564.
2. Baird DD, Weinberg CR, Schwingl P, Wilcox AJ. Selection bias associated with contraceptive practice in time-to-pregnancy studies. *Ann NY Acad Sci.* 1994;709:156-164.
3. Wilcox AJ, Weinberg CR, O'Connor JF, et al. Incidence of early loss of pregnancy. *N Engl J Med.* 1988;319(4):189-194.
4. Hertz-Picciotto I, Pastore L, Beaumont J. Timing and patterns of exposures during pregnancy and their implications for study methods. *Am J Epidemiol.* 1996;143(6):597-607.
5. Golding J, Pembrey M, Jones R, Team AS. ALSPAC--the avon longitudinal study of parents and children. I. Study methodology. *Paediatr Perinat Epidemiol.* 2001;15(1):74-87.
6. Vrijheid M, Casas M, Bergstrom A, et al. European birth cohorts for environmental health research. *Environ Health Perspect.* 2012;120(1):29-37.
7. Magnus P, Birke C, Vejrup K, et al. Cohort profile update: the Norwegian mother and child cohort study (MoBa). *Int J Epidemiol.* 2016;45(2):382-388.
8. Weinberg CR, Baird DD, Rowland AS. Pitfalls inherent in retrospective time-to-event studies: the example of time to pregnancy. *Stat Med.* 1993;12(9):867-879.
9. Basso O, Christensen K, Olsen J. Higher risk of pre-eclampsia after change of partner. An effect of longer interpregnancy intervals? *Epidemiology.* 2001;12(6):624-629.
10. Skjaerven R, Wilcox AJ, Lie RT. The interval between pregnancies and the risk of preeclampsia. *N Engl J Med.* 2002;346(1):33-38.
11. Weinberg CR, Hertz-Picciotto I, Baird DD, Wilcox AJ. Efficiency and bias in studies of early pregnancy loss. *Epidemiology.* 1992;3(1):17-22.
12. Cho SI, Goldman MB, Ryan LM, et al. Reliability of serial urine HCG as a biomarker to detect early pregnancy loss. *Hum Reprod.* 2002;17(4):1060-1066.
13. Harmon QE, Basso O, Weinberg CR, Wilcox AJ. Two denominators for one numerator: the example of neonatal mortality. *Eur J Epidemiol.* 2018;33(6):523-530.
14. Joffe M. Biases in research on reproduction and women's work. *Intl J Epidemiol.* 1985;14(1):118-123.
15. Lie R, Wilcox A, Skjaerven R. A population-based study of the risk of recurrence of birth defects. *New Engl J Med.* 1995;331(1):1-4.
16. Laurence K, Miller J, Tennant G, Campbell H. Double-blind randomised controlled trial of folate treatment before conception to prevent recurrence of neural-tube defects. *Br Med J (Clin Res Ed).* 1981;282(6275):1509-1511.
17. Weinberg CR. Toward a clearer definition of confounding. *Am J Epidemiol.* 1993;137(1):1-8.
18. Greenland S. Quantifying biases in causal models: classical confounding vs collider-stratification bias. *Epidemiology.* 2003;14(3):300-306.
19. Basso O, Wilcox AJ, Weinberg CR. Birth weight and mortality: causality or confounding? *Am J Epidemiol.* 2006;164(4):303-311.
20. Wilcox AJ, Weinberg CR, Basso O. On the pitfalls of adjusting for gestational age at birth. *Am J Epidemiol.* 2011;174(9):1062-1068.
21. Ananth CV, Schisterman EF. Confounding, causality, and confusion: the role of intermediate variables in interpreting observational studies in obstetrics. *Am J Obstet Gynecol.* 2017;217(2):167-175.
22. Snowden JM, Basso O. Causal inference in studies of preterm babies: a simulation study. *BJOG.* 2018;125(6):686-692.
23. Basso O, Olsen J, Bisanti L, Juul S, Boldsen J. Are seasonal preferences in pregnancy planning a source of bias in studies of seasonal variation in reproductive outcomes? The European Study Group on Infertility and Subfecundity. *Epidemiology.* 1995;6(5):520-524.
24. Weinberg CR, Shi M, DeRoo LA, Basso O, Skjaerven R. Season and preterm birth in Norway: a cautionary tale. *Int J Epidemiol.* 2015;44(3):1068-1078.
25. Weinberg CR, Shi M, Basso O, et al. Season of conception, smoking, and preeclampsia in Norway. *Environ Health Perspect.* 2017;125(6):067022.
26. Tomova A, Robeva R, Kumanov P. Influence of the body weight on the onset and progression of puberty in boys. *J Pediatr Endocrinol Metab.* 2015;28(7-8):859-865.

27. Gold E, Bromberger J, Crawford S, et al. Factors associated with age at natural menopause in a multiethnic sample of midlife women. *Am J Epidemiol*. 2001;153(9):865-874.

28. Marshall W, Tanner M. Variations in pattern of pubertal changes in girls. *Arch Dis Child*. 1969;44:291-303.

29. Marshall WA, Tanner JM. Variations in the pattern of pubertal changes in boys. *Arch Dis Child*. 1970;45:13-23.

30. Rockette J, Lynch C, Buck G. Biomarkers for assessing reproductive development and health: Part I - pubertal development. *Environ Health Perspect*. 2004;112:105-112.

31. Baird DD, McConnaughey DR, Weinberg CR, et al. Application of a method for estimating day of ovulation using urinary estrogen and progesterone metabolites. *Epidemiology*. 1995;6(5):547-550.

32. Treloar AE, Boynton RE, Borghild GB, Behn BG, Brown BW. Variation of the human menstrual cycle through reproductive life. *Int J Fertil*. 1967;12(1):77-126.

33. Harlow SD, Zeger SL. An application of longitudinal methods to the analysis of menstrual diary data. *J Clin Epidemiol*. 1991;44(10):1015-1025.

34. Hornsby PP, Wilcox AJ, Weinberg CR, Herbst AL. Effects on the menstrual cycle of in utero exposure to diethylstilbestrol. *Am J Obstet Gynecol*. 1994;170(3):709-715.

35. https://www. acog.org/Clinical-Guidance-and-Publications/Committee-Opinions/Committee-on-Adolescent-Health-Care/Menstruation-in-Girls-and-Adolescents-Using-the-Menstrual-Cycle-as-a-Vital-Sign. Accessed August 10, 2020.

36. Harlow S, Ephross S. Epidemiology of menstruation and its relevance to women's health. *Epidemiologic Rev*. 1995;17(2):265-286.

37. Murphy SA, Bentley GR, O'Hanesian MA. An analysis for menstrual data with time-varying covariates. *Stat Med*. 1995;14(17):1843-1857.

38. Lisabeth L, Harlow SD, Lin X, Gillespie B, Sowers M. Sampling strategies for prospective studies of menstrual function. *Am J Epidemiol*. 2004;159(8):795-802.

39. Baird DD, Weinberg CR, Wilcox AJ, McConnaughey DR, Musey PI. Using the ratio of urinary oestrogen and progesterone metabolites to estimate day of ovulation. *Stat Med*. 1991;10(2):255-266.

40. Lu Y, Bentles G, Gann P, Hodges K, Chatterton R. Salivary estradiol and progsterone levels in conception and nonconception cycles in women: evaluation of a new assay for salivary estradiol. *Fertil Sterility*. 1999;71(5):863-868.

41. Deeley K, Noel J, Vieira AR. Comparative study of five commercially available saliva collection kits for DNA extraction. *Clin Lab*. 2016;62(9):1809-1813.

42. Krailo MD, Pike MC. Estimation of the distribution of age at natural menopause from prevalence data. *Am J Epidemiol*. 1983;117(3):356-361.

43. Brambilla DJ, McKinlay SM. A prospective study of factors affecting age at menopause. *J Clin Epidemiol*. 1989;42(11):1031-1039.

44. Weinberg CR. Infertility and the use of illicit drugs. *Epidemiology*. 1990;1(3):189-192.

45. Boivin J, Bunting L, Collins JA, Nygren KG. International estimates of infertility prevalence and treatment-seeking: potential need and demand for infertility medical care. *Hum Reprod*. 2007;22(6):1506-1512.

46. Tietze C. Fertility after discontinuation of intrauterine and oral contraception. *Int J Fertil*. 1968;13(4):385-389.

47. Baird DD, Wilcox AJ. Cigarette smoking associated with delayed conception. *J Am Med Assoc*. 1985;253(20):2979-2983.

48. Weinberg CR, Gladen BC. The beta-geometric distribution applied to comparative fecundability studies. *Biometrics*. 1986;42:547-560.

49. Baird DD, Wilcox AJ, Weinberg CR. Use of time to pregnancy to study environmental exposures. *Am J Epidemiol*. 1986;124(3):470-480.

50. Wise LA, Rothman KJ, Wesselink AK, et al. Male sleep duration and fecundability in a North American preconception cohort study. *Fertil Steril*. 2018;109(3):453-459.

51. Baird DD, Weinberg CR, Rowland AS. Reporting errors in time-to-pregnancy data collected with a short questionnaire. Impact on power and estimation of fecundability ratios. *Am J Epidemiol*. 1991;133(12):1282-1290.

52. Weinberg CR, Gladen BC, Wilcox AJ. Models relating the timing of intercourse to the probability of conception and the sex of the baby. *Biometrics*. 1994;50(2):358-367.

53. Zhou H, Weinberg CR, Wilcox AJ, Baird DD. A random-effects model for cycle viability in fertility studies. *J Am Stat Assoc*. 1996;91(436):1413-1422.

54. Dunson DB, Weinberg CR. Accounting for unreported and missing intercourse in human fertility studies. *Stat Med*. 2000;19(5):665-679.

55. Dunson DB, Weinberg CR. Modeling human fertility in the presence of measurement error. *Biometrics*. 2000;56(1):288-292.

56. Schantz JS, Fernandez C, Jukic AMZ. Menstrual cycle tracking applications and the potential for epidemiological research: a comprehensive review of the literature. *Curr Epidemiol Rep*. In press.

57. Basso O, Juul S, Olsen J. Time to pregnancy as a correlate of fecundity: differential persistence in trying to become pregnant as a source of bias. *Int J Epidemiol.* 2000;29(5):856-861.

58. Jukic AM, McConnaughey DR, Weinberg CR, Wilcox AJ, Baird DD. Long-term recall of time to pregnancy. *Epidemiology.* 2016;27(5):705-711.

59. Nguyen RH, Baird DD. Accuracy of men's recall of their partner's time to pregnancy. *Epidemiology.* 2005;16(5):694-698. doi:10.1097/01.ede.0000173038.93237.b3.

60. Bolumar R, Olsen J, Boldsen J; The European Study Group on Infertility and Subfecundity. Smoking reduces fecundity: a European multicenter study on infertility and subfecundity. *Am J Epidemiol.* 1996;143(6):578-587.

61. Joffe M, Villard L, Li Z, Plowman R, Vessey M. Long-term recall of time to pregnancy. *Fertil Sterility.* 1993;60(1):99-104.

62. Keiding N, Kvist K, Hartvig H, Tvede M, Juul S. Estimating time to pregnancy from current durations in a cross-sectional sample. *Biostatistics.* 2002;3(4):565-578.

63. Slama R, Ducot B, Carstensen L, et al. Feasibility of the current-duration approach to studying human fecundity. *Epidemiology.* 2006;17(4):440-449.

64. Sheps MC, Mencken JA. *Mathematical Models of Conception and Birth.* Chicago, IL: University of Chicago Press; 1973.

65. Cox D, Oakes D. *Analysis of Survival Data.* New York, NY: Chapman and Hall; 1984.

66. Hernan MA. The hazards of hazard ratios. *Epidemiology.* 2010;21(1):13-15.

67. Eijkemans MJC, Leridon H, Keiding N, Slama R. A systematic comparison of designs to study human fecundity. *Epidemiology.* 2018;30(1):120-129.

68. Weinberg CR, Baird DD, Wilcox AJ. Bias in retrospective studies of spontaneous abortion based on the outcome of the most recent pregnancy. *Ann NY Acad Sci.* 1994;709:280-286.

69. Weinberg CR, Baird DD, Wilcox AJ. Sources of bias in studies of time to pregnancy. *Stat Med.* 1994;13(5-7):671-681.

70. Juul S, Keiding N, Tvede M. Retrospectively sampled time-to-pregnancy data may make age-decreasing fecundity look increasing. European Infertility and Subfecundity Study Group. *Epidemiology.* 2000;11(6):717-719.

71. Schwingl PJ. *Prenatal Smoking Exposure in Relation to Female Adult Fecundability [Ph.D.].* Chapel Hill, NC: Department of Epidemiology, University of North Carolina at Chapel Hill; 1992.

72. Robins J, Blevins D, Ritter G, Wulfsohn M. G-estimation of the effect of prophylaxis therapy for pneumocystis carinii pneumonia on the survival of AIDS patients. *Epidemiology.* 1992;3:319-336.

73. Machtinger R, Gaskins AJ, Mansur A, et al. Association between preconception maternal beverage intake and in vitro fertilization outcomes. *Fertil Steril.* 2017;108(6):1026-1033.

74. Machtinger R, Gaskins AJ, Racowsky C, et al. Urinary concentrations of biomarkers of phthalates and phthalate alternatives and IVF outcomes. *Environ Int.* 2018;111:23-31.

75. Carignan CC, Minguez-Alarcon L, Williams PL, et al. Paternal urinary concentrations of organophosphate flame retardant metabolites, fertility measures, and pregnancy outcomes among couples undergoing in vitro fertilization. *Environ Int.* 2018;111:232-238.

76. Bonde JP, Ernst E, Jensen TK, et al. Relation between semen quality and fertility: a population-based study of 430 first-pregnancy planners. *Lancet.* 1998;352(9135):1172-1177.

77. Larsen L, Scheike T, Jensen T, et al. Computer-assisted semen analysis parameters as predictors for fertility of men from the general population. *Hum Reprod.* 2000;15(7):1562-1567.

78. Selevan S, Borkovec L, Slott V, et al. Semen quality and reproductive health of young Czech men exposed to seasonal air pollution. *Environ Health Perspect.* 2000;108(9):887-894.

79. Whorton D, Krauss RM, Marshall S, Milby TH. Infertility in male pesticide workers. *Lancet.* 1977;2(8051):1259-1261.

80. Oldereid NB, Wennerholm UB, Pinborg A, et al. The effect of paternal factors on perinatal and paediatric outcomes: a systematic review and meta-analysis. *Hum Reprod Update.* 2018;24(3):320-389.

81. Abbasi J. The paternal epigenome makes its mark. *J Am Med Assoc.* 2017;317(20):2049-2051.

82. Soubry A, Guo L, Huang Z, et al. Obesity-related DNA methylation at imprinted genes in human sperm: results from the TIEGER study. *Clin Epigenetics.* 2016;8:51.

83. Jenkins TG, James ER, Alonso DF, et al. Cigarette smoking significantly alters sperm DNA methylation patterns. *Andrology.* 2017;5(6):1089-1099.

84. Wu H, Estill MS, Shershebnev A, et al. Preconception urinary phthalate concentrations and sperm DNA methylation profiles among men undergoing IVF treatment: a cross-sectional study. *Hum Reprod.* 2017;32(11):2159-2169.

85. Wilcox AJ, Baird DD, Weinberg CR. Time of implantation of the conceptus and loss of pregnancy. *N Engl J Med.* 1999;340(23):1796-1799.

86. Goldhaber MK, Fireman BH. The fetal life table revisited: spontaneous abortion rates in three Kaiser-Permanente cohorts. *Epidemiology.* 1992;2:33-39.

87. Baird DD. The gestational timing of pregnancy loss: adaptive strategy? *Am J Hum Biol.* 2009;21(6):725-727.

88. Promislow JH, Baird DD, Wilcox AJ, Weinberg CR. Bleeding following pregnancy loss before 6 weeks' gestation. *Hum Reprod.* 2007;22(3):853-857.

89. Nybo Andersen AM, Wohlfahrt J, Christens P, Olsen J, Melbye M. Maternal age and fetal loss: population based register linkage study. *Br Med J.* 2000;320(7251):1708-1712.

90. Susser E. Spontaneous abortion and induced abortion: an adjustment for the presence of induced abortion when estimating the rate of spontaneous abortion from cross-sectional studies. *Am J Epidemiol.* 1983;117(3):305-308.

91. Magnus MC, Wilcox AJ, Morken N-H, Weinberg CR, Håberg SE. The role of maternal age and pregnancy history in risk of miscarriage: a prospective register-based study. *Br Med J.* 2019;364:1869.

92. Kline J, Stein Z, Susser M. *Conception to Birth: Epidemiology of Prenatal Development.* New York, NY: Oxford University Press; 1989:108-109.

93. Hertz-Picciotto I, Swan SH, Neutra RR, Samuels SJ. Spontaneous abortions in relation to consumption of tap water: an application of methods from survival analysis to a pregnancy follow-up study. *Am J Epidemiol.* 1989;130(1):79-93.

94. Wilcox AJ, Gladen BC. Spontaneous abortion: the role of heterogeneous risk and selective fertility. *Early Hum Dev.* 1982;7:165-178.

95. Greenland S, Pearl J, Robins JM. Causal diagrams for epidemiologic research. *Epidemiology.* 1999;10(1):37-48.

96. Howards PP, Schisterman EF, Heagerty PJ. Potential confounding by exposure history and prior outcomes: an example from perinata epidemiology. *Epidemiology.* 2007;18(5):544-551.

97. Howards PP, Schisterman EF, Poole C, Kaufman JS, Weinberg CR. "Toward a clearer definition of confounding" revisited with directed acyclic graphs. *Am J Epidemiol.* 2012;176(6):506-511.

98. Hoffman E, Sen P, Weinberg C. Within-cluster resampling. *Biometrika.* 2001;88:1121-1134.

99. Williamson J, Datta S, Satten G. Marginal analysis of clustered data when cluster size is informative. *Biometrics.* 2003;59(1):36-42.

100. Watier L, Richardson S, Hemon D. Accounting for pregnancy dependence in epidemiologic studies of reproductive outcomes. *Epidemiology.* 1997;8(6):629-636.

101. Olsen J, Andersen P. RE: accounting for pregnancy dependence in epidemiologic studies of pregnancy outcomes. *Epidemiology.* 1998;9(3):363.

102. Gourbin C, Masuy-Stroobant G. Registration of vital data - are live births and still births comparable all over Europe? *Bull World Health Organ.* 1995;73(4):449-460.

103. Kowaleski J. *State Definitions and Reporting Requirements for Live Births, Fetal Deaths and Induced Terminations of Pregnancy (1997 Revision).* Hyattsville, MD: National Center for Health Statistics; 1997.

104. MacDorman MF, Gregory EC. Fetal and perinatal mortality: United States, 2013. *Natl Vital Stat Rep.* 2015;64(8):1-24.

105. Anderson B, Silver B. Infant mortality in the Soviet Union: regional differences and measurement issues. *Popul Dev Rev.* 1986;12(4):705-738.

106. Yudkin PL, Wood L, Redman CW. Risk of unexplained stillbirth at different gestational ages. *Lancet.* 1987;1(8543):1192-1194.

107. Harmon QE, Huang L, Umbach DM, et al. Risk of fetal death with preeclampsia. *Obstet Gynecol.* 2015;125(3):628-635.

108. Donald I, Macvicar J, Brown TG. Investigation of abdominal masses by pulsed ultrasound. *Lancet.* 1958;1(7032):1188-1195.

109. Campbell S. A short history of sonography in obstetrics and gynaecology. *Facts Views Vis Obgyn.* 2013;5(3):213-229.

110. Hadlock FP, Harrist RB, Sharman RS, Deter RL, Park SK. "Estimation of fetal weight with the use of head, body, and femur measurements – a prospective study. *Am J Obstet Gynecol.* 1985;151(3):333-337.

111. Papageorghiou AT, Ohuma EO, Altman DG, et al. International standards for fetal growth based on serial ultrasound measurements: the Fetal Growth Longitudinal Study of the INTERGROWTH-21st Project. *Lancet.* 2014;384(9946):869-879.

112. Villar J, Papageorghiou AT, Pang R, et al. The likeness of fetal growth and newborn size across non-isolated populations in the INTERGROWTH-21st project: the fetal growth longitudinal study and newborn cross-sectional study. *Lancet Diabetes Endocrinol.* 2014;2(10):781-792.

113. Salomon LJ, Bernard JP, Duyme M, Buvat I, Ville Y. The impact of choice of reference charts and equations on the assessment of fetal biometry. *Ultrasound Obstet Gynecol.* 2005;25(6):559-565.

114. Buck Louis GM, Grewal J, Albert PS, et al. Racial/ethnic standards for fetal growth: the NICHD Fetal Growth Studies. *Am J Obstet Gynecol.* 2015;213(4):449.e1-449.e41.

115. Lopez-Espinosa MJ, Murcia M, Iniguez C, et al. Organochlorine compounds and ultrasound measurements of fetal growth in the INMA cohort (Spain). *Environ Health Perspect*. 2016;124(1):157-163.

116. Campbell S, Thoms A. Ultrasound measurement of the fetal head to abdomen circumference ratio in the assessment of growth retardation. *Br J Obstet Gynaecol*. 1977;84(3):165-174.

117. Nieto A, Matorras R, Villar J, Serra M. Neonatal morbidity associated with disproportionate intrauterine growth retardation at term. *J Obstet Gynaecol*. 1998;18(6):540-543.

118. Cheung YB, Yip PS, Karlberg JP. Size at birth and neonatal and postneonatal mortality. *Acta Paediatr*. 2002;91(4):447-452.

119. Leitner Y, Fattal-Valevski A, Geva R, et al. Neurodevelopmental outcome of children with intrauterine growth retardation: a longitudinal, 10-year prospective study. *J Child Neurol*. 2007;22(5):580-587.

120. Lao TT, Wong W. The neonatal implications of a high placental ratio in small-for-gestational age infants. *Placenta*. 1999;20(8):723-726.

121. Khalil A, Morales-Rosello J, Khan N, et al. Is cerebroplacental ratio a marker of impaired fetal growth velocity and adverse pregnancy outcome? *Am J Obstet Gynecol*. 2017;216(6):606.e1-606.e10.

122. Wilcox AJ. *Fertility and Pregnancy: An Epidemiologic Perspective*. New York, NY: Oxford University Press; 2010.

123. Joseph KS, Kramer MS. The fetuses-at-risk approach: survival analysis from a fetal perspective. *Acta Obstet Gynecol Scand*. 2018;97(4):454-465.

124. https://www.cdc.gov/nchs/fastats/births.htm. Accessed August 12, 2020.

125. Jackson D, White IR, Seaman S, Evans H, Baisley K, Carpenter J. Relaxing the independent censoring assumption in the Cox proportional hazards model using multiple imputation. *Stat Med*. 2014;33(27):4681-4694.

126. Olsen J, Basso O. Reproductive epidemiology. In: Wolfgang A, Iris P, eds. *Handbook of Epidemiology*. Berlin Heidelberg, NY: Springer-Verlag; 2004:1043-1110.

127. Wilcox A, Skjaerven R. Birthweight and perinatal mortality: the effect of gestational age. *Am J Public Health*. 1992;82:378-382.

128. Matthews T, MacDorman M, Thoma ME. Infant mortality statistics from the 2013 period linked birth/infant death data set. *Natl Vital Stat Rep*. 2015;64(9):1-30.

129. Lubchenco LO, Hansman C, Dressler M, Boyd E. Intrauterine growth as estimated from liveborn birthweight data at 24 to 42 weeks of gestation. *Pediatrics*. 1963;32:793-800.

130. Wilcox A. Birthweight and perinatal mortality: the effect of maternal smoking. *Am J Epidemiol*. 1993;137:1098-1104.

131. Hernandez-Diaz S, Schisterman EF, Hernan MA. The birth weight "paradox" uncovered? *Am J Epidemiol*. 2006;164(11):1115-1120.

132. Hernandez-Diaz S, Wilcox AJ, Schisterman EF, Hernan MA. From causal diagrams to birth weight-specific curves of infant mortality. *Eur J Epidemiol*. 2008;23(3):163-166.

133. Basso O, Wilcox AJ. Intersecting birth weight-specific mortality curves: solving the riddle. *Am J Epidemiol*. 2009;169(7):787-797.

134. Wilcox AJ, Russell IT. Birthweight and perinatal mortality: III. Towards a new method of analysis. *Int J Epidemiol*. 1986;15(2):188-196.

135. Wilcox A. On the importance – and the unimportance – of birthweight. *Int J Epidemiol*. 2001;30(6):1233-1241.

136. Hoover RN, Hyer M, Pfeiffer RM, et al. Adverse health outcomes in women exposed in utero to diethylstilbestrol. *N Engl J Med*. 2011;365(14):1304-1314.

137. Barker DJ. Human growth and cardiovascular disease. *Nestle Nutr Workshop Ser Pediatr Program*. 2008;61:21-38.

138. Olsen J, Melbye M, Olsen SF, et al. The Danish National Birth Cohort – its background, structure and aim. *Scand J Public Health*. 2001;29(4):300-307.

139. Weinberg CR. Invited commentary: Barker meets Simpson. *Am J Epidemiol*. 2005;161(1):33-35; discussion 36-37.

140. Gregg N. Congenital cataract following German measles in the mother. *Trans Ophthalmol Soc Aust*. 1941;3:35-46.

141. Brent R, ed. *The Complexities of Solving the Problem of Human Malformations. Teratogen Update: Environmentally Induced Birth Defect Risks*. New York, NY, AR Liss, Inc; 1986.

142. Herbst A, Ulfelder H, Poskanzer D. Adenocarcinoma of the vagina: association of maternal stilbestrol therapy with tumor appearance in young women. *New Eng J Med*. 1971;284:878-881.

143. Kubon C, Sivertsen A, Vindenes HA, Abyholm F, Wilcox A, Lie RT. Completeness of registration of oral clefts in a medical birth registry: a population-based study. *Acta Obstet Gynecol Scand*. 2007;86(12):1453-1457.

144. Kalter H, Warkany J. Congenital malformations (second of two parts). *N Engl J Med*. 1983;308(9):491-497.

145. Kalter H, Warkany J. Medical progress. Congenital malformations: etiologic factors and their role in prevention (first of two parts). *N Engl J Med*. 1983;308(8):424-431.

146. Newman CG. Teratogen update: clinical aspects of thalidomide embryopathy – a continuing preoccupation. *Teratology*. 1985;32(1):133-144.
147. Svensson E, Ehrenstein V, Norgaard M, et al. Estimating the proportion of all observed birth defects occurring in pregnancies terminated by a second-trimester abortion. *Epidemiology*. 2014;25(6):866-871.
148. Mackenzie SG, Lippman A. An investigation of report bias in a case-control study of pregnancy outcome. *Am J Epidemiol*. 1989;129(1):65-75.
149. Werler M, Pober B, Nelson K, Holmes L. Reporting accuracy among mothers of malformed and nonmalformed infants. *Am J Epidemiol*. 1989;129:415-421.
150. Swan S, Shaw G, Shulman J. Reporting and selection bias in case-control studies of congenital malformations. *Epidemiology*. 1992;3:356-363.
151. Rockenbauer M, Olsen J, Czeizel A, Pedersen L, Sorensen H; EuroMap Group. Recall bias in a case-control surveillance system on the use of medicine during pregnancy. *Epidemiology*. 2001;12(4):461-466.
152. Khoury M, James L, Flanders W, Erickson J. Interpretation of recurring weak associations obtained from epidemiologic studies of suspected human teratogens. *Teratology*. 1992;46:69-77.
153. Khoury M, James L, Erickson J. On the use of affected controls to address recall bias in case-control studies of birth defects. *Teratology*. 1994;49:273-281.
154. MacLehose RF, Olshan AF, Herring AH, et al. Bayesian methods for correcting misclassification: an example from birth defects epidemiology. *Epidemiology*. 2009;20(1):27-35.
155. MacLehose RF, Bodnar LM, Meyer CS, Chu H, Lash TL. Hierarchical semi-bayes methods for misclassification in perinatal epidemiology. *Epidemiology*. 2018;29(2):183-190.
156. Basso O, Olsen J, Christensen K. Recurrence risk of congenital anomalies – the impact of paternal, social, and environmental factors: a population-based study in Denmark. *Am J Epidemiol*. 1999;150(6):598-604.
157. Bonde JPE, Wilcox A. Ratio of boys to girls at birth. *BMJ*. 2007;334(7592):486-487.
158. Macmahon B, Pugh TF. Sex ratio of white births in the United States during the second World war. *Am J Hum Genet*. 1954;6(2):284-292.
159. Hansen D, Moller H, Olsen J. Severe periconceptional life events and the sex ratio in offspring: follow up study based on five national registers. *Br Med J*. 1999;319(7209):548-549.
160. Davis DL, Gottlieb MB, Stampnitzky JR. Reduced ratio of male to female births in several industrial countries: a sentinel health indicator? *J Am Med Assoc*. 1998;279(13):1018-1023.
161. Ding QJ, Hesketh T. Family size, fertility preferences, and sex ratio in China in the era of the one child family policy: results from national family planning and reproductive health survey. *Br Med J*. 2006;333(7564):371-373.
162. Adams MM, Elam-Evans LD, Wilson HG, Gilbertz DA. Rates of and factors associated with recurrence of preterm delivery. *J Am Med Assoc*. 2000;283(12):1591-1596.
163. Trogstad L, Skrondal A, Stoltenberg C, Magnus P, Nesheim BI, Eskild A. Recurrence risk of preeclampsia in twin and; singleton pregnancies. *Am J Med Genet A*. 2004;126A(1):41-45.
164. Lie R, Wilcox A, Skjærven R. A population-based study of risk of recurrence of birth defects. *N Eng J Med*. 1994;331:1-4.
165. Tollanes MC, Wilcox AJ, Lie RT, Moster D. Familial risk of cerebral palsy: population based cohort study. *Br Med J*. 2014;349:g4294.
166. Dekker GA, Robillard PY, Hulsey TC. Immune maladaptation in the etiology of preeclampsia: a review of corroborative epidemiologic studies. *Obstet Gynecol Surv*. 1998;53(6):377-382.
167. McGue M. When assessing twin concordance, use the probandwise not the pairwise rate. *Schizophr Bull*. 1992;18(2):171-176.
168. Nordstrom ML, Cnattingius S. Smoking habits and birthweights in two successive births in Sweden. *Early Hum Dev*. 1994;37(3):195-204.
169. Jensen MS, Toft G, Thulstrup AM, et al. Cryptorchidism concordance in monozygotic and dizygotic twin brothers, full brothers, and half-brothers. *Fertil Steril*. 2010;93(1):124-129.
170. Frisell T, Oberg S, Kuja-Halkola R, Sjolander A. Sibling comparison designs: bias from non-shared confounders and measurement error. *Epidemiology*. 2012;23(5):713-720.
171. Sjolander A, Frisell T, Kuja-Halkola R, Oberg S, Zetterqvist J. Carryover effects in sibling comparison designs. *Epidemiology*. 2016;27(6):852-858.
172. Sjolander A, Zetterqvist J. Confounders, mediators, or colliders: what types of shared covariates does a sibling comparison design control for? *Epidemiology*. 2017;28(4):540-547.
173. Mitchell L. Differentiating between fetal and maternal genotypic effects, using the transmission test for linkage disequilibrium (letter). *Am J Hum Genet*. 1997;60:1006-1007.
174. Weinberg CR, Wilcox AJ, Lie RT. A log-linear approach to case-parent triad data: assessing effects of disease genes that act directly or through maternal effects, and may be subject to parental imprinting. *Am J Hum Gen*. 1998;62(4):969-978.
175. Spielman RS, McGinnis RE, Ewens WJ. Transmission test for linkage disequilibrium: the insulin gene region and insulin-dependent diabetes mellitus (IDDM). *Am J Hum Genet*. 1993;52(3):506-516.

176. Wilcox AJ, Weinberg CR, Lie RT. Distinguishing the effects of maternal and offspring genes through studies of "case-parent triads". *Am J Epidemiol.* 1998;148(9):893-901.

177. Weinberg CR. Allowing for missing parents in genetic studies of case-parent triads. *Am J Hum Genet.* 1999;64(4):1186-1193.

178. Weinberg CR. Methods for detection of parent-of-origin effects in genetic studies of case-parents triads. *Am J Hum Genet.* 1999;65(1):229-235.

179. Wacholder S, Rothman N, Caporaso N. Counterpoint: bias from population stratification is not a major threat to the validity of epidemiological studies of common polymorphisms and cancer. *Cancer Epidemiol Biomarkers Prev.* 2002;11(6):513-520.

180. Lee W. Genetic association studies of adult-onset diseases using case-spouse and case-offspring designs. *Am J Epidemiol.* 2003;158(11):1023-1032.

181. Kopsida E, Mikaelsson MA, Davies W. The role of imprinted genes in mediating susceptibility to neuropsychiatric disorders. *Horm Behav.* 2011;59(3):375-382.

182. Allen AS, Rathouz PJ, Satten GA. Informative missingness in genetic association studies: case-parent designs. *Am J Hum Genet.* 2003;72(3):671-680.

183. Chen YH. New approach to association testing in case-parent designs under informative parental missingness. *Genet Epidemiol.* 2004;27(2):131-140.

184. Sinsheimer J, Palmer C, Woodward J. Detecting genotype combinations that increase risk for disease: maternal-fetal genotype incompatibility test. *Genet Epidemiol.* 2003;24(1):1-13.

185. Palmer C, Turunen J, Sinsheimer J, et al. RHD maternal-fetal genotype incompatibility increases schizophrenia susceptibility. *Am J Hum Genet.* 2002;71:1312-1319.

186. Umbach DM, Weinberg CR. The use of case-parent triads to study joint effects of genotype and exposure. *Am J Hum Genet.* 2000;66(1):251-261.

187. Kistner EO, Shi M, Weinberg CR. Using cases and parents to study multiplicative gene-by-environment interaction. *Am J Epidemiol.* 2009;170(3):393-400.

188. Weinberg CR Umbach DM. A hybrid design for studying genetic influences on risk of diseases with onset early in life. *Am J Hum Genet.* 2005;77(4):627-636.

189. Kistner E, Weinberg CR. A method for identifying genes related to a quantitative trait, incorporating multiple siblings and missing parents. *Genet Epidemiol.* 2005;29(2):155-165.

190. Kistner EO, Weinberg CR. Method for using complete and incomplete trios to identify genes related to a quantitative trait. *Genet Epidemiol.* 2004;27(1):33-42.

191. Laird N, Lange C. Family-based designs in the age of large-scale gene-association studies. *Nat Rev Genet.* 2006;7:385-394.

192. Borgan Ø, Breslow N, Chatterjee N, Gail MH, Scott A, Wild CJ. *Handbook of Statistical Methods for Case-Control Studies.* Boca Raton; London; New York: Chapman and Hall/CRC; 2018.

CHAPTER 34

Psychiatric Epidemiology

Katherine M. Keyes, Sharon B. Schwartz, and Ezra S. Susser

Katherine M. Keyes, Sharon B. Schwartz, and Ezra S. Susser

PART I: WHAT IS A PSYCHIATRIC DISORDER?

Psychiatric epidemiology pertains primarily to the epidemiology of disorders that are manifest in disturbances of thoughts, feelings, and behaviors. Psychiatric epidemiologists seek to understand the distribution and determinants of such disorders in populations, how to prevent these disorders and mitigate their course. As psychiatric disorders are considered among the leading causes of disability worldwide[1] and are interwoven with so many other disorders,[2-4] these goals are significant for public health. Moreover, people with severe mental disorders are among the most disadvantaged and vulnerable populations across the globe; hence, these goals are also significant for the moral meter of society.

In terms of epidemiologic methods, the distinctive character of psychiatric epidemiology derives, in large part, from the challenge of defining and measuring psychiatric disorders. The response to this challenge shaped not only the history and present state of psychiatric epidemiology, but also the contributions it has made to theories and methods used in other fields of epidemiology. We begin, therefore, by posing the question: What is a psychiatric disorder?

As a starting point, we offer a current working definition from the most recent version of the *Diagnostic and Statistical Manual of Mental Disorders (DSM)*, p. 20-21[5]:

> "A mental disorder is a syndrome characterized by clinically significant disturbance in an individual's cognition, emotion regulation, or behavior that reflects a dysfunction in the psychological, biological, or developmental processes underlying mental functioning. Mental disorders are usually associated with significant distress in social, occupational, or other important activities. An expectable or culturally approved response to a common stressor or loss, such as the death of a loved one, is not a mental disorder. Socially deviant behavior (*e.g.*, political, religious, or sexual) and conflicts that are primarily between the individual and society are not mental disorders unless the deviance or conflict results from a dysfunction in the individual, as described above."

This excerpt highlights three key features of psychiatric disorders. First, these disorders are generally defined by symptom constellations without corresponding biological markers of psychological or physiological disruption. Second, the disorder symptoms are in domains popularly considered "of the mind" rather than "of the body." Third, to have diagnostic meaning, the symptoms must be contextualized within both their consequences for the individual as well as societal expectations. Although the *DSM* is but one nosology for psychiatric disorders and is primarily used in clinical practice in the United States, other nosologies have definitions with similar features. This includes, most notably, the International Classification of Disease used in most parts of the world outside of the United States.[6]

These features of psychiatric disorders make their diagnosis fraught with complexity and hazard. On the one hand, psychiatric disorders are accompanied by considerable suffering. They make it more difficult to function in central domains of work and relationships and are associated with risk for physical disorders, suicide, and other sources of mortality.[2-4] A diagnosis can provide comfort, a sense of control over baffling symptoms, and access to treatment. On the other hand, partly due to these features, a psychiatric diagnosis can also be a source of stigma and exclusion. Being labeled with a psychiatric diagnosis can lead to difficulties in employment and social relationships even in the absence of disabling psychiatric symptoms.[7] Psychiatric diagnoses can be wielded for social control, a way for those in power to punish individuals for socially deviant behavior.[8]

Differentiating the "Normal" From the "Abnormal"

Psychiatric disorders are currently diagnosed by signs and symptoms related to cognition, emotion regulation, and behavior that frequently overlap normal fluctuations across individuals and within persons over time. For example, sadness, a core feature of major depressive disorder, is also a normal human response to life events and circumstances. Distinguishing the boundaries of normal variation from those of disorder is difficult and value laden.[8] For example, responses to the death of a loved one, such as frequent crying, trouble sleeping, and loss of enjoyment in usual activities, could meet criteria for major depressive disorder. While recognizing the legitimacy of bereavement as an appropriate response, there is controversy about the normalcy of the length of the response and its severity. Such controversies about the delineation of the normal from the abnormal are both scientific (*e.g.*, controversies about the conditions under which the symptoms represent an underlying dysfunction) and value laden (*e.g.*, societal variability in bereavement norms). As global mental health increases in prominence, cross-cultural variations in values and norms loom large in these debates.

Furthermore, the core symptoms of psychiatric disorders—thoughts, feelings, and behaviors—are central to concepts of the self. In Western cultures, at least, it is often easier to think of a disease in our bodies as an affliction that falls upon us than a disease of our mind, which in some central way speaks to who we are. Therefore, individuals often resist the disorder label, contending that their symptoms are a different way of being, rather than a sign of disorder. For example, some individuals on the autism spectrum reframe their diagnosis, which includes assessments of the difficulty of social interaction and communication, as a label reflecting the hegemony of "neurotypicals" in defining what is normal. There are also movements to resist labels of schizophrenia, and defend anorexia as a "lifestyle choice."[9,10]

Such resistance is not unique to psychiatric disorders, as seen in debates about the role of cochlear implants in the Deaf Community, or limb-lengthening procedures for dwarfism.[11,12] Here too the boundaries between disorder and identity are powerful. However, these issues are far more central and pervasive for psychiatric disorders. Because psychiatric disorders can impair cognition and judgment, it is easier to discredit the opinions of psychiatric patients about their symptoms and treatments.

These debates about disorder boundaries arise between not only the labelers and those who are labeled, but also among prominent medical insiders. For example, the editors of the previous version of the *DSM* contend that they created an epidemic of attention-deficit disorder and childhood bipolar disorder through diagnostic criteria that were too liberal. The concept of "diagnostic creep" and the labeling of an ever-growing swath of behaviors as disordered is a concern within the profession.[13] Other leaders within the profession acknowledge this hazard but argue that the undertreatment of psychiatric disorders across the globe is presently the overriding concern.[14]

Differentiating the "Mad" From the "Bad"

Historically, a label of madness has been used to discredit, isolate, and punish those who were seen as threatening, different, or inconvenient.[15] For example, drapetomania, a disorder label given to enslaved people who try to escape their captivity, made the desire for freedom an indication of a mental illness. In a similar way, hysteria was a diagnostic label used to justify the institutionalization of women who rejected their confining social roles. Labeling political dissenters as mentally ill and controversies around "homosexuality" and forced treatment show how the power of a psychiatric label makes their boundaries extraordinarily consequential.

Diagnostic labels are also used to mitigate the consequences of one's actions. The impaired judgment assumed to arise from some psychiatric symptoms, such as those related to psychosis, mitigates the consequences of acts which would otherwise be attributed to criminality or the result of bad personality characteristics such as a lack of will or discipline. Advocacy for the recognition of posttraumatic stress disorder for war combatants is an example where the goal was not only to obtain treatment but also to shift the label from a personal deficit to a disorder.[15] The expansion of addictive disorders is another example where the mental disorder label is seen as potentially beneficial, by changing a label of "bad behavior" into a label of illness.

The *DSM* definition of psychiatric disorders is an attempt to navigate this perilous terrain of identifying and diagnosing psychiatric disorders. Core to the definition is a relatively objective medical component, that there must be an internal dysfunction. However, the requirement for distress or disability is a nod to the difficulty in identifying this component. Currently, no objective criteria delineate such internal dysfunctions; the careful language about distinguishing disorder from mere deviance is an attempt to avoid past abuses in the application of the disorder label to behavior that is merely socially unacceptable. A definitive operationalization of this definition and rules for distinguishing between normal and abnormal symptoms remain elusive.

PART II: EMERGENCE AND CONSOLIDATION OF PSYCHIATRIC EPIDEMIOLOGY

To establish psychiatric epidemiology as a field of research, investigators had to contend with two central challenges emphasized throughout this chapter: how to define and measure "psychiatric disorders," and how to identify people who have psychiatric disorders but have not been treated. Here we select a few key developments to illustrate the evolution of the field, focusing primarily though not exclusively on the United States.

Early History: Up to 1949

During the 19th century, "insanity" was a prominent concern in social reform, public health, and epidemiology.[16] Studies of insanity were, however, largely confined to people in asylums, and nosologies were in the early stages of differentiation.[17,18] Moreover, many people in asylums had conditions that are not currently classified as "psychiatric disorders," such as epilepsy, late-stage neurosyphilis (general paresis), and pellagra.[16] Nonetheless, a few pioneers began to lay a platform for psychiatric epidemiology, by ascertaining and studying people with "insanity" who were living outside of asylums, and following people after they left asylums.[19-25]

More differentiated psychiatric nosologies emerged in the 20th century.[16,18,26-28] In parallel, the population of asylums changed alongside advances in medicine, such as the introduction of a treatment for syphilis.[16] Between World War I and II, studies of mental disorders began to examine potential determinants such as social ecology, familial transmission, migration, and biological factors like infections and nutritional deficiencies.[17,29] In a classic example, sociologists Faris and Dunham, from the Chicago School of Social Ecology,[30] found that schizophrenia hospital admissions were more common in "disorganized" inner city Chicago neighborhoods and among people residing in neighborhoods where they were different from others (*e.g.*, Blacks living in mainly White areas, and Whites living in mainly Black areas). This work illustrates the discipline's roots in sociology and its early adoption of thinking about causes at multiple levels of organization. Indeed, their work was adumbrated by the work of sociologist Emile Durkheim, who framed the rate of suicide as a "social fact" that reflected the social characteristics of a particular society.[31]

Experiences during World War II also suggested that psychiatric disorders were more common and more treatable than previously recognized. Screening scales identified psychological impairment in a large proportion of potential recruits and frontline treatments for "war neuroses" enabled many soldiers to return to combat. These experiences provided a major impetus for psychiatric epidemiology in the United States and shifted the attention of psychiatrists toward mental disorders and stressful experiences in the general population.[32] By the late 1940s, the training of psychiatrists had accelerated, practice outside of asylums increased, and the National Institute of Mental Health had been established.[33] In this same period, the larger field of epidemiology was shifting its focus to noncommunicable diseases.

Against this backdrop, the subspecialty of psychiatric epidemiology began to form its identity. A signal event was a roundtable convened by the Milbank Memorial Fund in 1949, with the express purpose to help bring that about.[34] A key participant (Ernest Gruenberg) later remarked: "The best work which had been done previously had not been done in the name of 'epidemiology'…They were like the man in Moliere's play who had been speaking prose all his life and did not know it."[34]

Maturation of the Field: The 1950s to the 1980s

From the many lines of research that contributed to the maturation of psychiatric epidemiology, we select three: community surveys of psychiatric disorders, international studies of schizophrenia, and birth cohort studies of early brain development. These are chosen to illustrate different ways in which the central challenges were addressed and to represent distinct threads within psychiatric epidemiology. For a broader perspective of other areas of the discipline such as developmental, genetic, and lifecourse epidemiology, see referenced texts.[35-43]

Community Surveys of Mental Disorders

Recognizing that most people with psychiatric disorders are not treated, investigators turned to community surveys to describe the range, frequency, and severity of psychiatric disorders in populations. Sophisticated community surveys were fielded in the 1950s, using sampling methods and assessments that went far beyond those used in earlier studies. Most influential were the Midtown Manhattan Mental Health Study[44] and the Stirling County Study of Psychiatric Disorder and Sociocultural Environment conducted in Nova Scotia.[45] The Midtown Manhattan study, for example, drew a random sample of adult residents of a central area of Manhattan and used "allied professionals" (*e.g.*, social workers) to administer surveys and psychiatrists to rate current mental health across a spectrum of severity based on the interview and other available information (*e.g.*, records). Compatible with other studies at the time and later, about 23% were rated as having disabling mental health symptoms and being in need of professional help, but only a minority of these individuals had seen a mental health professional.

Both the Midtown Manhattan and Stirling County study were collaborations among psychiatrists, psychologists, sociologists, and anthropologists.[16,33] Thought leaders such as Alexander Leighton, who spearheaded the Stirling County Study,[45] theorized that sociocultural influences on mental health were paramount to their distributions in the population and argued that the focus of psychiatric epidemiology should be broad, encompassing the full range of mental health and illness in the general population. From the beginning, psychiatric epidemiology advanced a multilevel, community-oriented life course approach, making psychiatric epidemiology among the disciplines of epidemiology at the forefront of current approaches to understanding disease and illness from a social perspective.

The results of these community surveys were revealing, but often received with skepticism. Studies used different measures of symptoms and impairment, a major source of variability in their results.[46] Also, the absence of diagnoses ran counter to the trend in epidemiology and medicine. Increasingly, psychiatric epidemiologists perceived a need to align with other fields of epidemiology by defining discrete diagnoses as the dependent variable, and examining multiple independent variables as potential causes. By the 1970s, a paradigm shift was occurring in psychiatric epidemiology, heralded by an emphasis on specific diagnostic categories. In 1980, this shift was solidified when the American Psychiatric Association published the *DSM-III*.[47-50] Shortly thereafter, the shift found expression in the Epidemiologic Catchment Area (ECA) study of the 1980s.[51] Elaboration of the ECA and subsequent evolution of community surveys are described in Part III.

International Studies of Schizophrenia

Schizophrenia emerged in the 20th century as a hallmark psychiatric disorder, and two WHO studies were enormously influential in laying a foundation for the epidemiology of schizophrenia.[52] The first, the International Pilot Study of Schizophrenia (IPSS), launched in the 1960s, took up the challenge of defining and measuring schizophrenia.[53] The IPSS was preceded by the "US-UK study," which revealed a remarkable discrepancy between diagnoses made in the United States and the United Kingdom on patients with similar conditions; more affective disorders were diagnosed in the United Kingdom and more schizophrenia in the United States.[54] These results highlighted the need for diagnoses that were reliable across different raters. At the same time, a strong "antipsychiatry" movement was questioning the very existence of schizophrenia as a disorder rather than a label for deviant behaviors in Western cultures.[55] In this context, it was essential to test whether schizophrenia could be reliably identified using the same approach in a variety of cultures.

The IPSS was conducted across nine socioculturally diverse locales, including three in "developing" countries. At that time, terms such as global health, global mental health, and low-,middle-, high-income country, were not in use. In the field known as international health, it was common to label nonindustrialized countries (many of which were former colonies) as "developing" and industrialized countries as "developed". These terms fell into disfavor with the advent of global health. This was in part because of objections to the implication that developing countries were on the same path as developed countries but lagged behind. The "developing" countries in the WHO studies would now be considered low- and middle- income countries (LMIC) according to the World Bank Classification system. A detailed semistructured interview, the Present State Examination, was the centerpiece of an extensive diagnostic evaluation of psychiatric patients. Psychiatrists were trained to use it in comparable ways within as well as across locales. The results indicated that essentially the same syndrome could be identified as schizophrenia in all locales and that the diagnosis could be made with acceptable reliability by different psychiatrists. The IPSS also found that at 2-year follow-up, patients in developing countries with fewer resources were faring better than those in developed countries with more resources. The investigators recognized that this perplexing finding could be due to differential selection into treatment across settings, but it was consistent with some prior reports and could not simply be dismissed.

The IPSS was followed in the 1980s by the WHO Determinants of Outcome of Severe Mental Disorders, conducted across 13 locales in 10 countries, often referred to as the Ten Country Study.[56] The Ten Country Study sought to examine the determinants of variation in both incidence and outcome of schizophrenia across socioculturally diverse settings. The detection of causes in an incident sample would represent a leap toward alignment with other realms of epidemiology, but required major innovations in methods. Previously, studies of "incidence" relied on first hospital admissions (at best), but such admissions may have occurred long after the start of outpatient treatment or informal health care (*e.g.*, traditional healers). Still another dilemma was that the specific diagnosis was not always evident at first contact, but required longitudinal data. Accordingly, the Ten Country Study introduced a novel "first contact" method for estimating "treated incidence" of schizophrenia. People with possible psychoses were identified at all points of first contact with any kind of health services (including general practitioners and traditional healers) and then administered standardized diagnostic assessments by psychiatrists, at first contact and at 2-year follow-up.

Even now, this approach remains the gold standard for incidence studies of schizophrenia. It is, however, challenging to implement[57-59] and is not applicable to settings where most people with schizophrenia do not receive any kind of treatment.[60]

A surprising result from the Ten Country study was that incidence did not vary a great deal across diverse settings. Another was that 2-year outcomes were indeed better in developing than developed country settings. Although both results have been strongly critiqued, the innovation in methods has stood the test of time and is continually being refined for better application.

Birth Cohort Studies of Early Brain Development

Some areas of research in psychiatric epidemiology could not easily be brought into accord with the approach to defining mental disorders represented in the *DSM-III*. Among them were studies of causes that were theorized to manifest in a variety of ways, including but not limited to "psychiatric disorders." The manifestations of psychiatric disorders were sometimes classified as secondary to a medical condition, and research on these topics tended to migrate to other fields, such as neuroepidemiology or environmental epidemiology. Yet psychiatric epidemiologists did not relinquish their interest in such research, though it often fell outside the dominant focus of the field. Birth cohort studies of early brain development provide an example.

At another significant conference on psychiatric epidemiology in 1969, Ernest Gruenberg (also quoted above) proposed that many questions framed in terms of "mental disorders" in 1949 could now be approached "as part of a complex of consequences of certain types of infections… chromosomal abnormalities…nutritional deficiencies…" [34] Another renowned figure in the history of psychiatric epidemiology, Benjamin Pasamanick, took a similarly cross-cutting perspective.[61] He was concerned with neuropsychiatric outcomes ranging from intellectual disability to cerebral palsy to schizophrenia, and his work helped to motivate the Collaborative Perinatal Project, a >50,000 birth cohort born 1959 to 1966 across 13 sites in the United States, with follow-up starting in pregnancy and continuing up to age 7 years.[62] As a third example, Stein et al. (1975) focused on a range of neurodevelopmental outcomes in their study of prenatal effects of the Dutch Hunger Winter of 1944-1945 on military inductees' cognitive performance at age 18 years, as well as on congenital neural defects, personality disorders, and other outcomes.[63] This thread of research in psychiatric epidemiology emerged partly through connections to subfields of epidemiology that focused on sets of causes (*e.g.*, nutritional epidemiology) rather than specific outcomes. Nonetheless, for these investigators, the outcomes of interest were primarily (though not entirely) in the neuropsychiatric domain, broadly defined.

Psychiatric epidemiologists continue to engage in birth cohort studies of early brain development that encompass but are not limited to outcomes defined as mental disorders (see Part III). Sometimes these studies fit emerging paradigms that seek to identify an underlying pathophysiology and trace a range of resulting psychiatric and other manifestations, rather than focusing on causes of specific predefined symptom clusters (see Part V).

PART III: MEASURING FREQUENCY, CAUSES, AND CONSEQUENCES OF PSYCHIATRIC DISORDERS

The difficulties of demarcating psychiatric disorders, and the social consequences of a psychiatric diagnosis, have shaped the general contours of our field and also shape the specific methodological strategies used for measuring incidence and prevalence, identifying causes, and examining the secondary consequences of disorders.

One immediate manifestation of the general diagnostic problem, relevant to any study of psychiatric disorders, and certainly of incidence, is the difficulty in answering the question: When does a disorder begin? Is it the first appearance of symptoms, the combination of several symptoms, or a particular set of hallmark symptoms?

Accepted nosologies provide guideposts to answer these questions for specific disorders, yet are not always sufficient. Given high rates of comorbidity, is the incidence of a particular disorder relevant, or should we be assessing the beginning of any disorder? Often symptoms of severe psychological distress can be traced to childhood, even if the constellation of symptoms that constitute a diagnosis are not aggregated until adulthood. Furthermore, the demarcation between a risk factor for disorder and the start of disorder itself can be blurry (*e.g.*, childhood anxiety is a "risk factor" for adolescent depression, but could easily be conceptualized as part of the same underlying pathology). Like many issues in psychiatric epidemiology, these questions are not unique to psychiatric disorders. Indeed, throughout much of chronic disease epidemiology, the issue of when illness begins stymies research efforts. As with other disciplines, questions of disorder onset do not have single answers, and the problem driving a particular research effort will guide how and when to "count" a disorder as beginning. Consequently, research efforts to count cases use a wide variation of definitions for disorder onset, which are reflected in the different study designs deployed.

Measuring Incidence and Frequency

Three main study designs have been used to estimate incidence and prevalence: samples drawn from individuals in treatment for a particular disorder or set of disorders, longitudinal cohorts drawn from the community, and cross-sectional surveys of the population. The choice of design depends on the proportion of individuals who receive treatment for the disorder under investigation, the difficulty in assessing the disorder in the community, and whether the study goal requires measuring incidence, or if a prevalence measure would suffice.

Individuals in Treatment

Studies of individuals in treatment provide reasonable estimates of incidence and prevalence, as in many areas of medicine, only when most people with a disorder are treated. The proportion treated depends partly on access to treatment, which varies widely across countries, as well as within countries by region, socioeconomic status, and other factors. Treatment tends to be most accessible in high-income countries with universal health care and well-developed services for individuals with psychiatric disorders, and least accessible in low-income countries with minimal mental health services.[64] The proportion treated in "formal" mental health services also depends upon how disabling the disorder/s tends to be and upon attitudes toward being treated for the psychiatric disorder/s under study, which may be influenced by symptom severity, stigma associated with treatment, cultural concepts of mental illness, and preference for alternative modes of treatment such as traditional healers or informal family support.

   In countries where treatment is most accessible, the utility of treated samples for understanding incidence and prevalence is optimized when there are comprehensive registries of treatment contacts and diagnoses that can be linked across multiple registry systems, as is the case in an increasing number of countries.[57,65,66] These registries have been particularly illuminating for psychotic disorders, because people with these disorders—especially those with disabling or disruptive symptoms—are more likely to be channeled into formal medical systems. For estimates of treated incidence, "first contact" designs complement registry data with more in-depth information or substitute for it where there are no registry data (see Part II). Registries are also increasingly used for attention deficit hyperactivity disorder,[67] and for autism spectrum disorders,[68] with the caution that treatment utilization is changing rapidly and varies across countries, leaving potential for either over- or underascertainment.[69,70] Yet in virtually all countries, psychiatric disorders such as depression and anxiety remain substantially undertreated, and therefore, treatment registries yield underestimates of incidence and prevalence. While treatment utilization for such disorders has rapidly escalated in many countries in the past two decades,[71] attributable in part to the availability of antidepressant and antianxiety medications, the overall proportion of affected individuals who receive treatment remains low.

Longitudinal Cohorts

Alternative designs for estimating incidence and prevalence are those that assess disorders in the community, including longitudinal cohort studies. Conducting a longitudinal community study is difficult and expensive, requiring strong participation rates among individuals with disorders that are often associated with social withdrawal and housing transience. Long-term and intergenerational studies also depend upon sustaining a strong study team and funding source for long periods. Notwithstanding the difficulties, a wealth of high-quality cohorts have been established to assess incidence and monitor the course of disorders over time.

   Canonical studies of psychiatric disorders in the community often begin in the prenatal period, at birth, or in early childhood and follow individuals with regular assessments. Examples include the Dunedin Multidisciplinary Health and Development Study,[72] the Avon Longitudinal Study of Parents and Children,[73] and the Great Smoky Mountains Study.[74] Recently established cohorts are sometimes much larger in size and incorporate more biological and genetic data; for example, the Norwegian Mother and Child Cohort has been following more than 115,000 children since the prenatal period and has archived biological specimens on mother, father, and child.[75,76] Generally, these cohorts study a range of other health outcomes alongside psychiatric disorders as well as a continuum of psychiatric symptoms, harking back to our discussion of birth cohorts in Part II.

Well-replicated results from these cohorts confirm many conclusions from the mid-20th century studies: disabling psychiatric disorders are common, there is wide variation in the average age of onset among different disorders and symptoms, and there is considerable variation in the age of onset around the mean age for individual disorders. Disorders that commonly have onset in childhood include neurodevelopmental disorders such as autism and attention-deficit hyperactivity disorder, as well as many anxiety disorders including specific phobia and separation anxiety. In adolescence, mood disorders, such as major depression and dysthymia, tend to increase. Young adulthood is also a high-risk developmental period for many disorders, including substance use disorders. Notwithstanding these broad patterns, modal onset and course are not immutable characteristics of disorders and can vary across time and place.

Cross-Sectional Studies

Cross-sectional studies have been among the most widely used designs in psychiatric epidemiology. Cross-sectional studies generally provide prevalence estimates from a single time point of assessment, although some studies attempt to estimate onset through retrospective reporting, or estimate new episode onset by conducting follow-ups of the survey sample. For common psychiatric disorders that are often undertreated, assessments from cross-sectional surveys provide useful information about the distribution and correlates of psychiatric disorders in population settings. However, standard designs for cross-sectional studies (and indeed, community-based longitudinal studies) are traditionally not well suited to estimate prevalence for disorders that are less common and more difficult to assess via structured interviews (*e.g.*, schizophrenia, autism spectrum disorders) [77]; efforts are underway to develop surveys for this purpose.[78]

Among the first large-scale psychiatric epidemiological studies of the general population in the United States was the Epidemiologic Catchment Area (ECA) study. The ECA was developed across five study sites in geographically diverse cities.[79] It included sampling strategies to recruit participants from all accessible settings—including households, hospitals, and homeless shelters—and provided foundational information on the prevalence and distribution of diagnosed psychiatric disorders. In contrast, later US prevalence studies, such as the National Comorbidity Studies and the National Epidemiological Survey on Alcohol and Related Conditions, used complex survey designs.[80-82] In these studies, geographic areas of the United States are divided into segments, and then smaller geographic areas and households are sampled within those segments; hard to reach groups are often oversampled. One drawback is that the sampling frames for these studies include only individuals living in households, which may result in underestimates of people with psychotic disorders and other conditions who are overrepresented in institutional settings.[83] Increasingly, cross-sectional studies are conducted globally as well. The WHO World Mental Health Surveys, a prominent example, used sophisticated sampling strategies to assess prevalence of psychiatric disorders in 27 countries worldwide.[84]

A modification of the standard cross-sectional design, "two-stage" case ascertainment,[85] helps to address the difficulties in diagnosis of conditions such as schizophrenia and autism spectrum disorders. In this approach, individuals are screened to identify potential cases; a small sample of those who are screened negative and a larger sample of those screened positive (*i.e.*, potential cases) are then selected for a full diagnostic assessment. Although not used in the most prominent US studies, this design has been employed to good effect in global mental health research.[86,87]

Measurement of Disorder

The current paradigm for describing symptoms and assembling them into diagnoses involves nosologies such as the DSM and the ICD, and the validity of these classification systems is uncertain.[14,88] But even if one assumes that a classification system is valid, the task of collecting information about psychiatric symptoms in a reliable and valid manner remains. Here we will mainly discuss measurement in general population samples.

While measurement instruments for psychiatric disorders have a long history of development and application,[89] currently used instruments are largely rooted in the promise of increased reliability in the third revision of the DSM. Structured interviews administered by lay interviewers, and semistructured interviews administered by clinician interviewers, were designed to collect and assemble the symptoms described in the DSM and ICD with increased reliability. Structured interviews are most often used in population studies. One reason is that lay interviewers are much less expensive than clinician interviewers. Another potential benefit of structured interviews is that, in theory, they use standard predesigned questions that elicit sufficient information to identify disorder symptoms. Each respondent is asked the same series of questions and interviewers are often not allowed to deviate from the prescribed script. This reduces variation both in eliciting and interpreting the respondent report, compared with semistructured interviews where clinicians are allowed to probe to elicit and clarify responses and take account of cultural context. Disadvantages are that validity can be compromised if the structured interview does not accurately capture the clinical phenomena of interest. Furthermore, items are decontextualized and may not capture variation in the meaning of symptoms, especially when applied cross-culturally.[90-92]

A variety of strategies are used to assess the reliability and validity of these structured interviews. Among the most common is the test-retest design; the same respondent is interviewed twice over a relatively short period of time, and agreement between responses on the two test administrations is calculated. Cohen's kappa statistic is commonly used to estimate chance-adjusted agreement.[93] While there is no empirical cutoff to decide when a kappa is high enough to deem a measure "reliable," the typical rule-of-thumb is that kappas of >0.7 indicate excellent agreement, between 0.4 and 0.7 indicate fair agreement, and below 0.4 indicate poor agreement. Thus, a kappa of 0.7 would indicate that N assessments agree 70% of the time on the diagnosis above what we would expect by chance alone. It should be noted, however, that the cut points for acceptable reliability are debated, and depend upon what is required to address a particular research question.[94]

Studies using this design suggest that reliability is often low to moderate for many common disorders based on commonly used structured interviews.[95,96] There are many different reasons why a respondent may change answers from one administration to another: a true change in symptoms, forgetting, reinterpretation of situations and symptoms, or burden and annoyance with the length of the instrument. Reliability is often highest for disorders with necessary causes embedded in the diagnosis itself, such as posttraumatic stress disorder and substance use disorders, and is higher among patient samples than community samples.[97-99] Among children, assessment of psychiatric disorders often requires multiple informants (e.g., parents, teachers). But agreement is often low across informants,[100] as each informant may see different aspects of child behavior and/or give priority to different signs or symptoms. For example, a teacher may notice deficits in attention and focus more than a parent, as these cognitive skills are more salient in the school setting.[101]

The assessment of validity is also difficult and is severely hampered by the lack of a gold standard. Validity is often established through re-interview of a respondent by a clinician using a semistructured interview. But the reliability of semistructured interviews is far from perfect,[97,102] and disagreement between a (lay) structured interview and a (clinician) semistructured interview does not necessarily mean that the structured interview is invalid.[103]

Identifying Causes of Psychiatric Disorders

The search for causes in psychiatric epidemiology has often, though not always, built upon observed patterns of diagnoses within and across social groups. Despite the serious measurement issues described above, some patterns are clear. For example, when assessed across binary categories of gender, there are strong differences in many disorders. Girls and women are more likely to endorse symptoms of depression and anxiety, whereas boys and men have higher rates of autism and other neurodevelopmental disorders, substance use disorders, and antisocial personality. Such patterns often become the framework from which hypotheses are developed. Furthermore, across a wide variety of study designs, study populations, assessment instruments, and time-periods, studies find that most psychiatric disorders aggregate within families, have manifestations before adulthood, and are more common in contexts of severe adversity and among many marginalized social groups. This patterning suggests that causes of psychiatric disorders, like most disorders, are multileveled and span the life course. Indeed, symptoms and early indicators of psychiatric disorders, even those that are not diagnosable until midlife or later, can often (though, again, not always) be traced to early childhood.[104] Here we describe some of the causal investigations deriving from these observations, and the challenges to causal inference in investigating them. We acknowledge from the outset that our discussion of causes is necessarily incomplete and overlooks the wealth of neuroscientific data that has shaped our understanding of mediational processes that underlie dysfunction. Our focus here is on how psychiatric epidemiological studies have framed the study of causation, and some central issues that have arisen from these investigations.

Genetic Causes of Psychiatric Disorders

The vast majority of psychiatric disorders co-occur within families, at least to some degree. Familial aggregation may of course be due to familial environment as well as genetic transmission. Psychiatric epidemiology and the related field of behavioral genetics have a long history of methodological developments to try and tease apart genetic and environmental contributions to familial aggregation, including large twin, family, and adoption studies.[105,106] In most, though not all instances, genetic transmission appears to play an important role.

As in other fields of epidemiology, the rapid advance of genomic and other "omic" studies have transformed our ability to interrogate genetic causes and their interplay with the environment. Yet the notion that understanding the genetic architecture of psychiatric disorders would be straightforward once we understood more about the genome has not been borne out. As new methods and data emerge, a continuing lesson is that things are more complex than we had assumed. Two models of genetic causation are compatible with familial aggregation as well as with current genomic data on schizophrenia, autism spectrum disorder, and several other psychiatric disorders: (1) a polygenic model where thousands of common polymorphisms have very small individual effects; (2) a "private mutation" model where rare mutations have strong effects within individual families and collectively make an important contribution to genetic transmission. Though the models are quite different, both appear to play a role. In addition, evidence supports a significant role for *de novo* genetic mutations with strong effects that arise in the parental germ line or the early embryo, and therefore are present in the child but not in somatic cells of the biological parents.[107,108] This field is still evolving rapidly. For example, recent work suggests that rare variants in regions of DNA that do not code for proteins may play a role in autism spectrum disorder, due to previously unidentified regulatory functions of these regions.[109] Furthermore, under any scenario, an interplay between genetic risk and environment is likely and may involve complex epigenetic pathways.[110]

Perhaps most relevant to this chapter, the genomic findings have underscored the central challenge confronted by psychiatric epidemiology—defining and measuring psychiatric disorders. The same genetic mutations appear to confer risk for an array of disorders, and the same is true for polymorphisms.[111] This finding might suggest that we are looking for causes of disorders that are not meaningfully classified by current nosologies. Or it might simply suggest that different disorders share genetic causes to a much greater degree than anticipated, though they also have some distinct genetic causes. Although it is too early to reach strong conclusions, it is reasonable to anticipate that a deeper understanding of genetic pathways to psychiatric disorders will reveal much about their neurobiology, help to differentiate disorders in a meaningful way, and may aid in the search for nongenetic causes.

Prenatal Exposures

The early manifestations identifiable in people who later develop psychiatric disorders suggest a role for prenatal and early childhood environmental causes. Prenatal nutrition, infections, exposure to toxins and psychoactive substances, and other in utero experiences are among the most well-documented contributors to neurodevelopmental disorders, including many that have at some point been placed in the category of psychiatric disorders. For example, childhood exposure to lead is causally related to cognitive impairment and behavioral problems in children.[112,113] Prenatal exposure to heavy alcohol causes a cascade of neurodevelopmental consequences such that a disorder has been codified specifically for alcohol exposure (fetal alcohol syndrome).

In some instances, the effect of in utero exposure may be evident in disorder at birth or in early childhood, but in others, there may be a long latency period before a diagnosable disorder is apparent. Natural experiments based on the Dutch Famine of 1944-1945, and later the Chinese Famine of 1959-1961, demonstrated that malnutrition early in prenatal development increases the risk of schizophrenia and possibly other neurodevelopmental disorders in adulthood.[114-116] Ongoing efforts are evaluating the relation of various prenatal exposures to a wide range of psychiatric disorders, for example, the relation of prenatal maternal stress to offspring development.[117-119]

Childhood Adversity

Maltreatment, neglect, poverty, and unstable environments in childhood are associated with the development of most psychiatric disorders, suggesting that adverse childhood environments are a transdiagnostic cause that can unfurl in a multitude of ways. Studies such as the Bucharest Early Intervention Project, where orphaned children in Romania were randomly assigned high-quality foster care or institutional rearing, provide strong evidence for a causal role of early rearing in a range of outcomes including cognition, brain structure and function, and psychiatric disorders.[120,121] These results are in line with a wealth of much earlier theory and observational data on the effects of early childhood rearing environments.[122,123] They provide a solid empirical framework suggesting the plasticity of cognition and emotion across development and the role that strong emotional connections early in life play in normal development.[124]

Stress Exposure and Social Marginalization

More broadly, the social patterning of psychiatric disorders, with often a higher prevalence among those in marginalized social positions, has prompted a long tradition in psychiatric epidemiology of examining the role of stress exposure. Stressors, the stressful factors to which one is exposed, can be conceptualized in multiple ways, but definitions that explicitly refer to external stimuli that are negative in valence have proved most useful in psychiatric epidemiology. Stressors can also be categorized in terms of other dimensions, such as magnitude, duration, and predictability.[125] A dimension used to overcome ubiquitous problems of reverse causation is fatefulness, a measure of how much control the individual had over the occurrence of the stressor. Fateful stressors (e.g., sudden death of a parent in a plane crash) are less likely to arise from reverse causation because symptoms of psychiatric disorders may prompt the occurrence of stressors that are more likely to arise as a consequence of psychiatric disorder symptoms (e.g., divorce, job loss).

There are long-standing debates in psychiatric epidemiology regarding appropriate ways to measure stressors,[125-127] as the same stressor may have a different impact depending on the context in which it occurred and the way in which it was perceived by the individual. Indeed, some have suggested that measuring the subjective appraisal of stress in response to the stressor, rather than the stressor itself, offers a more direct path to understanding the causes of psychiatric disorders.[128] However, measuring subjective stress itself can also be difficult. Some prominent theories go beyond the concepts of stressor and subjective stress. For example, the theory of allostatic load links chronic stressors to changes in the neuroendocrine system.[129] These neuroendocrine changes are thought to have long-term effects upon the regulation (or dysregulation) of multiple systems, including physiological, immunological, and, indeed, psychological. Yet the measurement of allostatic load poses as much complexity as the measurement of stress.[130] It is important to note that these differing approaches to measurement are not mutually exclusive; each focuses on a different point in the process through which stressors cause disorder.

In addition to understanding how and why stressful circumstances produce psychiatric illness, it is increasingly clear that lack of social connectedness is an important stressor. For example, remarkably consistent findings have emerged from Europe that migrants who constitute certain ethnic minorities in the European countries to which they migrated have higher rates of schizophrenia than the "native" population.[131] This risk is even greater among ethnic minority migrants who live in neighborhoods with few members of their own ethnic group. It persists across generations, suggesting that it reflects ethnic minority status, not just migration per se. These results are compatible with the theory that alienation and marginalization, as well as lack of social connectedness, may be important determinants of schizophrenia and perhaps other disorders as well.[59] Such hypotheses have been posited for many decades[30] (see also Part II). Alternative hypotheses such as selective migration are not supported in the literature.[131] Furthermore, activities that are associated with lower risk of psychiatric disorders such as social support, entrance into marriage, and religious service attendance are hypothesized to operate by increasing social connectedness,[132,133] though selection into these activities is not random and the effects are heterogeneous (*e.g.*, by marital satisfaction and community norms), certainly complicating causal inference.

The social patterning of psychiatric disorders has provided a basis for causal hypotheses and investigations. Many of these hypothesized causes, as currently conceived, are not specific to one disorder but general across many disorders. This is in some ways a product of how psychiatry has developed as a field. When proximal biological causes of a specific disorder are identified, the disorder may lose its classification as a "psychiatric disorder." For example, when a vitamin B3 deficiency was identified as a cause of the psychiatric symptoms of pellagra, it was reclassified as a nutritional disorder. Other examples include epilepsy, mercury and lead poisoning, and many learning and cognitive disorders. Because of these disciplinary shifts, psychiatric disorders largely comprise those for which underlying mechanisms have not yet been firmly identified.

Establishing the Consequences of Disorders

Individuals with psychiatric disorders have a drastically shortened life span.[134] They have increased risk for a wide range of other chronic diseases, such as cardiovascular disease, and increased risk of death by suicide, homicide, or other injury.[3] These sequelae are not fully attributable to the disorder or its symptoms; they also reflect stigma, social exclusion, and other negative societal responses.[7] Medications for psychiatric disorders also play a role; for example, antipsychotic medications that cause obesity, metabolic disorders, and physical stigmata such as tardive dyskinesia.[135]

PART IV: ETHICAL, LEGAL, POLICY, AND SOCIAL ISSUES

Particularly salient in psychiatric epidemiology is the use (or misuse) of epidemiologic results to inform or justify health and social policies. This issue is also contentious in other fields of epidemiology, but in psychiatric epidemiology, it is greatly accentuated by the dilemmas we confront in defining psychiatric disorders (Part I).

Extension of Treatment for People With Mental Disorders

Epidemiologic research suggests that most people will meet diagnostic criteria for a psychiatric disorder at some point in their lifetime[136,137] and that psychiatric disorders are leading contributors to the global burden of disease.[1,3] Yet mental health receives much less attention than "physical" health in medical care, epidemiology, and public health.[138] The result of this neglect, together with stigma that reduces help-seeking, is that most people with psychiatric disorders are not treated. Estimates extrapolated from epidemiologic studies suggest that the proportion untreated, sometimes termed "the treatment gap," varies from over 50% in high-income countries to over 90% in many low-income countries.[138] These estimates provided a key foundation for launching a global movement to help close the treatment gap (Movement for Global Mental Health, 2018). A WHO Mental Health Action Plan provides guidelines for extending humane treatments in various contexts.[139] Initiatives such as task-shifting and internet therapy delivery are being examined as ways to extend treatment in underresourced settings.[140]

As we extend treatment, however, we need to keep in mind that it could be harmful to adopt an approach that is too broad. Given the limitations of psychiatric nosology applied in epidemiologic research, we cannot always differentiate people who have psychiatric disorders from those who are experiencing normative responses to life circumstances.[141] In primary care settings, screening for common mental disorders often captures transient distress in addition to disorder, and resources may not be sufficient to distinguish between them and assess the true need for treatment.[142] It is important to do so because psychiatric treatments are not always benign. Medications have side effects and costs; it can be hazardous to use them indiscriminately and without sufficient expertise. People treated for psychiatric disorders may be exposed to stigma and discrimination, limiting access to education and employment, and to internalized stigma that affects identity and social interactions. Another hazard of too broad an approach is that it might classify people as having a mental disorder when their behavior is socially unacceptable from one perspective but socially useful from another perspective. Finally, we might want to give priority to improving the lives of people with chronic severe mental disorders who are most vulnerable and socially marginalized.[78]

The dilemmas of differentiation become especially acute in efforts to progress toward early preventive interventions. For example, experiencing mild and/or transient psychotic symptoms is common among adolescents (prevalence estimates of 10%-15%) and predicts increased risk for common mental disorders and suicide as well as psychoses.[143] Youth might benefit from participation in treatments aimed at ameliorating these symptoms or learning to cope with them,[144] raising the tantalizing prospect that we could develop early interventions to reduce risk of mental disorders. Often an analogy is drawn to early interventions to prevent obesity and promote physical activity in youth. Yet psychiatric interventions need to consider carefully the potential harms described above. Creative efforts are underway to devise and implement preventive programs for youth that minimize the potential for these harms.[145]

Misuse of Diagnoses to Discredit Social Groups

Individuals who do not have psychiatric disorders have sometimes been discredited and harmed by being designated as mentally ill, for example, members of the LGBT community and political dissidents. Associations derived from psychiatric epidemiology can contribute to this problem. For example, some evidence suggests that the incidence of schizophrenia may be higher in Blacks than Whites. This difference might be due to diagnostic bias, but, if true, could be seen as another health disparity that should be addressed. There is also a danger, however, in reporting this association without great care, as associating a group with a stigmatized disorder can be used to cast aspersions on that group. Historical examples of this kind of misuse abound.[146]

Maltreatment of People With Chronic Severe Mental Disorders

Across historical time and across the globe, children and adults with chronic severe mental disorders have been subjected to inhumane living conditions and treatments. They have been socially marginalized, through explicit policy or malign neglect, and denied the opportunity to contribute to civil society and to participate in decisions about the care they receive. Some low- and middle-income countries offer little more than crowded custodial asylums where conditions are scandalous. Where community care is available, it is often inadequate, even in high-income countries. To its credit, the WHO Mental Health Action Plan emphasizes that treatments should be extended in tandem with policies to promote social integration (*e.g.*, access to work, education, housing) and a legal framework to protect civil rights for people with mental disorders.[139] These include the right to participate in decision-making about the nature of social and mental health services offered, as well as their own personal care.

Psychiatric epidemiologists did not produce these abuses, and many have worked to develop more humane treatments. Nonetheless, we are all prisoners of our historical moment and, on occasion, have contributed to these phenomena. The extermination of individuals with severe psychiatric disorders in Nazi Germany based on valid epidemiological data regarding familial aggregation is a horrific example of the way in which sound scientific findings can be used for extreme harm.[147-149]

PART V: FUTURE DIRECTIONS OF PSYCHIATRIC EPIDEMIOLOGY

Changes in disorder patterns draw our attention to emerging issues that inform future directions. Autism and autism spectrum disorders, for example, were historically considered relatively rare conditions with prevalence estimates around 5 per 10,000 throughout the mid-20th century. Beginning in the 1990s, however, autism incidence began exponentially increasing in many countries across the world. Some of this increase reflects better ascertainment and diagnosis, more awareness among parents and clinicians, and expanded criteria. Yet in our view, while existing studies suggest that these artifacts do explain a large part of the increase in diagnosis,[150] they are not sufficient to explain all of it.[151] Work is underway to identify underlying causes of true increase in the prevalence of autism; while there are many hypotheses, none, as of this writing, have been confirmed.

Other disorders also warrant close attention. Opioid disorders and overdose death remain at critically high levels,[152] and suicide has been increasing for over a decade, in both the United States and elsewhere.[153] Depression and other mood and anxiety disorders continue to contribute to global disability and death.[134]

Changing technology also affects our future. The move toward "big data" as a salvo for currently unsolvable problems is underway in psychiatric epidemiology. Large and detailed cohorts are being assembled, with massive repositories of biological and cognitive data. This effort includes consortia projects harmonizing data among hundreds of thousands of cases, as well as projects such as iPsych that are collecting extraordinary amounts of genomic and other biological data among tens of thousands of individuals with disorder as well as the population at large.[154] Integration of genomics and neuroscience with epidemiological and population-based studies are accelerating as technology advances to bring down costs. Indeed, compelling models for the neuroscience that underlies psychiatric disorders are becoming part of the converging evidence of mediational pathways to disorder risk and have been prominent models that guide psychiatric epidemiological studies. Nevertheless, foundations in social science and sociological theory, attention to measurement reliability and validity, and careful delineation of cause and consequence, remain vitally important for these technological advances in biology to hold promise in promoting public mental health.

The rapid growth of global psychiatric epidemiology reflects the transformation of societies as well as technologies across the globe, and is having a profound influence on understanding as well as treatment of mental disorders.[155,156] Until recently, our understanding of the social patterning of mental disorders was largely shaped by studies done in a few high-income societies, and it is increasingly apparent that the patterns evident in those societies often do not pertain to the much larger populations in low- and middle-income countries that are now being studied by psychiatric epidemiologists.[157,158] Genomic studies of mental disorders, too, have been largely based in the same few countries, and their current expansion by teams of geneticists and epidemiologists to African populations (which have greater genetic diversity) may reveal new relationships.[159-161] As a caution, global studies also can mislead us when differences in cultures and contexts are not taken into account.

The need for a broader perspective has been reinforced by the COVID-19 pandemic, which is presently reshaping social interactions across the globe. As we write this chapter, a panoply of effects on population mental health are unfolding alongside public health responses such as physical distancing and economic lockdowns, which are especially punishing in low-income countries. Many argue that control of the pandemic will require a coordinated global response, including attention to the vast inequities it has revealed within and across countries.

Among the most prominent emerging directions for the field of psychiatry is a response to the long-standing questions that we posed throughout this chapter—what is a psychiatric disorder? The dominant approach for the last several decades has been to draw boundaries around symptom clusters or prototypes and attempt to create reliable diagnoses, assess the patterns of these diagnoses and search for causes implicated in these patterns. The relationship between research and category has always been iterative—we begin with a collection of symptoms that seem to correlate in dysfunction and distress, and then refine the category as research identifies potential causes and correlates and better characterizes the underlying phenomenology. This process of refinement or reorganization is not based on scientific discovery alone, but also on utility, paradigmatic shifts, and values. Yet the dissatisfaction with binary categories of symptoms counts, as well as rapid progress in understanding neurocircuitry, has led to the development of new initiatives for assessing psychiatric symptoms and their causes. This is perhaps most notably seen in the building of Research Domain Criteria (RDoC) initiative,[6] which seeks to integrate information from across multiple disciplines to provide a more fruitful platform for the identification of the causes of psychiatric problems. Other approaches to reclassifying disorders have stemmed from long-standing movements in psychiatry toward more dimensional approaches to understanding population variation in disorder symptoms;[162] such movements have been catalyzed in recent years as high-quality data continue to emerge suggesting that binary categorizations of disorders obscure their underlying dimensionality.[104] Yet another approach that is rapidly gaining currency is "network theory," which postulates that the various symptoms of psychopathology are interconnected and cause one another, such that the process of spreading across a symptom network leads to a cluster of symptoms that is self-sustaining.[163] Although network theory presumes that biological or social experience can activate symptoms, the subsequent evolution to mental disorder depends upon their interaction.

The potentially radical implications of dimensional approaches as a future direction of the field are exemplified in the conceptualization of subclinical psychotic experiences in youth. Based on substantial (though not definitive) data, some leading psychiatric epidemiologists now conceptualize subclinical psychotic experiences in youth as part of a single underlying dimension of common mental distress that includes depressive, anxiety, and subclinical psychotic symptoms,[164-166] with early psychotic experiences as a potential marker of the severity of common mental distress. This paradigmatic shift has catalyzed broad efforts for early intervention and prevention for youth at risk for mental disorders. As previously discussed (see Part IV), such approaches are still in many ways controversial, and the optimal balance between treatment of symptoms that do not rise to the level of disorder versus early engagement with youth to monitor and follow them remains under discussion and development.

Along with these newly emerging and longstanding scientific challenges, and perhaps most critically, those with mental illness continue to be stigmatized, undertreated, and marginalized. The implicit, or explicit, value judgments in disorder definitions and their uses must continue to be questioned to ensure that the human rights and dignity of all individuals are maintained. One promising development that might help combat ongoing maltreatment is the growth of movements led by people who have diagnoses of psychiatric disorders. The slogan "nothing about us without us" captures their essence. Such movements have a long history but have never been as powerful or widespread as they are today. The most important advocacy group for global mental health, the Global Mental Health Movement, includes people in leadership who have a diagnosis of a psychiatric disorder. For psychiatric epidemiology, an open dialogue including people who have diagnoses of severe psychiatric disorders, and their family members, may help limit the use of research for unethical and harmful purposes. Because much of the burden of illness among those with psychiatric disorders may indeed stem from inequalities in treatment, stigma and rejection, social justice and advocacy remain important priorities, alongside scientific advances, to ameliorate the occurrence and consequences of psychiatric disorders.

References

1. Whiteford HA, Degenhardt L, Rehm J, et al. Global burden of disease attributable to mental and substance use disorders: findings from the Global Burden of Disease Study 2010. *Lancet*. 2013;382(9904):1575-1586.
2. Prince M, Patel V, Saxena S, et al. No health without mental health. *Lancet*. 2016;370(9590):859-877.
3. Vigo D, Thornicroft G, Atun R. Estimating the true global burden of mental illness. *Lancet Psychiatry*. 2016;3(2):171-178.
4. Liu NH, Daumit GL, Dua T, et al. Excess mortality in persons with severe mental disorders: a multilevel intervention framework and priorities for clinical practice, policy and research agendas. *World Psychiatry*. 2017;16(1):30-40.
5. American Psychiatric Association. *Diagnostic and Statistical Manual of Mental Disorders*. 5th ed. Washington, DC: 2013.
6. Clark LA, Cuthbert B, Lewis-Fernández R, Narrow WE, Reed GM. Three approaches to understanding and classifying mental disorder: ICD-11, DSM-5, and the national institute of mental health's research domain criteria (RDoC). *Psychol Sci Public Interest*. 2017;18(2):72-145.
7. Link BG, Phelan JC. *Mental Illness Stigma and the Sociology of Mental Health*. Cham: Springer; 2014.
8. Horwitz AV. *The Logic of Social Control*. New York, NY: Plenum Press; 1990.
9. Bobel C, Kwan S. *Embodied Resistance: Challenging the Norms, Breaking the Rules*. Nashville, TN: Vanderbilt University Press; 2011.
10. Grandin T, Panek R. *The Autistic Brain: Thinking Across the Spectrum*. New York, NY: Houghton Mifflin Harcourt; 2013.
11. Padden C, Humphries T. *Deaf in America: Voices From a Culture*. Cambridge: Harvard University Press; 1988.
12. Parens E. *Surgically Shaping Children: Technology, Ethics, and the Pursuit of Normality*. Baltimore, MD: Johns Hopkins University Press; 2006.
13. Frances A. *Saving Normal: An Insider's Revolt against Out-Of-Control Psychiatric Diagnosis, DSM-5, Big Pharma, and the Medicalization of Ordinary Life*. New York, NY: William Morrow; 2013.
14. Maj M. Why the clinical utility of diagnostic categories in psychiatry is intrinsically limited and how we can use new approaches to complement them. *World Psychiatry*. 2018;17:121-122.

15. Kutchins H, Kirk SA. *Making Us Crazy: DSM the Psychiatric Bible and the Creation of Mental Disorders*. New York, NY: Free Press; 1997.

16. Susser E, Schwartz S, Morabia A, Bromet EJ. *Psychiatric Epidemiology Searching for the Causes of Mental Disorders: Searching for the Causes of Mental Disorders*. Oxford, NY: Oxford University Press; 2006.

17. Grob GN. The origins of American psychiatric epidemiology. *Am J Public Health*. 1985;75(3):229-236.

18. Kendler KS. The transformation of American psychiatric nosology at the dawn of the twentieth century. *Mol Psychiatry*. 2016;21(2):152-158.

19. Davis JE. Family care of the mentally ill in Norway. *Am J Psychiatry*. 1962;119(2):154-158.

20. Elvbakken KT, Ludvigsen K. Medical professional practices, university disciplines and the state: a case study from Norwegian hygiene and psychiatry 1800-1940. *Hygiea Int*. 2016;12(2):7-28.

21. Grob GN. *Edward Jarvis and the Medical World of Nineteenth-Century America*. Knoxville, TN: University of Tennessee Press; 1978.

22. Holst F. *Beretning, Betænkning og Indstilling fra en til at undersøge de Sindssvages Kaar i Norge og gjøre Forslag til deres Forbedring i Aaret 1825 naadigst nedsat kgl. Commission*. Christiania: Jacob Lehmanns Enke, 1828.

23. Jarvis E. *Insanity and Idiocy in Massachusetts: Report of the Commission on Lunacy*. Cambridge, MA: Harvard University Press; 1855.

24. Mitchell A. *The Insane in Private Dwellings*. Edinburgh: Edmonston and Douglas; 1864.

25. Susser E, Baumgartner JN, Stein Z. Commentary: Sir Arthur Mitchell–pioneer of psychiatric epidemiology and of community care. *Int J Epidemiol*. 2010;39(6):1417-1425.

26. Kraeplin E, Diefendorf RA. *Clinical Psychiatry: A Text-Book for Students and Physicians. Abstracted and Adapted From the Sixth German Edition of Kraepelin's 'Lehrbuch der Psychiatrie'*. New York, NY: Macmillan Company, 1904.

27. Kraepelin E. *Ein Lehrbuch für Studirende un Aerzte*. 5th ed. Leipzig, Germany: JA Barth; 1896.

28. Report of the committee on statistics of the American Medico-Psychological Association. *Am J Insanity*. 1917;74:256-258.

29. Gruenberg EM. *Epidemiology of Mental Disorder*. New York: Milbank Memorial Fund; 1950.

30. Faris RE, Dunham HW. *Mental Disorders in Urban Areas: An Ecological Study of Schizophrenia and Other Psychoses*. American Psychological Association; 1939:38.

31. Durkheim E. *Le Suicide*. Spalding J, Simpson G, trans-eds. New York, NY: Free Press; 1897.

32. Pols H, Oak S. War and military mental health: the US psychiatric response in the 20th century. *Am J Public Health*. 2007;97(12):2132-2142.

33. March D, Oppenheimer GM. Social disorder and diagnostic order: the US Mental Hygiene Movement, the Midtown Manhattan study and the development of psychiatric epidemiology in the 20th century. *Int J Epidemiol*. 2014;43(suppl 1):29-42.

34. Gruenberg EM. Progress in psychiatric epidemiology. *Psychiatr Q*. 1973;47(1):1-11.

35. Susser M. *Community Psychiatry: Epidemiologic and Social Themes*. New York, NY: Random House; 1968.

36. Cooper B, Morgan HG. *Epidemiological Psychiatry*. Springfield, IL: Thomas; 1973.

37. Shepherd M. Psychiatric epidemiology and epidemiological psychiatry. *Am J Public Health*. 1985;75(3):275-276.

38. Gottesman I. *Schizophrenia Genesis, the Origins of Madness*. New York, NY: W.H. Freeman and Company; 1990.

39. Costello EJ, Angold A. Developmental epidemiology. In: Cicchetti D, Toth S, eds. *Developmental Psychopathology*. Lawrence Erlbaum and Associates; 1991;23-56.

40. Wadsworth MEJ. *The Imprint of Time: Childhood, History and Adult Life*. New York, NY: Oxford University Press; 1991.

41. Desjarlais R. *World Mental Health: Problems and Priorities in Low-Income Countries*. New York, NY: Oxford University Press; 1996.

42. Koenen K. *A Lifecourse Approach to Mental Disorders*. New York, NY: Oxford University Press; 2014.

43. Lovell AM, Susser E. History of psychiatric epidemiology. *Int J Epidemiol*. 2014;43(suppl 1):1-66.

44. Srole L. *Mental health in the metropolis: the Midtown Manhattan study*. In: *Thomas A C Rennie Series in Social Psychiatry V 1*. New York, NY: Blakiston Division, McGraw-Hill; 1962.

45. Leighton AH. *My Name Is Legion; Foundations for a Theory of Man in Relation to Culture. The Stirling County Study of Psychiatric Disorder & Sociocultural Environment*. New York, NY: Basic Books; 1959.

46. Dohrenwend BP, Dohrenwend BS. Perspectives on the past and future of psychiatric epidemiology. *Am J Public Health*. 1982;72(11):1271-1279.

47. Weissman MM, Klerman GL. Epidemiology of mental disorders: emerging trends in the United States. *Arch Gen Psychiatry*. 1978;35(6):705-712.

48. American Psychiatric Association. *Diagnostic and statistical manual of mental disorders*. In: *Diagnostic and Statistical Manual of Mental Disorders*. 3rd ed. Washington, DC: The American Psychiatric Association; 1980.

49. Srole L, Fischer AK. Debate on psychiatric epidemiology. *Arch Gen Psychiatry*. 1980;37(12):1424.

50. Weissman MM, Klerman GL. Debate on psychiatric epidemiology-reply. *Arch Gen Psychiatry*. 1980;37(12):1423.

51. Robins LN, Regier DA. Psychiatric disorders in America: the epidemiologic catchment area study. *J Psychiatry Neurosci*. 1991;17(1):34-36.

52. Lovell AM. The World Health Organization and the contested beginnings of psychiatric epidemiology as an international discipline: one rope, many strands. *Int J Epidemiol*. 2014;43(suppl 1):6-18.

53. Sartorius N, Shapiro R, Kimura M, Barrett K. WHO international pilot study of schizophrenia. *Psychol Med*. 1972;2(4):422-425.

54. Cooper JE, Kendell RE, Gurland BJ, Sartorius N, Farkas T. Cross-national study of diagnosis of the mental disorders: some results from the first comparative investigation. *Am J Psychiatry*. 1969;10 suppl:21-29.

55. Crossley N. R. D. Laing and the British anti-psychiatry movement: a socio–historical analysis. *Soc Sci Med*. 1998;47(7):877-889.

56. Jablensky A, Sartorius N, Ernberg G, et al. Schizophrenia - manifestations, incidence and course in different cultures - a World-Health-Organization 10-country study. *Psychol Med Monogr Suppl*. 1992;20:1-97.

57. Hogerzeil SJ, Susser E. Schizophrenia: learning about the other half. *Psychiatr Serv*. 2017;68(5):425.

58. Susser E, Martínez-Alés G. Putting psychosis into sociocultural context. *JAMA Psychiatry*. 2018;75(1):9.

59. Jongsma HE, Gayer-Anderson C, Lasalvia A, et al. Treated incidence of psychotic disorders in the multinational EU-GEI study. *JAMA Psychiatry*. 2018;75(1):36.

60. Kebede D, Alem A, Shibre T, et al. Onset and clinical course of schizophrenia in Butajira-Ethiopia. *Soc Psychiatry Psychiatr Epidemiol*. 2003;38(11):625-631.

61. Lilienfeld AM, Pasamanick B, Rogers M. Relationship between pregnancy experience and the development of certain neuropsychiatric disorders in childhood. *Am J Public Health Nations Health*. 1955;45(5 pt 1):637-643.

62. Broman SH. Prenatal risk factors for mental retardation in young children. *Public Health Rep*. 1987;102(suppl 4):55-57.

63. Stein Z, Susser M, Saenger G, Marolla F. *Famine and Human Development. The Dutch Hunger Winter of 1944-1945*. New York, NY: Oxford University Press; 1975.

64. Wang PS, Aguilar-Gaxiola S, Alonso J, et al. Use of mental health services for anxiety, mood, and substance disorders in 17 countries in the WHO world mental health surveys. *Lancet*. 2007;370(9590):841-850.

65. Andreassen OA. eHealth provides a novel opportunity to exploit the advantages of the Nordic countries in psychiatric genetic research, building on the public health care system, biobanks, and registries. *Am J Med Genet B Neuropsychiatr Genet*. 2018;177(7):625-629.

66. Initiative NLC. Nordic Life Course Research Initiative. Available at http://nordiclifecore.com/. Accessed July 31, 2020.

67. Ystrom E, Gustavson K, Brandlistuen RE, et al. Prenatal exposure to acetaminophen and risk of ADHD. *Pediatrics*. 2017;140(5):20163840.

68. Schendel DE, Bresnahan M, Carter KW, et al. The international collaboration for autism registry epidemiology (iCARE): multinational registry-based investigations of autism risk factors and trends. *J Autism Dev Disord*. 2013;43(11):2650-2663.

69. Liu K, King M, Bearman PS. Social influence and the autism epidemic. *AJS*. 2010;115(5):1387-1434.

70. Kim YS, Leventhal BL, Koh YJ, et al. Prevalence of autism spectrum disorders in a total population sample. *Am J Psychiatry*. 2011;168(9):904-912.

71. Olfson M, Marcus SC. National patterns in antidepressant medication treatment. *Arch Gen Psychiatry*. 2009;66(8):848-856.

72. Poulton R, Moffitt TE, Silva PA. The Dunedin multidisciplinary health and development study: overview of the first 40 years, with an eye to the future. *Soc Psychiatry Psychiatr Epidemiol*. 2015;50(5):679-693.

73. Fraser A, Macdonald-Wallis C, Tilling K, et al. Cohort profile: the avon longitudinal study of parents and children ALSPAC mothers cohort. *Int J Epidemiol*. 2013;42(1):97-110.

74. Costello EJ, Copeland W, Angold A. The great Smoky Mountains study: developmental epidemiology in the southeastern United States. *Soc Psychiatry Psychiatr Epidemiol*. 2016;51(5):639-646.

75. Olsen J, Melbye M, Olsen SF, et al. The Danish National Birth Cohort–its background, structure and aim. *Scand J Public Health*. 2001;29(4):300-307.

76. Magnus P, Birke C, Vejrup K, et al. Cohort profile update: the Norwegian mother and child cohort study (MoBa). *Int J Epidemiol*. 2016;45(2):382-388.

77. Kendler KS. Lifetime prevalence, demographic risk factors, and diagnostic validity of nonaffective psychosis as assessed in a US community sample. *Arch Gen Psychiatry*. 1996;53(11):1022.

78. Merikangas KR, Bromet EJ, Druss BG. Future surveillance of mental disorders in the United States count people: not disorders. *JAMA Psychiatry*. 2017;74(5):431-432.

79. Robins LN, Regier DA. *Psychiatric Disorders in America the Epidemiologic Catchment Area Study*. New York, NY: Free Press; 1991.

80. Kessler RC, McGonagle K., Zhao S, et al. Lifetime and 12-month prevalence of DSM-III-R psychiatric disorders in the United States. Results from the national comorbidity survey. *Arch Gen Psychiatry*. 1994;51(1):8-19.

81. Kessler RC, Berglund P, Demler O, Jin R, Merikangas KR, Walters EE. Lifetime prevalence and age-of-onset distributions of DSM-IV disorders in the national comorbidity survey replication. *Arch Gen Psychiatry*. 2005;62(6):593-602.

82. Grant BF, Hasin DS, Stinson FS, et al. Co-occurrence of 12-month mood and anxiety disorders and personality disorders in the US: results from the national epidemiologic survey on alcohol and related conditions. *J Psychiatr Res*. 2005;39(1):1-9.

83. Prins SJ. Prevalence of mental illnesses in U.S. State prisons: a systematic review. *Psychiatr Serv*. 2014;65(7):862-872.

84. Kessler RC, Ustun TB. *The WHO World Mental Health Surveys*. New York, NY: Cambridge University Press; 2008.

85. Dohrenwend B, Shrout PE. Toward the development of a two-stage procedure for case identification and classification in psychiatric epidemiology. *Res Community Ment Health*. 1981;2:295-323.

86. Zaman SS, Khan NZ, Islam S, et al. Validity of the "Ten Questions" for screening serious childhood disability: results from urban Bangladesh. *Int J Epidemiol*. 1990;19(3):613-620.

87. Phillips MR, Zhang J, Shi Q, et al. Prevalence, treatment, and associated disability of mental disorders in four provinces in China during 2001-05: an epidemiological survey. *Lancet*. 2009;373(9680):2041-2053.

88. Krueger RF, Markon KE. Reinterpreting comorbidity: a model-based approach to understanding and classifying psychopathology. *Annu Rev Clin Psychol*. 2006;2(1):111-133.

89. Robins LN. Psychiatric epidemiology-a historic review. *Soc Psychiatry Psychiatr Epidemiol*. 1990;25(1):16-26.

90. Rutter M, Nikapota A. Culture, ethnicity, society and psychopathology. In: Rutter M, Taylor E, eds. *Child and Adolescent Psychiatry*. Oxford: Blackwell Publishing; 2002:277-286.

91. Haroz EE. How is depression experienced around the world? A systematic review of qualitative literature. *Soc Sci Med*. 2017;183:151-162.

92. DeVylder JE, Kelleher I, Lalane M, Oh H, Link BG, Koyanagi A. Association of urbanicity with psychosis in low- and middle-income countries. *JAMA Psychiatry*. 2018;75(7):678-686.

93. Cohen J. A coefficient of agreement for nominal scales. *Educ Psychol Meas*. 1960;20(1):37-46.

94. Kirk SA, Kutchins H. *The Selling of DSM: The Rhetoric of Science in Psychiatry*. London: Routledge Taylor & Francis; 1992.

95. Hasin DS, Greenstein E, Aivadyan C, et al. The Alcohol Use Disorder and Associated Disabilities Interview Schedule-5 (AUDADIS-5): procedural validity of substance use disorders modules through clinical re-appraisal in a general population sample. *Drug Alcohol Depend*. 2015;148:40-46.

96. Wittchen HU. Reliability and validity studies of the WHO–composite international diagnostic interview (CIDI): a critical review. *J Psychiatr Res*. 1994;28(1):57-84.

97. Anthony JC, Folstein M, Romanoski AJ, et al. Comparison of the lay diagnostic interview schedule and a standardized psychiatric diagnosis: experience in eastern baltimore. *Arch Gen Psychiatry*. 1985;42(7):667-675.

98. Jensen P, Roper M, Fisher P, et al. Test-retest reliability of the diagnostic interview schedule for children (DISC 2.1). Parent, child, and combined algorithms. *Arch Gen Psychiatry*. 1995;52(1):61-71.

99. Kraemer HC. Charlie Brown and statistics: an exchange. *Arch Gen Psychiatry*. 1987;44(2):192-193.

100. Achenbach TM, McConaughy SH, Howell CT. Child/adolescent behavioral and emotional problems: implications of cross-informant correlations for situational specificity. *Psychol Bull*. 1987;101(2):213-232.

101. Narad ME, Garner AA, Peugh JL, et al. Parent-teacher agreement on ADHD symptoms across development. *Psychol Assess*. 2015;27(1):239-248.

102. Helzer JE, Robins LN, McEvoy LT, et al. A comparison of clinical and diagnostic interview schedule diagnoses. *Arch Gen Psychiatry*. 1985;42(7):657-666.

103. Robins LN. Epidemiology: reflections on testing the validity of psychiatric interviews. *Arch Gen Psychiatry*. 1985;42(9):918-924.

104. Caspi A, Houts RM, Belsky DW, et al. The p factor: one general psychopathology factor in the structure of psychiatric disorders? *Clin Psychol Sci*. 2014;2(2):119-137.

105. Plomin R, Rendell R. Human behavioral genetics. *Annu Rev Psychol*. 1991;42(1):161.

106. Schwartz S, Susser E. Chapter 31 Twin studies of heritability. In: Susser E, ed. *Psychiatric Epidemiology*. New York, NY: Oxford University Press; 2006: 1-38.

107. Smoller JW, Andreassen OA, Edenberg HJ, Faraone SV, Glatt SJ, Kendler KS. Psychiatric genetics and the structure of psychopathology. *Mol Psychiatry*. 2019;24(3):409-420.

108. Sullivan PF, Daly MJ, O'Donovan M. Genetic architectures of psychiatric disorders: the emerging picture and its implications. *Nat Rev Genet*. 2012;13(8):537-551.

109. Brandler WM. Paternally inherited cis-regulatory structural variants are associated with autism'. *Science*. 2018;360(6386):327-331.

110. Os J, Kenis G, Rutten BPF. The environment and schizophrenia. *Nature*. 2010;468(7321):203-212.

111. Lee SH, Ripke S, Neale BM, et al. Genetic relationship between five psychiatric disorders estimated from genome-wide SNPs. *Nat Genet*. 2013;45(9):984-994.

112. Bellinger DC. The protean toxicities of lead: new chapters in a familiar story. *Int J Environ Res Public Health*. 2011;8(7):2593-2628.

113. Lanphear BP, Hornung R, Khoury J, et al. Low-level environmental lead exposure and children's intellectual function: an international pooled analysis. *Environ Health Perspect*. 2005;113(7):894-899.

114. Susser E, Neugebauer R, Hoek HW, et al. Schizophrenia after prenatal famine. Further evidence. *Arch Gen Psychiatry*. 1996;53(1):25-31.

115. St Clair D, Xu M, Wang P, et al. Rates of adult schizophrenia following prenatal exposure to the Chinese famine of 1959-1961. *J Am Med Assoc*. 2005;294(5):557-562.

116. Susser E, St Clair D. Prenatal famine and adult mental illness: interpreting concordant and discordant results from the Dutch and Chinese Famines. *Soc Sci Med*. 2013;97:325-330.

117. Monk C, Spicer J, Champagne FA. Linking prenatal maternal adversity to developmental outcomes in infants: the role of epigenetic pathways. *Dev Psychopathol*. 2012;24(4):1361-1376.

118. Gelaye B, Koenen KC. The intergenerational impact of prenatal stress: time to focus on prevention? *Biol Psychiatry*. 2018;83(2):92-93.

119. MacKinnon N, Kingsbury M, Mahedy L, Evans J, Colman I. The association between prenatal stress and externalizing symptoms in childhood: evidence from the avon longitudinal study of parents and children. *Biol Psychiatry*. 2018;83(2):100-108.

120. Humphreys KL, Fox NA, Nelson CA, Zeanah CH. Psychopathology following severe deprivation: history, research, and implications of the Bucharest early intervention project. In: Rus A, Parris S, Stativa E, eds. *Child Maltreatment in Residential Care: History, Research, and Current Practice*. Springer; 2017:129-148.

121. Nelson CA, Zeanah CH, Fox NA, Marshall PJ, Smyke AT, Guthrie D. Cognitive recovery in socially deprived young children: the Bucharest early intervention project. *Science*. 2007;318(5858):1937-1940.

122. Bowlby J. *Child Care and the Growth of Love*. London: Penguin Books; 1953.

123. Harlow HF, Suomii SJ. Social recovery by isolation-reared monkeys. *Proc Natl Acad Sci USA*. 1971;68(7):1534-1538.

124. McLaughlin KA, Sheridan MA, Lambert HK. Childhood adversity and neural development: deprivation and threat as distinct dimensions of early experience. *Neurosci Biobehav Rev*. 2014;47:578-591.

125. Dohrenwend BP. Inventorying stressful life events as risk factors for psychopathology: toward resolution of the problem of intracategory variability. *Psychol Bull*. 2006;132(3):477-495.

126. Rabkin J, Struening E. Live events, stress, and illness. *Science*. 1976;194(4269):1013-1020.

127. Holmes TH, Rahe RH. The social readjustment rating scale. *J Psychosomatic Res*. 1967;11(2):213-218.

128. Lazarus RS. *Psychological Stress and the Coping Process*. New York, NY: McGraw-Hill; 1966.

129. McEwen BS, Gianaros PJ. Central role of the brain in stress and adaptation: links to socioeconomic status, health, and disease. *Ann New York Acad Sci*. 2010;1186:190-222.

130. Johnson SC, Cavallaro FL, Leon DA. A systematic review of allostatic load in relation to socioeconomic position:Poor fidelity and major inconsistencies in biomarkers employed. *Soc Sci Med*. 2017;192:66-73.

131. Radua J, Ramella-Cravaro V, Ioannidis JPA, et al. What causes psychosis? An umbrella review of risk and protective factors. *World Psychiatry*. 2018;17(1):49-66.

132. Berkman LF. From social integration to health: Durkheim in the new millennium. *Soc Sci Med*. 2000;51(6):843-857.

133. VanderWeele TJ. Association between religious service attendance and lower suicide rates among US women. *JAMA Psychiatry*. 2016;73(8):845-851.

134. Walker ER, McGee RE, Druss BG. Mortality in mental disorders and global disease burden implications. *JAMA Psychiatry*. 2015;72(4):334.

135. De Hert M, Detraux J, Van Winkel R, Yu W, Correll CU. Metabolic and cardiovascular adverse effects associated with antipsychotic drugs. *Nat Rev Endocrinol*. 2012;8:114-126.

136. Moffitt TE, Caspi A, Taylor A, et al. How common are common mental disorders? Evidence that lifetime prevalence rates are doubled by prospective versus retrospective ascertainment. *Psychol Med*. 2010;40(6):899-909.

137. Susser E, Shrout PE. Two plus two equals three? Do we need to rethink lifetime prevalence? *Psychol Med*. 2010;40(6):895-897.

138. Global Mental Health. [Special series]. Lancet. 2007:370.

139. World Health Organisation. *Comprehensive Mental Health Action Plan 2013-2020*. Geneva, Switzerland; 2013. Available at https://www.who.int/mental_health/action_plan_2013/en/.

140. Patel V. Global mental health: from science to action. *Harv Rev Psychiatry*. 2012;20(1):6-12.

141. Horwitz AV, Wakefield JC. *The Loss of Sadness: How Psychiatry Transformed normal Sorrow into Depressive Disorder*. Oxford: Oxford University Press; 2007.

142. Palmer SC, Coyne JC. Screening for depression in medical care: pitfalls, alternatives, and revised priorities. *J Psychosomatic Res*. 2003;54(4):279-287.

143. Kelleher I, Keeley H, Corcoran P, et al. Clinicopathological significance of psychotic experiences in non-psychotic young people: evidence from four population-based studies. *Br J Psychiatry*. 2012;201(1):26-32.

144. Rickwood DJ, Telford NR, Parker AG, Tanti CJ, McGorry PD. Headspace - Australia's innovation in youth mental health: who are the clients and why are they presenting? *Med J Aust*. 2014;200(2):108-111.

145. Headspace. *National Youth Mental Health Foundation*. 2018. Available at https://headspace.org.au. Accessed July 31, 2020.

146. Susser E, Bresnahan M. *Global mental health and social justice*. In: *Mental Health and Human Rights: Vision, Praxis and Courage*. New York, NY: Oxford University Press; 2012:195-206.

147. Torrey EF, Yolken RH. Psychiatric genocide: Nazi attempts to eradicate schizophrenia. *Schizophrenia Bull*. 2010;36(1):26-32.

148. Alexander L. Medical science under dictatorship. *New Engl J Med*. 1949;241(2):39-47.

149. Strous RD. Psychiatry during the Nazi era: ethical lessons for the modern professional. *Ann Gen Psychiatry*. 2007;6(1):8.

150. Hansen SN, Schendel DE, Parner ET. Explaining the increase in the prevalence of autism spectrum disorders. *JAMA Pediatr*. 2015;169(1):56.

151. Russell G, Collishaw S, Golding J, Kelly SE, Ford T. Changes in diagnosis rates and behavioural traits of autism spectrum disorder over time. *BJPsych Open*. 2015;1(2):110-115.

152. Rudd RA, Aleshire N, Zibbell JE, Matthew Gladden R. Increases in drug and opioid overdose deaths - United States, 2000-2014. *Am J Transplant*. 2016;16(4):1323-1327.

153. Hedegaard H, Warner M, Curtin SC. Increase in suicide in the United States, 1999-2014: *NCHS Data Brief*. 2016:241:1-8.

154. Bøcker Pedersen C, Bybjerg-Grauholm J, Gjørtz Pedersen M, et al. *The iPSYCH2012 Case-Cohort Sample: New Directions for Unravelling the Genetic and Environmental Architecture of Severe Mental Disorders*. 2017.

155. Patel V, Prince M. Global mental health: a new global health field comes of age. *JAMA*. 2010;303:1976-1977. doi:10.1001/jama.2010.616.

156. Susser E, Patel V. Psychiatric epidemiology and global mental health: joining forces. *Int J Epidemiol*. 2014;43:287-293. doi:10.1093/ije/dyu053.

157. Phillips MR, Li X, Zhang Y. Suicide rates in China, 1995-99. *Lancet*. 2002;359(9309):835-840.

158. Yang GH. Understanding the unique characteristics of suicide in China: national psychological autopsy study'. *Biomed Environ Sci*. 2005;18(6):379-389.

159. McClellan JM, Lehner T, King MC. Gene discovery for complex traits: lessons from africa. *Cell*. 2017;171(2):261-264.

160. Campbell MM, Susser E, Vries J, et al. Exploring researchers' experiences of working with a researcher-driven, population-specific community advisory board in a South African schizophrenia genomics study. *BMC Med Ethics*. 2015;16(45):1-9.

161. Gulsuner S, Stein DJ, Susser ES, et al. Genetics of schizophrenia in the South African Xhosa. *Science*. 2020;367(6477):569-573. doi:10.1126/science.aay8833.

162. Krueger RF. The structure of common mental disorders. *Arch Gen Psychiatry*. 1999;56(10):921-926.

163. Borsboom D. Λ network theory of mental disorders. *World Psychiatry*. 2017;16(1):5-13.

164. Os J, Guloksuz S. A critique of the "ultra-high risk" and "transition" paradigm. *World Psychiatry*. 2017;16(2):200-206.

165. Murray GK, Jones PB. Psychotic symptoms in young people without psychotic illness: mechanisms and meaning. *Br J Psychiatry*. 2012;201(1):4-6.

166. Stochl J, Khandaker GM, Lewis G, et al. Mood, anxiety and psychotic phenomena measure a common psychopathological factor. *Psychol Med*. 2015;45(7):1483-1493.

CHAPTER 35

Clinical Epidemiology

Jan P. Vandenbroucke and Henrik Toft Sørensen

INTRODUCTION

In this chapter, we introduce clinical epidemiology for epidemiologists and clinicians with little experience in the field and reflect on progress for experienced clinical epidemiologists. We first describe the history and the scope of clinical epidemiology to clarify the work and goals of its practitioners. We emphasize that clinical epidemiology is a rapidly evolving discipline, as medicine itself is evolving and posing ever different and greater challenges for research. We describe how clinical epidemiology may be considered a continuation of the tradition of "clinical science," *i.e.*, learning from patient observations. As such, it also encompasses etiology and pathogenesis. Second, we review the key clinical issues: diagnosis, prognosis, therapy, and risk. We elucidate how each is investigated, emphasizing some of the complex underlying theories. Third, we describe the role of case reports and case series, as they are ubiquitous in medicine and serve to address wide-ranging questions, from detection of new diseases to etiology and quality assurance. It is important for epidemiologists and clinicians to reflect on the strengths and weaknesses of case reports and case series and to understand their role in complementing formal study designs.

OBJECTIVES, HISTORY, AND SCOPE OF CLINICAL EPIDEMIOLOGY

As difficult as it is to define epidemiology as a science,[1,2] it is even harder to define "clinical epidemiology" to the satisfaction of practitioners in the field and others seeking an orderly demarcation of applications of epidemiology.[3] Even Feinstein (1925-2001) and Sackett (1934-2015), authors of two groundbreaking textbooks published in 1985 with "Clinical Epidemiology" in their titles,[4,5] disagreed on the definition. In the prologue to his book, Feinstein[4] described why he decided to include "Epidemiology" in its title: he was paying tribute to a Presidential Address presented by Paul to the Society of Clinical Investigation in 1938. In that address, Paul may have been the first to join the words "clinical" and "epidemiology." Feinstein used the combination of "epidemiology" and "clinical" because epidemiology denoted research in groups of people, but he posited that clinical epidemiology is *"enlarged epidemiology"*—enlarged beyond topics of interest for public health applications—to *"include clinical decisions in personal-encounter care for individual patients"*.[4]

In the preface to the second edition of their textbook, Sackett et al. explained how their view of clinical epidemiology originated in clinical practice: *"...we addressed the three challenges that face every clinician every day: ...the correct diagnosis, the correct management, and keeping up with the literature."* They refused to define clinical epidemiology, because they rejected the idea that each word should have "a single and formally correct definition," because that does not correspond to the uses of words in everyday life.[5]

We consider clinical epidemiology to encompass more than diagnosis and treatment and more than research conducted on patients. In their medical decisions and advice to patients, health care providers need etiologic and pathogenetic knowledge in addition to diagnostic, prognostic, and therapeutic knowledge. For instance, in treating and counseling patients with HIV, providers need information about the spread of HIV in the population (patterns and modes of spreading in the patient's community). In diagnosing and treating breast cancer patients, providers need knowledge about genetic risk factors or somatic mutations. Recent examples of etiologic and pathogenetic clinical epidemiologic research, which also involve general population data, are presented in Box 35-1.

In prognostic studies, databases containing information on patient populations of entire countries or regions now are commonly used, which allows comparisons with the general population or population subgroups. For example, a Danish nationwide population-based cohort study investigated 30-year mortality among venous thromboembolism patients.[11] The use of a population approach to study the natural history of diseases is not new; it was already advocated at the turn of the 19th century by Mackenzie.[12]

The boundaries between "clinical epidemiology" and other branches of epidemiology, such as "public health epidemiology" or "cancer epidemiology," are fluid. Clinicians make use of all types of information needed for patient care, including immunology, genetics, pathophysiology, epidemiology in the general population, and quantitative studies on patients. A distinction that seems to remain between "clinical epidemiology" and other branches of epidemiology is that clinical epidemiology is primarily directed toward knowledge needed for the theory and practice of clinical medicine,[13] while other branches of epidemiology are more directed toward knowledge needed to promote public health, especially by disease prevention. Thus, clinical epidemiology continues the long tradition of "clinical investigation"—research of the type described as "clinical science" by Lewis as early as 1934.[14] Clinical epidemiology often focuses on rare diseases affecting patients who present in tertiary care settings—diseases like Cushing disease, scleroderma, and IgA nephritis—which are often outside of the scope of general, public health-oriented epidemiology.

There is a strong link between clinical epidemiology and pharmacoepidemiology, (see Chapter 43) as clinical epidemiologists are interested in the beneficial as well as the adverse effects of medications. The study of adverse effects of medications is, in fact, a type of etiologic research, since medications can cause collateral (and sometimes new) types of illness.

> **BOX 35-1** Examples of Etiologic and Pathogenetic Research in Clinical Epidemiology
>
> - Roux-en-Y bariatric surgery and hypoglycemia
>   An investigation examined overall and cause-specific mortality after Roux-en-Y gastric bypass surgery for morbid obesity. It found that all-cause mortality was similar in patients who underwent Roux-en-Y gastric bypass surgery from 2006 to 2010 and in a 25-fold larger age- and gender-matched population comparison cohort. However, patients who underwent the procedure had increased mortality due to suicide, accidents, and gastrointestinal diseases, and lower mortality due to cancer. In addition, a medical record audit found that possibly 8% of deaths in the bariatric surgery group were hypoglycemia-related.[6]
> - Factor V Leiden
>   A case-control study into rare genetic and hemostatic causes of venous thrombosis, designed by clinical epidemiologists, coagulation researchers, and clinicians in the Netherlands, was the first to show that a newly discovered hemostatic abnormality, activated protein C resistance, was a major cause of venous thrombosis. The defect, originally detected in Swedish family studies,[7] was found to be present in about 1 in 5 consecutive patients with venous thrombosis treated in outpatient thrombosis centers[8] (see also the section on case reports). Later investigations, some using data from the case-control study, led to the discovery of Factor V Leiden.[9] Most importantly, interaction with several environmental factors was found to cause venous thrombosis, *e.g.*, long-haul air travel, obesity, hospitalizations, short immobilizations, other genetic factors, and medications such as oral contraceptives.[10]

Earlier Attempts to Base Medical Practice on Numerical Thinking

While the term "clinical epidemiology" was coined in 1938, the discipline did not have any major influence on medicine until the 1980s. Still, the idea of looking at groups of patients numerically (*i.e.*, counting patients as the unit of observation and drawing conclusions from those observations) is much older.

At least twice in the history of medicine, small groups of physicians advanced the use of numerical arguments to support insights about causes of disease or the benefits of treatment. A first movement consisted of "arithmetic observationalists and experimentalists" in 18th-century Britain.[15] Most were army and navy surgeons and provincial Scottish physicians, often dissenters like Quakers and Unitarians. In making elementary numerical observations on groups of patients, they deviated from the traditional methods and aphorisms of Galenus and Hippocrates that had dominated medicine for more than 1000 years, and also from Boerhaave's 18th-century writings. However, they remained outside the academic worlds of Oxford and London and left no real legacy of a "numerical school of thinking" about medicine.

In the 1830s, a second "numerical movement" emerged in Paris, which centered around the towering figure of Charles Pierre Alexandre Louis (1787-1872). Louis advocated the "numerical method" for the comparative study of the benefits of treatment and founded the "Societé de Médicine d'Observation." Members of the society distrusted "received wisdom" in the medical theory of their times—for example, the theory that the position of the stars in heaven should determine when to bleed a patient. Louis' fame endures because of his attempt to show that bloodletting was of no avail in patients with pneumonia, by comparing patients who were bled early versus late in the course of their disease.[16] Some famous debates took place in the French "Académie" about the value of the new numerical thinking, but again the approach did not take hold in clinical medicine.[17] At the London School of Hygiene and Tropical Medicine, Greenwood lamented in 1936 that the movement had failed, disappearing from the clinic[18]:

> The success of clinical medicine in the second half of the 19th century and first half of the 20th century was mainly based on knowledge accrued in pathology, microbiology, and pathophysiology in the spirit of the "experimental method" proposed by Claude Bernard in 1865,[19] with little regard for numerical observations on patients.

At the same time, however, the numerical method became a working tool for physicians, who wished to use data to improve public health. Such ideas were carried on by Louis' overseas students in Britain and the United States. Osler[a] listed 37 American students who came to listen to Louis' lectures in Paris in the 1830s,[17] when young US and UK medical doctors learned French and flocked to Paris to learn what was new. People directly influenced by Louis represent a lineage of epidemiology and the hygienist movements in the 19th century (see Figure 35-1), including the Shattuck family in the United States and Farr and Guy in London.[20] Around 1850, Farr and Guy, together with Snow, helped to found a society for the study of Asiatic Cholera that later became the "Epidemiological Society of London."

While some notable Boston clinicians attended Louis' lectures, including Oliver Wendell Holmes (1809-1894) (later Dean of the Harvard Medical School), a school of "Médecine d'Observation" did not arise in the United States. Louis' school of thought was initially lost to clinical medicine, but his numerical method lived on, grew, and amalgamated via the hygienist movement into public health and general epidemiology.

From Clinical Epidemiology to Evidence-Based Medicine and the Cochrane Collaboration

A revival of numerical reasoning took place in clinical medicine starting in the 1960s. Its sources and motivations were manifold. First was the advent of the randomized controlled trial (RCT). Forerunners of RCTs in the 18th and 19th centuries included clever schemes devised by physicians to compare "like with like" (such as asking patients to take a bean from an urn with different-colored beans to decide on treatment). However, these physicians were mostly bright loners. In the 1930s and 1940s, different forms of "alternation" of patient allocation to treatment were propagated. (A comprehensive historical collection can be found at the James Lind Library.[21]) Thus, the RCT was not suddenly invented in the mid-20th century "out of the blue." In the 1950s and 1960s, Hill initiated a systematic "school of thought" about the necessity of RCTs, leading to decades of books, papers, and courses about all elements of RCTs, which strongly anchored it in medicine. The US Food and Drug Administration (FDA) enshrined the randomized trial in medicine through its requirements, from the 1960s onward, for evidence on the safety and effectiveness of new drugs *"consisting of adequate and well-controlled investigations incorporating statistical methods"*—in short, RCTs—before drugs would be allowed to enter the marketplace.[22] Later, randomized trials with positive results became prerequisites for reimbursement of drug claims by insurance companies and/or government organizations.

A second impetus for the revival of numerical reasoning was a movement beginning in the 1960s and 1970s under the banner "epidemiology should return to the clinic." The need for such a "return" was a perception of a schism that had occurred between "Schools of Public Health" and "Schools of Medicine." Major schools of public health, founded in the 19th and the beginning of the 20th centuries, considered numerical thinking about the causes and evolution of frequencies of disease to be their province. Such numerical thinking had receded from schools of medicine, where pathophysiological research had become the main basis of scientific medicine. Proponents of the new movement argued that because medicine was becoming increasingly powerful, expensive, and complex, a numerical understanding was needed of the volume and the application of diagnoses, procedures, and therapies received by patients. Such information could provide the basis for guidelines for the practice of medicine and for an overall increase in health of populations, as described in a book with a telling title: *Healing the Schism: Epidemiology, Medicine, and the Public's Health.*[23] It was recognized that departments were needed within medical schools for the clinical application of epidemiology; initiatives to build such departments were supported by charities and research organizations.

A third push for the revival of numerical reasoning came from individual pioneers like Feinstein and Sackett, who apparently keenly sensed the needs of medical practitioners and the evolution of medicine, and started writing about "clinical epidemiology" in the 1960s.[3,24-27] In 1966, Sackett established the first clinical epidemiology unit at the State University of New York at Buffalo. By 1967, he moved to Hamilton, Canada, to establish the Department of Clinical Epidemiology and Biostatistics at McMaster University.[28] Feinstein, Sackett, and like-minded colleagues considered clinical epidemiology to be a new type of clinical investigation or clinical science, contrasting with existing pathophysiologic science rooted in laboratory sciences. As well, their work reflected a power struggle, in which clinicians reacted against the dominance of basic laboratory sciences in

---

[a]William Osler (1894-1919), one of the founding medical professors of Johns Hopkins Hospital, later Regius Professor of Medicine at Oxford, UK.

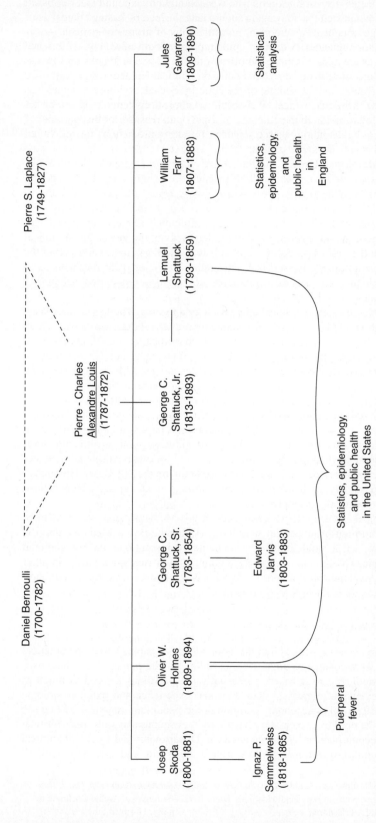

FIGURE 35-1 The influence of P.C.A. Louis on the development of statistics and epidemiology in the 19th century. (From Lilienfeld AM, Lilienfeld DE. What else is new? An historical excursion. Am J Epidemiol. 1977;105(3):169-179. doi:10.1093/oxfordjournals.aje.a112373. https://pubmed.ncbi.nlm.nih.gov/322476/.)

guiding medicine. It also reflected distrust of experts who were thought to expound theories based only on their experience. Clinicians felt that they again should take the lead by basing clinical decisions on objective knowledge obtained by numerical investigations of groups of patients—over and beyond the basic laboratory sciences. A dose of epidemiology would make clinical science more scientific. These motives are apparent in the subtitles of the two 1985 textbooks on Clinical Epidemiology cited earlier; the subtitle of Feinstein's book on Clinical Epidemiology was *"The Architecture of Clinical Research"* and the subtitle of the book by Sackett and his colleagues was *"A Basic Science for Clinical Medicine."* Later, Weiss defined clinical epidemiology, somewhat more narrowly, as the study of variation in the outcome of illness and reasons for this variation.[29] The Fletchers defined clinical epidemiology as the science of making predictions for individual patients by counting clinical events in similar patients.[30]

Such ideas did not only develop in Canada and the United States. In Denmark, Henrik Wulff published *Rational Diagnosis and Treatment* in 1973,[31] which went into several editions and English-language translations.[32] With today's eyes, Wulff's work reads like an introduction to "Evidence-Based Medicine," well before this concept became current. In the Netherlands, Wulff's book was translated into Dutch in 1980 and became widely influential. There were several reasons for these interests. Uneasiness was growing within academia about the low status of clinical investigation compared with the basic sciences. Critical self-reflection was increasing within the medical profession. At the same time, government health authorities longed for mechanisms to control the increasing complexity and costs of medicine, as described in a historical account of similar ideas in the Netherlands.[3]

In 1992, two conceptual descendants of clinical epidemiology appeared. The "Evidence-Based Medicine" movement, which favors basing medical practice on numerical data, was advanced by Sackett and his colleagues.[33] The Cochrane Collaboration,[b] which advocates evaluating numerical data in systematic literature reviews, particularly of RCTs, was proposed by Iain Chalmers in the United Kingdom and was enthusiastically embraced by the Evidence-Based Medicine movement. An initial rallying concept was the "Evidence Hierarchy" with the randomized trial on top and case reports and expert opinion at the bottom. Evidence-Based Medicine and the Cochrane Collaboration had little place for observational (*i.e.*, nonrandomized) research. Protracted discussions followed, examining whether this hierarchy was absolute or whether hierarchies might differ according to the research problem under study.[34-36] The healing of the old schism between public health epidemiology and clinical medicine somehow led to a new schism between observationalists and devotees of the RCT.[37] In the end, the emphasis of Evidence-Based Medicine on the "Evidence Hierarchy" relied somewhat too enthusiastically on the objectivity and validity of RCTs,[38] so the concept of hierarchies has since been substantially deemphasized.[36]

Both offshoots of clinical epidemiology, Evidence-Based Medicine and the Cochrane Collaboration, have been enormously influential worldwide. Evidence-Based Medicine and the Cochrane Collaboration have led to guideline-based medicine, to institutions like the National Institute of Clinical Excellence (NICE) in the United Kingdom, and to similar initiatives in other countries. They also led to development of numerous checklists to confirm the veracity and completeness of a piece of research (*e.g.*, the GRACE principles[39]).

Success in the 20th Century

At the end of the 20th century, general medical journals abounded with papers based on numerical research, in which patients were counted as units of observation, to examine etiology, diagnosis, prognosis, and treatment. Medical care is based increasingly on guidelines derived as much as possible from systematic reviews of numerical data. Personal experience and pathophysiologic reasoning have come to be regarded as secondary—although the pendulum may have swung too far.[40] In medical education, the need for systematic reviews and new numerical tools, like "Critical Appraisal Topics,"[41] have become standard items in curricula. Departments and Chairs of Clinical Epidemiology have been founded at medical schools around the world, and even at schools of

---

[b]Named after Archibald Cochrane (1909-1988), author of the influential book: *Effectiveness and Efficiency: Random Reflections on Health Services*, Nuffield Provincial Hospitals Trust, 1972. Biography of Archie Cochrane by Iain Chalmers. *J R Soc Med*. 2008;101:41-44.

public health. In less industrialized countries, clinical epidemiology departments were promoted by the early International Clinical Epidemiology Initiative (INCLEN).[42]

In the 21st century, medical editors have argued that the RCT, championed by the Evidence-Based Medicine movement, may have been encapsulated and transformed into a marketing instrument by the pharmaceutical industry.[43] It also has been stated that the Evidence-Based Medicine and Cochrane movements have lost some of their initial drive and credibility.[40] Several views about the achievements and prospects of Evidence-Based Medicine were published during 2017.[38,44-49] Interest in Evidence-Based Medicine has inspired important initiatives like the funding of the Patient-Centered Outcomes Research Institute program in the United States.

THE ROLE OF CLINICAL EPIDEMIOLOGY

The major roles for clinical epidemiology in the 21st century are to produce research that validly guides clinical care and to assure and sustain training of clinicians and others in the valid conduct and interpretation of this research.[50] Clinicians well informed about the conduct of research have a definite advantage in recognizing opportunities to solve clinical problems. Persons with both clinical and methodological expertise function as translators, who are able to talk to practicing clinicians as well as to methodologists, which will lead to better and more focused research. In addition, understanding why existing research methods will not work to solve a particular clinical problem spurs development of new methods. See Box 35-2 for an example concerning the clinical problem of hereditary coagulation disorders leading to venous thrombosis.

Persons with both clinical and methodological expertise play a key role in the adoption or rejection of clinical guidelines: they are able to adopt a critical attitude toward the research behind the guidelines, and understand from their own experience the way clinicians think, how clinical problems look, and the complex organization of health care.[53]

Defining and Delimiting the Research Question

Teaching state-of-the-art epidemiologic and statistical methods includes teaching how to transform a question about a particular clinical problem into a feasible study.[54] Clinicians focus on the overall clinical picture, but rarely is it possible to conduct useful quantitative research encompassing clinical complexity. Clear and specific comparisons between groups must be made, requiring sufficient numbers of subjects and availability of ancillary data. However, they should also learn, as Medawar explained, that *"Research is the art of the soluble."*[55]

BOX 35-2 Should Persons Who Carry Hereditary Coagulation Disorders That Predispose to Venous Thrombosis Be Treated for Life With Anticoagulation Medication?

Persons can carry a gene that predisposes to coagulation problems associated with venous thrombosis, but never had disease. The issue is whether they should be treated prophylactically for life with anticoagulation medications. Often these persons are family members of probands who carried one of more causal genes and who developed venous thrombosis (sometimes with severe consequences, including death). Because of the rarity of the mutations and the impossibility of doing a decades-long RCT to study unpredictable rare occurrences of venous thrombosis, the prospect of undertaking a study was daunting. It was known that continuous anticoagulation has an important adverse effect: during a year of treatment, close to half a percent of the patients develop severe (sometimes fatal) bleeding. The solution came to light through the realization that family pedigrees of probands could be reconstructed to study past survival in families. Thus, it would be possible to assign retroactively the probability of carrying the genes of these coagulation mutations, starting with the known probands. It was found that past survival of definite as well as potential carriers of the mutations was identical to that of the general population. The tentative conclusion was that permanent anticoagulation, with its annual risk of severe bleeding, is not indicated.[51] The same method was later applied to other hereditary conditions and proved highly useful.[52]

Feinstein described this process as the *"Preliminary Appraisal of the Outline."*[4] He emphasized the need for accuracy in defining the study objective, both stated and, perhaps more importantly, latent. He specified the questions to be asked of a clinician-researcher, as follows:

1. *What is the question,* i.e., what does the clinician propose as the problem that needs to be solved? While this question seems simple, the proposed problem frequently does not really coincide with the initial formulation of the proposed study design. Even more "delicate," writes Feinstein, is the situation in which the investigator does not readily state the basic question that the research needs to answer.

2. *What will be done with the answer*, once study data are obtained? This question reveals the "latent" objective of the investigator, which illuminates the importance of the research question, as well as the motivations behind it, *e.g.*, a competition between rival ideas. Addressing the latent objective may reveal that the originally stated objective or the originally proposed design does not align with the real intent. A thorough understanding of the latent motivation may lead to different stated objectives, or other research designs that are more convincing or feasible. To probe the latent objective in depth, it is often fruitful to "begin at the end": what conclusion or recommendation does the investigator think the research will yield? How will others with opposing views or vested interests react to the research if its results support or disprove a particular viewpoint? How will the research change prevailing views or medical practice?

Once a design is chosen that reconciles the stated with the latent objective, clinicians must learn to look at their study with the mindset of persons whose differing perspectives will affect the interpretation of the results in varying ways. For instance, cases of a disease may be identified from a registry, but the diagnoses may not have been validated and a sizable number of "cases" may not be true cases, which may lead to criticism. An example is a purely clinical diagnosis of venous thrombosis of the leg, which is known to be erroneous in a sizable percentage of patients and might sow doubt on the study's credibility.[56] To improve understanding of a study based on registered diagnoses, it is worthwhile, as part of a bias analysis, to spend extra time and resources to ascertain the validity of registry diagnoses for at least a sample of patients. As an example, a recent study showed that 12% to 30% of patients registered in the Danish National Patient Registry with a diagnosis of venous thromboembolism did not fulfill clinical criteria for the condition.[57]

When registry data are already available for a given exposure and outcome, it is tempting to jump immediately to data analysis, without considering the information really needed to solve the problem (such as data on possible confounders and biases). Even if data *seem* readily available, it pays to consider what data would be ideal if the study could be designed from scratch, without money or time constraints. Although optimal data might not be available in practice, this step identifies potential study shortcomings and is worthwhile in anticipating future discussions or designing analyses to examine potential biases (see Chapter 29).

A temptation is to consider clinical epidemiology as an "over-the-counter" research service for clinicians who need help with routine quantitative problems, such as calculating study size or responding to a reviewer's request for extra analyses or statistical tests. Often such services are requested *post hoc* by clinicians when their paper has been nearly completed or even after it has been rejected by a journal. A better strategy for clinical epidemiology is to collaborate with clinical departments interested in doing quantitative research, to learn from each other's skills and backgrounds, so that the proposed research undertaking is rooted in a deep understanding of its clinical, physiological, biochemical, and organizational ramifications—and becomes a continuing teaching opportunity for all practicing clinicians who are involved, and vice versa for clinical epidemiologists who learn about new problems to solve.

METHODOLOGIC CONCERNS SPECIFIC TO CLINICAL EPIDEMIOLOGY

Clinical and general epidemiologic scientific evidence is a prerequisite for providing safe, high-quality patient care and taking maximum advantage of advances in diagnostics, treatment, rehabilitation, and prevention. While clinicians use etiologic knowledge in their clinical decisions, and clinical epidemiologists often may conduct research into the causes of diseases, study designs addressing disease etiology are covered in other chapters of this book. Here, we limit our discussion to the type of evidence needed to answer four key clinical questions and some problems specific to clinical epidemiology. Evidence to guide clinical actions is best derived from continually updated answers to these questions[29,58]:

1. Which tests/examinations should be used to diagnose a disease and predict its course, while reducing false-positive and false-negative results so far as practical (**diagnosis**)?
2. What is the expected course of a disease, *e.g.*, spontaneous cure or progression without clinical intervention (*natural history*) or with treatment (*clinical course*) (**prognosis**)? Knowledge of the natural history of many diseases is limited for several reasons. Many have a long asymptomatic phase during which they are unrecognized. As well, most diagnosed diseases and their complications are treated, so we know their clinical course, but not their natural course.
3. To what extent will a specific clinical intervention be beneficial in terms of curing or preventing a disease, slowing its progression, or reducing its symptom burden (**interventions**)?
4. What are the risks—side effects, unintended adverse effects, or complications—of selected treatments and interventions, and the safety and quality of clinical care (**risk-harm**)?

In the following text, we review key concepts relevant to validity and interpretation of clinical epidemiological studies that address these four questions.

Question 1: Diagnosis

Accurate diagnosis of a disease is the first step in predicting the prognosis and optimizing therapy.[59] Clinicians begin the diagnostic process by obtaining a medical, social, and family history, assessing the frequency of potential risk factors, and performing an initial physical examination. They make decisions at each step of the process. Diagnostic tests are used to increase the likelihood of determining presence or absence of a disease and to predict prognosis. During the clinical course (please see below for definition) the tests can be used to monitor the effect of treatment.

The increasing availability of new and sensitive diagnostic tests has put the initial classical clinical physical examination under pressure. Often multiple tests are requested. No diagnostic test is perfect, and in clinical medicine it is common to reduce the results of a diagnostic test to a dichotomous outcome, such as positive or negative. Clinicians use many diagnostic strategies, based on experience, pattern recognition, and algorithms, to confirm or rule out a diagnosis.[59,60] The availability of diagnostic tests does not relieve clinicians from carefully observing and examining the patient.

Despite the important technological advances over the past 50 years in medicine, uncertainty remains a key feature of clinical care. Clinicians' perceptions of the risk of a malpractice suit may have major impact on the number of tests selected and are an important component of the concept of *defensive medicine*. It is beyond the scope of this chapter to discuss psychological aspects of diagnostic and therapeutic decision-making.

The accuracy of a diagnostic test is often said to be evaluated in relation to a "*gold standard*"—which would be an ideal diagnostic test with no false positives or negatives. With few exceptions, such a test does not exist, since almost all diagnostic procedures require interpretation and are subject to error. However, there might be a "*reference standard,*" which can be a single test or a combination of tests. The reference standard should be the best existing test to guide clinical action at the time that a new test is proposed.[61] The *sensitivity* (true positive rate) and *specificity* (true negative rate) are classical clinical epidemiological parameters that can be calculated to evaluate a diagnostic test. Table 35-1 shows the most commonly used measures of diagnostic test accuracy. The intricacies of diagnostic studies have been discussed in detail by several epidemiologists[29,62,63] and in the publications of the "Standards for Reporting Diagnostic Accuracy Studies" (STARD) initiative, which is a useful current guideline for reporting studies of diagnostic tests.[64]

Likelihood ratios combine elements of sensitivity and specificity and can be combined with pretest probability, or disease prevalence, to obtain posttest disease probability. Likelihood ratios are used to determine how probable it is for a diagnostic test result to be found in diseased versus nondiseased persons. The likelihood ratio thus indicates how much a given diagnostic test will raise or lower a pretest probability of the target disorder.[29,62] For a positive test, the likelihood

TABLE 35-1

Measures of Test Accuracy

Test Result	Gold Standard		
	Positive	Negative	*N*
Positive	*a*	*b*	*a + b*
Negative	*c*	*d*	*c + d*
	a + c	*b + d*	

Accuracy Term

Sensitivity	*a/(a + c)*
Specificity	*d/(b + d)*
Predictive value of a positive test (PV+)	*a/(a + b)*
Predictive value of a negative test (PV−)	*d/(c + d)*
Likelihood ratio for a positive test result	$\dfrac{\text{Sensitivity}}{1-\text{specificity}}$
Likelihood ratio for a negative test result	$\dfrac{1-\text{Sensitivity}}{\text{Specificity}}$

Example:

Measures of test accuracy in a hypothetical study of 2,000 patients undergoing a diagnostic test.

Test Result	Gold Standard		
	Positive	Negative	N
Positive	900	100	1,000
Negative	50	950	1,000
			2,000

Accuracy Term

Sensitivity	900/950 = 0.95
Specificity	950/1,050 = 0.90
Predictive value of a positive test	900/1,000 = 0.90
Predictive value of a negative test	950/1,000 = 0.95
Likelihood ratio of a positive test	$\dfrac{0.95}{1-0.90} = 9.95$
Likelihood for a negative test	$\dfrac{1-0.90}{0.95} = 0.11$

ratio is sensitivity/(1 − specificity). For a negative test, the corresponding likelihood ratio is (1 − sensitivity)/specificity. As examples, the positive likelihood ratio for an ECG for acute myocardial infarction is 28.5 and the negative likelihood ratio is 0.44. A CT scan for a brain tumor has a positive likelihood ratio of 31.7 and a negative likelihood ratio of 0.05.[65]

The pretest probability represents a clinician's estimate of the probability that a patient has a disease based on the patient's symptoms, frequency of risk factors, age, clinical findings, and published or other external data. This probability can be graphed as a *receiver operating characteristics* (ROC) *curve* (Figure 35-2). The curve expresses the sensitivity and the false-positive rate

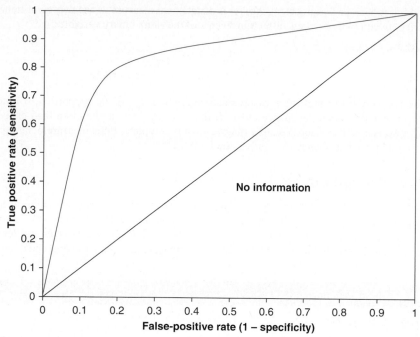

FIGURE 35-2 The receiver operator characteristic curve illustrates the relation between specificity and sensitivity. The closer to 1 for the area under the curve (AUC), the better the test. A good test normally has a 0.7 to 0.8 AUC.

for a given test. The true positives are shown on the *y*-axis and the false positives on the *x*-axis. The closer the ROC curve is to the upper left-hand corner of the graph, the more accurate are the test results. Clinicians often use many tests in parallel to reach a diagnosis quickly, a practice that increases the risk of false-positive diagnoses because a false-positive test for any one of the tests yields a false-positive diagnosis.[62]

Classification of Diseases

Much clinical epidemiological research, especially registry studies and studies using electronic medical records, rely on the WHO's *International Classification of Diseases* (ICD), a system used to code patient diagnoses and procedures. The ICD was originally developed as a uniform classification of causes of death. Validation studies of registry data have shown a potential risk of misclassification of almost every disease in the ICD,[66] along with other methodological challenges. For example, in ICD-10, laterality (right or left) in paired organs is not always recorded; it is recorded for breast cancer, but not for renal or lung cancer. Laterality might be important, *e.g.*, when an organ might suffer from previous therapeutic radiation on the right or left side of the body. Furthermore, changes in coding systems in succeeding versions of the ICD may introduce lack of comparability and detail; *e.g.*, venous thrombosis in the upper extremities had a specific code in ICD-8 but not in ICD-10. Moreover, the ICD often lacks information on disease severity. Another limitation is use of broad categories of diseases; thus it is not possible to separate amyotrophic lateral sclerosis from other motor neuron diseases in ICD-10. Diagnostic criteria also may change over time, new diseases might be added to the ICD, and known diseases might be split up into subgroups (see "Description of New Diseases").

Clinical Disagreement

Interpretation of findings is a key component of clinical care. It follows that disagreement over diagnosis and treatment decisions is common.[67,68] Disagreement may stem from history-taking or physical findings, such as hypertension. Even if a clinician examines the same patient twice, he or she may disagree with his or her own earlier assessment. This is called *clinical disagreement*. Interpretation of x-rays, ECGs, pathological specimens, and mammograms is especially subject to intra- and interobserver disagreement. *Kappa* is a statistical measure of the degree of nonrandom agreement between two observers or measurements of the same binary variables:

$$Kappa = \frac{A_{obs} - A_{exp}}{1 - A_{exp}} = \text{where}$$

A_{obs} is the proportion of times the measurements agree and A_{exp} is the proportion of times they would be expected to agree by chance alone. If the measurements agree more than expected by chance, Kappa is positive. Kappa equals 1 if agreement is complete. If the measurements agree less than expected by chance, Kappa is negative (Table 35-2).[69,70]

Question 2: Prognosis

Predicting the course of a disease and trying to improve its prognosis is a key goal of clinical care. For this reason, clinical epidemiology has an important focus on understanding prognosis.[59] *Prognostic research* is the investigation of the relation between patients' clinical characteristics and future outcomes.[61] Most patients wish to know the likelihood of obtaining relief from symptoms and discomfort.[71]

TABLE 35-2

Observer Reliability

The Kappa coefficient is a measure of the reliability of categorical measures designed to take chance agreement into consideration. Reliability is also termed reproducibility. A_{Obs} is relative observed agreement among the two observers. A_{Exp} is a probability that the agreement is due to chance alone. If measurements agree more than expected by chance, Kappa is positive. If agreement is perfect, Kappa is 1. If there is no agreement, Kappa is 0. Sometimes the strength of agreement using Kappa statistics is expressed as follows:

Kappa	Strength of Agreement
0.00	Poor
0.01-0.20	Slight
0.21-0.40	Fair
0.41-0.60	Moderate
0.61-0.80	Substantial
0.81-1.00	Almost perfect

Example:

Reliability evaluation in a hypothetical study based on two observers, for example a pathological specimen.

		Observer 2		
		Positive	Negative	Total
Observer 1	Positive	66	22	88
	Negative	24	80	104
	Total	90	102	192

$$A_{obs} = \frac{A+D}{A+B+C+D} = \frac{66+80}{66+22+24+80} = 0.76$$

$$A_{exp} = \frac{(66+24)(66+22)+(22+80)(24+80)}{(66+22+24+80)^2} = 0.50$$

$$Kappa = \frac{A_{obs} + A_{exp}}{1 - A_{exp}} = \frac{0.76-0.50}{1-0.50} = 0.52$$

From Glasser SP. *Essentials of Clinical Research.* New York: Springer; 2008.

In prognostic research, concepts of probability and risk are more important than measurement of relative association. A *risk factor* is associated with an increased risk of developing a disease or another outcome, while a *prognostic factor* is associated with an outcome of a disease.[62] A factor associated with increased risk of a disease does not necessarily imply poor prognosis once the disease occurs. A classic example is blood pressure: high blood pressure is a risk factor for developing acute myocardial infarction, while low blood pressure after myocardial infarction is a strong prognostic factor for mortality.

The severity, aggressiveness, and spread of the *underlying disease*, often referred to as the *index disease*, and *comorbid diseases* (presence of diseases other than the index disease) are important predictors of outcome.[72] Hemingway and colleagues proposed the four distinct, but interrelated, themes of prognostic research:[73]

1. *Fundamental prognostic research* on medical conditions in the context of the nature and quality of current care.
2. *Prognostic factor research* on specific factors (such as biomarkers) associated with prognosis.
3. *Prognostic model research* focusing on development, validation, and impact of statistical models for predicting individual risk and future outcomes.
4. *Tailoring treatment decisions on medicines* focusing on use of prognostic information to help stratify treatment decisions to an individual or a group of individuals with similar characteristics (also called "personalized medicine").

Endpoints or outcomes are used to describe the natural or clinical course of a disease. These include[74]:

1. *Hard endpoints.* Examples are mortality, recurrence, complications, or remission. Remission is defined as a phase in which the disease is no longer detectable. In-hospital mortality is commonly used as an endpoint, but this measure is vulnerable to bias because patients can be transferred between hospitals or because early death after discharge is not captured.
2. *Surrogate endpoints.* Examples are changes in lab values, blood pressure, or reduction of tumor size, which indicate response to treatment. Surrogate and hard endpoints do not always correlate, as shown in the well-known CAST trial.[75] The trial focused on premature ventricular depolarizations (arrhythmias), which are predictors of sudden death in survivors of acute myocardial infarction. CAST examined the effect of antiarrhythmic treatment with encainide, flecainide, and placebo on risk of death in 1,498 patients with asymptomatic or mildly symptomatic ventricular arrhythmia after myocardial infarction. After an average of 10 months of follow-up, patients treated with an antiarrhythmic agent had fewer arrhythmias but higher mortality than those not receiving treatment (7.7% vs. 3%) and the trial was discontinued. The mechanisms behind the findings were not clear.[75]
3. *Soft endpoints.* Examples are measures of quality of life or functional status. Functional status is a primary concern both for patients and their clinical providers.[76] *Patient-reported outcome* (PRO) instruments assess outcomes from the patient perspective. PRO instruments often include a defined list of items to which patients respond using standardized options. Examples are the Short Form 36 general health questionnaire and the Stroke Impact Scale.[76-78]
4. *Composite endpoints.* Composite endpoints are a set of endpoints treated as a single endpoint.[28] For example, in some cardiac trials, all-cause mortality, myocardial infarction, revascularization, and stroke are combined into a single endpoint called MACE.[79-81] Arguments have been made for the use of composite endpoints. First, the distinction between different endpoints might be unnecessary because they have the same consequences, such as ischemic and hemorrhagic stroke. Second, combining endpoints will increase a study's statistical power by increasing the number of events, and hence decreasing the variance of the estimates of effect. On the other hand, if some included endpoints are unrelated to the intervention, composite outcomes may reduce study power because the effect of the intervention on the related part of the composite outcome is diluted by the null effect of the intervention on the unrelated part of the composite outcome.[28,82-84] Lauer and Topol have provided a number of questions to be considered when reporting composite endpoints.[85] The most important questions are:
   a. Are the endpoints of clinical interest or only surrogates for clinically meaningful endpoints?[86]

    b. How are nonfatal endpoints measured? Endpoints requiring a measurement that involves human judgment are inherently subject to bias and hence warrant an endpoints committee, a core laboratory, or both, and these should be blinded to treatment information.[87-90]

    c. How many individual endpoints are considered part of a composite endpoint and how are they reported? When composite endpoints are analyzed, the individual endpoints are by default treated to be of equal clinical importance, which is evidently wrong whenever death is included alongside a nonfatal event.

    d. It is important to clarify how nonfatal events are analyzed. A composite endpoint that includes death as well as nonfatal events may be subject to biases related to competing risks.[91,92] Obviously, patients who die cannot later experience other nonfatal or fatal events.

5. A *primary* endpoint is the main endpoint in a study, either an observational study or an RCT. Studies are often designed based on primary endpoints. Other endpoints are called *secondary endpoints*.

6. *Health economic endpoints* include health care utilization and expenditures. The main types of cost analyses include:

    a. Cost-benefit analysis, examining the trade-off between the cost of caring for a patient and the overall benefit.

    b. Cost-effectiveness analysis, examining the trade-off between the cost of caring for a patient and the level of efficacy of a treatment.

    c. Cost utility analysis, examining the trade-off between costs and measures of utility, including efficacy, increased life expectancy, and productivity.

Follow-Up in Prognostic Studies

In prognostic research, it is important to specify whether cases are incident (new) or prevalent (existing) or a mixture. Moreover, it is important to clearly define when follow-up time starts, *e.g.*, at the onset of symptoms, at time of diagnosis, at treatment initiation, or at hospital discharge, and make sure that no follow-up time is included before the last event required to meet enrollment criteria. Depending on the study design, use of prevalent cases or inclusion of person-time before the last event required to meet enrollment criteria may result in inclusion of immortal person-time and its resulting biases (see Chapter 7). While researchers should always be cautious about this bias, it does not rule out the use of prevalent exposures, *e.g.*, for etiologic research[93] or when using "period analysis" for prognosis (see below).

    The type of study population being examined is another important consideration. Is the study drawn from primary care, drawn from tertiary care, or population-based? The prognosis might vary considerably within the clinical spectrum represented in various study populations. A classic example is Ellenberg and Nelson's 1980 study investigating adverse outcomes following febrile convulsions. Risks ranged from a low value of 1.5% in population-based studies to almost 60% in clinic-based studies.[94]

    Prognostic studies can be comparative and, as mentioned in the introduction to this chapter, may straddle traditional population epidemiology and clinical epidemiology. For example, a cohort study of multisystem morbidity and mortality in Cushing syndrome compared all Danish patients diagnosed with benign Cushing syndrome of adrenal or pituitary origin during 1980 to 2010 with a matched comparison cohort drawn from the general population. The study found that the multimorbidity risk was increased even before diagnosis, but also that mortality and risk of myocardial infarction remained elevated during long-term follow-up—when most patients were cured from an endocrinological point of view. The prolonged excess mortality was likely due to the long period of hypercorticism *before* diagnosis, which has lasting effects.[95]

    Calculation of patient survival based on past studies may seriously underestimate survival, because medicine continues to improve, and older findings, particularly for early-stage disease, may no longer apply. For example, 30-day mortality after myocardial infarction declined from 31% in 1981-1988 to 14.8% in 2004-2008.[96] For this reason, the method of "period analysis"[97] can be used. In this method, a recent calendar time period is defined and the follow-up of patients diagnosed during that calendar time is tallied. The follow-up of patients who were diagnosed before that recent calendar time period, but who were still alive at the beginning of that period, is also tallied and only the person-time of follow-up during that recent calendar time period is used. For example, suppose an investigator wants to examine 20-year survival among persons who have undergone colon cancer surgery. Using a cancer registry, the investigator would identify all persons who were alive after such surgery at a certain date, for example, January 1, 2009. All these patients would be enrolled for follow-up, but stratified according to the length of time since their surgery. Patients who underwent this surgery after January 2009 also would be enrolled in the study. All patients would be followed until a given date, for example, December 31, 2012. The 2009 to 2012 period represents different time windows of follow-up since surgery for different patients. For each time window of follow-up since surgery, incidence rates of death can be calculated for this 4-year period; the incidence rates of death can then be transformed into a life table, starting with recent follow-up and ending with long-term follow-up, up to 20 years after surgery. This amounts to "left-censoring" and staggered entry in a life table (this approach is how population life tables are calculated: from birth to age 100 in the same calendar year). The 20-year cohort experience reconstructed in this way is *not* the same as that obtained when follow-up begins at the time of surgery among patients who were treated 20 years ago. The life table for the latter complete cohort is of little interest for future patients, however, since it reflects past surgical and medical practice, rather than present practice. The experience of those in their earlier years of follow-up during the 2009 to 2012 time period coupled with the experience of long-time survivors who have the benefits of recent medical care has the advantage of representing a more contemporary state of health care. The most recent experience may be of greatest value for decisions about future health care for individuals as well as for society.[97]

Clinical Scales, Prognostic Scores, Comorbidity, Complications, and Multimorbidity

Clinical scales are summary measures of a state of disease or health. Examples are scales describing functional status, quality of life, or symptoms. They typically combine several medical measurements into a single index. The TNM cancer staging system developed by the American Joint Committee on Cancer to predict cancer prognosis,[98,99] the Framingham Risk Score to predict risk of cardiovascular disease,[100] the American Society of Anesthesiologists (ASA) physical status classification system to predict physical function of patients prior to receiving anesthesia,[101] and the APGAR score to predict the physical function of newborns[102] are well-known examples.

The outcome of most diseases is affected by the presence of other diseases (*comorbidity*).[72] The scientific and clinical importance of comorbidity is underestimated in clinical medicine, as clinicians and researchers in given medical specialties have a preference for focusing on diseases subsumed within their own specialty. Many scales have been developed to quantify the impact of comorbidity by estimating the prognostic effect of the most prevalent comorbid diseases on mortality and compiling these effects into an index. One of the most widely used indices is the Charlson Comorbidity Index (CCI).[103] Charlson et al. examined the prognostic impact of 19 selected chronic diseases on 1-year mortality among patients in hospital medical wards.[103] Based on the regression coefficients, an individual disease was allocated a score reflecting its prognostic effect. For instance, previous acute myocardial infarction received a score of 1 and previous stroke with hemiplegia received a score of 2. One should be aware that CCI scores were developed 30 years ago and their relevance to the current state of medicine is becoming attenuated. Still, the CCI score remains useful to predict risk of death for a given group of patients and to adjust for the influence of diseases other than the index disease in prognostic studies.

Other indices include the Index of Coexisting Disease[104] and the Cumulative Illness Rating Scale (CIRS).[105] The Index of Coexisting Disease (ICED) consists of two dimensions, one measuring the disease severity of 14 categories of comorbid diseases (ICED-DS) and one measuring "overall functional severity" (disability) caused by comorbidity (ICED-FS). Scores are based on an explicit list of symptoms, signs, and laboratory tests.[106,107] The CIRS attempts to address all relevant body systems without using specific diagnoses. It rates 13 conceptually valid body systems (supporting content validity) on a five-point (pathophysiologic) severity scale.[108,109]

Comorbidity exists independently of the index disease, whereas *complications* are conditions that are a consequence of the index disease or its treatment.[72] For example, diabetes may be a comorbid condition in patients undergoing fracture surgery, but venous thromboembolism may be a complication of the fracture surgery.

Case *mix* is a term often used in clinical practice, but the term was originally used for measuring hospital performance.[110] "Diagnosis Related Groups" is a system that classifies patients according to diagnosis, age, and treatment. It is used to inform the payment system, in which hospitals are reimbursed a set fee for a given patient category regardless of the actual cost of care.

The health care systems of many countries are facing the aging of the population in conjunction with pressure to contain costs. The proportion of people aged 65 years or more in Western Europe and North America is expected to increase from 18% in 2012 to 26% in 2025. Diagnostics and chronic disease treatment have improved, and the threshold for initiating preventive treatment of asymptomatic conditions has been lowered.[111] Consequently, the number of patients with multimorbidity will increase dramatically. This development has several important implications. For example, elderly patients with comorbidity benefit only to a limited extent from recent breakthroughs in areas such as cancer treatment.[112] This issue has been the focus of editorials in major journals, such as *BMJ, JAMA*, and *The Lancet*, with a call for innovative approaches.[112-115] In addition, as individuals live longer with multiple chronic diseases, each requiring treatment with evolving medical interventions, major clinical challenges of polypharmacy and iatrogenic harms emerge. Research and treatment will remain suboptimal if they focus only on single diseases or illness episodes, individual treatments, or mortality, without attention to quality of life.[111]

Question 3: Interventions

After diagnostic tests, application of interventions is the key responsibility of clinicians. Knowledge of the benefit and risk of interventions, provided by clinical epidemiology, is central to their decisions. Interventions may include drugs, surgery, vaccinations, lifestyle changes, and rehabilitation. Human trials are divided broadly into four phases (Table 35-3). In the following, we review the major aspects of clinical trials, focusing on the ability of an experimental design to reduce the risks of bias and confounding.

In clinical trials the investigator applies an intervention and observes the outcome. Trials may be considered a type of cohort study, with assignment of the exposure and structured follow-up. The clinical course observed after an intervention may be a consequence of a combination of the intervention itself, the placebo effect, the effect of co-medications, and the natural course of the disease.[62]

TABLE 35-3

Phase I to Phase IV Clinical Trials

Phase I trial	First test of a drug (or a candidate vaccine) in a small group of humans to determine its safety and mode of action. It usually involves fewer than 100 healthy volunteers. The focus is on safety and pharmacological profits; it may also assess dose and route of administration.
Phase II trial	Pilot efficacy studies. Initial trial to examine efficacy, usually in 200 to 500 volunteers; with vaccines, the focus is on immunogenicity, and with drugs, on demonstration of safety and efficacy in comparison to existing regimens. Usually, but not always, subjects are randomly allocated to the study and control groups.
Phase III trial	Extensive clinical trial. This phase is intended for complete assessment of safety and efficacy. It involves large numbers of patients with the disease or condition of interest, sometimes thousands. It uses random allocation to study and control groups.
Phase IV trial	Conducted after the regulatory authority has approved registration and marketing begins. The common aim is to estimate the incidence of rare adverse reactions and other potential effects of long-term use in real life. It may also study new uses and indications. It is part of postmarketing surveillance, which also includes observational studies.

From Porta M. *A Dictionary of Epidemiology*. 5th ed. Oxford: Oxford University Press; 2008.

Clinical trials are often described as either *efficacy* or *effectiveness* trials.[116] Efficacy pertains to whether an intervention works in highly selected patients who actually receive it. An efficacy trial is also called an *explanatory* trial. An effectiveness trial evaluates whether an intervention with proven efficacy works in routine clinical circumstances. An effectiveness trial is also called a *pragmatic* trial. The outcome in the intervention group is compared with the outcome in a comparison (or control) group exposed to another treatment already shown to be effective, or to a placebo in the absence of an alternative intervention.

Clinicians are, of course, interested in the specific effect of an intervention, but this may be difficult to ascertain in studies using a *nonexperimental design*. For instance, a classic problem is *regression toward the mean,* a common, often unrecognized, consequence of measurement variability. In statistical terms, the phenomenon of regression toward the mean is seen if a variable is by chance extreme on its first measurement. It will tend to be closer to the average at the second measurement. For example, patients with high blood pressure will be treated, yet, even without treatment, their blood pressure may be closer to the normal level when measured again. A lower blood pressure on the second measurement is a combination of the treatment benefit and the regression toward the mean.[117] In clinical settings, with many repeated unstructured measurements, regression toward the mean can lead to false impressions of treatment effectiveness and a distorted understanding of the natural history of disease, because treatment is only given to persons with particularly high or particularly low values. To avoid this common pitfall, it is often imperative to conduct a randomized trial in such persons; regression toward the mean will, of course, also be present in a trial setting, but the problem is corrected by the comparison group that estimates its magnitude.

Confounding by Indication

Confounding by indication is a key problem in evaluation of clinical therapeutics. The term was introduced in 1980 by Greenland and Neutra[118] in the context of a study on the benefit of fetal monitoring during labor. Fetal monitoring seemed to lead to a twofold increase in Cesarean sections. Greenland and Neutra argued that fetal monitoring during labor is initiated, among other reasons, because the delivery process appears to slow at some point. Thus, they concluded that more Caesarean sections were to be expected in the group of women receiving monitoring.[119] That is, deliveries with indications for fetal monitoring also have indications for Caesarean section.

All interventions are undertaken with the express intention to avoid particular outcomes. It follows that all medical actions and interventions are guided by the risk of one or more particular outcomes in a patient. Pregnant women with a high-risk delivery will receive monitoring, a patient with more severe hypertension and existing vascular damage will receive more therapy than a patient with mild uncomplicated hypertension, and a patient with an advanced stage of cancer will receive different treatment than the patient with localized disease.

Because interventions rarely completely reverse a high risk of an undesired outcome, a group of patients with advanced disease will almost always fare more poorly than a group of patients with more moderate disease, even if the former group receives cutting-edge therapy. "Channeling" is a term used in the literature to describe this phenomenon.[120] Whether confounded by indication or by channeling, when different groups of patients are followed up and compared, the therapy provided to those at low risk will almost always appear superior and that given to patients at high risk will appear inferior. Proper medical care purposefully tailors therapy to prognosis, which in turn makes nonrandomized research on the effectiveness of therapies difficult. The problem might be worse for new therapies, which are often first used in patients with a poor prognosis, for whom no other therapy is available. Some therapies might first be tested in persons with a good prognosis because they are "ideal candidates." Either way, it will be difficult to assess the effect of the new therapy, unless the therapeutic benefit is extreme (see section on case reports).

Confounding by indication has been called an "intractable" bias,[121,122] because the choice of treatment is guided foremost by the risk of a particular outcome. The degree of confounding by indication is difficult to assess, because it is based on "expected" prognosis, and that expectation is formed in the mind of a physician dealing with an individual patient. It might be argued that if we were to know all the factors on which the judgment of the prognosis is based, then we might select similar patients or adjust the analysis. However, it is almost impossible to identify a sufficient set of prognostic variables to control for the confounding analytically or by design features such as matching or restriction. The grading of prognosis by physicians is subjective and affected by measurable factors and intangible factors. For example, grading of a patient's cardiovascular disease might include "degree of ankle edema" or "degree of exhaustion after (mild) exertion," but such judgments are often not available to the data analyst because they were observed by the doctor but not recorded, or recorded only in "free text fields" of a medical file. Even if captured in clinical records, the grading remains subjective. The subjectivity of the judgment is increased by intangibles, such as the way a patient looks and behaves. A 70-year-old with a past myocardial infarction might express worry about her exhaustion on mild exercise by gesticulating forcefully that she wants to go golfing next summer with a group of friends. She will be judged to have a different prognosis and will be approached differently than a 70-year-old with a similar medical history who shuffles in, sits with stooped shoulders, looks dejected, and indicates that things outside of his immediate home environment no longer interest him much.

"Making a prognosis" is an important aim of clinical care.[71] Physicians are in general good prognosticators and rely heavily on intangibles. It has been shown that a clinician's judgment about poor short-term survival in an intensive care unit is superior to a numerical score based on hard estimates.[123] As well, if physicians are good at short-term prognostication, groups of patients treated differently may show little overlap in prognosis—putting a nonrandomized comparison between different therapies out of reach.

There have been some methodological advances in design and analysis, but these still generally fail to address fully the problem of confounding by indication. The resistance of confounding by indication to standard statistical adjustment, to propensity scoring, and to instrumental variable analysis has led to it being described as the "most stubborn bias."[122] Clinical epidemiologists have been warning in the strongest terms how and why it still causes problems, despite analytic and methodologic advances.[82]

Randomization: What Does It Do and What Does It Not Do?

Randomized trials are cohort studies in which investigators randomly allocate patients to an intervention. Randomization is a technique used to break the link between perceived prognosis and the medical actions that follow that perception (whether these actions are increased monitoring, administering drugs, doing surgery, etc.). The aim is to eliminate confounding by indication and to compare "like with like." Randomization provides several benefits when it can be ethically implemented. First, it provides a baseline expectation of exchangeability of treatment groups (see Chapter 5). Second, it allows valid assignment of a probability distribution to the set of possible data arrangements (outcomes), which lends meaning to conventional inferential statistics. Finally, randomization breaks the link between prognosis and therapy because the allocation to treatment is concealed.

To understand how randomization works, it is necessary to trace the history of randomization. Chalmers argues that before randomization was widely employed, and even before Fisher introduced this method in agricultural experiments, physicians knew that a fair comparison between similar patients was needed to test interventions.[124] In the 1930s and 1940s, the concept of "alternation" was applied: the first patient encountered who was eligible in a treatment trial received therapy A, the second received therapy B, the third therapy A, and so on in the sequence that patients were seen. The first edition of Hill's *Principle of Medical Statistics* published in 1937 advocated this method for allocating treatment "to rule out conscious and unconscious bias."[125] However, Hill changed his mind when he saw that it led to lopsided distributions of baseline characteristics. The reason was that physicians who enrolled patients in a trial *knew beforehand* which therapy a patient would receive. The result was all too human behavior in which the physician apparently thought that some patients were better candidates for treatment A than for B; thus if a patient showed up for the "wrong" treatment, that patient was not entered in the trial. Because they enrolled the patients knowing what treatment they would receive, they recreated the situation in which physicians choose a therapy because of patient characteristics. This led Hill to propose randomization (instead of alternation) in the British Medical Research Council's landmark clinical trial of streptomycin for pulmonary tuberculosis, published in 1948.[124]

Randomization was *proposed to make the allocation unpredictable*. While Hill is considered the "father of the randomized trial" in medicine, it is often felt that he borrowed the idea from Fisher. However, Hill's reasons for introducing randomization in medicine had little to do with statistical theory—which motivated Fisher. Rather, Hill intended to prevent "conscious and unconscious bias" in the allocation of an intervention.[126] However, to make it possible for randomization to work in that way, it is essential that the patient be enrolled in the trial before the physician is informed about the random allocation. This is called *"concealed allocation."* Without concealment, randomization would not work at all, as can be seen in the following scenario: a table of random numbers is used to allocate patients to treatment A or B, and the physician is instructed to follow the table, but the table is open on the desk when seeing patients. This would not differ from alternation, because whenever the physician encountered a potentially eligible patient, she would know whether the patient would get treatment A or B, and on this basis decide whether to enroll the patient in the trial. This would again produce lopsided comparison groups.

That concealment is actually as important as randomness is evident in a second theoretical scenario: suppose that in a large randomized trial with many centers participating, one treatment allocation office serves all centers. After enrolling a patient in the trial, a physician receives a treatment allocation through a telephone call to the central office. It would not matter if the allocation office used "alternation" in an ABABABABA scheme since a physician in one center would not know whether the previous patient in another center had received treatment A or B. In this case, alternation would be as good as randomization, because the allocation is concealed and pseudorandomized.

Myths About Randomization

Concealed randomization guarantees that there is no bias in the *mechanism* of the allocation to treatment arms. However, this is only a guarantee about the *mechanism*, not about the outcome of randomization. It is often taught that "by randomization the two groups become alike in all known and unknown characteristics." This is impossible because randomization is a game of chance. Human beings have innumerable characteristics (from their DNA sequences to the length of the toenail of their right little toe, or the color of their socks). When a few hundred or even a few thousand persons are randomized, it is inescapable that several of these innumerable characteristics will be distributed in an unbalanced way, including some potential confounders. What randomization guarantees is that any incomparability of *known* or *unknown* prognostic factors is *due to chance*.

Thus, after randomization, confounding can remain.[127] For *known* characteristics that are potential confounders, potential differences following randomization can be evaluated in a table of baseline characteristics. Some differences *should* appear, as randomization does not provide perfectly balanced groups. For *unknown* or unmeasured characteristics, randomization provides a type of statistical control: confidence intervals and other statistics derived solely from the randomization assumption will incorporate uncertainty about the net effect of these characteristics given their probable degree of imbalance (assuming that randomization was carried out as stated, without violations).[127] Unfortunately, typical settings will hold problems that can undermine these statistics, much as in nonexperimental studies. Biased loss to follow-up (informative censoring), improper adjustment for posttreatment events, nonadherence to assigned treatment, and other complications will undermine randomization and may bring in the need for adjustments like nonrandomized studies (see "Generalizability and Principles of Analysis").

Often it is said that the comparability of treatment groups is better in large trials. Very large trials (so-called megatrials) are conducted to evaluate small effects or rare outcomes. For instance, 10,000 patients may be enrolled to evaluate an effect smaller than a percentage point. In such trials, known baseline characteristics often will look nearly the same in the treatment groups, *i.e.*, with less than a percentage point of difference. However, if several small differences occur by chance in the same direction as the prognosis, the results of a trial designed to detect small differences will be biased.

Randomization allows valid assignment of probability distributions to the event space (possible outcomes of the trial).[127] One can then validly compute the probability of the observed result, or results more extreme, and make an inference by choosing between the assumption that the observed result emanates from a treatment benefit or the assumption that the observed result emanates from the combined impact of biases, including chance imbalances from the expected exchangeability. Senn provides a more technical exposition about this and other myths about randomization.[128]

When Comparison Groups Are Not Necessary

Evaluation of the *intended effects of treatment* almost always requires a comparison group and randomization. Some exceptions do exist. Comparison groups (and randomization) are unnecessary if knowledge of an expected outcome without treatment is secure, and the outcome observed after treatment deviates greatly from the expected outcome without treatment. In this case, confounding by indication can be ruled out by logic. For instance, a comparison is not required to evaluate the necessity of parachutes for persons jumping from an airplane.[129] A comparative study is also unnecessary if it is observed that out of eight insulin-dependent patients with diabetes who received pancreatic islet cell transplantation, five did not require insulin for more than a year; this could not occur spontaneously.[130] Furthermore, a comparative study is not needed if it is observed that only 1 out of 62 persons with a known highly toxic dose of paracetamol poisoning develops liver damage after treatment with intravenous acetylcysteine.[131] Similarly, no comparison group is needed to study a topical treatment of strawberry angiomas on the skin, if a topically treated lesion that existed for years disappears in a fortnight. While such skin lesions can disappear spontaneously, the odds of this occurring at the time of topical treatment seem remote.

Judgments about the effectiveness of treatments, based on persons receiving the intervention without a control group, are often based on common sense. For example, a "mother's kiss" may dislodge a bean stuck in the nose of a toddler (the mother blows on the child's mouth, while closing the child's other nostril). It is too much of a stretch of imagination to believe that beans would repeatedly pop out spontaneously at the moment the mother blows.[132] Moreover, like the parachute effect, the mechanism is obvious, due to the open airway connection between mouth and nose. And even if the technique does not always work, it is good to give it a try before a physician tries to dislodge the bean with calipers. In day-to-day medical decision-making, still other types of background knowledge justify introduction of a procedure, *e.g.*, when there are no alternatives for a severe condition and a new procedure seems to offer hope of improvement. Here, mechanistic reasoning often is coupled with some early quantitative results.[133]

The Need for Randomization Differs by Medical Discipline

The principles described earlier regarding randomization were developed mostly in the sphere of drug treatment. Disciplines using other treatments may have separate requirements because of different development trajectories and background knowledge.

Drug treatments usually rely on extensive basic science and preclinical data, and their application is uniform, with probabilistic benefits. The physician prescribing a drug is not tailoring its chemistry or adjusting its metabolism to an individual patient. This contrasts with surgery, where slight deviations and improvisations are always needed, given the different anatomy and physiology of individual patients. As such, surgical innovation may occur during a procedure in a patient with an unexpected problem. A surgeon may be forced to try a new approach when a complication occurs or because standard procedures cannot be used. Still, for many new technical procedures in surgery, a prolonged preclinical phase is pursued using animal models. As well, a surgical procedure is performed by a particular surgeon and is affected by individual characteristics such as surgical skills, decision-making style, preferences, and experience. Delivery of a surgical intervention also depends on other members of the team (*e.g.*, anaesthetists, nurses, and technicians) and preoperative and postoperative care (*e.g.*, access to emergency departments and imaging). The complexity of many procedures makes it difficult and costly to conduct clinical trials in the field of surgery. In addition, masking of patients, surgeons, and other caregivers is difficult and often impossible in surgical trials. Not surprisingly, less than 1% of surgical patients are enrolled in RCTs.

A continuing controversy is whether procedures or surgeons should be randomized, since individual surgeons might be better at some procedures than at others. In intensive care medicine, a particular problem is exposure of patients to multiple interventions over a short time period. In addition, many of the patients are unconscious and unable to provide informed consent.

Although randomized trials for surgical procedures are often impossible, the introduction of new surgical treatments should follow rigorous procedures based on principles that are continuously reassessed.[134] For more information on this topic, see the IDEAL Collaboration (Idea, Development, Exploration, Assessment in Surgery).[135-137]

Ascertainment Bias

Ascertainment bias occurs when the results of a trial are distorted by knowledge of the intervention received by each study participant.[62,138] *Blinding* of the exposure to the intervention reduces the risk of biased ascertainment. *Double blinding* is achieved when both the patient and the researcher are blinded. If only one of the two is blinded, the term *single blinding* is used. A trial without blinding is called an *open label trial*.

In some disciplines, it is difficult to conduct blinded RCTs. As mentioned, this is especially difficult or even impossible in studies examining the effect of surgical procedures.[139]

Inclusion and Exclusion Criteria—Generalizability and Principles of Analysis

Inclusion and exclusion criteria are used to describe clearly the characteristics of study participants. They also represent a restriction technique to increase the homogeneity of the study population and thereby reduce confounding, improve study efficiency, and increase adherence to the intervention. There is a gain in statistical power and internal validity by focusing the intervention on a homogenous study population and excluding patients who are unlikely to follow the intervention or complete the follow-up. However, narrow inclusion criteria may restrict the generalizability of a study, to the extent that important segments of the patient population, such as elderly persons, those with severe comorbidity, and those with mental illness, are excluded.

To preserve the advantages of randomization in balancing risk factors between groups, analysis of clinical trial data needs to be based on the original randomized treatment groups, including subjects in each group who drop out or cross over to another treatment group.[140,141] In some contexts, *e.g.*, when proof of principle of a therapeutic effect is needed, the goal is to include only patients who will adhere to the protocol and actually receive the intervention. A *prerandomization run-in period* can be used to exclude patients who are less compliant.[142]

Depending on the extent of noncompliance, an *intent-to-treat* analysis usually provides an underestimate of the magnitude of treatment effects.[143] This type of analysis does not take into account compliance with treatment or treatment crossover during the follow-up period. In studies with long follow-up, it can be difficult to maintain compliance or to avoid changes in treatment for serious conditions. A drawback of the intent-to-treat analysis is that even study subjects who never received the assigned intervention are included in the estimate of the intervention's effect. In contrast, a *per protocol* analysis includes only participants who received the intervention, such as study medications, and who incurred no major protocol violations.

New techniques are being applied to remedy the biases that occur in intent-to-treat analyses, by G-estimation[144] or marginal structural models. These methods were first developed to handle analytic problems such as selection bias and time-varying confounding in observational studies. However, randomized trials can be analyzed using the same techniques to adjust for selective dropout from treatment or crossovers during the trial. These studies become randomized trials analyzed as observational studies. One example is a study that examined possible outcomes if women on hormone replacement therapy continued using these medications for years, instead of stopping early, as often occurs in daily practice. The study showed that the women would experience greater harms with continued use.[145,146]

Clinical and Statistical Significance

In clinical medicine, the *effect* of a treatment, including side effects and relevant endpoints, has major relevance for patient outcomes. Based on the estimated difference in the effect of two treatments (or screening procedures), it is possible to estimate the *number needed to treat* (NNT) and the *number needed to harm* in relation to a treatment. This is the reciprocal of the risk difference and denotes the number of subjects who need to be treated on average to avoid one endpoint (Table 35-4).[147] While the measure NNT is popular, NNTs cannot be interpreted without knowing at least the baseline risk (preferably the risk in each group), and the time interval over which it is calculated; in addition it is a nonadditive effect measure, which complicates its use for prediction.[148,149]

An effect size considered important for clinical decisions is termed *clinically significant* (the term *clinically relevant* is also used).[150] However, when large numbers of subjects are studied, as in many trials, differences may be *statistically significant* although the effect size is small.[150]

The difference between statistical and clinical significance underscores a continuing problem in the clinical decision-making process. In clinical journals, associations are still too often reported using *P*-values only (linked to the concept of the null hypothesis) or *P*-values accompanying effect estimates. While *P*-values and confidence intervals are related, there remains considerable

TABLE 35-4

Measures of Effect and Harm in a Hypothetical Clinical Trial of Two Treatments With Potential Side Effects in Patients With a Serious Disease in a Study Population of 2,000 Patients

	Survived	Died	Side Effects
Treatment A	800	200	100
Treatment B	750	250	60

Measures of therapeutic effect

Measure of effect	Formula
Relative risk	(Event risk in intervention group) − (event risk in control group)
Absolute risk reduction	(Event risk in intervention group) − (event risk in control group)
Number needed to treat	1/(absolute risk reduction)

Risk difference = 800/1000 − 750/1000 = 0.05

$$\text{Risk ratio} = \frac{800/1000}{750/1000} = 1.07$$

$$\text{Number needed to treat} = \frac{1}{0.80 - 0.75} = 20 \text{ patients}$$

$$\text{Number needed to harm} = \frac{1}{0.1 - 0.06} = 25 \text{ patients}$$

controversy regarding the utility of the information conveyed by P-values.[151] The "Uniform Requirements for Manuscripts Submitted to Biomedical Journals" recommends against relying only on statistical hypothesis-testing, *i.e.*, depending on P-values,[152] and the American Statistical Association has advised the same.[153,154] See Chapter 15 for further discussion of the many ways in which use of statistical significance for inference can be badly misleading.

In designing a study, investigators are often obliged by funders to address the so-called Type 1 and Type 2 error risk (and thus the statistical power) as the main parameters determining necessary study size. From a clinical point of view, another potentially more relevant key parameter is the smallest effect size an investigator wishes to measure in a study. This is also called *minimal relevant important difference* (MIREDIF) or *inferiority margin*[155] and is closely related to the concept of clinical significance. Another obligation, for ethical concerns, but also often enforced by funders and data safety monitoring boards, is to conduct *interim analyses* of the primary endpoint with a predefined *stopping rule* to be implemented if the data indicate clear superiority of an intervention,[142] or when prolongation of the trial would be futile, *e.g.*, evidence of harm without benefit.

Variants of Randomized Trials and Variant Analyses

Studies undertaken to detect a difference between two treatments are called *superiority trials*. They also may aim to identify a cheaper treatment or one with fewer adverse effects. *Equivalence or noninferiority trials* aim to test whether treatments have equal efficacy. They require large study sizes. This design may be problematic, due to problems with the validity of the subjective choice of the margin and the uncertainty of expected efficacy based on previous trials. Guidelines from the FDA and the European Medicines Agency warn about the intricacies of noninferiority trials.[156-158]

The term *effect measure modification* refers to a situation in which the effect of a risk or prognostic factor differs depending on other factors (see Chapter 26). In clinical trials, the concept of effect measure modification is closely related to *subgroup analysis*.[159] Subgroup analyses are defined as comparisons between randomized groups in a subset of trial participants. While they can provide useful information, they also can lead to incorrect conclusions, due to small sample sizes within strata. Thus, subgroup analyses are generally approached with extra caution.[160] An exception might be the use of prognostic stratification where the results of the trial are stratified according to baseline prognostic variables.[161] As well, subgroup analyses based on characteristics that develop after randomization do not preserve the randomization balance. For example, per protocol analysis, comparing groups based on adherence to assigned treatment schedules, is a postrandomization subgroup analysis and may be a biased comparison.

A trial with a *factorial design* compares two or more interventions in a single study. Typically, subjects are randomized to "no treatment," to "treatment A," to "treatment B," or to both "treatment A and treatment B" in a 2 × 2 factorial design, which assigns patients with equal probability to each of the four groups.

In the experimental design called a *crossover trial,* patients function as their own controls. This design is in principle only possible if the prognosis of the patient returns completely to baseline rather soon after stopping an intervention—otherwise, a second crossover intervention is no longer possible. Consider weight loss: after a person has lost weight, it is no longer reasonable to try out another intervention to lose weight. The main limitation of this design remains the need to account for any residual effects of one treatment before initiating the next treatment. Such residual effects have been found, for example, in crossover trials examining the effect of estrogen treatment on postmenopausal symptoms.

"N of 1" trials, sometimes also called a crossover study in a single patient, are occasionally used to identify effective treatments or side effects for individual subjects.[162,163] Such trials combine the features of experiments with case-report logic. As in other trials, treatment should be blinded and the order of treatment should vary randomly. The design is especially useful when it is vital to assess the extent to which benefits outweigh side effects. Despite initial enthusiasm, the design remains infrequently used.[164]

Roles of Randomized Controlled Trials

Well-designed randomized studies that are sufficiently large are time- and cost-intensive. They are often conducted when strong economic incentives exist. Thus, many treatments of great clinical importance, which fail to attract attention from commercial interests, have not been investigated with trials. Those that are carried out may have serious limitations, such as relying on surrogate measures, being small and thus inconclusive, failing to include all relevant patient populations, or the intervention is out of date when the study is completed.[143]

Other concerns are that compliance can be harder to maintain in a preventive than in a therapeutic trial. Furthermore, complicated protocols are associated with poorer compliance than simple ones. Furthermore, few randomized studies are able to assess the long-term effects of treatment, leaving unanswered the question of outcomes if study participants had been followed longer. Randomized trials also have been criticized for having limited relevance in real-world clinical decision-making for patients with multimorbidity and co-medications, who are often excluded from trials.

In some circumstances, studies based on large databases and registries have proven to be a valuable population-based alternative to randomized controlled studies.[165] Large databases and registries make it possible to study rare exposures, diseases, and effects quickly and inexpensively. Strengths of using databases include reduction in problems with nonresponse, lack of follow-up, and recall bias compared with other data collection methods. In Scandinavia, population-based hospital registries even have been used as an inexpensive source to identify outcomes in randomized trials[143,166] However, existing registries collect data for administrative or other purposes unrelated to a specific research question. Thus, studies relying on such registries have limitations, as elucidated by Sørensen et al.[143]

The CONsolidated Standards of Reporting Trials (CONSORT) guidelines for reporting RCTs can be found at http://www.consort-statement.org/. Guidelines for reporting database studies (RECORD) can be found at http://www.record-statement.org/.[167]

Question 4: Risk-Harm

Side effects, clinical quality, safety, and *adherence*—important influences on disease outcomes—are underprioritized in clinical medicine. A clinician's skills and motivation determine whether an accurate medical history is obtained and relevant diagnostic tests and treatments are provided. In

everyday clinical practice, access to new treatments, dissemination of updated guidelines, maintenance of competence and provision of continuing medical education, stress levels, and institutional
barriers (such as long waiting times) play essential roles in patients' exposure to harm. The study of
side effects of drug therapy is covered in Chapter 43. In this section, we review some key concepts
of harm relevant for clinical epidemiology.

Side Effects

In general, detection and quantification of side effects, *i.e.*, adverse effects of treatments, are not
handled well in randomized trials. Detection of adverse events is suboptimal because only "per
protocol" events are documented, and quantification of adverse events is unsatisfactory because
RCTs often are based on selected small populations without comorbidities, and with short follow-up.[143] Randomized trials can be biased in their analyses of adverse effects, either by lumping
adverse effects together or by splitting them up excessively.[168]

Fortunately, randomization often is not needed to study adverse effects. In contrast to desired
effects of treatment, there is little or no confounding by indication in many, if not most, studies
of adverse effects of treatments.[169-171] Adverse effects of treatments are usually diseases different
than the treated disease, with different risk factors. Thus, the prognostic reasons for providing the
treatment are unrelated to the prognostic factors and mechanisms for developing adverse effects.

Some data collected during follow-up of treated versus untreated patients cannot be used to
investigate the intended (desired) effect. However, such data could be useful for investigating
unintended (undesired, adverse) effects. An example is treatment of hypertension with the aim of
decreasing cardiovascular disease. In many countries, the strategy is for a physician to prescribe a
diuretic for mild hypertension and to add an ACE inhibitor for more severe or complicated hypertension (with clinical vascular damage). The groups treated with diuretics only and with diuretics plus ACE inhibitors cannot be compared in studying the outcome of cardiovascular disease.
Randomization would be needed for this purpose. However, a major but rare adverse effect of ACE
inhibitors is angioneurotic edema and a mild common adverse effect is cough.[172] The occurrence of
cough and/or angioneurotic edema is unpredictable at the time of prescribing the medication, and
no risk factors for these events can be considered in practice. Thus, comparison of their frequencies
between people treated for mild and more severe hypertension is possible. Angioneurotic edema
with ACE inhibitors seems to occur more often in carriers of a variant of an aminopeptidase gene.
This condition is not checked before initiation of hypertension treatment, because it is neither a
risk factor for hypertension nor a prognostic factor for cardiovascular disease. Other examples are
provided in the literature.[170]

Adverse effects of treatment thus can be investigated reasonably in case-control or cohort studies. Confounding still could occur, but this confounding is more remediable than confounding by
indication.[173] The difference in confounding between desired and undesired effects of treatment has
been addressed several times in the literature, leading to new concepts and terminology over recent
decades. Examples include:

1. The difference between "intended" versus "unintended" effects.[121]
2. The concept of "ignorability of allocation," which can be conditional, dependent on stratification of other variables (weak), or unconditional, independent of other variables (strong).[174,175]
3. The need for "idiopathic cases," *i.e.*, cases without known risk factors. The difference in
   occurrence of venous thrombosis with different types of oral contraceptives provides one
   example. In general, oral contraceptives are prescribed routinely to young women without taking risk factors into account. Most young women do not have risk factors for venous thrombosis, and known risk factors are not strong predictors. However, it has become standard practice
   in many pharmacoepidemiologic studies for investigators to exclude persons with major risk
   factors at the time of a given adverse event, since they might have harbored these risk factors
   at the time the prescription was issued.[176] The subtlety of this approach has been highlighted
   by Rothman and Ray[177] in that it is only appropriate to exclude persons with "known" causes
   if they can be excluded from numerator and denominator (*e.g.*, studying the effects of radon
   exposure on lung cancer in nonsmokers).

It remains a judgment that randomization is unnecessary because confounding by indication is
absent or limited in a study of unintended adverse effects. In addition, one should each time also

envisage the possibility of "confounding by contraindication,"[178] which suggests that physicians might take a known and predictable adverse effect into account when deciding which drug to prescribe. For example, deaths caused by a drug used to treat cardiac failure in routine medical care decreased dramatically after it was found in a randomized trial that the drug caused deaths in persons with severe cardiac failure, but not in those with mild cardiac failure.[178,179]

Even more complex are situations in which the adverse effect is the same as the intended effect. For example, cardiac arrhythmias can be caused by antiarrhythmic drugs that suppress conductivity in the heart. Persons who are given antiarrhythmic drugs to treat arrhythmias can develop (and even die of) arrhythmias caused by the drug. There may be a delay in recognizing the adverse effect, as it could appear that the drug did not work adequately in some patients. A randomized trial could address the problem, as in the CAST trial for antiarrhythmic drugs.[75] In contrast, when a cytostatic drug prescribed for cancer treatment is found to cause arrhythmias, this is not an issue. The idea that adverse effects can be studied observationally thus rests on two underlying assumptions: (1) Different risk profiles exist for disease outcomes and adverse effects, and (2) the treated disease and the adverse effect are different diseases.

Empirical Evaluation of the Theory that Randomization Is Not Needed to Examine "Adverse Effects"

To date, a few studies have assessed whether observational studies of adverse effects might yield the same results as randomized trials. Such evaluations can only be conducted when both types of studies exist, which is not often. For frequent adverse events occurring early in treatment, single, large RCTs might suffice. For rare effects occurring early in treatment, systematic reviews of RCTs are needed to conduct this assessment. Almost no trials, or meta-analyses of trials, have information about long-term effects.

Papanikolaou et al. compared large meta-analyses of randomized trials (with more than 4,000 patients included in an individual review or observational study) and found no systematic differences between RCTs and observational studies.[180] The observational analyses were more conservative; *i.e.*, they detected a lower relative frequency of adverse effects, than the randomized analyses. This is to be expected because adverse effects are evaluated using a strict protocol in RCTs, while in observational studies, analyses are restricted to data available in databases—which invariably contain more noise and missing values.[181]

In a similar but larger study, Golder et al. found that the correspondence between RCTs and observational studies and/or systematic reviews of observational studies was a matter of precision: outliers were seen mainly in small studies, as illustrated in Figure 35-3.[182]

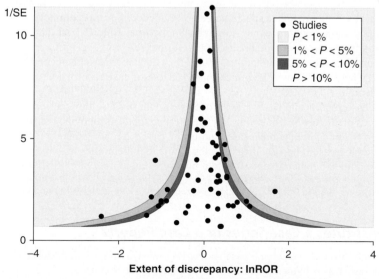

FIGURE 35-3 Contour funnel plot: discrepancy (lnROR [ROR = risk odds ratio]) between RCTs and observational studies in relation to precision of estimates (1/SE [standard error]).[182]

Clinical Quality and Patient Safety

Clinical quality has been defined as "the degree to which health services for individuals and populations increase the likelihood of desired health outcomes and are consistent with current professional knowledge."[183] *Patient safety* was defined by Vincent in 2006 as "the avoidance, prevention and amelioration of adverse outcomes or injuries stemming from the profession of health care."[184]

Hippocrates said "first, do no harm" 2000 years ago, but clinical medical errors and patient safety have received attention in the medical literature for only a few decades.[185] Wennberg and colleagues found large variations in care among hospitals for the same problem or procedure.[186] The landmark Harvard Medical Practice Study reported in 1991 that 44,000 to 98,000 Americans die each year from medical errors.[187,188] Based on more than 400 evidence-based measures of quality, McGlynn et al. showed that practice was consistent with evidence only 54% of the time.[185] Preventable iatrogenic infections and venous thromboembolism are common causes of death associated with hospitalization. Many thousands of deaths are also associated with diagnostic errors.[189,190] Most quality and safety research to date has focused on iatrogenic infections, ulcers, venous thromboembolism, communication errors, diagnostic errors, medication errors, and errors during surgical procedures.[179] In 2000, *The BMJ* devoted an entire issue to medical errors.[191] Overall, adherence to evidence-based care has been found to be associated with better clinical outcomes.[192]

Adherence

Patients' *adherence (*or *compliance) to diagnostics* and *treatment, i.e.*, the extent to which they follow medical advice, also may influence the course of disease.[193] Educational level and frailty are known predictors of the association between a physician's recommendations and a patient's willingness and ability to follow the recommendations. These factors determine level of adherence, which often fluctuates and most often declines over time. However, the complexity of treatment (multiple doses, diet change) and side effects also are important predictors of compliance. Several methods have been suggested to examine and monitor compliance in clinical trials,[193,194] including (1) pill counts, (2) prescription refill rate, (3) electronic monitoring (whereby the frequency and timing of doses taken by the patient are recorded by special software,[195] and (4) monitoring of blood samples. For vitamin K antagonists and some antibiotic drugs, the amount of drug remaining unused is compared with the amount that should be left, based on the prescription. Frequency of prescription refills also can be compared with the frequency expected from physicians' records.

CASE REPORTS AND CASE SERIES

At the height of the Evidence-Based Medicine movement described earlier in this chapter, case reports and case series became suspect sources of evidence. Several editors vowed to weed out case reports and case series from their journals. One journal editorialized that "more often than not" new ideas from case reports do not hold up to further research, that case reports contain "misleading elements" in clinical presentation, and that they do "more harm than good" by emphasizing the bizarre.[196] These criticisms were aimed mostly at use of case reports and case series to show efficacy of therapies.

However, case reports and case series proved resilient, because they perform several important functions in medicine. Not only did they reappear in medical journals, but new journals have been launched specifically to publish case reports and case series for general medicine. Thus, after severely criticizing case reports and case series, clinical epidemiologists have learned to defend their use. One clinical epidemiologist wrote a book on this topic, noting that *"Case reports and case series may be the "lowest" or the "weakest" level of evidence, but they often remain the first line of evidence".... "This is where everything begins."*[197]

What Constitutes a Case Series or a Case Report?

It is surprisingly difficult to define a case series. Previously, we provided examples in which the effect of a therapy was convincing without a comparison group. Such studies are often described as case series, but they are not. Rather they are a cohort study in which all patients receiving a particular intervention are enrolled and followed up over time. While there is no unexposed comparison group, such a group is not essential to conduct a cohort study. In fact, the hallmark of an epidemiologic cohort study is that an incidence rate or risk can be calculated. Therefore, the aforementioned examples, such as the pancreatic islet transplantation study, were cohort studies.[198]

A proper case series is more like the case group in a case-control study. It might consist of a series of persons who have a particular disease (or a particular outcome of a disease) and concurrently a particular exposure history, or a series of persons with a particular disease (or a particular outcome of the disease) *regardless* of exposure history. In case-control studies, one expects the cases to meet certain selection criteria. This requirement is relaxed for case series: it might be a series of patients that struck one or more doctors as noteworthy. For a case report, the issues are easier, since it concerns only a single patient. The defining characteristic is therefore that the single case or group of cases share both their disease history and an exposure history that is viewed as noteworthy. An exposure history of cases would be compared against the exposure history of controls in a conventional case-control design. Since the reported cases are often limited to those with the exposure, and no controls are available for a case report or case series, the evaluation of the exposure history as noteworthy depends on the observer's experiences and not on a measurement in a comparison group.[198]

The Uses of Case Reports and Case Series

The way case reports and case series are used in medicine is diverse, ranging from discovery to education to quality control.[199-201]

Description of New Diseases

New diseases are continuously detected and new subcategories of diseases are differentiated.[202] New diseases may have existed already for some time but not been hitherto described, or they may be truly new conditions caused by new agents. The former includes infectious diseases occurring in places where they were not previously described, and hence are thought to be discovered for the first time at a new place. Examples include the epidemic of *Rickettsia akari* in New York in 1946[203] and the epidemic of West Nile encephalitis in New York in 1999.[204] New diseases also can arise from a new interaction of humans with their environment. For example, epidemics of Legionnaires' disease are caused by a bacterium that rests innocuously in the soil or on surface water until it spreads into people's lungs by air conditioning. Examples of truly new conditions include respiratory distress syndromes, retroperitoneal fibrosis, retrolental fibroplasia, and, in part, AIDS. Respiratory distress syndromes came to light in intensive care units with improved survival among premature infants and adults surviving major trauma. Retroperitoneal fibrosis arose from administration of practolol, and retrolental fibroplasia arose from administration of oxygen to newborns (although there might have been rare descriptions of these conditions beforehand). AIDS belongs to an intermediate category. The virus may have existed for a long time in apes and may have been occasionally transferred to humans by eating meat from infected animals. It is a disease of animals that spread to humans (a zoonosis), and then spread explosively in the late 20th century due to travel and sexual behaviors. Covid-19 is also a recent example of a new disease.

Demarcating new diseases by differentiating subgroups is a well-established process in medicine.[202] In the Middle Ages, people died of "dropsy" (generalized edema). In the 19th century, Bright differentiated between cardiac and renal causes of dropsy and attached his name to the latter (Bright disease). Presumably, most of these patients had end-stage renal failure, later found to be an end stage of several forms of glomerulonephritis, some of which were only differentiated in the 1960s. Similarly, in the 19th century, infants died of "fever," which was later differentiated into several infectious diseases. This process is ongoing: "mitochondrial diabetes" as a subgroup of diabetes was discovered in the 1990s. It must have existed for thousands of years, but was never determined to be a separate entity until shrewd clinical observation, initiated by making of a pedigree of a large family with many cases of diabetes—which showed that the condition was only inherited via mothers—coupled with modern genetics.[205,206] New forms of hepatitis continue to be detected: first hepatitis A and non-A were distinguished; later this became hepatitis A and B; and now we are up to hepatitis E.

Interestingly, there are no rules for detecting new diseases or for proposing to split an existing disease entity. Almost invariably, such events are based on a description of a case series that is striking to one or more astute doctors. The new entity is accepted if it makes medical sense, *i.e.*, if it has a reasonably different etiology, diagnosis, prognosis, and possibly a different therapy from existing conditions.

Causes of Disease

Side Effects

Detecting new adverse effects of treatments, diagnostics, drugs, and devices is an activity similar to detecting new diseases. It relies heavily on detection by astute doctors. The "Yellow Card Scheme" was introduced in the United Kingdom in 1964 after the Thalidomide disaster, in order to capture and report unexpected events recognized by physicians. Electronic submission now has replaced the "Yellow Cards."[207,208] It became the inspiration for all voluntary reporting systems of adverse effects in medicine worldwide. Since its beginning, this system has been criticized for being unsystematic and prone to subjective reporting, *i.e.*, known adverse effects fail to be reported, but a media storm about a side effect results in increased reporting. On one hand, it has been argued that the success score of spontaneous detection is rather good: 35 of 47 anecdotical reports that were published have been found to be clearly correct on further investigation.[209,210] On the other hand, Loke and also Various noted that 56 of 63 case reports on adverse reactions were cited at least once, but these follow-up publications were only accepted as a validation when there had been additional investigations, which happened only in 11 of the 63 cases.[211,212]

There have been attempts to mine the Yellow Card Scheme and similar systems by continuously calculating proportional reporting ratios: the ratio between the frequency with which a specific adverse event is reported for one drug (relative to all reported events for the drug) and the frequency with which the same adverse event is reported for all drugs in a comparison group (relative to all reported events in the comparison group).[213] It has been pointed out that an odds ratio would be a better measure.[214,215]

The background conditions for detecting adverse effects by the naked eye also have received little attention. The common opinion is that adverse effects will be seen spontaneously by the astute physician when there is *a large increase of a rare disease* and/or when a new drug becomes available and is not yet commonly used.[216-218]

Because small increases in common diseases are not detected spontaneously, *e.g.*, a small effect of an infrequently used drug on the incidence of myocardial infarction,[216] and because of the subjective nature of the Yellow Card Scheme, it was proposed in the 1960s that continuous and systematic monitoring be instituted. The principles were set forth by Finney[219] and have become the basis of almost all follow-up systems for drug monitoring worldwide. Intriguingly, there is an abundance of anecdotes about adverse effects of drugs detected by case reports and case series, but a lack of anecdotes about adverse effects discovered by continued routine drug monitoring. Formal drug and medical device monitoring systems with a clear underlying epidemiologic design seem mostly useful to verify the notifications of astute practitioners of medicine or patients. New systems continue to be invented to allow more or less automatic detection, which poses new challenges, such as the problem whether the data that generated a signal can also be used for a subsequent in-depth studies.[220]

Occupational Hazards

Occupational hazards are detected often by astute observers. The "rule of four" has been proposed: spontaneous detection happens whenever four or more patients are seen over a relatively short time by one or a small group of doctors, with a condition that has a relative risk of four or more relative to persons not exposed to this occupation.[221] This capitalization on chance events in spontaneous detection has led to calls for monitoring systems to aid astute observation in occupational and environmental health. The role of epidemiology in occupational health is the subject of Chapter 41.

Mechanisms of Disease

The discovery of mitochondrial diabetes, as described earlier, represented a new mechanism of disease. Another example is provided by the discovery of an important coagulation disorder;

a basic science researcher[7] had been intrigued for years by a particular family with familial venous thrombosis, whose members did not have one of the known familial coagulation defects. In a series of discoveries, this led to the detection of the Factor V Leiden mutation[9,222] (see also Box 35-1).

Detection of New Therapies

The lowering of blood sugar observed in patients taking sulfa drugs, intended as antibiotics, led to the development of oral hypoglycemics. The improvement observed in patients taking a tuberculostatic drug led to antidepressants.[223] A review of case reports and case series with proposals for innovative or unusual treatment, published in *The Lancet*, found that 17% of case reports and 33% of case series were followed by a clinical trial, which points to their importance.[224]

The discovery that sildenafil could lead to an erection was an unplanned event. The sildenafil compound was originally developed for treatment of hypertension and angina pectoris. During a clinical trial, researchers discovered that the drug was more effective at inducing erection than treating angina. It was realized that there was an unmet medical need, and in 1998 the FDA approved Viagra as the first oral treatment for erectile dysfunction.[225,226]

Education and Quality Assurance

Case reports continue to be used for education and quality assurance in pathology conferences (discussions about autopsies of patients) and clinical grand rounds. By confronting intriguing cases in the course of their professional life, physicians develop pattern recognition for rare manifestations or rare diagnoses. An example is the presentation at a clinical conference at a hospital in the Netherlands of the case of a young man who developed scurvy (vitamin C deficiency), a disease that had all but disappeared in past centuries. The diagnosis of an unusual and unseen coagulation problem became evident after hearing about the decade-long refusal of the young man to eat vegetables. In clinical demonstrations, the question is often asked whether a diagnosis might have been made more speedily, or treatment might have been initiated more aggressively. These are informal quality control moments.

Why Do Case Reports or Case Series Work?

Case reports and case series work because they appeal to surprise, deduction, and induction.

The recognition of the unexpected is the point at which all case reporting begins, both in clinical care and in the laboratory. According to Popper, casual observations are striking when they refute our previously held beliefs or expectations, and they lead to new conjectures—new ideas and new theories.[227] As in the example of encephalitis in New York, a clustering of an unknown type of encephalitis in a specific area of a large metropolis is not expected. Likewise, a young man is not expected to have the scurvy that plagued sailors in previous centuries.

Similar to therapeutic cohorts that can be convincing in themselves, case series often have a "mental control group." A "mental control group" can point to the rarity of a combination of occurrences. Even if it is poorly understood how this works, the jump from unexpected findings to generalizations is crucial in the development of new scientific ideas.

Can Case Reports or Case Series Convince on Their OWN?

Case reports or case series can be convincing in themselves, much like the exposure-only reports noted earlier regarding treatments. In studying mechanisms of disease, medical practitioners are accustomed to generalizing from a few patients with the same disease.

Can case reports or case series also lead to action? In the area of side effects, they certainly can. An example is the sudden unexpected deaths observed during or immediately after intravenous infusion of high dosages of an antiemetic.[228] A few such deaths, reported independently by physicians who saw no reason for the sudden intractable arrhythmias in their patients, sufficed to alarm the authorities. The intravenous form was withdrawn from the market. A review found that most decisions to take drugs off the market were based on case reports.[229] Of course, this primarily happens in the context of severe immediate adverse effects that are clearly strange and totally unexpected.

Sensitivity and Specificity of Case Reports

As a rule, case reports and case series have high sensitivity but poor specificity. They are good at detection, but the message that they convey might be an overestimation. Moreover, there are many associations that case reports and case series have not detected.

Pocock and Hughes described why randomized trials that are stopped prematurely because of extremely high benefit (*i.e.*, much larger than expected) will more often than not represent a random high: the direction of the effect is correct, the magnitude is indeed large, but there is a distinct possibility that mere chance added an extra benefit that made the effect so striking as to stop the trial.[230] In a similar vein, the report that OKT3 antibody treatment in a series of transplantation patients induced a surprising number of lymphoreticular disorders early in therapy[231] certainly contains truth, but the magnitude of the effect might reflect bad luck in these patient series. This leads to an intriguing paradox: on the one hand, we only see the effect because of the fortuitous random high; on the other hand, the magnitude of the effect is almost certainly overestimated. However, if this accidental high does not happen or is not noted, an association is not seen spontaneously.

How to Report Case Reports and Case Series?

Given that the idea for case reports and case series arises after the fact, the key point of their presentation is the reason for surprise or the learning point, which needs to be communicated to the medical community.[200,201] Guidelines and checklists for reporting case reports "*with an emphasis on a single priority message*" have been proposed[232,233] and called the CARE guidelines (see http://www.care-statement.org/).[234]

The Place of Case Reports and Case Series in Medicine

The role of case reports and case series is old. In his *Introduction á la médecine expérimentale (1856),* Bernard wrote: "Medical observations often happen haphazardly... the initiative of the medical doctor consists in not letting escape the facts that chance has offered him and his merit consists in observing them painstakingly."[19] They are a unique source of progress in clinical medicine: knowledge that originates at the bedside of one patient and is applied either directly at the bedside of the next patient, or sparks further clinical, biological, or epidemiological investigation.

THE FUTURE OF CLINICAL EPIDEMIOLOGY

Clinical medicine meets rapidly evolving challenges, and clinical epidemiology as a discipline should be able to address these challenges in a clinical context. In the following, we briefly review some of these key clinical challenges and new concepts related to new opportunities based on access to large health care data and new statistical tools. The population in many countries is aging, which results in an increasing burden of comorbidity and polypharmacy. A substantial proportion of patients do not receive recommended therapies, and preventable iatrogenic harms are common. Modern research brings the possibility of new treatments that may be effective, but with unknown long-term side effects. Improved diagnostics may allow earlier disease detection, but at unknown cost and long-term benefit. The trajectory of health care costs is most likely unsustainable in many countries. The quality of clinical care and the efficiency of health care delivery must improve to overcome problems brought on by demographic changes, rapidly changing and complex technologies, and limited economic resources.

Personalized medicine (now more often called *precision medicine)* is a fast advancing concept, entailing medical decision-making and treatment customized to individual patients using genetic or other clinical information.[235] This approach was taken long before the term "personalized medicine" was introduced. Oncology has a long history of adjusting treatment according to tumor stage and anatomical and pathological findings.[236,237] In many situations, data as straightforward as age,

---

c *"Les Observations médicales se font généralement par hasard....l'initiative du médecin consiste à voir et à ne pas laisser échapper le fait que le hasard lui a offert et son mérite se réduit à l'observer avec exactitude."*

body mass index, or renal function are used to adjust treatment regimens. In recent years, the idea to use a patient's proteomic, genetic, and metabolic profile to tailor medical care has led to recognition of this "personalizing" aspect of medicine.[238]

Pharmacogenetics uses genetic variation in response to medications to tailor drug therapy and maximize efficacy and safety.[239] A crucial element for personalized medicine in the future is a comprehensive description of patients' phenotypes (observed physical/biological characteristics) since changes in phenotype are one of the most valid manifestations of altered gene function.[240]

The cost, complexity, and biases often associated with primary data collection, together with the need for long-term follow-up, have led to use of disease registries and databases as alternative sources for studying many epidemiological and clinical questions[143] because much larger sources of electronic, clinical and health care data, and faster computers have become available over the past decades. It is relatively well-established that medical databases can be used efficiently to evaluate utilization, effectiveness, and safety of medical interventions.[241,242]

However, medical information stored in registry databases has not always been subject to systematic quality control.[243] In many databases, the level of clinical detail is insufficient for high-quality clinical research purposes. Information is often incomplete, missing, or incorrectly coded for important elements such as comorbidity, disease severity, and treatments. Many data elements are not standardized, well defined, or clearly documented.[243]

With the increasing use of electronic medical records, a massive amount of clinical and phenotype and genetic data will be collected in the coming years, also called "*big data.*" This might be a threat to the interest in primary data collection. However, only rarely are electronic medical record systems designed in collaboration with clinical researchers, as research is not the primary goal of these record systems. Thus, there will always remain a need for collecting primary clinical data for research purposes in many contexts; moreover, many clinical questions cannot be addressed without conducting RCTs.

The availability of large datasets and new analytical methods are the background for the concepts of big data, machine learning, data mining, and the use of artificial intelligence. We know very little of the clinical utility of these methods in patient care,[244] but the data and new methods represent an opportunity. Recently, it has been shown that a deep learning algorithm was capable of detecting diabetic retinopathy from retinal photographs equally or even better than ophthalmologists.[245,246] Moreover, social media platforms like Google and Facebook have recently been used as tools in epidemiology.[247,248]

Now, perhaps more than ever, we need clinicians with training in epidemiology, working in tandem with interested methodologists, for a sober assessment of the usefulness of the new data and data-analytic capacities in the context of the four clinical questions described in this chapter—in order to meet the challenges of the future of medicine in a scientifically appropriate way.

References

1. Miettinen OS. On progress in epidemiologic academia. *Eur J Epidemiol.* 2017;32(3):173-179.
2. Galea S. On the potential of academic epidemiology. *Eur J Epidemiol.* 2017;32(3):169-171.
3. Bolt T. *A Doctor's Order. The Dutch Case of Evidence-Based Medicine (1970-2015)* [PhD dissertation]. Garant-Uitgevers; 2015.
4. Feinstein A. *Clinical Epidemiology: The Architechture of Clinical Research.* Philadelphia, PA: W.B. Saunders Company; 1985.
5. Sackett DL, Haynes RB, Guyatt GH, Tugwell P. *Clinical Epidemiology: A Basic Science for Clinical Medicine.* 2nd ed. Boston: Little, Brown; 1991.
6. Gribsholt SB, Thomsen RW, Svensson E, Richelsen B. Overall and cause-specific mortality after Roux-en-Y gastric bypass surgery: a nationwide cohort study. *Surg Obes Relat Dis.* 2017;13(4):581-587.
7. Dahlbäck B. Thrombophilia: the discovery of activated protein C resistance. *Adv Genet.* 1995;33:135-175.
8. Koster T, Rosendaal FR, de Ronde H, Briet E, Vandenbroucke JP, Bertina RM. Venous thrombosis due to poor anticoagulant response to activated protein C: Leiden Thrombophilia Study. *Lancet.* 1993;342(8886-8887):1503-1506.
9. Bertina RM, Koeleman BP, Koster T, et al. Mutation in blood coagulation factor V associated with resistance to activated protein C. *Nature.* 1994;369(6475):64-67.
10. Vandenbroucke JP, Koster T, Briet E, Reitsma PH, Bertina RM, Rosendaal FR. Increased risk of venous thrombosis in oral-contraceptive users who are carriers of factor V Leiden mutation. *Lancet.* 1994;344(8935):1453-1457.

11. Sogaard KK, Schmidt M, Pedersen L, Horvath-Puho E, Sorensen HT. 30-year mortality after venous thromboembolism: a population-based cohort study. *Circulation*. 2014;130(10):829-836.
12. Mackenzie J. *The Future of Medicine*. Oxford Medical Publications. London: H. Frowde; 1919.
13. Vandenbroucke JP. Clinical epidemiology: a daydream? *Eur J Epidemiol*. 2017;32(2):95-101.
14. Lewis T. *Clinical Science, Illustrated by Personal Experiences*. London: Shaw and Sons; 1934.
15. Tröhler U. *Quantification in British Medicine and Surgery 1750-1830, With Special Reference to its Introduction Into Therapeutics*. University of London; 1978.
16. Morabia A. P. C. A. Louis and the birth of clinical epidemiology. *J Clin Epidemiol*. 1996;49(12):1327-1333.
17. Ackerknecht E. *Medicine at the Paris Hospital*. Johns Hopkins Press; 1967:1794-1848.
18. Greenwood M Louis and the numerical method. In: Hill AB, ed. *The Medical Dictator and Other Biographical Studies*. London: Williams and Norgate/The Keynes Press, British Medical Association; 1936/1986:123-142.
19. Bernard C. *Introduction à l'étude de la médecine expérimentale (1865) Herdruk*. Paris: Flammarion; 1966.
20. Lilienfeld AM, Lilienfeld DE. What else is new? An historical excursion. *Am J Epidemiol*. 1977;105(3):169-179.
21. http://www.jameslindlibrary.org/.
22. Marks HM. *The Progress of experiment: Science and Therapeutic Reform in the United States, 1900-1990*. Cambridge History of Medicine. Cambridge, England/New York: Cambridge University Press; 1997.
23. White K. *Healing the Schism: Epidemiology, Medicine, and the Public's Health*. New York: Springer; 1991.
24. Feinstein AR. Clinical epidemiology. I. The populational experiments of nature and of man in human illness. *Ann Intern Med*. 1968;69(4):807-820.
25. Feinstein A. Clinical epidemiology. II. The identification of rates of disease. *Ann Intern Med*. 1968;968(69):1037-1061.
26. Feinstein AR. Clinical epidemiology. 3. The clinical design of statistics in therapy. *Ann Intern Med*. 1968;69(6):1287-1312.
27. Sackett DL. Clinical epidemiology. *Am J Epidemiol*. 1969;89(2):125-128.
28. Schünemann H, Guyatt G. Clinical epidemiology and evidence in health care. In: Ahrens W, Pigeot I, eds. *Handbook of Epidemiology*. 2nd ed. New York: Springer; 2014:1813-1873.
29. Weiss NS. *Clinical Epidemiology: the Study of the Outcome of Illness*. Monographs in Epidemiology and Biostatistics. 3rd ed. Oxford/New York: Oxford University Press; 2006.
30. Fletcher RH, Fletcher SW, Wagner EH. *Clinical Epidemiology: The Essentials*. Baltimore: Williams & Wilkins; 1982.
31. Wulff HR, Frølund F. *Rationel klinik: Grundlaget for diagnostiske og terapeutiske beslutninger*. Scandinavian University Books. København: Munksgaard; 1973.
32. Wulff HR, Gøtzsche PC. *Rational Diagnosis and Treatment: Evidence-Based Clinical Decision-Making*. 3rd ed. Oxford: Blackwell Science; 2000.
33. Guyatt G, Cairns J, Chruchill D. Evidence-based medicine. A new approach to teaching the practice of medicine. *J Am Med Assoc*. 1992;268(17):2420-2425.
34. Vandenbroucke JP. Observational research, randomised trials, and two views of medical science. *PLoS Med*. 2008;5(3):e67.
35. Sørensen HT. Case-control studies & the hierarchy of study design. *Curr Epidemiol Rep*. 2016;3(4):262-264.
36. Rothman KJ. Six persistent research misconceptions. *J Gen Intern Med*. 2014;29(7):1060-1064.
37. Lash TL, Vandenbroucke JP. Should preregistration of epidemiologic study protocols become compulsory? Reflections and a counterproposal. *Epidemiology*. 2012;23(2):184-188.
38. Djulbegovic B, Guyatt GH. Progress in evidence-based medicine: a quarter century on. *Lancet*. 2017;390(10092):415-423.
39. Grace Principles: Good ReseArch for Comparative Effectiveness. https://www.graceprinciples.org/.
40. Greenhalgh T, Howick J, Maskrey N; Evidence Based Medicine Renaissance Group. Evidence based medicine: a movement in crisis? *BMJ*. 2014;348:g3725.
41. Sadigh G, Parker R, Kelly AM, Cronin P. How to write a critically appraised topic (CAT). *Acad Radiol*. 2012;19(7):872-888.
42. Halstead SB, Tugwell P, Bennett K. The International Clinical Epidemiology Network (INCLEN): a progress report. *J Clin Epidemiol*. 1991;44(6):579-589.
43. Smith R. Medical journals are an extension of the marketing arm of pharmaceutical companies. *PLoS Med*. 2005;2(5):e138.
44. Guyatt G. EBM has not only called out the problems but offered solutions. *J Clin Epidemiol*. 2017;84:8-10.
45. Fava GA. Evidence-based medicine was bound to fail: a report to Alvan Feinstein. *J Clin Epidemiol*. 2017;84:3-7.

46. Richardson WS. The practice of evidence-based medicine involves the care of whole persons. *J Clin Epidemiol.* 2017;84:18-21.

47. Horwitz RI, Singer BH. Why evidence-based medicine failed in patient care and medicine-based evidence will succeed. *J Clin Epidemiol.* 2017;84:14-17.

48. Ioannidis JPA. Hijacked evidence-based medicine: stay the course and throw the pirates overboard. *J Clin Epidemiol.* 2017;84:11-13.

49. Knottnerus JA, Tugwell P. Evidence-based medicine: achievements and prospects. *J Clin Epidemiol.* 2017;84:1-2.

50. Vandenbroucke JP. On the new clinical fashion in epidemiology. *Epidemiol Infect.* 1989;102(2):191-198.

51. Allaart CF, Rosendaal FR, Noteboom WM, Vandenbroucke JP, Briet E. Survival in families with hereditary protein C deficiency, 1820 to 1993. *BMJ.* 1995;311(7010):910-913.

52. Hille ET, Siesling S, Vegter-van der Vlis M, Vandenbroucke JP, Roos RA, Rosendaal FR. Two centuries of mortality in ten large families with Huntington disease: a rising impact of gene carriership. *Epidemiology.* 1999;10(6):706-710.

53. Hirsh J, Guyatt G. Clinical experts or methodologists to write clinical guidelines? *Lancet.* 2009;374(9686):273-275.

54. Vandenbroucke JP, Pearce N. From ideas to studies: how to get ideas and sharpen them into research questions. *Clin Epidemiol.* 2018;10:253-264.

55. Medawar PB. *Advice to a Young Scientist.* The Alfred P Sloan Foundation Series. 1st ed. New York: Harper & Row; 1979.

56. Vandenbroucke JP. Alvan Feinstein and the art of consulting: how to define a research question. *J Clin Epidemiol.* 2002;55(12):1176-1177.

57. Sundboll J, Adelborg K, Munch T, et al. Positive predictive value of cardiovascular diagnoses in the Danish National Patient Registry: a validation study. *BMJ Open.* 2016;6(11):e012832.

58. Hróbjartsson A, Sørensen HT. Evidensbaseret medicin og klinisk epidemiologi. In: Schaffalitzky de Muckadell OB, Svendsen JH, Vilstrup H, eds. *Medicinsk Kompendium.* 19th ed. Copenhagen: Munksgaard; 2019.

59. Steyerberg EW. *Clinical Prediction Models: A Practical Approach to Development, Validation, and Updating.* Statistics for Biology and Health. New York, NY: Springer; 2009.

60. Kasper D, Fauci A, Hauser S, Longo D, Jameson J, Loscalzo J. *Harrison's Principle of Internal Medicine.* Vol 1. New York: McGraw Hill; 2015.

61. Grobbee DE, Hoes AW. *Clinical Epidemiology: Principles, Methods, and Applications for Clinical Research.* 2nd ed. Burlington, Massachusetts: Jones & Bartlett Learning, 2015.

62. Fletcher RH, Fletcher SW, Fletcher GS. *Clinical Epidemiology: The Essentials.* 5th ed. Philadelphia, PA: Wolters Kluwer/Lippincott Williams & Wilkins Health; 2014.

63. Riegelman RK. *Studying a Study and Testing a Test: How to Read the Medical Evidence.* 4th ed. Philadelphia, PA: Lippincott Williams & Wilkins; 2000.

64. http://www.stard-statement.org/.

65. Kestenbaum B. *Epidemiology and Biostatistics: An Introduction to Clinical Research.* Dordrecht/New York: Springer; 2009.

66. Schmidt M, Schmidt S, Sandegaard J, Ehrenstein V, Pedersen L, Sørensen H. The Danish National Patient Registry: a review of content, data quality, and research potential. *Clin Epidemiol.* 2015;7:449-490.

67. Department of Clinical Epidemiology and Biostatistics, McMaster University, Hamilton, Ontario. Clinical disagreement: I. How often it occurs and why. *Can Med Assoc J.* 1980;123(6):499-504.

68. Department of Clinical Epidemiology and Biostatistics, McMaster University, Hamilton, Ontario. Clinical disagreement: II. How to avoid it and how to learn from one's mistakes. *Can Med Assoc J.* 1980;123(7):613-617.

69. Cohen J. A coefficient of agreement for nominal scales. *Educ Psychol Meas.* 1960;20:37-46.

70. Fleiss JL. *Statistical Methods for Rates and Proportions.* Wiley Series in Probability and Mathematical Statistics. 2d ed. New York: Wiley; 1980.

71. Curtis LH, Rao SV. Putting prognosis into perspective. *Circ Cardiovasc Qual Outcomes.* 2017;10(6):e003956.

72. Ording AG, Cronin-Fenton D, Ehrenstein V, et al. Challenges in translating endpoints from trials to observational cohort studies in oncology. *Clin Epidemiol.* 2016;8:195-200.

73. Hemingway H, Croft P, Perel P, et al. Prognosis research strategy (PROGRESS) 1: a framework for researching clinical outcomes. *BMJ.* 2013;346:e5595.

74. Machin D, Day S, Green S.. *Textbook of Clinical Trials.* Chichester: John Wiley & Sons; 2006.

75. Echt DS, Liebson PR, Mitchell LB, et al. Mortality and morbidity in patients receiving encainide, flecainide, or placebo. The Cardiac Arrhythmia Suppression Trial. *N Engl J Med.* 1991;324(12):781-788.

76. Katzan IL, Thompson NR, Lapin B, Uchino K. Added value of patient-reported outcome measures in stroke clinical practice. *J Am Heart Assoc.* 2017;6(7):e005356.

77. Duncan PW, Lai SM, Bode RK, Perera S, DeRosa J. Stroke Impact Scale-16: a brief assessment of physical function. *Neurology*. 2003;60(2):291-296.

78. Moriello C, Byrne K, Cieza A, Nash C, Stolee P, Mayo N. Mapping the stroke impact scale (SIS-16) to the international classification of functioning, disability and health. *J Rehabil Med*. 2008;40(2):102-106.

79. Goldberg R, Gore JM, Barton B, Gurwitz J. Individual and composite study endpoints: separating the wheat from the chaff. *Am J Med*. 2014;127(5):379-384.

80. Tyler KM, Normand SL, Horton NJ. The use and abuse of multiple outcomes in randomized controlled depression trials. *Contemp Clin Trials*. 2011;32(2):299-304.

81. Raungaard B, Christiansen EH, Botker HE, et al. Comparison of durable-polymer zotarolimus-eluting and biodegradable-polymer biolimus-eluting coronary stents in patients with coronary artery disease: 3-year clinical outcomes in the randomized SORT OUT VI trial. *JACC Cardiovasc Interv*. 2017;10(3):255-264.

82. Freemantle N, Marston L, Walters K, Wood J, Reynolds MR, Petersen I. Making inferences on treatment effects from real world data: propensity scores, confounding by indication, and other perils for the unwary in observational research. *BMJ*. 2013;347:f6409.

83. Freemantle N, Calvert M, Wood J, Eastaugh J, Griffin C. Composite outcomes in randomized trials: greater precision but with greater uncertainty? *J Am Med Assoc*. 2003;289(19):2554-2559.

84. Ahrens W, Pigeot I. *Handbook of Epidemiology*. 2nd ed. New York, NY: Springer Reference; 2014.

85. Lauer MS, Topol EJ. Clinical trials--multiple treatments, multiple end points, and multiple lessons. *J Am Med Assoc*. 2003;289(19):2575-2577.

86. Topol EJ, Califf RM, Van de Werf F, et al. Perspectives on large-scale cardiovascular clinical trials for the new millennium. The Virtual Coordinating Center for Global Collaborative Cardiovascular Research (VIGOUR) Group. *Circulation*. 1997;95(4):1072-1082.

87. Holmvang L, Hasbak P, Clemmensen P, Wagner G, Grande P. Differences between local investigator and core laboratory interpretation of the admission electrocardiogram in patients with unstable angina pectoris or non-Q-wave myocardial infarction (a Thrombin Inhibition in Myocardial Ischemia [TRIM] substudy). *Am J Cardiol*. 1998;82(1):54-60.

88. Mahaffey KW, Harrington RA, Akkerhuis M, et al. Disagreements between central clinical events committee and site investigator assessments of myocardial infarction endpoints in an international clinical trial: review of the PURSUIT study. *Curr Control Trials Cardiovasc Med*. 2001;2(4):187-194.

89. Mahaffey KW, Roe MT, Dyke CK, et al. Misreporting of myocardial infarction end points: results of adjudication by a central clinical events committee in the PARAGON-B trial. Second platelet IIb/IIIa antagonist for the reduction of acute coronary syndrome events in a global organization network trial. *Am Heart J*. 2002;143(2):242-248.

90. Naslund U, Grip L, Fischer-Hansen J, Gundersen T, Lehto S, Wallentin L. The impact of an end-point committee in a large multicentre, randomized, placebo-controlled clinical trial: results with and without the end-point committee's final decision on end-points. *Eur Heart J*. 1999;20(10):771-777.

91. Cole BF, Gelber RD, Anderson KM. Parametric approaches to quality-adjusted survival analysis. International breast cancer study group. *Biometrics*. 1994;50(3):621-631.

92. Shen Y, Thall PF. Parametric likelihoods for multiple non-fatal competing risks and death. *Stat Med*. 1998;17(9):999-1015.

93. Vandenbroucke J, Pearce N. Point: incident exposures, prevalent exposures, and causal inference. Does limiting studies to persons who are followed from first exposure onward damage epidemiology? *Am J Epidemiol*. 2015;182(10):826-833.

94. Ellenberg JH, Nelson KB. Sample selection and the natural history of disease. Studies of febrile seizures. *J Am Med Assoc*. 1980;243(13):1337-1340.

95. Dekkers OM, Horvath-Puho E, Jorgensen JO, et al. Multisystem morbidity and mortality in Cushing's syndrome: a cohort study. *J Clin Endocrinol Metab*. 2013;98(6):2277-2284.

96. Schmidt M, Jacobsen JB, Lash TL, Botker HE, Sorensen HT. 25 year trends in first time hospitalisation for acute myocardial infarction, subsequent short and long term mortality, and the prognostic impact of sex and comorbidity: a Danish nationwide cohort study. *BMJ*. 2012;344:e356.

97. Brenner H, Hakulinen T. Up-to-date long-term survival curves of patients with cancer by period analysis. *J Clin Oncol*. 2002;20(3):826-832.

98. Abarca JF, Casiccia CC, Zamorano FD. Increase in sunburns and photosensitivity disorders at the edge of the Antarctic ozone hole, southern Chile, 1986-2000. *J Am Acad Dermatol*. 2002;46(2):193-199.

99. Sobin LH. TNM, sixth edition: new developments in general concepts and rules. *Semin Surg Oncol*. 2003;21(1):19-22.

100. Wilson PW, D'Agostino RB, Levy D, Belanger AM, Silbershatz H, Kannel WB. Prediction of coronary heart disease using risk factor categories. *Circulation*. 1998;97(18):1837-1847.

101. Haynes SR, Lawler PG. An assessment of the consistency of ASA physical status classification allocation. *Anaesthesia*. 1995;50(3):195-199.

102. American Academy of Pediatrics Committee on Fetus and Newborn, American College of Obstetricians and Gynecologists Committee on Obstetric Practice. The Apgar score. *Pediatrics*. 2015;136(4):819-822.

103. Charlson ME, Pompei P, Ales KL, MacKenzie CR. A new method of classifying prognostic comorbidity in longitudinal studies: development and validation. *J Chronic Dis*. 1987;40(5):373-383.

104. de Groot V, Beckerman H, Lankhorst GJ, Bouter LM. How to measure comorbidity. a critical review of available methods. *J Clin Epidemiol*. 2003;56(3):221-229.

105. Hudon CFM, Vanasse A. Cumulative Illness Rating Scale was a reliable and valid index in a family practice context. *J Clin Epidemiol*. 2005;58(6):603-608.

106. Imamura K, McKinnon M, Middleton R, Black N. Reliability of a comorbidity measure: the index of Co-existent disease (ICED). *J Clin Epidemiol*. 1997;50(9):1011-1016.

107. Greenfield S, Apolone G, McNeil BJ, Cleary PD. The importance of co-existent disease in the occurrence of postoperative complications and one-year recovery in patients undergoing total hip replacement. Comorbidity and outcomes after hip replacement. *Med Care*. 1993;31(2):141-154.

108. Linn BS, Linn MW, Gurel L. Cumulative illness rating scale. *J Am Geriatr Soc*. 1968;16(5):622-626.

109. Waldman E, Potter JF. A prospective evaluation of the cumulative illness rating scale. *Aging (Milano)*. 1992;4(2):171-178.

110. Roberts RF, Reid BA, Irwin AL. Case-mix grouping and DRGs: making the principal diagnosis. *Med J Aust*. 1985;143(6):243-245.

111. Starfield B. Point: the changing nature of disease. Implications for health services. *Med Care*. 2011;49(11):971-972.

112. Tinetti ME, Fried TR, Boyd CM. Designing health care for the most common chronic condition--multimorbidity. *J Am Med Assoc*. 2012;307(23):2493-2494.

113. Pronovost PJ, Goeschel CA. Time to take health delivery research seriously. *J Am Med Assoc*. 2011;306(3):310-311.

114. Salisbury C. Multimorbidity: redesigning health care for people who use it. *Lancet*. 2012;380(9836):7-9.

115. Whitty CJM, MacEwen C, Goddard A et al. Rising to the challenge of multimorbidity. *BMJ*. 2020;368:l6964.

116. Jadad AR, Enkin M. *Randomized Controlled Trials: Questions, Answers, and Musings*. 2nd ed. Malden, MA.: Blackwell Publisher; 2007.

117. Bland JM, Altman DG. Some examples of regression towards the mean. *BMJ*. 1994;309(6957):780.

118. Greenland S, Neutra R. Control of confounding in the assessment of medical technology. *Int J Epidemiol*. 1980;9(4):361-367.

119. Neutra RR, Greenland S, Friedman EA. Effect of fetal monitoring on cesarean section rates. *Obstet Gynecol*. 1980;55(2):175-180.

120. Petri H, Urquhart J. Channeling bias in the interpretation of drug effects. *Stat Med*. 1991;10(4):577-581.

121. Miettinen OS. The need for randomization in the study of intended effects. *Stat Med*. 1983;2(2):267-271.

122. Bosco JL, Silliman RA, Thwin SS, et al. A most stubborn bias: no adjustment method fully resolves confounding by indication in observational studies. *J Clin Epidemiol*. 2010;63(1):64-74.

123. Rocker G, Cook D, Sjokvist P, et al. Clinician predictions of intensive care unit mortality. *Crit Care Med*. 2004;32(5):1149-1154.

124. Chalmers I. Statistical theory was not the reason that randomisation was used in the British Medical Research Council's clinical trial of streptomycin for pulmonary tuberculosis. In: Jorland G, Opinel A, Weisz G, eds. *Body Counts: Medical Quantification in Historical and Sociological Perspectives*. Montreal: McGill-Queens University Press; 2005.

125. Hill A. *Principles of Medical Statistics*. London: Lancet; 1937.

126. Chalmers I. Explaining the unbiased creation of treatment comparison groups. *Lancet*. 2009;374(9702):1670-1671.

127. Greenland S. Randomization, statistics, and causal inference. *Epidemiology*. 1990;1(6):421-429.

128. Senn S. Seven myths of randomisation in clinical trials. *Stat Med*. 2013;32(9):1439-1450.

129. Smith GC, Pell JP. Parachute use to prevent death and major trauma related to gravitational challenge: systematic review of randomised controlled trials. *BMJ*. 2003;327(7429):1459-1461.

130. Hering BJ, Kandaswamy R, Ansite JD, et al. Single-donor, marginal-dose islet transplantation in patients with type 1 diabetes. *J Am Med Assoc*. 2005;293(7):830-835.

131. Prescott LF, Illingworth RN, Critchley JA, Stewart MJ, Adam RD, Proudfoot AT. Intravenous N-acetylcystine: the treatment of choice for paracetamol poisoning. *BMJ*. 1979;2(6198):1097-1100.

132. Glasziou P, Chalmers I, Rawlins M, McCulloch P. When are randomised trials unnecessary? Picking signal from noise. *BMJ*. 2007;334(7589):349-351.

133. Rawlins M. De testimonio: on the evidence for decisions about the use of therapeutic interventions. *Lancet*. 2008;372(9656):2152-2161.

134. http://www.ideal-collaboration.net/the-collaboration/.

135. Ergina PL, Cook JA, Blazeby JM, et al. Challenges in evaluating surgical innovation. *Lancet*. 2009;374(9695):1097-1104.

136. Barkun JS, Aronson JK, Feldman LS, et al. Evaluation and stages of surgical innovations. *Lancet*. 2009;374(9695):1089-1096.

137. McCulloch P, Altman DG, Campbell WB, et al. No surgical innovation without evaluation: the IDEAL recommendations. *Lancet*. 2009;374(9695):1105-1112.

138. Sackett DL, Gent M. Controversy in counting and attributing events in clinical trials. *N Engl J Med*. 1979;301(26):1410-1412.

139. Friedman L, Furberg C, DeMets D, Reboussin D, Granger C. *Fundamentals of Clinical Trials*. 5th ed. Cham: Springer; 2015.

140. Brody T. *Clinical Trials: Study Design, Endpoints and Biomarkers, Drug Safety, FDA and ICH Guidelines*. 2nd ed. Amsterdam/Boston: Elsevier/AP; 2016.

141. Liao JM, Stack CB, Griswold ME, Localio AR. Annals understanding clinical research: intention-to-treat analysis. *Ann Intern Med*. 2017;166(9):662-664.

142. Matthews JNS. *Introduction to Randomized Controlled Clinical Trials*. Texts in Statistical Science. 2nd ed. Boca Raton: Chapman & Hall/CRC, 2006.

143. Sørensen HT, Lash TL, Rothman KJ. Beyond randomized controlled trials: a critical comparison of trials with nonrandomized studies. *Hepatology*. 2006;44(5):1075-1082.

144. Greenland S, Lanes S, Jara M. Estimating effects from randomized trials with discontinuations: the need for intent-to-treat design and G-estimation. *Clin Trials*. 2008;5(1):5-13.

145. Toh S, Hernandez-Diaz S, Logan R, Robins JM, Hernan MA. Estimating absolute risks in the presence of nonadherence: an application to a follow-up study with baseline randomization. *Epidemiology*. 2010;21(4):528-539.

146. Hernan MA, Hernandez-Diaz S, Robins JM. Randomized trials analyzed as observational studies. *Ann Intern Med*. 2013;159(8):560-562.

147. Haynes B, Sackett D, Guyatt G, Tugwell P. *Clinical Epidemiology: How to Do Clinical Practice Research*. Philadelphia, PA: Lippincott Williams & Wilkins; 2006.

148. Senn S, Julious S. Measurement in clinical trials: a neglected issue for statisticians? *Stat Med*. 2009;28(26):3189-3209.

149. Wald NJ, Morris JK. Two under-recognized limitations of number needed to treat. *Int J Epidemiol*. 2020;49(2):359-360. doi:10.1093/ije/dyz267.

150. Parfrey P, Barrett B. *Clinical Epidemiology*. 2nd ed. New York: Humana Press; 2015.

151. Amrhein V, Greenland S, McShane B. Scientists rise up against statistical significance. *Nature*. 2019;567(7748):305-307. doi:10.1038/d41586-019-00857-9.

152. International Committee of Medical Journal Editors. Uniform requirements for manuscripts submitted to biomedical journals. *N Engl J Med* 1997;336(4):309-315.

153. Wasserstein RL, Lazar NA. ASA statement on statistical significance and P-values. *Am Statist*. 2016;70(2):131-133.

154. Wasserstein RL, Schirm AL, Lazar NA. Moving to a world beyond "p<0.05". *Am Statist*. 2019;73(suppl 1):1-19.

155. Gøtzsche PC, Wulff HR. *Rational Diagnosis and Treatment: Evidence-Based Clinical Decision-Making*. 4th ed. Chichester, England/Hoboken, NJ: John Wiley & Sons; 2007.

156. Agency EM. http://www.ema.europa.eu/docs/en_GB/document_library/Scientific_guideline/2009/09/WC500003636.pdf.

157. U.S. Department of Health and Human Services, Food and Drug Administration, Center for Drug Evaluation and Research (CDER), Center for Biologics Evaluation and Research (CBER). Non-Inferiority Clinical Trials to Establish Effectiveness Guidance for Industry https://www.fda.gov/downloads/Drugs/Guidances/UCM202140.pdf.

158. Hulley SB, Cummings SR, Browner WS, Grady DG, Newman TB. *Designing Clinical Research*. 3rd ed. Philadelphia, PA: Lippincott Williams & Wilkins; 2007.

159. VanderWeele TJ. On the distinction between interaction and effect modification. *Epidemiology*. 2009;20(6):863-871.

160. Hopewell S, Clarke M, Moher D, et al. CONSORT for reporting randomised trials in journal and conference abstracts. *Lancet*. 2008;371(9609):281-283.

161. Pocock SJ, Lubsen J. More on subgroup analyses in clinical trials. *N Engl J Med*. 2008;358(19):2076; author reply 2076-7.

162. Guyatt G, Sackett D, Taylor DW, Chong J, Roberts R, Pugsley S. Determining optimal therapy--randomized trials in individual patients. *N Engl J Med*. 1986;314(14):889-892.

163. McLeod RS, Taylor DW, Cohen Z, Cullen JB. Single-patient randomised clinical trial. Use in determining optimum treatment for patient with inflammation of Kock continent ileostomy reservoir. *Lancet*. 1986;1(8483):726-728.

164. Porta M, Bolumar F, Hernandez I, Vioque J. N of 1 trials. Research is needed into why such trials are not more widely used. *BMJ*. 1996;313(7054):427.

165. Baron JA, Weiderpass E. An introduction to epidemiological research with medical databases. *Ann Epidemiol*. 2000;10(4):200-204.

166. Calltorp J, Adami HO, Astrom H, et al. Country profile: Sweden. *Lancet*. 1996;347(9001):587-594.

167. Benchimol EI, Smeeth L, Guttmann A, et al. The REporting of studies Conducted using Observational Routinely-collected health Data (RECORD) statement. *PLoS Med.* 2015;12(10):e1001885.
168. Ioannidis JP, Contopoulos-Ioannidis DG. Reporting of safety data from randomised trials. *Lancet.* 1998;352(9142):1752-1753.
169. Vandenbroucke JP. When are observational studies as credible as randomised trials? *Lancet.* 2004;363(9422):1728-1731.
170. Vandenbroucke JP, Psaty BM. Benefits and risks of drug treatments: how to combine the best evidence on benefits with the best data about adverse effects. *J Am Med Assoc.* 2008;300(20):2417-2419.
171. Vandenbroucke JP. Why do the results of randomised and observational studies differ? *BMJ.* 2011;343:d7020.
172. Johnsen SP, Jacobsen J, Monster TB, Friis S, McLaughlin JK, Sorensen HT. Risk of first-time hospitalization for angioedema among users of ACE inhibitors and angiotensin receptor antagonists. *Am J Med.* 2005;118(12):1428-1429.
173. Jick H, Garcia Rodriguez LA, Perez-Gutthann S. Principles of epidemiological research on adverse and beneficial drug effects. *Lancet.* 1998;352(9142):1767-1770.
174. Rosenbaum P, Rubin D. The central role of the propensity score in observational studies for causal effects. *Biometrika.* 1983;70(1):41-55.
175. Rubin D. Bayesian inference for causal effects: the role of randomization. *Ann Stat.* 1978;6(1):34-58.
176. Jick H, Vessey MP. Case-control studies in the evaluation of drug-induced illness. *Am J Epidemiol.* 1978;107(1):1-7.
177. Rothman KJ, Ray W. Should cases with a 'known' cause of their disease be excluded from study? (commentary). *Pharmacoepidemiol Drug Saf.* 2002;11(1):11-14.
178. Feenstra H, Grobbee RE, in't Veld BA, Stricker BH. Confounding by contraindication in a nationwide cohort study of risk for death in patients taking ibopamine. *Ann Intern Med.* 2001;134(7):569-572.
179. Hampton JR, van Veldhuisen DJ, Kleber FX et al. Randomised study of effect of ibopamine on survival in patients with advanced severe heart failure. Second Prospective Randomised Study of Ibopamine on Mortality and Efficacy (PRIME II) Investigators. *Lancet.* 1997;349(9057):971-977.
180. Papanikolaou PN, Christidi GD, Ioannidis JP. Comparison of evidence on harms of medical interventions in randomized and nonrandomized studies. *Can Med Assoc J.* 2006;174(5):635-641.
181. Vandenbroucke JP. What is the best evidence for determining harms of medical treatment? *Can Med Assoc J.* 2006;174(5):645-646.
182. Golder S, Loke YK, Bland M. Meta-analyses of adverse effects data derived from randomised controlled trials as compared to observational studies: methodological overview. *PLoS Med.* 2011;8(5):e1001026.
183. Wachter R. *Understanding Patient Safety.* 2nd ed. New York: McGraw Hill Medical; 2012.
184. Vincent C. *Patient Safety.* Edinburgh/New York: Churchill Livingstone; 2006.
185. McGlynn EA, Asch SM, Adams J, et al. The quality of health care delivered to adults in the United States. *N Engl J Med.* 2003;348(26):2635-2645.
186. Wennberg J, Freeman J, Culp W. Are hospital services rationed in New Haven or over-utilised in Boston? *Lancet.* 1987;1(8543):1185-1189.
187. Brennan T, Leape L, Laird N, et al. Incidence of adverse events and negligence in hospitalized patients. Results of the Harvard Medical Practice Study I. *N Engl J Med.* 1991;324(6):370-376.
188. Leape L, Brennan T, Laird N, et al. The nature of adverse events in hospitalized patients. Results of the Harvard Medical Practice Study II. *N Engl J Med.* 1991;324(6):377-384.
189. Newman-Toker DE, Pronovost PJ. Diagnostic errors—the next frontier for patient safety. *J Am Med Assoc.* 2009;301(10):1060-1062.
190. Landrigan CP, Parry GJ, Bones CB, Hackbarth AD, Goldmann DA, Sharek PJ. Temporal trends in rates of patient harm resulting from medical care. *N Engl J Med.* 2010;363(22):2124-2134.
191. Leape LL, Berwick DM. Safe health care: are we up to it? *BMJ.* 2000;320(7237):725-726.
192. Higashi T, Shekelle P, Adams J, et al. Quality of care is associated with survival in vulnerable older patients. *Ann Intern Med.* 2005;143(4):274-281.
193. Acri T, Gross R. *Studies of medication adherence.* In: *Pharmacoepidemiology. Chichester*: John Wiley & Sons; 2005.
194. Cutler DM, Everett W. Thinking outside the pillbox--medication adherence as a priority for health care reform. *N Engl J Med.* 2010;362(17):1553-1555.
195. Urquhart J. The electronic medication event monitor. Lessons for pharmacotherapy. *Clin Pharmacokinet.* 1997;32(5):345-356.
196. Hoffman JR. Rethinking case reports. *West J Med.* 1999;170(5):253-254.
197. Jenicek M. *Clinical Case Reporting in Evidence Based Medicine.* 2nd ed. London: Hodder Arnold Publication; 2001.
198. Dekkers OM, Egger M, Altman DG, Vandenbroucke JP. Distinguishing case series from cohort studies. *Ann Intern Med.* 2012;156(1 pt 1):37.

199. Crombie IK, Davies HTO. *Case Reports and Case Series. Research in Health Care: Design, Conduct, and Interpretation of Health Services Research.* Chichester/New York: Wiley; 1996:288.
200. Vandenbroucke JP. Case reports in an evidence-based world. *J R Soc Med.* 1999;92(4):159-163.
201. Vandenbroucke JP. In defense of case reports and case series. *Ann Intern Med.* 2001;134(4):330.
202. Anonymous. Rise and fall of diseases. *Lancet.* 1993;341(8838):151-152.
203. Wikipedia. https://en.wikipedia.org/wiki/Rickettsialpox.
204. Mostashari F, Bunning ML, Kitsutani PT, et al. Epidemic West Nile encephalitis, New York, 1999: results of a household-based seroepidemiological survey. *Lancet.* 2001;358(9278):261-264.
205. Ballinger SW, Shoffner JM, Hedaya EV, et al. Maternally transmitted diabetes and deafness associated with a 10.4 kb mitochondrial DNA deletion. *Nat Genet.* 1992;1(1):11-15.
206. van den Ouweland JMW, Lemkes HH, Ruitenbeek W, et al. Mutation in mitochondrial tRNA(Leu) (UUR) gene in a large pedigree with maternally transmitted type II diabetes mellitus and deafness. *Nat Genet.* 1992;1(5):368-371.
207. UK TMHpRA. https://yellowcard.mhra.gov.uk/.
208. Wikipedia. https://en.wikipedia.org/wiki/Yellow_Card_Scheme.
209. Chalmers I. Evaluating the effects of care during pregnancy and childbirth. In: Chalmers I, Enkin M, Keirse M, eds. *Effective Care in Pregnancy and Childbirth.* Oxford: Oxford University Press; 1989.
210. Venning GR. Validity of anecdotal reports of suspected adverse drug reactions: the problem of false alarms. *BMJ.* 1982;284(6311):249-252.
211. Loke YK. Case reports of suspected adverse drug reactions--systematic literature survey of follow-up. *BMJ.* 2006;332(7537):335-339.
212. Various. Debate proofs adverse effect. *BMJ.* 2006;(332):488.
213. Evans SJW, Waller PC, Davis S. Use of proportional reporting ratios (PRRs) for signal generation from spontaneous adverse drug reaction reports. *Pharmacoepidemiol Drug Saf.* 2001;10(6):483-486.
214. Rothman KJ, Lanes S, Sacks ST. The reporting odds ratio and its advantages over the proportional reporting ratio. *Pharmacoepidemiol Drug Saf.* 2004;13(8):519-523.
215. Waller P, van Puijenbroek E, Egberts A, Evans S. The reporting odds ratio versus the proportional reporting ratio: 'deuce'. *Pharmacoepidemiol Drug Saf.* 2004;13(8):525-526; discussion 527-8.
216. Jick H. The discovery of drug-induced illness. *New Engl J Med.* 1977;296(9):481-485.
217. Begaud B, Moride Y, Tubert-Bitter P, Chaslerie A, Haramburu F. False-positives in spontaneous reporting: should we worry about them? *Br J Clin Pharmacol.* 1994;38(5):401-404.
218. Tubert P, Bégaud B, Péré J-C, Haramburu F, Lellouch J. Power and weakness of spontaneous reporting: a probabilistic approach. *J Clin Epidemiol.* 1992;45(3):283-286.
219. Finney DJ. The design and logic of a monitor of drug use. *J Chronic Dis.* 1965;18(1):77-98.
220. Toh S, Avorn J, D'Agostino RB, et al. Re-using Mini-Sentinel data following rapid assessments of potential safety signals via modular analytic programs. *Pharmacoepidemiol Drug Saf.* 2013;22(10):1036-1045.
221. Lee JAH, Vaughan TL, Diehr PH, Haertle RA. *The recognition of new kinds of occupational toxicity.* In: *Epidemiology and Quantitation of Environmental Risk in Humans from Radiation and Other Agents.* Springer US; 1985:307-337.
222. Vandenbroucke J. *Factor V Leiden.* In: *Human Genome Epidemiology: A Scientific Foundation for Using Genetic Information to Improve Health and Prevent Disease.* Oxford/New York: Oxford University Press; 2004.
223. Goodwin JS. The empirical basis for the discovery of new therapies. *Perspect Biol Med.* 1991;35(1):20-36.
224. Albrecht J, Meves A, Bigby M. Case reports and case series from Lancet had significant impact on medical literature. *J Clin Epidemiol.* 2005;58(12):1227-1232.
225. Burls A, Gold L, Clark W. Systematic review of randomised controlled trials of sildenafil (Viagra) in the treatment of male erectile dysfunction. *Br J Gen Pract.* 2001;51(473):1004-1012.
226. Lue TF. Erectile dysfunction. *N Engl J Med.* 2000;342(24):1802-1813.
227. Popper KR. *Conjectures and Refutations: The Growth of Scientific Knowledge.* 4th rev ed. London: Routledge and Kegan Paul; 1972.
228. Joss R, Goldhirsch A, Brunner K, Galeazzi R. Sudden death in cancer patients on high-dose domperidone. *Lancet.* 1982;319(8279):1019.
229. Arnaiz JA, Carne X, Riba N, Codina C, Ribas J, Trilla A. The use of evidence in pharmacovigilance. Case reports as the reference source for drug withdrawals. *Eur J Clin Pharmacol.* 2001;57(1):89-91.
230. Pocock SJ, Hughes MD. Practical problems in interim analyses, with particular regard to estimation. *Controlled Clin Trials.* 1989;10(4):209-221.
231. Swinnen LJ, Costanzo-Nordin MR, Fisher SG, et al. Increased incidence of lymphoproliferative disorder after immunosuppression with the monoclonal antibody OKT3 in cardiac-transplant recipients. *New Engl J Med.* 1990;323(25):1723-1728.
232. Gagnier JJ, Kienle G, Altman DG, et al. The CARE guidelines: consensus-based clinical case reporting guideline development. Case Reports. *BMJ Case Rep.* 2013;2013:bcr2013201554.

233. Riley DS, Barber MS, Kienle GS, et al. CARE guidelines for case reports: explanation and elaboration document. *J Clin Epidemiol.* 2017;89:218-235.

234. Baker G. *An Essay Concerning the Cause of the Endemial Colic of Devonshire.* Theatre of the College of Physicians in London. London: J Hughs, near Lincoln's-Inn-Fields; 1767.

235. Dandona S, Roberts R. Personalized cardiovascular medicine: status in 2012. *Can J Cardiol.* 2012;28(6):693-699.

236. Baron JA. Screening for cancer with molecular markers: progress comes with potential problems. *Nat Rev Cancer.* 2012;12(5):368-371.

237. Cho SH, Jeon J, Kim SI. Personalized medicine in breast cancer: a systematic review. *J Breast Cancer.* 2012;15(3):265-272.

238. Chen R, Mias GI, Li-Pook-Than J, et al. Personal omics profiling reveals dynamic molecular and medical phenotypes. *Cell.* 2012;148(6):1293-1307.

239. Whirl-Carrillo M, McDonagh EM, Hebert JM, et al. Pharmacogenomics knowledge for personalized medicine. *Clin Pharmacol Ther.* 2012;92(4):414-417.

240. Pathak J, Kho AN, Denny JC. Electronic health records-driven phenotyping: challenges, recent advances, and perspectives. *J Am Med Inform Assoc.* 2013;20(e2):e206-e211.

241. Wang SV, Schneeweiss S, Gagne JJ, et al. Using real world data to extrapolate evidence from randomized controlled trials. *Clin Pharmacol Ther.* 2019;105(5):1156-1163.

242. Schneeweiss S, Avorn J. A review of uses of health care utilization databases for epidemiologic research on therapeutics. *J Clin Epidemiol.* 2005;58(4):323-337.

243. Sørensen HT, Baron JA. Registries and medical databases. In: Olsen J, Saracci R, Trichopoulos D, eds. *Teaching Epidemiology.* 3rd ed. Oxford/New York: Oxford University Press; 2010:551,xiii.

244. Wang SV, Maro JC, Baro E, et al. Data mining for adverse drug events with a propensity score matched tree-based scan statistic. *Epidemiology.* 2018;29(6):895-903.

245. Beam AL, Kohane IS. Big data and machine learning in health care. *J Am Med Assoc.* 2018;319(13):1317-1318.

246. Gulshan V, Peng L, Coram M, et al. Development and validation of a deep learning algorithm for detection of diabetic retinopathy in retinal fundus photographs. *J Am Med Assoc.* 2016;316(22):2402-2410.

247. Thiebaut R, Thiessard F. Public health and epidemiology informatics. *Yearb Med Inform.* 2017;26(1):248-251.

248. Mikkelsen EM, Riis AH, Wise LA, et al. Alcohol consumption and fecundability: prospective Danish cohort study. *BMJ.* 2016;354:i4262.

CHAPTER 36

Molecular Epidemiology

Claire H. Pernar, Konrad H. Stopsack, and Lorelei Mucci

INTRODUCTION

Molecular epidemiology has played a prominent role in public health discoveries over the past decades. It joins an understanding of disease at a molecular level with population-based study designs and approaches. Its value lies in the interdisciplinary approach that links epidemiology with laboratory sciences to study states of health using biomarkers. These markers need not be measured within the individual; they can span a continuum of sources from an individual's cells to their environment. The major objectives of molecular epidemiology are to integrate biomarkers into epidemiologic studies to understand how biological processes explain, contribute, or serve as markers for disease susceptibility, risk, early detection, and progression. The goal is to translate this understanding to interventions or prevention strategies that address the spectrum of public health challenges. Molecular epidemiology has close ties to many other disciplines, such as clinical epidemiology, toxicology, environmental health, and cancer and nutritional epidemiology. The principles of molecular epidemiology are critical also in the context of clinical trials, in which biomarkers are often used.

One of the earliest mentions of the term "molecular epidemiology" appeared in a 1973 publication that applied a novel understanding of influenza viral variants and subtype-specific immunity to explain variation in influenza pandemic severity.[1] Several earlier examples of molecular epidemiology exist. One classic example is the identification of cholesterol levels as a risk factor for coronary heart disease in the Framingham Heart Study, a prospective cohort established in 1948 among residents of Framingham, Massachusetts. Blood-based measures of serum cholesterol measured before diagnosis were positively associated with the risk of heart disease.[2]

Molecular epidemiology studies are often translational, both "forward" translational to clinical trials and "reverse" translational for testing in experimental models. For example, the results on cholesterol from the Framingham Heart Study together with other early studies catalyzed a large body of work to disentangle the relationship between low- and high-density lipoproteins and cardiovascular disease using experimental models.[3] Ultimately, this research led to randomized trials of lipid lowering drugs, including statins, in both primary and secondary cardiovascular disease prevention.[3]

Particularly in cancer epidemiology, biomarker-focused approaches have been central since Perera and Weinstein applied the term "molecular cancer epidemiology" when studying DNA adducts as a biomarker in carcinogenesis.[4] For example, DNA adduct biomarkers helped solidify the link between the chemical carcinogen benzo(a)pyrene, present in tobacco smoke and occupational environments, and the risk of lung cancer. Integration of these biomarkers helped move beyond job-based exposure measures, establishing a mechanistic relationship between benzo(a)pyrene and lung cancer, and further supporting public health policies to protect individuals from exposure to benzo(a)pyrene.

The successful implementation of molecular epidemiology requires expertise in epidemiology and in diverse fields such as medicine, basic science, chemistry, genetics, biostatistics, and others. A major source of evolution in the field of molecular epidemiology has been in new technologies, such as novel bioassays and a growing list of -omics technologies. While sometimes defined and dominated by such technological advances, molecular epidemiology can only contribute valid and reproducible findings if epidemiologists critically integrate core methodological concepts of epidemiology. Indeed, there are unique epidemiologic issues in the discipline of molecular epidemiology that need to be integrated to generate valid and reproducible research. Specifically, the collection and storage of biospecimens and the measurements of biomarkers can influence the validity and reproducibility of a molecular epidemiology study. These factors should be considered at the design stage, as they will ultimately have implications for study validity, expertise in the investigator team, and expense of assaying biomarkers.

This chapter will provide an introduction to the theory and practice of molecular epidemiology, including integration of biospecimens into study design, methodological challenges, and social and ethical considerations. It complements the chapter on genetic epidemiology (see Chapter 37), which shares many of its guiding principles.

METHODOLOGIES AND CHALLENGES IN MOLECULAR EPIDEMIOLOGY

Fundamental Principles and Terminology

Molecular epidemiology has unique aspects stemming from specific methodologic issues in biospecimen collections, the biomarkers that can (and cannot) be measured in them, approaches to assessing validity, and issues critical to study design. The following terminology will lay a foundation for discussing these features (listed in alphabetical order).

Assay. In molecular epidemiology, an assay refers to the test or procedures used to measure a biomarker. (See also *Intra-Assay Variability* and *Inter-Assay Variability*.) Assays are critical components of the validity of molecular epidemiology studies, and there are three primary considerations. First, whether the assay is reproducible, that is, if the assay was conducted in the same samples over and over, would it provide the same measure of the biomarker. Second, whether the assay is valid, that is, does the assay measure what it intends to measure. Third, whether the assay performs well on the available biospecimen in terms of the type of biospecimen, its storage, or other features.

Batch. A batch in the laboratory setting refers to the group of samples analyzed together on the same instrument, under a particular set of conditions. The size of the batch is a function of the assay technology as well as the ability of the laboratory staff to group certain runs. For example, blood-based assays are often conducted on 96-well plates, and thus a batch size is 96 samples. A batch for RNA sequencing often includes 4 to 24 samples, while a tissue microarray may contain a few hundred samples. As molecular epidemiology studies often include hundreds or thousands of study participants or biospecimens, each assay may need to be conducted in multiple batches. A key challenge is to avoid or reduce any sources of variability within and across batches, which can otherwise lead to different forms of measurement error. A laboratory should try to replicate the conditions as much as possible, including using the same reagents, staff, and machine settings. (See also *Intra-Assay Variability* and *Inter-Assay Variability*.)

Biomarker. In 1998, the Biomarkers Definitions Working Group of the National Institutes of Health (NIH) defined a biomarker as "a characteristic that is objectively measured and evaluated as an indicator of normal biological processes, pathogenic processes, or pharmacologic responses to a therapeutic intervention."[5] The World Health Organization (WHO) has defined a biomarker as "any substance, structure, or process that can be measured in the body or its products and influence or predict the incidence of outcome or disease."[6]

An even broader definition of a biomarker takes into account not just the disease and its outcomes, but also environmental and lifestyle exposures and measures of the effect of interventions, such as treatments. An expanded definition of biomarkers includes "almost any measurement reflecting an interaction between a biological system and a potential hazard, which may be chemical, physical, or biological. The measured response may be functional and physiological, biochemical at the cellular level, or a molecular interaction."[6] Figure 36-1 represents the diversity of biomarker categories and their uses. Of note, a biomarker need not be measured directly in an individual. For example, sampling of water or dust in an individual's environment can be used to identify biomarkers of pollutants, infectious agents, and other compounds.

Biospecimen. A biospecimen refers to a sample of biological material used to measure a biomarker. As described in the National Cancer Institute's Best Practices for Biospecimen Research,[7] a biospecimen can include fluids (*e.g.*, blood, saliva, sweat, lymph, tears), waste products (*e.g.*, urine, stool, hair, nail clippings), tissues (*e.g.*, bone, muscle, organs, tumor), and cells. Different biospecimens may be used to measure the same biomarker, but its interpretation in diverse specimens may vary as a function of what each biospecimen implies in terms of time integration. For example, a biomarker measured in urine may reflect an exposure that occurred over the past 24 hours whereas that same marker measured in blood may reflect an exposure over the past 2 months. The selection of the biospecimen for a study should reflect the epidemiologic hypothesis that is being tested and an understanding of the interpretation of the marker in that biospecimen. Table 36-1 presents an overview of the types of biospecimens used in molecular epidemiology, as well as examples of biomarkers often measured in such specimens.

Coefficients of Variation (CVs). Measurement error in biomarkers can arise from multiple sources (also see the terms *Batch*, *Intra-Assay Variability*, and *Inter-Assay Variability*). One method for assessing the extent of measurement error is through the calculation of the CV, which considers *Technical Replicates* (see below), that is, repeated laboratory measurements of the same biological specimen. It is calculated as the standard deviation of the measurements divided by the mean of the measurements and then often expressed in percent. The greater the standard deviation is relative to the mean values of the assay, the greater the extent of the measurement error deriving from the laboratory protocol. While interpretation depends critically on the exact biomarker and its intended use, a CV% greater than 15% or 20% is often considered to be poor. CV% can be assessed as intra-assay CV and thus measure variance between data points within an assay, referring to the sample replicates within the same assay batch (see below, *Intra-Assay Variability*). CV% can also be assessed as inter-assay CV, measuring variance between sample replicates in different batches that can be used to assess batch-to-batch consistency of an assay (see below, *Inter-Assay Variability*).

Inter-Assay Variability. Inter-assay variability, also referred to as batch-to-batch variability, is the extent to which measurement error occurs across batches (Box 36-1). Such an error can result when extraneous variability in a biomarker is introduced due to variability in procedures, methods,

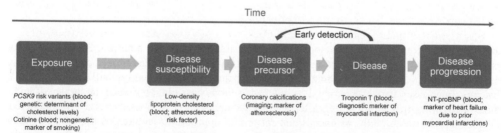

FIGURE 36-1 **The spectrum of biomarkers in molecular epidemiology.** Biomarkers can serve as proxies of events along the exposure-outcome spectrum (*e.g.*, cotinine as a proxy for smoking status) or for more specific subtyping (*e.g.*, coronary calcium scoring for cardiovascular disease risk stratification). Example biomarkers from cardiovascular epidemiology are listed below the boxes with commonly used biospecimens for assessing them. Note that the same biomarker can serve multiple purposes at different time points along the pathway. For example, highly-sensitive troponin T can be used for assessing disease risk and as a biomarker to diagnose disease. One of the key features of biomarkers is time, which is a function both of the biomarker itself and the biospecimen used to measure it.

TABLE 36-1

Types of Biospecimens That May Be Collected in a Molecular Epidemiology Study

Biospecimen	Common Examples of Biomarkers[a]
Blood	Genetics, sex hormones, metabolomics, methylation, cytokines, proteomics, infections, toxicants
Bone marrow	Proteins, transcriptome, mutations, adipocytes, histology
Breast milk	Pesticides, nutrients, hormones, cytokines, growth factors, breast cells
Breath (exhaled air)	Volatile organic compounds, hydrogen, carbon dioxide, isoprene, ethanol
Bronchoalveolar lavage	Immune cell counts, cytokines, pH, oxidative stress, toxicants
Emesis	Infections, toxicants
Hair	Cortisol, heavy metals, alcohol, toxicants
Muscle	RNA, morphology, methylation
Nail clippings	Heavy metals, selenium, arsenic, nicotine
Nasopharyngeal swabs	Infections, protein, RNA
Placenta, meconium, cord blood	Sex hormones, pollutants, heavy metals, immune markers, oxidative stress, cotinine
Saliva	Cortisol, drugs, alcohol, amino acids, environmental toxins, zinc, toxicants
Semen	Sperm quality and morphology, reactive oxygen species, proteomics, sex hormones
Skin	Microbiome, proteins, cytokines, histology
Sputum	Infections, inflammation, immune cells
Stool	Microbiome, bacterial species, DNA mutations, metabolomics, proteins
Sweat	Electrolytes, proteins, lipids, metabolic output, ion concentrations, immunoglobulin, musk
Tissue (FFPE or fresh frozen)	Transcriptome, genomics, protein expression, methylation, metabolomics, histologic markers
Urine	Hormones, proteins, microbiome, cotinine, metabolomics, toxicants

FFPE, formalin-fixed, paraffin embedded.

[a]Many biomarkers may be collected from more than one type of biospecimen. However, it is critical to assess reliability and validity across these biospecimens as well as the time period a specific biospecimen may reflect.

and standards from one batch to another when an assay is done. In addition, it can also occur due to variability in the quality of samples between batches. When the number of samples being assayed is large relative to the sample size of the batch, biomarker assays will require multiple batches. Inter-assay variability should be reduced as far as possible. To reduce the impact of inter-assay variability that is remaining after careful standardization of how the assay is conducted, batches should be carefully balanced with respect to appropriate features of the study population to decrease the potential for differential misclassification. For example, in a study where the biomarker assesses an exposure, if some batches contained a higher proportion of samples from participants with the disease outcome than other batches, then inter-assay variability could result in some extent of differential misclassification of the exposure and in bias of the estimated exposure-disease relationship. (See also *Batch* and *Coefficients of Variation*.)

Intra-Assay Variability. Also referred to as within-batch variability, intra-assay variability is a measure of the variability of measurement values within a batch of samples. (Compare to

---

BOX 36-1   An Example Illustrating Terminology and Concepts of Molecular Epidemiology

In 2002, the Swedish National Food Administration found high levels of the compound acrylamide in commonly baked and fried foods (including cakes, cookies, and potatoes), coffee, and olives.[8] Acrylamide formation occurred naturally during the cooking and heating of foods, and the amount of acrylamide generated within a food depended on the cooking time and temperature as well as specific components of the foods. The identification of acrylamide in commonly consumed foods raised public health concern given that the World Health Organization had labeled acrylamide as a Group 2A human carcinogen.[9] In addition, acrylamide exposure has been linked to an array of neurological conditions including peripheral neuropathy. A key question to assess the potential for public health harm was whether there was a reproducible and valid biomarker of acrylamide exposure through diet. Molecular epidemiologists undertook a study of women who were participants in the Nurses' Health Study 2 to assess the validity of biomarkers of acrylamide exposure in diet.[10] First, they studied 45 women who had given two blood specimens at least 10 months apart to assess the reproducibility of two potential biomarkers, hemoglobin adducts to acrylamide (AA-Hb) and to its main metabolite glycidamide (GA-Hb). These adducts reflect acrylamide exposure over approximately the previous 4 months, which is the lifetime of red blood cells, and estimate the average dose across time. The ICCs were 0.78 for AA-Hb and 0.80 for GA-Hb, which are high and suggest that the variability in acrylamide biomarkers was stable across time and thus reproducible. Next, the researchers assayed AA-Hb and GA-Hb on 296 women including technical replicates. The assays were run on 12 batches. The intra-assay CV (assessing variability within a batch) was 13% for AA-Hb and 14% for GA-Hb while the inter-assay CV (assessing variability across batches) was 9.8% for AA-Hb and 10.9% for GA-Hb, suggesting that the biomarker assays were reproducible and the extent of measurement error was low.

Inter-Assay Variability.) On one hand, intra-assay variability is a consequence of measurement error in an assay, its performance, or the biospecimen used. This error is commonly assumed to be random and to result in nondifferential misclassification, resulting at minimum in decreased precision in effect estimates. On the other hand, it can reflect true biological variability in the study population. For example, sex hormone levels among postmenopausal women would show higher intra-assay variability than among premenopausal women sampled on the same day of their menstrual cycle, since the mean levels will be quite low in postmenopausal women and consequently within-assay variability may seem high if assessed via a *CV*.

Intra-Class Correlation Coefficients (ICCs). Even a perfect assay without measurement error will give different values on biospecimens if done repeatedly because the extent to which a biomarker is reproducible is a function of the biology of an individual and inherent in physiological processes. ICCs can be calculated as the ratio of between-person variance over the sum of within-person and between-person variance, for example, using mixed-effects models. ICCs are useful measures of how consistently a biomarker measurement can be repeated. For example, biospecimens from a given person could be assayed for the same marker at multiple time points, or multiple samples could be taken from the same person at the same time. The ICC will set the variability within a group of measurements within a person (*e.g.*, how much do circulating vitamin D levels change in time for one person) in contrast to the variability between individuals (*e.g.*, how do vitamin D levels differ, on average, between groups of people with common characteristics). The former is typically a nuisance and the latter the quantity of interest in epidemiologic studies.

Omics. The term *omics* refers to the broad category of technologies or approaches that provide an assessment of multiple biomarkers of the same molecule type, up to a comprehensive quantification of all molecular data of that type. Many of these omics stem from measuring components based on the Central Dogma of Molecular Biology (Figure 36-2). For example, genomics refers to an assessment of multiple DNA molecules, *transcriptomics* refers to RNA transcripts, *proteomics* refers to protein expression, *metabolomics* refers to the detection of metabolites, and *epigenomics* refers to epigenetic modifications to DNA. While the study of individual biomarkers

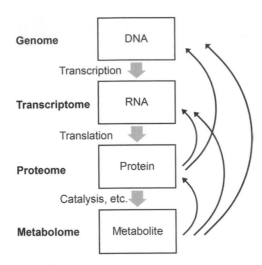

FIGURE 36-2 The central dogma of molecular biology states unidirectionally that protein is encoded by RNA, which is encoded by DNA. However, molecular epidemiology studies need to consider many of the additional mechanisms invoked on the right side of the scheme on a cellular level, individual level, and population level. For example, DNA and how it is transcribed is not static, with the entirety of these modifications being termed the "epigenome."

typically relies on *a priori* specified hypotheses, omics studies are high dimensional and undertake discovery-based approaches to identify novel biomarkers. Core principles of epidemiology methods, design, and analysis remain critical to the valid interpretation of study findings (see *New Directions in Molecular Epidemiology*, below).

Technical *Versus* Biological Replicate. *Technical and biological replicates* of a biospecimen are critical to quality control to assess the reproducibility and validity of a biomarker. Technical replicates refer to repeated measurements on samples for which the biological sample is the same but the technical steps that are used to assay the sample are repeated. Biological replicates are repeated measurements done on biologically distinct samples from the sample individual and where the technical steps are repeated on each biological sample. Consider a validation study for RNA sequencing of tissue specimens. With a technical replicate, the team would use the same sample of tissue and extract RNA and then perform the RNA sequencing assay on multiple aliquots of the RNA from the same tissue. In contrast, with a biological replicate, the team would sample two or more, perhaps adjacent, tissue specimens, extract RNA independently from each, and then conduct the assay on each RNA aliquot. How technical and biological replicates are distinguished is strongly dependent on context. In the example, RNA extraction could also be considered part of technical replication.

Selection of Biospecimen

Biospecimens may be collected at study baseline, for example, at the time of enrollment in a study or during follow-up intervals. In addition, biospecimens may be retrieved after the sample has been collected as part of routine clinical care, such as tumor tissue specimens following a cancer diagnosis or mammography images, and then integrated into the epidemiology study. The timing of collection is important to consider when addressing the window of exposure or outcome the study intends the biomarker to reflect (see Figure 36-1).

The source of collection is important since it may lead to variability in sample collection, handling, and storage that is outside the scope of an investigator. Ultimately, these collection factors may affect the validity of the biomarker. As a corollary, it is critical to understand whether there is any variability in procedures that is differential with respect to the outcome of interest. There are a range of resources that describe best practices for the collection and storage of biospecimens, and these are summarized in Table 36-2. The investigator team has control over the standardization of biospecimens that are collected as part of a molecular epidemiology study. In contrast, samples collected as part of routine clinical care may have significant heterogeneity across clinic sites. For example, with tumor tissue materials, a pathology department may have different procedures for the time between surgery and processing, different durations of fixation, and may use different fixation methods for tissue preservation.

TABLE 36-2

Molecular Epidemiology References for Biomarker and Biospecimen Research Best Practices

Title	Source	Year	URL or PMID
Biospecimen Storage, Tracking, Sharing, and Disposal within the NIH Intramural Program	NIH	2019	https://oir.nih.gov/sites/default/files/uploads/sourcebook/documents/ethical_conduct/guidelines-biospecimen.pdf
Best Practices for Biospecimen Resources	NCI	2016	https://biospecimens.cancer.gov/bestpractices/index.asp
Molecular Epidemiology: Principles and Practices	IARC	2011	https://publications.iarc.fr/_publications/media/download/1390/1a8a810e5a30e-326be59857acf30c55a8ec78a34.pdf
UK Biobank sample handling and storage validation studies	UK Biobank	2008	*Int J Epidemiol.* 2008;37(2):234-244; PMID:18381398
Tissue banking for biomedical research	National Cancer Center/Singapore	2001	https://www.bioethics-singapore.org/files/publications/others/tissue-banking-for-biomedical-research.pdf
Biospecimens and biorepositories: from afterthought to science	NCI	2013	*Cancer Epidemiol Biomarkers Prev.* 2012;21(2):253-255. PMID 22313938
NIH Human Microbiome Project, clinical sampling	NIH	2020	https://www.hmpdacc.org/hmp/micro_analysis/microbiome_analyses.php

IARC, International Agency for Research on Cancer; NCI, National Cancer Institute; NIH, National Institutes of Health.

Table 36-1 summarizes the plethora of biospecimen types in molecular epidemiology studies. Below are detailed descriptions of commonly used biospecimens in molecular epidemiology studies: blood, urine, tissue, and nails.

<u>Blood:</u> Blood is perhaps the most commonly used biospecimen in molecular epidemiology studies, because of the diversity of biomarkers that can be measured in its multiple derivatives as well as its relative ease of collection and storage. After its collection, blood is often centrifuged resulting in multiple fractions. Figure 36-3 illustrates several of the key components and derivatives of blood that are subsequently used in molecular epidemiology studies, as well as the types of biomarkers that can be assayed in each fraction.

DNA is most abundant in whole blood or the buffy coat, although small amounts of DNA known as "cell-free DNA" can be extracted from other fractions as well. Cell-free DNA is a biomarker in reproductive epidemiology studies of pregnancy to determine molecular alterations in the fetus as well as in cancer epidemiology studies to capture DNA from tumors. Blood is used to assess an array of biomarkers. Red blood cells can, for example, be used to assess the presence of DNA adducts or fatty acid concentrations. Plasma and serum biomarkers are quite diverse and include dietary markers such as carotenoids, growth factors, sex hormones, vitamin D, adipokines, inflammatory markers, stress hormones, and many others.

An alternate blood collection method uses dried blood spots, in which blood droplets produced via skin prick are collected onto absorbent cards. This collection mode results in samples of whole blood minus water, which remains stable on the absorbent matrix. In principle, study participants experienced in performing skin pricks can provide dried blood specimens from home, without a need for study personnel to conduct venipunctures. Shipping, processing, and storage are easy and efficient. Many of the biomarkers that can be measured in whole blood samples, including DNA, proteins, hormones, and infectious agents, can be quantified on dried blood spots or detected in a semiquantitative fashion.

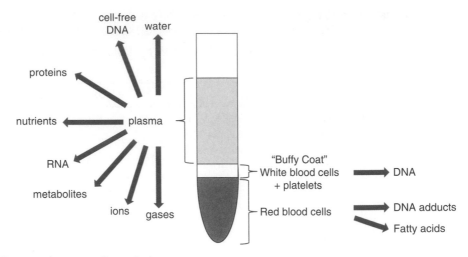

Serum = plasma − anticoagulant

FIGURE 36-3 Components and derivatives of blood.

Before beginning a molecular epidemiology study using any biospecimen, it is critical to first conduct pilot studies to assess how well the selected assay works on the biospecimen available. In the case of blood, this can include assessing reproducibility and validity of the biomarker: in plasma versus serum; whether or not the blood sample was collected at fasting; whether heparin, EDTA, or another preservative was used, how long is the time between when the sample was collected and processed, what the storage temperature has been, or whether the aliquot of blood has been previously thawed. Each of these aspects of blood collection and storage may or may not have an effect on measured concentrations of individual biomarkers. As an example, the freezing and thawing of blood samples can influence both the pH and ionic balance, with the downstream effect of degradation of some biomarkers, while others may not be influenced.[11]

Urine: While less commonly collected in molecular epidemiology studies, urine has a number of advantages compared to blood in terms of ease of collection and processing as well as its utility for measuring specific biomarkers. Urine is noninvasive, and collection kits can be sent to study participants at home with instructions on the collection process. The samples can then be stored under refrigeration until ready for shipment. Urine also has the advantage of being a more limitless sample given the potential volume produced and relative ease of collection.

There are three primary modes of sample collection: first morning void; timed void; and random (spot) urines collected without timing. First morning void urines are collected immediately upon waking, collecting the entire urine void. Because the total volume is collected, first morning voids have the advantage to allow concentration of a biomarker to be measured. It is also a useful sample to capture biomarkers with diurnal variation. A timed urine collection, such as 24-hour, involves the collection of all urine output over that time period. As with first morning void, this type of collection provides a total volume of output for a day and thus allows for biomarker concentration as well as for capturing diurnal variation. While having the advantage of complete capture of urine output, it adds some burden to study participants. Spot urines represent the easiest of collections but pose challenges in determining concentrations of analytes, such as protein excretion.

Urine is a useful biospecimen to assay a diversity of biomarkers, including hormones, renal markers, medications and illicit drugs, and pesticides. Urine production occurs as a function of plasma filtration, selective reabsorption and secretion, and shedding of proteins from both the kidney and the urinary tract.[12] Blood composition is highly regulated to maintain homeostasis and is a reflection of what the body is exposed to but also what is not excreted. While its proteome is not as diverse as blood, urine has the advantage of being less homeostatically regulated and may reflect a better estimate of exposure for some biomarkers. However, the higher variability in urine volume production, with a physiologic range greater than an order of magnitude, inherently poses challenges if analytes are measured in terms of concentrations but their masses are of interest.

Before undertaking a new biospecimen collection, it may be useful to consider adding urine as an additional biospecimen. It also would be of interest to compare the same biomarker measured in blood and urine, in order to understand the potential implications of interpretation of that marker.

Tissue: In molecular epidemiology studies, the primary sources of tissue are biopsy or surgery. The materials may be collected per study protocol, in which case study investigators have input on standardizing procedures for collecting, processing, and storing the tissue specimens. There are also opportunities to leverage tissue specimens that were collected as part of routine clinical care. For example, breast tissue can be obtained from women undergoing mammoplasty, breast biopsy after mammography screening, or surgery following lumpectomy or mastectomy for breast cancer treatment. In another example, a molecular epidemiology study of HPV16 viral load and cervical cancer leveraged serial Papanicolaou tests (Pap smears) that were collected among Swedish women attending cervical cancer screening over time. In a nested case control design, women with high HPV16 viral load in Pap smears were at 30 times greater risk of cervical cancer during 13 years of median follow-up.[13]

The types of biomarkers that can be measured in tissue are diverse and include RNA, DNA, protein, metabolites, and epigenetics. In addition, histologic biomarkers may be gleaned through review of hematoxylin and eosin slides (H&E), sections stained with dyes to differentiate the cytoplasm and nuclear components of cells. The quality of tissue-based biomarkers in tissue is influenced by the two primary modes of tissue preservation to prevent degradation, fresh frozen preservation or formalin fixation followed by paraffin embedding (FFPE) (Table 36-3). When tissue is being collected prospectively and biobanked as part of a molecular epidemiology study, freezing tissue may be preferable, as the downstream measurement of most biomarkers is more straightforward. However, freezing tissue and storing frozen tissue are more expensive. The majority of pathology banking of tissues in clinical care that might be leveraged is FFPE-preserved tissue with its superior histological quality, also allowing for storage at room temperature. In terms of biomarker research, the FFPE process leads to cross-linking of proteins as well as degradation of the nucleic acids. Immunohistochemical protocols to measure protein biomarkers account for the cross-linking via antigen retrieval steps. Newer technologies to undertake transcriptomic or genomic approaches in tissue have accounted for the degradation and allowed for reproducible measures of RNA and DNA.[14]

Molecular epidemiology is a transdisciplinary field, and this is particularly so with respect to tissue as a biospecimen and tissue-based biomarkers. Studies integrating tissue should partner with a pathologist from the study inception.

Nails: Nail clippings, particularly from toenails, are a straightforward biospecimen to collect. One advantage of nail clippings is that the nail tips represent a relatively long-term assessment of

TABLE 36-3

Effect of Preservation on Storage and Biomarker Quality for Tissue Biospecimens

	Frozen	Formalin-Fixed, Paraffin-Embedded
Storage	Stored in liquid nitrogen; expensive	Stored and "stable" at room temperature
Morphology	Mediocre morphology	Excellent morphology
Protein expression: detection	Antigenicity is excellent	Cross-links mask antigens; antigen retrieval to address cross-links eliminates issue
Protein expression: localization	Challenging	Excellent
RNA	Excellent	Degradation; covalent modification of RNA
DNA	Excellent	Degradation; preserved DNA sequence
Metabolites	Excellent	Some metabolites washed away during fixation; others detectable

many exposures, up to 1 year in toenails depending on the nails' growth rate. As an example, arsenic is common in the environment and can leech into water supplies causing high levels in some populations. Arsenic is quickly metabolized after exposure and excreted through urine. Blood concentrations of arsenic would capture only the most recent exposure, while toenail concentration will capture longer-term exposure. Another advantage is that toenail collections can be completely self-administered by study participants and can be stored stably at room temperature.

Because of their composition, nails can be a reliable source of trace elements from dietary or other exposures as well as environmental contaminants including heavy metals.[15] Toenails have been used in molecular epidemiology studies to examine potential health benefits of selenium through diet or supplementation in relation to health outcomes ranging from birth outcomes, cancer, neurologic conditions, and other chronic diseases. Toenails may also be useful to capture diverse exposures from nicotine in cigarette smokers,[16] to illicit drugs, and to cortisol as a measure of stress.

Although different biomarkers can be measured across different biospecimens, it is critical to understand: (1) how reproducible the biomarkers are across these biospecimens; (2) what time period of exposure the biomarker reflects in different biospecimens; and (3) how reproducible a biomarker is in that particular biospecimen. As a corollary, pilot studies are essential to evaluating these three features.

Categories of Biomarkers

This section describes categories of biomarkers and provides examples to demonstrate how biomarkers can be used to address different types of epidemiologic research questions. While it can be useful to categorize biomarkers, there is no single way to define these categories. Furthermore, a given biomarker may fit into more than one category, as shown in an example below. Figure 36-1 depicts the wide spectrum of ways in which biomarkers may be applied to study exposure-disease relationships and how they may be integrated in time. This framework may be applied in study design and in decisions regarding when it is most appropriate to collect a biomarker.

Exposure

Biomarkers can be categorized by grouping those used to assess the *exposure*. This category can include a direct measure of a substance or action, or a biomarker that provides a measure of biological change caused by the exposure. If information is known about the relevant time period of exposure, this information should be used in selection of an appropriate biomarker. For example, cotinine is a metabolite of nicotine, a component of tobacco products, and can be measured in the blood, urine, and saliva with a half-life of 3 to 4 days,[17] and in hair. Cotinine is a both sensitive and specific biomarker for tobacco exposure, including environmental exposure to tobacco smoke in nonsmokers.[18]

Biomarkers of exposure can be used to calibrate questionnaire-based exposures or other methods of exposure assessment. This calibration can be useful in settings where a biomarker can be feasibly measured only in a subset of the study population. For example, self-reported diet from food frequency questionnaires was used to create a dietary index of hyperinsulinemia based on a prediction model for fasting levels of C-peptide, a measure of pancreas β-cell secretion, measured in a subset of participants.[19] This empirically derived dietary index then could be applied to the full set of study participants to examine associations with disease risk, or indeed applied to epidemiologic studies that lack biospecimens altogether.

Biomarkers of exposure need not always be measured in an individual. A biomarker of exposure measured in an individual may provide a more accurate measure of the internal dose of the exposure. A biomarker from the environment may help elucidate a mechanism for an exposure-disease relationship of interest. For example, disruption of circadian rhythm has been shown to increase risk for several health outcomes, including sleep disorders, cancer, and premature death.[20,21] Melatonin is a biomarker of circadian rhythm that is measured at the individual level in urine samples. This biomarker provides information about the internal or biological effects of circadian disruption. Exposure to light at night, which can be conceptualized as an environmental biomarker, is also used to measure circadian disruption. One such way to measure light at night is using satellite image data that captures the amount of nighttime illumination in a defined geographic area and is linked with an individual's geocoded home or work address.[22]

Disease Susceptibility

Biomarkers of disease susceptibility in molecular epidemiology studies may include biomarkers that provide information about disease risk or biomarkers of an intermediate biological effect of the exposure of interest. A biomarker of susceptibility may be detectable long before the disease itself is present. This preclinical information can be an advantage in studies when follow-up of study participants is not long enough to observe disease development and the biomarker of disease susceptibility has been validated as being closely linked to a meaningful disease precursor or as an intervention target on its own right. Biomarkers of susceptibility may also allow for study of effect modification by allowing comparison of the exposure-disease association among individuals with and without a biomarker of susceptibility, and for the study of mediation, assessing to what extent the effect of exposure is mediated through a particular mechanism reflected by the biomarker of susceptibility.

An example of a biomarker of susceptibility for atherosclerosis is low-density lipoprotein (LDL) cholesterol as measured in the blood. Evidence from cohort studies shows that elevated LDL cholesterol levels are associated with a higher risk of developing atherosclerotic cardiovascular disease.[2] LDL is also an intermediate biomarker between dietary saturated fat intake and heart disease.

Disease Precursor

Biomarkers of disease precursors are markers of a biological state that precedes or leads to a disease. This category of biomarker can provide important information about the pathogenesis of a disease. These biomarkers may also provide opportunities for early detection or secondary prevention. As an example, colon polyps are preneoplastic precursors of colon cancer. Specific features of polyps, including histologic (high-grade dysplasia, sessile serrated) and molecular biomarkers, can be used to risk stratify future colon cancer risk. Coronary calcifications are a disease precursor for atherosclerosis and can be assessed through imaging techniques, such as computed tomography. Scoring of coronary artery calcifications has also been combined with the Framingham Risk Score, based on traditional risk factors, to modify risk prediction of coronary heart disease.[23] This example also illustrates how biomarkers of disease precursors have the potential to identify asymptomatic individuals who may benefit from prevention strategies.

Disease

Biomarkers of disease in molecular epidemiology studies may serve as objective measures of disease occurrence, differentiate between disease subtypes, or indicate severity or extent of disease. A biomarker of disease may be a gold standard method of assessing the presence of a disease and could be used to validate another assessment method, such as a diagnosis self-reported by a study participant.

As an example, troponin T is part of the troponin complex in heart and skeletal muscle that is released into the blood stream after a myocardial infarction. Troponin T as measured in blood is a highly sensitive and specific biomarker used in the diagnosis of myocardial infarction (Figure 36-1).[24] An example of a biomarker of disease subtype is estrogen receptor expression in tissue. Identification of the presence or absence of estrogen receptor expression in tumor tissue of women with breast cancer has profoundly influenced disease treatment and management, including use of estrogen receptor–targeted drugs such as tamoxifen, and aided in understanding of breast cancer etiology.[25,26]

Disease Progression

There are different ways that biomarkers of disease progression are applied in the treatment and management of disease. Biomarkers may provide information about individuals' likely response to a treatment of interest. They can be used to tailor a patient's disease follow-up procedures or treatment strategy in terms of prognosis and reduction of adverse treatment side effects. When a biomarker is an effect modifier in the association of treatment (exposure) and disease progression or death (outcome), it is often referred to as "predictive" in clinical literature; a biomarker is described as "prognostic" when it is assessed as the exposure and not as an effect modifier.[27] In other words, a prognostic biomarker is one that indicates poor outcomes or worse survival, regardless of the treatment. For example, estrogen receptor expression is both prognostic, with presence of expression indicating a better prognosis, and predictive of tamoxifen response in breast cancer; its expression modifies the effectiveness of the drug.

> **BOX 36-2**   **Example of When to Use Biomarkers in Epidemiology Research**
>
> Aflatoxin is a metabolite of *Aspergillus* fungus, a mold that grows on peanuts, corn, and grains in hot and humid climates. High rates of primary liver cancer overlap with areas of high aflatoxin exposure, which raised concern that dietary intake of foods on which this fungus grows could increase the risk of primary liver cancer. Epidemiologic studies until the 1990s had primarily relied on food frequency questionnaires together with food sampling to assess potential exposure to aflatoxin and association with primary liver cancer. Using a prospective cohort from Shanghai, Qian et al.[28] assessed aflatoxin exposure and risk of primary liver cancer using both questionnaires and two biomarkers of aflatoxin: urinary aflatoxin B1 (AFB1) and DNA adducts of acrylamide (AFB1-N-Gua) in red blood cells. Table 36-4 summarizes the study results. Using dietary intake as assessed by food frequency questionnaires, there was no association between higher intake and risk of primary liver cancer. In contrast, dietary exposure based on biomarker positivity showed strong positive associations of aflatoxin assessed in urine and DNA adducts. This study highlights an example for which assessing exposure to aflatoxin was not possible using questionnaire data, as there was too much variability in whether or not specific foods were contaminated by *Aspergillus* fungus. In this setting, the use of the biomarker reduced misclassification and increased specificity of the actual exposure. Moreover, it provided a more valid assessment of the association between exposure and outcome.

TABLE 36-4

Rate Ratios and 95% Confidence Intervals of the Association Between Exposure to Aflatoxin and Risk of Primary Liver Cancer Based on Dietary Food Frequency Questionnaire (FFQ) Compared to Urinary and Blood-Based Biomarkers[28]

Aflatoxin Assessed Through FFQ		Aflatoxin Assessed Through Biomarker	
Dietary Intake	Rate Ratio (95% Confidence Interval)	Biomarker	Rate Ratio (95% Confidence Interval)
Low	1 (Reference)	Negative	1 (Reference)
Medium	1.6 (0.8, 3.1)	Urinary AFB1+	3.5 (1.2, 9.9)
High	0.9 (0.4, 1.9)	DNA adduct+	9.1 (2.9, 29.2)

Aflatoxin B1 (AFB1) is considered the most toxic of aflatoxins.

It is possible for a biomarker to serve for multiple purposes at different time points along the exposure-disease pathway. For example, mammograms can be used for assessing disease susceptibility (breast density; a risk factor for breast cancer), for screening and detecting disease precursors (ductal carcinoma in situ), when diagnosing disease (breast cancer), and as part of assessments for disease progression (local recurrence after therapy). Prostate-specific antigen is similarly used in prostate cancer screening and diagnosis among men, and as a biomarker of disease progression (Box 36-2).

Epidemiologic Concepts in Molecular Epidemiology

Integration of Time

The integration of time is an essential feature of molecular epidemiology studies, as time may influence the interpretation and validity of biomarker research. There are three main elements that drive the determination of the exposure time window associated with a biomarker: the biospecimen used to measure the biomarker, the timing of biospecimen collection, and the half-life of a biomarker.

Different biospecimens capture different windows of exposure to internal or external substances. Because of the half-life of red blood cells, biomarkers in this biospecimen ordinarily reflect the past half year of exposure. Plasma-based markers such as hormones may reflect exposure that occurred in the past 1 to 3 months. Urine generally reflects more recent exposures, and hormones and other markers likely reflect levels during the prior 12 to 24 hours. Biomarkers measured in tissue, such as protein or RNA, may reflect only that point in time or may capture earlier time points, for example, if there is gene methylation.

In many studies, a blood, urine, or tissue sample is collected per participant (or subset of participants) at a single point in time. Depending on what the biomarker is measuring, its measurement at one point in time may not reflect sufficient duration that is relevant to the study question. Some biomarkers vary considerably by time of day (cortisol), season (25-hydroxyvitamin D), within a woman's menstrual cycle (estrogens), or may have little regular variation over time (specific fatty acids). As a corollary, if the biospecimen is collected at or near the time of disease diagnosis, the disease itself may influence biomarker levels. If the goal of the molecular epidemiology study is to assess causation, then concerns of reverse causation must be addressed. Instead, if the goal is to identify an early detection biomarker, such timing of the collection could actually be an asset.

One advantage of nesting a study within a prospective cohort is the ability to examine latency. For example, a hypothetical cohort study collects baseline bloods in 2000, in which the biomarker of interest (*e.g.*, C-peptide) is measured. Incident cases of the disease of interest (*e.g.*, diabetes) are identified between 2000 and 2020, and a measure of effect is estimated. The etiologic question is whether circulating C-peptide levels, as a marker of hyperinsulinemia, is associated with an increased risk of diabetes. To address latency effects of a biomarker, sensitivity analyses can be conducted to assess whether C-peptide levels are more strongly associated with disease risk during the first decade or whether there are longer latency effects.

There is variability in the half-life of a biomarker in humans, ranging from a median of 8 to 10 hours for phytoestrogens, phthalates, and organophosphates to 200 hours for metals such as lead and cadmium to 360 hours for 25-hydroxyvitamin D to more than 20,000 hours for dioxins and polychlorinated biphenyls in the blood. Unless there is continuous exposure, the levels detectable in blood will vary over time as a function of the half-life. Half-life of biomarkers varies also as a function of the biospecimen. As such, an understanding of the half-life of biomarkers in different settings is essential to determining which research questions can (and cannot) be answered with the study (Box 36-3).

Sampling and Selection Bias

Study designs commonly used in molecular epidemiology typically use some form of efficient sampling designs (see Chapter 8). Potential study designs and features relevant to molecular epidemiology studies are described below.

Determining the size of the study requires specific considerations. The number of individuals that may be included is limited by costs of biospecimen collection, storage, and laboratory assays. In addition, use of biomarkers in studies, particularly of chronic diseases, may require long periods of participant follow-up and biospecimen storage. Participation in studies that involve collection of biospecimens may also be lower than in other studies, due to issues such as time commitment, the invasiveness or acceptability of the procedure required to collect the biospecimen, or concerns about privacy. Consideration of these factors in the study design can reduce the burden on participants. For example, saliva and urine can be collected by a study participant using written instructions and returned by mail, whereas blood collection typically requires a visit to a trained health professional.[30] Even if collection of biospecimens adds little to no burden to participants, it is important to consider issues of selection bias due to the use of biomarkers. For example, in studies of solid tumors, it is possible that more cancer tissue is available for biomarker studies from participants with larger tumors of advanced stage.[31]

Commonly Used Study Designs

Prospective Cohort Studies. As described in Chapter 7, an advantage of a prospective cohort study design, or studies nested in prospective cohorts, is that it can assure the temporal relationship

BOX 36-3   **Example of Time Integration in Molecular Epidemiology: Environmental Exposure to Lead and Risk of Amyotrophic Lateral Sclerosis**

Lead is ubiquitous in the environment. Lead exposure can occur through lead-based paints, contaminated water, occupational exposures, exhaust from combustion of lead-based gasoline, and other sources. When the body is exposed to lead, 95% of absorbed lead is ultimately sequestered primarily in bone and teeth, leaving little in circulation. Bone lead levels determined through x-ray fluorescence are thought to estimate cumulative lead exposure over an individual's lifetime. Blood lead levels generally indicate current lead exposure, although with aging and other conditions, lead is released from bone to blood. The half-life of lead in blood is 6 to 8 weeks, whereas the half-life in bone is 10 to 30 years. High levels of lead are associated with an increased risk of a number of health conditions. Fang et al.[29] investigated the hypothesis that high blood lead levels were associated with an increased risk of amyotrophic lateral sclerosis (ALS), a neurodegenerative disease. Cases ($N = 184$) were identified through the National Registry of Veterans with ALS, diagnosed between 2003 and 2007 who provided a blood specimen in 2007. Controls ($N = 194$) were sampled from a parallel Veteran's Administration study (GENEVA) and provided a blood sample between 2007 and 2008. The investigators focused on veterans because of their potentially higher exposure to lead in the military setting. Lead levels were measured in blood using mass spectrometry, and the blood lab was blinded to the case-control status. Quality control specimens were included across all batches, and CV% was <5% for almost all of the batches, suggesting excellent reproducibility and minimal batch to batch variation. In multivariable models, a twofold higher blood lead level was associated with a higher risk of ALS (odds ratio, 2.6; 95% CI, 1.9-3.7). The odds ratio was 1.7 (95% CI, 1.2-2.5) after excluding cases diagnosed more than 2 years before the blood collection. There appeared to be little difference between timing between ALS diagnosis and blood lead levels, although all blood specimens were taken after diagnosis. There remained a possibility that results were partially explained by reverse causation, because cases with ALS may have had greater bone turnover from lower physical activity, resulting in a higher release of lead into the blood. However, the investigators were able to address this issue to some extent by additionally measuring biomarkers of bone turnover.

between the exposure and outcome of interest. This advantage is an important consideration in studies of biomarkers, which can reflect different time periods of exposure—from exposure in the previous 24 hours to cumulative lifetime exposure. Cohort studies also have challenges due to the (1) high cost of enrolling a cohort for prospective follow-up; (2) recruitment of a large study population; and (3) possibly lengthy follow-up. Biomarker measurements in cohort studies therefore often employ efficient sampling designs, such as nested case-control studies or case-cohort studies.

The number of epidemiologic cohort studies that integrate collection of biospecimens and measurement of biomarkers has grown rapidly along with emerging technologies (Table 36-5). For example, the UK Biobank is a population-based cohort study of approximately 500,000 men and women across the United Kingdom beginning in 2006 and designed to study many health outcomes. In addition to questionnaire data on lifestyle, environment, and health history, biospecimens including blood and urine were collected to ascertain biomarkers associated with a wide range of cancer, cardiovascular disease, diabetes, and other disease-related biomarkers. An imaging substudy in the UK Biobank aims to collect magnetic resonance imaging scans of vital organs from 100,000 participants for imaging biomarker studies.

Case-Control Studies. Case-control studies are commonly employed in molecular epidemiology research because they are well suited to the study of uncommon diseases. A frequently used variation of this design is the nested case-control study, which requires the existence of an enumerated underlying cohort from which to sample (see Chapter 8). It is important to consider in a given study how the biomarker of interest changes over time and the estimated length of the induction period. A nested case-control design that allows for measurement of biomarkers of exposure before the disease of interest has been diagnosed is generally advantageous over a design that measures

TABLE 36-5

Examples of Epidemiologic Cohort Studies and Tissues or Biospecimens Collected

Cohort	Country	Population	Examples of Tissues or Biospecimens Collected
Melbourne Collaborative Cohort Study	Australia	41,500 people (24,500 women and 17,000 men) between 1990 and 1994 between the ages of 40 and 69	Blood
Breast Cancer Family Registry (BCFR)	United States, Canada, and Australia	Over 30,000 women and men from nearly 12,000 families	DNA (lymphocytes, cell lines, buccal cells), cell lines, plasma, tumor tissue (archived blocks, slides, and tissue microarrays)
Canadian Partnership for Tomorrow Project (CPTP)	Canada	Over 300,000 participants aged 30-74 between 2009 and 2016	Blood, urine, toenail, saliva
Shanghai Men's Health Study (SMHS) and Shanghai Women's Health Study (SWHS)	China	61,500 men between the ages of 40 and 74 between the years of 2001 and 2006; 75,000 Chinese women recruited between 1997 and 2000	Blood, urine, buccal cells
European Prospective Investigation into Cancer and Nutrition (EPIC)	10 Western European countries	520,000 people 20 y of age or older living in 10 European countries between 1993 and 1999	Plasma, serum, leukocytes, and erythrocytes
Atherosclerosis Risk in Communities Cohort-Cancer (ARIC-Ca)	United States	15,792 individuals from Maryland, Minnesota, North Carolina, and Mississippi	Blood, urine
Black Women's Health Study (BWHS)	United States	59,000 Black women aged 21 to 69	Buccal cells
California Teachers Study (CTS)	United States	133,479 California public school teachers, administrators, and other school professionals	Blood, saliva, urine, toenail clippings
Sister Study	United States	50,884 sisters of women who had breast cancer between ages of 35 and 74 enrolled 2003-2009	Whole blood, lymphocytes, plasma, serum, urine, toenail clippings, and household dust collected with alcohol wipes
Southern Community Cohort Study (SCCS)	United States	90,000 residents of southeastern United States aged 40-79 of which over two-thirds are African American	Blood, buccal cells, urine
Women's Health Study (WHS)	United States	39,876 female health professionals enrolled between 1992 and 1995 living in the United States	Blood

(Continued)

TABLE 36-5   (Continued)

Examples of Epidemiologic Cohort Studies and Tissues or Biospecimens Collected

Cohort	Country	Population	Examples of Tissues or Biospecimens Collected
RERF Life Span Study, Adult Health Study, and F1 Cohorts (Hiroshima and Nagasaki)	Japan	Life Span Study: 120,000 people of all ages and sex. 90,000 were exposed to atomic bomb radiation. Adult Health Study: 23,000 individuals, In Utero Study: 3,600 individuals	Blood, urine
Mexican Teacher's Cohort (MTC)	Mexico	115,315 female teachers from 12 state areas in Mexico recruited between 2006 and 2008	Blood, urine
Growing Up Today Study (GUTS) I and II	United States	GUTS I: 16,882 girls and boys aged 9-14 in 1996; GUTS II: 10,923 girls and boys aged 10-17 in 2004	Blood, saliva, semen
Nurses Health Studies I-III	United States	NHS I: 121,000 US female nurses aged 30-55 in 1976; NHS II: 116,430 US nurses aged 25-42 in 1989; NHS III: nurses and nursing students aged 20-46 in the United States and Canada in 2010	Blood, urine, tissue blocks and slides, cheek cells, toenails, mammograms

Also see the Cancer Epidemiology Descriptive Cohort Database (CEDCD) for a searchable list of biospecimens in cancer cohorts: https://cedcd.nci.nih.gov/biospecimen

biomarkers among cases after a diagnosis of the disease. In the setting of a prospective cohort study, the nested case-control design often carries the advantage of prospectively collected questionnaire or interview data on demographic, health, and lifestyle factors. This information may be used to address confounding and to evaluate effect modification.

Matching can be a useful technique at the design stage to improve efficiency in biomarker-related studies. Matching factors should typically be biomarker-related factors that could introduce measurement error and that are not of scientific interest for the study. Such factors may include the time of day and date of sample collection, fasting status, length of time between collection and processing, storage temperature, freeze-thaw cycle, and others.[30] While the causal role of a biomarker may not be entirely clear, care should be taken to avoid matching on potential causal intermediates (overmatching).

As in prospective cohort studies, a nested case-control design can establish the temporal relationship between an exposure and outcome of interest. As noted above, however, biomarker studies are susceptible to reverse causation, and that possibility should ideally be considered in the study design. This may be of particular concern in studies of outcomes with long latency periods or for diseases with a subclinical phase. For example, the potentially bidirectional relationship between type 2 diabetes and pancreatic cancer presents a challenge in studying the etiologic role of diabetes in development of this cancer. Long-term diabetes is associated with an increased risk of pancreatic cancer.[32] However, subclinical pancreatic cancer can disrupt metabolic pathways leading to new onset of diabetes. Use of biomarkers of metabolism, such as glucose and insulin levels, has been important in gaining understanding of the causal mechanisms underlying this complex relationship.[33,34]

Additional advantages of the nested case-control design for molecular epidemiology include its practicality, given that collection and analysis of biospecimens in a full cohort may be infeasible due to cost. Appropriate sampling of cases and controls, for example, from the underlying cohort, allows for measurement of biomarkers in a restricted number of individuals while optimizing power of the study. An example of this in practice is a case-control study nested in the Framingham Heart Study that examined the association between metabolites and risk of type 2 diabetes over 12 years of follow-up.[35] Metabolite profiling was performed using specimens stored for most cohort members in only a subset of individuals who developed diabetes ($N = 188$) and matched controls ($N = 188$). These analyses were therefore much less expensive than had they been assayed in all participants and assaying only a small proportion of biospecimens also allowed conservation of the rare biospecimen resources. Of 70 metabolites studied, 2-aminoadipic acid had the strongest association with risk of diabetes, more than a four-fold elevated risk comparing the highest with the lowest quarter of the population. This case-control design retains its prospective nature, but in a more cost-efficient approach to examining the association.

Case-Cohort Studies. A variant of the case-control design that is especially advantageous in molecular epidemiology is the case-cohort study. As described in Chapter 8, this design enjoys the advantage of efficient sampling common to case-control designs. In addition, it allows for cohort-type analyses by using the subcohort, such as for estimates of prevalence and etiologic analyses where the biomarker is the outcome of interest. It also allows for studying multiple outcomes by adding more than one case series. These advantages simultaneously reduce costs and allow for a more comprehensive characterization of the causes and consequences of the biologic process measured by the biomarker. Considerations particularly relevant for molecular epidemiology have been central to the development of the case-cohort design.[36,37]

An important consideration in case-cohort studies is the potential for differences in timing of biospecimen collection between the cases and controls in the subcohort, depending on whether a case-cohort study is conducted nested in a cohort study or as a stand-alone prospective study. For example, if blood samples are collected among the subcohort at baseline and among cases over a period of several years, there may be differences between cases and controls with regard to sample degradation or other factors related to collection and storage of samples. In some situations, time- and batch-related factors can potentially outweigh the clear advantages of case-cohort studies as compared with case-control studies.[38] Many of these challenges can be addressed through typical assay design and analytical strategies that are generally recommended in biomarker studies (see below). For example, the investigator can randomize the cases and comparators to batches in the design phase if assays are conducted at once after enrollment and sample collection are finished. Moreover, there are analytic approaches to adjust for potential batch effects in the analysis phase. A pilot study is a useful way to identify how such factors may affect the assays used in a particular study.[30] Since subcohort samples can be used as comparators for multiple studies of different disease endpoints, it is also important to anticipate depletion of biospecimen samples over time in the subcohort due to repeated use.[17]

Randomized Controlled Trials. Elements of molecular epidemiology are increasingly integrated in randomized controlled trials (RCTs), particularly those that aim to deliver "precision medicine" treatments. Biomarkers are typically integrated into RCTs by (1) restricting the study population to those with a particular biomarker, (2) randomization to treatments based on a biomarker, (3) using a biomarker as a primary trial endpoint, or (4) using a biomarker for exposure assessment in observational analyses integrated in RCTs. Clinical trials are referred to as "umbrella trials" if biomarkers are used to identify molecular disease subtypes among patients with one disease and then test different targeted treatments according to the molecular subtype.[39] In contrast, "basket trials" use biomarkers to identify one molecular subtype across different diseases and then test the same targeted treatment among patients with the molecular subtype.

A common question asked in RCTs is whether patients have better outcomes on average with the experimental treatment relative to a comparator. Integration of biomarkers in RCTs allows research questions that address effect-measure modification, where biomarkers identify subsets of patients, for example with molecularly different disease subtypes, who are more likely to benefit from the experimental treatment. For example, a biomarker-stratified design may address the question of whether treatment is better for patients who are biomarker-positive than for those who are biomarker-negative.[40] If a biomarker is predictive of treatment response, then efficacy of different treatments in biomarker-defined subgroups may differ. For example, phase 3 randomized-controlled trials have evaluated whether mutations in the *EGFR* gene, encoding for the epidermal growth factor receptor, could be used to guide treatment choice for patients with non–small-cell lung cancer. In some of the trials, patients were stratified based on whether their tumors tested positive for *EGFR* mutations and were then randomized to either an EGFR-targeted therapy or an alternative therapy.

Importantly, confounding, including by post-baseline confounders, must be considered, and all other considerations described for nonexperimental studies apply, such as issues regarding selection bias, measurement error, and sources of variability, as well as substantial costs incurred by integrating of biomarkers. A particular challenge with biomarker studies within RCTs is selection bias in the setting of narrow inclusion criteria, which may select participants with specific biomarker profiles that may in turn be associated with the outcome of interest.

Challenges in Design and Practice of Biomarker Studies

Confounding

As usual in nonexperimental epidemiologic research, it is critically important to consider the role of confounding in molecular epidemiology studies. The interpretation of confounding may depend on the study goal. For example, if the goal of a molecular epidemiology study is to use biomarkers to understand etiology, then accounting for confounders of the biomarker-disease association is essential. Instead, if the goal is to identify prognostic biomarkers, then controlling confounding is less a concern because the focus is to identify biomarkers that most strongly predict the outcome, whether causal or not. An approach to address confounding should be tailored to the specific research question and study setting (Chapter 12).

Measurement Error

Unique aspects of biospecimens and biomarkers in molecular epidemiology studies can result in considerable error leading to spuriously null or non-null results. An error can result from variability across the continuum from biospecimen sample collection, processing, storage, as well as factors that influence the assay conduct. This error often leads to nondifferential misclassification. However, molecular epidemiology studies are not immune from differential misclassification. For example, if all cases are distributed on one assay batch and all controls are on a second, there will be differential measurement error of the biomarkers, which will be a function of the extent of batch-to-batch variation.

There are four broad categories of potential sources of measurement error that should be considered in the design and analysis of biomarkers in molecular epidemiology studies. In addition, the role of heterogeneity in tissue-based studies is discussed. Some of these errors are preventable during the design phase and others may be corrected during data analysis. Pilot studies and validation studies are valuable in identifying sources of error, and potential solutions, before undertaking a larger investigation. Below are specific categories of measurement error specific to biomarker research.

Errors that arise due to variables in biospecimen collection, processing, and storage. Errors in biomarker measurements can arise from factors occurring during the biospecimen collection phase, before an assay being conducted. For example, small delays in the time between blood collection and processing can have big effects on some biomarkers, and little effect on others.[41,42] Delays in fixation after tissue removal can lead to degradation of many phospho-proteins, whereas other proteins remain stable. Fasting status can influence a range of biomarkers. For example, C-peptide, insulin, and free insulin-like growth factor 1 (IGF-1) levels are influenced by the fasting state, while total IGF-1 is not affected.[43] Collecting blood-based samples when fasting may not be uniformly feasible in a large epidemiology or clinical study, but capturing information on time from last meal, as well as other preanalytic variables, will allow for these variables to be integrated into the design and analysis stage of a study.

Sample preservation can affect biomarker quality. The section above on tissue biospecimens describes the effect of formalin fixation on proteins, RNA, and DNA. The reproducibility of some biomarkers may be influenced by the blood preservative, generally heparin or EDTA.[44]

Prospectively collected biobanks are often leveraged decades later. The time in storage or temperature conditions should be considered as a preanalytic variable. Long-term storage of stool samples at $-80°C$ for microbiome had little effect on microbiota composition if the samples were processed quickly after collection.[45] The quality of nucleic acids extracted from tissue specimens was improved when tissue blocks were stored at $-4°C$ versus room temperature, although reproducible RNA transcriptome data can be generated even from tissue blocks stored at room temperature up to 30 years.[14]

The standardization of collection procedures and best practices at the stage of biospecimen collection are essential features to reduce measurement error.[46] Given the range of sensitivity of biomarkers to different preanalytic features, the ultimate goal should be to have a collection protocol that optimizes validity for the greatest number of biomarkers as well as practicality of implementation of the protocol. The success of biospecimen collection can be enhanced with regular trainings with research staff as well as instructional videos demonstrating study staff successfully completing each of the study tasks.

Intra-assay and inter-assay laboratory errors. Laboratory errors can lead to substantial misclassification errors of a biomarker due to assay variability in the laboratory. This variability can arise from both within-batch (intra-assay) and across-batches (inter-assay) issues, resulting potentially in nondifferential and differential misclassification. There are some issues that can be anticipated and prevented, some design features that can help reduce the bias, and analytic strategies to account for the laboratory errors after the fact. Core definitions related to laboratory errors are detailed in the Fundamental Principles section.

Analytic factors can affect the performance of testing procedures, and these should be limited to the extent possible and documented as they arise for consideration in the analysis phase. Examples from early RNA microarray studies found that the temperature and humidity in the laboratory had a substantial effect on reproducibility of transcriptomic biomarkers. Changes in reagent lots, laboratory staff, and machine calibration can lead to inter-assay variability.

Several factors in the design phase can be integrated to reduce these errors. For example, if undertaking a nested case-control study, cases and controls can be run on adjacent wells within a batch and placed in a random order to maintain blinding. The random assignment of cases within batches (*e.g.*, not adjacent wells) and between batches (consider stratified block randomization if small batch size) is helpful to reduce potential laboratory error.

The inclusion of technical replicates within and across batches is essential to evaluate laboratory errors by comparing the concordance of the biomarker on the same sample. Additionally, the inclusion of known quality control measures—for example, samples that have been assayed previously using a "gold standard assay" or that are known positive or negative controls—is also useful to assess potential for measurement error. The blinding of laboratory personnel to disease status or other variables is essential to avoid the potential for the disease state to influence the results or data interpretation.

After the biomarker measurements are completed, calculation of CV% within and across batches will provide information on the reproducibility. Batches with high CV% could be excluded from the study or reassayed. A comparison of biomarker results on quality control specimens with the prior results from a gold standard assay can be useful as a benchmark for biomarker and assay validity. For example, if a positive control sample tests negative on the biomarker assay, this would suggest potentially large misclassification.

Errors due to variability of a biomarker over time within an individual. One way in which molecular epidemiology diverges from genetic epidemiology, in particular the study of germline genetics, is that molecular biomarkers generally change over time and may be affected by a wide range of biological, behavioral, and environmental factors. Depending on the substantive question, these changes can be a form of measurement error, for example, by increasing within-person variability, can be a reflection of confounding, or can even be the phenomenon of interest (*e.g.*, the extent of within-person variation in melatonin levels as a readout of circadian rhythm). The design and approach of a molecular epidemiology study must integrate this knowledge for variability over time to be a variable of interest rather than an error. For example, in the case of melatonin, the ideal biospecimen would be a timed 24-hour urine, which would capture the entire circadian output of melatonin throughout a 24-hour cycle as well as the total volume of urine to determine concentration. If instead melatonin was assayed on untimed spot urines, where each individual provided a sample at different points in the day, considerable measurement error would result. The concept of time as a potential source of measurement error is described in detail earlier in the chapter (page 946).

Errors that arise due to the effect of subclinical or clinical disease on the biomarker. There are numerous examples for which disease or its preclinical manifestation can influence biomarker levels, whether measured in blood, tissue, urines, or other biospecimen. Whether or not such an effect is considered measurement error in a study is a function of the study design and the research question. If the goal is etiology, then the biomarker measured in subclinical disease is different from the causal level of the biomarker. This is not a measurement error per se, but an error due to reverse causation as a form of selection bias. Studies using prospectively banked biospecimens collected years before a disease diagnosis allow the investigator to test whether subclinical disease biases effect estimates by probing if results are sensitive to different lag times between biomarker collection and start of follow-up for the outcome of interest. Moreover, even if subclinical disease is influencing the biomarker levels, this influence may be an asset if the goal of biomarker research is to identify disease earlier than current clinical practice. Similarly, if more aggressive forms of a disease lead to greater alterations of a biomarker at diagnosis, such a relationship may prove useful in developing prognostic biomarkers.

Errors that arise due to tissue heterogeneity. Tissue-based biomarker studies pose an additional layer of potential error due to tissue and biomarker heterogeneity. Pathologists describe tissues as "complex cities," composed of not only the tissue cell of origin but also the surrounding microenvironment, which is layered with immune cells, blood vessels, fibroblasts, and connective tissue. For in situ assays, those performed directly on a tissue section or slide, a pathologist is critical to ensure the biomarker is present (expressed) where it should be and absent where it should not and aid in the quantification of the biomarker of interest. *Ex situ* assays are performed on extracted components of tissue, primarily RNA or DNA, which require the pathologist to dissect tissue for biomarker analysis. Laser capture microdissection provides for precise dissection of the specific tissue area for biomarker analysis. However, it is a time intensive procedure, often prohibitively so in larger studies. Macrodissection involves pathologists first identifying an area of interest for tissue sampling with high homogeneity and then coring or scraping that area for biomarker extraction (*e.g.*, nucleic acids). The validity of the biomarker to assess a specific tissue of interest depends on the degree of contamination, or tissue heterogeneity, with other cell types. At the same time, tissue heterogeneity might sometimes be considered an asset in biomarker studies as it better reflects the complex interactions of cells.

An additional layer of heterogeneity is the variability in tissue markers across a single tissue. As an example, mutation or copy number loss of the tumor suppressor gene *PTEN* is common in many types of cancer. However, tumors including prostate cancer often display intra-tumor heterogeneity, such that *PTEN* loss is found only in a portion of the tumor.[47] Indeed, many tumor types display intra-tumoral heterogeneity for a range of biomarkers. *Ex situ* assays may result in false-negative findings or a misrepresentation of the biomarker profile for a biomarker depending on where the tumor is sampled. One way to reduce such measurement error is to sample multiple areas of tissue to evaluate the possibility of intra-tumoral heterogeneity, even for a subset of cases.

Figure 36-4 provides an overview of potential sources of measurement error in tissue biomarker studies as a function of heterogeneity, sample processing, and the assay itself. Before beginning any tissue-based biomarker evaluation, each stage of potential error should be evaluated with a pilot study as well as consideration of prior studies.

Pilot Studies

Pilot studies are essential to the successful conduct of molecular epidemiologic studies as well as any observational study using biomarkers. Pilot studies should address the broad spectrum of potential sources of error to estimate the potential impact that measurement error would have on the study. The goal should be to reduce measurement error to optimize the validity and reproducibility of the biomarker research. Key considerations when conducting pilot studies were outlined by Tworoger and Hankinson.[30]

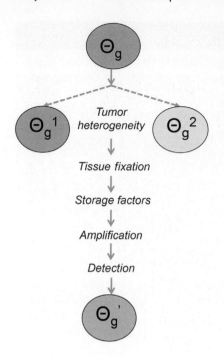

FIGURE 36-4 Potential sources of biomarker measurement error in omics technologies in formalin-fixed, paraffin-embedded tissue. Θ_g is the true value of the biomarker (in this case, g refers to gene expression) and Θ_g' is the measured value. If there is intra-tumoral heterogeneity, then the "true" biomarker value may be more challenging to determine without multiple sampling, as the biomarker values taken from one area of sample tissue (Θ_g^1) may vary from those of another area of tissue (Θ_g^2).

Pilot studies should be conducted for any new biomarker, biospecimen, or assay. They should always be performed with samples from the same study population and biorepository, even if the laboratory or other investigators have previously shown high reproducibility and validity of quantifications using the same biospecimen, biomarker, or assay. As throughout biomarker studies, a close communication with the laboratory is critical when conducting pilot studies. Nevertheless, blinding is a critical component of pilot studies, such that the laboratory needs to be unaware of technical replicates selected by the investigator and of the expected values for quality control samples for which biomarker levels have been determined from a different assay or a different laboratory. Pilot studies need to be conducted early during any study and repeated as necessary until satisfactory performance is achieved. In addition, unless not feasible, such as for tissue specimens, quality control samples should be included in the main study as well to assess for laboratory drift over time and for batch effects. Repeat pilot studies are typically necessary when established assays or biospecimen-related factors such as the mode of specimen collection or preservation change during conduct of a study.

STROBE-ME Recommendations

A key issue in the ultimate translation of biomarkers from molecular epidemiology into public health or clinical practice is reproducibility and replication of findings across studies. To address these issues, a group of epidemiologists, biostatisticians, and laboratory scientists developed recommendations known as *STROBE-ME*: STrengthening Reporting of OBservational studies in Epidemiology-Molecular Epidemiology.[11] The goal was to provide a cohesive set of recommendations and principles for the reporting of molecular epidemiology studies with the purpose of enhancing the quality, validity, and reproducibility of studies. The general considerations set forth by STROBE-ME should be supplemented with and, as appropriate, superseded by subject matter–specific considerations in each study (Box 36-4).

ETHICAL, LEGAL, AND SOCIAL ISSUES

The use of biospecimens in molecular epidemiology research has enormous potential to reduce disease burden and enhance human health. However, it also poses ethical challenges that require

---

BOX 36-4   Examples of Measurement in Biomarkers: COVID-19 and SARS-CoV-2 Virus

The global COVID-19 pandemic caused by infection with the SARS-CoV-2 virus highlighted key issues in molecular epidemiology. Molecular epidemiology–oriented questions concerning COVID-19 included biomarkers of disease susceptibility (*e.g.*, risk factors for SARS-CoV-2 infection), disease outcome (*e.g.*, cancer patients at greater risk of death following COVID-19), and disease progression (*e.g.*, SARS-CoV-2 viral load, a marker of progression). Addressing such questions using biomarkers was necessary to understand prevalence, spread, severity, and many other features of a novel infection. One challenge in this area was selection of the optimal COVID-19 biomarker and establishing what aspects of time course the biomarker captured. If the goal was to study a measure of disease progression, then the optimal biomarker would be the presence of SARS-CoV-2 in nasopharyngeal swabs during the initial phase of infection. Such an approach would have required widespread testing of asymptomatic individuals in order to avoid potential selection bias by focusing only on individuals showing COVID-19 symptoms. If instead the goal was to study susceptibility, serologic detection of past infection would be assessed by the presence of IgM or IgG antibodies in blood samples. Each biomarker approach was susceptible to measurement error. While detecting SARS-CoV-2 using nucleic acid testing is highly specific (*i.e.*, the rate of false positives is very low), false negatives occurred due to insufficient sampling of the nasopharynx or if the sampling was done too early in the disease course. With serologic testing, false positives can occur if the antibodies detected in the assay cross-react with antibodies to other coronaviruses. Even if the specificity of the assay was high, the resulting number of false positives could be substantial if the overall prevalence of infection in the population was low. These factors and others illustrate the critical role of molecular epidemiology in understanding pandemics such as that of COVID-19 and in informing public health decision-making.

---

consideration by researchers and their institutions, funding agencies, and the larger public. Fortunately, many of these issues can be anticipated and ways to address them integrated into the design and execution of molecular epidemiology investigations. While molecular epidemiology faces many of the same ethical issues as other scientific disciplines, this section focuses on issues relevant to the use of biospecimens and biomarkers in particular.

One such challenge is the protection of the privacy and confidentiality of individuals who provide biological samples used in research. In the United States, privacy in scientific research is governed by the Common Rule and the Privacy Rule of HIPAA.[48] In the European Union, privacy is overseen by the 2018 General Data Protection Regulation. Risk of loss of privacy and confidentiality is particularly relevant to biospecimen research because human-derived materials may inherently contain individual-identifying information or result in identifiability when combined with other data.[49,50] For example, since each person's genetic sequence is unique, genetic information has potential to identify an individual or family. DNA sequencing of tumors excised from cancer patients also has this issue. While linkage of biological samples to other information, such as demographic or medical history, can enhance research, there is an accompanying trade-off of added risk to the participant. For these reasons, ethical review boards at research institutions are tasked with careful review of proposed studies that involve biospecimen collection to ensure that appropriate procedures are in place to obtain informed consent, secure storage of specimens and data, and communication of relevant results and findings to participants and the larger public.

A related issue is that results from molecular epidemiology studies may translate into the development of intellectual property and patent applications. The informed consent process for biomarker research should include information about intellectual property.

Increasingly, samples are placed for long-term storage in biorepositories for future use. This storage requires researchers to anticipate and establish protections to mitigate future risk, which is a challenge in the context of rapidly developing technology. The process of informed consent is central to meeting ethical obligations to participants. Key issues to address in the informed consent process include how data will be used, who will have access to the data, and whether or not a participant will be notified of any results related to analysis of their biological material.[51] The latter point is important given the growing role molecular epidemiology plays in the discovery of biomarkers that are actionable in the treatment setting, such as tumor biomarkers that could affect a cancer patient's optimal treatment or family members' future risk.[48] Indeed, it is imperative that the informed consent process can anticipate not only what researchers propose today but also how the samples might be used in the future as new assay technologies develop and as partnerships between academia and biotechnology companies become more common. Although rare, legal controversy over consent to use biological specimens can result in destruction of samples, as exemplified by the destruction of five million blood samples at a Texas biobank following a 2009 lawsuit.[52]

Ethical and social concerns also include responsibilities to communicate findings to, and share data with, the public. For certain types of research, this sharing may be required by the funding agency, and increasingly molecular epidemiologists are drawn to share research findings and original data with the broader research community. In 2014, the NIH established the Genomic Data Sharing Policy to promote sharing of genomic data resulting from NIH-funded research. Part of the impetus was the recognition that genomic data are expensive to collect, so unlikely to be generated without public support in multiple large studies. These resources should therefore be available to researchers outside of the group that generated them. A primary consideration of data sharing efforts is the importance of maintaining confidentiality of data deposited in the registries. Two benefits to data sharing are to optimize statistical power of molecular epidemiology studies and to provide opportunities for validation of epidemiologic findings in additional cohorts. Table 36-6 highlights several of the resources that exist to enable researchers to access publicly available data for molecular epidemiology studies.

NEW DIRECTIONS IN MOLECULAR EPIDEMIOLOGY

Classic molecular epidemiology studies typically focus on unidimensional biomarkers, such as a single protein biomarker measured in a large number of study participants after a validation study for the assay has been conducted. Biomarkers are chosen such that prior knowledge exists on the mechanisms that influence the biomarker and on the performance of the assay used to quantify the biomarker. This integration of biomarker-specific prior knowledge has contributed to inferential validity in molecular epidemiology studies. In contrast, omics studies typically assess several hundreds to thousands of biomarkers at once using methods such as microarrays, sequencing techniques, or mass spectrometry. The promise of these technological advances is that such large collections of biomarkers may provide a more granular assessment of the biological state of interest. In addition, these efforts allow for "discovery" of new biomarkers that may not have been identified by assessing single markers at a time. Moreover, such omics approaches allow for assessing biomarkers in combination or as a pathway, which may hold greater information.

The advent of omic technologies also poses a significant challenge, because the high dimensionality of the biomarker measurements makes it more difficult to assess threats to validity. For better interpretability, inferences are typically not drawn on a per-biomarker level, but often involve data-driven summarizations such as clustering. Clustering itself may be susceptible to analytical issues in typical datasets.[53] Even before such final steps of summarization, data preprocessing often involves multiple "hidden" steps of statistical inference. For example, DNA sequencing studies of tumor tissue may only report a DNA mutation as present in a tumor sample if mutations at the same DNA position have a statistically significant higher prevalence than a certain threshold in a reference database of nontumor DNA sequences.

High-dimensional omics biomarkers would be oversimplified if thought of as many measurements of identical biomarkers, since individual elements of the omic may be influenced differently by threats to validity. For example, in an etiologic study assessing the plasma metabolome as a disease risk factor, certain classes of metabolites may not be measurable reliably in samples stored or preprocessed differently, potentially leading to exclusion of participants with certain characteristics from analyses of metabolite classes (selection bias); batch effects may affect certain metabolites more strongly than others (measurement error); upstream causal factors, such as physical activity, may specifically alter some metabolite levels (confounding); and preclinical disease may alter some but not all metabolite classes (reverse causation).[44,54,55]

TABLE 36-6

Publicly Available Resources of Biomarker Data for Molecular Epidemiology

Resource	Description	Website
The Cancer Genome Atlas (TCGA); Pan-Cancer Atlas	Cancer genomics project that profiled 20,000 tumors from 33 cancer types. Available biomarker data include transcriptomic, copy number alterations, DNA mutations, proteomics, and histology	https://portal.gdc.cancer.gov/
cBioPortal	Cancer genomics portal that brings together a broad array of tumor profiling studies across tumor types, including TCGA. Data visualization as well as access to original data.	https://www.cbioportal.org/
UK Biobank	Cohort of 500,000 individuals from the UK. Diverse biomarkers measured in blood and urine including germline genetics, sex hormones, renal markers, growth factors; imaging data and other biomarkers in process	http://www.ukbiobank.ac.uk/
All of Us	Aiming to recruit 1 million US participants and develop biorepository of blood, urine, and saliva linked with clinical and lifestyle data	https://allofus.nih.gov/about
ENCODE	Database of functional elements of human genome including RNA, protein, ChIP-Seq	https://genome.ucsc.edu/ENCODE/
Gene Expression Omnibus (GEO)	NIH repository for depositing microarray- and sequencing-based gene expression and functional genomics data, together with associated clinical data	https://www.ncbi.nlm.nih.gov/geo/
Genotype-Tissue Expression (GTex)	Detailed genomic data generated on 1,000 individuals across 54 nondiseased tissues including whole genome sequencing, whole exome sequencing, RNA-sequencing, as well as histology images	https://gtexportal.org/home/
NHANES	Program of studies in nationally representative samples of US adults and children with interviews, physical exams, and blood- and urine-based biomarker data	https://www.cdc.gov/nchs/nhanes/index.htm

A blurring of boundaries between genetic and molecular epidemiology has resulted from high-dimensional, high-resolution studies of the genome. The germline genetic makeup of an individual is static by definition, and DNA from blood cells has typically been regarded as a measure of germline DNA, regardless of when a blood sample was obtained during a lifetime. However, at least a fraction of blood cells undergoes somatic DNA changes during a lifetime.[56] Detectable with DNA sequencing techniques from the early 2010s, such DNA alterations, for example, termed chromosomal mosaicism and clonal hematopoiesis, occur in a sizable proportion of the population. These DNA alterations are strongly associated with age at biospecimen collection and other exposures such as cigarette smoking. Further connections between these genetic alterations with human disease and as a biomarker of the aging process will need to be made. Taken another way, some DNA biomarkers should be viewed through a lens of molecular epidemiology in addition to aspects of genetic epidemiology.

Some new types of biomarkers are gaining prominence. Wearable sensors are used to obtain biomarker data and are being integrated into epidemiology studies. With these approaches, data on exposures (*e.g.*, physical activity) and disease precursors (*e.g.*, heart rhythm) can be captured at an unprecedented level of detail in terms of temporal and spatial resolution. An additional area of innovation is imaging-based biomarkers, such as mammogram texture features[57] or photographs of the eye fundus.[58] The development of these imaging-based biomarkers is occurring in parallel to advances in machine-learning techniques often used to analyze them.

New derivatives of biospecimens are also emerging. For example, extracellular vesicles are a family of vesicles that are commonly excreted by different cell types and can be found commonly in blood and urine samples. Exosomes are a subset of extracellular vesicles that are excreted from cells by endocytosis, contain nucleic acids, proteins, and lipids from the originating cells, and thus can be leveraged to measure cellular biomarkers. In cancer, blood-based exosomes are being explored to assess tumor biomarkers of aggressiveness. In cardiovascular disease, the study of exosomes holds promise as a potential early diagnosis biomarker.

With the ubiquitous use of biomarkers for screening, diagnosis, prognosis, and treatment selection in clinical medicine, the number of observational studies using biomarkers is growing rapidly. Many of these studies are conducted in hospital-based populations, in patients already diagnosed with a specific disease, or are exploring within-person variability such as that due to intratumoral heterogeneity. Biomarkers are also incorporated into prevention studies in an attempt of precision prevention to identify subsets of the population who would potentially benefit most from a lifestyle, chemoprevention, or other prevention strategy.[59]

Many biomarker studies have little to no expertise in epidemiology as part of the study team, even though considerations of molecular epidemiology principles are critical in all biomarker studies. Diverse and transdisciplinary teams bring complementary expertise needed to tackle biomarker research. Molecular epidemiology studies should rely on team science approaches to maximize the ultimate impact of this type of research.

References

1. Kilbourne ED. The molecular epidemiology of influenza. *J Infect Dis*. 1973;127:478-487.
2. Kannel WB, Dawber TR, Friedman GD, Glennon WE, McNamara PM. Risk factors in coronary heart disease. An evaluation of several serum lipids as predictors of coronary heart disease; the Framingham study. *Ann Intern Med*. 1964;61:888-899.
3. Goldstein JL, Brown MS. A century of cholesterol and coronaries: from plaques to genes to statins. *Cell*. 2015;161:161-172.
4. Perera FP, Weinstein IB. Molecular epidemiology and carcinogen-DNA adduct detection: new approaches to studies of human cancer causation. *J Chronic Dis*. 1982;35:581-600.
5. Biomarkers Definitions Working Group. Biomarkers and surrogate endpoints: preferred definitions and conceptual framework. *Clin Pharmacol Ther*. 2001;69:89-95.
6. World Health Organization. *Biomarkers in Risk Assessment: Validity and Validation*. 2001. Available at http://www.inchem.org/documents/ehc/ehc/ehc222.htm.
7. National Cancer Institute. *NCI Best Practices for Biospecimen Resources*. Bethesda, MD: National Institutes of Health; 2016. Available at https://biospecimens.cancer.gov/bestpractices/index.asp.
8. Tareke E, Rydberg P, Karlsson P, Eriksson S, Tornqvist M. Analysis of acrylamide, a carcinogen formed in heated foodstuffs. *J Agric Food Chem*. 2002;50:4998-5006.
9. IARC. *Monographs on the Evaluation of Carcinogen Risk to Humans: Some Industrial Chemicals*. Lyon, France: International Agency for Research on Cancer; 1994.
10. Wilson KM, Vesper HW, Tocco P, et al. Validation of a food frequency questionnaire measurement of dietary acrylamide intake using hemoglobin adducts of acrylamide and glycidamide. *Cancer Causes Control*. 2009;20:269-278.
11. Gallo V, Egger M, McCormack V, et al. STrengthening the reporting of OBservational studies in epidemiology--molecular epidemiology (STROBE-ME): an extension of the STROBE statement. *PLoS Med*. 2011;8:e1001117.
12. Harpole M, Davis J, Espina V. Current state of the art for enhancing urine biomarker discovery. *Expert Rev Proteomics*. 2016;13:609-626.
13. Ylitalo N, Sorensen P, Josefsson AM, et al. Consistent high viral load of human papillomavirus 16 and risk of cervical carcinoma in situ: a nested case-control study. *Lancet*. 2000;355:2194-2198.
14. Tyekucheva S, Martin NE, Stack EC, et al. Comparing platforms for messenger RNA expression profiling of archival formalin-fixed, paraffin-embedded tissues. *J Mol Diagn*. 2015;17:374-381.
15. He K. Trace elements in nails as biomarkers in clinical research. *Eur J Clin Invest*. 2011;41:98-102.
16. Al-Delaimy WK, Mahoney GN, Speizer FE, Willett WC. Toenail nicotine levels as a biomarker of tobacco smoke exposure. *Cancer Epidemiol Biomarkers Prev*. 2002;11:1400-1404.
17. Rothman N, Hainaut P, Schulte P, Smith M, Boffetta P, Perera F. *Molecular Epidemiology: Principles and Practices*. Lyon, France: International Agency for Research on Cancer; 2011.
18. Benowitz NL. Biomarkers of environmental tobacco smoke exposure. *Environ Health Perspect*. 1999;107(suppl 2):349-355.

19. Tabung FK, Wang W, Fung TT, et al. Development and validation of empirical indices to assess the insulinaemic potential of diet and lifestyle. *Br J Nutr*. 2016;16:1787-1798.

20. Garcia-Saenz A, Sanchez de Miguel A, Espinosa A, et al. Evaluating the association between artificial light-at-night exposure and breast and prostate cancer risk in Spain (MCC-Spain study). *Environ Health Perspect*. 2018;126:047011.

21. Zuurbier LA, Luik AI, Hofman A, Franco OH, Van Someren EJ, Tiemeier H. Fragmentation and stability of circadian activity rhythms predict mortality: the Rotterdam study. *Am J Epidemiol*. 2015;181:54-63.

22. James P, Bertrand KA, Hart JE, Schernhammer ES, Tamimi RM, Laden F. Outdoor light at night and breast cancer incidence in the nurses' health study II. *Environ Health Perspect*. 2017;125:087010.

23. Greenland P, LaBree L, Azen SP, Doherty TM, Detrano RC. Coronary artery calcium score combined with Framingham score for risk prediction in asymptomatic individuals. *J Am Med Assoc*. 2004;291:210-215.

24. Jaffe AS, Babuin L, Apple FS. Biomarkers in acute cardiac disease: the present and the future. *J Am Coll Cardiol*. 2006;48:1-11.

25. Tamoxifen for early breast cancer: an overview of the randomised trials. Early Breast Cancer Trialists' Collaborative Group. *Lancet*. 1998;351:1451-1467.

26. Barnard ME, Boeke CE, Tamimi RM. Established breast cancer risk factors and risk of intrinsic tumor subtypes. *Biochim Biophys Acta*. 2015;1856(1):73-85.

27. Ballman KV. Biomarker: predictive or prognostic? *J Clin Oncol*. 2015;33:3968-3971.

28. Qian GS, Ross RK, Yu MC, et al. A follow-up study of urinary markers of aflatoxin exposure and liver cancer risk in Shanghai, People's Republic of China. *Cancer Epidemiol Biomarkers Prev*. 1994;3:3-10.

29. Fang F, Kwee LC, Allen KD, et al. Association between blood lead and the risk of amyotrophic lateral sclerosis. *Am J Epidemiol*. 2010;171:1126-1133.

30. Tworoger SS, Hankinson SE. Use of biomarkers in epidemiologic studies: minimizing the influence of measurement error in the study design and analysis. *Cancer Causes Control*. 2006;17:889-899.

31. Liu L, Nevo D, Nishihara R, et al. Utility of inverse probability weighting in molecular pathological epidemiology. *Eur J Epidemiol*. 2018;33:381-392.

32. Huxley R, Ansary-Moghaddam A, Berrington de Gonzalez A, Barzi F, Woodward M. Type-II diabetes and pancreatic cancer: a meta-analysis of 36 studies. *Br J Cancer*. 2005;92:2076-2083.

33. Gapstur SM, Gann PH, Lowe W, Liu K, Colangelo L, Dyer A. Abnormal glucose metabolism and pancreatic cancer mortality. *J Am Med Assoc*. 2000;283:2552-2558.

34. Li D. Diabetes and pancreatic cancer. *Mol Carcinog*. 2012;51:64-74.

35. Wang TJ, Ngo D, Psychogios N, et al. 2-Aminoadipic acid is a biomarker for diabetes risk. *J Clin Invest*. 2013;123:4309-4317.

36. Prentice RL, Self SG. Aspects of the use of relative risk models in the design and analysis of cohort studies and prevention trials. *Stat Med*. 1988;7:275-287.

37. Wacholder S. Practical considerations in choosing between the case-cohort and nested case-control designs. *Epidemiology*. 1991;2:155-158.

38. Rundle AG, Vineis P, Ahsan H. Design options for molecular epidemiology research within cohort studies. *Cancer Epidemiol Biomarkers Prev*. 2005;14:1899-1907.

39. Woodcock J, LaVange LM. Master protocols to study multiple therapies, multiple diseases, or both. *N Engl J Med*. 2017;377:62-70.

40. Freidlin B, McShane LM, Korn EL. Randomized clinical trials with biomarkers: design issues. *J Natl Cancer Inst*. 2010;102:152-160.

41. Jones ME, Folkerd EJ, Doody DA, et al. Effect of delays in processing blood samples on measured endogenous plasma sex hormone levels in women. *Cancer Epidemiol Biomarkers Prev*. 2007;16:1136-1139.

42. Murphy JM, Browne RW, Hill L, et al. Effects of transportation and delay in processing on the stability of nutritional and metabolic biomarkers. *Nutr Cancer*. 2000;37:155-160.

43. Murphy N, Falk RT, Messinger DB, et al. Influence of fasting status and sample preparation on metabolic biomarker measurements in postmenopausal women. *PLoS One*. 2016;11:e0167832.

44. Townsend MK, Clish CB, Kraft P, et al. Reproducibility of metabolomic profiles among men and women in 2 large cohort studies. *Clin Chem*. 2013;59:1657-1667.

45. Tap J, Cools-Portier S, Pavan S, et al. Effects of the long-term storage of human fecal microbiota samples collected in RNAlater. *Sci Rep*. 2019;9:601.

46. White E. *Measurement error in biomarkers: sources, assessment, and impact on studies*. In: *Molecular Epidemiology: Principals and Practices*. Lyon, France: International Agency for Research on Cancer; 2011.

47. Ahearn TU, Pettersson A, Ebot EM, et al. A prospective investigation of PTEN loss and ERG expression in lethal prostate cancer. *J Natl Cancer Inst*. 2016;108(2):djv346.

48. Schulte P, Smith A. Ethical issues in molecular epidemiologic research. In: Rothman N, Hainaut P, Schulte P, Smith M, Boffetta P, Perera F eds, *Molecular Epidemiology: Principal and Practices* Lyon, France: International Agency for Research in Cancer; 2011:chap 2.

49. Cambon-Thomsen A, Rial-Sebbag E, Knoppers BM. Trends in ethical and legal frameworks for the use of human biobanks. *Eur Respir J*. 2007;30:373-382.

50. Colditz GA. Constraints on data sharing: experience from the nurses' health study. *Epidemiology*. 2009;20:169-171.

51. Chin WW, Wieschowski S, Prokein J, Illig T, Strech D. Ethics reporting in biospecimen and genetic research: current practice and suggestions for changes. *PLoS Biol*. 2016;14:e1002521.

52. Beleno v Texas Department of State Health Services Case 5:2009cv00188. U.S. District Court for the Western District of Texas in San Antonio, March 3, 2009.

53. Lusa L, McShane LM, Reid JF, et al. Challenges in projecting clustering results across gene expression-profiling datasets. *J Natl Cancer Inst*. 2007;99:1715-1723.

54. Ding M, Zeleznik OA, Guasch-Ferre M, et al. Metabolome-wide association study of the relationship between habitual physical activity and plasma metabolite levels. *Am J Epidemiol*. 2019;188:1932-1943.

55. Mayers JR, Wu C, Clish CB, et al. Elevation of circulating branched-chain amino acids is an early event in human pancreatic adenocarcinoma development. *Nat Med*. 2014;20:1193-1198.

56. Machiela MJ, Chanock SJ. The ageing genome, clonal mosaicism and chronic disease. *Curr Opin Genet Dev*. 2017;42:8-13.

57. Manduca A, Carston MJ, Heine JJ, et al. Texture features from mammographic images and risk of breast cancer. *Cancer Epidemiol Biomarkers Prev*. 2009;18:837-845.

58. Gulshan V, Peng L, Coram M, et al. Development and validation of a deep learning algorithm for detection of diabetic retinopathy in retinal fundus photographs. *J Am Med Assoc*. 2016;316:2402-2410.

59. Rebbeck TR, Burns-White K, Chan AT, et al. Precision prevention and early detection of cancer: fundamental principles. *Cancer Discov*. 2018;8(7):803-811.

CHAPTER 37

Genetic Epidemiology

John S. Witte and Duncan C. Thomas

INTRODUCTION

Genetic epidemiology marries the fields of human genetics and epidemiology. It covers detection of the genetic origin of phenotypic variability in humans,[1] inquiry into the genetic components that contribute to the development or progression of diseases or traits, and evaluation of environmental or other risk factors that may modify the effects of genetic factors.

The first reference to the term "genetic epidemiology" was in a 1954 textbook,[2] but it was not until the founding of the International Genetic Epidemiology Society in 1983 that the term came to be widely used. In an editorial accompanying the inaugural issue of the society's official journal, Rao wrote[3]:

> Genetic epidemiology differs from epidemiology by its explicit consideration of genetic factors and family resemblance; it differs from population genetics by its focus on disease; it also differs from medical genetics by its emphasis on population aspects.

Rao's is just one interpretation of the term "genetic epidemiology." In a second editorial, Neel[4] commented on genetic epidemiology investigating the multifactorial nature of many chronic diseases and highlighted a concern about environmental mutagens. Later, Thomas[5] summarized three distinguishing characteristics of the field: a focus on population-based research; joint consideration of genes and the environment; and incorporation of biological processes into its conceptual models. Only by large-scale appraisal of genetics, environment, and their interaction can a full understanding of the etiology of complex traits be achieved.

Genetic epidemiology is closely related to molecular epidemiology (see Chapter 36), but the former has historically focused on germline and somatic genetic factors, while the latter has focused on cellular and molecular biomarkers.[6] This distinction has become increasingly blurred as both fields have transitioned into an era of *integrative genomics*. Investigators are using a range of measurements (*e.g.*, epigenetics, transcription, metabolism, protein synthesis) to understand complex pathways involving both genetic and environmental exposures. Emerging high-volume and high-density omics technologies, as discussed later, have made these evaluations possible.

Genetic epidemiology research relied heavily on the development of novel statistical methods and has been critical to our understanding of human diseases. Most early successes involved the discovery of single genes that caused rare Mendelian disorders such as cystic fibrosis[7] and Huntington disease.[8] Even these seemingly simple etiologies were soon recognized as more complex, however, with the discovery of multiple mutations within causal genes[9] and modifier genes affecting severity.[10] It has become clear that many diseases and traits are complex—such as cancer or height—in that they are attributable to a large number of genetic variants, each with a small effect on risk.[11] Deciphering the genetic basis of such polygenic[12,13]—or even *omnigenic*[14]—traits may require very large populations and novel analytic approaches.[15]

The incorporation of environmental factors into studies of genetics has been slower-moving. While some complex diseases have long been recognized as having both environmental and familial components, our understanding of their interaction is only in its infancy. Early insights in breast cancer, for example, include the potential interaction of cigarette smoking with the *NAT2* gene[16] and of ionizing radiation with the *ATM* gene.[17] However, a full understanding of how genes and environment affect breast cancer remains elusive.[18] While genetic epidemiology has detected many important associations between genetic variants and a broad range of diseases and traits, much more remains to be understood.

METHODOLOGIES AND CHALLENGES IN GENETIC EPIDEMIOLOGY

Fundamental Principles

An understanding of key terminology is fundamental to comprehension of genetic epidemiology studies. It is also critical to appreciate the basic principles of the transmission of genetic information to later generations and across populations. In addressing these fundamental concepts, we emphasize binary disease traits (*e.g.*, cancer) for simplicity, but the general principles are equally applicable to continuous quantitative traits (*e.g.* blood pressure) with appropriate model specification.

General Terminology

The *genome* can be defined as the complete collection of an individual's genetic material. It consists of *chromosomes*, which are long strands of deoxyribonucleic acid (DNA) present in most cells. The human genome is *diploid*, whereby chromosomes are paired. Every human cell contains 22 *autosomal* pairs (which are *homologous*) and one pair of sex chromosomes (X and Y). During *meiosis*, a diploid chromosome set is reduced to a *haploid* chromosome set of a germ cell, the *gamete*.

A *gene* is a piece of a chromosome that codes for a function. Regions that encompass genes (~1%-2% of the genome) and nongenes (~98%-99% of the genome) can have important effects on disease. A *locus* is a position along the chromosome that denotes the location of a *genetic marker*. For simplicity's sake, we refer to any piece of DNA as a marker, whether it is in a genic or nongenic region. Regions in the genome exhibiting variation across individuals are said to contain *variants*, the different versions of which are called *alleles*. The smallest variant is a *single nucleotide polymorphism* (SNP), or if rare, called a *single nucleotide variant* (SNV). Each pair of autosomal chromosomes contains the same markers, with possibly different alleles, at the same locations. The pair of an individual's alleles at a marker is called a *genotype*. If the alleles are identical, the individual is called *homozygous* at the marker; otherwise the individual is called *heterozygous*. When considering several loci simultaneously, the multilocus alleles inherited from the same parent constitute a *haplotype*.

Genetic Transmission

Genetic information is transmitted from each generation to the next according to the fundamental laws of Mendelian inheritance. One copy of each pair of chromosomes is randomly transmitted from each parent's respective gametes (sperm or ova), which upon fertilization form a complete genotype.

Segments that have identical DNA sequences in two or more individuals are called *identical by state (IBS)*. Such segments are considered to be *identical by descent (IBD)* if the individuals inherited them from a common ancestor without recombination. *IBS* segments can alternatively result from the same mutation arising multiple times in the past. Any two individuals can share 0, 1, or 2 alleles IBD with probabilities that depend upon their familial relationship. For example, full siblings have IBD probabilities equal to ¼, ½, and ¼ for sharing 0, 1, or 2 alleles, respectively. In contrast, parent-offspring pairs always share exactly one allele IBD. The selection of which allele is transmitted from a parent to his or her offspring is purely random; this phenomenon is termed Mendel's *law of segregation*.

The relationship between a genotype and disease is termed *penetrance* and defined by Mendel's *law of dominance*. If only one of the two alleles determines the phenotype, that allele is called *dominant* and the other *recessive*. If both alleles have an effect on disease risk, inheritance is said to be *codominant*, and when the effect of two different alleles on disease is midway between the effect of homozygotes for either of the two alleles, inheritance is said to be *additive*.

Markers on separate chromosomes or located far apart on the same chromosome segregate independently; this is Mendel's *law of independent assortment*. However, markers located nearby on the same chromosome may be transmitted together, a process known as *genetic linkage*, with a probability that depends upon the distance between them (the *recombination fraction, θ*). This phenomenon underlies linkage analysis, a method for mapping disease genes by studying the cosegregation of the disease with markers in families.

Linkage Disequilibrium

Markers far apart or on different chromosomes will generally be independently distributed in a homogeneous population, a situation known as *linkage equilibrium*. Associations at neighboring loci, known as *linkage disequilibrium* (LD)[19,20] can arise when new mutations appear or populations with differing allele frequencies mix. Such associations among alleles will gradually decay over generations at a rate that depends upon the physical distance between loci and underlies the most widely used approach to mapping disease genes: association studies. LD can result in associations between marker alleles and alleles of a causal variant, such that certain marker alleles will be present more often in affected individuals than in a random sample of individuals from the population. Thus, one can estimate the association between specific alleles and disease status; when an association is observed, the locus may be causal, or more likely be in LD with a putative disease locus. Another important mechanism for the appearance of LD at unlinked loci, even on different chromosomes, is *population stratification*, which can lead to spurious associations (discussed further later).

Investigating the Potential Genetic Basis of Disease

Familial Aggregation and Recurrence Risks

Often the first step to investigating a possible genetic etiology of a disease is establishing whether it "runs in the family" (*familial aggregation*). Clustering within families suggests genetic and/or shared environmental risk factors for a disease. A simple evaluation of aggregation may entail a standard case-control comparison of family history of a disease. Based on such a design, it can be determined whether cases are more likely than controls to have one or more close relatives affected. There are many ways to define family history and more sophisticated tests to assess familial aggregation. Some permit calculation of the recurrence risk of disease, the ratio of the risk for an individual with an affected relative to the baseline risk of disease in the general population. Recurrence risks are most commonly calculated for siblings, with larger values supporting a genetic basis for disease. However, familial aggregation and increased recurrence risks do not themselves indicate a genetic etiology, as they could be due in part to sharing of environmental factors for disease.

Twin Studies and Heritability

The study of twins also permits evaluation of genetic involvement in disease. If a disease occurs more often among both identical (*monozygotic*, MZ) twins than both fraternal (*dizygotic*, DZ) twins or siblings, then genetics likely play a role (assuming environmental factors are shared equally by MZ and DZ pairs). One can calculate *narrow sense heritability*, which is the proportion of phenotypic variance attributable to additive genetic effects (excluding dominance, epistasis, and gene-environment interactions). A classic example is a study of 4,840 male twin pairs tracked by the Swedish Twin Registry and Swedish Cancer Registry.[21] The authors observed 458 occurrences of prostate cancer. Sixteen MZ but only six DZ twin pairs were concordant for prostate cancer, yielding proband concordance rates of 0.192 and 0.043, respectively, suggesting that genetics may play a substantial role in the development of the disease. In a similar study of Finnish twins, 12,941 same-sexed twin pairs were investigated for the incidence of primary cancers. Based on 1,613 malignant neoplasms, the authors found that the cotwins of MZ twins with cancer had a 50% greater risk of developing cancer themselves than dizygotic cotwins.[22] Nevertheless, a subsequent, much larger study of 44,768 of Swedish, Danish, and Finnish twins[23,24] concluded that environmental factors may have a larger effect on most cancer sites than germline genetics.

In addition to estimating heritability, twin studies can be used in other ways. Comparison of twins reared apart versus twins reared together allows one to estimate both genetic and shared environmental effects, thereby overcoming one of the most important challenges to the classical twin design.[25] MZ twin pairs discordant for disease can also be viewed as genetically matched pairs for study of environmental risk factors and also provides a different perspective on risk factors by asking each about both their own and their cotwin's histories.[26] For disease-discordant twins, one might compare the case-spouse to the cotwin-spouse. Shared environmental factors can be compared between disease-concordant and discordant twin pairs, treating the pair as the unit of observation: factors that are more common among concordant pairs would be interpreted as risk factors, while differences in relative risks between MZ and DZ pairs would be evidence of an interaction effect. Twin-family[27] and cotwin-control[28] designs allow one to study even more complex hypotheses.

Segregation Analysis

Segregation analysis also does not require DNA from study subjects as it is aimed at determining the mode of inheritance for a disease. It seeks to establish the potential genetic basis of disease, whether a single or multiple loci are involved in disease, and whether they act in a dominant, recessive, or codominant fashion. Segregation analysis also estimates allele frequencies and penetrances by fitting parametric models to familial phenotype data using maximum likelihood.

To establish a genetic etiology with segregation analysis, one tests the various Mendelian inheritance models against a more general alternative that might mimic environmental transmission, such as the *ousiotype* model in which risk also clusters into three categories like genotypes, but their probabilities are independent across generations.[29] A challenge to segregation analysis of disease traits (and particularly rare diseases) is that families are not generally randomly sampled from the population. More often, they are ascertained through one or more affected *probands*. One must account for this ascertainment through a likelihood calculation that conditions on family selection. This requires that families be ascertained according to a well-defined statistical sampling scheme, which may not be possible when families are derived from genetic counseling clinics, for example.

In addition to testing the major gene inheritance models, segregation analysis generally tests for *polygenic* models. Here, the disease is assumed to be caused by many genes, each of which has small effects, so one can assume that their aggregate effect is normally distributed in the population. Then each individual's polygene has an expectation midway between that of the two parents and a variance half that of the population variance. To compare major gene and polygenic models, both are nested within the general mixed model that includes both.

Linkage Analysis

Given evidence of a genetic basis of a disease, the location of the relevant genes may be sought using linkage analysis. This approach searches for genetic markers that are transmitted through families in a manner closely paralleling the transmission of the disease. The approach requires DNA from affected pairs of relatives or extended pedigrees and relies on the phenomenon of chromosomal recombination.

Parametric linkage models require specification of a genetic inheritance model (allele frequencies and penetrances), often obtained from a prior segregation analysis. These models use likelihoods that involve two loci, the marker locus and an unobserved disease locus, separated by a recombination fraction θ that will be estimated. To avoid the difficulties of ascertainment correction (since heavily loaded pedigrees with many diseased individuals are generally used), a conditional likelihood is formed for the probability of the marker data given the phenotype data; conditioning on the phenotypes renders the method of ascertainment irrelevant. The results from such models are given in terms of the *lod score*, which provides evidence in support of or against linkage. In the latter case, the region around the marker locus might be excluded from further consideration as containing a causal variant.

Nonparametric or model-free linkage analysis uses affected pairs of relatives, generally sibling pairs. It does not require specification of a genetic inheritance model or extensive likelihood calculations. Instead, one searches for markers that are shared by affected pairs IBD more frequently than expected by chance. Sibling pairs, as noted earlier, are expected to share 50% of their alleles IBD, so a greater percentage would be evidence of linkage. One can apply a test of the 50% value and estimate the actual sharing using simple methods for proportions, but the approach does not provide an estimate of the recombination fraction.

The heyday of linkage analysis was the last two decades of the 20th century, when dense panels of hundreds of highly polymorphic multiallelic markers became available that made scans across the genome possible. Once a region was identified as possibly containing a disease-causing genetic variant, additional flanking markers would be tested and *multipoint linkage analysis* methods[30] would be used to further localize the variant. Nevertheless, the resolution of linkage analysis for most realistic sample sizes was only about 1% recombination or 1 cM ($\theta = .01$), corresponding to about 1 million base pairs. This is a large region for trying to identify a potential causal genetic variant.

Association Studies

Association studies can be more powerful than linkage analyses and can delineate more manageable regions potentially harboring disease-causing variants. As a result, association studies have displaced linkage as the primary approach in genetic epidemiology. The aim of association studies is to provide evidence for association between markers and disease. These studies can be undertaken among unrelated individuals or within families.

Unrelated Individuals

Most commonly, association studies use cohort or case-control designs to compare marker allele or genotype frequencies between a group of unrelated affected individuals and a group of unrelated unaffected individuals. Association studies can also evaluate continuous traits, studying entire groups of subjects or selecting subjects at the extremes of the trait distribution to increase the statistical information (power and precision).[31] Whatever the phenotype, study subjects should be representative of their respective source populations to allow for generalization of results and to help address issues of potential population stratification bias.[32] In a case-control study, this implies that controls should be individuals who, if diseased, would have been cases (see Chapter 8). Controls are also commonly selected to match cases with respect to ethnicity, age, sex, and other potential confounders. Nevertheless, many association studies have been successful without overly rigorous control selection. In fact, due to the high cost of subject recruitment and genotyping, there is a growing movement toward using genotype information among controls recruited into previous studies or large publicly available population surveys like the UK Biobank.[33,34] The potential bias arising from using "convenience" controls is tempered by the low potential for important confounding or selection effects—since external factors seldom affect the genotype "assigned" at conception. There is also low potential for measurement error in SNP genotyping, lack of recall bias when studying inherited variants, large sample sizes, and potential for rigorous replication of findings.

In addition, using such controls can result in population stratification bias—confounding of associations between particular genetic characteristics and the outcome by the rest of the genome—and overdispersion of test statistics, due to case-control differences in genetic ancestry.[35] This can be addressed analytically using a large panel of genetic markers to characterize and adjust for genetic ancestry.[36-39]

Family-Based Association Studies

Family-based association study designs have the appeal of providing protection from confounding by population stratification because all the subjects within a family are likely to have similar ancestry. There are two basic modes of this design, one comparing affected and unaffected relatives as matched case-control sets, and one leveraging transmission of alleles from parents to affected offspring. The former mode is straightforward when using full siblings as controls, as matched sets will have the same parents and hence identical ancestries. However, if the marker under analysis is not the causal genetic variant, then the results must be interpreted as referring to linkage and association. Furthermore, if multiple cases or multiple controls from the same sibship are included, then the usual conditional likelihood for matched sets is no longer valid because transmissions to each subject are not independent conditional on their allele sharing. In this situation, a robust variance estimator must be used.[40] If more distant relatives are included, then their ancestries may not be identical, so protection from confounding is incomplete.

The second family-based association study design compares the alleles transmitted from parents to affected offspring with those not transmitted, which can be done using methods for matched-pair analysis (see Chapter 19), such as a form of the McNemar test of alleles known as the *transmission-disequilibrium test.*[41] In this design, only the case and parents are genotyped and the disease status of the parents is not used. Equivalently, the design can be thought of as a 1:3 matched case-control comparison of the case to the "pseudosibs" carrying the other possible genotypes the case could have inherited.

Studying families can be statistically less efficient than studying unrelated subjects.[42] This is because the genetic similarity among family members can result in fewer discordant genotypes sets for analyzing main effects than in studies of unrelated individuals. On the other hand, for analyzing gene-environment interactions, power or precision may be enhanced, essentially because the most informative comparisons are genotype-concordant exposure-discordant pairs, which tend to be enriched despite their potential "overmatching" on exposure precisely because of their greater concordance in genotype. Moreover, selecting unrelated cases with a positive family history of disease can increase the information in association studies.[43]

Analyzing Associations

Whatever the design, the association between genetic variants and disease is most commonly evaluated using a trend test across the number of variant alleles. This allelic trend test is relatively robust to model misspecification (*e.g.*, if the true mode of inheritance is recessive or dominant rather than additive). Investigators generally use a regression model for the variant-disease association that adjusts for confounders. An unbiased, systematic association has at least two interpretations.[44] First, the disease-associated variant might be the susceptibility allele itself. Second, the associated allele might be in LD with the susceptibility allele at the disease locus. In the first case, the marker and disease locus are one in the same, so LD is complete and the association is expected to occur in all populations harboring the allele. In the second case, the marker and disease locus are very close to each other, but differences in LD may lead to different associations across populations. For this reason, association studies can narrow the region potentially containing a disease-causing marker. Multiethnic studies provide a valuable approach to distinguishing these possible explanations by exploiting differences in LD structure across populations.

Genome-Wide Association Studies

Most early association studies among unrelated individuals focused on specific *candidate genes* with suspected functionality on a pathway to the phenotype. In the late 1990s, however, emerging microarray chip technologies began to enable the interrogation of all the common variants across the genome for association with disease or quantitative traits. Investigators quickly realized that clusters of variants on the same chromosome (haplotypes) could effectively tag many other variants, so that it was really only necessary to genotype a modest number of variants at any locus to capture most of the common variation. The advent of the genomics era in genetic epidemiology can be dated to a seminal paper in *Science* by Risch and Merikangas,[45] in which they predicted it would soon become possible to search for disease genes in an agnostic fashion by testing hundreds of thousands of such "tag SNPs" for association with disease.

Two major advances soon made this vision a reality. Further improvements in genotyping technologies brought down the cost of assaying SNPs genome-wide to a few thousand dollars per sample (a trend mirroring the Moore law in computing that by 2018 had lowered the cost for millions of variants to less than 100 $). Then, with the creation of the International Haplotype Mapping Project (HapMap),[46] investigators began systematically cataloging haplotype tagging SNPs across the entire genome in multiple populations.[46-50] Less than a decade after Risch and Merikangas' paper, the first genome-wide association study (GWAS) was published[51] along with two confirmatory studies,[52,53] reporting an association of age-related macular degeneration with the complement factor H gene *CFH*. This association helped localize a gene within a previously known linkage region, demonstrating the power of GWAS.

In the early days of GWAS, the high cost of genotyping motivated the use of multistage designs.[54] In the first stage, part of the sample was genotyped using a GWAS array. In the second stage, the remaining samples were genotyped for the most strongly associated markers using a less expensive custom panel. Information from the two stages was then combined in a final analysis. With declining genotyping costs for GWAS compared with custom panels and the recognition that genome-wide data are useful for many other purposes, such as testing for gene-environment and gene-gene interactions, most studies conducted at present aim to obtain GWAS data on an entire sample.[55]

The number of GWAS undertaken has expanded rapidly since 2005. The association results from these studies with $P < 1 \times 10^{-5}$ have been catalogued by the National Human Genome Research Institute and European Molecular Biology Institute.[56] As of November 2017, the searchable database (http://www.ebi.ac.uk/gwas/home) contained 187,409 unique SNP-trait associations from 4,582 publications. The vast majority are weak associations, with relative risks between 1.1 and 1.3.

Very large sample sizes are required to study associations with ever-smaller effect sizes, which has motivated the creation of large consortia, often comprising tens of thousands of cases and controls. Although sharing of raw data at the individual level across a consortium, each with their own consent and data sharing rules, can be problematic, a joint analysis can often be conducted by meta-analysis of summary statistics, at least for genetic main effects.

To date, for most complex diseases, the proportion of the estimated heritability explained by SNPs detected in GWAS is somewhat limited, as is the area under the curve (AUC) of receiver operating characteristic (ROC) curves for these SNPs. For example, even for height—a highly heritable trait that is easily and accurately measured—an early meta-analysis of almost 200,000 individuals found 180 associated loci, but together they accounted for only 10% of the phenotypic variation.[57] The authors estimated that as many as 600 loci with similar effect sizes might be detectable with sample sizes of 500,000 subjects, but the explained variation would still be only 16%. Chatterjee and Park[58] described the AUCs for available genetic loci of complex diseases, with and without including family history and nongenetic risk factors, and for most cancers they were under 0.65 (with 0.5 being the expected value for a risk index that is no better than chance). Inclusion of SNPs predicted to be discovered in the future only increased the estimates by a modest degree. Only for Crohn disease and type I diabetes were AUCs greater than 0.75. That said, there is a growing appreciation that combining GWAS risk variants into a polygenic risk score might offer some "translational" value for predicting risk to guide screening and prevention strategies or for stratification in therapeutic studies and treatment planning.[59]

There has been considerable discussion about the "hidden" or "missing" heritability that remains to be explained.[60] With regard to what is "hidden," a much larger proportion of heritability can be explained when looking at all variants genotyped or tagged by GWAS arrays (*e.g.*, up to 80% for height).[57,61] For example, Purcell et al.[13] showed that risk indices comprising increasing numbers of the "top" SNPs (up to as much as half the genome) produced better and better prediction of the risk of schizophrenia and bipolar disorder (but not for heart disease, rheumatoid arthritis, hypertension, Crohn disease, or diabetes). "Missing" heritability might be explained with larger studies focused on rare variants with larger effect sizes that are not covered by current GWAS panels, or considering gene-gene or gene-environment interactions. Whole genome sequencing may provide some of these clues (discussed further below).

Imputation of Genetic Markers

Most associations discovered via GWAS are unlikely to be directly causal, because only a limited fraction of the genetic variation in the genome is directly measured. Marker associations are instead expected to reflect indirect relationships with nearby causal variants in LD. With the availability of extensive reference panels of variation from projects such as the Haplotype

Reference Consortium,[62] it has become possible to infer genotypes for most variants in the genome with >1% minor allele frequency (MAF) by using imputation techniques.[63,64] Although some programs provide the most likely genotype at each untyped locus, the use of best guess genotypes in association analysis fails to account for the uncertainty, thereby leading to biased tests. A more appropriate procedure is therefore to use the estimated genotype probabilities or (under an additive model) the expected "geneotype dosage" as a continuous variable in regression models.[65] Prior to imputation, quality control of genotyping data is essential for valid results.[66] Standard practice involves eliminating samples with undue numbers of loci that fail certain quality control filters and eliminating markers with low genotype call rates and departures from Hardy-Weinberg equilibrium.

Population Stratification

In the analysis of association study data, one must account for potential confounding due to population stratification. If variant allele frequencies and disease risks vary across ancestral populations, genetic associations at a particular locus can be confounded by the genetic associations in the rest of the genome. Such confounding can lead to bias in statistical results, even within apparently homogeneous populations. Various methods have been developed to account for such population stratification using the entire distribution of associations. The most widely used method today is to adjust for principal components of genetic ancestry.[36] Alternatives are to adjust for estimates of the proportion of the genome inherited from different ancestries,[67] or to use mixed models that combine features of both approaches and can be applied to family-based or case-control studies.[39] A typical diagnostic used to assess potential population stratification is to plot the observed cumulative distribution of P-values against its expected uniform distribution (a Q-Q plot) and verify that its median is close to $\frac{1}{2}$ ($\lambda = 1$). When using ancestry estimation, it may be important to adjust not just for global ancestry, but also for the local ancestry in each region of the genome, particularly in admixed populations like Hispanics or African Americans.[68]

Statistical Testing for GWAS Studies

To obtain valid tests in GWAS analyses, one must address the issue of multiple comparisons arising from evaluating millions of associations. Pe'er et al.[69] have estimated that for modern high-density genotyping chips with imputation to reference panels or next generation sequencing (NGS), which may allow one to assess tens of millions of genetic variants, the linkage disequilibrium structure translates to approximately 1 million effectively independent comparisons in Europeans or about 2 million in Africans. The simplest approach is then to use a Bonferroni correction, in which α is divided by the number of effectively independent tests performed, for example, with $\alpha = .05$ and a million independent associations, the new cut point is $0.05/1,000,000 = 5 \times 10^{-8}$. More refined methods have better performance and more scientific relevance, however.[70] Some GWAS also calculate the false discovery rate (FDR) or use permutation testing to assess the strength of associations.[71-73] Note that while adhering to strict "significance" cut points may help address issues of multiple comparisons, the cut points are somewhat arbitrary and do not reflect the potential clinical or biological importance of associations,[74] nor do they account for the costs of false negatives. A case in point is the increase in heritability explained when considering all variants measured by a GWAS array, and not just those reaching genomewide significance. Furthermore, an important aspect of GWAS findings is not simply "statistical significance" but also their validity, as examined by replication studies on independent samples.[75-78]

Recent Advances in Association Methods

Next Generation Sequencing

GWAS usually assay known genetic variants with MAF greater than 5%. Other common SNPs are well tagged by SNPs on GWAS arrays, as are "uncommon" variants with MAF from 1% to 5%. To measure rare variants (<1% frequency), one can attempt to impute them, add custom genotyping content to a GWAS array, or undertake NGS. NGS also allows for the measurement of genetic variants that are not known or not amenable to measurement or imputation by genotyping, such as *copy number variants* (CNVs). Thus, the appeal of NGS is the ability to discover *all* the variants in a gene, in the entire exome, or even the entire genome, and not just the common variants. A popular hypothesis is that these rare variants may have larger effect sizes than common variants,[79] but note that some of the purported evidence for this hypothesis may be due simply to the lower power for rare variants, so that only those with large effect sizes are detectable!

To perform NGS, one randomly breaks samples of DNA from each chromosome into many small overlapping fragments, such that any given locus is spanned by a random number of fragments. These fragments are then sequenced and aligned against a reference sequence to report the number of copies of each nucleotide base at each location. A sample that is heterozygous at a given location may or may not be correctly called as such; the call depends upon whether both alleles are covered by one or more fragments, which in turn depends upon the *depth of sequencing* (the average number of copies across the genome). Because sequencing is less than perfect, one might want to dismiss an observation of only one or two copies of the variant allele as a false positive, so that greater depth of sequencing would be needed.

Due to the expense of NGS, there is a trade-off between average depth of sequencing and the number of samples that can be sequenced. If the goal is to discover rare alleles (which would occur predominately in the heterozygous state), then the number of samples tested is far more important than depth, suggesting one might prefer large-scale low-coverage studies.[80,81] An alternative is to combine or "pool" DNA samples. Here one could use either a two-stage design, initially using pooling to identify sets of samples containing variants of interest followed by individual sequencing to identify specific samples containing those variants,[82] or directly use a test of association comparing estimated allele frequencies in case and control pools.[83]

Rare Variant Analyses

Conventional approaches to assessing association are inefficient when studying rare variants. This has given rise to numerous novel statistical tests for rare variant association, generally falling into two main categories: burden tests and variance component kernel machine tests. Burden tests aim not at testing association with individual variants but rather with the number of variants or some weighting of their aggregate effect in a gene region.[84,85] Since their introduction in 2011, a more widely used approach has been the variance component sequence kernel association test (SKAT), which tests for some measure of genetic similarity in a region between pairs of subjects with similar phenotypes (*e.g.*, greater genetic similarity between case-case than case-control pairs).[86] Burden approaches are more powerful if all of the rare variants under study have association effects in the same direction. Conversely, variance component approaches are more powerful when some rare variants are positively associated and others are negatively associated. One can also use an approach that compromises between the burden and variance component approaches (SKAT-O).[87]

Another important development in the study of rare variants has been a resurgence of interest in family-based designs. These have three advantages: first, by focusing on families with multiple cases, the frequency of causal variants is likely to be enhanced; second, they allow for more powerful tests of causality by identifying variants that cosegregate within families along with the inheritance of the disease; third, they provide a way to get lots of "free" genotyping by imputing the genotypes of untested family members based on those of their close relatives. Variations on SKAT and other rare variant tests have been developed for family data.[88] A particularly appealing design is a two-stage family-based design in which a subset of the most informative family members (based on their disease status and prior linkage or GWAS markers) is sequenced and used to prioritize a subset of variants most likely to be causal for testing in an independent sample.[89] This contrasts with a "two-phase" design for case-control samples of unrelated individuals,[90] in which a subsample of individuals is chosen for sequencing based on their disease status and associated markers, and then used to impute genotypes for the remaining sample in a joint analysis of the main study and subsample.

Evaluating Multiple Risk Factors

Interactions

Following an initial scan for main effects of SNPs from GWAS or rare variants from NGS, much more remains to be explored. One possibility is that there could be gene-environment or gene-gene interaction effects that do not involve markers producing important marginal effects. (We caution that we are here following the traditional genetic use of "interaction" to mean modification of a multiplicative measure, rather than some biological interaction; see Chapter 26). A challenge to evaluating interaction is that the number of possible interactions is much larger than the number of main effects. For example, a GWAS of 1 million SNPs will have a half a trillion possible pairwise interactions. A simple Bonferroni correction for multiple comparisons would thus require an alpha level of 1×10^{-13}, and interaction tests require much larger sample sizes than main effects even at the same alpha level.[91]

The study of interactions can be enhanced by "case-only" analyses (see Chapter 8) that assume independence of the interacting factors in the source population. For example, a reanalysis of cleft palate data obtained narrower confidence limits for the interaction between smoking and the *TGFα* gene (an odds ratio [OR] of 5.14 with 95% confidence limits [CL] of 1.68 and 15.7 for the case-only analysis compared with an OR of 6.57 with CL of 1.72 and 25.0 for the case-control analysis), equivalent to a 30% reduction in sample size required for the same precision.[92] Case-only analyses are, however, biased if the independence assumption is violated, as might arise due to LD among nearby pairs of variants, population stratification, or behavioral factors that induce an association between genes and environmental factors. Unlike the case-control design, the case-only design can only measure interaction on a multiplicative scale (see later).

To overcome these concerns, various staged and hybrid approaches have been introduced.[93-97] Although power will still be much lower for interactions than for main effects, these methods generally yield much better power than a simple exhaustive search.[98,99] Moreover, for future studies of gene-environment interactions, it is essential that investigators planning new GWAS studies design them to have appropriate environmental measurements and population-based sampling schemes. For example, the NIH post-GWAS "GAME-ON" initiative aimed at synthesizing all available data on five cancer sites, replicating findings, and characterizing genetic risks and their modification by environmental exposures[100] has been limited by many of the available studies not having collected any environmental exposure data. Even those studies that did collect such data did so in a highly variable manner; the data range from very crude to very detailed, such that they often require considerable efforts at harmonization across studies.[101]

It has long been recognized that any statement about interaction is necessarily scale dependent. The dominance of the logistic model and odds ratios for estimating associations has led to a focus of interaction measuring departures from the multiplicative model, but it has also been recognized that the public health concept of "synergy" is often better captured by departure from the additive model and that the simplest biological models of interaction produce departures from additivity, not multiplicativity.[102] For example, while radiation exposure has been shown to have a greater-than-multiplicative effect with the *ATM* gene on the risk of second breast cancers following radiotherapy,[17] its interaction with *BRCA1* and *BRCA2* was not shown to be different from multiplicative although it may be somewhat greater than additive.[103] Thus, while carriers of these mutations are at considerably increased baseline risk, radiation exposure could still further enhance their risk.

Pathways

Another way to consider multiple risk factors is to recognize that SNPs that individually fail to reach genome-wide significance may jointly contribute to a common pathway. A variety of methods have been developed for identifying subsets of genes in known pathways that are collectively overrepresented among the top GWAS associations.[104,105] The first and perhaps best known method is Gene Set Enrichment Analysis (GSEA).[106] GSEA and other approaches entail some way of combining the study data, say from a GWAS or eQTL study, with external information. The external information is typically highly structured using expert systems approaches to organizing information in a computable format, known as an "ontology." The Gene Ontology[107] is an example of such a database aimed at characterizing gene products in terms of cellular component, biological process, and molecular function. Entries in the Gene Ontology are manually curated by a small army of biological experts using phylogenetic relationships among members of a gene family across species. Other ontologies include the Kyoto Encyclopedia of Genes and Genomes[108] and Ingenuity Pathway Analysis.[109] Our understanding of pathways is continually curated into various databases in particular biological domains (*e.g.*, genomic, pathway, or functional). Other systems, like the GRAIL program,[110] use statistical techniques based on expert systems to mine the database of PubMed abstracts to identify functional relationships among a set of genes.

Hierarchical Modeling

Yet another approach to incorporating additional information in genetic epidemiology is Bayesian hierarchical modeling.[111-117] Unlike other methods that require prior specification of the importance of external information, hierarchical modeling uses a higher-level regression model to infer from the study data the utility of such information (*e.g.*, annotations) across the entire set of associations under consideration. The inclusion of relatively uninformative annotations in the second-level model produces very little loss of power because such variables received little or no weight, whereas including truly informative annotations greatly improves power.[118,119] In contrast, standard methods with prespecified weights lead to substantial loss of power when the weights are incorrectly specified. For example, Minelli et al.[120] compared the weights for 15 types of knowledge about SNPs elicited from 10 experts using a Delphi survey versus empirical estimates of their predictive values for seven diseases; they found some agreement but also some disagreement (*e.g.* the empirical evidence did not support the importance of a gene encoding a protein in a pathway or interactions relevant to a trait that were ascribed by experts). A companion paper[121] showed how both kinds of external information could be used to estimate the probability of association in a hierarchical modeling framework. For example, data from an epidemiologic study of gene-environment interactions in asthma were combined with an experimental challenge study using model air pollutants in a panel of allergic subjects in a multivariate hierarchical model, along with external pathway information from Ingenuity Pathway Analysis.[122]

Mendelian Randomization

In 2004, George Davey Smith and Shan Ebrahim[123] reprinted a 1986 letter to the editor of *The Lancet* by Martijn Katan[124] in the *International Journal of Epidemiology*. It proposed a way to evaluate the causality of the observed association between serum cholesterol and cancer by relating both variables to the *ApoE* genotype. Although the approach was never performed, it appears to be an early reference in the medical literature to a technique long used in econometrics[125] known as "instrumental variables." In the context of genetic epidemiology, the basic idea is to indirectly analyze an association between some exposure "biomarker" (*e.g.*, serum cholesterol) and disease by examining the extent to which a genotype that is strongly related to the biomarker is also related to disease risk solely through that intermediate variable. Here, genotype functions as the instrumental variable[126] (see Chapter 28).

This approach, now known as Mendelian randomization (MR), attempts to address two well-known problems in directly testing associations of a biomarker with a disease or trait in case-control or cohort studies. The first is reverse causation, whereby the disease process or its treatment alters the biomarker, rather than the biomarker affecting the risk of disease. This problem is more severe in retrospective case-control studies, but could affect cohort studies using stored biospecimens if the disease has a long presymptomatic period. The second problem is uncontrolled confounding, a near-universal problem in observational epidemiology. Because constitutional genotypes are immutable, there is no possibility for reverse causation, and because genes are transmitted randomly from parents to offspring, confounding is avoided, at least within families, although spurious gene-biomarker or gene-disease associations can arise in comparisons across populations. MR does require certain key assumptions,[127] the most important being that there is no pathway from the genetic marker to disease other than through the biomarker (no "pleiotropic" effects). For any given gene, this can be essentially impossible to know with certainty.

There has been growing enthusiasm for applying MR in the context of GWAS, scanning first for a subset of genes that are predictive of the biomarker and then analyzing their association with disease. This can be done using separate samples for testing the two associations ("two-sample MR") and in the context of large-scale consortia for greater power.[128] However, the no-pleiotropy assumption becomes less convincing as many variants are included for which little is known about function. As a result, methods such as weighted median regression[129] have been developed that only require half of the variants to be valid instrumental variables. In GWASs, the expectation is that few of the variants would actually be causally related to a phenotype, so even if some might have pleiotropic effects through mechanisms unrelated to the biomarker under study and hence would not be valid instrumental variables, it is unlikely that the majority of them would be invalid.

Thus, the median of the ratios of the regressions of individual SNPs associations on the biomarker and the phenotype should be a valid estimator of the effect of the biomarker on the phenotype. Greater precision can be obtained by using a weighted estimate of the median, giving more weight to the more precise estimates of the ratios.

ETHICAL, LEGAL, AND SOCIAL ISSUES

The field of genetic epidemiology raises a number of important ethical, legal, and social issues (ELSI). These include the potential value of genetic testing, the possibility of genetic discrimination, reporting research findings to study subjects and their family members, and incorporating genetics into treatment and prevention. Results of genetic epidemiology research can thus impact individuals who carry markers for disease, their families, and society as a whole.

The growing number of discoveries from genetic epidemiologic research and decreases in genotyping and sequencing costs have resulted in increasing availability of genetic testing. Such tests range from those ordered by a physician for high-risk disease genes to those marketed direct-to-consumer for modest- or low-risk variants that span the entire genome.[130] Clinical genetic tests are generally coupled with genetic counseling to help individuals understand the risk of disease associated with carrying disease markers. Such tests can, however, also detect incidental findings such as genetic mutations from sequencing that are not directly related to the disease originally under study. Determining how to report such results to individuals has important ELSI implications.

In addition to informing treatment decisions, genetic testing has potential implications for both primary and secondary prevention.[131,132] For example, should carriers of a mutation that increases susceptibility to a particular chemical be barred from occupational exposure or should they have a right to choose once properly informed? Should disease screening programs be designed to target individuals with high genetic risk scores?

Some tests include information about the genetic basis of drug response, which is now being studied using GWAS.[133] Pharmacogenomics has important near-term implications for what drug and dose an individual should receive. For example, GWAS confirmed that variants in the gene *CYP2C9* impact metabolism of the anticoagulant drug warfarin[134]; such findings suggest that individuals who carry the *CYP2C9* variant could be prescribed lower doses of warfarin, reducing potential side effects of severe bleeding and unnecessary healthcare costs. In light of such results, precision medicine is commonly touted as a major potential benefit of pharmacogenomics and GWAS—albeit with some reservations.[135,136]

Direct-to-consumer testing generally offers individuals the opportunity to have variation in their genomes assayed with the same genotyping arrays used in GWAS. Results from these assays are returned to the consumer along with additional information such as their genetic ancestry and estimated health risks. Understanding the implications of risk is challenging when the effect estimates are modest. This raises the question of how to regulate recommendations about behavior modification from direct-to-consumer testing services to ensure they are based on sound science. Concerns here have led the Food and Drug Administration to restrict what information can be provided by direct-to-consumer genetic testing companies to their customers. However, the Food and Drug Administration has approved direct-to-consumer testing of high-risk *BRCA* mutations, which raises a number of concerns about overtesting and false assurances from negative results in low-risk populations.[137]

There are also a number of ELSI issues surrounding altering disease genes to treat or prevent disease. Gene therapy—whereby genes are therapeutically inserted to an individual's cells—has had many failures until very recently. The gene editing technology, CRISPR-Cas9, shows promise for altering disease genes, including the ability to not only edit genes but also to impact expression without altering the structure of an existing gene.[138,139]

NEW DIRECTIONS IN GENETIC EPIDEMIOLOGY

Advances in genetic, genomic, and other omic technologies over the past decade have yielded stunning progress in our understanding of the biological basis of disease. An obvious manifestation is the success of GWAS at discovering thousands of unforeseen loci related to hundreds of diseases.[140] While individually these risk loci typically have very small effect sizes, in aggregate they account for an increasing proportion of disease heritability.[60,141,142] Moreover, we can now assess uncommon and rare variants that will help decipher an increasing proportion of the genetic basis of disease.[143]

Gene Expression and GWAS

The study of disease etiology and prognosis benefits from the rich spectrum of potential biomarkers that are rapidly becoming available. These include gene expression, epigenetics, and proteomics. With regard to gene expression, arrays and RNA-Seq can be combined with GWAS data to undertake agnostic scans for expression quantitative trait loci (eQTL) and their role in disease.[144-146] eQTLs are loci that influence expression in the same or nearby genes (*cis*) or anywhere in the genome (*trans*). A salient example is a result based on RNA samples from 175 individuals across 43 tissues as part of the Genotype-Tissue Expression (GTEx) project[146] highlighting tissue-specific and shared regulatory eQTLs and subsequently linking them to GWAS variants. One can impute expression levels from GTEx into genotyped GWAS data,[147] providing an important avenue for assessing the relation between gene expression and disease without having directly measured expression. Related methods are also now being applied to identify epigenetic effects of environmental exposures and their role in mediating gene expression and ultimately disease phenotypes.[148] These methods include measuring high-density panels, making Epigenome-Wide Association Studies feasible.[149] Proteomics techniques are just beginning to mature to the point of providing insight into the biological processes in disease etiology and ultimately sensitive early markers of disease or progression.[150]

Exposome and Microbiome

High-throughput, highly sensitive, multiplex metabolomics methods such as mass spectrometry may provide advances for studying essentially all environmental exposures (the "Exposome")[151] and to facilitate agnostic Environment-Wide Association Studies.[152] There remain numerous methodological challenges before the EWAS concept can be considered a real companion to GWAS.[153] Unlike the genome, environments are dynamic and the appropriate critical periods of exposure for etiology may occur in the distant past, so current measurements taken may not reflect earlier exposures. To avoid the problem of reverse causation, a cohort or nested case-control design is needed. In GWAS, confounding by population substructure may be addressable by genomic control techniques, but there is no obvious parallel for controlling host and environmental confounders of exposures. The measurement of exposures is fraught with measurement error (*e.g.*, temporal variability, instrument error, and identification of unknown chemicals). The advent of EWAS also opens the possibility of Gene-Environment-Wide Interaction Studies (GEWIS)-agnostic scanning of all possible gene-environment interactions.[154]

One key component of the exposome, disruptions of the incredible diversity of microorganisms that inhabit the body, has been increasingly recognized as important in numerous chronic diseases.[155,156] There is an emerging view that a host and microbiota form a "superorganism" in a symbiotic relationship that plays a role in risk of disease by mediating immune response. Dramatic examples include improvement in symptoms of inflammatory bowel disease with a change in flora after antibiotic and probiotic use,[157] the use of fecal transplants from healthy subjects to cure *Clostridium difficile* infections,[158] and weight loss in obese subjects.[159] Evidence is mounting to link tumor promotion in many cancer types to the effects of bacterial microbiota.[155,156,160]

Although the gut microbiome is thought to be largely set by age 3, exposures and interventions later in life, including diet, antibiotics, and other lifestyle characteristics, may affect the structure of microbial communities.[161-163] Alterations of the microbiome in turn affect local and systemic host physiology and thus risk of disease and response to therapy. There is a dearth of sophisticated statistical methods for relating complex microbial community structure to the metabolome and disease.[164] Microbiome research raises many of the same methodological challenges as the exposome and is further complicated by community-level effects like diversity and resilience and rarely occurring species. By jointly considering the microbiome and environmental exposures, investigators will have an opportunity to examine host-microbial[165] and microbiome-metabolome[166] interactions, topics that have been largely neglected, in part due to their staggering methodological complexity.

Integrative Genomics

All of the aforementioned omics measures should be analyzed in a comprehensive manner to develop a fuller understanding of the disease process, but the methodological challenges are numerous.[153] With the explosion of high-density omics platforms and the enthusiasm for agnostic association testing, genetic epidemiology has had to seriously confront the inference problems posed by high-dimensional data. Doing so is the ultimate goal of the emerging field of *integrative genomics*.[167,168]

A key challenge of high-dimensional data is that the number of variables P is much larger than the number of observations n (the "$P > n$" problem). This issue arises in both the frequentist and Bayesian contexts and various approaches have been taken to address it. For frequentists, Bonferroni adjustment of acceptable type 1 error rates and modifications thereof that allow for the correlation between tests[169] have become conventional. In the gene expression field, the use of the FDR has become conventional, as the expectation is that there will be many noteworthy findings.[72] Bayesian versions of the FDR concept have also been proposed.[71,170,171]

Beyond testing for associations one-at-a-time, the real challenge for integrative genomics is variable selection in model building. It has long been appreciated that the importance of variables selected by some stepwise or greedy algorithms (*e.g.*, in a conventional regression model) cannot be interpreted at face value, nor can confidence intervals on the parameters of a "best" model. A variety of approaches have been taken to address this problem in a frequentist framework, such as splitting the analysis into a discovery and testing step, cross-validation, or penalized regression (*e.g.*, LASSO[172] or elastic net[173]). By itself, however, LASSO does not provide a formal significance test, only a sparse selection of variables, although there have been important developments in frequentist inference.[174,175]

Bayesian variable selection has also been a viable approach since the seminal work of George and colleagues on "stochastic search variable selection" (SSVS) using a "spike and slab" normal mixture model.[176,177] Although not originally proposed for the $P > n$ problem, Bayesian methods of variable selection have recently been extended for that purpose.[178-180] An example in the context of rare variant association modeling is the Bayesian Risk Index[181]—and extensions using Bayes model averaging in the Bayesian Model Uncertainty method[119]—as well as incorporating external information as priors in the iBMU approach.[118] These methods allow valid inference on both the set of variables and the set of alternative models via Bayes factors.

Machine Learning

Another emerging theme in the systems biology and genomics literatures has been the development of machine learning approaches to "big data," for example, as a nonparametric approach to discovering high-dimensional interactions.[182-186] Such methods simply look for patterns in the data in an agnostic manner. While there have been some notable discoveries using such techniques, it remains somewhat unclear how useful they will be for building interpretable biologically based models. Given the high-dimensionality of genome-scale problems, the use of parametric models, starting with relatively simple linear main effects models and adding in two-way or higher-order interaction terms as needed, may be a more promising strategy for finding biologically interpretable and reproducible models. This strategy risks missing some complex interactions that could exist in biology[187]; however, it is less clear whether such effects extensively carry over into epidemiologic data.

CONCLUSIONS

Genetic epidemiology has evolved at a rapidly increasing rate over the last two decades, mirroring and largely driven by technological advancements and "big science" collaborations. These trends are likely to continue, with further novel techniques developed to interrogate the genetic and environmental processes underlying disease. This expansion will undoubtedly improve our ability to relate different types of information in ever-larger sample sizes while exploiting the wealth of biological knowledge available in public databases. Hopefully, improving our understanding of the genetic and environmental causes of disease will result in personalized prevention and treatment strategies that improve the public's health.

References

1. Vogel W. Genetische Epidemiologie oder zur Spezifität von Subdisziplinen der Humangenetik. *Med Genet.* 2000;4:395-399.
2. Neel JV, Schull WJ. *Human Heredity.* Chicago, IL: University of Chicago Press; 1954.
3. Rao D. Editorial comment. *Genet Epidemiol.* 1984;1:3.
4. Neel J. Editorial. *Genet Epidemiol.* 1984;1:5-6.
5. Thomas D. Genetic epidemiology with a capital "E". *Genet Epidemiol.* 2000;19:289-3000.
6. Thomas DC. *Statistical Methods in Genetic Epidemiology.* Oxford: Oxford University Press; 2004.
7. Kerem B, Rommens J, Buchanan J, et al. Identification of the cystic fibrosis gene: genetic analysis. *Science.* 1989;245:1073-1080.
8. MacDonald M, Lin C, Srinidhi L, et al. Complex patterns of linkage disequilibrium in the Huntington's disease region. *Am J Hum Genet.* 1991;49:723-734.
9. Cordovado SK, Hendrix M, Greene CN, et al. CFTR mutation analysis and haplotype associations in CF patients. *Mol Genet Metab.* 2012;105(2):249-254.
10. Wright FA, Strug LJ, Doshi VK, et al. Genome-wide association and linkage identify modifier loci of lung disease severity in cystic fibrosis at 11p13 and 20q13.2. *Nat Genet.* 2011;43(6):539-546.
11. Fisher RA. *The Correlation Between Relatives on the Supposition of Mendelian Inheritance.* Vol 52. Edinburgh: Royal Society of Edinburgh; 1918:399-433.
12. Dudbridge F. Polygenic epidemiology. *Genet Epidemiol.* 2016;40(4):268-272.
13. Purcell SM, Wray NR, Stone JL, et al. Common polygenic variation contributes to risk of schizophrenia and bipolar disorder. *Nature.* 2009;460(7256):748-752.
14. Boyle EA, Li YI, Pritchard JK. An expanded view of complex traits: from polygenic to omnigenic. *Cell.* 2017;169(7):1177-1186.
15. Thun MJ, Hoover RN, Hunter DJ. Bigger, better, sooner – scaling up for success. *Cancer Epidemiol Biomarkers Prev.* 2012;21(4):571-575.
16. Ambrosone CB, Freudenheim JL, Graham S, et al. Cigarette smoking, N-acetyltransferase 2 genetic polymorphisms, and breast cancer risk. *J Am Med Assoc.* 1996;276(18):1494-1501.
17. Bernstein JL, Haile RW, Stovall M, et al; WECARE Study Collaborative Group. Radiation exposure, the ATM Gene, and contralateral breast cancer in the women's environmental cancer and radiation epidemiology study. *J Natl Cancer Inst.* 2010;102(7):475-483.
18. Fejerman L, Stern MC, John EM, et al. Interaction between common breast cancer susceptibility variants, genetic ancestry, and non-genetic risk factors in Hispanic women. *Cancer Epidemiol Biomarkers Prev.* 2015;24(11):1731-1738.
19. Weiss KM. *Genetic Variation and Human Disease: Principles and Evolutionary Approaches.* Cambridge: Cambridge University Press; 1993.
20. Ott J. *Analysis of Human Genetic Linkage.* 3rd ed. Baltimore, MD: Johns Hopkins; 1999.
21. Gronberg H, Damber L, Damber JE. Studies of genetic factors in prostate cancer in a twin population. *J Urol.* 1994;152(5 pt 1):1484-1487; discussion 1487-1489.
22. Verkasalo PK, Kaprio J, Koskenvuo M, Pukkala E. Genetic predisposition, environment and cancer incidence: a nationwide twin study in Finland, 1976-1995. *Int J Cancer.* 1999;83(6):743-749.
23. Lichtenstein P, Holm NV, Verkasalo PK, et al. Environmental and heritable factors in the causation of cancer--analyses of cohorts of twins from Sweden, Denmark, and Finland. *N Engl J Med.* 2000;343(2):78-85.
24. Mucci LA, Hjelmborg JB, Harris JR, et al. Familial risk and heritability of cancer among twins in nordic countries. *J Am Med Assoc.* 2016;315(1):68-76.
25. Heston LL. Psychiatric disorders in foster home reared children of schizophrenic mothers. *Br J Psychiatry.* 1966;112(489):819-825.
26. Hamilton AS, Mack TM. Use of twins as mutual proxy respondents in a case-control study of breast cancer: effect of item nonresponse and misclassification. *Am J Epidemiol.* 2000;152(11):1093-1103.
27. Laitinen T, Rasanen M, Kaprio J, Koskenvuo M, Laitinen LA. Importance of genetic factors in adolescent asthma: a population-based twin-family study. *Am J Respir Crit Care Med.* 1998;157(4 pt 1):1073-1078.
28. Duffy DL, Mitchell CA, Martin NG. Genetic and environmental risk factors for asthma: a cotwin-control study. *Am J Respir Crit Care Med.* 1998;157(3 pt 1):840-845.
29. Hopper JL. Modelling sibship environment in the regressive logistic model for familial disease. *Genet Epidemiol.* 1989;6(1):235-240.
30. Lander ES, Green P. Construction of multilocus genetic linkage maps in humans. *Proc Natl Acad Sci.* 1987;84:2363-2367.
31. Huang BE, Lin DY. Efficient association mapping of quantitative trait loci with selective genotyping. *Am J Hum Genet.* 2007;80(3):567-576.
32. Wacholder S, McLaughlin JK, Silverman DT, Mandel JS. Selection of controls in case-control studies. I: Principles. *Am J Epidemiol.* 1992;135(9):1019-1028.

33. Luca D, Ringquist S, Klei L, et al. On the use of general control samples for genome-wide association studies: genetic matching highlights causal variants. *Am J Hum Genet*. 2008;82(2):453-463.

34. Thompson SG, Willeit P. UK Biobank comes of age. *Lancet*. 2015;386(9993):509-510.

35. Thomas DC, Witte JS. Point: population stratification. A problem for case-control studies of candidate-gene associations? *Cancer Epidemiol Biomarkers Prev*. 2002;11(6):505-512.

36. Price AL, Patterson NJ, Plenge RM, Weinblatt ME, Shadick NA, Reich D. Principal components analysis corrects for stratification in genome-wide association studies. *Nat Genet*. 2006;38(8):904-909.

37. Devlin B, Roeder K. Genomic control for association studies. *Biometrics*. 1999;55(4):997-1004.

38. Pritchard JK, Rosenberg NA. Use of unlinked genetic markers to detect population stratification in association studies. *Am J Hum Genet*. 1999;65(1):220-228.

39. Zhu X, Li S, Cooper RS, Elston RC. A unified association analysis approach for family and unrelated samples correcting for stratification. *Am J Hum Genet*. 2008;82(2):352-365.

40. Siegmund KD, Gauderman WJ. Association tests in nuclear families. *Hum Hered*. 2001;52:66-76.

41. Spielman RS, McGinnis RE, Ewens WJ. Transmission test for linkage disequilibrium: the insulin gene region and insulin-dependent diabetes mellitus (IDDM). *Am J Hum Genet*. 1993;52:506-516.

42. Witte JS, Gauderman WJ, Thomas DC. Asymptotic bias and efficiency in case-control studies of candidate genes and gene-environment interactions: basic family designs. *Am J Epidemiol*. 1999;149(8):693-705.

43. Antoniou AC, Easton DF. Polygenic inheritance of breast cancer: implications for design of association studies. *Genet Epidemiol*. 2003;25(3):190-202.

44. Lander ES, Schork NJ. Genetic dissection of complex traits. *Science*. 1994;265:2037-2048.

45. Risch N, Merikangas K. The future of genetic studies of complex human diseases. *Science*. 1996;273:1616-1617.

46. Gibbs RA, Belmont JW, Hardenbol P, et al. The international HapMap project. *Nature*. 2003;426(6968):789-796.

47. Daly MJ, Rioux JD, Schaffner SF, Hudson TJ, Lander ES. High-resolution haplotype structure in the human genome. *Nat Genet*. 2001;29(2):229-232.

48. Gabriel SB, Schaffner SF, Nguyen H, et al. The structure of haplotype blocks in the human genome. *Science*. 2002;296(5576):2225-2229.

49. Frazer KA, Ballinger DG, Cox DR, et al. A second generation human haplotype map of over 3.1 million SNPs. *Nature*. 2007;449(7164):851-861.

50. International HapMap Consortium. A haplotype map of the human genome. *Nature*. 2005;437(7063):1299-1320.

51. Klein RJ, Zeiss C, Chew EY, et al. Complement factor H polymorphism in age-related macular degeneration. *Science*. 2005;308:385-389.

52. Edwards AO, Ritter R III, Abel KJ, Manning A, Panhuysen C, Farrer LA. Complement factor H polymorphism and age-related macular degeneration. *Science*. 2005;308(5720):421-424.

53. Haines JL, Hauser MA, Schmidt S, et al. Complement factor H variant increases the risk of age-related macular degeneration. *Science*. 2005;308:419-421.

54. Satagopan JM, Verbel DA, Venkatraman ES, Offit KE, Begg CB. Two-stage designs for gene-disease association studies. *Biometrics*. 2002;58(1):163-170.

55. Thomas DC, Casey G, Conti DV, Haile RW, Lewinger JP, Stram DO. Methodological issues in multi-stage genome-wide association studies. *Stat Sci*. 2009;24(4):414-429.

56. MacArthur J, Bowler E, Cerezo M, et al. The new NHGRI-EBI Catalog of published genome-wide association studies (GWAS Catalog). *Nucleic Acids Res*. 2017;45(D1):D896-D901.

57. Lango Allen H, Estrada K, Lettre G, et al.. Hundreds of variants clustered in genomic loci and biological pathways affect human height. *Nature*. 2010;467(7317):832-838.

58. Chatterjee N, Park J-H, Caporaso N, Gail MH. Predicting the future of genetic risk prediction. *Cancer Epidemiol Biomarkers Prev*. 2011;20(1):3-8.

59. Dudbridge F, Pashayan N, Yang J. Predictive accuracy of combined genetic and environmental risk scores. *Genet Epidemiol*. 2017;42(1):4-19.

60. Eichler EE, Flint J, Gibson G, et al. Missing heritability and strategies for finding the underlying causes of complex disease. *Nat Rev Genet*. 2010;11(6):446-450.

61. Yang J, Benyamin B, McEvoy BP, et al. Common SNPs explain a large proportion of the heritability for human height. *Nat Genet*. 2010;42(7):565-569.

62. Iglesias AI, van der Lee SJ, Bonnemaijer PWM, et al. Haplotype reference consortium panel: practical implications of imputations with large reference panels. *Hum Mutat*. 2017;38(8):1025-1032.

63. Li Y, Willer CJ, Ding J, Scheet P, Abecasis GR. MaCH: using sequence and genotype data to estimate haplotypes and unobserved genotypes. *Genet Epidemiol*. 2010;34(8):816-834.

64. Marchini J, Howie B. Genotype imputation for genome-wide association studies. *Nat Rev Genet*. 2010;11(7):499-511.

65. Hu YJ, Lin DY. Analysis of untyped SNPs: maximum likelihood and imputation methods. *Genet Epidemiol*. 2010;34(8):803-815.

66. Pluzhnikov A, Below JE, Konkashbaev A, et al. Spoiling the whole bunch: quality control aimed at preserving the integrity of high-throughput genotyping. *Am J Hum Genet*. 2010;87(1):123-128.

67. Pritchard JK, Stephens M, Rosenberg NA, Donnelly P. Association mapping in structured populations. *Am J Hum Genet*. 2000;67:170-181.

68. Zhang J, Stram DO. The role of local ancestry adjustment in association studies using admixed populations. *Genet Epidemiol*. 2014;38(6):502-515.

69. Pe'er I, Yelensky R, Altshuler D, Daly MJ. Estimation of the multiple testing burden for genomewide association studies of nearly all common variants. *Genet Epidemiol*. 2008;32(4):381-385.

70. Efron B, Hastie T. *Computer Age Statistical Inverence: Algorithms, Evidence and Data Science. Institute of Mathematical Statistics Monographs*. Cambridge: Cambridge University Press; 2016.

71. Wacholder S, Chanock S, Garcia-Closas M, El Ghormli L, Rothman N. Assessing the probability that a positive report is false: an approach for molecular epidemiology studies. *J Natl Cancer Inst*. 2004;96(6):434-442.

72. Storey JD, Tibshirani R. Statistical significance for genomewide studies. *Proc Natl Acad Sci USA*. 2003;100(16):9440-9445.

73. Thomas DC, Clayton DG. Betting odds and genetic associations. *J Natl Cancer Inst*. 2004;96(6):421-423.

74. Witte JS, Elston RC, Schork NJ. Genetic dissection of complex traits. *Nat Genet*. 1996;12(4):355-356; author reply 357-358.

75. Kraft P, Zeggini E, Ioannidis JPA. Replication in genome-wide association studies. *Stat Sci*. 2009;24(4):561-573.

76. Ioannidis JP, Thomas G, Daly MJ. Validating, augmenting and refining genome-wide association signals. *Nat Rev Genet*. 2009;10(5):318-329.

77. Ioannidis JP, Ntzani EE, Trikalinos TA, Contopoulos-Ioannidis DG. Replication validity of genetic association studies. *Nat Genet*. 2001;29(3):306-309.

78. Ioannidis JP, Boffetta P, Little J, et al. Assessment of cumulative evidence on genetic associations: interim guidelines. *Int J Epidemiol*. 2008;37(1):120-132.

79. Bodmer W, Bonilla C. Common and rare variants in multifactorial susceptibility to common diseases. *Nat Genet*. 2008;40(6):695-701.

80. Li Y, Sidore C, Kang HM, Boehnke M, Abecasis G. Low coverage sequencing: implications for the design of complex trait association studies. *Genome Res*. 2011;21(6):940-951.

81. Ionita-Laza I, Laird NM. On the optimal design of genetic variant discovery studies. *Stat Appl Genet Mol Biol*. 2010;9(1):033.

82. Xu C, Wu K, Zhang J-G, Shen H, Deng H-W. Low-, high-coverage, and two-stage DNA sequencing in the design of the genetic association study. *Genet Epidemiol*. 2017;41(3):187-197.

83. Liang WE, Thomas DC, Conti DV. Analysis and optimal design for association studies using next-generation sequencing with case-control pools. *Genet Epidemiol*. 2012;36(8):870-881.

84. Bansal V, Libiger O, Torkamani A, Schork NJ. Statistical analysis strategies for association studies involving rare variants. *Nat Rev Genet*. 2010;11(11):773-785.

85. Basu S, Pan W. Comparison of statistical tests for disease association with rare variants. *Genet Epidemiol*. 2011;35(7):606-619.

86. Lee S, Wu MC, Lin X. Optimal tests for rare variant effects in sequencing association studies. *Biostatistics*. 2012;13(4):762-775.

87. Lee S, Emond MJ, Bamshad MJ, et al. Optimal unified approach for rare-variant association testing with application to small-sample case-control whole-exome sequencing studies. *Am J Hum Genet*. 2012;91(2):224-237.

88. Schifano ED, Epstein MP, Bielak LF, et al. SNP set association analysis for familial data. *Genet Epidemiol*. 2012;36(8):797-810.

89. Thomas DC, Yang Z, Yang F. Two-phase and family-based designs for next-generation sequencing studies. *Front Genet*. 2013;4:276.

90. Breslow NE, Chatterjee N. Design and analysis of two-phase studies with binary outcome applied to Wilms tumor prognosis. *Appl Statist*. 1999;48:457-468.

91. Marchini J, Donnelly P, Cardon LR. Genome-wide strategies for detecting multiple loci that influence complex diseases. *Nat Genet*. 2005;37(4):413-417.

92. Umbach DM, Weinberg CR. Designing and analysing case-control studies to exploit independence of genotype and exposure. *Stat Med*. 1997;16(15):1731-1743.

93. Murcray CE, Lewinger JP, Conti DV, Thomas DC, Gauderman WJ. Sample size requirements to detect gene-environment interactions in genome-wide association studies. *Genet Epidemiol*. 2011;35(3):201-210.

94. Kooperberg C, Leblanc M. Increasing the power of identifying gene x gene interactions in genome-wide association studies. *Genet Epidemiol*. 2008;32:255-263.

95. Mukherjee B, Chatterjee N. Exploiting gene-environment independence for analysis of case-control studies: an empirical Bayes-type shrinkage estimator to trade-off between bias and efficiency. *Biometrics*. 2008;64(3):685-694.

96. Li D, Conti DV. Detecting gene-environment interactions using a combined case-only and case-control approach. *Am J Epidemiol*. 2009;169(4):497-504.

97. Evans DM, Marchini J, Morris AP, Cardon LR. Two-stage two-locus models in genome-wide association. *PLoS Genet*. 2006;2(9):e157.

98. Cornelis MC, Tchetgen Tchetgen EJ, Liang L, et al. Gene-environment interactions in genome-wide association studies: a comparative study of tests applied to empirical studies of type 2 diabetes. *Am J Epidemiol*. 2012;175(3):191-202.

99. Mukherjee B, Ahn J, Gruber SB, Chatterjee N. Testing gene-environment interaction in large-scale case-control association studies: possible choices and comparisons. *Am J Epidemiol*. 2012;175(3):177-190.

100. Fehringer G, Kraft P, Pharoah PD, et al. Cross-cancer genome-wide analysis of lung, ovary, breast, prostate, and colorectal cancer reveals novel pleiotropic associations. *Cancer Res*. 2016;76(17):5103-5114.

101. Bookman EB, McAllister K, Gillanders E, et al. Gene-environment interplay in common complex diseases: forging an integrative model – recommendations from an NIH workshop. *Genet Epidemiol*. 2011;35(4):217-225.

102. Rothman KJ, Greenland S, Walker AM. Concepts of interaction. *Am J Epidemiol*. 1980;112(4):467-470.

103. Bernstein JL, Thomas DC, Shore RE, et al; WECARE Study Collaborative Group. Contralateral breast cancer after radiotherapy among BRCA1 and BRCA2 mutation carriers: a WECARE Study Report. *Eur J Cancer*. 2013;49(14):2979-2985.

104. Thomas DC. Some surprising twists on the road to discovering the contribution of rare variants to complex diseases. *Hum Hered*. 2012;74(3-4):113-117.

105. Wang K, Li M, Hakonarson H. Analysing biological pathways in genome-wide association studies. *Nat Rev Genet*. 2010;11(12):843-854.

106. Subramanian A, Tamayo P, Mootha VK, et al. Gene set enrichment analysis: a knowledge-based approach for interpreting genome-wide expression profiles. *Proc Natl Acad Sci USA*. 2005;102(43):15545-15550.

107. Gene Ontology C, Blake JA, Dolan M, et al. Gene Ontology annotations and resources. *Nucleic Acids Res*. 2013;41(Database issue):D530-D535.

108. Kanehisa M, Araki M, Goto S, et al. KEGG for linking genomes to life and the environment. *Nucleic Acids Res*. 2008;36(Database issue):D480-D484.

109. Kramer A, Green J, Pollard J Jr, Tugendreich S. Causal analysis approaches in ingenuity pathway analysis. *Bioinformatics*. 2014;30(4):523-530.

110. Raychaudhuri S, Plenge RM, Rossin EJ, et al. Identifying relationships among genomic disease regions: predicting genes at pathogenic SNP associations and rare deletions. *PLoS Genet*. 2009;5(6):e1000534.

111. Wilson MA, Baurley JW, Thomas DC, Conti DV. Complex system approaches to genetic analysis Bayesian approaches. *Adv Genet*. 2010;72:47-71.

112. Lewinger JP, Conti DV, Baurley JW, Triche TJ, Thomas DC. Hierarchical Bayes prioritization of marker associations from a genome-wide association scan for further investigation. *Genet Epidemiol*. 2007;31(8):871-882.

113. Conti DV, Lewinger JP, Swan GE, Tyndale RF, Benowitz NL, Thomas PD. Using ontologies in hierarchical modeling of genes and exposures in biologic pathways. In: Swan GE, ed. *Phenotypes and Endophenotypes: Foundations for Genetic Studies of Nicotine Use and Dependence*. Vol 20. Bethesda, MD: NCI Tobacco Control Monographs; 2009:539-584.

114. Conti DV, Witte JS. Hierarchical modeling of linkage disequilibrium: genetic structure and spatial relations. *Am J Hum Genet*. 2003;72(2):351-363.

115. Capanu M, Concannon P, Haile RW, et al. Assessment of rare BRCA1 and BRCA2 variants of unknown significance using hierarchical modeling. *Genet Epidemiol*. 2011;35(5):389-397.

116. Hung RJ, Baragatti M, Thomas D, et al. Inherited predisposition of lung cancer: a hierarchical modeling approach to DNA repair and cell cycle control pathways. *Cancer Epidemiol Biomarkers Prev*. 2007;16(12):2736-2744.

117. Capanu M, Orlow I, Berwick M, Hummer AJ, Thomas DC, Begg CB. The use of hierarchical models for estimating relative risks of individual genetic variants: an application to a study of melanoma. *Stat Med*. 2008;27(11):1973-1992.

118. Quintana MA, Schumacher FR, Casey G, Bernstein JL, Li L, Conti DV. Incorporating prior biologic information for high-dimensional rare variant association studies. *Hum Hered*. 2012;74(3-4):184-195.

119. Quintana MA, Conti DV. Integrative variable selection via Bayesian model uncertainty. *Stat Med*. 2013;32(28):4928-4953.

120. Minelli C, De Grandi A, Weichenberger CX, et al. Importance of different types of prior knowledge in selecting genome-wide findings for follow-up. *Genet Epidemiol*. 2013;37(2):205-213.

121. Thompson JR, Gögele M, Weichenberger CX, et al. SNP prioritization using a Bayesian probability of association. *Genet Epidemiol*. 2013;37(2):214-221.

122. Li R, Conti DV, Diaz-Sanchez D, Gilliland F, Thomas DC. Joint analysis for integrating two related studies of different data types and different study designs using hierarchical modeling approaches. *Hum Hered*. 2013;74(2):83-96.

123. Davey Smith G, Ebrahim S. Mendelian randomization: prospects, potentials, and limitations. *Int J Epidemiol*. 2004;33(1):30-42.

124. Katan MB. Apolipoprotein E isoforms, serum cholesterol, and cancer. *Lancet*. 1986;1(8479):507-508.

125. Wright S. Appendix. In: Wright PG, ed. *The Tariff on Animal and Vegetable Oils*. New York, NY: Macmillan; 1928.

126. Greenland S. An introduction to instrumental variables for epidemiologists. *Int J Epidemiol*. 2000;29(4):722-729.

127. Didelez V, Sheehan N. Mendelian randomization as an instrumental variable approach to causal inference. *Stat Methods Med Res*. 2007;16(4):309-330.

128. Burgess S, Butterworth A, Thompson SG. Mendelian randomization analysis with multiple genetic variants using summarized data. *Genet Epidemiol*. 2013;37(7):658-665.

129. Bowden J, Davey Smith G, Haycock PC, Burgess S. Consistent estimation in mendelian randomization with some invalid instruments using a weighted median estimator. *Genet Epidemiol*. 2016;40(4): 304-314.

130. Kaye J. The regulation of direct-to-consumer genetic tests. *Hum Mol Genet*. 2008;17(R2):R180-R183.

131. Rebbeck TR. Precision prevention of cancer. *Cancer Epidemiol Biomarkers Prev*. 2014;23(12):2713-2715.

132. Thomas DC. What does "precision medicine" have to say about prevention? *Epidemiology*. 2017;28(4):479-483.

133. Rieder MJ, Livingston RJ, Stanaway IB, Nickerson DA. The environmental genome project: reference polymorphisms for drug metabolism genes and genome-wide association studies. *Drug Metab Rev*. 2008;40(2):241-261.

134. Takeuchi F, McGinnis R, Bourgeois S, et al. A genome-wide association study confirms VKORC1, CYP2C9, and CYP4F2 as principal genetic determinants of warfarin dose. *PLoS Genet*. 2009;5(3):e1000433.

135. Nebert DW, Zhang G, Vesell ES. From human genetics and genomics to pharmacogenetics and pharmacogenomics: past lessons, future directions. *Drug Metab Rev*. 2008;40(2):187-224.

136. Omenn GS. From human genome research to personalized healthcare. *Issues Sci Technol*. 2009;25:55-61.

137. Gill J, Obley AJ, Prasad V. Direct-to-Consumer genetic testing: the implications of the US FDA's first marketing authorization for BRCA mutation testing. *J Am Med Assoc*. 2018;319(23):2377-2378.

138. Cong L, Ran FA, Cox D, et al. Multiplex genome engineering using CRISPR/Cas systems. *Science*. 2013;339(6121):819-823.

139. Mali P, Yang L, Esvelt KM, et al. RNA-guided human genome engineering via Cas9. *Science*. 2013;339(6121):823-826.

140. Welter D, MacArthur J, Morales J, et al. The NHGRI GWAS Catalog, a curated resource of SNP-trait associations. *Nucleic Acids Res*. 2014;42(Database issue):D1001-D1006.

141. Zaitlen N, Kraft P. Heritability in the genome-wide association era. *Hum Genet*. 2012;131(10):1655-1664.

142. Manolio TA, Collins FS, Cox NJ, et al. Finding the missing heritability of complex diseases. *Nature*. 2009;461(7265):747-753.

143. Casey G, Conti D, Haile R, Duggan D. Next generation sequencing and a new era of medicine. *Gut*. 2013;62(6):920-932.

144. He X, Fuller CK, Song Y, et al. Sherlock: detecting gene-disease associations by matching patterns of expression QTL and GWAS. *Am J Hum Genet*. 2013;92(5):667-680.

145. Mele M, Ferreira PG, Reverter F, et al. Human genomics. The human transcriptome across tissues and individuals. *Science*. 2015;348(6235):660-665.

146. GTEx_Consortium. Human genomics. The Genotype-Tissue Expression (GTEx) pilot analysis: multitissue gene regulation in humans. *Science*. 2015;348(6235):648-660.

147. Gamazon ER, Wheeler HE, Shah KP, et al. A gene-based association method for mapping traits using reference transcriptome data. *Nat Genet*. 2015;47(9):1091-1098.

148. Cortessis VK, Thomas DC, Levine AJ, et al. Environmental epigenetics: prospects for studying epigenetic mediation of exposure-response relationships. *Hum Genet*. 2012;131(10):1565-1589.

149. Rakyan VK, Down TA, Balding DJ, Beck S. Epigenome-wide association studies for common human diseases. *Nat Rev Genet*. 2011;12(8):529-541.

150. Stunnenberg H, Hubner N. Genomics meets proteomics: identifying the culprits in disease. *Hum Genet*. 2014;133(6):689-700.

151. Wild CP. The exposome: from concept to utility. *Int J Epidemiol*. 2012;41(1):24-32.

152. Patel CJ, Bhattacharya J, Butte AJ. An environment-wide association study (EWAS) on type 2 diabetes mellitus. *PLoS One*. 2010;5(5):e10746.

153. Chadeau-Hyam M, Campanella G, Jombart T, et al. Deciphering the complex: methodological overview of statistical models to derive OMICS-based biomarkers. *Environ Mol Mutagen.* 2013;54(7):542-557.

154. Thomas D. Gene-environment-wide association studies: emerging approaches. *Nat Rev Genet.* 2010;11(4):259-272.

155. Cho I, Blaser MJ. The human microbiome: at the interface of health and disease. *Nat Rev Genet.* 2012;13(4):260-270.

156. Schwabe RF, Jobin C. The microbiome and cancer. *Nat Rev Cancer.* 2013;13(11):800-812.

157. Morgan XC, Tickle TL, Sokol H, et al. Dysfunction of the intestinal microbiome in inflammatory bowel disease and treatment. *Genome Biology.* 2012;13(9):R79.

158. van Nood E, Vrieze A, Nieuwdorp M, et al. Duodenal infusion of donor feces for recurrent *Clostridium difficile. N Engl J Med.* 2013;368(5):407-415.

159. Ridaura VK, Faith JJ, Rey FE, et al. Gut microbiota from twins discordant for obesity modulate metabolism in mice. *Science.* 2013;341(6150):1241214.

160. Gargano LM, Hughes JM. Microbial origins of chronic diseases. *Annu Rev Public Health.* 2014;35(1):65-82.

161. O'Sullivan O, Coakley M, Lakshminarayanan B, et al. Alterations in intestinal microbiota of elderly Irish subjects post-antibiotic therapy. *J Antimicrob Chemother.* 2013;68(1):214-221.

162. Arumugam M, Raes J, Pelletier E, et al. Enterotypes of the human gut microbiome. *Nature.* 2011;473(7346):174-180.

163. Pepper JW, Rosenfeld S. The emerging medical ecology of the human gut microbiome. *Trends Ecol Evol.* 2012;27(7):381-384.

164. Li K, Bihan M, Yooseph S, Methe BA. Analyses of the microbial diversity across the human microbiome. *PLoS One.* 2012;7(6):e32118.

165. Kinross JM, Darzi AW, Nicholson JK. Gut microbiome-host interactions in health and disease. *Genome Med.* 2011;3(3):14.

166. Ursell LK, Haiser HJ, Van Treuren W, et al. The intestinal metabolome: an intersection between microbiota and host. *Gastroenterology.* 2014;146(6):1470-1476.

167. Kristensen VN, Lingjærde OC, Russnes HG, Vollan HKM, Frigessi A, Børresen-Dale AL. Principles and methods of integrative genomic analyses in cancer. *Nat Rev Cancer.* 2014:14(5):299-313.

168. Schadt EE, Lamb J, Yang X, et al. An integrative genomics approach to infer causal associations between gene expression and disease. *Nat Genet.* 2005;37(7):710-717.

169. Conneely KN, Boehnke M. So many correlated tests, so little time! Rapid adjustment of P values for multiple correlated tests. *Am J Hum Genet.* 2007;81(6):1158-1168.

170. Wakefield J. A Bayesian measure of the probability of false discovery in genetic epidemiology studies. *Am J Hum Genet.* 2007;81(2):208-227.

171. Whittemore AS. A Bayesian false discovery rate for multiple testing. *J Appl Stat.* 2007;34(1):1-9.

172. Tibshirani R. Regression shrinkage and selection via the lasso. *J R Stat Soc Ser B (Methodological).* 1996;58(1):267-288.

173. Zou H, Hastie T. Regularization and variable selection via the elastic net. *J R Stat Soc Ser B.* 2005;67(2):301-320.

174. Lockhart R, Taylor J, Tibshirani RJ, Tibshirani R. A significance test for the lasso. *Ann Stat.* 2014;42(2):413-468.

175. Meinshausen N, Bühlmann P. Stability selection. *J R Stat Soc Ser B (Statistical Methodology).* 2010;72(4):417-473.

176. George EI, Foster DP. Calibration and empirical Bayes variable selection. *Biometrika.* 2000;87:731-747.

177. George EI, McCulloch RE. Variable selection via Gibbs sampling. *J Am Stat Assoc.* 1993;88:881-889.

178. Bottolo L, Richardson S. Evolutionary stochastic search for Bayesian model exploration. *Bayesian Anal.* 2010;5(3):508-610.

179. Bottolo L, Chadeau-Hyam M, Hastie DI, et al. GUESS-ing polygenic associations with multiple phenotypes using a GPU-based evolutionary stochastic search algorithm. *PLoS Genet.* 2013;9(8):e1003657.

180. Ročková V, George EI. EMVS: the EM approach to Bayesian variable selection. *J Am Stat Assoc.* 2013;109(506):828-846.

181. Quintana MA, Berstein JL, Thomas DC, Conti DV. Incorporating model uncertainty in detecting rare variants: the Bayesian risk index. *Genet Epidemiol.* 2011;35(7):638-649.

182. McKinney BA, Reif DM, Ritchie MD, Moore JH. Machine learning for detecting gene-gene interactions: a review. *Appl Bioinformatics.* 2006;5(2):77-88.

183. Greene CS, White BC, Moore JH. Ant colony optimization for genome-wide genetic analysis. In: Dorigo M, ed. *Ant Colony Optimization and Swarm Intelligence. Lecture Notes in Computer Science.* Vol 5217. Berlin: Springer; 2008:37-47.

184. Moore JH, Gilbert JC, Tsai CT, et al. A flexible computational framework for detecting, characterizing, and interpreting statistical patterns of epistasis in genetic studies of human disease susceptibility. *J Theor Biol.* 2006;241(2):252-261.

185. Motsinger-Reif AA, Dudek SM, Hahn LW, Ritchie MD. Comparison of approaches for machine-learning optimization of neural networks for detecting gene-gene interactions in genetic epidemiology. *Genet Epidemiol*. 2008;32(4):325-340.
186. Romualdi C, Campanaro S, Campagna D, et al. Pattern recognition in gene expression profiling using DNA array: a comparative study of different statistical methods applied to cancer classification. *Hum Mol Genet*. 2003;12(8):823-836.
187. Moore JH. The ubiquitous nature of epistasis in determining susceptibility to common human diseases. *Hum Hered*. 2003;56(1-3):73-82.

CHAPTER 38

Injury and Violence Epidemiology

Stephen W. Marshall and Guohua Li

Injury and violence epidemiology encompasses a diverse array of topics. Motor vehicle crashes, opioid overdose, falls in older adults, sports-related concussion and other traumatic brain injury, firearm-related violence, child maltreatment, sexual violence, homicide and assault, suicide and self-harm, and acts of warfare are all conditions of considerable public health significance that lie within the general domain of injury and violence. The epidemiologic study of injury and violence addresses the distribution, determinants, and prevention of this heterogeneous group of incidents and their adverse health outcomes.

At least two major commonalities link together this group of incidents and outcomes. The most obvious commonality is that the onset of the forces that generate injury and violence is external to the human body. The second major commonality is the vigorous scientific focus on prevention efforts. As in all areas of epidemiology, risk factor studies play an important role in injury and violence epidemiology. Additionally, injury and violence epidemiology has historically placed substantial emphasis on research that develops, implements, and evaluates interventions.

FOUNDATIONS

Injury is defined as physical damage to tissues, organs, and systems of the human body as a result of sudden or cumulative transfer of energy (*e.g.*, concussion resulting from impact in a car crash), or the sudden absence of an essential agent (*e.g.*, oxygen in the case of drowning and suffocation).[1] Injury is most commonly associated with a one-time sudden transfer of kinetic energy (*e.g.*, a blow to the head). However, injury can also result from the cumulative effects of multiple transfers (repetitive motion injury in workers; overuse injury in athletes). Furthermore, the external energy is not always kinetic (*e.g.*, a burn arises from thermal energy). The term *trauma* is often used clinically to refer to severe injury that requires hospitalization or admission to a trauma center from one-time sudden transfer of kinetic energy (as in a car crash).

The Energy Transfer Model of Injury Causation

The foundational concept underlying this definition of injury is that there are biomechanically derived injury criteria that specify the threshold or tolerance level of a given human tissue. Above that threshold, an impact (or other external force) results in injury. This model is called the energy transfer model of injury causation. Fundamental to the model is the concept that energy is the etiologic agent of injury, or proximal cause of injury.

The energy transfer model originated from the application of the classical epidemiologic triad of agent, host, and environment.[2,3] The energy transfer model extends the concept of the epidemiologic triad into a dynamic model of injury causation that unifies a diverse group of incidents and outcomes. Framed in terms of the epidemiologic triad,[2] the host is the human body that will be disrupted by the damaging energy transfer, the environment is the physical and social context in which the damaging energy transfer takes place, and the vector or vehicle refers to the various pathways by which the damaging energy is delivered to the host body.[3] Note that, in road safety, a common vehicle for the delivery of damaging energy is (ironically) motor vehicles.

Consistent with the definition of injury presented in the first paragraph of this section, there are two main pathways linking energy to tissue and organ injury in humans.[4] The first is that energy is transmitted to the human body in an amount that exceeds the tolerance level of specific human tissues, organs, and systems (*i.e.*, the injury threshold). This pathway represents the mechanism underlying the majority of mechanical injuries, such as those resulting from vehicle crashes, falls, burns, and firearms. The second pathway does not involve sudden energy transfer to the human body, but rather interferes with normal energy exchange necessary for maintaining physiological functions, such as drowning, suffocation, overdose, and carbon monoxide poisoning.

One important implication of the energy transfer model is that any measure that prevents or mitigates energy transfers provides an opportunity for injury or violence prevention.[3] The energies involved in injury can present in many different forms, such as mechanical, thermal, radiant, electrical, and chemical.[4] This concept is expanded in detail in the section on Haddon Matrix and Countermeasures below.

Another key implication from the energy transfer model is that the injury or violence outcome (*e.g.*, suicide, homicide, overdose) will depend on the type of energy transferred (*e.g.*, mechanical, thermal, radiant, electrical, or chemical), the modality of the energy transfer (*e.g.*, sudden-onset or cumulative), the body component affected (*e.g.*, tissue, organ, or system), and the intentionality of the mechanism of energy transfer (*e.g.*, self-harm, violence against another, or unintentional). Each of these concepts is illustrated below.

Energy Type: There are five types of energy that result in injury: mechanical, thermal, radiant, electrical, and chemical. Each energy-tissue combination has its own set of tolerances, some of which have been extensively studied in animal and human models.[4] For example, early 20th century studies of full thickness burns of the skin determined that the time to burn decreases more than linearly as the temperature applied to the skin increases. This explains why reducing household water temperature is a highly effective countermeasure for preventing scalds.

Modality: Injury events usually result from a single, sudden-onset energy transfer event (such as a car crash). However, injury can also result from the cumulative effect of multiple transfers over time (such as lower back injury in workers who lift excessive loads throughout their workday).

Body Component: Energy may result in damage to specific tissues or organs (traumatic injury) or may disrupt an essential body system (systemic injury). Consider, for example, the case of thermal energy. Traumatically, immersion of one's hand in hot water generates scalding and searing damage to the dermal and subdermal tissues. Systemically, excessive ambient thermal energy, such as vigorous physical activity for an extended period in hot humid conditions, may disrupt the body's thermal autoregulation system, resulting in exertional heatstroke.

Intentionality: Intent also has an effect on the type of injury. Injurious mechanical energy, for example, may be delivered unintentionally (*e.g.*, loss of balance resulting in a fall) or intentionally. Intentional injury and violence are synonyms. Violence may be directed toward one's self (suicide and self-harm), toward others (assault and homicide), or a combination of both.

Violence outcomes are best understood by extending the energy transfer model to include the social context in which perpetrators and victims interact and the violence occurs. It is important to frame the forces exchanged in violence within the social context of power and advantage. For example, violence in relationships is often one endpoint on a continuum of coercive and power-over behaviors. A sexual assault in marital and other intimate partner relationships often reflects a need for control and dominance by a male partner.[5] This behavior pattern may be reinforced by repeated viewing of controlling and violent sexual acts, such as those commonly depicted in online pornography.[5]

Community violence has been framed in the context of infectious disease epidemiology.[6,7] In this model, violence is conceptualized as a socially contagious phenomenon that spreads through communities when key influencers endorse resolution of conflict by force, rather than through negotiation. This model has led to the development of violence prevention programs.[6] As with unintentional injuries, recognizing the preventability of violence is paramount. A number of trials have demonstrated that violence is a learned behavior that can be unlearned, given sufficient time and resources.

Magnitude and Burden of Injury and Violence

Globally, more than 5 million people die each year from injury and violence, accounting for 9% of the world's deaths.[8] Approximately one-quarter of these deaths are suicide and homicide, while road traffic injuries account for nearly another quarter.[8] Globally, one-third of women experience sexual violence or violence inflicted by an intimate partner, and 20% of girls and 10% of boys are sexually abused at some point in their childhood.[8] From 1990 to 2017, despite increases in the absolute number of injury cases and deaths, global age-standardized death rates from injuries actually decreased.[9] This decrease likely represents the combined effects of improvements in healthcare systems, investments in injury prevention programs, and safety improvements due to enhanced infrastructure.[9]

In the United States, injury claims nearly a quarter of a million lives and results in over 30 million emergency department visits annually, including about two million hospital admissions (Table 38-1). The estimated annual economic cost of injury in the United States is about $1.85 trillion.[10] In contrast to later life outcomes such as cardiovascular disease and cancer, injury or violence affects predominantly people under the age of 65 years and is the leading cause of death in the United States between ages 1 and 45 years.[11] Because injury and violence affect people during the most economically and culturally productive years of life, the disability-adjusted life years lost are high, accounting for 10% of lost global disability-adjusted life years.[12]

These statistics, while startling, only provide a partial picture of the impact of injury and violence. Estimates of the numbers of deaths and hospitalizations are good at capturing the effect of acute conditions that pose an imminent threat to life but tend to under-represent the burden of long-term conditions and their social ramifications. Even measures such as disability-adjusted life years fail to capture the burden of rehabilitation and care borne by family members who are caregivers. They also do not capture the destructive effect of violence that involves repetitive demeaning and corrosive assaults, such as child abuse and neglect, or long-term intimate partner violence. The long-term sequalae of interpersonal violence has a profound effect on self-esteem and ultimately limit the ability of survivors to realize their full intellectual and creative potential.[13-15] Interpersonal violence compromises the integrity and order of our whole society, not only through the damage inflicted on survivors, but also through reinforcement of the negative behavior patterns associated with coercion and resolution of conflict through force.

History and Evolution of Injury Epidemiology

Although injury has been a major cause of death throughout human history, it did not garner the attention of epidemiologists until the 1930s. From the 1840s to 1930s, epidemiology was primarily focused on studies of infectious diseases, such as tuberculosis, influenza, typhoid, and diphtheria. By the 1940s, many of the infectious diseases had been brought under control in industrialized countries through vaccines, antibiotics, and improved sanitary and housing conditions. While the death rates from infectious diseases declined considerably during the first four decades of the

TABLE 38-1

Frequencies and Rates of Fatal and Nonfatal Injuries by Intent and Mechanism (United States, 2017)

	Fatally Injured		Injury Treated in Emergency Departments	
	Number	Rate per 100,000 Population	Number	Rate per 1,000 Population
Unintentional	169,936	52.2	28,027,606	86.2
Poisoning (incl. overdose)	64,795	19.9	1,755,044	5.4
Transportation-related	42,159	12.9	3,700,456	11.3
Falls	36,338	11.2	8,591,683	26.4
Others	26,644	8.2	13,980,423	42.9
Intentional	67,299	20.7	2,292,945	7.0
Suicide/self-inflicted	47,173	14.5	492,037	1.5
Homicide/assault	19,510	6.0	1,718,208	5.3
Legal intervention	616	0.2	82,700	0.2
Intent Undetermined	5,799	1.8	n/a	n/a
Total	*243,034*	*74.6*	*30,320,552*	*93.1*

From Web-based Injury Statistics Query and Reporting System (WISQARS), National Center for Injury Prevention and Control, Centers for Disease Control and Prevention.

20th century, morbidity and mortality from injury, particularly injury from motor vehicle crashes, increased markedly and became the number one cause of death for children and young adults in the United States.[16] The shift in mortality patterns prompted public health researchers to explore the utility of epidemiologic methods for studying injuries and noncommunicable diseases. Godfrey (1937)[17] and Armstrong et al. (1945)[16] were among the first to recognize the importance of "accidents" as a major public health problem, and Press (1948),[18] Gordon (1949),[19] and King (1949)[20] were among the first to apply epidemiologic methods in studying the causes and prevention of "accidents." Since then, injury epidemiology and prevention has gone through major evolutions and emerged as a vibrant, prevention-focused specialty that is widely accepted in the academic and practice-based public health communities.[21]

The single most important conceptual breakthrough in the evolution of injury epidemiology was the genesis of the energy transfer model of injury causation described above, *i.e.*, the identification of transfer of energy that exceeds the tolerance of the human body as the common etiologic agent for most injuries. This concept was first published in 1961 by experimental psychologist James Gibson.[22] However, the foundation for this conceptual breakthrough was Gordon's systematic application of the epidemiologic triad to analyzing the causes of injuries and accidents.[19] Although he did not distinguish the agent from the vector in the context of injury and accident causation, Gordon[19] stated aptly that the etiologic agents of injuries and accidents were "of physical, chemical, and biologic nature."

Around the same time, King posited that injuries and accidents were caused by external stresses (*e.g.*, physical, chemical, and biological stresses) exceeding the human tolerance level.[20] However, Gordon and King, both trained epidemiologists, did not make the fundamental discovery of the common etiologic agent for most injuries, partly because they viewed injury and accident as the same. The key conceptual breakthrough was made by Gibson, who stated "injuries to a living organism can be produced only by some energy interchange."[22] Gibson's discovery built on findings from intense research on occupant protection in aviation and automobiles through dynamic crash testing pioneered by Hugh DeHaven, John P. Stapp, and others.[21] Stapp's contributions to understanding the prevention of car crash injuries are particularly notable for the use of his own body, which he subjected to repeated standardized impacts, as an experimental tool.[23] This mode of research would now be viewed as unethical.

TABLE 38-2

Characteristic Differences Between Injury and Disease

Characteristic	Injury	Disease
Main etiologic agent	Energy (physical, chemical, electrical, thermal, and nuclear)	Biological pathogens (microbes, gene mutations, environmental and chemical toxins)
Latency	Instant	Hours to years
Intentionality	Unintentional and intentional	Unintentional
Susceptibility	Universal	Individual- and disease-specific
Preventability	High	Varied
Medical approach	Emergency medical services, trauma care, and rehabilitation	Screening, diagnosis, and treatment

Another milestone in the evolution of injury epidemiology was the explicit separation of injury (health consequence) from "accident" (event), following the recognition of vectors (or vehicles) carrying the etiologic agent of injury (energy). This development is mainly due to the innovative work of William Haddon Jr, who clarified that objects directly involved in injury causation, such as motor vehicles and bullets, are vectors that carry the etiologic agent of injury,[24] akin to mosquitos carrying the Zika virus. Because vectors carrying the etiologic agent of injury are mostly man-made and can be modified through design, engineering, and regulation, they represent an important target for interventions to decrease the incidence and severity of injury.

A public health physician, Haddon is widely credited with laying the foundation for the scientific discipline of injury epidemiology. He separated injury from event ("accident") and described the characteristic differences in etiologic agent, latency, intentionality, susceptibility, and preventability between injury and disease (Table 38-2). Additionally, he extended the epidemiologic triad—agent, host, and environment—into an organizational model known today as the Haddon Matrix. Susan P. Baker recognized the significance of the Haddon Matrix and widely popularized its use.[25] Haddon also utilized the energy transfer model to develop a conceptual framework for preventing and mitigating injury, the Haddon Countermeasures.[3,26] These innovations solidified the conceptual basis of the field into tangible and pragmatic tools, which are discussed in detail below.

Since the 1960s, injury epidemiology has developed into an established academic specialty, making injury prevention and control an important realm for public health research and practice.[27] Early in 1980, the Epidemiology Section of the American Public Health Association recognized advances in injury epidemiology as one of the 10 landmark achievements in American Epidemiology.[26] The subsequent decades have witnessed remarkable growth in injury epidemiology. This growth has included the development of innovative research methods, such as the spatiotemporally matched case-control design,[28-30] injury severity scaling,[31,32] the case-crossover design,[33,34] the pair-matched induced exposure method,[35,36] and the decomposition method.[37-39] Additionally, this period has witnessed the establishment of injury surveillance systems that allow public health to quantify the incidence and burden of injury, such as the Fatality Reporting Analysis System, the National Violent Death Reporting System, and the National Electronic Injury Surveillance System.[32,40] Finally, this period also saw the establishment of academic injury research and training programs, such as the injury control research centers and the occupational health and safety education and research centers. Much of this growth was precipitated by the publication of *Injury in America*,[41] which provided a comprehensive review of injury epidemiology and outlined an action plan for a public health approach to injury control. As a result, the US congress passed the Injury Control Act in 1990, the Centers for Disease Control and Prevention (CDC) established the National Center for Injury Prevention and Control in 1992, and many state health departments evolved to incorporate some form of injury control activity into their core functions. On the global level, the World Health Organization in 2000 created the

Department of Injury and Violence Prevention to provide leadership, coordination, and technical assistance to member states for the development and implementation of evidence-based injury and violence prevention programs.

KEY METHODOLOGIC CONCEPTS

The methodologic concepts that underlie injury epidemiology arise from the key concepts introduced in the previous section: the energy transfer model of injury causation, and the realization, due to Haddon, of the importance of conceptually separating the injury event from the resulting physical harm (*i.e.*, injuries).

Injury Events Are Predictable and Preventable

This key milestone in the evolution of injury epidemiology separated the injury from the precipitating event (aka "accident").[26] The distinction between "injury" and "accident" is much more than semantic. Rather, it represents a seminal starting place for injury epidemiology as a scientific discipline. Starting in the early 1980s, this differentiation between injury and event represents a profound change that fostered increasing acceptance of the view that the word "accident" should be discontinued in scientific discussions of injury and violence.[42] For centuries, injuries have been perceived to be "accidents," malevolent events deemed to be unpredictable and unpreventable, and have been attributed to "bad luck" or "acts of god." Epidemiologic research over a period of decades has provided compelling evidence that injury is predictable and preventable and that the public health approach is applicable and effective for injury prevention and control.[21,43-45] The occurrence of an "accident" does not necessarily produce injury and the undesirable connotations of accidents that they are unpredictable and unavoidable should not be applied to injury prevention and control. Even if an injury occurs, the severity and outcome of the injury can be mitigated through interventions. The discontinuation of the word "accident" in scientific discourse has been instrumental to differentiating injury from event and instilling a prevention-focused academic research discipline.

Haddon Matrix and Haddon Countermeasures

As noted above, Haddon developed two fundamental organizational models for injury prevention, the Haddon Matrix and the Haddon Countermeasures.[26] Haddon's most notable contribution to the field was extending the epidemiologic triad—agent, host, and environment—into a dynamic model known today as the Haddon Matrix.[25] Specifically, Haddon added a time dimension (*i.e.*, preinjury, injury, and postinjury) to the epidemiologic triad (agent, host, and environment) to create a 3×3 matrix. Over time, it became convention to divide the environment column into two separate columns, physical environment and social environment, to emphasize the importance of regulatory and policy processes in injury prevention (these are placed in the social environment column). Susan Baker encouraged the broad application of the Haddon Matrix across all areas of injury and violence.[25] Carol Runyan extended the Matrix to add a third dimension (acceptability and feasibility of the intervention) to create the Haddon-Runyan cube.[46]

The genius of the Haddon Matrix is that it codifies the field's conceptual foundation (the energy transfer model of injury causation model) into a practical tool for guiding the development of injury prevention strategies.[1,46] To illustrate the use of the Haddon Matrix, consider the problem of a male-on-female sexual assault that occurs while two teenagers are on a date (Table 38-3). In this example, the injury event is the sexual assault, the host is the young woman, and the vector is the young man. Examples of prevention strategies include education programs and behavioral programs that set norms for dating behavior (pre-event, host and vector), strategies for resisting assault, such as calling for emergency assistance (event, host), ensuring that high schools and other public institutions have policies and strategies for responding to disclosure of a sexual assault (social, postevent), and facilities and supplies to ensure physical and verbal evidence can be collected postassault (physical, postevent).

The Haddon Matrix is a useful tool for conceptualizing a diverse range of prevention strategies and for understanding the interplay between prevention strategies. By convention, a prevention strategy is placed in the row in which the strategy becomes active. For example, programs to

TABLE 38-3

Haddon Matrix Applied to Male-on-Female Adolescent Dating Violence

	Host (Adolescent Female)	Agent/Vehicle (Adolescent Male)	Physical Environment (Setting Where the Assault Occurred)	Social Environment (Community Norms, Policies, Rules)
Pre-event (before the assault)	Role models and education that stress the importance of respectful romantic relationships	Education and role models that stress the importance of respectful romantic relationships	Venues that provide dating adolescents with a safe and supervised group environment	Laws and norms that provide zero tolerance for sexual assault
Event (during the assault)	Training in how to resist sexual assault	Education that use of force during a sexual encounter is wrong and causes great pain and harm to others	Emergency phone stations readily available	Norms and training programs that support bystander intervention
Postevent (after the assault)	Encourage seeking support services immediately following a sexual assault	Judicial systems that require perpetrators to confront and acknowledge the harms done to the violence survivors	Provide appropriate facilities for support services and collection of physical evidence for prosecution	Support services for disclosing and recovering from sexual assault

educate women about how to seek emergency assistance during an assault take place before the event has occurred (pre-event phase), but this strategy does not become active until during the assault. Therefore, by convention, it is considered an event phase strategy.

As noted previously, the energy transfer model of injury causation implies that any intervention aimed at preventing or limiting energy flow represents an important opportunity for injury prevention. In addition to his Matrix, Haddon also published a list of ten countermeasures for preventing injury via energy containment and mitigation.[3] The 10 countermeasures represent a more academic application of the energy transfer model than the pragmatic Matrix. An example of the application of the countermeasure to handgun-related injury, adapted from Runyan,[47] is provided in Table 38-4.

Partitioning Person-Time Into Activity-Time

In chronic disease epidemiology, person-time at risk is usually conceptualized as a continuous stream of time for each individual. For example, in an occupational cohort of work-related cancer mortality, study subjects typically contribute time-at-risk in a continuous manner between cohort entry and exit dates. In contrast, in injury or violence epidemiology, person-time at risk can frequently be usefully partitioned into discrete episodes. Consider a cohort study of motor vehicle drivers that examines cellphone use while driving as a risk factor for motor vehicle crash. It is reasonable to condition accrual of person-time at risk on the act of driving, *i.e.*, to exclude nondriving person-time from the study. Conditioning on activity (limiting person-time at risk to driving-time), provided appropriate design considerations are observed,[48,49] can facilitate scientific inference (see Control Selection in Case-Control Studies below).

Partitioning of person-time into discrete activity episodes (hereafter, activity-time) poses a problem for epidemiologists, in that they must decide among alternative forms of denominator when computing incidence rates. For example, suppose we wish to quantify population-based motor vehicle crash rates in the United States. The numerator of the rate is clearly the number of

TABLE 38-4

Haddon Countermeasures Applied to Firearm Injury

	Countermeasure	Application
1	Prevent the creation of the hazard	Eliminate all firearms
2	Reduce the amount of hazard brought into existence	Reduce the number of firearms that are manufactured
3	Prevent the release of the hazard	All firearms are securely stored in a location that is inaccessible to people
4	Modify the rate of release of the hazard from its source	Eliminate automatic and semiautomatic firing mechanisms
5	Separate the hazard from that which is to be protected by time and space	Eliminate home storage of firearms
6	Separate the hazard from that which is to be protected by a physical barrier	Store firearms in locked containers
7	Modify relevant basic qualities of the hazard	Modify bullets to do less damage on impact
8	Make what is to be protected more resistant to damage from the hazard	Create and market bulletproof garments
9	Begin to counter damage done by the hazard	Provide good access to emergency care in the prehospital period
10	Stabilize, repair, and rehabilitate the object of damage	Provide high-quality trauma care in hospitals

Adapted with permission from Runyan CW. Introduction: back to the future—revisiting Haddon's conceptualization of injury epidemiology and prevention. *Epidemiol Rev.* 2003;25(1):60-64.

injuries occurring from crashes, but there are several options for the denominator: population of the United States, population of the United States of driving age, number of licensed drivers, miles driven in the United States, miles traveled in the United States (which is greater than miles driven because it includes miles traveled as a nondriving passenger), number of motor vehicle trips, hours spent traveling in motor vehicles, etc. Sports injury studies also have a range of potential denominators, including players on the team roster, players participating in competition and practice, team-competitions, and player-minutes of training and competition, among others.[50] None of these alternative denominators can be deemed universally correct in every situation. Rather, the choice of denominator will depend on the scientific question to be addressed.

Ongoing advances in technology are providing researchers with new, scientifically important activity-time measurements. In road safety, studies of young drivers use mobile devices (smartphones) to capture trip start and end times. In sports injury epidemiology, the use of helmet-based head impact telemetry permits the computation of concussion incidence rates per 1000 head impacts.

Decomposition of Rates

An important application of activity-time denominators is the decomposition of mortality rates. Consider the rate of fatal crashes per 100,000 drivers. This mortality rate is actually the product of three components: activity prevalence (number of miles per driver), the crash rate (number of crashes per mile driven), and the case fatality proportion (proportion of crashes resulting in fatality). Partitioning or "decomposing" the overall mortality rate in this manner has permitted significant epidemiologic investigation of age and gender differences in crash mortality.[37,39,51]

As an illustration of the decomposition method, Li et al.[37] studied gender differences in mortality from motor vehicle crashes in the United States. The rate of fatal crashes per 10,000 drivers in males is three times the rate in females. Application of the decomposition method (Table 38-5)

TABLE 38-5

Decomposition of the Fatal Crash Involvement Rate Into Components (Age 16 years and Older, United States, 1990)

	Fatal Crash Involvement Rate	=	Case Fatality Proportion	×	Crash Incidence Rate	×	Driving Prevalence
	(Fatal Crashes per 10,000 Drivers)		(Fatal Crashes per 1000 Crashes)		(Crashes per Million Person-Miles)		(Average Annual Miles Driven per Driver in thousands)
	# Fatal crashes divided by #drivers	=	# Fatal crashes divided by #all crashes	×	#All crashes divided by #miles driven	×	#Miles driven divided by #drivers
Male	5.31		6.29		5.09		16.54
Female	1.73		3.20		5.68		9.53
Male:female	3.07		1.97		0.90		1.74

Reproduced with permission from Li G, Baker SP, Langlois JA, Kelen GD. Are female drivers safer? An application of the decomposition method. *Epidemiology*. 1998;9(4):379-384.

demonstrated that this excess results from two sources: males drive more than females (gender ratio of 1.7) and males have more fatal crashes per 1000 crashes than females (gender ratio of 2.0).[37] This suggests the potential for tailoring road safety messaging to address risk factors for crashes among males.

To date, the public health significance of the decomposition method has been largely underappreciated. However, the relevance of the decomposition method is likely to grow in the future, as advances in technology facilitate the capture of novel activity-time data. An example is the use of GPS signals from smartphones to capture data on movement and mobility.

SPECIAL CONSIDERATIONS IN STUDY DESIGN AND ANALYSIS

Injury epidemiology has unique features that raise issues pertinent to epidemiologic study design and analysis. Here we summarize some of these issues.

Interrupted Time Series Designs

Injury epidemiologists are frequently interested in assessing the effects of various laws and regulations. Interrupted time series designs are a useful method for quantifying the effect of state, regional, municipal, or institutional policy change. For example, researchers have studied whether laws requiring cigarettes to be self-extinguishing ("firesafe" cigarette laws) prevent residential fire deaths,[52,53] whether laws limiting access to firearms reduce firearm-related mortality,[54] and whether laws limiting alcohol sales reduce alcohol-related motor vehicle crashes.[55] Note that policy can be defined and modified at a level of healthcare facilities, prisons, neighborhoods, workplaces, and local municipalities. However, in the United States, analyses of state-level legislation are particularly germane in the field of injury epidemiology.

Quasi-experimentation[56] is a term that refers to cohesive set of observational designs that can be used to examine the effects of policy change (see Chapter 28). Quasi-experiments typically involve an aggregated and longitudinal ("time series") set of measurements of an injury outcome, *e.g.*, the rate of housefire death per 100,000 population per year per state. The strongest types of quasi-experiments combine time series from multiple locations (*e.g.*, cities or states), some of which experienced a policy change ("interruption") while others did not. The interrupted time series design is a common means of analyzing quasi-experimental surveillance data.

As an example, a study of firesafe cigarette laws utilized the time series of the annual rate of housefire deaths for all 50 states and DC from 2000 to 2010.[53] The "interruption" variable (main exposure) was the date of implementation of firesafe cigarette legislation in each state. States that passed firesafe cigarette laws during 2000 to 2010 contributed both unexposed prelegislation person-time and exposed postlegislation person-time to the analysis. States that did not pass a firesafe cigarette law during 2000 to 2010 contributed only unexposed time.

Important threats to validity in an interrupted time series analysis[56] include (1) heterogeneity between the geographical units and (2) unmeasured temporal trends and other unmeasured changes over time. For example, nationally there is linearly decreasing trend in housefire mortality[57] and failing to account for such a trend could create bias from temporal confounding. Therefore, a key challenge in interrupted time series analysis is to remove temporal sources of bias, without inducing bias by over-controlling and masking intervention effects.[58]

An additional consideration in any evaluation of policy change is obtaining access to data on implementation intensity and compliance with the new policy. Such data can help identify areas in which the policy change was implemented with greater rigor. For example, enforcement of firesafe cigarette laws in some states involved purchasing cigarettes from randomly selected retailers and laboratory testing to ensure cigarettes met the new self-extinguishing standard. Incorporating implementation data into interrupted time series models can help evaluate whether greater intensity of enforcement is associated with a stronger protective effect.

Cluster-Randomized Trials

Some injury and violence interventions operate or are delivered at an aggregate level, rather than at an individual level, making random assignment of individual interventions impossible. Cluster-randomized studies are trials in which randomization occurs at an aggregate level (see Chapter 6), such as when an intervention program is delivered or operates at a community level.

As an example, Coker et al.[59] developed a campus-wide sexual violence prevention program focused on changing social norms around interpersonal violence in colleges and universities. This program was designed to be implemented campus-wide, and therefore randomization had to occur at the level of the institution, rather than at the level of the individual student. As another example, Gilchrist et al. examined the effect of a training program designed to prevent serious knee injuries in collegiate women's soccer.[60] Because the program was delivered within the context of a collegiate team's soccer practice, the trial had to be randomized by team, rather than by individual.

Cluster-randomization requires special considerations in the design, implementation, and analysis of the trial.[61-63] Typically, the size of a cluster-randomized trial will be larger than the size of an equivalent individual-randomized trial.[61,62] The statistical power for these trials is often estimated using the increase in variance associated with cluster-randomization, relative to a hypothetical version of the study in which individual-randomization was possible. This ratio is the "design effect" or DEFF in short. As DEFF increases, so does the required size for a cluster-randomized trial, relative to the same study with individual-level randomization. DEFF can be estimated as[61,62]

$$\text{DEFF} = 1 + \left(m_a - 1 \right) \rho$$

where $m_a = \sum m_i^2 / \sum m_i$, m_i is the size of each cluster and ρ is the intra-cluster correlation coefficient. Statistical analysis of cluster-randomized trials needs to account for the fact that treatment arm is assigned at an aggregate level but outcome is observed at a personal level. Methods for analysis of clustered data include generalized estimating equations and generalized linear mixed models. Cluster-randomized trials in injury epidemiology frequently are unblinded.

Cluster-Crossover Designs

The cluster-crossover study is a variation of the cluster-randomized design that is highly useful for injury research. In the cluster-crossover design, an environmental intervention is alternately installed and removed at a physical site location. This creates clustering by site over time.

This design cannot be used unless the exposure can be completely removed, *i.e.*, there are no "carryover effects" of the intervention. For example, Ranapurwala et al. randomly allocated, by day of the week, scuba divers on charter boats to the presence or absence of a predive safety checklist.[64] Sometimes the allocation to treatment arm may be systematic, rather than being random. As an example, Girasek et al. assessed the efficacy of safety and warning signs on exposure to drowning risks in a state park by placing and removing safety signs on altering weekends.[65] Statistical design and power considerations for this design are described by Giraudeau et al.[66] and Crespi.[67] The case-crossover design (see below) is the nonrandomized individual-level analog of this design.

Control Selection in Case-Control Studies

The choice of control selection strategy is an important aspect of designing a case-control study (see Chapter 8). As noted earlier in this chapter, a key conceptual breakthrough in the history of injury epidemiology was the separation of injury from event and the development of the Haddon Matrix.[26] It logically follows that, for a given series of injured cases, the investigator may choose to select controls that sample the population *at risk for the event* (pre-event controls) or may choose to select controls that sample the population *at risk for injury*, given that the event has occurred (event-phase controls).[49]

The choice of controls should be driven by the research question of interest. To illustrate, consider a case-control study of the protective effect of ski helmets.[68] Cases are a group of skiers who crashed while skiing and sustained a head injury. Suppose a researcher seeks to estimate whether wearing a ski helmet reduces the risk of head injury *while skiing*? In this case, the study base is all skiers. Accordingly, controls should be selected at random from the population of skiers who were using the same ski fields, at the same time, as the cases. We refer to these controls as sampled from the "pre-event" base, meaning that they are skiers, but do not need to have sustained a skiing crash to enter the study.

Suppose that another researcher seeks to estimate the effect for a related, but subtly different, scientific question: does wearing a ski helmet reduce the risk of head injury *in the event of a skiing crash*? In this case, the base is all skiing crashes, not all skiers. Controls should be selected at random from the population of skiing crashes that occurred on same ski fields, at the same time, as the cases. In other words, these controls are drawn from the "event phase" base. Note that the "event phase" base is a population of events (crashes), whereas the "pre-event" base is a population of people (skiers).

The two researchers are addressing two scientific questions that are distinct but complementary.[49] Neither one is wrong nor right. The first study is examining the total protective effect of the helmet to the skier. This is important because, although helmets are protective in crash event, they may also potentially precipitate crashes through reduced visibility or altered safety behavior.[68] The first study captures the net benefit of the helmet-wearing behavior. The second study, on the other hand, isolates the pure protective effect of the helmet *in a crash event*. This provides an important real-world observational analog to laboratory-based experimental testing of helmets.

Under some assumptions, the second study's controls can be used to answer the first study's research objective.[48] In other words, it is sometimes possible to extrapolate beyond the base from which the controls were selected to a broader population, by letting controls from one base serve as proxies for another base. This requires that the underlying exposure prevalence in the two bases (the underlying hypothetical cohorts from which the events or cases arose) be the same. As an example, a classic case-control study of the effectiveness of bicycle helmets in preventing head and face injury used head or face-injured bicyclists presenting in Seattle-area Emergency Department (EDs) as cases.[69] This study sampled control subjects from nonhead injuries presenting in the same EDs. Let us assume that the prevalence of helmet-wearing in these controls is a reasonable proxy for the prevalence of helmet-wearing in general cycling population. If this is true, then pre-event research questions can be answered using event-phase controls.[48,49] In the Seattle case-control study, the researchers verified this assumption by enrolling a second control group that sampled the general cycling population of Seattle cycleways. Results from the population-based control group were similar to those obtained using the ED-based control group.[69]

Case-Crossover Studies

Case-crossover studies are observational analogs to the randomized clinical cross-over trial. Subjects in case-crossover studies contribute both case (injury) and control (noninjury) time periods. The conceptual "units of analysis" in this design are not people, but periods of time that are nested within people (see Chapter 8). This study design is well suited to exposures that are intermittent and have an effect on risk that is immediate and transient and when the outcome is abrupt.[70] Thus, this design is highly applicable to epidemiologic studies of injury and violence. In fact, this design was used by injury researchers in the 1970s[34] before being formalized in the early 1990s.[71]

A number of variations of the design have evolved.[70] In the interests of brevity, this discussion focuses on the original design,[71] in which injured people would contribute case and control time periods. We refer to this design as the "classical" case-crossover study. One appealing aspect of this design is that subjects "serve as their own controls." Time-independent confounders (confounders that do not change over time) can therefore be assumed to be implicitly controlled.[70] Furthermore, a classical case-crossover study has the potential to considerably simplify study logistics. Injured subjects can be enrolled in clinical settings and contribute both case and control time periods, removing the need to locate control subjects. Additionally, if we can assume that the outcome does not affect the exposure, then control windows can be drawn from postinjury person-time, and control exposures can be obtained *after* the injured subject is enrolled in the study.[70] Logistically, this represents a major efficiency.

Case-crossover studies offer important advantages, but investigators who fail to note the limitations of this design run the risk of obtaining biased results. One frequent challenge in case-crossover studies is accurate exposure assessment. As with case-control studies, exposure data should be obtained in a manner that yields comparable data for cases and controls,[70,72] see also qualifications of this guidance in Chapter 8. In addition to accurate quantification of the *magnitude* of exposures, case-crossover studies also demand accuracy in measuring the *timing* of exposure. One means of overcoming this issue is to obtain exposure information from some automated or administrative source. Even then, challenges can still persist.

To illustrate this point, consider a Toronto case-crossover study of whether cellphone use while driving is associated with an increased risk of motor vehicle crash.[73] To obtain accurate data on cellphone use, the researchers obtained billing records from mobile phone carriers for drivers who reported crashes. This source provided accurate information on the timing of calls and their duration. However, the data on the timing of crashes was less accurate, since it depended on driver (or law enforcement) recall. Unfortunately, it is common to use one's phone immediately after a crash (*e.g.*, to summon emergency assistance or to report the crash). Misclassification of the relative ordering of events in time (a call following a crash that was misclassified as a call that preceded a crash) has the potential to introduce information bias that would spuriously create the illusion of a risk association.

Another frequent limitation relates to temporal confounders. Temporal confounding arises when exposed and unexposed time periods lack exchangeability due to the presence of a third factor that is temporally associated with both exposure and outcome. Let us assume that we are interested in the effect of marijuana consumption on driving crash risk. Further, assume that marijuana use is highly correlated in time with the use of alcohol, a known risk factor for crashing one's car. Isolating the time-dependent effect of marijuana use will require measuring and controlling for alcohol use as a covariate. If the two exposures are collinear (*i.e.*, marijuana users who drive tend to be intoxicated from alcohol), isolating the effect of marijuana use becomes difficult.

A third limitation pertains to the definition of the "hazard window," a key concept in case-crossover design.[70] The hazard window is the time period during which the risk of injury is elevated because of exposure. This window is not necessarily equivalent to the time of exposure. In general, exposures can elevate risk well after the exposure itself is gone, and the same is true in injury settings. For example, the excess crash risk associated with conducting a telephone conversation does not return to zero immediately following termination of the call. A residual risk "footprint" persists for some time after the call, due to postcall cognitive processing of the information exchange during the call. Bias can arise if the hazard window is too narrowly or too broadly defined. In practice, the hazard window must be hypothesized, and the hypothesis should take into account the duration, and shape over time, of any excess risk related to the exposure. Based on this hypothesis, the investigator can define the duration of case and control time periods.

A classical case-crossover study requires special formulas to estimate power, and the analysis uses stratified methods.[70] There are several variants of the classic case-crossover study (see Chapter 8). One useful variant, which is under-utilized in injury epidemiology, is the cluster-crossover[67] (see above).

Matched Designs

The previous sections on control selection and case-crossover studies noted the logistical efficiency of using control data obtained from comparison groups composed of injured individuals. A related topic is the use of matched designs, which are discussed for cohort and case-control designs in Chapter 6. These cost-effective designs often use pre-existing data collected for administrative or surveillance purposes. Although these designs have mainly been applied in road safety research, they have also been applied to injuries from boxing and mixed martial arts,[74,75] where pair matching is inherent in the nature of the contest.

A major data resource for epidemiologists working in the area of road safety is the Fatal Analysis Reporting System (FARS). FARS is a census of all fatal motor vehicle crashes in the United States. It provides detailed data on the circumstances and events of these crashes, including environment, human, and vehicular details. While FARS represents a rich source of "case" data, it provides limited "denominator data" on vehicles and individuals not involved in fatal crashes. Matched designs have been used to overcome this limitation, by making use of the fact that FARS includes complete information on both decedents and nondecedents involved in these fatal crashes. Unlike boxing matches, vehicle crashes may involve more than two occupants, allowing for N to M matching of N decedents with M nondecedents.

In studies assessing factors influencing injury severity and occupant survival (*e.g.*, seatbelt use and seating), the idea underlying the application of matched designs to FARS data is that nondecedents in fatal crashes essentially provide a sample from the underlying population of all motor vehicle occupants. These designs either make use of the data on other occupants of the same motor vehicle,[35] or the other vehicles that were involved in the same crash.[76] In addition to being an efficient use of pre-existing data, such designs also have potential to implicitly control for crash and/or vehicles characteristics, such as crash speed or make and model of a vehicle.[77] However, caution is required, since bias can result if researchers do not appreciate the importance of potential confounders such as seating position within the vehicle.[78]

METHODOLOGIC CHALLENGES

Some areas of injury and violence epidemiology pose methodologic challenges. Below we highlight a few of those challenges.

Unintentional Injury

The topic of *sports-related concussion* has seen enormous scientific progress over the past two decades, partially due to the advent of large-scale multisite studies in this area.[79,80] Such studies, in part, resulted in a surge in public recognition of the problem and led to a call for the establishment of a national surveillance system for youth sports-related concussion.[81] However, there remains a pressing need for high-quality epidemiologic studies that define the short-term and long-term neurologic sequalae of concussion. Additionally, in both research and clinical settings, concussion identification largely relies on athlete self-report of symptomology. Better methods for identification of concussion are urgently needed.

In the field of *road safety*, fatality rates have trended steadily downwards for decades in high income countries. However, pedestrians in the United States have been experiencing rising fatality rates.[82] The United States lacks a national system for tracking pedestrian travel and exposure to motor vehicles, hindering research in this area. Law enforcement and transportation officials collect data on traffic crashes in each state, and probabilistic data linkage is used to integrate injury details and health outcomes with these crash records.[83] However, this linkage is not universally established and ongoing in all 51 US jurisdictions, creating gaps in knowledge of nonfatal injury outcomes from motor vehicle crashes. Globally, epidemiologists and others have championed the incorporation of system perspectives into research studies, prevention programs, and transportation planning decisions.[84,85] This approach has contributed to reductions in traffic fatalities in many developed countries but has not yet been widely adopted in the United States.[86]

Violence

Gender-based violence is a conceptual framework that unifies multiple forms of violence (sexual assault, partner violence, adolescent dating violence) and provides a linkage between injury and non-injury issues (such as sexual harassment and human trafficking).[87] Recent randomized trials demonstrate that gender-based violence is amenable to behavioral interventions that modify the cultural constructs and social norms that undergird violence.[14,88,89] Methodologic development is needed to lay the groundwork for large-scale trials of these interventions. As an example, it remains unclear how to best evaluate intervention programs that educate and support bystanders to intervene on sexual assaults and/or recognizable events that precede sexual assaults. The metrics for evaluating such programs, and methods for measuring these metrics, require methodologic development.[90]

The United States has higher rates of *firearm-related homicide and suicide* than most other developed countries.[91] Unfortunately, political lobby groups have limited federal funding for public health action and epidemiologic research in this area.[92-94] Recently, growing public concern over mass casualty events in public settings (such as schools) has resulted in increases in research funding, but the federal support for research remains small relative to the total magnitude and burden of firearm-related violence.[95,96] As a result, there is a dearth of studies of risk and protective factors that could inform intervention development and evaluation of legislative and regulatory approaches.[93] As with road safety, law enforcement and health data sources are frequently disconnected from one another, limiting the potential for addressing analytical research questions using pre-existing data sources.

Structural racism acts through deep-rooted direct and indirect mechanisms to generate profound disparities in the risk of violence. There is a need to strengthen the evidence base for addressing these disparities by incorporating measures of racial inequalities into violence prevention research. There is also a need for study designs that use mixed methods and other techniques to document racial inequalities in the events and pathways that lead to violence perpetration and victimization.

Cross-Cutting Topics

Over the past two decades, the rate of *opioid-related overdose* has steadily risen in the United States.[97,98] Between 1999 and 2018, opioids were involved in nearly 450,000 deaths in the United States.[97] The initial escalation derived from excessive prescribing of prescription opioids stemming from manipulation of pain management practice by United States pharmaceutical companies. Over time, the epidemic evolved to include heroin[99] and illicit fentanyl[100] from international sources. From a research perspective, response to the opioid epidemic has been hampered by the limited surveillance for fatal and nonfatal overdose events in the United States.[101] Ascertaining overdose deaths can be complex, costly, and time-consuming, particularly when toxicological testing is involved. As a result, both vital statistics data and analytical epidemiologic studies have lagged the rapidly evolving epidemic by several years, forcing federal agencies to formulate policy guidelines[102] based on information that was not timely[103] and studies that have methodologic limitations.[104,105] In response to the escalating deaths, all states have established prescription drug monitoring programs. However, the limits imposed on sharing of these data for research purposes have hindered efforts to provide more timely and comprehensive population-based studies.

Injury surveillance data provide descriptive information that is critical for informing prevention efforts. These data are also a rich source of epidemiologic data for researchers, particularly when used in combination with other databases. The past 50 years have seen tremendous growth in the number and sophistication of injury surveillance systems in the United States, including those addressing emergency department-attended injuries,[106] fatal motor vehicle crashes,[107] homicide and suicide,[108] opioid overdose,[109] and sports injuries.[110] Going forward, there is an ongoing need for innovation and evolution in injury surveillance systems, partly in response to the technological and information changes in modern society. Crowdsourcing of surveillance systems using social media platforms presents new opportunities to engage communities in both data collection and prevention-focused action using the tools of community-based participatory research and community mobilization.[111,112] Despite advancements in modern informatics, and technological advances in the platforming data in an interactive manner, much of our nation's injury and violence surveillance data remains inaccessible to nonacademic audiences.

FUTURE DIRECTIONS IN INJURY AND VIOLENCE RESEARCH

The field of injury epidemiology will continue to evolve in the coming years. There are three areas that offer important potential to transform the landscape of injury epidemiology.

First, research on physical injury and psychological trauma is converging. Traditionally, injury epidemiologists have focused on physical injuries while psychological trauma (*e.g.*, adverse childhood experiences and post-traumatic stress disorder) has traditionally been studied by psychologists and psychiatrists. In recent years, the boundary between physical injury and psychological trauma has become increasingly blurred, as we have come to understand the intersectionality of these domains to the survivors of injury and violence. The convergence of the two fields will likely foster interdisciplinary collaboration and growth.

Second, violence is increasingly recognized by the general public as a public health problem and has become a priority area in injury epidemiology. Violence results from behaviors involving intimidation or physical force intended to do harm. Physical injury resulting from violence, *i.e.*, intentional injury whether self-inflicted or assaultive, is an integral part of the domain of injury epidemiology. Violence as a behavior, however, has traditionally been seen as an area of interest for behavioral scientists, sociologists, and criminologists. More recently, growing numbers of epidemiologists are active in this area. The politically charged polemic concerning firearms in the United States has hindered epidemiologic research on firearm-related injuries for decades, in part through severe limitations in research funding.[92-94] The growing impact of mass casualty events, particularly those in elementary and high schools, has stimulated research investment in this area by private foundations and has led to renewed interest in this topic from federal funding agencies. Integration with community-based violence prevention efforts will help expand the scope of injury epidemiology and further strengthen its role in public health.

Finally, the opioid epidemic represents an unprecedented challenge for injury epidemiology. As noted above, the opioid epidemic was initially driven by overconsumption and misuse of prescription opioids and subsequently fueled by surges in illicit opioids, in particular, heroin and fentanyl. Since 2009, drug overdose has overtaken motor vehicle crashes to become the leading cause of injury mortality in the United States (Figure 38-1). In 2017, the US federal government

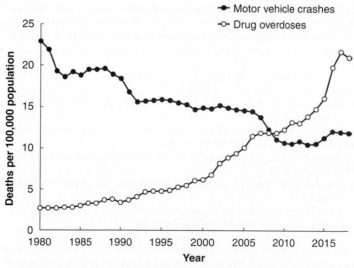

FIGURE 38-1 Annual death rates from motor vehicle crashes and drug overdoses in the United States, 1980 to 2017. (Data from National Center for Health Statistics [NCHS], US Centers for Disease Control and Prevention. See NCHS Data Briefs No. 81 and No. 329.)

declared the opioid epidemic a national public health emergency, paving the way for the deployment of substantial financial and other resources to control this man-made crisis. Injury epidemiologists, particularly those working at the US Center for Disease Control and Prevention, have played an instrumental role in monitoring and intervening on the opioid epidemic. Responding to this national public health emergency presents both a challenge to, and an opportunity to bolster, the foundations of injury epidemiology.

References

1. Li G, Baker SP. Epidemiologic methods. In: Li G, Baker SP, eds. *Injury Research: Theories, Methods, and Approaches*. New York, NY: Springer; 2012:203-220.
2. Frost WH. Some conceptions of epidemics in general (Lecture at Harvard University on February 2, 1928). *Am J Epidemiol*. 1976;103(2):141-151.
3. Haddon W Jr. Energy damage and the ten countermeasure strategies. *J Trauma*. 1973;13(4):321-331.
4. Waller JA. *Injury Control: A Guide to the Causes and Prevention of Trauma*. Lexington, MA: Lexington Books; 1985.
5. National Research Council. *Understanding Violence against Women*. Washington, DC: National Academies Press; 1996.
6. Butts JA, Roman CG, Bostwick L, Porter JR. Cure violence: a public health model to reduce gun violence. *Annu Rev Public Health*. 2015;36:39-53.
7. Slutkin G, Ransford C, Zvetina D. How the health sector can reduce violence by treating it as a contagion. *AMA J Ethics*. 2018;20(1):47-55.
8. World Health Organization. *Injuries and Violence: The Facts 2014*. Geneva, Switzerland: WHO. 2014. Report No. 9241508019.
9. James SL, Castle CD, Dingels ZV, et al. Global injury morbidity and mortality from 1990 to 2017: results from the global burden of disease study 2017. *Inj Prev*. 2020:Published Online First: 24 April 2020. doi: 2010.1136/injuryprev-2019-043494.
10. Zonfrillo MR, Spicer RS, Lawrence BA, Miller TR. Incidence and costs of injuries to children and adults in the United States. *Inj Epidemiol*. 2018;5(1):37.
11. National Center for Injury Prevention and Control. *10 Leading Causes of Death by Age Group, United States, 2018*. Atlanta, GA: Centers for Disease Control and Prevention. Available at https://www.cdc.gov/injury/wisqars/LeadingCauses.html. 2020. Accessed Janury 15, 2020.
12. Global Burden of Disease 2017 DALYs and HALE Collaborators. Global, regional, and national disability-adjusted life-years (DALYs) for 359 diseases and injuries and healthy life expectancy (HALE) for 195 countries and territories, 1990-2017: a systematic analysis for the Global Burden of Disease Study 2017. *Lancet*. 2018;392(10159):1859-1922.
13. Fortson BL, Klevens J, Merrick MT, et al. Preventing child abuse and neglect: A technical package for policy, norm, and programmatic activities. Atlanta, GA: Division of Violence Prevention, National Center for Injury Prevention and Control, Centers for Disease Control and Prevention; 2016.
14. Niolon PH, Kearns MC, Dills J, et al. *Preventing Intimate Partner Violence across the Lifespan: A Technical Package of Programs, Policies, and Practices*. Atlanta, GA: Division of Violence Prevention, National Center for Injury Prevention and Control, Centers for Disease Control and Prevention; 2017.
15. David-Ferdon C, Vivolo-Kantor AM, Dahlberg LL, Marshall KJ, Rainford N, Hall JE. *A Comprehensive Technical Package for the Prevention of Youth Violence and Associated Risk Behaviors*. Atlanta, GA: Division of Violence Prevention, National Center for Injury Prevention and Control, Centers for Disease Control and Prevention; 2016.
16. Armstrong DB, Bauer WW, Dukelow DA. Accident prevention—an essential public health service. *Am J Public Health Nations Health*. 1945;35(3):216-218.
17. Godfrey ES. Role of the health department in the prevention of accidents. *Am J Public Health Nations Health*. 1937;27(2):152-155.
18. Press E. Epidemiological approach to accident prevention. *Am J Public Health Nations Health*. 1948;38(10):1442-1445.
19. Gordon JE. The epidemiology of accidents. *Am J Public Health Nations Health*. 1949;39(4):504-515.
20. King BG. Accident prevention research. *Public Health Rep*. 1949;64(12):373-382.
21. Baker SP. Injury science comes of age. *J Am Med Assoc*. 1989;262(16):2284-2285.
22. Gibson JJ. The contribution of experimental psychology to the formulation of the problem of safety – a brief for basic research. In: Jacobs HH, ed. *Behavioral Approaches to Accident Research*. New York, NY: Association for the Aid of Crippled Children; 1961.
23. Ryan C. *Sonic Wind: The Story of John Paul Stapp and How a Renegade Doctor Became the Fastest Man on Earth*. New York, NY: Liveright; 2015.

24. Haddon W Jr. A note concerning accident theory and research with special reference to motor vehicle accidents. *Ann N Y Acad Sci.* 1963;107:635-646.

25. Baker SP, Haddon W Jr. Reducing injuries and their results: the scientific approach. *Milbank Mem Fund Q Health Soc.* 1974;52(4):377-389.

26. Haddon W Jr. Advances in the epidemiology of injuries as a basis for public policy. *Public Health Rep.* 1980;95(5):411-421.

27. Hemenway D. Building the injury field in North America: the perspective of some of the pioneers. *Inj Epidemiol.* 2018;5(1):47.

28. Holcomb RL. Alcohol in relation to traffic accidents. *J Am Med Assoc.* 1938;111(12):1076-1085.

29. Haddon W Jr, Valien P, Mc CJ, Umberger CJ. A controlled investigation of the characteristics of adult pedestrians fatally injured by motor vehicles in Manhattan. *J Chronic Dis.* 1961;14:655-678.

30. Li G, Baker SP, Smialek JE, Soderstrom CA. Use of alcohol as a risk factor for bicycling injury. *J Am Med Assoc.* 2001;285(7):893-896.

31. Baker SP, O'Neill B, Haddon W Jr, Long WB. The injury severity score: a method for describing patients with multiple injuries and evaluating emergency care. *J Trauma.* 1974;14(3):187-196.

32. Warner M, Chen LH. Surveillance of injury mortality. In: Li G, Baker SP, eds. *Injury Research: Theories, Methods, and Approaches.* New York, NY: Springer; 2012:2-22.

33. Wintemute GJ, Kraus JF, Teret SP, Wright MA. Death resulting from motor vehicle immersions: the nature of the injuries, personal and environmental contributing factors, and potential interventions. *Am J Public Health.* 1990;80(9):1068-1070.

34. Wright P, Robertson L. Priorities for roadside hazard modification. *Traffic Eng.* 1976;46:24-30.

35. Perneger T, Smith GS. The driver's role in fatal two-car crashes: a paired "case-control" study. *Am J Epidemiol.* 1991;134(10):1138-1145.

36. Li G, Chihuri S, Brady JE. Role of alcohol and marijuana use in the initiation of fatal two-vehicle crashes. *Ann Epidemiol.* 2017;27(5):342-347.e341.

37. Li G, Baker SP, Langlois JA, Kelen GD. Are female drivers safer? An application of the decomposition method. *Epidemiology.* 1998;9(4):379-384.

38. Goldstein GP, Clark DE, Travis LL, Haskins AE. Explaining regional disparities in traffic mortality by decomposing conditional probabilities. *Inj Prev.* 2011;17(2):84-90.

39. Li G, Baker SP. Exploring the male-female discrepancy in death rates from bicycling injury: the decomposition method. *Accid Anal Prev.* 1996;28(4):537-540.

40. Chen LH, Warner M. Surveillance of injury morbidity. In: Li G, Baker SP, eds. *Injury Research: Theories, Methods, and Approaches.* New York, NY: Springer; 2012:23-44.

41. Committee on Trauma Research. *Injury in America: A Continuing Public Health Problem.* Washington, DC: National Academies Press; 1985.

42. Langley JD. The need to discontinue the use of the term "accident" when referring to unintentional injury events. *Accid Anal Prev.* 1988;20(1):1-8.

43. Kraus JF, Anderson BD, Mueller CE. The effectiveness of a special ice hockey helmet to reduce head injuries in college intramural hockey. *Med Sci Sports.* 1970;2(3):162-164.

44. Robertson LS, Kelley AB, O'Neill B, Wixom CW, Eiswirth RS, Haddon W Jr. A controlled study of the effect of television messages on safety belt use. *Am J Public Health.* 1974;64(11):1071-1080.

45. Waller PF, Stewart JR, Hansen AR, Stutts JC, Popkin CL, Rodgman EA. The potentiating effects of alcohol on driver injury. *J Am Med Assoc.* 1986;256(11):1461-1466.

46. Runyan CW. Using the Haddon matrix: introducing the third dimension. *Inj Prev.* 1998;4(4):302-307.

47. Runyan CW. Introduction: back to the future—revisiting Haddon's conceptualization of injury epidemiology and prevention. *Epidemiol Rev.* 2003;25(1):60-64.

48. Cummings P, Rivara FP, Thompson DC, Thompson RS. Misconceptions regarding case-control studies of bicycle helmets and head injury. *Accid Anal Prev.* 2006;38(4):636-643.

49. Marshall SW. Injury case-control studies using "other injuries" as controls. *Epidemiology.* 2008;19(2):277-279.

50. Kerr ZY, Roos KG, Djoko A, et al. Epidemiologic measures for quantifying the incidence of concussion in national collegiate athletic association sports. *J Athl Train.* 2017;52(3):167-174.

51. Dellinger AM, Langlois JA, Li G. Fatal crashes among older drivers: decomposition of rates into contributing factors. *Am J Epidemiol.* 2002;155(3):234-241.

52. Bonander C, Jakobsson N, Nilson F. Are fire safe cigarettes actually fire safe? Evidence from changes in US state laws. *Inj Prev.* 2018;24(3):193-198.

53. Yau RK, Marshall SW. Association between fire-safe cigarette legislation and residential fire deaths in the United States. *Inj Epidemiol.* 2014;1(1):10.

54. Sivaraman JJ, Ranapurwala SI, Moracco KE, Marshall SW. Association of state firearm legislation with female intimate partner homicide. *Am J Prev Med.* 2019;56(1):125-133.

55. Villaveces A, Cummings P, Koepsell TD, Rivara FP, Lumley T, Moffat J. Association of alcohol-related laws with deaths due to motor vehicle and motorcycle crashes in the United States, 1980-1997. *Am J Epidemiol.* 2003;157(2):131-140.

56. Kontopantelis E, Doran T, Springate DA, Buchan I, Reeves D. Regression based quasi-experimental approach when randomisation is not an option: interrupted time series analysis. *Br Med J*. 2015;350:h2750.

57. Kegler SR, Dellinger AM, Ballesteros MF, Tsai J. Decreasing residential fire death rates and the association with the prevalence of adult cigarette smoking—United States, 1999-2015. *J Saf Res*. 2018;67:197-201.

58. Ranapurwala SI. Identifying and addressing confounding bias in violence prevention research. *Curr Epidemiol Rep*. 2019;6(2):200-207.

59. Coker AL, Bush HM, Fisher BS, et al. Multi-College bystander intervention evaluation for violence prevention. *Am J Prev Med*. 2016;50(3):295-302.

60. Gilchrist J, Mandelbaum BR, Melancon H, et al. A randomized controlled trial to prevent noncontact anterior cruciate ligament injury in female collegiate soccer players. *Am J Sports Med*. 2008;36(8):1476-1483.

61. Klar N, Donner A. Current and future challenges in the design and analysis of cluster randomization trials. *Stat Med*. 2001;20(24):3729-3740.

62. Campbell MJ, Donner A, Klar N. Developments in cluster randomized trials and Statistics in Medicine. *Stat Med*. 2007;26(1):2-19.

63. Donner A, Klar N. Pitfalls of and controversies in cluster randomization trials. *Am J Public Health*. 2004;94(3):416-422.

64. Ranapurwala SI, Denoble PJ, Poole C, Kucera KL, Marshall SW, Wing S. The effect of using a pre-dive checklist on the incidence of diving mishaps in recreational scuba diving: a cluster-randomized trial. *Int J Epidemiol*. 2016;45(1):223-231.

65. Girasek DC. Evaluating a novel sign's impact on whether park visitors enter a dangerous river. *Inj Epidemiol*. 2019;6:46.

66. Giraudeau B, Ravaud P, Donner A. Sample size calculation for cluster randomized cross-over trials. *Stat Med*. 2008;27(27):5578-5585.

67. Crespi CM. Improved designs for cluster randomized trials. *Annu Rev Public Health*. 2016;37:1-16.

68. Mueller BA, Cummings P, Rivara FP, Brooks MA, Terasaki RD. Injuries of the head, face, and neck in relation to ski helmet use. *Epidemiology*. 2008;19(2):270-276.

69. Thompson RS, Rivara FP, Thompson DC. A case-control study of the effectiveness of bicycle safety helmets. *N Engl J Med*. 1989;320(21):1361-1367.

70. Maclure M, Mittleman MA. Should we use a case-crossover design? *Annu Rev Public Health*. 2000;21:193-221.

71. Maclure M. The case-crossover design: a method for studying transient effects on the risk of acute events. *Am J Epidemiol*. 1991;133(2):144-153.

72. Wacholder S, McLaughlin JK, Silverman DT, Mandel JS. Selection of controls in case-control studies. I. Principles. *Am J Epidemiol*. 1992;135(9):1019-1028.

73. Redelmeier DA, Tibshirani RJ. Association between cellular-telephone calls and motor vehicle collisions. *N Engl J Med*. 1997;336(7):453-458.

74. Bledsoe GH, Hsu EB, Grabowski JG, Brill JD, Li G. Incidence of injury in professional mixed martial arts competitions. *J Sports Sci Med*. 2006;5(CSSI):136-142.

75. Bledsoe GH, Li G, Levy F. Injury risk in professional boxing. *South Med J*. 2005;98(10):994-998.

76. Cummings P, Rivara FP. Car occupant death according to the restraint use of other occupants: a matched cohort study. *J Am Med Assoc*. 2004;291(3):343-349.

77. Cummings P, McKnight B, Weiss NS. Matched-pair cohort methods in traffic crash research. *Accid Anal Prev*. 2003;35(1):131-141.

78. Cummings P, Wells JD, Rivara FP. Estimating seat belt effectiveness using matched-pair cohort methods. *Accid Anal Prev*. 2003;35(1):143-149.

79. Register-Mihalik JK, Guskiewicz KM, Marshall SW, et al. Methodology and implementation of a randomized controlled trial (RCT) for early post-concussion rehabilitation: the Active Rehab study. *Front Neurol*. 2019;10:1176.

80. Broglio SP, McCrea M, McAllister T, et al. A national study on the effects of concussion in collegiate athletes and US military service academy members: the NCAA-DoD Concussion Assessment, Research and Education (CARE) Consortium structure and methods. *Sports Med*. 2017;47(7):1437-1451.

81. Institute of Medicine and National Research Council. *Sports-Related Concussions in Youth: Improving the Science, Changing the Culture*. Washington, DC: The National Academies Press; 2014.

82. National Highway Traffic Safety Administration. *Traffic Safety Facts 2013 Data — Pedestrians*. Washington, DC: U.S. Department of Transportation; 2015. Publication DOT-HS-812-375.

83. Sauber-Schatz EK, Thomas AM, Cook LJ. Motor vehicle crashes, medical outcomes, and hospital charges among children aged 1-12 Years - crash outcome data evaluation system, 11 states, 2005-2008. *MMWR Surveill Summ*. 2015;64(8):1-32.

84. Naumann RB, Kuhlberg J, Sandt L, et al. Integrating complex systems science into road safety research and practice, part 1: review of formative concepts. *Inj Prev*. 2020;26(2):177-183.

85. Ludvigsson JF, Stiris T, Del Torso S, Mercier JC, Valiulis A, Hadjipanayis A. European Academy of Paediatrics Statement: Vision zero for child deaths in traffic accidents. *Eur J Pediatr*. 2017;176(2):291-292.

86. Evenson KR, LaJeunesse S, Heiny S. Awareness of vision zero among United States' road safety professionals. *Inj Epidemiol*. 2018;5(1):21.

87. Russo NF, Pirlott A. Gender-based violence: concepts, methods, and findings. *Ann N Y Acad Sci*. 2006;1087:178-205.

88. Coker AL, Bush HM, Cook-Craig PG, et al. RCT testing bystander effectiveness to reduce violence. *Am J Prev Med*. 2017;52(5):566-578.

89. Basile KC, DeGue S, Jones K, et al. *STOP SV: A Technical Package to Prevent Sexual Violence*. Atlanta, GA: Division of Violence Prevention, National Center for Injury Prevention and Control, Centers for Disease Control and Prevention; 2016.

90. Bush HM, Bell SC, Coker AL. Measurement of bystander actions in violence intervention evaluation: opportunities and challenges. *Curr Epidemiol Rep*. 2019;6(2):208-214.

91. Global Burden of Disease Injury Collaborators. Global mortality from firearms, 1990-2016. *J Am Med Assoc*. 2018;320(8):792-814.

92. Kellermann AL, Rivara FP. Silencing the science on gun research. *J Am Med Assoc*. 2013;309(6):549-550.

93. Sacks CA. In memory of Daniel—reviving research to prevent gun violence. *N Engl J Med*. 2015;372(9):800-801.

94. Hemenway D. *Private Guns, Public Health*. Ann Arbor, MI: University of Michigan Press; 2017.

95. Spitzer SA, Staudenmayer KL, Tennakoon L, Spain DA, Weiser TG. Costs and financial burden of initial hospitalizations for firearm injuries in the United States, 2006-2014. *Am J Public Health*. 2017;107(5):770-774.

96. Cunningham RM, Ranney ML, Goldstick JE, Kamat SV, Roche JS, Carter PM. Federal funding for research on the leading causes of death among children and adolescents. *Health Aff (Millwood)*. 2019;38(10):1653-1661.

97. Wilson N, Kariisa M, Seth P, Smith H IV, Davis NL. Drug and opioid-involved overdose deaths—United States, 2017-2018. *MMWR Morb Mortal Wkly Rep*. 2020;69:290-297.

98. Scholl L, Seth P, Kariisa M, Wilson N, Baldwin G. Drug and opioid-involved overdose deaths—United States, 2013-2017. *MMWR Morb Mortal Wkly Rep*. 2019;67(5152):1419.

99. Rudd RA, Paulozzi LJ, Bauer MJ, et al. Increases in heroin overdose deaths—28 states, 2010 to 2012. *MMWR Morb Mortal Wkly Rep*. 2014;63(39):849.

100. Gladden RM, Martinez P, Seth P. Fentanyl law enforcement submissions and increases in synthetic opioid–involved overdose deaths—27 states, 2013-2014. *MMWR Morb Mortal Wkly Rep*. 2016;65(33):837-843.

101. Slavova S, Delcher C, Buchanich JM, Bunn TL, Goldberger BA, Costich JF. Methodological complexities in quantifying rates of fatal opioid-related overdose. *Curr Epidemiol Rep*. 2019;6(2):263-274.

102. Dowell D, Haegerich TM, Chou R. CDC guideline for prescribing opioids for chronic pain—United States, 2016. *J Am Med Assoc*. 2016;315(15):1624-1645.

103. Ward PJ, Rock PJ, Slavova S, Young AM, Bunn TL, Kavuluru R. Enhancing timeliness of drug overdose mortality surveillance: a machine learning approach. *PLoS One*. 2019;14(10):e0223318.

104. Ranapurwala SI, Naumann RB, Austin AE, Dasgupta N, Marshall SW. Methodologic limitations of prescription opioid safety research and recommendations for improving the evidence base. *Pharmacoepidemiol Drug Saf*. 2019;28(1):4-12.

105. Staffa J, Meyer T, Secora A, McAninch J. Commentary on "Methodologic limitations of prescription opioid safety research and recommendations for improving the evidence base. *Pharmacoepidemiol Drug Saf*. 2019;28(1):13-15.

106. National Center for Injury Prevention and Control. *Web-based Injury Statistics Query and Reporting System (WISQARS)*. Atlanta, GA: Centers for Disease Control and Prevention. Available at https://www.cdc.gov/injury/wisqars/index.html. 2020. Accessed January 15, 2020.

107. National Highway Traffic Safety Administration. *Fatality Analysis Reporting System (FARS) Analytical User's Manual, 1975-2018*. Washington, DC: US Department of Transportation;2019. Report DOT-HS-812-827.

108. Blair JM, Fowler KA, Jack SPD, Crosby AE. The national violent death reporting system: overview and future directions. *Inj Prev*. 2016;22(suppl 1):i6-i11.

109. Hargrove SL, Bunn TL, Slavova S, et al. Establishment of a comprehensive drug overdose fatality surveillance system in Kentucky to inform drug overdose prevention policies, interventions and best practices. *Inj Prev*. 2018;24(1):60-67.

110. Ekegren CL, Gabbe BJ, Finch CF. Sports injury surveillance systems: a review of methods and data quality. *Sports Med*. 2016;46(1):49-65.

111. Ising A, Proescholdbell S, Harmon KJ, Sachdeva N, Marshall SW, Waller AE. Use of syndromic surveillance data to monitor poisonings and drug overdoses in state and local public health agencies. *Inj Prev*. 2016;22(suppl 1):i43-i49.

112. Dasgupta N. "He is the object of information": the intersection of big data and the opioid crisis. *Am J Public Health*. 2018;108(9):1122-1123.

CHAPTER 39

Social Epidemiology

Jay S. Kaufman

WHAT IS SOCIAL EPIDEMIOLOGY?

Social epidemiology is the study of relations between social factors and disease in populations. It may be broadly interpreted to subsume differential occurrence of any risk factor or health outcome across groups categorized according to any of a number of socially defined dimensions. Primary among the axes of social distinction in contemporary Western societies are race/ethnicity, gender, and socioeconomic class/position.[1,2] Social epidemiology therefore embraces a large number of questions about exposures and outcomes, and indeed one might question whether there is any epidemiology that is *not* social epidemiology. The practical distinction appears to be that social epidemiology is characterized by explicit inclusion of social, economic, or cultural quantities in the exposure definition or the analytic model, or by explicit reference to social science theory in the interpretation.[3] Therefore, any exposure-disease relation can be studied from the point of view of social epidemiology to the extent that the relation is modeled in light of social variation in the quantities under study or interpreted in the context of a social theory or sociohistorical paradigm such as "social stratification," "urbanization," or "colonialism."[4]

As in all of epidemiology, there are at least three distinct types of scientific activity, all well represented in the social epidemiologic literature: (1) surveillance, (2) prediction, and (3) etiologic inference. In surveillance, we seek to describe accurately what the real world looks like. A typical social epidemiologic example describes the racial and social class distribution of coronary disease.[5,6] Although we often seek to generalize beyond an observed sample, the purpose is entirely descriptive. The focus is on occurrence of an outcome, perhaps in relation to a scaled axis—such as time, age, or social class—but without regard to a specific exposure. The epidemiologic quantity of interest is generally a frequency measure itself, such as prevalence or incidence, rather than a causal effect contrast.

In prediction exercises, the goal is not the description of the current landscape, but forecasting how the target condition will evolve over time, extrapolating or modeling into the future. An example is projecting the racial/ethnic disparities in cardiovascular mortality that will be observed in the United States in 2030 based on current demographic trends.[7] This sort of estimate requires modeling under specified assumptions, but again, no explicit exposure intervention contrast is considered.

The third class of epidemiologic activity is etiologic inference, in which one seeks to understand the causal relation between a defined exposure and outcome, or the mechanistic pathway through which this effect occurs. This analysis is designed not to describe the world as it exists, but rather how it would change under some unambiguous hypothetical intervention.[8] A typical social epidemiologic example estimates the causal effect of socioeconomic status on mortality and how much of this effect is relayed through measured health behaviors.[9] Despite the many philosophic and methodologic dilemmas associated with causal inference, etiologic investigations constitute the bulk of published work in social epidemiology. This result follows naturally from the fact that epidemiology is situated within the larger domain of public health, a disciplinary identity that fixes population intervention as the primary focus of research and practice.[10]

CAUSATION AND CONFOUNDING IN SOCIAL EPIDEMIOLOGY

Because a causal effect is defined on the basis of contrasts between potential outcomes under distinct intervention regimens, many authors have argued that we must immediately exclude nonmanipulable factors, such as individual race/ethnicity and gender, from consideration as causes in this sense.[8,11] This conclusion does not imply that a construct such as race/ethnicity is not a valid focus of social epidemiologic research, only that the study design and analytic approach must correspond to a substantively meaningful conceptualization of the exposure and of the hypothesized intervention. For example, the effect of a patient's racial classification on a clinician's diagnostic judgment is a well-defined causal quantity because the exposure can be physically manipulated in a real or imagined experiment.[12] In contrast, the effect of a patient's racial classification on that same patient's risk of incident coronary disease is more vague as a causal exposure, since this quantity has no unambiguous interventional analogue. Nonetheless, even within causal models, nonmanipulable quantities such as race/ethnicity and gender can be employed sensibly as stratification variables or effect-measure modifiers.[13] They may be also be adjusted for as confounders in order to reduce error in the estimated exposure effects of interest.[14] When a racial/ethnic health disparity is the focus of research, the manipulable intermediates that explain this disparity may also be modeled causally.[15,16]

Common modifiable exposures of interest in social epidemiology include factors such as income, education, and housing. Although the observed values of these exposures usually result from complex interactions of social stratification and individual volition, they are potentially modified through public policy via governmental programs of income supplementation, educational loans, and housing assistance. Etiologic interest then lies in the contrast between outcome distributions under various intervention regimens that fix the level (or distribution) of the exposure in the target population.[17] For example, consider binary outcome $Y = 1$, defined as an incident asthma attack within the period of observation, and the social exposure of interest, defined as residence in privately owned housing ($X = 1$) versus residence in a public housing project ($X = 0$) during a defined exposure period. A simple generalization would allow X to represent the proportion of the population assigned to privately owned housing, rather than just the extremes of 1 and 0.[18] One causal effect of housing type on asthma would be the contrast (*e.g.*, difference, ratio) between the average risks of an asthma attack in the target population during the specified time period if all households were assigned to public housing versus if all were assigned to private housing, $\Pr[Y = 1|\text{Set}(X = 1)]$ versus $\Pr[Y = 1|\text{Set}(X = 0)]$.

Confounding arises when the associational measure in the source population, $\Pr(Y = 1|X = 1)$ versus $\Pr(Y = 1|X = 0)$, does not correspond to the effect measure that would be observed under hypothetical manipulations of the social exposure in that population, actively setting X rather than passively observing X (Chapter 12). For example, the hypothesis of a causal relation between housing type and asthma attacks is plausible, but subject-matter knowledge suggests other influences on this health outcome from quantities—such as poverty—that also potentially influence residential housing type. This prior knowledge implies that some part of the empirical association observed between housing type and incident asthma attack may arise not from the causal link between them, but rather from their mutual response to other material or psychosocial manifestations of poverty. The crux of the problem in observational data is that we do not have the opportunity to assign any of the exposures to the population, and so we must employ the observed quantities in some way to estimate more validly the causal effect of interest.[19]

The traditional epidemiologic solution is to condition on measured aspects of poverty status. The logic behind this strategy is that within the categorizations of poverty (e.g., poor and nonpoor if poverty is dichotomous and homogeneous within categories), there can be no confounding by this quantity.[20] To the extent that we have enumerated and accurately measured a sufficient set of common causes of exposure and outcome, this conventional solution is adequate for the specification of the desired causal effect from observational data in point-exposure studies.[21] Indeed, this strategy for the estimation of causal effects dominates epidemiologic analysis of observational data and has enjoyed some undeniable success. For social exposures, however, this strategy seems much less realistic, because the enumeration and accurate measurement of common causes for multifactorial disease outcomes and complex behaviors such as residential housing choices is a daunting task. Behaviors with dominating economic and social inputs have often proven quite difficult to model in the social sciences.[22] Even if we know all the factors that determine where a person would choose to live, the task of obtaining accurate measures of these many variables in a real dataset is formidable. For example, one must decide on some measurable characterization of "poverty" in the preceding example, by obtaining reported information on a limited number of material factors considered likely to influence both housing type and exposure to other causes of an asthma attack.

To surmount this challenge, social epidemiologists have long relied on social theory to construct realistic causal diagrams,[23] but increasingly turn to econometric methods or other identification strategies that do not rely on covariate sufficiency.[24] These include natural experiments that approximate random assignments and instrumental variable methods that seek at least some component of exogenous variation in the exposure to leverage, replacing the need for measured confounders with other structural assumptions that may be more credible in specific circumstances[25] (Chapter 28). This new trend has led to a diverse and dynamic subfield, with ongoing and vociferous disagreements about theory, methods, and inferences. As psychology, sociology, economics, and other social science and humanistic disciplines intersect with social epidemiology, they each imprint their distinctive traditions and perspectives. Some embrace this methodological plurality,[26] while others decry a surfeit of associations dressed up as evidence of causality on the basis of little more than wishful thinking.[27] Social epidemiology continues to evolve rapidly, with a panorama that looks radically different from the one that prevailed just a decade ago.

EXPOSURE AND COVARIATE ASSESSMENT IN SOCIAL EPIDEMIOLOGY

Social epidemiology is characterized primarily by the nature of the exposures that are investigated, and techniques for defining and measuring exposures and covariates are therefore a major component of social epidemiologic methodology. Throughout the history of the subfield, measurement has involved a wide array of constructs. The majority of studies have considered exposures related in some way to the primary axes of social discrimination cited previously: race/ethnicity, gender, and social class/position. But many other studies have explored alternative quantities at the individual level, such as marital status, material deprivation, social support, or status incongruity. Additionally, many social epidemiologic exposures have also been defined at the aggregate level, including constructs such as social networks, economic inequality, social capital, and neighborhood deprivation. Not only have a staggering number of diverse exposures been considered, many of these have in turn been defined and assessed in myriad different ways across a multitude of studies. Some representative and popular methodologic approaches are described in the following.

Social Factors Defined and Measured at the Individual Level

Race/Ethnicity

Racial/ethnic status is central to personal and social identity in cosmopolitan societies and serves as an important determinant of material and social status as well as influencing social networks, residential patterns, and behaviors. Although race and ethnicity are ostensibly designated in terms of ancestry and physical characteristics, the nature of these quantities as aspects of personal identity means that ultimately the "gold-standard" assessment is based on self-report.[28] Although analysis of highly variable regions of DNA can now apportion continental ancestry with considerable accuracy,[29] this is not the quantity of social epidemiologic interest. The dominating influences on life chances and social status arise not from biologic ancestry, but rather from the racial/ethnic categorization perceived by others, and as a consequence, adopted by the individual as a foundation for social affiliation and self-definition.

The continual evolution of racial and ethnic categorizations and their administrative management is itself a methodologic morass.[30] Epidemiologic studies in the United States have traditionally accepted the binary classification system of "white" and "black" that reflects the history of slavery and de jure segregation in these terms. More recently, categorization has generally followed definitions established for administrative purposes by the US government for census data and other demographic monitoring.[31,32] For the year 2000 US census, respondents were for the first time permitted to report two or more racial identities, leading to 63 possible combinations of six basic racial categories: American Indian and Alaska Native, Asian, Black or African American, Native Hawaiian and Other Pacific Islander, White, and "Some Other Race." In addition, individuals could define their ethnicity as Hispanic or non-Hispanic.[33] The situation is even more complicated globally, where a chaotic plethora of variations exist in racial or ethnic nomenclature and categorization.[34,35] Study of racial and ethnic variation has been further complicated in recent years by the advent of molecular methods that estimate components of continental ancestry, and which are increasingly used in studies to classify participants continuously by ancestry rather than categorically by self-defined race or ethnicity.[36]

Sex/Gender

As in the case of race/ethnicity, gender serves as an important determinant of social, environmental, and material circumstances in all human societies and is therefore a key quantity in any social epidemiologic analysis as a covariate, effect-measure modifier, or stratification variable.[37] Although gender is the social expression of biologic sex, which is ostensibly designated in terms of genotypic and phenotypic traits, its implications and manifestations are highly dependent on culture and therefore vary substantially with time and place.[38] Nonetheless, common practice for assessment of gender is self-report into a binary categorization, although recent decades have witnessed the increasing tendency to refer to this quantity more accurately as "gender" as opposed to "sex." Both theoretical work and increased awareness of substantial natural variability in physiology and behavior have also led to growing recognition that this traditional dichotomy is a convenient fiction originating in historical convention.[39,40] Recent developments in social epidemiology have also seen increasing focus on sexuality as a distinct concern beyond sex and gender, and their intersection with race/ethnicity.[41]

Educational Attainment

Level of achieved education is one of the oldest and most commonly used social epidemiologic quantities and has the practical advantages of having a naturally ordered scaling and a value that is often fixed early in adult life and reported consistently. The widespread use of this quantity also derives from its presence in a great variety of administrative databases and other common data sources. Educational attainment also has substantive relevance as a mechanism for achievement of social position, as it facilitates advantageous behaviors and occupational advancement and is therefore highly predictive of income and wealth.[42]

Nonetheless, the variable also has several disadvantages, both practical and theoretical. Typical educational attainment and the economic and social benefits that accrue as a result have changed over time, so comparison between age cohorts or across geographic regions is difficult.[43] Similar incommensurabilities also complicate comparisons across gender and racial/ethnic groups.[44] There are also inherent discontinuities in the education scale corresponding to completion of degrees and certifications.[45] For example, completion of an additional year of high school beyond 10th grade may confer little social advantage, whereas completion of an additional year beyond 11th grade may confer substantial advantage. This distinction leads some analysts to categorize education according to these milestones—for example, into three categories corresponding to less than, equal to, or greater than 12 years of education, which a common standard for secondary school diploma. Given the uncertain connection between educational content and years of schooling, as well as the overriding socioeconomic significance of degree completion, the graded relationship that is observed for many health outcomes with years of completed education may be interpreted as evidence of the endogenous assignment of years of schooling as a function of family resources and other personality and environmental factors.[46]

Annual Individual or Family Income

Annual individual income is a key variable in social epidemiologic analyses for the obvious reason that health is a commodity in market economies, and therefore financial resources are logically expected to have a causal effect on health outcomes. Income also functions, like education, as a sensitive marker of social position and therefore as an indicator not only of financial resources but also of status and its social and material consequences, such as access to institutions and connections to individuals with power and influence.[47] Unlike attained education, income is fluid over time and is therefore more responsive to changes in status over the life-course. Potentially dynamic patterns of annual income also present an analytic challenge, however, especially for measuring the status and resources of the retired.[48] Changing income over the life-course also makes it sensitive to "reverse causality"; whereas low income facilitates negative health transitions, it is also true that failing health lowers earnings.[49] Indeed, the volatility of annual income itself has been an exposure of interest, under the hypothesis that drastic changes in financial resources, such as those associated with job loss or divorce, may be more salient for health outcomes.[50]

Measurement of income is often by self-report in surveys, although the data may also be drawn secondarily from administrative records.[51,52] For self-reported data, the data are often queried in broad categories in order to minimize respondent discomfort. Even so, item nonresponse for income is considerably higher than for education or occupation, with more than 20% often declining to answer.[53] Use of empirical categories may limit the ability to compare studies if these categorization boundaries differ, but the implications of absolute income values are contextually dependent in any case, so comparison across populations may often be tenuous, even for studies with common categorizations. For statistical analysis, natural-log transformation of income is often warranted because of the rightward skew of the distribution and the observation that effects on health outcomes appear more log-linear than linear.[54] Nonlinearity in this relation is intuitively reasonable, because income changes are inherently relative: A change of $1,000 has a much bigger impact on someone who is destitute than it does on a millionaire.

Because families tend to share both material resources and social prestige, it is common practice to assess not individual income, but rather household income.[55] This quantity could be construed to subsume all financial compensation received during the relevant period, including paid employment and value of employee benefits. Survey respondents may need to be specifically directed to consider less obvious sources of income, including Social Security payments, capital gains from sales of assets, interest and dividends received, receipt of rent payments, child support and alimony payments, and receipts from government aid programs. Measurement error can be substantial, and the error cannot be assumed to be uncorrelated with the true value.[56] The ascertained value may often be scaled to the number of people relying on the specified income, although "economies of scale" exist such that the accounting for family size might not involve a simple division.[57]

A related concept is "poverty," a state of insufficient income to meet basic material needs. This designation is a dichotomization of household income on the basis of some assessment of what is a minimally sufficient quantity for sustaining the dependent individuals. The determination of this value has been controversial. In the United States, it has relied heavily on a method devised in 1963 by an economist at the Social Security Administration.[58] This definition was revised in 1969 to allow the threshold to be linked to the Consumer Price Index and has been subject to further incremental modifications in subsequent years. The definition accounts for household income, household size, and ages of individuals in the household, creating 48 distinct threshold values. Although many critics maintain that the definition remains inadequate, it has remained a fixture of US government and public health statistics for four decades.[59] In addition to modeling income as a continuous quantity or as a dichotomy at the poverty line, this definition also allows each income to be modeled in proportion to the poverty line with respect to the specific household size and composition, solving the problem of having to scale the income to the number of people supported. On the other hand, poverty thresholds remain undefined for many individuals outside of households, including those in prisons, nursing homes, college dormitories, and military barracks.

Household Wealth

Whereas income represents a flow of material resources to an individual or family, wealth represents the accumulated stock of these resources and therefore has relevance to health outcomes as both an indicator of achieved social position as well as a measure of the total resources that can be mobilized in the service of health and well-being. Lower levels of assets also make individuals and families vulnerable to income fluctuations and to periods of unemployment that disrupt health insurance coverage.[60] Incommensurabilities between income and wealth are particularly striking when comparing men and women, or when comparing racial/ethnic groups.[61] For example, models that contrast outcome risks between racial/ethnic groups while adjusting for income and education in order to control for social position leave the racial/ethnic contrast heavily confounded by wealth differences.[62,63]

Though traditionally absent from many health surveys, wealth data are now increasingly available, albeit often in the form of a few crude indicators. Whereas assets may exist in a variety of financial instruments (*e.g.*, stocks, bonds, retirement accounts) and material repositories (*e.g.*, home, vehicles, jewelry), the largest amount of wealth in the United States is held in the value of real estate and vehicles, comprising >50% of privately held assets in 2000.[64] Therefore, questions as simple as "Do you own your home?" can be quite informative for distinguishing low from high asset levels. Surveys that query the home value are even more useful in this regard, although respondents are unlikely to distinguish between home value and equity actually held. An increasing proportion of personal wealth is held in individual retirement accounts, stocks, and mutual fund shares, but survey protocols for the accurate collection of these data are laborious and exist in only a few large health surveys. Where these have been analyzed with respect to health outcomes, however, they have been shown to be highly predictive of endpoints, even after conditioning on education and income and other socioeconomic covariates.[63] Methodologic obstacles include the potential for substantial measurement error and item nonresponse, as well as the challenges posed by the large proportion of households with no assets, and the very extended right tail of the distributions. For example, median household assets for Blacks and non-Hispanic Whites in 2016 were $17,000 and $171,000, respectively, whereas mean household assets for the same two groups were $138,200 and $933,700.[66]

Occupation/Unemployment

Another historically important indicator of social class or social position has been an individual's current employment status, occupation, or occupational class. These measures provide not only an indication of social prestige and the functional consequences of education and social connections, but also a direct reflection of the circumstances relevant to health through the physical and psychologic environment of the workplace itself.[67] Many countries, such as the United Kingdom, continue to base their standard socioeconomic position measure on occupational class, as opposed to the education and income measures that dominate in the United States. The British Registrar General's Scale, used for almost 100 years, was a hierarchy of six categories: Social Class I (professional), Social Class II (intermediate), Social Class III-NM (skilled nonmanual), Social Class III-M (skilled manual), Social Class IV (partly skilled), and Social Class V (unskilled).[68] As of 2001, this schema has been revised to include eight categories, including a new category for the long-term unemployed, a subdivision of professionals into higher and lower managerial positions, and a change in terminology from "unskilled" to "routine" occupations.[69]

Previously in the United States, occupational categories were commonly combined with achieved educational level or other socioeconomic quantities to generate a summary socioeconomic index. Various of these indices, such as the one developed by Hollingshead, experienced periods of popularity in sociology and epidemiology,[70] although they are used to a much lesser extent in the contemporary epidemiologic literature. Among the most influential of these combined measures was the Duncan Socioeconomic Index (SEI), which required analysts to map all reported occupations onto US census occupation score codes, a laborious and often frustrating task because of the ambiguity of many self-reported job descriptions.[71]

Like income, occupation and employment status can by dynamic throughout the life-course, and therefore these measures share the advantages and disadvantages of this potential volatility, including the "reverse causality" of declining health leading to a diminution in occupational prestige. Occupation also shares the problem of incommensurability of prestige and remuneration across gender or racial/ethnic groups or across geographically distinct populations, as well as changes over time in the social and material significance of various occupations. Furthermore, occupational category is difficult to assign for individuals functioning outside of the wage economy, including unpaid domestic labor and those performing informal or illegal activities.[72]

One distinct conceptualization of occupation is as an indicator of economic relations between groups of people rather than as a measure of the characteristics of individuals considered in terms of a continuous social hierarchy. A contemporary operationalization of this approach is to categorize occupations in relation to the economic classes that define capitalist production.[73] This entails collection of information about power relations in the workplace, as well as the assets that allow craftspersons or artisans to control their own production, or managers to control the process of production involving larger groups of workers in factories or office blocks.

Discrimination and Racism

Whereas dimensions of individual identity such as race/ethnicity, gender, and sexual orientation are not manipulable through public health interventions, the consequences of these categories as social labels are entirely malleable and therefore have causal meaning as exposures in the sense described above.[14] The key distinction is that the causal quantity is not the identity of the individual per se, but rather the perception of this identity by others, and the role this perception plays in influencing the behavior of individuals and institutions that the person encounters.[74] Differential behavior of individuals and institutions on the basis of perceived social categorization is broadly described as "discrimination," including the forms of discrimination corresponding to specific dimensions of identity, such as "racism."[75]

Methodology for assessment of discrimination in surveys has most often focused on self-report of interpersonal affronts and experiences of perceived injustice.[76] An obvious limitation of this approach is that discrimination need not be perceived by the respondent in order to be consequential, and indeed, structural and institutional discrimination may often be invisible to the individual. One innovation to achieve greater sensitivity in this regard is to query individuals not about their own experiences, but rather about the experiences faced by others who share their identity.[77]

Another approach is to use experimental or quasi-experimental designs to isolate the effect of perceived identity on the decision-making of an individual or institutional process. For example, "audit studies" of medical or economic encounters, such as referral for surgical procedures or application for employment, involve comparison of cases matched (observationally or experimentally) on individual characteristics with the exception of social category of interest (usually race and/or gender) in order to isolate the causal effect of perceived group membership on the decision process.[78,79] When real subjects are matched on observed covariates, the possibility exists that imbalance persists in unmeasured attributes.[80] When actors are used in place of real subjects, or when case vignettes or medical charts or job applications are artificially created to be completely identical except for the group identifier, then the causal discrimination effect is directly identifiable.[81]

Stress

The social epidemiology of the 20th century was dominated by a psychosocial paradigm in which most effects were thought to operate through affective states such as anger and stress. The field was led largely by researchers with formation in psychology and sociology, and maintained strong connections to psychosomatic theories in physiology and medicine.[82] Indeed, the classic theories of 20th century psychosocial epidemiology were constructs such as type A behavior,[83] stress,[84] and the demand-control dimensions of job strain.[85] The highly influential Whitehall Study in Great Britain, for example, took an overtly psychologistic stance on the social gradient among civil servants, arguing that the perception of a lower social rank was enough to drive physiological responses.[68,86] This dominance of psycho-physiological theories led to some backlash in the 21st century, as materialists argued for a greater attention to economic factors operating in pathways other than affective status.[87] Nonetheless, psychosocial epidemiology remains alive and well as a subfield, focused on the measurement of affective states and their implications for population health.[88]

The study of affective states and their impact on health includes both transient emotions and more stable personality types and is often situated in a life-course perspective. Measurement is often influenced by a voluminous literature in psychology, including experimental and observational work in animals, such as the seminal work of Sapolsky on the health implications for social status in primates.[89] Assessment has traditionally been accomplished with self-reported scales, such as the widely used Cohen Stress Scale.[90] Recently, attention has shifted to trying to find biomarkers of stress response, to avoid the inconvenience and potential error of self-report. For stress response, one popular possibility has been measurement of plasma or salivary cortisol,[91] but research has been plagued by difficulties in assessment and interpretation, for example, wide intra-individual variation in measured values.[92] To date, no consensus has emerged on a biomarker approach to assessment of psychological stress that addresses these concerns.[93]

Social Support

From the same psychosocial epidemiology tradition that focused on affective states came a robust literature oriented around connections to others, broadly subsumed under various notions of "social support."[94] This literature has a strong theoretical foundation in both psychology and sociology, for example, the work of Émile Durkheim. The classic era of psychosocial epidemiology in the 1970s led by scholars such as John Cassel, Sidney Cobb, and Leonard Syme prioritized epidemiologic investigation into the buffering role of social networks in avoiding or alleviating stress.[95] The seminal paper by Berkman and Syme from 1979, which examined survival as a function of number of social ties, has now been cited almost 7,000 times.[96] Social connection was long understood to operate through instrumental and emotional pathways, leading to a diversity of constructs, measures, and techniques. Indeed, a recent review by Berkman and Krishna[97] notes over 50 distinct scales and indices. The contemporary literature has prioritized social network analysis as one potent and robust analytic approach to describing the pattern of social connections and their specific arrangements.[98] But related concepts of social isolation, social integration, and aspects of social functioning probe the quality of these ties, not only their number or pattern. The concept of social support blends readily into the broader health psychology literature on the salubrious impact of positive psychological states,[99] but it should also be remembered that people with greater social connections can also face burdens, expectations, and other harmful consequences of their ties to others.[100]

Social Factors Defined and Measured at the Aggregate Level

A number of important quantities in social epidemiology are defined not at the individual or household level, but at the level of some larger aggregation, often neighborhoods, counties, states, or nations. Neighborhoods, in particular, have been of long-standing interest in social epidemiology,[101] despite the fact that no consensus on an operational definition for what constitutes a neighborhood has been achieved.[102] Because of the frequent dependence on routine census data for characterizing aggregations of individuals, administrative boundaries such as census block groups and tracts in the United States (and census enumeration districts in the United Kingdom) are the most widely used proxies for neighborhood boundaries, even though the locations of these boundaries are generally unknown to the inhabitants.

Deprivation

Just as the material resources of individuals and households characterize their socioeconomic position, a neighborhood's material resources may be used to characterize the community's degree of deprivation. These material resources may be aggregates of individual-level data, such as the average income or average educational level, or they may be resources that are defined only at the neighborhood level, such as population density, the presence of health clinics or sidewalks, the prevalence of broken windows or graffiti, or the magnitude of some summary quantity such as "social disorganization" or "neighborhood efficacy."[102] When summary scores are created from a number of social variables, factor-analytic or latent-variable methods are often employed in order to find weights for the component quantities.[103,104] Several scales have been defined in the literature and have gained widespread use, such as the Townsend and Carstairs deprivation indices that were developed in the United Kingdom, the EPICES score in France, or the Pampalon Index in

Canada.[105,106] The variables employed to characterize neighborhoods are most often those available from census and other administrative data, but direct observation of neighborhoods has also been employed in order to provide a richer assessment of the social and material environment.[107] Direct observation can be expensive and time-consuming, but recent innovations in image processing have suggested ways to automate this approach.[108]

Segregation

Residential segregation is a measure of the systematic physical arrangement of individuals with respect to some dimension of social identity, most often race/ethnicity, within communities or larger spatial units such as cities or counties.[109,110] Segregation emerges from a complex mix of factors, including voluntary choices and involuntary constraints such as discrimination in the housing market and economic barriers to mobility. Massey and Denton[111] identified 20 statistical indices of residential segregation and grouped these into five distinct dimensions: evenness, exposure, concentration, centralization, and clustering.

Evenness is simply the degree to which a minority group is distributed uniformly over space and can be assessed statistically by the dissimilarity index, which measures the percentage of the minority group's population that would have to change residence for each spatial unit to have the same percentage of that group as the population has overall, with the index ranging from 0 (no segregation) to 1 (complete segregation). An alternative index of evenness is the Gini coefficient, which is the average absolute difference between minority-group proportions weighted across all pairs of spatial units, expressed as a proportion of the maximum weighted average difference. The Gini coefficient also varies from 0 to 1. There are additional evenness measures, including Theil entropy (or information index) and the Atkinson index.[112]

Exposure is the dimension of segregation that pertains to the extent of potential contact or interaction between members of diverse social groups. Evenness and exposure are correlated but distinct, because unlike evenness measures, exposure measures take into account the relative sizes of the groups being compared. The two measures of exposure that were identified by Massey and Denton[111] represent the probability that a minority chosen at random will share a spatial unit with a majority person (interaction index) or another minority person (isolation index). When only two groups are considered, these two measures sum to unity.[113]

These evenness and exposure measures of segregation have been found to be more closely associated with health outcomes than other segregation domains defined by Massey and Denton.[114] Nonetheless, the other three dimensions are concentration, centralization, and clustering. Concentration describes the relative amount of physical space occupied by each social group. In considering two minority groups that have equal representation in the total population, the group that occupies the smaller physical space may be considered more highly segregated. One such measure is Hoover "delta," which represents the proportion of minorities in spatial units that have above-average density of minorities. The fourth dimension of segregation is centralization, which refers to the location of the minority population with respect to the geographic center of the larger area under consideration.[115] A relative measure of centralization represents the proportion of the minority population that would have to change spatial units in order to be distributed like the majority population, whereas an absolute measure of centralization considers the spatial distribution of the minority group alone, without reference to the majority group. Both relative and absolute measures range from -1 to 1, with negative numbers indicating residence distant from the geographic center of the larger area and positive numbers indicating residence near the center. The centralization dimension may be considered increasingly irrelevant, as megacities make a residential location in relation to a single geographic metropolitan center less significant. Finally, clustering is the dimension of segregation that represents whether or not minorities live in contiguous spatial units.[116] An absolute index of clustering measures the average number of minorities in adjacent spatial units as a proportion of the total denominator population of these units. Alternatively, a relative clustering measure compares the expected distance between any two minority individuals chosen at random with the expected distance between any two majority members chosen at random. Massey and Denton also proposed "distance-decay interaction" and "distance-decay isolation" measures, which represent the probabilities that the person a minority next encounters is also member of the majority or minority group, respectively.

Inequality

Residential segregation is merely one dimension of inequality, but the differential distribution of social and material resources in the society may be considered along any of a number of other dimensions as well. Greatest interest has centered on economic inequality—for example, the unequal distribution in a population of income or wealth. A research agenda relating economic inequality to population health has been a primary focus of social epidemiologic activity for the last two decades,[117,118] spurred in part by increasing levels of income and wealth inequality in industrialized societies since the 1970s. Whereas earlier papers focused on variation in income distribution between wealthy nations, the literature quickly expanded to include comparisons of smaller political entities such as states and provinces, as well as counties and metropolitan areas.[119] Studies have pursued a wide variety of health outcomes, with an emphasis on various measures of all-cause or cause-specific mortality risk. Most studies also adjusted for some measure of absolute wealth or poverty, such as per-capita income. This adjustment was motivated by the concern that if individuals with low incomes have higher risk of adverse outcomes and live disproportionately in areas with greater income inequality, then the causal effect of inequality may be confounded. This potential confounding has been described as a problem of disentangling the "compositional" from the "contextual" effects of income inequality and has led to widespread use of multilevel regression modeling in order to address this concern.[120,121] Nonetheless, misspecification of the model (*e.g.*, using linear regression though the true relationship is nonlinear) will still leave inequality and health outcomes associated, even if there is no true causal effect of inequality.[122]

Several popular measures of income or wealth inequality are derived from the well-known curve introduced by Lorenz in 1905.[123] To construct the Lorenz curve, rank-order the n individuals in the population according to the quantity of interest y—say, income—such that $y_1 \leq y_2 \leq y_3 \leq \ldots \leq y_n$, and pass through the population from smallest income value to largest value. The horizontal axis of the Lorenz curve measures the cumulative proportion of individuals passed at any point, $F(y)$, so it runs from 0 at the left to 1 at the right. The cumulative share of income accounted for by the ranked individuals, $\Phi(y)$, is similarly recorded on the vertical axis: as one reaches an income y_i while passing from left to right across the income values, the corresponding cumulative income proportion, p, held by the individuals to the left of y_i is plotted. The resulting graph of $F(y)$ versus $\Phi(y)$ is the Lorenz curve (Figure 39-1). Because the individuals are rank-ordered, the curve must always either lie along the 45° diagonal (in the case of perfect equality) or be strictly convex under the diagonal (if there is any inequality).

The Gini coefficient described in the previous section is the most common inequality measure, and it has the attractive property of being the proportion of the area under the diagonal that is above the Lorenz curve. Therefore, when there is perfect equality, this area disappears, and the Gini coefficient is 0. When there is complete inequality (the richest unit y_n holds 100% of the income in the population), then 100% of the area under the diagonal is above the Lorenz curve, and the Gini coefficient equals unity. Despite its widespread use, the classic Gini coefficient has the notable

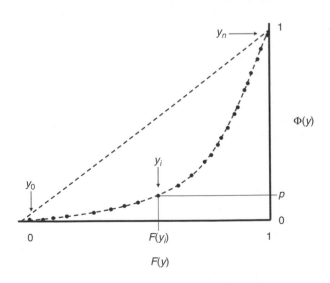

FIGURE 39-1 The Lorenz curve.

disadvantage that it entails differential weighting of transfers that occur at various locations in the distribution. For example, a transfer of a fixed amount of income that occurs between a richer and a poorer individual has a much larger effect on the Gini coefficient if the two individuals are near the center of the rankings than if they are at the extremes.[124] Some novel formulations of the Gini coefficient seek to overcome these limitations.[125]

A variety of other inequality measures have been applied in the social epidemiologic literature, and these are reviewed in detail in Harper and Lynch.[126] For example, the Robin Hood index is the maximum vertical distance between the 45° diagonal representing perfect equality and the Lorenz curve. This can be interpreted as the proportion of the total income in the population that would have to be transferred from individuals above the mean to individuals below the mean in order to achieve equality in the distribution of incomes. Computation of Atkinson index requires specification of a social-welfare constant representing the society's aversion to inequality. Theil entropy index was introduced in the late 1960s and is based on information theory. It is also derived from general measures of entropy through an explicit aversion parameter that, like Atkinson index, reflects some assumptions about social norms.

Finally, three rank-based indices are of growing importance in the literature of the past several decades: the concentration index, the slope index of inequality, and the relative index of inequality.[127] The concentration index is conceptually related to the Gini coefficient, representing the joint distribution of health outcome and social ranking.[128] Consider a population ordered by social status, rather than by health outcome. To obtain the concentration curve, plot the cumulative percent of the population on the horizontal axis against proportion of the population with the adverse health outcome on the vertical axis. The concentration index is then defined as twice the area between this curve and the horizontal line, ranging from −1 to 1, with perfect equality at 0.

The slope index of inequality (SII) and relative index of inequality (RII) are both regression-based measures, but on absolute and relatives scales, respectively.[129] The SII is obtained simply as the estimated slope coefficient from the linear regression of the health outcome on the social ranking variable. The ranking variable varies by definition from 0 to 1, so the estimated regression slope represents the change in the mean health outcome associated with moving from the lowest to the highest rank of the social distribution. Confusingly, there are two distinct formulations for the relative scale version, the RII. The first is to simply take the value of the fitted regression line at the highest rank and divide by the value of the fitted line at the lowest rank. The alternate method, which provides a distinct numerical value, is obtained by dividing the SII by the mean health value in the population.

Social Capital

Another characteristic of a community, neighborhood, or other natural aggregation of individuals is the level of "social capital": the totality of social organization, including networks and relationships of trust and obligation that function to the mutual benefit or detriment of the inhabitants.[130] This communitarian conceptualization, which dominates contemporary epidemiologic applications, is often attributed to work by Putnam, and contrasts with an alternate conceptualization attributed to Bourdieu that sees social capital primarily as an attribute of individuals.[131] According to the dominant interpretation of social capital in public health research, bonding between individuals and the bridging and linking of subgroups within the larger community act to produce society-wide attributes of collective trust and result in an elevated level of functionality and cohesion. Commensurate with this viewpoint, the common measures of social capital in health research have involved measures of civic participation such as voting or survey responses concerning the levels of membership in voluntary organizations and levels of reported "interpersonal trust."[132]

Closely linked to the concept of social capital is the study of social networks, which has established methodology within sociology and yet has been applied less consistently in public health research.[133] This analytic approach adopts a view of social capital more heavily influenced by Coleman, focusing on social structure and exchange of material and information. Related concepts can be found in earlier work in psychosocial epidemiology around constructs such as "social support" and "instrumental support," often based on scales summed from Likert-scale survey questions.[134] But in contrast to these earlier methods, analysis of social networks is at the aggregate level, considering the structure of the links between individuals in the population and how they function to transmit information, material assistance, or even infectious agents.[135] Networks are represented as directed arcs between nodes, which give rise to parameters such as density, centralization, and clustering (or segmentation) and facilitate statistical modeling for static or dynamic networks, such as decision-making structures, patterns of mutual assistance, or sexual relationship structures.[136] Notably, social network analysis explicitly permits the potential responses of a unit to an exposure to depend on the treatments assigned to other units, thus allowing violations of the noninterference assumption invoked in most applications of potential-outcome models.[137] Such analyses require significantly greater investment in data collection, but they are obviously better suited to the task of providing realistic models of social phenomena than are the static, individually focused survey questions of past eras.[138]

ANALYTIC APPROACHES

Multilevel Modeling

Alongside the growth of quantitative social epidemiology over the past 30 years, multilevel regression modeling emerged as an intimately related statistical technique. This marriage of method and application arose in the early 1990s with roughly coincident revolutions in theory and technology. The theoretical revelation was that social epidemiology could not move forward without explicit accounting for hierarchical structures, a need articulated forcefully by Susser's metaphor of "Chinese boxes."[139] The "Chinese boxes" paradigm was intended to extend the traditional epidemiologic "black box" to encompass multiple and nested levels of organization, from the molecular to the individual to the societal. On the technological side, the innovation was the advent of regression methods for clustered data in popular statistical software, with rapid progress in the 1980s and 1990s in the development and implementation of both random-coefficient and population-average models. Early work by Mason et al.[140] introduced these methods to sociology, although it was another decade or more before they became common in social epidemiologic applications.[141]

The term *multilevel model* is now used so broadly as to include any statistical technique that accommodates clustered data, but the random-coefficient model became the common form in social epidemiologic applications.[142,143] Regression is the most popular statistical technique for conditioning on multiple covariates without creating sparse cells. But standard model-fitting methods assume independent observations, an assumption that will be false under study designs such as cluster randomized trials or cohort studies with repeated measures, or when data are collected at several levels of a natural hierarchy, such as individuals within neighborhoods. If, after control of covariates, the cluster variable (such as neighborhood) still predicts the outcome, then an analysis that ignores this variable will produce biased variance estimates for estimated coefficients of neighborhood-level predictors, and therefore lead to invalid tests and intervals (Chapter 24).

To illustrate the multilevel concept, consider continuous outcomes Y_{ij} for $i = 1,\ldots, n$ individuals living in $j = 1,\ldots, m$ neighborhoods, where Y is normally distributed within each neighborhood with mean β_{0j} and variance σ^2. The random-coefficient concept applied to the intercept, or "random-intercept model," assumes that the neighborhood-specific means β_{0j} can also be described by a random distribution of known form—for example, that they are normally distributed with mean γ_{00} and variance τ_{00}. These assumptions give rise to a two-level model:

$$Y_{ij} = \beta_{0j} + \varepsilon_{ij} \left(\text{Level 1} \right)$$

$$\beta_{0j} = \gamma_{00} + \mu_{0j} \left(\text{Level 2} \right)$$

where $\varepsilon_{ij} \sim N(0, \sigma^2)$, $\mu_{0j} \sim N(0, \tau_{00}^2)$, and $\text{COV}(\varepsilon_{ij}, \mu_{0j}) = 0$.

The combined model, replacing β_{0j} in level 1 with its components from level 2, is:

$$Y_{ij} = \gamma_{00} + \mu_{0j} + \varepsilon_{ij}$$

which expresses each outcome as the sum of an individual deviation (ε_{ij}) and a neighborhood-specific deviation (μ_{0j}) from a grand mean (γ_{00}). This model is also known as a one-way random-effects ANOVA because it partitions variability into a component due to individuals (σ^2) and a component due to neighborhoods (τ_{00}^2). The relative contribution of the variance components to the total variance may be represented by the intraclass (or intracluster) correlation coefficient, the proportion of the variability in Y that occurs between neighborhoods, rather than between individuals within neighborhoods[142]:

$$\text{ICC} = \rho = \frac{\tau_{00}^2}{\sigma^2 + \tau_{00}^2}$$

Multilevel models can be expanded to include fixed-coefficient and random-coefficient terms at the individual level, at the neighborhood level, or both. A fixed coefficient takes the same value for all neighborhoods. For example, the model:

$$Y_{ij} = \beta_{0j} + \beta_1 X_{ij} + \varepsilon_{ij} \, (\text{Level 1})$$

$$\beta_{0j} = \gamma_{00} + \mu_{0j} \text{ and } \beta_1 = \gamma_{10} \, (\text{Level 2})$$

implies that the expected change in Y per unit increase in X is β_1 for all neighborhoods. A random coefficient for an individual-level covariate X, which allows a distribution of X effects rather than a single effect, could be modeled as:

$$Y_{ij} = \beta_{0j} + \beta_{1j} X_{ij} + \varepsilon_{ij} \, (\text{Level 1})$$

$$\beta_{0j} = \gamma_{00} + \mu_{0j} \text{ and } \beta_{1j} = \gamma_{10} + \mu_{1j} \, (\text{Level 2})$$

where $\mu_{0j} \sim N(0, \tau_{00})$, $\mu_{1j} \sim N(0, \tau_{11})$, and $\text{COV}(\mu_{0j}, \mu_{1j}) = \tau_{01}$.
One can also add neighborhood-level covariates to the level 2 equations:

$$\beta_{0j} = \gamma_{00} + \mu_{0j} Z_j + \mu_{0j} \text{ and } \beta_{1j} = \gamma_{10} + \gamma_{11} Z_j + \mu_{1j} \, (\text{Level 2})$$

This model implies cross-level product (interaction) terms between covariates X and Z, as well as a product between X and random effect μ_{1j}, as can be seen by replacing the coefficients in the level 1 model with their equations in the level 2 models to form a single combined equation:

$$Y_{ij} = \gamma_{00} + \gamma_{01} Z_j + \mu_{0j} + \left(\gamma_{10} + \gamma_{11} Z_j + \mu_{1j}\right) X_{ij} + \varepsilon_{ij}$$
$$= \gamma_{00} + \gamma_{01} Z_j + \gamma_{10} X_{ij} + \gamma_{11} Z_j X_{ij} + \mu_{1j} X_{ij} + \mu_{0j} + \varepsilon_{ij}$$

Therefore, according to this model, the effect of X on the outcome Y in a given neighborhood j will depend on the level of Z in that neighborhood and on the random effect (level 2 error term) μ_{1j}. For units with $Z = 0$, this random effect μ_{1j} is the deviation of the X effect in neighborhood j from the average X effect in all neighborhoods, γ_{10}. If only β_{0j} is treated as random, then the cross-level product involves only Z and X:

$$Y_{ij} = \gamma_{00} + \gamma_{01} Z_j + \mu_{0j} + \left(\gamma_{10} + \gamma_{11} Z_j\right) X_{ij} + \varepsilon_{ij}$$
$$= \gamma_{00} + \gamma_{01} Z_j + \gamma_{10} X_{ij} + \gamma_{11} Z_j X_{ij} + \mu_{0j} + \varepsilon_{ij}$$

For example, for binary X, the expected difference between exposed ($X = 1$) and unexposed ($X = 0$) groups is $(\gamma_{10} + \gamma_{11} Z_j)$, and so depends on the value of Z in neighborhood j.

This framework may be applied to generalized linear modeling. For example, for binary Y_{ij}, the level 1 model could be logistic while the level 2 models could remain linear. More than two levels can be used, although applications with three or more levels are uncommon in practice. Regardless of the model form or number of levels, however, a key point is that the regression coefficients in random-effects models represent within-cluster (*i.e.*, cluster-conditional) relations. In this respect, their interpretation parallels those in stratified analysis and ordinary regression. For example, in the ordinary linear model $Y = \beta_0 + \beta_1 X + \beta_2 Z + \varepsilon$, the coefficient β_1 in the fitted model is interpreted as the expected change in Y per unit change in X, *holding Z fixed*. Similarly, in a model with a random effect such as μ_{0j} in $Y_{ij} = \gamma_{00} + \beta_1 X_{ij} + \mu_{0j} + \varepsilon_{ij}$, the interpretation of β_1 is similarly conditional on all other variables in the model held constant including μ_{0j}, a neighborhood-specific quantity that is not directly observable. Rearranging the model as $Y_{ij} = (\gamma_{00} + \mu_{0j}) + \beta_1 X_{ij} + \varepsilon_{ij}$, it can be more readily seen that within neighborhood j, the regression of Y on X is linear with intercept $(\gamma_{00} + \mu_{0j})$ and X coefficient β_1. Note that this model assumes that the X coefficient is constant across neighborhoods. Considering the clusters as analysis strata, this assumption is just a regression version of the homogeneity (uniformity) assumption made by summary estimators such as Mantel-Haenszel. Interpreting β_1 causally, which requires absence of bias as well as correct specification of the model, this corresponds to assuming a uniform effect of X across clusters when effects are measured by estimated coefficients.

When a coefficient is treated as random, the cluster-specific estimates of effect are "shrunk" toward the mean value that corresponds to what would have been estimated had the coefficient been treated as fixed.[144] For example, consider again the simplest model with a random intercept, $Y_{ij} = \gamma_{00} + \mu_{0j} + \varepsilon_{ij}$. We observe neighborhood-specific sample means $\widehat{\beta}_{0j} = \overline{Y}_j$, as well as the observed marginal (total) sample mean $\widehat{\gamma}_{00} = \overline{Y}$. In a valid cohort study, the neighborhood-specific sample means are unbiased estimates of the population values of β_{0j}, but fitting the random-intercept model instead produces estimates that are biased by being "shrunk" toward the grand sample mean $\widehat{\gamma}_{00} = \overline{Y}$. The extent to which they are shrunk is a function of their precision: A neighborhood with many observations has a more stable estimate of its mean and therefore takes a value close to $\widehat{\beta}_{0j} = \overline{Y}_j$, whereas a neighborhood with fewer observations has a more unstable estimate of its population mean and therefore takes a value close to $\widehat{\gamma}_{00} = \overline{Y}$. The inverse-variance weighted average of these two values produces estimates that minimize mean-squared error (between the estimates and population means) and is also known as empirical-Bayes estimates.[145]

Frequently, the application of multilevel models in social epidemiology is oriented around the random-effects ANOVA interpretation, partitioning the variance that is due to community-level factors (contextual effects) from that due to individual-level factors (compositional effects). For example, the conditional level 2 variance τ_{00}^2 approaching 0, and thus ICC = 0, is generally considered to imply that differences in outcome means between communities are accounted for by the covariates included in the model. Nonetheless, omitted covariates can account for residual variability at either level. For example, there can be large effects of neighborhood characteristics even when ICC is small.[142] Furthermore, if ICC > 0 even after inclusion of individual-level characteristics, there is no logical way to assert that the residual between-neighborhood variability is therefore contextual in nature (*i.e.*, due to omitted neighborhood-level factors). Assertions of contextual effects should therefore be based on the estimated coefficients of measured neighborhood-level variables, rather than on variability that remains after individual-level variables have been included in the model.[146]

An important assumption of the multilevel model that is necessary for causal interpretation of the estimated coefficients is that there is no residual correlation between individual-level predictors and neighborhood-level random effects (*i.e.*, level 2 error terms), essentially an assumption of no-residual confounding. Interestingly, while concern over the validity of this assumption has preoccupied economists for decades,[147] it still receives considerably less attention in biostatistics and epidemiology. Econometricians generally test for violations of this assumption with a specification test and revert to a fixed-effects analysis if there is evidence of such a violation.[145] Another option is a hybrid model, in which a random intercept model is fit after centering the exposure or other covariates. This approach retains the greater efficiency of the random effects formulation while avoiding the bias from confounding between the exposure and the random effects.[148]

Marginal Models

The models described above describe the relation of Y to covariates among subjects *within* clusters and are therefore referred to as "subject-specific" or "cluster-specific" models. A different class of models, marginal models, considers the change in the mean of Y *across* clusters, and hence is labeled "population-average" or "marginal" models. Instead of entering cluster effects as random terms, these models account for cluster effects by introducing parameters for within-cluster correlations, and the most popular form of this model employs generalized estimating equations as the fitting method to allow for these correlations.

Marginal models can be viewed as multilevel insofar as they permit inclusion of predictors from both levels of aggregation. Unlike within-cluster models, however, they do not directly model distributions of effects across clusters.[149]

Suppose there are neighborhood effects beyond those captured by the modeled covariates, and one fits a model for the outcome that is neither linear nor log-linear (*e.g.*, a logistic regression model). In this case, the parameters and hence estimates from marginal models will tend to differ from the corresponding parameters and estimates from within-cluster models, especially if the outcome Y is binary and $Y = 1$ is common.[150] The difference between the within-cluster and population-average parameters is just a general case of the noncollapsibility phenomenon for odds ratios illustrated in Chapter 5, and like that phenomenon it can lead to great confusion of interpretation and usage. The choice of approach should follow from consideration of the causal question at hand, however. Within-cluster models are suitable for estimating the effect on Y of changes in X within clusters, albeit they may assume that those effects are homogeneous across clusters. In contrast, marginal models are suitable for estimating the effect on Y of a change in X in the total population (*i.e.*, the effect on the mean of Y of a unit change in X over all clusters), conditional on other covariates in the model. In this respect, marginal models are just generalizations of standardization.[151]

Life-Course SES Concepts

Another key social epidemiologic concept that has evolved rapidly over the past decades is the life-course model, which seeks to account for the dynamic trajectory of social exposures over the lifetime of the individual, rather than the simple cross-sectional association between adult social status and adult health that is so often modeled.[152] Interest in this model was spurred by accumulating evidence of social conditions in early life having an effect on adult risk for chronic disease, as posited, for example, by Barker hypothesis, which suggests that deprivation during the fetal or infant periods of life "programs" the individual to a higher level of susceptibility to cardiovascular and metabolic diseases in adulthood.[153] The life-course model soon expanded, however, to include not just a consideration of perinatal and adult conditions, but combinations, accumulation, and interactions of different conditions and experiences throughout all phases of life.

Several specific analytic models to address life-course effects have been described in the literature. A "latent effects" model focuses on early-life social exposures—for example, parental social position—often with control for adult social status. This latter control is motivated by an interest in estimating the direct effect of these early life conditions on later outcomes, ignoring the indirect effect that occurs because parental social position is a determinant of offspring's social position. Another conceptualization is a "pathway model" that focuses not merely on the direct effects of early-life deprivation, but rather on the total effects of this advantage by precipitating a "social chain of risk" or "life trajectory" in which one disadvantageous exposure predisposes to another through the life-course.[154] Sometimes this "life trajectory" total effect is modeled through a "social mobility model" in which the analysis considers contrasting patterns of upward or downward social movement, such as the contrast between those who are at a lower category of social position at each measured point in the life-course contrasted with those who rose from a lower category to a higher category, or alternatively from a higher category to a lower category. This analytic design allows the consideration of health selection (*i.e.*, sick individuals declining in their social position as a consequence of their illness) and of interaction between timepoints, such as in Forsdahl hypothesis that the joint exposure to early-life deprivation and adult overnutrition is a particularly potent determinant of cardiovascular disease.[155] The "social mobility" model may be contrasted with a "cumulative model" that, like the "pathway model" described previously, considers the total cumulative effect of deprivation throughout the life-course, without regard to critical periods or specific patterns of mobility.[156]

Experiments and Quasi-Experiments

Given the potential for strong confounding in observational social epidemiology, it is natural to consider randomized study designs. A number of successful randomized social interventions have been conducted and reported, such as the Moving to Opportunity (MTO) study, in which residents in poverty housing were randomly assigned to receive vouchers for nonpoverty housing.[51,52] Researchers may reap the benefits of randomization through a variety of designs other than traditional controlled experiments, however (Chapter 28). In particular, investigators may take advantage of a random assignment that is predictive of the exposure, even when the exposure of interest has not itself been randomly assigned. Educational attainment, for example, is hopelessly confounded by unmeasurable aspects of personality, ability, and environment, but a policy change that impacts educational attainment provides variation in the exposure that is not a function of these confounders. Banks and Mazzonna[157] therefore exploited a 1947 policy change that required English school children to be 1 year older before they could quit school, and thereby obtained an unconfounded estimate for the effect of education on cognitive ability. This technique is referred to as "instrumental variable analysis" and has a long tradition in econometrics.[158] In many other examples investigators have been able to find data in which nature had been so kind as to assign the exposure of interest in an essentially random fashion, as when researchers tested competing theories of social causation versus social selection in the etiology of child psychopathology by making use of a fortuitous financial windfall that affected a portion of the children in a longitudinal study.[159] In another example, investigators used the random distance between survey respondents and the epicenter of a 2010 earthquake in Chile to explore effects of the disaster on mental health.[160]

There are several variations on and extensions to the instrumental variable approach, including the regression discontinuity design.[161] The logic of this design is that when an arbitrary cutpoint is used to assign treatment, then individuals just slightly to one side or the other of this cutpoint are essentially randomized, and their confounding covariates are balanced in expectation. For example, to estimate the effect of HPV (human papillomavirus) vaccination on the sexual behavior of girls, researchers exploited a birthdate cutpoint of January 1 for entering children into kindergarten.[162] When a program of free, voluntary school-based vaccination was initiated for eighth grade girls, the difference between a girl ending up in seventh grade (no vaccine offered) or eighth grade (vaccine offered) for those girls born around January 1 was just the random chance of having been born a few days earlier or later, creating an essentially random split for those close to the cutpoint.

Another common variation on this theme is Mendelian randomization, in which a genetic variant or a polygenic risk score (*i.e.*, a collection of variants) is used as the instrumental variable.[163] The idea is that there is random assignment of the allele from the mother or from the father at the moment of conception, and that when a genetic variant affects an exposure of interest, this can therefore serve as an instrumental variable. The technique has been widely applied, but a major challenge in social epidemiology is that the effects of single polymorphisms on social exposures of interest tend to be very modest in magnitude, and therefore require huge sample sizes. In one recent social epidemiology example, this was surmounted by assembling a polygenetic score of over 1,200 variants for the prediction of educational attainment.[164] While this improves the prediction of the exposure and therefore the power of the instrumental variable analysis, it also raises doubts about potential violations of key assumptions, for example, that none of these many variants have any effects on outcomes except through their effects on education.[165]

A primary weakness of randomized designs is one of generalizability, because participants in trials usually differ from nonparticipants. For example, studying lottery winners may be an ideal way to estimate the effects of income supplementation because the winners and losers will differ only randomly with respect to potential confounders. Nonetheless, individuals self-select to be in the experiment by purchasing a lottery ticket, and so any generalization to a population that includes nonparticipants may be faulty.[166] Interpretation is further complicated because of "noncompliance," meaning that some participants elect not to adhere to their assigned treatment regimen, or if the random assignment changes the behavior of the participants in other ways besides the receipt of treatment of interest.[19] These problems can to some extent be addressed analytically if information on all those assigned is available, but often that is not the case. For example, if some lottery winners fail to claim their prizes, or if nonwinners become rich through some other means, this noncompliance generally introduces bias in the comparison of interest. This is because we could not expect noncompliance mechanisms such as losing the winning ticket or inheriting a windfall to be unassociated with confounding personality or socioeconomic traits, and we will not typically have any idea who in the population is noncompliant with their assignment or why.

In the case of randomized social interventions, changes in individual conditions may also affect the entire social context, thus violating the assumption made by most statistical methods that one individual's treatment does not affect others. This would be the case if an intervention such as randomly assigning individuals in poverty housing to receive vouchers for nonpoverty housing were to change the characteristics of the various neighborhoods involved in ways that would affect the outcomes.[167] There are numerous other limitations to the conduct and interpretation of randomized studies, especially for the complex interventions of interest to social epidemiology. Therefore, observational studies will undoubtedly remain a mainstay of social epidemiology.[19]

Narrative Historical Approach

The oldest and most widely used approach for examining the effect of social exposures on health is the one that is least often used by epidemiologists: the narrative historical approach. This method involves telling the story about exposures and outcomes in the specific sociohistorical context in which they actually occurred, rather than in the abstract and idealized context defined by statistical models. Narrative historical depictions can be quantitative, in that they may involve numerical summaries of what happened. They may involve causal assertions, in arguing that events are the results of specific conditions that, had these conditions not pertained, would have come out differently. What this method avoids, however, is the seductive generality of statistical models, the results of which are often described in universal terms, devoid of the specific context in which the data were realized. Narrative historical accounts also present causal assertions qualitatively as opposed to quantitatively, which avoids the illusion of numerical precision for observations that fall outside the realm of the observed data.[168]

For example, Braun and Kisting explored asbestos-related disease in South Africa in relation to work environment, labor policies, and racial inequality.[169] The arguments are quantitative, but no regression models are used and no statistical tests are conducted, and to the extent that causality is asserted, it is argued substantively rather than statistically. Many other deeply insightful and persuasive works of this nature have made great contributions to the social epidemiology of a variety of conditions, from ethnic disparities in diabetes[170] to the origins and dynamics of the opioid epidemic.[171] In some cases, statistical and historical accounts work side by side to illuminate the unique nuances that each paradigm can provide, as in the epidemiological and historical foundations of the John Henryism phenomenon.[172,173]

Regrettably, this approach appears to suffer a distinct lack of respect within epidemiology as a whole, as judged, for example, by the dearth of this sort of work in epidemiologic journals, which enforce formatting and length standards that are inconsistent with this methodology. Other social sciences recognize the narrative historical approach as an essential tool in understanding the complex relations between human social arrangements and their biologic consequences.[174] If social epidemiology is to thrive in the 21st century, we must also accept that some scientific questions will not be answered best by treating observational data as though they arose from an experimental trial. The complexity of social arrangements may often surpass our ingenuity to model these arrangements with the quantitative precision demanded by statistical methodology, while at the same time validly reflecting the social system under study. Narrative methods provide a source of theories whose richness provides a valuable counterpoint to the Spartan oversimplifications that typify the parsimony-driven models of statistics.

SUMMARY

Rudolf Virchow, the founder of the "social medicine" movement, famously declared that "Medicine is a social science, and politics is nothing else but medicine on a large scale."[175] What are the causes of the causes, the nodes furthest to the left-hand side of a complete DAG? For randomized clinical trials there may be just a lone coin flip, but for any real, free-living, human population, the left-hand size of the DAG will always comprise social and historical variables. This makes social epidemiology the bedrock of all honest population research. What distinguishes epidemiology from medicine is the very concept of a population, which is itself a social and historical construct. This realization suggests that the term "social epidemiology" may therefore be redundant. As stated at the outset, these variables are always present, but we call our work social epidemiology when they are brought into view, as the focus of inference rather than being merely a nuisance. The concepts and methods necessary for working fruitfully with these social and historical variables have evolved over time, with generous input from various social science disciplines. We now have a rich set of designs, measures, and analytic techniques available for use. Subject matter knowledge is a crucial prerequisite for meaningful inference, as is a clear scientific question in terms of description, prediction, or etiology. Social epidemiology remains one of the most challenging branches of our field, but also among the most essential.

References

1. Krieger N, Rowley DL, Herman AA, Avery B, Phillips MT. Racism, sexism, and social class: implications for studies of health, disease, and well-being. *Am J Prev Med*. 1993;9(6 suppl):82-122. Review. PMID: 8123288.
2. Berkman LF, Kawachi I. A historical framework for social epidemiology: social determinants of population health. In: Berkman LF, Kawachi I, Glymour MM, eds. *Social Epidemiology*. 2nd ed. New York, NY: Oxford University Press;2014:1-16.
3. Krieger N. Theories for social epidemiology in the 21st century: an ecosocial perspective. *Int J Epidemiol*. 2001;30(4):668-677. Review. PMID: 11511581.
4. Kaplan GA. What's wrong with social epidemiology, and how can we make it better? *Epidemiol Rev*. 2004;26:124-135. PMID: 15234953.
5. Vaughan AS, Quick H, Pathak EB, Kramer MR, Casper M. Disparities in temporal and geographic patterns of declining heart disease mortality by race and sex in the United States, 1973-2010. *J Am Heart Assoc*. 2015;4(12):e002567. PMID: 26672077.
6. Singh GK, Siahpush M, Azuine RE, Williams SD. Widening socioeconomic and racial disparities in cardiovascular disease mortality in the United States, 1969-2013. *Int J MCH AIDS*. 2015;3(2):106-118. PMID: 27621991.
7. Pearson-Stuttard J, Guzman-Castillo M, Penalvo JL, et al. Modeling future cardiovascular disease mortality in the United States: National trends and racial and ethnic disparities. *Circulation*. 2016;133(10):967-978. PMID: 26846769.
8. Kaufman JS, Cooper RS. Seeking causal explanations in social epidemiology. *Am J Epidemiol*. 1999;150(2):113-120. PMID: 10412955.
9. Nandi A, Glymour MM, Subramanian SV. Association among socioeconomic status, health behaviors, and all-cause mortality in the United States. *Epidemiology*. 2014;25(2):170-177. PMID: 24487200.
10. Galea S. An argument for a consequentialist epidemiology. *Am J Epidemiol*. 2013;178(8):1185-1191. PMID: 24022890.
11. Holland PW. Statistics and causal inference. *J Am Statist Assoc*. 1986;81(396):945-960.
12. Kaufman JS. Epidemiologic analysis of racial/ethnic disparities: some fundamental issues and a cautionary example. *Soc Sci Med*. 2008;66(8):1659-1669. PMID: 18248866.
13. Holland PW. The false linking of race and causality: lessons from standardized testing. *Race Soc*. 2001;4:219-233.
14. Kaufman JS, Cooper RS. Commentary: considerations for use of racial/ethnic classification in etiologic research. *Am J Epidemiol*. 2001;154(4):291-298. PMID: 11495850.
15. VanderWeele TJ, Robinson WR. On the causal interpretation of race in regressions adjusting for confounding and mediating variables. *Epidemiology*. 2014;25(4):473-484. PMID: 24887159.
16. Naimi AI, Schnitzer ME, Moodie EE, Bodnar LM. Mediation analysis for health disparities research. *Am J Epidemiol*. 2016;184(4):315-324. PMID: 27489089.
17. Maldonado G, Greenland S. Estimating causal effects. *Int J Epidemiol*. 2002;31(2):422-429. PMID:11980807.
18. Westreich D. From exposures to population interventions: pregnancy and response to HIV therapy. *Am J Epidemiol*. 2014;179(7):797-806. doi:10.1093/aje/kwt328.
19. Kaufman JS, Kaufman S, Poole C. Causal inference from randomized trials in social epidemiology. *Soc Sci Med*. 2003;57(12):2397-2409. PMID: 14572846.

20. Greenland S, Morgenstern H. Confounding in health research. *Annu Rev Public Health*. 2001;22:189-212. Review. PMID: 11274518.

21. VanderWeele TJ. Principles of confounder selection. *Eur J Epidemiol*. 2019;34(3):211-219. PMID: 30840181.

22. Angrist JD, Krueger AB. *Empirical strategies in labor economics*. In: *Handbook of Labor Economics*. Vol 3. New York: Elsevier; 1999:1277-1366.

23. Krieger N. History, biology, and health inequities: emergent embodied phenotypes and the illustrative case of the breast cancer estrogen receptor. *Am J Public Health*. 2013;103(1):22-27. PMID: 23153126.

24. Angrist JD, Pischke JS. *Mostly Harmless Econometrics: An Empiricist's Companion*. Princeton, NJ: Princeton University Press; 2009.

25. Imbens GW. Instrumental variables: an econometrician's perspective. *Stat Sci*. 2014;29(3):323-358.

26. Lawlor DA, Tilling K, Davey Smith G. Triangulation in aetiological epidemiology. *Int J Epidemiol*. 2016;45(6):1866-1886. PMID: 28108528.

27. Harper S, Strumpf EC. Social epidemiology: questionable answers and answerable questions. *Epidemiology*. 2012;23(6):795-798. PMID: 23038109.

28. Kaufman JS. How inconsistencies in racial classification demystify the race construct in public health statistics. *Epidemiology* 1999;10:101-103. PMID: 10069240.

29. Royal CD, Novembre J, Fullerton SM, et al. Inferring genetic ancestry: opportunities, challenges, and implications. *Am J Hum Genet*. 2010;86(5):661-673. PMID: 20466090.

30. Williams DR. Race and health: basic questions, emerging directions. *Ann Epidemiol*. 1997;7(5):322-333. PMID: 9250627.

31. Office of Management and Budget. *Directive Number 15: Race and Ethnic Standards for Federal Statistics and Administrative Reporting*. Washington, DC: Off. Fed. Stat. Policy Standards, US Dep. Comm.; 1977.

32. Office of Management and Budget. Revisions to the standards for classification of Federal data on race and ethnicity. *Fed Regist*. 1997;62:58781-58790.

33. Mays VM, Ponce NA, Washington DL, Cochran SD. Classification of race and ethnicity: implications for public health. *Annu Rev Public Health*. 2003;24:83-110. PMID: 12668755.

34. Villarroel N, Davidson E, Pereyra-Zamora P, Krasnik A, Bhopal RS. Heterogeneity/granularity in ethnicity classifications project: the need for refining assessment of health status. *Eur J Public Health*. 2019;29(2):260-266. PMID: 30260371.

35. Muniz JO, Bastos JL. Classificatory volatility and (in)consistency of racial inequality. *Cad Saude Publica*. 2017;33(suppl 1):e00082816. PMID: 28562697.

36. Mersha TB, Abebe T. Self-reported race/ethnicity in the age of genomic research: its potential impact on understanding health disparities. *Hum Genomics*. 2015;9:1. PMID: 25563503.

37. Phillips SP. Including gender in public health research. *Public Health Rep*. 2011;126(suppl 3):16-21. PMID: 21836732.

38. Krieger N. Genders, sexes, and health: what are the connections—and why does it matter? *Int J Epidemiol*. 2003;32(4):652-657. doi:10.1093/ije/dyg156.

39. Dreger AD. "Ambiguous sex"—or ambivalent medicine? Ethical issues in the treatment of intersexuality. *Hastings Cent Rep*. 1998;28(3):24-35. PMID: 9669179.

40. Sanz V. No way out of the binary: a critical history of the scientific production of sex. *Signs: J Women Cult Soc*. 2017;43(1):1-27.

41. Cherng H-YS. The color of LGB: racial and ethnic variations in conceptualizations of sexual minority status. *Popul Rev*. 2017;56(1):46-67.

42. Conti G, Heckman J, Urzua S. The education-health gradient. *Am Econ Rev*. 2010;100(2):234-238. PMID: 24741117.

43. Goldring T, Lange F, Richards-Shubik S. Testing for changes in the SES-mortality gradient when the distribution of education changes too. *J Health Econ*. 2016;46:120-130. PMID: 26830225.

44. Case A, Deaton A. Rising morbidity and mortality in midlife among White non-Hispanic Americans in the 21st century. *Proc Natl Acad Sci USA*. 2015;112(49):15078-15083. PMID: 26575631.

45. Liu SY, Buka SL, Kubzansky LD, Kawachi I, Gilman SE, Loucks EB. Sheepskin effects of education in the 10-year Framingham risk of coronary heart disease. *Soc Sci Med*. 2013;80:31-36. PMID: 23415589.

46. Raudenbush SW, Eschmann RD. Does schooling increase or reduce social inequality? *Annu Rev Sociol*. 2015;41:443-470.

47. Oakes JM, Rossi PH. The measurement of SES in health research: current practice and steps toward a new approach. *Soc Sci Med*. 2003;56(4):769-784. PMID: 12560010.

48. Formosa M, Higgs P. *Social Class in Later Life: Power, Identity and Lifestyle*. Bristol, UK: Policy Press; 2015.

49. Stauder J. Unemployment, unemployment duration, and health: selection or causation? *Eur J Health Econ*. 2019;20(1):59-73.

50. Elfassy T, Swift SL, Glymour MM, et al. Associations of income volatility with incident cardiovascular disease and all-cause mortality in a US cohort. *Circulation*. 2019;139(7):850-859. PMID: 30612448.

51. Chetty R, Stepner M, Abraham S, et al. The association between income and life expectancy in the United States, 2001-2014. *J Am Med Assoc*. 2016;315(16):1750-1766. PMID: 27063997.

52. Chetty R, Hendren N, Katz LF. The effects of exposure to better neighborhoods on children: new evidence from the Moving to Opportunity experiment. *Am Econ Rev*. 2016;106(4):855-902. doi:10.1257/aer.20150572.

53. Valet P, Adriaans J, Liebig S. Comparing survey data and administrative records on gross earnings: nonreporting, misreporting, interviewer presence and earnings inequality. *Qual Quantity*. 2019;53(1):471-491.

54. Backlund E, Sorlie PD, Johnson NJ. The shape of the relationship between income and mortality in the United States. Evidence from the National Longitudinal Mortality Study. *Ann Epidemiol*. 1996;6(1):12-20. PMID: 8680619.

55. Beblo M, Beninger D. Do husbands and wives pool their incomes? A couple experiment. *Rev Econ Household*. 2017;15(3):779-805.

56. Gottschalk P, Huynh M. Are earnings inequality and mobility overstated? The impact of nonclassical measurement error. *Rev Econ Stat*. 2010;92(2):302-315.

57. Iceland J, Bauman KJ. Income poverty and material hardship. *J Socio-Econ*. 2007;36(3):376-396.

58. Fisher GM. The development and history of the poverty thresholds. *Social Security Bull*. 1992;55:3-14.

59. Meyer BD, Mittag N. Using linked survey and administrative data to better measure income: implications for poverty, program effectiveness, and holes in the safety net. *Am Econ J Appl Econ*. 2019;11(2):176-204.

60. Pool LR, Burgard SA, Needham BL, Elliott MR, Langa KM, Mendes de Leon CF. Association of a negative wealth shock with all-cause mortality in middle-aged and older adults in the United States. *J Am Med Assoc*. April 3, 2018;319(13):1341-1350. PMID: 29614178.

61. Sykes BL, Maroto M. A wealth of inequalities: mass incarceration, employment, and racial disparities in US household wealth, 1996 to 2011. *RSF: The Russell Sage Found J Social Sci*. 2016;2(6):129-152.

62. Kaufman JS, Cooper RS, McGee DL. Socioeconomic status and health in Blacks and Whites: the problem of residual confounding and the resiliency of race. *Epidemiology*. 1997;8(6):621-628. PMID: 9345660.

63. Nuru-Jeter AM, Michaels EK, Thomas MD, Reeves AN, Thorpe RJ Jr, LaVeist TA. Relative roles of race versus socioeconomic position in studies of health inequalities: a matter of interpretation. *Annu Rev Public Health*. 2018;39:169-188. PMID: 29328880.

64. Killewald A, Pfeffer FT, Schachner JN. Wealth inequality and accumulation. *Annu Rev Sociol*. 2017 43:379-404.

65. Makaroun LK, Brown RT, Diaz-Ramirez LG, et al. Wealth-associated disparities in death and disability in the United States and England. *JAMA Intern Med*. 2017;177(12):1745-1753. PMID: 29059279.

66. Oliver ML, Shapiro TM. Disrupting the racial wealth gap. *Contexts*. 2019;18(1):16-21.

67. Berkman LF, Kawachi I, Theorell T. Working conditions and health. In: Berkman LF, Kawachi I, Glymour MM, eds. *Social Epidemiology*. 2nd ed. New York: Oxford University Press; 2014:153-181.

68. Marmot MG, Smith GD, Stansfeld S, et al. Health inequalities among British civil servants: the Whitehall II study. *Lancet*. 1991;337(8754):1387-1393. PMID: 1674771.

69. Rose D, Pevalin DJ, O'Reilly K. *The National Statistics Socio-Economic Classification: Origins, Development and Use*. Basingstoke: Palgrave Macmillan; 2005.

70. Liberatos P, Link BG, Kelsey JL. The measurement of social class in epidemiology. *Epidemiol Rev*. 1988;10:87-121. PMID: 3066632.

71. Hauser RM, Warren JR. Socioeconomic indexes for occupations: a review, update, and critique. *Sociol Methodol*. 1997;27:177-298.

72. Bukodi E, Dex S, Goldthorpe JH. The conceptualisation and measurement of occupational hierarchies: a review, a proposal and some illustrative analyses. *Qual Quantity*. 2011;45(3):623-639.

73. Wright EO. *Approaches to Class Analysis*. Cambridge: Cambridge University Press; 2005.

74. Paradies Y, Ben J, Denson N, et al. Racism as a determinant of health: a systematic review and meta-analysis. *PLoS One*. 2015;10(9):e0138511. PMID: 26398658.

75. Williams DR, Lawrence JA, Davis BA. Racism and health: evidence and needed research. *Annu Rev Public Health*. 2019;40:105-125. PMID: 30601726.

76. Black LL, Johnson R, VanHoose L. The relationship between perceived racism/discrimination and health among Black American women: a review of the literature from 2003 to 2013. *J Racial Ethn Health Disparities*. 2015;2(1):11-20. PMID: 25973361.

77. Taylor DM, Wright SC, Moghaddam FM, Lalonde RN. The personal/group discrimination discrepancy perceiving my group, but not myself, to be a target for discrimination. *Personal Soc Psychol Bull*. 1990;16(2):254-262.

78. Darity WA Jr. Employment discrimination, segregation, and health. *Am J Public Health*. 2003;93(2):226-231. PMID: 12554574.

79. Quillian L, Pager D, Hexel O, Midtbøen AH. Meta-analysis of field experiments shows no change in racial discrimination in hiring over time. *Proc Natl Acad Sci USA*. 2017;114(41):10870-10875. PMID: 28900012.

80. Neumark D, Burn I, Button P. Experimental age discrimination evidence and the Heckman critique. *Am Econ Rev*. 2016;106(5):303-308.

81. Bertrand M, Mullainathan S. Are Emily and Greg more employable than Lakisha and Jamal? A field experiment on labor market discrimination. *Am Econ Rev*. 2004;94(4):991-1013.

82. Everson-Rose SA, Lewis TT. Psychosocial factors and cardiovascular diseases. *Annu Rev Public Health*. 2005;26:469-500. PMID: 15760298.

83. Syme SL. Coronary artery disease: a sociocultural perspective. *Circulation*. 1987;76(1 pt 2):I112-I116. Review. PMID: 3297393.

84. Medalie JH, Stange KC, Zyzanski SJ, Goldbourt U. The importance of biopsychosocial factors in the development of duodenal ulcer in a cohort of middle-aged men. *Am J Epidemiol*. 1992;136(10):1280-1287. PMID: 1476150.

85. Theorell T, Karasek RA. Current issues relating to psychosocial job strain and cardiovascular disease research. *J Occup Health Psychol*. 1996;1(1):9-26. PMID: 9547038.

86. Marmot MG, Smith GD. Socio-economic differentials in health. *J Health Psychol*. 1997;2(3):283-296. PMID: 22013023.

87. Muntaner C, Lynch J, Oates GL. The social class determinants of income inequality and social cohesion. *Int J Health Serv*. 1999;29(4):699-732. Review. PMID: 10615570.

88. Kubzansky LD, Winning A, Kawachi I. Affects states and health. In: Berkman LF, Kawachi I, Glymour MM, eds. *Social Epidemiology*. 2nd ed. Oxford, UK: Oxford University Press; 2014:320-364.

89. Sapolsky RM. The influence of social hierarchy on primate health. *Science*. 2005;308(5722):648-652. PMID: 15860617.

90. Cohen S, Kamarck T, Mermelstein R. A global measure of perceived stress. *J Health Soc Behav*. 1983;24(4):385-396. PMID: 6668417.

91. Schlotz W. Investigating associations between momentary stress and cortisol in daily life: what have we learned so far? *Psychoneuroendocrinology*. 2019;105:105-116 PMID: 30503527.

92. Segerstrom SC, Sephton SE, Westgate PM. Intraindividual variability in cortisol: approaches, illustrations, and recommendations. *Psychoneuroendocrinology*. 2017;78:114-124. PMID:28192775.

93. Johnson SC, Cavallaro FL, Leon DA. A systematic review of allostatic load in relation to socioeconomic position: poor fidelity and major inconsistencies in biomarkers employed. *Soc Sci Med*. 2017;192:66-73. PMID: 28963986.

94. Holt-Lunstad J, Smith TB, Layton JB. Social relationships and mortality risk: a meta-analytic review. *PLoS Med*. 2010;7(7):e1000316. PMID: 20668659.

95. Cassel J. The contribution of the social environment to host resistance. *Am J Epidemiol*. 1976;104(2):107-123. PMID: 782233.

96. Berkman LF, Syme SL. Social networks, host resistance, and mortality: a nine-year follow-up study of Alameda County residents. *Am J Epidemiol*. 1979;109(2):186-204. PMID: 425958.

97. Berkman LF, Krishna A. Social network epidemiology. In: Berkman LF, Kawachi I, Glymour MM, eds. *Social Epidemiology*. 2nd ed. Oxford, UK: Oxford University Press; 2014:235-289.

98. Smith KP, Christakis NA. Social networks and health. *Annu Rev Sociol*. 2008;34(1):405-429.

99. VanderWeele TJ, Chen Y, Long K, Kim ES, Trudel-Fitzgerald C, Kubzansky LD. Positive epidemiology? *Epidemiology*. 2020;31(2):189-193. PMID: 31809344.

100. Brooks KP, Dunkel Schetter C. Social negativity and health: conceptual and measurement issues. *Social Personal Psychol Compass*. 2011;5(11):904-918.

101. Duncan DT, Kawachi I, eds. *Neighborhoods and Health*. 2nd ed. New York, NY: Oxford University Press; 2018.

102. O'Campo P, O'Brien Caughy M. Measures of residential community contexts. In: Oakes JM, Kaufman JS, eds. *Methods in Social Epidemiology*. 2nd ed. San Fransisco, CA: John Wiley & Sons; 2017:158-176.

103. Raudenbush SW, Sampson RJ. Ecometrics: toward a science of assessing ecological settings, with application to the systematic social observation of neighborhoods. *Sociological Methodology*. 1999;29(1):1-41.

104. Messer LC, Laraia BA, Kaufman JS, et al. The development of a standardized neighborhood deprivation index. *J Urban Health*. 2006;83(6):1041-1062. PMID: 17031568.

105. Labbe E, Blanquet M, Gerbaud L, et al. A new reliable index to measure individual deprivation: the EPICES score. *Eur J Public Health*. 2015;25(4):604-609. PMID: 25624273.

106. Pampalon R, Hamel D, Gamache P, Philibert MD, Raymond G, Simpson A. An area-based material and social deprivation index for public health in Québec and Canada. *Can J Public Health*. 2012;103(8 suppl 2):S17-S22. PMID: 23618066.

107. Lafontaine SJ, Sawada M, Kristjansson E. A direct observation method for auditing large urban centers using stratified sampling, mobile GIS technology and virtual environments. *Int J Health Geogr*. 2017;16(1):6. PMID: 28209210.

108. Marco M, Gracia E, Martín-Fernández M, López-Quílez A. Validation of a Google Street View-based neighborhood disorder observational scale. *J Urban Health*. 2017;94(2):190-198. PMID: 28236183.

109. Galster G, Sharkey P. Spatial foundations of inequality: a conceptual model and empirical overview. *RSF: The Russell Sage Found J Social Sci*. 2017;3(2):1-33.

110. Reardon SF. A conceptuial framework for measuring segregation and its association with population health. In: Oakes JM, Kaufman JS, eds. *Methods in Social Epidemiology*. 2nd ed. San Fransisco, CA: John Wiley & Sons; 2017:132-157.

111. Massey DS, Denton NA. The dimensions of residential segregation. *Social Forces*. 1988;67(2):281-315.

112. Yao J, Wong DW, Bailey N, Minton J. Spatial segregation measures: a methodological review. *Tijds voor Econ en Soc Geog*. 2019;110:235-250. doi:10.1111/tesg.12305.

113. Williams AD, Wallace M, Nobles C, Mendola P. Racial residential segregation and racial disparities in stillbirth in the United States. *Health Place*. 2018;51:208-216. PMID: 29715639.

114. Yang TC, Matthews SA. Death by segregation: does the dimension of racial segregation matter? *PLoS One*. 2015;10(9):e0138489. PMID: 26398346.

115. Fennie KP, Lutfi K, Maddox LM, Lieb S, Trepka MJ. Influence of residential segregation on survival after AIDS diagnosis among non-Hispanic Blacks. *Ann Epidemiol*. 2015;25(2):113-119. PMID:25542342.

116. Ard K. By all measures: an examination of the relationship between segregation and health risk from air pollution. *Popul Environ*. 2016;38(1):1-20. doi: 10.1007/s11111-015-0251-6.

117. Lynch J, Smith GD, Harper S, et al. Is income inequality a determinant of population health? Part 1. A systematic review. *Milbank Q*. 2004;82(1):5-99. PMID: 15016244.

118. Marmot MG. The health gap: the challenge of an unequal world. *Lancet*. 2015;386(10011):2442-2444. PMID: 26364261.

119. Hosseinpoor AR, Bergen N. Area-based units of analysis for strengthening health inequality monitoring. *Bull World Health Organ*. 2016;94(11):856-858. PMID: 27821889.

120. Greenland S Ecologic versus individual-level sources of bias in ecologic estimates of contextual health effects. *Int J Epidemiol*. 2001;30(6):1343-1350. PMID: 11821344.

121. Kondo N, Sembajwe G, Kawachi I, van Dam RM, Subramanian SV, Yamagata Z. Income inequality, mortality, and self rated health: meta-analysis of multilevel studies. *Br Med J*. 2009;339:b4471. PMID: 19903981.

122. Wagstaff A, van Doorslaer E. Income inequality and health: what does the literature tell us? *Annu Rev Public Health*. 2000;21:543-567. Review. PMID: 10884964.

123. Cowell F. Measuring Inequality. 3rd ed. Oxford, UK: Oxford University Press; 2011.

124. Gastwirth JL. Is the Gini index of inequality overly sensitive to changes in the middle of the income distribution? *Stat Public Policy*. 2017;4(1):1-11. doi:10.1080/2330443X.2017.1360813.

125. Bowles S, Carlin W. Inequality as experienced difference: a reformulation of the Gini coefficient. *Econ Lett*. 2020;186:108789.

126. Harper S, Lynch J. Health inequalities: measurement and decomposition. In: Oakes JM, Kaufman JS, eds. *Methods in Social Epidemiology*. 2nd ed. San Fransisco, CA: John Wiley & Sons; 2017:91-131.

127. Moreno-Betancur M, Latouche A, Menvielle G, Kunst AE, Rey G. Relative index of inequality and slope index of inequality: a structured regression framework for estimation. *Epidemiology*. 2015;26(4):518-527. PMID: 26000548.

128. Koolman X, van Doorslaer E. On the interpretation of a concentration index of inequality. *Health Econ*. 2004;13(7):649-656. PMID: 15259044.

129. King NB, Harper S, Young ME. Use of relative and absolute effect measures in reporting health inequalities: structured review. *Br Med J*. 2012;345:e5774. PMID: 22945952.

130. Rodgers J, Valuev AV, Hswen Y, Subramanian SV. Social capital and physical health: an updated review of the literature for 2007-2018. *Soc Sci Med*. 2019;236:112360. PMID: 31352315.

131. Manning P. Putnam and radical socio-economic theory. *Int J Social Econ* 2010;37(3):254-269. doi: 10.1108/03068291011018794.

132. Villalonga-Olives E, Kawachi I. The measurement of social capital. *Gac Sanit*. 2015;29(1):62-64. PMID: 25444390.

133. Lin N. Building a network theory of social capital. In: Lin N, Cook K, Burt R, eds. *Social Capital*. New York: Routledge; 2001.

134. Gottlieb BH, Bergen AE. Social support concepts and measures. *J Psychosom Res*. 2010;69(5):511-520. PMID: 20955871.

135. Christakis NA, Fowler JH. Social contagion theory: examining dynamic social networks and human behavior. *Stat Med*. 2013;32(4):556-577. PMID: 22711416.

136. Shoham DA, Messer LC. Social network analysis for epidemiology. In: *Methods in Social Epidemiology*, 2nd ed. Oakes JM, Kaufman JS, eds., John Wiley & Sons; 2017:212-238.

137. Tchetgen Tchetgen EJ, VanderWeele TJ. On causal inference in the presence of interference. *Stat Methods Med Res*. 2012;21(1):55-75. PMID: 21068053.

138. Cerdá M, Keyes KM. Systems modeling to advance the promise of data science in epidemiology. *Am J Epidemiol*. 2019;188(5):862-865. doi:10.1093/aje/kwy262.

139. Susser M, Susser E. Choosing a future for epidemiology: II. From black box to Chinese boxes and eco-epidemiology. *Am J Public Health*. 1996;86(5):674-677. PMID: 8629718.

140. Mason WM, Wong GY, Entwisle B. Contextual analysis through the multilevel linear model. In: Leinhardt S, ed. *Sociological Methodology*. San Francisco: Jossey-Bass; 1983:72-103.

141. O'Campo P, Xue X, Wang MC, Caughy M. Neighborhood risk factors for low birthweight in Baltimore: a multilevel analysis. *Am J Public Health*. 1997;87(7):1113-1118. PMID: 9240099.

142. Bingenheimer JB, Raudenbush SW. Statistical and substantive inferences in public health: issues in the application of multilevel models. *Annu Rev Public Health*. 2004;25:53-77. PMID: 15015912.

143. Merlo J, Wagner P, Austin PC, Subramanian SV, Leckie G. General and specific contextual effects in multilevel regression analyses and their paradoxical relationship: a conceptual tutorial. *SSM Popul Health*. 2018;5:33-37. PMID: 29892693.

144. Greenland S Principles of multilevel modelling. *Int J Epidemiol*. 2000;29(1):158-167. PMID: 10750618.

145. Hirai AS, Kaufman JS. Fixed versus random effects models for multilevel and longitudinal data. In: Oakes JM, Kaufman JS, eds. *Methods in Social Epidemiology*. 2nd ed. San Fransisco, CA: John Wiley & Sons; 2017:369-397.

146. Oakes JM. The (mis)estimation of neighborhood effects: causal inference for a practicable social epidemiology. *Soc Sci Med*. 2004;58(10):1929-1952. PMID: 15020009.

147. Hausmann JA, Taylor WE. Panel data and unobservable individual effects. *Econometrica*. 1981;49:1377-1398.

148. Twisk JWR, de Vente W. Hybrid models were found to be very elegant to disentangle longitudinal within- and between-subject relationships. *J Clin Epidemiol*. 2019;107:66-70. PMID: 30500406.

149. Gardiner JC, Luo Z, Roman LA. Fixed effects, random effects and GEE: what are the differences? *Stat Med*. 2009;28(2):221-239. PMID: 19012297.

150. Burgess S. Estimating and contextualizing the attenuation of odds ratios due to non-collapsibility. *Commun Stat - Theor Methods*. 2017;46(2):786-804. doi: 10.1080/03610926.2015.1006778.

151. Sato T, Matsuyama Y. Marginal structural models as a tool for standardization. *Epidemiology*. 2003;14(6):680-686. PMID: 14569183.

152. Lynch J, Smith GD. A life course approach to chronic disease epidemiology. *Annu Rev Public Health*. 2005;26:1-35. PMID: 15760279.

153. Wells JC. A critical appraisal of the predictive adaptive response hypothesis. *Int J Epidemiol*. 2012;41(1):229-235. PMID: 22422458.

154. Pollitt RA, Rose KM, Kaufman JS. Evaluating the evidence for models of life course socioeconomic factors and cardiovascular outcomes: a systematic review. *BMC Public Health*. 2005;5:7. PMID: 15661071.

155. Almond D, Currie J. Killing me softly: the fetal origins hypothesis. *J Econ Perspect*. 2011;25(3):153-172. doi: 10.1257/jep.25.3.153.

156. Heraclides A, Brunner E. Social mobility and social accumulation across the life course in relation to adult overweight and obesity: the Whitehall II study. *J Epidemiol Community Health*. 2010;64(8):714-719. PMID: 19737739.

157. Banks J, Mazzonna F. The effect of education on old age cognitive abilities: evidence from a regression discontinuity design. *Econ J*. 2012;122(560):418-448. doi: 10.1111/j.1468-0297.2012.02499.x.

158. Glymour MM, Walter S, Tchetgen Tchetgen EJ. Natural experiments and instrumental variables analyses in social epidemiology. In: Oakes JM, Kaufman JS, eds. *Methods in Social Epidemiology*. 2nd ed. San Fransisco, CA: John Wiley & Sons; 2017:493-538.

159. Costello EJ, Erkanli A, Copeland W, Angold A. Association of family income supplements in adolescence with development of psychiatric and substance use disorders in adulthood among an American Indian population. *J Am Med Assoc*. 2010;303(19):1954-1960. PMID: 20483972.

160. Zubizarreta JR, Cerdá M, Rosenbaum PR. Effect of the 2010 Chilean earthquake on posttraumatic stress: reducing sensitivity to unmeasured bias through study design. *Epidemiology*. 2013;24(1):79-87. PMID: 23222557.

161. Bor J, Moscoe E, Mutevedzi P, Newell ML, Bärnighausen T. Regression discontinuity designs in epidemiology: causal inference without randomized trials. *Epidemiology*. 2014;25(5):729-737. PMID: 25061922.

162. Smith LM, Kaufman JS, Strumpf EC, Lévesque LE. Effect of human papillomavirus (HPV) vaccination on clinical indicators of sexual behaviour among adolescent girls: the Ontario Grade 8 HPV Vaccine Cohort Study. *Can Med Assoc J*. 2015;187(2):E74-E81. PMID: 25487660.

163. Evans DM, Davey Smith G. Mendelian randomization: new applications in the coming age of hypothesis-free causality. *Annu Rev Genomics Hum Genet*. 2015;16:327-350. PMID: 25939054.

164. Carter AR, Gill D, Davies NM, et al. Understanding the consequences of education inequality on cardiovascular disease: mendelian randomisation study. *Br Med J*. 2019;365:1855. PMID: 31122926.

165. Swanson SA. Can we see the forest for the IVs?: mendelian randomization studies with multiple genetic variants. *Epidemiology*. 2017;28(1):43-46. PMID: 27662595.

166. Stuart EA, Bradshaw CP, Leaf PJ. Assessing the generalizability of randomized trial results to target populations. *Prev Sci*. 2015;16(3):475-485. PMID: 25307417.

167. VanderWeele TJ, Christakis NA. Network multipliers and public health. *Int J Epidemiol*. 2019;48(4):1032-1037. PMID: 30793743.

168. King G, Zeng L. When can history be our guide? The pitfalls of counterfactual inference. *Int Stud Q*. 2007;51(1):183-210. doi: 10.1111/j.1468-2478.2007.00445.x.

169. Braun L, Kisting S. Asbestos-related disease in South Africa: the social production of an invisible epidemic. *Am J Public Health*. 2006;96(8):1386-1396. PMID: 16809596.

170. Montoya M. *Making the Mexican Diabetic: Race, Science, and the Genetics of Inequality*. Berkeley, CA: University of California Press; 2011.

171. Kolodny A, Courtwright DT, Hwang CS, et al. The prescription opioid and heroin crisis: a public health approach to an epidemic of addiction. *Annu Rev Public Health*. 2015;36:559-574. PMID: 25581144.

172. Bennett GG, Merritt MM, Sollers JJ, et al. Stress, coping, and health outcomes among African-Americans: a review of the John Henryism hypothesis. *Psychol Health*. 2004;19(3):369-383. doi: 10.1080/0887044042000193505.

173. James SA. John Henryism and the health of African-Americans. *Cult Med Psychiatry*. 1994;18(2):163-182. doi: 10.1007/BF01379448.

174. Ermakoff I. Causality and history: modes of causal investigation in historical social sciences. *Annu Rev Sociol*. 2019;45:29.1-29.26. doi: 10.1146/annurev-soc-073117-041140.

175. Ashton JR. Virchow misquoted, part-quoted, and the real McCoy. *J Epidemiol Community Health*. 2006;60(8):671.

CHAPTER 40

Environmental Epidemiology

Irva Hertz-Picciotto and Stephanie M. Engel

DOMAIN OF ENVIRONMENTAL EPIDEMIOLOGY

One of the earliest published environmental epidemiology studies was Baker's report on the "Endemial Colic of Devonshire" (1767). Physicians had puzzled for 50 years about why those who drank cider in Devonshire became seriously ill, experienced seizures, and sometimes died whereas cider-drinkers elsewhere drank with impunity. Baker concluded that "the cause of this Colic is not …in the pure Cyder; but in some, either fraudulent, or accidental adulteration." Inspections of the presses revealed abundant use of lead in Devonshire, but not elsewhere. Baker then chemically tested the cider and found lead precipitated only in Devonshire samples. Like many environmental epidemiology studies, the investigation began with observations of regional differences in disease rates, proceeded to a more careful examination of symptoms and circumstances and discovery of a suspect cause, and finally confirmed the cause acting in the high-incidence county, but not the low-incidence counties.

For our purposes, the *environment* will be defined as factors that are external to the body and to which humans are unintentionally exposed. It therefore includes physical, chemical, and biologic agents, as well as social, political, cultural, and engineering or architectural factors affecting human contact with such agents. Because environmental exposures are involuntary, the presence or magnitude of such exposures may be subject to legal restrictions or influenced by political or economic pressures. Industrial or commercial parties may in some cases be responsible for the pollution, and therefore the policy or legal liability implications of environmental epidemiology studies may lead to results being contested. In some cases, studies may be used as evidence in litigation or as the basis for risk assessment and regulatory policy decisions. Epidemiologists may contribute to or conduct quantitative risk assessments to assist policy-makers in establishing a regulatory framework for a chemical or family of chemicals[1-3]. Therefore, the need for the work to withstand intense scientific and public scrutiny underscores the importance of rigorous methodology.

Most environmental epidemiology studies fall into one of two types. The first is when the epidemiologist seeks to characterize the health effects of a *known* exposure. Conversely, a disease pattern may be observed, and the epidemiologist sets out to determine the as yet *unknown causes*. In either case, definitiveness of the findings will depend on the quality of the exposure assessment. Evidence can be strengthened by distinguishing persons receiving high versus low levels of exposure or by identifying a susceptible window when exposure can affect the relevant tissue, organ, or outcome. Prior to the 20th century, environmental epidemiology focused primarily on biologic agents and factors such as water distribution systems, sewage collection, and food handling. The delivery of sanitary water, construction of comprehensive sewage systems, and passage of laws governing the handling of food were environmental measures that substantially reduced morbidity and mortality from infectious agents. In many developing countries as well as some communities in the United States, most often those with a primarily Black, Hispanic, or immigrant population or increasingly in rural areas, these basic issues are still a primary environmental health concern.

Around the middle of the 20th century, the focus of environmental epidemiology largely shifted to chemical and physical agents such as metals, particulate matter and other air pollutants, pesticides, volatile organic compounds, and radiation. The continual and rapid introduction of new chemicals, many with limited safety data, to the global marketplace fuels concern by the lay, clinical, and scientific communities.[4] Example sources of exposure to environmental agents include industrial facility and motor vehicle emissions; hormones added to animal feed; pesticide residues in food and in run-off reaching drinking water reservoirs; chemical spills during production or transportation; hazardous waste sites; radon from naturally occurring geologic sources; minerals in groundwater—both naturally occurring (*e.g.*, arsenic) and added through human activity (*e.g.*, lead, fluoride)—plasticizers in building materials, medical tubing, food and beverage packaging, and enteric coatings on medications; household cleaning products and air fresheners; and personal care products such as cosmetics, soaps, shampoos, lotions, and hair dyes. Many environmental agents come to attention after health effects are observed at relatively high levels in an occupational setting or as a result of an accidental release. For example, respiratory problems from workplace exposures such as dust in mines raise the possibility of analogous though potentially less severe effects at community-level exposures. Environmental epidemiology also examines patterns of disease in populations struck by disasters, including war, floods, tsunamis, and earthquakes, and most recently has begun tackling the "built" environment.

Additionally, the health effects of global climate change, increasing transport of species outside their ecologic niches, inappropriate fire management strategies, and expansion of urban/suburban development into wildland spaces pose critical threats to human health. Extreme weather events such as more intense hurricanes and hotter, longer heat waves have led to environmental health disasters and have appropriately emerged as a major focus of modern environmental epidemiology research (see below, Environmental Disaster Epidemiology).

Toxicology and environmental epidemiology are interconnected; hypotheses may be generated by or tested in experimental systems, but only an epidemiologic study can establish relevance to humans. Alternatively, when epidemiologic associations precede traditional toxicity testing, plausibility is often questioned until a controlled experiment demonstrates similar outcomes, or an in vitro study uncovers a pathogenic mechanism. Recently, high-throughput toxicity testing has emerged as paradigm-shifting approach for chemical hazard characterization, which had previously relied on time consuming and laborious whole-animal experimental models.[5] Leveraging computational bioinformatics, systems biology, high-throughput in vitro bioassays, and efforts such as Tox21 are poised to transform our current approach to chemical risk assessment, as well as the manner in which epidemiologists prioritize and group putative chemical risk factors in studies.[6] For more discussion on high-throughput toxicity testing in relation to environmental epidemiology, see Future Directions below.

Exposure to environmental agents is frequently affected by where one lives, works, socializes, or buys food, which, in turn, are determined by social and economic factors, such as race, ethnicity, class, and wealth. Thus, socioeconomic attributes are determinants of exposure, as established by environmental justice research.[7-10] These contexts, which are integral to most environmental epidemiology problems, have been understudied. Moreover, the field of environmental epidemiology has largely considered socioeconomic characteristics as confounders, which they can be, but often, these factors alter susceptibility, thereby influencing the impact of other physical and chemical insults. In other words, they are effect modifiers. Consequently, the goal of disentangling contributions of social, economic, and cultural factors from those of environmental chemicals and pollutants may require a more nuanced approach that integrates the contributions from chemical and social stressors, acknowledges neighborhood and the broader milieu, and emphasizes multifactorial causation and mixtures from the conceptual stage through the analysis, interpretation, and translation toward policy.

This chapter does not seek to cover a litany of environmental exposures and what has been learned through epidemiologic research. Instead, it focuses on key methodologic issues currently facing the field and problems that feature more prominently in environmental epidemiology than in other substantive areas; additionally, it provides a flavor of how the field has made progress over time, its relationship to public health policy, and major new challenges. The remainder of this chapter is organized as follows: we begin with exposure assessment because of the critical role it plays; next, study designs and issues related to investigations of environmental factors are discussed; then, analytic methods for such investigations are addressed, including Poisson regression, time-space analyses, and clustering. The chapter continues with discussions of environmental health surveillance, vulnerable populations, some historical examples, and an exposition of new environmental epidemiology challenges and concludes with brief remarks about future needs, both practical and conceptual.

ENVIRONMENTAL MONITORING AND EXPOSURE ASSESSMENT

Human exposure to environmental agents may be either directly measured or inferred. Sources of environmental exposure information include (1) databases on sales or use of products or proximity to an agent of concern; (2) interviews, questionnaires, and structured diaries; (3) measurements in external media (macroenvironment) either from passive monitoring devices (*e.g.*, air pollutants as mandated by federal and sometimes also regional or state authorities) or conducted expressly for the epidemiologic investigation (*e.g.*, criteria pollutants or levels of chlorination by-products measured at the water company's reservoir); (4) concentrations in the personal or microenvironment (*e.g.*, carbon monoxide in indoor air or trihalomethanes in tap water); (5) individual doses (*e.g.*, using personal air monitors, or combining measurements at the tap with self-reported water consumption and hot shower use); (6) biological measurements of concentrations in human tissues (*e.g.*, blood lead or polychlorinated biphenyls [PCBs] in breast milk) or metabolic products (*e.g.*, dimethylarsinic acid in urine after arsenic exposure or phthalate metabolites in urine or meconium); and (7) biological markers of physiologic effects (*e.g.*, protein adducts), which are often the most critical determinant of the validity of an environmental epidemiology study. There is, however, no universal hierarchy for assessing quality, as it will depend on the persistence of the exposure, the duration of the exposure period, whether it is episodic or consistent in magnitude, its timing, induction period and latency to health outcome, length of follow-up of study participants, and type of outcome of interest—acute, chronic, cumulative, etc.—and the organ system(s) affected.

A distinction should be made between an agent measured in the external environment and a *dose* measured either in the human tissue or at the point of contact between the subject and the environment (*e.g.*, using a personal monitor or breath sampler). The difference between the two depends on the extent and nature of the contact between the agent and human tissue, which is dependent on human activity patterns, physiologic characteristics, and variation in the external exposures themselves over time and space. However, for an environmental agent to be an "exposure," at a minimum, there needs to be contact between that agent and the individual.

In the following sections, we will describe features of environmental monitoring, exposure assessment, and relationships of exposure timing to disease. These, in turn, play a fundamental role in the design and analysis of environmental epidemiology studies.

Monitoring of Exposure to Environmental Agents

Environmental monitoring is central to the timely identification of prevalent environmental threats; required to track changes in concentrations of environmental agents over time; and useful for the examination of the impact of environmental policy and compliance with existing environmental regulations. Environmental monitoring may be mandated by federal or state law, or implemented for research purposes, and may include measurements of air, water, soil, or biological media. One of the most widely used sources of monitoring data for epidemiology research is ambient concentrations of federally regulated criteria air pollutants (ozone, carbon monoxide, lead, particulate matter, sulfur dioxide, and nitrogen dioxide) obtained from monitoring stations dispersed across the United States. Monitoring is an essential component of the implementation of the Clean Air Act,[11] the Toxic Substances Control Act,[12] and its amendments, including the Frank R. Lautenberg Chemical Safety for the 21st Century Act.[13] Placement of air quality monitors is designed to maximize the density of measurements within population centers, meaning that there may be less resolution of exposure in less populous areas. Other sources of national, regional, or local monitoring data include emissions monitoring, designed to ascertain the air pollution output of specific stationary sources, pesticide use reporting in some regions, and water quality monitoring. Across all types of monitoring systems, the principles and purpose of exposure monitoring are the same: namely, to provide objective information about the quantities and sources of chemicals in the environment and any changes in their concentrations over time. For many of these monitoring programs, the data produced are useful to agencies that are required to meet legal standards.

Nationally representative human biomonitoring efforts, such as the US National Health and Nutrition Examination Survey (NHANES) biomonitoring program,[14] have emerged as key sources of exposure information for environmental chemicals.[15] Human biomonitoring is the measurement of chemicals, or their metabolites or adducts, in biological media, most commonly, urine or blood.[16] These biomarker measurements, often conducted in representative samples over time, permit the examination of temporal trends in human exposure, as well as the identification of subpopulations that may have a higher prevalence of exposure. Biomonitoring has another inherent advantage over ambient exposure monitoring for human health research, in that it reflects the amount of that chemical that is absorbed by the human body, integrated across all routes of exposure (inhalation, dermal, ingestion, or other) and sources,[17] while accounting for bioaccumulation, excretion, half-life, and other toxicokinetic parameters.[15] Additionally, the exquisitely sensitive assays in many cases permit measurement of concentrations down to trace levels, often far below what would be expected to result in any human health effects. By leveraging human biomonitoring data, environmental epidemiologists can prioritize chemicals for health research both based on their toxicity profiles, as well as their internal dose. Unfortunately, even the largest biomonitoring efforts currently in place only measure on the order of hundreds of chemicals or their metabolites,[18] a small fraction of the tens of thousands of chemicals in common use.[19] Furthermore, some segments of the population that may have heightened susceptibility to chemical agents may not be routinely captured in population-based surveillance efforts, for example, pregnant women, infants, and young children.

Exposure Assessment

When George Box opined "*All models are wrong but some are useful,*"[20] he could have been describing exposure assessment strategies. Optimally, we strive to maximize accuracy while minimizing cost within the landscape of what is feasible to do, but it is always the case that we have misclassified or mischaracterized an individual's relevant biologic exposure to some extent. Measurements in external media yield an ecologic measure and are useful when the exposures are high or widespread in some but not all geographic areas or time periods under study or, more specifically, when group differences outweigh interindividual differences. If trihalomethanes or arsenic in the drinking water are 10 times higher in one community than in others, interindividual variation in doses based on water consumption might be far outweighed by the between-community differences, and the benefit of collecting extensive water consumption data would then be small. Macroenvironment measures are also useful when the overall exposure setting rather than individual pollutants are of concern, for instance, if regulatory action levels are to be determined and the pollutants derive from the same sources. Direct methods of external exposure measurement must be validated through both a quality control or quality assurance program, and a sampling strategy that is based on the biodynamics of the pollutant in the environment.[21] In addition, population-level or aggregate estimates of exposure may do a poor job of capturing individual-level exposure if activity patterns in the population vary and are related to exposure.[22] Characterizing those activity patterns, if not the individual exposures directly, would be needed.

Whether planning a study or evaluating a body of literature, epidemiologists must grapple with uncertainty regarding the best estimate of relevant exposure and the extent of measurement error in that estimate. To that end, three features of exposure assessment capture the quality of the exposure measure: (1) the validity of the measurement, (2) the reliability of the measurement, and (3) the extent to which the measurement relates to a putative susceptible window for the disease in question. The first two are discussed in this section. The third is elaborated in the subsection "Exposure timing and relationship to disease outcome."

Among the first challenges faced in environmental epidemiology research is how to optimize the *validity* and *reliability* of the chosen estimate of exposure. We are using *validity* to mean the extent to which that measurement reflects the actual exposure of interest. We note, however, that chemists may use the term *validity* to denote various aspects of uncertainty in their methods, including batch effects, sensitivity and specificity, the extent to which that biomarker can be distinguished from analytic noise, and its reliability. Validity also applies to metrics other than chemical quantitation. Estimation of cumulative exposure, for example, requires reconstruction of past exposures, which, in the absence of intensive monitoring or complete historical specimens, is often a process fraught with problems of recall, incomplete measurements in external or biological media, or inaccurate records that can no longer be validated. Both biomarkers and environmental measurements frequently provide a more accurate picture of exposure in circumstances where individuals are unlikely to be able to report exposures.

Reliability captures a different feature of exposure assessment, specifically, how repeatable an exposure measurement is over time. If the exposure is constant and the same measurement were taken on a given individual a week, a month, or a year later, how similar would the estimates of exposure be? In the setting of biomarkers, these estimates of *reliability* are closely related to the half-life of the compound in question, half-life being the time it takes for the concentration to reduce by half. Biomarkers of chemicals with long half-lives tend to have higher estimates of reliability over a given period than biomarkers of chemicals with short half-lives. Reliability may also apply to questionnaire responses: if you asked the same study participant about a specific exposure a day, a month, a year, or 5 years later, would they report their exposure similarly? The difficulty of measuring an exposure increases if the exposure changes over time through long-term trends, seasonal effects, or shifts in behaviors. Such changes require more time points to be sampled, or questions asked, to obtain an accurate measure of a changing exposure. Alternatively, one can measure all participants at the same time.

Biological markers, or "biomarkers," encompass a broad range of measurements in a variety of tissues, including both endogenously produced and exogenous compounds, as well as biomarkers of susceptibility and markers of early disease.[23] In the context of environmental epidemiology and exposure assessment, we are typically most concerned with measurements that reflect exposure to environmental chemicals or their impact on biological systems. As such, biomarkers of exposure may be viewed as a snapshot of the absorbed dose of that chemical agent integrated across all routes and sources of exposure,[16,24,25] thus providing a considerable advantage over external exposure measurements when estimating total exposures for chemicals that have multiple sources. A range of biological media may be used for the measurement of exposure biomarkers, including most commonly blood and urine, but also deciduous teeth, hair, nails, saliva, breast milk, amniotic fluid, meconium, adipose tissue, and feces. A major caveat for biomarkers, however, is that depending on the half-life of the chemical in the selected biologic tissue, the biomarker may represent exposures only during a brief time period.

While exposure biomarkers may be found in many different tissues, the proper measurement matrix for any specific compound, as well as the meaning of that measurement, is governed by its chemical disposition and toxicokinetic properties.[16] Polar compounds are most validly measured in aqueous matrices (such as urine),[26] whereas lipophilic compounds are most validly measured in blood or adipose tissue.[27] Polar compounds measured in urine are often metabolites of chemical compounds that are rapidly metabolized and excreted, thereby providing information on relatively short-term windows of exposure.[26] Blood biomarkers, in contrast, may sometimes reflect temporally recent exposures (for example, blood concentrations of benzene dissipate in a matter of hours [28]) and other times reflect stable, long-term exposures to compounds with long half-lives that partition into adipose tissue, such as organochlorine pesticides, PCBs, or polybrominated diphenyl ethers (PBDEs).[27] These differences in the persistence and reliability of exposure biomarkers critically impact our ability to infer causal mechanisms for biomarker-disease associations. Because biomarkers inherently integrate exposures from all sources, generally yield quantitative estimates of intensity, and are unaffected by information biases like preferential recall, they are often the preferred exposure assessment method. However, biomarker-based exposure assessment is not always possible or even optimal for a variety of reasons: specimens may not have been collected in the appropriate time period or covering the entire window of relevance; validated assays may not be available for your exposure or may be too costly; the chemicals or their metabolites may represent a short time interval such as minutes or hours (which for episodic exposures may result in highly unrepresentative measurements); or biological sample collection or storage protocols that were used during fieldwork may not conform to the assay requirements for that specific biomarker.

When measurements on each individual are infeasible, a surrogate can be constructed using dosimetric modeling.[29] Measurements at the source of exposure are combined with information about physicochemical properties and often also with field measurements in multiple locations. Examples include dispersion models for air pollutants, hydrogeologic modeling of waterborne exposures, and isopleth modeling of soil contaminants. Since a model is simply a set of structured assumptions, dosimetric models should be validated before being introduced into epidemiologic studies.[21] For example, estimated individual measures could be a poor surrogate for individual absorbed doses because of variability by breathing rate, age, sex, medical conditions, and so on. The pertinent dose at the target tissue further depends on pharmacokinetics, that is, distribution to various body compartments (bloodstream, kidney, brain, etc.), metabolic rates and pathways that could either produce the active compound, or detoxify it, storage or retention times, and elimination. Individual differences in pharmacokinetics influence the dose at the target site and its time course. Tissue concentrations may be better than external measures and activity data but, in some situations, could be a poor indication of long-term exposure. For advantages and disadvantages of various exposure measurement methods, see Armstrong et al.[30] and Nieuwenhuijsen.[31]

Errors in measurement of exposure introduce both bias and imprecision into the estimates of their health effects.[32] Repetition of measurements can improve precision in exposure estimates, thereby reducing bias in effect measures.[32,33] Note also that when intraindividual variability is great, macro-level exposure measures may be preferred over personal or biologic measures since they will tend to give better estimates of average exposures.[34] Sheppard and colleagues point out that in time series studies of air pollution, when nonambient sources of pollution are ignored, if they are independent of the ambient sources, the resulting error in exposure assessment will not introduce bias in the estimation of effect.[35,36] The literature on measurement error is abundant,[37-39] with entire textbooks devoted to this topic, ranging to levels that are highly technical (e.g.,[40]).

Other perspectives on improving exposure assessment focus on the integration of a wide range of variables through geographic information systems (GIS), software that provides data management, mapping, and statistical analysis capabilities for incorporating spatial attributes of data.[41] These systems can superimpose maps of topographic (e.g., land cover, soil type, watershed), meteorologic, sociodemographic, health services infrastructure, and other data. Applications have included analysis of childhood cancer incidence at the level of census tracts in relation to hazardous air pollutant exposures from mobile, area, and point sources[42]; residential magnetic field exposures in relation to risk of childhood leukemia[43]; and identification of the areas within a county where children with high lead levels were concentrated, in order to plan targeted screening.[44] Geographic information can take a variety of forms in epidemiologic investigation, from simply locating the residential address of study subject, to using information on proximity to agents of concern over time and space as a surrogate metric of exposure. Leveraging historical geographic information, for example, residential history, can enable researchers to construct long-term estimates of exposure over time, which is particularly useful for diseases with long induction periods or for exposures that are episodic or have short half-lives. For example, an association between lifetime exposure to paraquat and maneb, two agricultural pesticides, and Parkinson disease was detected using California Pesticide Use Reports to estimate historical exposures to pesticides proximate to residences going as far back as 1974.[45] The strength of this approach is underscored by the recent validation of this database of pesticide applications. In a year-long monitoring study, weekly measurements of individual pesticides in ambient air of a nearby town were highly correlated with the amount of those same pesticides applied during that week within 8 km^2 of the monitors.[46] Both spatial and temporal aspects of exposure are addressed, as illustrated in a study of prenatal organophosphate exposures and diagnosis of autism spectrum disorder (ASD).[47] Mothers of cases with ASD and controls with neither ASD nor other cognitive impairments provided their residential histories, and once their addresses were geocoded, residential proximity to applications of chlorpyrifos revealed a higher exposure to nearby applications in those with ASD children versus those whose children were developing more typically.

Additionally, locating environmental hazards in geographic space in relation to the census-level descriptors of communities (race/ethnicity, income, mean educational level) can provide evidence of environmental injustice or better elucidate structural contributors to health disparities in low-income communities or populations of color (see below, "Vulnerable Populations"). The sophisticated use of mapping data in combination with information on individual behaviors or health outcomes has been a critical factor in the explosion of research on health consequences of the "built environment." For example, see research on residential proximity to natural environments and physical activity[48] and the neighborhood food environment and obesity.[49]

In study planning, the utility of existing measurements from administrative or surveillance databases and the decisions of how many and what kind of measurements to make are critical. Both require a close examination of variability within and across individuals over time, as well as sources of error and uncertainty. Exposure may be measured using sophisticated instruments, or it may be inferred from databases or questionnaires about the presence or use of the agents of concern. Crude categorization (yes/no or high/low) is often not adequate because of uncertainty in the assignment and the wide variability within groups. Ordinal categories provide the opportunity to assess dose-response relations. Optimally, the quantification on a continuous scale of exposure from the relevant time period will endow a study with the greatest sensitivity. Quantified measures also allow researchers to assess comparability across studies and can provide the basis for regulatory decision-making.

It is useful to distinguish among an exposure setting, a complex mixture, and a single agent. An exposure setting involves a specific situation and a mix of exposures that may change over time or from place to place. Coal burning produces a different mix of air pollutants than combustion of automotive fuel. Pollutants from automotive exhaust vary by type of fuel, air temperature, and sunshine; the fuel composition has itself changed over time. Sidestream and mainstream smoke, and e-cigarettes, differ in composition, both vary by source of tobacco and additives. In particularly, they produce a highly variable chemical mixture, which also is influenced by solvent, temperature, and puffing behavior.[50,51] The investigator should be clear on whether the hypothesis concerns a setting, a mix, or a single exposure and should select the appropriate study design and exposure assessment strategy. Inferences about a mix of exposures or a specific setting can be equally valid as those pertaining to individual agents. They may also have more predictive and public health value, since interventions frequently affect an overall exposure scenario rather than a single agent.

Relationship of Exposure Timing to Health Outcome

The relevant timing for an exposure assessment is specific to the etiologic hypothesis and disease outcome. Thus, additional considerations for selecting the exposure metric for a given study pertain to the timing of the exposure and its relationship to the occurrence of the disease. A first concept in timing of exposure and relation to disease is that of the critical window. Susceptibility for some conditions is related to a specific period in gestation, growth or development, such as the time when major organs are forming, when neural networks are emerging in the cerebral cortex, when infant production of IgG begins, when breast development is taking place, or when an adolescent growth spurt is occurring. Other factors may influence the critical window of susceptibility for specific types of chemical compounds, such as the maturation of detoxification mechanisms that might protect the fetus by reducing the toxic exposure. Thus, cofactors may magnify or reduce the effect of the exposure and alter the window of susceptibility. When the timing for initiation of pathogenesis is confined to a well-defined developmental period, the latency until the time of onset of clinical disease may nonetheless still vary widely.

The timing between the action of an exposure in a susceptible person and the occurrence of clinically detectable disease, which may occur much later, comprises two distinct periods.[52] The first is the induction period, which we consider to be the time between exposure and the initiation of disease or pathogenesis. During the induction period, the causal mechanism is being completed and is still subject to being interrupted. Following the induction period is the latency period, which represents the time from actual disease initiation to the point in time when the disease is clinically detectable. However, because the precise time of disease detectability is almost always unknown, in practice, latency is usually defined as the time from disease initiation to actual detection of disease. The induction period could be minutes or hours for acute poisonings, hours or days for respiratory symptoms such as asthma exacerbations, months or years for developmental disorders, or decades for cancer, cardiovascular effects, or neurodegenerative disorders. The latency period will depend on the nature of the disease and the stage at which the exposure plays a role, as well as individual-level susceptibility and defense mechanisms including detoxification and immune responses. In developing a plan for exposure assessment, epidemiologists will need to consider the lengths of both the induction and latency periods or, at least, their combined duration.

For protracted exposures, the combined induction and latency periods span from the time when exposure reaches a critical threshold until the time when disease is clinically manifest. The point when exposure reaches such a threshold will not usually be known: it will be a function of the exposure intensity or cumulative exposure and the individual's protective capacity. Interestingly, the induction period can extend beyond the period of external exposure: if the chemical agent has a long retention time, then the internal stores of the exogenous exposure or its toxic metabolites may continue to "expose" the target tissues—for compounds like dioxin (2,3,7,8-tetrachlorodibenzodioxin, or TCDD), with a half-life in the body of 7-10 years, internal exposures can continue for decades[53,54] (see Retention times, below). Both the induction and latency periods can vary by individual susceptibilities.

Protracted exposures present a challenge for epidemiologists whenever the critical window of susceptibility is unknown and could be an extended interval. Past and/or even distant past exposures are relevant for studying diseases that have long induction periods or are caused by long-term chronic insults; when biological specimens have not been collected, biomarker-based exposure assessment may be impossible. Extensive investigations of leukemia clustering around the Sellafield nuclear facility in West Cumbria, England, found an excess among children born in the village but not among those who moved into the area, suggesting that if an exposure was responsible, it operated before birth.[55,56] Some biomarkers can capture long-term or distant past exposures, including measurements in bone and teeth. Cognitive function in the elderly might be related to lifetime lead exposure, which is better assessed by bone lead (with a half-life of 10-15 years) than blood lead (half-life of 45 days) measurements. In contrast, for a study of the effect of in utero lead exposure on the fetus, the mother's cumulative exposure is less relevant than the amount reaching fetal circulation; hence, maternal blood lead during pregnancy (which readily crosses the placenta) might be superior to a single measurement of bone lead.

For acute or moderately short-term effects, the critical period may be easier to identify (*e.g.*, air pollution-induced asthma episodes, certain adverse reproductive outcomes, and in some cases, developmental or behavioral disorders), and the pay-off from collection of detailed timing information may be great. Bell et al.[57-59] found that the strength of association between pesticides and late fetal deaths from congenital anomalies was greatest for weeks 3 to 8, the period of organogenesis. This study took advantage of the known critical window for that outcome. However, if the time period chosen for exposure assessment is not the biologically relevant one, the resulting misclassification could cause biased estimates of association.[60] When information on timing of exposure is collected but the critical time window is not known, analyses with several different choices may be instructive, as long as there is variability in exposure between time periods and across persons. For example, a number of studies have implicated maternal fever during pregnancy with increased risk for autism. Among these, two independent reports on timing converged on an elevated risk from a second trimester episode,[61,62] while a separate investigation linked ASD to lengthy febrile episodes in the first or second trimester.[63]

A related issue is that of retention time. Even though external exposures may have ended years earlier, a compound with a long half-life will continue to be present in certain organs. The tragic incidents known as Yusho ("oil disease") in Japan and Yu-Cheng in Taiwan involved consumption of cooking oil contaminated with PCB compounds.[64,65] Children born years later to women who had been poisoned suffered severe developmental deficits due to their prenatal exposures to the mother's accumulated and stored "body burden"[64] (see Environmental Disasters section). The persistence of organochlorine pesticides in fat tissue results in highly reliable biomarkers of exposure, which enables inferences about exposures in earlier periods, an advantage for case-control studies.

Duration of contact (or potential contact) may be employed as a surrogate quantitative exposure measure. This measure, however, can be problematic if intensity of exposure varies across individuals and across time and is a strong determinant of the effect. In this case, real associations could be obscured. A lack of data on how exposure—either prevalence or concentration—changes over time is difficult to overcome. When external measurements are available, they can be combined with duration and timing of residence and activity-pattern information (for example, the time spent indoors and outdoors or the quantity of water ingested) to assign quantitative or semiquantitative exposure estimates for individuals.

Environmental Health Surveillance

Environmental health surveillance involves the systematic collection, linkage, and analysis of both environmental and health data, in order to identify those exposures that are adversely affecting the well-being of the population so that rational public policy can be developed. However, existing surveillance systems are limited by the availability of high-quality health data that can be linked with environmental exposures. In the absence of adequate prerelease testing, systematic monitoring for adverse health effects is rational and appropriate. Disease surveillance is discussed extensively in Chapter 9, but surveillance for environmental hazards requires additional elements.[66]

An ideal surveillance system for environmentally induced disease would have the following elements: (1) high-quality mortality and morbidity data with residence information; (2) timely population data for denominators to calculate rates with adjustment for migration between censuses; (3) timely, high-quality emissions and environmental monitoring data for air, water, soil, and food, and other exposure media, characterized geographically and temporally; (4) personal monitoring, biomonitoring, and exposure modeling data to capture transport and transmission; (5) tools to link these various types of data; (6) compatible standards across data sources and standardized vocabularies; (7) fine enough resolution to be useful for observing effects of localized exposures on small communities; and (8) systems for dissemination of such data.[66,67] Although costly, the benefits of such a surveillance system would include information on long-term trends; an early warning capability, that is, the ability to detect unusually high incidence of diseases covered by the system; ready linkage to potential causative agents; avoidance of public anxiety and costly investigations of situations where no excess risk is ascertained; and the potential for increased public confidence in the commitment of government and health scientists to protect the population's health.

Initiatives in the United States and other countries have begun to address the need for integrated surveillance systems. In the United States, the Pew Environmental Health Commission[68] called for establishment of a Nationwide Health Tracking Network that would monitor and establish relations between environmental hazards and disease. The report cited the absence of information on autoimmune diseases, developmental disabilities, diabetes and other endocrinologic disorders, asthma, and birth defects. In 2002, the Centers for Disease Control and Prevention[69] established a national Environmental Public Health Tracking program, which has included more than half the States and New York City, and integrates health data, human biomonitoring, census-level population data, and ambient exposure monitoring.[70] The California program "CalEnviroScreen"[71] has become a model (*e.g.*, see version 3.0) through development of a risk score based on a range of environmental (air pollution, water contaminants, pesticide use, traffic density, industrial toxic releases, groundwater threats, waste facilities), sociodemographic (education, poverty, unemployment, housing, and linguistic isolation), and health indicators of sensitive populations (asthma, cardiovascular disease, and low birth weight). Every census tract is scored on each indicator, and the resulting data can be viewed in maps and data files in various formats. Most significantly, the scores are used to identify disadvantaged communities to which the state designates a portion of its revenue from specific sources.

These resources have increasingly been utilized for environmental health research, leveraging information on health in relation to lead exposure, air quality, climate data, and exposure biomonitoring.[72] The Environmental Protection Agency created EJSCREEN,[73] a mapping tool designed to promote transparency in how the agency takes into consideration environmental justice in its programs, activities, including outreach and engagement; implementation of permitting and enforcement; to assist stakeholders in their decision-making about pursuing environmental justice; and to create a common understanding between the agency and the public when examining issues related to environmental justice. Similar to CalEnviroScreen, EJSCREEN combines environmental and census-level demographic data.

These surveillance systems are useful for identifying and describing environmental health hazards and can facilitate design of epidemiological studies by geographically locating high-risk populations (*e.g.*, high exposure and high disease burdens); however, care must be taken when making etiological inferences. Current surveillance systems are blind to issues such as induction period and latency and therefore may suggest associations between exposure and outcome that are noncausal and/or may miss important causal associations for diseases with long induction periods or latencies.

STUDY DESIGNS IN ENVIRONMENTAL EPIDEMIOLOGY

Environmental epidemiology uses all of the standard study designs: cohort, cross-sectional, case-control, ecologic, community intervention, natural experiments, and randomized trials with individual or group (*e.g.*, place-based) randomization. Whereas replication with similar designs can establish consistency, use of multiple different designs can provide broad evidence for coherence and avoid replicating biases across multiple studies.

Environmental epidemiology has also provided impetus for a wide range of methodologic developments to address key issues of the field. The major challenges of exposure assessment for environmental epidemiology, sometimes viewed as its "Achilles Heel," have been described above. Beyond exposure assessment, additional challenges for environmental epidemiology relate to both study designs and analytic methods. These issues include time trends in exposures, outcomes, or confounders; rare outcomes; unknown lag between exposures and development of diseases; short-term versus long-term effects; and confounding from strong risk factors such as social class, smoking, or other lifestyle factors. Natural, man-made, or combined disasters frequently result in extreme levels of exposure, sometimes with both acute and chronic components (see below, Disasters in Environmental Epidemiology). Two examples below illustrate how multiple study designs—some common and some more specialized—can be leveraged to build a case for causation; in subsequent sections, we highlight two specific designs that have featured prominently in some areas of environmental epidemiology.

1) Cholera and contamination of drinking water: The classic work of John Snow (1855), "On the Mode of Communication of Cholera," presented an array of evidence that fecal matter from infected patients carried the "morbid poison," that ingestion of small quantities was the mode of transmission, and that mixing of sewage and drinking water sources enabled such transmission on a wide scale. His focus on the gastrointestinal tract was in contrast to prevailing views that disease was carried in the air by infective material, termed miasma. Snow's method proceeded from an initial case series tracing the introduction of the epidemic into a municipality involving person-to-person contact; to mapping of cases and ecologic comparisons across districts of London for the 1832, 1849, and 1853 outbreaks; and finally to a natural experiment (a cohort design in which exposure occurs effectively at random, with no preference as to confounding factors [see Chapter 6]). The ecologic intercommunity comparisons of districts in London were accompanied by property value data to show the lack of correspondence between water source and wealth, thereby providing evidence that the association was not due to social class. The natural experiment was a serendipitous occurrence, but Snow strengthened the findings by incorporating individual confirmation of exposure by visiting homes of all cholera victims to obtain documentation of the water supplier. If this was not available, Snow collected a vial of tap water. Although he could not test for the as yet unidentified microorganism, London's sewage-contaminated downstream water had 40 times higher sodium chloride, which precipitated with the addition of silver nitrate. Thus Snow could determine each case's household water source with high accuracy.[74]

Snow's accounts addressed apparent inconsistencies of various types of information with his hypothesized mode of transmission. He noted that wherever the general water supply was not contaminated, cholera was primarily seen in crowded areas where the poor and laboring classes lived, but that in districts near the Broad Street pump, the disease had struck the wealthier and poorer houses equally. While it may be difficult for today's epidemiologists to appreciate the skepticism with which Snow's theory of epidemic transmission was received for decades, Snow's clarity and unrelenting thoroughness as he sought to reconcile each detail of the cholera epidemics with his unpopular theory of oral-fecal transmission serve as a model for present-day environmental epidemiology that similarly faces skeptics both by medical professions and the lay public.

2) Lead exposure and neurodevelopment: Early studies of chronic low-level lead exposure and mental development in children included cohort[75] and case-control[76] designs, and in a classic cross-sectional study with a biomarker of historical exposure, Needleman et al.[77] estimated cumulative childhood exposure by measuring the dentin lead content of their deciduous teeth: this seminal study established that, after adjustment for many confounders, higher cumulative lead exposure (from conception to the age of tooth shedding) was associated with lower IQ and more behavior problems.

Methodologically, this landmark study also highlights how standard rankings of study quality (*e.g.*, Newcastle Ottawa Scale[78]), which place cohort studies above other nonrandomized designs, can fail to capture the core strength or superiority of a given study[79]: evidence from a cross-sectional study with an objective exposure marker that accurately captures exposures in a relevant time window can be less biased than results of a cohort study, *e.g.*, one that used error-prone methods for exposure assessment, such as self-reports for common exposures that might be easily forgotten or overlooked, or measurements taken at a single time point when exposures vary widely, especially when the vulnerable window might be an extended time period or a short period not including that single time point.

Longitudinal follow-up of those children whose teeth were analyzed produced evidence that tooth lead exposure predicted failure to complete high school, and poorer scores on reading, vocabulary, hand-eye coordination, and reaction time tests.[80] Bellinger et al.[81] similarly found dentin lead in deciduous teeth was associated with problem behaviors in 8-year-old children, while prenatal exposure, measured by cord blood lead, was not. In adolescents, executive function and self-regulation were found to be adversely affected by lead exposures.[82] Thus, a series of studies of different designs revealed neurologic, cognitive, and behavioral impacts of lead, suggested that cumulative exposure was responsible for these adverse outcomes, and built a compelling body of literature that supported coherence of evidence around aberrant development of the central nervous system functions.

Two specific designs are frequently used by environmental epidemiologists: case-crossover[83,84] and ecologic studies.[85,86] A third design, the community intervention, has been less commonly used, but has strong potential for helping to move the science on environmental etiologic factors into appropriate policy changes. These interventions may be ad hoc, with the research capitalizing on implementation of new policies or practices that change the environmental exposures, or may be planned community trials with real or quasi-randomization.

Case-Crossover Design

Case-crossover designs were introduced in the early 1990s[87] (see Mittleman and Mostofsky on exchangeability in the case-crossover design[88]) for estimating a short-term, transient effect of intermittent exposures on acute-onset diseases. This exposure-outcome model corresponds to scenarios in environmental epidemiology, such as asthma exacerbations in relation to air pollutants or eye irritation from wildfire smoke. In a case-crossover study, for each event occurrence, the exposure preceding it (case period) is compared with exposures of the same person in one or more other control or referent periods. Confounding from individual time-invariant characteristics is completely controlled, as the individual supplies his or her own referent periods. This design can be used for both one-time events (death) and recurrent events (asthma episodes, otitis media, acute respiratory illnesses). The analysis may be done using person-time methods if exposure is recorded continuously or by using defined risk windows if exposure is known only at sampled times, given the matching of cases to their own "controls"; see Chapter 8 for further discussion of the design. In the last decade, this design has been commonly applied to air pollution health effect studies.[89-91]

Ecologic Studies

Ecologic studies utilize group-level data on outcomes (*e.g.*, rates of disease, prevalence proportions, or mean measurements) in relation to group-level data on exposures (proportions exposed, mean or median exposure concentrations, *e.g.*, in air or water). These studies are distinct from studies that have individual-level data on outcomes but assign exposure at a group level. Ecologic studies are often conducted when exposures are already measured at the group level (monitoring data, for example) or when limited resources for conducting the study prohibit collection of individual-level data.

For exposures that are not homogeneous or well distributed within the groups, or in other words, for which interindividual differences predominate within a group, ecologic studies are a particularly weak study design. This is because they are subject to group-level confounding, individual-level confounding, and cross-level confounding, also known as ecologic bias (see Chapter 30). This bias arises if, within the groups having higher average levels of exposure X, a subset of those with low or absent exposure X are at higher risk for disease. In this scenario, the average exposure, or the aggregate exposure assigned to the group, does not represent those who are primarily afflicted with the disease. The key is the heterogeneity of the exposure, for which a group summary statistic is the exposure metric. The ecologic bias leads to an incorrect conclusion, and, for this reason, results from ecologic studies should be viewed critically, and investigators conducting such studies need to take account all possible sources of confounding. Having some evidence that exposure is not highly heterogeneous within groups could be reassuring. Nevertheless, environmental exposures can easily be confounded by socioeconomic factors; higher affluence leads to different behaviors, greater access to healthy foods and higher quality health care, and an ability to afford living in areas with less air pollution, noise, and other types of stressors. Ecologic comparisons across regions must take account such factors. Another way to think about this problem is to view ecologic study results as a first pass at generating hypotheses or gathering preliminary, crude support for funding a more accurate individual-level study.

That said, ecologic studies may be the best or only study design for addressing many policy questions, for example, to evaluate health impacts of environmental regulations or of a new technology. If regulations result in reduced emissions from tailpipes of motor vehicles, or zero-emission vehicles become widespread for economic or other reasons, then ambient air pollutant levels may be reduced throughout a state region, and one may seek to determine if health is improved population-wide in those areas. Between the 2003 heat wave in western Europe[85,92] and the subsequent one in 2006, authorities in France implemented multiple interventions designed to reduce mortality. Indeed, predictive models indicated that 4,400 deaths were averted, suggesting that the combination of greater awareness and specific measures taken was successful.[86] Additionally, if policies are implemented at different time points in different locations, before-vs-after studies may be less susceptible to confounding from other time trends that might be more uniform across areas.

A common study design used in environmental epidemiology compares disease rates in communities having high exposure with rates in lower exposure communities. This design is appropriate when exposures are spread throughout a community but not where point sources pollute small areas within a community. Intercommunity comparisons are particularly useful for evaluating the impact of chronic ongoing exposures that vary primarily between rather than within communities. However, social, cultural, and economic factors may similarly vary across communities, introducing serious difficulty in achieving complete control for confounding (see next section, Social Class discussion).

Note that if *only the exposure* is measured at the group level, while the outcome and confounders are both measured at the level of the individual, the analysis can be conducted at the individual-level and therefore the study design would not be ecologic (see *e.g.*,[93]). Intercommunity comparisons with group-level indices of exposure but individual data on covariates and outcome are superior to an ecologic study. It is an individual-level study with group-level exposure metrics, which may engender potential measurement error depending on dispersion of those exposures. The approach of group-level exposure assignment with individual data on outcome and confounders has frequently been used in air pollution epidemiology, for which most exposures of concern (particles, NOx) disperse over fairly wide areas. Unfortunately, these studies have been widely mischaracterized as being ecologic. This erroneous characterization has hampered the field, clouded discussion of the health consequences with unwarranted skepticism, and possibly delayed translation of air pollution research findings into regulation to protect public health.

A four-level hierarchy for ecologic studies by Susser[94] provides a useful framework for illustrating circumstances in which this design is (1) "obligate and apt," (2) "optional and apt" (3) "optional, not apt, but convenient," and (4) maladroit. At the top are studies for which the goal is to determine the effectiveness of programs, policies, or regulations that are implemented at the ecologic level, as described above. Generally, the exposure is homogeneous across individuals, and the outcomes are meaningful primarily for the group as a whole. In the second category, one might place studies in which exposure itself can be defined at the group level even though related behaviors or factors can also be assessed at the individual level, such as neighborhood density of liquor stores versus individual intake of alcohol, median income or percent employment in the census block versus employment status of the individual, or green space versus personal physical activity. The investigator's perspective on different types of intervention approaches might dictate which level to study. Ecologic studies can also be useful when a field is new and the goal is to screen hypotheses inexpensively (time trend, birth cohort, and mapping studies might apply) or when interindividual variation is outweighed by between-group differences (see example concerning trihalomethanes in drinking water, "Exposure Assessment: subsection above). These examples fall in Susser's third group, where it would be convenient to do such studies at the ecologic level, even though an individual-level study would be more convincing.

Common ecologic approaches include exploration of regional variations in health outcomes and exposures, to examine how they covary either geographically or in their time trends. These approaches include: Mapping, trend or time series analyses, and either differences in time trends across regions or changes in spatial patterns over time. Tools that link space and time variation in exposure, with space and time variation in health outcomes, have become highly accessible through GIS that permit overlay of numerous, diverse databases with spatially referenced variables. As described above (*Environmental Health Surveillance*), environmental health monitoring systems such as the EJSCREEN and CalEnviroScreen provide interactive mapping with numerous well-defined indicators of exposure burden, population vulnerability, and vital statistics and other health outcomes. As more "big data" resources and EMR (electronic medical records) have become available for research purposes, opportunities for environmental epidemiology expand.

Community Studies and Intervention Trials

While not unique to environmental epidemiology, community studies can be ideal for assessing impacts of social or environmental policies or interventions that are more feasible at the group than the individual level. A recent analysis evaluated the effect of bans, in some parts of Ireland, on the marketing, sale, and distribution of coal. These policies were followed by a decrease in both particulate black smoke and respiratory disease mortality,[95] suggesting a measurable benefit to the population.

An historical example of community-level intervention trials was the planned fluoridation of certain public water supply systems. Ast[96] summarized their results: Comparing post- with pre-fluoridation figures, the number of decayed, missing, or filled (DMF) teeth per child was reduced dramatically, *i.e.*, by -48% to -70%. These trials demonstrated that addition of fluoride had the same effect as was known to be associated with naturally occurring fluoride in the prevention of dental caries.

METHODOLOGICAL CHALLENGES AND ANALYSIS CONSIDERATIONS IN ENVIRONMENTAL EPIDEMIOLOGY

Models for Applications to Environmental Epidemiology

When environmental exposures are characterized by high temporal or spatial variability, the epidemiologist studying their effects will want to adjust for multivariable confounding and may want to model exposure-response relations quantitatively. Besides typical models used in epidemiologic cohort and case-control studies, such as multiple logistic regression and proportional hazards models, environmental epidemiologic research that focuses on long-term effects or trajectories of health or development or that examines spatial aspects of exposure and health may call for more complex designs and analytic methods. In longitudinal studies with repeated measures, adjustment for autocorrelation will usually be necessary, and geographic studies may require special methods such as empirical Bayes,[97] or kriging,[98] adjacency,[99] and distance-based techniques. Generalized linear models provide an overall framework that can encompass both group-level and individual-level data, or both simultaneously, and can accommodate cross-sectional, longitudinal, or spatial data. This class of models also permits outcomes from various distributions: binomial, multinomial, or continuous Normal, log-Normal and Poisson.

For disease rates aggregated into categories, Poisson regression (see Chapter 20) is frequently the method of choice[100] and can be applied to data in which time and space are central factors defining the units of observation. For risk data, especially when the disease is common, binomial regression or survival analysis is more appropriate. The interrelationships among these three methods are discussed by Pearce et al.[101] In Poisson regression, either counts or rates of events are a function of exposure, spatial, time-period, demographic, and other variables. The method is commonly used with categorical (nominal or ordinal) predictors but need not be limited to such variables, as maximum likelihood estimation for Poisson modeling is consistent with sparse cells and can be used for continuous data as well. Within cells constructed by cross-classification across predictor variables, events are enumerated, and, in most cases, it will also be necessary to obtain the person-time or expected count associated with each cell. The data collected from time series or geographic regions can be organized into cells such as days, weeks, years, etc.; counties, states, regions of the world, etc.; or space-time units such as county-years, etc.

In typical exponential (log-linear) Poisson regression models, assumptions include the following: (1) the logarithm of the disease rate changes linearly with equal-increment increases in the exposure variable; (2) changes in the rate from the combined effects of different exposures or risk factors are multiplicative; (3) at each level of the covariates, the number of cases has variance equal to its mean; and (4) observations are independent. Methods to detect and deal with violations of assumptions (1) and (2) are similar to those used for other exponential models (*e.g.*, logistic, proportional hazards).[102] Methods to identify violations of assumption (3), that is, to determine whether there is overdispersion (variances are too large) or underdispersion (too small), include plots of residuals versus the mean at different levels of the predictor variable. Methods for dealing with violation of the Poisson assumptions are discussed in Breslow[103] and McCullagh and Nelder.[104]

Social Class and Its Multiple Roles Relative to Environmental Health

Environmental exposures with deleterious effects on health tend to be higher in communities already burdened by low wealth, political capital, and other resource deficits. These community characteristics tend to disproportionately include members from disadvantaged racial and ethnic group. The exposures that are disproportionately found in such communities include air pollutants from traffic and industrial emissions, water contamination, hazardous waste sites, a lack of green space, and older housing stock more likely to be affected by legacy lead paint, along with a host of other unhealthy conditions. The convergence of social, cultural, and economic factors with exposures that lead to poorer health, a problem referred to as environmental justice—that is, the lack of it—is both an ethical concern and an epidemiologic challenge. When communities of color or low resources are more likely to have polluting industries sited in their midst, two issues arise. The first is the serious difficulty in achieving complete control for confounding. The second is the need to address effect measure modification; specifically, a growing body of evidence suggests that the health impacts arising from similar levels of air pollution, household chemicals, breastfeeding, and other risk or protective factors may differ according to the socioeconomic and other resources available to an individual or a community; this heterogeneity of effect may exacerbate the already elevated disease burden in underserved areas (see below, Vulnerable Populations).

Social class is strongly and consistently associated with a broad range of diseases,[105] and systematic inequities in environmental pollution with regard to poverty or race are well documented.[106-108] These disparities have been documented for decades. The concentrations of dichlorodiphenyltrichloroethane (DDT), its metabolites, and PCBs in San Francisco Bay Area residents were substantially higher among African Americans than among Whites during the 1960s.[109] Similarly, data collected in 1976 to 1980 for the Second NHANES demonstrated much higher levels of blood lead among African Americans and among those of low education, as compared with Whites and those of higher education.[110]

Given strong associations of socioeconomic status (SES) with both environmental exposures and health outcomes, the potential for confounding to distort the impact of environment is great. As information on income is difficult to collect (many people decline to report it), epidemiologists typically use education or sometimes occupation to capture social class. Adjustment for these factors may be inadequate due to residual confounding arising in multiple ways, including the use of broad categories for education or SES,[111] and lack of data on resources or social capital, factors that operate at the individual, household, family, or neighborhood level, and that influence host susceptibility and access to medical or preventive care.

However, beyond the socioeconomics lies a trove of other health-related attributes. A recent analysis of NHANES urine and blood measurements for several hundred analytes found that 20% of measurements were strongly associated with household income after consideration of multiple comparisons and validation on a split sample: these included many environmental chemicals or their metabolites; nutrients or other biochemical analytes; anthropometric variables; and infectious agents.[112] This analysis demonstrates how pervasive the effects of SES are—they are literally in our bodies—and how challenging it is to adjust adequately for the diverse pathways through which SES influences health and well-being.

In addition to these internal aspects, neighborhood characteristics appear to predict health even after controlling for individual-level factors.[113-115] Potentially relevant census-derived neighborhood factors include percentage unemployed, percent owner-occupied housing, and median income. Others are the availability of supermarkets with fresh produce,[116] density of liquor stores,[117] and crime rates.[118]

In light of complex relationships of sociodemographic and economic variables with environment and health, use of directed acyclic graphs[119-121] in conjunction with the existing literature can help clarify the factors involved and how they fit into a conceptual causal model, which in turn provides a valid way to select covariates appropriate for adjustment purposes. Inadequately measured confounders can result in biased estimates of associations between the main exposure and outcome, even after adjustment for these confounders (see Chapter 12). Such errors can be substantial but would not be detectable in standard analysis that lacks data on the degree of measurement error of the confounder (social class). Moreover, even when the misclassification (of confounders) is nondifferential, the adjusted measure could be more biased than the crude one.[122] Hence, one may need to go beyond the usual surrogates, especially for socioeconomic determinants.

Moreover, despite the fact that socioeconomics, at both the individual and the neighborhood level, is a profound predictor of health, treating it as a confounder could be inappropriate for perhaps three reasons: (1) if some of the disparities in health outcomes attributed to socioeconomics are actually due to shared variance between socioeconomic factors and environmental exposures[123]; (2) if instead the socioeconomic factors are (in part) a consequence of environmental exposures and hence potentially on the causal pathway; or (3) if the effect of an environmental exposure varies by socioeconomic level. As an example of (2) could occur when environmental conditions can serve to perpetuate disparities in education and wealth, as for example, when lead exposures impair intellectual development. In this scenario, SES may be an intermediate, for which adjustment could introduce bias, and in both (1) and (2), adjustment could result in underestimates of the effect of lead on neurobehavioral development.

With regard to effect modification, a growing body of literature describes heterogeneity by race, ethnicity, and other correlates of social class for associations between environmental chemicals and health outcomes. Specifically, those exposures have a greater effect on communities of color or of low resources. Examples are elaborated below (see below, Vulnerable Populations). Investigators need to address social class in the design, data collection, and analysis phases of a study and should consider various roles that sociodemographic and economic variables could play in the causal web leading from environmental injustice to health disparities.

Analysis of High-Dimensional and Mixed Exposures

Humans are exposed to more than one chemical at a time.[124] Our ability to measure an increasingly wide array of environmental exposures (see below "Exposure Mixtures & The Exposome") presents "big data" challenges to environmental epidemiology that necessitate increasingly sophisticated statistical methods.[125,126] Recently, statistical methods have been developed for assessing the effects of mixtures as a whole and for teasing out which compounds might be the main drivers of the overall association.[127-130] Major statistical problems in exposome research include nonindependence (across environmental factors) and mixtures. Hierarchical regression and Bayesian methods have addressed nonindependence across a large set of explanatory variables[131] and machine learning algorithms accounting for nonindependence have been developed.[132] For real-world scenarios of simultaneous exposures, various tools address different questions: principal components can identify clusters of correlated items, reducing them to a few principal components that maximize orthogonality; weighted quantile sum regression (WQSR) can estimate the effect of the whole mixture on an outcome and apportion the relative contributions of the parts;[133] and elastic net addresses correlated covariates and allows the number of predictors to be larger than the number of observations. Network and pathway models can characterize overlapping and/or interchangeable functionality and also suggest potential synergistic effects produced by chemicals acting on different steps along the same or converging pathways. There is no single method that is optimal for all scenarios and all research questions, but thoughtful comparisons among methods and across their applications can guide biostatisticians and epidemiologists toward the best approach for their research question (See e.g.,[128]). An NIEHS workshop emphasized the need for toxicologists, statisticians, and epidemiologists to work collaboratively, bringing their respective knowledge bases to the mixture problem.[134] This will become increasingly essential over the next decade, as environmental epidemiologists begin to integrate modern exposomics platforms into our research studies (see below, Special Topics in Environmental Epidemiology).

Searching for Patterns

Time Patterns

Three main types of time-related exposure-disease patterns can be useful to discovering relationships of health conditions with environmental factors: time clustering, longitudinal trends, and cyclic patterns. Time clustering usually occurs when an agent is newly introduced into the human environment, when a human behavior suddenly brings the population into contact with an exposure or pathogen not commonly encountered on as large a scale, or when a disaster strikes. Although one might be tempted to distinguish human-induced events such as shipwrecks, plane crashes, and mass shootings from natural occurrences such as hurricanes and wildfires, in the current Anthropocene era,[135,136] the intensity and magnitude of many of these "natural" disasters have been amplified by human activities that have led to global climate changes and major alterations in ecosystems from molecular, cellular, and microscopic to continental, oceanic, and planetary scales.

For other types of health outcome clusters, the purpose of the investigation may be to identify the cause(s). Several disease cluster investigations of grave neurologic problems succeeded in a definitive determination that the cause was mercury poisoning, which had resulted from decades of industrial waste disposal into Minimata Bay, Japan, and from shorter episodes of grain contamination in Iraq.[137-139] The cause in Minimata was identified only after thousands of people had been affected by severe physical and mental disabilities. More recently, a policy disaster that switched the source of residential water from a safe one to a river with highly corrosive water exposed thousands to high lead levels in Flint, Michigan.[140] (See section: Environmental Disasters and Health, below.)

When the cause is known, the focus of epidemiologic studies may be on documenting the attributable fraction or identifying cofactors associated with higher than typical risk, that is, the more vulnerable subgroups. An analysis of deaths from the 1999 earthquake in Taiwan demonstrated, for instance, that those with mental illness, physical disability, or low SES were at highest risk.[141] Mortality from the 2003 heat wave in France was close to 15,000 deaths, concentrated in elderly persons[85] and those with more socioeconomic vulnerability.[142] In the 2017 wildfires in northern California, which broke out in the middle of the night and rapidly spread through urban areas, deaths were also highest among the elderly (average age of victims, 79 years).[143]

Both sudden surges and slower long-term trends can easily be confounded or can arise from artifacts of diagnosis. For example, a new diagnostic test or a change or reorganization of data collection procedures/practices can lead to the appearance of a rapid or gradual change in incidence. Similarly, prevalence can change when new treatments are adopted or healthcare access is increased (or reduced) based on new policies. An example is the steady rise in both the prevalence proportions and incidence rates for ASD for over more than a decade[144] following changes from DSM (Diagnostic and Statistical Manual) version III to IV (1994). Nevertheless, the magnitude of the rise had been much larger than could be explained by those diagnostic changes or by other artifacts.[144,145] The full explanations for ~10% average increase per year for ~20 years are still unknown, although—beyond artifacts of ascertainment—suggestive clues have emerged from various strands of research. Teasing out heterogeneity of time trends by different subsets of the population can be informative: gender differences in time trends imply factors on which men and women tend to differ (*e.g.*, occupations, alcohol, etc.). Conversely, when little or no gender difference is observed, exposures shared by all are more plausible explanations. If the exposures are prenatal, genetic or intrauterine hormones may be implicated.

Although time trends may reveal etiologic clues, confounding factors may also undergo time trends. Our modern era of rapid changes in all aspects of human activity presents a particular challenge for time-trend analysis, *e.g.*, increased consumption of sweetened beverages[146]; rise in intake of high fructose corn syrup from <10 g to nearly 100 g per person per day[147]; introduction in the early 1980s of ultrasound equipment for fetal imaging that delivered an eightfold higher thermal dose than the previous technology[148]; increasing C-section deliveries[149]; and the rising use of brominated flame retardants in household products.[150] Additional changes include massive globalization of commerce and human travel bringing many new viruses across borders; the advent of the internet and cell phones along with accompanying lifestyle changes; the introduction of e-cigarettes; the pervasive incorporation of phthalates in scented air fresheners, personal care products, building materials, medical plastic tubing, and food packaging; the opioid epidemic; changes in prescribing patterns for psychotropic medications and blood pressure control, among others; legalization of marijuana in some states; and the recent appearance of antimicrobial chemicals in soaps, toothpaste, socks, and other clothing, followed by new regulations now limiting these.

Thus, in a society marked by fast changes in all sectors of life, any single change is likely confounded by a multiplicity of others. Not surprisingly, many parallel trends turn out to be coincidences, as data mining readily shows.[151] Thus, parallel trends, by themselves, cannot be construed as evidence of causality and are generally far more likely to be chance occurrences. Moreover, multiple factors are most likely involved in virtually all disease conditions, and, hence, the problem of mixtures, in its broadest sense, becomes central to the challenge of making sense from time trends.

In this light, a fresh perspective on time trends and their causes is to consider multiple health outcomes that are all rising during the same time period. These may offer insights into upstream causes that might not be noticed in traditional medical disciplines organized around specific organs or organ systems. The last few decades have seen unusually rapid, consistent rises in obesity, diabetes, asthma, autoimmune conditions, attention-deficit hyperactivity disorder (ADHD), autism, and some mental health conditions, as well as certain cancers, for example, thyroid and malignant melanoma. One might ask: could some common exposures and/or biologic pathways provide a link tying together at least some of these similar trends in quite disparate diseases and disorders?

Cyclic patterns of exposure often reflect changes in the physical environments of human activity and may in turn alter physiologic functions and behaviors. Hence, seasonal patterns of disease are clues to underlying etiology. It has long been established that cardiovascular, cerebrovascular, and respiratory disease deaths rise in winter and decline in summer,[152,153] but extreme heat waves also increase deaths, usually peaking over only a few days.[92,154] Cyclic incidence is often viewed as evidence for a possible infectious etiology, but many potential causes such as temperature, sunlight, air pollutants, time spent outdoors, other behaviors, fruit and vegetable availability/consumption, fertility, use of pesticides, and even magnetic fields are also cyclic. Some evidence of seasonality of birth or conception for schizophrenia[155] and for autism[156] may plausibly indicate infectious etiology or the maternal response to infection, *e.g.*, fever,[61,62,157-159] although associations have also been observed with other factors that have seasonal patterns, such as air pollution[160] and pesticides.[47]

On the flip side, many constructs that typically confound environmental exposure-disease relationships, such as age, SES, and smoking habits, tend to vary little by season, and hence rarely confound analyses of seasonal exposures, although they could be effect-measure modifiers. This phenomenon and the stability of denominators across seasons simplify these analyses, but replication of results may be difficult due to climatic and other differences across regions.

Time series analyses follow the population of a given community or region through time, often without covariate data on individuals; this approach is especially useful to address highly variable exposures and their short-term effects, such as pulmonary function or rates of events (death, hospital admission, symptoms). Within-community comparisons, in contrast to spatial comparisons, obviate the need for denominator data when the population composition and size do not change over the time period of interest. This approach is particularly advantageous if the catchment area is unclear, say, for hospital-based studies in densely populated areas where not all hospitals can be included, yet counts of admissions or outpatients might be comparable for high versus low pollution days if there are no changes that would alter the population base for the included hospitals (*i.e.*, closure of one of the nonincluded ones). Thus, comparisons across time within a population are convenient to assess acute effects from community-wide exposures and may provide more valid estimates of potential environmental effects than comparisons between communities.

Although individual-level confounders are not a problem in such studies, confounding can occur as a result of infectious agents, correlated pollutants, seasonal factors and associated behavioral changes (see "Cyclic patterns" above), time trends in competing risks, and variation in meteorological factors. Temperature, humidity, and seasonal fluctuations may correlate with both pollution and health outcomes. High correlations among individual pollutants (particulates, acid aerosols, ozone, etc.) can be a problem but not if the mixture is of interest.

Long-term trends in mortality can also be a problem in time series analyses of environmental exposures. Adjustment for such trends, however, should be undertaken with caution. If there has been a long-term trend in the exposure (increases or declines in pollution levels), then adjustment could introduce bias toward the null in measures of pollution effects. Confounding of the effect of environmental exposures on long-term disease trends can come from patterns of migration, shifting diagnostic practices, changes in behavior, and other important sources of drift or bias.

Mapping

Mapping of disease rates serves a similar function as time-trend or birth-cohort analysis and has played a role in identifying environmental factors contributing to disease. As early as the 1790s, spot maps of yellow fever cases along the eastern seaboard of the United States played a role in the debate between contagionists and anticontagionists.[161] Snow's map of cholera cases surrounding the Broad Street pump illuminated the proximate cause.[74] Mapping of endemic disease came later. For a history of disease mapping and its use in the study of 19th and 20th century epidemics, see[161]. For more detailed treatment of current methods for mapping and spatial analysis, see[162-164].

Methodologic challenges to disease and exposure mapping arise from variability in population density and population characteristics. Standardization can resolve the differences in characteristics such as age (see Chapter 5). However, small population sizes remain a problem, especially in rural areas. The resulting instability of rates can lead to misleading maps for rare diseases and large but imprecise relative risks for exposures. One solution involves "shrinkage" using empirical Bayes methods. This approach combines some form of "prior" information with the empirical data to derive an improved posterior estimate. For example, in the mapping of both the exposure and the disease, the overall prevalence or rate for the total map can serve as the prior information. The term "shrinkage" refers to replacing each observed small area rate with an adjusted rate that is partially based on the mean rate for all locations—a shrinkage or adjustment toward the overall mean.

For disease mapping, variation in population sizes is a nuisance source of heterogeneity, and empirical Bayes methods function as smoothing techniques, based on three assumptions: (1) the overall rate is unbiased and should not be altered; (2) shrinkage of an individual rate should increase as the variance of that rate increases; and (3) the variation of incidence rates follows a theoretical distribution.[41] Elliott et al.[165] show how mapping rates that have been stabilized via empirical Bayes techniques can stabilize rates, filter out noise, and highlight noteworthy geographic patterns (see color plate 4 in Elliott et al.). If exposure is monitored or measured at the ecologic level, there may also be variability in, for example, the number of readings or monitoring sites. However, models based on monitoring can be used to assign exposures at the individual level (when, *e.g.*, address data are available) of disease. Although not all artifacts of mapping can be removed,[166] these methods offer major advantages over maps of crude rates.[167] For more information on Bayesian mapping methods, see textbooks cited above; or for a detailed account, see[168].

Historically, maps have helped stimulate etiologic research, including focused case-control or cohort studies. The US county-specific maps published by the National Cancer Institute (NCI) in the 1970s[169] were used for surveillance and led to targeted case-control studies that ultimately identified high mortality rates from nasal cancer in areas with furniture-manufacturing industries,[170] lung cancer in counties with petrochemical manufacturing,[171] and bladder cancer where chemical industries were located.[172]

Even for studies of environmental determinants of disease that are not obviously spatial in nature, geographic location may need to be controlled because important confounders that are hard or infeasible to measure may cluster spatially. Examples include physician diagnostic practices or local customs that propel persons to seek medical attention. Cressie demonstrates the use of techniques to remove spatial trends in data and thereby control spatially related confounders.[173]

In spatial or time-trend studies, the assumption of independence may be violated. In time series, the numbers of events (*e.g.*, deaths, hospital admissions, etc.) occurring on a given day, i, may be correlated with the numbers of events on days i-1, i-2, etc. Such correlation may occur because of time clustering in explanatory variables (cold weather) but also for unknown or unmeasured reasons. Similar lack of independence can occur with spatial data. Similarity of disease rates in a given geographic region and those rates in contiguous regions could be due to person-to-person transmission, the presence of the same vectors or sources of exposure, or the influence of physician diagnostic practices. Autocorrelation models can incorporate these nonindependent outcomes.

Analysis of Clustering Around Point Sources

A conventional approach to address clustering around known pollutant sources involves drawing boundaries around the site of the exposure source(s) to include a nearby exposed population, calculation of the disease rate, and comparison with state or national rates. Problems with this approach include (1) indeterminate population sizes, (2) arbitrariness of the boundaries, and (3) difficulties if the area chosen is too large (effect is swamped) or too small (low precision).[173] Another problem can be a lack of sociodemographic comparability between the exposed and referent populations.

Some of these problems are overcome by distance-measure methods, which may examine distances between cases and similarly between randomly selected controls. This approach avoids arbitrary definitions of the affected area and does not require equal population sizes. The method of Besag and Newell[174] involves creation of zones ordered by distance from an exposure source. The source need not be a point; it could be a river or a coastline, with distance defined appropriately.

General Considerations in the Investigation of Clusters

Reports of perceived clusters are frequently made to local, state, and federal agencies by concerned citizens, physicians, or other health practitioners, sometimes overwhelming local, state, or federal agencies. The Centers for Disease Control and Prevention[175] guidelines for investigation of clusters call for an integrated approach that seeks to be responsive to community concern and, at the same time, recognizes that most such reports do not lead to identification of a common causal exposure for the events of interest. Frequently, there simply is no excess of cases. Second, the reported cases may be too diverse to be reasonably suspected of arising from the same cause, *e.g.*, many chemical carcinogens primarily affect a few rather than all cancers. Third, even if there is an excess, the number of cases may be too small for meaningful statistical analysis. Fourth, there may be no identified suspect exposure, or the exposure(s) suggested by the community may not be a plausible cause or set of causes for the outcome reported.

Disease clusters are often reported by small communities, but these are difficult to confirm. If confirmed, two research issues arise. First is the question of whether the disease cluster is part of a general pattern of space-time or space clustering of the disease in question. Specialized studies aimed at evaluating time-space clustering may be undertaken to address that issue. If there is space-time or space clustering, it focuses attention on either environmental or infectious agents that vary geographically or move through populations. A second research question is whether the cause of a single observed disease cluster can be identified. Cluster investigations aimed at explaining a local epidemic are most fruitful when (1) the outcome is rare and occurs primarily by a single mechanism or (2) the rate of disease has increased rapidly.[176] Health professionals who communicate with the lay public need to recognize the culture gap between scientists and nonscientists in how evidence is evaluated. This gap can only be bridged through two-way communication: listening to the concerns and ideas of those outside the profession and respectfully explaining the rationale for choices made. Bringing the community into the process of evaluating health and exposure information will go a long way toward overcoming the differences in perspectives.

SPECIAL TOPICS IN ENVIRONMENTAL EPIDEMIOLOGY

Vulnerable Populations

Children's Environmental Health

Children have greater exposure to toxic chemicals than adults—relative to their body weight: at 6 months, infants consume seven times more water for their size than an adult and take in twice as much air; children consume three times more calories than adults and many times more fruit, vegetables, and dairy products[177]; importantly, air, water, and diet are major sources of toxicant exposures. For this reason, chemicals like pesticides, which contaminate conventionally grown produce and animal feed, may be disproportionately consumed by children. Behaviors like crawling and mouthing of objects render children vulnerable to chemicals that reside in dust that settles on surfaces. Such chemicals may include lead, residential insecticides, and cleaning products. Children also have immature metabolic pathways that interfere with their ability to metabolize and excrete certain toxicants.[178,179]

A considerable body of evidence has linked exposure to environmental toxicants during vulnerable stages of development with neurodevelopmental disorders,[180-182] asthma,[181,182] and somatic growth.[183] Stages of development, from the in utero period through adolescence, constitute unique windows of vulnerability that may be more or less susceptible to specific toxicant exposures.[184] Several examples of periods of susceptibility in early life have been described, including adolescent soot exposure to chimney sweepers and cancer of the scrotum[185]; in utero exposure to methylmercury and damage to the fetal nervous system[186]; and early-life radiation exposure and pediatric thyroid cancer.[187]

The Elderly

Social, physiologic, and metabolic changes associated with aging make the elderly particularly vulnerable to the effects of environmental hazards.[188] Decreased functionality of organ systems, layered on top of preexisting health conditions, could have important implications on susceptibility. Enzymes responsible for the detoxification and subsequent elimination of chemical contaminants have decreased efficacy among the elderly,[189-191] which could amplify the impacts from chemical exposures. Similarly, poorer absorption of nutrients can reduce the protection that a high-quality diet might confer.[192] Outdoor pollution (traffic related and wildfire) exposure has been associated with increased mortality among the elderly,[193,194] who also have a decreased capacity to regulate body temperature, rendering them more vulnerable to heat stress.[195-197] The physiological vulnerabilities posed by aging may be exacerbated by social vulnerabilities. Following the Fukushima disaster, evacuation and long-term displacement were associated with an increased risk of death among hospital inpatients and elderly people at nursing facilities, which persisted for several months after the accident. Causes of death included hypothermia, deterioration of existing medical conditions, and dehydration.[198] The overlapping burdens of declining health, an accumulation of lifetime exposures, and physiological changes such as reduced enzyme efficacy, increasing social isolation, and a high prevalence of poverty render the elderly a particularly vulnerable population.

Communities of Color, Poor, or Rural Populations

"Environmental justice" is a term coined to draw attention to the extra burden borne by communities already at risk due to their socioeconomics, race, and/or ethnicity, as they additionally face disproportionately high exposures to chemical or other pollutants. In their classic 1993 paper, Bullard and Wright[9] compellingly document the systematic siting of hazardous waste sites, chemical plants, smelters, and other polluting industries in neighborhoods populated by people perceived to be the least likely to resist: those of low-income families and communities of color. Supporting the lack of environmental justice, a recent NHANES analysis demonstrated high correlations of household income with scores of urinary and blood markers for micronutrients, environmental contaminants, and infectious agents.[112] This intersection of family/social, chemical, and food-related vulnerabilities magnifies health inequities and can be self-perpetuating through replication in subsequent generations. Public health practitioners need look no further than Flint, Michigan, to see a tragic, contemporary example of environmental injustice,[199] with echoes of history.[200] The health consequences of a protracted period of lead contamination in municipal water in Flint may well be long lasting—an enduring tragedy in an already socioeconomically depressed population.[140,201]

Yet the "double jeopardy" lies not only in the intersection of socioeconomic disadvantage and environmental pollution but also pertains to how they synergistically increase health risks. Several studies demonstrate such interactions for birth outcomes or infant growth/habitus relative to air pollution and the SES of families or Census tracts[202,203]; PCB exposures and ethnicity[204]; lead exposure and zinc status[205]; and second-hand smoke and exclusive breastfeeding.[206] Systematic reviews provide strong evidence that organophosphate pesticides are associated with poorer cognitive scores in various populations,[207,208] including Hispanic farmworker families and urban immigrant and racially/ethnically diverse communities,[209-211] but not in affluent largely White populations.[212,213] And prenatal PCB exposures have been shown to result in deficits for individuals with less optimal family and home characteristics, while those with more optimal circumstances are not affected.[214] Climate change is the new frontier in environmental justice, given that, globally, the lowest income countries that have historically generated the least greenhouse gases are being disproportionately affected[197] (see below, Globalization, the Anthropocene, and climate change: ultimate challenges for environmental epidemiology").

Genetic Susceptibility

There may be individuals in a population that are at increased risk for adverse effects from toxicant exposures as a result of their genetic makeup. The investigation of gene-environment interactions can help to identify these uniquely susceptible individuals and, in some cases, provide important evidence on the biological mechanism underlying toxicant-induced disease and/or identify points of intervention.[215] Classic examples in environmental epidemiology focus on genes that encode enzymes responsible for the metabolism of that toxicant and have demonstrated in a number of cases that individuals who are "slow" metabolizers of a compound tend to be at higher risk of adverse effects arising from exposure. Examples of this paradigm include the interaction of paraoxonase 1 genotype or enzyme expression and the effects of organophosphate pesticide exposure,[209,216-220] and variants that affect arsenic metabolism capacity, arsenic exposure, and skin lesions.[221-225] Whereas the majority of the existing gene-toxicant interaction literature employs this "candidate gene" philosophy, modern genetic epidemiology resides in a much more high-dimensional space, leveraging our analytic capacity to measure millions of markers across the genome. This presents challenges and opportunities for environmental epidemiologists: the opportunity is the capacity to *discover* important interactions that may not currently be known; the challenge is the risk of false positives and the need for a large population—at least in the tens of thousands—to reduce the proportion of false positives. For further discussion of gene-environment interaction see Chapter 37.

Environmental Disaster Epidemiology

Environmental disasters have played a special role and bring unique issues for environmental epidemiology. They embody the concept of a space-time cluster, with the spatial reach ranging from a small neighborhood or community to worldwide. Disaster is a term most often used for sudden events, but the time span for a disaster can extend for decades or longer. They often wreak death and destruction, taking a heavy toll on life and health. Although volcanoes, earthquakes, and floods predate our species, humans have also contributed to environmental disasters leading to serious or widespread losses, injuries, and chronic human health effects.

Specific Chemical Agent– or Physical Agent–Induced Disasters

Examples of localized environmental disasters occurred when high levels of PCBs (PCBs, an industrial chemical) were mistakenly introduced into cooking oil in two separate incidents, one in Japan and one in Taiwan.[65,226] Those exposed in utero were the most severely affected, with physical deformities and mental disabilities. Because PCBs are persistent (half-lives in humans are years and even longer in the environment), even those children born to exposed mothers many years after the incident suffered similar impairments.[64] Numerous incidents of PCB contamination have been documented.[230] At far lower prenatal levels, PCBs appear to disrupt thyroid hormones, immune function, hearing, and early childhood neurobehavioral outcomes,[228,229] potentially through the ryanodine receptor.[254] Although PCBs were banned virtually worldwide by the mid-1980s,[231] exposures continue as a result of prior widespread uses and their persistence in the environment.[232,233]

More than a century ago, leaded paint was determined to be the cause of severe physical and mental impairments in young children.[234] Early studies of exceedingly high exposures prompted regulations to reduce lead exposures in many settings, and clinically evident lead poisoning declined. Decades later, however, a landmark investigation by Needleman established, for the first time, behavioral alterations and intellectual deficits even at levels that had previously been considered safe.[77] At levels current at that time, lead exposure is not necessarily accompanied by clinical symptoms, and therefore, these effects have been characterized as a "silent" epidemic. Forty years later, the ongoing failure to clean up legacy lead exposures (e.g., replace lead pipes for water distribution, clean up soil contaminated from leaded paint in low-income housing) or to abandon its continuing uses (e.g., aviation fuels) continues to harm children during vulnerable periods of brain development.[235] In 2014, the city of Flint, Michigan, with an aging distribution system of 10%-80% lead pipes, changed its water source from one with low corrosiveness to the Flint River, with high corrosiveness, resulting in increased levels of lead in water and in children's blood.[140] An outbreak of Legionnaire disease in the elderly also coincided with the switch to corrosive, low-chlorine water.[236,237]

Some disasters like the Minimata mercury poisonings are slow to be recognized, while others are immediately identified. In 1976, an explosion at a chemical plant led to contamination in the area of Seveso, Italy, with dioxins, chemicals known to be highly toxic at extremely low levels. Toxic plumes immediately blanketed the area and over 160 children developed chloracne, a skin condition indicative of high dioxin exposure.[238] Soil contamination continued for years, and dozens of research reports have documented longer-term impacts spanning alterations in liver, immune, thyroid, and reproductive (varying by age at exposure).[239]

Workplaces also incur exposures that often are higher than typical environmental levels and sometimes disastrous. Occupational studies have also been a major source for insights into potential risks, at lower concentrations, to the general population. For both disasters and workplace exposures, the question of high-to-low dose extrapolation of health effects is one of the key challenges in applying environmental epidemiology to chemical regulatory policy.

Chemical and Infectious Threats to Health: Overlapping or Competing?

Infectious diseases are reemerging as major threats to public health, sometimes linked in complex ways to problematic chemical toxins and physical hazards. For instance, hundreds of thousands of tube wells dug during the 1970s in India, Bangladesh, and elsewhere to combat waterborne diseases has resulted in high arsenic exposure for millions of people, at levels that increase risks for cancer and possibly also for respiratory and other adverse effects.[240-245] More recently, an outbreak of Zika virus in Brazil in 2015, transmitted by mosquitoes, was found to be responsible for a cluster of microcephaly defects among infants whose mothers were exposed during pregnancy and Guillain-Barré syndrome among infected adults.[246] The severity of the defects, along with the rapid transmission of Zika throughout the Americas, resulted in urgent public health efforts to control the mosquito vector. Among these efforts included aerial spraying of Naled, an organophosphate pesticide, in population centers.[247] While the concentrations of Naled sprayed were estimated to be low enough to not pose a significant threat to humans,[247] prenatal exposure to organophosphate pesticides have been linked with neurodevelopmental impairments in both urban and agricultural populations.[209,248,249] Therefore, the risk of widespread population exposure to a potentially toxic pesticide, albeit at low levels, must be balanced against the threat of a devastating birth defect.

A similar debate is underway as some countries reintroduce DDT for mosquito control to reduce malaria transmission; unlike organophosphate pesticides, DDT can persist in the environment for decades and bioaccumulate. While DDT has been associated with several different cancers in humans[250] and is classified as a "possible carcinogen" by the International Agency for Research on cancer,[251] globally, hundreds of millions of malaria cases and hundreds of thousands of malaria deaths (*e.g.*, 435,000 in 2017[252]) occur every year. Although a large trial of a partially effective vaccine against malaria has just been launched—the first breakthrough in the decades-long search for a malaria vaccine—the tensions between the need for effective vector control to reduce incidence of devastating/deadly communicable diseases and concerns about potential long-term health impacts of chemicals deployed for this purpose will continue and may intensify in coming years.

Beyond Individual Chemicals

Accidents such as shipwrecks, plane crashes, and fires; natural disasters such as earthquakes, heat waves, floods, or tsunamis; and political and social upheaval such as war and forced migration may also produce time-space clusters of injury and death. Weapons of mass destruction are exactly that the atomic bombs that were dropped on Hiroshima and Nagasaki destroyed over 90% of the buildings[253] and resulted in several hundred thousand deaths from the immediate casualties. Many more deaths occurred from cancer and other conditions with longer induction periods, as was documented by the Atomic Bomb Casualty Commission and, later, the Radiation Effects Research Foundation, which led a large research program on survivors.[254,255] Other large-scale disasters include meltdowns at nuclear power plants (Three Mile Island, Chernobyl, Fukushima), which contaminate wide areas with radioactive nucleotides that induce high cancer rates, particularly of the thyroid gland. For instance, in the first 5 years after the 2011 Fukushima meltdown, rates of thyroid cancer in youth have increased 63-fold in those aged 15 to 17 years and 50-fold in those aged 18 to 20 years.[256] Data from the British Petroleum (BP) *Deepwater Horizon* Oil spill in the Gulf of Mexico resulted in enormous devastation of the marine ecology and wildlife, while health effects in cleanup workers and coastal communities have also been documented.[257-262] It is also not uncommon for disasters to have a greater impact on disadvantaged communities, particularly for long-term recovery.

In addition to injuries and increases in chronic diseases, many disasters have major impacts on mental well-being, including increased depression, anxiety, and posttraumatic stress both in the short-term and extending for years,[263-266] though some individuals experiencing seriously traumatic events achieve greater personal growth (*i.e.*, enhanced appreciation for life, increased personal strength, improved interpersonal relationships).[266] To reduce mental health stress during the postdisaster recovery period, Shultz and colleagues emphasize the critical role of broad efforts, including by governments, to provide resources for the rebuilding of housing and other infrastructure, the regaining of economic vitality of the community, and the sustenance for individuals and households.[267]

Horney et al.[268] and Zubizarreta et al.[269] discuss methodologic challenges of disaster epidemiology, including the difficulty in obtaining unbiased predisaster data, in capturing variation in the severity of the disaster experience across individuals, and avoiding recall biases for persons who have experienced serious mental trauma. Unbiased predisaster data such as vital statistics or hospital admissions, for example, can permit studies that compare outcomes at the same time of year in the previous year or previous years, if a heat wave, wildfire, or flooding did not occur in the same region in those previous years (valid for outcomes without long-term trends). Long-term follow-up studies are still rather rare. Interindividual variation in the stress of the disaster will entail a subjective element to the experience and therefore may be more difficult to overcome but still may be roughly approximated by objective measures such as complete loss of home and belongings or deaths of family members or close friends.

As human activity has altered the ecology from the upper atmosphere to the bottom of the oceans, the distinction between anthropogenic and natural disasters has blurred. Many "natural" disasters today are increasingly linked to and influenced by human activities, which have intensified hurricanes, fires, and flooding, causing damages on an unprecedented scale. An example is Pakistan, where 90% of their natural disasters over the past 40 years—primarily flooding—was triggered by climate change.[270] Greenhouse gas emissions, mostly from the burning of fossil fuels, into the atmosphere have been the primary cause of global warming; 30% of CO_2 emissions have been absorbed by oceans, warming the surface waters, and increasing the size and intensity of hurricanes[271] (see below, Globalization, the Anthropocene, and climate change: ultimate challenges for environmental epidemiology).

Regrettable Substitution

Environmental epidemiologists typically focus on the measurement of environmental exposures at the time of disease susceptibility, which may be months, years, or even decades before the study began, and may have uncertain relevance to the contemporary constellation of toxic exposures. Temporal changes in population exposure to chemicals may result from governmental policy changes, corporate-initiated responses to evidence of hazards, or consumer pressure, but regardless of the impetus, the common practice of substitution with chemical alternatives that often have limited safety data means epidemiologists are frequently playing catch-up. The term "regrettable substitution" has been coined to describe chemical replacements that have equal or worse effects on health than their predecessor.[272] Contemporary examples of it are numerous, including 1-bromopropane,[273] flame retardants,[272] bisphenols,[274-276] fluorinated compounds,[277] pyrethroid pesticides,[278] and phthalates.[275,279] As epidemiologists, we are often utilizing studies, or leveraging biorepositories, that were started many years before. These resources represent the constellation of exposures that were prevalent at the time the study was assembled and may not represent the current constellation of exposures, particularly for diseases that have long induction periods (*e.g.*, cancer). Regrettable substitution requires a strategic reevaluation of both our research and regulatory approach; at a minimum, it seems inevitable that the one-chemical-at-a-time research strategy may need to be retired in favor of an alternative, such as grouping similar chemicals by biological activity or human exposure potential using external toxicity and biomonitoring data.[280]

Exposure Mixtures and the Exposome

We simultaneously receive exposure to multiple chemicals through the air we breathe; the food we eat; the water we drink, bathe and wash our dishes in; the homes we live in; and the products we use. By studying one chemical at a time, which is typical of most epidemiologic analyses, we are making the explicit assumption that these chemicals are independent. And yet we have good evidence to support that many are at least correlated by source, and chemical structure or toxicity data may further suggest similar biological activity. The problem of exposure mixtures could be viewed as a problem of confounding (measured or unmeasured). Specifically, the association of chemical A with disease is residually confounded by chemical B, which is correlated with chemical A (perhaps by a common source), and independently associated with disease. It could also be viewed as a problem of unspecified interaction. Specifically, chemical A may act differently in the presence of chemical B—perhaps they have a common toxicity profile and their effects are additive, or perhaps they act on different enzymes along a detoxification pathway and their effects are synergistic or antagonistic. In any case, whether viewed as confounding or interaction, or most likely, both, the one-chemical-at-a-time paradigm that dominates the majority of epidemiological studies is inadequate for identifying the environmental factors that are influencing health, and more diverse approaches are needed. This is also a key to developing strategies for intervention. Under the concept of "sufficient sets of causes," where there may be dozens of such sets for any given disease, the most effective preventive strategy would focus on those single exposures that are common to many sufficient sets that apply to large numbers of people. If, in fact, most diseases are multifactorial, there is no need to tackle all the contributing factors. We need only to dismantle each of the sufficient sets by eliminating at least one of its components. Yet little attention has been paid to mixtures or even to two-way or three-way interactions. Added to this, our ability to consider extrapolation of synergistic/antagonistic effects observed in toxicologic studies is hampered by the fact that the majority of such studies are similarly based on a one-chemical-at-a-time experimental paradigm.[281] Clearly, this is an area in need of development from the perspective of design and analysis.

Taking lessons from genome-wide studies, environmental health scientists have begun to explore moving from candidate exposures to more comprehensive analyses of the universe of human exposures. Although genetics is exceedingly complex, the DNA code is, for the most part, fixed for life. In contrast, environment has the additional feature (curse, for researchers!) of being in constant change. The "exposome" represents a fundamental shift in priorities, whereby we are less focused on the minute characterization of a single agent and instead focused on characterizing the totality of human exposure over time and across all sources.[282] At its most ambitious, this life-course approach to exposure assessment is inclusive of both endogenous and exogenous compounds, physical and climatic exposures, nutritional and psychological factors, as well as macroscale economic and social exposures that come together to influence health.[283] Exposome-scale research requires substantial advancements in both measurement and statistical analysis approaches to accommodate multidimensional and hierarchical data structures; however, innovative technologies such as environmental sensors, in combination with existing geospatial and ambient monitoring systems, human biomonitoring, and untargeted metabolomics analysis, suggest the realization of exposome-scale research may not be far off.[284]

Increasingly, our ability to measure multiple compounds within a mixture is being realized through methods that leverage high-resolution mass spectrometry.[285] Nontargeted chemical analyses, *e.g.*, via gas (or liquid) chromatography with quantitative time-of-flight mass spectrometry, are identifying an increasingly large array of chemicals in various media: food packaging,[286] river water for pharmaceuticals,[287] and breast milk for organics.[288] Wearable sensors being deployed for exogenous chemicals include silicone wristbands,[289] skin patches,[290] or handheld breathalyzers[291] for children or adults.[289] Sensor technology has begun to make its way into clinical medicine and monitoring and offers high-dimensional data collection that can dramatically advance the field of environmental epidemiology.

Early examples of exposome-scale research are appearing in the literature, and generating novel insights on the relationship of chemical and nonchemical stressors on health and disease. Nieuwenhuijsen and colleagues examined the urban exposome, inclusive of air pollution, road traffic and associated noise, the built environment and natural space, as well as meteorology, in relation to birth weight among 32,000 pregnant women from extant European cohorts. They observed that green space was positively associated with increased birth weight.[292] Agier et al.[293] examined 85 prenatal and 125 postnatal exposures in relation to childhood lung function among 1,033 mother-child dyads from the European HELIX cohort, finding several notable associations between perfluoroalkyl substances, phthalates, as well as social determinants and the built environment.[293]

GLOBALIZATION, THE ANTHROPOCENE, AND CLIMATE CHANGE: ULTIMATE CHALLENGES FOR ENVIRONMENTAL EPIDEMIOLOGY

The Anthropocene is the term now commonly used to describe the current geologic epoch of the planet, in which human intervention has altered and now widely dominates all major ecosystems including a high proportion of the land mass, water bodies, and atmosphere. Among the results of human activity are massive losses of biodiversity and unprecedentedly rapid and accelerating warming of earth. Globalization has been used to describe the ways in which practices (economic, food production, communications, etc.) and products (technology, culture) once limited to certain countries or regions of the world have now spread, frequently overtaking local initiative, and individual control and autonomy. Some of its earliest ramifications for environmental epidemiology are not difficult to see.[294] First, issues that were of high priority only in Western countries are now on the agendas of less industrialized nations (*e.g.*, motor vehicle exhaust, industrial emissions). Second, pollution does not respect state or national borders, as the industrial waste poured into the rivers, lakes, and oceans of one locale washes up on the shores of many others, and toxins released into the air are deposited thousands of miles away (chlorinated hydrocarbons). Third, travel and transport of disease vectors, pathogenic viruses, and predator species into all corners of the world have had a major impact in wiping out thousands of species in the last few decades. Fourth, destruction of undeveloped wilderness has contributed further to reduced global capacity to support large animals, leading to further extinctions and degradation of ecosystems. As habitats are lost, various wildlife species are forced to survive within close range of human populations, promoting spillover of viral and other microbes pathogenic to our species. Additionally, localized problems are frequently repeated in one region after the next, such as overuse of fertilizers or genetically modified organism (GMO) crops that severely suppress native species. Finally, the development and economic gains of transitional economies has only increased our global dependency on fossil fuels, the major driver of climate change. Fossil fuels and the consequences of pumping them out of the ground and transporting, spilling, and burning them have seriously harmed local water and other resources, as well as massively impacted planetary health, with global warming the most irreversible of the products of human activity. Global climate change is the single biggest environmental threat ever faced by humanity, with all major ecosystems—prairies, oceans, permafrost, polar ice, atmospheres, forests of all types, and the plants and animals they support—at risk. Climate change has already brought shifting patterns of precipitation leading to intensified droughts and a resulting loss of arable land. Increasingly uncontrollable wildfires, more intense hurricanes, catastrophic floods, changing endemicity of disease vectors such as mosquitoes, melting of the polar ice, and threats to island countries are just a few of the known consequences.[294] Current estimates are that at least a million species are likely to go extinct, as a result of land degradation, exploitation of organisms, climate change, pollution, and invasive species introduced into new regions.[295]

Human activity has resulted in the release of large amounts of CO_2 and methane into the atmosphere. Although concentrations of these greenhouse gases in the earth's atmosphere have varied through different geologic periods and given rise to different climatic conditions, they have now risen to be outside the variability of the last half million years. Thus, earth's climate is changing at an unprecedented rate, with human activity the dominant cause.[296] A rise in global mean temperature between 1 and 3.5°C by the year 2100 is currently predicted. By the early 2010s, the earth was regularly experiencing more frequent extreme climate events (heavy rains and storms, more intense hurricanes, drought, and heat waves), with the greatest changes at highest latitudes, where melting of sea ice and permafrost rapidly began to accelerate.

Regarding health impacts, according to the Intergovernmental Panel on Climate Change (IPCC), Fifth Assessment Report,[271] the anticipated public health impacts of medium to high confidence include "greater risk of injury, disease, and death due to more intense heat waves and fires," "increased risk of undernutrition resulting from diminished food production in poor regions," "consequences for health from lost work capacity and reduced labor productivity in vulnerable populations," and "increased risks of food- and waterborne diseases."[297] Changes in the incidence and transmission of vector-borne diseases were an early warning of climate change because the vectors themselves are particularly sensitive to environmental stressors, including temperature, moisture, and land cover.[298] In addition, the IPCC and the World Health Organization[270] both recently highlighted near-term health consequences of climate altering pollutants. For example, interactions between extreme heat and exposure to high ozone and particulate matter, contributed to excess mortality during the 2003 European heat wave.[299,300] Similarly, a 44-day heat wave in Moscow, Russia, during 2010 and a coincident wildfire that led to significant particulate matter exposure and loss of one-third of the country's wheat production during this same period, together resulted in a greater than additive effect of 2,000 excess deaths.[301,302] The clear conclusion is that reducing greenhouse gas emissions will benefit population health virtually immediately, as well as help to avert some of the more extreme consequences of global climate change, including other health-related effects of climate change.

Community preparedness is now a primary concern in many areas of the world, including in the United States. Even with little specific attention to climate-induced disasters, existing infrastructure—such as well-trained professional firefighters, air conditioning, community cooling centers, and community alert systems—has saved lives. After the 2017 wildfires in both northern and southern California, local, county, and state agencies began overhauling their emergency preparations, developing coordinated systems for issuing alerts. In France, a heavy death toll from the 2003 heat wave prompted the Directorate General of Health to adopt a National Heat Wave Plan, which included setup of a real-time health surveillance system, compiling recommendations on prevention and treatment of heat-related illnesses, installation of air conditioning in hospitals and retirement homes, censuses to identify the isolated and vulnerable followed by visits to those people during the alert period, and setup of a heat health-watch warning system for summer months. These measures along with overall increased awareness likely contributed to 4,400 fewer deaths than expected when the next heat wave hit.[86] However, there may also be unintended consequences of community preparedness programs for imminent weather-related threats. For example, public school closures in the Mississippi Harrison County School District, enacted in preparation for Hurricane Isaac, resulted in lost income among adults working outside the home and increased reporting of food insecurity among families participating in the subsidized school lunch program.[303] Existing underlying health inequities are likely to exacerbate environmental health consequences of global climate change. Already, a disproportionate burden of adverse effects is being shouldered by countries and communities that are resource-poor and lack adequate infrastructure, *e.g.*, the Phillippines and Puerto Rico. Low-income countries (including, *e.g.*, island countries) and vulnerable subpopulations such as the elderly, women, and children, communities of color, and other economically or socially disadvantaged groups, people with existing chronic illnesses, both mental and physical, and residents in areas with a high likelihood of extreme weather events are at the greatest risk.[197,270]

Deforestation of a large proportion of the earth's land mass is predicted to change weather patterns, adding to the toll of greenhouse gas emissions. Overuse of freshwater and longer droughts are lowering water tables in many areas of the world. This lack of water poses a real threat to sustainable food production and has prompted mass migrations from affected areas. These "climate refugees" are seeking to migrate to regions with greater infrastructure and food sources, initially to cities in less developed regions of the world, which are swelling far beyond the capacity of the infrastructure to provide clean water, adequate housing, and sanitation.[304] Massive changes in both physical and social environments[305] and, increasingly, pressures from drought brought about by deforestation and increased temperatures, declining food production, and, in some cases, exacerbation of all of these forces by political conflict and social upheaval may significantly alter patterns of health and disease.

The major drivers of health risks from climate change are thought to arise from the impacts on environmental systems and social conditions that affect food yields, water supplies, stability of infectious disease patterns, and the integrity of natural and human-built protections against natural disasters and from social disruption, population displacement, and political/social/military conflict.[294] Demographic changes and mass migrations are already occurring in response to climatic changes that are rendering large regions of land nonarable. The battles over water are likely to increase in intensity as agriculture requires a larger portion of water in drought-prone areas. The loss of biodiversity due to rapid species extinctions that are expected to accelerate as the planet heats up is a serious loss for *Homo sapiens*. Concentrations of CO_2 continue to increase not only in the atmosphere but also in the oceans, resulting in acidification that is predicted to alter ocean ecology and threaten many species of fish that have been an essential component of the human diet for millennia.

Roles for Environmental Epidemiologists

Efforts aimed at tracking the health effects of climate change are underway (see, for example, the annual Lancet Countdown[306]). Surveillance systems are being used to document changes in time and space of both health outcomes and climate change–related exposures. For example, extreme precipitation events were found to be associated with increased risk of campylobacteriosis in a clever analysis that leveraged the Maryland Foodborne Diseases Active Surveillance Network data in relation to daily climate data from 2002 to 2012.[307] Creative epidemiologic methods that enable us to both understand these phenomena and devise policies that can prevent potentially catastrophic effects on human health and well-being are needed. Studies of health effects from specific events, such as those cited above in relation to heat waves, are of great value and can be useful to public health practitioners and agencies seeking to serve their constituencies. As some adverse health effects of "global change" have not yet been observed, forward-looking strategies may include "scenario epidemiology" that may allow us to make reliable, quantitative forecasts of the effects on population health from future global changes in climate, land use, and social conditions.[1,308] For example, groundwater vulnerability to pollution was modeled in relation to potential climate change scenarios, in an effort to guide future water quality management.[309] Although future-oriented models are more frequently used in infectious disease epidemiology where they play a role in policy and planning by State and Federal agencies, the time may be ripe for their incorporation into environmental epidemiology.

Predictive modeling has played a major role in laying out climate scenarios for periods of the next few decades into the next century. Predictions of the rates of change and the impacts, however, have been outstripped by actual temperature rises and unforeseen consequences. An example is the melting of the permafrost, which was predicted to become noticeable around 2090: instead, it is already well underway 75 years ahead of schedule. The occurrence of wildfires on massive scales in western North America, some parts of Europe, and Australia emerged in the 2010s. As testimony to how unexpected these were, an authoritative report on human health in the face of global degradation of natural systems essential to human civilization, which was published in 2015 in *The Lancet*, made no mention of wildfires. Even further uncertainty arises when attempting to understand and quantify the relationship of climate events to consequences for human health. Nevertheless, predictive modeling can be used to help agencies and medical facilities prepare for a changing climate and the human health needs. These models can assist in highlighting ways in which we can adapt and build community resilience.

Another area in which epidemiology can contribute to the science on health impacts from climate change is known as attribution science (PMID: 28483866).[310] The goal is to attribute effects stemming from a particular event or type of ecosystem change (*e.g.*, a heat wave, wildfire, hurricane, or the clearing of a forest). There are two components to this exercise: (1) estimating the impact of climate change on the occurrence or magnitude of the event and (2) determining the amount of disease that is estimated to be attributed to the climate-induced portion of the event. Because these relationships may be governed by nonlinear dynamics, the attribution can be subject to large uncertainties. However, spatial models on climate change have been improving and new methods for downscaling may increase accuracy of climate change-related attribution applied to extreme weather events.

Extrapolating outside the range of experience is fraught and nonlinearities or breakpoints may characterize much of the changes. Positive feedback loops are being identified in many of the ecosystems, suggesting extreme and accelerating changes for which adaptations now being planned may be inadequate. Furthermore, needs and abilities to adapt vary widely by socioeconomic factors, as well as prior health. Models that assume homogeneity across populations may also fail to capture the risks and experiences of large regions or subsets of people where the highest risks may reside. Hence, use of empirical studies are needed to verify predictive models but have a much broader role to play as well: *e.g.*, to demonstrate the assumptions that are not supported, understand variability across populations, and identify the drivers of that heterogeneity.

Lest we leave the reader crushed by the apparent intractability of our current climate and ecosystem crisis, there is scientific evidence that global cooperation can positively affect these dire projections. Earlier, we described the depletion of stratospheric ozone from use of chlorofluorocarbons. This ozone depletion was expected to increase exposure to ultraviolet B (UVB) radiation, which in turn was expected to increase rates of skin cancer and cataracts, as well as change immune function.[311] In a recent study by Langston and colleagues, temporal trends in UVB radiation from 1978 to 2014 within the continental United States were examined.[312] They identified only small changes in UVB radiation over this 30-year period. The stabilization of these trends in ultraviolet radiation is attributed largely to the Montreal Protocol, a global agreement that phased-out the production of ozone depleting substances and was implemented beginning in 1987. Although we are heartened by signs of ozone recovery, the relationship between stratospheric ozone and climate change is as yet uncertain.[311] We also acknowledge that ozone recovery may be regional, whereas the interconnectedness across climate and multiple other ecosystems spans the entire globe.

FUTURE DIRECTIONS

Environmental epidemiology stands at the crossroads of multiple public health fields. Themes likely to be of continued importance include advances in environmental exposure assessment, integration of biologic markers, and understanding of time-related issues such as critical windows, induction, and latency. The development of sensor technologies capable of assessing both the xeno- and endobiotic space isincreasingly called for. The continued development and refinement of analytic tools and statistical methods for assessing the combined effects from exposure mixtures is an urgent need. And transdisciplinary engagement between epidemiologists, anthropologists, toxicologists, wildlife biologists, environmental scientists, sociologists, climatologists, oceanographers, molecular biologists, and geneticists, to name a few, would benefit global public health.

Traditional epidemiology is slow. It can take years to assemble cohorts and potentially many more years to observe the occurrence of disease in these populations. These studies tend to be designed to assess the health effects of candidate exposures identified when the study was initiated. How these candidate exposures are identified varies, but oftentimes the existence of validated assays for a set of exposures forms the bounds within which candidates are selected. This is a type of bias, in which only the exposures that are the easiest to study (which may have no relationship with their potential toxicity) are examined and is frequently referred to in environmental epidemiology as "Looking under the lamppost." While it remains infeasible (currently) to incorporate markers for the more than 80,000 chemicals that may be present in commerce today, it is essential that we contribute to novel approaches that may enable us to move beyond the lamppost. One such approach leverages high-throughput computational toxicology data such as ToxCast. Auerbach and colleagues demonstrated an approach for chemical prioritization for obesity and diabetes research that began with identifying the assay targets for biological processes that contribute to obesity/diabetes and then filtering the 1,860 chemicals in the ToxCast chemical library for activity on these prespecified assays.[313] Using their approach, the most highly ranked chemicals were, for the most part, not currently being studied for metabolic effects. However, there are several challenges with a broader dissemination of this approach into the epidemiological literature. Among them, the set of assays included in ToxCast may not represent all biological process of interest for all health endpoints, the activity on these assays may not perfectly translate to human health effects or demonstrate poor reproducibility, the doses tested may not represent typical human exposure levels, and prioritizing solely on biological activity ignores the importance of exposure prevalence in the population. However, computational toxicology is much quicker and less expensive than epidemiology and at some point may play a leading role in the regulatory environment going forward. Epidemiologists must engage and help to address these challenges in order to ensure that the integration of these disciplines is a net positive for population health.

Good public policies require scientific input from epidemiologists to help those outside our field distinguish real from imagined hazards, and important from negligible risks, and can pave the way for a more rational allocation of intervention resources to reduce environmentally induced disease. We began this chapter with a description of George Baker's investigation of lead in the cider of Devonshire. Baker (1767) went on to disseminate his report to the people of Devonshire in order to provide them "the earliest intimation of their danger; in order that they may take the proper steps to preserve their health." This example of engagement between a scientist and the community he served remains a model for all public health professionals. Rational public health policy and chemical regulations require the active engagement of researchers with regulators and the community they serve.

References

1. Cifuentes L, Borja-Aburto VH, Gouveia N, Thurston G, Davis DL. Climate change. Hidden health benefits of greenhouse gas mitigation. *Science*. 2001;293(5533):1257-1259.
2. Hertz-Picciotto I, Talbott EO, Craun GF. *Environmental Risk Assessment. Introduction to Environmental Epidemiology*. New York, NY: CRC Lewis Publishers; 1995:23-38.
3. Kunzli N, Kaiser R, Medina S, et al. Public-health impact of outdoor and traffic-related air pollution: a European assessment. *Lancet*. 2000;356(9232):795-801.
4. Coucil on Environmental Health. Chemical-management policy: prioritizing children's health. *Pediatrics*. 2011;127(5):983-990.
5. Schroeder AL, Ankley GT, Houck KA, Villeneuve DL. Environmental surveillance and monitoring – The next frontiers for high-throughput toxicology. *Environ Toxicol Chem*. 2016;35(3):513-525.
6. Huang R, Xia M, Sakamuru S, et al. Modelling the Tox21 10 K chemical profiles for in vivo toxicity prediction and mechanism characterization. *Nat Commun*. 2016;7:10425.
7. Institute of Medicine Committee on Environmental Justice. *Toward Environmental Justice: Research, Education, and Health Policy Needs*. Washington, DC: National Academy Press; 1999.

8. Brulle RJ, Pellow DN. Environmental justice: human health and environmental inequalities. *Annu Rev Public Health*. 2006;27:103-124.

9. Bullard RD, Wright BH. Environmental justice for all: community perspectives on health and research needs. *Toxicol Ind Health*. 1993;9(5):821-841.

10. Morello-Frosch R, Lopez R. The riskscape and the color line: examining the role of segregation in environmental health disparities. *Environ Res*. 2006;102(2):181-196.

11. US Environmental Protection Agency. *Clean Air Act*. Washington, DC: Environmental Protection Agency; 1970. NumberSection 7401.

12. *An Act to Regulate Commerce and Protect Human Health and the Environment by Requiring Testing and Necessary Use Restrictions on Certain Chemical Substances, and for Other Purposes*. Washington, DC: US GPO; 1976: 2601-2629.

13. United States. *Frank R Lautenberg Chemical Safety for the 21st Century Act*. Washington, DC: US Government Publishing Office; 2017. Number2601.

14. Centers for Disease Control and Prevention. *Fourth Report on Human Exposure to Environmental Chemicals*. 2009. Available at https://www.cdc.gov/exposurereport/.

15. Smolders R, Schramm KW, Stenius U, et al. A review on the practical application of human biomonitoring in integrated environmental health impact assessment. *J Toxicol Environ Health B Crit Rev*. 2009;12(2):107-123.

16. Calafat AM, Ye X, Silva MJ, Kuklenyik Z, Needham LL. Human exposure assessment to environmental chemicals using biomonitoring. *Int J Androl*. 2006;29(1):166-171; discussion 181-185.

17. Angerer J, Ewers U, Wilhelm M. Human biomonitoring: state of the art. *Int J Hyg Environ Health*. 2007;210(3-4):201-228.

18. Paustenbach D, Galbraith D. Biomonitoring and biomarkers: exposure assessment will never be the same. *Environ Health Perspect*. 2006;114(8):1143-1149.

19. Wilson MP, Schwarzman MR. Toward a new US chemicals policy: rebuilding the foundation to advance new science, green chemistry, and environmental health. *Environ Health Perspect*. 2009;117(8):1202-1209.

20. Box GEP. Robustness in the strategy of scientific model building. In: Launer RL, Wilkinson GN, eds. *Robustness in Statistics*. New York, NY: Academic Press; 1979: 201-236.

21. Seifert B. Validity criteria for exposure assessment methods. *Sci Total Environ*. 1995;168(2):101-107.

22. Nuckols JR, Ward MH, Jarup L. Using geographic information systems for exposure assessment in environmental epidemiology studies. *Environ Health Perspect*. 2004;112(9):1007.

23. Vineis P, Perera F. Molecular epidemiology and biomarkers in etiologic cancer research: the new in light of the old. *Cancer Epidemiol Biomarkers Prev*. 2007;16(10):1954-1965.

24. Lowry LK. Role of biomarkers of exposure in the assessment of health risks. *Toxicol Lett*. 1995;77(1-3):31-38.

25. Watson WP, Mutti A. Role of biomarkers in monitoring exposures to chemicals: present position, future prospects. *Biomarkers*. 2004;9(3):211-242.

26. Calafat AM, Longnecker MP, Koch HM, et al. Optimal exposure biomarkers for Nonpersistent chemicals in environmental epidemiology. *Environ Health Perspect*. 2015;123(7):A166-A168.

27. National Research Council (US) Committee on National Monitoring of Human Tissues. *Monitoring Human Tissues for Toxic Substances*. Washington, DC: National Academy Press; 1991.

28. Weisel CP. Benzene exposure: an overview of monitoring methods and their findings. *Chem Biol Interac*. 2010;184(0):58-66.

29. Lebret E. Models of human exposure based on environmental monitoring. *Sci Total Environ*. 1995;168(2):179-185.

30. Armstrong BK, White E, Saracci R. *Principles of Exposure Measurement in Epidemiology*. Oxford, New York: Oxford University Press; 1992. Monographs in epidemiology and biostatistics 21.

31. Nieuwenhuijsen M. *Exposure Assessment in Occupational and Environmental Epidemiology*. Oxford: Oxford University Press; 2003.

32. Brunekreef B, Noy D, Clausing P. Variability of exposure measurements in environmental epidemiology. *Am J Epidemiol*. 1987;125(5):892-898.

33. Liu K, Stamler J, Dyer A, McKeever J, McKeever P. Statistical methods to assess and minimize the role of intra-individual variability in obscuring the relationship between dietary lipids and serum cholesterol. *J Chronic Dis*. 1978;31(6-7): 399-418.

34. Rappaport S, Symanski E, Yager J, Kupper L. The relationship between environmental monitoring and biological markers in exposure assessment. *Environ Health Perspect*. 1995;103(suppl 3):49.

35. Sheppard L, Burnett RT, Szpiro AA, et al. Confounding and exposure measurement error in air pollution epidemiology. *Air Qual Atmos Health*. 2012;5(2):203-216.

36. Sheppard L, Slaughter JC, Schildcrout J, Liu LJ, Lumley T. Exposure and measurement contributions to estimates of acute air pollution effects. *J Expo Anal Environ Epidemiol*. 2005;15(4):366-376.

37. Spiegelman D, Zhao B, Kim J. Correlated errors in biased surrogates: study designs and methods for measurement error correction. *Stat Med*. 2005;24(11):1657-1682.

38. Sturmer T, Thurigen D, Spiegelman D, Blettner M, Brenner H. The performance of methods for correcting measurement error in case-control studies. *Epidemiology*. 2002;13(5):507-516.

39. Thurigen D, Spiegelman D, Blettner M, Heuer C, Brenner H. Measurement error correction using validation data: a review of methods and their applicability in case-control studies. *Stat Methods Med Res*. 2000;9(5):447-474.

40. Carroll RJ, Ruppert D, Stefanski LA, Crainiceanu CM. *Measurement Error in Nonlinear Models: A Modern Perspective*. Boca Raton, FL: CRC Press; 2006.

41. Cromley EK, McLafferty SL. *GIS and Public Health*. New York, NY: Guilford Publications; 2011.

42. Reynolds P, Von Behren J, Gunier RB, Goldberg DE, Hertz A, Smith DF. Childhood cancer incidence rates and hazardous air pollutants in California: an exploratory analysis. *Environ Health Perspect*. 2003;111(4):663-668.

43. Kheifets L, Crespi CM, Hooper C, Cockburn M, Amoon AT, Vergara XP. Residential magnetic fields exposure and childhood leukemia: a population-based case-control study in California. *Cancer Causes Control*. 2017;28(10):1117-1123.

44. Reissman DB, Staley F, Curtis GB, Kaufmann RB. Use of geographic information system technology to aid Health Department decision making about childhood lead poisoning prevention activities. *Environ Health Perspect*. 2001;109(1):89-94.

45. Costello S, Cockburn M, Bronstein J, Zhang X, Ritz B. Parkinson's disease and residential exposure to maneb and paraquat from agricultural applications in the central valley of California. *Am J Epidemiol*. 2009;169(8):919-926.

46. Wofford P, Segawa R, Schreider J, Federighi V, Neal R, Brattesani M. Community air monitoring for pesticides. Part 3: using health-based screening levels to evaluate results collected for a year. *Environ Monit Assess*. 2014;186(3):1355-1370.

47. Shelton JF, Geraghty EM, Tancredi DJ, et al. Neurodevelopmental disorders and prenatal residential proximity to agricultural pesticides: the CHARGE study. *Environ Health Perspect*. 2014;122(10):1103-1109.

48. Triguero-Mas M, Donaire-Gonzalez D, Seto E, et al. Living close to natural outdoor environments in four European cities: Adults' contact with the environments and physical activity. *Int J Environ Res Public Health*. 2017;14(10):1162.

49. Rundle A, Neckerman KM, Freeman L, et al. Neighborhood food environment and walkability predict obesity in New York City. *Environ Health Perspect*. 2009;117(3):442-447.

50. Bitzer ZT, Goel R, Reilly SM, et al. Effects of solvent and temperature on free Radical formation in Electronic cigarette aerosols. *Chem Res Toxicol*. 2018;31(1):4-12.

51. Lee YO, Nonnemaker JM, Bradfield B, Hensel EC, Robinson RJ. Examining daily electronic cigarette puff topography among established and nonestablished cigarette smokers in their natural environment. *Nicotine Tob Res*. 2018;20(10):1283-1288.

52. Rothman KJ. "Induction and latent periods." *Am J Epidemiol*. 1981;114(2):253-259.

53. Hertz-Picciotto I. How scientists view causality and assess evidence: a study of the Institute of medicine's evaluation of health effects in vietnam veterans and agent orange. *J L Policy*. 2005;13(2):553-591.

54. Hertz-Picciotto I, Berhane KT, Bleecker ML, et al. *Committee to Review the Health Effects in Vietnam Veterans of Exposure to Herbicides (Fourth Biennial Update). I O M. (IOM)*. Washington, DC: National Academy Press; 2004.

55. Gardner MJ, Hall AJ, Downes S, Terrell JD. Follow up study of children born elsewhere but attending schools in Seascale, West Cumbria (schools cohort). *Br Med J (Clin Res Ed)*. 1987a;295(6602):819-822.

56. Gardner MJ, Hall AJ, Downes S, Terrell JD. Follow up study of children born to mothers resident in Seascale, West Cumbria (birth cohort). *Br Med J (Clin Res Ed)*. 1987b;295(6602):822-827.

57. Bell EM, Hertz-Picciotto I, Beaumont JJ. Case-cohort analysis of agricultural pesticide applications near maternal residence and selected causes of fetal death. *Am J Epidemiol*. 2001a;154(8):702-710.

58. Bell EM, Hertz-Picciotto I, Beaumont JJ. A case-control study of pesticides and fetal death due to congenital anomalies. *Epidemiology*. 2001b;12(2):148-156.

59. Bell EM, Hertz-Picciotto I, Beaumont JJ. Pesticides and fetal death due to congenital anomalies: implications of an erratum. *Epidemiology*. 2001c;12(5):595-596.

60. Hertz-Picciotto I, Pastore LM, Beaumont JJ. Timing and patterns of exposures during pregnancy and their implications for study methods. *Am J Epidemiol*. 1996;143(6):597-607.

61. Hornig M, Bresnahan MA, Che X, et al. Prenatal fever and autism risk. *Mol Psychiatry*. 2018;23(3):759-766.

62. Zerbo O, Iosif AM, Walker C, Ozonoff S, Hansen RL, Hertz-Picciotto I. Is maternal influenza or fever during pregnancy associated with autism or developmental delays? Results from the CHARGE (CHildhood Autism Risks from Genetics and Environment) study. *J Autism Dev Disord*. 2013;43(1):25-33.

63. Atladottir HO, Henriksen TB, Schendel DE, Parner ET. Autism after infection, febrile episodes, and antibiotic use during pregnancy: an exploratory study. *Pediatrics*. 2012;130(6):e1447-1454.

64. Chen Y, Yu M, Rogan WJ, Gladen BC, Hsu CC. A 6-year follow-up of behavior and activity disorders in the Taiwan Yu-cheng children. *Am J Public Health.* 1994;84(3):415-421.

65. Kuratsune M, Yoshimura T, Matsuzaka J, Yamaguchi A. Epidemiologic study on Yusho, a poisoning caused by ingestion of rice oil contaminated with a commercial brand of polychlorinated biphenyls. *Environ Health Perspect.* 1972;1:119.

66. Hertz-Picciotto I. Towards a coordinated system for surveillance of environmental health hazards (Commentary). *Am J Public Health Nations Health.* 1996;86:638-641.

67. McGeehin MA, Qualters JR, Niskar AS. National environmental public health tracking program: bridging the information gap. *Environ Health Perspect.* 2004;112(14):1409-1413.

68. Pew Environmental Health Commission. *Transition Report to the New Administration: Strengthening Our Public Health Defense Against Environmental Threats.* Baltimore, MD: Pew Environmental Health Commission; 2001a.

69. National Environmental Public Health Tracking Program Strategic Plan, Fiscal Years 2016-2020. Atlanta, GA: Centers for Disease Control and Prevention. Available at https://www.cdc.gov/nceh/tracking/pdfs/cdc_eph_tracking_program_2016-2020_strategic_plan_508.pdf.

70. Centers for Disease Control and Prevention. *National Environmental Public Health Tracking Network.* Available at https://ephtracking.cdc.gov. Accessed January 29, 2018.

71. California Environmental Protection Agency. Available at http://oehha.ca.gov/calenviroscreen. Accessed May 21, 2019.

72. Kearney GD, Namulanda G, Qualters JR, Talbott EO. A decade of environmental public health tracking (2002-2012): progress and challenges. *J Public Health Manag Pract.* 2015;21(suppl 2):S23-S35.

73. EPA EJSCREEN. *Environmental Justice Screening and Mapping Tool.* Available at https://www.epa.gov/ejscreen. Accessed January 29, 2018.

74. Snow J. *On the Mode of Communication of Cholera.* 2nd ed. London: John Churchill; 1860.

75. de la Burdé B, Choate MS. Early asymptomatic lead exposure and development at school age. *J Pediatr.* 1975;87(4):638-642.

76. Youroukos S, Lyberatos C, Philippidou A, Gardikas C, Tsomi A. Increased blood lead levels in mentally retarded children in Greece. *Arch Environ Health.* 1978;33(6):297-300.

77. Needleman HL, Gunnoe C, Leviton A, et al. Deficits in psychologic and classroom performance of children with elevated dentine lead levels. *New Engl J Med.* 1979;300(13):689-695.

78. Wells GA, Shea B, O'Connell D, Peterson J, Welch V, Losos M, Tugwell P. *The Newcastle-Ottawa Scale (NOS) for assessing the quality of nonrandomised studies in meta-analyses.* 2013. Available at http://www.ohri.ca/programs/clinical_epidemiology/oxford.asp.

79. Bae JM. A suggestion for quality assessment in systematic reviews of observational studies in nutritional epidemiology. *Epidemiol Health.* 2016;38:e2016014.

80. Needleman HL, Schell A, Bellinger D, Leviton A, Allred EN. The long-term effects of exposure to low doses of lead in childhood. An 11-year follow-up report. *N Engl J Med.* 1990;322(2):83-88.

81. Bellinger D, Leviton A, Allred E, Rabinowitz M. Pre- and postnatal lead exposure and behavior problems in school-aged children. *Environ Res.* 1994b;66(1):12-30.

82. Bellinger D, Hu H, Titlebaum L, Needleman HL. Attentional correlates of dentin and bone lead levels in adolescents. *Arch Environ Health.* 1994a;49(2):98-105.

83. Janes H, Sheppard L, Lumley T. Overlap bias in the case-crossover design, with application to air pollution exposures. *Stat Med.* 2005;24(2):285-300.

84. Levy D, Lumley T, Sheppard L, Kaufman J, Checkoway H. Referent selection in case-crossover analyses of acute health effects of air pollution. *Epidemiology.* 2001;12(2): 186-192.

85. Fouillet A, Rey G, Laurent F, et al. Excess mortality related to the August 2003 heat wave in France. *Int Arch Occup Environ Health.* 2006;80(1):16-24.

86. Fouillet A, Rey G, Wagner V, et al. Has the impact of heat waves on mortality changed in France since the European heat wave of summer 2003? A study of the 2006 heat wave. *Int J Epidemiol.* 2008;37(2):309-317.

87. Maclure M. The case-crossover design: a method for studying transient effects on the risk of acute events. *Am J Epidemiol.* 1991;133(2):144-153.

88. Mittleman MA, Mostofsky E. Exchangeability in the case-crossover design. *Int J Epidemiol.* 2014;43(5):1645-1655.

89. Buteau S, Goldberg MS, Burnett RT, et al. Associations between ambient air pollution and daily mortality in a cohort of congestive heart failure: case-crossover and nested case-control analyses using a distributed lag nonlinear model. *Environ Int.* 2018;113:313-324.

90. Jaakkola JJ. Case-crossover design in air pollution epidemiology. *Eur Respir J Suppl.* 2003;40:81s-85s.

91. Montresor-Lopez JA, Yanosky JD, Mittleman MA, et al. Short-term exposure to ambient ozone and stroke hospital admission: a case-crossover analysis. *J Expo Sci Environ Epidemiol.* 2016;26(2):162-166.

92. Poumadere M, Mays C, Le Mer S, Blong R. The 2003 heat wave in France: dangerous climate change here and now. *Risk Anal.* 2005;25(6):1483-1494.

93. Windham GC, Zhang L, Gunier R, Croen LA, Grether JK. Autism spectrum disorders in relation to distribution of hazardous air pollutants in the San Francisco Bay area. *Environ Health Perspect.* 2006;114(9):1438-1444.

94. Susser M. The logic in ecological: II. The logic of design. *Am J Public Health.* 1994;84(5):830-835.

95. Clancy L, Goodman P, Sinclair H, Dockery DW. Effect of air-pollution control on death rates in Dublin, Ireland: an intervention study. *Lancet.* 2002;360(9341):1210-1214. doi:10.1016/S0140-6736(02)11281-5.

96. Ast DB, Fitzgerald B. Effectiveness of water fluoridation. *J Am Dent Assoc.* 1962;65(5):581-587.

97. Greenland S, Poole C. "Empirical-Bayes and semi-Bayes approaches to occupational and environmental hazard surveillance. *Arch Environ Health.* 1994;149(1):9-16.

98. Alexeeff S, Schwartz J, Kloog I, Chudnovsky A, Koutrakis P, Coull BA. Consequences of kriging and land use regression for PM2.5 predictions in epidemiologic analyses: insights into spatial variability using high-resolution satellite data. *J Expo Sci Environ Epidemiol.* 2015;25(2):138-144.

99. Anderson C, Lee D, Dean N. Bayesian cluster detection via adjacency modelling. *Spat Spatiotemporal Epidemiol.* 2016;16(1):11-20.

100. Checkoway H, Pearce N, Kriebel D. *Research Methods in Occupational Epidemiology, Monographs in Epidemiology and Biostatistics.* Oxford: Oxford University Press; 2004.

101. Pearce N, Checkoway H, Dement J. Exponential models for analyses of timerelated factors, illustrated with asbestos textile worker mortality data. *J Occup Environ Med.* 1988;30(6):517-522.

102. Greenland S. Modeling and variable selection in epidemiologic analysis. *Am J Public Health.* 1989;79(3):340-349.

103. Breslow NE. Extra-Poisson variation in log-linear models. *Appl Stat.* 1984;33(1):38-44.

104. McCullagh P, Nelder J. *Generalized Linear Models.* 2nd ed. New York, NY: Chapman and Hall; 1989.

105. Krieger N, Fee E. Social class: the missing link in US health data. *Int J Health Serv.* 1994;24(1):25-44.

106. United States Environmental Protection Agency. *Environmental Equity: Reducing Risk for All Communities.* Washington, DC: US Environmental Protection Agency; 1992.

107. Evans GW, Kantrowitz E. Socioeconomic status and health: the potential role of environmental risk exposure. *Annu Rev Public Health.* 2002;23:303-331.

108. United Church of Christ Commission for Racial Justice. *Toxic Wastes and Race in the United States: A National Report on the Racial and Socio-Economic Characteristics of Communities With Hazardous Waste Sites.* 1987.

109. James RA, Hertz-Picciotto I, Willman E, Keller JA, Charles MJ. Determinants of serum polychlorinated biphenyls and organochlorine pesticides measured in women from the child health and development study cohort, 1963-1967. *Environ Health Perspect.* 2002;110(7):617-624.

110. Mahaffey KR, Annest JL, Roberts J, Murphy RS. National estimates of blood lead levels. United States, 1976-1980: association with selected demographic and socioeconomic factors. *N Engl J Med.* 1982;307(10):573-579.

111. Kaufman JS, Cooper RS, McGee DL. Socioeconomic status and health in Blacks and Whites: the problem of residual confounding and the resiliency of race. *Epidemiology.* 1997;8(6):621-628.

112. Patel CJ, Ioannidis JP, Cullen MR, Rehkopf DH. Systematic assessment of the correlations of household income with infectious, biochemical, physiological, and environmental factors in the United States, 1999-2006. *Am J Epidemiol.* 2015;181(3):171-179.

113. DeRouen MC, Schupp CW, Koo J, et al. Impact of individual and neighborhood factors on disparities in prostate cancer survival. *Cancer Epidemiol.* 2018;53:1-11.

114. Fernandez RM, Kulik JC. A multilevel model of life satisfaction: effects of individual characteristics and neighborhood composition. *Am Sociol Rev.* 1981;46:840-850.

115. Fox AJ, Jones DR, Goldblatt PO. Approaches to studying the effect of socio-economic circumstances on geographic differences in mortality in England and Wales. *Br Med Bull.* 1984;40(4):309-314.

116. Fitzgibbon ML, Stolley MR. Environmental changes may be needed for prevention of overweight in minority children. *Pediatr Ann.* 2004;33(1):45-49.

117. LaVeist TA, Wallace JM Jr. Health risk and inequitable distribution of liquor stores in African American neighborhood. *Soc Sci Med.* 2000;51(4):613-617.

118. Cinat ME, Wilson SE, Lush S, Atkins C. Significant correlation of trauma epidemiology with the economic conditions of a community. *Arch Surg.* 2004;139(12):1350-1355.

119. Greenland S, Pearl J, Robins JM. Causal diagrams for epidemiologic research. *Epidemiology.* 1999;10(1):37-48.

120. Hernan MA, Hernandez-Diaz S, Werler MM, Mitchell AA. Causal knowledge as a prerequisite for confounding evaluation: an application to birth defects epidemiology. *Am J Epidemiol.* 2002;155(2):176-184.

121. Pearl J. *Causality.* Cambridge, New York: Cambridge University Press; 2000.

122. Brenner H. Bias due to non-differential misclassification of polytomous confounders. *J Clin Epidemiol.* 1993;46(1):57-63.

123. Bellinger DC. Assessing environmental neurotoxicant exposures and child neurobehavior: confounded by confounding? *Epidemiology*. 2004;15(4):383-384.

124. Carpenter DO, Arcaro KF, Bush B, Niemi WD, Pang S, Vakharia DD. Human health and chemical mixtures: an overview. *Environ Health Perspect*. 1998;106(suppl 6):1263-1270.

125. Manrai AK, Cui Y, Bushel PR, et al. Informatics and data analytics to support exposome-based discovery for public health. *Annu Rev Public Health*. 2017;38:279-294.

126. Patel CJ. Analytic complexity and challenges in identifying mixtures of exposures associated with phenotypes in the exposome era. *Curr Epidemiol Rep*. 2017;4(1):22-30.

127. Carrico C, Gennings C, Wheeler DC, Factor-Litvak P. Characterization of weighted quantile sum regression for highly correlated data in a risk analysis setting. *J Agric Biol Environ Stat*. 2015;20(1):100-120.

128. Davalos AD, Luben TJ, Herring AH, Sacks JD. Current approaches used in epidemiologic studies to examine short-term multipollutant air pollution exposures. *Ann Epidemiol*. 2017;27(2):145-153.e1.

129. Hastie T, Tibshirani R, Friedman JH. *The Elements of Statistical Learning: Data Mining, Inference, and Prediction*. New York, NY: Springer; 2009.

130. Hastie T, Tibshirani R, Wainwright M. *Statistical Learning With Sparsity: The Lasso and Generalizations*. Boca Raton: CRC Press, Taylor & Francis Group; 2015.

131. Witte JS, Greenland S, Haile RW, Bird CL. Hierarchical regression analysis applied to a study of multiple dietary exposures and breast cancer. *Epidemiology*. 1994;5(6):612-621.

132. Bobb JF, Claus Henn B, Valeri L, Coull BA. Statistical software for analyzing the health effects of multiple concurrent exposures via Bayesian kernel machine regression. *Environ Health*. 2018;17(1):67.

133. Czarnota J, Gennings C, Wheeler DC. Assessment of weighted quantile sum regression for modeling chemical mixtures and cancer risk. *Cancer Inform*. 2015;14(suppl 2):159-171.

134. Taylor KW, Joubert BR, Braun JM, et al. Statistical approaches for assessing health effects of environmental chemical mixtures in epidemiology: lessons from an innovative workshop. *Environ Health Perspect*. 2016;124(12):A227-A229.

135. Crutzen PJ. Geology of mankind. *Nature*. 2002;415(6867):23.

136. Kolbert E. *The Sixth Extinction: An Unnatural History*. New York, NY: Henry Holt and Company, LLC; 2014.

137. Al-Mufti AW, Copplestone JF, Kazantzis G, Mahmoud RM, Majid MA. Epidemiology of organomercury poisoning in Iraq. I. Incidence in a defined area and relationship to the eating of contaminated bread. *Bull World Health Organ*. 1976;53(suppl):23-36.

138. Harada M. Congenital Minamata disease: intrauterine methylmercury poisoning. *Teratology*. 1978;18(2):285-288.

139. Harada M. Minamata disease: methylmercury poisoning in Japan caused by environmental pollution. *Crit Rev Toxicol*. 1995;25(1):1-24.

140. Hanna-Attisha M, LaChance J, Sadler RC, Champney Schnepp A. Elevated blood lead levels in children associated with the Flint drinking water crisis: a spatial analysis of risk and public health response. *Am J Public Health*. 2016;106(2):283-290.

141. Chou YJ, Huang N, Lee CH, Tsai SL, Chen LS, Chang HJ. Who is at risk of death in an earthquake? *Am J Epidemiol*. 2004;160(7):688-695.

142. Rey G, Fouillet A, Bessemoulin P, et al. Heat exposure and socio-economic vulnerability as synergistic factors in heat-wave-related mortality. *Eur J Epidemiol*. 2009;24(9):495-502.

143. Tchekmedyian A, Bermudez E. *California Firestorm Takes Deadly Toll on Elderly; Average Age of Victims Identified So Far Is 79*. Los Angeles, Ross Levinsohn: Los Angeles Times; 2017.

144. Hertz-Picciotto I, Delwiche L. The rise in autism and the role of age at diagnosis. *Epidemiology*. 2009;20(1):84-90.

145. King M, Bearman P. Diagnostic change and the increased prevalence of autism. *Int J Epidemiol*. 2009;38(5):1224-1234.

146. Bleich SN, Wang YC, Wang Y, Gortmaker SL. Increasing consumption of sugar-sweetened beverages among US adults: 1988-1994 to 1999-2004. *Am J Clin Nutr*. 2009;89(1):372-381.

147. Bray GA, Nielsen SJ, Popkin BM. Consumption of high-fructose corn syrup in beverages may play a role in the epidemic of obesity. *Am J Clin Nutr*. 2004;79(4):537-543.

148. Webb SJ, Garrison MM, Bernier R, McClintic AM, King BH, Mourad PD. Severity of ASD symptoms and their correlation with the presence of copy number variations and exposure to first trimester ultrasound. *Autism Res*. 2017;10(3):472-484.

149. Osterman MJ, Martin JA. Trends in low-risk cesarean delivery in the United States, 1990-2013. *Natl Vital Stat Rep*. 2014;63(6):1-16.

150. Lorber M. Exposure of Americans to polybrominated diphenyl ethers. *J Expo Sci Environ Epidemiol*. 2008;18(1):2-19.

151. Spurious Correlations. Available at http://tylervigen.com/page?page=2. Accessed May 21, 2019.

152. Anderson T, Le Riche W. Cold weather and myocardial infarction. *Lancet*. 1970;295(7641):291-296.

153. Bull GM, Morton J. Relationships of temperature with death rates from all causes and from certain respiratory and arteriosclerotic diseases in different age groups. *Age Ageing*. 1975;4(4):232-246.
154. Gover M. Mortality during periods of excessive temperature. *Public Health Rep*. 1938;53(2):1122-1143.
155. Cheng C, Loh EW, Lin CH, Chan CH, Lan TH. Birth seasonality in schizophrenia: effects of gender and income status. *Psychiatry Clin Neurosci*. 2013;67(6):426-433.
156. Lee BK, Gross R, Francis RW, et al. Birth seasonality and risk of autism spectrum disorder. *Eur J Epidemiol*. 2019;34(8):785-792.
157. Al-Haddad BJS, Jacobsson B, Chabra S, et al. Long-term risk of neuropsychiatric disease after exposure to infection in utero. *JAMA Psychiatry*. 2019;76(6):594-602.
158. Brown AS, Begg MD, Gravenstein S, et al. Serologic evidence of prenatal influenza in the etiology of schizophrenia. *Arch Gen Psychiatry*. 2004;61(8):774-780.
159. Zerbo O, Iosif AM, Delwiche L, Walker C, Hertz-Picciotto I. Month of conception and risk of autism. *Epidemiology*. 2011;22(4):469-475.
160. Kalkbrenner AE, Schmidt RJ, Penlesky AC. Environmental chemical exposures and autism spectrum disorders: a review of the epidemiological evidence. *Curr Probl Pediatr Adolesc Health Care*. 2014;44(10):277-318.
161. Howe GM. Historical evolution of disease mapping in general and specifically of cancer mapping. *Recent Results Cancer Res*. 1989;114:1-21.
162. Banerjee S, Carlin BP, Gelfand AE. *Hierarchical Modeling and Analysis for Spatial Data*. Boca Raton, FL: CRC Press; 2014.
163. Cressie N. *Statistics for Spatial Data*. New York, NY: Wiley; 1991.
164. Waller LA, Gotway CA. *Applied Spatial Statistics for Public Health Data*. Hoboken, New Jersey: John Wiley & Sons, Inc; 2004.
165. Elliott P, Kleinschmidt I, Westlake AJ. Use of routine data in studies of point sources of environmental pollution. In: Elliott P, Cuzick J, English D. Stern R, eds. *Geographical and Environmental Epidemiology: Methods for Small-Area Studies*. New York, NY: Oxford University Press; 1992: 106-114.
166. Gelman A, Price PN. All maps of parameter estimates are misleading. *Stat Med*. 1999;18(23):3221-3234.
167. Moulton LH, Foxman B, Wolfe RA, Port FK. Potential pitfalls in interpreting maps of stabilized rates. *Epidemiology*. 1994;5(3):297-301.
168. Blangiardo M, Cameletti M. *Spatial and Spatio-Temporal Bayesian Models with R - INLA*. Chichester, United Kingdom: John Wiley & Sons, Ltd; 2015.
169. Mason TJ, McKay FW, Hoover R, Blot WJ, Fraumeni JF. *Atlas of Cancer Mortality for US Counties: 1950-1969*. 1st ed. DHEW Publication No. NIH 75-780. Washington, DC: US Department of Health, Education and Welfare, Public Health Service, National Institutes of Health; 1975.
170. Brinton LA, Blot WJ, Stone B, Fraumeni JF. A death certificate analysis of nasal cancer among furniture workers in North Carolina. *Cancer Res*. 1977;37(10):3473-3474.
171. Blot WJ, Fraumeni JF Jr. Geographic patterns of lung cancer: industrial correlations. *Am J Epidemiol*. 1976;103(6):539-550.
172. Hoover R, Mason TJ, McKay FW, Fraumeni JF Jr. Cancer by county: new resource for etiologic clues. *Science*. 1975;189(4207):1005-1007.
173. Bithell JF, Stone RA. On statistical methods for analysing the geographical distribution of cancer cases near nuclear installations. *J Epidemiol Community Health*. 1989;43(1):79-85.
174. Besag J, Newell J. The detection of clusters in rare diseases. *J R Stat Soc Ser A Stat Soc*. 1991;154(1):143-155.
175. National Center for Environmental Health. Investigating suspected cancer clusters and responding to community concerns: guidelines from CDC and the Council of State and Territorial Epidemiologists. *MMWR Recomm Rep*. 2013;62(RR-08):1-24.
176. Rothman KJ. A sobering start for the cluster busters' conference. *Am J Epidemiol*. 1990;132(suppl 1):S6-S13.
177. Landrigan PJ, Goldman LR. Children's vulnerability to toxic chemicals: a challenge and opportunity to strengthen health and environmental policy. *Health Aff (Millwood)*. 2011;30(5):842-850.
178. Atterberry TT, Burnett WT, Chambers JE. Age-related differences in parathion and chlorpyrifos toxicity in male rats: target and nontarget esterase sensitivity and cytochrome P450-mediated metabolism. *Toxicol Appl Pharmacol*. 1997;147(2):411-418.
179. Chen J, Kumar M, Chan W, Berkowitz G, Wetmur JG. Increased influence of genetic variation on PON1 activity in neonates. *Environ Health Perspect*. 2003;111(11):1403-1409.
180. Lanphear BP. The impact of toxins on the developing brain. *Annu Rev Public Health*. 2015;36:211-230.
181. Wigle DT, Arbuckle TE, Turner MC, et al. Epidemiologic evidence of relationships between reproductive and child health outcomes and environmental chemical contaminants. *J Toxicol Environ Health B Crit Rev*. 2008;11(5-6):373-517.
182. Wigle DT, Arbuckle TE, Walker M, Wade MG, Liu S, Krewski D. Environmental hazards: evidence for effects on child health. *J Toxicol Environ Health B Crit Rev*. 2007;10(1-2):3-39.

183. Lichtveld K, Thomas K, Tulve NS. Chemical and non-chemical stressors affecting childhood obesity: a systematic scoping review. *J Expo Sci Environ Epidemiol*. 2018;28(1):1-12.

184. Landrigan PJ, Etzel RA, eds. *Textbook of Children's Environmental Health*. New York, NY: Oxford University Press; 2014.

185. Brown JR, Thornton JL. Percivall Pott (1714-1788) and chimney sweepers' cancer of the scrotum. *Br J Ind Med*. 1957;14(1):68-70.

186. Rice KM, Walker EM Jr, Wu M, Gillette C, Blough ER. Environmental mercury and its toxic effects. *J Prev Med Public Health*. 2014;47(2):74-83.

187. Miyakawa M. Radiation exposure and the risk of pediatric thyroid cancer. *Clin Pediatr Endocrinol*. 2014;23(3):73-82.

188. Lopez R, Goldoftas B. The urban elderly in the United States: health status and the environment. *Rev Environ Health*. 2009;24(1):47-57.

189. Hunt CM, Westerkam WR, Stave GM. Effect of age and gender on the activity of human hepatic CYP3A. *Biochem Pharmacol*. 1992a;44(2):275-283.

190. Hunt CM, Westerkam WR, Stave GM, Wilson JA. Hepatic cytochrome P-4503A (CYP3A) activity in the elderly. *Mech Ageing Dev*. 1992b;64(1-2):189-199.

191. Schmucker DL. Liver function and phase I drug metabolism in the elderly: a paradox. *Drugs Aging*. 2001;18(11):837-851.

192. Soenen S, Rayner CK, Jones KL, Horowitz M. The ageing gastrointestinal tract. *Curr Opin Clin Nutr Metab Care*. 2016;19(1):12-18.

193. Simoni M, Baldacci S, Maio S, Cerrai S, Sarno G, Viegi G. Adverse effects of outdoor pollution in the elderly. *J Thorac Dis*. 2015;7(1):34-45.

194. Youssouf H, Liousse C, Roblou L, et al. Non-accidental health impacts of wildfire smoke. *Int J Environ Res Public Health*. 2014;11(11):11772-11804.

195. Benmarhnia T, Deguen S, Kaufman JS, Smargiassi A. Review article: vulnerability to heat-related mortality. A systematic review, meta-analysis, and meta-regression analysis. *Epidemiology*. 2015;26(6):781-793.

196. Davido A, Patzak A, Dart T, et al. Risk factors for heat related death during the August 2003 heat wave in Paris, France, in patients evaluated at the emergency department of the Hopital Europeen Georges Pompidou. *Emerg Med J*. 2006;23(7):515-518.

197. Levy BS, Patz JA. Climate change, human rights, and social justice. *Ann Glob Health*. 2015;81(3):310-322.

198. Hasegawa A, Tanigawa K, Ohtsuru A, et al. Health effects of radiation and other health problems in the aftermath of nuclear accidents, with an emphasis on Fukushima. *Lancet*. 2015;386(9992):479-488.

199. Campbell C, Greenberg R, Mankikar D, Ross RD. A case study of environmental injustice: the failure in Flint. *Int J Environ Res Public Health*. 2016;13(10):951.

200. Rosner D. Flint, Michigan: a century of environmental injustice. *Am J Public Health*. 2016;106(2):200-201.

201. Kennedy C, Yard E, Dignam T, et al. Blood lead levels among children aged <6 years - Flint, Michigan, 2013-2016. *MMWR Morb Mortal Wkly Rep*. 2016;65(25):650-654.

202. Ponce NA, Hoggatt KJ, Wilhelm M, Ritz B. Preterm birth: the interaction of traffic-related air pollution with economic hardship in Los Angeles neighborhoods. *Am J Epidemiol*. 2005;162(2):140-148.

203. Zeka A, Melly SJ, Schwartz J. The effects of socioeconomic status and indices of physical environment on reduced birth weight and preterm births in Eastern Massachusetts. *Environ Health*. 2008;7:60.

204. Sonneborn D, Park HY, Petrik J, et al. Prenatal polychlorinated biphenyl exposures in eastern Slovakia modify effects of social factors on birthweight. *Paediatr Perinat Epidemiol*. 2008;22(3):202-213.

205. Cantoral A, Tellez-Rojo MM, Levy TS, et al. Differential association of lead on length by zinc status in two-year old Mexican children. *Environ Health*. 2015;14:95.

206. Moore BF, Sauder KA, Starling AP, Ringham BM, Glueck DH Dabelea D. Exposure to secondhand smoke, exclusive breastfeeding and infant adiposity at age 5 months in the Healthy Start study. *Pediatr Obes*. 2017;12(suppl 1):111-119.

207. Gonzalez-Alzaga B, Lacasana M, Aguilar-Garduno C, et al. A systematic review of neurodevelopmental effects of prenatal and postnatal organophosphate pesticide exposure. *Toxicol Lett*. 2014;230(2):104-121.

208. Munoz-Quezada MT, Lucero BA, Barr DB, et al. Neurodevelopmental effects in children associated with exposure to organophosphate pesticides: a systematic review. *Neurotoxicology*. 2013;39:158-168.

209. Engel SM, Wetmur J, Chen J, et al. Prenatal exposure to organophosphates, paraoxonase 1, and cognitive development in childhood. *Environ Health Perspect*. 2011;119(8):1182-1188.

210. Eskenazi B, Marks AR, Bradman A, et al. Organophosphate pesticide exposure and neurodevelopment in young Mexican-American children. *Environ Health Perspect*. 2007;115(5):792-798.

211. Rauh V, Arunajadai S, Horton M, et al. Seven-year neurodevelopmental scores and prenatal exposure to chlorpyrifos, a common agricultural pesticide. *Environ Health Perspect*. 2011;119(8):1196-1201.

212. Cartier C, Warembourg C, Le Maner-Idrissi G, et al. Organophosphate insecticide metabolites in prenatal and childhood urine samples and Intelligence scores at 6 years of age: results from the mother-child PELAGIE cohort (France). *Environ Health Perspect*. 2016;124(5):674-680.

213. Donauer S, Altaye M, Xu Y, et al. An observational study to evaluate associations between low-level gestational exposure to organophosphate pesticides and cognition during early childhood. *Am J Epidemiol.* 2016;184(5):410-418.

214. Vreugdenhil HJ, Lanting CI, Mulder PG, Boersma ER, Weisglas-Kuperus N. Effects of prenatal PCB and dioxin background exposure on cognitive and motor abilities in Dutch children at school age. *J Pediatr.* 2002;140(1):48-56.

215. Gaffney A, Christiani DC. Gene-environment interaction from international cohorts: impact on development and evolution of occupational and environmental lung and airway disease. *Semin Respir Crit Care Med.* 2015;36(3):347-357.

216. Andersen HR, Wohlfahrt-Veje C, Dalgard C, et al. Paraoxonase 1 polymorphism and prenatal pesticide exposure associated with adverse cardiovascular risk profiles at school age. *PLoS One.* 2012;7(5):e36830.

217. Engel SM, Berkowitz GS, Barr DB, et al. Prenatal organophosphate metabolite and organochlorine levels and performance on the Brazelton Neonatal Behavioral Assessment Scale in a multiethnic pregnancy cohort. *Am J Epidemiol.* 2007;165(12):1397-1404.

218. Eskenazi B, Kogut K, Huen K, et al. Organophosphate pesticide exposure, PON1, and neurodevelopment in school-age children from the CHAMACOS study. *Environ Res.* 2014;134:149-157.

219. Harley KG, Huen K, Aguilar Schall R, et al. Association of organophosphate pesticide exposure and paraoxonase with birth outcome in Mexican-American women. *PLoS One.* 2011;6(8):e23923.

220. Morahan JM, Yu B, Trent RJ, Pamphlett R. A gene-environment study of the paraoxonase 1 gene and pesticides in amyotrophic lateral sclerosis. *Neurotoxicology.* 2007;28(3):532-540.

221. Gao J, Tong L, Argos M, et al. The genetic architecture of arsenic metabolism efficiency: A SNP-based Heritability study of Bangladeshi adults. *Environ Health Perspect.* 2015;123(10):985-992.

222. Pierce BL, Kibriya MG, Tong L, et al. Genome-wide association study identifies chromosome 10q24.32 variants associated with arsenic metabolism and toxicity phenotypes in Bangladesh. *Plos Genet.* 2012;8(2):e1002522.

223. Pierce BL, Tong L, Argos M, et al. Arsenic metabolism efficiency has a causal role in arsenic toxicity: Mendelian randomization and gene-environment interaction. *Int J Epidemiol.* 2013;42(6):1862-1871.

224. Pierce BL, Tong L, Dean S, et al. A missense variant in FTCD is associated with arsenic metabolism and toxicity phenotypes in Bangladesh. *Plos Genet.* 2019;15(3):e1007984.

225. Valenzuela OL, Drobna Z, Hernandez-Castellanos E, et al. Association of AS3MT polymorphisms and the risk of premalignant arsenic skin lesions. *Toxicol Appl Pharmacol.* 2009;239(2):200-207.

226. Hsu ST, Ma CI, Hsu SK, et al. Discovery and epidemiology of PCB poisoning in Taiwan: a four-year followup. *Environ Health Perspect.* 1985;59:5-10.

227. Hens B, Hens L. Persistent threats by persistent pollutants: chemical nature, concerns and future policy regarding PCBs-what are we heading for? *Toxics.* 2017;6(1):1.

228. Jacobson JL, Jacobson SW. Dose-response in perinatal exposure to polychlorinated biphenyls (PCBs): the Michigan and North Carolina cohort studies. *Toxicol Ind Health.* 1996;12(3-4):435-445.

229. Winneke G, Bucholski A, Heinzow B, et al. Developmental neurotoxicity of polychlorinated biphenyls (PCBS): cognitive and psychomotor functions in 7-month old children. *Toxicol Lett.* 1998;102-103:423-428.

230. Sethi S, Morgan RK, Feng W, et al. Comparative analyses of the 12 most abundant PCB congeners detected in human maternal serum for activity at the thyroid hormone receptor and ryanodine receptor. *Environ Sci Technol.* 2019;53(7):3948-3958.

231. UNEP. *Resolution of the Stockholm Convention on Persistent Organic Pollutants.* Geneva, Switzerland: United Nations Environment Programme; 2001b.

232. Osterberg D, Scammell MK. PCBs in schools – where communities and science come together. *Environ Sci Pollut Res Int.* 2016;23(3):1998-2002.

233. Xu P, Wu L, Chen Y, et al. High intake of persistent organic pollutants generated by a municipal waste incinerator by breastfed infants. *Environ Pollut.* 2019;250:662-668.

234. Gibson JL. A plea for painted railings and painted walls of rooms as the source of lead poisoning amongst Queensland children. *Australasian Medical Gazette.* 1904;23:149-153.

235. Bellinger DC, Chen A, Lanphear BP. Establishing and achieving national goals for preventing lead toxicity and exposure in children. *JAMA Pediatr.* 2017;171(7):616-618.

236. Craft-Blacksheare M. The growing impact of Legionella in the Flint water crisis. *J Natl Black Nurses Assoc.* 2018;29(1):44-50.

237. Rhoads WJ, Garner E, Ji P, et al. Distribution system operational deficiencies coincide with reported Legionnaires' disease clusters in Flint, Michigan. *Environ Sci Technol.* 2017;51(20):11986-11995.

238. Caramaschi F, del Corno G, Favaretti C, Giambelluca SE, Montesarchio E, Fara GM. Chloracne following environmental contamination by TCDD in Seveso, Italy. *Int J Epidemiol.* 1981;10(2):135-143.

239. Eskenazi B, Warner M, Brambilla P, Signorini S, Ames J, Mocarelli P. The Seveso accident: a look at 40years of health research and beyond. *Environ Int.* 2018;121(pt 1):71-84.

240. Chowdhury AM. Arsenic crisis in Bangladesh. *Sci Am.* 2004;291(2):86-91.

241. Mazumder DN, Das Gupta J, Santra A, Pal A, Ghose A, Sarkar S. Chronic arsenic toxicity in West Bengal – the worst calamity in the world. *J Indian Med Assoc*. 1998;96(1):4-7, 18.

242. Smith GD. Classics in epidemiology: should they get it right? *Int J Epidemiol*. 2004;33(3):441-442.

243. von Ehrenstein OS, Mazumder DN, Yuan Y, et al. Decrements in lung function related to arsenic in drinking water in West Bengal, India. *Am J Epidemiol*. 2005;162(6):533-541.

244. Wasserman GA, Liu X, Parvez F, et al. Water arsenic exposure and intellectual function in 6-year-old children in Araihazar, Bangladesh. *Environ Health Perspect*. 2007;115(2):285-289.

245. Wasserman GA, Liu X, Parvez F, et al. Water arsenic exposure and children's intellectual function in Araihazar, Bangladesh. *Environ Health Perspect*. 2004;112(13):1329-1333.

246. Baud D, Gubler DJ, Schaub B, Lanteri MC, Musso D. An update on Zika virus infection. *Lancet*. 2017;390(10107):2099-2109.

247. Likos A, Griffin I, Bingham AM, et al. Local mosquito-borne transmission of Zika virus - Miami-Dade and Broward counties, Florida, June-August 2016. *MMWR Morb Mortal Wkly Rep*. 2016;65(38):1032-1038.

248. Gunier RB, Bradman A, Harley KG, Kogut K, Eskenazi B. Prenatal residential proximity to agricultural pesticide use and IQ in 7-year-old children. *Environ Health Perspect*. 2017;125(5):057002.

249. Rauh VA, Perera FP, Horton MK, et al. Brain anomalies in children exposed prenatally to a common organophosphate pesticide. *Proc Natl Acad Sci USA*. 2012;109(20):7871-7876.

250. Longnecker MP, Rogan WJ, Lucier G. The human health effects of DDT (dichlorodiphenyltrichloroethane) and PCBS (polychlorinated biphenyls) and an overview of organochlorines in public health. *Annu Rev Public Health*. 1997;18:211-244.

251. IARC. DDT and associated compounds. *IARC Monogr Eval Carcinog Risks Hum*. 1991;53:179-249.

252. BBC. *Malaria Vaccine Rolled Out for Tens of Thousands of Children*. London, United Kingdom: British Broadcasting Corporation; 2019.

253. Atomic Heritage Foundation. *Bombings of Hiroshima and Nagasaki - 1945*. Available at https://www.atomicheritage.org/history/bombings-hiroshima-and-nagasaki-1945. Accessed May 29, 2019.

254. Putnam FW. The atomic bomb casualty commission in retrospect. *Proc Natl Acad Sci USA*. 1998;95(10):5426-5431.

255. RERF. *Radiation Effects Research Foundation - A Cooperative Japan-US Research Organization*. Available at https://www.rerf.or.jp/en/about/. Accessed May 29, 2019.

256. Ohtsuru A, Midorikawa S, Ohira T, et al. Incidence of thyroid cancer among children and young adults in Fukushima, Japan, screened with 2 rounds of ultrasonography within 5 years of the 2011 Fukushima Daiichi nuclear power station accident. *JAMA Otolaryngol Head Neck Surg*. 2019;145(1):4-11.

257. D'Andrea MA, Reddy GK. Health consequences among subjects involved in Gulf oil spill clean-up activities. *Am J Med*. 2013;126(11):966-974.

258. D'Andrea MA, Reddy GK. The development of long-term adverse health effects in oil spill cleanup workers of the deepwater horizon offshore drilling rig disaster. *Front Public Health*. 2018;6:117.

259. Gam KB, Kwok RK, Engel LS, et al. Lung function in oil spill response workers 1-3 years after the deepwater horizon disaster. *Epidemiology*. 2018;29(3):315-322.

260. McGowan CJ, Kwok RK, Engel LS, Stenzel MR, Stewart PA, Sandler DP. Respiratory, dermal, and eye irritation symptoms associated with Corexit EC9527A/EC9500A following the deepwater horizon oil spill: findings from the GuLF STUDY. *Environ Health Perspect*. 2017;125(9):097015.

261. Shenesey JW, Langhinrichsen-Rohling J. Perceived resilience: examining impacts of the deepwater horizon oil spill one-year post-spill. *Psychol Trauma*. 2015;7(3):252-258.

262. Strelitz J, Sandler DP, Keil AP, et al. Exposure to total hydrocarbons during cleanup of the deepwater horizon oil spill and risk of heart attack across 5 years of follow-up. *Am J Epidemiol*. 2019;188(5):917-927.

263. Cerda M, Bordelois PM, Galea S, Norris F, Tracy M, Koenen KC. The course of posttraumatic stress symptoms and functional impairment following a disaster: what is the lasting influence of acute versus ongoing traumatic events and stressors? *Soc Psychiatry Psychiatr Epidemiol*. 2013a;48(3):3 85-395.

264. Cerda M, Paczkowski M, Galea S, Nemethy K, Pean C, Desvarieux M. Psychopathology in the aftermath of the Haiti earthquake: a population-based study of posttraumatic stress disorder and major depression. *Depress Anxiety*. 2013b;30(5):413-424.

265. Galea S, Ahern J, Tracy M, et al. Longitudinal determinants of posttraumatic stress in a population-based cohort study. *Epidemiology*. 2008;19(1):47-54.

266. Lowe SR, Manove EE, Rhodes JE. Posttraumatic stress and posttraumatic growth among low-income mothers who survived Hurricane Katrina. *J Consult Clin Psychol*. 2013;81(5):877-889.

267. Shultz JM, Galea S. Mitigating the mental and physical health consequences of Hurricane Harvey. *J Am Med Assoc*. 2017;318(15):1437-1438.

268. Horney JA, Casillas GA, Baker E, et al. Comparing residential contamination in a Houston environmental justice neighborhood before and after Hurricane Harvey. *PLoS One*. 2018;13(2):e0192660.

269. Zubizarreta JR, Cerda M, Rosenbaum PR. Effect of the 2010 Chilean earthquake on posttraumatic stress: reducing sensitivity to unmeasured bias through study design. *Epidemiology*. 2013;24(1):79-87.

270. World Health Organization. *COP24 Special Report: Health and Climate Change.* 2018.

271. Intergovernmental Panel on Climate Change..*AR5 Synthesis Report: Climate Change 2014.* Geneva: IPCC; 2014.

272. Howard GJ. Chemical alternatives assessment: the case of flame retardants. *Chemosphere.* 2014;116:112-117.

273. Jacobs MM, Malloy TF, Tickner JA, Edwards S. Alternatives assessment frameworks: research needs for the informed substitution of hazardous chemicals. *Environ Health Perspect.* 2016;124(3):265-280.

274. Eladak S, Grisin T, Moison D, et al. A new chapter in the bisphenol A story: bisphenol S and bisphenol F are not safe alternatives to this compound. *Fertil Steril.* 2015;103(1):11-21.

275. Gyllenhammar I, Glynn A, Jonsson BA, et al. Diverging temporal trends of human exposure to bisphenols and plastizisers, such as phthalates, caused by substitution of legacy EDCs? *Environ Res.* 2017;153:48-54.

276. Rosenmai AK, Dybdahl M, Pedersen M, et al. Are structural analogues to bisphenol a safe alternatives? *Toxicol Sci.* 2014;139(1):35-47.

277. Wang Z, Cousins IT, Scheringer M, Hungerbuehler K. Hazard assessment of fluorinated alternatives to long-chain perfluoroalkyl acids (PFAAs) and their precursors: status quo, ongoing challenges and possible solutions. *Environ Int.* 2015;75:172-179.

278. Williams MK, Rundle A, Holmes D, et al. Changes in pest infestation levels, self-reported pesticide use, and permethrin exposure during pregnancy after the 2000-2001 US Environmental Protection Agency restriction of organophosphates. *Environ Health Perspect.* 2008;116(12):1681-1688.

279. Forner-Piquer I, Maradonna F, Gioacchini G, et al. Dose-specific effects of di-isononyl phthalate on the endocannabinoid system and on liver of female zebrafish. *Endocrinology.* 2017;158(10):3462-3476.

280. Ring CL, Pearce RG, Setzer RW, Wetmore BA, Wambaugh JF. Identifying populations sensitive to environmental chemicals by simulating toxicokinetic variability. *Environ Int.* 2017;106:105-118.

281. McCarty LS, Borgert CJ. Review of the toxicity of chemical mixtures: theory, policy, and regulatory practice. *Regul Toxicol Pharmacol.* 2006;45(2):119-143.

282. Wild CP. Complementing the genome with an "exposome": the outstanding challenge of environmental exposure measurement in molecular epidemiology. *Cancer Epidemiol Biomarkers Prev.* 2005;14(8):1847-1850.

283. Wild CP. The exposome: from concept to utility. *Int J Epidemiol.* 2012;41(1):24-32.

284. Turner MC, Nieuwenhuijsen M, Anderson K, et al. Assessing the exposome with external measures: commentary on the state of the science and research recommendations. *Annu Rev Public Health.* 2017;38:215-239.

285. Andra SS, Austin C, Patel D, Dolios G, Awawda M, Arora M. Trends in the application of high-resolution mass spectrometry for human biomonitoring: an analytical primer to studying the environmental chemical space of the human exposome. *Environ Int.* 2017;100:32-61.

286. Cherta L, Portoles T, Pitarch E, et al. Analytical strategy based on the combination of gas chromatography coupled to time-of-flight and hybrid quadrupole time-of-flight mass analyzers for non-target analysis in food packaging. *Food Chem.* 2015;188:301-308.

287. Martinez Bueno MJ, Ulaszewska MM, Gomez MJ, Hernando MD, Fernandez-Alba AR. Simultaneous measurement in mass and mass/mass mode for accurate qualitative and quantitative screening analysis of pharmaceuticals in river water. *J Chromatogr A.* 2012;1256:80-88.

288. Baduel C, Mueller JF, Tsai H, Gomez Ramos MJ. Development of sample extraction and clean-up strategies for target and non-target analysis of environmental contaminants in biological matrices. *J Chromatogr A.* 2015;1426:33-47.

289. Hammel SC, Hoffman K, Webster TF, Anderson KA, Stapleton HM. Correction to measuring personal exposure to organophosphate flame retardants using silicone wristbands and hand Wipes. *Environ Sci Technol.* 2016;50(18):10291.

290. Romanyuk AV, Zvezdin VN, Samant P, Grenader MI, Zemlyanova M, Prausnitz MR. Collection of analytes from microneedle patches. *Anal Chem.* 2014;86(21):10520-10523.

291. Gouma PI, Wang L, Simon SR, Stanacevic M. Novel isoprene sensor for a flu virus breath monitor. *Sensors (Basel).* 2017;17(1).

292. Nieuwenhuijsen MJ, Agier L, Basagana X, et al. Influence of the urban exposome on birth weight. *Environ Health Perspect.* 2019;127(4):47007.

293. Agier L, Basagana X, Maitre L, et al. Early-life exposome and lung function in children in Europe: an analysis of data from the longitudinal, population-based HELIX cohort. *Lancet Planet Health.* 2019;3(2):e81-e92.

294. McMichael AJ. Globalization, climate change, and human health. *N Engl J Med.* 2013;368(14):1335-1343.

295. UN. *UN Report: Nature's Dangerous Decline 'Unprecedented'; Species Extinction Rates 'Accelerating'.* 2019. Available at https://www.un.org/sustainabledevelopment/blog/2019/05/nature-decline-unprecedented-report/. United Nations Sustainable Development Report. Accessed May 29, 2019.

296. Cook J, Oreskes N, Doran PT, et al. Consensus on consensus: a synthesis of consensus estimates on human-caused global warming. *Environ Res Lett.* 2016;11(4):048002.

297. Field CB, Barros VR, Mach K, Mastrandrea M. *Climate Change 2014: Impacts, Adaptation, and Vulnerability.* Cambridge, New York: Cambridge University Press; 2014.

298. Randolph SE. Perspectives on climate change impacts on infectious diseases. *Ecology.* 2009;90(4):927-931.

299. Analitis A,s Michelozzi P, D'Ippoliti D, et al. Effects of heat waves on mortality: effect modification and confounding by air pollutants. *Epidemiology.* 2014;25(1):15-22.

300. Filleul L, Cassadou S, Medina S, et al. The relation between temperature, ozone, and mortality in nine French cities during the heat wave of 2003. *Environ Health Perspect.* 2006;114(9):1344-1347.

301. Hernandez MA, Robles M, Torero M. *Fires in Russia, Wheat Production and Volatile Markets: Reasons To Panic?* Washington, DC: International Food Policy Research Institute; 2010. Available at http://www.ifpri.org/sites/default/files/wheat.pdf.

302. Shaposhnikov D, Revich B, Bellander T, et al. Mortality related to air pollution with the moscow heat wave and wildfire of 2010. *Epidemiology.* 2014;25(3):359-364.

303. Zheteyeva Y, Rainey JJ, Gao H, et al. Unintended costs and consequences of school closures implemented in preparation for hurricane Isaac in Harrison county school district, Mississippi, August-September 2012. *PLoS One.* 2017;12(11):e0184326.

304. McMichael AJ. The urban environment and health in a world of increasing globalization: issues for developing countries. *Bull World Health Organ.* 2000;78(9):1117-1126.

305. McMichael AJ, Patz J, Kovats RS. Impacts of global environmental change on future health and health care in tropical countries. *Br Med Bull.* 1998;54(2):475-488.

306. Watts N, Amann M, Arnell N, et al. The 2018 report of the Lancet Countdown on health and climate change: shaping the health of nations for centuries to come. *Lancet.* 2018;392(10163):2479-2514.

307. Soneja S, Jiang C, Romeo Upperman C, et al. Extreme precipitation events and increased risk of campy-lobacteriosis in Maryland, USA. *Environ Res.* 2016;149:216-221.

308. Sieswerda LE, Soskolne CL, Newman SC, Schopflocher D, Smoyer KE. Toward measuring the impact of ecological disintegrity on human health. *Epidemiology.* 2001;12(1):28-32.

309. Li R, Merchant JW. Modeling vulnerability of groundwater to pollution under future scenarios of climate change and biofuels-related land use change: a case study in North Dakota, USA. *Sci Total Environ.* 2013;447:32-45.

310. Ummenhofer CC, Meehl GA. Extreme weather and climate events with ecological relevance: a review. *Philos Trans R Soc Lond B Biol Sci.* 2017;372(1723):20160135.

311. Bais AF, Lucas RM, Bornman JF, et al. Environmental effects of ozone depletion, UV radiation and inter-actions with climate change: UNEP Environmental Effects Assessment Panel, update 2017. *Photochem Photobiol Sci.* 2018;17(2):127-179.

312. Langston M, Dennis L, Lynch C, Roe D, Brown H. Temporal trends in satellite-derived erythemal UVB and implications for ambient sun exposure assessment. *Int J Environ Res Public Health.* 2017;14(2).

313. Auerbach S, Filer D, Reif D, et al. Prioritizing environmental chemicals for obesity and diabetes out-comes research: a screening approach using ToxCast high-throughput data. *Environ Health Perspect.* 2016;124(8):1141-1154.

CHAPTER 41

Occupational Epidemiology

David Richardson

MAJOR OBJECTIVES AND HISTORICAL DEVELOPMENT OF OCCUPATIONAL EPIDEMIOLOGY

Occupational epidemiology is the study of workers, the conditions that they experience in the workplace, and associated illnesses and injuries. Occupational epidemiologists undertake research to improve worker health and safety and to inform compensation decisions for sick and injured workers. Occupational epidemiology has contributed to identification of a variety of hazards in the workplace, including aniline dyes, asbestos, benzene, carbon disulfide, carbon monoxide, hydrogen sulfide, lead, mercury, radium, radon, silica, and vinyl chloride. Many of these were subsequently understood to be environmental hazards as well. While the methods used in occupational epidemiology are similar to those used in other substantive areas, there are some important strengths of epidemiological studies that are conducted in occupational settings, as well as some notable challenges commonly encountered when doing research on working populations, that have led to the emergence of occupational epidemiology as a distinct research area. This chapter reviews some major contributions of occupational epidemiology, discusses some of the strengths and limitations of occupational studies, and discusses how these influenced decisions about study design and analysis in this research area.

Historical Development of Occupational Epidemiology

Recognition of work-related disease often has been spurred by the observation of a seemingly unusual occurrence of disease among workers employed in a particular occupation or industry. In fact, clinicians have named a number of diseases after the occupation held by the workers among whom the condition was identified or the presumed causative agent, including Hatters' shakes, Baker's lung, popcorn lung, silicosis, asbestosis, anthracosis, and byssinosis. The naming of such diseases reflects a history of clinical observation about occupational diseases that has served as a basis for etiological inference. Hippocrates emphasized the importance of occupational factors in the etiology of disease and encouraged physicians to ask about the patient's occupational history to inform the diagnosis of disease.[1] Bernardino Ramazzini compiled a description of many work-related diseases in a treatise "De Morbis Artificum Diatriba" further strengthening diagnosis of occupational diseases and their attribution to specific occupational exposures.[2]

It is not just clinicians who have recognized clusters of disease among workers; workers themselves often help to recognize occupational health problems. Alice Hamilton, a physician and progressive activist, stressed the importance of the perceptions of workers and the insights that they could provide about occupational hazards, as she documented in *Industrial poisons in the United States* (1925).[3] Labor organizations, industrial hygienists, and community members also have played a role in recognition of clusters of disease among workers.[4-8]

In what is often regarded as the first recognized occupational carcinogen, Percivall Pott (1775) reported on the occurrence of scrotal cancer among chimney sweeps and posited that exposure to soot caused the disease.[9] Pott noted, "The fate of these people seems singularly hard: in their early infancy, they are most frequently treated with great brutality, and almost starved with cold and hunger; they are thrust up narrow, and sometimes hot chimneys, where they are bruised, burned and almost suffocated; and when they get to puberty, become peculiarly liable to a most noisome, painful, and fatal disease... The disease, in these people, seems to derive its origin from a lodgement of soot in the rugae of the scrotum, and at first not to be a disease of the habit ... but here the subjects are young, in general good health, at least at first; the disease brought on them by their occupation, and in all probability local; which last circumstance may, I think, be fairly presumed from its always seizing the same parts; all this makes it (at first) a very different case from a cancer which appears in an elderly man." The rarity of scrotal cancer and the early onset among chimney sweeps helped in its recognition. In general, case reports tend to be valuable for identifying occupational hazards that cause, or exacerbate, diseases that are rare in the general population (and are particularly useful if the relative risk among the occupationally exposed is large). Reports on other occupational carcinogens followed Potts report. Examples include Ayrton Paris' 1822 report on scrotal cancers among copper and tin smelters,[10] and Von Volkmann's (1874) and Bell's (1876) reports on scrotal cancer among paraffin workers.[11-14] In more contemporary examples, case reports have also played an important role in recognition of occupational diseases; the literature includes case reports on bone cancer among radium dial painters, on bladder cancer among rubber workers, and on cholangiocarcinoma, an extremely rare cancer, among workers in the printing industry.[4,15,16] In many of these more contemporary examples, case reports were complemented by formal epidemiological investigations that strengthened understanding of a potential occupational exposure-disease association and examined the association in a larger population. In the example of cholangiocarcinoma among printers, the initial case series led to an investigation in the printing facility at which the case cluster was identified[16] and in the broader printing industry.[17,18]

In contrast to episodic case reports, more systematic approaches to recognition of occupational disease frequently begin with examination of incidence or mortality rates in an occupation or industry. The statistical methods used for such investigations draw heavily upon the development of actuarial methods in the late 18th and early 19th centuries.[19] Laplace's 1814 *A Philosophical Essay on Probabilities,*" offers an early expression of the innovations in thinking about analyses of occupational disease in terms of rates in these actuarial "life table" calculations, "So many variable causes influence mortality that the tables which represent it ought to be changed according to place and time. The diverse states of life offer in this regard appreciable differences relative to the fatigues and the dangers inseparable from each state and of which it is indispensable to keep account in the calculations founded upon the duration of life. But these differences have not been sufficiently observed. Some day they will be and then will be known what sacrifice of life each profession demands and one will profit by this knowledge to diminish the dangers" (page 143).[20]

Pioneering work in the 19th century on the collection and coding of the occupational information of decedents by William Farr, the Superintendent of the Statistical Department of the General Register Office in Great Britain, laid groundwork for many studies of relationships between occupation and cause of death, and mortality differentials by sociodemographic and occupational factors.[21] Farr wrote "The deaths and causes of death are scientific facts which admit of numerical analysis; and science has nothing to offer more inviting in speculation than the laws of vitality, the variations of those laws in the two sexes at different ages, and the influence of civilization, occupation, locality, seasons, and other physical agencies, either in generating diseases and inducing death, or in improving the public health." Farr noted, for example, "The earthenware manufacture is one of the unhealthiest trades in the country. At the age of joining it is low, but the mortality after age 35 years approaches double the average; it is excessively high; it exceeds the mortality of publicans (bar keepers). What can be done to save the men dying so fast in the potteries and engaged in one of our most useful manufactures?" There are, of course, important limitations to investigations relying on death certificate–based information, as Major Greenwood subsequently noted, "Wishing to study the influence of occupational environment upon health, he adopted the simple plan of relating the deaths in the census year to the population as enumerated in occupational groups. Any critically minded man could point out objections to this method. The occupation recorded in a death certificate is the occupation known to the dead man's relations who from ignorance or snobbishness may report a designation altogether different from that which the living man would return in the census form." Other objections were noted, such as the departure of the disabled from an occupation before they died, so that their deaths were assigned to some other occupation (or no occupation at all).[22] Yet, despite these limitations, Farr's findings were notable as early occupational analyses that served to illustrate a pragmatic approach to investigation of occupational causes of mortality using data derived from death certificates. Contemporaries of Farr's, notably Edwin Chadwick, in his 1842 report from the Poor Law Commissioners on an Inquiry into the Sanitary Conditions of the Labouring Population of Great Britain,[23] and Fredrich Engels, in his 1845 report on The Condition of the Working Class in England,[24] also made use of information from the General Registrar of Births and Deaths. Among Farr and his contemporaries, there can be found examples of work that presaged the analytical designs and methods employed in 20th-century occupational epidemiology[25] and laid the groundwork for studies based on routine collection and coding of occupational information.[26,27]

Occupational epidemiology as a distinct academic discipline with a formalized set of methods owes much to the development of methods for chronic disease epidemiology in the 1950s. Many of the early academic faculty in the discipline of occupational epidemiology were working in the areas of chronic disease epidemiology, with attention on occupational chronic diseases. Within academic departments, occupational epidemiology began to be constituted as a distinct subdiscipline of epidemiology and occupational medicine, and specific programs in occupational epidemiology developed. In the 1950s, the research of occupational epidemiologists led to some notable results, including the identification of occupational hazards such as asbestos, nickel, coal tar, aniline dyes, and chromate.[28-33]

Over time, occupational epidemiologists broadened the scope of their investigations beyond studies of chronic diseases, and subsequently some epidemiologists began to explore application of epidemiological methods to other occupational health problems, such as occupational injury prevention[34-37] and reproductive health.[38,39]

Of course, the research agendas and directions for the discipline were not set just by the interests of researchers. Labor and social activism was an important driver of occupational epidemiology as well. For example, labor activists in the coal mining industry played an important role in shaping occupational research on respiratory disease and their efforts eventually helped to establish specialized research units and otherwise promoted research in this area.[22,40-42] Although coal miners' lung disease was well established by the 19th century, epidemiological work demonstrating the prevalence of the condition among coal workers was important in guiding public policy for insurance for the miners in the United Kingdom, and their example led to similar efforts in other countries to press for epidemiological studies of the coal industry.[42,43] Similarly, in the cotton textile manufacturing industry, labor activists drew upon occupational studies of UK cotton workers[44] to press for epidemiological research among cotton workers in other countries.[45-48]

Harmful exposures often cannot be completely removed from the work environment; therefore, much of occupational epidemiology is aimed at quantifying risks associated with different levels of exposure to an occupational hazard. This means that contemporary occupational epidemiology contributes not just to the recognition of novel causes of disease and injury (i.e., hazard identification) but also to risk quantification. The latter helps inform decision-making about adequate control of occupational hazards, risk assessments, and ultimately program evaluation to monitor improvements in worker health. The demands for quantitative answers to questions about the magnitude of the hazard and the exposure-risk association coincided with postwar institutions and labor efforts to strengthen worker protection. Developments in modern epidemiology and their application to study of occupational causes of disease have found a place within this regulatory model, providing quantitative results to inform risk assessments and decision-making.[49,50] This extends to decision-making in areas outside of regulation of contemporary workplaces, as occupational epidemiology plays an important role in contributing to the setting of exposure limits for exposures that occur in nonoccupational settings, as well as legal decisions and compensation schemes for such exposures.[51]

METHODOLOGIC TOPICS OF SPECIAL RELEVANCE TO OCCUPATIONAL EPIDEMIOLOGY

Occupational Study Designs

Many of the landmark studies in occupational epidemiology are facility-based or industry-based cohort studies that have involved enumeration of large cohorts of workers, often unionized, for whom it was possible to explicitly assemble rosters based on employer, trade union, or professional association records.[28,52-54] The occupational cohort study design is a logical choice when the exposure of interest is uncommon outside a specific workplace or industry; it is reasonable for a researcher to commence an investigation by enumeration of a study population based on the workplace or industry in which people who were exposed are found (as opposed, for example, to commencing with a hospital-based or population-based roster of cases of a specific disease). This focus of occupational epidemiologists on large cohorts has been influential on thinking about methods for assessment of exposures and outcomes that are well suited to such studies. In teaching about the general logic and design of epidemiological cohort studies, occupational cohort studies have often served as a benchmark for how cohort studies should be done.[55] In fact, there are a number of notable epidemiological studies, such as the British Doctors Study,[56] the US Nurses Health Study, and the California Teachers Study, that were enumerated from occupational or professional rosters, but are not usually considered as examples of occupational epidemiology because they were undertaken without the primary objective being to improve understanding of the health effects of workplace exposures or conditions. Nonetheless, the investigators recognized a general strength of the cohort study design is that it begins with a well-enumerated cohort and recognized the value of using occupational records for such a purpose.

Occupational cohort studies can be costly in terms of time and resources. To improve efficiency in data collection, or permit more in-depth exposure assessments on a subsample of the full cohort, occupational epidemiologists may undertake a nested case-control study within the enumerated study cohort. Efficiency in ascertainment of exposure and covariate information has been one motivation for nested case-control designs in occupational epidemiology. Another motivation for use of nested case-control designs has been computational efficiency; in an early example of this, Liddell, Thomas, and colleagues illustrated how case-control sampling within a cohort study of underground miners offered a computationally efficient approach to estimation of parameters describing the underlying model for the disease hazard.[57-62]

In occupational health research, population-based case-control designs (and case-crossover designs) are well suited to settings where the underlying occupational cohort is not explicitly enumerated. For example, while a sizable cohort of industrial workers may be enumerated from records assembled for a single employer or facility, it may be difficult to enumerate a sizable cohort of migrant workers or a cohort of self-employed workers or a cohort of those employed in small numbers at any particular worksite, such as nonunionized residential construction workers. In such settings, a population-based case-control study design may be appealing. A similar issue arises when the disease of interest is exceedingly rare; it may be difficult, or impossible, to assemble an occupational cohort large enough to yield adequate cases of the disease among those employed at a single facility or industry. In a population-based or hospital-based case-control study, the investigator commences with a registry of cases (rather than an explicit roster of workers in a particular occupation or industry) and attempts to assemble an appropriate control series. The approach is particularly well suited to investigations in which the occupational exposure of interest tends to be relatively common in the population surveilled by the disease registry so that a case-control study is likely to identify a reasonable number of exposed cases. Useful examples of this approach include case-control studies of the association between agricultural exposures and multiple myeloma among farmers, of wood dust and nasal cancer among carpenters, and of benzene exposure and leukemia among gas station attendants.[63-68] In occupational injury research, useful examples include case-crossover investigations of factors influencing injuries due to slips and falls among restaurant workers and of factors influencing lacerations among slaughterhouse workers.[69-72]

Cross-sectional study designs, in which exposures and health outcomes are assessed at a single point in time among workers currently employed at a facility or worksite, can be conducted quickly; however, there are important limitations of such studies for understanding exposure-disease associations. For example, in occupational settings, injury, symptoms, disease, or disability can lead to termination of employment, and therefore a cross-sectional study of currently employed workers may be susceptible to a form of collider stratification bias caused by conditioning on active employment status. Sometimes, an investigator will complement an initial cross-sectional collection of data (*e.g.*, collection and analysis of exposure-disease prevalence associations in a baseline interview) with subsequent follow-up information collected from either a registry or follow-up interviews.[73,74]

Occupational Exposure Assessment

One advantage of studies of occupational exposures, as compared to environmental exposures, is that the intensity of exposure to an agent in an occupational setting is often presumed to be greater than the exposure intensities typically encountered in nonoccupational settings. This presumption serves as the basis for one approach to exposure assessment employed in occupational epidemiology (albeit the least informative approach): the fact of employment in an industry or occupation defines the exposed population and is taken as an indication of occupational exposure potential. Often comparisons are drawn between the occupational cohort and an external reference population. A simple extension of this approach, possible to implement when workers' dates of employment are known, is to draw comparisons between workers who are classified according to duration of employment. The fact of employment is taken as a proxy for exposure, which ceases with termination of work. Under such an approach, individuals' durations of employment may offer a reasonable approximation of their cumulative exposures if average intensities of exposures at work are similar between workers and over time.

There are a variety of approaches to improve an occupational exposure assessment beyond the fact of employment or duration of employment. For example, one relatively simple method for exposure assessment is for workers to perform a self-assessment of their exposures. Self-assessments may be conducted by questionnaires, face-to-face interviews with workers, or focus group discussions. Types of information derived from self-assessment of exposure may range from information regarding the presence or absence of exposure to an agent, to assessments of the frequency, intensity, duration of exposure, or timing of exposure (*e.g.*, calendar years in which exposures occurred). Often in self-assessments, researchers will provide prompts, such as historical floor plans or photos of a worksite, that can aid in recall during the assessments.[75-77]

An important advantage of occupational studies is that the distribution and relative intensities of workplace hazards often can be predicted based upon information about production processes. The types of information routinely collected by employers and industrial hygienists for management, production, compliance, and regulatory purposes often are valuable resources for occupational exposure assessment that are rarely available in nonoccupational settings. Occupational studies often can draw upon descriptions of processes and production levels and information on agents present in the workplace, as well as engineering and personal controls (*e.g.*, use of protective clothing and respiratory protection) and changes in these controls over time. In addition, in contemporary industrial settings, jobs or tasks often are broken into small, simple repetitive activities (*i.e.*, Taylorism) resulting in workers performing routine tasks in defined work areas. For exposure assessment, this arrangement implies that there is often the ability to distinguish between jobs, areas, and time periods with respect to potential exposure to agents or hazards of interest. Consequently, it is often more feasible to derive individual exposure estimates with some accuracy in occupational studies than in environmental studies. An expert assessment of exposure may follow from an expert's (*e.g.*, industrial hygienist's) evaluation of this type of information on processes, engineering designs, and other factors influencing exposure concentrations (such as dates during which a particular agent was used). Such methods are well suited to studies of industrial workers, and, historically, the focus of many occupational epidemiological studies on cohorts of industrial workers has led to a substantial attention to development of methods suited to this kind of exposure assessment, often in collaboration with professionals in disciplines such as industrial hygiene, ergonomics, and health physics. This type of expert assessment often is preferred to self-assessment of occupational exposures,[78] and collaborative work across the disciplines of epidemiology and industrial hygiene has led to insights about exposure assessment methods that strengthen occupational exposure assessments and their application in epidemiological exposure-disease analyses.[79]

A widely used form of expert assessment involves construction of a multiway table defined by jobs or tasks cross-classified by other factors, such as areas or departments, and calendar periods, called a Job Exposure Matrix.[80] Drawing upon historical records, as well as expert judgment, an assessment can be made of important characteristics of exposure to an agent (or agents) of interest, such as intensity of exposure and frequency of exposure; a unique assessment is made for each cell of the multiway table defined by the job, departments, and other factors that define the dimensions of the matrix. Often a Job Exposure Matrix will include indications of the confidence of the assessor about their evaluations. This structure provides one widely used approach to synthesis of information and professional judgment regarding scenarios of exposure.

The information from a Job Exposure Matrix may be linked to an individual worker's employment history information. This requires individual employment history records that indicate a worker's dates of employment, ideally for each job and department title. Typically, a first step needed is to standardize the information in these records to assemble a set of all job titles and departments or work area designations observed during the study period. Such data provide information about workers' dates of employment in specific jobs or tasks and areas or departments that define the dimensions of the matrix. When employment history data are linked with the matrix, the linkage provides a basis for deriving individual time-varying exposure estimates. Sometimes researchers are able to assign scores to the cells of a Job Exposure Matrix that are supported by measurement data (*e.g.*, air sampling data, historical industrial hygiene reports) or use of a model relating workplace concentrations to determinants of exposure concentrations (*e.g.*, production volumes, the use of exhaust ventilation systems, agent volatility, and work activity).[81] Measures of the concentration of an agent of concern in the workplace may be monitored for compliance or protection purposes, providing a basis for characterizing occupational exposures derived from area monitoring. Records from area monitoring may provide information about concentration of an agent and its variation over time. There are many examples of such quantitative Job Exposure Matrices developed and used in epidemiological studies, in conjunction with information on time spent in different jobs and departments, to derive quantitative time-varying exposure histories.[82,83] Of course, attention to uncertainty and sensitivity to model assumptions is warranted, although, historically, such assessments are rare in the occupational literature.[84] In addition, when using company records to reconstruct exposures, it is important to recognize that such records were compiled for administrative or management purposes rather than for scientific purposes, and practices that influence recording and collection of information for managerial purposes may differ from those practices that would motivate data collection for a scientific study.

In population-based case-control studies and population-based studies using registry-based data, investigators rarely have access to company employment history files; this poses a different type of challenge for occupational exposure assessments.[85,86] In the absence of detailed employment history information derived from company records or union files, population-based case-control studies often elicit self-reported work histories, while register-based studies frequently use information on occupation and industry derived from administrative records such as those assembled for a national census.[87] Although Job Exposure Matrices are used in population-based studies, a difficulty is that the investigator typically is not focused on a specific facility, industry, or trade, and, unlike a facility-based cohort study, exposure assessment proceeds without historical knowledge regarding facility-specific changes in processes, engineering controls, or production levels. Consequently, the exposure characterization in a population-based study typically is less detailed than the exposure characterization possible in a facility-based study where the Job Exposure Matrix was tailored to the specific facility under study. Instead, population-based case-control and register-based studies have typically used qualitative or quantitative job exposure matrices derived for workers in a nation or region.[87-90] Sometimes in population-based case-control studies, researchers collect detailed employment histories through personal interview and, after assembling employment information, undertake expert evaluation of likely exposures to specific agents on a case-by-case basis, allowing the exposure assessment to be tailored to the study region and the jobs identified in the study sample.[91,92]

Individual exposure monitoring, which involves direct measurements of the exposure at the point of contact while the exposure is taking place, overcomes many of the limitations of exposure assessment approaches, such as Job Exposure Matrices, which assign an average or "typical" exposure score to all workers in a job, department, or area. Individual exposure monitoring may provide a quantitative measure of exposure concentration and an indication of time of contact or cumulative exposure over a measurement period. Although in some occupational studies, the investigator may individually monitor workers included in a study; examples of this are quite limited as it requires contemporaneous access to workers and workplaces, and when available, such data are often limited because collection of such data is often expensive, and the time period of sampling is typically short. However, for some agents, individual exposure measurements are routinely collected in the workplace for compliance or protection purposes. For example, individual monitoring for exposure to ionizing radiation often is routinely conducted for medical and dental staff, radiographers, some underground miners, and workers in the nuclear industry.[93,94] In these settings, records may exist at the time an epidemiological study is being planned, providing a historical record of exposure based on individual monitoring. Of course, such records should be reviewed for completeness and quality because these records are typically assembled and maintained for compliance purposes rather than scientific research purposes, and monitoring policies and techniques may change over time. Problems related to missing data, bias, and uncertainties in individual exposure estimates may be addressed analytically or by additional data collection. Another way to derive individual estimates of exposure is by biomonitoring of workers. Individual biomonitoring shares some of the strengths and limitations of individual measurement of exposure in the ambient environment. Biomonitoring consists of measurements taken in biological samples such as blood, urine, exhaled breath, hair, adipose tissue, or nails. Measurement can be made in vivo, as is done for example with whole body counting for incorporated radionuclides[95] or made in assays of collected biological samples that are subsequently analyzed in a laboratory for the substance of interest itself, a metabolite, or some other associated molecular, biochemical, or cellular alteration that can be measured in biological media. Biomonitoring can offer occupational epidemiologists extremely useful information for assessing workers' exposures. A biomarker may integrate exposure from all routes of exposure (inhalation, dermal, ingestion), which is useful in settings where multiple routes of exposure are possible (*e.g.*, inhalation and skin absorption), and important exposure may be missed if a study focused solely on one route (*e.g.*, inhalation).[96] In contrast to exposure assessment approaches based on typical, or average, exposure conditions in a job or area, a biomarker may be useful when conditions of exposure are unpredictable or personal protective equipment is worn intermittently. An investigator can initiate a biomonitoring program specifically for the purposes of an epidemiological study's exposure assessment; however, this requires access to workers, can be expensive, and the time period over which the investigator can feasibly biomonitor exposure is typically short. Occasionally, historical records of biomonitoring results may be collected and archived. For example, certain occupational hazards, such as lead and tritium, are sometimes assessed for regulatory compliance through biomonitoring. Use of such records requires understanding of historical practices with regards to collection and analytical methods, recording practices, and the completeness of such records. Interpretation of biomonitoring results can be complicated by small numbers of monitored workers, small numbers of samples per worker, long half-lives of materials, and unmeasured factors (such as ambient temperature, diet, physical activity, comorbid conditions) that lead to substantial inter- and intraindividual variability in results.

Outcome Assessment in Occupational Studies

In some settings, the investigator can work with the employer to directly ascertain outcome information among currently employed workers. Longitudinal data on disease symptoms, or impairments in physiological function, are sometimes collected in occupational studies. When available, these can provide a basis for extremely useful panel designs. However, prospective collection of health outcome information at a worksite requires access to workers and their informed consent. Collection of such data can be expensive, participation rates may be low, and occupational health studies are often concerned with effects of historical exposures on disease risk in the past, for which no specific outcome monitoring was undertaken. Moreover, when collection of information is cross-sectional, it characterizes the prevalence of the condition at the time of contact with the investigator and may be affected by health-related selection out of employment.

One advantage of epidemiological studies conducted in occupational settings is that occupational epidemiologists may have access to types of information about the occurrence of disease that are rarely available in many other cohort studies. The ability to collect information from interactions with employers, and employer-based services, often provides occupational epidemiologists indications of health, vital status, and information from work-related medical screening and care. For example, employer records, compensation records, trade union or professional association files, and pension systems can offer occupational epidemiologists access to information on health-related outcomes. Annual screenings, fit testing for respirator use, chest examinations, blood lead measures, and other information from employer-based medical providers can provide an important source of outcome information in occupational studies. Even payroll information can be used to establish that workers remained employed, an indication of vital status. In some settings, investigators have found ways to work with these types of historical records for epidemiological research purposes with ethical board approval and without the need to obtain individual informed consent.

However, after retirement, there are often limitations to information derived because of employment. Some types of information used to inform outcome ascertainment is contingent upon employment, and the accumulation of this information stops when a person terminates employment. For conditions that tend to occur after retirement (*e.g.*, chronic disease) or diseases with symptoms that may preclude or reduce the likelihood of continued employment, employer-based information sources may be of limited value. Nonetheless, medical records from occupational health services and direct measurements of clinical conditions are used in occupational epidemiology and can provide valuable information.[97]

Data derived from claims filed for workers' compensation can provide information about the occurrence of disease or injury; however, like information derived from employer-based medical care, compensation claim information often is contingent upon employment status, and investigators have noted the poor sensitivity of workers' compensation records as a tool for ascertainment of occupational injury and disease.[98,99] More severe conditions may be more likely to lead to claims than less severe conditions, and acute injuries that occur on the job as a direct consequence of work may be more likely to lead to claims for worker compensation than chronic conditions that occur after a long induction and latency period. The availability of such outcome data is conditional on filing a claim, and obstacles to filing workers' compensation are recognized as potential limitations of such data (for example, workers with greater job security may be more likely to file claims than those with less job security). Consequently, analyses based on such data may be susceptible to bias.

Direct contact with workers, for example, via a professional association, trade union, or licensing requirement, offers another approach to collecting health outcome information. With ethical board approval and after receipt of informed consent, information may be solicited through questionnaires, interviews or self-assessments, and direct contact with former workers, which can provide information about conditions experienced after employment termination. For example, an investigator might attempt to ascertain self-reported information on results of a clinical assessments or diagnoses or self-reported information regarding perceived conditions ("have you experienced shortness of breath?"). In the Agricultural Health Study, for example, one mechanism for ascertaining information about respiratory diseases (such as asthma, chronic bronchitis, and emphysema) was self-report,[73] and, in the US Radiologic Technologists study, one mechanism for ascertaining cancers was self-reported diagnoses.[100] Of course, the accuracy and completeness of self-reported information may be poorer than record-based information.

Given limitations, cost, and obstacles to direct access to workers, much of the occupational epidemiological literature relies upon sources of registry-based information external to the employer. Most notable among these for occupational epidemiology is information derived from the death certificate that has been assembled in state and national registries of deaths and can often be accessed with ethical board approval but without the need to obtain individual informed consent. Information derived from the death certificate is not contingent upon employment status (*i.e.*, it continues to be recorded regardless of whether a person terminates employment), and unlike workers' compensation, the worker does not have to take any action to file a claim. In fact, death certificates have been adapted over time to facilitate research on occupational diseases. Recording of information on the death certificate to associate decedents with their primary occupation and industry has allowed surveillance of occupational causes of death and comparative mortality studies.

For example, the US death certificate includes information on the decedent's usual industry and occupation (*i.e.*, the job and industry that the person held for longest during their lifetime), as well as an indicator of whether the death occurred at work.

However, the occurrence of injuries, diseases, and conditions that are rarely fatal are difficult to study using death certificate–based information because the death certificate provides such limited information. Some investigators have made use of multiple cause coding of the death certificate to improve the sensitivity of death certificate–based ascertainment of diseases that are less often fatal, although it is recognized that the death certificate may have poor sensitivity and specificity for ascertainment of many conditions, and factors such as medical care, place of death, region, and historical period can influence what gets recorded on it.[101,102] Complementary sources of registry-based information are increasingly used in occupational epidemiology, such as information derived from healthcare registries (particularly when a national patient registry is available), disease-specific registries (such as cancer registries), or, in studies of reproductive outcomes, registries of birth defects. For example, in countries with nationwide registration of hospital visits, such as Denmark, a patient register has been used to ascertain information on emergency department visits for nonfatal injuries among workers.[103] However, such registries tend to span shorter and more recent periods of time than registries of deaths.

Statistical Methods in Occupational Studies

Occupational epidemiologists draw upon a wide range of analytical approaches; however, certain methods of analysis have played an important role in the analysis of occupational studies and are well suited to the strengths and limitations of occupational epidemiology. Occupational cohort mortality studies often involve many workers followed over long periods, leading to large amounts of person-time under analysis. Tabulation of person-time and events in a multiway tabulation allows for a substantial reduction of information into a simple analytical data structure that facilitates summarization and statistical analysis. Consequently, methods based upon grouped data, in the form of tabulations of person-time and events, have had an important place in occupational epidemiology.[59,104-106]

Given occupational cohort data tabulated as person-time and events, one classical approach to analysis is calculation of the standardized mortality ratio (SMR),[29,107] in which comparisons are drawn between the observed mortality in an occupational cohort and that in a reference population. The approach is often used when there is limited information about individual workers' exposures, so internal comparisons of cumulative exposure or duration of exposure are difficult or impossible. SMRs are frequently calculated for an occupational group as a form of screening tool, comparing cause-specific mortality ratios for a list of categories of cause of death to investigate whether any outcome appears in excess.[106] The SMR has been described as an estimator of cumulative incidences, specifically the observed and expected numbers of deaths at the end of study follow-up, although this requires the condition that the occupational exposures have not meaningfully affected the person-time distribution in the exposed population, a condition guaranteed only at the null.[108] Nonetheless, under certain conditions, the SMR does have a useful interpretation as an estimate of the ratio of adjusted rates and remains widely used for that purpose.[109]

The proportionate mortality ratio (PMR) has been used in a variety of occupational cohort studies as well. Like the SMR, the PMR may be used when there is limited information about individual workers' exposures; the fact of employment at a study facility may be taken as indication of exposure potential. One setting well suited to analysis using the PMR is when information exists on cause-specific mortality (or incidence) for a roster of workers, but it is not possible to enumerate person-time at risk. This may occur, for example, if death certificates are available for deceased employees of a company or members of a union, but information needed to calculate person-time at risk is not.[110,111] For a PMR analysis, the observed cause-specific proportions of death are compared to expected values derived based on reference proportions of death, and the comparison is framed as relative proportions of causes of death among the worker cohort compared with corresponding proportions in the reference population. Under certain assumptions, it may be viewed as an estimator of rate ratios obtained assuming the data-generating model underlying the rates conforms to a Poisson model. A limitation is that an excess of deaths from one set of causes necessarily results in a deficit of deaths from a second set of causes, at least once all members of the cohort have died. To overcome this shortcoming, one may reconfigure the PMR study as a case-control study, as noted in Chapter 6.

Classical tabular methods for analyses of person-time and events have proven sufficient for identification of many occupational hazards.[55] However, given a multiway tabulation of person-time and events, multivariable regression modeling also is possible and offers a useful approach for summarizing and smoothing information in a multiway table and quantifying exposure-response associations. Regression models can be developed using internal or external reference populations. Poisson regression methods are widely used in occupational epidemiology for analysis of rates in a multiway table of person-time and events; the approach involves specifying a model for the mean of the observed number of events as a function of covariates. If the expected number of events (*i.e.*, the product of the person-time at risk and associated reference rate) serves as an offset, the estimated coefficients from the Poisson regression model fitting can be interpreted as estimates of the log SMR and its dependence upon explanatory variables.[112] Alternatively, and more commonly in contemporary occupational cohort studies, if the person-time at risk serves as an offset, a Poisson regression model for the observed number of events can be developed allowing a summary rate ratio to be estimated, as well as allowing comparisons of rate ratios between groups defined by strata of the multiway table yielding estimates of change in log rate ratio with change in explanatory variables.[105,112]

Summarization of cohort study data into a grouped data structure comes with limitations to analysis. An important consideration arises in analyses in which the goal is to evaluate the association between disease rates and a study factor that was originally measured on a continuous scale. Tabulation of person-time and events requires forming groups from underlying variables that were originally measured on a continuous scale. Furthermore, if an investigator subsequently wishes to model an explanatory variable as a continuous variable, this requires assigning scores to categories. When analyzing information in a grouped data structure, to derive an estimate of an exposure-response trend, an investigator needs to make decisions about how to form exposure categories (*i.e.*, choice of the number of categories formed and the cut points between categories), as well as how to assign scores to exposure categories, and the approach to assignment of scores may be influential on results. For example, category midpoints are sometimes used as the score assigned to a continuous explanatory variable that was grouped for the purposes of tabulation of person-time and events, although the highest exposure category is often open-ended and the midpoint (*e.g.*, the range between the lower boundary and highest observed dose) may not reflect the distribution of individual exposure levels observed for most of the person-time accrued in that category.[55] Assigning scores based on the mean or median value for a category often is a better approach to assign scores that reflect the distribution of exposures accrued by individuals at risk.[113] These limitations need not be overstated, however, because often analyses of grouped data yield quantitatively similar results to those obtained using methods of analysis for ungrouped data. The occupational literature includes numerous examples of relatively detailed exposure-response modeling of associations between metrics of occupational exposure and disease rates conducted using multiway tables of person-time and events.[50,114,115]

One approach to avoiding categorizing explanatory variables that were originally measured on a continuous scale involves creating a data structure with one record for each person-period of observation (*e.g.*, a record for each person-year at risk).[116] Unlike a multiway table, such a data structure does not require the analyst to summarize and categorize information on other continuous explanatory variables into groups because the person-periods and events are not cross-classified into a table whose dimensions are defined by categories of covariates. This approach can lead to data structures with extremely large numbers of records because the number of records is the product of the cohort size, average length of follow-up, and the resolution of the person-period enumeration (*i.e.*, the size of the structure increases as the length of the person-periods enumerated decreases, for example, from person-years to person-days) to reduce coarsening of the originally recorded time-varying information. Using such a data structure, fitting a discrete time model—whether based on Poisson, logistic, or other regression model forms—allows analyses of rates as a function of a history of exposure information.

The detailed, continuous, longitudinal data collected in some large occupational cohort studies can be used in analyses that are based on individual, rather than grouped, data methods,[117] such as proportional hazards regression.[118] The proportional hazards model allows analyses of rates as a function of a history of exposure information without discretizing time or any of the other measured covariates. The data structure may include one record per worker or may be structured based on risk sets enumerated at failure times for a given outcome. Alternatively, data derived from density sampled nested case-control designs can be analyzed using the same likelihood as the full cohort Cox proportional hazards regression.[119] The recognition that the parameters of a Cox regression model could be efficiently estimated with just a sample of the members of each risk set led to a quite rapid increase in the use of continuous time methods for analysis of occupational cohort data, facilitated by the computational reduction afforded by sampling risk set information.[57,120] The design, referred to as density-sampled nested case-control studies, employs a sample-based approach to fitting the proportional hazards model; for analyses modeling exposure-time-response associations, this approach has often been used.

Exposure-Response Analyses in Occupational Studies

A relatively unique feature of occupational studies is the ability, in many study settings, to reconstruct workers' exposures in terms of the intensity of exposure to the agent and the duration of exposure to it. The availability of quantitative, time-varying individual occupational exposure history data has allowed occupational epidemiologists to address questions about exposure-response functions for a number of important occupational agents. Notable examples arise in studies of arsenic-exposed smelter workers,[121] radon-exposed uranium miner cohorts,[59,122,123] gamma radiation–exposed nuclear worker cohorts,[124,125] benzene-exposed rubber workers,[126] and asbestos-exposed textile workers.[127] Exposure-response analyses can potentially strengthen an assessment of the credibility of overall study findings and utility of results for more general risk assessment purposes.

Investigators typically summarize detailed exposure histories by deriving a summary metric of exposure that can be used in an analysis of the exposure's effects. In selecting a summary exposure metric, attention may be given to considerations regarding retention and bioaccumulation of the agent.[128] The characteristics of the exposure history that are most relevant to an epidemiological investigation depend upon the presumed etiological mechanism involved in the exposure-disease association of interest. Acute peak exposure to an agent may be more relevant for an investigation of a prompt irritant response, for example, than a long-term average exposure intensity.[129] The hypothesized mechanism should be considered when choosing how to model exposure-response information. Depending on the nature of the study and the health outcomes of interest, evaluation of peak, average intensity, cumulative, or lagged exposures may be desirable. Clearly, the utility of a summary exposure measure is determined by the respective weight it attributes to either duration or concentration of exposure or both. Ideally, the summary measure selected should be based on a set of defensible assumptions regarding the postulated biological mechanism for the agent or disease association under study.[128]

A common approach to summarizing information about a protracted exposure history is to calculate a cumulative metric of exposure that is the product of intensity and duration of exposure and may be integrated over time for a history of exposures. Implicit in the use of a cumulative exposure metric is the assumption that the effects of exposures are additive, and the assumption that the impact of a unit of exposure on disease risk is the same regardless of when it occurred. These assumptions, however, can be loosened through various modeling approaches. Consider the assumption that the effects of exposures are additive, such that a history of exposures of varying intensities can be summed without meaningful loss of information.[123] This would not hold, for example, if a protracted, low-intensity exposure leads to a different risk than a short, high-intensity exposure for the same cumulative exposure. A notable form of variation in the effect of exposure arises if exposure tends to have little or no effect at exposure rates below some threshold but does have an effect when the exposure rate exceeds that threshold. There is interest in evaluation of such threshold functions for analyses of the health effects of exposure to many hazards because they might be posited to occur if a detoxification pathway, or a biologic repair mechanism, is overwhelmed when the accumulated exposure exceeds a certain level. Such a threshold model for intensity can be evaluated empirically as long as the detailed exposure history information is retained (and not summarized).[130]

The assumption that the impact of a unit of exposure on disease risk is the same regardless of when it occurred is also a strong assumption; it is an assumption that often is empirically evaluated in occupational cohort studies. For example, under the premise that there is typically an induction period (the period between exposure and irreversible onset of disease) and latency period (the period between the induction of disease and its detection) between exposure and its observed impact on disease,[131] a summary exposure metric is often "lagged" by excluding exposures that occurred in the months or years immediately preceding the outcome. Often an epidemiologist will evaluate several exposure lag assumptions and select the lag that maximizes the magnitude of the resultant effect estimate or the model goodness-of-fit;[132] alternatively, one can directly estimate the best lag jointly with the other parameters describing the exposure-response association.[133]

The standard approach to the practice of lagging exposure treats the interval as a constant, although in theory one could allow the length of the interval to depend on unmeasured individual characteristics, such that the interval can be viewed as a random variable. Of course, a lag between exposure and effect, reflecting an induction and latency interval, is only one consideration about temporal variation in the effect of an occupational exposure that can be explored. A related assumption embedded in a cumulative metric of exposure is that the effect of exposures accrue over time, and the effect per unit exposure is equivalent regardless of when it occurred; however, this assumption may be relaxed to permit an investigator to evaluate whether the effect of exposure on disease risk persists, increases over time, or eventually diminishes. Time-since-exposure is not the only time scale over which the magnitude of an occupational exposure-disease association may vary. People may be employed over a wide range of ages; therefore, it is reasonable to consider that the effect of exposure may also depend upon the ages at which exposures occur.[134] Variation with age in susceptibility to an occupational hazard's effect often is plausible and could reflect processes of maturation and senescence over a working life.

One common analytical approach to address such questions is to use exposure time-window analyses to describe variation in the magnitude of a protracted occupational exposure-disease association as a function of time-since-exposure or age-at-exposure. An exposure history is partitioned into intervals; the data analyst then examines separate estimates of the association between disease risk and exposures received in a series of time intervals prior to the current age. Of course, reliable estimation of exposure effects may be difficult when exposure is partitioned into multiple time-windows, and evidence of a temporal pattern may be sensitive to decisions about the number of time-windows and the boundary points between them. The approaches for lagging and exposure time-window analysis are two simple examples of a more general approach to framing the empirical description of variation over time in the etiological relevance of prior exposures as a time-varying weight function. A weighted cumulative exposure can be derived by summing the product of a time-varying intensity of exposure and a time-varying exposure weighting function. For example, suppose that this weighting function describes the variation in the exposure's effect with time-since-exposure, conforming to a 5-year exposure lag assumption. To classify a unit of person-time or death according to cumulative exposure under a 5-year lag, this implies a function that applied a weight of 0 in the 5 years immediately prior. However, there is a much richer variety of time-varying weight functions including smooth functions, such as a lognormal function that describes a rise and subsequent fall in the effect of exposure with time-since-exposure. Estimation of the parameters describing the time-varying weight function allows investigation regarding time-varying exposure effects. Examples of this approach have been developed in analyses of associations between occupational exposure to radon and subsequent lung cancer mortality.[135] Similarly, such empirical weight functions may allow for age-related changes in potency-of-exposure. In studies of occupational cancers, there is a long history of attention to potential importance of age-at-exposure and time-since-exposure, and this interest has been reinforced by multistage theories of carcinogenesis that predict that the impact of an increment of exposure to a carcinogen may depend upon the timing of exposure.[136,137] Armitage and Doll, for example, proposed a multistage model that can be viewed as a special case of time-dependent exposure weighting.[138] Such models draw attention to temporal factors, such as age-at-exposure, that may be overlooked in more standard cumulative exposure-response analyses of cohort data.[139]

While summarizing a potentially long and complex exposure history into a cumulative exposure metric is a common, and useful, analytical strategy, it implies assumptions about the etiological importance of timing, duration, and intensity of exposure. Ideally, a summary measure should be based on a set of defensible assumptions regarding the postulated biological mechanism for the agent or disease association under study.[128] Hypotheses about mechanisms can strengthen statistical modeling and inference; to evaluate such hypotheses, it is useful to have a general mathematical framework that encompasses a range of possible mechanistic models for such associations and allows for comparison of alternatives in a formal framework. As the above discussion suggests, occupational epidemiologists have been able to draw upon flexible empirical models for exposure-time-response functions as well as some biomathematical stochastic models of disease under which age-at-exposure and time-since-exposure are modeled (*e.g.*, defined by stage of action of the agent and number of stages in the disease process). The findings of such analyses can have practical implications for worker protection. Considerations about changes in susceptibility to an occupational hazard's effects with age, and persistence of effects over time, have relevance for worker protection, risk assessment, and compensation.

METHODOLOGIC CHALLENGES PERTINENT TO OCCUPATIONAL EPIDEMIOLOGY

Workers and management are seldom blinded to exposure. More often, they are aware of exposures. Workers and management may have incentives to increase hours worked and consequently occupational exposure, and there are often factors leading employees to persist working despite reaching safety limits (or despite perceiving harmful effects). One reason is that compliance with exposure-related regulations or rules may affect worker's income. However, there also are nonfinancial factors that may affect accrual of exposure at work, despite recognizing their potential danger. James et al. (1987), for example, proposed the term "John Henryism" to describe a potentially maladaptive active coping strategy in response to environmental stressors; workers may recognize potentially hazardous conditions and attempt to cope with them by working even harder work, expending high levels of effort, and resulting in increased risk of disease.[140]

Another challenging aspect of studying occupational exposures is that the person diagnosing disease, or certifying cause of death, is not necessarily blinded to a worker's exposure status. To the contrary, clinicians are often trained to inquire about a patient's vocation in the process of forming a diagnosis. Recording biases could affect death certificate–based information if the death certificate is completed by someone who knows the decedent's occupational history or place of death and is concerned about an employer's liability, burden of compensation, or reputation. Classically, the "company town" refers to a setting in which a single employer or industry was responsible for much of the economic activity in the community. In a company town, the industry may employ or contract with local medical providers. If quality of diagnosis of disease (or assignment of cause of death) in a company town differs from that in other towns, this could bias epidemiological analyses because place of diagnosis (or death) may be related to fact of employment and length of employment in the industry. Such concerns are not just theoretical; there are examples in which employer-affiliated medical providers influenced diagnosis of occupational disease and certification of causes of death. In coal mining communities, for example, sick miners often found themselves pitted against doctors who aggressively defended the mining industry and downplayed any harmful effects of mines or coal dust.[22] Employer influence on diagnosis of occupational disease is not limited to small company towns; for example, at the urging of the radium industry in Orange, New Jersey, diagnoses and deaths due to necrosis of the jaw among female radium dial painters were hidden and attributed to other causes, such as syphilis, in attempts to smear the reputations of workers who were litigants seeking compensation.[15]

A potential difficulty in interpreting epidemiological results is that workers at a facility often differ from the general population because being hired into a job tends to favor people fit enough to work. A person's health status and behavior may influence their decision to seek employment, particularly in a job that is physically demanding, and an employer may consider a job applicant's health status, for example, by means of a preemployment physical examination, before hiring someone to do a job. A difference in health status at baseline (*i.e.*, date of hire) between an occupational cohort and reference population, reflected by a relative advantage in terms of mortality or disease occurrence in the working populations when compared with a reference population, is sometimes referred to as a healthy worker hire effect.[141] Often, in occupational cohort studies, the working population differs from the general population in baseline characteristics associated with fitness and lower mortality risk, as might happen if preemployment medical screening or health-related behaviors led to selection into employment of people in good health (compared to the general population). Analyses of standardized mortality ratios have played an important role in occupational cohort mortality studies, and a common concern in such analyses is that interpretation of the SMR may be biased due to the healthy worker hire effect (*i.e.*, the reference population does not satisfy the assumption that the disease rates experienced by the reference population represent the expected rate of the outcome in the study population in the absence of exposure).[142]

An advantage in terms of health of an occupational cohort compared to the general population is not guaranteed of course. Some industries may be more selective than others, and some periods may have tighter labor markets (and hence less ability to be selective in hiring) than others.[52] Social class, race, and age can affect the presence and direction of this form of bias.[143,144] However, there is a general impression that occupational populations tend to be healthier than the population as a whole, because they comprise individuals healthy enough to be employed, and whose mortality risk is therefore, at least initially, lower than the general population. While often referred to as a healthy worker bias, the more general term confounding may be used as well.

Some authors have noted that no advantage in mortality is necessarily observed among employees in dirty trades that are poorly compensated.[52] Certain jobs deemed highly unpleasant or socially stigmatized may have little or no health-related selection into employment and no baseline advantage in terms of mortality of those hired compared to the general population.[145] Within a cohort, some subgroups may exhibit evidence of relatively better health than the general population while other subgroups do not. Assignment to dirty or unpleasant jobs or tasks may be based on social hierarchies, power relations, racial discrimination, and economic incentives. Black workers are employed in hazardous occupations more frequently than white workers, and black men experienced higher occupational fatal injury rates than white men employed in the same jobs.[146] Examples abound of black workers, recent immigrant workers, and women, moving into jobs that they did not previously hold, getting assigned jobs with greater exposure potential, and even dirtier tasks despite holding similar job titles. Evidence of relatively better health among recent hires than the general population may also depend upon labor markets, as employers may be less selective in recruitment when labor markets are tighter; a notable example relates to military conscription of healthy males during World War II, which has been posited to have led to increased hiring of men judged unfit for military service into employment in industries, so that any bias associated with baseline differences in health status for the cohort of men hired during this period may have differed from the bias expected in other hire cohorts.[147-149]

Different approaches to reduce or eliminate these problems of confounding bias have been discussed.[106,150] It has been suggested that initial selection or preemployment screening may be effective for conditions with easily detected clinical precursors or symptoms, such as deficits in pulmonary function or hypertension, but less so for diseases such as cancer. Therefore, different causes of death are likely to exhibit different magnitudes of such bias.[143] Some investigators have calculated a relative SMR, the ratio of the cause-specific SMR to the SMR for all causes except the cause of interest, as an approach to reduce bias.[151,152] Others have suggested that selection of a reference cause of death, indicative of the bias due to noncomparability between the study cohort and reference population and unaffected by the occupational hazard of primary concern, might be used as an indirect adjustment for such bias; this would be obtained by subtracting the log of the cause-specific SMR from the log of the reference SMR and taking the antilog of the resultant difference. This leads to a quantity, sometimes termed the mortality odds ratio (MOR), that can be viewed in a general framework of use of a negative control outcome.[153]

It also has been suggested that any effects of initial selection related to baseline health status would diminish over time, so that analyses focused on comparisons of a cohort to general population several years after initial hire should be less impacted.[154,155] In fact, often the person-time and events in the period immediately after hire are discounted from occupational cohort analysis, which has the potential to reduce any effects of initial selection related to baseline health status compared to the general population. The motivation for discounting observations in the period immediately after hire, however, may relate to defining a minimum length of employment criterion for the study cohort (*i.e.*, exclusion of short-term workers, thereby defining the study cohort as people who had at least some defined minimum period of employment). Specifying a cohort definition based on a minimal duration of employment necessarily implies that the start of follow-up begins only after that condition is met (*e.g.*, in a cohort defined as people who were employed at least 365 days, follow-up would not start until the 366th day of employment). There are often practical reasons for excluding short-term workers; very short-term workers often have lower quality (and less complete) information and higher loss-to-follow-up.

The most common remedy to the problem of bias due to initial baseline differences in health status between workers and the general population is to conduct internal comparisons, which can be done if there is information available to identify subgroups of the occupational cohort defined by differences in occupational exposure.[141] Occupational epidemiologists can compare rates between groups within the study cohort with one group (*e.g.*, the lowest exposed group) serving as an internal reference population. This is a strong argument in favor of comparisons between workers within a cohort as opposed to drawing comparisons to an external reference population. Of course, factors that lead to initial baseline differences between a working population and the general population may also operate within a cohort, albeit perhaps at a lesser degree. Initial hire into or assignment to dirtier or more unpleasant tasks in an industry or facility may be related to socioeconomic factors that are independent risk factors for disease. One way to adjust for such concerns in internal analyses of occupational cohort data is to adjust, when possible, for baseline socioeconomic and employment factors that are independent risk factors for the outcomes of interest.[106]

There may be ongoing processes related to selection or retention of workers based on physical fitness or tolerance for challenging work conditions (*e.g.*, noxious fumes). Tatham, in 1902, noted that "miners are a picked class of men ... their labor is so arduous that those only who possess exceptional endurance are able to continue at it."[156] Remaining employed in a job tends to favor people fit enough to work, with self-selection out of employment, as well as employer selection out of the workplace (or reassignment to a different task or job) based on physical fitness or tolerance for the working conditions. In cross-sectional occupational studies, in which health outcomes and exposures are measured at a single point in time, health-related selection out of employment can lead to a form of collider stratification bias (a form of selection bias sometimes termed survivor bias) if the investigator focuses only on currently employed workers (since the association between an exposure and disease is examined conditional on being employed). Similarly, in cohort studies that commence with a group of long-term workers employed at a factory (*i.e.*, prevalent workers as opposed to new hires), health-related selection out of employment can lead to bias; such bias also can operate in studies in which the cohort is a mixture of incident and prevalent hires. While typically investigators would like to start with an inception cohort, defined as newly hired workers who enter follow-up at the start of employment, it is not unusual to find that cohort studies involve a mixture of long-term employees, currently working at an administrative date defining the study's start of follow-up, and new hires who commence employment on, or after, that administrative date.[157] Failure to recognize such bias can lead to spectacularly incorrect conclusions; Harrington, for example, suggested that selection out of the coal mining industry of disabled or injured miners explained the "half-baked statements and misinterpreted statistics, largely of English origin, that ... coal mining is one of the most healthful of occupations."[158]

Even in occupations less hazardous than mining, workers in poor health, or with low tolerance for strenuous or irritating working conditions, may shift to less physically demanding jobs or less exposed work locations. Like health-related termination of employment, health-related changes in job assignment (possibly affected by prior exposure) is a mechanism through which bias in estimates of exposure-response associations may occur. Such disease-associated task shifting has been reported, for example, among nurses. Those with respiratory conditions are more likely to transition from jobs with high disinfectant exposure to jobs with lower exposure.[159]

In cohort studies in which questions arise regarding the effect of a protracted or repeated exposure, bias may arise because unhealthy, or poorly adaptive, people tend to leave work earlier than healthier or more adaptive people and thus cease the accrual of exposure. The fact that exposures that occur at work may be contingent upon continued employment and fitness, and that maintaining good health may be necessary for continued employment, leads to potential for bias. The term "healthy worker survivor effect" has been used to describe bias that may occur in standard analyses of occupational cohort studies if prior exposure affects employment status, and employment status affects both subsequent exposure and disease risk.[141]

To address questions regarding protracted effects of occupational exposures on disease, particularly chronic disease, occupational epidemiologists developed a number of methods for addressing bias due to a "healthy worker survivor effect."[141,147]. The healthy worker survivor effect has been framed as a problem of confounding by ongoing employment status,[147,160] noting that those who are actively employed tend to have lower mortality than is observed post termination of employment. This led some investigators to employ standard regression methods to control for potential bias due to the healthy worker survivor effect through adjustment for employment status (or duration of employment). However, if employment status is both a time-varying confounder and a causal intermediate, then such an approach will not yield an unbiased estimate of the exposure's effect.[161] Rather, it will be distorted because the fitted model adjusts for part of the effect of exposure. It is possible to assess whether the conditions under which standard methods will yield an unbiased estimate of the exposure's effect hold; these conditions can be assessed using standard regression modeling methods.[162]

Interest in the healthy worker survivor effect motivated seminal developments in methods for occupational analyses of protracted exposure effects on chronic disease that were subsequently adopted by, and applied in, other substantive areas of epidemiological research.[163,164] Robins proposed a set of methods, known as the g-methods, to control bias in this setting. The parametric g-formula can be employed in occupational settings to estimate exposure effects on disease that are not confounded by employment status; this involves fitting parametric models for time-varying explanatory variables (including employment status) and outcome and deriving results expected under different exposure conditions.[165]

ETHICAL AND SOCIAL ISSUES PERTINENT TO OCCUPATIONAL EPIDEMIOLOGY

The types of workplaces most often studied by occupational epidemiologists have been industrial settings, often unionized, for which large rosters could readily be assembled. Such settings have been conducive to study, often having maintained payroll and production records and having well-established work locations and processes. However, the field of occupational epidemiology is not limited to concern with the health of industrial workers; it also encompasses the study of self-employed workers, migrant and transient workers, and employees in small businesses that are not easily studied using the approaches often well-suited for studying industrial cohorts. In addition, the concerns of some occupational epidemiologists also encompass people working in the informal economy (*e.g.*, people working without contract or formal legal rights), people working in settings where remuneration may not occur (*e.g.*, on a family farm), and people working for pay in activities that are not legally sanctioned (*e.g.*, sex workers). It is often challenging to study such workers; however, it is also often challenging to conduct studies of people employed by large corporations, simply because employers pose barriers to investigators who wish to access the worksite, making it difficult to characterize the workplace and workers.[166] Standard occupational epidemiological methods require creative extensions and, in some cases, tradeoffs in terms of study designs and logistics to address study questions pertinent to the health and safety of non-industrial workers.[166]

Occupational epidemiological studies have often focused exclusively on male workers.[167] In part, this may reflect a historical focus on manufacturing and extractive industries in occupational epidemiology where, historically, fewer women than men were employed (although there are important exceptions to this[168,169]). However, even when women were employed in these industries, often women were excluded a priori from occupational cohort studies.[54,125,127] Similarly, historically, fewer nonwhite workers have been included in occupational cohort studies than white workers; in fact, historically, nonwhite workers often were excluded a priori in occupational cohort studies. The limited occupational research on women and nonwhite workers should not be taken as indication of their limited potential for occupational exposure (or occupational disease); rather, it reflects historical practice in the research area and, to some extent, decisions regarding whose problems were studied and whose were ignored. In fact, there are some dramatic examples of major industrial disasters involving black workers that were never systematically studied by epidemiologists; one example is the Hawks Nest Tunnel disaster that led to hundreds of deaths due to acute silicosis among mostly black, migrant underground miners during construction of a tunnel through Gauley Mountain in West Virginia.[170]

Many occupational epidemiological studies have been carried out in industrialized nations where regulation and control of recognized occupational hazards have tended to reduce exposures over time. In some cases, such regulations have resulted in transfer of hazardous industries and processes to the industrializing world.[171] Such global shifts in industry, and industrial hazards, have increasingly drawn attention of occupational epidemiologists to international studies of occupational hazards and to global assessments of the burden of occupational disease.

Use of data regarding workers who were exposed to, and potentially harmed by, an agent, suggests that the interests of those workers should be considered in research undertaken using their information. Ethical considerations about occupational research therefore relate to who frames the research questions, for example, the employer, the employee, the researcher, a labor union, or an industry-affiliated association. Often questions in occupational epidemiology concern the health effects of specific workplace agents or hazards. An industry- or employer-affiliated researcher may be interested in health effects of occupational exposure of an agent, particularly if the agent of interest is a commercial product intentionally manufactured and sold by the industry. Litigation or regulation also may spur studies to evaluate, reanalyze, or conduct novel studies of a specific industrial agent or product. However, workers may be interested in a broader range of hazards encountered on-the-job, including production intermediates, cleaning agents, asbestos in a facility's infrastructure, fumes and dusts, physical hazards, and complex waste streams. The former type of investigation, which focuses on a single agent, is often paradigmatic for training and thinking about methodological issues. However, the latter questions concern the complexity of working conditions in a particular facility or industry; focus groups or informal discussion with workers also frequently point to research questions that encompass organizational and managerial factors such as use of shift work, decisions regarding line speed, and factors that affect employee's autonomy and control on-the-job; these are also clearly germane to occupational epidemiology, and there are notable examples of studies of these factors' impacts on worker health.[172,173] In fact, when studies are undertaken with community and labor partners from the outset, helping to frame research questions in occupational epidemiology, such research can contribute to worker empowerment and organizing,[174] so that the conduct of research itself can contribute to well-being of the workers or community under study. Such examples underscore the connection between labor and social justice movements and epidemiological research on relationships between working conditions and disease or injury.

ANTICIPATED DIRECTIONS FOR OCCUPATIONAL EPIDEMIOLOGY

Occupational epidemiology is evolving to reflect economic and technological changes. In many countries, people are retiring at older ages, leading to changes in the demographics of working populations and increasing interest in the health of aging workers and better understanding of the occupational hazards that they face. There is growing attention to characterizing occupational hazards encountered by older workers (*e.g.*, workers who start a second career late in life), as well as attention to age-related changes in susceptibility to the effects of occupational exposures (*i.e.*, differences in the effects of exposures accrued at older adult ages compared to those exposures accrued at younger ages). A notable trend in the occupational literature is a growing focus not on classical chemical and physical hazards encountered in workplace (*i.e.*, industrial hygiene and safety), but rather on organization and managerial factors in the workplace. Occupational epidemiologists are investigating changes in the types of work being done, and the way that it is organized. Changes in employment conditions mean that few workers have a career connected to a single employer; rather many workers have employment that is characterized by greater precariousness of employment, and nontraditional work patterns (*e.g.*, flexible contracts, part-time work, and short-term gigs). Such changes pose challenges for occupational epidemiologists and also point to the growing importance for occupational epidemiology for attention to study of the impacts of different work conditions. The questions posed by such changes relate to health effects of different work organizations; however, they also relate to changing employment patterns in postindustrial economies, transformations in management and organization of work, and growing number of workers employed in service sector jobs. Growing employment in the service sector has led to increasing attention to research questions about shift work, ergonomics, sedentary work settings, circadian rhythm disruption, and job demand, and to nonfatal conditions, such as disability and nonfatal violence. Such research questions require epidemiologists to give greater attention to recurrent conditions and novel approaches to outcome assessments.

Innovations in the types of information and analytical methods available to occupational epidemiologists are also leading to new types of statistical analyses. The methods used in occupational epidemiology increasingly involve use of panel designs, and analytical methods for repeated measures, reflecting the increasing attention to questions related to nonfatal events and physiologic changes. Changes in computational power are having a large impact on occupational epidemiology. For example, many of the commonly used methods for analysis of occupational cohort data commenced with approaches based on data reduction. These approaches are increasingly set aside because of the feasibility of analyses without such reduction, foregoing the need to coarsen and categorize information. There are increasing examples of occupational cohort analyses using g-methods that are computationally intensive but offer an approach for addressing longstanding concerns regarding healthy worker survivor effects in occupational cohort studies. The types of data used in occupational epidemiology are increasingly drawing on computerized data resources from administrative records, such as residential history information that can facilitate cancer incidence studies,[175] and employer-affiliated insurance and medical information.[176,177] As opposed to assembling data *de novo*, administrative data are increasingly used; clearly, there are limitations to studies that rely solely upon routinely collected administrative data. Use of administrative data tends to imply reliance on less detailed information (*e.g.*, about exposures or employment histories) than one might obtain from direct interaction with workers, individual exposure monitoring, or reconstruction based upon company records. Yet it is likely that occupational epidemiologists will increasingly use methods for mining and pooling of data relevant to occupational health and disease by leveraging methods data from large data consolidators and administrative sources. An important role for occupational surveillance will remain because hazard control and protection will continue to require surveillance efforts. Surveillance based on routinely collected administrative data has been an important aspect of occupational health and safety for over two centuries. It contributes to identification of newly emerging hazards, recognition of reemergence of old hazards, and evaluation of health and safety efforts. There are also directions for future occupational epidemiology that suggest new opportunities. Methods and resources for surveillance and direct interaction with workers are likely to change and adapt; examples include methods that draw upon new forms of self-report and new tools for individual monitoring of occupational exposures, and outcomes. Assessments may be increasingly informed through interconnected devices for everything from environmental and physiological monitoring to self-reporting of conditions.[178]

The connection of occupational epidemiology to environmental health is likely to strengthen. Methodological questions are shared, such as an interest in complex mixtures of exposures over long durations and with different intensities. Historically, occupational studies have tended to focus on quantitative measures of one, or a very small number, of agents, but increasingly investigations address multiple agents present in the workplace. These agents may be correlated in the work environment posing similar analytical problems to those encountered in environmental studies. Over time, the legal, policy, and social relevance of occupational epidemiology has increasingly become intertwined with broader environmental concerns as well because the exposures or conditions encountered at work also may be encountered outside the workplace. For example, epidemiological investigations of many high-profile public health crises, from the Chernobyl accident, to the World Trade Center bombings, to the release of perfluorooctanoic acid from a plant in Parkersburg, West Virginia, to the Deep Water Horizon oil spill, include occupational and environmental investigations undertaken at the same time. There are examples, as well, of how exposures generated at work can be brought into the home, leading to childhood exposure to occupational hazards.[179,180] In the context of hazard evaluations and risk assessments, occupational epidemiology has come to play an important role in directly informing occupational safety and more generally informing evaluations regarding recognition of hazards (*e.g.*, identification of carcinogens) and protecting the environment.

Occupational epidemiology will continue to play an important role in epidemiological studies of the determinants of disease and injury in human populations, evolving as a discipline to address the changing nature of work, the shifting global distribution of hazards, the emergence of novel hazards associated with technological changes (and novel data resources). For hazard evaluations undertaken by governmental and nongovernmental agencies, and for public health responses to disaster, occupational epidemiology remains a key source of information about human health effects of exposure, leveraging the strengths of occupational study designs and the opportunities for exposure assessment in work settings.

References

1. Hippocrates. *Airs, Waters, and Places*. Baltimore: Williams & Wilkins Co.; 1938.
2. Ramazzini B. *De Morbis Artificum Bernardini Ramazzini Diatriba = Diseases of Workers: The Latin Text of 1713 Revised, with Translation and Notes*. Birmingham, AL: Classics of Medicine Library, a division of Gryphon Editions, Inc.; 1983.
3. Fee E, Brown TM. Alice Hamilton: settlement physician, occupational health pioneer. *Am J Public Health*. 2001;91(11):1767.
4. Ward E, Carpenter A, Markowitz S, Roberts D, Halperin W. Excess number of bladder cancers in workers exposed to ortho-toluidine and aniline. *J Natl Cancer Inst*. 1991;83(7):501-506.
5. Nelkin D, Brown MS. *Workers at Risk: Voices From the Workplace*. Chicago, IL: Univerisity of Chicago Press; 1984.
6. Watterson A. Whither lay epidemiology in UK public health policy and practice? Some reflections on occupational and environmental health opportunities. *J Public Health Med*. 1994;16(3):270-274.
7. Brown P. Popular epidemiology Revisited. *Curr Sociol*. 1997;45(3):137-156.
8. Sheehan HE, Wedeen RP. *Toxic Circles: Environmental Hazards From the Workplace Into the Community*. New Jersey: Rutgers; 1993.
9. Brown JR, Thornton JL. Percivall Pott (1714-1788) and chimney sweepers' cancer of the scrotum. *Br J Ind Med*. 1957;14(1):68-70.
10. Bishop C, Kipling MD. Dr J Ayrton Paris and cancer of the scrotum: 'Honour the physician with the honour due unto him'. *J Soc Occup Med*. 1978;28(1):3-5.
11. Bell J. Paraffin epithelioma. *Edinb Med J*. 1876;22:135-137.
12. Von Volkmann R. Ueber Theer- und Russkrebs. *Berliner Klinische Wochenschrift*. 1874;11:218.
13. Clayson DB. *Chemical Carcinogenesis*. London: JA Churchill; 1962.
14. McKinnell RG. *The Understanding, Prevention and Control of Human Cancer: The Historic Work and Lives of Elizabeth Cavert Miller and James A. Miller*. Leiden, Boston: Brill; 2016.
15. Mullner RM. *Deadly Glow: The Radium Dial Worker Tragedy*. Washington, DC: American Public Health Association; 1999.
16. Kumagai S, Kurumatani N, Arimoto A, Ichihara G. Cholangiocarcinoma among offset colour proof-printing workers exposed to 1,2-dichloropropane and/or dichloromethane. *Occup Environ Med*. 2013;70(7):508-510.
17. Vlaanderen J, Straif K, Martinsen JI, et al. Cholangiocarcinoma among workers in the printing industry: using the NOCCA database to elucidate the generalisability of a cluster report from Japan. *Occup Environ Med*. 2013;70(12):828-830.
18. Driscoll TR. Cholangiocarcinoma among workers in the printing industry. *Occup Environ Med*. 2013;70(12):827.
19. Keiding N. The method of expected number of deaths, 1786-1886-1986. *Int Stat Rev*. 1987;55(1):1-20.
20. Laplace PS. *A Philosophical Essay on Probabilities*. New York, NY: John Wiley and Sons; 1902.
21. Farr W. *Vital Statistics: A Memorial Volume of Selections From the Reports and Writings of William Farr With an Introduction by Mervyn Susser and Abraham Adelstein*. Metuchen, NJ: Scarecrow Press; 1975.
22. Derickson A. *Black Lung: Anatomy of a Public Health Disaster*. Ithaca, NY: Cornell University Press; 1998.
23. Chadwick E. *The Health of Nations. A Review of the Works of Edwin Chadwick. With a Biographical Dissertation by Benjamin Ward Richardson*. London: Longmans, Green &Co.; 1887.
24. Engels F. *The Condition of the Working Class in England Friedrich Engels; Edited With an Introduction and Notes by David McLellan*. Oxford, NY: Oxford University Press; 2009.
25. Axelson O. Some recent developments in occupational epidemiology. *Scand J Work Environ Health* 1994;20(special issue):9-18.
26. Kennaway NM, Kennaway EL. A study of the incidence of cancer of the lung and larynx. *J Hyg (Lond)*. 1936;36(2):236-267.
27. Milham S Jr. Leukemia and multiple myeloma in farmers. *Am J Epidemiol*. 1971;94(4):307-310.
28. Doll R. The causes of death among gas-workers with special reference to cancer of the lung. *Br J Ind Med*. 1952;9(3):180-185.
29. Doll R. Mortality from lung cancer in asbestos workers. *Br J Ind Med*. 1955;12(2):81-86.

30. Mancuso RF. Occupational cancer and other health hazards in a chromate plant: a medical appraisal. II. Clinical and toxicologic aspects. *Ind Med Surg*. 1951;20(9):393-407.

31. Mancuso TF, Hueper WC. Occupational cancer and other health hazards in a chromate plant: a medical appraisal. I. Lung cancers in chromate workers. *Ind Med Surg*. 1951;20(8):358-363.

32. Case RA, Hosker ME, Mc DD, Pearson JT. Tumours of the urinary bladder in workmen engaged in the manufacture and use of certain dyestuff intermediates in the British chemical industry. I. The role of aniline, benzidine, alpha-naphthylamine, and beta-naphthylamine. *Br J Ind Med*. 1954;11(2):75-104.

33. Case RA, Hosker ME. Tumour of the urinary bladder as an occupational disease in the rubber industry in England and Wales. *Br J Prev Soc Med*. 1954;8(2):39-50.

34. Coleman PJ. Epidemiologic principles applied to injury prevention. *Scand J Work Environ Health*. 1981;7(suppl 4):91-96.

35. Kraus JF. Fatal and nonfatal injuries in occupational settings: a review. *Annu Rev Public Health*. 1985;6:403-418.

36. Kraus JF. A journey to and through injury epidemiology. *Inj Epidemiol*. 2014;1(1):3.

37. Stout NA, Linn HI. Occupational injury prevention research: progress and priorities. *Inj Prev*. 2002;8(suppl 4):IV9-IV14.

38. Savitz DA, Sonnenfeld NL, Olshan AF. Review of epidemiologic studies of paternal occupational exposure and spontaneous abortion. *Am J Ind Med*. 1994;25(3):361-383.

39. Savitz DA, Whelan EA, Kleckner RC. Effect of parents' occupational exposures on risk of stillbirth, preterm delivery, and small-for-gestational-age infants. *Am J Epidemiol*. 1989;129(6):1201-1218.

40. Botsch RE. *Organizing the Breathless: Cotton Dust, Southern Politics, and the Brown Lung Association*. Lexington, Kentucky: University Press of Kentucky; 1993.

41. Derickson A. Down solid: the origins and development of the black lung insurgency. *J Public Health Policy*. 1983;4(1):25-44.

42. Derickson A. The United Mine Workers of American and the recognition of occupational respiratory diseases, 1902-1968. *Am J Public Health*. 1991;81(6):782-790.

43. Kerr LE. Coal workers' pneumoconiosis in an affluent society. *Public Health Rep*. 1970;85(10):847-852.

44. Schilling RS, Hughes JP, Dingwall-Fordyce I, Gilson JC. An epidemiological study of byssinosis among Lancashire cotton workers. *Br J Ind Med*. 1955;12(3):217-227.

45. McKerrow CB, Schilling RS. A pilot enquiry into byssinosis in two cotton mills in the United States. *J Am Med Assoc*. 1961;177:850-853.

46. Schilling RS. Epidemiological studies of chronic respiratory disease among cotton operatives. *Yale J Biol Med*. 1964;37:55-74.

47. Bouhuys A, Wolfson RL, Horner DW, Brain JD, Zuskin E. Byssinosis in cotton textile workers. Respiratory survey of a mill with rapid labor turnover. *Ann Intern Med*. 1969;71(2):257-269.

48. Merchant JA, Kilburn KH, O'Fallon WM, Hamilton JD, Lumsden JC. Byssinosis and chronic bronchitis among cotton textile workers. *Ann Intern Med*. 1972;76(3):423-433.

49. Stayner L, Smith R, Bailer AJ, Luebeck EG, Moolgavkar SH. Modeling epidemiologic studies of occupational cohorts for the quantitative assessment of carcinogenic hazards. *Am J Ind Med*. 1995;27(2):155-170.

50. Stayner L, Smith R, Bailer J, et al. Exposure-response analysis of risk of respiratory disease associated with occupational exposure to chrysotile asbestos. *Occup Environ Med*. 1997;54(9):646-652.

51. National Research Council. *Committee on Health Risks of Exposure to Radon (BEIR VI). Health Effects of Exposure to Radon*. Washington, DC: National Academy Press; 1999.

52. Wilcosky T, Wing S. The healthy worker effect. Selection of workers and work forces. *Scand J Work Environ Health*. 1987;13(1):70-72.

53. Checkoway H, Pearce N, Dement JM. Design and conduct of occupational epidemiology studies: I. Design aspects of cohort studies. *Am J Ind Med*. 1989;15(4):363-373.

54. Delzell E, Monson R. Mortality among rubber workers. IV. General mortality patterns. *J Occup Med*. 1981;23(12):850-856.

55. Breslow NE, Day NE. *Statistical Methods in Cancer Research: The Design and Analysis of Cohort Studies*. Vol II. Lyon: International Agency for Research on Cancer; 1987.

56. Doll R, Peto R, Boreham J, Sutherland I. Mortality in relation to smoking: 50 years' observations on male British doctors. *BMJ*. 2004;328(7455):1519.

57. Langholz B, Thomas DC. Nested case-control and case-cohort methods of sampling from a cohort: a critical comparison. *Am J Epidemiol*. 1990;131(1):169-176.

58. Liddell FDK, McDonald JC, Thomas DC, Cunliffe SV. Methods of cohort analysis:appraisal by application to asbestos mining. *J R Stat Soc*. 1977;140(4):469-491.

59. Whittemore AS. Methods old and new for analyzing occupational cohort data. *Am J Ind Med*. 1987;12(3):233-248.

60. Thomas D. General relative risk models for survival time and matched case-control analysis. *Biometrics*. 1981;37(4):673-686.

61. Langholz B, Goldstein L. Risk set sampling in epidemiologic cohort studies. *Stat Sci.* 1996;11(1):35-53.

62. Langholz B, Richardson D. Are nested case-control studies biased? *Epidemiology.* 2009;20(3):321-329.

63. Siemiatycki J, Richardson L, Gerin M, et al. Associations between several sites of cancer and nine organic dusts: results from an hypothesis-generating case-control study in Montreal, 1979-1983. *Am J Epidemiol.* 1986;123(2):235-249.

64. Cantor KP, Blair A. Farming and mortality from multiple myeloma: a case-control study with the use of death certificates. *J Natl Cancer Inst.* 1984;72(2):251-255.

65. Demers PA, Vaughan TL, Koepsell TD, et al. A case-control study of multiple myeloma and occupation. *Am J Ind Med.* 1993;23(4):629-639.

66. Olsson AC, Xu Y, Schuz J, et al. Lung cancer risk among hairdressers: a pooled analysis of case-control studies conducted between 1985 and 2010. *Am J Epidemiol.* 2013;178(9):1355-1365.

67. Kendzia B, Behrens T, Jockel KH, et al. Welding and lung cancer in a pooled analysis of case-control studies. *Am J Epidemiol.* 2013;178(10):1513-1525.

68. Behrens T, Kendzia B, Treppmann T, et al. Lung cancer risk among bakers, pastry cooks and confectionary makers: the SYNERGY study. *Occup Environ Med.* 2013;70(11):810-814.

69. Sorock GS, Lombardi DA, Hauser RB, Eisen EA, Herrick RF, Mittleman MA. A case-crossover study of occupational traumatic hand injury: methods and initial findings. *Am J Ind Med.* 2001;39(2):171-179.

70. Lander L, Sorock GS, Stentz TL, et al. A case-crossover study of occupational laceration injuries in pork processing: methods and preliminary findings. *Occup Environ Med.* 2010;67(10):686-692.

71. Lombardi DA, Sorock GS, Holander L, Mittleman MA. A case-crossover study of transient risk factors for occupational hand trauma by gender. *J Occup Environ Hyg.* 2007;4(10):790-797.

72. Mittleman MA, Maldonado G, Gerberich SG, Smith GS, Sorock GS. Alternative approaches to analytical designs in occupational injury epidemiology. *Am J Ind Med.* 1997;32(2):129-141.

73. Hoppin JA, Umbach DM, Long S, et al. Respiratory disease in United States farmers. *Occup Environ Med.* 2014;71(7):484-491.

74. Rinsky JL, Hoppin JA, Blair A, He K, Beane Freeman LE, Chen H. Agricultural exposures and stroke mortality in the agricultural health study. *J Toxicol Environ Health A.* 2013;76(13):798-814.

75. Hu YA, Smith TJ, Xu X, Wang L, Watanabe H, Christiani DC. Comparison of self-assessment of solvent exposure with measurement and professional assessment for female petrochemical workers in China. *Am J Ind Med.* 2002;41(6):483-489.

76. Borton EK, Lemasters GK, Hilbert TJ, Lockey JE, Dunning KK, Rice CH. Exposure estimates for workers in a facility expanding Libby vermiculite: updated values and comparison with original 1980 values. *J Occup Environ Med.* 2012;54(11):1350-1358.

77. Baumgarten M, Siemiatycki J, Gibbs GW. Validity of work histories obtained by interview for epidemiologic purposes. *Am J Epidemiol.* 1983;118(4):583-591.

78. Fritschi L, Nadon L, Benke G, et al. Validation of expert assessment of occupational exposures. *Am J Ind Med.* 2003;43(5):519-522.

79. Kromhout H. Design of measurement strategies for workplace exposures. *Occup Environ Med.* 2002;59(5):349-354; quiz 354,286.

80. Seixas NS, Checkoway H. Exposure assessment in industry specific retrospective occupational epidemiology studies. *Occup Environ Med.* 1995;52(10):625-633.

81. Couch JR, Petersen M, Rice C, Schubauer-Berigan MK. Development of retrospective quantitative and qualitative job-exposure matrices for exposures at a beryllium processing facility. *Occup Environ Med.* 2011;68(5):361-365.

82. Utterback DF, Rinsky RA. Benzene exposure assessment in rubber hydrochloride workers: a critical evaluation of previous estimates. *Am J Ind Med.* 1995;27(5):661-676.

83. Lubin JH, Pottern LM, Stone BJ, Fraumeni JF Jr. Respiratory cancer in a cohort of copper smelter workers: results from more than 50 years of follow-up. *Am J Epidemiol.* 2000;151(6):554-565.

84. Greenland S, Fischer HJ, Kheifets L. Methods to explore uncertainty and bias introduced by job exposure matrices. *Risk Anal.* 2016;36(1):74-82.

85. Hemon D, Clavel J. Retrospective assessment of occupational exposures in the context of community-based case-control studies. *Med Lav.* 1995;86(2):152-167.

86. McGuire V, Nelson LM, Koepsell TD, Checkoway H, Longstreth WT Jr. Assessment of occupational exposures in community-based case-control studies. *Annu Rev Public Health.* 1998;19:35-53.

87. Pukkala E, Guo J, Kyyronen P, Lindbohm ML, Sallmen M, Kauppinen T. National job-exposure matrix in analyses of census-based estimates of occupational cancer risk. *Scand J Work Environ Health.* 2005;31(2):97-107.

88. Peters S, Vermeulen R, Olsson A, et al. Development of an exposure measurement database on five lung carcinogens (ExpoSYN) for quantitative retrospective occupational exposure assessment. *Ann Occup Hyg.* 2012;56(1):70-79.

89. Pannett B, Coggon D, Acheson ED. A job-exposure matrix for use in population based studies in England and Wales. *Br J Ind Med*. 1985;42(11):777-783.

90. Olsson AC, Gustavsson P, Kromhout H, et al. Exposure to diesel motor exhaust and lung cancer risk in a pooled analysis from case-control studies in Europe and Canada. *Am J Respir Crit Care Med*. 2011;183(7):941-948.

91. Siemiatycki J, Wacholder S, Richardson L, Dewar R, Gerin M. Discovering carcinogens in the occupational environment. Methods of data collection and analysis of a large case-referent monitoring system. *Scand J Work Environ Health*. 1987;13(6):486-492.

92. Stewart PA, Stewart WF, Heineman EF, Dosemeci M, Linet M, Inskip PD. A novel approach to data collection in a case-control study of cancer and occupational exposures. *Int J Epidemiol*. 1996;25(4):744-752.

93. Thierry-Chef I, Marshall M, Fix JJ, et al. The 15-country collaborative study of cancer risk among radiation workers in the nuclear industry: study of errors in dosimetry. *Radiat Res*. 2007;167(4):380-395.

94. Thierry-Chef I, Pernicka F, Marshall M, Cardis E, Andreo P. Study of a selection of 10 historical types of dosemeter: variation of the response to Hp(10) with photon energy and geometry of exposure. *Radiat Prot Dosimetry*. 2002;102(2):101-113.

95. Palmer HE, Rieksts GA, Icayan EE. 1976 Hanford americium exposure incident: in vivo measurements. *Health Phys*. 1983;45(4):893-910.

96. Gaines LG, Fent KW, Flack SL, et al. Urine 1,6-hexamethylene diamine (HDA) levels among workers exposed to 1,6-hexamethylene diisocyanate (HDI). *Ann Occup Hyg*. 2010;54(6):678-691.

97. Wing S, Richardson DB, Wolf S, Mihlan G, Crawford-Brown D, Wood J. A case control study of multiple myeloma at four nuclear facilities. *Ann Epidemiol*. 2000;10(3):144-153.

98. Rosenman KD, Gardiner JC, Wang J, et al. Why most workers with occupational repetitive trauma do not file for workers' compensation. *J Occup Environ Med*. 2000;42(1):25-34.

99. Kica J, Rosenman KD. Multi-source surveillance for work-related crushing injuries. *Am J Ind Med*. 2018;61(2):148-156.

100. Freedman DM, Sigurdson A, Rao RS, et al. Risk of melanoma among radiologic technologists in the United States. *Int J Cancer*. 2003;103(4):556-562.

101. Steenland K, Nowlin S, Ryan B, Adams S. Use of multiple-cause mortality data in epidemiologic analyses: US rate and proportion files developed by the National Institute for Occupational Safety and Health and the National Cancer Institute. *Am J Epidemiol*. 1992;136(7):855-862.

102. Richardson DB. Use of multiple cause of death data in cancer mortality analyses. *Am J Ind Med*. 2006;49(8):683-689.

103. Nielsen HB, Larsen AD, Dyreborg J, et al. Risk of injury after evening and night work - findings from the Danish Working Hour Database. *Scand J Work Environ Health*. 2018;44(4):385-393.

104. Monson RR. Analysis of relative survival and proportional mortality. *Comput Biomed Res*. 1974;7(4):325-332.

105. Frome EL. The analysis of rates using Poisson regression models. *Biometrics*. 1983;39(3):665-674.

106. Checkoway H, Pearce N, Dement JM. Design and conduct of occupational epidemiology studies: II. Analysis of cohort data. *Am J Ind Med*. 1989;15(4):375-394.

107. Case RA, Lea AJ. Mustard gas poisoning, chronic bronchitis, and lung cancer; an investigation into the possibility that poisoning by mustard gas in the 1914-18 war might be a factor in the production of neoplasia. *Br J Prev Soc Med*. 1955;9(2):62-72.

108. Richardson DB, Keil AP, Cole SR, MacLehose RF. Observed and expected mortality in cohort studies. *Am J Epidemiol*. 2017;185(6):479-486.

109. Armstrong BG. Comparing standardized mortality ratios. *Ann Epidemiol*. 1995;5(1):60-64.

110. Milham S Jr. Mortality in workers exposed to electromagnetic fields. *Environ Health Perspect*. 1985;62:297-300.

111. Clapp RW. Mortality among US employees of a large computer manufacturing company: 1969-2001. *Environ Health*. 2006;5:30.

112. Frome EL, Checkoway H. Epidemiologic programs for computers and calculators. Use of Poisson regression models in estimating incidence rates and ratios. *Am J Epidemiol*. 1985;121(2):309-323.

113. Richardson D, Loomis D. The impact of exposure categorization for grouped analyses of cohort data. *Occup Environ Med*. 2004;61:930-935.

114. Lubin JH, Boice JD Jr, Edling C, et al. *Radon and Lung-Cancer Risk: A Joint Analysis of 11 Underground Miners Studies*. Washington, D.C.: National Institutes of Health, National Cancer Institute; 1994.

115. Tomasek L. Effect of age at exposure in 11 underground miners studies. *Radiat Prot Dosimetry*. 2014;160(1-3):124-127.

116. Richardson DB. Discrete time hazards models for occupational and environmental cohort analyses. *Occup Environ Med*. 2010;67(1):67-71.

117. Steenland K, Deddens JA. A practical guide to dose-response analyses and risk assessment in occupational epidemiology. *Epidemiology*. 2004;15(1):63-70.

118. Steenland K, Deddens J, Piacitelli L. Risk assessment for 2,3,7,8-tetrachlorodibenzo-p-dioxin (TCDD) based on an epidemiologic study. *Am J Epidemiol.* 2001;154(5):451-458.

119. Langholz B, Richardson DB. Fitting general relative risk models for survival time and matched case-control analysis. *Am J Epidemiol.* 2010;171(3):377-383.

120. Langholz B, Thomas DC. Efficiency of cohort sampling designs:some surprising results. *Biometrics.* 1991;47(4):1563-1571.

121. Lubin JH, Moore LE, Fraumeni JF Jr, Cantor KP. Respiratory cancer and inhaled inorganic arsenic in copper smelters workers: a linear relationship with cumulative exposure that increases with concentration. *Environ Health Perspect.* 2008;116(12):1661-1665.

122. Lubin JH. Models for the analysis of radon-exposed populations. *Yale J Biol Med.* 1988;61(3):195-214.

123. Thomas D. New techniques for the analysis of cohort studies. *Epidemiol Rev.* 1998;20(1):122-134.

124. Gilbert ES, Buchanan JA. An alternative approach to analyzing occupational mortality data. *J Occup Med.* 1984;26(11):822-828.

125. Wing S, Shy CM, Wood JL, Wolf S, Cragle DL, Frome EL. Mortality among workers at Oak Ridge National Laboratory. Evidence of radiation effects in follow-up through 1984. *J Am Med Assoc.* 1991;265(11):1397-1402.

126. Rinsky RA, Smith AB, Hornung R, et al. Benzene and leukemia: an epidemiologic risk assessment. *New Engl J Med.* 1987;316(17):1044-1049.

127. Dement JM, Harris RL Jr, Symons MJ, Shy CM. Exposures and mortality among chrysotile asbestos workers. Part II: mortality. *Am J Ind Med.* 1983;4(3):421-433.

128. Smith TJ, Kriebel D. *A Biologic Approach to Environmental Assessment and Epidemiology.* Oxford: Oxford University Press; 2010.

129. Checkoway H, Rice CH. Time-weighted averages, peaks, and other indices of exposure in occupational epidemiology. *Am J Ind Med.* 1992;21(1):25-33.

130. Richardson DB, Cole SR, Langholz B. Regression models for the effects of exposure rate and cumulative exposure. *Epidemiology.* 2012;23(6):892-899.

131. Rothman KJ. Induction and latent periods. *Am J Epidemiol.* 1981;114(2):253-259.

132. Salvan A, Stayner L, Steenland K, Smith R. Selecting an exposure lag period. *Epidemiology.* 1995;6(4):387-390.

133. Richardson DB, Cole SR, Chu H, Langholz B. Lagging exposure information in cumulative exposure-response analyses. *Am J Epidemiol.* 2011;174(12):1416-1422.

134. Stewart AM, Kneale GW. Relations between age at occupational exposure to ionising radiation and cancer risk. *Occup Environ Med.* 1996;53:225-230.

135. Langholz B, Thomas D, Xiang A, Stram D. Latency analysis in epidemiologic studies of occupational exposures: application to the Colorado Plateau uranium miners cohort. *Am J Ind Med.* 1999;35(3):246-256.

136. Armitage P, Doll R. The age distribution of cancer and a multistage theory of carcinogenesis. *Br J Cancer.* 1954;8(1):1-12.

137. Moolgavkar SH, Dewanji A, Venzon DJ. A stochastic two-stage model for cancer risk assessment. I. The hazard function and the probability of tumor. *Risk Anal.* 1988;8(3):383-392.

138. Pearce N. Multistage modelling of lung cancer mortality in asbestos textile workers. *Int J Epidemiol.* 1988;17(4):747-752.

139. Richardson DB. Temporal variation in the association between benzene and leukemia mortality. *Environ Health Perspect.* 2008;116(3):370-374.

140. James SA, Strogatz DS, Wing SB, Ramsey DL. Socioeconomic status, John Henryism, and hypertension in blacks and whites. *Am J Epidemiol.* 1987;126(4):664-673.

141. Arrighi HM, Hertz-Picciotto I. The evolving concept of the healthy worker survivor effect. *Epidemiology.* 1994;5(2):189-196.

142. Carpenter LM. Some observations on the healthy worker effect [editorial]. *Br J Ind Med.* 1987;44(5):289-291.

143. McMichael AJ. Standardized mortality ratios and the "healthy worker effect": Scratching beneath the surface. *J Occup Med.* 1976;18(3):165-168.

144. Choi BC. Definition, sources, magnitude, effect modifiers, and strategies of reduction of the healthy workers effect. *J Occup Med.* 1992;34(10):979-988.

145. Cole P, Green LC, Lash TL. Lifestyle determinants of cancer among Danish mastic asphalt workers. *Regul Toxicol Pharmacol.* 1999;30(1):1-8.

146. Loomis DL, Richardson DB. Race and risk of fatal injury at work. *Am J Public Health.* 1998;88(1):40-44.

147. Gilbert ES. Some confounding factors in the study of mortality and occupational exposures. *Am J Epidemiol.* 1982;116(1):177-188.

148. Frome EL, Cragle DL, McLain RW. Poisson regression analysis of the mortality among a cohort of World War II nuclear industry workers. *Radiat Res.* 1990;123(2):138-152.

149. Steenland K. Mortality of workers hired during world war II. *Am J Ind Med.* 1993;23(5):823-827.

150. Arrighi HM, Hertz-Picciotto I. Definitions, sources, magnitude, effect modifiers, and strategies of reduction of the healthy worker effect. *J Occup Med.* 1993;35(9):890-892.

151. Park RM, Maizlish NA, Punnett L, Moure-Eraso R, Silverstein MA. A comparison of PMRs and SMRs as estimators of occupational mortality. *Epidemiology.* 1991;2(1):49-59.

152. Waggoner JK, Kullman GJ, Henneberger PK, et al. Mortality in the agricultural health study, 1993-2007. *Am J Epidemiol.* 2011;173(1):71-83.

153. Richardson DB, Keil AP, Tchetgen Tchetgen E, Cooper G. Negative control outcomes and the analysis of standardized mortality ratios. *Epidemiology.* 2015;26(5):727-732.

154. Fox AJ, Collier PF. Low mortality rates in industrial cohort studies due to selection for work and survival in the industry. *Br J Prev Soc Med.* 1976;30(4):225-230.

155. Monson RR. Observations on the healthy worker effect. *J Occup Med.* 1986;28(6):425-433.

156. Oliver T. *Dangerous Trades; the Historical, Social, and Legal Aspects of Industrial Occupations as Affecting Health, by a Number of Experts.* New York, NY: E.P. Dutton/London: J. Murray; 1902.

157. Applebaum KM, Malloy EJ, Eisen EA. Reducing healthy worker survivor bias by restricting date of hire in a cohort study of Vermont granite workers. *Occup Environ Med.* 2007;64(10):681-687.

158. Harrington D. Is coal industry blind to health hazards of mine? *Coal Age* 1924;29:759.

159. Dumas O, Varraso R, Zock JP, et al. Asthma history, job type and job changes among US nurses. *Occup Environ Med.* 2015;72(7):482-488.

160. Steenland K, Deddens J, Salvan A, Stayner L. Healthy worker effect and cumulative exposure [letter; comment]. *Epidemiology.* 1995;6(3):339-341.

161. Buckley JP, Keil AP, McGrath LJ, Edwards JK. Evolving methods for inference in the presence of healthy worker survivor bias. *Epidemiology.* 2014;26(2):204-212.

162. Naimi AI, Cole SR, Hudgens MG, Brookhart MA, Richardson DB. Assessing the component associations of the healthy worker survivor bias: occupational asbestos exposure and lung cancer mortality. *Ann Epidemiol.* 2013;23(6):334-341.

163. Robins J. A new approach to casual inference in mortality studies with A sustained exposure period-application to control of the healthy worker survivor effect. *Math Model.* 1986;7(9-12):1393-1512.

164. Robins J. A graphical approach to the identification and estimation of causal parameters in mortality studies with sustained exposure periods. *J Chron Dis.* 1987;40(suppl 2):139S-161S.

165. Keil AP, Edwards JK, Richardson DB, Naimi AI, Cole SR. The parametric g-formula for time-to-event data: intuition and a worked example. *Epidemiology.* 2014;25(6):889-897.

166. Lipscomb HJ, Argue R, McDonald MA, et al. Exploration of work and health disparities among black women employed in poultry processing in the rural south. *Environ Health Perspect.* 2005;113(12):1833-1840.

167. Artazcoz L, Borrell C, Cortes I, Escriba-Aguir V, Cascant L. Occupational epidemiology and work related inequalities in health: a gender perspective for two complementary approaches to work and health research. *J Epidemiol Community Health.* 2007;61(suppl 2):ii39-ii45.

168. Dement JM, Brown DP, Okun A. Follow-up study of chrysotile asbestos textile workers: cohort mortality and case-control analyses. *Am J Ind Med.* 1994;26(4):431-447.

169. Fry S. Studies of U.S. Radium dial workers: an epidemiological classic. *Radiat Res.* 1998;150:S21-S29.

170. Cherniack M. *The Hawk's Nest Incident: America's Worst Industrial Disaster.* New Haven: Yale University Press; 1986.

171. Samuels SW. The international context of carcinogen regulation. *Banbury Rep.* 1981;9:497-512.

172. Greenlund KJ, Elling RH. Capital sectors and workers' health and safety in the United States. *Int J Health Serv.* 1995;25(1):101-116.

173. James SA, LaCroix AZ, Kleinbaum DG, Strogatz DS. John Henryism and blood pressure differences among black men. II. The role of occupational stressors. *J Behav Med.* 1984;7(3):259-275.

174. Wing S, Grant G, Green M, Stewart C. Community based collaboration for environmental justice: southeast Halifax environmental reawakening. *Environ Urbanization.* 1996;8:129-140.

175. Bender TJ, Beall C, Cheng H, et al. Methodologic issues in follow-up studies of cancer incidence among occupational groups in the United States. *Ann Epidemiol.* 2006;16(3):170-179.

176. Hamad R, Modrek S, Kubo J, Goldstein BA, Cullen MR. Using "big data" to capture overall health status: properties and predictive value of a claims-based health risk score. *PLoS One.* 2015;10(5):e0126054.

177. Neophytou AM, Costello S, Brown DM, et al. Marginal structural models in occupational epidemiology: application in a study of ischemic heart disease incidence and PM2.5 in the US aluminum industry. *Am J Epidemiol.* 2014;180(6):608-615.

178. Mitchell DC, Castro J, Armitage TL, et al. Recruitment, methods, and descriptive results of a physiologic assessment of Latino Farmworkers: the California heat illness prevention study. *J Occup Environ Med.* 2017;59(7):649-658.

179. Chisolm JJ Jr. Fouling one's own nest. *Pediatrics.* 1978;62(4):614-617.

180. Rinsky JL, Higgins S, Angelon-Gaetz K, et al. Occupational and take-home lead exposure among lead oxide manufacturing employees, North Carolina, 2016. *Public Health Rep.* 2018;133(6):700-706.

CHAPTER 42

Nutritional Epidemiology

Walter C. Willett and Frank B. Hu

OBJECTIVES AND BACKGROUND

The primary objective of nutritional epidemiology has been to describe relations between dietary factors and the occurrence of specific diseases, functional health outcomes, and overall health, including total mortality. As research has identified specific aspects of diet that are important for health, more recent work has used dietary variables as the outcome to identify determinants, including interventions, that can influence diet. Nutritional epidemiology has also become engaged in many aspects of policy that relate to food and diets.

Going back to the time of Hippocrates, and probably long before, observation and clinical experience led to the recognition that diet was an important factor in preventing and treating disease. In the early 20th century, short-term intervention studies documented that diseases such as scurvy and rickets were caused by specific nutritional deficiencies.[1] During that century, noncommunicable diseases emerged as the dominant sources of mortality in industrialized countries, and the investigation of these required epidemiologic approaches because they developed over many decades and result from many contributing factors. The formal, quantitative study of diet and health, nutritional epidemiology, has been a recent development. For many years, nutritionists and epidemiologists had believed that difficulties of assessing the diets of free-living human beings over extended periods of time made large-scale studies of diet and health impossible. Since the 1970s, however, methods for assessing dietary intake have been developed and validated, thus providing the underpinning for what became a rapidly expanding field. Largely because of this effort, the importance of diet in the cause and prevention of nearly all major diseases has come to be appreciated. For example, diseases as diverse as birth defects, most types of cancer, cardiovascular diseases (CVDs), infertility, and cataracts have important dietary determinants. Important findings include that low intakes of fruits, vegetables, and whole grains have been related to increased risk of CVD and low intake of fiber from grains has been associated with higher risk of type 2 diabetes. Also, replicated epidemiologic evidence has supported replacing saturated and trans fats with unsaturated fats for prevention of coronary heart disease (CHD) and type 2 diabetes. Evidence is now conclusive that specific overall dietary patterns, such as the Mediterranean diet, can importantly reduce risks of CVD and premature death. These and other findings from nutritional epidemiology have been incorporated into national and international dietary guidelines and policies. For example, in many countries, production of trans fat has been banned, resulting in reductions in rates of CHD.

In general, nutritional epidemiologists have not felt constrained by any formal definition of nutrition and are broadly concerned about health as it is related to food and its components, whether they be essential nutrients, other natural constituents of food, chemicals created in the cooking and preservation of food, or noninfectious food contaminants. Because a major distinction between nutritional epidemiology and other areas of epidemiology is that dietary exposures are an extremely complex set of variables—much of this chapter is devoted to the assessment of dietary intake. Before doing so, however, the classic epidemiologic approaches—ecologic, case-control, and cohort studies—are discussed in the context of issues that are particularly germane to the study of nutritional exposures. Because many of the topics considered in this chapter can be discussed only briefly, readers are referred to a full text on the topic of nutritional epidemiology[1] and to cited references for more detailed treatment.

METHODOLOGIES

Study Designs

Ecologic Studies

With few exceptions,[2] epidemiologic investigations of diet and disease before 1980 consisted largely of *ecologic* or *correlational* studies, that is, comparisons of disease rates in populations with the population per capita consumption or disappearance of specific dietary constituents. Perhaps, the most well known is the Seven Countries Study by Keys and colleagues,[3] which documented an ecological correlation between intake of saturated fat and rates of CHD. Usually, the dietary information in such studies is based on "disappearance" data, meaning the national figures for food produced and imported minus the food that is exported, fed to animals, or otherwise not available for humans. Many of the correlations based on such information have been remarkably strong; for example, the correlation between meat intake and incidence of colon cancer among countries was 0.85 for men and 0.89 for women.[4]

The use of international ecologic studies to evaluate the relation between diet and disease has several strengths. Most important, the contrasts in dietary intake are typically very large. For example, in the United States, most individuals consumed between 30% and 45% of their calories from fat,[5] whereas the *mean* fat intake for populations in various other countries has varied from approximately 15% to 42% of calories.[6] Also, the average of diets for persons residing in a country are likely to be more stable over time than are the diets of individual persons within the country; for most countries, the changes in per capita dietary intakes over a decade or two are relatively small. Finally, the disease rates on which international studies are based are usually derived from relatively large populations and are therefore subject to only small random errors.

A major limitation of such ecologic studies is that many potential determinants of disease other than the dietary factor under consideration may covary between areas with a high and low incidence of disease. Such confounding factors can include other dietary factors, including the availability of total food energy, other environmental or lifestyle practices, and genetic predisposition. For example, with few exceptions, such as Japan, countries with a low incidence of colon cancer tended to be economically undeveloped. Therefore, any variable related to industrialization was correlated with incidence of colon cancer to the same degree as dietary patterns typical of industrialization. Indeed, the correlation between gross national product and colon cancer mortality rate was 0.77 for men and 0.69 for women.[4] More complex analyses of such ecologic data can be conducted that control for some of the potentially confounding factors. For example, McKeown-Eyssen and Bright-See[7] found that an inverse association of per capita dietary fiber intake and national colon cancer mortality rates decreased substantially after adjustment for fat intake.

Another major limitation of ecologic studies is their reliance on population rather than individual characteristics (see Chapter 30). Aggregate data for a geographic unit may be only weakly related to the diets of those individuals at risk of disease. As an extreme example, the interpretation of ecologic data regarding alcohol intake and breast cancer is complicated because, in some cultures, most of the alcohol is consumed by men, but it is the women who develop breast cancer. In addition, ecologic studies of diet are often limited using disappearance data that are only indirectly related to intake and are likely to be of variable quality. For example, the higher "disappearance" of calories per capita for the United States compared with most countries is probably related largely to wasted food. These problems of ecologic associations and issues of data quality can potentially be addressed by collecting information on actual dietary intake in a uniform manner from the population subgroups of interest.[8,9] This strategy was applied in the Seven Countries Study and in a study conducted in 65 geographic areas in China.[10]

Another serious limitation of the international ecologic studies is that they cannot be reproduced independently, which is an important part of the scientific process. Although the dietary information can be improved and the analyses can be refined, the data will not really be independent even as more information becomes available over time; the populations, their diets, and the confounding variables will be similar. Thus, it is not likely that many new insights will be obtained from further ecologic studies among countries.

The role of ecologic studies in nutritional epidemiology has been controversial. Clearly, these analyses have stimulated much of the current research on diet in relation to cancer and CVD, and they have emphasized the major differences in rates of these diseases among countries. Traditionally, such studies have been considered weak evidence, primarily owing to the potential for confounding by factors that are difficult to measure and control.[11] Others have felt that such studies provide strong evidence for evaluating hypotheses relating diet to cancer.[12,13] On balance, ecologic studies have clearly been useful, but they are far from conclusive regarding the relations between dietary factors and disease and may sometimes be totally misleading.[14]

Special Exposure Groups

Subgroups within a population that consume unusual diets provide an additional opportunity to learn about the relation of dietary factors and disease. These groups are often defined by religious or ethnic characteristics and provide many of the same strengths as ecologic studies. In addition, the special populations often live in the same general environment as the comparison group, which may somewhat reduce the number of alternative explanations for any differences that might be observed. For example, the observation that colon cancer mortality in the largely vegetarian Seventh-Day Adventists was only about half that expected[15] has been taken as support for the hypothesis that meat consumption is a cause of colon cancer.

Findings based on special exposure groups are subject to many of the same confounding issues as ecologic studies. Many factors, both dietary and nondietary, are likely to distinguish these special groups from the comparison population. Thus, another possible explanation for the lower colon cancer incidence and mortality among the Seventh-Day Adventist population is that differences in rates are attributable to a lower intake of alcohol, lower rates of smoking, or higher intake of vegetables. Given the many possible alternative explanations, such studies may be particularly useful when a hypothesized association is *not* observed. For example, the finding that the breast cancer mortality rate among the Seventh-Day Adventists is not appreciably different from the rate among the general US population suggests that eating meat is not a major cause of breast cancer.

Migrant Studies and Secular Trends

Migrant studies have been particularly useful in addressing the possibility that the correlations observed in the ecologic studies are due to genetic factors. For most cancers, populations migrating from an area with its own pattern of cancer incidence rates acquire rates characteristic of their new location,[16-19] although, for a few tumor sites, this change occurs only after several generations.[20,21]

Therefore, genetic factors cannot be primarily responsible for the large differences in cancer rates among these countries. Migrant studies may also be useful for examining the induction time, that is, the timing of exposure most relevant to disease onset.

Major changes in the rates of a disease within a population over time provide evidence that non-genetic factors play an important role in the etiology of that disease. In Japan, for example, rates of colon cancer have risen dramatically since 1950.[22] These secular changes clearly demonstrate the role of environmental factors, possibly including diet. The effects of environmental factors do not preclude simultaneous effects of genetic factors, which may influence who becomes affected within a population.

Case-Control and Cohort Studies

Many weaknesses of ecologic studies are potentially avoidable in case-control studies or cohort investigations. In such studies, the confounding effects of other factors can be controlled either in the design or in the analysis if good information has been collected on these variables. Furthermore, dietary information can be obtained for the individuals in the study, rather than using the average intake of the population.

Unfortunately, consistently valid results are difficult to obtain from case-control studies of dietary factors and disease because of the inherent potential for methodologic bias in those of retrospective design. This potential for bias is not unique for diet but is likely to be unusually serious for several reasons. Owing to the limited range of variation in diet within most populations and some inevitable error in measuring intake, realistic relative risks in most studies of diet and disease are likely to represent modest associations, within the range of 0.5 to 2.0, even for extreme categories of intake. These relative risks may seem to reflect modest effects, but the public-health impact may be substantial because the prevalence of exposure is often high. Given typical distributions of dietary intake, these relative risks are usually based on differences in means for cases and controls of only about 5%.[23] Thus, a systematic error of even 2% or 3% can seriously distort such a relation. In retrospective case-control studies, biases (due to selection or recall) of this magnitude could easily occur, and it is extremely difficult to exclude the possibility that this degree of bias has occurred in any specific study. Hence, it is not surprising that retrospective case-control studies of dietary factors have often provided inconsistent findings.

The selection of an appropriate control group for a study of diet and disease is also usually problematic. One common practice in hospital-based case-control studies is to use patients with another disease to provide the controls, with the assumption that the exposure under study is unrelated to the condition of this control group. Because diet may influence the incidence of many diseases, it is often difficult to identify disease groups that are, with confidence, unrelated to the aspect of diet under investigation. A common alternative is to use a sample of persons from the general population as the control group. In many areas, particularly large cities, participation rates are low; it is common for only 60% or 70% of eligible population controls to complete an interview.[24] Since diet is particularly associated with general health consciousness, the diets of those who participate are likely to differ substantially from those who do not, introducing an important bias even before the data are collected.

The potential opportunities for bias in case-control studies of diet raise a concern that spurious associations may frequently occur. To assess the magnitude of bias due to a case-control design, in two large prospective cohort studies of diet and cancer, the diets of breast cancer cases and a sample of controls were also assessed retrospectively. In one study, no evidence of recall bias was observed,[25] but in the other, the combination of recall and selection bias seriously distorted associations with fat intake.[26] Even if many studies arrive at correct conclusions, distortion of true associations in a substantial percentage would produce an inconsistent body of published data, making a coherent synthesis difficult or impossible for a specific diet and cancer relation. Additional sources of inconsistency may also be present in nutritional epidemiology owing to the inherent biologic complexity resulting from nutrient-nutrient interactions. Because the effect of one nutrient may depend on the level of another (which can differ between studies and may not have been measured), interactions may result in apparently inconsistent findings in epidemiologic studies. Thus, biologic complexity compounded with methodologic inconsistency may result in a literature that is a challenge to interpret.

Prospective cohort studies reduce most of the potential sources of methodologic bias associated with retrospective case-control investigations. Because the dietary information is collected before the diagnosis of disease, illness should not affect the recall of diet. Although losses to follow-up that vary by level of dietary factors can result in distorted associations in a cohort study, follow-up rates tend to be high because participants have already provided evidence of willingness to participate. Also, in prospective studies, participants may be followed passively by means of disease registries and vital statistics listings,[27] although information on time-dependent variables (which might include diet) would be lost with only registry-based follow-up. A sufficient number of prospective cohort studies have now been published to compare their results with those of case-control investigations of the same relations. For total dietary fat and breast cancer, the associations in case-control studies have been heterogeneous, but, in a meta-analysis,[28] a small but precisely estimated positive association was seen (see Figure 42-1A). In contrast, prospective cohort studies on the same topic have consistently found little relation between total fat intake and breast cancer risk, and a pooled analysis of primary data showed no overall association.[29] Even more strikingly, total fat intake had been positively associated with risk of lung cancer in several case-control studies, but the findings were highly inconsistent (see Figure 42-1B). In contrast, findings from prospective cohort studies have been consistently null.[35] As another example, an apparent protective effect of fruits and vegetables had been seen so frequently in case-control studies and lung cancer that this relation was thought to be established.[36] In prospective cohort studies, however, the findings have been far weaker, and, in a pooled analysis, there was little overall association.[37] The available evidence now strongly suggests that retrospective case-control studies of the effects of dietary factors on the risks of disease are often misleading.

In addition to being less susceptible to recall and selection bias, prospective studies provide the opportunity to obtain repeated assessments of diet over time and to examine the effects of diet on a wide variety of diseases, including total mortality, simultaneously. The primary constraints on prospective cohort studies of diet are practical. Even for common diseases such as CHD or breast cancer, it is necessary to enroll tens of thousands of subjects to have reasonable precision to measure effects. The use of structured, self-administered questionnaires has made studies of this size possible, although still expensive. For diseases of somewhat lower frequency, however, even very large cohorts will not accumulate a sufficient number of cases within a reasonable amount of time. Therefore, case-control studies will continue to play some role in nutritional epidemiology but should be designed and interpreted with the preceding limitations in mind.

Experimental Studies

The most rigorous evaluation of a dietary hypothesis is the randomized trial, optimally conducted as a double-blind experiment. The principal strength of a randomized trial is that risk factors other than the intervention variable should be distributed at random between the treatment and control groups, thus permitting reliable calculation of the probability that any observed relation is due to chance. The investigator can reduce this probability below any threshold he or she desires by increasing the study size, thereby reducing the possibility of confounding by extraneous factors to an acceptable level. In addition, it is sometimes possible to create a larger dietary contrast between the groups being compared by use of an active intervention. Such experiments among humans, which are almost always costly, are best justified after considerable nonexperimental data have been collected to ensure that benefit is reasonably probable and that an adverse outcome is unlikely. Experimental studies are particularly practical for evaluating hypotheses that minor components of the diet, such as trace elements or vitamins, can prevent cancer because these nutrients can be formulated into pills or capsules.

Even if feasible, randomized trials of dietary factors and disease are likely to encounter several limitations. The time between change in the level of a dietary factor and any expected change in the incidence of disease is typically uncertain. Therefore, if an effect is not found, it will usually be difficult to eliminate the possibility that the follow-up was of insufficient duration. Compliance with the treatment diet is likely to decrease during an extended trial, particularly if treatment involves a real change in food intake, and the comparison group may well adopt the dietary behavior of the treatment group if the treatment diet is thought to be beneficial. Such trends, which were found in

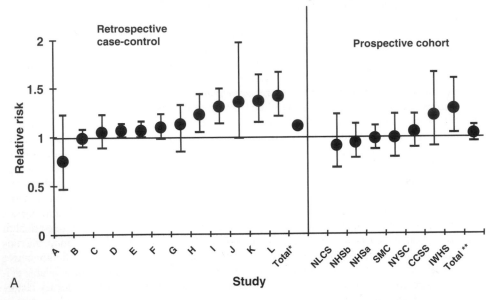

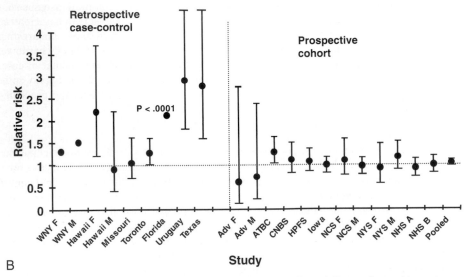

FIGURE 42-1 Comparison of results for case-control studies of total dietary fat and breast cancer (A) and of dietary fat and lung cancer (B). Retrospective case-control studies of breast cancer were summarized by Howe et al.,[28] and prospective cohort studies were summarized by Hunter et al.[29] Retrospective case-control studies of lung cancer included those by Byers et al.,[30] Goodman et al.,[31] Mohr et al.,[32] De Stefani et al.,[33] and Alavanja et al.[34] Prospective cohort studies of lung cancer were summarized by Smith-Warner et al.[35]

the Multiple Risk Factor Intervention Trial of coronary disease prevention,[38] may obscure a real benefit of the treatment.

The more recent case of the Women's Health Initiative low-fat dietary trial provides an additional example of the difficulty of maintaining a substantial contrast in diet between groups.[39] The investigators expected a 14% of energy difference in fat intake between groups, but the difference based on self-reported intake was only 9% of energy. Further, this difference is almost certainly greater than the reality because of the general tendency of humans to over-report compliance with interventions.[1] Notably, two biomarkers that would be expected to change with reductions in dietary fat, plasma levels of triglycerides and high-density lipoprotein (HDL) cholesterol, were not much different between the dietary groups during follow-up, which provides strong evidence of little difference in dietary fat between the randomized groups.

A related potential limitation of trials is that participants who enroll in such studies tend to be highly selected based on health consciousness and motivation. Therefore, it is likely that the subjects at highest potential risk because of their diet, and who are thus susceptible to intervention, are seriously underrepresented. For example, if low β-carotene intake is thought to be a risk factor for lung cancer and a trial of β-carotene supplementation is conducted among a health-conscious population that includes few individuals with low β-carotene intake, one might see no effect simply because many persons in the study population were already receiving the maximal benefit of this nutrient through their usual diet. In such an instance, it would be useful to measure dietary intake of β-carotene before starting the trial. Because the effect of supplementation is likely to be greatest among those with low dietary intakes, it would be possible either to exclude those with high intakes (for whom supplementation would likely have little effect) either before randomization or in subanalyses after the study. This approach requires a reasonable measurement of dietary intake at the study's outset.

Trials are sometimes said to provide a better quantitative measurement of the effect of an exposure or treatment because the difference in exposure between groups is better measured than in a nonexperimental study. Although this contrast may at times be better defined in a trial (it is usually clouded by some degree of noncompliance; see Chapter 6), trials still usually produce an imprecise measure of the effect of exposure on the outcome, owing to marginally adequate study sizes and ethical considerations that require stopping a trial after interim analyses showing benefit. For example, were a trial stopped with a P-value close to 0.05, the corresponding 95% confidence interval would likely extend from a lower bound of no effect to an upper bound indicating an implausibly strong effect. In a nonexperimental study, interim analyses do not create an ethical imperative to stop the study early so long as the interim results are published. Continued accumulation of data can therefore improve the precision of the estimated relation between exposure and disease. On the other hand, a trial can provide information on the induction period between change in an exposure and change in diet, whereas estimation of induction periods for dietary effects will usually be difficult in nonexperimental studies because spontaneous changes in diet are typically not clearly demarcated in time.

Practical or ethical reasons often preclude randomized trials in humans. For example, our knowledge of the effects of cigarette smoking on risk of lung cancer is based entirely on observational studies, and it is similarly unlikely that randomized trials could be conducted to examine the effect of alcohol use on human breast cancer risk. It is unlikely that cancer-prevention trials of sufficient size, duration, and degree of compliance can be conducted to evaluate many hypotheses that involve major behavioral changes in eating patterns. For these hypotheses, nonexperimental studies will continue to provide the best available data to understand the relation between diet and disease.

Measurement of Diet in Epidemiologic Studies

The complexity of the human diet represents a daunting challenge to anyone contemplating a study of its relation to chronic diseases such as cancer. The foods we consume each day contain literally thousands of specific chemicals, some known and well quantified, some characterized only poorly, and others completely undescribed and presently unmeasurable. In human diets, intakes of various components tend to be correlated. With few exceptions, all individuals are exposed; for example, everyone eats fat, fiber, and vitamin A. Thus, dietary exposures can rarely be characterized as present or absent; rather, they are continuous variables, often with rather limited range of variation between persons with a common culture or geographic location. Furthermore, individuals are generally not aware of the composition of the foods that they eat; hence, the consumption of nutrients is usually determined indirectly.

Nutrients, Foods, and Dietary Patterns

Throughout nutrition in general and in much of the existing nutritional epidemiology literature, diet has usually been described in terms of its nutrient content. Alternatively, diet can be described in terms of foods, food groups, or overall dietary patterns. The primary advantage of representing diets as specific compounds, such as nutrients, is that such information can be related directly to our fundamental knowledge of biology. From a practical perspective, the exact structure of a compound must usually be known if it is to be synthesized and used for supplementation or fortification. Also, measurement of total intake of a nutrient (as opposed to using the contribution of only one food at a time) provides the most powerful test of a hypothesis, particularly if many foods each contribute only modestly to intake of that nutrient. For example, in a particular study, it is quite possible that total fat intake could be clearly associated with risk of disease, whereas none of the contributions to fat intake by individual foods would be strongly related to disease on their own.

On the other hand, the use of foods to represent diet also has several practical advantages when examining relations with disease. Particularly when suspicion exists that some aspect of diet is associated with risk but a specific hypothesis has not been formulated, an examination of the relations of foods and food groups with risk of disease will provide a means to explore the data. Associations observed with specific foods may lead to a hypothesis relating to a defined chemical substance. For example, observations that higher intakes of green and yellow vegetables were associated with reduced rates of lung cancer led to the hypothesis that β-carotene might protect DNA from damage due to free radicals and singlet oxygen.[40] The finding by Graham et al.[41] that intake of cruciferous vegetables was inversely related to risk of colon cancer suggested that indole compounds contained in these vegetables may be protective.[42]

A problem even more serious than the lack of a well-formulated hypothesis, the premature focus on a specific nutrient that turns out to have no relation with disease, may lead to the erroneous conclusion that diet has no effect. Mertz[43] pointed out that foods are not fully represented by their nutrient composition, noting as an example that milk and yogurt produce different physiologic effects despite a similar nutrient content. Furthermore, the valid calculation of a nutrient intake from data on food consumption requires reasonably accurate food composition information, which markedly constrains the scope of dietary chemicals that may be investigated, because such information exists for only several dozen commonly studied nutrients. Even then, there can be considerable variation in nutrient composition that is not captured in standard food tables that have a single value for each food. If extreme, as in the case of selenium, which can vary in concentration several hundred-fold in different samples of the same food, calculated intake may be of no value.[23]

Epidemiologic analyses based on foods, as opposed to nutrients, are generally most directly related to dietary recommendations because individuals and institutions ultimately determine nutrient intake largely by their choice of foods. Even if the intake of a specific nutrient is convincingly shown to be related to risk of a disease, this relation is not sufficient information on which to make dietary recommendations. Because foods are an extremely complex mixture of different chemicals that may compete with, antagonize, or alter the bioavailability of any single nutrient contained in that food, it is not possible to predict with certainty the health effects of any food solely on the basis of its content of one specific factor. For example, there is concern that high intake of nitrates may be deleterious, particularly with respect to gastrointestinal cancer. However, the primary sources of nitrates in our diets are green, leafy vegetables which, if anything, appear to reduce risk of cancer at several sites. Similarly, because of the high cholesterol content of eggs, their avoidance has received particular attention in diets aimed at reducing the risk of CHD; per capita consumption of eggs declined by 25% in the United States between 1948 and 1980.[44] But eggs are more than cholesterol capsules; they provide a rich source of essential amino acids and micronutrients and are relatively low in saturated fat. It is thus difficult to predict the net effect of egg consumption on risk of CHD, much less the effect on overall health, without empirical evidence.

Given the strengths and weaknesses of using nutrients or foods to represent diet, an optimal approach to epidemiologic analyses will employ both. In this way, a potentially important finding is less likely to be missed. Moreover, the case for causality is strengthened when an association is observed with overall intake of a nutrient and with more than one food source of that nutrient, particularly when the food sources are otherwise different. This situation provides, in some sense, multiple assessments of the potential for confounding by other nutrients; if an association was observed for only one food source of the nutrient, other factors contained in that food would tend to be similarly associated with disease. As an example, the hypothesis that alcohol intake causes breast cancer was strengthened by observing an overall association between alcohol intake and breast cancer risk and by independent associations with both beer and liquor intake, thus making it less likely that some factor other than alcohol in these beverages is responsible for the increased risk.

One practical drawback of using foods to represent diet is their large number and the complex, often reciprocal, correlations among intakes of different foods that are due largely to individual behavioral patterns. Many reciprocal relations emerge upon perusal of typical datasets; for example, dark-bread eaters tend not to eat white bread, margarine users tend not to eat butter, and skim-milk users tend not to use whole milk. This complexity is one of the reasons to compute nutrient intakes that summarize the contributions of all foods.

An intermediate solution to the problem posed by the complex interrelations among foods is to use food groups or to compute the contribution of nutrient intake from various food groups. For example, Manousos et al.[45] combined the intakes of foods from several predefined groups to study the relation of diet with risk of colon cancer. They observed increased risk among subjects with high meat intake and with low consumption of vegetables. The computation of nutrient intakes from different food groups is illustrated by a prospective study among British bank clerks conducted by Morris et al.,[46] who observed an inverse relation between overall fiber intake and risk of CHD. It is well recognized that fiber is an extremely heterogeneous collection of substances and that the available food composition data for specific types of fiber are incomplete. Therefore, these authors computed fiber intake separately from various food groups and found that the entire protective effect was attributable to fiber from grains; fiber from fruits or vegetables was not associated with risk of disease. This analysis circumvents the inadequacy of food composition databases and provides information in a form that is directly useful to individuals faced with decisions regarding choices of foods.

In general, maximal information will be obtained when analyses are conducted at the levels of nutrients, foods, food groups, and dietary patterns. Dietary patterns take into account the complex interrelations of food consumption and are usually derived by empirical methods such as factor analysis or by creating a priori indices. The latter approach, for example, has been used to develop a Mediterranean diet index based on specific aspects of diet; this index was then found to predict lower mortality.[47] Dietary patterns are potentially useful because they combine multiple aspects of diet into one or two variables, but they lack direct biologic interpretation. It is also possible to enter the distinct levels of nutrients, foods, food groups, and dietary patterns into the same analysis through the use of hierarchical (multilevel) analysis, which allows some degree of adjustment for effects at one level (*e.g.*, the food level) when estimating effects at another level (*e.g.*, the nutrient level) and which produces more stable effect estimates.[48]

Temporal Relationships

The assessment of diet in epidemiologic studies is further complicated by the dimension of time. Because our understanding of the pathogenesis of cancers and many other diseases is limited, considerable uncertainty exists about the period of time before diagnosis for which diet might be relevant. For some cancers and CVD, diet may be important during childhood, even though the disease is diagnosed decades later. For other diseases, diet may act as a late-stage promoting or inhibiting factor; thus, intake near the time before diagnosis may be important. Ideally, data on dietary intake at different periods before diagnosis could help to resolve these issues, which have great practical importance in study design and when considering interventions. Individuals rarely make clear changes in their diet at identifiable points in time; more typically, eating patterns evolve over periods of years. Thus, in case-control studies, epidemiologists often direct questions about diet to a period several years before diagnosis of disease with the hope that diet at this point in time will represent, or at least be correlated with, diet during the critical period in cancer development. In long-term cohort studies, especially with repeated measures of diet, relative risks for different induction periods between assessment of diet and diagnosis of disease can be evaluated directly.[49]

Fortunately, diets of individuals do tend to be correlated from year to year, so that some imprecision in identification of critical periods of exposure may not be serious. For most nutrients, correlations for repeated assessments of diet at intervals from 1 year to about 5 years tend to be of the order of 0.6 to 0.7,[1,50,51] with decreasing correlations over longer intervals.[52] For scientists accustomed to measurements made under highly controlled conditions in a laboratory, this correlation may seem like a low degree of reproducibility. Nevertheless, these correlations are similar to correlations of other biologic measurements made in free-living populations over equivalent time intervals, such as serum cholesterol[53] and blood pressure.[54]

Even though diets of individuals have a strong element of consistency over intervals of several years, they are characterized by marked variation from day to day.[1,55] This variation differs from nutrient to nutrient, being moderate for total energy intake but extremely large for cholesterol and vitamin A. For this reason, even perfect information about diet on any single day or the average of a small number of days will poorly represent long-term average intake, which is likely to be more relevant to etiology of most diseases.

General Methods of Dietary Assessment

Three general approaches have been used to assess dietary intake: information about intake of foods that can be used directly or to calculate intake of nutrients, biochemical measurements using blood or other body tissues that provide indicators of diet, and measures of body dimensions or composition that reflect the long-term effects of diet. Because the interpretation of data on diet and disease is heavily influenced by the methods used to assess diet, features of these methods and their limitations will be considered.

Methods Based on Food Intake

Short-Term Recall and Diet Records

The 24-hour recall, in which subjects are asked to report their food intake during the previous day, has been the most widely used dietary assessment method. It has been the basis of most national nutrition surveys and many cohort studies of CHD. Interviews are conducted by nutritionists or trained interviewers, usually using visual aids such as food models or shapes to obtain data on quantities of foods, and are now often computer-assisted to standardize the technique and facilitate data entry. The 24-hour recall requires about 10 to 20 minutes for an experienced interviewer. Although it has traditionally been conducted in person, it has also been done by telephone using a visual aid that is mailed beforehand to assist in the estimation of portion sizes.[56] This method has the advantages of requiring no training or literacy and little effort on the part of the participant. More recently, interactive web-based methods have been developed that require no interviewer[57]; this approach greatly reduces the cost of data collection but increases the burden on the participant, including the time commitment.

Dietary records or food diaries are detailed meal-by-meal recordings of types and quantities of foods and beverages consumed during a specified period, typically 3 to 7 days. Ideally, subjects weigh each portion of food before eating, although doing so is frequently impossible for all meals, as many are eaten away from home. Alternatively, household measures can be used to estimate portion sizes. The method places a considerable burden on the subject, thus limiting its application to those who are literate and highly motivated. In addition, the effort involved in keeping diet records may increase awareness of food intake and induce an alteration in diet. Nevertheless, diet recording has the advantages of not depending on memory and allowing direct measurements of portion sizes.

The validity of 24-hour recalls has been assessed by observing the actual intake of subjects in a controlled environment and interviewing them the next day. In such a study, Karvetti and Knuts[58] observed that subjects both erroneously recalled foods that were not actually eaten and omitted foods that were eaten; correlations between nutrients calculated from observed intakes and calculations from the recalled information ranged from 0.58 to 0.74. In a similar study among elderly persons, Madden et al.[59] found correlations ranging from 0.28 to 0.87. These validation methods evaluate the reporting of what is eaten on the specific day of assessment but do not address the validity of the method as a representation of long-term intake, which is centrally important to epidemiologists. As described below, the validity of long-term intake has recently been evaluated by comparisons of intakes with "recovery" biomarkers, biomarkers using 24-hour urine samples that reflect absolute intakes of energy, protein, nitrogen, and sodium. In an analysis pooling data from several studies,[60-62] for potassium, potassium density (absolute intake divided by energy intake), sodium, sodium density, and the potassium/sodium ratio, correlation coefficients between a single 24-hour recall and "true" intake assessed by biomarkers were 0.47, 0.46, 0.32, 0.31, and 0.46, respectively. When the average of three 24-hour recalls was used, these correlations increased to 0.56, 0.53, 0.41, 0.38, and 0.60. The correlations were probably overestimated because, in some studies, the intake and biomarker assessments were close in time; to assess the ability to measure longer term intake, these measurements should be at least several months apart. In a large study in which the 24-hour recalls and biomarker assessments were by design separated in time, the correlations were somewhat weaker for sodium.[63]

The most serious limitation of the 24-hour recall method is that dietary intake is highly variable from day-to-day. Diet records reduce the problem of day-to-day variation because the average of a number of days is used. For nutrients that vary substantially, however, even 3 or 4 days of recording may not provide an accurate estimate of an individual's average intake.[55,63-66] The variability in intake of specific foods is even greater than for nutrients,[67,68] so only commonly eaten foods can be studied by this method. The problem of day-to-day variation is not an issue if the objective of a study is to estimate a mean intake for a population, as might be the goal in an ecologic study. In case-control or cohort investigations, however, accurate estimation of individual intakes is necessary.

Practical considerations and issues of study design further limit the application of short-term recall and diet-record methods in epidemiologic studies. Because they provide information on current diet, their use will typically be inappropriate in case-control studies because the relevant exposure will have occurred earlier and diet may have changed because of the disease or its treatment. A few exceptions may occur, as in the case of very early tumors or premalignant lesions. Although the average of multiple days of 24-hour recalls or diet recording could theoretically be used in prospective cohort studies of diet, the costs are usually prohibitive because of the large numbers of subjects required and the substantial expense involved in collecting this information and processing it. These methods, however, can play an important role in the validation or calibration of other methods of dietary assessment that are more practical for epidemiologic studies.[66] With much lower costs of obtaining 24-hour recall data by interactive web-based methods, it is possible that combining results from a few days of 24-hour recalls with those from other methods may provide additional independent information.[69]

Food-Frequency Questionnaires

Because short-term recall and diet-record methods are generally expensive, unrepresentative of usual intake, and inappropriate for assessment of past diet, investigators have sought alternative methods for measuring long-term dietary intake. Burke[70] developed a detailed dietary history interview that attempted to assess an individual's usual diet; this assessment included a 24-hour recall, a menu recorded for 3 days, and a checklist of foods consumed over the preceding month. This method was time-consuming and expensive because a highly skilled professional was needed for both the interview and processing of information. The checklist, however, was the forerunner of the more structured dietary questionnaires in use today. During the 1950s, Wiehl and Reed,[71] Heady,[72] Stephanik and Trulson,[73] and Marr[74] developed food-frequency questionnaires and evaluated their role in dietary assessment. In diet records collected from British bank clerks, the *frequencies* with which foods were used correlated well with the total *weights* of the same foods consumed over a several-day period, thus providing the theoretical basis for the food-frequency method.[72] Similar findings were seen in a US population.[75] Use of food-frequency questionnaires has emerged as the method of dietary assessment best suited for most epidemiologic studies. During recent years, substantial refinements, modifications, cultural customizations, and evaluations of food-frequency questionnaires have occurred, so that data derived from their use have become considerably more interpretable.

A food-frequency questionnaire consists of two main components: a food list and a frequency-response section for subjects to report how often each food was eaten (see Figure 42-2). Questions related to further details of quantity and composition may be appended, such as the types of cooking oil used or breakfast cereal usually consumed. A fundamental decision in designing a questionnaire is whether the objective is to measure intake of a few specific foods or nutrients or whether to obtain a comprehensive assessment of diet. A comprehensive assessment is generally desirable whenever possible. It is often impossible to anticipate at the beginning of a study all the questions

Foods and amounts	Never or less than once per month	1-3 per mo	1 per wk	2-4 per wk	5-6 per wk	1 per day	2-3 per day	4-5 per day	6+ per day
A Eggs (1)	○	○	Ⓦ	○	○	●	○	○	○
B Whole milk (8-oz glass)	○	○	Ⓦ	○	○	Ⓓ	●	○	○
C Ice cream (1/2 cup)	○	○	Ⓦ	○	●	Ⓓ	○	○	○

FIGURE 42-2 Section from a food-frequency questionnaire completed by several large cohorts of men and women. For each food listed, participants were asked to indicate how often, on average, they had used the amount specified during the past year. Example of calculation of daily cholesterol intake: From a food composition table, the cholesterol contents are: 1 egg = 274 mg; 1 glass of milk = 33 mg; ½ cup of ice cream = 29.5 mg. Thus, the average daily cholesterol intake for the person completing this abbreviated questionnaire would be (274 mg × 1) + (33 mg × 2.5) + (29.5 mg × 0.8) = 380.1 mg/d. (Reproduced with permission from Sampson L. Food frequency questionnaires as a research instrument. *Clin Nutr.* 1985;4:171-178.)

regarding diet that will appear important at the end of data collection; a highly restricted food list may not have included an item that is, in retrospect, important. Furthermore, as described later in this chapter, total food intake, represented by total energy consumption, may confound the effects of specific nutrients or foods or create extraneous variation in specific nutrients; being able to adjust for energy intake is thus a great advantage. Nevertheless, epidemiologic practice is usually a compromise between the ideal and reality, and it may simply be impossible to include a comprehensive diet assessment in an interview or questionnaire, especially if diet is not the primary focus of the study.

Because diets tend to be reasonably correlated from year to year, most investigators have asked subjects to describe the frequency of their using foods in reference to the preceding year. This interval provides a full cycle of seasons so that, in theory, the responses should be independent of the time of year. In case-control studies, the time frame could be in reference to a period of a specified number of preceding years.

Typically, investigators have provided a multiple-choice response format, with the number of options usually ranging from 5 to 10 (Figure 42-2). Another approach is to use an open-ended format and provide subjects the option of answering in terms of frequency per day, week, or month.[77] In theory, an open-ended frequency-response format might provide for some enhanced precision in reporting, because the frequency of use is truly a continuous rather than a categorical variable. Nevertheless, it is unlikely that the overall increment in precision is large because the estimation of the frequency of use of a food is inherently an approximation.

Several options exist for collecting additional data on serving sizes. The first is to collect no additional information on portion sizes at all—that is, to use a simple frequency questionnaire. A second possibility is to specify a portion size as part of the question on frequency—for example, to ask how often a glass of milk is consumed rather than only how often milk is consumed. This technique has been termed a *semiquantitative* food-frequency questionnaire. A third alternative is to include an additional question for each food to describe the usual portion size in words,[73] using food models,[78] or using pictures of different portion sizes.[79] Because most of the variation in intake of a food is explained by frequency of use rather than differences in serving sizes, portion-size data are relatively unimportant.[80-82] Cummings et al.[83] found that adding questions on portion sizes to a simple frequency questionnaire only slightly improved estimation of calcium intake, and others have found that the use of food models in an in-person interview did not increase the validity of a self-administered semiquantitative food-frequency questionnaire.[84] These findings have practical implications because the cost of data collection by mail or telephone is far less than the cost of personal interviews, which are necessary if food models are to be used for assessing portion sizes. Cohen et al.[85] also found that the portion-size information included in the Block questionnaire added only slightly to agreement with diet records (average correlation of 0.41 without portion sizes and 0.43 with portion sizes).

Food-frequency questionnaires are extremely practical in epidemiologic applications because they are easy for subjects to complete, often as a self-administered form that can be optically scanned. Processing is readily computerized and inexpensive, so that their use in prospective studies involving repeated assessments of diet among many tens of thousands of subjects is feasible.

Validity of Dietary Assessment Methods

The interpretation of epidemiologic data on diet and disease depends directly on the validity of the methods used to measure dietary intake, particularly when no association is found, because one possible explanation could be that the method used to measure diet was not able to discriminate among study participants. A substantial body of evidence has accumulated regarding the validity of dietary assessment method—especially food-frequency questionnaires—because of their widespread use.

In evaluating the validity of a dietary assessment method, the choice of a standard for comparison is a critical issue because no perfect standard exists. A desirable feature for the comparison method is that its errors be independent of the method being evaluated, so that an artificial correlation will not be observed. For this reason, biochemical indicators of diet are probably the optimal standard. Their greatest limitation is that specific markers of diet do not exist for most of the nutrients of current interest, such as total fat, fiber, and sucrose intake. Moreover, the available biochemical indicators of diet are likely to be imprecise measures of diet because they are influenced by many factors, such as differences in absorption and metabolism, short-term biologic variation, and laboratory measurement error. Even biochemical measures that specially reflect dietary intake are subject to within-person variation over time because of variation in diet. Despite these limitations, for biochemical indicators that are sensitive to intake, a correlation between a questionnaire estimate of nutrient intake and the indicator can provide a useful qualitative measure of the validity of the questionnaire estimate. Such correlations have been reported for questionnaire estimates of a variety of nutrients.[86-97] For example, in controlled feeding studies, dietary fat reduces blood triglyceride levels; thus, documentation that total fat intake assessed by a food-frequency questionnaire was inversely associated with blood triglycerides provides important support for the validity of the questionnaire assessment.[98] For a small number of nutrients, including total energy, protein, sodium, and potassium, measurements of 24-hour urinary samples can provide a good estimate of absolute intakes and have been termed "recovery biomarkers." The issue of within-person variation can be addressed by collecting multiple 24-hour urine samples and using statistical techniques to correct for this source of variation to obtain an estimate of "true" intake. Because of the high cost of these measurements, they have mainly been used as gold standards in studies to evaluate the validity of other measures of intake.

Because of the cost of collecting and analyzing samples for biomarkers of diet, most validation studies have instead compared intakes assessed by standardized questionnaires with intakes based on other dietary assessment methods. Among the possible comparison methods, diet records are particularly attractive because they do not depend on memory, and, when weighing scales are used to assess portion sizes, do not depend on perception of amounts of foods eaten. These characteristics tend to reduce correlated errors; because 24-hour recalls share many cognitive demands with food-frequency questionnaires, they are, in principle, less than ideal. Despite this, in a recent validation study, similar correlations were obtained when nutrients calculated from a semiquantitative food-frequency questionnaire were compared with both diet records and multiple 24-hour recalls.[66] Although the detail of questionnaires and the populations studied have varied substantially, the correlation between nutrients assessed by food-frequency questionnaires and the comparison methods, when adjusted for total energy intake, has consistently varied between 0.4 and 0.7.[1] Four comprehensive validation studies that compared questionnaires completed at about a 1-year interval with multiple diet records collected during the intervening months reported similar degrees of correlation.[64,65,86,99,100] For questionnaires completed at the end of the 1-year recording of diet (which corresponds to the time frame of the questionnaires), correlations adjusted for total energy intake tended to be mainly between 0.5 and 0.7. Although the food supply and eating habits have evolved since these validation studies were conducted, a 2017 validation study conducted among 632 participants in the Nurses' Health Study found almost identical results as those seen in the 1980s.[66] Although these studies assessed the validity of a single dietary question over a 1-year period, the time frame of interest in most epidemiologic studies encompasses multiple years. In the Nurses' Health Study, 90 women participated in two validation studies 6 years apart; the validity of the average of three food-frequency questionnaires to represent this longer period was substantially higher than seen in the validation studies using just one questionnaire, supporting the value of obtaining repeated dietary questionnaires in cohort studies.

Subar et al.[101] used doubly labeled water and urinary nitrogen as biomarkers of energy and protein intake to assess the validity of a food-frequency questionnaire and 24-hour dietary recalls. The authors concluded errors in the 24-hour recalls and food-frequency questionnaires are correlated, and therefore that earlier studies using 24-hour recalls and food-frequency questionnaires as comparison methods have seriously overstated validity. Subar et al. did not, however, obtain a realistic measure of the within-person variation in their biomarkers (*e.g.*, at an interval of 6-12 months), and failure to account for this variation may have created the false impression of correlated error.[102]

In the 2017 Nurses' Health validation study, energy-adjusted protein intake assessed by food frequency questionnaire was similarly correlated with intake assessed by these biomarkers or by weighed diet records, indicating that correlated errors have not seriously overstated validity when diet records were used as the gold standard. Because this study included both recovery biomarkers and extensive plasma biomarkers that reflect dietary intake and also intakes assessed by 24-hour recall (4 days), weighed diet records (two 1-week records), and food-frequency questionnaire, it was possible to compare each of these dietary assessment methods with the corresponding biomarkers.[63] Because these biomarkers are also influenced by many factors in addition to diet, these correlations do not represent correlations with true intake but do provide an evaluation of the *relative validity* of these three measures of diet (see Figure 42-3 for example). Overall, for energy-adjusted intakes, the best measure was 2 weeks of weighed diet record and 1 week was

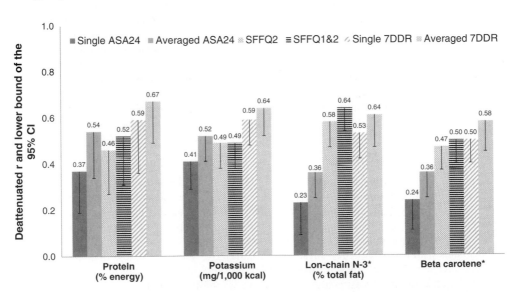

*Subgroups of women who did not take supplements for this nutrient (N= 363 for long-chain N-3 fatty acids, and 335 for beta-carotene).

FIGURE 42-3 Deattenuated Spearman correlation coefficients (and lower bound of the 95% CI) between diet assessed by FFQ's, 24-hour recalls, and 1-week diet records and biomarkers of diet (n = 627 US female nurses aged 45-80 years)[63]. FFQ, food-frequency questionnaire. (From Yuan C, Spiegelman D, Rimm EB, et al. Relative validity of nutrient intakes assessed by questionnaire, 24-hour recalls, and diet records compared with urinary recovery and plasma concentration biomarkers: findings for women. *Am J Epidemiol*. 2018;187(5):1051-1063.)

only slightly inferior. For most nutrients, the food-frequency measures were similar to 1 week of weighed diet record. For nutrients with lower within-person variation (*e.g.*, protein and potassium), the multiple 24-hour recalls were similar to the food-frequency questionnaire, and a single 24-hour recall was the least valid. For nutrients with higher within-person variation, such as beta-carotene and n-3 fatty acids, the multiple 24-hour recalls were inferior to the food-frequency questionnaire. Because most foods have relatively high within-person variation, the data for beta-carotene and n-3 fatty acids are probably representative of relative validity of the different dietary assessment methods for these foods.

Although the degree of measurement error associated with nutrient estimates calculated from food-frequency questionnaires appears to be similar to that for many epidemiologic measures, measurement errors from using a single questionnaire can result in important underestimates of relative risks, and errors in confounding nutrients tend to lead to loss of control for confounding (see Chapter 13). Less commonly appreciated, the errors will also result in observed confidence intervals that are inappropriately narrow, as the confidence intervals reflect only random error and fail to account for the biases from misclassification. To form inferences properly cautioned by data limitations, one should consider the entire range of possible relative risks that are reasonably compatible with the data (see Chapter 29). In part, generated by the interest in diet and cancer and the recognized issue of measurement error in assessing dietary intake, considerable effort has been directed to the development of methods that provide bias-adjusted estimates of relative risks and confidence intervals based on quantitative assessments of measurement error.[103] Thus, validation studies of dietary questionnaires can provide important estimates of error that can be used to interpret quantitatively the influence of error on observed associations. Based on such analyses, it can be shown that important associations will generally not be missed by typical dietary questionnaires,[104,105] although study sizes will need to be several times larger than those estimated assuming that measurement error did not exist.[106] As noted above, one valuable way to improve measurement of diet in a longitudinal study is to repeat the dietary assessments over time. This repetition will tend to dampen random (nonsystematic) error and will also account for true changes in intake.[107] The repeated questionnaires, with adequate follow-up time, will also provide the ability to assess the effects of changes in diet.

Technological advancements have already contributed greatly to dietary assessment by allowing more efficient and accurate collection and analysis of dietary data using optical scanning, computer-assisted interviewing, and web-based interactive programs. Much interest exists in newer methods such as optical recognition of foods using smartphones or wearable sensors to assess food intake. Whether these approaches will provide important improvements beyond existing methods remains an open question. Important barriers include the difficulties of making important distinctions visually, for example, between a diet soda versus a regular soda or the content of beef burger versus a vegetarian burger. These new approaches will need rigorous evaluation, including a comparison with currently available methods.

Biochemical Indicators of Diet

The use of biochemical measurements made on blood or other tissues as indicators of nutrient intake is attractive because such measurements do not depend on the memory or knowledge of the subject. Furthermore, they can be made in retrospect, for example, using blood specimens that have been collected and stored for other purposes. As noted above, they can also serve as the reference method when evaluating the validity of dietary intake methods.

Choice of Tissues for Analysis

Most commonly, serum or plasma has been used in epidemiologic studies to measure biochemical indicators of diet. Consideration should also be given, however, to red blood cells, subcutaneous fat, hair, and nails. The choices should be governed by the ability of the tissue to reflect dietary intake of the factor of interest; the time-integrating characteristics of the tissue; practical considerations in collecting, transporting, and storing the specimen; and cost. These considerations are examined in detail elsewhere for a number of dietary factors[108]; some general comments are provided here.

Red Blood Cells

For some dietary factors, red cells are less sensitive to short-term fluctuations in diet than plasma or serum and may thus provide a better index of long-term exposure. Nutrients that can be usefully measured in red cells include fatty acids, folic acid, and selenium.

Subcutaneous Fat

Composed primarily of fatty acids, the adipose tissue turns over slowly among individuals with relatively stable weight. For at least some fatty acids, the half-life is of the order of 600 days, making this an ideal indicator of long-term diet in epidemiologic studies. Fat-soluble vitamins such as retinol, vitamin E, and carotenoids are also measurable in subcutaneous fat, but these measurements may not be superior to food-frequency questionnaires as a measure of intake.[109]

Hair and Nails

Hair and nails incorporate many elements into their matrix during formation, and, for many heavy metals, these may be the tissues of choice because these elements tend to be cleared rapidly from the blood. Nails appear to be the optimal tissue for the assessment of long-term selenium intake owing to their capacity to integrate exposure over time.[110] Because the hair and nails can be cut at various times after formation (a few weeks for hair close to the scalp and approximately 1 year for the great toe), an index of exposure can be obtained that may be little affected by recent experiences. This information can be an advantage in the context of a case-control study of diet and cancer because they do not rely on participant self-report. Contamination poses the greatest problem for measurements in hair owing to its intense exposure to the environment and very large surface area; these problems are generally much less for nails but still need to be considered.

Limitations of Biochemical Indicators

Although the use of biochemical indicators for assessing diet is attractive, no practical indicator exists for many dietary factors. Even when tissue levels of a nutrient can be measured, these levels are often highly regulated and thus poorly reflect dietary intake; blood retinol and cholesterol are good examples. Just as with dietary intake, the blood levels of some nutrients fluctuate substantially over time, so one measurement may not provide a good reflection of long-term intake. Furthermore, experience has provided sobering evidence that the tissue levels of many nutrients can be affected by the presence of cancer or other chronic diseases, even several years before diagnosis,[111] rendering the use of many biochemical indicators invalid in most retrospective case-control studies. Despite these limitations, careful application of biochemical indicators can provide important information about dietary intake, particularly for nutrients or food contaminants that cannot be accurately calculated from data on food intake.

Anthropometry and Measures of Body Composition

Energy balance at various times in life has important effects on the incidence of many diseases. Energy balance is better reflected by measurements of body size and composition than by assessments based on the difference between energy intake and expenditure (largely physical activity) because both of these variables are measured with considerable error.[1]

The most common use of anthropometric measurements in epidemiology is to calculate estimates of adiposity using either indices such as body mass index (BMI, also called Quetelet index) (weight in kilograms divided by the second power of height in meters) or relative weight (weight standardized for height). Remarkably valid estimates of weight and height can be obtained even by questioning,[112] including their recall several decades earlier.[113,114] Thus, good assessments of adiposity can be obtained easily for large prospective investigations or retrospectively in the context of case-control studies. The major limitation of adiposity estimates based on height and weight is that they cannot differentiate between fat and lean body mass. Studies of the validity of the BMI as a measure of obesity have commonly used as a "gold standard" body fat expressed as a percentage of total weight, usually determined by underwater weighing, or more recently by dual x-ray absorptiometry (DEXA). BMI, however, is actually a measure of fat mass adjusted for height rather than a measure of percentage body fat. When fat mass determined from densitometry is adjusted for height and used as the standard, the correlation with BMI is approximately 0.90 among young and middle-aged adults, indicating a substantially higher degree of validity than has generally been appreciated.[115] Moreover, in the same study, fat mass adjusted for height correlated more strongly with biologically relevant variables such as blood pressure and fasting blood glucose than did percentage body fat. Similar findings were seen when DEXA was used as the "gold standard."[116] BMI may be less valid as an index of adiposity among the elderly, however, because variation in loss of lean body mass contributes more importantly to weight during this period of life.

The use of one or a small number of skin-fold thicknesses does not appear to be appreciably more accurate than weight and height in the estimation of overall adiposity among young and middle-aged adults, but it can provide additional information on the distribution of body fat. The ratio of waist to hip circumference, or waist circumference alone, provides information on adiposity that adds independently, beyond BMI alone, to predictions of obesity-related conditions.[117] This additional prediction may be, in part, because central fat functions metabolically differently from peripheral fat and also because these circumference measurements help distinguish fat mass from muscle mass.

Height has often been ignored as a variable of potential interest in epidemiologic studies, perhaps because analysts fail to recognize that it is not addressed by control for BMI. Height can, however, provide unique information on energy balance during the years before adulthood, a time period that may be important in the development of some cancers that occur many years later. For example, in many studies, height has been positively associated with risk of breast and other cancers.[118,119] Furthermore, this information can be valid even in the context of case-control studies, because height will usually be unaffected even if illness has caused recent weight loss. Therefore, height should not be excluded from consideration just because BMI or another weight-for-height-based index is included in the analysis.[120]

CENTRAL METHODOLOGIC ISSUES IN NUTRITIONAL EPIDEMIOLOGY

Between-Person Variation in Dietary Intake

In addition to the availability of a sufficiently precise method for measuring dietary intake, an adequate degree of variation in diet is necessary to conduct observational studies within populations. If no variation in diet exists among persons, no association can be observed. Some have argued that the diets in populations such as the United States are too homogeneous to study relations with disease.[6,12,13] The true between-person variation in diet is difficult to measure directly and generally cannot be measured by the questionnaires used by epidemiologists because the observed variation will combine true differences with those due to measurement error; more quantitative methods must be used for this purpose. The fat content of the diet varies less among persons compared with most other nutrients[55]; for women in one prospective study,[121] the mean fat intake assessed by the mean of four 1-week diet records for those in the top quintile was 44% of calories, while for those in the bottom quintile, it was 32% of calories. This range of fat intake is smaller than the variation among countries, but nevertheless it is of considerable interest because this difference (12% absolute difference) corresponds closely to changes that were recommended by many organizations.[122] Other nutrients vary much more within populations than total fat intake,[1,55] and, for many nutrients and foods, the variation within a population can be much greater than the variation between populations.

Evidence that measurable and informative variation in diet exists within the US population is provided by several sources. First, the strong correlations between food-frequency questionnaires and independent assessments of diet found in the validation studies noted previously would not have been observed if variation in diet did not exist. For the same reason, the correlations between questionnaire estimates of nutrient intakes and biochemical indicators of intake provide solid evidence of measurable variation. In addition, the ability to find associations between dietary factors and incidence of disease (particularly when based on prospective data) indicates that measurable and biologically relevant variation exists. For example, reproducible inverse associations have been observed between fiber intake and risks of CHD[122] and diabetes.[123]

Although accumulated evidence has indicated that informative variation in diets exists within the US population and that these differences can be measured, it is important that findings be interpreted in the context of that variation. For example, a lack of association with fat intake within the range of 32% to 44% of energy should not be interpreted to mean that fat intake has no relation to risk of disease under any circumstance. It is possible that the relation is nonlinear and that risk changes at lower levels of fat intake (*e.g.*, <20% of total energy) or that diet has an influence much earlier in life.

Implications of Total Energy Intake

Energy balance is likely to have important associations with some cancers; however, this relation cannot be studied directly because energy intake largely reflects factors other than over- or undereating in relation to requirements.[1,124] The implications of total energy intake can be appreciated by realizing that variation among persons is to a large degree secondary to differences in body size and physical activity. Persons also appear to differ in metabolic efficiency (inefficient persons requiring higher energy intake for the same level of function); however, these differences in metabolic efficiency are not practically measurable in epidemiologic studies. Because virtually all nutrient intakes tend to be correlated with total energy intake, much of the variation in intake of specific nutrients is secondary to factors that may be unrelated to risk of disease. Nutrient intakes adjusted for total energy can be viewed conceptually as measures of nutrient composition rather than as measures of absolute intake. Measures of dietary composition are more relevant to personal decisions and public-health policy than are absolute intakes because individuals must alter nutrient intakes primarily by manipulating the composition of their diets rather than their total energy intake. Thus, for most purposes, measures of dietary composition, meaning nutrients adjusted for total energy intake, are the appropriate focus of epidemiologic studies.

When total energy intake is related to risk of disease, failure to consider total energy intake in the analysis can be particularly serious because it can confound associations with specific nutrients. For example, total energy intake increases with physical activity, so when physical activity is protective, total energy intake will also appear protective. The example of CHD is instructive. Risk of CHD is inversely related to physical activity and so also to total energy intake. Specific nutrients, such as saturated fat, that are strongly correlated with total energy intake also tend to be inversely related to risk of CHD. Several statistical methods can be used to adjust for total energy intake, which is necessary to avoid the misleading conclusion that saturated fat intake protects against CHD. The most common method, division of saturated fat intake by total energy intake, which is also called nutrient density, is not an adequate solution because the division can introduce confounding by the inverse of energy intake. For example, if energy intake is positively associated with risk of disease, any random variable divided by energy intake will be inversely associated with risk. Instead, total energy intake could be included in a multiple-regression model together with the nutrient density. Alternatively, nutrient intake residuals standardized for total energy intake will not be confounded by total energy intake. Appropriate adjustment for energy intake can be a nontrivial issue in some studies. Without such an adjustment, the direction of association with a specific nutrient can be reversed, such as with the relation between saturated fat intake and myocardial infarction[125] and with the relation between fiber intake and risk of colon cancer.[126] If total energy intake has not been measured or adjusted appropriately, a useful interpretation of a finding may not be possible.

Adjustment of nutrient intakes (N) for total energy intake (E) will often reduce measurement error (e), which can be seen as higher correlations in validation studies or stronger associations with biomarkers,[127] although this is not the primary rationale for energy adjustment. The reason for the reduction in error can be appreciated by considering that the observed nutrient density is $(N + e_N)/(E + e_E)$. e_N and e_E will tend to be highly correlated because they are calculated from many of the same foods; for example, if meat is overreported, both fat and total energy will be overreported. Thus, these errors will largely cancel out, leaving an improved estimate of N/E. Jakes et al.[128] have suggested that adjusting for physical activity and body size may provide a better adjustment for total energy intake itself than measured energy intake. This approach will not, however, necessarily result in better control for confounding, and it will fail to reduce measurement errors that are correlated with those in total energy intake.[129]

The Substitution Principle

In designing a controlled feeding trial to evaluate the effect of a nutrient or food, a first principle is that the diets being compared should be isocaloric; otherwise any observed effect could be just due to the difference in energy intake rather than the specific aspect of diet being evaluated. A second basic consideration is the composition of comparison diet; for example, if fat intake is being reduced, what is being substituted for fat in the comparison diet? The apparent effect of fat may depend strongly on whether calories from protein or carbohydrate are substituted for calories from fat. Although this principle has long been appreciated in experimental nutrition, until recently the specific substitution was ignored in epidemiologic analyses. If ignored and the analysis is appropriately adjusted for total energy intake, the nutrient included in the model is by default compared with the mix of calories from all other sources. Because a large proportion of the calories in the typical US diet are rather unhealthy, mainly refined starch, sugar, potatoes, and (until recently) partially hydrogenated oil, the finding of a null association only means that the dietary factor included in the model is about as bad as the rest of the diet.

A more informative analysis can be obtained by examining specific substitutions for the nutrient of interest.[130] For example, if a model includes total energy, fat, protein, and alcohol (carbohydrate being the contribution to energy left out), the effect of fat observed represents carbohydrate substituting for fat. The effect of protein substituting for fat can be estimated by leaving protein (instead of fat) out of the model, or by calculating the difference in coefficients for fat and protein, using the same units (percent of energy) for all macronutrients. This analytic approach was first used by Hu et al. to examine the relation of type of fat to risk of CHD[131]; in this analysis, intake of saturated fat was only weakly associated with risk of CHD if compared iso-calorically with carbohydrate intake, but was strongly associated with risk if compared with polyunsaturated fat intake.

The substitution approach also applies to foods that contribute substantially to energy intake. These substitutions can reflect options that consumers often consider. For example, intake of red meat was only weakly associated with risk of CHD if no specific substitution was specified but was strongly associated with risk if compared with intakes of fish, poultry, or nuts.[132]

OBESITY EPIDEMIOLOGY

Obesity has become a global epidemic. Worldwide between 1975 and 2014, the age-standardized mean body mass index (BMI) increased from 21.7 to 24.2 kg/m^2 in men and from 22.1 to 24.4 kg/m^2 in women.[133] In conjunction with the rise in BMI, the prevalence of overweight and obesity is increasing globally, in both children and adults.[134] In 2015, a total of 107.7 million children (5.0%) and 603.7 million adults (12.0%) were obese.[134] In the United States during 2013 to 2014, the prevalence of obesity among children (defined by growth curves from the Centers for Disease Control and Prevention) was 17.2%, and the prevalence among adults (defined as BMI ≥30 Kg/m^2) was 37.7%[135]; by 2017 to 2018, the prevalence in adults had increased to 42%.[136]. Another one-third of US adults are overweight (defined as BMI 25-29.9 Kg/m^2). Obesity rates are notably higher in non-Hispanic blacks, Hispanics, and Mexican American adults than in non-Hispanic white adults.

Dietary Determinants of Weight Gain and Obesity

Nutritional epidemiologic studies have contributed substantially to our understanding of dietary determinants of weight gain and obesity.[136,137] Although dietary fat has long been considered the main culprit behind obesity, large prospective cohort studies have not demonstrated that total dietary fat intake plays a major role. In contrast, types of dietary fat appear to be more important. In particular, increased energy intake from animal, saturated, and, notably, trans fats is positively associated with greater weight gain, while higher consumption of polyunsaturated fats is associated with lower weight gain.[138] A comprehensive analysis of food intake changes and weight changes indicates that increased intake of potato chips and potatoes, refined grains, sweets or desserts, sugar-sweetened beverages (SSBs), processed and unprocessed red meats, or fried foods is associated with greater weight gain, while increased intake of vegetables, fruits, whole grains, nuts, or yogurt is associated with less weight gain.[139] Greater adherence to healthy dietary patterns based on the Alternate Healthy Eating Index is also associated with less weight gain.[140] Recent large epidemiologic studies and longer term trials have failed to confirm the beneficial effects of dairy (except yogurt) or calcium on weight.[141,142] Many epidemiologic studies have shown that light to moderate alcohol consumption is not associated with weight gain in men and may be beneficial in women.[143] Heavy alcohol consumption, however, increases energy intake and results in greater weight gain.[143] Recent evidence indicates that poor dietary and lifestyle habits, such as higher intake of sugar-sweetened beverages or fried foods, more time spent watching television, or physical inactivity exacerbate genetic predispositions to obesity.[144-146]

Cumulative epidemiologic and clinical-trial evidence indicates that there is no "magic bullet" for weight control. Rather, many individual dietary factors each exerts a modest effect on body weight, and, over time, cumulative effects of small changes in daily energy balance lead to weight gain and obesity. Current evidence suggests that altering macronutrient composition is unlikely to have an appreciable effect on body weight. However, the combined effects of multiple dietary factors (including individual foods and beverages and various eating patterns) can accumulate over time to have a substantial long-term impact on body weight.

Health Consequences of Obesity

Numerous epidemiologic studies have demonstrated that being overweight or obese is an important risk factor for type 2 diabetes, CVDs, certain types of cancers, and premature death.[147-150] The causal relationship between higher BMI and cardiometabolic diseases has been further confirmed by Mendelian randomization analyses of BMI-raising genetic variants and these outcomes.[151] Overweight and obesity among adolescents were also found to be strongly associated with increased cardiovascular mortality in adulthood during 40 years of follow-up.[152] In addition, even modest amounts of weight gain from young adulthood (age 18 years for women and age 21 years for men) to middle adulthood (age 55 years) were associated with considerably elevated risk of chronic diseases and premature death.[147] In particular, for each 5-kg weight gain, the risk ratios were 1.31 (95% confident interval [CI]: 1.28%~1.33%) for type 2 diabetes, 1.14 (95% CI: 1.10~1.17) for hypertension, 1.08%~1.09% for CVD, 1.06 (95% CI: 1.02~1.09) for obesity-related cancer, and 1.05 (95% CI: 1.04~1.07) for dying prematurely (which was 1.07~1.08 among never smokers).[147] These findings indicate that prevention of weight gain through healthy diet and lifestyle during young and middle adulthood is of paramount importance.

The relationship between body weight and mortality has been controversial. Some studies have suggested that excess weight is protective against mortality,[153] but this "obesity paradox" appears to be mainly due to confounding by smoking and existing or preclinical conditions that lead to weight loss preceding death, *i.e.*, reverse causation. Reverse causation increases with older age because of the accumulation of chronic illness, making the relationship between BMI and mortality less clear among the elderly than among middle-aged adults.[150] In studying obesity and mortality, age appears to be the most important effect modifier. Typically, the positive association of mortality with increasing BMI tends to decline with age. The declining relative impact of BMI on mortality with increasing age may reflect several methodological issues: (1) greater bias due to higher prevalence of existing and occult chronic diseases in the elderly; (2) lower validity of BMI in measuring excess body fat in older people; or (3) survival bias or depletion of the susceptibles, which relates to the deaths of those most vulnerable to obesity-related complications. Another explanation for the "obesity paradox" is referred to as "index event bias," a form of selection bias when the analysis of BMI and mortality is conducted among individuals with specific obesity-related conditions such as type 2 diabetes.[154] This bias tends to exacerbate residual confounding by smoking and reverse causation by occult chronic diseases.

To address these methodological issues, the best estimates of the impact of obesity on mortality should derive from large cohort studies with long follow-up periods from midlife or earlier. In fact, many large studies that were conducted among middle-aged subjects have shown a monotonic relationship between increasing BMI and elevated mortality risk, especially when analyses were restricted to healthy participants who had never smoked. In these studies, BMI values associated with the lowest mortality were clearly below 25. A recent individual-level meta-analysis based on 10,625,411 participants from 239 prospective studies indicated that all-cause mortality was lowest at a BMI of 20.0 to 25.0 kg/m^2, and both overweight and obesity were associated with considerably elevated all-cause mortality risk.[155] The relationship between BMI and mortality was consistently observed across populations from multiple continents (North America, Europe, and Asia-Pacific). It was estimated that in 2015, excess body weight accounted for about 4 million deaths and 120 million disability-adjusted life-years worldwide,[134] and nearly 70% of the deaths attributable to high BMI were due to CVD.[134]

Existing evidence suggests that various measurements of fat distribution, including waist circumference, waist to hip ratio, and waist to height ratio, provide similar predictions of type 2 diabetes, CVD, and mortality.[156] Because waist circumference measurement is more practical and easier to interpret than other measures of fat distribution, it should be monitored routinely for most people, even for those who are normal weight. All three variables in the "adiposity triad" (BMI, waist circumference, and weight gain since young adulthood) are important in assessing the relationship between adiposity and health risk because each adds information to the risk prediction and indicates the potential for prevention.[154]

INTEGRATING OMICS TECHNOLOGIES INTO NUTRITIONAL EPIDEMIOLOGY

The past two decades have seen remarkable advances in "omics" technologies, which include a collection of high-throughput methods for assessing many genomic, epigenomic, transcriptomic, proteomic, metabolomic, and microbiomic traits from biological specimens. The integration of such technologies into epidemiological studies, referred to as "systems epidemiology,"[157] can enhance our understanding of biological mechanisms underlying diet and human health. This approach can also enable us to achieve better assessment of diet and nutritional status in free-living populations by identifying novel biomarkers of dietary intakes. Analogous to the concept of precision medicine, precision nutrition or personalized nutrition aims to use the systems epidemiology approach to tailor nutrition interventions and recommendations to individual genetic backgrounds and metabolic profiles for more effective dietary prevention of diseases.[158]

Gene-Diet Interactions

The advent of genome-wide association studies (GWAS), and more recently exome sequencing studies, has enabled researchers to identify numerous genetic loci for obesity, type 2 diabetes, and other chronic diseases. Most of the identified loci are common but have a modest effect size. GWAS have also uncovered genetic variants associated with intake of macronutrients, alcohol, coffee, and other dietary components.[159-161] These findings have provided the rationale and tools for examining gene-diet interactions to identify individuals who are more susceptible or responsive to certain dietary exposures. These tools may lead to more effective dietary interventions based on genetic testing of disease risk or nutrient and food metabolism.

Recent work on gene-environment interactions suggests that the adverse effects of obesity, diabetes, and other disease loci can be attenuated by high physical activity levels or healthy lifestyles. On the other hand, low physical activity and a Western dietary pattern may augment these effects.[162] For example, healthy dietary patterns were found to mitigate the effects of genetic variants on type 2 diabetes[163] and CHD,[164] whereas unhealthy dietary habits such as regular consumption of SSBs, fried food, and saturated fat, were found to exacerbate the effects of genetic variants on obesity.[144,145,165,166] These findings suggest that individuals with greater genetic predispositions may benefit more from interventions to improve diet quality. There is evidence that individuals carrying the homozygous FTO obesity-predisposing allele may lose more weight through diet and lifestyle interventions than noncarriers, although the difference in the amount of weight loss induced by the interventions was small between the genotypes.[167] Nonetheless, gene-diet interaction analyses may provide evidence to partially explain large individual variability in response to diet and lifestyle interventions on weight loss.

Despite some progress in characterizing gene-diet interactions underlying chronic disease risk, major challenges remain, particularly regarding inconsistencies and nonreplication of published results. Nonreplication can result from false-positive results, false-negative results, or true heterogeneity across populations. Additionally, lack of statistical power and measurement errors for dietary factors can contribute to nonreplication.

Mendelian Randomization

Nutritional epidemiologic studies have applied the Mendelian randomization method to examine the causal effect of dietary intakes as predicted by genotypes, on health outcomes. Because various genotypes are assigned to individuals randomly at birth, Mendelian randomization analysis mimics a randomized intervention trial, by which it could theoretically eliminate unmeasured confounding and reverse causation. The genotype can serve as a surrogate of long-term dietary exposure either because it alters dietary behaviors, affects the absorption or metabolism of a dietary factor, or modifies receptor response to a dietary factor.[168] The relationship among ALDH2 genotypes, alcohol intake, and risk of esophageal cancer provides an example of Mendelian randomization analysis.[169] Individuals who carry the ALDH2 *2*2 genotype are unable to metabolize acetaldehyde and are therefore less tolerant of alcohol drinking. A meta-analysis found that compared with wild-type homozygotes, *2*2 homozygotes had a considerably lower risk of esophageal cancer, whereas heterozygotes, which can partially metabolize acetaldehyde, had an increased risk. This analysis provides evidence to support a causal relationship between alcohol or its principal metabolite acetaldehyde and risk of esophageal cancer.[169] Evidence for an interaction was found between ALDH2/ADH1B (alcohol dehydrogenase-1B) genotypes and alcohol drinking in relation to esophageal cancer, in that drinkers with both of the ADH1B and ALDH2 risk alleles had a fourfold increased risk for esophageal cancer compared with drinkers without these risk alleles; risk was increased by about 1.5 with this genotype among nondrinkers and by only about 1.2 among drinkers without this genotype.[170]

So far only a small number of genetic variants have been found to strongly predict and thus can serve as proxies for dietary intake and nutritional status. A key assumption of Mendelian randomization analysis is that the observed associations between genotype and disease risk are not likely to be confounded by other aspects of diet or lifestyle because individuals are in essence randomized to various genotypes at conception and are usually unaware of those genotypes. However, this assumption is likely to apply less to genotypes that alter behavior. For example, the polymorphisms in the lactase gene that are associated with lactose intolerance are associated with reduced consumption of milk but may therefore be associated with increased consumption of soda and other dietary factors, which could complicate a causal interpretation of the association between milk consumption and disease risk.[168]

Metabolomics

High-throughput metabolomics can measure thousands of small-molecule metabolites in various biospecimens, which integrate information from food and nutrient metabolism, genetic variation, microbial activity, and environmental exposures. In recent years, this technology has enabled researchers to identify metabolites that predict future risk of type 2 diabetes, CVD, and some cancers. For example, higher plasma levels of branched chain amino acids (BCAAs, including leucine and valine) and aromatic amino acids (AAAs, including tyrosine and phenylalanine) but lower plasma levels of glycine and glutamine were found to predict risk of type 2 diabetes,[171] CVD,[172] and pancreatic cancer.[173] Although the biological mechanisms underlying these associations are not completely understood, because the concentrations of these metabolites are influenced by both dietary intake and metabolism, they can be considered as potential nutritional intervention targets for disease prevention.

Metabolomics holds some promise for the development of objective biomarkers for measuring diet. To date, many plasma or urinary metabolites have been associated with dietary patterns as well as intakes of specific nutrients and foods.[174] However, most identified metabolites are not sensitive or specific to dietary intakes. Also, many metabolites have a short half-life and thus may not represent usual intake, the most relevant exposure in nutritional epidemiology. In addition, metabolomics assays are expensive, rendering it infeasible to analyze hundreds and thousands of participants in large cohort studies. Therefore, metabolomics biomarkers are unlikely to replace traditional dietary assessments using self-reported methods. Biomarkers identified from metabolomics should be used in conjunction with self-reported methods such as validated FFQs and traditional biomarkers of nutrient intakes as described above.

Recent advances in omics technologies have offered promising opportunities to assess individuals' characteristics including the genome, epigenome, metabolome, and microbiome, which can be integrated into nutritional epidemiologic studies through the systems epidemiology approach.

In addition, the use of mobile apps and wearable devices has the potential to improve real-time assessment of dietary intakes, although the validity of these methods remains to be established. Despite these advances, major challenges still exist, including nonreplication of study results, difficulty in translation of research findings into practice, and high cost. Although commercial companies have promoted personalized nutrition assessment and genetic testing, there is little evidence on the benefits of these approaches for improving diet and preventing disease.

Unhealthy dietary habits are shaped not only by individuals' characteristics but also by the food environment and public policies. In recent years, although overall food quality has improved modestly in the US population, the gap between the rich and poor has widened, contributing to increased disparity in diet quality and health.[175] In addition, the current food systems have not only contributed substantially to poor human health but also have negatively affected the environment, which in turn adversely affects nutrient contents and food production.[176] Therefore, it is essential to balance the investment in precision nutrition, which targets individual characteristics, with public-health nutrition, which aims to improve the health of populations. Public-health approaches such as food and agricultural policies, legislation and regulations, and evidence-based dietary guidelines should continue to be the fundamental approaches to changing unhealthy food systems and improving human and planetary health.

Translation of Nutritional Epidemiologic Evidence into Policies

Randomized controlled trials (RCTs) with disease end points are typically considered the highest level of evidence to inform health policies. However, RCTs in general and dietary factors in particular are limited by multiple methodological issues such as short follow-up, poor compliance, high drop-out rate, high cost, and ethical considerations.[177] Thus, nutritional epidemiologic studies of hard disease end points through well-conducted prospective cohort studies, together with evidence from intervention studies on intermediate biomarkers, can often provide the best available evidence to inform health policies and dietary recommendations.[178]

A successful example of translating evidence from nutritional epidemiologic studies into policies is the dramatic reduction of partially hydrogenated vegetable oils, the predominant dietary source of *trans* fatty acids, in the US food supply. In the early 20th century, partial hydrogenation of vegetable oils was widely adopted by the food industry to turn liquid oils into solid fats that mimicked lard and butter. In 1993, the Nurses' Health Study (NHS) first reported a meaningful positive association between a higher intake of trans fatty acids and risk of CHD.[179] Meanwhile, controlled feeding studies documented the adverse effects of trans fat intake on blood lipids and other CVD risk factors.[180] These findings were further confirmed in subsequent prospective cohort studies and controlled feeding studies.[131,181-184] Based on this evidence, in 2003 Denmark became the first country to restrict the use of *trans* fat in the food supply[185] and was followed by others including Austria, Hungary, Norway, Switzerland, Iceland, Sweden, Canada, Brazil, Chile, Argentina, and South Africa.[186,187] In 2005, the US Dietary Guidelines recommended limiting intake of *trans* fats.[188] Beginning in 2006, the FDA required that food manufacturers disclose *trans* fat amounts on food labels.[189] Following the FDA's rule, many states and cities took legislative/regulatory actions to limit *trans* fat use in restaurants and other food outlets. For example, New York City banned *trans* fat from restaurant foods in 2006[190] and California did the same in 2008.[191] In the meantime, food manufacturers reformulated products to reduce the amount of *trans* fat.[192,193] In 2015, the FDA released its final determination that partially hydrogenated oils were not "generally recognized as safe" (GRAS) for use in food. This series of policy changes has led to a dramatic reduction in *trans* fat in the US diet, contributing substantially to the improvement of overall dietary quality[194] and the reduction in the burden of chronic disease, in particular CVD.[195]

Legislation and regulations regarding SSBs provide another example of the influence of nutritional epidemiologic evidence on policy. Numerous prospective cohort studies have documented that higher consumption of SSBs is associated with an increased risk of weight gain, obesity, type 2 diabetes, CHD, and stroke.[196-198] In addition, RCTs found that decreasing SSB consumption reduced weight gain and fat accumulation in children and adolescents.[199,200] These consistent findings have provided a strong evidence base for policies to reduce SSB consumption. Early policy actions included local- and state-level policies in the United States that required/recommended removing SSBs from vending machines in public schools[201] and a ban on SSB sales in schools and other public properties in Boston, MA.[189] In 2013, Mexico passed an excise tax on SSBs and a sales tax on several foods with high energy density.[202] Following the implementation of the SSB tax, purchases of taxed beverages in Mexico decreased 5.5% in 2014 and 9.7% in 2015, yielding an average reduction of 7.6% over 2 years.[203] More recently, US cities, including Philadelphia, Seattle, Boulder, Cook County, Berkeley, San Francisco, Oakland, and Albany, CA passed excise taxes on SSBs.[204] One year after implementation of the SSB tax in Berkeley, a striking decline in SSB sales was observed.[205] It has been estimated that if implemented nationally, an SSB tax would avert 101,000 disability-adjusted life-years and gain 871,000 quality-adjusted life-years, leading to $23.6 billion in healthcare cost savings from 2015 to 2025. In the meantime, the tax would generate $12.5 billion in annual revenue,[206] which could be used for education and obesity prevention initiatives.

Nutritional epidemiologic studies have also played a central role in the development of the Dietary Guidelines for Americans (DGAs), which are intended to serve as a basis for federal policies related to food. For example, large cohort studies have found that specific types of dietary fat rather than total amount of fat were associated with risk of CVD and mortality.[39,131,207-210] Controlled feeding trials have also shown the divergent effects of different types of fat on blood lipids.[211] Both of these findings provided strong support for the 2015 to 2020 DGAs to remove the upper limit on total dietary fat and instead recommend replacing saturated and trans fats with unsaturated fats, especially polyunsaturated fats.[212] In addition, the 2015 to 2020 DGAs put a greater emphasis on recommending healthy dietary patterns, including the healthy US-style pattern, the Mediterranean-style pattern, and the healthy vegetarian pattern. This shift was based on the evidence that healthy dietary patterns were strongly associated with a lower risk of major chronic disease and mortality in prospective cohort studies, corroborated by some evidence from RCTs.[213]

In most situations, RCTs of dietary factors and hard end points are not feasible and thus policy decisions have to be made based on existing observational evidence. In this scenario, the Hill criteria (see Chapter 2) may provide useful considerations for causal inference from observational data and making timely policy decisions that could avert preventable morbidity and mortality in the population[214]. Observational data are also important in demonstrating lack of hypothesized harm, *e.g.*, in the cases of total fat in the diet and omega-6 fatty acid intake on CHD, and thus can play a key role in resolving ongoing controversies.[214]

In summary, nutritional epidemiology has played an indispensable role in developing and shaping nutrition policy and will continue to contribute to policy-making. However, scientific evidence itself will not automatically lead to policy change. The translation of evidence into policies also requires leadership and political will, education, and advocacy. Nevertheless, building a strong evidence base through sound epidemiologic studies and intervention trials is the foundation for effective policy changes.

CONCLUSION

The last four decades have seen enormous progress in the development of nutritional epidemiology methods. Work by many investigators has provided clear support for the essential underpinnings of this field. Substantial between-person variation in consumption of most dietary factors in populations has been demonstrated, methods to measure diet applicable to large epidemiologic studies have been developed, and their validity has been documented. Based on this evidence, many large prospective cohort studies have been established that are now providing a wealth of data on many outcomes. In addition, methods to account for errors in measurement of dietary intake have been developed and are beginning to be applied in reporting findings from studies of diet and disease.

Nutritional epidemiology has contributed importantly to understanding the etiology of many diseases. Low intake of fruits and vegetables has been shown to be related to increased risk of CVD. Also, a substantial amount of epidemiologic evidence has accumulated indicating that replacing saturated and trans fats with unsaturated fats can play an important role in the prevention of CHD and type 2 diabetes. Diseases—as diverse as cataracts, neural-tube defects, and macular degeneration—that were not thought to be nutritionally related have been found to have important dietary determinants. Many findings from nutritional epidemiology have been translated into national policies and guidelines. Nonetheless, much more needs to be learned regarding other diet and disease relations, especially cognitive decline and other neurodegenerative conditions, and the dimensions of time and ranges of dietary intakes need to be expanded further for outcomes that have already been studied. Furthermore, new products are constantly being introduced into the food supply, which will require continued epidemiologic vigilance. The development and evaluation of additional methods to measure dietary factors, particularly those using biochemical methods to assess long-term intake, can contribute substantially to improvements in the capacity to assess diet and disease relations. The capacity to identify persons at genetically increased risk of disease is allowing the study of gene-nutrient interactions, although the paucity of strong genetic variants has meant that very large studies are needed. The development of other new technologies, including metabolomics and the ability of characterize the microbiome genetically and metabolically, is creating new opportunities to understand mechanisms underlying diet and disease relationships. Conversely, integration of nutritional epidemiology into epidemiologic studies using these technologies will be necessary to make them fully informative because diet can strongly modify genetic risk and metabolic pathways. The challenges posed by the complexities of nutritional exposures are likely to spur methodologic developments, as has already happened in the field of measurement error that will contribute to the parent field of epidemiology.

Although many adverse consequences of overweight and obesity are now well documented, the prevalence of obesity continues to increase relentlessly and threatens to reverse gains in health that have been achieved in the United States and globally. Some modifiable aspects of diet and lifestyle have been identified that can mitigate weight gain during young and middle adulthood, but more research is needed, including randomized trials of specific interventions lasting at least a year or two. Also, further research should include studies on the upstream social and environmental determinants of diet and physical activity.

Much is now known about the elements of a healthy diet, but a large gap exists between current and optimal dietary patterns, and considerable effort is needed to bridge this gap. The methods developed by nutritional epidemiologists will be important in developing priorities, interventions, and policies and in monitoring trends and the effects of policies.

References

1. Willett WC. *Nutritional Epidemiology*. 3rd ed. New York, NY: Oxford University Press; 2013.
2. Dawber T, Kannel W, Pearson G. Assessment of diet in the Framingham study, methodology and preliminary observations. *Health News*. 1961;38:4-6.
3. Keys A, ed. Coronary heart disease in seven countries. American heart association monograph number 29. *Circulation*. 1970;41,(suppl I):1-211.
4. Armstrong B, Doll R. Environmental factors and cancer incidence and mortality in different countries, with special reference to dietary practices. *Int J Cancer*. 1975;15:617-631.
5. Willett W. Nutritional epidemiology: issues and challenges. *Int J Epidemiol*. 1987;16:312-317.
6. Goodwin PJ, Boyd NF. Critical appraisal of the evidence that dietary fat intake is related to breast cancer risk in humans. *J Natl Cancer Inst*. 1987;79:473-485.
7. McKeown-Eyssen GE, Bright-See E. Dietary factors in colon cancer: international relationships. An update. *Nutr Cancer*. 1985;7:251-253.
8. Navidi W, Thomas D, Stram D, Peters J. Design and analysis of multilevel analytic studies with applications to a study of air pollution. *Environ Health Perspect*. 1994;102(suppl 8):25-32.
9. Sheppard L, Prentice RL. On the reliability and precision of within- and between-population estimates of relative rate parameters. *Biometrics*. 1995;51(3):853-863.
10. Chen J, Campbell TC, Junyao L, Peto R. *Diet, Life-Style, and Mortality in China: A Study of the Characteristics of 65 Chinese Counties*. Oxford, England: Oxford University Press; 1990.
11. Kinlen LJ. Fat and cancer. *Br Med J (Clin Res Ed)*. 1983;286:1081-1082.
12. Hebert JR, Miller DR. Methodologic considerations for investigating the diet-cancer link. *Am J Clin Nutr*. 1988;47:1068-1077.
13. Prentice RL, Kakar F, Hursting S, Sheppard L, Klein R, Kushi LH. Aspects of the rationale for the women's health trial. *J Natl Cancer Inst*. 1988;80:802-814.
14. Greenland S, Robins J. Invited commentary: ecologic studies - biases, misconceptions, and counterexamples. *Am J Epidemiol*. 1994;139:747-760.
15. Phillips RL, Garfinkel L, Kuzma JW, Beeson WL, Lotz T, Brin B. Mortality among California Seventh-day Adventists for selected cancer sites. *J Natl Cancer Inst*. 1980;65:1097-1107.
16. Staszewski J, Haenszel W. Cancer mortality among the Polish-born in the United States. *J Natl Cancer Inst*. 1965;35:291-297.
17. Adelstein AM, Staszewski J, Muir CS. Cancer mortality in 1970-1972 among polish-born migrants to england and wales. *Br J Cancer*. 1979;40:464-475.

18. McMichael AJ, Giles GG. Cancer in migrants to Australia: extending the descriptive epidemiological data. *Cancer Res*. 1988;48:751-756.

19. Shimizu H, Ross RK, Bernstein L, Yatani R, Henderson BE, Mack TM. Cancers of the prostate and breast among Japanese and white immigrants in Los Angeles County. *Br J Cancer*. 1991;63:963-966.

20. Haenszel W, Kurihara M, Segi M, Lee RKC. Stomach cancer among Japanese in Hawaii. *J Natl Cancer Inst*. 1972;49:969-988.

21. Buell P. Changing incidence of breast cancer in Japanese-American women. *J Natl Cancer Inst*. 1973;51:1479-1483.

22. Ferlay J, Bray F, Pisani P, Parkin DM. *GLOBOCAN 2000: Cancer Incidence, Mortality and Prevalence Worldwide. Version 1.0*. Lyon: IARCPress, 2001. IARC CancerBase No. 5.

23. Willett WC. *Nutritional Epidemiology*. 2nd ed. New York, NY: Oxford University Press; 1998.

24. Hartge P, Brinton LA, Rosenthal JFA, Cahill JI, Hoover RN, Waksberg J. Random digit dialing in selecting a population-based control group. *Am J Epidemiol*. 1984;120:825-833.

25. Friedenreich CM, Howe GR, Miller AB. An investigation of recall bias in the reporting of past food intake among breast cancer cases and controls. *Ann Epidemiol*. 1991;1:439-453.

26. Giovannucci E, Stampfer MJ, Colditz GA, et al. A comparison of prospective and retrospective assessments of diet in the study of breast cancer. *Am J Epidemiol*. 1993;137:502-511.

27. Stampfer MJ, Willett WC, Speizer FE, et al. Test of the national death index. *Am J Epidemiol*. 1984;119:837-839.

28. Howe GR, Hirohata T, Hislop TG, et al. Dietary factors and risk of breast cancer: combined analysis of 12 case-control studies. *J Natl Cancer Inst*. 1990;82:561-569.

29. Hunter DJ, Spiegelman D, Adami HO, et al.. Cohort studies of fat intake and the risk of breast cancer: a pooled analysis. *N Eng J Med*. 1996;334:356-361.

30. Byers TE, Graham S, Haughey BP, Marshall JR, Swanson MK. Diet and lung cancer risk: findings from the Western New York Diet Study. *Am J Epidemiol*. 1987;125:351-363.

31. Goodman MT, Kolonel LN, Yoshizawa CN, Hankin JH. The effect of dietary cholesterol and fat on the risk of lung cancer in Hawaii. *Am J Epidemiol*. 1988;128:1241-1255.

32. Mohr DL, Blot WJ, Tousey PM, Van Doren ML, Wolfe KW. Southern cooking and lung cancer. *Nutr Cancer*. 1999;35:34-43.

33. De Stefani E, Deneo-Pellegrini H, Mendilaharsu M, Carzoglio JC, Ronco A. Dietary fat and lung cancer: a case-control study in Uruguay. *Cancer Causes Control*. 1997;8:913-921.

34. Alavanja MC, Brown CC, Swanson C, Brownson RC. Saturated fat intake and lung cancer risk among nonsmoking women in Missouri. *J Natl Cancer Inst*. 1993;85:1906-1916.

35. Smith-Warner SA, Ritz J, Hunter DJ, et al. Dietary fat and risk of lung cancer in a pooled analysis of prospective studies. *Cancer Epidemiol Biomarkers Prev*. 2002;11(10):987-992.

36. World Cancer Research Fund, American Institute for Cancer Research. *Food, Nutrition and the Prevention of Cancer: A Global Perspective*. Washington, DC: American Institutue for Cancer Research; 1997.

37. Smith-Warner SA, Spiegelman D, Yaun SS, et al. Fruits, vegetables and lung cancer: a pooled analysis of cohort studies. *Int J Cancer*. 2003;107(6):1001-1011.

38. Multiple Risk Factor Intervention Trial Research Group. Multiple risk factor intervention trial: risk factor changes and mortality results. *J Am Med Assoc*. 1982;248:1465-1477.

39. Prentice RL, Caan B, Chlebowski RT, et al. Low-fat dietary pattern and risk of invasive breast cancer: the women's health initiative randomized controlled dietary modification trial. *J Am Med Assoc*. 2006;295(6):629-642.

40. Peto R, Doll R, Buckley JD, Sporn MB. Can dietary beta-carotene materially reduce human cancer rates? *Nature*. 1981;290:201-208.

41. Graham S, Dayal H, Swanson M, Mittelman A, Wilkinson G. Diet in the epidemiology of cancer of the colon and rectum. *J Natl Cancer Inst*. 1978;61:709-714.

42. Wattenberg LW, Loub WD. Inhibition of polycyclic aromatic hydrocarbon-induced neoplasia by naturally occurring indoles. *Cancer Res*. 1978;38:1410-1413.

43. Mertz W. Food and nutrients. *J Am Diet Assoc*. 1984;84:769-770.

44. Welsh SO, Marston RM. Review of trends in food use in the United States, 1909 to 1980. *J Am Diet Assoc*. 1982;81:120-128.

45. Manousos O, Day NE, Trichopoulos D, Gerovassilis F, Tzanou A, Polychronopoulou A. Diet and colorectal cancer: a case-control study in Greece. *Int J Cancer*. 1983;32:1-5.

46. Morris JN, Marr JW, Clayton DG. Diet and heart: a postscript. *Br Med J*. 1977;2:1307-1314.

47. Trichopoulou A, Costacou T, Bamia C, Trichopoulos D. Adherence to a Mediterranean diet and survival in a Greek population. *N Engl J Med*. 2003;348:2599-2608.

48. Greenland S. Principles of multilevel modelling. *Int J Epidemiol*. 2000;29(1):158-167.

49. Lee JE, Willett WC, Fuchs CS, et al. Folate intake and risk of colorectal cancer and adenoma: modification by time. *Am J Clin Nutr*. 2011;93(4):817-825.

50. Rohan TE, Potter JD. Retrospective assessment of dietary intake. *Am J Epidemiol*. 1984;120:876-887.
51. Byers T, Marshall J, Anthony E, Fiedler R, Zielezny M. The reliability of dietary history from the distant past. *Am J Epidemiol*. 1987;125:999-1011.
52. Byers TE, Rosenthal RI, Marshall JR, Rzepka TF, Cummings KM, Graham S. Dietary history from the distant past: a methodological study. *Nutr Cancer*. 1983;5:69-77.
53. Shekelle RB, Shryock AM, Paul O, et al. Diet, serum cholesterol, and death from coronary heart disease: the Western Electric Study. *N Engl J Med*. 1981;304:65-70.
54. Rosner B, Hennekens CH, Kass EH, Miall WE. Age-specific correlation analysis of longitudinal blood pressure data. *Am J Epidemiol*. 1977;106:306-313.
55. Beaton GH, Milner J, Corey P, et al. Sources of variance in 24-hour dietary recall data: implications for nutrition study design and interpretation. *Am J Clin Nutr*. 1979;32:2546-2549.
56. Posner BM, Borman CL, Morgan JL, Borden WS, Ohls JC. The validity of a telephone-administered 24-hour dietary recall methodology. *Am J Clin Nutr*. 1982;36:546-553.
57. Subar AF, Thompson FE, Potischman N, et al. Formative research of a quick list for an automated self-administered 24-hour dietary recall. *J Am Diet Assoc*. 2007;107:1002-1007.
58. Karvetti R-L, Knuts LR. Validity of the 24-hour dietary recall. *J Am Diet Assoc*. 1985;85:1437-1442.
59. Madden JP, Goodman SJ, Guthrie HA. Validity of the 24-hour recall. Analysis of data obtained from elderly subjects. *J Am Diet Assoc*. 1976;68:143-147.
60. Freedman LS, Commins JM, Willett W, et al. Evaluation of the 24-hour recall as a reference instrument for calibrating other self-report instruments in nutritional cohort studies: evidence from the validation studies pooling project. *Am J Epidemiol*. 2017;186(1):73-82.
61. Freedman LS, Commins JM, Moler JE, et al. Pooled results from 5 validation studies of dietary self-report instruments using recovery biomarkers for potassium and sodium intake. *Am J Epidemiol*. 2015;181(7):473-487.
62. Freedman LS, Commins JM, Moler JE, et al. Pooled results from 5 validation studies of dietary self-report instruments using recovery biomarkers for energy and protein intake. *Am J Epidemiol*. 2014;180(2):172-188.
63. Yuan C, Spiegelman D, Rimm EB, et al. Relative validity of nutrient intakes assessed by questionnaire, 24-hour recalls, and diet records compared with urinary recovery and plasma concentration biomarkers: findings for women. *Am J Epidemiol*. 2018;187(5):1051-1063.
64. Rimm EB, Giovannucci EL, Stampfer MJ, Colditz GA, Litin LB, Willett WC. Reproducibility and validity of a expanded self-administered semiquantitative food frequency questionnaire among male health professionals. *Am J Epidemiol*. 1992;135:1114-1126.
65. Rimm EB. Authors' response to "Invited commentary: some limitations of semiquantitative food frequency questionnaires. *Am J Epidemiol*. 1992;135:1133-1136.
66. Yuan C, Spiegelman D, Rimm EB, et al. Validity of a dietary questionnaire assessed by comparison with multiple weighed dietary records or 24-hour recalls. *Am J Epidemiol*. 2017;185(7):570-584.
67. Salvini S, Hunter DJ, Sampson L, et al. Food-based validation of a dietary questionnaire: the effects of week-to-week variation in food consumption. *Int J Epidemiol*. 1989;18:858-867.
68. Feskanich D, Rimm EB, Giovannucci EL, et al. Reproducibility and validity of food intake measurements from a semiquantitative food frequency questionnaire. *J Am Diet Assoc*. 1993;93:790-796.
69. Carroll RJ, Midthune D, Subar AF, et al. Taking advantage of the strengths of 2 different dietary assessment instruments to improve intake estimates for nutritional epidemiology. *Am J Epidemiol*. 2012;175(4):340-347.
70. Burke BS. The dietary history as a tool in research. *J Am Diet Assoc*. 1947;23:1041-1046.
71. Wiehl DG, Reed R. Development of new or improved dietary methods for epidemiological investigations. *Am J Pub Health*. 1960;50:824-828.
72. Heady JA. Diets of bank clerks. Development of a method of classifying the diets of individuals for use in epidemiologic studies. *J R Stat Soc*. 1961;124:336-361.
73. Stephanik PA, Trulson MF. Determining the frequency of foods in large group studies. *Am J Clin Nutr*. 1962;2:335-343.
74. Marr JW. Individual dietary surveys: purposes and methods. *World Rev Nutr Diet*. 1971;13:105-164.
75. Humble CG, Samet JM, Skipper BE. Use of quantified and frequency indices of vitamin A intake in a case-control study of lung cancer. *Int J Epidemiol*. 1987;16:341-346.
76. Sampson L. Food frequency questionnaires as a research instrument. *Clin Nutr*. 1985;4:171-178.
77. Block G, Hartman AM, Dresser CM, Carroll MD, Gannon J, Gardner L. A data-based approach to diet questionnaire design and testing. *Am J Epidemiol*. 1986;124:453-469.
78. Morgan RW, Jain M, Miller AB, et al. A comparison of dietary methods in epidemiologic studies. *Am J Epidemiol*. 1978;107:488-498.
79. Hankin JH, Nomura AM, Lee J, Hirohata T, Kolonel LN. Reproducibility of a dietary history questionnaire in a case-control study of breast cancer. *Am J Clin Nutr*. 1983;37:981-985.

80. Samet JM, Humble CG, Skipper BE. Alternatives in the collection and analysis of food frequency interview data. *Am J Epidemiol*. 1984;120:572-581.

81. Pickle LW, Hartman AM. Indicator foods for vitamin A assessment. *Nutr Cancer*. 1985;7:3-23.

82. Block G, Woods M, Potosky A, Clifford C. Validation of a self-administered diet history questionnaire using multiple diet records. *J Clin Epidemiol*. 1990;43:1327-1335.

83. Cummings SR, Block G, McHenry K, Baron RB. Evaluation of two food frequency methods of measuring dietary calcium intake. *Am J Epidemiol*. 1987;126:796-802.

84. Hernandez-Avila M, Master C, Hunter DJ, et al. Influence of additional portion size data on the validity of a semi-quantitative food frequency questionnaire (abstract). *Am J Epidemiol*. 1988;128:891.

85. Cohen NL, Lans MJ, Ferris AM, et al. *The Contributions of Portion Size Data to Estimating Nutrient Intakes of Food Frequency Questionnaires*. Amherst, MA: Massachusetts Agriculture Experiment Station, University of Massachusetts; 1990. Research Bulletin 730.

86. Willett WC, Sampson L, Stampfer MJ, et al. Reproducibility and validity of a semiquantitative food frequency questionnaire. *Am J Epidemiol*. 1985;122:51-65.

87. Willett WC, Stampfer MJ, Underwood BA, Speizer FE, Rosner B, Hennekens CH. Validation of a dietary questionnaire with plasma carotenoid and alpha-tocopherol levels. *Am J Clin Nutr*. 1983;38:631-639.

88. Russell-Briefel R, Bates MW, Kuller LH. The relationship of plasma carotenoids to health and biochemical factors in middle-aged men. *Am J Epidemiol*. 1985;122:741-749.

89. Sacks FM, Handysides GH, Marais GE, Rosner B, Kass EH. Effects of a low-fat diet on plasma lipoprotein levels. *Arch Intern Med*. 1986;146:1573-1577.

90. Stryker WS, Kaplan LA, Stein EA, Stampfer MJ, Sober A, Willett WC. The relation of diet, cigarette smoking, and alcohol consumption to plasma beta-carotene and alpha-tocopherol levels. *Am J Epidemiol*. 1988;127:283-296.

91. Silverman DI, Reis GJ, Sacks FM, Boucher TM, Pasternak RC. Usefulness of plasma phospholipid N-3 fatty acid levels in predicting dietary fish intake in patients with coronary artery disease. *Am J Cardiol*. 1990;66:860-862.

92. Coates RJ, Eley JW, Block G, et al. An evaluation of a food frequency questionnaire for assessing dietary intake of specific carotenoids and vitamin E among low-income black women. *Am J Epidemiol*. 1991;134:658-671.

93. London SJ, Sacks FM, Caesar J, Stampfer MJ, Siguel E, Willett WC. Fatty acid composition of subcutaneous adipose tissue and diet in post-menopausal US women. *Am J Clin Nutr*. 1991;54:340-345.

94. Ascherio A, Stampfer MJ, Colditz GA, Rimm EB, Litin L, Willett WC. Correlations of vitamin A and E intakes with the plasma concentrations of carotenoids and tocopherols among American men and women. *J Nutr*. 1992;122:1792-1801.

95. Hunter DJ, Rimm EB, Sacks FM, et al. Comparison of measures of fatty acid intake by subcutaneous fat aspirate, food frequency questionnaire, and diet records in a free-living population of US men. *Am J Epidemiol*. 1992;135:418-427.

96. Jacques PF, Sulsky SI, Sadowski JA, Phillips JC, Rush D, Willett WC. Comparison of micronutrient intake measured by a dietary questionnaire and biochemical indicators of micronutrient status. *Am J Clin Nutr*. 1993;57:182-189.

97. Selhub J, Jacques PF, Wilson PWF, Rush D, Rosenberg IH. Vitamin status and intake as primary determinants of homocysteinemia in an elderly population. *J Am Med Assoc*. 1993;270:2693-2698.

98. Willett WC, Stampfer M, Chu N, Spiegelman D, Holmes M, Rimm E. Assessment of questionnaire validity for measuring total fat intake using plasma lipid levels as criteria. *Am J Epidemiol*. 2001;154:1107-1112.

99. Pietinen P, Hartman AM, Haapa E, et al. Reproducibility and validity of dietary assessment instruments II. A qualitative food-frequency questionnaire. *Am J Epidemiol*. 1988;128:667-676.

100. Goldbohm RA, van den Brandt PA, Brants HAM, et al. Validation of a dietary questionnaire used in a large-scale prospective cohort study on diet and cancer. *Eur J Clin Nutr*. 1994;48:253-265.

101. Subar AF, Kipnis V, Troiano RP, et al. Using intake biomarkers to evaluate the extent of dietary misreporting in a large sample of adults: the OPEN study. *Am J Epidemiol*. 2003;158(1):1-13.

102. Willett W. Invited commentary: OPEN questions. *Am J Epidemiol*. 2003;158(1):22-24.

103. Spiegelman D, McDermott A, Rosner B. Regression calibration method for correcting measurement – error bias in nutritional epidemiology. *Am J Clin Nutr*. 1997;65(suppl 4):1179S-1186S.

104. Rosner B, Willett WC, Spiegelman D. Correction of logistic regression relative risk estimates and confidence intervals for systematic within-person measurement error. *Stat Med*. 1989;8:1051-1069.

105. Rosner B, Spiegelman D, Willett WC. Correction of logistic regression relative risk estimates and confidence intervals for measurement error: the case of multiple covariates measured with error. *Am J Epidemiol*. 1990;132:734-745.

106. Walker AM, Blettner M. Comparing imperfect measures of exposure. *Am J Epidemiol*. 1985;121:783-790.

107. Hu FB, Stampfer MJ, Rimm E, et al. Dietary fat and coronary heart disease: a comparison of approaches for adjusting total energy intake and modeling repeated dietary measurements. *Am J Epidemiol*. 1999;149:531-540.

108. Van Dam RM, Hunter D. Biochemical indicators of dietary intake. In: Willett WC, ed. *Nutritional Epidemiology*. 3rd ed. New York, NY: Oxford University Press; 2013:150-212.

109. Kabagambe EK, Baylin A, Allan DA, Siles X, Spiegelman D, Campos H. Application of the method of triads to evaluate the performance of food frequency questionnaires and biomarkers as indicators of long-term dietary intake. *Am J Epidemiol*. 2001;154(12):1126-1135.

110. Longnecker MP, Stram DO, Taylor PR, et al. Use of selenium concentration in whole blood, serum, toe-nails, or urine as a surrogate measure of selenium intake. *Epidemiology*. 1996;7:384-390.

111. Wald N, Boreham J, Bailey A. Serum retinol and subsequent risk of cancer. *Br J Cancer*. 1986;54:957-961.

112. Stunkard AJ, Albaum JM. The accuracy of self-reported weights. *Am J Clin Nutr*. 1981;34:1593-1599.

113. Rhoads GG, Kagan A. The relation of coronary disease, stroke, and mortality to weight in youth and middle age. *Lancet*. 1983;1:492-495.

114. Must A, Willett WC, Dietz WH. Remote recall of childhood height, weight, and body build by elderly subjects. *Am J Epidemiol*. 1993;138:56-64.

115. Spiegelman D, Israel RG, Bouchard C, Willett WC. Absolute fat mass, percent body fat, and body-fat distribution: which is the real determinant of blood pressure and serum glucose? *Am J Clin Nutr*. 1992;55:1033-1044.

116. Sun Q, van Dam RM, Spiegelman D, Heymsfield SB, Willett WC, Hu FB. Comparison of dual-energy x-ray absorptiometric and anthropometric measures of adiposity in relation to adiposity-related biologic factors. *Am J Epidemiol*. 2010;172(12):1442-1454.

117. Snijder MB, Zimmet PZ, Visser M, Dekker JM, Seidell JC, Shaw JE. Independent and opposite associations of waist and hip circumferences with diabetes, hypertension and dyslipidemia: the AusDiab Study. *Int J Obes Relat Metab Disord* 2004;28(3):402-409.

118. van den Brandt PA, Spiegelman D, Yaun SS, et al. Pooled analysis of prospective cohort studies on height, weight, and breast cancer risk. *Am J Epidemiol*. 2000;152:514-527.

119. American Institute for Cancer Research; World Cancer Research Fund International. *Second Expert Report. Food, Nutrition, Physical Activity, and the Prevention of Cancer: A Global Perspective*. Washington, DC: WCRF/AICR; 2007.

120. Michels KB, Greenland S, Rosner BA. Does body mass index adequately capture the relation of body composition and body size to health outcomes? *Am J Epidemiol*. 1998;147(2):167-172.

121. Willett WC, Reynolds RD, Cottrell-Hoehner S, Sampson L, Browne ML. Validation of a semi-quantitative food frequency questionnaire: comparison with a 1-year diet record. *J Am Diet Assoc*. 1987;87:43-47.

122. Hu FB, Willett WC. Optimal diets for prevention of coronary heart disease. *J Am Med Assoc*. 2002;288:2569-2578.

123. Schulze MB, Hu FB. Primary prevention of diabetes: what can be done and how much can be prevented? *Ann Rev Public Health*. 2005;26:445-467.

124. Willett WC, Stampfer MJ. Total energy intake: implications for epidemiologic analyses. *Am J Epidemiol*. 1986;124:17-27.

125. Gordon T, Kagan A, Garcia-Palmieri M, et al. Diet and its relation to coronary heart disease and death in three populations. *Circulation*. 1981;63:500-515.

126. Lyon JL, Mahoney AW, West DW, et al. Energy intake: its relationship to colon cancer risk. *J Natl Cancer Inst*. 1987;78:853-861.

127. Willett W. Isocaloric diets are of primary interest in experimental and epidemiological studies. *Int J Epidemiol*. 2002;31(3):694-695.

128. Jakes RW, Day NE, Luben R, et al. Adjusting for energy intake--what measure to use in nutritional epidemiological studies? *Int J Epidemiol*. 2004;33:1382-1386.

129. Rhee JJ, Cho E, Willett WC. Energy adjustment of nutrient intakes is preferable to adjustment using body weight and physical activity in epidemiological analyses. *Public Health Nutr*. 2014;17(5):1054-1060.

130. Willett WC. Will it be cheese, bologna, or peanut butter? *Eur J Epidemiol*. 2017;32(4):257-259.

131. Hu F, Stampfer MJ, Manson JE, et al. Dietary fat intake and the risk of coronary heart disease in women. *N Engl J Med*. 1997;337:1491-1499.

132. Bernstein AM, Sun Q, Hu FB, Stampfer MJ, Manson JE, Willett WC. Major dietary protein sources and risk of coronary heart disease in women. *Circulation*. 2010;122(9):876-883.

133. NCD Risk Factor Collaboration. Trends in adult body mass index in 200 countries from 1975 to 2014: a pooled analysis of 1698 population-based measurement studies with 19.2 million participants. *Lancet*. 2016;387:1377-1396.

134. Afshin A, Forouzanfar MH, et al; GBD 2015 Obesity Collaborators. Health effects of overweight and obesity in 195 countries over 25 years. *N Engl J Med*. 2017;377(1):13-27.

135. Ogden CL, Carroll MD, Fryar CD, Flegal KM. Prevalence of obesity among adults and youth: United States, 2011-2014. *NCHS Data Brief*. 2015;219:1-8.

136. Hu FB. Diet, nutrition, and obesity. In: Hu FB, ed. *Obesity Epidemiology*. New York, NY: Oxford University Press; 2008:275-300.

137. Hruby A, Manson JE, Qi L, et al. Determinants and consequences of obesity. *Am J Public Health.* 2016;106(9):1656-1662.
138. Field AE, Willett WC, Lissner L, Colditz GA. Dietary fat and weight gain among women in the Nurses' Health Study. *Obesity (Silver Spring).* 2007;15(4):967-976.
139. Mozaffarian D, Hao T, Rimm EB, Willett WC, Hu FB. Changes in diet and lifestyle and long-term weight gain in women and men. *N Engl J Med.* 2011;364(25):2392-2404.
140. Fung TT, Pan A, Hou T, et al. Long-term change in diet quality is associated with body weight change in men and women. *J Nutr.* 2015;145(8):1850-1856.
141. Schwingshackl L, Hoffmann G, Schwedhelm C, et al. Consumption of dairy products in relation to changes in anthropometric variables in adult populations: a systematic review and meta-analysis of cohort studies. *PLoS One.* 2016;11(6):e0157461.
142. Chen M, Pan A, Malik VS, Hu FB. Effects of dairy intake on body weight and fat: a meta-analysis of randomized controlled trials. *Am J Clin Nutr.* 2012;96(4):735-747.
143. Bendsen NT, Christensen R, Bartels EM, et al. Is beer consumption related to measures of abdominal and general obesity? A systematic review and meta-analysis. *Nutr Rev.* 2013;71(2):67-87.
144. Qi Q, Chu AY, Kang JH, et al. Fried food consumption, genetic risk, and body mass index: gene-diet interaction analysis in three US cohort studies. *Br Med J.* 2014;348:g1610.
145. Qi Q, Chu AY, Kang JH, et al. Sugar-sweetened beverages and genetic risk of obesity. *N Engl J Med.* 2012;367(15):1387-1396.
146. Qi Q, Li Y, Chomistek AK, et al. Television watching, leisure time physical activity, and the genetic predisposition in relation to body mass index in women and men. *Circulation.* 2012;126(15):1821-1827.
147. Zheng Y, Manson JE, Yuan C, et al. Associations of weight gain from early to middle adulthood with major health outcomes later in life. *J Am Med Assoc.* 2017;318(3):255-269.
148. Hu FB. Obesity and cardiovascular disease. In: Hu FB, ed. *Obesity Epidemiology.* New York, NY: Oxford University Press; 2008:174-195.
149. Calle EE. Obesity and cancer. In: Hu FB, ed. *Obesity Epidemiology.* New York, NY: Oxford University Press; 2008:196-215.
150. Hu FB. Obesity and mortality. In: Hu FB, ed. *Obesity Epidemiology.* New York, NY: Oxford University Press; 2008:216-233.
151. Lyall DM, Celis-Morales C, Ward J, et al. Association of body mass index with cardiometabolic disease in the UK biobank: a mendelian randomization study. *JAMA Cardiol.* 2017;2(8):882-889.
152. Twig G, Yaniv G, Levine H, et al. Body-mass index in 2.3 million adolescents and cardiovascular death in adulthood. *N Engl J Med.* 2016;374(25):2430-2440.
153. Flegal KM, Kit BK, Orpana H, Graubard BI. Association of all-cause mortality with overweight and obesity using standard body mass index categories: a systematic review and meta-analysis. *J Am Med Assoc.* 2013;309(1):71-82.
154. Hu FB. Measurement of adiposity and body composition. In: Hu FB, ed. *Obesity Epidemiology.* New York, NY: Oxford University Press; 2008:53-83.
155. Di Angelantonio E, Bhupathiraju S, Wormser D, et al; Global BMI Mortality Collaboration. Body-mass index and all-cause mortality: individual-participant-data meta-analysis of 239 prospective studies in four continents. *Lancet.* 2016;388(10046):776-786.
156. Hu FB. *Obesity Epidemiology.* New York, NY: Oxford University Press; 2008.
157. Cornelis MC, Hu FB. Systems epidemiology: a new direction in nutrition and metabolic disease research. *Curr Nutr Rep.* 2013;2(4).
158. Bhupathiraju SN, Hu FB. One (small) step towards precision nutrition by use of metabolomics. *Lancet Diabetes Endocrinol.* 2017;5(3):154-155.
159. Tanaka T, Ngwa JS, van Rooij FJ, et al. Genome-wide meta-analysis of observational studies shows common genetic variants associated with macronutrient intake. *Am J Clin Nutr.* 2013;97(6):1395-1402.
160. Cornelis MC, Kacprowski T, Menni C, et al. Genome-wide association study of caffeine metabolites provides new insights to caffeine metabolism and dietary caffeine-consumption behavior. *Hum Mol Genet.* 2016;25(24):5472-5482.
161. Chu AY, Workalemahu T, Paynter NP, et al. Novel locus including FGF21 is associated with dietary macronutrient intake. *Hum Mol Genet.* 2013;22(9):1895-1902.
162. Cornelis MC, Hu FB. Gene-environment interactions in the development of type 2 diabetes: recent progress and continuing challenges. *Annu Rev Nutr.* 2012;32:245-259.
163. Qi L, Cornelis MC, Zhang C, van Dam RM, Hu FB. Genetic predisposition, Western dietary pattern, and the risk of type 2 diabetes in men. *Am J Clin Nutr.* 2009;89(5):1453-1458.
164. Do R, Xie C, Zhang X, et al. The effect of chromosome 9p21 variants on cardiovascular disease may be modified by dietary intake: evidence from a case/control and a prospective study. *PLoS Med.* 2011;8(10):e1001106.
165. Brunkwall L, Chen Y, Hindy G, et al. Sugar-sweetened beverage consumption and genetic predisposition to obesity in 2 Swedish cohorts. *Am J Clin Nutr.* 2016;104(3):809-815.

166. Olsen NJ, Angquist L, Larsen SC, et al. Interactions between genetic variants associated with adiposity traits and soft drinks in relation to longitudinal changes in body weight and waist circumference. *Am J Clin Nutr.* 2016;104(3):816-826.

167. Xiang L, Wu H, Pan A, et al. FTO genotype and weight loss in diet and lifestyle interventions: a systematic review and meta-analysis. *Am J Clin Nutr.* 2016;103(4):1162-1170.

168. Willett W Genetics in dietary analysis. In: Willett W, ed. *Nutritional Epidemiology.* 3rd ed. New York, NY: Oxford University Press; 2013. p. 334-343.

169. Lewis SJ, Smith GD. Alcohol, ALDH2, and esophageal cancer: a meta-analysis which illustrates the potentials and limitations of a Mendelian randomization approach. *Cancer Epidemiol Biomarkers Prev.* 2005;14(8):1967-1971.

170. Wu C, Kraft P, Zhai K, et al. Genome-wide association analyses of esophageal squamous cell carcinoma in Chinese identify multiple susceptibility loci and gene-environment interactions. *Nat Genet.* 2012;44(10):1090-1097.

171. Guasch-Ferre M, Hruby A, Toledo E, et al. Metabolomics in prediabetes and diabetes: a systematic review and meta-analysis. *Diabetes Care.* 2016;39(5):833-846.

172. Ruiz-Canela M, Toledo E, Clish CB, et al.. Plasma branched-chain amino acids and incident cardiovascular disease in the PREDIMED trial. *Clin Chem.* 2016;62(4):582-592.

173. Mayers JR, Wu C, Clish CB, et al. Elevation of circulating branched-chain amino acids is an early event in human pancreatic adenocarcinoma development. *Nat Med.* 2014;20(10):1193-1198.

174. Scalbert A, Brennan L, Manach C, et al. The food metabolome: a window over dietary exposure. *Am J Clin Nutr.* 2014;99(6):1286-1308.

175. Wang DD, Leung CW, Li Y, et al. Trends in dietary quality among adults in the United States, 1999 through 2010. *JAMA Intern Med.* 2014;174(10):1587-1595.

176. Nelson ME, Hamm MW, Hu FB, Abrams SA, Griffin TS. Alignment of healthy dietary patterns and environmental sustainability: a systematic review. *Adv Nutr.* 2016;7(6):1005-1025.

177. Frieden TR. Evidence for health decision making - beyond randomized, controlled trials. *N Engl J Med.* 2017;377(5):465-475.

178. Satija A, Yu E, Willett WC, Hu FB. Understanding nutritional epidemiology and its role in policy. *Adv Nutr.* 2015;6(1):5-18.

179. Willett WC, Stampfer MJ, Manson JE, et al. Intake of trans fatty acids and risk of coronary heart disease among women. *Lancet.* 1993;341:581-585.

180. Mensink RPM, Katan MB. Effect of dietary trans fatty acids on high-density and low-density lipoprotein cholesterol levels in healthy subjects. *N Engl J Med.* 1990;323:439-445.

181. Oh K, Hu FB, Manson JE, Stampfer MJ, Willett WC. Dietary fat intake and risk of coronary heart disease in women: 20 years of follow-up of the Nurses' Health Study. *Am J Epidemiol.* 2005;161(7):672-679.

182. Ascherio A, Rimm EB, Giovannucci EL, Spiegelman D, Stampfer MJ, Willett WC. Dietary fat and risk of coronary heart disease in men: cohort follow up study in the United States. *Br Med J.* 1996;313:84-90.

183. Pietinen P, Ascherio A, Korhonen P, et al. Intake of fatty acids and risk of coronary heart disease in a cohort of Finnish men: the ATBC Study. *Am J Epidemiol.* 1997;145:876-887.

184. Xu J, Eilat-Adar S, Loria C, et al. Dietary fat intake and risk of coronary heart disease: the Strong Heart Study. *Am J Clin Nutr.* 2006;84(4):894-902.

185. Restrepo BJ, Rieger M. Denmark's policy on artificial trans fat and cardiovascular disease. *Am J Prev Med.* 2016;50(1):69-76.

186. Coombes R. Trans fats: chasing a global ban. *Br Med J.* 2011;343:d5567.

187. World Health Organization Regional Office for Europe. *Eliminating Trans Fats in Europe.* Copenhagen: World Health Organization Regional Office for Europe; 2015.

188. US Department of Health and Human Services. *Dietary Guidelines for Americans, 2005.* Washington, DC: US Department of Health and Human Services; 2005. Available at https://www.dietaryguidelines.gov/about-dietary-guidelines/previous-editions/2005-dietary-guidelines-americans. Accessed September 23, 2010

189. Food labeling: trans. *Fed Regist.* 2003;21(101):41433-41506.

190. Angell SY, Cobb LK, Curtis CJ, Konty KJ, Silver LD. Change in trans fatty acid content of fast-food purchases associated with New York City's restaurant regulation. *Ann Intern Med.* 2012;157(2):81-86.

191. Assaf RR. Overview of local, state, and national government legislation restricting trans fats. *Clin Ther.* 2014;36(3):328-332.

192. Dietz WH, Scanlon KS. Eliminating the use of partially hydrogenated oil in food production and preparation. *J Am Med Assoc.* 2012;308(2):143-144.

193. Mozaffarian D, Jacobson MF, Greenstein JS. Food reformulations to reduce trans fatty acids. *N Engl J Med.* 2010;362(21):2037-2039.

194. Wang DD, Li Y, Chiuve SE, Hu FB, Willett WC. Improvements in US diet helped reduce disease burden and lower premature deaths, 1999-2012; overall diet remains poor. *Health Aff (Millwood).* 2015;34(11):1916-1922.

195. Brandt EJ, Myerson R, Perraillon MC, Polonsky TS. Hospital admissions for myocardial infarction and stroke before and after the trans-fatty acid restrictions in New York. *JAMA Cardiol*. 2017;2(6):627-634.

196. Bernstein AM, de Koning L, Flint AJ, Rexrode KM, Willett WC. Soda consumption and the risk of stroke in men and women. *Am J Clin Nutr*. 2012;95(5):1190-1199.

197. Fung TT, Malik V, Rexrode KM, Manson JE, Willett WC, Hu FB. Sweetened beverage consumption and risk of coronary heart disease in women. *Am J Clin Nutr*. 2009;89(4):1037-1042.

198. Schulze MB, Manson JE, Ludwig DS, et al. Sugar-sweetened beverages, weight gain, and incidence of type 2 diabetes in young and middle-aged women. *J Am Med Assoc*. 2004;292(8):927-934.

199. de Ruyter JC, Olthof MR, Seidell JC, Katan MB. A trial of sugar-free or sugar-sweetened beverages and body weight in children. *N Engl J Med*. 2012;367(15):1397-1406.

200. Ebbeling CB, Feldman HA, Chomitz VR, et al. A randomized trial of sugar-sweetened beverages and adolescent body weight. *N Engl J Med*. 2012;367(15):1407-1416.

201. Centers for Disease Control and Prevention. *Competitive Foods and Beverages in US Schools: A State Policy Analysis*. Atlanta, GA: US Department of Health and Human Services; 2012.

202. Cámara de Diputados del Congreso de la Unión. *Ley de Impuesto Especial sobre Producción y Servicios. [Law of special tax on production and services]*. 2013.

203. Colchero MA, Rivera-Dommarco J, Popkin BM, Ng SW. In Mexico, evidence of sustained consumer response two years after implementing A sugar-sweetened beverage tax. *Health Aff (Millwood)*. 2017;36(3):564-571.

204. The Center for Science in the Public Interest. Soda Tax.

205. Silver LD, Ng SW, Ryan-Ibarra S, et al. Changes in prices, sales, consumer spending, and beverage consumption one year after a tax on sugar-sweetened beverages in Berkeley, California, US: a before-and-after study. *PLoS Med*. 2017;14(4):e1002283.

206. Long MW, Gortmaker SL, Ward ZJ, et al. Cost effectiveness of a sugar-sweetened beverage excise tax in the US. *Am J Prev Med*. 2015;49(1):112-123.

207. Willett WC, Stampfer MJ, Colditz GA, Rosner BA, Hennekens CH, Speizer FE. Dietary fat and the risk of breast cancer. *N Engl J Med*. 1987;316:22-28.

208. Willett WC, Hunter DJ, Stampfer MJ, et al. Dietary fat and fiber in relation to risk of breast cancer: an 8-year follow-up. *J Am Med Assoc*. 1992;268:2037-2044.

209. Smith-Warner SA, Spiegelman D, Adami HO, et al.. Types of dietary fat and breast cancer: a pooled analysis of cohort studies. *Int J Cancer*. 2001;92:767-774.

210. Wang DD, Hu FB. Dietary fat and risk of cardiovascular disease: recent controversies and advances. *Ann Rev Nutr*. 2017;37:423-446.

211. Mensink RP, Zock PL, Kester AD, Katan MB. Effects of dietary fatty acids and carbohydrates on the ratio of serum total to HDL cholesterol and on serum lipids and apolipoproteins: a meta-analysis of 60 controlled trials. *Am J Clin Nutr*. 2003;77(5):1146-1155.

212. US Department of Health and Human Services; US Department of Agriculture. *2015-2020 Dietary Guidelines for Americans*. New York, NY: Skyhorse Publishing; 2015.

213. US Department of Agriculture; US Department of Health and Human Services. Scientific Report of the 2015 Dietary Guidelines Advisory Committee. Washington, DC: U.S. Gov't Printing Offices.

214. Satija A, Yu E, Willett WC, Hu FB. Objective measures are complementary to, rather than a replacement for, self-reported methods. *Int J Obes (Lond)*. 2015;39(7):1179.

CHAPTER 43

Pharmacoepidemiology

Sebastian Schneeweiss and Krista F. Huybrechts

PHARMACOEPIDEMIOLOGY

Pharmacoepidemiology, the study of medical product use and the resulting health outcomes in clinical practice, provides information on under- and overutilization of medications and on the safety and effectiveness of medical products in routine care. The field integrates clinical pharmacology and medicine with epidemiology. Results of pharmacoepidemiology studies inform decisions made by physicians and their patients, regulators, policy-makers, and payer organizations. Given the growing availability of diverse and increasingly large and clinically detailed data sources that can be used for pharmacoepidemiology studies, the field has developed rapidly over the past decades. With that, the methodological understanding of how to mitigate biases commonly occurring when using secondary data sources and nonrandomized study designs has evolved.

Pharmacoepidemiology has successfully helped to identify and quantify the risk of adverse drug reactions for many years. The typical methodology, when applied appropriately, has proven robust in discovering unexpected outcomes of medication treatment. In recent years, pharmacoepidemiology has been increasingly used to study beneficial drug effects, evidence that had earlier mostly been obtained from randomized controlled trials (RCTs). Such studies have also been described as comparative effectiveness research and real-world evidence.

Professional societies and regulatory agencies have issued multiple guidance documents on how to conduct medication safety studies. As part of the expanded use of pharmacoepidemiology coinciding with the growth of suitable longitudinal data sources, there have been statements of ambition from regulators on how to study beneficial effects of drugs and from professional societies on how to conduct pharmacoepidemiology studies transparently.[1-3]

Pharmacoepidemiology applies the same principles of epidemiologic research as any other type of noninterventional study, and all principles of causal inference and other technical aspects of study design and data analysis described in this book pertain. Pharmacoepidemiology builds on our understanding of clinical pharmacology and the practice of medicine that provides the context for the study design and analysis. Some issues particular to pharmacoepidemiology originate from working with longitudinal healthcare databases that were not created for answering the research question at hand. Working with these databases leads to workarounds that were developed to mitigate biases that may arise from working with such data.

This chapter gives a structured overview of the considerations when conducting or interpreting pharmacoepidemiology studies. The chapter focuses on comparative analyses of the safety and effectiveness of medical products. Much is written on drug utilization studies, but these are covered here only in passing. We build on the previous chapters and specifically refer to the chapter on secondary data sources, which are an important resource for pharmacoepidemiology studies.

APPLICATIONS OF PHARMACOEPIDEMIOLOGY

Pharmacoepidemiology answers a wide range of study questions using a variety of data sources and analytic methodologies. Findings are used to inform decisions by physicians and their patients, by policy-makers contemplating insurance coverage and quality improvement measures, by regulators who are concerned with the safety of medications and the population-based benefit-harm balance, and by payer organizations evaluating how to cover medication cost.

Typical applications include:

- Drug utilization research: Understanding the prevalence and incidence of medication use is an essential tool for monitoring the care of populations. It uncovers under- and overuse of medications, and it describes medication use outside of the labeled indication, often for good reasons but sometimes against medical evidence. Drug utilization research may identify clusters of unusual prescribing patterns (*e.g.*, prescribing of opioids) and may highlight how much medical practice lags behind new evidence from well-conducted randomized trials (*e.g.*, the persistent use of sulfonylureas in patients with type-2 diabetes despite safer and more effective alternatives for second-line use). Last, utilization studies often uncover a frustratingly low level of adherence and persistence with medication use and the medical and behavioral factors that influence such suboptimal use patterns.[4] Drug utilization studies are thus highly valuable to monitor the access to and quality of medication prescribing for large populations.
- Drug policy analyses: Pharmacoepidemiology analyses of medication use data have been instrumental in uncovering unintended and sometimes detrimental health effects of coverage policy changes. For example, an insurance policy change limiting coverage to three medications dispensed per month led to a dramatic drop in the use of essential medications in vulnerable Medicaid beneficiaries.[5] Expanding drug coverage and reducing patient copayment, on the contrary, resulted in improved medication adherence and health outcomes.[6]
- Drug safety analyses: Most randomized trials presented to regulators for approval decisions are limited in size and unable to rule out uncommon adverse reactions. From its inception, pharmacoepidemiology focused on studying the safety of medications in large and broad populations, including those excluded from trials, such as pregnant women, multimorbid patients, or older adults. Regulators now routinely ask for such pharmacoepidemiology studies as postmarketing requirements or postapproval safety studies. They aim to quantify the risk of unintended harms of medications often in relevant user populations and enable

a comprehensive benefit-risk assessment. Prominent examples were the increased risk of myocardial infarction associated with rofecoxib, a pain medication,[7] the risk of bladder cancer in patients using pioglitazone,[8] and the risk of psychosis in children and adolescents starting stimulant medications.[9]

- Comparative drug effectiveness research: While randomized control trials can establish the efficacy of medications, they leave open many questions on the effectiveness of drugs that are relevant for prescribers and patients in clinical practice. Firstly, an RCT may have focused on a narrow population segment, while prescribers treat a much broader population in terms of comorbidities, comedications, age, and other characteristics that might influence how well the drugs work and how safe they are. Second, an RCT typically compares an experimental drug against a placebo while providers wish to know the incremental benefit compared to an agent currently in use. Third, a provider organization or insurance plan may wish to know the medication's impact on use patterns observed in typical care delivery settings. Pharmacoepidemiologic studies can address these questions, and we discuss below the challenges in overcoming confounding that may arise from strong patient selection to treatment based on their underlying risk. More recently, regulatory agencies are interested in understanding to what extent RCTs can be augmented or even replaced in select settings to inform approval of supplemental indications or approval of drugs in rare disease.[10,11]

- RCT planning and augmentation: Pharmacoepidemiology has been used to help understand variation in background incidence rates of trial end points by baseline risk factors and help enrich RCTs with patients with high event risks and free of serious comorbid conditions to improve the efficiency of a trial.[12] Participants of trials are sporadically followed beyond the trial period to understand long-term end points in pharmacoepidemiology analyses.[13] Linkage with claims data helps generalize RCT findings to broader insured populations.[12]

- Drug repurposing: It is an ongoing promise that some of the marketed medications may have additional effects beyond those for which they were initially developed and marketed. There is a range of in vitro and in silico approaches that generate hypotheses of novel drug-outcome associations in specific populations that one may wish to test in humans. It is impractical to move all these hypotheses directly to RCTs. Pharmacoepidemiology has emerged as an intermediate step to test the potential repurposed drug effects. By definition, the drugs of interest are already marketed, so that data on their use and outcomes are available. With a scalable pharmacoepidemiology infrastructure based on epidemiologic principles, one can now investigate multiple hypotheses and either refute or further characterize an effect before embarking on human experiments and eventually relabeling.[14]

In this chapter, we focus mostly on studies and methodologies to assess the comparative safety and effectiveness of medications used in routine care.

DATA SOURCES IN PHARMACOEPIDEMIOLOGY AND ANALYSIS IMPLICATIONS

Pharmacoepidemiology applies principles of epidemiologic research the same way as any other type of noninterventional study. The majority of pharmacoepidemiology studies are conducted using longitudinal healthcare databases, opting for the advantage of large study populations with extended follow-up while sacrificing the controlled and detailed data capture characteristic of primary data collection. In such studies, it is essential to understand the data generating process.

Modern healthcare systems generate a wealth of electronically stored information on individual patients producing ongoing data streams that can be connected longitudinally through patient identifiers. Today most pharmacoepidemiology studies use such electronic longitudinal data on medication use and health events captured during the routine operation of a healthcare system. These data include insurance claims data, electronic health records (EHRs), and specific disease registries. There are several reasons why such data have gained popularity in pharmacoepidemiology. First, they cover populations more representative than trials of all patients taking the drug, and even when restricted to patients who initiate a newly marketed medication, there are often reasonable numbers of users. Second, they include prospective recording of prescribing or prescription filling with great details and do not rely on patient consent to participation and recall to record use. Third,

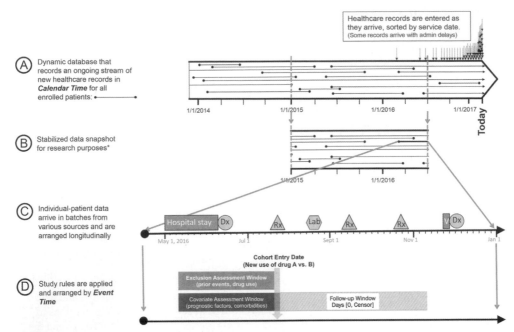

FIGURE 43-1 From electronic health data to a longitudinal study. (Adapted from Schneeweiss S. Automated data-adaptive analytics for electronic healthcare data to study causal treatment effects. *Clin Epidemiol.* 2018;10:771-788. © 2018 Dove Medical Press.)

they are more timely and less expensive than most primary data collection mechanisms. Chapter 11 on secondary data sources provides an introduction to the many different data sources available to researchers, including their strengths and weaknesses. Here, we focus on electronic healthcare databases used specifically to study medication use and health outcomes.

Healthcare databases are transactional databases that collect clinical and administrative information related to the delivery and administration of health care. As encounters occur and services are provided, records are generated and added to an ever-growing database. Each service provided comes with a service date stamp and patient identifier, generating longitudinal patient records of increasing duration (Figure 43-1A). As a first step in the implementation of a study, one identifies and sets aside a section of the dynamic data stream that covers the calendar time period of interest (Figure 43-1B). This data snapshot is a prerequisite for making results from a study replicable at a later time point. It produces an enumerable set of longitudinal patient records, each with a start and end date in calendar time. Encounters and services are recorded with diagnostic and procedural information on each patient's timeline (Figure 43-1C). The rules and algorithms that define a specific study design implementation are applied to each patient's longitudinal data stream (Figure 43-1D).

Dates and Time Windows

Certain principles guide the design and implementation of studies in healthcare data streams. One of the most important is longitudinality of measurement. Many measurements in healthcare databases are made by reviewing the information recorded during multiple healthcare encounters over time. In primary data collection, a study subject's health state is established at a point in time when the patient is thoroughly interviewed or examined during a study visit. In healthcare databases, there is no defined interview date with the investigator team. Instead, studies rely on the occurrence of visits and other healthcare encounters to collect information that was recorded while providing care. Thus, information that we often conceptualize as being captured at a particular point in time, such as baseline patient characteristics before the start of exposure, is recorded during a defined time window through a series of encounters.[15]

Anchors in Patient Event Time

When implementing a study of the effectiveness or safety of medications, the time scale shifts from calendar time to patient event time. Specific algorithms define events in the patient timeline. As in RCTs, where the randomization date is the most critical anchor date for subsequent analyses, the cohort entry date (CED, also referred to as the index date) is the primary anchor in a noninterventional database study (Figure 43-1D). The CED is the date when subjects enter the analytic study population.

Secondary temporal anchors are defined relative to the first-order anchor, the CED. Similar to the temporal ordering in a randomized trial, we wish to assess all patient characteristics before the start of exposure to avoid adjusting for causal intermediates.[16] We, therefore, define an exclusion assessment window (EXCL) and the covariate assessment window (Figure 43-2). In many applications, we want to make sure that the outcome of interest has not yet occurred at the time of study entry and the beginning of medication exposure. To study such newly occurring events, investigators can require an outcome washout window. Similarly, an exposure washout window of defined duration determines the new use of a drug or other treatment. For example, to identify new users of direct oral anticoagulants, we can require the index dispensing to be preceded by 6 or 12 months during which there was no evidence of anticoagulant use.

The follow-up window, during which the study population is at risk for developing the outcome of interest, begins after study entry. It may begin on the CED or after an assumed induction window before which there is no biologically plausible effect of exposure on the outcome. The maximum duration of the follow-up window is defined by one or more censoring criteria, *e.g.*, end of enrollment, death, maximum causal time window, or end of data stream. In case-based sampling designs nested in cohorts of patients, like the case-control and case-crossover sampling, the study entry can be additionally defined by an event date. Figure 43-2 exemplifies the longitudinal design choices in a cohort study and a case-control sampling of the same cohort. Next, we will turn to the specifics of how to estimate treatment effects that may support causal conclusions. The process has three layers establishing a fairly linear workflow: a data layer, a measurement layer, and an analysis layer. Figure 43-3 provides a summary of the considerations and tasks, which we explain in greater detail in the following sections.

STUDY DESIGN CONSIDERATIONS

The study question informs study design choices. In pharmacoepidemiology, the design choice is further influenced by the reality of the underlying data sources. When studying the effect of medication treatment, considerations about the sources for exposure variation—such as whether the drug exposure varies within a patient, between patients, or between providers who treat groups of patients—lead to fundamental decisions on the appropriate study design, whether it is a noninterventional study or a randomized experiment.

In a hypothetical counterfactual experiment, one would expose a patient to an agent and observe the occurrence or nonoccurrence of the health outcome. Then, counterfactually, one would rewind time and repeat while leaving the patient unexposed (or exposed to a different agent), keeping all other factors constant to establish a counterfactual experience. To approximate this thought experiment, we introduce or observe exposure variation within the same patient at different times or between different patients at the same time or between providers (Figure 43-4).

If we observe fluctuations of exposure status within a patient over time, *e.g.*, headache medication, and if that drug has a short hypothesized duration of action, and if the event of interest has a rapid onset, *e.g.*, liver toxicity, then we may consider a case-crossover design or self-controlled case series. While such designs inherently control for time-invariant risk factors by comparing a patient's experience with himself or herself at different times, within-person confounding may nonetheless occur if the disease state changes with time and with its treatment.[17]

Most pharmacoepidemiology studies exploit naturally occurring variation in medication exposure between patients and therefore use a cohort study design with concurrent controls. Historical control groups have had a renaissance mainly because highly targeted treatments reduce the size of the available study population, and investigators resort to observing past experiences to increase the useable data. Within cohorts, efficient sampling designs like the case-control, case-cohort, or two-stage sampling can be used when information gathering is time-consuming or expensive.[18]

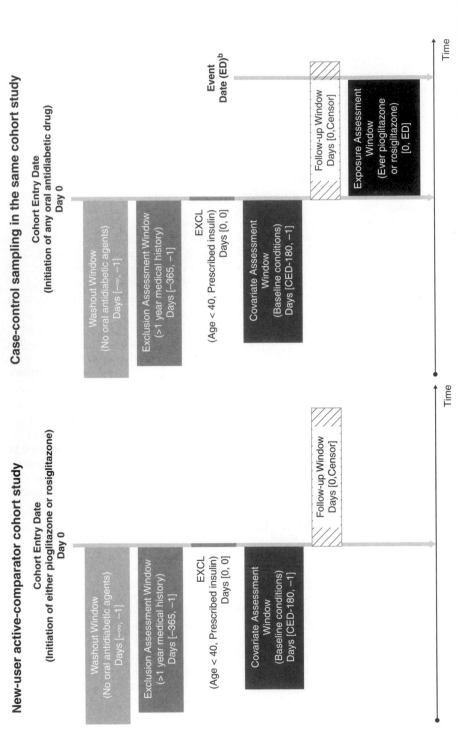

FIGURE 43-2 Illustration of typical longitudinal study design choices in pharmacoepidemiology. The diagrams use a comparative analysis of new users of pioglitazone versus new users of rosiglitazone on some health outcome to illustrate how time windows are used to identify key markers and variables. (© 2019 Harvard Medical / Brigham Division of Pharmacoepidemiology.)

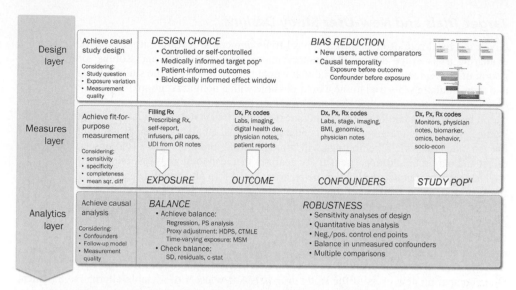

FIGURE 43-3 From electronic healthcare data to estimating medication treatment effects.

Medication exposure variation among higher-level entities, *i.e.*, between physicians, hospitals, health plans, regions, etc., which cover groups of patients, can be exploited using instrumental variable analyses. The instrument, which corresponds to the reason for the group-level exposure variation, must be unrelated to patient characteristics either directly or indirectly (see Chapter 28 on quasi-experimental designs).[19] Selecting a comparator group is arguably the most fundamental choice in a pharmacoepidemiology study design and may influence results substantially. The comparator needs to be relevant in the clinical context and a viable alternative to the study drug. Ideally, we want to restrict the comparison population to patients who, in clinical practice, have the same indication as the users of the study agent. The oral antidiabetic drugs rosiglitazone and pioglitazone are an example of such a medication pair. They were marketed around the same time, were both indicated for second-line treatment of diabetes, come from the same class of compound, and, in the early marketing phase, were thought to have similar effectiveness and safety profiles. This should make treatment choice largely random with regard to patient characteristics and should therefore make treatment groups comparable by design, resulting in little confounding.

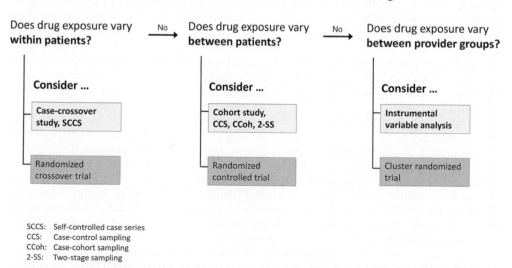

SCCS: Self-controlled case series
CCS: Case-control sampling
CCoh: Case-cohort sampling
2-SS: Two-stage sampling

FIGURE 43-4 Aspects of the study question and sources of exposure variation guide fundamental design choices. (Adapted from Schneeweiss S. A basic study design for expedited safety signal evaluation based on electronic healthcare data. *Pharmacoepidemiol Drug Saf*. 2010;19:858-868.)

Target Trials and New-User Study Designs

Given the focal role of randomized control trials in medical research, it was natural to consider emulating trials in the design of noninterventional studies. Hernan and Robins formalized this notion of conceptualizing a target trial that would be able to answer the study question accurately and then emulating this trial to the extent possible with a noninterventional study.[20] Attempting to do this highlights the compromises needed, given the reality of the underlying data source, medication use patterns, and other medical context-specific issues not controllable in nonexperimental studies. Specifying a target trial and its noninterventional emulation often provides clarity regarding the extent to which the findings will provide causal interpretations of an observed treatment effect and may spur additional sensitivity analyses that lead to more measured interpretations.

The target trial conceptualization helps bring to the fore and avoid design flaws like immortal time bias, adjustment for causal intermediates, reverse causation, and dealing with time-varying hazards and depletion of susceptibles.[21] In the cohort study setting, the target trial conceptualization guides users to the new-user study design, as that is what occurs in a typical randomized clinical trial. Studying ongoing users who have "survived" on the drug of interest until cohort entry has produced misleading findings.[22,23]

There are several advantages to studying new users in pharmacoepidemiology, particularly when comparing new users of the study drug versus new users of a viable alternative treatment. As patients in both treatment groups are newly started on medications, they have been evaluated by a physician who concluded that these patients would benefit from starting therapy with a newly prescribed drug. This process produces compared treatment groups that are similar with respect to characteristics that are both observable and unobservable in a given data source.[24] The clear temporal sequence of measuring confounders before treatment begins avoids the mistake of adjusting for the consequences of treatment (causal intermediates). Because of the well-defined starting point of new-user cohorts, it is possible to assess how hazards vary with duration of treatment. Because the new-user cohort study design emulates the standard parallel-group randomized trial closely, it is easier to understand by general readers. This cogency should not be underestimated in an era where decision-makers ignore noninterventional studies because they seem too complicated and the validity of the study seems obscure.[25] Examples of such new-user cohort studies are of the risk of psychosis in children and adolescents starting stimulant medications[9] or the relationship of statin use on a range of health outcomes.[26]

The new-user design also has clear benefits when studying newly marketed medications: it avoids comparing populations composed of first-time users of a newly marketed drug with a population comprising mainly prevalent users of an existing comparator drug.[27] Such a comparison would be prone to bias because patients who stay on treatment tend to be those who tolerate the treatment, experience its benefits, and are less susceptible to the event of interest. The same phenomenon plays out when comparing patients who switch a medication versus those who stay on their medication. This is an essential clinical question in most chronic conditions, but because patients with treatment failure are more likely to switch to an alternative treatment, confounding may be substantial. In the setting of studying newly marketed medication to treat chronic conditions, most patients starting on the new medication have already been using an alternative medication, often one of the comparator drugs. Given the temporal sequence that patients first were new users of the comparison drug and subsequently switch treatment to become a new user of the study drug, the standard new-user design that excludes drug switchers would lead to a small cohort of study drug users. To accommodate this setting, there is an alternative to the new-user design, which is the prevalent new-user design, that allows study drug users to have previously used the comparison agent.[28] Although this design increases the number of study-drug users, which is frequently the limiting factor to study size, it increases the risk of confounding by allowing drug switchers to be included in the analysis. In studies of outcomes with long induction times, such as diethylstilbestrol (DES) and vaginal cancer,[29] the outcome risk may be falsely attributed to the study drug although it was already induced by the preceding comparator drug.

Comparing two active treatment groups not only leads to more comparable patient groups but also further reduces the chance of immortal time bias, a problem that emerges if future information is used to define earlier exposure status in healthcare databases. A typical example of immortal time bias is to define nonusers as patients who do not use the study medication during the first

12 months of follow-up. By definition, these nonuser patients cannot die during the first 12 months of follow-up or else they could not be included. As their mortality rate must be zero during the first 12 months of follow-up, the inclusion of their 12 months of follow-up needed to establish the exposure definition will bias mortality findings.[30]

Nonuser comparisons that are conducted in an attempt to emulate placebo-controlled trials often suffer from strong treatment selection. Persons prescribed the drug are different from persons not prescribed the drug in ways that are difficult to completely measure and control analytically. Such strong confounding also occurs when comparing two different treatment modalities, *e.g.*, oral antipsychotic treatment versus injectable depot antipsychotics or medical treatment versus surgery. An example of such uncontrollable confounding is the comparison of medication treatment versus implantable cardioverter-defibrillators in patients with heart failure and the risk of sudden cardiac death.[31] The frailest patients will not undergo surgery because of its risks, and yet these patients are at the highest risk for the outcome of interest, biasing the comparison.

MEASUREMENT CONSIDERATIONS

Working with secondary data in pharmacoepidemiology studies makes data completeness and quality a paramount concern for drawing causal conclusions.

In order to study a causal treatment effect, the following four features need to be measured: (1) the population inclusion and exclusion criteria to characterize the study population and clinically relevant patient subgroups, (2) the exposure status, (3) the postexposure outcome, and (4) the pre-exposure confounding factors that influence both the treatment decision and the outcome (Figure 43-5). The measurement of each of those features comes with specific measurement characteristics that can be quantified by metrics like sensitivity and specificity for binary variables or mean squared difference and proportion missing for continuous variables. For example, accuracy of measurement of diabetes based on the presence of a relevant diagnosis code is characterized with sensitivity, specificity, and positive predictive value (PPV). Accuracy of a continuous measurement, such as HbA1c, is characterized by the proportion of patients who have the measurement of interest in the time period relevant for the study, for example, during the 3 months before treatment initiation and by the error in the measurement.

Study features:	Examples of ways to improve measurement characteristics	Typical proxies for data quality in secondary data	Actual measurement characteristics[1]
1) Population characteristics, subgroups	Require two diagnosis codes to increase specificity of underlying condition	Prior experience with a data source, publications Availability of validation studies	Binary data, e.g., diagnostic codes present: • Sensitivity • Specificity • PPV
2) Exposure measurement	Use dispensing information instead of prescribing data to increase completeness	Detailed documentation of data generation mechanism	
3) Outcome measurement	Use serious events, e.g., that require hospitalizations to increase specificity of outcome measurement	Detailed description of data curating process Detailed description of mapping to medical constructs (if any)	Continuous data, e.g., lab test values: • % missing • Mean squared deviation Time-to-event: • Accuracy of onset
4) Confounder measurement	Screen a wide range of potential confounders and their proxies to limit unobserved confounding	Documentation of coding shift over time	

1) These metrics are relevant for quantifying potential bias and assessing the likelihood of a causal drug-outcome relationship vs. spurious findings.

FIGURE 43-5 Measurement considerations for pharmacoepidemiology database studies. (Adapted from Franklin JM, Glynn RJ, Martin D, Schneeweiss S. Evaluating the use of nonrandomized real world data analyses for regulatory decision making. *Clin Pharm Ther.* 2019;105:867-877. © 2019 Harvard Medical/Brigham Division of Pharmacoepidemiology.)

In a specific study, most of these measurement characteristics are unknown and approximated from prior experience in the same or similar data sources. When constructing measures, investigators often apply general principles that increase the likelihood that the measurement characteristics will improve in the desired direction. For example, we typically want to increase the specificity of an outcome measure.[32] This can be achieved by requiring two visits with a diagnosis to indicate the disease onset, *e.g.*, diabetes, instead of just one visit, the purpose of which could have been simply to rule out diabetes.[33] But even if the exact measurement characteristics of the four study features are perfectly known, it is not obvious how good is good enough for unbiased treatment effect estimation. Even randomized trials using primary data collection have imperfect measurements. The goal is to have measurements that are as complete and accurate as possible and have known measurement characteristics to put findings in context of the underlying data quality.

Often, the values of the measurement characteristics that are required depend on the setting. For illustration, if one wishes to estimate a risk ratio, it is advisable to have the highest possible specificity of the outcome measurements, while if the estimate of interest is the risk difference, a high sensitivity is equally important to reduce bias.[32,34]

The Consequences of Mismeasurement in Pharmacoepidemiology Studies

The same principles of measurement error that were discussed in earlier chapters apply to pharmacoepidemiology. Most mismeasurement in pharmacoepidemiology stems from insufficient surveillance and, most worrisome, differential surveillance. As pointed out earlier, information on diagnoses and procedures is recorded when interacting with the professional healthcare system. The more the contacts, the more likely the health state of a patient is recorded fully during a covariate assessment window and the more likely outcomes are captured completely and timely during follow-up. This situation is fundamentally different from primary data collection. For example, in most RCTs, a large battery of tests and examinations are performed for every patient at enrollment and in defined follow-up intervals. A strategy to mitigate this issue is to adjust for the number of preexposure healthcare encounters as a proxy measure for information completeness and surveillance.[35] Differential surveillance is often a concern when physicians prescribe newly marketed medications with which they have less experience and ask the patient to visit more frequently for follow-up or if early symptoms of an outcome of interest lead to intensified medical workup. Generally, it is recommended to engage in bias modeling to understand the consequences of suboptimal data quality on the study findings.

Drug Exposure Misclassification and its Consequences

For almost all pharmacoepidemiology studies, it is fundamental to measure the start and end of a given drug exposure. Electronic pharmacy dispensing records are considered largely accurate in recording the start of a drug exposure because pharmacists fill prescriptions with little room for interpretation and are reimbursed by insurers based on detailed, complete, and accurate claims submitted electronically. Since patients need to go to the pharmacy and typically pay a copayment, it is considered highly likely that they will take the medication. Therefore, pharmacy dispensing information is seen as a reliable measure of drug exposure information, more so than patient-reported information or physician records.

Often a drug claim contains a field for the number of *days supply* representing the number of days a dispensing is intended to cover. Alternatively, one can multiply the number of dispensed pills by their strength and divide by a typical dosing like that described by *defined daily doses* or other estimates. To assess the overall duration of medication use, the individual dispensings need to be strung together. While this is a reasonable approach, it may cause exposure misclassification in two ways. If the calculated or pharmacist-recorded days supply is too short or if patients decide to stretch a prescription by using a lower dose, *e.g.*, by tablet splitting, some person-time will be classified as unexposed, whereas it truly is exposed. Most drugs treating chronic conditions are used for extended periods resulting in multiple refills. A patient can thus be classified as being unexposed intermittently despite continuous exposure (Figure 43-6). Many investigators, therefore, extend the calculated days supply by some fraction called a grace period, *e.g.*, 10 days per prescription, to avoid this misclassification. However, this strategy can also lead to unexposed time

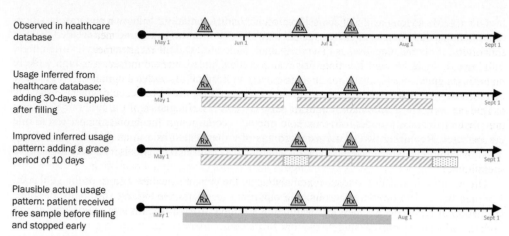

Observed in healthcare database

Usage inferred from healthcare database: adding 30-days supplies after filling

Improved inferred usage pattern: adding a grace period of 10 days

Plausible actual usage pattern: patient received free sample before filling and stopped early

FIGURE 43-6 Longitudinal drug exposure as observed in healthcare databases. (© 2019 Harvard Medical / Brigham Division of Pharmacoepidemiology.)

being classified as exposed if a patient discontinues drug use without finishing the supply. The right balance between improved sensitivity versus specificity of drug exposure assessment depends on how well the days supply is calculated, which in turn depends on the type of drug, the underlying disease, and eventually how regularly it is taken.[36]

Exposure to drugs taken sporadically is particularly challenging to model accurately. For example, the dose of warfarin, a blood thinner, is frequently modified depending on a lab test result. When the dose is reduced, the supply is stretched longer beyond the initially planned days supply and vice versa. It violates an epidemiologic principle to assess the time to the next refill and assume that the days between were continuously exposed because the knowledge of a future drug dispensing means that this person-time is immortal time—if a patient dies, there is no next refill. This immortal time may cause bias, especially if estimating mortality or events that have a high risk of dying. The difficulty in precisely defining the end of drug exposure in individual patients is a common issue in most data sources. Preplanned sensitivity analyses can explore the effect of the misclassification on validity by varying the duration of the grace period added to the days supply.

The addition of a grace period is intended to improve the measure of patient time on treatment. This issue is conceptually different from the exposure risk window, the time period during which an event might be causally attributed to the study drugs. The latter is defined by pharmacokinetic parameters and the underlying biology of the condition.

Physicians may hand out a free medication sample at the time they write the first prescription. Such samples will not be recorded in pharmacy dispensing databases and are another potential source of bias by misclassification. Since samples usually cover a brief period of time, rarely longer than 14 days, such misclassification produces meaningful bias only in extreme cases of substantial free sample distribution and when studying effects that occur immediately after starting a new drug. Similarly, medications that cost less than a required copayment may be purchased without involving the insurance, and therefore, no electronic record is generated in claims data.

In summary, there rarely is a perfect algorithm to classify exposure 100% correctly in healthcare databases, although data quality is still considered better than self-report and physician notes. The choice of the measurement strategy depends on whether one needs to be more concerned about falsely classifying person-time as exposed or unexposed, as well as on the pharmacology of the hypothesized drug effect.

Outcome Misclassification and its Consequences

Utilization databases often lack detailed clinical information and, one must consider the possible effect of outcome misclassification. Generally, a lack of specificity of the outcome measurement is worse than a lack of sensitivity. A relative risk estimate is unbiased by outcome misclassification if the specificity of the outcome assessment is 100%, even if the sensitivity is substantially less than 100% as long as the misclassification is nondifferential.[32] Studies on the misclassification of claims data diagnoses using medical records review as the gold standard revealed that the sensitivity of claims diagnoses is often less than moderate, while their specificity is often high. This pattern arises because if a diagnosis was recorded, coded, and submitted, it is highly likely that this diagnosis was actually made, particularly in hospital discharge summaries.[34] For many conditions, specificity can be further improved by requiring the occurrence of disease-specific procedure codes or a minimum length of stay. By contrast, diagnoses for ambulatory services may include diagnostic codes for services to rule out a condition, *e.g.*, a blood glucose test to rule out diabetes. Requiring two or more recordings of a diagnosis made in an ambulatory setting, possibly combined with a procedure claim specific to a confirmed diagnosis, can help to increase specificity.

The results of validation studies conducted using the patient's medical record as the gold standard can be used to optimize the outcome algorithm to ensure the highest specificity possible. Validation of all events is superior to validating a sample if the availability of validation records itself is associated with the study exposure or outcome. Identifying, retrieving, and abstracting medical record information is time-consuming. Sampling designs, such as case-control sampling (see case-control studies, Chapter 8), can be considered as useful strategies to reduce time and cost.[37]

Confounder Misclassification and its Consequences

Misclassified or completely missing confounder information leads to residual confounding, which is addressed in the next section.

ANALYSIS CONSIDERATIONS

As in any noninterventional study, the analysis of treatment effects in pharmacoepidemiology is concerned with choosing the appropriate analysis method that fits the disease model, research hypothesis, data, and study design. Two aspects stand out in pharmacoepidemiology and deserve specific attention. First, for most chronic conditions, medication treatment varies over time according to changes in the disease state. Even if the clinical strategy is to continue using a medication, patients need to fill prescriptions repeatedly, providing occasions to reconsider and discontinue treatment against advice. This circumstance has implications for choosing the causal effect of interest that best fits the study question. Second, given the nonrandomized treatment choice, there is specific attention given to adjusting for the selective entering into the medication exposure groups as well as the selective discontinuation of the initial treatment.

Causal Effects of Interest in Pharmacoepidemiology Studies

There is a range of causal parameters that can be estimated in longitudinal studies. Here, we focus on those most relevant in pharmacoepidemiology. Deciding on which approach to use is a trade-off between the clinical relevance of the different target parameters for the given question and feasibility in being able to obtain unbiased estimates of the targeted parameter.

The "On-Treatment" Effect Similar to a Simple Per-Protocol Effect in RCTs

The on-treatment effect is the effect of initiating the study treatment and continuing to receive it. Patients' follow-up time is censored at discontinuation of the initial treatment. The numerical value of the on-treatment effect from a given study takes into account the duration of treatment persistence.

The on-treatment effect is in most situations of great interest to patients and physicians because it informs about the expected treatment effect, while the patient is actually using the medication. On-treatment analyses need to take informative censoring into account, as discontinuation of the initial treatment may be informed by early signs of the outcome of interest or be otherwise associated with the study end point. In many situations, treatment discontinuation is a quasi-random process, and predictors of discontinuation are not obvious. In other situations, discontinuation and switching to another treatment or dose is part of a clinical strategy.

Dynamic Treatment Strategies Following a Complex Protocol

In many chronic conditions, it is recommended to start, stop, switch therapy, or change dose depending on clinical markers. One may therefore be interested in estimating the effect of a treatment strategy instead of analyzing the effect of treatment with a single drug. The on-treatment effect in such situations is defined as following a specific strategy, and censoring occurs if a patient deviates from following that strategy. These analyses can become complex and require dynamic control for confounding beyond baseline factors because future treatment choices depend on clinical markers and health states that change over time. Such time-varying confounding can be addressed with time-varying propensity score weighting approaches embedded in marginal structural models or G-estimation (see Chapters 25). Well-publicized examples are the treatment of human immunodeficiency virus (HIV) infection with antiretroviral therapy that may be intensified based on CD4 counts or viral load, which are blood markers for disease activity.[38] Data sources for such studies need to contain frequent measurements of the clinical markers determining treatment choice over time.

The "As-Started" Effect

The as-started effect is the effect of the initial treatment choice regardless of whether that treatment was continued over a given period of time. It is similar to the intention-to-treat effect in RCTs. The magnitude of the as-started effect from a given pharmacoepidemiology study depends on the specific patterns of deviation from the initial treatment choice during the follow-up time. As patients discontinue treatment, their exposure status will still be categorized according to the initial treatment. This handling avoids issues arising from informative censoring but leads to exposure-misclassified person-time. Two studies of the same treatment strategies, conducted in the same population, could have different as-started effects if persistence patterns differ between the studies but would have the same on-treatment effect in the absence of time-varying hazards. If discontinuation is nondifferential between compared groups, it will lead to increasingly smaller effect sizes with decreasing on-treatment durations and resulting increasing exposure mischaracterization. The more person-time that is mischaracterized, the more the as-started effect estimate will differ from the on-treatment estimate. Given that persistence patterns are often less than optimal in clinical practice even for life-extending medications,[4] this mischaracterization can be a major concern, particularly if the intended estimate of interest is really the on-treatment effect.

The on-treatment and as-started effects are the same for one-time exposures, like some vaccines, medical device implantation, or very long-lasting medications like some osteoporosis medications administered once a year. In these settings, adherence beyond the first exposure is much less or not at all relevant. Depending on the medication of interest and the biologic disease model, the as-started effect may be more informative than an on-treatment effect. For example, there was a concern that tumor necrosis factor (TNF)-alpha blocking agents in the treatment of rheumatic diseases could be associated with an increased risk of B-cell lymphoma. The postulated disease model was that even fairly short-term exposure to the agents could induce damage, and it would take years for the lymphoma to become apparent. An on-treatment effect estimate would not fit this disease model well.[39]

In summary, the on-treatment effect is often the clinically most relevant effect, while the as-started analysis requires the fewest assumptions to obtain an unbiased causal estimate.

Understanding Channeling of Treatments to Patients

Physicians prescribe drugs in light of disease severity and prognostic information available at the time of prescribing. The factors influencing this decision vary by physician and with time and frequently involve clinical, functional, or behavioral characteristics of patients that may not be completely recorded in healthcare databases. If such prognostic factors are imbalanced among drug users and comparator patients, then failing to control for such factors may lead to confounding bias. The same mechanism applies to treatments other than drugs, like surgical interventions and medical devices. Because treatment selection according to disease severity and prognosis is an integral part of practicing medicine, the resulting bias can be strong. The confounding arising through selective treatment decisions in medicine is sometimes more specifically called confounding by indication, confounding by contraindication, channeling, healthy-user bias, or sick-stopper bias, all of which address the same underlying challenge.

A first step in resolving potential confounding is understanding the channeling process. This is done by consulting physicians to understand the factors practitioners consider when making treatment decisions for a specific disease state, by reviewing treatment guidelines and by empirically describing the actual prescribing behavior in the study population. The latter often results in long tables listing tens or hundreds of observable patient characteristics by the treatment groups of interest. If meaningful imbalances in key prognostic factors raise concerns, investigators may limit the study to more homogeneous patient subgroups or consider alternative comparison groups. Both strategies may result in more balanced patient characteristics, indicative of equipoise in the clinical decision. If extreme imbalances persist, one should reconsider the feasibility of the study with noninterventional designs.

This book describes many design and analysis options for reducing confounding that are available to epidemiologists. If confounders are measured in a particular data source, then the usual strategies for controlling confounding can be applied: restriction, stratification, standardization, matching, and multivariable modeling. These techniques can be directly applied to database studies with the usual caveats. Figure 43-7 gives a pragmatic overview of the tools commonly used in pharmacoepidemiology to reduce confounding bias.

Focusing on the Analysis of Comparable Patients

Restriction is a common and effective analytic tool to make treatment groups more comparable and therefore to reduce residual confounding. Some restrictions are obvious since they are made by explicit criteria, such as, for example, limiting the study population to patients 65 years of age and with dementia to study the safety of antipsychotic medications used to control behavioral disturbances in this population. Other restrictions, like matching on a confounder summary score, either a propensity score or a disease risk score, are frequently used in pharmacoepidemiology. It is important to understand the specific reasons for restrictions and their implications for the generalizability of findings.

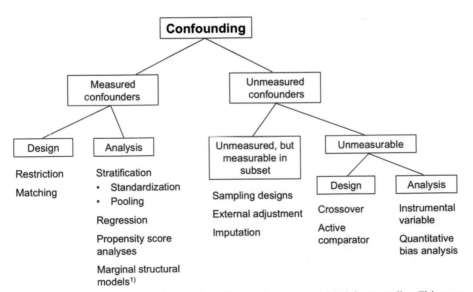

FIGURE 43-7 Approaches to minimize confounding in pharmacoepidemiology studies. This serves as a practical guide not as a technical taxonomy in the absence of random treatment assignment. 1) Mostly used to study complex treatment strategies with time-varying exposures. (Adapted from Schneeweiss S Sensitivity analysis and external adjustment for unmeasured confounders in epidemiologic database studies of therapeutics. *Pharmacoepidemiol Drug Saf.* 2006;15:291-303.)

Restricting to New Users

Restricting the study population to new users of the study agent or a comparator agent implicitly requires that both groups have recently been evaluated by a physician. Based on this evaluation, the physician has decided that the indicating condition has reached a state where a treatment should be initiated. Therefore, such patients are likely to be more similar in observable and unobservable characteristics than nonusers or ongoing users of another treatment.

Restricting to Well-Matched Patients

Matching by a summary confounder score has become frequent in pharmacoepidemiology studies that use secondary healthcare data. Most matching strategies lead to a group of exposed patients that have been paired with comparator patients who are similar with regard to the matching variable or score and a remainder group for whom there were no good matches in the comparison group. The latter group, lacking comparators, will not contribute to the analysis.

While restriction is an important tool to improve internal validity, it may make more difficult the generalization of study findings to the patient groups excluded from the analysis. Given that pharmacoepidemiology studies inform decisions that will affect patient care, we place high value on internal validity even if that comes at the price of reduced external validity. Investigators need to be aware of this trade-off and justify their choices accordingly.

Propensity Score Analyses

Propensity scores (PS) are known as a multivariable balancing tool that can efficiently balance large numbers of covariates, even if the study outcome is rare, which is frequently the case in pharmacoepidemiology. PS analyses have, therefore, emerged as a convenient and effective tool for adjusting large numbers of potential confounders in pharmacoepidemiology studies. They fit the target trial paradigm alluded to earlier as the PS emulates the randomization process based on observed data. In a new-user cohort design, a PS is the estimated probability of starting treatment A versus starting treatment B, conditional on all observed pretreatment patient characteristics. Estimating the PS using logistic regression is uncomplicated, and strategies for variable selection are well described.[40] Once a PS is estimated based on observed covariates, there are several options to use it in a second step to reduce confounding. Typical strategies include adjustment for quintiles or deciles of the score with or without trimming, matching, fine stratification, or weighting by PS.

Matching on PS in a cohort study has several advantages that may outweigh its drawback of not using the full dataset in situations where not all eligible patients match. Matching excludes patients in the extreme PS ranges where there is little clinical ambivalence in treatment choice. These tails of the PS distribution often harbor extreme patient scenarios caused by unobserved characteristics in patients who are not representative of the majority of patients in clinical practice. Dropping such patients from the analysis reduces residual confounding and may lead to clinically more relevant findings. In contrast to traditional outcome models, PS analyses allow the investigator to demonstrate the covariate balance achieved in the final study sample. Postmatching c-statistics or standardized differences of covariates have gained popularity in PS matching analyses.[41] Fixed-ratio matching in cohort studies, such as the frequently used 1:1 matching on PS, does not require matched analyses to obtain an unbiased result. The simplicity of the analysis when the matching is ignored is attractive but comes at a cost because taking the matching into account in the analysis will produce narrower confidence intervals. In settings with very few events 1:r matching or fine stratification may be preferred.[42]

If a rational treatment decision process can be predicted well with the observed patient characteristics, a resulting PS may lead to substantial or even full separation of exposed and comparator patients. If that occurs, comparatively few patients initiated on a comparison treatment would have the same propensity score as patients starting the study treatment. In this situation, treatment choice is almost deterministic; there is little random treatment variation left in the treatment decision that can be exploited for inference about the treatment effect. Consider the comparison of a fixed combination of two lipid-lowering drugs, ezetimibe with simvastatin, versus simvastatin alone, and their effect on coronary events. Suppose that a health plan that provides the study data covers the ezetimibe-simvastatin combination only if the low-densitylipoprotein (LDL) cholesterol serum level has crossed a certain threshold. Every patient below that threshold uses simvastatin alone. The LDL level, therefore, becomes a strong if not perfect determinant of treatment choice and including it in the PS estimation will lead to substantial or complete separation of the PS distributions for the two treatment groups. If such a strong separation of PS distributions is observed, it indicates that the specific comparison cannot be made validly in the study population. In the above example, all ezetimibe-simvastatin combination users have high LDL level, and hardly any simvastatin users have a comparable LDL level. Therefore, very few comparable patients are available for valid inference. This is not a limitation of the method but rather an insightful multivariable diagnostic describing the limitations inherent in a study population. Investigators may want to reconsider the comparator agent and choose a drug that physicians consider a reasonable alternative to the study drug or use another study population where there is less treatment separation in clinical practice. When substantial separation in the PS distribution is observed, it is advisable to verify that no instruments, *i.e.*, variables that are predicting the exposure but not the outcome, have erroneously been included in the PS. Including instrumental variables in confounding adjustment increases bias instead of decreasing it.[43]

As the ezetimibe-simvastatin combination continues to be marketed, it may, over time, be prescribed less selectively and the coverage restriction may be loosened. Consequently, as time goes on and as the prescribers' treatment decisions are increasingly preference based, the PS distributions may overlap more as more patients are subject to clinical treatment equipoise.

In summary, PS analyses are convenient tools to adjust for many covariates when study outcomes are rare. Extensive confounding adjustment is central in most pharmacoepidemiology applications using secondary healthcare databases. We can often identify many covariates that can serve as proxies for unobserved or misclassified patient characteristics. Combined with the fact that most safety outcomes in pharmacoepidemiology are rare, PS analyses fit the needs well. It is important to remember, however, that PS analyses only adjust for measured variables.

Reducing Confounding by Unobserved Patient Characteristics Through Proxy Measures

Longitudinal electronic healthcare databases may lack critical details on health state and risk factors for the outcome, which leads to residual confounding if left unadjusted. An analysis of such data identifies the research constructs through the lenses of medical practice patterns and recording practices under financial constraints. The characteristics of the patient health status that we wish to adjust for may not always be directly observed, but it may be observed through a set of proxies. For example, old age serves as a proxy for many factors including comorbidity, frailty, and cognitive decline; use of an oxygen canister is a sign of very frail health, including advanced chronic obstructive pulmonary disease or advanced heart failure; having regular annual checkups is indicative of a health-seeking lifestyle and increased adherence. The degree to which a proxy is related to an unobserved or imperfectly observed confounder is proportional to the degree to which adjustment can be achieved. For effective confounder control, one does not need an exact interpretation of each proxy variable.

Proxy adjustment can be exploited by algorithms that systematically search through recorded codes for diagnoses, procedures, equipment purchases, and drug dispensings to identify factors that empirically feature the characteristics of confounders.[44] The hundreds of proxies that can be empirically identified are then adjusted for in a large PS model. This high-dimensional PS approach has been empirically shown to perform as well as or better than investigator-selected covariate adjustment. While such data-adaptive proxy adjustment strategies are remarkably robust, issues may arise in small studies with few exposed patients and rare outcomes. Unknowingly adjusting for collider variables or variables that are only related to the exposure and not to the outcome may theoretically increase bias. The effect of this potential "overadjustment" is minimal in most practical pharmacoepidemiology scenarios and needs to be weighed against the genuine threat of failing to adjust for true confounders.[45]

Variation in Prescribing Preference for Instrumental Variable Analysis

Confounding arising from unmeasured risk factors can be reduced using instrumental variable analyses (see Chapter 28). One may be able to identify naturally occurring quasi-random treatment choices in routine care. Factors that determine such quasi-random treatment choices are called instrumental variables (IVs).

An IV is an observed variable that causes, or is a marker of, variation in the exposure that is unrelated to any risk factors for the outcome and therefore correspondent to random treatment choice. An instructive example of an IV is a hospital drug formulary. Some hospitals use only drug A for a given indication, and other hospitals that are comparable in their patient case mix use only drug B. It is a reasonable assumption that patients do not choose their hospital based on its formulary preference but instead on location and recommendation. Therefore, the choice of drug A versus drug B should be independent of patient characteristics in the hospitals with these restricted formularies. If no disease state–related factors lead to preferential admission to one of the hospitals, comparing patient outcomes from drug A hospitals with patient outcomes from drug B hospitals should result in an unbiased estimate of the effects of drug A versus drug B. An example is a study on the risk of death from aprotinin, an antifibrinolytic agent given to reduce bleeding during cardiac surgery.[46] The study identified hospitals that always used aprotinin and compared their outcomes to hospitals that always used aminocaproic acid, an alternative drug. If physician skill level and performance are on average equal between institutions, independent of drug use, this results in valid treatment effect estimates. Such an assumption may be violated, however, if, for example, academic hospitals allow less restrictive formularies, are more likely to see sicker patients, and have more specialized physicians.

In noninterventional research, identifying valid instruments is difficult and valid IV analyses of drug effects are infrequent. In principle, treatment preference can be influenced by time if treatment guidelines change rapidly and substantially. A comparison of patient outcome rates before versus after a sudden change in treatment patterns may then be a reasonable instrument.[47] More commonly, IV analyses utilize individual, clinic/hospital, or regional treatment preferences. For example, one may use physician-prescribing preference to study the effect of analgesic treatment with COX-2 selective inhibitors versus nonselective nonsteroidal anti-inflammatory drugs (NSAIDs) on the risk of upper gastrointestinal bleed. A study demonstrated that such preference is a fairly strong and valid instrument.[47] Others used regional variation in the rate of cardiac catheterization to estimate its effect on mortality after myocardial infarction.[48] While this regional preference instrument was weaker than the physician-prescribing preference, it was argued that the instrument was more valid as it is less likely that patients would move to another region to receive the preferred care, but they may more readily switch their physician.

The price of potentially unbiased estimation in IV analyses is the ultimately untestable assumptions that the authors need to argue based on substantive knowledge and some empirical data. Because of the two-stage estimation, IV analyses are generally less precise, which can severely reduce their utility for decision-making. Users should also be cautioned that IV inference is based on those "marginal" patients whose treatment decision is influenced by the IV status. This concept is somewhat similar to PS analyses, where only patients in the overlapping area of PS distributions contribute to the analysis. In contrast to PS analyses, the marginal patients in an IV analysis cannot be enumerated and characterized.

Pharmacoepidemiology Database Studies Combined With Detailed Confounding Data

If unmeasured patient characteristics that are deemed important confounders remain unobserved, then additional information can be collected in a subset of patients. A common version thereof is the case-control sampling or the case-cohort sampling where only a sample of controls or a sample of exposed and unexposed will be used to collect detailed confounder information.[49] Eng et al. conducted a case-cohort analysis embedded in a much larger claims-based cohort to assess the impact of unobserved risk factors of thromboembolic events in women using oral contraceptives, by interviewing a subset of women on their body mass index (BMI), smoking status, and exercise.[50] The two-stage sampling approach is even more efficient. It samples patients according to their exposure and outcome status simultaneously.[37] These approaches are resource intensive even though only a subset of patients is interrogated for additional health status information.

Increasingly, it is possible to link information-rich EHRs or registry data to large subsets of population-based claims data studies. Such linkage can be used to demonstrate the balance achieved in patient characteristics that were unobserved in claims data. In a new-user active-comparator cohort study of oral antidiabetic medications with PS matching, it was demonstrated that laboratory test results, BMI, and duration of diabetes were well balanced although these parameters were only observable in the subset of EHR-linked patients and not part of the claims data analysis.[51] In the right data environment, such data linkage is possible and one can routinely check the achieved balance of baseline factors unmeasured in the main study.

There are multiple strategies to incorporate additional detailed information on confounding factors that is available in a subset into the main study and adjust the initial observed effect estimate for any residual confounding. Simple algebraic solutions are available to adjust for individual binary factors as was demonstrated in a study of older adults and missing quantifications of the limitations in activities of daily living, cognitive impairment, and physical impairments.[52] PS calibration extends this simple adjustment to multiple confounders on any scale.[53] The basic concept of PS calibration is to estimate two multivariable PS in the information-rich subset data. One PS mimics the information available in the main study and is seen as an error-prone PS. The second PS uses all available information and is called the complete PS. By regressing the error-prone PS on the complete PS, a calibration factor is estimated. With this factor, the error-prone PS-adjusted result in the main study will be calibrated to produce results that are adjusted for the additional factors only available in the more detailed survey data.

Sensitivity Analyses and Bias Modeling

A series of prespecified and posthoc sensitivity analyses can help investigators to understand better how robust a study's findings are to structural assumptions. Some of the sensitivity analyses suggested below are specific to pharmacoepidemiology database analyses and others are generic to study causal relationships. In Figure 43-8, we list several frequently used sensitivity analyses in pharmacoepidemiology. Some of those are variations of key study design parameters that can be incorporated in the planning and implementation of the study, and others are "back-end" analyses that are based on the actual study finding.

In most pharmacoepidemiology studies based on large patient databases, new users of the drugs of interest are identified empirically by a drug prescribing/dispensing that was not preceded by a prescribing/dispensing of the same drug for a defined time period. The validity of this washout window depends on all patients being enrolled in the plan or part of the EHR system during the time window so that the information can be captured. The length of the window should be identical for all patients across treatment groups. A typical choice of the washout window duration is 6 months; a sensitivity analyses could extend the window to 9 and 12 months. In a study on the comparative safety of antidepressant agents in children in British Columbia, this interval was extended from 1 year to 3 years to ensure that the children in the study were treatment naive before

"Front end": Study validity issues that can be explored by varying design choices	Suggested sensitivity analysis
1) Incomplete covariate assessment	Extend covariate assessment window further to the past to increase information capture
2) Reverse causation	Lengthen induction time to sharpen temporality
3) Misspecified follow-up model	On-treatment vs. as-started
4) Misspecified exposure risk window	Vary start and end date of risk window
5) Differential surveillance bias	Adjust for healthcare utilization intensity
"Back end": Explore alternative explanations of the study findings	
6) Imperfect outcome measurement	Quantitative bias analysis
7) Imperfect exposure measurement (see #4)	Quantitative bias analysis
8) Residual confounding due to imperfect measurement	Quantitative bias analysis

FIGURE 43-8 Potential sources for bias that are addressed by sensitivity analyses.

their first use.[54] Although increasing the length of the washout window increases the likelihood that patients are truly new users, it may reduce the number of patients eligible for the study in left-censored data because the longer eligibility requirement excludes some patients. This trade-off is particularly worth noting in health plans with high enrollee turnover. Analogously, the covariate assessment window could be extended in sensitivity analyses in order to capture more information that defines the study patients' health state.

There is often uncertainty about the correct definition of the exposure risk window based on the clinical pharmacology of the study agent and the current understanding of the biology and physiology. Varying the exposure risk window is, therefore, insightful and easy to accomplish in cohort studies.

Another sensitivity analysis concerns the potential for informative censoring. Patients change and discontinue treatment because there is a disappointing treatment effect or they experience early signs of a side effect. The stronger such nonpersistence is associated with the outcome, the more an on-treatment analysis, which censors at the point of discontinuation, is biased. Alternatively, the as-started analysis follows all patients for a fixed time period disregarding any changes in treatment status over time. It will avoid informative censoring but suffers from increasing exposure mischaracterization with time. In most cases, though not all, such mischaracterization will bias effects toward the null, similar to intention-to-treat analyses in randomized trials. Viewed separately, these two analysis types trade different strengths and weaknesses, and together, they bound a range of plausible effect estimates.

An important yet underutilized diagnostic tool for the impact of unobserved confounding on the validity of findings in noninterventional studies is quantitative bias analysis (see Chapter 29). Basic bias analyses of residual confounding try to determine how strong and how imbalanced a confounder would have to be among exposure groups to explain the observed effect.[52] Lash and Fox proposed an approach that considers several systematic errors simultaneously, allowing sensitivity analyses for confounding, misclassification, and selection bias in one process.[55]

DEVELOPMENTS

The enrichment of existing data environments with supplemental clinical or patient-reported data is increasingly common. This enrichment can occur by linking with electronic medical records, disease registries, patient surveys, laboratory test result repositories, wearable devices, and digital health devices. While this information will provide an opportunity for improved confounding adjustment, it comes with methodological challenges, as information is collected in routine care and may have been requested or recorded selectively in patients who were thought to benefit most.

EHRs are now standard practice in modern healthcare systems. They store not only physician-recorded observations but laboratory test results, imaging studies, genetic or biomarker test, and much other structured and unstructured information. Use of natural language processing and machine learning is increasingly common to identify patient phenotypes and record changes in health state over time. Medical devices, wearable devices, mobile phones, and many other technologies that are now ubiquitous will increasingly be used for collecting high-fidelity information on patient behavior, disease state, etc. from the patient directly and prospectively. In order to take full advantage of these massive influx of additional information on patients and their care, automated data-adaptive algorithms will be useful to identify and optimize confounder selection. We mentioned already HDPS as an algorithm well-fitting the medical data landscape.[45] Similar techniques, like collaborative targeted maximum likelihood estimation, are equally data adaptive and optimize learning and effect estimation in a causal framework.[56]

As analyses become increasingly complex, new processes may be needed for efficient and reproducible research. Confidence in pharmacoepidemiology study findings is based on transparency of the research process and study implementation that allows assessing the validity of the study findings. The use of software platforms that are connectable to any healthcare database and allow investigators to design studies, implement feasibility analyses, register study protocols, and analyze data for comprehensive reports in one validated environment will become increasingly common. They satisfy the needs of decision-makers to understand fully a study implementation and to be able to trace a finding back to the raw data, as is done for randomized trials with primary data collection with approval decisions resting on the review.

References

1. The International Society of Pharmacoepidemiology. Guidelines for good pharmacoepidemiology practices (GPP). *Pharmacoepidemiol Drug Saf.* 2008;17(2):200-208.
2. Langan SM, Schmidt SA, Wing K, et al. The reporting of studies conducted using observational routinely collected health data statement for pharmacoepidemiology (RECORD-PE). *BMJ.* 2018;363:k3532.
3. Wang SV, Schneeweiss S, Berger ML, et al. Reporting to improve reproducibility and facilitate validity assessment for healthcare database studies V1.0. *Pharmacoepidemiol Drug Saf.* 2017;26(9): 1018-1032.
4. Benner JS, Glynn RJ, Mogun H, Neumann PJ, Weinstein MC, Avorn J. Long-term persistence in use of statin therapy in elderly patients. *J Am Med Assoc.* 2002;288(4):455-461.
5. Soumerai SB, Ross-Degnan D, Avorn J, McLaughlin T, Choodnovskiy I. Effects of Medicaid drug-payment limits on admission to hospitals and nursing homes. *N Engl J Med.* 1991;325(15):1072-1077.
6. Choudhry NK, Avorn J, Glynn RJ, et al. Full coverage for preventive medications after myocardial infarction. *N Engl J Med.* 2011;365(22):2088-2097.
7. Ray WA, Stein CM, Daugherty JR, Hall K, Arbogast PG, Griffin MR. COX-2 selective non-steroidal anti-inflammatory drugs and risk of serious coronary heart disease. *Lancet.* 2002;360(9339):1071-1073.
8. Azoulay L, Yin H, Filion KB, et al. The use of pioglitazone and the risk of bladder cancer in people with type 2 diabetes: nested case-control study. *BMJ.* 2012;344:e3645.
9. Moran LV, Ongur D, Hsu J, Castro VM, Perlis RH, Schneeweiss S. Psychosis with methylphenidate or amphetamine in patients with ADHD. *N Engl J Med.* 2019;380(12):1128-1138.
10. U.S. Food and Drug Administration. *Framework for FDA's Real-World Evidence Program.* Washington, DC: US FDA; 2018.
11. Franklin JM, Schneeweiss S. When and how can real world data analyses substitute for randomized controlled trials? *Clin Pharmacol Ther.* 2017;102(6):924-933.
12. Najafzadeh M, Gagne JJ, Schneeweiss S. Synergies from integrating randomized controlled trials and real-world data analyses. *Clin Pharmacol Ther.* 2017;102(6):914-916.
13. McConnachie A, Walker A, Robertson M, et al. Long-term impact on healthcare resource utilization of statin treatment, and its cost effectiveness in the primary prevention of cardiovascular disease: a record linkage study. *Eur Heart J.* 2014;35(5):290-298.
14. Cheng F, Desai RJ, Handy DE, et al. Network-based approach to prediction and population-based validation of in silico drug repurposing. *Nat Commun.* 2018;9(1):2691.
15. Schneeweiss S, Rassen JA, Brown JS, et al. Graphical depiction of longitudinal study designs in health care databases. *Ann Intern Med.* 2019;170(6):398-406.
16. VanderWeele TJ. Principles of confounder selection. *Eur J Epidemiol.* 2019;34(3):211-219.
17. Maclure M. The case-crossover design: a method for studying transient effects on the risk of acute events. *Am J Epidemiol.* 1991;133(2):144-153.
18. Schneeweiss S. A basic study design for expedited safety signal evaluation based on electronic healthcare data. *Pharmacoepidemiol Drug Saf.* 2010;19(8):858-868.
19. Brookhart MA, Wang PS, Solomon DH, Schneeweiss S. Evaluating short-term drug effects using a physician-specific prescribing preference as an instrumental variable. *Epidemiology.* 2006;17(3):268-275.
20. Hernan MA, Robins JM. Using big data to emulate a target trial when a randomized trial is not available. *Am J Epidemiol.* 2016;183(8):758-764.
21. Hernan MA, Sauer BC, Hernandez-Diaz S, Platt R, Shrier I. Specifying a target trial prevents immortal time bias and other self-inflicted injuries in observational analyses. *J Clin Epidemiol.* 2016;79:70-75.
22. Hernan MA, Alonso A, Logan R, et al. Observational studies analyzed like randomized experiments: an application to postmenopausal hormone therapy and coronary heart disease. *Epidemiology.* 2008;19(6):766-779.
23. Suissa S. Immortal time bias in observational studies of drug effects. *Pharmacoepidemiol Drug Saf.* 2007;16(3):241-249.
24. Ray WA. Evaluating medication effects outside of clinical trials: new-user designs. *Am J Epidemiol.* 2003;158(9):915-920.
25. Malone DC, Brown M, Hurwitz JT, Peters L, Graff JS. Real-world evidence: useful in the real world of US payer decision making? How? When? And what studies? *Value Health.* 2018;21(3):326-333.
26. Smeeth L, Douglas I, Hall AJ, Hubbard R, Evans S. Effect of statins on a wide range of health outcomes: a cohort study validated by comparison with randomized trials. *Br J Clin Pharmacol.* 2009;67(1):99-109.
27. Johnson ES, Bartman BA, Briesacher BA, et al. The incident user design in comparative effectiveness research. *Pharmacoepidemiol Drug Saf.* 2013;22(1):1-6.
28. Suissa S, Moodie EE, Dell'Aniello S. Prevalent new-user cohort designs for comparative drug effect studies by time-conditional propensity scores. *Pharmacoepidemiol Drug Saf.* 2017;26(4):459-468.
29. Hatch EE, Palmer JR, Titus-Ernstoff L, et al. Cancer risk in women exposed to diethylstilbestrol in utero. *J Am Med Assoc.* 1998;280(7):630-634.

30. Suissa S. Immortal time bias in pharmaco-epidemiology. *Am J Epidemiol*. 2008;167(4):492-499.

31. Setoguchi S, Warner Stevenson L, Stewart GC, et al. Influence of healthy candidate bias in assessing clinical effectiveness for implantable cardioverter-defibrillators: cohort study of older patients with heart failure. *BMJ*. 2014;348:g2866.

32. Rothman KJ, Poole C. A strengthening programme for weak associations. *Int J Epidemiol*. 1988;17(4):955-959.

33. Glynn RJ, Monane M, Gurwitz JH, Choodnovskiy I, Avorn J. Agreement between drug treatment data and a discharge diagnosis of diabetes mellitus in the elderly. *Am J Epidemiol*. 1999;149(6):541-549.

34. Funk MJ, Landi SN. Misclassification in administrative claims data: quantifying the impact on treatment effect estimates. *Curr Epidemiol Rep*. 2014;1(4):175-185.

35. Schneeweiss S, Seeger JD, Maclure M, Wang PS, Avorn J, Glynn RJ. Performance of comorbidity scores to control for confounding in epidemiologic studies using claims data. *Am J Epidemiol*. 2001;154(9):854-864.

36. Schneeweiss S, Avorn J. A review of uses of health care utilization databases for epidemiologic research on therapeutics. *J Clin Epidemiol*. 2005;58(4):323-337.

37. Collet JP, Schaubel D, Hanley J, Sharpe C, Boivin JF. Controlling confounding when studying large pharmacoepidemiologic databases: a case study of the two-stage sampling design. *Epidemiology*. 1998;9:309-315.

38. Hernán MA, Brumback B, Robins JM. Marginal structural models to estimate the causal effect of zidovudine on the survival of HIV-positive men. *Epidemiology*. 2000;11(5):561-570.

39. Solomon DH, Lunt M, Schneeweiss S. The risk of infection associated with tumor necrosis factor alpha antagonists: making sense of epidemiologic evidence. *Arthritis Rheum*. 2008;58(4):919-928.

40. Brookhart MA, Schneeweiss S, Rothman KJ, Glynn RJ, Avorn J, Stürmer T. Variable selection for propensity score models. *Am J Epidemiol*. 2006;163(12):1149-1156.

41. Franklin JM, Rassen JA, Ackermann D, Bartels DB, Schneeweiss S. Metrics for covariate balance in cohort studies of causal effects. *Stat Med*. 2014;33(10):1685-1699.

42. Desai RJ, Rothman KJ, Bateman BT, Hernandez-Diaz S, Huybrechts KF. A propensity-score-based fine stratification approach for confounding adjustment when exposure is infrequent. *Epidemiology*. 2017;28(2):249-257.

43. Myers JA, Rassen JA, Gagne JJ, et al. Effects of adjusting for instrumental variables on bias and precision of effect estimates. *Am J Epidemiol*. 2011;174(11):1213-1222.

44. Schneeweiss S, Rassen JA, Glynn RJ, Avorn J, Mogun H, Brookhart MA. High-dimensional propensity score adjustment in studies of treatment effects using health care claims data. *Epidemiology*. 2009;20(4):512-522.

45. Schneeweiss S. Automated data-adaptive analytics for electronic healthcare data to study causal treatment effects. *Clin Epidemiol*. 2018;10:771-788.

46. Schneeweiss S, Seeger JD, Landon J, Walker AM. Aprotinin during coronary-artery bypass grafting and risk of death. *N Engl J Med*. 2008;358(8):771-783.

47. Brookhart MA, Rassen JA, Schneeweiss S. Instrumental variable methods in comparative safety and effectiveness research. *Pharmacoepidemiol Drug Saf*. 2010;19(6):537-554.

48. Stukel TA, Fisher ES, Wennberg DE, Alter DA, Gottlieb DJ, Vermeulen MJ. Analysis of observational studies in the presence of treatment selection bias: effects of invasive cardiac management on AMI survival using propensity score and instrumental variable methods. *J Am Med Assoc*. 2007;297(3):278-285.

49. Wacholder S. Practical considerations in choosing between the case-cohort and nested case-control designs. *Epidemiology*. 1991;2(2):155-158.

50. Eng PM, Seeger JD, Loughlin J, Clifford CR, Mentor S, Walker AM. Supplementary data collection with case-cohort analysis to address potential confounding in a cohort study of thromboembolism in oral contraceptive initiators matched on claims-based propensity scores. *Pharmacoepidemiol Drug Saf*. 2008;17(3):297-305.

51. Patorno E, Gopalakrishnan C, Franklin JM, et al. Claims-based studies of oral glucose-lowering medications can achieve balance in critical clinical variables only observed in electronic health records. *Diabetes Obes Metab*. 2018;20(4):974-984.

52. Schneeweiss S. Sensitivity analysis and external adjustment for unmeasured confounders in epidemiologic database studies of therapeutics. *Pharmacoepidemiol Drug Saf*. 2006;15(5):291-303.

53. Sturmer T, Schneeweiss S, Avorn J, Glynn RJ. Correcting effect estimates for unmeasured confounding in cohort studies with validation studies using propensity score calibration. *Am J Epidemiol*. 2005;162:279-289.

54. Schneeweiss S, Patrick AR, Solomon DH, et al. Comparative safety of antidepressant agents for children and adolescents regarding suicidal acts. *Pediatrics*. 2010;125(5):876-888.

55. Lash TL, Fox MP, MacLehose RF, Maldonado G, McCandless LC, Greenland S. Good practices for quantitative bias analysis. *Int J Epidemiol*. 2014;43(6):1969-1985.

56. van der Laan MJ, Rose S. *Targeted Learning: Causal Inference for Observational and Experimental Data*. Berlin/Heidelberg/New York: Springer; 2011.

Index

Note: Page numbers followed by "f" indicate figures, "t" indicate tables, and "b" indicate boxes.